Directions to the Student

The nursing actions listed below underlie safe, competent nursing and as such have been omitted in some procedures to avoid repetition.

- Before implementing any interventions, refer to the agency's specific protocols for further information and recommendations.
- Many agencies require a signed, informed consent for certain invasive procedures. Please refer to specific agency policies for this information.
- Some procedures refer to a physician performing some diagnostic and therapeutic procedures (eg, thoracentesis and paracentesis). In some agencies and settings, individuals practicing in expanded roles including nurse practitioners and physician assistants may be responsible for performing these procedures.
- Wash the hands before gathering any clean or sterile supplies, before gloving, before implementing a procedure, after contact with a client, and after removing gloves to avoid transmission of microorganisms to clients and others.
- Implement appropriate blood and body fluid precautions (see inside back cover). The authors suggest wearing gloves for most procedures that involve direct contact with any body fluid.
- Identify the client appropriately by reading the client's wrist band and asking the client their name.
- Explain the procedure to the client and, in some instances, to support persons, adjusting your explanation to their needs. Explaining what you plan to do reassures people by letting them know what to expect. Explanations are provided in some procedures.
- Provide privacy for the client when any aspect of the procedure could be embarrassing to the client or others and as an indication of respect even when the client is not conscious.
- Elevate the client's bed to a working level and lower the near side rail before starting a procedure. These actions help the nurse maintain good body mechanics.
- Recheck an abnormal reading or measurement (eg, blood pressure) and if it is still abnormal, report and record it immediately.
- Procedures pertinent to intravenous therapy may include the use of needles. In many agencies, use of a "needleless" system has replaced traditional needles. Familiarize yourself with an agency's policies and practices regarding the use of needles during IV therapy.
- Following a procedure, lower the bed and raise the near side rail for clients requiring these precautions. These actions are taken for the client's safety.
- Ensure that the client is comfortable following the procedure.
- Dispose of used and unused supplies according to agency practice. This step includes cleaning and/or disinfecting equipment as necessary.

We dedicate this book to

Barbara's parents, the late Luella and Bertie Blackwood

Glen's brother and sister, Don and Val

Kathy's son, David

Judy's parents, Hubert and Vera Mason, and sons, Todd, Bryan, and Chris

Occupational Strategies	Commonalities A	Commonalities B
Sec I Chp 1 & 3	Sec I – Chp 33	Sec I, Chp 37
Sec II " 4-13-15-16-18	Sec II – 35, 36	Sec II Fecal Chp 40 urine Chp 41
Sec III " 2-11-12	Sec III – 34	Sec III – 39
Sec IV " 5, 6, 7, 8, 9, 10, 20	Sec IV –	Sec IV – 38
	Sec V –	
	Sec VI – 18, 19	
	Sec VII	

FUNDAMENTALS OF NURSING

CONCEPTS, PROCESS, AND PRACTICE

UPDATED FIFTH EDITION

BARBARA KOZIER RN, MN

GLENORA ERB RN, BSN

KATHLEEN BLAIS RN, EdD
School of Nursing
Florida International University
Miami, Florida

JUDITH M. WILKINSON RNC, MA, MS
Nursing Program
Johnson County Community College
Overland Park, Kansas

Updated material contributed by
KAREN VAN LEUVEN, RN, PhD
Department of Nursing
Samuel Merritt College
Oakland, California

ADDISON-WESLEY

An Imprint of Addison Wesley Longman, Inc.

Menlo Park, California • Reading, Massachusetts • New York • Harlow, England
Don Mills, Ontario • Sydney • Mexico City • Madrid • Amsterdam

Senior Editor: *Erin Mulligan*
Managing Editor: *Wendy Earl*
Production Supervisor: *David Rich*
Text and Page Designers: *Juan Vargas and Edie Williams*
Cover Designer: *Yvo Riezebos Design*
Manufacturing Supervisor: *Merry Free Osborn*

Library of Congress Cataloging-in-Publication Data

Fundamentals of nursing : concepts, process, and practice / Barbara Kozier ... [et al.]. — Updated 5th ed.
p. cm.
Includes bibliographical references and index.
ISBN 0-8053-7472-8
1. Nursing. I. Kozier, Barbara.
[DNLM: 1. Nursing Process. 2. Nursing Care. WY 100 F97984 1998]
RT41.F8813 1998
610.73—dc21
DNLM/DLC
for Library of Congress 97-26045
CIP

ISBN 0-8053-7472-8
2 3 4 5 6 7 8 9 10-RNV-01 00 99 98 97

Addison Wesley Longman, Inc.
2725 Sand Hill Road
Menlo Park, California 94025

Photographic and art credits begin on page 1450.

The authors and publisher thank the following California institutions for their kind permission to photograph many of the nurses and clients who appear in this book:

Alta Bates Hospital, Berkeley
Children's Hospital of Oakland
Eden Medical Center, Castro Valley
Family Planning Clinic, San Francisco
Jewish Home for the Aged, San Francisco
Kaiser Medical Center of San Francisco
Laguna Honda Hospital, San Francisco
St. Luke's Hospital, San Francisco
St. Mary's Hospital, San Francisco
Samuel Merritt College, Oakland
San Francisco General Hospital
Stanford University Medical Center, Palo Alto
University of California at San Francisco Medical Center
University of California at San Francisco School of Nursing
Valencia Pediatric Clinic, San Francisco
Veteran's Administration Hospital of San Francisco
Visiting Nurses Association of San Francisco
Well Baby Clinic, San Francisco

Care has been taken to confirm the accuracy of information presented in this book. The authors, editors, and the publisher, however, cannot accept any responsibility for errors or omissions or for consequences from application of the information in this book and make no warranty, express or implied, with respect to its contents.

The authors and publisher have exerted every effort to ensure that drug selections and dosages set forth in this text are in accord with current recommendations and practice at time of publication. However, in view of ongoing research, changes in government regulations, and the constant flow of information relating to drug therapy and drug reactions, the reader is urged to check the package inserts of all drugs for any change in indications of dosage and for added warnings and precautions. This is particularly important when the recommended agent is a new and/or infrequently employed drug.

The cover illustration is from a quilt designed by Merrill Mason and photographed by Erik Landsberg.

Contributors

Leslie Atkinson, RN, MSN
School of Nursing
Normandale Community College
Bloomington, Minnesota
Contributed selected material for:
Chapter 17 Sexuality
Chapter 18 Helping and Communicating
Chapter 19 Teaching and Learning
Chapter 36 Comfort and Pain
Chapter 38 Fluid, Electrolyte, and Acid-Base Balance

Suzanne C. Beyea, RN, CS, PhD
Department of Nursing
Saint Anselm College
Manchester, New Hampshire
Contributed Critical Pathways in Chapters 4, 31, 34 through 42, 44, and 45

Evelyn L. Brooks, RN, MN
University of Kansas Medical Center
Kansas City, Kansas
Contributed to Chapter 42, Sensory Perception and Cognition

Susan S. Fairchild, RNC, EdDc, CNOR
Barry University School of Nursing
Miami Shores, Florida
Contributed to Chapter 45, Perioperative Nursing

Suzanne Phillips, ARNP, EdD
School of Nursing
Florida International University
Miami, Florida
Revised Chapter 24, Infancy Through Late Childhood, and Chapter 25, Adolescence Through Middle Adulthood

Jean Smith Temple, RN, MSN
College of Nursing
University of South Alabama
Mobile, Alabama
Revised Chapter 27, Preventing the Transfer of Microorganisms

Karen Van Leuven, RN, PhD
Department of Nursing
Samuel Merritt College
Oakland, California
Revised Chapter 43, Medications
Provided all updated material

Reviewers

Joanne Anfinson, RN, PhD
Capital Community Technical College
Hartford, CT

Mary Auterman, RN, DNS
Department of Nursing
Augustana College
Sioux Falls, SD

Janet Craig Azar, RN, MNEd
Nursing Program
Tidewater Community College
Portsmouth, VA

Sheri L. Banovic, RN, MSN
Allied Health
Lewis and Clark Community College
Godfrey, IL

Audrey Berman, RN, PhD, OCN
Department of Nursing
Samuel Merritt College
Oakland, CA

Marjorie T. Burkett, RN, PhD
School of Nursing
Florida International University
Miami, FL

Patricia A. Burks, RN, BSN
School of Nursing
Western Oklahoma State College
Altus, OK

Tonya L. Buttry, RN, MSN
College of Nursing
Southeast Missouri Hospital
Cape Girardeau, MO

Robert L. Campbell, RN, MN
Department of Nursing
Bloomsburg University
Bloomsburg, PA

Shirley Cashio, RN, MSN
Division of Nursing
Northwestern State University
Shreveport, LA

Stephanie Catron, RN, MSN
Nursing Department
Northern Montana College
Great Falls, MT

Bonita Morrow Cavanaugh, RN, PhD
School of Nursing
University of Colorado
Denver, CO

Norma L. Cole, RN, MA
Nursing Program
Johnson County Community College
Overland Park, KS

Patricia S. Crose, RN, MS
School of Nursing
Saint Francis Hospital and Medical Center
Hartford, CT

Sandra K. Croyle, RN, PhD
Nursing Division
Butler County Community College
Butler, PA

Patricia Cryer, RN, MS
Texas Eastern School of Nursing
Tyler Junior College
Tyler, TX

Marilyn E. Cunningham, RN, MSN, C
Department of Nursing
Miami University
Middletown, OH

Patricia A. Diehl, RN, MA
School of Nursing
West Virginia University
Morgantown, WV

John Drury, RN, BAppSc, PGDip, HSc
Edith Cowen University
Perth, Australia

Edward J. Edwards, RN, EdD, CHES
Department of Nursing and Allied Health Professions
Indiana University of Pennsylvania
Indiana, PA

Madge Ellis, RN, BScN, MEd
Durham College
Ottawa, Canada

Bonita Fae Fador, RN, MSN
School of Nursing
Belmont Technical College
St. Clairsville, OH

Nancy Ferguson, RN, MS, CNS
College of Nursing
Houston Community College
Houston, TX

Melba Leroux Figgins, RN, MSN
Department of Nursing
University of Tennessee
Martin, TN

Chloe Hammons Findley, RN, MA, MS
School of Nursing
Southern Nazarene University
Bethany, OK

Lisa Fiorentino, RN, MS, CRNP
Department of Nursing
University of Pittsburgh
Bradford, PA

Cheryl P. Franklin, RN, MN
School of Nursing
Nicholls State University
Thibodaux, LA

Jane H. Freeman, RN, EdD
College of Nursing
Jacksonville State University
Jacksonville, AL

Patricia B. Graham, RN, MN
School of Nursing
Medical College of Georgia
Augusta, GA

Gloria J. Green, RN, PhD
Department of Nursing
Southeast Missouri State University
Cape Girardeau, MO

Marian S. Gustafson, RN, MSN
Nursing Division
Butler County Community College
Butler, PA

H. June Heaven, RN, BSc, MEd
Health Sciences Division
Humber College
Toronto, Canada

Tana W. Hunter, RN, MS, CS
College of Nursing
Brigham Young University
Provo, UT

Marguerite Jackson, RN, MS, CIC, FAAN
University of California
UCSD Medical Center
San Diego, CA

Alva Jordan, RN, MSN
School of Nursing
Alcorn State University
Natchez, MS

Mary M. Lambert, RN, BS, MSEd
School of Nursing
Western Oklahoma State College
Altus, OK

Margie Bentch Landson, RN, MSN
Associate Degree Nursing Program
Houston Community College
Houston, TX

Susan G. Larson, RN, MS
School of Nursing
Mid-America Nazarene College
Olathe, KS

Sarah V. Latham, RN, DSN
College of Nursing
Jacksonville State University
Jacksonville, AL

Rita J. Lourie, RN, MSN
Department of Nursing
Temple University
Philadelphia, PA

Marilyn Lowe, RN, MSN
Nebraska Methodist Hospital
Omaha, NE

Paula Lisa Mastrilli, RN, BScN, MScN
Faculty of Nursing
University of Toronto
Toronto, Canada

Jane McAteer, RN, MN
Department of Nursing
College of San Mateo
San Mateo, CA

Marycarol McGovern, RN, MSN
College of Nursing
Villanova University
Villanova, PA

Rebecca Merriam, RN, MSN
Division of Nursing
Olympic College
Bremerton, WA

Carol Ann Mitchell, EdD, NP, CS
College of Nursing
East Tennessee State University
Johnson City, TN

Dorothy Dark Mixon, RN, MS, MSN
Coosa Valley Medical Center School of Nursing
Sylacauga, AL

Sheila Money, RN, BA, MEd
Health Sciences Division
Humber College
Toronto, Canada

Janet G. Mooney, RN, MS
Health Science Department
Rock Valley College
Rockford, IL

Kathleen Mulryan, RN, MS
Nursing Program
LaGuardia Community College
Long Island City, NY

Irene Oswald, RN, BSN, MA
Health Sciences Division
Humber College
Toronto, Canada

Kathleen T. Patterson, MSN, CS
School of Nursing
University of Pittsburgh
Bradford, PA

Lynne Peterson, RN, MSN, MEd
Hocking College
Nelsonville, OH

Jennifer Reilly, RN, MSN, MEd
Hocking College
Nelsonville, OH

Jane Richard, RN, MS
Department of Nursing
Houston Community College
Houston, TX

Laura R. Romero, RN, MSN, CNM
Department of Nursing
East Los Angeles College
Monterey Park, CA

Judith Ruland, RN
Department of Nursing
Hartwick College
Oneonta, NY

Marjorie Ryan, RN, MSN
Department of Nursing
Miami University
Oxford, OH

Mary E. Sampel, RN, MSN
School of Nursing
St. Louis University
St. Louis, MO

Gladys L. Simenc, RN, MS
Department of Nursing
Bradley University
Peoria, IL

Darlene S. Smikahl, RN, MSN, CS
Department of Nursing
Ft. Scott Community College
Ft. Scott, KS

Golden T. Soileau, RN, MA, MSN
College of Nursing
McNeese State University
Lake Charles, LA

Irene Stein, BA, BAppSci, DipNEd, MA
University of Wollongong
Wollongong, NSW, Australia

Ruby L. Steele, RN, PhD, CS
Director of Nursing Program
Fort Valley State College
Fort Valley, GA

Saundra L. Theis, RN, PhD
College of Nursing
University of Illinois
Chicago, IL

Margaret Kittman-Thomas, RN, MEd, MSN
School of Nursing
Western Oklahoma State University
Altus, OK

Linda Tozer-Johnston, RN, BScN, MEd
School of Health Sciences
Sault College
Sault Ste. Marie, Canada

Sandra McSherry Waguespack, RN, MSN
School of Nursing
Louisiana State University
New Orleans, LA

Dorothy Ann Walker, RN, MSN
School of Nursing
Indiana University
Kokomo, IN

Karen Watson, RN, DipT, BEd, PGHthAdm
University of Southern Australia
Adelaide, Australia

Shirley A. Watts, RN, BSN
Faculty of Nursing
University of Manitoba
Winnipeg, Canada

Dorothy Windsor, RN, BEd
Diploma Nursing Faculty
Saskatchewan Institute of Applied Science and Technology
Regina, Canada

Jean H. Woods, RN, CS, THD
College of Allied Health Professionals
Temple University
Philadelphia, PA

Preface for the Updated Fifth Edition

No matter where care is delivered, no matter what the pathophysiologic process, no matter how many lines, medications, or pieces of equipment are involved, nursing's unique role is to care for the person.

Sarah Sanford

Nursing's unique role demands a blend of sensitivity, caring, commitment, and skill based on broad knowledge and its application in practice. This text provides a foundation on which students can build their professional repertoire of knowledge as well as their interpersonal and clinical expertise.

In this updated edition of *Fundamentals of Nursing*, selected content has been replaced to reflect the latest nursing research and current health care delivery realities. Many of the changes are in response to suggestions and comments from reviewers, nurses, and students using the text.

The updated fifth edition is **not** a new edition. This version incorporates the many recent changes in health care to keep your students as informed as possible. The page numbers are the same as the original fifth edition so there is no need to change class notes extensively. Also, there are no new instructor or student supplements and all existing supplements are still available.

New Updated Fifth Edition Features

Three Updated Chapters

The following chapters underwent major revision and updating:

Chapter 4 Health Care Delivery Systems
Chapter 15 Ethnicity and Culture
Chapter 27 Preventing the Transfer of Microorganisms

One New Chapter

A new chapter, Individuals and Families in the Home and Community, replaces the fifth edition Chapter 14, Individuals, Families, and Community Health.

Other Updates

The updated fifth edition has been carefully constructed to reflect current health care realities. The updated edition features include the following:

- Updated information throughout the text on community health settings, home health care delivery, managed care realities, outcomes measurement, and the role of the case manager in health care.
- New information on the changing role of the nurse, changing demands for nurses, and new job opportunities for nurses.
- New information on preventing the transfer of microorganisms that reflects the most current CDC guidelines for infection control. (See Chapter 27 and the inside back cover of the text.)
- Updated information on providing culturally sensitive care.
- Selected new research boxes, which reflect current studies.
- Introductory information on holistic health and alternative health care providers.
- New NANDA diagnoses as appropriate.
- Updated statistics throughout the book.

What will not change in the updated edition:

- Page numbering in the text will remain the same as it was in the original fifth edition.
- The Supplemental Teaching/Learning Package, available to qualified instructors, will remain the same. Some package items may not be available to adopters outside the United States.

Fifth Edition Features

Full-Color Design

The fifth edition of *Fundamentals of Nursing* uses full color throughout the book, making the text more appealing and easier to use.

Critical Pathways

Critical Pathways prepared by a clinical expert have replaced the Nursing Care Plans at the end of each chapter in the fourth edition. The Critical Pathways concept is introduced in Chapter 4, Health Care Delivery.

Time Line of Nursing History

A colorful pictorial history of nursing is presented in a time line format across the top of most pages in Chapter 1.

Student Profiles
Student profiles occur throughout the book in each unit opener. The profiles include photos of nursing students and information about why they chose nursing, their most gratifying moment in nursing, advice for other students, and more.

Wellness Teaching Boxes
These boxes are designed to help students focus on wellness information that will help clients live healthier, happier lives.

Critical Thinking Boxes
Many chapters present a potential clinical problem that could arise when providing care. Entitled, "What Would You Do?", they are designed to stimulate critical thinking. Topics to consider when responding to the dilemmas posed in the boxes are available in the Instructor's Guide that accompanies the text. They may be used as a basis for post-clinical conference discussions or in a classroom setting.

Nursing Diagnoses Boxes
Selected NANDA nursing diagnoses with definitions, defining characteristics, and related factors are presented in the following chapters:

- Spirituality and Sexuality in Unit 4
- Helping/Communicating and Teaching/Learning in Unit 5
- All chapters in Units 8, 9, and 10

Care Planning Guides
Care Planning Guides, provided in tabular format in each of the chapters mentioned above, include *outcome criteria* for a specified nursing diagnosis, as well as related *nursing interventions* and *rationales*.

NIC Taxonomy Structure
The six domains of the Nursing Intervention Taxonomy (independent nursing actions) developed by the Iowa Intervention Project are presented in Chapter 8, Implementing and Evaluating, in the Nursing Process Unit.

Procedures
All procedures are written in the three-column procedure format used in the fourth edition. Each procedure contains purposes, an assessment focus, a list of equipment, a list of step-by-step interventions describing how to perform each procedure, and an evaluation focus. The purposes, the assessment focus at the beginning of each procedure, and the evaluation focus at the end of each procedure were new to the fifth edition. New procedures included:

Using an Ambularm Safety Monitoring Device

Using a Pulse Oximeter

Managing Pain with a Patient-Controlled Analgesia Pump (PCA)

Special Learning Aids

- Safety alert logos indicating when safety precautions are essential
- Blood and body fluid alert logos to reinforce awareness of CDC body fluid precautions
- Wellness logos to emphasize the nurse's role in health promotion
- A full-color section showing common skin disorders, including decubitus ulcers

Retained in this Edition
The updated fifth edition of *Fundamentals of Nursing* retains many of the features that have been well received by the users of this book.

- Table of Contents, organized so that it can be used with various nursing theories and conceptual frameworks.
- Use of the nursing process as a framework for nursing care in all clinically oriented chapters.
- Nursing process application to nursing practice. The client (Luisa Sanchez), is used as a frame of reference for applying content in all phases of the nursing process in Chapters 5, 6, 7, and 8.
- Emphasis on the elderly. Eighteen boxes in Chapter 22, Assessing Health Status, show normal physical changes; an entire chapter (Chapter 26, Late Adulthood) is devoted to promoting the health of the elderly.
- Emphasis on wellness (Chapter 13 and Unit 7). See also Special Learning Aids.
- Clinical Guidelines boxes—instant-access summaries of clinical do's and don'ts.
- Client teaching boxes—quick reference displays that focus on the client's learning needs.
- Updated nursing research notes that describe relevant studies and relate them to clinical practice.
- A detailed table of contents, glossary, and index to enhance use of the book.

SUPPLEMENTAL TEACHING/ LEARNING PACKAGE

The Clinical Companion. The Companion, which includes pertinent information students will use in a clinical setting, eg, assessment guides, safety information, medical terminology, and communication tips, was compiled with the assistance of nursing students.

Study Guide. This guide with learning exercises, written by Karen Van Leuven, helps students apply and extend knowledge.

Procedures Manual and Checklists. This supplement, compiled by Suzanne Beyea, provides approximately 80 additional procedures, and includes checklists to document student progress.

Fluid and Electrolyte Module. This module provides additional information to help students apply this content in the clinical area.

Checklists for Procedures in the Text. This tool, prepared by Cari Boatright Cagle, provides key steps in procedures in *Fundamentals of Nursing*. These checklists can be used to help students evaluate their learning performance.

Set of Full-Color Transparency Acetates. These acetates provide visual support for classroom instruction.

Instructor's Guide. This guide, prepared by Audrey Berman, provides chapter outlines, objectives, discussion questions, suggestions for audiovisual materials, and learning activities for classroom and clinical conferences.

Test Bank. Prepared by Judith M. Wilkinson, this supplement provides over 1000 test items.

IBM Testing Software. This material is available in 3½ or 5¼ format.

We have tried to prepare a book that reflects our values about nursing, and we are, indeed, enthusiastic about the updated fifth edition of *Fundamentals of Nursing*. In the words of Virginia Henderson:

> *The complete, mature, or excellent nurse . . . is the one who remains compassionate and sensitive to patients, who has thoroughly mastered nursing's technical skills, but who uses—and has the opportunity to use—her emotional and technical responses in a unique design that suits the peculiar needs of the person she serves and the situation in which she finds herself.*
>
> *Virginia Henderson*
> "Excellence in Nursing"
> American Journal of Nursing,
> October, 1969

Barbara E. Kozier
Glenora L. Erb
Kathleen K. Blais
Judith M. Wilkinson
Karen Van Leuven

Acknowledgments

We wish to extend a sincere thank you to the committed and talented team involved in the book. Each of you has made a very important contribution in this revision.

- The two additional authors for this edition, **Kathleen Koernig Blais** and **Judith M. Wilkinson** revised many chapters in this edition and wrote the chapter on Critical Thinking, Problem Solving, and Decision Making. Also, Kathleen Blais created the fascinating historical time line in Chapter 1. Our association with them has been a most enriching experience.
- The **contributors** who provided content in their areas of expertise: Leslie Atkinson, Suzanne Beyea, Evelyn Brooks, Susan Fairchild, Suzanne Phillips, Jean Temple, and Karen Van Leuven.
- All **reviewers,** who provided so many valuable comments.
- The **nursing students** and **teachers** who used previous editions of *Fundamentals of Nursing* and who sent us many helpful suggestions for this edition.
- ***Patti Cleary,*** executive and sponsoring editor. Her continued dedication and leadership has been a guiding light during the preparation of this edition. We greatly appreciate her commitment to an excellent product and her vision for this text. Her ideas stimulate thought and we continue to value her support and editorial expertise.
- ***Wendy Earl,*** managing editor. As always, she makes the impossible appear easy. In particular, Wendy has contributed to the book's style and visual appeal. We are also grateful for her organizational ability in coordinating the work of all the production staff and the authors.
- ***David Rich,*** production supervisor. His cheerful disposition, energy, flexibility, and sense of humor have often transformed work into pleasure. His attention to detail and to the appearance of the pages has been greatly appreciated.
- ***Juan Vargas,*** text designer. His great talent has made the fifth edition the best looking ever.
- ***Michele Mangelli,*** art coordinator. Her calm, capable, professional manner and detective's eye for detail provided consistency and accuracy in the line drawings. She has been a pleasure to work with.
- ***Bradley Burch,*** production coordinator. Bradley assisted in art and photo development, and coordinated all supplements for this edition. We feel fortunate to have had this large package of nine supplements in such capable hands.
- ***Elena Dorfman,*** photo coordinator and photographer and ***Richard Tauber,*** photographer, for their creative, realistic, and sensitive photographs, even though they were often difficult to obtain in a busy clinical setting.
- ***Chris Burke, Nea Hanscomb, Linda Harris,*** and ***Precision Graphics,*** principal artists. Their explicit line drawings confirm the saying that "one picture is worth a thousand words."
- ***Suzanne Rotondo,*** editorial assistant. She graciously helped whenever it was needed.
- ***Sally Peyrefitte,*** copy editor. Sally provided many suggestions on style and syntax. Her patience with the complexities of the manuscript was greatly appreciated.
- ***Edie Williams,*** page designer. Edie's expertise is seen in the visual appeal of each page.
- ***Katherine Pitcoff,*** indexer. Her meticulous reading of each page is evident in the comprehensive index.
- ***Grace Wong,*** project editor. Her careful attention to detail while coordinating the content of the Clinical Companion has enhanced the usefulness of this handbook for students in the clinical area.
- ***Mary Tobin,*** typist. Mary made miracles come true in meeting schedules. We continue to value her skills and flexibility for yet another manuscript.
- ***Library Personnel: Joan Andrews, Carole MacFarlane,*** and staff; in particular, ***Linda Edge*** at the Registered Nurses Association of British Columbia and ***Daniel Tan*** at the Florida International University Library. They never failed to obtain the many reference materials the authors requested.

Finally, we thank our understanding families and friends who, once again, were patient and supportive throughout yet another writing schedule.

Barbara Kozier

Glenora Erb

Contents

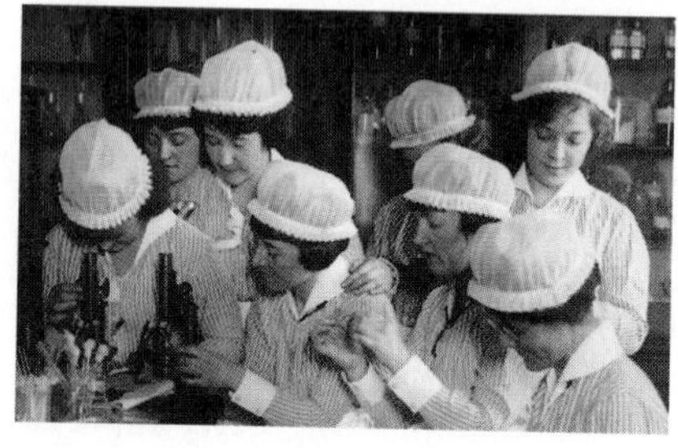

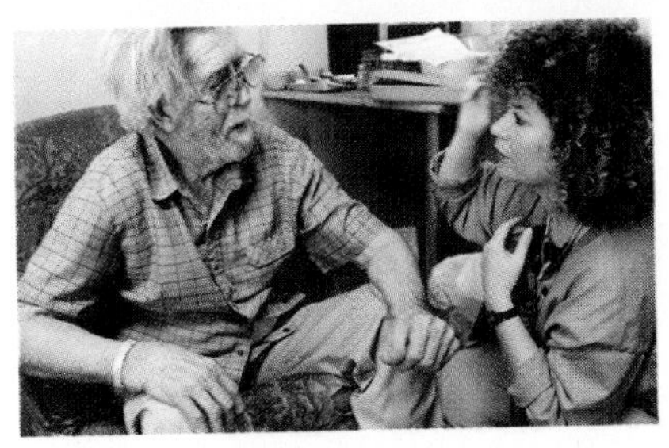

UNIT 2 THE NURSING PROCESS 81

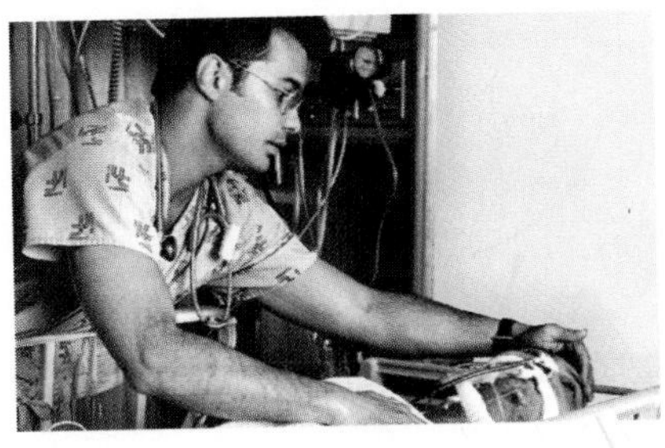

UNIT 3 PROFESSIONAL ACCOUNTABILITY AND ADVOCACY 199

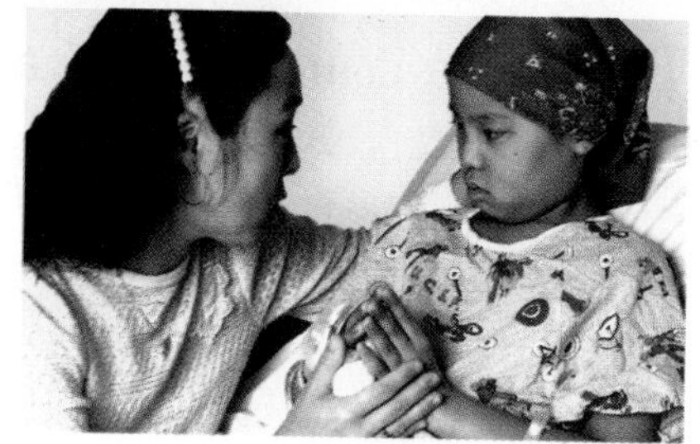

UNIT 4
ELEMENTS OF HOLISTIC CARE 243

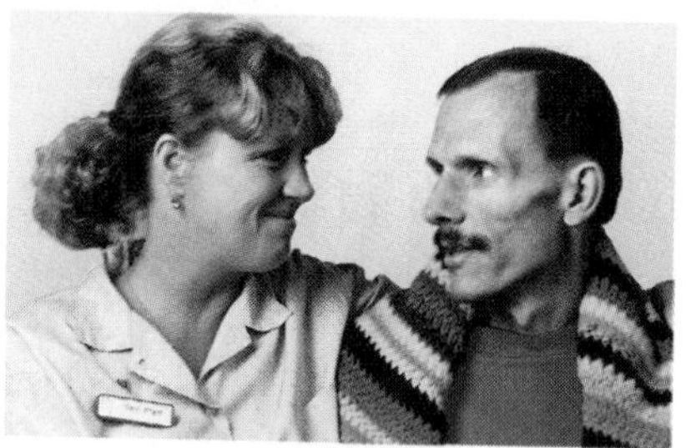

UNIT 5
INTEGRAL COMPONENTS OF CLIENT CARE 351

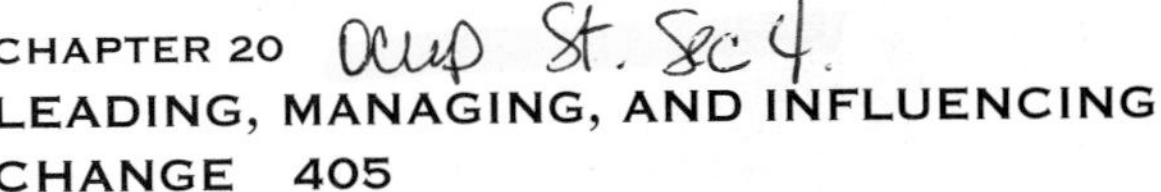

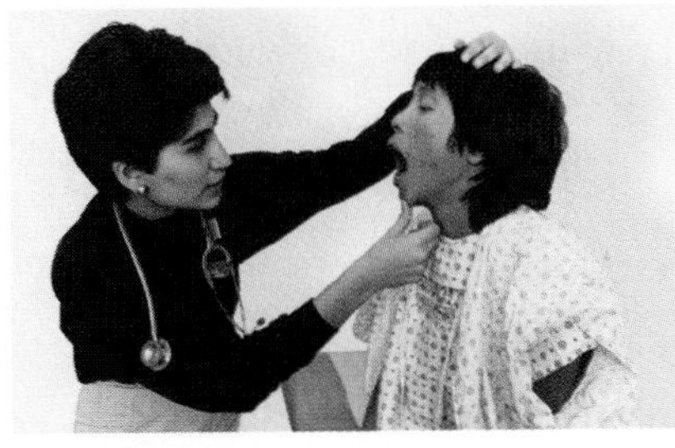

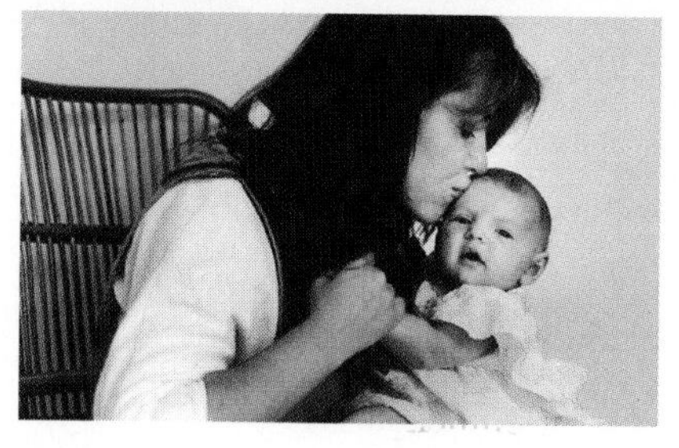

UNIT 7
PROMOTING WELLNESS THROUGH THE LIFE SPAN 567

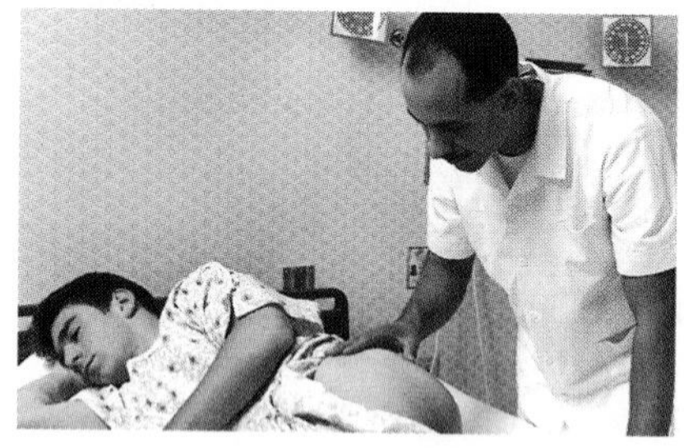

UNIT 8
PROTECTING HEALTH 661

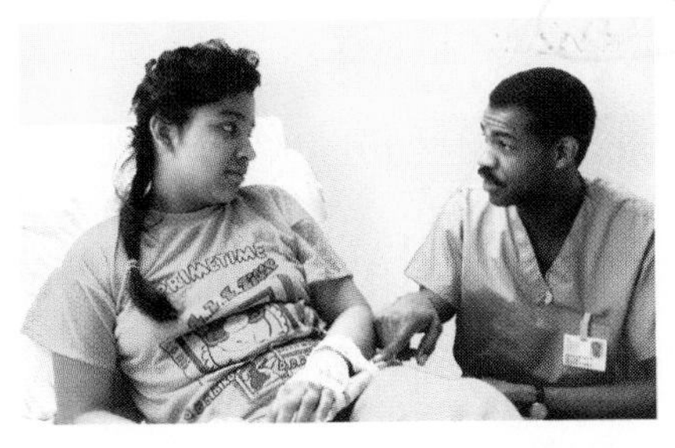

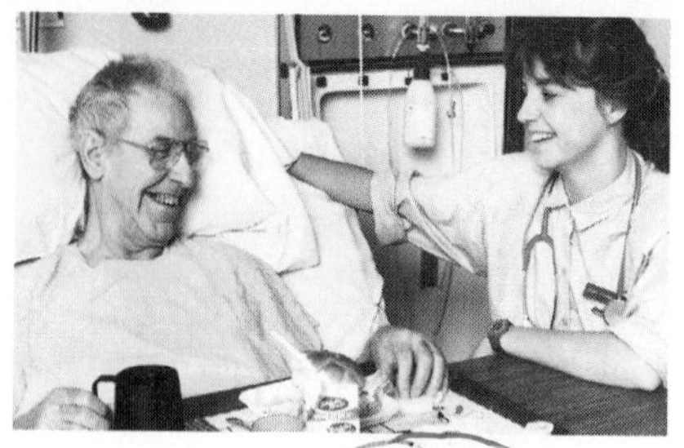

UNIT 10

PROMOTING PHYSIOLOGIC HEALTH 877

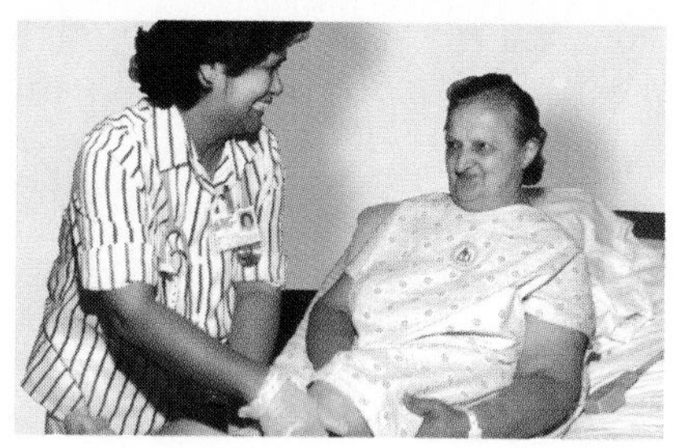

UNIT 11
IMPLEMENTING SPECIAL NURSING MEASURES 1293

CHAPTER 43
MEDICATIONS 1294

CHAPTER 44
WOUND CARE 1358

CHAPTER 45
PERIOPERATIVE NURSING 1397

APPENDICES 1425

Special Features

Critical Thinking Challenges

Critical Pathways

Clinical Assessment/Assessment Interview

Client/Wellness Teaching

NURSING DIAGNOSES

CARE PLANNING GUIDES

CLINICAL GUIDELINES

RESEARCH NOTES

Blood and Body Fluid Precautions

This logo draws attention to the need for blood and body fluid precautions. These precautions are intended to protect the nurse and others from infection. See the Universal Precautions on the inside back cover, and check with your instructor regarding agency protocol to determine which precautionary measures to implement.

Safety Precautions

This logo highlights nursing actions that are of particular significance for maintaining client and nurse safety. If you require clarification, consult your instructor or check agency protocol to ensure safe practice.

Wellness

This logo alerts students to pertinent information about maintaining and promoting wellness.

UNIT 1

Contemporary Nursing Practice

STUDENT PROFILE

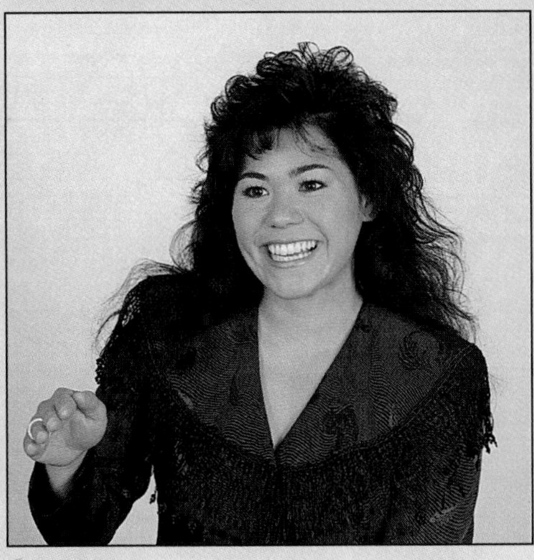

NAME	Kathy Evans
SCHOOL OF NURSING	University of New Mexico, Albuquerque, New Mexico
HOMETOWN	Albuquerque

WHY DID YOU ENTER THE FIELD OF NURSING?
I want to do more for my community, and I'd like to help change the nursing image to a more professional role. It is a great feeling to know you are helping others in their time of illness or need.

WHAT QUALITIES DO YOU THINK ARE NECESSARY TO BE A GOOD NURSE?
Being a caring person, having empathy—as well as sympathy—and good communication skills.

WHAT HAS BEEN YOUR MOST GRATIFYING MOMENT AS A STUDENT NURSE?
It was my third week in my Med-Surg unit and I was taking care of a man who had spinal cancer. I spent a lot of time with him and learned a lot about his life. He was really grateful to me for spending the time to talk to him and care about him. It really touched my heart.

WHAT ADVICE WOULD YOU GIVE A NEW STUDENT?
Try to get as much experience as possible. Take some time for yourself and enjoy nursing school. Take advantage of all the opportunities available to you, including volunteer work.

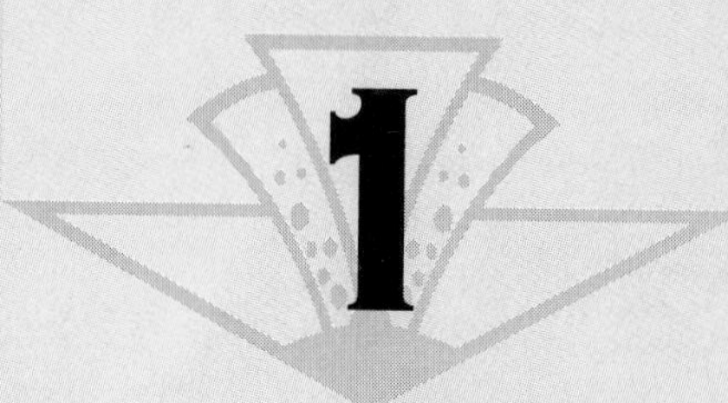

1 Introduction to Nursing

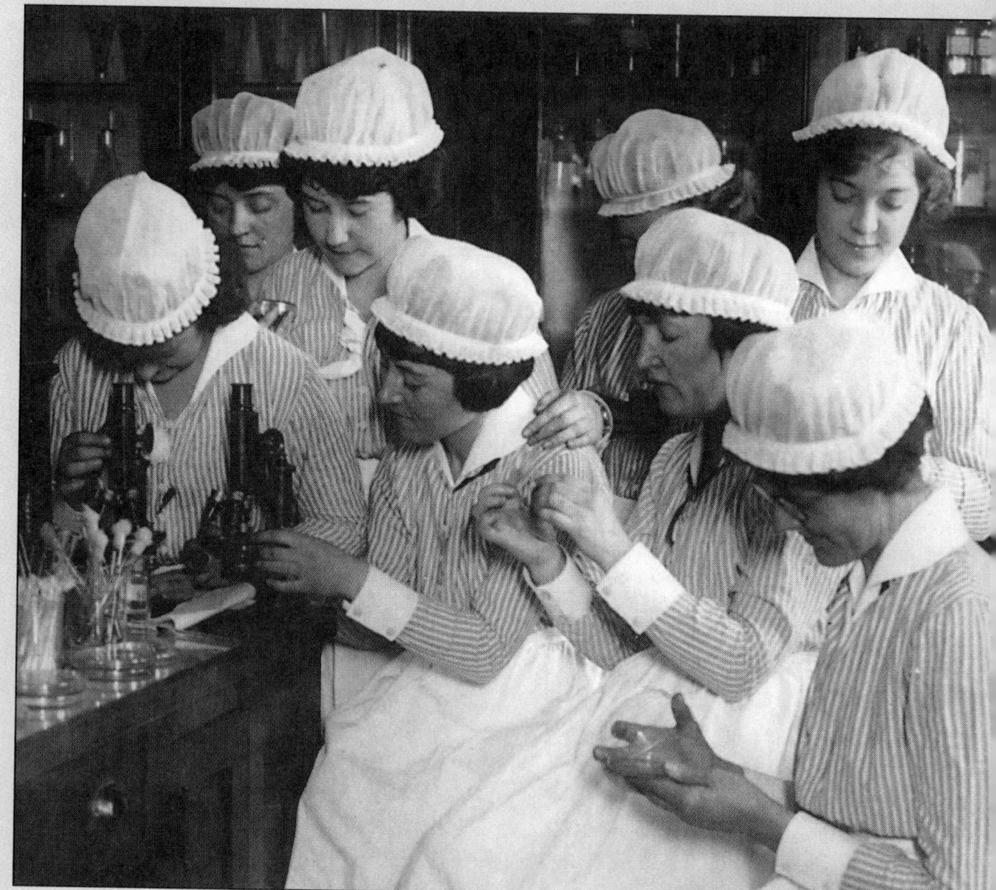

Objectives

- Identify the essential aspects of nursing.
- Discuss the historical development of nursing.
- Explain the professional growth within nursing.
- Describe the five behaviors of the professional nurse as identified by Miller.
- Discuss the critical components of professionalism: specialized education, knowledge base, ethics, and autonomy.
- Identify the critical attributes of professionalism in nursing.
- Identify Styles's beliefs about the nature and purpose of nursing.
- Identify nursing's "patterns of knowing."
- Discuss Benner's levels of nursing proficiency.
- Describe the roles of the professional nurse.
- Describe the expanded nursing roles of nurse clinician, clinical nurse specialist, and advanced nurse practitioner.
- Explain the functions of the national nurses' associations.

Nursing today is far different from nursing as it was practiced 50 years ago, and it takes a vivid imagination to envision how the nursing profession will change as we move forward into the 21st century. To comprehend present-day nursing and at the same time prepare for the future, one must understand not only past events but also contemporary nursing practice and the sociologic factors affecting it.

AN EMERGING DEFINITION OF NURSING

To understand what nursing is, one must first define the word. However, many definitions exist, and some misrepresent the complex knowledge and skill of professional nursing. Common dictionary definitions, for example, still refer to the nurse as "a person, usually a woman, trained to care for the sick" (*The New Lexicon Webster's Dictionary of the English Language*). Today, however, many men are choosing to become nurses, and nurses also provide preventive care to well clients through immunization programs and health teaching.

Florence Nightingale defined nursing over 100 years ago as "the act of utilizing the environment of the patient to assist him in his recovery" (Nightingale 1860). Nightingale considered a clean, well-ventilated, and quiet environment essential for recovery. Often considered the first nurse theorist, Nightingale raised the status of nursing through education. Nurses were no longer untrained housekeepers but people trained in the care of the sick.

Virginia Henderson was one of the first modern nurses to define nursing. In 1960, she wrote, "The unique function of the nurse is to assist the individual, sick or well, in the performance of those activities contributing to health or its recovery (or to peaceful death) that he would perform unaided if he had the necessary strength, will, or knowledge, and to do this in such a way as to help him gain independence as rapidly as possible" (Henderson 1966, p. 3). Like Nightingale, Henderson described nursing in relation to the client and the client's environment. Unlike Nightingale, Henderson saw the nurse as concerned with both well and ill individuals, acknowledged that nurses interact with clients even when recovery may not be feasible, and mentioned the teaching and advocacy roles of the nurse.

Professional nursing associations have also examined nursing and developed their definitions of nursing. The American Nurses Association (ANA) describes nursing practice as "direct, goal oriented, and adaptable to the needs of the individual, the family, and community during health and illness" (ANA 1973, p. 2). In 1980, the ANA published this definition of nursing: "Nursing is the diagnosis and treatment of human responses to actual or potential health problems" (ANA 1980, p. 9). In its 1987 House of Delegates, the ANA adopted a statement on the scope of nursing practice: "There is one scope of clinical nursing practice. The core, or essence, of that practice is the nursing diagnosis and treatment of human responses to health and to illness" (ANA 1987a, p. 76). The new statement further describes the differences between professional and technical nurses: The "depth and breadth to which the individual nurse engages in the total scope of the clinical practice of nursing are defined by the knowledge base of the nurse, the role of the nurse, and the nature of the client population within a practice environment" (ANA 1987a, p. 76). The Canadian Nurses Association (CNA) published a definition in 1984 that serves as the professional standard for nurses in Canada.

> "Nursing" or "the practice of nursing" means the identification and treatment of human responses to actual or potential health problems and includes the practice of and supervision of functions and services that, directly or indirectly, in collaboration with a client or providers of health care other than nurses, have as their objectives the promotion of health, prevention of illness, alleviation of suffering, restoration of health and optimum development of health potential and includes all aspects of the nursing process (CNA Connection 1984, p. 8).

In the latter half of the 20th century, a number of nurse theorists developed their own theoretical definitions of nursing. Theoretical definitions are important because they go beyond simplistic common definitions. They describe what nursing is and the interrelationship between nurses, nursing, the client, and the intended client outcome—health. They try to answer the question, "If nursing disappeared and there were no nurses, what would be missing?" Certain themes are common to many of these definitions:

- Nursing is caring.
- Nursing is an art.
- Nursing is a science.
- Nursing is client centered.
- Nursing is holistic.
- Nursing is adaptive.
- Nursing is concerned with health promotion, health maintenance, and health restoration.
- Nursing is a helping profession.

MILESTONES IN NURSING HISTORY

Ancient Civilizations

3000 BC

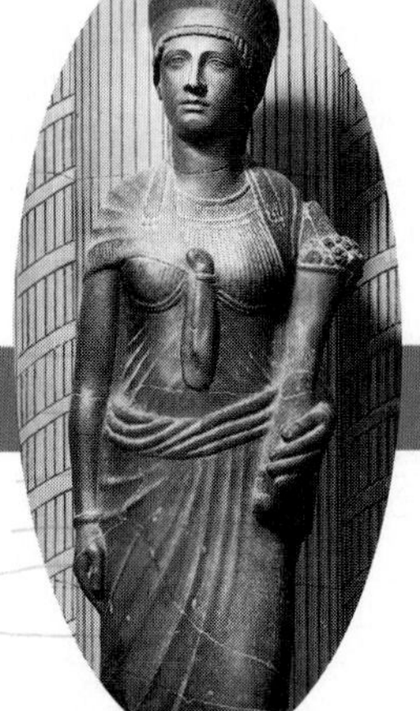

Egypt
The Egyptian goddess Isis and her son Horus were regarded as creators of the medical arts. They used the medium of dreams to minister to the sick.

1900 BC

Babylonia
In a Babylonian sickroom, healers and assistants followed the Code of Hammurabi to cure and to provide care.

50 BC

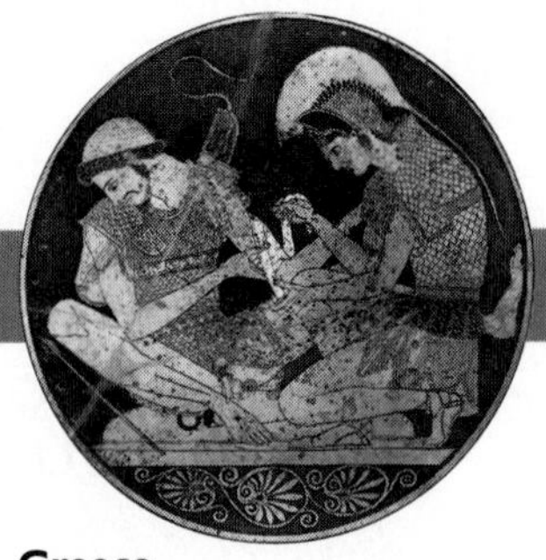

Greece
The ancient Greek gods were believed to have special healing powers. In this detail from the bowl of Sosias, Achilles bandages the wounds of Patroclus.

Chapter 3 provides more detailed information about nursing theorists and discusses their beliefs about the interrelationship between the nurse, the client, health, and the environment in which the interaction occurs.

HISTORICAL PERSPECTIVES OF NURSING

The nursing profession has a proud history. Traditional female roles of wife, mother, daughter, and sister have always included the care and nurturing of other family members. Artifacts in earliest primitive societies establish the existence of individuals, both men and women, who comforted and cared for the sick and those unable to care for themselves. There are also artistic representations of individuals who assisted the society's healers in curing. The traditional nursing role was one of humanistic caring, nurturing, comforting, and supporting.

NURSING IN ANCIENT CIVILIZATIONS

The early recordings of ancient civilizations offer little information about those who cared for the sick. During this time, beliefs about the cause of disease were embedded in superstition and magic, and thus treatment often involved magical cures. As these societies evolved, however, practical theories of medical care emerged as nonmagical causes of disease were observed. It is known that midwives provided care for the mother and infant during birthing and that wet nurses often suckled and cared for infant children of wealthy families. Often these roles were filled by female slaves. The slave-nurse was dependent on the master, healer, or priest for instruction or direction in the care of her charge. Often the care provided for the sick was related to physical maintenance and comfort.

The earliest recording of healing practices is a 4000-year-old clay tablet attributed to the Sumerian civilization. It contains healing prescriptions but, unfortunately, neglects to describe the illnesses for which they were prescribed. The earliest documentation of law governing the practice of medicine is the Code of Hammurabi, attributed to the Babylonians and dating to 1900 BC. The code recorded regulations related to sanitation and public health, the practice of surgery, the differentiation between the practice of human medicine and veterinary medicine, a table of fees for operations, and penalties for violators of the code. There is no specific record of nursing in the Babylonian civilization; however, there are references to tasks and practices traditionally provided by nurses. Medical illustration from that period often includes a nurselike figure providing patient support or comfort. Nurses are mentioned occasionally in the Old Testament as women who provided care for infants and children, for the sick

The Common Era

Roman Benefactors
Wealthy Roman matrons like Fabiola—viewed by some as the patron saint of early nursing—used position and wealth to establish hospitals for the sick.

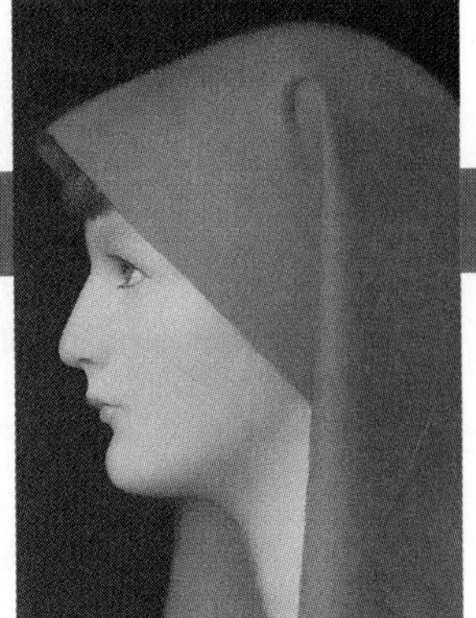

400 AD

1096 AD

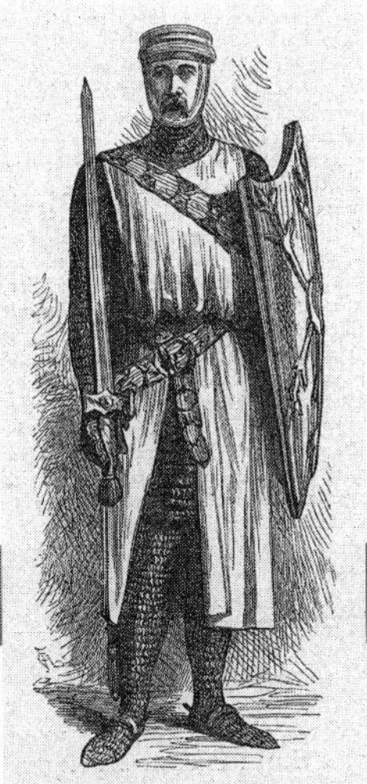

Crusaders
During the Crusades, military Knighthood orders were established to provide care to soldiers and pilgrims to the Holy Land. This may be the first recognition of men providing nursing care.

1099 AD

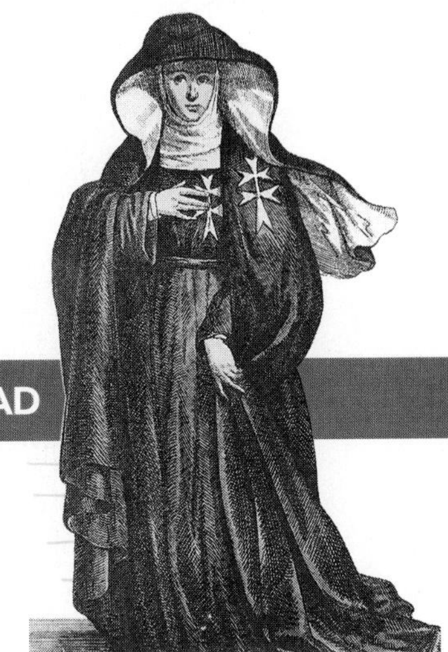

Christians
Sisters of the Order of the Knights Hospitallers of St. John of Jerusalem embroidered the cross on their tunics to represent their Christian charity.

and dying, and as midwives who assisted during pregnancy and at delivery.

In ancient Greece and Rome, care of the sick and injured was advanced in mythology and reality. The Greek god Asklepios was the chief healer; his wife, Epigone, was the soother. Hygeia, daughter of Asklepios, was goddess of health and was revered by some as the embodiment of the nurse. After they conquered Greece in 200 BC, the Romans borrowed gods from the Greeks, including Aesculapius (Asklepios) and Hygeia.

In ancient African cultures, the nurturing functions of the nurse included roles as midwife, herbalist, wet nurse, and carer for children and the elderly. In ancient India, early hospitals were staffed by male nurses who were required to meet four qualifications: "(1) knowledge of the manner in which drugs should be prepared for administration, (2) cleverness, (3) devotedness to the patient, and (4) purity of mind and body" (Donahue 1985, p. 61). Indian women served as midwives and nursed ill family members.

The Role of Religion in the Development of Nursing

Many of the world's religions encourage benevolence, but it was the Christian value of "love thy neighbor as thyself" that had a significant impact on the development of Western nursing. The principle of caring was established with Christ's parable of the Good Samaritan providing care for a tired and injured stranger. Converts to Christianity during the third and fourth centuries included several wealthy matrons of the Roman Empire, including Marcella, Fabiola, and Paula, who used their wealth to provide houses of care and healing (the forerunner of hospitals) for the poor, the sick, and the homeless.

Women were not the sole providers of nursing services; in the third century in Rome there was an organization of men called the Parabolani Brotherhood. This group of men provided care to the sick and dying during the great plague in Alexandria. During the Crusades, several knighthood orders—such as the Knights of Saint John of Jerusalem (also known as the Knights Hospitalers), the Teutonic Knights, and the Knights of Lazarus—formed, composed of brothers in arms who provided nursing care to their sick and injured comrades. These orders were responsible for building great hospitals, the organization and management of which set a standard for the administration of hospitals throughout Europe at that time. As the Christian church grew, more hospitals were built, as were specialized institutions providing care for orphans, widows, the elderly, the poor, and the sick. During the Middle Ages (AD 500–1500), male and female religious, military, and secular orders with the primary purpose of caring for the sick were formed. Conspicuous among them were the aforementioned Knights of Saint John (Knights Hospitalers); the Alexian Brotherhood

The Middle Ages

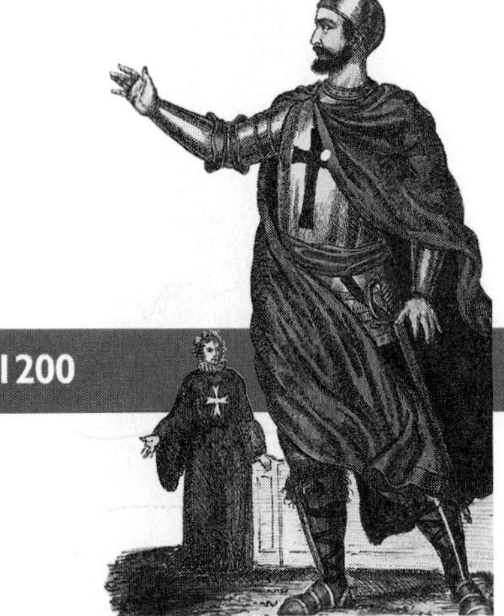

Charitable Nursing
Camillus DeLellis, considered the patron saint of nurses, was the founder of the Nursing Order of Ministries of the Sick. His first efforts focused on preparing nurses to provide care for the poor, the imprisoned, and the dying.

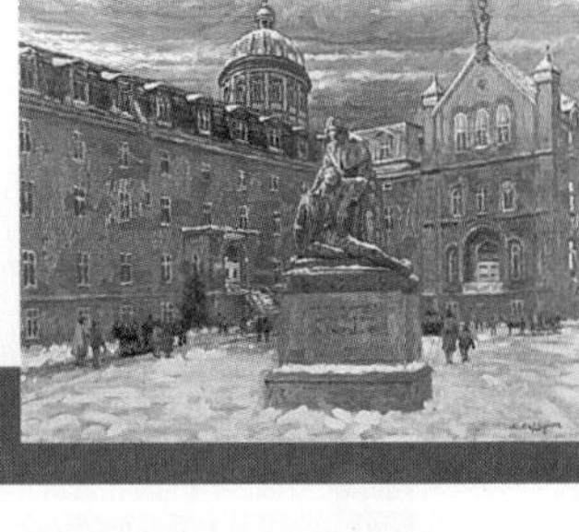

1200 — 1550 — 1639

Nursing Care of Outcasts
The Knights of St. Lazarus dedicated themselves to the care of people with leprosy, syphilis, and chronic skin conditions. From the time of Christ to the mid-thirteenth century, leprosy was viewed as an incurable and terminal disease.

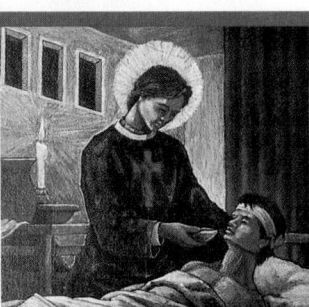

Early Canadian Hospitals
The Hotel Dieu Hospital in Quebec, founded by the Duchesse d'Aiguillon and staffed by three hospital Sisters from the Order of St. Augustine, is considered the first hospital in Canada. In 1644, Jeanne Mance, known as the Florence Nightingale of Canada, founded the Hotel Dieu in Montreal.

(organized in 1431); and the Augustinian sisters, which was the first purely nursing order.

In the late 16th century, Camillus DeLellis, later sainted for his work of Christian charity, founded a nursing order to provide care for the poor, the sick, the dying, and those in prisons. In 1633, the Sisters of Charity were founded by Saint Vincent de Paul in France. It was the first of many such orders organized under various Roman Catholic church auspices and largely devoted to caring for the sick. The Order of the Sisters of Charity sent nursing sisters to provide care in the New World, establishing hospitals in Canada, the United States, and Australia.

The deaconess groups, composed of women who provided care, had their origins in the Roman Empire of the third and fourth centuries but were suppressed during the Middle Ages by the Western churches. However, these groups of nursing providers resurfaced occasionally throughout the centuries, most notably in 1836, when Theodor Fliedner reinstituted the Order of Deaconesses and opened a small hospital and training school in Kaiserswerth, Germany. Florence Nightingale received her "training" in nursing at the Kaiserswerth School.

The Development of Modern Nursing

The intellectual revolution of the 18th and 19th centuries led to a scientific revolution. With the discovery and exploration of new continents, an economic revolution evolved, after which nations became more interdependent through trade. The Industrial Revolution displaced workers from cottage craftsmen to factory laborers. With these changes came stressors to health. New illnesses, transmitted in the holds of ships by seamen and stowaway rodents, jumped national boundaries and continents. The closeness of factory work, the long hours, and the unhealthy working conditions led to the rapid transmission of communicable diseases such as cholera and plague. Lack of prenatal care, inadequate nutrition, and poor delivery techniques resulted in a high rate of maternal and infant mortality. Many orphaned children died in workhouses of neglect or cruelty.

During this time, a "proper" woman's role in life was to maintain a gracious and elegant home for her family. The common women worked as servants in private homes or were dependent on their husbands' wages. The provision of care for the sick in hospitals or private homes fell to the uncommon women—often prisoners or prostitutes who had little or no training in nursing. Because of this, nursing had little acceptance and no prestige. The only acceptable nursing role was within a religious order where services were provided as part of Christian charity.

The creation of the Institute of Protestant Deaconesses at Kaiserswerth, Germany, changed all this. Associated with a religious organization, the Order of Deaconesses ignited recognition of the need for the services of

Early Nineteenth Century

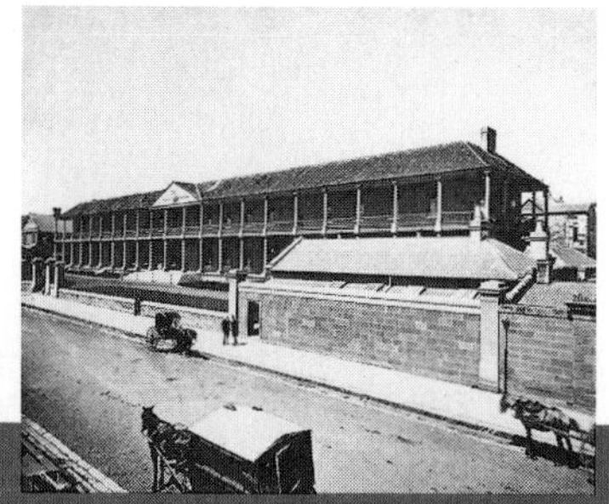

1812

Early Australian Hospitals
In Sydney, Australia's first hospital was named for its designer and builder, Governor Lachlan Macquarie.

1854

Mary Grant Seacole
Jamaican nurse Mary Grant Seacole (1805-1881) worked with Florence Nightingale to provide care to the soldiers of the Crimean War.

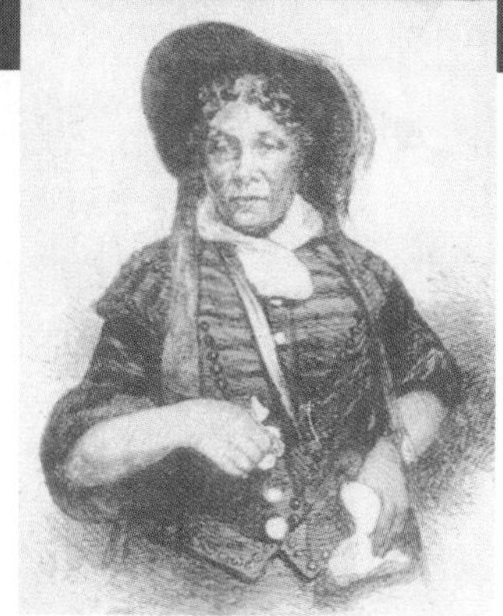

1859

Florence Nightingale
Considered the founder of modern nursing, Nightingale (1820-1910) was influential in developing nursing education, practice, and administration. Her 1859 publication, *Notes on Nursing: What it Is and What it Is Not*, was intended for all women.

women in the care of the sick, the poor, children, and female prisoners. The training school for nurses at Kaiserswerth included care of the sick in hospitals, instruction in visiting nursing, instruction in religious doctrine and ethics, and pharmacy. The deaconess movement eventually spread to four continents, including North America, North Africa, Asia, and Australia.

Florence Nightingale, the most famous Kaiserswerth pupil, was born to a wealthy and intellectual family. Her education included the mastery of several ancient and modern languages, literature, philosophy, history, science, mathematics, religion, art, and music. It was expected that she would follow the usual path of a wealthy and intelligent woman of the day: marry, bear children, and maintain an elegant home. Nightingale believed she was "called by God to help others . . . [and] to improve the well-being of mankind" (Schuyler 1992, p. 4). She was determined to become a nurse, in spite of opposition from her family and the restrictive societal code for affluent young English women. As a well-traveled young woman of the day, she visited Kaiserswerth in 1847, where she received three months' training in nursing. In 1853, she studied in Paris with the Sisters of Charity, after which she returned to England to assume the position of superintendent of a charity hospital for ill governesses.

During the Crimean War, the inadequacy of care for the soldiers led to public outcry. Florence Nightingale was asked by Sir Sidney Herbert of the British War Department to recruit a contingent of female nurses to provide care to the sick and injured in the Crimea. Nightingale and her nurses transformed the military hospitals by setting up diet kitchens, a laundry, recreation centers, and reading rooms, and organizing classes for orderlies. Mary Grant Seacole, a Jamaican born and trained nurse also went to the Crimean to assist Nightingale's nurses in their care of the injured.

When she returned to England, Nightingale was given an honorarium of £4500 by a grateful English public. She later used this to develop the Nightingale Training School for Nurses, which opened in 1860. The school served as a model for other training schools. Its graduates traveled to other countries to manage hospitals and institute nurse training programs. The efforts of Florence Nightingale and her nurses changed the status of nursing to a respectable occupation for women.

The Development of Nursing in America

In North America, nursing and health services were slow to be established before the American Revolution (1775–1783). One notable organization was the Nurse Society of Philadelphia, which gave women minimal instruction in obstetrics to enable them to provide maternity nursing services in home settings.

The American Civil War

1861

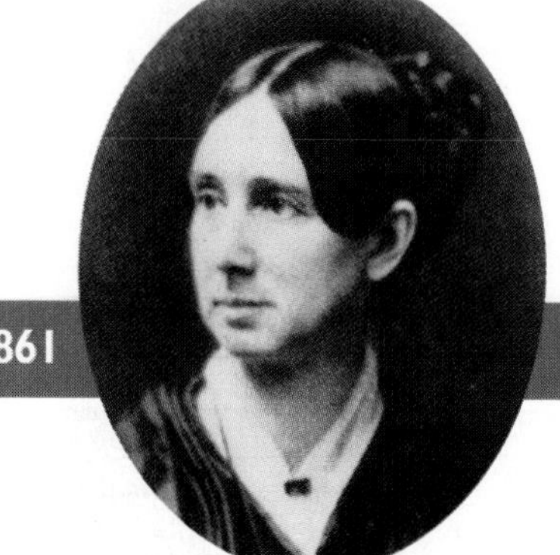

Dorothea Lynde Dix
Dix (1802-1887) was over 60 when she was appointed Superintendant of the Female Nurses of the Union Army in 1861 during the Civil War. After the war, she returned to her work with the mentally ill.

1862-1863

Louisa May Alcott
Noted author Alcott (1832-1888) worked as a nurse at the Union Hospital in Washington, D.C. during the Civil War, and documented the work of Civil War volunteer nurses in her book, *Hospital Sketches*.

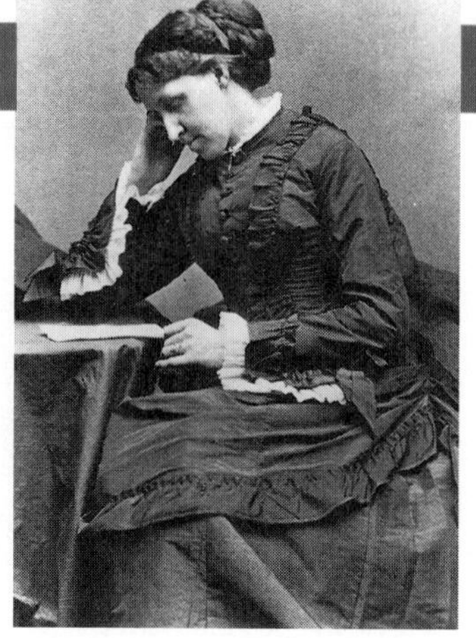

1861-1865

Harriet Tubman
Tubman (1820-1913) was known as "The Moses of her People" for her work with the Underground Railroad. During the Civil War, she nursed the sick and suffering of her own race.

During the American Civil War, several nurses emerged who were notable for their contributions to a country torn by internal strife. Harriet Tubman and Sojourner Truth provided care and safety to slaves fleeing to the North on the "Underground Railroad." Mother Bickerdyke and Clara Barton (who is credited with founding the American Red Cross) searched the battlefields and gave care to injured and dying soldiers. Noted authors Walt Whitman and Louisa May Alcott volunteered as nurses to give care to injured soldiers in military hospitals. They chronicled their experiences in their writings as a permanent record of nursing's contribution during this time.

The late 1800s was a time of rapid reform of nursing services in the United States and Canada. Schools of nursing with planned educational programs were founded. A number of their graduates became the early leaders in the profession. Isabel Hampton Robb is one example. A young school-teacher in Canada, Robb decided to change her profession and entered the Bellevue Hospital Training School in New York. After graduation, she nursed in Rome for 2 years, and then she became superintendent of the Illinois Training School at 26 years of age. Three years later, she went to Baltimore to organize a new school in connection with Johns Hopkins Hospital. Among her many accomplishments was to author a nursing textbook, which became the standard text for nursing schools in America.

Mary Adelaide Nutting, also from Canada, was in the first class at Johns Hopkins. After graduation, she established a course of training for students prior to ward experience at Johns Hopkins. Later, she reduced the nursing students' hours from 12 to 8 and lengthened the nurses training to 3 years.

Mary Agnes Snively graduated from Bellevue Hospital Training School and returned to Canada to take charge of the nurses' training at Toronto General Hospital. She is credited largely with the direction of Canadian nursing education and was the first president of the Canadian Nurses Association.

Two American graduates of the New York Hospital, Lillian D. Wald and Mary Brewster, were the first to offer trained nursing services to the poor in the New York slums. Their home among the poor on the upper floor of a tenement is now famous as a center of public health nursing: the Henry Street Settlement. Soon after the founding of the Henry Street Settlement, school nursing was established as an adjunct to visiting nursing. Again, Wald was involved, along with Lina L. Rogers.

Linda Richards, who graduated in 1873 from the New England Hospital for Women and Children Training School for Nurses in Boston, is cited by many historians as America's first trained nurse. She is credited with reforming nursing in 12 major hospitals, some of which were specialized mental hospitals. She also founded the first training school for nurses in Japan.

1862-1865

Walt Whitman
Writer and poet Whitman (1819-1882) was a volunteer nurse during the Civil War, and chronicled the care of the ill in his collection of poetry, *Drum Taps*, and in his diary, *Specimen Days*.

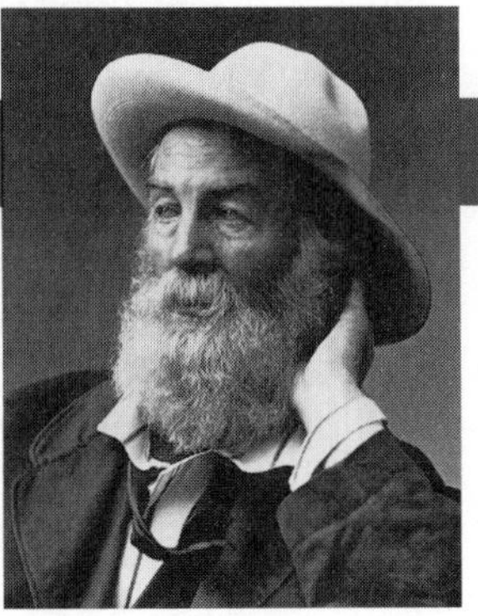

1862-1865

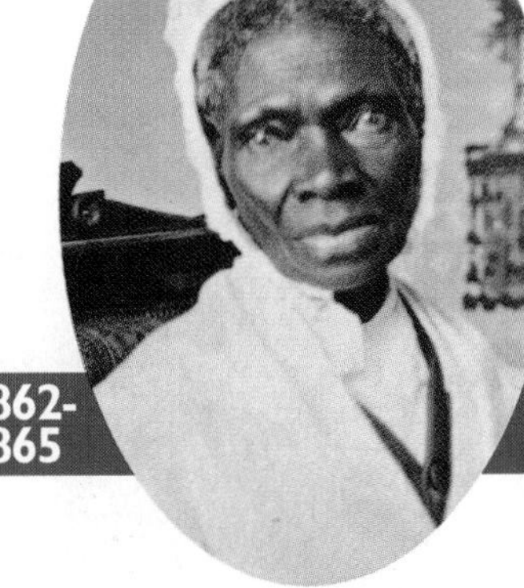

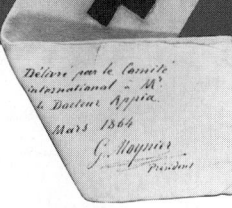

Sojourner Truth
Sojourner Truth (1797-1883), abolitionist, underground railroad agent, preacher, and women's rights advocate, was a nurse for over four years during the Civil War and worked as a nurse/counselor for the Freedmen's Relief Association after the war.

1864

The International Red Cross
During the Geneva Convention, Jean Henri Dunant of Switzerland organized the international conference that founded the Red Cross, for the relief of suffering in war.

Some, however, dispute that Richards was the first trained nurse. Evidence in a series of reports of Women's Hospital of Philadelphia suggests that Harriet Newton Phillips was the first trained nurse to receive a certificate from that hospital in 1864 (Large 1976, p. 50). Phillips is also considered the first trained nurse in America to do community nursing, to do missionary service, and to take postgraduate training.

America's first trained black nurse was Mary Mahoney. She trained at the same hospital as Linda Richards and graduated in 1879.

The need for concerted action by nurses was first felt in England during the late 1800s. In 1894, the Matron's Council of Great Britain and Ireland was organized, followed by the American Society of Superintendents of Training Schools for Nurses of the United States and Canada. Alumnae associations joined to form the Nurses Associated Alumnae of the United States and Canada in 1897. These North American organizations were the predecessors of current national groups. The Society of Superintendents divided nationally and ultimately became the Canadian National Association of Trained Nurses in 1908—now the Canadian Nurses Association (CNA)—and the National League of Nursing Education in 1912. The Nurses Associated Alumnae became the American Nurses Association (ANA) in 1911. (See the section on nursing organizations, later in this chapter.) In 1908, the National Association of Colored Graduate Nurses was founded by a group of nurses who felt such an association could further not only the nursing cause but also their own interests.

In 1893, the Nightingale Pledge was written and administered to the graduating class of the Farrand (Nurse) Training School in Detroit, Michigan. At that time, the pledge reflected the nurse's commitment to moral and ethical values and principles in the practice of nursing. Despite modern criticisms of the pledge as portraying the nurse as subservient to the physician, it continues to provide "a framework for clarifying moral and ethical values and principles needed for delivering health care and promoting the standards of nursing" (Calhoun 1993, p. 130).

After World War I, the Frontier Nursing Service (FNS) was established by a notable pioneer nurse, Mary Breckinridge. In 1918, she worked with the American Committee for Devastated France, distributing food, clothing, and supplies to rural villages in France and taking care of sick children. In 1921, Breckinridge returned to the United States with plans to provide health care to the people of rural America. She had initially prepared herself by taking courses at Teacher's College in New York (where she met Mary Adelaide Nutting and gained her approval) and midwifery training in London and by developing prominent social contacts for fund-raising. In 1925, Breckinridge and two other nurses began the FNS in Leslie County, Kentucky. Within this organization,

Early Nursing Education

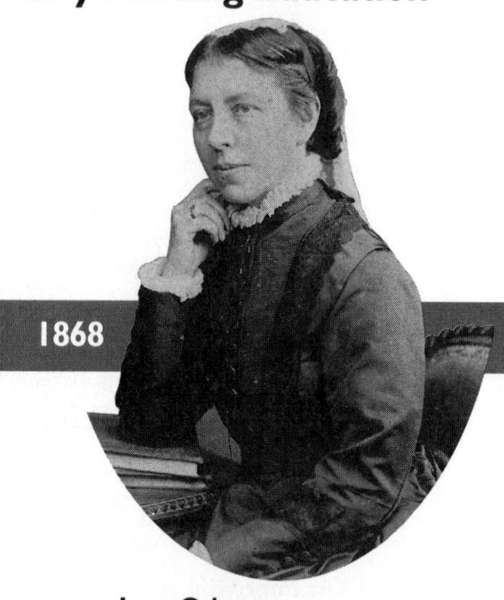

1868

Lucy Osborne
Osborne (1835-1891) trained under Nightingale at St.Thomas Hospital in London, then became Superintendent at Sydney Hospital and developed Australia's first school for nurses.

1872

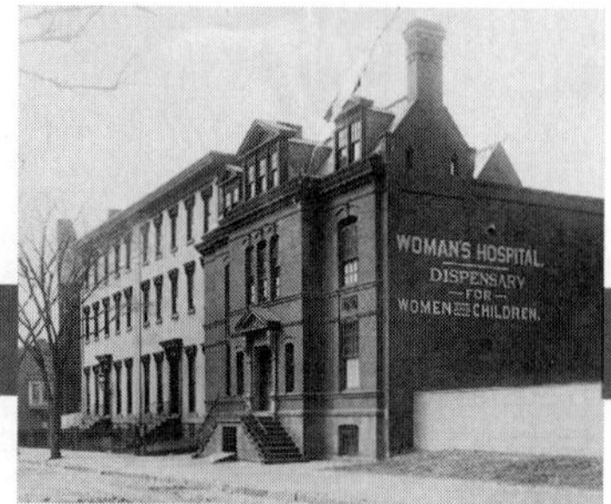

Early Nursing Schools
Woman's Hospital in Philadelphia (pictured above) and New England Hospital for Women and Children in Boston opened training programs for nurses.

1873

Linda Richards
Richards (1841-1930) graduated from New England Hospital for Women and Children training school for nurses, and is considered America's first trained nurse.

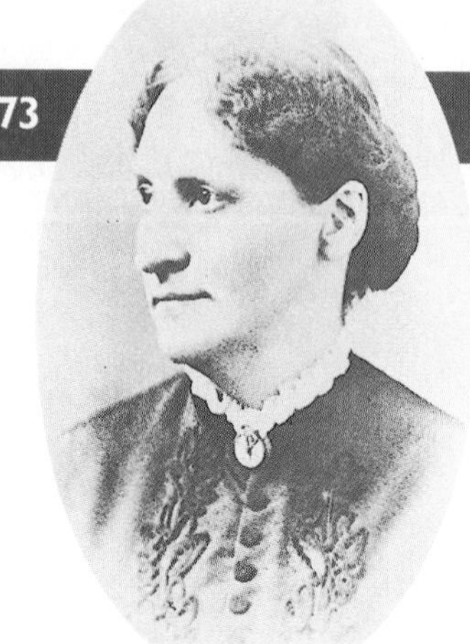

Breckinridge started one of the first midwifery training schools in the United States.

From the beginning of formal organization of nursing of the late 1800s to the end of World War I, the general trend was rapid expansion in the establishment of hospitals, with nursing schools dependent on them for support. Hospitals in turn depended on the schools to carry the chief nursing load. During the war, greater numbers of young women were accepted for entrance, and less consideration was given to selection requirements. Most schools by this time had adopted 3-year programs, but the 8-hour day originally proposed with those programs was less quickly adopted.

By 1920, the hospital system of educating nurses was coming under increasing criticism. In addition, the effectiveness of having nurses teach other nurses was being questioned. Thus, a special post-basic course was offered at Teachers College, Columbia University, New York, to prepare nurses to be teachers. A post-basic public health nursing program was also developed, in response to the postwar influenza epidemic and the medical profession's new emphasis on teaching the principles of healthful living to individuals, families, and community groups.

During the early 1920s, the Rockefeller Survey (Committee for the Study of Nursing Education) recommended that nursing schools be independent of hospitals and on a college level. As a result, two university schools of nursing were set up, one at Yale University, New Haven, Connecticut, the other at Western Reserve University, Cleveland, Ohio. The purpose of these experimental schools was to prove the feasibility of planning both classroom instruction and ward practice in accordance with the educational needs of the students. These schools emphasized the social welfare and health aspects of nursing and demonstrated the value of university standards in the nursing field.

Another far-reaching result of the Rockefeller Survey was the National League of Nursing Education's comprehensive study of nursing education (1926–1934), which led to the grading of nursing schools. It was believed that grading would establish standards for education in these schools. This was the beginning of the accreditation function now carried out by the National League for Nursing (NLN).

During this period, the concept of the clinical nurse specialist arose. In the early decades of the 20th century, hospitals started to segregate patients according to their disease process. Nurses were called upon to acquire expert knowledge in the care of specific patient types. These nursing roles were called extended or expanded roles. In the early 1940s, it was thought that more emphasis needed to be placed on the clinical specialties in the advanced professional curricula of colleges and universities. Most advanced nursing curricula were preparing special-

1879

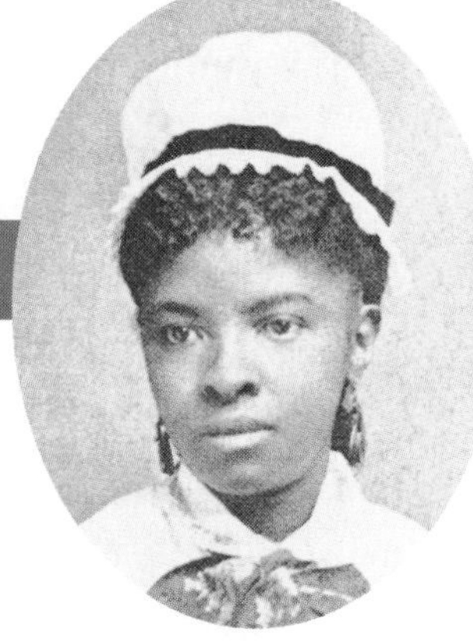

Mary Mahoney
Mary Mahoney (1819-1882) became America's first trained black nurse when she graduated from New England Hospital for Women and Children training school for nurses.

1882

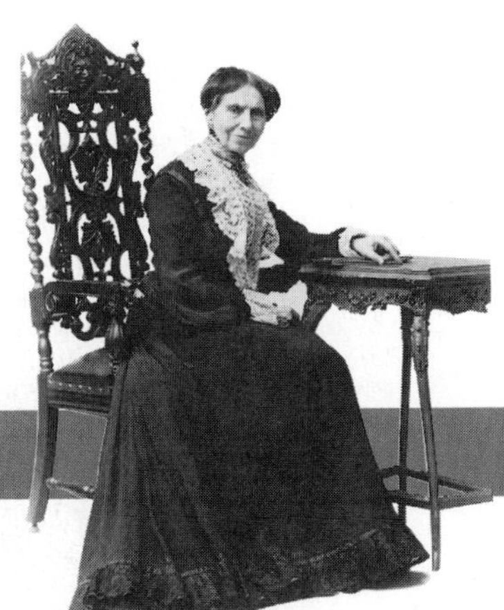

Clara Barton and the American Red Cross
Barton (1812-1912) organized the American National Red Cross, which linked with the international Red Cross when the United States Congress ratified the Geneva Convention.

1884

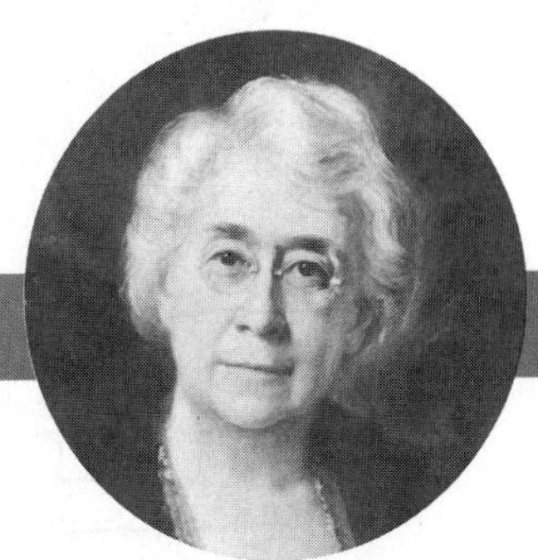

Mary Agnes Snively
Canadian born Mary Agnes Snively (1847-1933), a graduate of the Bellevue Hospital Training School for Nurses in New York, returned to Canada to develop the Toronto General Hospital School of Nursing. She was the first president of the Canadian Nurses Association.

ists in nursing school administration, teaching, and supervision in public health and in hospital administration but were not emphasizing clinical specialties. These specialties gained prominence in the post–World War II society. Nurses returning from overseas were required to work in clinical areas not familiar to them. One such area was psychiatric nursing, which helped individuals readjust to civilian life. By 1946, many nursing programs in the United States were providing more clinical content. Today the clinical nurse specialist is a graduate of a master's or doctoral program in nursing with a major in a clinical specialty. These nurses are responsible for increasing their own clinical knowledge and competence and for enhancing the quality of nursing care and the quality of the organizational climate for learning and research.

From its early days to the present, nursing has undergone change in every area. Rapid strides have been made in nursing education programs and in a wide variety of hospital and community nursing services. Throughout these changes, nursing has continued to provide a stable service to help people. Nurses have also been part of the larger societal changes that have influenced nursing. Twentieth-century nursing leaders in the United States have been active in women's suffrage, civil rights, and health care reform movements. Nurses have been elected to office at local and state levels. In 1992, Eddie Bernice Johnson from Texas became the first nurse elected to the United States House of Representatives. The time line running throughout this chapter highlights selected people and events in nursing's history, demonstrating that nursing is a profession for and influenced by women and men of all cultural backgrounds and all socioeconomic levels.

Growth of Professionalism

A **profession** is a calling that requires special knowledge, skill, and preparation. A profession is generally distinguished from other kinds of occupations by (a) its requirement of prolonged, specialized training to acquire a body of knowledge pertinent to the role to be performed and (b) an orientation of the individual toward service, either to a community or to an organization. The standards of education and practice for the profession are determined by the members of the profession, rather than by outsiders. The education of the professional involves a complete socialization process, more far-reaching in its social and attitudinal aspects and its technical features than is usually required in other kinds of occupations.

Miller states that the critical attributes of professionalism in nursing are the following:

Late Nineteenth Century

1893

THE NIGHTINGALE PLEDGE
I solemnly pledge myself before God, and in the presence of this assembly, to pass my life in purity and to practice my profession faithfully. I will abstain from whatever is deleterious and mischievous and will not take or knowingly administer any harmful drug. I will do all in my power to elevate the standard of my profession, and will hold in confidence all personal matters committed to my keeping, and all family affairs coming to my knowledge in the practice of my calling. With loyalty will I endeavor to aid the physician in his work and devote myself to the welfare of those committed to my care.

The Nightingale Pledge was written and administered for the first time to graduates of the Farrand Training School of Harper Hospital in Detroit, Michigan.

1893

Lillian Wald
Lillian Wald (1867-1940) founded the Henry Street Settlement and Visiting Nurse Service, which provided nursing services, social services, and organized educational and cultural activities. She is considered the founder of public health nursing.

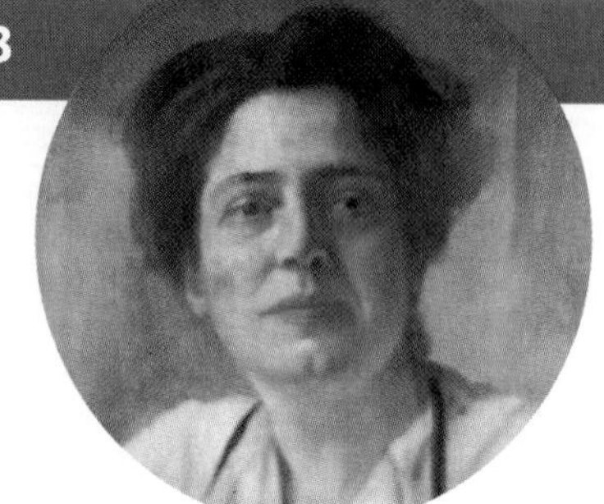

1897

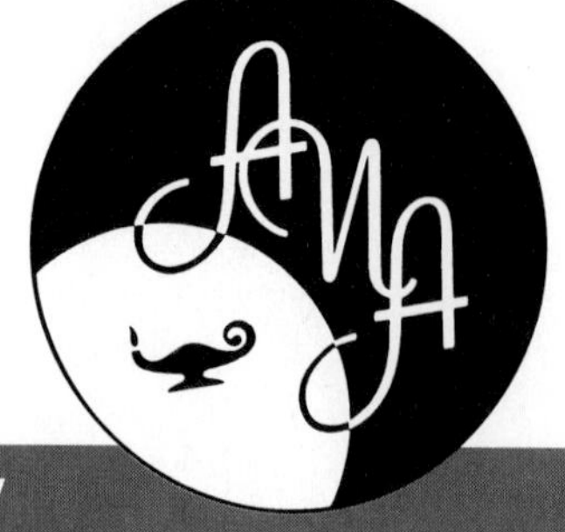

The ANA
The Nurses Alumnae Association of the United States and Canada, later renamed the American Nurses Association, was organized.

- Gaining a body of knowledge in a university setting and a science orientation at the graduate level in nursing
- Attaining competence derived from the theoretical base wherein the "diagnosis and the treatment of human responses to actual or potential health problems" (ANA 1980) can be accomplished
- Delineating and specifying the skills and competencies that are the boundaries of expertise (Miller 1985, p. 25)

The growth of professionalism in nursing can be viewed in relation to specialized education, knowledge base, ethics, and autonomy.

Specialized Education

Specialized education is an important aspect of professional status. Historically, nurses were educated in hospitals. In modern times, the trend has shifted toward nursing education programs in colleges and universities. Many nursing educators believe that the undergraduate nursing curriculum should include liberal arts education in addition to the biologic and social sciences and the nursing discipline. The ANA's *Standards for Professional Nursing Education* (1984, p. 1) states that the "education for those preparing to become nurses as well as those already licensed to practice nursing should take place in institutions of higher education." In 1983, the National League for Nursing (NLN) voted at its convention to retain the baccalaureate degree as the minimal academic preparation for the professional nurse (Lewis 1983, p. 246).

In the United States today, there are five levels of entry into registered nursing: hospital diploma, associate degree, baccalaureate degree, master's degree, and doctoral degree. These programs are discussed in Chapter 2.

Body of Knowledge

As a profession, nursing is establishing a well-defined body of knowledge and expertise. A number of nursing conceptual frameworks (discussed in Chapter 3) contribute to the knowledge base of nursing and give direction to nursing practice, education, and ongoing research.

Increasing research in nursing is contributing to this body of knowledge. In the 1940s, nursing research was at a very early stage of development. In the 1950s, increased federal funding and professional support helped establish centers for nursing research. Most early research was directed to the study of nursing education. In the 1960s studies were often related to the nature of the knowledge base underlying nursing practice. Since the 1970s, nursing research has focused on practice-related issues. Nursing research as a dimension of the nurse's role is discussed further in Chapter 2.

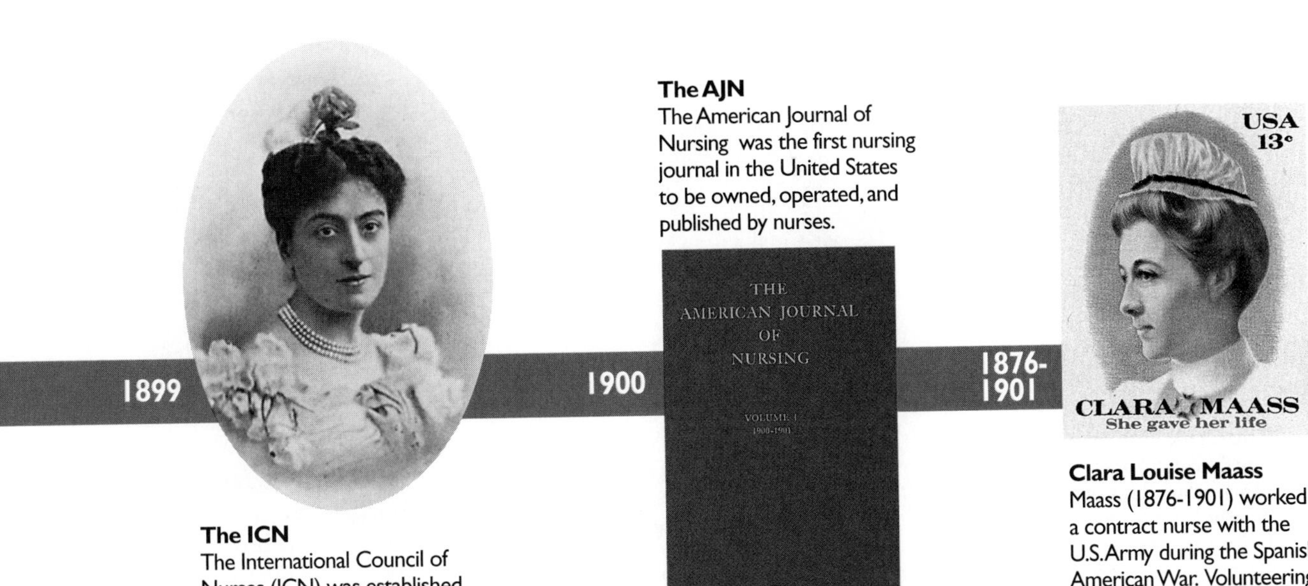

The ICN
The International Council of Nurses (ICN) was established by Mrs. Bedford Fenwick of Great Britain. Nurses from the United States and Canada were among the founders, and their national associations among the first admitted to membership.

The AJN
The American Journal of Nursing was the first nursing journal in the United States to be owned, operated, and published by nurses.

Clara Louise Maass
Maass (1876-1901) worked as a contract nurse with the U.S. Army during the Spanish American War. Volunteering to nurse victims of yellow fever in Cuba, she died after allowing herself to be bitten by a mosquito as an experiment on immunity.

ETHICS

Nurses have traditionally placed a high value on the worth and dignity of others. The nursing profession requires integrity of its members; that is, a member is expected to do what is considered right regardless of the personal cost. Nurses must respect the professional judgment of others and must develop nursing standards and establish mechanisms for identifying and dealing with unethical behavior.

Ethical codes change as the needs and values of society change. Nursing has developed its own codes of ethics and in most instances has set up means to monitor the professional behavior of its members. See Chapter 11 for additional information on ethics.

AUTONOMY

A profession is autonomous if it regulates itself and sets standards for its members. Providing autonomy is one of the purposes of a professional association. If nursing is to have professional status, it must function autonomously in the formation of policy and in the control of its activity. To be autonomous, a professional group must be granted legal authority to define the scope of its practice, describe its particular functions and roles, and determine its goals and responsibilities in delivery of its services. The amount of autonomy a professional group possesses depends on its effectiveness at governance. **Governance** is the establishment and maintenance of social, political, and economic arrangements by which practitioners control their practice, their self-discipline, their working conditions, and their professional affairs. Nurses, therefore, must work within their professional organizations.

To practitioners of nursing, autonomy means independence at work, responsibility, and accountability for one's actions.

The ANA statement on the scope of practice describes the accountability of professional and technical nurses:

> Professional nurses develop nursing policies, procedures, and protocols and set standards for nursing care for all client populations in all practice settings. . . . Technical nurses use policies, procedures, and protocols developed by professional nurses in implementing an individual's plan of care. Technical nurses are accountable for practicing within these guidelines (ANA 1987b, p. 77).

Autonomy is more easily achieved and maintained from a position of authority. Therefore, many nurses seek administrative positions rather than expanded clinical competence as a means to ensure their autonomy in the workplace.

Early Twentieth Century

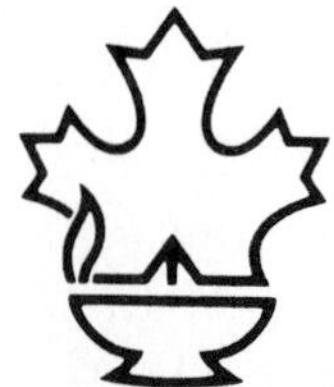

1908

The CNA
The Canadian Society of Superintendants of Training Schools for Nurses and the Canadian National Association for Trained Nurses joined to become the Canadian Nurses Association.

1912

The NLN
The National League for Nursing Education, the forerunner of the National League for Nursing, was established for the development of nursing education standards. Today, the NLN is the accrediting body for all schools of nursing in the United States.

1916

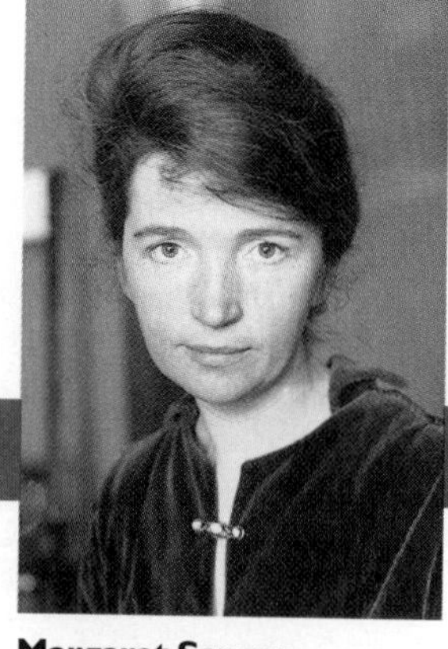

Margaret Sanger
Nurse activist Margaret Sanger, considered the founder of Planned Parenthood, was imprisoned for opening the first birth control information clinic in Baltimore.

Professional Behaviors of Nurses

Miller states that the degree to which a nurse behaves as a professional is reflected in the following five behaviors. The professional

1. Assesses, plans, implements, and evaluates theory, research, and practice in nursing. These behaviors are reflected in the entire nursing process. See also Chapters 5 through 8.
2. Accepts, promotes, and maintains the interdependence of theory, research, and practice. These three elements make nursing a profession and not a task-centered activity (Miller 1985, p. 26).
3. Communicates and disseminates theoretical knowledge, practical knowledge, and research findings to the nursing community. Professionalism must be demonstrated by supporting, counseling, and assisting other nurses (Miller 1985, p. 26).
4. Upholds the service orientation of nursing in the eyes of the public. This orientation differentiates nursing from an occupation pursued primarily for profit. Many consider altruism (selfless concern for others) the hallmark of a profession. Nursing has a tradition of service to others. This service, however, must be guided by certain rules, policies, or code of ethics (Miller 1985, p. 26). The nursing code of ethics is formulated by national nursing associations. In addition, society is protected by licensure and accreditation of nurses. These self-regulatory provisions give nurses the autonomy to function in the public's best interests rather than in the best interests of an institution or other profession.
5. Preserves and promotes the professional organization as the major referent. Operation under the umbrella of a professional organization differentiates a profession from an occupation (Miller 1985, p. 26). In nursing, the American Nurses Association in the United States and the Canadian Nurses Association in Canada perform the self-regulatory functions.

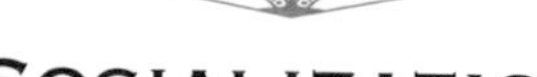

Socialization

Socialization is a process by which a person learns the ways of a group or society in order to become a functioning participant. Although the student may bring some knowledge of nursing through past experiences, socialization to nursing starts when the student makes the decision to become a nurse, and it continues throughout the nurse's professional career. Socialization is a reciprocal learning process that occurs through interaction with other people. This learning can be conscious or unconscious, formal or informal. The nursing student becomes socialized to the nursing profession through interaction

Lavinia Dock
Nursing leader and suffragist Lavinia L. Dock (1858-1956) was active in the protest movement for women's rights that resulted in the United States Constitution amendment allowing women to vote.

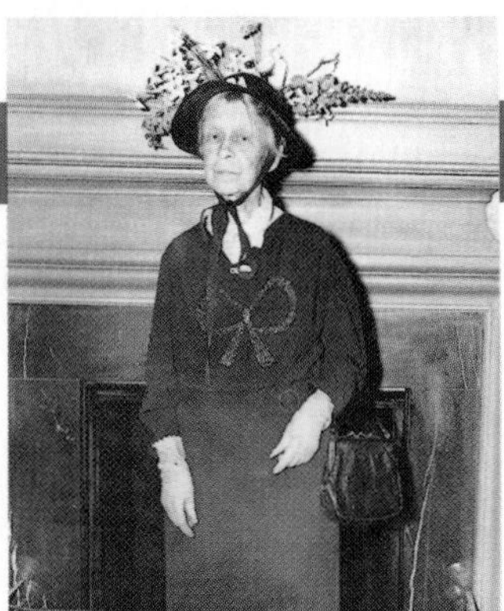

1920

1922

Sigma Theta Tau
Sigma Theta Tau, the international honor society that promotes nursing research and leadership, was founded at the Indiana University School of Nursing.

1925

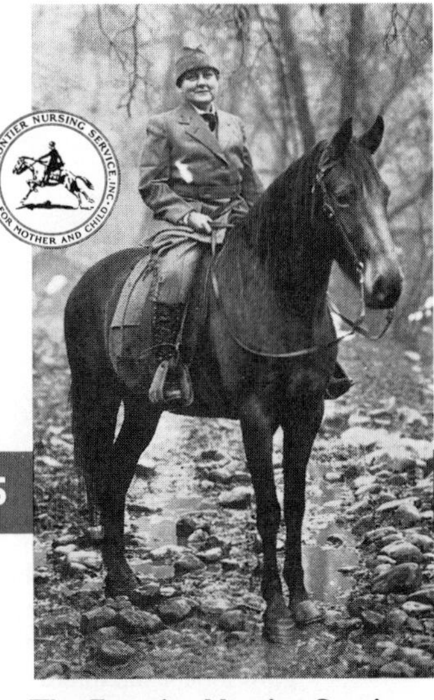

The Frontier Nursing Service
Mary Breckenridge, a nurse who practiced midwifery in England, Australia, and New Zealand, founded the Frontier Nursing Service in Kentucky to provide family-centered primary health care to rural populations.

with nursing faculty, practicing nurses, nursing student colleagues, and media portrayals of nursing. Through this interaction, the nurse learns the knowledge required to practice as an effective nurse.

Types of Nursing Knowledge

Carper (1978) identifies four "patterns of knowing" that make up the basic core of nursing knowledge: nursing science, nursing esthetics, nursing ethics, and personal knowledge.

Nursing science or scientific knowledge is the "cognitive brain" of nursing and includes knowledge obtained through nursing research and research done in other disciplines. For example, the nurse learns to determine the effectiveness of specific nursing interventions through nursing research, but the underlying knowledge of the body's physiologic and psychologic functioning has been obtained through research conducted by physiologists and psychologists. Scientific knowledge includes the facts and information necessary for performing technical skills—that is, the principles of the skill, the steps of the procedure, and knowledge of the equipment. When nursing procedures are done skillfully, nursing actions are more likely to be successful.

Because nursing takes place in the context of an interactive relationship between nurse and client, knowledge about interpersonal relationships and communication is a part of the nurse's scientific knowledge. Nurses must understand the nature of a helping relationship and how to use verbal and nonverbal communication techniques with clients, families, groups, and other health professionals. Scientific knowledge also includes an understanding of the ways in which sociocultural and developmental factors affect client behavior (for example, understanding how a client's religious or cultural beliefs may influence compliance or willingness to cooperate with treatment plans).

Finally, nursing science includes knowledge of change theory and motivational theory. Nurses call upon this knowledge when they work directly with clients or supervise other nursing personnel. This text presents information based on nursing scientific knowledge.

Nursing esthetics is the way in which nursing knowledge is expressed. It is the "art" or "heart" of nursing. Unlike scientific knowledge, which is acquired by research, esthetics involves feelings gained by subjective experience. It is through the art of nursing that nurses express caring; therefore, esthetics includes attitudes, beliefs, and values. Sensitivity and empathy (the ability to imagine what another person is feeling) are important facets of this type of knowing. They enable the nurse to be aware of the client's perspective and to be attentive to verbal and nonverbal cues to the client's psychologic state. A nurse who is highly skilled in empathizing with clients has a wider range of interventions for providing effective, satisfying nursing care (Carper 1978, pp. 17–18).

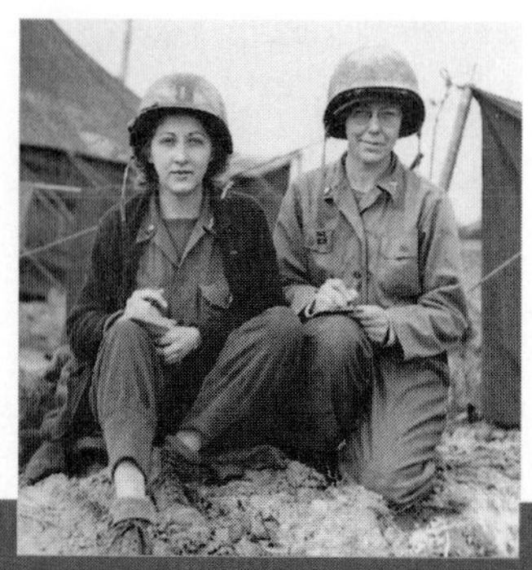

1943-1945

WWII: The Cadet Nurse Corps
Through the United States Cadet Nurse Corps, the federal government subsidized the cost of nursing education for all students agreeing to serve in civilian or military nursing services for the duration of the war. The Corps was discontinued in 1945.

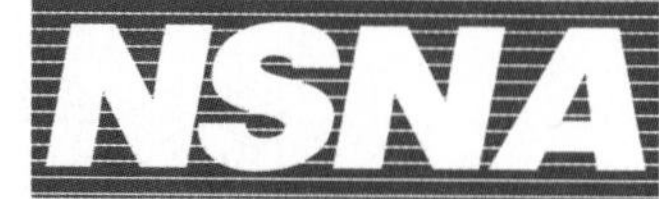

1953

The NSNA
The National Student Nurses Association was founded to promote professionalism among students and prepare them for membership in ANA.

1963-1975

The Vietnam War
More than 5,000 nurses served in Vietnam, and a 1966 Congressional bill allowed the appointment of male nurses to the Army, Navy, and Air Force Nurse Corps.

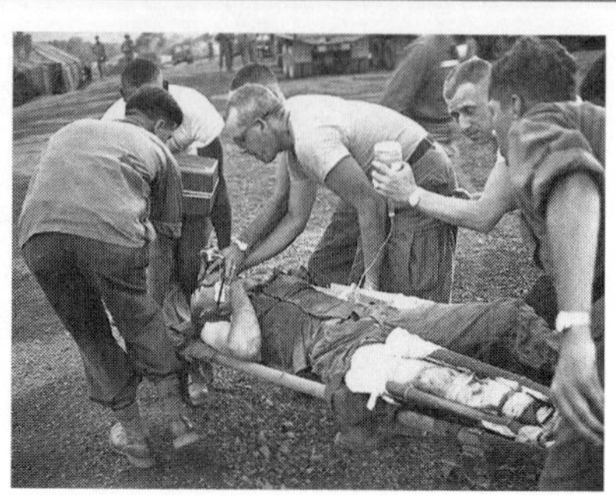

Nursing ethics refers to the knowledge of accepted professional standards of conduct. It is concerned with matters of obligation, or what ought to be done; it consists of information about basic moral principles and processes for determining "right" actions. Nurses are accountable to consumers and to each other for the ethical performance of their work. Whether developed formally (by a written code of ethics) or informally, the ethics of a profession represents the traditions and values of the groups. See Chapter 11 for more information about nursing ethics.

Personal knowledge is concerned with knowing oneself, that is, having a conscious awareness of one's own values, beliefs, attitudes, and abilities. Further, it involves the knowing of self in relation to another and interacting on a person-to-person, rather than a role-to-role, basis. This pattern of knowing enables nurses to treat clients as persons rather than as objects. Nurses with highly developed self-awareness and self-knowledge generally have a better self-concept and are more attuned to their clients (Carper 1978, pp. 18–19).

Socialization for Professional Nursing Practice

Each student enters a nursing education program with knowledge and values that reflect the student's individual experiences. Many students enter nursing with a perception that nurses are individuals who do things that help *sick* people recover. However, the professional nurse is one whose scope has broadened, interacting with clients and other health professionals to promote, maintain, and restore the client's health.

The socialization process therefore involves changes in perceptions, knowledge, skills, attitudes, and values. Benner (1984) describes five levels of proficiency as the nurse progresses and acquires the knowledge, skills, attitudes, and values of nursing. These levels of proficiency are novice, advanced beginner, competent, proficient, and expert.

Stage 1: Novice A novice may be a nursing student or any nurse entering a clinical setting where that person has no experience. Because novices have no experience, their ability is extremely limited, inflexible, and governed by structured rules and protocols.

Stage 2: Advanced Beginner The advanced beginner can demonstrate marginally accepted performance. The beginner has had experience with enough real situations to be aware of the meaningful aspects of a situation. An example is the ability to recognize a client's readiness to learn how to manage a treatment plan.

Stage 3: Competent Competence is manifested by the nurse who has been on the job in a similar situation for 2

Diversity in the 70's

1971

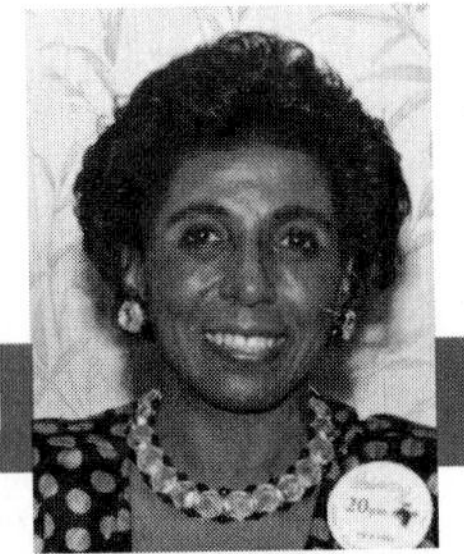

The NBNA
Dr. Lauranne Sams served as first president of the National Black Nurses Association.

Independent Practitioners
M. Lucille Kinlein became the first nurse to hang out her shingle as an independent practitioner.

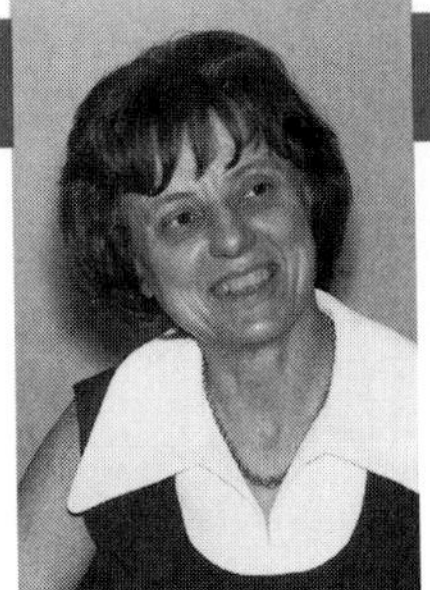

1973

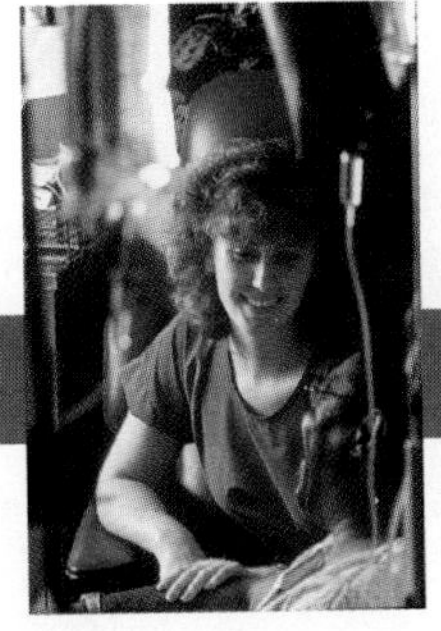

ANA Specialty Certification
The ANA began a certification program for nurses in speciality practice. Medical-Surgical nursing was the first speciality to be recognized in this program.

1974

THE NHNA
Dr. Ildaura Murillo-Rohde, JMR, PhD, ND, FAAN, served as the first president of the National Hispanic Nurses Association.

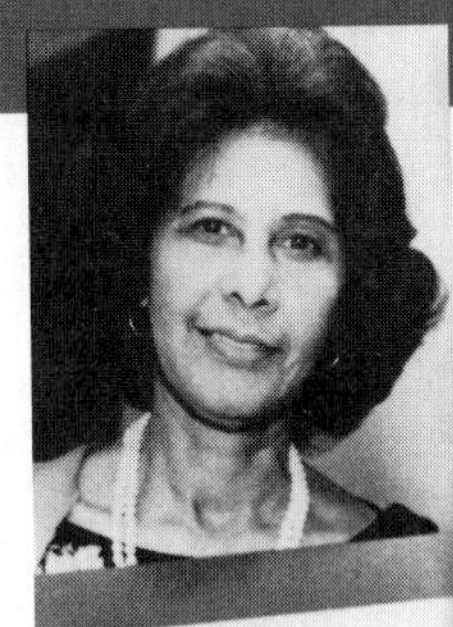

or 3 years. Competence develops when the nurse consciously and deliberately plans nursing care and coordinates multiple complex care demands. The nurse at this stage demonstrates organizational ability but lacks the speed and flexibility of the proficient nurse. The competent nurse knows how to prioritize care requirements for an individual or groups of clients. For example, the competent nurse will ensure that intravenous infusions are running, that clients are receiving required medications, and that a client's urgent physical needs are met before other needs are dealt with.

Stage 4: Proficient The proficient nurse perceives a situation as a whole rather than just its individual aspects. The nurse focuses on long-term goals and is oriented toward managing the nursing care of a client rather than performing specific tasks. This holistic understanding improves the decision making of the proficient nurse.

The proficient nurse uses maxims as guides but applies them only after acquiring a deep understanding of the situation. For example, a nurse weaning a client from a respirator assesses the client's vital signs to discover any significant finding, but even then the nurse is aware that elevated readings may indicate anxiety. The nurse weighs the decision to medicate to calm the client down against the knowledge that the medication may impair breathing. The nurse makes the decision according to the demands of the situation and the lessons of past experience.

Stage 5: Expert The expert performer no longer relies on rules, guidelines, or maxims to connect an understanding of the situation to an appropriate action. The expert nurse intuitively grasps each situation and focuses on the accurate area of the problem without wasteful consideration of large ranges of unnecessary alternative diagnoses and solutions. The expert nurse may be inclined to say that a certain action was taken because "it felt right." Expert nurses have highly developed perceptual acuity or recognitional ability, and their performance is fluid, flexible, and highly proficient. The nurse's highly skilled analytic ability can be transferred to situations with which the nurse has had no previous experience.

Nursing students can enhance their own socialization process by seeking out learning experiences with the help of nursing faculty and by discussing clinical and classroom learning experiences with faculty, student colleagues, and practicing nurses.

Roles of the Professional Nurse

The following nurse roles are ways of describing the nurse's activities in practice. Each role is described as a separate entity for the sake of clarity. However, the roles are not in actuality exclusive of one another. In practice,

Impact on Government

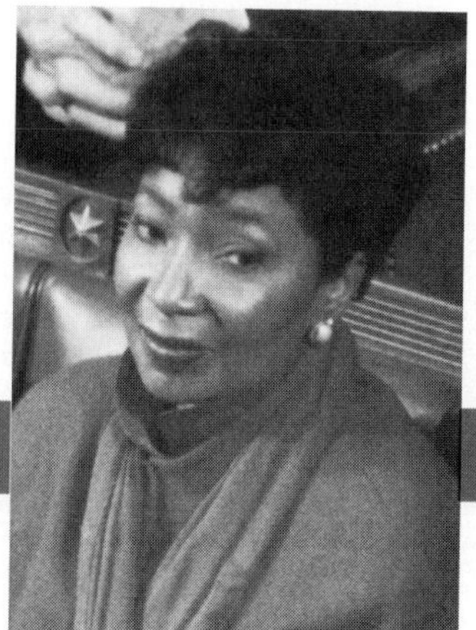

1992

The U.S. House of Representatives
Eddie Bernice Johnson of Texas became the first nurse to be elected to the United States House of Representatives.

1992

US Public Health Service
As Chief Nurse Officer, Rear Admiral Julia R. Plotnick, RN, BSN, MPH is an active leader in policy coordination for the U.S. Surgeon General and provides leadership to 6500 nurses within the Public Health Service.

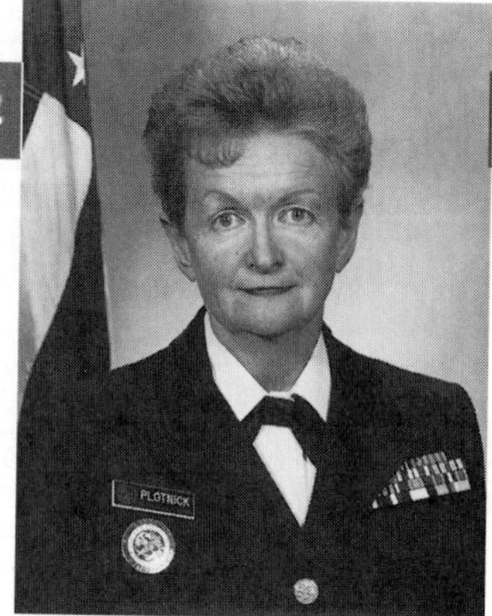

1993

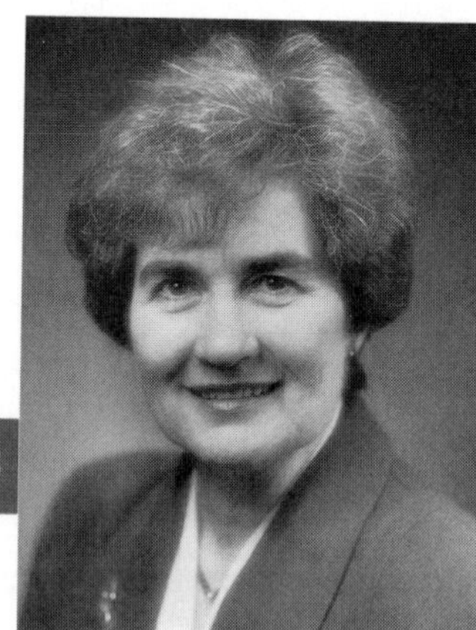

The NIH
Under the directorship of Ada Sue Hinshaw, PhD, RN, FAAN, the National Center for Nursing Research became the National Institute for Nursing Research within the National Institutes for Health.

several roles often coincide. For example, the nurse may act as a client advocate while also caring, communicating, teaching or counseling, and acting as a change agent and leader.

Care Provider

The caring/comforting role of the nurse has traditionally included those activities that preserve the dignity of the individual and those often referred to as the "mothering actions" in nursing. However, caring involves knowledge and sensitivity to what matters and what is important to clients. (See caring theories in Chapter 3, page 53.) The caring role is difficult to define specifically. It is the role of human relations. The chief goal of the nurse in this role is to convey understanding about what is important and to provide support. The nurse supports the client by attitudes and actions that show concern for client welfare and acceptance of the client as a person, not merely a mechanical being.

Benner and Wrubel (1989, p. 4) state that "caring is central to effective nursing practice. . . . Nursing can never be reduced to mere technique and scientific knowledge because humor, anger, 'tough love,' administering medications, and even client teaching have different effects in a caring context than a noncaring one." Caring is central to most nursing interventions and an essential attribute of the expert nurse.

Communicator/Helper

Effective communication is an essential element of all helping professions, including nursing. Communication shapes relationships between nurses and clients, nurses and support persons, and nurses and colleagues. It plays a role in every action the nurse undertakes. The communication process, listening and responding skills, and ways to establish helping relationships are discussed in detail in Chapter 18.

Communication facilitates all nursing actions. The nurse communicates to other health care personnel the nursing interventions planned and implemented for each client. Planned nursing interventions are written on the client's care plan. Once the interventions are implemented, the nurse documents them on the client's record, recording assessment findings, procedures implemented, and the client's responses. Nurses communicate pertinent information verbally at change-of-shift reports, when clients are transferred to another unit, at client rounds, and when clients are discharged to another health care agency. This type of communication needs to be concise, clear, and relevant. See Chapter 9 for details of reporting and recording.

Teacher

Teaching refers to activities by which the teacher helps the student to learn. It is an interactive process between a

Contemporary Nursing Leaders

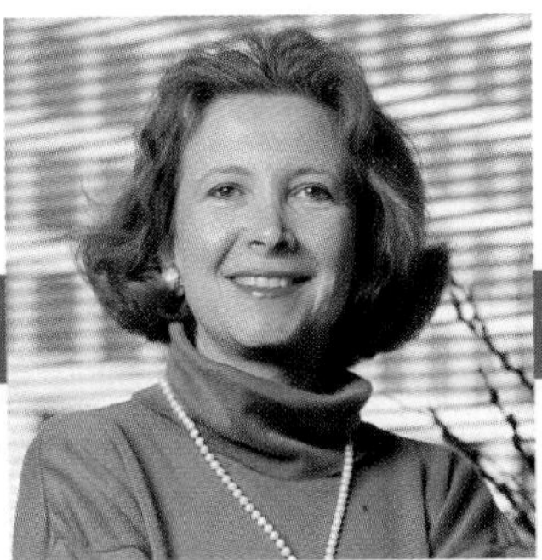

Virginia Trotter Betts, JD, RN, MSN. President of ANA, nursing and health policy expert, member of President Clinton's Health Care Reform Task Force.

Margretta Styles, RN, EdD Former president of ANA and current president of ICN.

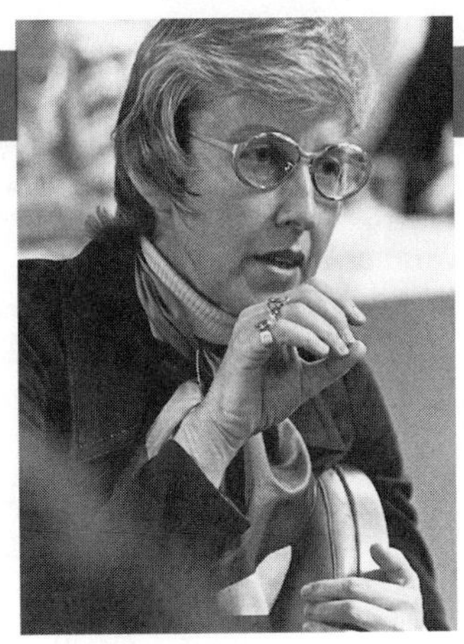

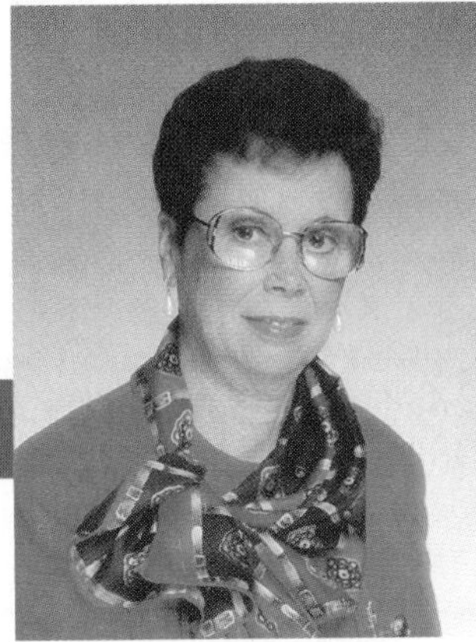

Fay Bower, RN, DNSc, FAAN Twentieth president of Sigma Theta Tau International Honor Society of Nursing.

teacher and one or more learners in which specific learning objectives or desired behavior changes are achieved (Redman 1993, p. 8). The focus of the behavior change is usually the acquiring of new knowledge or technical skills.

The teaching process has four components—assessing, planning, implementing, and evaluating—which can be viewed as parallel to the parts of the nursing process. In the assessment phase, the nurse determines the client's learning needs and readiness to learn. During planning, the nurse sets specific learning goals and teaching strategies. During implementation, the nurse enacts teaching strategies and, during evaluation, measures learning. See Chapter 19 for detailed information about the teaching/learning process.

Many factors have increased the need for health teaching by nurses. Today, there is a new emphasis on health promotion and health maintenance rather than on treatment alone; as a result, people desire and require more knowledge. Shortened hospital stays mean that the clients must be prepared to manage convalescence at home. The increase in long-term illnesses and disabilities often requires that both the client and the family understand the illness and its treatment.

COUNSELOR

Counseling is the process of helping a client to recognize and cope with stressful psychologic or social problems, to develop improved interpersonal relationships, and to promote personal growth. It involves providing emotional, intellectual, and psychologic support. In contrast to the psychotherapist, who counsels individuals with identified problems, the nurse counsels primarily healthy individuals with normal adjustment difficulties. The nurse focuses on helping the person develop new attitudes, feelings, and behaviors rather than on promoting intellectual growth. The nurse encourages the client to look at alternative behaviors, recognize the choices, and develop a sense of control.

Counseling can be provided on a one-to-one basis or in groups. Often nurses lead group counseling sessions. For example, on the individual level, the nurse counsels clients who need to decrease activity levels, stop smoking, lose weight, accept changes in body image, or cope with impending death. At the group level, the nurse may be a leader, member, or resource person in any self-help group in which the nurse may assume the role of structuring activities and fostering a climate conducive to group interaction and productive work.

Obviously, counseling requires therapeutic communication skills. In addition, the nurse must be a skilled leader able to analyze a situation, synthesize information and experiences, and evaluate the progress and productivity of the individual or group. The nurse must also be willing to model and teach desired behaviors, to be sincere when caring in the welfare of others. The nurse-leader needs an inventive mind, a flexible attitude, and a sense of humor to deal with the varied experiences of people. Essential to leadership abilities is self-awareness, self-assurance, and self-understanding.

CLIENT ADVOCATE

An **advocate** pleads the cause of another or argues or pleads for a cause or proposal. Advocacy involves concern for and defined actions in behalf of another person or organization to bring about a change. A **client advocate** is an advocate of clients' rights. According to Disparti (1988, p. 140), advocacy involves promoting what is best for the client, ensuring that the client's needs are met, and protecting the client's rights. **Social advocacy** entails advocating on behalf of a population or a community to effect positive change. Nurses engaged in this form of advocacy can create healthy environments through political action, community education, and involvement in professional organizations. See Chapter 11 for further discussion of the nurse as client advocate and Chapter 14 for further discussion of the nurse as social advocate.

CHANGE AGENT

A **change agent** is a person or group who initiates changes or who assists others in making modifications in themselves or in the system (Kemp 1986). Marriner-Tomey (1992, p. 162) describes a change agent as one who identifies the problem, assesses the client's motivations and capacities for change, determines alternatives, explores the possible outcomes of the alternatives, assesses resources, determines appropriate helping roles, establishes and maintains a helping relationship, recognizes the phases of the change process, and guides the client through these phases.

The promotion of change is an essential component of nursing care. By using the nursing process, the nurse helps the client to propose, implement, and maintain changes (eg, knowledge, skill, feelings, attitudes) that promote the client's health. Types, theories, and the process of change are discussed in Chapter 20.

LEADER

The leadership role can be applied at many different levels: individual, family, groups, communities, or the larger society. At the client level, **nursing leadership** is defined as a mutual process of interpersonal influence through which the nurse helps a client make decisions in establishing and achieving goals to improve the client's well-being. Leadership validates the professional nurse's practice and enhances professional growth (Leddy & Pepper 1993, p. 384).

The purposes of leadership vary according to the level of application and include (a) improving the health status and potential of individuals or families, (b) increasing the effectiveness and level of satisfaction among professional colleagues providing care, and (c) raising citizens' and legislators' attitudes toward and expectations of the nursing profession (Leddy & Pepper 1993, p. 384). The leadership role of the nurse is further discussed in Chapter 20.

MANAGER

Management is often confused with leadership, because in much of the literature, leadership is associated with group interaction within an organizational setting. Tappen (1989, p. 101) defines **management** as "planning, giving direction, developing staff, monitoring operations, giving rewards fairly, and representing both staff members and administration as needed." Management, therefore, occurs within an organizational environment. Leadership, by contrast, may or may not require delegated authority within a formal organization.

The nurse manages the nursing care of individuals, groups, families, and communities. The nurse-manager also delegates nursing activities to ancillary workers and other nurses and supervises and evaluates their performance. In addition, the nurse uses principles of management and leadership when functioning as a **case manager.** Case management involves coordination among disciplines and with ancillary personnel to deliver care to the client in the most appropriate setting and in a cost-efficient manner. Whether functioning as a manager of employees, clients, or services, the nurse must have knowledge of organizational structure and dynamics, authority and accountability, group process, leadership, change theory, advocacy, delegation, and supervision and evaluation. See Chapter 20 for further discussion of the nurse as manager.

RESEARCHER

The majority of researchers in nursing are prepared at the doctoral and postdoctoral level, although an increasing number of clinicians with master's degrees are beginning to participate in research activity as part of the advanced practice role. The ANA's *Standards of Clinical Nursing Practice* (1991, p. 16) states that all nurses should select nursing interventions that are substantiated by research and, further, that all nurses may participate in research activities based on their level of education, their position, and their practice setting. If nursing is to develop as a research-based practice, it is not unreasonable to expect the nurse in the clinical area to (a) have some awareness of the process and language of research, (b) be sensitive to issues related to protecting the rights of human subjects, (c) participate in identifying significant researchable problems, and (d) be a discriminating consumer of research findings.

Nursing students, therefore, must learn the investigative role of the nurse early in their careers so that they acquire the tools to bridge the research-practice gap effectively. As the body of nursing knowledge increases, the science of nursing and the art of nursing coalesce, resulting in more effective nursing care. In 1989, the ANA published its *Education for Participation in Nursing Research*, which specifies the expected research competence of nurses with associate, bachelor's, master's, and doctoral degrees. Additional information about the nurse's role in research can be found in Chapter 2.

Expanded Nursing Roles

A role is a pattern of behavior expected of individuals in specific social situations. An **expanded role** is one that a nurse assumes by virtue of education and experience. The nurse who assumes an expanded role has increased responsibilities and, usually, greater autonomy. Nurses are assuming expanded roles in both hospital and community settings.

Nurse Generalist The ANA conducts nurse generalist certification programs that issue certificates in eleven areas: general nursing practice, medical-surgical nursing, gerontologic nursing, pediatric (child and adolescent) nursing, perinatal nursing, college health nursing, school nursing, community health nursing, psychiatric and mental health nursing, nursing continuing education and staff development, and home health nursing. According to the report of the American Nurses Credentialing Center (ANCC) to the 1993 ANA House of Delegates (ANCC 1993, p. 1), more than 95,000 nurses had been certified by January 1, 1993. The certification designation is RN, C (Registered Nurse, Certified).

Nurse Clinician The term *nurse clinician* was first used by Frances Reiter in 1966. Nurse clinicians provide bedside or direct care in a specialty area. They may or may not have advanced educational preparation. They may be certified through the American Nurses Credentialing Center or through specialty nursing organization certifying programs such as the Association of Operating Room Nurses or the Emergency Nurses Association.

Nurse Practitioner The role of the nurse practitioner is an extension of the nurse's basic caregiving role; it prepares nurses for an expanded role in the provision of primary care. Nurse practitioners who wish to become certified through the ANA must have graduate education and practice experience at the advanced level. As of January 1, 1992, 13,552 nurses had been certified as nurse practitioners (ANCC 1992, p. 5). Additionally, the American Association of Nurse Anesthetists certifies nurse anesthetists, and the American Association of Nurse Midwives certifies the advanced practice of nurse-midwifery.

Nurse practitioners may be generalists (eg, family nurse practitioners) or specialists (eg, geriatric nurse practitioners). Nurse practitioners in a community may be employed in health maintenance organizations, health centers, schools, and physicians' offices. They are usually skilled at making nursing assessments, performing physical assessments, counseling, teaching, and treating minor, self-limiting illnesses or stable, long-term illness. Nurse practitioners in hospitals are often employed in specialty areas, such as geriatric nursing.

Nurse Specialist The nurse specialist has advanced knowledge and skills in a particular area of nursing. An educational prerequisite is a master's degree in nursing. The ANA's certification designation for both the nurse practitioner and the nurse specialist is CS (certified specialist). Clinical specialist certification is available through the ANA in the following areas: medical-surgical nursing, gerontologic nursing, community health nursing, psychiatric and mental health nursing, and child and adolescent psychiatric and mental health nursing. By January 1992, 16,391 nurses had been certified as nurse specialists (ANCC 1992, p. 5). These nurses practice in hospitals or communities. In the hospital, such nurses give direct client care, advise other nurses, and coordinate nursing given by others. The clinical nurse specialist is a role model and is expected to keep abreast of new developments in the field.

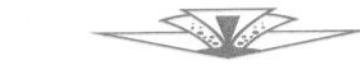

Nursing Organizations

One way nurses can demonstrate professional commitment is active involvement in a nursing organization. There are two types of organizations: professional and nonprofessional. "A professional organization is an organization of practitioners who judge one another as professionally competent and who have banded together to perform social functions which they cannot perform in their separate capacities as individuals" (Merton 1958, p. 50).

Styles (1983) writes that nursing organizations must perform the following five functions for the preservation and development of the profession:

1. Defining and regulating the profession through setting and enforcing standards of education and practice for the generalist and the specialist. In the United States and Canada, regulation is achieved largely through the licensure of individual nurses, certification, and accreditation. (See the section on credentialing of nurses in Chapter 12.) Regulation is also achieved through the adoption of codes of ethics and norms of conduct (Styles 1983, p. 570).
2. Developing the knowledge base for practice in its broadest and narrowest components. Various theorists have made major contributions to the development of

nursing knowledge. The challenge for nurses in the future is to generate questions and formulate hypotheses from these published theories and then test those hypotheses through nursing research. Because only research can determine the usefulness of a theory, research makes a major contribution to the development of nursing knowledge. Another significant contribution to nursing knowledge is the work of the North American Nursing Diagnosis Association (NANDA) (see Chapter 6). This group is generating and expanding a taxonomy of nursing diagnoses. Research is required to determine the validity and reliability of these diagnoses.

3. Transmitting values, norms, knowledge, and skill to nursing students, new graduates, and members of the profession for application in practice. This function is largely performed through the education of nurses and the socialization process.
4. Communicating and advocating the values and contributions of the field to several publics and constituencies. This function requires that nursing organizations speak for nurses from a position of broad agreement. It is essential for nurses to participate actively in formulating health legislation and policy.
5. Attending to the social and general welfare of their members. Professional associations give their members social and moral support to perform their roles as professionals and to cope with professional problems. Association journals disseminate updated knowledge, new ideas, and professional concerns. By participating in the collective bargaining process, nurses can improve their economic and working conditions.

Nursing organizations are established at local, national, and international levels. Selected nursing organizations are discussed below. See also Appendix A for other nursing organizations.

NATIONAL STUDENT NURSES ASSOCIATION (NSNA)

The National Student Nurses Association (NSNA) is the official preprofessional organization for nursing students. Formed in 1953 and incorporated in 1959, the NSNA originally functioned under the aegis of the ANA and NLN; however, in 1968 the NSNA became an autonomous body, although it communicates with the NLN and the ANA. To qualify for membership in the NSNA, a student must be enrolled in a state-approved nursing education program. The official organ of the NSNA is *Imprint* magazine.

In Canada, nursing students have a similar organization, the Canadian University Student Nurses Association. The provincial student nurses' associations also have programs related to the needs of nursing students and concerns within the health field in general.

AMERICAN NURSES ASSOCIATION (ANA)

The American Nurses Association (ANA) is the national professional organization for nursing in the United States. It was founded in 1896 as the Nurses Associated Alumnae of the United States and Canada. In 1911, the name was changed to the American Nurses Association. It was a charter member of the International Council of Nurses, along with Great Britain and Germany, in 1899. The purposes of the ANA are to foster high standards of nursing practice and to promote the educational and professional advancement of nurses so that all people may have better nursing care. The ANA is composed of the nurses' associations from the 50 states, Guam, the Virgin Islands, Puerto Rico, and the District of Columbia. These state associations are in turn divided into regional and local chapters.

In 1982, the organization became a federation of state nurses' associations. Individuals can no longer belong to the ANA, but they participate by joining their state nurses' associations. Each state nurses' association is entitled to representation as a member of the federation. The number of seats allocated to each state's delegation depends on the number of members in each state organization. The official journal of the ANA is the *American Journal of Nursing*, and *American Nurse* is the official newspaper. The functions of the ANA are shown in the box on page 23.

CANADIAN NURSES ASSOCIATION (CNA)

The Canadian Nurses Association (CNA) is the national nursing association of Canada. Nurses do not join the CNA independently but obtain membership by paying a fee to the provincial chapters. In November 1985, the Ordre des infirmières et infirmiers du Quebec (the Quebec Nurses Association) withdrew from the CNA.

The CNA has developed national standards and a code of ethics, and it offers support to all provincial associations. Through the National Testing Services, the CNA prepares licensure examinations. These examinations are available to all provinces and territories and provide a national standard for licensure of registered nurses. Through the Canadian Nurses Foundation, research grants, fellowships, and scholarships are offered to Canadian nurses. The official journal of the CNA, *Canadian Nurse*, is published monthly and sent to each nurse member.

INTERNATIONAL COUNCIL OF NURSES (ICN)

The International Council of Nurses (ICN) was established in 1899. Nurses from Great Britain, the United

FUNCTIONS OF THE AMERICAN NURSES ASSOCIATION (ANA)

- Establish standards of nursing practice, nursing education, and nursing services
- Establish a code of ethical conduct for nurses
- Ensure a system of credentialing in nursing
- Initiate and influence legislation, governmental programs, national health policy, and international health policy
- Support systematic study, evaluation, and research in nursing
- Serve as the central agency for the collection, analysis, and dissemination of information relevant to nursing
- Promote and protect the economic and general welfare of nurses
- Provide leadership in national and international nursing
- Provide for the professional development of nurses
- Conduct an affirmative action program
- Ensure a collective bargaining program for nurses
- Provide services to constituent members
- Maintain communication with members through official publications
- Assume an active role as consumer advocate
- Represent and speak for the nursing profession with allied health groups, national and international organizations, governmental bodies, and the public
- Protect and promote the advancement of human rights related to health care and nursing

Source: American Nurses Association, *American Nurses Association Bylaws,* as revised June 30, 1991 (Washington, DC: American Nurses Association, 1991). Used by permission.

States, and Canada were among the founding members. The council is a federation of national nurses' associations, such as the ANA and CNA. In 1993, 111 national nurses associations representing 1.4 million nurses worldwide were affiliated with the ICN.

The ICN provides an organization through which member national nursing associations can work together to promote the health of people and the care of the sick. The objectives of ICN are (1) to improve the standards and status of nursing, (2) to promote the development of strong national nurses' associations, and (3) to serve as the authoritative voice for nurses and the nursing profession worldwide (Backus 1990, p. 168). The official journal of the ICN is *International Nursing Review.*

In 1987, the governing body of the ICN set the following priorities for its future:

- To continue efforts to strengthen the effectiveness of the constituent national nurses' associations.
- To support the work of national nurses' associations to improve employment conditions for nurses in all settings and to promote the social and economic welfare of all nursing personnel.
- To strengthen the ICN and the national nurses' associations in ways oriented to promote participation in effective relationships with interdisciplinary, interprofessional, and international government agencies, for the purposes of improving the health of the public.
- To review changes and adjustments in the organizational components and relationships of the ICN.
- To encourage national nurses' associations to be more active in selling and enforcing standards for nursing education and nursing practice, leadership, and management in their countries.
- To assist national nurses' associations and others in bringing about more appropriate regulatory mechanisms for nursing practice, thus making it possible for the knowledge and skills of nurses to be utilized more effectively and recognized within the health system.
- To orient national nurses' associations to promote and assist as feasible with health personnel planning and development for nursing in all its areas of practice.
- To ensure that the ICN Code for Nurses continues to provide the ethical guidance required by nurses in a rapidly changing world with constant social, technologic, genetic, and pharmacologic advances.
- To work with national nurses' associations to encourage and facilitate the development of research in nursing by nurses and the dissemination of research findings.

NATIONAL LEAGUE FOR NURSING (NLN)

The National League for Nursing, formed in 1952, is an organization of both individuals and agencies. Its objective is to foster the development and improvement of all nursing services and nursing education. People who are not nurses but have an interest in nursing services, for example, hospital administrators, can be members of the league. This feature of the NLN—involving nonnurse members, consumers, and nurses from all levels of practice—is unique.

The purposes of the NLN are to strengthen and support nursing services, to promote research for widening the knowledge base of nursing education and practice, to maintain responsiveness to its membership, to promote public understanding and support of nursing, and to explore new avenues for promoting nursing, such as alternative health care settings (NLN 1991). The NLN has traditionally offered a wide range of services, including continuing education workshops and seminars, consultation, and educational aid. In terms of schools of nursing, the NLN offers two major services: (a) voluntary accreditation for educational programs in nursing, and (b) testing services, including preadmission testing for potential students, achievement testing throughout the program, and state board examinations for licensure. The NLN also conducts yearly surveys of nursing schools, newly registered nurses, and post-basic graduates. These surveys serve as a primary source of research data about nursing education in the United States. The official journal of the NLN up to 1979 was *Nursing Outlook;* in 1980, the official magazine became *Nursing and Health Care.*

INTERNATIONAL HONOR SOCIETY: SIGMA THETA TAU

Sigma Theta Tau, the international honor society in nursing, was founded in 1922 and is headquartered in Indianapolis, Indiana. The greek letters stand for the Greek words *storga, tharos,* and *tima,* meaning love, courage, and honor. The society is a member of the association of college honor societies. The society's purpose is professional rather than social. Membership is attained through academic achievement. Students in baccalaureate programs in nursing and nurses in master's, doctoral, and postdoctoral programs are eligible to be selected for membership.

The official journal of Sigma Theta Tau, *Image: Journal of Nursing Scholarship,* is published quarterly. The journal publishes scholarly articles of interest to nurses. The society also publishes *Reflections,* a quarterly newsletter that provides information about the organization and its various chapters.

CHAPTER HIGHLIGHTS

- There are many definitions and descriptions of nursing, but the essence of nursing is caring for and caring about people as holistic beings in matters related to health promotion, health maintenance, health restoration, and dying.
- Nursing as a humanistic, caring, nurturing, comforting, and supporting profession has evolved over centuries.
- Modern nursing in the Western Hemisphere finds its education and professional practice origins with Florence Nightingale in 19th-century England.
- A desired goal of nursing is professionalism, which necessitates specialized education; a unique body of knowledge, including specific skills and abilities; autonomous regulation; and a code of ethics.
- Socialization is a lifelong process by which people become functioning participants of a society or a group. It is a reciprocal learning process brought about by interaction with other people and establishes boundaries of behavior. Socialization to professional nursing practice is the process whereby the values and norms of the nursing profession are internalized into the nurse's own behavior and self-concept. The nurse acquires the knowledge, skills, and attitudes characteristic of the profession.
- Nursing's types of knowledge include nursing science, nursing esthetics, nursing ethics, and personal knowledge.
- Nurses function in a variety of roles that are not exclusive of one another; in reality, they often occur together and serve to clarify the nurse's activities. These roles include care provider, communicator/helper, teacher, counselor, client advocate, change agent, leader, manager, and researcher.
- Nurses are fulfilling expanded nursing roles, for example, those of the nurse generalist, the nurse clinician, the nurse specialist, and the advanced nurse practitioner.
- Both professional and nonprofessional nursing organizations and associations fulfill essential functions for the nursing profession and for individual nurses.
- Participation in the activities of nursing associations enhances the growth of involved individuals and helps nurses collectively influence policies affecting nursing practice.

READINGS AND REFERENCES

SUGGESTED READINGS

Backer, BA. 1993. Lillian Wald: Connecting caring with activism. *Nursing and Health Care* 14(3):122–29.
As nurses today become involved in professional advocacy for health care and social reform, they would do well to study the history of Lillian Wald. Between the years 1893 and 1915, Wald created and developed the Visiting Nurse Service of New York and the Henry Street Settlement House. Backer provides a history of Lillian Wald, desribing how she "transformed her nursing and her caring into establishing health and social policies."

Diers, D. January 1990. Learning the art and craft of nursing. *American Journal of Nursing* 90:65–66.
Diers writes about the art of nursing, which is characterized in part as self-discipline. The tool of the nurse in this context is the intellect. Diers describes the discipline of nursing as the constant attention to difference and unpredictability.

Donahue, PM. 1985. *Nursing: The Finest Art: An Illustrated History.* St Louis: Mosby.
This book, in Donahue's own words, is the "demonstration of the historical development of nursing from primitive times to the present through an integration of a variety of selected illustrations and written text."

SELECTED REFERENCES

American Journal of Nursing. September 1993. ICN '93: A call to "fight, in unity, for nurses' rights." *American Journal of Nursing* 93: 74, 82.

American Nurses Association. 1973. *Standards of Nursing Practice.* Kansas City, MO: ANA.

______. 1980. *Nursing: A Social Policy Statement.* Washington, DC: ANA.

______. 1984. *Standards for Professional Nursing Education.* Washington, DC: ANA.

______. 1987a. *Facts about Nursing 86–87.* Washington, DC: ANA.

______. 1987b. *Proceedings of the 1987 House of Delegates.* Washington, DC: ANA.

______. 1989. *Education for Participation in Nursing Research.* Washington, DC: ANA.

______. 1991a. *American Nurses Association Bylaws.* Washington, DC: ANA.

______. 1991b. *Standards of Clinical Nursing Practice.* Washington, DC: ANA.

American Nurses Association, Commission of Nursing Research. 1981. *ANA Guidelines for Investigative Function of Nurses.* Washington, DC: ANA.

American Nurses Credentialing Center. 1992. *American Nurses Credentialing Center Certification Catalog.* Washington, DC: ANA.

______. 1993. *Report to the House of Delegates.* Washington, DC: ANA.

Backer, B. 1993. Lillian Wald: Connecting caring with activism. *Nursing and Health Care* 14(3):122–29.

Backus, K. 1990. *Medical and Health Information Directory.* 5th ed. Vol. 1: *Organizations, Agencies, and Institutions.* Detroit: Gale Research Inc.

Benner, P. 1984. *From Novice to Expert: Excellence and Power in Clinical Nursing Practice.* Redwood City, CA: Addison-Wesley Nursing.

Benner, P and Wrubel, J. 1989. *The Primacy of Caring: Stress and Coping in Health and Illness.* Redwood City, CA: Addison-Wesley Nursing.

Calhoun, J. 1993. The Nightingale Pledge: A commitment that survives the passage of time. *Nursing and Health Care* 14(3):130–36.

Carper, B. 1978. Fundamental patterns of knowing in nursing. *Advances in Nursing Science* 1(3):13–23.

CNA Connection. April 1984. Canada health act: CNA appears before commons committee. *Canadian Nurse* 80:8–9.

Disparti, J. 1988. Nutrition and self care. In Caliandro, G and Judkins, BL, editors. *Primary Nursing Practice.* Glenview, IL: Scott, Foresman.

Dolan, J, Fitzpatrick, ML, and Hermann, E. 1983. *Nursing in Society: A Historical Perspective.* 15th ed. Philadelphia: Saunders.

Donahue, B. 1985. *Nursing: The Finest Art: An Illustrated History.* St Louis: Mosby.

Flaherty, MJ. 1979. The characteristics and scope of professional nursing. *Journal for Nursing Leadership and Management* 1:61, 63, 69.

Henderson, V. 1966. *The Nature of Nursing: A Definition and Its Implications for Practice, Research, and Education.* New York: Macmillan.

International Council of Nurses. 1973. *Constitution and Regulations.* Geneva: International Council of Nurses.

Kelly, LY. 1985. *Dimensions of Professional Nursing.* 5th ed. New York: Macmillan.

Kemp, VH. 1986. An overview of change and leadership. In Hein, EC and Nicholson, MJ, editors. *Contemporary Leadership Behavior: Selected Readings.* 2d ed. Boston: Little, Brown.

Large, JT. October 1976. Harriet Newton Phillips, the first trained nurse in America. *Image: Journal of Nursing Scholarship* 8:49–51.

Leddy, S and Pepper, JM. 1993. *Conceptual Bases of Professional Nursing.* 2d ed. Philadelphia: Lippincott.

Lewis, EP. September/October 1983. News outlook: The issue that won't go away. A report on the 1983 NLN convention. *Nursing Outlook* 31:246–47.

Marriner-Tomey, A. 1992. *Guide to Nursing Management.* 4th ed. St Louis: Mosby.

Merton, RK. January 1958. The function of the professional organization. *American Journal of Nursing* 58:50–54.

Miller, BK. April 1985. Just what is a profession? *Nursing Success Today* 2:21–27.

National League for Nursing. 1991. *NLN Mission and Goals, 1991–93.* New York: NLN.

The New Lexicon Webster's Dictionary of the English Language, S.V. "nursing."

Nightingale, F. 1860. *Notes on Nursing: What It Is, and What It Is Not.* Commemorative Edition. Philadelphia: Lippincott.

Ohlson, VM. 1990. The role of the International Council of Nurses and the World Health Organization. In McCloskey, JC and Grace, HK, editors. pp. 330–37. *Current Issues in Nursing.* St Louis: Mosby.

Polit, DF and Hungler, BP. 1989. *Essentials of Nursing Research: Methods, Appraisal, and Utilization.* 2d ed. Philadelphia: Lippincott.

Quinn, S. 1981. *What About Me? Caring for the Careers.* Geneva: International Council of Nurses.

Redman, BK. 1993. *The Process of Patient Education.* 7th ed. St Louis: Mosby.

Schuyler, CB. 1992. Florence Nightingale. In Nightingale, F. *Notes on Nursing: What It Is, and What It Is Not.* Commemorative Edition. Philadelphia: Lippincott.

Styles, MM. 1978. Why publish? *Image: Journal of Nursing Scholarship* 10:28–32.

______. 1982. *On Nursing: Toward a New Endowment.* St Louis: Mosby.

______. November 1983. The anatomy of a profession. *Heart and Lung* 12:570–75.

Tappen, RM. 1989. *Nursing Leadership and Management: Concepts and Practice.* Philadelphia: FA Davis.

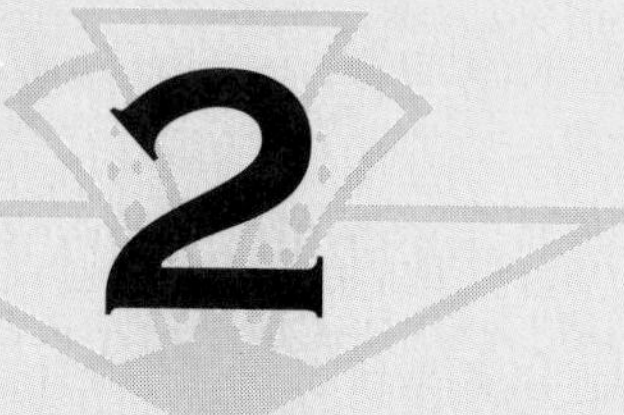

Dimensions of Nursing: Practice, Education, and Research

Objectives

- Describe the recipients of nursing.
- Identify the various settings for nursing.
- Identify the purpose of nurse practice acts.
- Identify the standards of clinical nursing practice.
- Identify the factors influencing nursing practice.
- Explain how nursing education affects nursing practice.
- Discuss the titling and licensure of registered nurses.
- Describe the different types of nursing education.
- Describe the importance of continuing education.
- Describe the role of nursing research as it influences current and future nursing practice.
- Describe the role of the nurse in protecting the rights of clients.
- Discuss the role of nursing in participating in research activities.
- Discuss future trends in nursing.

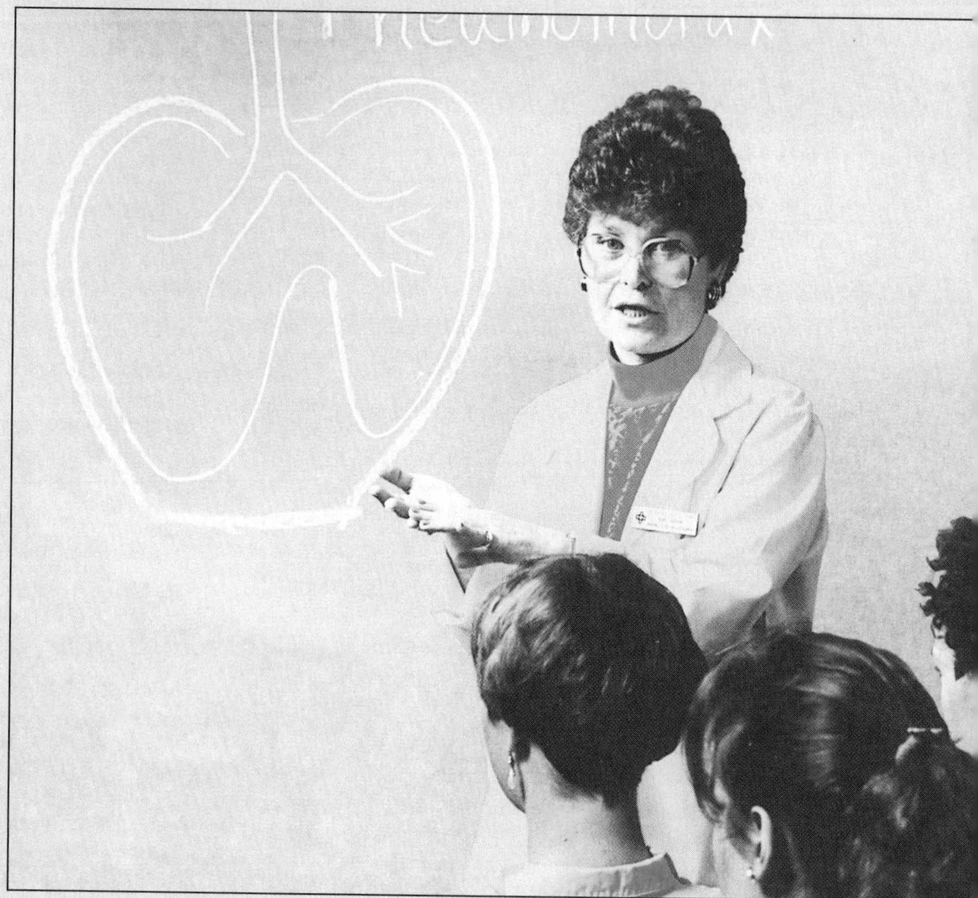

Nurses practice in an ever-increasing variety of ways and settings. The focus of all nursing practice is the client, who may be an individual, a family, a group, or a community. The practice of an individual nurse is determined largely by the setting and the needs of the clients served by the setting. For example, in the school health setting, the client focus is the schoolchildren and their families. The nurse practicing in this setting must have special knowledge of pediatric growth and development and the health needs of school children. Other practice settings include hospitals, clinics, industry, extended care facilities, and home health. All nursing practice is defined by the standards of the professional organization and regulated by the nurse practice acts of the area in which the nurse works.

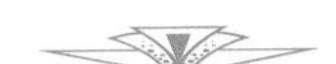

Nursing Practice

Recipients of Nursing

The recipients of nursing are sometimes called *consumers*, sometimes *patients*, and sometimes *clients*. A **consumer** is an individual, a group of people, or a community that uses a service or commodity. A family that uses electricity in their home is a consumer of electricity. People who use health care products or services are consumers of health care.

A **patient** is a person who is waiting for or undergoing medical treatment and care. The word *patient* comes from a Latin word meaning to suffer or to bear. Traditionally, the person receiving health care has been called a patient. Usually, people become patients when they seek assistance because of illness or for surgery. Some nurses believe that the word *patient* implies passive acceptance of the decisions and care of health professionals. Additionally, with the emphasis on health promotion and prevention of illness, many recipients of nursing care are not ill. Moreover, nurses interact with family members and significant others in addition to the persons actually receiving nursing care.

For these reasons, nurses are increasingly referring to recipients of health care as clients. A **client** is a person who engages the advice or services of another who is qualified to provide this service. The term *client* presents the receivers of health care less as passive recipients and more as collaborators in the care, that is, as persons who are also responsible for their health. Thus, the health status of a client is the responsibility of the individual in collaboration with health professionals. In this book, *client* is the preferred term, although *consumer* and *patient* are used in some instances.

Focus of Nursing

Nursing involves an interrelationship of many people concerned with a client's responses to potential or actual health problems. Today, nursing emphasizes the whole person; people are seen not merely as physical beings but as biopsychosocial beings. Nursing practice involves a complex of knowledge and skills applied to the whole client. Nurses are also involved with support persons and the community as a whole. For this reason, nurses must be aware of how the support persons and community affect the client's well-being and consider the well-being of these support persons and the community.

Nursing practice involves four areas related to health (health is discussed in Chapter 13):

1. *Health promotion.* Health promotion means helping people develop resources to maintain or enhance their health and well-being. The focus of health promotion is "directed toward maintaining or improving the general health of individuals, families, and communities" (Edelman & Mandle 1990, p. 10). Examples of nursing actions that promote health include explaining the benefits of good nutrition and exercise to a client and encouraging a client to stop smoking. Health promotion is discussed in more detail in Chapter 13.
2. *Health maintenance.* Health maintenance nursing activities are those actions that help clients to maintain their health status. For example, an elderly person in a long-term care facility can be taught and encouraged to exercise to maintain muscle strength and mobility.
3. *Health restoration.* Health restoration means helping people to improve health following health problems or illness. Examples of activities that help restore health are teaching a client to protect an incision and to change a surgical dressing, and assisting handicapped individuals to attain the highest level of physical strength of which they are capable.
4. *Care of the dying.* This area of nursing practice involves comforting and caring for people of all ages while they are dying. Nurses carrying out these activities work in homes, hospitals, and extended care facilities. Some agencies, called hospices, are specifically designed for this purpose.

Settings for Nursing

In the past, the acute care hospital was the only practice setting open to most nurses. Today, however, nurses work not only in acute and long-term chronic or rehabilitation hospitals but also in clients' homes, community agencies, ambulatory clinics or health maintenance organizations (HMOs), and nursing practice centers, for example. Table 2–1 shows areas of registered practice in the United States and Canada. Figure 2–1 shows nurses practicing in a variety of settings.

Nurses have different degrees of nursing autonomy and nursing responsibility in the various settings. Today, nurses have a variety of career choices and can pursue any number of interests. They may specialize, for example, in intensive care nursing or respiratory nursing. In addition to providing direct care, they teach clients and support persons, serve as nursing advocates and agents of change, and help determine health policies affecting consumers in the community and in hospitals. For information about the models for delivery of nursing, see Chapter 20, page 410.

Table 2–1 Areas of Registered Nurse Employment in the United States: Contemporary Changes

Practice Setting	United States 1991 (percentage*)	United States 1996 (percentage*)
Hospitals	67.9	60.0
Nursing homes/homes for the aged	6.6	8.1
Community health/ public health	6.8	17.0
Ambulatory care	7.7	8.5
Nursing education, schools, occupational health, and other (self-employed, insurance claims reviewers)	10.7	6.4

* Rounded to the first decimal

Sources: American Nurses Association, *Nursing and the American Nurses Association* (Washington, DC: ANA, 1991) and Health Resources and Services Administration, *Advance Notes from the National Sample Survey of Registered Nurses* (Rockville, MD: Division of Nursing Bureau of Health Professions, 1996).

NURSE PRACTICE ACTS

Nurse practice acts, or acts for professional nursing practice, regulate the practice of nursing in the United States and Canada. Each state in the United States and each province in Canada has its own act. Although nurse practice acts differ in various jurisdictions, they all have a common purpose: to protect the public. Nurse practice acts are a formalized contract between society and the profession. They serve a public purpose and also meet the needs of the profession. Nurse practice acts grant the public a mechanism to ensure minimum standards for entry into the profession and to distinguish the unqualified. The profession maintains standards in practice in part through appropriate entry credentialing. During the past 10 years, many states have revised their nurse practice acts to permit expanded nursing roles. For additional information, see Chapter 12.

STANDARDS OF CLINICAL NURSING PRACTICE

Establishing and implementing standards of practice are major functions of a professional organization. The purpose of **standards of clinical nursing practice** is to describe the responsibilities for which nurses are accountable. The standards (a) reflect the values and priorities of the nursing profession, (b) provide direction for professional nursing practice, (c) provide a framework for the evaluation of nursing practice, and (d) define the profession's accountability to the public and the client outcomes for which nurses are responsible (ANA 1991c, p. 3). In 1991, the American Nurses Association (ANA) developed standards of clinical nursing practice that are generic in nature and provide for the practice of nursing regardless of area of specialization. See the box on page 30. Various specialty nursing organizations have further developed specific standards of nursing practice related to the practice of nursing in a specialty area.

In *Standards of Clinical Nursing Practice*, the ANA comments on the responsibility of the nursing profession to society in developing standards that include outcome criteria:

> Increases in health care costs, competition, and regulation are forcing health care providers to define their practice in a measurable way and to identify the client outcomes to which they contribute. Additionally, federal and private sector initiatives are focusing on the development of methods to evaluate the quality, appropriateness, and effectiveness of health care services. The nursing profession continues to closely monitor the evolving external environment and analyze the

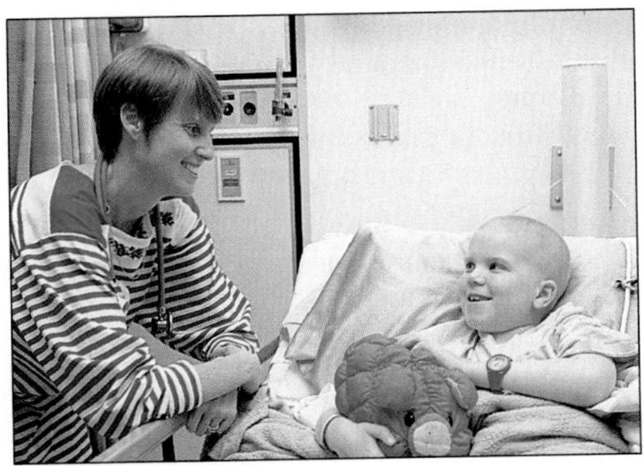

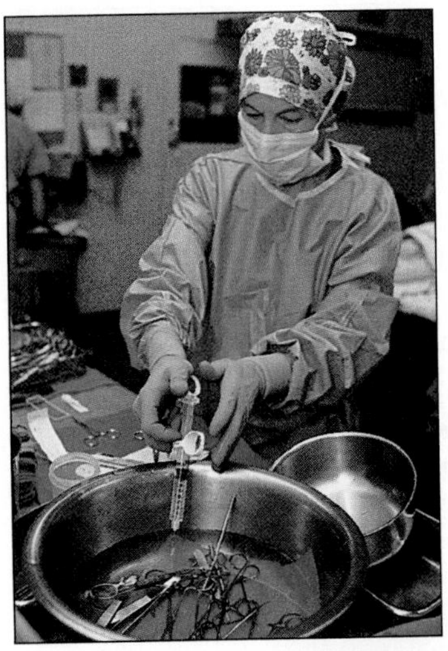

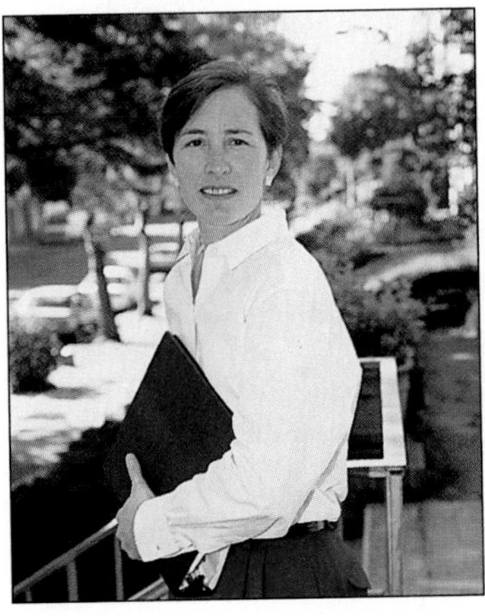

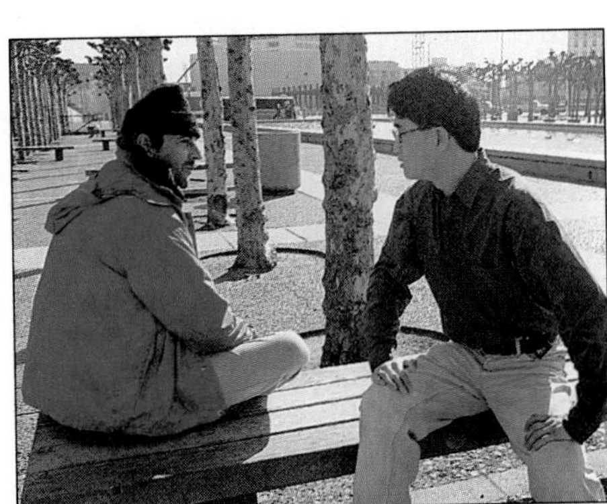

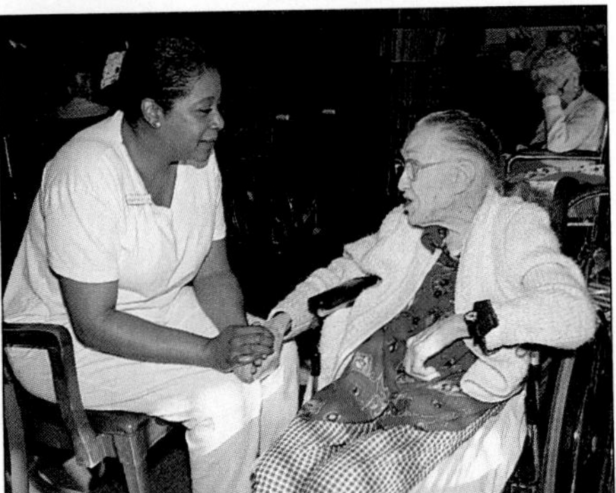

Figure 2–1 Nurses practice in a variety of settings. Clockwise from top left: pediatric nursing, operating room nursing, geriatric nursing, community nursing, and home nursing.

need to modify existing standards or develop new standards for all areas of nursing practice. Standards must receive ongoing attention by the profession to assure that they remain timely and reflect advances in nursing knowledge and clinical technology. (ANA 1991c, p. 1)

The profession's responsibilities inherent in establishing and implementing standards of practice include (a) to establish, maintain, and improve standards, (b) to hold members accountable for using standards, (c) to educate the public to appreciate the standards, (d) to protect the public from individuals who have not attained the standards or willfully do not follow them, and (e) to protect individual members of the profession from each other (Phaneuf & Lang 1985, p. 2).

Nursing standards clearly reflect the specific functions and activities that nurses provide, as opposed to the functions of other health workers. The ANA's standards of clinical nursing practice consist of standards of care and standards of professional performance, which are listed in the box on page 30. Standards of care describe the competence of nursing care demonstrated by the components of the nursing process. Standards of professional performance describe the competence level of professional role behaviors. The complete standards of clinical nursing practice, including measurement criteria, can be obtained from the ANA. The standards of practice of the Canadian Nurses Association (CNA) are summarized in the box on page 31.

When standards of professional practice are implemented, they serve as yardsticks for the measurements used in licensure, certification, accreditation, quality assurance, peer review, and public policy (Phaneuf & Lang

ANA STANDARDS OF CLINICAL NURSING PRACTICE

Standards of Care

I. Assessment
The Nurse collects client health data.

II. Diagnosis
The Nurse analyzes the assessment data in determining diagnoses.

III. Outcome Identification
The Nurse identifies expected outcomes individualized to the client.

IV. Planning
The Nurse develops a plan of care that prescribes interventions to attain expected outcomes.

V. Implementation
The Nurse implements the interventions identified in the plan of care.

VI. Evaluation
The Nurse evaluates the client's progress toward attainment of outcomes.

Standards of Professional Performance

I. Quality of Care
The Nurse systematically evaluates the quality and effectiveness of nursing practice.

II. Performance Appraisal
The Nurse evaluates his/her own nursing practice in relation to professional practice standards and relevant statutes and regulations.

III. Education
The Nurse acquires and maintains current knowledge in nursing practice.

IV. Collegiality
The Nurse contributes to the professional development of peers, colleagues, and others.

V. Ethics
The Nurse's decisions and actions on behalf of clients are determined in an ethical manner.

VI. Collaboration
The Nurse collaborates with the client, significant others, and health care providers in providing client care.

VII. Research
The Nurse uses research findings in practice.

VIII. Resource Utilization
The Nurse considers factors related to safety, effectiveness, and cost in planning and delivering client care.

Source: American Nurses Association, *Standards of Clinical Nursing Practice* (Washington, DC: ANA, 1991). Used with permission.

1985, p. 7). Licensure, certification, and accreditation are discussed in Chapter 12. Quality assurance and peer review are discussed in Chapter 8.

CAREER MOBILITY

The public image of the nurse is often that of a hospital staff nurse. Many laypeople are unaware of the variety of roles and educational backgrounds of nurses. Two kinds of mobility are open to the nurse: vertical and horizontal. Vertical mobility means advancing upward within a hierarchy, for example, from staff nurse to head nurse. Horizontal mobility refers to ability to change practice setting, such as from a nursing home to a community health agency.

Recognizing that nurses require encouragement, motivation, and recognition, some settings provide clinical ladder models for career development. Traditionally, a nurse's clinical competence was rewarded by moving the nurse away from client care into administrative roles. Clinical ladders provide nurses with recognition of their clinical competence, at the same time permitting them to continue clinical nursing practice.

FACTORS INFLUENCING NURSING PRACTICE

To understand nursing as it is practiced today and as it will be practiced tomorrow requires not only a historical perspective of nursing's evolution but also an understanding of some of the social forces currently influencing this profession. These forces usually affect the entire health care system, and nursing, as a major component of that system, cannot avoid the effects. See Chapter 1 for the historical development of nursing.

Economics The economic climate of health care has changed dramatically because of sharply escalating health care costs due to a growing aging population, an expanding number of uninsured and under-insured persons, and increased use of technology. Cost containment efforts have resulted in hospital closures, mergers among previously competing facilities, and a shift in the site of care away from the hospital setting. These system-wide changes have resulted in a move toward community-based care as well as changes in the skill-mix of providers.

CANADIAN NURSES ASSOCIATION STANDARDS FOR NURSING PRACTICE

I. Nursing practice requires that a conceptual model(s) for nursing be the basis for that practice.

II. Nursing practice requires the effective use of the nursing process.

III. Nursing practice requires that the helping relationship be the nature of the client-nurse interaction.

IV. Nursing practice requires nurses to fulfill professional responsibilities.

Source: Canadian Nurses Association, *A Definition of Nursing Practice: Standards for Nursing Practice* (Ottawa: CNA, 1987), Pub No. ISBN 0-919 108-51-2. Reprinted with permission.

Table 2-2 Average Nursing Salaries 1986–1994

	Average Starting Salary	Average Maximum Salary
1994	$29,384	***
1992	$27,625	$41,559
1991	$26,500	$40,000
1990	$24,768	$37,168
1989	$23,488	$35,300
1988	$22,416	$32,160
1987	$20,964	$29,088
1986	$20,340	$27,744

*** Previous data has been based on hospital nursing salaries. In 1994, however, 40% of nurses worked in a variety of roles outside of acute care for which average salary data is unavailable.

Sources: American Nurses Association, *Nursing and the American Nurses Association* (Washington, DC: ANA, 1991), P Brider, Annual nursing salary survey: Where did the jobs go? *American Journal of Nursing*, April 1993, 93:31–40, D Louden, L Crawford & S Trotman, Profiles of the newly licensed nurse. *NLN*, 1996.

The cost of health care has increased greatly over the past two decades. In 1982, the Medicare payment system to hospitals and physicians was revised to establish fees according to **diagnostic related groups (DRGs)**. With the implementation of this legislation, more clients in hospitals are more acutely ill than before, and clients once considered sufficiently ill to be hospitalized are now treated at home. In spite of these efforts, health care costs continue to rise, totaling almost 15% of the gross domestic product in 1994.

Paradoxically, rising health care costs have been accompanied by an increasing number of uninsured persons. In 1995, an estimated 39 million people in the United States did not have health insurance; a similar number of people are estimated to be under-insured (Bodenheimer & Grumbach, 1995). These clients often delay seeking medical treatment until problems become more severe. The National Leadership Coalition for Health Care Reform (1991, p. 2) predicts that without significant health care reform, the cost of health care will reach $2.7 trillion by the year 2000. Due to the increasing costs and decreasing coverage, the United States is struggling to reform its health care system.

These changes present challenges to nurses. Currently, the health care industry is shifting its emphasis from inpatient to outpatient care with preadmission testing, increased outpatient same-day surgery, posthospitalization rehabilitation, home health care, health maintenance, physical fitness programs, and community health education programs. As a result, more nurses are being employed in community-based health settings, such as home health agencies, hospices, and community clinics.

These changes in employment for nurses have implications for nursing education, nursing research, and nursing practice.

Changing Demands for Nurses The rapid social, political, and economic changes in health care have caused marked shifts in nursing employment. As health care costs rise, hospitals—once considered the major employment site for registered nurses—have experienced down-sizing and closures. A significant amount of care has shifted to nontraditional sites such as outpatient service centers, subacute care units within long-term care facilities, and the home. As a result, the employment of nurses in community and home health care, ambulatory care, and long-term care has expanded.

Of the 2.5 million registered nurses in the United States, 83% are working, and of those who are working, 60% are employed by hospitals. The remaining 40% work in a variety of health care settings (Bureau of Health Professions, 1996, p 1). Based on projections of the National Commission on Nursing Implementation Project (NCNIP), Fagin (1990, pp. 191–92) suggests that the future demands for nursing will include the following:

- An increased number of nurses outside acute care settings

- Traditional settings requiring a greater proportion of nurses with advanced preparation to manage the needs of clients with more acute or specialized problems
- An increased need for highly technically skilled nurses in acute care settings
- Nurses who move with clients across the various health care settings
- Nurses managing and coordinating care, consulting with self-help groups, advocating, teaching and directing, and providing direct care and referral

One anticipated outcome of health care reform will be an increased need for nurses providing care in primary care facilities such as community based clinics, schools, and industrial and occupational settings.

Consumer Demands Consumers of nursing services (the public) have become an increasingly effective force in changing nursing practice. On the whole, people are better educated and have more knowledge about health and illness than in the past. Consumers also have become more aware of others' needs for care. The ethical, moral, and health issues raised by poverty and neglect have stimulated discussion about the needs of minority groups and the poor.

The public's concepts of health and nursing have also changed. The media emphasize the message that individuals must assume responsibility for their own health by obtaining a physical examination regularly, checking for the seven danger signals of cancer, and maintaining their mental well-being by balancing work and recreation. Interest in health and nursing services is therefore greater than ever. Furthermore, many people now want more than freedom from disease—they want energy, vitality, and a feeling of wellness.

Increasingly, the consumer has become an active participant in making decisions about health and nursing care. Planning committees concerned with providing nursing services to a community usually have active consumer membership. Recognizing the legitimacy of public input, many state and provincial nursing associations and regulatory agencies have consumer representatives on their governing boards.

Family Structure New family structures are influencing the need for and provision of nursing services. More people are living away from the extended family and the nuclear family, and the family breadwinner is no longer necessarily the husband.

Today, many single men and women rear children, and in many two-parent families both parents work. It is also common for young parents to live at great distances from their own parents. This separation among generations has created a void in care available to the young and the old. In response, new services—such as adult day health care and multigenerational day care services—have emerged. For additional information about the family, see Chapter 14.

Adolescent mothers also need specialized nursing services, both while they are pregnant and after their babies are born. McAnarney and Hendee (1989, p. 78) state that one million pregnancies occurred in 15- to 19-year-old adolescents. Forty-nine percent of these pregnancies resulted in live births. These young mothers usually have the normal needs of teenagers as well as those of new mothers. Many teenaged mothers are raising their children alone with little, if any, assistance from the child's father. This type of single-parent family is especially vulnerable because motherhood compounds the difficulties of adolescence. And because many of these families live in poverty, the children often do not receive preventive immunizations and are at increased risk for nutritional and other health problems.

Science and Technology Advances in science and technology affect nursing practice. For example, people with **acquired immune deficiency syndrome (AIDS)** are receiving new drug therapies to prolong life and delay the onset of AIDS-associated diseases. Nurses must be knowledgeable about the action of such drugs and the needs of clients receiving them. As physicians expand their knowledge base and technical skills, nurses acquire complementary knowledge and skills as they adapt to meet the new needs of clients.

In some settings, technologic advances have required that nurses become highly specialized. Nurses frequently have to use sophisticated computerized equipment to monitor or treat clients. As technologies change, nursing education changes, and nurses require increasing education to provide effective, safe nursing practice.

The space program has developed advanced technologies for space travel based on the need for long-distance monitoring of astronauts and space craft, lighter materials, and miniaturization of equipment. Health care has benefited as this new technology has been adapted in such health care aids as Viewstar (an aid for the visually impaired), the insulin infusion pump, the voice-controlled wheelchair, magnetic resonance imaging, laser surgery, filtering devices for intravenous fluid control devices, and intensive care monitoring systems (Haggerty 1989).

Advances in technology are exemplified by the many machines now used to help clients maintain life. There seems to be no end to the discoveries and the knowledge explosion of the twentieth century. With this knowledge explosion has come the charge that medical services—and some health professionals—have become dehumanized. Yet the understanding of the psychologic, emotional, and spiritual aspects of care has also increased, balancing the technologic advances. As science and technology create methods of treating disease, all health professionals, and nurses in particular, have a responsibility to remember that clients are human beings requiring warmth, care, and acknowledgment of self-worth. Medical equipment is often frightening to clients and their support persons; medical vocabulary appears mysterious and is frequently misunderstood. The nurse who deals with clients daily is in an ideal situation to humanize technology as much as possible. To humanize highly technical care, nurses can offer explanations, communicate their support, and recognize the clients' needs to understand and to be supported. This is the "high touch" aspect of a "high tech" environment.

Health care providers must also consider the ethical and financial cost of using technology. For example, ever-improving knowledge and equipment now allow many people to survive serious injury or disease; however, these changes do not ensure quality of life and may not be affordable to all. Most developed countries are grappling with the balance between science and technology, quality of life, individual choice, and the cost of providing these services. Efforts to control costs have prompted review of many expensive therapies, and there is fear that cost-containment strategies may stifle research and innovation.

Legislation Legislation about nursing practice and health matters affects both the public and nursing. Legislation related to nursing is discussed in Chapter 12. Changes in legislation relating to health also affect nursing. For example, in 1991 the **Patient Self Determination Act (PSDA)** went into effect requiring that every competent adult be informed in writing upon admission to a health care institution about his or her rights to accept or refuse medical care and to use advance directives. See Chapter 20 for more information about the PSDA and advance directives. This law, which in many institutions is implemented by nurses, affects the nurse's role in supporting clients and their families.

Demography Demography is the study of population, including statistics about distribution by age and place of residence, mortality (death), and morbidity (incidence of disease). From demographic data, needs of the population for nursing services can be assessed. For example:

- The total population in North America has increased since 1900. The proportion of elderly people has also increased, creating an increased need for nursing services for this group.
- The population is shifting from rural to urban settings. This shift signals increased needs for nursing related to problems caused by pollution and by the effects on the environment of concentrations of people. Thus, most nursing services are now provided in urban settings.
- Mortality and morbidity studies reveal the presence of "risk factors." Many of these "risk factors" (eg, smoking) are major causes of death and disease that can be prevented through changes in life-style. The nurse's role in assessing risk factors and helping clients make healthy life-style changes is discussed in Chapter 13.

The Women's Movement The women's movement has brought public attention to human rights. Persons are seeking equality in all areas, particularly educational, political, economic, and social equality. Because the majority of nurses are women, this movement has altered nurses' perspectives on economic and educational needs. As a result, nurses are increasingly asserting themselves as professional people who have a right to equality with men in health professions and are demanding more autonomy in client care.

Sampselle (1990, p. 243) suggests that "incorporating feminist philosophy into practice can make it more likely for women to become full partners in sexual, social, and economic relationships and to be valued for a wide range of contributions to society." Nurses who integrate feminist philosophy into their practice may also view their female clients from a feminist perspective, challenging stereotypical characteristics of women in relation to ability, beauty, and health.

The women's movement has empowered nurses to identify "the commonality and interconnectedness of nurses' experience as women and men and as health care workers." This enables nurses to develop a greater sense of autonomy and group consciousness that can lead to greater empowerment and involvement in effective political action (Mason et al 1993, p. 107). Recently, the federal government has been challenged in its funding of research in women's health problems. As a result, a new concern for women's issues has emerged.

Collective Bargaining The ANA has participated in collective bargaining on behalf of nurses for more than 40 years through its economic and general welfare programs. Today, some nurses are joining other labor organizations that represent them at the bargaining table. In both the United States and Canada, nurses have gone on strike over certain demands and concerns. Often these concerns go beyond economic reward to issues about safe care for clients and safety for nursing staff.

The ANA Commission on Economic and Professional Security (ANA-CEPS 1993a) has identified the following specific issues related to workplace safety: compensation issues related to occupational human immunodeficiency virus (HIV) infection, tuberculosis, and hepatitis; workplace violence; back injuries and other ergonomic hazards; and stress in the workplace. Compensation issues of concern to nurses include wage compression and the availability of portable pension plans to provide for adequate retirement income (ANA-CEPS 1993b, 1993c).

Nursing Associations Professional nursing associations have provided leadership that affects many areas of nursing. Voluntary accreditation of nursing education programs by the National League for Nursing (NLN) and by mandatory accreditation licensing boards in each state have also influenced nursing. Many programs have steadily improved to meet the standards for accreditation over the years. As a result, nurse graduates are better prepared to meet the demands of society.

In 1979, the ANA published findings of a committee on credentialing, which recommended the establishment of a center for credentialing in nursing (ANA 1979, p. 682). **Credentialing** is the process of determining and maintaining competence in nursing. The credentialing of expanded nursing roles, such as that of the nurse practitioner, is carried out by the ANA and certain other nursing specialty organizations. Nurse anesthetists, for example, are certified through the American Association of Nurse Anesthetists.

To influence health care policy-making, a group of professional nurses organized formally to promote political action in the nursing and health care arenas. Nurses for Political Action (NPA) formed in 1971 and became an arm of the ANA in 1974, when its name changed to Nurses Coalition for Action in Politics (N-CAP). In 1986, the name was changed to ANA-PAC. Through this group, nurses have lobbied actively for legislation affecting health care. A number of nursing leaders hold positions of authority in government. Attaining such positions is essential if nurses hope to exert ongoing political influence.

The drive for increased autonomy comes from the nursing profession itself. During the past 20 years, the increased autonomy of nurses has been evidenced by their function in specialty care units, such as intensive care units, and in their expanded roles, such as that of the nurse practitioner. Many states have rewritten their nurse practice acts to reflect such changes in nursing practice.

NURSING EDUCATION

The future of nursing lies not with the leaders of the past or present but rather with today's and tomorrow's nursing students. Although current scientific, social, and economic influences may affect the utilization of nursing services, they do not determine nursing practice. The nursing profession is therefore particularly interested in the educational preparation of nurses for the future. This interest is reflected in documents such as the ANA's *Standards for Professional Nursing Education* (1984) and the NLN's *Criteria and Guidelines for the Evaluation of Diploma Programs in Nursing* (1992b), *Associate Degree Programs in Nursing* (1991a), and *Baccalaureate Degree and Higher Degree Programs in Nursing* (1992a), which set forth the profession's beliefs about, goals of, and evaluation criteria for nursing education programs.

Nursing and the education of nurses is controlled from within the profession through state and provincial boards of nursing and national accrediting bodies. The traditional focus of nursing education was to teach the knowledge and skills to enable the nurse to practice in the hospital setting. However, as nursing responds to new scientific knowledge and technologic, cultural, political, and socioeconomic changes in society, nursing education curricula need to be reviewed and revised to meet the needs of nurses working in a changing environment. Programs of nursing study are increasingly based on a broad knowledge of biologic, social, and physical sciences as well as the liberal arts and humanities. As a result, nursing curricula now have a greater focus on critical thinking and the application of nursing and supporting knowledge to health promotion and health restoration as provided in both community and hospital settings.

It is not possible for nurses to acquire a safe level of skill through empiric means (experience and observation) alone. They require specific knowledge and skills that can be gained only through an organized nursing curriculum that includes classroom and laboratory instruction and clinical application of knowledge and skill. Nurses also need to learn the professional values and attitudes that enable them to practice in an ethically responsible way in a rapidly changing world.

TITLING AND LICENSURE

The designations **registered nurse (RN)** and **licensed practical** or **vocational nurse (LPN, LVN)** have been used since licensure laws were first enacted. In 1985, the ANA endorsed the baccalaureate degree in nursing as the entry level for professional practice, with the baccalaureate graduate licensed under the legal title registered nurse (RN). The graduate with an associate degree in nursing would be considered a technical nurse and be licensed under the legal title **associate nurse (AN)**. A timetable for implementation was established by the National Commission on Nursing Implementation Project (NCNIP 1987). However, the ANA, as a professional organization, cannot legislate these changes. It is the responsibility of each state to define the legal boundaries of nursing practice and to designate the titles to be used by those practitioners who meet the individual state's criteria for licensure. If this proposal is to be accepted nationally, therefore, each state will need to adopt the proposal and implement its own changes in its licensure law. Such changes have major implications for diploma nurses and LPNs, because their status is not discussed in the proposal. In addition, this proposal means that new standardized examinations must be developed to test the two levels of competence. This has become a controversial issue in nursing, debated at state and national levels and among nurses of different educational backgrounds, nursing specialties, and clinical levels. In addition, there are nurses who believe that the appropriate entry level for nursing should be at the master's or doctoral level. In Canada, in 1982, the board of directors of the Canadian Nurses Association (CNA) endorsed the recommendation of the Committee on Entry to Practice that the baccalaureate degree be the minimum entry level for professional nursing practice by the year 2000.

However, changes in the practice environment are beginning to reward the nurse who holds a baccalaureate degree with greater autonomy, responsibility, participation in institutional decision making, and career advancement. These changes provide an incentive for nurses with diplomas and associate degrees to continue their formal preparation in baccalaureate completion (transition) programs.

At the present time, state laws in the United States and provincial laws in Canada recognize two types of nurses: the licensed practical (vocational) nurse (LPN or LVN) and the registered nurse (RN). Various types of programs prepare nurses to enter practice. In some states, advanced nursing practice, such as nurse anesthetist, nurse-midwife, or family nurse practitioner, requires a third type of nurse licensure, **advanced nurse practitioner (ANP)** or **advanced registered nurse practitioner (ARNP).**

TYPES OF EDUCATIONAL PROGRAMS

Licensed Practical Nursing Approved practical or vocational nursing programs are provided by high schools, community colleges, vocational schools, hospitals, and a variety of health agencies. These programs usually last 1 year and provide both classroom and clinical experiences. At the end of the program, the graduate takes National Council Licensing Examination (NCLEX) examinations to obtain a license as a practical or vocational nurse. Licensed practical nurses work in structured care settings, such as hospitals and long-term care agencies. Their skills are basically those required for bedside nursing under the guidance of a registered nurse, who has the knowledge and skills to make more sophisticated nursing judgments. In some areas of the United States, LPN programs are being expanded to the associate degree level.

Registered Nursing In the United States, most basic education for registered nurses is provided in three types of programs: diploma, associate degree, and baccalaureate programs. In Canada, the 2-year diploma, 3-year (or more) diploma, and baccalaureate programs prepare registered nurses.

Diploma Nursing education originated in hospital-based programs. First developed by Florence Nightingale (circa 1860), these programs were operated by hospitals as "training" schools for nurses, to ensure a source of qualified nurses. Today's diploma nursing programs have changed markedly from the original Nightingale model, becoming hospital-based educational programs that provide a rich clinical experience for nursing students. These programs may last 2 or more years and are often associated with colleges or universities. Though the number of diploma nursing programs has declined since the ANA resolution in 1965, the 119 existing programs are still providing one avenue for students desiring an education in nursing (NLN 1996).

Associate Degree Associate degree programs in nursing were suggested in 1951 by Mildred L. Montag (1980) as a solution to the acute shortage of nurses that came about because of World War II. Associate degree programs are offered in the United States in junior colleges as well as in colleges and universities. In 1996, there were 876 associate degree programs in nursing in the United States (NLN 1996). The graduating student receives an associate degree in nursing (ADN) or an associate of arts (AA), associate of science (AS), or associate in applied science (AAS) degree with a major in nursing. In Canada, associate degrees are not offered, but similar programs confer a diploma upon graduation.

Although ADN programs relieved the post–World War II nursing shortage, the utilization of ADN graduates in hospital practice did not fulfill Montag's original intent; ADN and BSN graduates are often used interchangeably. This creates a discrepancy between the competence expected of new graduates and their actual competence. In an effort to resolve this discrepancy, differentiated competence statements were developed during two projects sponsored by the Midwest Alliance in Nursing and funded by the W. K. Kellogg Foundation (Primm 1986, pp. 135–37). Because ADN- and BSN-prepared nurses currently function under the same practice acts, "these differentiated statements provide a basis for discussion of collaborative ADN and BSN nursing practice" (Primm 1986, p. 136). The National Organization of ADN Educators has been formed to address issues in modern ADN education.

Baccalaureate Degree Although baccalaureate nursing education programs were established in universities in both the United States and Canada in the early 1900s, it was not until the 1960s that the number of students enrolled in these programs increased markedly. By 1996 there were 521 baccalaureate programs of nursing and 144 baccalaureate transition programs for nurses with diplomas or associate degrees (NLN 1996).

Most baccalaureate programs also admit registered nurses who have diplomas or associate degrees. Some programs have special curricula to meet the needs of these students. Some universities also offer nursing students the opportunity to pursue a self-paced or independent study program. Many accept transfer credits from other accredited colleges and universities and offer students the opportunity to take challenge examinations when they believe they have the knowledge or skills taught in a course.

Graduate Programs Most graduate programs are conducted by departments within the graduate school of a university, and the applicant must first meet requirements established by the graduate school. Although all graduate schools have somewhat different requirements, common requirements for admission to graduate programs in nursing include the following:

- The applicant must be a registered nurse and licensed or eligible for licensure within the program's state.
- The applicant must hold a baccalaureate degree in nursing from an approved college or university and have had an acceptable upper division major in nursing at the baccalaureate level.
- The applicant must give evidence of scholastic ability (usually a minimum grade point average of 2.7 to 3.0 on a 4.0 scale).
- The applicant must demonstrate satisfactory achievement on a qualifying examination, such as the Graduate Record Examination (GRE) or the Miller Analogy Test (MAT).
- Letters of recommendation from supervisors, nursing faculty, and/or nursing colleagues indicating the applicant's ability for graduate study.

Master's Programs Master's programs generally take from 1½ to 2 years to complete. Degrees granted are the Master of Arts (MA), Master in Nursing (MN), Master of Science in Nursing (MSN), and Master of Science (MS).

Master's degree programs may focus on an area of advanced clinical practice, such as psychiatric mental health nursing, or on areas such as administration or nursing management.

The number of nurses obtaining master's degrees has increased. In 1995, 35,707 students were pursuing master's study, as compared to 22,908 who obtained master's degrees in 1990 (ANA 1991a, NLN 1996).

Doctoral Programs Doctoral programs in nursing, which award the degrees of doctor of philosophy (PhD), doctor of nursing science (DNS or DNSc), or nursing doctorate (ND), began in the 1960s in the United States. These programs further prepare the nurse for advanced clinical practice, administration, education, and research. Before 1960, nurses acquired doctoral degrees in such related fields as psychology, sociology, physiology, and education.

Content and approach vary among doctoral programs. One may focus on usual clinical areas, such as medical-surgical nursing, while others emphasize such nontraditional areas as transcultural nursing. Some programs emphasize theory development, but all emphasize research. In 1995, 3,230 nurses were pursuing doctoral degrees (NLN 1996).

Ladder Programs The ladder concept fosters progression of an individual from one educational level to another. The nurse who wishes to progress "up the ladder" can often obtain credit for experience and/or courses at an earlier level. Other terms used are BSN completion, BSN transition, 2 + 2, or RN-BSN programs. Many universities now grant academic credit toward a baccalaureate degree for the years spent in the associate degree program.

Often, baccalaureate programs emphasize independent learning and self-pacing. External degree programs, such as the New York State Regents Program and the California Statewide Nursing Program, provide alternatives to traditional university programs to allow for this independent, self-paced learning.

CONTINUING EDUCATION

The term **continuing education** refers to formalized experiences designed to enlarge the knowledge or skills of practitioners. Compared to advanced education programs, which result in an academic degree, continuing education courses tend to be more specific and shorter. Participants may receive certificates of completion or specialization.

Continuing education is the responsibility of each practicing nurse. Constant updating and growth are essential to keep abreast of scientific and technologic change and changes within the nursing profession. A variety of educational and health care institutions conduct continuing education programs. They are usually designed to meet one or more of the following needs: (a) to keep nurses abreast of new techniques and knowledge; (b) to help nurses attain expertise in a specialized area of practice, such as intensive care nursing; and (c) to provide nurses with information essential to nursing practice, for example, knowledge about the legal aspects of nursing.

Some state laws require nurses to obtain a certain number of continuing education credits to renew their licenses. In these states, required continuing education (CE) contact hours vary from 15 to 30 hours for every

2-year relicensure period. All, some, or none of these hours may be acquired through home study. Some home study courses are offered through professional journals. A few regions also require a certain number of hours of practice, either independently or in lieu of study hours, before license renewal.

IN-SERVICE EDUCATION

An **in-service education** program is administered by an employer; it is designed to upgrade the knowledge or skills of employees. For example, an employer might offer an in-service program to inform nurses about a new piece of equipment, about specific isolation practices, or about methods of implementing a nurse theorist's conceptual framework for nursing.

NURSING RESEARCH

Nursing research is more than just scientific investigations conducted by a person educated and credentialed as a nurse. Rather, nursing research has been defined by the ANA Commission on Nursing Research (1981) as research that develops knowledge about the following:

- Health and the promotion of health over the full life span
- Care of persons with health problems and disabilities
- Nursing actions to enhance people's ability to respond effectively to actual or potential health problems

Nursing research includes investigation into health promotion and health restoration of individuals, families, groups, and communities. Nurse researchers also investigate issues related to nursing education, nursing administration, and nursing's role in health policy formation.

THE NURSE'S ROLE IN RESEARCH

The ANA's *Standards of Clinical Nursing Practice* encourages nurses to be involved in the research process. (See Chapter 10 for further discussion of the research process.) Standard VII of the professional performance standards for nurses states, "The Nurse uses research findings in practice" (1991c, p. 16). The measurement criteria for this standard identify ways in which the clinical nurse might utilize research findings and participate in research activity. These criteria include the following:

- Identify clinical problems suitable for nursing research.
- Participate in data collection
- Participate in a unit, organization, or community research committee or program
- Share research activities with others
- Conduct independent or collaborative research
- Critique research for application to practice
- Use research findings in the development of policies, procedures, and guidelines for client care

Polit and Hungler (1991) suggest that Florence Nightingale, while caring for the wounded of the Crimean War, conducted nursing research as she maintained detailed recorded observations about the effects of nursing actions. On the basis of her observations, she subsequently changed aspects of nursing care. Early nursing research studied nursing education and nursing manpower issues. In the 1950s, research about nursing activities began to appear in the literature. In 1952, *Nursing Research*, a professional journal devoted to the publication of nursing research, was first published.

Nursing research gained greater significance in 1985, when the United States Congress passed a bill creating a Center for Nursing Research in the National Institutes of Health (NIH) to house the research activities conducted by the Division of Nursing of the Department of Health and Human Services (DHHS). In 1993, the Center for Nursing Research was promoted to the Institute for Nursing Research, gaining equal status with other institutes within the NIH. Initially, the research priorities of the 1988 Center for Nursing Research included low birth weight, HIV infection, long-term care, symptom management, nursing informatics, health promotion, and technology dependency. In 1993, nursing scientists recommended that research priorities for the years 1995 to 1999 be updated to include developing community-based nursing models, promoting behaviors that prevent AIDS in women, devising ways to remedy cognitive impairment, and helping patients cope with chronic illness (American Journal of Nursing 1993a, p. 70).

The examples in the box on page 38 suggest the diversity of subjects, topics, and settings of actual nursing studies. The sample of contemporary nursing studies in this box only begins to show the diversity of fascinating and ultimately valuable research projects being conducted in the field of nursing.

Findings from nursing studies are being incorporated into textbooks such as this one. Clinical journals such as the *American Journal of Nursing*, *Heart and Lung*, and *Gerontological Nursing* are increasingly publishing the results of studies about nursing practice. Nursing journals such as *Advances in Nursing Science*, *Image: Journal of Nursing Scholarship*, the *Journal of Research in Nursing and Health*, *Nursing Research*, the *Western Journal of Nursing Research*,

EXAMPLES OF NURSING STUDIES

Acorn, Ratner, and Crawford (1997) tested a theoretical model relating decentralization, autonomy, organizational commitment, and job satisfaction among nurse managers.

Brown and Olshansky (1997) explored the transition experience of nurse practitioner graduates during their first year of practice. By examining NPs at 1, 6, and 12 months after graduation, they developed a model to explain this role transition.

Coffman (1997) investigated the boundaries of practice and family-nurse relationships as nurses move from the hospital into the home setting.

Matthiesen et al (1996) described the knowledge, practice, and attitudes of hospital nursing staff in the use of physical restraints with elderly patients in multiple clinical settings.

Ott and Hardie (1997) examined the ease of reading and understanding of advance directive documents and the implications for autonomy in end-of-life care.

and the *International Journal of Nursing Studies* have editorial policies that stress science, research, and nursing scholarship and publish current research studies.

The *Cumulative Index to Nursing and Allied Health Literature*, the *International Nursing Index*, and the *Cumulative Medical Index* are excellent resources for locating research published on a topic or problem of interest. Computerized literature searches, such as Medline and MEDLARS, are available through many school libraries. They, too, help the student or researcher find relevant study reports. Since 1983, research on a variety of topics has been collected in yet another valuable resource, the *Annual Review of Nursing Research*.

Bridging the research-practice gap, that is, bringing research into the clinical practice arena, is a key strategy in uniting the scholarly, scientific, and caring aspects of nursing in the future. Table 2–3 summarizes this position in the ANA's *Guidelines for the Investigative Function of Nurses* (1981a). The steps in the research process are listed in the accompanying box.

STEPS IN THE RESEARCH PROCESS

1. Stating a research question or problem
2. Defining the purpose of a study
3. Reviewing related literature
4. Formulating hypotheses and defining variables
5. Selecting the research design
6. Selecting the population, sample, and setting
7. Conducting a pilot study
8. Collecting the data
9. Analyzing the data
10. Communicating conclusions and implications

In February 1985, the CNA published a statement on research in nursing:

> The Canadian Nurses Association believes systematic investigation of the needs of individuals, groups and society forms an essential component of total health care. Research in nursing is needed to improve the quality of nursing care and to contribute to the efficiency and effectiveness of health care and the quality of life of Canadians. . . .
>
> Nursing research is central to the development of theories for nursing practice. It stimulates growth of the body of knowledge upon which the practice of nursing is built.
>
> Nursing research focuses on the ways individuals and families maintain, promote or restore their health, and examines the process of adaptation to life situations, the caring for and the well-being of individuals.

In 1983, the CNA published similar guidelines in *Ethical Guidelines for Conducting Nursing Research with Human Subjects*.

PROTECTING THE RIGHTS OF HUMAN SUBJECTS

Because nursing research usually focuses on humans, a major nursing responsibility is to be aware of and advocate clients' rights. All clients must be informed about the consequences of consenting to serve as research subjects. The client needs to be able to assess whether an appropriate balance exists between the risks of participating in a study and the potential benefits, either to the client or to the development of knowledge.

Research ethics not only protect the rights of human subjects but also encompass a broader list of characteristics. Most of these characteristics are reflected in the ANA's *Human Rights Guidelines for Nursing in Clinical and Other Research*. These guidelines are based on historic documents, such as the Nuremberg Code and the Declaration of Helsinki, and United States federal regulations,

Table 2–3 Investigative Functions of a Nurse at Various Educational Levels

Educational Level	Investigative Functions
Associate Degree in Nursing	1. Demonstrates awareness of the value or relevance of research in nursing
	2. Assists in identifying problem areas in nursing practice
	3. Assists in collecting data within an established, structured format
Baccalaureate in Nursing	1. Reads, interprets, and evaluates research for applicability to nursing practice
	2. Identifies nursing problems that need to be investigated and participates in the implementation of scientific studies
	3. Uses nursing practice as a means of gathering data to refine and extend practice
	4. Applies established findings of nursing and other health-related research to nursing practice
	5. Shares research findings with colleagues
Master's Degree in Nursing	1. Analyzes and reformulates nursing practice problems so that scientific knowledge and scientific methods can be used to find solutions
	2. Enhances the quality and clinical relevance of nursing research by providing expertise in clinical problems and by providing knowledge about the way in which these clinical services are delivered
	3. Facilitates investigations of problems in clinical settings through such activities as contributing to a climate supportive of investigative activities, collaborating with others in investigations, and enhancing nursing's access to clients and data
	4. Conducts investigations for the purpose of monitoring the quality of the practice of nursing in a clinical setting
	5. Assists others to apply scientific knowledge in nursing practice
Doctoral Degree in Nursing or a Related Discipline	1. Provides leadership for the integration of scientific knowledge with other sources of knowledge for the advancement of practice
	2. Conducts investigations to evaluate the contribution of nursing activities to the well-being of clients
	3. Develops methods to monitor the quality of the practice of nursing in a clinical setting and to evaluate contributions of nursing activities to the well-being of clients
Graduate of a Research-Oriented Doctoral Program	1. Develops theoretical explanations of phenomena relevant to nursing by empiric research and analytic processes
	2. Uses analytic and empiric methods to discover ways to modify or extend existing scientific knowledge so that it is relevant to nursing
	3. Develops methods for scientific inquiry of phenomena relevant to nursing

Source: American Nurses Association, Commission on Nursing Research, *Guidelines for the Investigative Function of Nurses* (Kansas City, MO: ANA, 1981). Reprinted with permission.

all of which set standards governing the conduct of research involving human subjects. The ANA Guidelines are presented in Appendix B.

THE NURSE'S ROLE IN PROTECTING SUBJECTS' RIGHTS

All nurses who practice in settings where research is being conducted with human subjects or who participate in such research as data collectors or collaborators play an important role in safeguarding the following rights:

Right to Not Be Harmed The Department of Health and Human Services defines **risk of harm** to a research subject as exposure to the possibility of injury going beyond everyday situations. The risk can be physical, emotional, legal, financial, or social. For instance, withholding standard care from a client in labor for the purpose of studying the course of natural childbirth clearly poses a potential physical danger. Risks can be less overt and involve psychologic factors, such as exposure to stress or anxiety, or social factors, such as loss of confidentiality, loss of privacy, and the like.

Right to Full Disclosure Even though it may be possible to collect data about a client as part of everyday care without the client's particular knowledge or consent, to do so is considered unethical. **Full disclosure** is a basic right. It means that deception, either by withholding information about a client's participation in a study or by giving the client false or misleading information about what participating in the study will involve, will not occur.

Right of Self-Determination Many clients in dependent positions, such as people in nursing homes, feel pressured to participate in studies. They feel that they must please those doctors and nurses who are responsible for their treatment and care. The **right of self-determination** means that subjects should feel free from constraints, coercion, or any undue influence to participate in a study. Masked inducements, for instance, suggesting that they might become famous by making an important contribution to science or get special attention by taking part in the study, must be strictly avoided. Nurses must be assertive in advocating this essential right as well.

Right of Privacy and Confidentiality Privacy enables a client to participate without worrying about later embarrassment. The anonymity of a study is ensured if even the investigator cannot link a specific subject to the information reported. **Confidentiality** means that any information a subject relates will not be made public or available to others. Investigators must inform research subjects about the measures that provide for these rights. Such measures may include using pseudonyms, code numbers, or reporting only aggregate or group data in published research.

Nurses who participate in scientific investigations that involve human subjects are in a key position to serve as advocates for research subjects.

TRENDS IN NURSING

A **trend** is a general direction or a prevailing tendency or inclination. Several trends are apparent in the nursing profession today. Some trends in nursing are subtle and emerge slowly, whereas others are obvious and seem to surface quickly. Not all trends complement one another; some may seem divergent, if not in conflict. Over time, some aspects of nursing become prevailing trends, whereas others may be modified by social forces or disappear altogether. A number of trends are apparent today: the broadening focus and increasingly scientific basis of nursing practice (including nursing research), the increasing use of technology, a renewed focus on the caring aspect of nursing, and an increased involvement of nurses in health policy decision making at all levels.

BROADENING FOCUS

The focus of nursing has broadened from the care of the ill person to the care of people in illness and health, and from care of only the patient to care of the client, the family or support persons, and, in some instances, the community. In the past, nursing, like medicine, was oriented toward disease and illness. Today, there is increasing recognition of people's need for health care as distinct from illness care and of the nurse's independent functions in this area.

A holistic philosophy is evident in modern nursing care. Today's nurse deals with clients as emotional and social beings as well as physical beings. Care is directed not toward a particular health problem but toward the response of the total person, the health of the whole person. The broadened focus of care requires an integration of skills and concepts.

Another aspect of the broader nursing focus is the movement of nursing practice into the community. In a sense, this is a return to the beginnings of nursing, that is, before it became a recognized occupation. Throughout much of this century, however, nurses worked only in institutions; increasingly, nursing services are provided in the community, often in homes and in clinics. These nursing activities not only assist those who are ill but also help those who are healthy to maintain or enhance their health.

SCIENTIFIC BASIS

In the past, nursing largely was either intuitive or relied on experience or observation rather than on research. Through trial and error, the individual nurses discovered which measures would assist the client, and many nurses became highly skilled in providing care through experience. The past 20 years have brought an increased emphasis on nursing research and on the use of scientific data at the bedside. The authorization of a National Institute for Nursing Research and the increasing levels of funding for nursing research from private and public sources demonstrate the value given to nursing research.

TECHNOLOGY

Technology or mechanization is being applied in the health field extensively. Certain areas of a hospital (eg, intensive care units and coronary care units) are more technologic than others. Nurses find themselves in the midst of this rapidly changing, increasingly technologic environment in hospitals and in clients' homes. Indicators of increasing technology include (a) the proliferation of technologic equipment used in the care of clients in hospitals and homes, (b) the increasing costs of home and self-care equipment, and (c) the use of computers in many areas of health care. Many nurses feel they need more education to obtain the knowledge and skills necessary to use the new technology.

Computers are being used at the bedside to enable nurses and other health care workers to access client information more readily and input client assessment data more quickly and accurately. Community health and home health nurses are using portable "laptop" computers to increase the speed and accuracy of documenting client care and to decrease the amount of paperwork previously required in these work settings. See Chapter 9 for more information about how nurses are using computers in their documenting and recording.

High technology has enabled nurses to gather client assessment data through noninvasive techniques (eg, pulse oximetry) rather than through the costly invasive procedures of the past.

RENEWED FOCUS ON CARING

The increasing use of technology in hospitals and homes has created an increasing need to humanize care. Nursing has traditionally been a caring and humanizing profession. Today there is a renewed focus on the caring aspects of nursing. Indicators of this trend include (a) the increasing number of professional articles and books about balancing caring and technical skills, (b) many studies regarding caring as an aspect of nursing, and (c) increasing recognition in nursing of the needs of clients in technologic environments.

INVOLVEMENT IN HEALTH POLICY DECISION MAKING

Nurses and professional nursing organizations are becoming more involved in the political process and more influential in health care policy planning and decision making. With the publication of *Nursing's Agenda for Health Care Reform* (ANA 1991b), nurses demanded a voice in shaping a new health care system for the United States. Nurses have become more involved in political action campaigns, asking discerning questions of candidates before making voting decisions. Nurses have been elected and appointed to political office at local, state, and national levels. Eddie Bernice Johnson of Texas was elected to the United States House of Representatives in 1992, and in 1993, Kristine Gebbie of Washington State was appointed "AIDS Czar" to take charge of the federal response to the AIDS epidemic. Additionally, nurses who have interest in the area of health care policy are obtaining advanced degrees in public policy and public administration in order to exert greater influence on health policy decisions.

CHAPTER HIGHLIGHTS

- Although the majority of nurses today are employed in hospital settings, more nurses are working in other areas, such as home health care and community clinics.
- Nurse practice acts vary among states and provinces, and nurses are responsible for knowing the act that governs their practice.
- Standards of clinical nursing practice provide criteria against which the effectiveness of nursing care and professional performance behaviors can be evaluated.
- The career mobility of nurses increases with their education and experience.
- Nursing practice is influenced by economics, changing demands for nurses, consumer demand, family structure, science and technology, legislation, demographic and social changes, and nursing associations.
- Nursing education focuses on preparing today's nursing students to fulfill current and future expectations and roles.
- Educational programs for nurses must reflect the health care demands and needs of a changing society, accommodate changes in the health care delivery system, adhere to professional standards, yet be responsible to concerns about rising cost of health care.
- Nursing research is having an increasing impact on nursing education, administration, and practice.
- Nurses at all levels are participating in nursing research activities.
- All nurses practicing in settings where research is conducted have a role in safeguarding their client's rights.
- Apparent trends in nursing today are the broadening focus of nursing practice, the increasingly scientific basis of nursing practice, the increasing use of technology in nursing, a renewed focus on the caring aspect of nursing, and increased involvement in health policy decision making.

READINGS AND REFERENCES

SUGGESTED READINGS

Fagin, CM. 1990. The visible problems of an "invisible" profession: The crisis and challenge for nursing. In Lee, PR and Estes, CL, editors. pp. 190–200. *The Nation's Health.* Boston: Jones and Bartlett.

The author discusses ongoing issues in nursing, including the supply of nurses versus the potential demand, entry-level education requirements and other issues related to nursing education, the impact on nursing of changes in the health care delivery system, the need for more nurses with advanced degrees, interprofessional tensions between nurses and physicians, and the emerging role of the nurse in the next century.

Nornhold, P. January 1990. 90 predictions for the 90's. *Nursing 90* 34–41.

The author predicts that historic changes will take place in the health care industry in the 1990s. Nursing will obtain increased autonomy, with increased responsibility for maintaining quality in a cost-effective manner. More men will enter nursing, and nurses will become more politically aware and involved. There will be new opportunities in critical and emergency care, with new technologies to support clients and personnel. The author also details specific changes in different specialty areas.

RELATED RESEARCH

Stevens, KA and Waldker, EA. January 1993. Choosing a career: Why not nursing for more high school seniors? *Journal of Nursing Education* 32:13–17.

Young, WB, Lehrer, EL, and White, WD. Summer 1991. The effect of education on the practice of nursing. *Image: Journal of Nursing Scholarship* 23: 105–8.

SELECTED REFERENCES

Aiken, LH. March 1988. Solutions to the nursing shortage bear repeating. *American Nurse* 20:4.

Aiken, LH and Mullinix, CF. 1990. The nurse shortage: Myth or reality? In Lee, P and Estes, C, editors. pp. 181–89. *The Nation's Health.* 3d ed. Boston: Jones and Bartlett.

American Academy of Nursing. 1993. *Health Care Access: Problems and Policy Recommendations: Working Paper.* Washington, DC: American Academy of Nursing.

American Journal of Nursing. August 1993a. Nursing research center is reborn as an institute. *American Journal of Nursing* 93:69–70.

———. September 1993b. Headlines: The nation's RN population now tops 2.2 million. *American Journal of Nursing* 93:9.

American Nurses Association. April 1979. Credentialing in nursing: A new approach. Report of the Committee for the Study of Credentials in Nursing. *American Journal of Nursing* 79:674–83.

———. 1980. *Nursing: A Social Policy Statement.* Kansas City, MO: ANA.

———. 1981a. *ANA Guidelines for the Investigative Function of Nurses.* Kansas City, MO: ANA.

———. 1981b. *The Nursing Practice Act: Suggested State Legislation.* Kansas City, MO: ANA.

———. 1984. *Standards for Professional Nursing Education.* Washington, DC: ANA.

———. 1985. *Facts about Nursing 84–85.* Washington, DC: ANA.

———. 1991a. *Nursing and the American Nurses Association.* Washington, DC: ANA.

———. 1991b. *Nursing's Agenda for Health Care Reform.* Washington, DC: ANA.

———. 1991c. *Standards of Clinical Nursing Practice.* Washington, DC: ANA.

———. 1993. *Proceedings of the 1993 House of Delegates.* Washington, DC: ANA.

American Nurses Association, Commission on Economic and Professional Security. 1993a. *Informational Report: Health and Safety in the Workplace.* Washington, DC: ANA-CEPS.

———. 1993b. *Informational Report: Pension Portability/Reform Project.* Washington, DC: ANA-CEPS.

———. 1993c. *Informational Report: Wage Compression.* Washington, DC: ANA-CEPS.

American Nurses Association, Commission on Nursing Research. 1981. *Priorities for the 1980s.* Kansas City, MO: ANA.

Brider, P. April 1993. Annual nursing salary survey: Where did the jobs go? *American Journal of Nursing* 93:31–40.

Burkhardt, MA. Winter 1993. Characteristics of spirituality in the lives of women in a rural Appalachian community. *Journal of Transcultural Nursing* 4:12–17.

Canadian Nurses Association. February 1985. *CNA Position Statements.* Ottawa: CNA.

———. 1995. *Employment of Canadian RNs–1995.* Ottowa: CNA.

DeBack, V. 1990. Debate: Entry into practice: Will the 1985 proposal ever happen? In McCloskey, JC and Grace HK, editors. *Current Issues in Nursing.* 3d ed. St Louis: Mosby.

Dugas, BW. May 1985. Baccalaureate for entry to practice: A challenge that universities must meet. *Canadian Nurse* 81:17–19.

Edelman, CL and Mandle, CL. 1990. *Health Promotion Throughout the Life Span.* 2d ed. St Louis: Mosby.

Fagin, CM. 1990. The visible problems of an "invisible" profession: The crisis and challenge for nursing. In Lee, PR and Estes, CL, editors. pp. 190–200. *The Nation's Health.* 3d ed. Boston: Jones and Bartlett.

Graham, NO and Sheppard, C. 1990. Realities in retention and recruitment. In Chaska, NL, editor. *The Nursing Profession: Turning Points.* St Louis: Mosby.

Haggerty, JJ. 1989. *Spinoff. National Aeronautics and Space Administration.* Washington DC: US Government Printing Office.

Hall, L. November 1963. A center for nursing. *Nursing Outlook* 11:805–6.

Hartweg, DL. July/August 1993. Self-care actions of health: Middle-aged women to promote well-being. *Nursing Research.* 42:221–27.

Health Resources and Services Administration. 1996. *Advance Notes from the National Sample Survey of Registered Nurses.* Rockville, MD: Division of Nursing Bureau of Health Professions.

Kerr, J. May 1985. Taking the campus to the student. *Canadian Nurse* 81:30–31.

Lambertson, E. 1953. *Nursing Team Organization and Functioning.* New York: Teacher's College Press.

McAnarney, E and Hendee, W. July 1989. The prevention of adolescent pregnancy. *Journal of the American Medical Association* 262:78–82.

Maloni, JA, Chance, B, Zhang, C, Cohen, A, Betts, D, and Gange, SJ. July/August 1993. Physical and psychosocial side effects of antepartum hospital bed rest. *Nursing Research* 42:197–203.

Mason, DJ, Backer, BA, and Georges, CA. Spring 1993. Feminism and nursing: Toward a feminist model for the political empowerment of nurses. *Revolution: The Journal of Nurse Empowerment* 3:62–65, 68, 70–71, 106–7.

Meek, SS. Spring 1993. Effects of slow stroke back massage on relaxation in hospice clients. *Image: Journal of Nursing Scholarship* 25:17–21.

Monheim, BJ. January/February 1989. Encouraging the growth of computer applications in nursing. *Computers in Nursing* 7:35, 34.

Montag, ML. 1980. Looking back: Associate degree nursing education in perspective. *Nursing Outlook* 28:248–50.

Mosher, C, Cronk, P, Kidd, A, McCormick, P, Stockton, S, and Sulla, C. January 1992. Upgrading practice with critical pathways. *American Journal of Nursing* 92:41–44.

National Commission on Nursing Implementation Project. 1987. *Timeline for Transition into the Future: Nursing Education System for Two*

Categories of Nurse. Milwaukee: National Commission on Nursing Implementation Project.

National Leadership Coalition for Health Care Reform. 1991. *A Comprehensive Reform Plan for the Health Care System.* Washington, DC: National Leadership Coalition for Health Care Reform.

National League for Nursing. 1991a. *Criteria and Guidelines for the Evaluation of Associate Degree Programs in Nursing.* New York: NLN.

______. 1991b. *Differentiated Nursing Practice: Position Statement.* New York: NLN.

National League for Nursing. 1992a. *Criteria and Guidelines for the Evaluation of Baccalaureate and Higher Degree Programs in Nursing.* New York: NLN.

National League for Nursing. 1992b. *Criteria and Guidelines for the Evaluation of Diploma Programs in Nursing.* New York: NLN.

Nyberg, J. May 1990. The effects of care and economics on nursing practice. *Journal of Nursing Administration* 20:13–18.

Phaneuf, MC and Lang, M. 1985. *Issues in Professional Nursing Practice 7: Standards of Nursing Practice.* Washington, DC: ANA.

Polit, DF and Hungler, BP 1991. *Nursing Research: Principles and Methods.* 4th ed. Philadelphia: Lippincott.

Poteet, GW and Hodges, LE. 1990. How to choose a graduate program. In McCloskey, JC and Grace, HD, editors. *Current Issues in Nursing.* 3d ed. St Louis: Mosby.

Powell, DJ. January/February 1984. Nurses—"High touch" entrepreneurs. *Nursing Economics* 2:33–36.

Primm, PL. May/June 1986. Entry into practice: Competency statements for BSN's and ADN's. *Nursing Outlook* 34:135–37.

Rogers, ME. 1985. High touch in a high-tech future. Paper presented at the National League for Nursing convention, San Antonio, Texas.

Sampselle, CM. Winter 1990. The influence of feminist philosophy on nursing practice. *Image: Journal of Nursing Scholarship* 22:243–47.

Sayles-Cross, S. Summer 1993. Perceptions of familial caregivers of elder adults. *Image: Journal of Nursing Scholarship* 25:88–91.

Stevens, KR. May/June 1985. Does the 1985 education proposal make economic sense? *Nursing Outlook* 33:124–27.

Tanner, CA and Lindeman, CA. 1989. *Using Nursing Research.* NLN Pub No. 15-22-32-1-513. New York: NLN.

US Congressional Record Service (USCRS). 1988. *Health Insurance and the Uninsured: Background Data and Analysis.* Washington, DC: US Congress.

US Department of Commerce. 1991. Health and medical services. In *U.S. Industrial Outlook 1991.* Chapter 44. Washington, DC: US Department of Commerce.

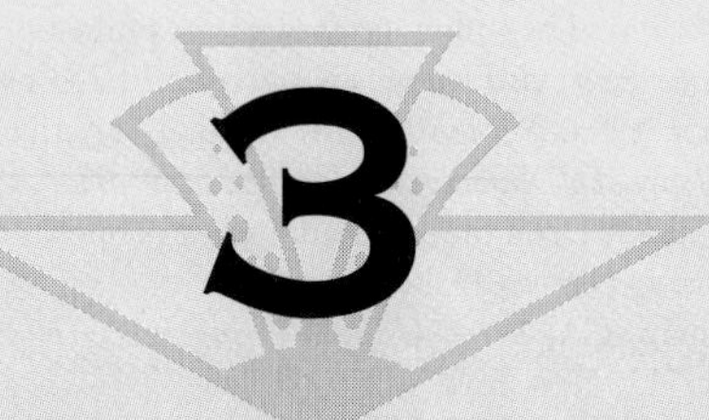

3 Nursing Theories and Conceptual Frameworks

Objectives

- Identify the purposes of nursing theories.
- Define the terms *concept*, *conceptual framework*, *proposition*, *theory*, *construct*, and *hypothesis*.
- Differentiate a theory from a conceptual framework.
- Identify three essential elements of a theory.
- Identify the four major concepts that nursing theories address.
- Compare selected theories and conceptual models for nursing.
- Identify essential aspects of caring.
- Describe the seven major units of a conceptual model of nursing.
- Describe the relationship of the nursing process to conceptual models of nursing.
- Describe the relationship of nursing theory to nursing research.

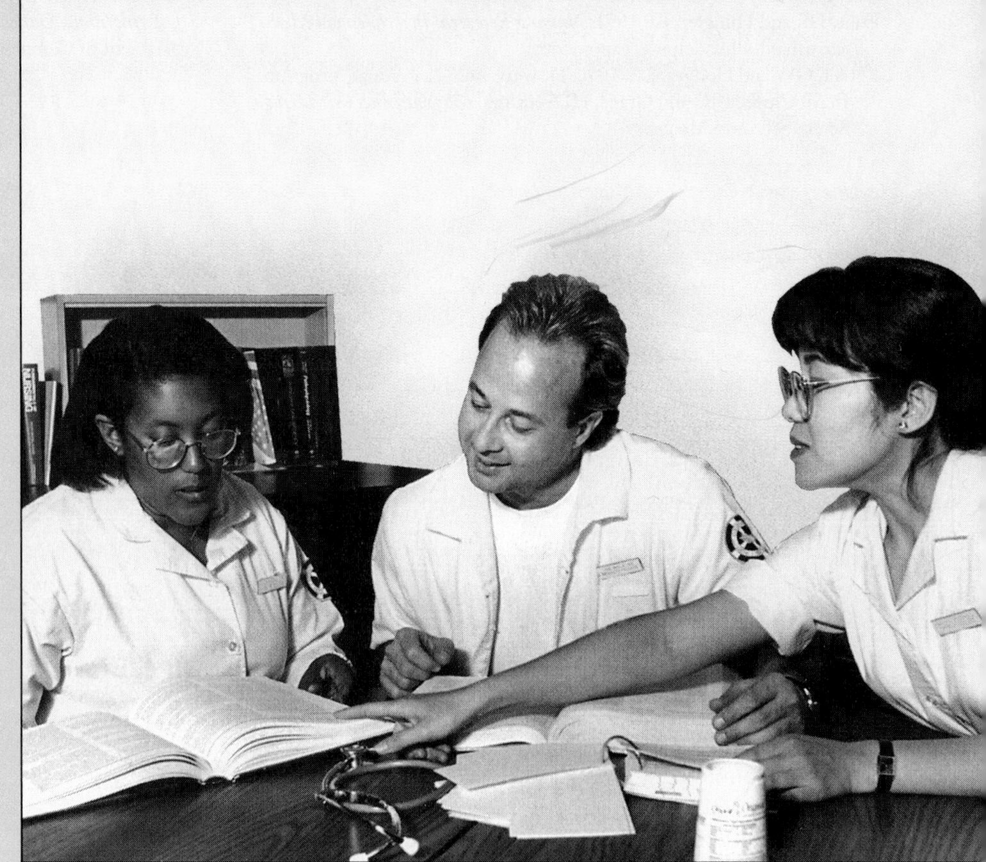

Theory development is considered by many nurses to be one of the most crucial tasks facing the profession today. Historically, knowledge used by nurses has been derived from the physical and behavioral sciences. As an increasingly emerging profession, nursing is now deeply involved in identifying its own unique knowledge base—that is, the body of knowledge essential to nursing practice, or a so-called nursing science. For this knowledge base to be identified, concepts and theories specific to nursing must be developed and recognized.

Theories offer ways of looking at (conceptualizing) a discipline (eg, nursing) in clear, explicit terms that can be communicated to others. Although most nurses have a clear idea of what nursing is, its uniqueness needs to be clearly stated to other health care workers and the public. Professionalism and a desire for collegial status with other health professionals have made the need for conceptual frameworks of nursing to be explicit. If nurses are to be considered health professionals, they must communicate exactly what makes their place in the interdisciplinary team unique and important.

Nursing theories serve several essential purposes. See the accompanying box at the right.

Theory development gained momentum in the 1960s and has progressed markedly since then through the work of several nurse theorists and the participation of nurses in theory conferences and in research to refine or validate the theories. Because opinions on the nature and structure of nursing vary, theories continue to be developed. Each theory bears the name of the person or group who developed it and reflects the beliefs of the developer.

Purposes of Nursing Theories and Conceptual Frameworks

- Provide direction and guidance for (a) structuring professional nursing practice, education, and research; and (b) differentiating the focus of nursing from other professions.

In Practice

- Assist nurses to describe, explain, and predict everyday experiences.
- Serve to guide assessment, intervention, and evaluation of nursing care.
- Provide a rationale for collecting reliable and valid data about the health status of clients, which are essential for effective decision making and implementation.
- Help to establish criteria to measure the quality of nursing care.
- Help build a common nursing terminology to use in communicating with other health professionals. Ideas are developed and words defined.
- Enhance autonomy (independence and self-governance) of nursing through defining its own independent functions.

In Education

- Provide a general focus for curriculum design.
- Guide curricular decision making.

In Research

- Offer a framework for generating knowledge and new ideas.
- Assist in discovering knowledge gaps in the specific field of study.
- Offer a systematic approach to identify questions for study, select variables, interpret findings, and validate nursing interventions.

Definition of Terms

Before specific theories and conceptual frameworks can be understood, the terms *concept*, *framework*, *conceptual framework* (or *model*), and *theory* must be clarified. **Concepts,** the building blocks of theory, are abstract ideas or mental images of phenomena or reality. Concepts are words that bring forth mental pictures of the properties and meanings of things. Concepts may be concrete ideas (eg, chair, table, dog) or abstract ideas (eg, equilibrium, adaptation, powerlessness, nursing). Many concepts apply to nursing: concepts about human beings, health, helping relationships, and communication. Nursing theories address and specify relationships among four major concepts:

1. *Person* or *client*, the recipient of nursing care (includes individuals, families, groups, and communities)
2. *Environment*, the internal and external surroundings of the client
3. *Health/illness*, the client's state of well-being
4. *Nursing*, a discipline from which client care interventions are provided

Each nurse theorist's definitions of these four major concepts vary in accordance with personal philosophy, scientific orientation, experience in nursing, and how that experience has affected the theorist's view of nursing. For example, while working as a pediatric staff nurse, Sister Callista Roy, a nurse and sociologist, noticed the great resilience of children and their ability to adapt to major physical and psychologic changes. Adaptation thus forms the basis of Roy's conceptual framework for nursing. In contrast, Martha Rogers used a broad knowledge base that included multiple scientific disciplines to develop a theory of unitary human beings and the environment as an energy field integral to the life process. Her theory was influenced by Einstein's theory of relativity, which introduced the four coordinates of space-time; Burr and Northrop's electrodynamic theory of life, which revealed the pattern and organization of the electrodynamic field; and von Bertalanffy's general systems theory. See Table 3–1 for selected theorists' definitions and descriptions of person, environment, health, and nursing.

A **framework** is a basic structure supporting anything. A **conceptual framework,** viewed simply, is a group of related concepts. It provides an overall view or orientation to focus our thoughts. A conceptual framework can be visualized as an umbrella under which many theories can exist (Creasia & Parker 1991, p. 7). For example, theories about the concept of client differ (see Table 3–1). The term *conceptual framework* is often used interchangeably with **conceptual model,** although the term *model* usually refers to a graphic illustration of relationships.

The concepts in a conceptual framework are linked together to form propositions. A **proposition** is a statement that expresses the relationship between concepts and is capable of being tested, believed, or denied. An example of a proposition is "People and their environments are open systems." (Systems theory is discussed in Chapter 14, page 277.)

A **theory,** like a conceptual model, is made up of concepts and propositions; however, a theory accounts for phenomena with much greater specificity. The literature contains numerous definitions of *theory*. Most definitions include three elements:

1. A set of well-defined constructs or concepts. A **construct** is a concept that has been invented to suit a special purpose. It is measurable and can be observed in relation to other constructs. For example, "id," "ego," and "super ego" are constructs Sigmund Freud developed to explain the concept of personality. To use a nursing example, the constructs in Imogene King's (1981) theory of goal attainment include perception, communication, interaction, transaction, self, role, growth and development, stress, time, and space.
2. A set of propositions that specify the relationships among the constructs. For example, one of the eight propositions King developed to describe the relationship among the concepts in her theory of goal attainment is "If perceptual accuracy is present in nurse-client interactions, transactions (goal attainment) will occur."
3. **Hypotheses,** conjectures that test the relationships between the constructs and propositions. Because the theory is abstract, it cannot be applied to practice. Instead, hypotheses derived from the theory are tested. For example, a testable hypothesis derived from King's goal-attainment theory is the following: "Perceptual accuracy in nurse-client interactions increases mutual goal setting" (King 1981).

The major distinction between a theory and a conceptual framework or model is the level of *abstraction*, with the conceptual framework being more abstract than the theory. A conceptual model is a system of related concepts or a conceptual diagram. Its major purpose is to give clear and explicit direction to the three areas of nursing: practice, education, and research. See major units of nursing models on page 55. A theory, in contrast, is more limited in scope. Its primary purpose is to generate knowledge in a field. A theory explores phenomena, expresses relationships between facts, generates a hypotheses, and predicts future events and relationships.

Because the primary purpose of nursing theory is to generate scientific knowledge, nursing theory and nursing research are closely related. Scientific knowledge is derived from testing hypotheses (assumptions) generated by theories for nursing. Research determines the utility of those hypotheses, and research findings may be developed into theories for nursing. In the research process, comparisons are made between the observed outcomes of research and the relationship predicted by the hypotheses.

OVERVIEW OF SELECTED NURSING THEORIES

The theories and conceptual models included in this section are categorized as general theories, systems theories, and interpersonal theories. They are presented in chronologic order as a means of organization only. Only brief summaries of the theorist's central theme and basic assumptions are included; for the theorist's definition and description of client, environment, health, and nursing, see Table 3–1. Theories vary considerably in (a) their level of abstraction, (b) their conceptualization of the client, health/illness, and nursing, and (c) in their ability to describe, explain, or predict. Some theories are broad in scope; others are limited.

GENERAL THEORIES

Nightingale's Environmental Theory Florence Nightingale, the "mother of modern nursing," considered nursing to be a religious calling to be fulfilled only by women. Her theory focused on the environment, although this term never appeared in her writings. She linked health with five environmental factors: (1) pure or

Table 3–1 Theorists' Definitions/Descriptions of Four Major Concepts

Theorist		Definitions/Descriptions
Florence Nightingale (1860) Environmental theory	Person/Client	An individual with vital reparative processes to deal with disease and desirous of health but passive in terms of influencing the environment or nurse.
	Environment	The major concepts for health are ventilation, warmth, light, diet, cleanliness, and absence of noise. Although the environment has social, emotional, and physical aspects, Nightingale emphasized the physical aspects.
	Health	Being well and using one's powers to the fullest extent. Health is maintained through prevention of disease via environmental health factors. Disease is a reparative process nature institutes because of some want of attention.
	Nursing	Provision of optimal conditions to enhance the person's reparative processes and prevent the reparative process from being interrupted.
Virginia Henderson (1955, 1966, 1969, 1978) Definition of nursing	Person/Client	A whole, complete, and independent being who has 14 fundamental needs to breathe, eat and drink, eliminate, move and maintain posture, sleep and rest, dress and undress, maintain body temperature, keep clean, avoid danger, communicate, worship, work, play, and learn.
	Environment	The aggregate of the external conditions and influences affecting the life and development of an organism.
	Health	Viewed in terms of the individual's ability to perform 14 components of nursing care unaided (eg, breathe normally, eat and drink adequately). Health is a quality of life basic to human functioning and requires independence and interdependence. It is the quality of health rather than life itself that allows people to work most effectively and to reach their highest potential level of satisfaction in life. Individuals will achieve or maintain health if they have the necessary strength, will, or knowledge.
	Nursing	The unique function of the nurse is to assist clients, sick or well, in performing those activities contributing to health, its recovery, or peaceful death—activities that clients would perform unaided if they had the necessary strength, will, or knowledge. Also, to do so in such a way as to help clients gain independence as rapidly as possible.
Martha E. Rogers (1970, 1980, 1983, 1986, 1989) Unitary human beings as an energy field	Person/Client	A unified whole possessing integrity and manifesting characteristics that are more than and different from the sum of its parts; an organized patterned energy field that continually exchanges matter and energy with the environmental energy field, resulting in continuous repatterning. The human being has the capacity for abstraction and imagery, language and thought, and sensation and emotion.
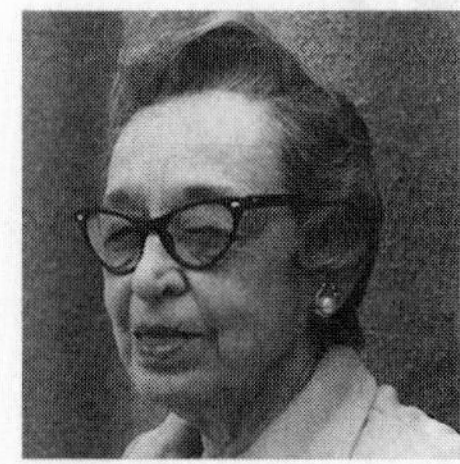	Environment	The irreducible, four-dimensional energy field identified by pattern and manifesting characteristics different from those of the parts. Each environmental field is specific to its given human field. They are identified by wave patterns manifesting continuous change, and both change continuously and creatively.
	Health	Positive health symbolizes wellness. It is a value term defined by the culture or individual. Health and illness are considered "to denote behaviors that are of high value and low value."
	Nursing	A humanistic science dedicated to compassionate concern with maintaining and promoting health, preventing illness, and caring for and rehabilitating the sick and disabled. Nursing seeks to promote symphonic interaction between the environment and the person, to strengthen the coherence and integrity of the human beings, and to direct and redirect patterns of interaction between the person and the environment for the realization of maximum health potential.

Table 3–1 Theorists' Definitions/Descriptions of Four Major Concepts *continued*

Theorist	Definitions/Descriptions	
Sister Callista Roy (1970, 1976, 1980, 1984, 1989, 1991) Adaptation model	Person/Client	A biopsychosocial being who is in constant interaction with the environment and who has four modes of adaptation, based on *physiologic needs, self-concept* (physical self, moral-ethical self, self-consistency, self-ideal and expectancy, and self-esteem), *role function*, and *interdependence relations*.
	Environment	All the conditions, circumstances, and influences surrounding and affecting the development and behavior of persons or groups; the input into the person as an adaptive system involving both internal and external factors.
	Health	A state and a process of being and becoming an integrated and whole person. Lack of integration represents lack of health.
	Nursing	A theoretical system of knowledge that prescribes a process of analysis and action related to the care of the ill or potentially ill person. As a science, nursing is a developing system of knowledge about persons used to observe, classify, and relate the processes by which persons positively affect their health status. As a practice discipline, nursing's scientific body of knowledge is used to provide an essential service to people, that is, to promote ability to affect health positively.
Dorothea E. Orem (1971, 1980, 1985, 1991) Self-care deficit theory	Person/Client	A unity who can be viewed as functioning biologically, symbolically, and socially and who initiates and performs self-care activities on own behalf in maintaining life, health, and well-being; self-care activities deal with air, water, food, elimination, activity and rest, solitude and social interaction, prevention of hazards to life and well-being, and promotion of human functioning.
	Environment	The environment is linked to the individual, forming an integrated and interactive system.
	Health	Health is a *state* that is characterized by soundness or wholeness of developed human structures and of bodily and mental functioning. It includes physical, psychologic, interpersonal, and social aspects. *Well-being* is used in the sense of individuals' perceived condition of existence. Well-being is a state characterized by experiences of contentment, pleasure, and certain kinds of happiness; by spiritual experiences; by movement toward fulfillment of one's self-ideal; and by continuing personalization. Well-being is associated with health, with success in personal endeavors, and with sufficiency of resources.
	Nursing	A helping or assisting service to persons who are wholly or partly dependent—infants, children, and adults—when they, their parents, guardians, or other adults responsible for their care are no longer able to give or supervise their care. A creative effort of one human being to help another human being. Nursing is deliberate action, a function of the practical intelligence of nurses, and action to bring about humanely desirable conditions in persons and their environments. It is distinguished from other human services and other forms of care by its focus on human beings.
Imogene King (1971, 1981, 1986, 1987, 1989) Goal attainment theory	Person/Client	Three interacting systems: individuals (personal systems), groups (interpersonal systems), and society (social systems); the personal system is a unified, complex, whole self who perceives, thinks, desires, imagines, decides, identifies goals, and selects means to achieve them.
	Environment	Adjustments to life and health are influenced by an individual's interactions with environment. The environment is constantly changing.
	Health	A dynamic state in the life cycle; illness is an interference in the life cycle. Health implies continuous adaptation to stress in the internal and external environment through the use of one's resources to achieve maximum potential for daily living.
	Nursing	A helping profession that assists individuals and groups in society to attain, maintain, and restore health. If this is not possible, nurses help individuals die with dignity.

Table 3–1 *continued*

Theorist		Definitions/Descriptions
Imogene King *continued*		Nursing is perceiving, thinking, relating, judging, and acting vis-à-vis the behavior of individuals who come to a nursing situation. A nursing situation is the immediate enBvironment, spatial and temporal reality, in which nurse and client establish a relationship to cope with health states and adjust to changes in activities of daily living if the situation demands adjustment. It is an interpersonal process of action, reaction, interaction, and transaction whereby nurse and client share information about their perceptions in the nursing situation.
Betty Neuman (1972, 1974, 1980, 1982, 1989) Health care systems model 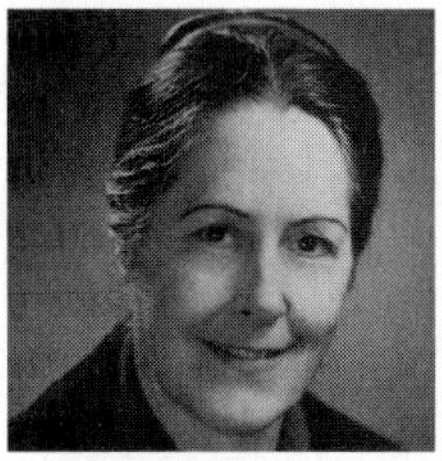	Person/Client	Open system consisting of a basic structure or central core of survival factors surrounded by concentric rings that are bounded by lines of resistance, a normal line of defense, and a flexible line of defense. The total person is a composite of physiologic, psychologic, sociocultural, and developmental variables.
	Environment	Both internal and external environments exist and a person maintains varying degrees of harmony and balance between them. It is all factors affecting and affected by the system.
	Health	Wellness is the condition in which all parts and subparts of an individual are in harmony with the whole system. Wholeness is based on interrelationships of variables that determine the resistance of an individual to any stressor. Illness indicates lack of harmony among the parts and subparts of the system of the individual. Health is viewed as a point along a continuum from wellness to illness; health is dynamic (ie, constantly subject to change). Optimal wellness or stability indicates that all a person's needs are being met. A reduced state of wellness is the result of unmet systemic needs. The individual is in a dynamic state of wellness-illness, in varying degrees, at any given time.
	Nursing	A unique profession in that it is concerned with all of the variables affecting an individual's response to stressors, which are intra-, inter-, and extrapersonal in nature. The concern of nursing is to prevent stress invasion, or, following stress invasion, to protect the client's basic structure and obtain or maintain a maximum level of wellness. The nurse helps the client, through primary, secondary, and tertiary prevention modes, to adjust to environmental stressors and maintain client system stability.
Dorothy E. Johnson (1959, 1968, 1974, 1980) Behavioral system model 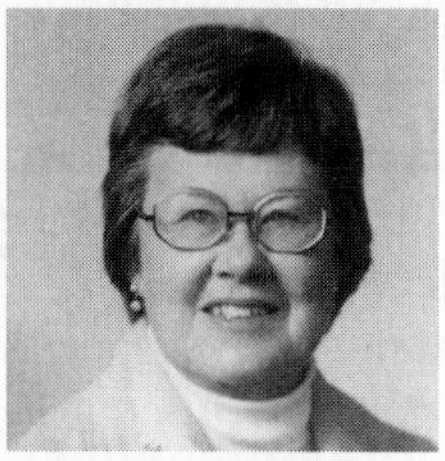	Person/Client	A behavioral system composed of seven subsystems: affiliative, achievement, dependence, aggressive, eliminative, ingestive, and sexual.
	Environment	Consists of all factors that are not part of the individual's behavioral system but that influence the system and some of which can be manipulated by the nurse to achieve the health goal of the client. The individual links to and interacts with the environment.
	Health	Health is an elusive, dynamic state influenced by biologic, psychologic, and social factors. Health is reflected by the organization, interaction, interdependence, and integration of the subsystems of the behavioral system. Humans attempt to achieve a balance in this system; this balance leads to functional behavior. A lack of balance in the structural or functional requirements of the subsystems leads to poor health.
	Nursing	An external regulatory force that acts to preserve the organization and integration of the client's behavior at an optimal level under those conditions in which the behavior constitutes a threat to physical or social health or in which illness is found.

fresh air, (2) pure water, (3) efficient drainage, (4) cleanliness, and (5) light, especially direct sunlight. Deficiencies in these five factors produced lack of health or illness.

The above factors attain significance when one considers that sanitation conditions in hospitals of the mid 1800s were extremely poor, and the women working in the hospitals were unreliable, uneducated, and incompetent to care for the ill.

In addition to the factors above, Nightingale also stressed the importance of keeping the patient warm, maintaining a noise-free environment, and attending to the patient's diet in terms of assessing intake, timeliness of the food, and its effect on the person.

Nightingale set the stage for further work in the development of nursing theories. Her general concepts about ventilation, cleanliness, quiet, warmth, and diet remain integral parts of nursing and health care today.

Henderson's Definition of Nursing In 1955, Virginia Henderson formulated a definition of the unique function of nursing. This definition was a major stepping-stone in the emergence of nursing as a discipline separate from medicine (see Table 3–1). Basic to her definition are various assumptions about the individual: namely, that the individual (a) needs to maintain physiologic and emotional balance, (b) requires assistance to achieve health and independence or a peaceful death, and (c) needs the necessary strength, will, or knowledge to achieve or maintain health. These needs give direction to the nurse's role.

Henderson conceptualized the nurse's role as assisting sick or well individuals in a supplementary or complementary way. The nurse needs to be a partner with the patient, a helper to the patient, and, when necessary, a substitute for the patient. The nurse's focus is to help individuals and families (which she viewed as a unit) to gain independence in meeting 14 fundamental needs (Henderson 1966):

1. Breathing normally
2. Eating and drinking adequately
3. Eliminating body wastes
4. Moving and maintaining a desirable position
5. Sleeping and resting
6. Selecting suitable clothes
7. Maintaining body temperature within normal range by adjusting clothing and modifying the environment
8. Keeping the body clean and well-groomed to protect the integument
9. Avoiding dangers in the environment and avoiding injuring others
10. Communicating with others in expressing emotions, needs, fears, or opinions
11. Worshiping according to one's faith
12. Working in such a way that one feels a sense of accomplishment
13. Playing or participating in various forms of recreation
14. Learning, discovering, or satisfying the curiosity that leads to normal development and health, and using available health facilities

Henderson has published many works and continues to be cited in current nursing literature. Her emphasis on the importance of nursing's independence from, and interdependence with, other health care disciplines is well recognized.

Rogers's Science of Unitary Human Beings Martha Rogers first presented her theory of unitary human beings in 1970. It contains complex conceptualizations related to Einstein's theory of relativity, Burr and Northrop's electrodynamic theory of life, von Bertalanffy's general systems theory, and many other social sciences. Rogers views the person as an irreducible whole, the whole being greater than the sum of its parts. *Whole* is differentiated from *holistic*, the latter often being used to mean only the sum of all the parts. She states that humans are dynamic energy fields in continuous exchange with environmental fields, both of which are infinite. Both human and environmental fields are characterized by pattern, a universe of open systems, and four-dimensionality. According to Rogers, *unitary man*

- Is an irreducible, four-dimensional energy field identified by pattern.
- Manifests characteristics different from the sum of the parts.
- Interacts continuously and creatively with the environment.
- Behaves as a totality.
- As a sentient being, participates creatively in change.

Key concepts Rogers uses to describe the individual and the environment are energy fields, openness, pattern and organization, and multidimensionality. *Energy fields* are the fundamental level of humans and the environment (all that is outside a given human field). Energy fields are dynamic, constantly exchanging energy from one to the other. The concept of *openness* holds that the energy fields of humans and the environment are open systems, that is, infinite, integral with one another, and in continuous process. *Pattern* refers to the unique identifying behaviors, qualities, and characteristics of the energy fields that change continuously and innovatively. Rogers defines *four-dimensionality* as a nonlinear domain without temporal or spiritual attributes. All reality is considered to be four-dimensional.

To Rogers, the life process in humans is homeodynamic, involving continuous and creative change. She provides three principles of homeodynamics to offer a way of perceiving how unitary human beings develop: integrality (formerly complementarity), resonancy, and helicy. According to the principle of *integrality*, the human and environmental fields interact mutually and simultaneously. *Resonancy* means the wave pattern in the fields change continuously and from lower- to higher-frequency patterns. *Helicy* postulates that the field changes are innovative, probabilistic, and characterized by increasing diversity of field patterns and repeating rhythmicities.

Some find Rogers's concepts difficult to understand, but a specific example can help clarify them. Nurses' use of therapeutic touch is based on the concept of human energy fields (see Chapter 32, page 848). The human energy field is identified by pattern. The qualities of the field vary from person to person and are affected by pain and illness. Although the field is infinite, realistically it is most clearly "felt" within several feet of the body. The trained nurse can assess and feel the energy field and manipulate it to help a person manage pain.

Orem's Self-Care Deficit Theory Dorothy Orem's self-care deficit theory, published first in 1971, has been widely accepted by the nursing community. It includes three related theories of self-care, self-care deficit, and nursing system. *Self-care theory* postulates that self-care and the self-care of dependents are learned behaviors that individuals initiate and perform on their own behalf to maintain life, health, and well-being. The individual's ability to perform self-care is called *self-care agency*. Adults care for themselves, whereas infants, the aged, the ill, and the disabled require assistance with self-care activities.

There are three kinds of self-care requisites:

1. *Universal requisites,* common to all people, include the maintenance of air, water, food, elimination, activity and rest, solitude, and social interaction; prevention of hazards to life and well-being; and the promotion of human functioning.
2. *Developmental requisites* are those associated with conditions that promote known developmental processes throughout the life cycle.
3. *Health deviation requisites* relate to defects and deviations from normal structure and integrity that impair an individual's ability to perform self-care.

Self-care deficit theory asserts that people benefit from nursing because they have health-related limitations in providing self-care. Limitations may result from illness, injury, or from the effects of medical tests or treatments. Two variables affect these deficits: self-care agency (ability) and *therapeutic self-care demands* (the measures of care required to meet existing requisites). *Self-care deficit* results when self-care agency is not adequate to meet the known self-care demand.

Nursing system theory postulates that nursing systems form when nurses prescribe, design, and provide nursing that regulates the individual's self-care capabilities and meets therapeutic self-care requirements. Three types of nursing systems are identified:

1. *Wholly compensatory* systems are required for individuals unable to control and monitor their environment and process information.
2. *Partially compensatory* systems are designed for individuals who are unable to perform some (but not all) self-care activities.
3. *Supportive-educative (developmental)* systems are designed for persons who need to learn to perform self-care measures and need assistance to do so.

SYSTEMS THEORIES

Systems theories include Roy's adaptation model, King's goal attainment theory, Neuman's health care systems model, and Johnson's behavioral systems model. **Systems** consist of interrelated parts functioning together to form a whole. (See systems theory in Chapter 14, page 277.)

Roy's Adaptation Model Sister Callista Roy's adaptation model, originating in 1970, is widely used by nurse educators, researchers, and practitioners. Roy focuses on the individual as a biopsychosocial adaptive system. Both the individual and the environment are sources of stimuli that require modification to promote adaptation, an ongoing purposive response. Adaptive responses contribute to health, the process of being and becoming integrated; ineffective or maladaptive responses do not.

As an open system, an individual receives inputs or stimuli from both the self and the environment. Roy identifies three classes of stimuli:

1. *Focal stimulus:* the internal or external stimulus most immediately confronting the person and contributing to behavior
2. *Contextual stimuli:* all other internal or external stimuli present
3. *Residual stimuli:* beliefs, attitudes, or traits having an indeterminate effect on the person's behavior but whose effects are not validated

Roy's adaptive system consists of two interrelated subsystems. The *primary subsystem* is a functional or internal control process that consists of the regulator and the cognator. The *regulator* processes input automatically through neural-chemical-endocrine channels. The *cognator* processes input through cognitive pathways, such as perception, information processing, learning, judgment, and emotion. Roy views the regulator and cognator as methods of coping.

The *secondary subsystem* is an effector system that manifests cognator and regulator activity. It consists of four adaptive modes:

1. The *physiologic mode* involves the body's basic physiologic needs and ways of adapting in regard to fluid and electrolytes, activity and rest, circulation and oxygen, nutrition and elimination, protection, the senses, and neurologic and endocrine function.
2. The *self-concept mode* includes two components: the *physical* self, which involves sensation and body image, and the *personal* self, which involves self-ideal, self-consistency, and the moral-ethical self.
3. The *role function mode* is determined by the need for social integrity and refers to the performance of duties based on given positions within society.
4. The *interdependence mode* involves one's relations with significant others and support systems that provide help, affection, and attention.

King's Goal Attainment Theory Imogene King's theory of goal attainment, first published in 1971, was derived from a conceptual framework of three dynamic interacting systems: (a) personal systems (individuals), (b) interpersonal systems (groups), and (c) social systems (society). Key concepts are identified for each system as follows:

1. Personal system concepts: perception, self, body image, growth and development, space, and time
2. Interpersonal system concepts: interaction, communication, transaction, role, and stress
3. Social system concepts: organization, authority, power, status, and decision making

The client and nurse are personal systems or subsystems within interpersonal and social systems. To identify problems and to establish goals, the nurse and client perceive one another, act and react, interact, and transact. *Transactions* are defined as purposeful interactions that lead to goal attainment. Transactions have the following characteristics:

- They are basic to goal attainment and include social exchange, bargaining and negotiating, and sharing a frame of reference toward mutual goal setting.
- They require perceptual accuracy in nurse-client interactions and congruence between role performance and role expectation for nurse and client.
- They lead to goal attainment, satisfaction, effective care, and enhanced growth and development.

King postulates seven hypotheses in goal attainment theory:

1. Perceptual congruence in nurse-client interactions increases mutual goal setting.
2. Communication increases mutual goal setting between nurses and clients and leads to satisfactions.
3. Satisfactions in nurses and clients increase goal attainment.
4. Goal attainment decreases stress and anxiety in nursing situations.
5. Goal attainment increases client learning and coping ability in nursing situations.
6. Role conflict experienced by clients, nurses, or both decreases transactions in nurse-client interactions.
7. Congruence in role expectations and role performance increases transactions in nurse-client interactions.

King's theory highlights the importance of the participation of all individuals in decision making and deals with the choices, alternatives, and outcomes of nursing care. The theory offers insight into nurses' interactions with individuals and groups within the environment.

Neuman's Health Care Systems Model Betty Neuman's systems model, first published in 1972, is based on the individual's relationship to stress, the reaction to it, and reconstitution factors that are dynamic in nature. *Reconstitution* is the state of adaptation to stressors.

Neuman views the client as an open system consisting of a basic structure or central core of energy resources (physiologic, psychologic, sociocultural, developmental, and spiritual) surrounded by two concentric boundaries or rings referred to as *lines of resistance*. The two lines of resistance represent internal factors that help the client defend against a stressor. The inner or *normal line of defense* represents the person's state of equilibrium or the state of adaptation developed and maintained over time and considered normal for that person. The *flexible line of defense* is dynamic and can be rapidly altered over a short period of time. It is a protective buffer that prevents stressors from penetrating the normal line of defense.

The nurse's focus is all the variables affecting an individual's response to stressors. Nursing interventions are carried out on three preventive levels:

1. *Primary prevention* identifies risk factors, attempts to eliminate the stressor, and focuses on protecting the normal line of defense and strengthening the flexible line of defense. A reaction has not yet occurred, but the degree of risk is known.
2. *Secondary prevention* relates to interventions or active treatment initiated after symptoms have occurred. The focus is to strengthen internal lines of resistance, reduce the reaction, and increase resistance factors.

3. *Tertiary prevention* refers to intervention following that in the secondary stage. It focuses on readaptation and stability and protects reconstitution or return to wellness following treatment. The nurse emphasizes educating the client in strengthening resistance to stressors and ways to help prevent recurrence of reaction or regression.

Betty Neuman's model of nursing has been widely accepted by the nursing community, nationally and internationally. It is applicable to a variety of nursing practice settings involving individuals, families, groups, and communities.

Johnson's Behavioral System Model Dorothy Johnson used her observations of behavior over many years to formulate a general theory of man as a behavioral system. The theory was originally presented orally in 1968 but was not published until 1980. Johnson defines a system as a whole that functions as a whole by virtue of the interdependence of its parts. Individuals strive to maintain stability and balance in these parts through adjustments and adaptations to the forces that impinge on them. A behavioral system is patterned, repetitive, and purposeful.

Johnson's key concepts describe the individual as a behavioral system composed of seven subsystems:

1. The *attachment-affiliative* subsystem provides survival and security. Its consequences are social inclusion, intimacy, and the formation and maintenance of a strong social bond.
2. The *dependency* subsystem promotes helping behavior that calls for a nurturing response. Its consequences are approval, attention or recognition, and physical assistance.
3. The *ingestive* subsystem satisfies appetite. It is governed by social and psychologic considerations as well as biologic.
4. The *eliminative* subsystem excretes body wastes.
5. The *sexual* subsystem functions dually for procreation and gratification.
6. The *achievement* subsystem attempts to manipulate the environment. It controls or masters an aspect of the self or environment to some standard of excellence.
7. The *aggressive* subsystem protects and preserves the self and society within the limits imposed by society.

Each of the above subsystems has the same functional requirements: protection, nurturance, and stimulation. The subsystems' responses are developed through motivation, experience, and learning and are influenced by biopsychosocial factors.

Other concepts associated with Johnson's model are *equilibrium*, a stabilized but more or less transitory resting state in which the individual is in harmony with the self and the environment; *tension*, a state of being stretched or strained; and *stressors*, internal or external stimuli that produce tension and result in a degree of instability.

INTERPERSONAL/CARING THEORIES

Interpersonal/psychodynamic theories seek to develop the nurse's skill in relationships with clients, compassion, the helping process, and caring. Interpersonal theories include Peplau's psychodynamic nursing theory, Leininger's transcultural care theory, Watson's philosophy and science of caring, and Benner's primacy of caring.

Peplau's Psychodynamic Nursing Theory Hildegard Peplau is one of the first theorists since Nightingale to present a theory for nursing. She introduced her interpersonal concepts in 1952 and based them on available theories at the time: psychoanalytic theory, principles of social learning, and concepts of human motivation and personality development. *Psychodynamic nursing* is defined as understanding one's own behavior to help others identify felt difficulties and applying principles of human relations to problems arising during the experience.

Peplau views nursing as a maturing force that is realized as the personality develops through educational, therapeutic, and interpersonal processes. Nurses enter into a personal relationship with an individual when a felt need is present. This nurse-patient relationship evolves in four phases:

1. *Orientation.* During this phase, the patient seeks help, and the nurse assists the patient to understand the problem and the extent of need for help.
2. *Identification.* During this phase, the patient assumes a posture of dependence, interdependence, or independence in relation to the nurse (relatedness). The nurse's focus is to assure the person that the nurse understands the interpersonal meaning of the patient's situation.
3. *Exploitation.* In this phase, the patient derives full value from what the nurse offers through the relationship. The patient uses available services on the basis of self-interest and needs. Power shifts from the nurse to the patient.
4. *Resolution.* In this final phase, old needs and goals are put aside and new ones adopted. Once older needs are resolved, newer and more mature ones emerge.

During the nurse-patient relationship, nurses assume many roles: stranger, teacher, resource person, surrogate, leader, and counselor. Today, Peplau's model continues to be used by clinicians when working with individuals who have psychologic problems.

Leininger's Transcultural Care Theory Madeleine Leininger's theory, which first appeared in 1978, postulates that caring and culture are inextricably linked. Educated in cultural and social anthropology, Leininger observed a marked number of differences between Western and non-Western cultures in caring and health practices. She defines *transcultural nursing* as a major area of nursing that focuses on comparative study and analysis of different cultures and subcultures in the world, with respect to their caring behavior, nursing care, and health values, beliefs, and patterns. The goal of transcultural nursing is to develop a scientific and humanistic body of knowledge in order to provide culture-specific and culture-universal nursing practices. She believes culture is the broadest and the most holistic means to conceptualize, understand, and be effective with people.

Leininger states that *care* is the essence of nursing and the dominant, distinctive, and unifying feature of nursing. She says that there can be no cure without caring, but that there may be caring without curing. She emphasizes that human caring, although a universal phenomenon, varies among cultures in its expressions, processes, and patterns; it is largely culturally derived. These differences in caring values and behaviors lead to differences in the expectations of those seeking care. For example, cultures that perceive illness primarily as a personal and internal body experience—caused by physical, genetic, and intrabody stresses—tend to use more medications and physical techniques than cultures that view illness as an extrapersonal experience.

Leininger identifies many caring constructs (see the accompanying box). Leininger believes that the goal of health care personnel should be to work toward an understanding of care and the values, health beliefs, and lifestyles of different cultures, which will form the basis for providing culture-specific care.

LEININGER'S DESCRIPTIONS OF CARE AND CARING

- Caring includes assistive, supportive, and facilitative acts toward or for another individual or group with evident or anticipated needs.
- Caring serves to ameliorate or to improve human conditions or life ways. It emphasizes healthful, enabling activities of individuals and groups that are based on culturally defined, ascribed, or sanctioned helping modes.
- Caring is essential to human development, growth, and survival.
- Caring behaviors include comfort, compassion, concern, coping behavior, empathy, enabling, facilitating, interest, involvement, health consultative acts, health instruction acts, health maintenance acts, helping behaviors, love, nurturance, presence, protective behaviors, restorative behaviors, sharing, stimulating behaviors, stress alleviation, succor, support, surveillance, tenderness, touching, and trust.

Watson's Philosophy and Science of Caring Jean Watson's theory of the science of caring was first published in 1979. She believes the practice of caring is central to nursing; it is the unifying focus for practice. Two major assumptions underlie human care values in nursing: (a) care and love constitute the primal and universal psychic energy, and (b) care and love are requisite for our survival and the nourishment of humanity. Watson's major assumptions about caring are shown in the box on page 55.

Nursing interventions related to human care are referred to as *carative factors*. Watson outlines the following ten factors:

1. Forming a *humanistic-altruistic system of values*. This factor relates to satisfaction through giving and extending the sense of self. Although the values are learned early in life, they can be greatly influenced by educators.
2. Instilling *faith and hope*. Feelings of faith and hope promote wellness by helping the client to adopt health-seeking behaviors. By developing an effective nurse-client relationship, the nurse facilitates feelings of optimism, hope, and trust.
3. Cultivating *sensitivity to one's self and others*. Nurses who are able to recognize and express their feelings are better able to allow others to express theirs.
4. Developing a *helping-trust (human care) relationship*. This kind of relationship involves effective communication, empathy, and nonpossessive warmth. It promotes and accepts the expression of positive and negative feelings.
5. Expressing *positive and negative feelings*. Sharing feelings of sorrow, love, and pain is a risk-taking experience. The nurse must be prepared for negative feelings.
6. Using a *creative problem-solving caring process*. Caring linked to the nursing process contributes to a creative problem-solving approach to nursing care.
7. Promoting *transpersonal teaching-learning*. This factor separates caring from curing and shifts responsibility for wellness to the client.
8. Providing a *supportive, protective, or corrective mental, physical, sociocultural, and spiritual environment*. Be-

WATSON'S ASSUMPTIONS OF CARING

- Human caring in nursing is not just an emotion, concern, attitude, or benevolent desire. *Caring* connotes a personal response.
- Caring is an intersubjective human process and is the moral ideal of nursing.
- Caring can be effectively demonstrated only interpersonally.
- Effective caring promotes health and individual or family growth.
- Caring promotes health more than does curing.
- Caring responses accept a person not only as they are now, but also for what the person may become.
- A caring environment offers the development of potential while allowing the person to choose the best action for the self at a given point in time.
- Caring occasions involve action and choice by nurse and client. If the caring occasion is transpersonal, the limits of openness expand, as do human capacities.
- The most abstract characteristic of a caring person is that the person is somehow responsive to another person as a unique individual, perceives the other's feelings, and sets one person apart from another.
- Human caring involves values, a will and a commitment to care, knowledge, caring actions, and consequences.
- The ideal and value of caring is a starting point, a stance, and an attitude that has to become a will, an intention, a commitment, and a conscious judgment that manifests itself in concrete acts.

cause the client can experience change in any aspect of the internal and external environments, the nurse must assess and facilitate the client's abilities to cope with mental, emotional, and physical changes.

9. Assisting with *gratification of human needs.* Caring is conveyed by recognizing and attending to the physical, emotional, social, and spiritual needs of the client.
10. Being sensitive to *existential-phenomenologic-spiritual force.* Phenomenology describes data of the immediate situation that help people understand the phenomena in question. The *phenomenal field* is the individual's frame of reference; this field can be known only to the person. Existential psychology is a science of human existence that employs the method of phenomenologic analysis. Persons possess three spheres of being: mind, body, and soul. Allowing for expression of these forces leads to a better understanding of self and others.

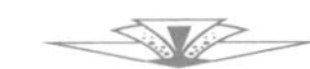

MAJOR UNITS OF NURSING MODELS

Each nursing education program is based on a conceptual framework selected or developed by the program's faculty to guide student learning and to provide a nursing model for graduates. In addition to clearly stated assumptions and values or beliefs, seven elements or units are necessary to meet the requirements for an effective conceptual model for nursing. These units, which relate to the broad conceptualizations of nursing and client, are (a) goal of nursing, (b) client (patient), (c) role of the nurse, (d) source of difficulty of the client, (e) intervention focus, (f) modes of intervention, and (g) consequences of nursing activity. A summary of these units in the major conceptual models is given in Table 3–2, page 56. Some theorists have developed certain units more than others.

Goal of Nursing The goal is the end or aim of nursing, what nursing is trying to achieve. This goal has to agree with the goals common to all health professionals—to improve health, to maintain health, to prevent health problems, to restore health, and so on. However, each health discipline has a goal distinct enough to justify the presence of that discipline on the health team. Specific nursing goals vary from model to model, depending on its assumptions about people. Goals need to be broad enough (a) to indicate what end the nursing profession is working toward, (b) to indicate what to teach future practitioners, and (c) to apply to nursing practice in all practice settings (community, hospital, home, health center, and so on). Before the 20th century, Florence Nightingale believed the goal of nursing was to make the patient as comfortable as possible and to put the patient in the best possible condition for nature to act and for the physician's treatment to take effect. For current goals of nursing, see Table 3–2, page 56.

Client The client unit refers not only to the intended recipient(s) of nursing service but also to conceptions about that person or group. Most models indicate that the client is a biopsychosocial being, but they differ in exactly how the client is conceptualized as such. Henderson views the client as a whole, complete, independent being who has 14 fundamental needs, whereas Johnson views the client as a behavioral system composed of seven subsystems. For further information, see the discussion of human needs in Chapter 14.

Table 3–2 Summary of Major Units from Selected Conceptual Models for Nursing*

Theorist	Goal of Nursing	Client	Role of the Nurse
Virginia Henderson (1955, 1966, 1969, 1978): Complementary-supplementary model	Independence in the satisfaction of human beings' 14 fundamental needs	A whole, complete and independent being who has 14 fundamental needs to breathe, eat and drink, eliminate, move, sleep and rest, avoid danger, communicate, worship, and so on (see Table 3–1, pp. 47–49)	A complementary-supplementary role to maintain or restore independence in the satisfaction of clients' 14 fundamental needs
Dorothy E. Johnson (1980): Behavioral system model	Behavioral system equilibrium and dynamic stability	A behavioral system composed of seven subsystems: affiliative, achievement, dependence, aggressive, eliminative, ingestive, and sexual	A regulator and controller of behavioral system stability and equilibrium
Imogene King (1971, 1981, 1986, 1987, 1989): Systems interaction model	Attainment, maintenance, or restoration of health to allow clients to achieve maximum potential for daily living	Three interacting systems: individuals (personal systems), groups (interpersonal systems), and society (social systems); the personal system is a unified, complex, whole self who perceives, thinks, desires, imagines, decides, identifies goals, and selects means to achieve them	An interaction process
Betty Neuman (1972, 1974, 1980, 1982, 1989): Health care systems model	Attainment and maintenance of client system equilibrium	Open system consisting of a basic structure or central core of survival factors surrounded by concentric rings that are bounded by lines of resistance, a normal line of defense, and a flexible line of defense (see Table 3–1, pp. 47–49)	To identify intrapersonal, interpersonal, and extrapersonal stressors and assist the individual to respond to stressors
Dorothea E. Orem (1971, 1980, 1985, 1991): Self-care model	Achievement of optimal client self-care so that clients can achieve and maintain an optimal health state	A unity who can be viewed as functioning biologically, symbolically, and socially and who initiates and performs self-care activities on own behalf in maintaining life, health, and well-being	To provide assistance to influence clients' development in achieving an optimal level of self-care
Martha E. Rogers (1970, 1980, 1983, 1986, 1989): Science of unitary human beings	Achievement of maximum health potential	A unified whole possessing integrity and manifesting characteristics that are more than and different from the sum of its parts; an organized patterned energy field that continually exchanges matter and energy with the environmental energy field, resulting in continuous repatterning. (see Table 3–1, pp. 47–49)	To help clients develop patterns of living that accommodate environmental changes rather than conflict with them
Sister Callista Roy (1970, 1976, 1980, 1984, 1989, 1991): Adaptation model	Adaptation in each of the four adaptive modes in situations of health and illness	A biopsychosocial being who has four modes of adaptation, based on: physiologic needs, self-concept (physical self, moral-ethical self, self-consistency, self-ideal and expectancy, and self-esteem), role function, and interdependence relations	To promote clients' adaptive behaviors by manipulating focal, contextual, and residual stimuli

* The models are listed in alphabetical order.

Source of Client Difficulty	Intervention Focus	Modes of Intervention	Consequences of Nursing Activity
Lack of strength, will, or knowledge	The deficit that is the source of client difficulty	Actions to replace, complete, substitute, add, reinforce, or increase strength, will, or knowledge	1. Increased independence in satisfaction of the client's 14 fundamental needs, or 2. Peaceful death
Functional or structural stress; inadequate input to the system; breakdown in regulatory system; exposure to noxious influences	1. The mechanisms of control and regulation 2. The functional requirements	Imposing external regulatory control mechanisms; fulfilling functional requirements; helping to regulate subsystem balance	Efficient and effective client behavior
Stressors in the internal and external environment	Perception of client difficulty and goal setting through communication	Interaction process in which both client and nurse set goals, explore and agree on the means to achieve them, and make transactions	Goal attainment
Intrapersonal, interpersonal, and extrapersonal stressors in the internal and external environments	Strengthening normal and flexible lines of defense and reducing stress factors	Primary, secondary, and tertiary prevention (a) strengthening the person's flexible line of defense; (b) strengthening internal lines of resistance; and (c) maintaining the person's existing energy resources	Reconstitution (ie, movement from a variance of wellness to the desired level of wellness and client system stability)
Any interference with self-care, by a person, object, condition, event, circumstance, or any combination of interferences	Inability to maintain self-care (a deficit in the self-care agency)	Five general ways of assisting: acting for or doing for, guiding, supporting, providing a developmental environment, and teaching	Achievement of the client's optimal level of self-care
Unharmonious person-environment interactions that are determined by social values	Coordinating environmental field and human field rhythmicities	Actions to promote harmonious interaction between the client and environment, to strengthen the integrity of the human field, and to direct and redirect patterning of the human and environmental fields	Maximum health potential, unity, and increasing complexity of organization
Coping activity that is inadequate to maintain integrity in the face of a need deficit or excess	The focal, contextual, and residual stimuli	Manipulation of the stimuli by increasing, decreasing, and/or maintaining them	Adaptive responses to stimuli by the client

Role of the Nurse The role of the nurse must be wanted, needed, and accepted by society just as the physician's curative role or the lawyer's defending role is wanted and accepted. Many nurses consider their role to be one of "caring"; however, caring is a vague concept that is difficult to operationalize. In Orem's self-care model, the role of the nurse is to provide assistance to influence the client's development in achieving an optimal level of self-care; in Roy's adaptation model, the nurse's role is to promote the client's adaptive behaviors by manipulating stimuli. See also Table 3–2 on pages 56–57.

Source of Difficulty The source of difficulty resides with the client, not the nurse. In other words, it is the nursing diagnosis or probable origin or cause of any client problems amenable to nursing intervention. Clients in health care agencies have health problems that may be subcategorized as medical, psychologic, dietary, nursing, and so on. The physician deals with medical problems, the psychologist or psychiatrist with psychologic problems, the dietitian with dietary problems, and the nurse with nursing problems. The source of difficulty is an explicit statement of the nursing problem. For example, in Henderson's model, the origin of the client's problem is lack of strength, will, or knowledge; in Johnson's model, it is functional or structural stress. Table 3–2, pp. 56–57, lists sources of difficulty identified by other theorists.

Intervention Focus Another unit of each model is the target or focus of nursing intervention. The universally accepted intervention focus for the physician is the client's pathology. In Orem's self-care model, the intervention focus for nurses is a deficit in the client's ability to maintain self-care; in Roy's adaptation model, it is the stimuli the client is having difficulty adapting to. See Table 3–2 on pages 56–57 for additional information.

Modes of Intervention The modes of intervention unit clarifies the means at the nurse's disposal when intervening. It is closely allied to the intervention focus and spells out specific ways in which the nurse helps the client. For example, in Roy's adaptation model the intervention focus is stimuli, and the mode of intervention is manipulation of the stimuli. In contrast, Florence Nightingale believed the mode of intervention was manipulation of the environment. This was done by providing warmth, fresh air, light, food, and sanitation. See Table 3–2 on pages 56–57, for other intervention modes.

Consequences The last unit states the expected consequences of nursing actions. It reflects the nursing goal and the concept of the client. See Table 3–2, pages 56–57, for consequences identified by specific models.

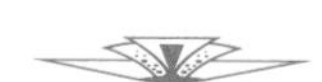

ONE MODEL VERSUS SEVERAL MODELS

Many nurses believe that having a single, universal model for nursing offers the following advantages:

- It would further the development of nursing as a profession.
- It would give all nurses a common framework, enhancing communication and research.
- It would promote understanding about the nurse's role in nontraditional nursing settings, such as independent nurse practitioner practice, self-help clinics, and health maintenance organizations (HMOs), correcting the common misconception that nurses provide care only for sick persons.

In contrast, advocates of several different conceptual models point out the following:

- Most disciplines have several conceptual models, which allow members to explore phenomena in different ways and from different viewpoints.
- Several models increase an understanding of the nature of nursing and its scope.
- Several models foster development of the full scope and potential of the discipline.

It is possible that in the 21st century many more models for nursing will be developed or that existing ones will be refined in accordance with societal needs and with their tested usefulness.

RELATIONSHIP OF THEORIES TO THE NURSING PROCESS

Conceptual models for nursing are abstractions that are operationalized or made real by the use of the nursing process. See Chapters 5 through 8 for detailed information on the nursing process. This systematic process, similar to the scientific or problem-solving process, consists of five steps:

1. *Assessing.* The specific data collected about a client's health needs relate directly to the second unit of the conceptual model for nursing, the client. For example, if the client is seen as having 14 fundamental needs, the nurse collects data about these 14 needs.
2. *Diagnosing.* In this step, the nurse analyzes assessment data to identify actual, potential, and possible nursing

diagnoses. The nurse outlines or writes the client's actual or potential health problems as a nursing diagnostic statement in accordance with the nursing model used.

3. *Planning.* Planning also relates directly to the conceptual nursing model. The nurse establishes goals for resolution of client problems, nursing interventions aimed at achieving those goals, and outcome criteria by which the nurse can evaluate whether or not the goals are met. These goals, interventions, and criteria are established in accordance with the modes of intervention outlined in the conceptual model.
4. *Implementing.* Implementing the planned interventions draws on scientific knowledge that is not part of the nursing model. The nursing model instructs the nurse what to do and directly influences what nursing interventions are planned, but it does not tell the nurse how to do it.
5. *Evaluating.* Evaluating is a continuous nursing function. How is the client adjusting and reacting? What does the client see as needs? How does the client see these needs changing? Has the client achieved the desired consequences? The answers to these questions help the nurse evaluate the effectiveness of the total nursing process and the nursing model.

CHAPTER HIGHLIGHTS

- As an increasingly emerging profession, nursing is now deeply involved in identifying its own unique knowledge base—that is, the body of knowledge essential to nursing practice, or a so-called nursing science.
- If nurses are to be considered health professionals, they must communicate exactly what makes their place in the interdisciplinary team unique and important.
- Theories offer ways of conceptualizing a discipline in clear, explicit terms that can be communicated to others.
- Because opinions about the nature and structure of nursing vary, theories continue to be developed. Each nursing theory bears the name of the person or group who developed it and reflects the beliefs of the developer.
- Nursing theories serve several essential purposes, some of which are to differentiate the focus of nursing from other professions; to structure professional nursing practice, education, and research; to help build a common nursing terminology to use in communicating with other health professionals; and to enhance autonomy of nursing through defining its own independent functions.
- Nursing theories address and specify relationships among four major concepts, the building blocks of theory: person or client, environment, health/illness, and nursing.
- Each nurse theorist's definitions of these four major concepts vary in accordance with personal philosophy, scientific orientation, experience in nursing, and how that experience has affected the theorist's view of nursing.
- Concepts in a conceptual framework are linked together to form a proposition, a statement that expresses the relationship between concepts and is capable of being tested, believed, or denied.
- Nursing theories included three elements: (a) a set of well-defined constructs, (b) a set of propositions, and (c) hypotheses.
- The major distinction between a theory and a conceptual framework or model is the level of abstraction, with the conceptual framework being more abstract than the theory. A conceptual model is a system of related concepts or a conceptual diagram. Its major purpose is to give clear and explicit direction to the three areas of nursing: practice, education, and research. A theory, in contrast, is more limited in scope. Its primary purpose is to generate knowledge in a field.
- Because the primary purpose of nursing theory is to generate scientific knowledge, nursing theory and nursing research are closely related. Scientific knowledge is derived from testing hypotheses generated by theories for nursing. Research determines the utility of those hypotheses, and research findings may be developed into theories for nursing.

- A number of theories have been developed by nurse theorists. The theories vary considerably in (a) their level of abstraction; (b) their conceptualization of the client, health/illness, and nursing; and (c) their ability to describe, explain, or predict. Some theories are broad in scope; others are limited.
- Definitions and a clear understanding of the terms *care* and *caring* are being developed. The major theorists involved to date are Leininger and Watson.
- To be effective in guiding nursing education and practice, conceptual frameworks include seven major elements: goal of nursing, view of client, role of the nurse, source of difficulty of the client,intervention focus, modes of intervention, and consequences of nursing activity.
- Conceptual models for nursing relate to the nursing process in that they are operationalized or made real by the use of the nursing process. How nurses view human beings influences how they assess and intervene.
- It is possible that in the 21st century many more models for nursing will be developed or that existing ones will be refined in accordance with societal needs and with their tested usefulness.

READINGS AND REFERENCES

SUGGESTED READINGS

Anderson, KH. Spring 1992. The family health system as an emerging paradigmatic view for nursing. *Image: Journal of Nursing Scholarship* 24:57–63.

This author explores the phenomena of family health from a nursing perspective by comparing the view of health in the discipline of nursing with the view of family health in multiple disciplines. Anderson proposes a holistic definition of family health for nursing, which includes five realms of family experience that make up the family health system. Anderson offers the proposed classification as a beginning model to organize the generation of knowledge for use in the practice of family nursing.

Nevin-Hass, M. February 1992. Checking the fit . . . nursing models: Are we buying or just looking? *Canadian Nurse* 88:33–34.

Nevin-Hass outlines the four hierarchic types of theories: factor-isolating, factor-relating, situation-relating, and situation-producing. The author then presents steps to analyze a nursing model, advising nurses that as "consumers" of these models, they must take time when "buying."

RELATED RESEARCH

von Essen, L and Sjoden, P. November 1991. Patient and staff perceptions of caring: Review and replication. *Journal of Advanced Nursing* 16:1363–74.

SELECTED REFERENCES

Chinn, PL, editor. 1991. *Anthology on Caring.* New York: NLN.
Chinn, PL and Kramer, MK. 1991. *Theory and Nursing.* 3d ed. St Louis: Mosby-Year Book.
Creasia, JL and Parker, B. 1991. *Conceptual Foundations of Professional Nursing Practice.* St Louis: Mosby-Year Book.
Doheny, M, Cook, C, and Stopper, C. 1992. *The Discipline of Nursing: An Introduction.* 3d ed. Norwalk, CT: Appleton & Lange.
George, JB, editor. 1990. *Nursing Theories: The Base for Professional Nursing Practice.* 3d ed. Norwalk, CT: Appleton & Lange.
Harmer, B and Henderson, V. 1955. *Textbook of the Principles and Practice of Nursing.* 5th ed. Riverside, NJ: Macmillan.
Henderson, V. 1966. *The Nature of Nursing: A Definition and Its Implications for Practice, Research, and Education.* Riverside, NJ: Macmillan.
———. October 1969. Excellence in nursing. *American Journal of Nursing* 69:2133–37.
———. 1978. The concept of nursing. *Journal of Advances in Nursing* 3:113–30.
Henderson, V and Nite, G. 1978. *The Principles and Practice of Nursing.* 6th ed. Riverside, NJ: Macmillan.
Johnson, DE. 1980. The behavioral system model for nursing. In Riehl, JP and Roy C, editors. pp. 207–16. *Conceptual Models for Nursing Practice.* 2d ed. Norwalk, CT: Appleton-Century-Crofts.
King, IM. 1971. *Toward a Theory for Nursing: General Concepts of Human Behavior.* New York: Wiley.
———. 1981. *A Theory for Nursing: Systems, Concepts, Process.* New York: Wiley.
———. 1987. King's theory of goal attainment. In Parse, RR, editor. *Nursing Science: Major Paradigms, Theories, and Critiques.* Philadelphia: WB Saunders.
———. 1989. King's general systems framework and theory. In Riehl-Sisca, J, editor. pp. 149–58. *Conceptual Models for Nursing Practice.* 3d ed. Norwalk, CT: Appleton & Lange.
Leininger, MM. 1978. *Transcultural Nursing: Concepts, Theories, and Practices.* New York: Wiley.
———. October 1980. Caring: A central focus of nursing and health care services. *Nursing and Health Care* 1(3): 135–43.
———. 1981. The phenomenon of caring: Importance, research questions and theoretical considerations. In *Caring: An Essential Human Need.* Proceedings of the three national caring conferences. pp. 3–15. Thorofare, NJ: Charles B. Slack.
———. 1984. *Care: The Essence of Nursing and Health.* Thorofare, NJ: Charles B. Slack.
———. November 1988. Leininger's theory of nursing: Cultural care, diversity and universality. *Nursing Science Quarterly* 1 (4):152–60.
Mariner-Tomey, A. 1989. *Nursing theorists and their work.* 2d ed. St Louis: Mosby.
Neuman, B. 1974. The Betty Neuman health-care systems model: A total person approach to patient problems. In Riehl, JP and Roy, C, editors. *Conceptual Models for Nursing Practice.* New York: Appleton-Century-Crofts.

______. 1980. The Betty Neuman health-care systems model: A total person approach to patient problems. In Riehl, JP and Roy, C, editors. pp. 119–31. *Conceptual Models for Nursing Practice.* 2d ed. New York: Appleton-Century Crofts.

______. 1982. *The Neuman Systems Model: Applications to Nursing Education and Practice.* New York: Appleton-Century-Crofts.

______. 1989. *The Neuman Systems Model: Applications to Nursing Education and Practice.* 2d ed. Norwalk, CT: Appleton & Lange.

Neuman, BM and Young, RJ. May/June 1972. A model for teaching total person approach to patient problems. *Nursing Research* 21:264–69.

Nicoll, LH. 1992. *Perspectives on Nursing Theory.* 2d ed. Philadelphia: Lippincott.

Nightingale, F. [originally published 1860] 1957. *Notes on Nursing.* Philadelphia: Lippincott.

Orem, DE. 1971. *Nursing: Concepts of Practice.* Hightstown, NJ: McGraw-Hill.

______. 1980. *Nursing: Concepts of Practice.* 2d ed. Hightstown, NJ: McGraw-Hill.

______. 1985. *Nursing: Concepts of Practice.* 3d ed. Hightstown, NJ: McGraw-Hill.

______. 1991. *Nursing: Concepts of Practice.* 4th ed. St Louis: Mosby-Year Book.

Parker, ME, editor. 1990. *Nursing Theories in Practice.* New York: NLN.

Peplau, HE. 1952. *Interpersonal Relations in Nursing.* New York: Putnam.

______. October/November 1963. Interpersonal relations and the process of adaptations. *Nursing Science* 1(4): 272–79.

______. 1980. The Peplau developmental model for nursing practice. In Riehl, JP and Roy, C, editors. pp. 53–73. *Conceptual Models for Nursing Practice.* 2d ed. New York: Appleton-Century-Crofts.

Rogers, ME. 1970. *An Introduction to the Theoretical Basis of Nursing.* Philadelphia: FA Davis.

______. 1980. Nursing: A science of unitary man. In Riehl, JP and Roy, C, editors. pp. 329–37. *Conceptual Models for Nursing Practice.* 2d ed. New York: Appleton-Century-Crofts.

______. 1983. Science of unitary human beings: A paradigm for nursing. In Clements, IW and Roberts, FB, editors. pp. 219–28. *Family Health: A Theoretical Approach to Nursing Care.* New York: Wiley.

______. 1986. Science of unitary human beings. In Malinski, VM, editor. pp. 3–8. *Exploration on Martha Rogers' Science of Unitary Human Beings.* Norwalk, CT: Appleton-Century-Crofts.

______. 1989. Nursing: A science of unitary human beings. In Riehl-Sisca, J. editor. pp. 181–88. *Conceptual models for nursing practice.* 3d ed. Norwalk, CT: Appleton & Lange.

Roy, C. March 1970. Adaptation: A conceptual framework in nursing. *Nursing Outlook* 18:42–45.

______. 1976. *Introduction to Nursing: An Adaptation Model.* Englewood Cliffs, NJ: Prentice Hall.

______. 1980. The Roy adaptation model. In Riehl, JP and Roy, C, editors. pp. 179–88. *Conceptual Models for Nursing Practice.* 2d ed. New York: Appleton-Century-Crofts.

______. 1984. *Introduction to Nursing: An Adaptation Model.* 2d ed. Englewood Cliffs, NJ: Prentice Hall.

______. 1989. The Roy adaptation model. In Riehl-Sisca, J, editor. pp. 105–14. *Conceptual Models for Nursing Practice.* 3d ed. Norwalk, CT: Appleton & Lange.

Roy, C and Andrews, HA. 1991. *The Roy Adaptation Model: The Definitive Statement.* Norwalk, CT: Appleton & Lange.

Sarter, B. 1988. *The Stream of Becoming: A Study of Martha Rogers' Theory.* NLN Pub No. 15-2205. New York: NLN.

Watson, J. 1979. *Nursing: The Philosophy and Science of Caring.* Boston: Little, Brown.

______. 1985. *Nursing: Human Science and Human Care.* Norwalk, CT: Appleton-Century-Crofts.

______. 1988. *Nursing: Human Science and Human Care. A Theory of Nursing.* NLN Pub No. 15-2236. New York: NLN.

______. 1989. Watson's philosophy and theory of human caring. In Riehl-Sisca, J, editor. pp. 219–36. *Conceptual Models for Nursing Practice.* 3d ed. Norwalk, CT: Appleton & Lange.

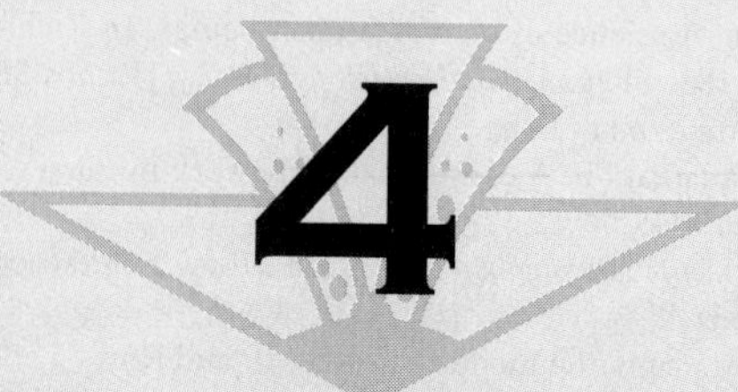

Health Care Delivery Systems

Objectives

Differentiate primary, secondary, and tertiary health care delivery services.

Describe the functions and purposes of the health care agencies outlined in this chapter.

Identify the roles of various health care professionals.

Discuss health care as a right and the essentials of the Patient's Bill of Rights.

Describe the effects of specific social, legislative, and technologic changes on health care delivery.

Identify ways in which the nurse can help people make the best use of health care services when seeking health care.

Compare various systems of payment for health care services.

Discuss contemporary issues and problems in the health care system.

Identify the basic components of nursing's "core of care" as developed by the American Nurses Association in *Nursing's Agenda for Health Care Reform.*

Describe the concept of case management and critical pathways.

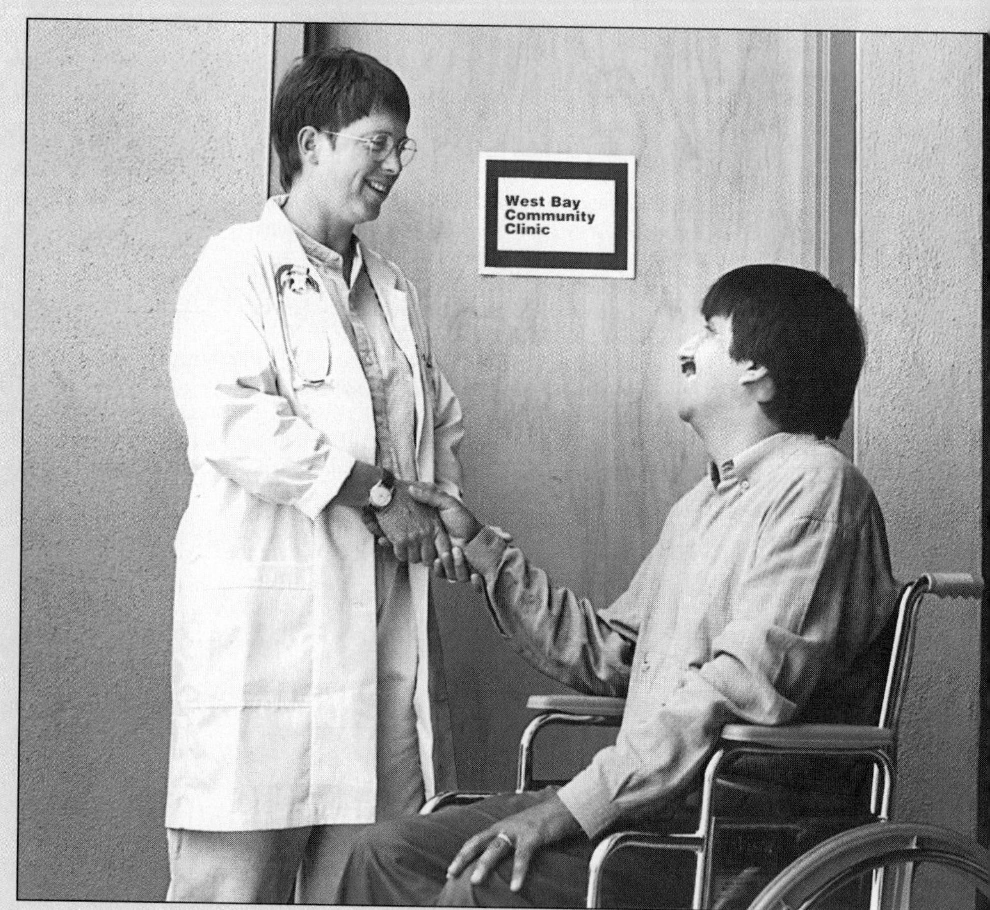

A health care system is the totality of services offered by all health disciplines. Traditionally, the primary purpose of a health care system had been to offer care to the ill and the injured; for this reason, the health care system of the past might be more accurately described as an "illness care system." However, it has been undergoing considerable change in recent years. The awareness of health promotion and disease prevention is increasing, as is the emphasis on the role of nurses in these areas.

Today's health care system is large and highly complex. It has a multilevel organizational structure involving a variety of agencies and a myriad of health professionals. The specialization of knowledge has resulted in the specialization of health professionals, health agencies, and hospital units.

Currently, nurses and other health professionals—and governments—are helping people become more aware of health as a way of life. For example, the health care system is doing more to alert people to the ill effects of smoking, excessive alcohol consumption, illicit drug use, and the overuse of prescribed and over-the-counter medications, rather than focusing only on treating the consequences of these activities. The health care system is also putting greater emphasis on measures to prevent disease or reduce risks. Examples of such measures include immunizing children; reducing the incidence of road accidents, particularly among adolescents; and preventing accidents in the home, especially among children and older people.

Rights of Health Care

The movement for clients' rights in health care arose in the late 1960s. At that time, the broad goals of the movement were to improve the quality of health care and to make the health care system more responsive to clients' needs. Today, clients are also seeking more self-determination and control over their own bodies when they are ill. Informed consent, confidentiality, and the right of the client to refuse treatment are all aspects of this self-determination. The need for clients' rights is largely the result of two circumstances: the vulnerability of the client because of illness and the complexity of the relationships in the health care setting.

When people are ill, they are frequently unable to assert their rights as they would if they were healthy. Asserting rights requires energy and an underlying awareness of one's rights in the situation.

Today, the goals of health include the return of autonomy and independence to the client and the acceptance of good health as a responsibility of the client, the care providers, and society. These goals cannot be met unless clients accept active responsibility for their health and health care and unless clients and care providers have mutual respect.

In 1973, the American Hospital Association (AHA) published "A Patient's Bill of Rights" to promote the rights of hospitalized clients. These were revised in 1992.

Included in this Bill of Rights are the right of a client to considerate and respectful care; consideration of privacy for the client, including confidentiality of all records and communications regarding their care; and the right to make decisions about their care, including the right to refuse a treatment or plan of care. In addition, a client has a right to make a statement such as a living will, which should be followed by the agency as permitted by law.

The AHA Bill of Rights states that a client has the right to review all their medical records and have them explained; to receive requested care and services, provided these are reasonable; and to be informed of any business arrangements among institutions or people involved in their care. In addition, a client has the right to be informed of resources that can be used to resolve a dispute or grievance and of hospital policies and practices that relate to client care, treatment, and responsibilities, and to be informed of hospital charges and available payment methods. Furthermore, the AHA bill states that a client has the right to refuse to participate in any research study, to expect a reasonable continuity of care, and to have options explained when hospital care is no longer appropriate.

This Bill of Rights also states that health care agencies must advise clients of their rights, under state laws and hospital policy, to make informed choices about their treatment. The client should be asked about any advance directive (eg, not to be resuscitated in event of a cardiac arrest), and this information must be on the client's record. If the hospital's policy limits its ability to implement any advance directive, the client has a right to be informed of this before any problem arises.

If a client lacks decision-making capacity, is legally incompetent, or is a minor, these rights can be exercised on their behalf by a designated surrogate or proxy decision-maker.

Types of Health Care Delivery Services

A great variety of health care services is available to clients. Health care delivery services can be categorized according to the complexity of the services provided; primary, secondary, or tertiary (Table 4–1, p. 64). Generally,

Table 4–1 Types of Health Care Service Classified According to Increasing Complexity

Type	Service
Primary Care	Health promotion
	Preventive care
	Continuing care for common health problems
	Integrates and explains client's or family's overall health problems
	Gives adequate attention to psychologic and social dimensions
	Refers clients to specialists
Secondary Care	Surgery and services by specialists, such as cardiologists and endocrinologists
Tertiary Care	Advanced specialized diagnostic, therapeutic, and rehabilitative care

health care services can also be grouped according to the type of service: (1) health promotion and illness prevention, (2) diagnosis and treatment, and (3) rehabilitation. See also Levels of Prevention in Chapter 13, page 260.

Health Promotion and Illness Prevention Health promotion was slow to develop until the 1980s. Since that time, more and more people are recognizing that keeping healthy is preferable to treating injury and illness. Health promotion programs address healthy eating, weight control, stress reduction, and stopping smoking, for example. These activities take place in a variety of settings, including hospitals and community centers, and nurses are active in many of these programs. See Chapter 13.

The health care system also offers illness prevention programs. They may be directed at the client or the community and involve such practices as providing immunizations, identifying risk factors for illnesses (eg, cardiovascular disease), and helping people take measures to prevent these illnesses from occurring. Illness prevention also includes environmental programs that can reduce the incidence of illness or disability. Examples are restricting burning to decrease air pollution and requiring inspections to ensure acceptable levels of fumes from automobile exhaust systems. Environmental protective measures are frequently legislated by governments.

Diagnosis and Treatment Traditionally, the largest segment of the health care system has been dedicated to the diagnosis and treatment of illness. Hospitals and physicians' offices are the major agencies offering these services. More recently, community clinics have also provided these services. For example, clinics in some communities provide mammograms and education about early detection of cancer of the breast. Some shopping malls and shopping centers have walk-in clinics that provide selected diagnostic tests, such as screening for cholesterol levels and blood sugar levels.

Rehabilitation Rehabilitation is a process of restoring people to useful function in physical, mental, social, economic, and vocational areas of their lives. Rehabilitation, then, is a process of restoring people to their previous level of health (ie, to their previous capabilities) or to the level that is possible for them. Rehabilitation, as distinct from maintenance, is an active concept and can be considered largely an educational function.

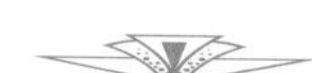

PROVIDERS OF HEALTH CARE

The providers of health care, also referred to as the health care team or health professionals, are health personnel from different disciplines who coordinate their skills to assist a client and/or support persons. Their mutual goal is to restore a client's health and promote wellness. The choice of personnel for a particular client depends on the needs of the client. In the present system of health care in North America, health teams commonly include nurses, advanced practice nurses, physicians, physicians' assistants, dentists, pharmacists, dietitians, physiotherapists, respiratory therapists, occupational therapists, paramedical technologists, social workers, and chaplains.

Nurse The role of the nurse varies with the needs of the situation. As nursing roles have expanded, new dimensions for nursing practice have been established. See Chapter 1 for the roles of the nurse. Nurses can pursue a variety of practice specialties (eg, critical care, pediatrics) in a multitude of settings.

Various nursing personnel often participate actively on a health team. Nursing assistants and vocational (practical) nurses are often important members of the nursing group. Registered nurses often coordinate the health care team, and may work with advanced practice nurses (APNs) in the care of clients. APNs may be **Certified Nurse Midwives (CNM), Nurse Anesthetists (CRNA), Nurse Practitioners (NP),** or **Clinical Nurse Specialists (CNS).**

Physician A physician is a person who has successfully completed a course of medical studies and is licensed to practice medicine in a particular jurisdiction. In a hospital setting, the physician is responsible for medical diagnosis and for determining the therapy required by a person who has a disease or injury. The traditional role of the physician is the treatment of disease and trauma (injury). However, many physicians, especially family practice physicians, are now including health promotion and disease prevention in their practice. Some physicians are specialists in surgery and are referred to as surgeons. An example is a neurosurgeon or an orthopedic surgeon. Some physicians extend their roles by employing a **physician's assistant (PA)** who is educated to perform certain tasks and authorized to practice under the direction of the physician. In many states, nurses are not legally permitted to follow a PA's orders unless they are co-signed by a physician. PAs do not practice in Canada at the time of writing.

Dentist Dentists diagnose and treat dental problems. Dentists are also actively involved in preventive measures to maintain healthy oral structures (eg, teeth and gums).

Pharmacist A pharmacist prepares and dispenses pharmaceuticals in hospital and community settings. The role of the pharmacist in monitoring and evaluating the actions and effects of medications on clients is becoming increasingly prominent. Pharmacists are also actively involved in preparing individual dosages for clients in hospitals that employ the unit dose system. In some settings, pharmacists prepare medications for intravenous therapy. A **clinical pharmacist** is a specialist who guides physicians in prescribing medications. A **pharmacy assistant** is also recognized in some states. This person administers medications to clients or works in the pharmacy under the direction of the pharmacist.

Dietitian or Nutritionist When dietary and nutritional services are required, the dietitian or nutritionist may be a member of a health team. A **dietitian,** often a registered dietitian (RD), has special knowledge about the diets required to maintain health and to treat disease. A **nutritionist** is a person who has special knowledge about nutrition and food. Dietitians and nutritionists may work in a hospital or in the community to educate clients about therapeutic diets, assist with preparation of special diets, or promote health and prevent disease by advising families about balanced diets.

Physiotherapist The physiotherapist (PT), or physical therapist, assists clients with musculoskeletal problems. Physiotherapists treat the body by means of heat, water, exercise, massage, and electric current. They provide physical therapy in response to a physician's order. The physiotherapist's functions include assessing clients' mobility and strength, providing therapeutic measures (eg, exercises and heat applications to improve mobility and strength), and teaching new skills (eg, how to walk with an artificial leg). Most physiotherapists provide their services in hospitals; however, independent practitioners establish offices in communities and serve clients either at the office or in the home.

Respiratory Therapist A respiratory therapist (RT) is skilled in therapeutic measures used in the care of clients with respiratory problems. These therapists are knowledgeable about oxygen therapy devices, intermittent positive pressure breathing respirators, artificial mechanical ventilators, and accessory devices used in inhalation therapy. Respiratory therapists are able to administer many of the pulmonary function tests.

Occupational Therapist An occupational therapist (OT) assists clients with some impaired function to gain the skills to perform activities of daily living. For example, an occupational therapist might teach a man with severe arthritis in his arms and hands how to adjust his kitchen utensils so that he can continue to cook. The therapist also teaches skills that are therapeutic and at the same time provide some satisfaction. For example, weaving is a recreational activity but also exercises the arthritic man's arm and hands.

Paramedical Technologists Laboratory technologists, radiologic technologists, and nuclear medicine technologists are just three kinds of paramedical technologists in an expanding field of medical technology. **Paramedical** means having some connection with medicine. Laboratory technologists examine specimens such as urine, feces, blood, and discharges from wounds to provide exact information that facilitates the medical diagnosis and the prescription of a therapeutic regimen. The radiologic technologist assists with a wide variety of X-ray film procedures, from simple chest radiography to more complex fluoroscopy. The nuclear medicine technologist uses radioactive substances to provide diagnostic information, for example, about a client's liver, and can administer therapeutic doses of radioactive materials as part of a therapeutic regimen. These technologists have highly specialized skills and knowledge important to client care.

Social Worker A social worker counsels clients and support persons about social problems, such as finances, marital difficulties, and adoption of children. It is not unusual for health problems to produce problems in living and vice versa. For example, an elderly woman who lives alone and has a stroke resulting in impaired walking may find it impossible to continue to live in her third-floor apartment. Finding a more suitable living arrangement can be the responsibility of the social worker if the client has no support network in place.

Chaplains Hospital chaplains serve as part of the health care team by attending to the spiritual needs of clients. In most facilities, local clergy volunteer their services on a regular or "on-call" basis. Hospitals affiliated with specific religions, as well as many large medical centers, have full-time chaplains on staff. The nurse is often instrumental in identifying the client's desire to see a chaplain.

Case Managers The case manager's role is to ensure fiscally sound, appropriate care in the best setting. This role is often filled by the member of the health care team who is most involved in the client's care. Depending on the nature of the client's concerns, the case manager may be a nurse, a social worker, an occupational therapist, a physical therapist, or any member of the health care team.

Alternative Providers Chiropractors, herbalists, acupuncturists, and other nontraditional health care providers are playing increasing roles in the contemporary health care system. These providers may practice alongside traditional health care providers, or clients may use their services in conjunction with, or in lieu of, traditional therapies.

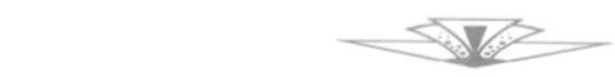

HEALTH CARE AGENCIES

Health care agencies in the United States and Canada are both varied and numerous. In addition, the same services may be found in several agencies. For example, hospice services may be provided in the home by a community agency, in a hospice unit of a hospital, or in an institution devoted solely to hospice care. With such an array of health care services and agencies, the nurse often needs to help clients choose a service that best suits their needs.

Agencies can be categorized in various ways, such as inpatient or outpatient, institutional or community. Hospitalization is an inpatient service. Care given in a physician's office or ambulatory care center is an outpatient service.

Hospitals Hospitals traditionally have provided restorative care to the ill and injured. They vary in size from the 12-bed rural hospital to the 1500-bed metropolitan hospital with a 50-bed day-surgery center. Hospitals can be classified according to their ownership or control as governmental (public) and nongovernmental (private). In the United States, governmental hospitals are either federal, state, city, or county hospitals; in Canada, they are federal or provincial hospitals. In both countries, federal governments have traditionally provided hospital facilities for veterans and merchant mariners. Military hospitals provide care to military personnel and their families. Private hospitals are often operated by churches, companies, communities, and charitable organizations. Private hospitals may be for-profit or not-for-profit.

Although hospitals are chiefly viewed as institutions that provide care, they have other functions, such as providing resources for health-related research and teaching.

Hospitals also are classified by the services they provide. General hospitals admit clients requiring a variety of services, such as medical, surgical, obstetric, pediatric, and psychiatric services. Other hospitals offer only specialty services, such as psychiatric or pediatric care.

Hospitals can be further described as acute care or chronic (long-term) care. An acute care hospital provides assistance to clients who are acutely ill or whose illness and need for hospitalization are relatively short-term, for example, 2 days. Long-term care hospitals provide health services for longer periods, sometimes for years or the remainder of the client's life.

Hospitals in the United States have undergone massive change. Some hospitals have merged or been sold to large multihospital for-profit corporations (eg, Humana, Inc., and Hospital Corporation of America).

Another change that has occurred relates to the client population. Most clients in hospitals are seriously ill; others less ill are treated outside the hospital setting. Because so many of the seriously ill are elderly, some general hospitals are becoming acute care hospitals solely for the elderly. Because of the increasing acuity of illness among clients, general hospitals have virtually become intensive care centers.

Hospitals provide a variety of health care services. The large urban hospital usually has inpatient beds, emergency facilities, diagnostic facilities, day-surgery, pharmacy services, and intensive care and coronary care units. Some large hospitals have other specialized services, such as a spinal cord injury unit, burn unit, and oncology unit. In addition, some hospitals have added substance abuse treatment units and health promotion units. Small rural hospitals are often limited to inpatient beds, radiologic and laboratory services, and emergency services. The number of services a rural hospital provides is usually directly related to its size and its distance from an urban center.

Long-Term Care Facilities Traditionally, all long-term care facilities were called nursing homes. Long-term care facilities now include skilled nursing facilities for extended care, intermediate care, and personal care for those who are chronically ill or are unable to care for themselves without assistance. Because clients are being discharged earlier from acute care hospitals, some clients require supplemental care in a long-term care facility before they return home.

Because long-term illness occurs most often in the elderly, many long-term care facilities have programs that are oriented to the needs of this age group. Long-term care facilities are intended for people who require not only personal services (such as meal preparation and assistance in bathing and dressing) but also some regular nursing care and occasional medical attention. However, the type of care provided varies considerably. Some facilities admit and retain only residents who can dress themselves and are ambulatory. Other long-term care facilities provide bed care for clients who are more incapacitated. These facilities can, in effect, become the client's home, and consequently the people who live there are frequently referred to as residents rather than patients or clients.

In 1987, as part of the Omnibus Budget Reconciliation Act (OBRA), the Congress of the United States passed legislation to bring a measure of quality assurance to the nursing home industry. In response to growing concern about whether minimal essential standards were being met in many nursing home facilities, OBRA instituted requirements for nurse's aide training. Specific requirements include a 75-hour training program for nurse's aides and competence evaluation of nurse's aides.

Retirement Centers Another type of extended care facility is the retirement center or community, which comprises separate houses, condominiums, or apartments for its residents. Residents live relatively independently; however, many of these facilities offer meals, laundry service, nursing care, transportation, and social activities. Some centers have a separate hospital to care for residents with short-term or long-term illness. The retirement center is intended to meet the needs of people who are unable to remain at home but do not need nursing home care.

Rehabilitation Centers Rehabilitation centers usually are independent community centers or special units in hospitals. However, because rehabilitation ideally starts the moment a client enters the health care system, nurses who are employed on pediatric, psychiatric, or surgical units of hospitals also help rehabilitate clients. Today, the concept of rehabilitation is applied to all illness (physical and mental), to injury, and to chemical addiction. Drug and alcohol rehabilitation centers, for example, help free clients of drug and alcohol dependence.

Hospice Services Traditionally, a hospice was a place for travelers to rest. Recently, the term has come to mean a health care facility for the dying. The hospice movement subsumes a variety of services given to the terminally ill, their families, and support persons. The movement sprang initially from dissatisfaction with the health care community's preoccupation with technologic care and insufficient emphasis on caring and psychologic support. In the 1970s, the movement gained momentum. It derived impetus from new attitudes toward death and from the work of such people as Elisabeth Kübler-Ross, whose books challenged prevailing attitudes, and Cicely Saunders, founder of St. Christopher's Hospice in London, England. Saunders believed that the physical and social environments of dying people are as important as medical interventions on their behalf. The central concept of the hospice movement, as distinct from the acute care model, is not saving life but improving or maintaining the quality of life until death. For additional information, see Chapter 33, page 869.

Physicians' Offices In North America, the physician's office is a traditional primary care setting. The majority of physicians either have their own offices or work with several other physicians in a group practice. People usually go to a physician because they consider themselves ill, because a relative thinks the client is ill, or because the client needs medical advice.

Nurses employed in physicians' offices have a variety of roles. Some nurses carry out the traditional functions of registering the client, preparing the client for an examination or treatment, and providing information. Other nurses function as nurse practitioners and are responsible for providing primary care to clients in stable health.

Ambulatory Care Centers Ambulatory care centers are being used more frequently in many communities. Most ambulatory care centers have diagnostic and treatment facilities providing medical, nursing, laboratory, and radiologic services, and they may or may not be attached to or associated with an acute care hospital. Some ambulatory care centers provide services to people who require minor surgical procedures that can be performed outside the hospital. After surgery, the client returns home the same day. These centers offer two advantages: They permit the client to live at home while obtaining needed health care, and they free costly hospital beds for seriously ill clients. Nurses in ambulatory care centers frequently function as nurse practitioners or clinical nurse specialists, for example, in gastroenterology or urology.

The term *ambulatory care center* has replaced the term *clinic* in many places. The term *clinic* can refer to a department in a hospital or a group practice of physicians. Traditionally, a hospital clinic was called an outpatient clinic, serving only outpatients, as opposed to inpatients (those admitted to the hospital). The role of the nurse in a clinic may be similar to that of a nurse practitioner or a nurse in a physician's office.

Industrial Clinics The industrial clinic is gaining importance as a setting for primary care. Employee health has long been recognized as important to productivity. Today, more companies recognize the value of healthy employees and encourage healthy life-styles by providing exercise facilities and healthy snacks, such as fruit, instead of coffee. Also, more businesses are prohibiting smoking in the work setting.

Community health nurses in the occupational setting have a variety of roles. Worker safety has been a traditional concern of occupational nurses. Today, nursing functions include health education, screening for such health problems as hypertension and obesity, counseling, and initial care after accidents.

Health Maintenance Organizations A health maintenance organization (HMO) is a group health care agency that provides basic and supplemental health maintenance and treatment services to voluntary enrollees. A fee is set without regard to the amount or kind of services received.

The HMO plan stresses wellness; the better the health of the person, the less HMO services are needed and the greater the agency's profit. Because the emphasis is on health promotion and prevention of illness, nurses in HMOs focus on these aspects of care, frequently as nurse practitioners, client educators, and consultants.

HMOs have been established across the United States. The largest HMO, the Kaiser Permanente Medical Care Program, serves clients in 15 states plus Washington DC. Whereas a person with private health insurance can obtain services in most hospitals, clients of an HMO must use its facilities except under specific provisions such as extreme emergencies. Consequently, many HMOs offer a full range of services, including acute and long-term care. Services not offered directly by the HMO are often provided through cooperative arrangements with other facilities.

Preferred Provider Organizations and Preferred Provider Arrangements The preferred provider organization (PPO), which has emerged as another alternative in the health care delivery system, consists of a group of physicians and/or a hospital that provides an insurance company or employer with health services at a discounted rate. Hospitals, physicians, and insurance companies are the major sponsors of PPOs. Physicians can belong to one or several PPOs, and the client can choose among the physicians belonging to that PPO. PPOs were first established in 1980 in the United States.

Preferred provider arrangements (PPAs) are similar to PPOs. The main difference is that PPAs can be contracted with *individual* health care providers, whereas PPOs involve an organization of health care providers. A PPA plan can be limited or unlimited. A limited PPA restricts the client to use only preferred providers of health care; an unlimited PPA permits the client to use any health care provider in the area who accepts the contractual agreement of the plan.

Independent Practice Associations Independent practice associations (IPAs) are somewhat like HMOs and PPOs. The IPA provides care in offices, just as the providers belonging to a PPO do. The difference is that clients pay a fixed prospective payment to the IPA, and the IPA pays the provider. In some instances, the health care provider bills the IPA for services; in others, the provider receives a fixed fee for services given. At the end of the fiscal year, any surplus money is divided among the providers; any loss is assumed by the IPA.

Crisis Centers Crisis centers provide emergency services to clients experiencing life crises. These centers may operate out of a hospital or in the community, and most provide 24-hour telephone service. Some also provide direct counseling to people at the center or in their homes. The primary purpose of a crisis center is to help people cope with an immediate crisis and then provide guidance and support for long-term therapy.

Nurses working in crisis centers need well-developed communication and counseling skills. The nurse must immediately identify the person's problem, offer assistance to help the person cope, and perhaps later direct the person to resources for long-term support.

Home Health Care Agencies Home health care agencies are rapidly becoming major tertiary care providers. Home care is one aspect of comprehensive health care. Its purposes include promoting, maintaining, and restoring health—specifically, maximizing independent functioning and minimizing the disabling effects of illness, including terminal illness. Services appropriate to the needs of clients and their families are planned, coordinated, and delivered by providers organized for the delivery of home health care. The implementation of prospective payment (discussed later in this chapter on page 70) and the resulting earlier discharge of clients from hospitals have made home care an essential aspect of the health care delivery system.

As concerns about the cost of health care have escalated, the use of the home as a care delivery site has increased. In addition, the scope of services offered in the home has broadened. Home health care agencies offer education to clients and families, as well as provide comprehensive care to acute, chronic, and terminally ill clients. Often clients are referred to home health agencies for follow-up care after discharge from the hospital, or for skilled care that will allow the client to remain at home. Self-care and care given by health professionals and allied health personnel in the home account for the majority of health care provided in the United States today. The time a person spends in a hospital receiving care for acute conditions is generally a very small percentage of the person's life. The need for home care services is increasing as the population of the United States ages and the incidence of chronic illness increases correspondingly.

The scope of home care services has broadened to include both acute, short-term care as well as long-term monitoring of problems associated with chronic illness.

Community Health Agencies Community health agencies provide services to either geographic regions or specific populations. They may be independent agencies or they may be associated with other health facilities or affiliated with church or fraternal organizations. Examples of community health agencies include parish nursing services, senior centers, homeless food/health centers, or clinics designed for specific ethnic groups.

Mutual Support and Self-Help Groups In North America today, there are more than 500 mutual support or self-help groups that focus on nearly every major health problem or life crisis people experience. Such groups arose largely because people felt their needs were not being met by the existing health care system. Alcoholics Anonymous, which formed in 1935, served as the model for many of these groups. The National Self-Help Clearinghouse provides information on current support groups and guidelines about how to start a self-help group. The nurse's role in self-help groups is discussed in Chapter 18, page 376.

Day-Care Centers Day-care centers serve many functions and many age groups. Some day-care centers provide care for infants and children while parents work. Other centers provide care for adults who cannot be left at home alone but do not need to be in an institution. Elder care centers often provide care involving socializing, exercising programs, and stimulation. Some centers provide counseling and physical therapy. Nurses who are employed in day-care centers may provide medications, treatments, and counseling, thereby facilitating continuity with care in the home.

Rural Primary Care Rural primary care hospitals (RPCH) were created as a result of the 1987 Omnibus Budget Reconciliation Act (OBRA). They provide emergency care to clients in rural areas who require stabilization before transfer to a larger hospital. Usually, basic laboratory and radiologic services are also available.

Public Health Government (official) agencies are established at the local, state (or provincial), and federal levels to provide public health services. Health agencies at the state, county, or city level vary according to the need of the area. Their funds, generally from taxes, are administered by elected or appointed officials. Local health departments (county, bicounty, or tricounty) traditionally have responsibility for developing programs to meet the health needs of the people, providing the necessary staff and facilities to carry out these programs, continually evaluating the effectiveness of the programs, and monitoring changing needs. State health organizations are responsible for assisting the local health departments. In some remote areas, state departments also provide direct services to people.

The Public Health Service (PHS) of the United States Department of Health and Human Services is an official agency at the federal level. Its functions include conducting research and providing training in the health field, providing assistance to communities in planning and developing health facilities, and assisting states and local communities through financing and provision of trained personnel. Also at the national level in the United States are research institutions such as the National Institutes of Health (NIH). The National Institute on Drug Abuse, the National Institute on Alcohol Abuse and Alcoholism, and the National Institute of Mental Health work with federal, regional, and state agencies. The Centers for Disease Control (CDC) in Atlanta, Georgia, administer a broad program related to surveillance of diseases. By means of laboratory and epidemiologic investigations, data are made available to appropriate authorities. The CDC also publish recommendations about the prevention and control of infections and administer a national health program. The federal government also administers a number of Veterans Administration (VA) services in the United States.

The Canadian Department of Health and Welfare (CDHW) administers such federal programs as native health in the north and health care in the territories. However, provincial governments generally have responsibility for administering health services to the people of each province.

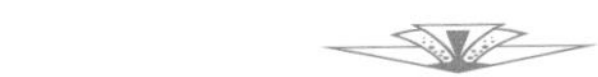

FINANCING HEALTH CARE

Because health care is so expensive, few people can afford to pay for their own health care from their resources. Therefore, government agencies and private organizations have developed health care insurance, prepaid plans, and federally funded programs to meet health care costs.

FEDERAL GOVERNMENT INSURANCE PLANS

Federal funding is largely through the social insurance programs Medicare and Medicaid in the United States, and the National Medical Care Insurance program in Canada.

United States In the United States, the 1965 **Medicare** amendments (Title 18) to the Social Security Act provided a national and state health insurance program for the aged. By the mid 1970s, virtually everyone over 65 years was protected by hospital insurance under Part A, which also includes posthospital extended care and home health benefits. Medicaid was established the same year under Title 19 of the Social Security Act. **Medicaid** is a federal public assistance program paid out of general taxes to people who require financial assistance, such as low-income groups.

In 1972, Congress directed the Department of Health, Education, and Welfare to create professional standards review organizations (PSROs) to monitor the appropriateness of hospital use under the Medicare and Medicaid programs. In 1974, the National Health Planning and Resources Development Act established health systems agencies (HSAs) throughout the United States for comprehensive health planning. In 1978, the Rural Health Clinics Act provided for the development of health care in medically underserved rural areas. This act opened the door for nurse practitioners to provide primary care.

In addition, disabled or blind persons may be eligible for special payments called **Supplemental Security Income (SSI)** benefits. These benefits are also available to people not eligible for Social Security, and payments are not restricted to health care costs. Clients often use this money to purchase medicines or to cover costs of extended health care.

Medicare Medicare covers people 65 years of age and older and people of any age who have kidney failure or other selected disabling conditions.

Medicare clients pay a deductible and coinsurance. **Coinsurance** is the 20% share of a payment that is paid by the client; the other 80% is paid by the government.

Medicare is divided into two parts: Part A is available to the disabled and people 65 years and over. It provides insurance toward hospitalization, home care, and hospice care. Part B is voluntary and provides partial coverage of physician services to people eligible for Part A. Clients pay a monthly premium for this coverage.

When Medicare was instituted in 1965, it was intended to provide care to the elderly. In 1972, its coverage was broadened to include permanently disabled workers and their dependents who are eligible for disability insurance under Social Security. In 1988, Congress expanded Medicare to include extremely expensive hospital care, "catastrophic care," and expensive drugs. This cost was initially borne by the elderly who could afford to pay, but as a result of their protests, this coverage was repealed.

Medicare does not cover dental care, dentures, eyeglasses, hearing aids, or examinations to prescribe and fit hearing aids. Most preventive care, including routine physical examinations and associated diagnostic tests, is also not included. Recently, there has been extensive debate in the United States about options to curtail Medicare expenses.

Medicaid Medicaid is a public assistance program paid out of general taxes for people who require financial assistance (ie, low-income groups). Medicaid is paid by federal and state governments. Each state program is distinct. Some states provide very limited coverage, whereas others pay for dental care, eyeglasses, and prescription drugs.

Prospective Payment System To curtail health care costs in the United States, Congress in 1983 passed legislation putting the prospective payment system (PPS) into effect. This legislation limits the amount paid to hospitals that are reimbursed by Medicare. Reimbursement is made according to a classification system known as **diagnostic related groups (DRGs).**

Under this system, the hospital is paid a predetermined amount for clients with a specific diagnosis. For example, a hospital that admits a client with a diagnosis of uncomplicated asthma is reimbursed a specified amount, such as $1300, regardless of the cost of services, the length of the stay, or the acuity or complexity of the client's illness. Prospective payment or billing is formulated before the client is even admitted to the hospital; thus, the record of admission, rather than the record of treatment, now governs payment. As a result, hospitals have attempted to decrease costs by limiting inpatient length of stay and increasing use of nonacute care services, such as outpatient surgery, ambulatory care, and home health care.

Canada The Canadian National Hospital Insurance program was started in 1958, and the National Medical Care Insurance program (Medicare) began in 1968. Through these programs, every Canadian can obtain health insurance. Not all hospital and medical services are covered by provincial hospital insurance or Medicare plans; there are slight differences between provinces. The Canada Health Act was passed in 1984 by Parliament to provide federal government reimbursement to provincial governments for health services they provide. This act replaced two acts: the Hospital Insurance and Diagnostic Services Act and the Medical Care Act. The new act penalizes provinces that permit extra billing of clients by physicians by a levy of a dollar-for-dollar assessment. The act also creates incentives for home care, community health clinics, and health promotion.

Through this act, Canadians can be hospitalized without client cost; the hospitals are financed through taxation. Medical services are provided through an insurance program partially funded by clients and/or employers. In 1992, people living in British Columbia paid a $420 (Cdn) annual fee to the provincial government for medical coverage. In this plan, Canadians can choose their own physician.

The Canadian Nurses Association (CNA) is actively lobbying for health care reform. It continues to advocate a greater emphasis on health promotion, illness prevention, and community participation in decisions regarding health care. Although nurse practitioners at time of writing are not practicing in Canada, the possibility of their becoming an access point to the health care system is under discussion.

Australia Australia's Medicare system provides health care for all who are legally permanent residents of Australia or are visitors from countries with which Australia has a health care agreement. The Medicare system consists of three parts: (1) free or subsidized treatment by a general practitioner, medical specialist, or optometrist, (2) free treatment as public patients in a public hospital, and (3) subsidized prescription medicines. Clients may choose their own general practitioner; however, treatment by a specialist requires referral by a general practitioner.

The Medicare system is funded through the Australian tax system and pays 85% of the Schedule fee, which is set by the government. If a client or client family spends in excess of a government-set amount on health care costs within a given year (A$247.90 in 1993), the Medicare system will pay 100% of Schedule fees for the remainder of that year through the Medicare Safety Net. This entitlement is designed to protect individuals and families from high medical expenses.

Australia's public hospital system is funded jointly by the Commonwealth, State, and Territory governments and is administered by the State/Territory Health Departments. Medicare does not pay for private accommodation in either a public or private hospital, so individuals who choose to be treated as private patients must pay the difference between the amount Medicare subsidizes and the cost of service. Medicare pays 75% of the Schedule fee for private physician services. Private patient services can also be paid for through private insurance such as Medibank Private.

GROUP PLANS

Health care group plans provide blanket medical service in exchange for a predetermined monthly payment.

A variety of group plans have come into existence to finance health care in the United States. These include health maintenance organizations (HMOs), preferred provider organizations (PPOs), and preferred provider arrangements (PPAs). See earlier in this chapter, page 68.

Each group plan offers different options for consumers to consider when choosing a prepaid health care program.

PRIVATE INSURANCE

In the United States, numerous commercial health insurance carriers offer a wide range of coverage plans. There are two types of private health insurance: not-for-profit (eg, Blue Cross–Blue Shield) and for-profit (eg, commercial companies such as Metropolitan Life, Travelers, and Aetna). Private health insurance is known as *third-party* reimbursement because the insurance company pays either the entire bill or, more often, 80% of the costs.

With these plans, insurance may be purchased either as an individual plan or as part of a group plan through a person's employer, union, student association, or similar organization. The individual usually pays a monthly premium to obtain this protection. Group plans offer premiums at lower cost. Some employers share the costs of the premiums, and this benefit is often a major item in labor contracts. About one-third of all personal health services were paid for by private health insurance in 1988, and about 80% of private health insurance is provided by employers for employees (Jonas 1992, p. 129).

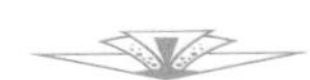

ISSUES AND PROBLEMS IN HEALTH CARE DELIVERY

Major advances in medicine and technology have meant better care for many. With this improved care, however, have come such problems as fragmentation of care and high costs.

Other issues and problems have always existed with health care delivery systems and are present today. Some of these are unmet needs of low-income people and the special needs of the homeless and the elderly. Another problem is uneven national distribution of health care services; limited resources are available in rural and inner-city areas, whereas more services are available in more prosperous urban and suburban areas. The consumer is becoming more aware of these problems and is exerting increasing pressure to have them corrected, but corrections are gradual and must accommodate to economic and political realities.

The following are some of the issues and problems that currently impact the health care delivery system.

THE CONSUMER

A **consumer** is a person who uses a product or a service. Today's health care consumers have greater knowledge about their health than in previous years and they are increasingly influencing health care delivery. Formerly, people expected a physician to make decisions about their care; today, however, consumers expect to be involved in making any decisions.

Consumers have also become aware of how life-style affects health. As a result, they desire more information and services related to health promotion and illness prevention. Legislation requiring that clients give informed consent before receiving many treatments has encouraged both consumers' desire for knowledge and their influence on health care. See Chapter 12, page 228, for more information about informed consent.

LEGISLATION

Legislation continually affects health care. For example, political decisions have a great impact on health insurance programs, health care funding, and the allocation of resources such as money, people, and equipment.

In the United States, legislation was passed in 1983 to bring about the *prospective payment system* (PPS), which limits the amount of money paid to hospitals that are reimbursed by Medicare. See Prospective Payment System on page 70.

THE WOMEN'S MOVEMENT

The women's movement has been instrumental in changing health care practices. Examples are the provision of childbirth services in more relaxed settings, such as birthing centers, and the provision of overnight facilities for parents in children's hospitals. The literature on the health concerns of women and research into women's unique health experiences are growing.

FAMILY CHARACTERISTICS

The characteristics of the North American family have changed considerably in the last few decades. The number of single-parent families has increased markedly. Most single-parent families are headed by women, many of whom work and require assistance when a child is ill at home.

Recognition of the cultural diversity of the United States and Canada is also increasing. Health care services are aware of this diversity and employing means to meet the challenges it presents. For example, more agencies are employing nurses who can communicate with non-English-speaking clients in their own language.

NUMBER OF ELDERLY

In 1988, 12.4% of the population in the United States was elderly. By the year 2000 it is estimated that it will be 13%, with the highest increase among people 85 years and older (US DHHS 1991, p. 23). Longterm illnesses are prevalent among this group and frequently require special housing, treatment services, financial support, and social networks.

In Canada a similar increase in the number of older people is anticipated: from 3.9 million in the year 2000 to 4.9 million by 2011 (Statistics Canada 1991, pp. 139, 150). Because only 5% of older people are institutionalized with health problems, substantial home management and nursing support services are required to assist those in their homes and communities.

The frail aged population over age 85 are projected to be the fastest growing population in North America and will constitute 14% of the elderly by 2030 (Lee & Estes 1990, p. 77).

The elderly also need to feel they are still part of a community even though they are approaching the end of their lives. The feeling of being a useful, wanted, and productive citizen is essential to every person's health. Special programs are being designed in communities so that the talents and skills of this group will be used and not lost to society. These programs—partial employment, for example—are designed especially for the elderly person.

ADVANCES IN KNOWLEDGE AND TECHNOLOGY

Scientific knowledge and technology related to health care are rapidly increasing. Improved diagnostic procedures permit early recognition of diseases that might otherwise have remained undetected. New antibiotics are continually being manufactured to treat infections. Surgical procedures involving the heart, lungs, and liver that were nonexistent 20 years ago are common today.

These discoveries have changed the profile of the hospital client. People who have pneumonia, for example, are rarely hospitalized, and poliomyelitis, smallpox, and diphtheria—diseases that people were routinely hospitalized for—are now rarely encountered. Thirty years ago, a person having cataract surgery had to remain in bed in the hospital for 10 days; today, most cataract removals are performed in day surgery. However, present-day hospitals have clients who undergo intricate surgical procedures and are seriously ill during hospitalization.

ECONOMIC FACTORS

The health care delivery system is very much affected by a country's total economic status. Inflation and the economic recession of the 1980s and early 1990s brought increasing concern about escalating health care costs. The United States spends $1 billion a day on health care, and costs are still rising. Medical care costs have increased more than 400% since 1965. They increased an average of 12.6% annually between 1970 and 1984 and currently account for about 11.1% of the gross national product (GNP) (Jonas 1992, p. 1). In Canada, health care expenditures have increased at a similar rate. In 1988, health care costs were 8.7% of the GNP (Deber et al 1991, p. 72). Some reasons for this sizable increase are advanced techniques and technology, inflation, increased utilization of health services, and the system of payment for hospitals and physicians.

Unemployment and poverty affect which health services are offered and used. Because the unemployed do not receive employment-based health insurance, they do not use health care services to the same extent as the general population. Even though some government aid is available, eligibility for government insurance programs and benefits varies considerably from state to state. Canada's economic problems are similar to those of the United States; however, the overall effects are not always as apparent because Canada has a smaller population.

FRAGMENTATION OF CARE

Because of the highly specialized techniques and new knowledge that have emerged during the past 30 years of research, an increasing number of health care personnel provide specialized services. They may be highly specialized technicians or technologists who have relatively narrow but exacting jobs, such as respiratory technologists, biomedical electronic technologists, and nuclear medicine technologists. Increased specialization is evident also among physicians. The largest physician specialities are general and family practice and internal medicine. This specialization leads to fragmentation of care and, often, increased cost of care. To clients, it may mean receiving care from 5 to 30 people during their hospital experience. This seemingly endless stream of personnel is often confusing and frightening.

INCREASED COST OF SERVICES

The problem of financing health care services is becoming increasingly severe. There are five major reasons for increased costs:

1. Existing equipment and facilities are continually becoming obsolete as research uncovers new and better methods in health care.
2. Additional sophisticated equipment is required to provide the newest diagnostic and treatment methods, and staff must be educated in its use.
3. Inflation increases all costs.
4. The total population has increased, and the demand for services has changed. Increasingly health care is directed at chronic illness management.
5. The relative number of people who provide health care services has increased.

HEALTH CARE FOR THE HOMELESS

The number of homeless people in towns and cities continues to grow. Estimates vary widely, but advocates of the homeless estimate this number at 2 million to 3 million in the United States. Reasons for this increase include the following (Lindsay 1989, p. 78):

- Rising cost of housing.
- Reduction in federal subsidies for low-income housing.
- Economic recessions resulting in continued low or minimum wages, plant closures, and unemployment.
- Alcohol and drug abuse.
- Deinstitutionalization of mental health facilities and a change in the laws governing commitment of the mentally ill. About 30% to 40% of the homeless are mentally ill.

FACTORS CONTRIBUTING TO POOR HEALTH OF THE HOMELESS

- Poor physical environment resulting in increased susceptibility to infections
- Inadequate rest and privacy
- Improper nutrition
- Poor access to facilities for personal hygiene
- Exposure to the elements
- Lack of social support
- Few personal resources
- Questionable personal safety (physical assault is a constant threat)
- Inadequate health care
- Poor compliance with treatment plans

The homeless differ from those who are poor: They are alone, lack some type of permanent residence, and are disaffiliated from family and friends. Because of the conditions in which homeless people live (in shelters, on the streets, in parks, in tents, under scrap material covers, under viaducts, in all-night movie theaters, in transportation terminals, or in cars), their health problems are often exacerbated and sometimes become chronic. Major health problems of the homeless include the following (Lindsay 1989, p. 79):

- Chronic health problems, such as diabetes, hypertension, and drug and alcohol abuse
- Risk of communicable diseases, such as tuberculosis, scabies, lice, and AIDS
- Hypothermia in the winter
- Malnutrition
- Dental problems
- Peripheral vascular problems
- Traumatic injuries and risk of assault
- Children at risk of abuse, neglect, and missing immunizations, making them vulnerable to disease

The 1987 Report of the Panel on Health Goals for Ontario has suggested several basics to good health (Spasoff 1987): "peace; an adequate income; adequate housing and food; a valued role to play in family, work, and community; a safe environment; and a healthy lifestyle." These basics, however, are beyond the reach of the homeless population, many of whom are multiply handicapped by physical, mental, social, and emotional problems. Several factors contribute to poor health among the homeless (see the box above).

NURSING'S AGENDA FOR HEALTH CARE REFORM (EXECUTIVE SUMMARY)

The basic components of nursing's "core of care" include

- A restructured health care system which
  - Enhances consumer access to services by delivering primary health care in community-based settings.
  - Fosters consumer responsibility for personal health, self-care, and informed decision making in selecting health care services.
  - Facilitates utilization of the most cost-effective providers and therapeutic options in the most appropriate settings.
- A federally defined standard package of essential health care services available to all citizens and residents of the United States, provided and financed through an integration of public and private plans and sources:
  - A public plan, based on federal guidelines and eligibility requirements, will provide coverage for the poor and create the opportunity for small businesses and individuals, particularly those at risk because of preexisting conditions and those potentially medically indigent, to buy into the plan.
  - A private plan will offer, at a minimum, the nationally standardized package of essential services. This standard package could be enriched as a benefit of employment, or individuals could purchase additional services if they so choose. If employers do not offer private coverage, they must pay into the public plan for their employees.
- A phase-in of essential services, in order to be fiscally responsible:
  - Coverage of pregnant women and children is critical. This first step represents a cost-effective investment in the future health and prosperity of the nation.
  - One early step will be to design services specifically to assist vulnerable populations who have had limited access to our nation's health care system. A "Healthstart Plan" is proposed to improve the health status of these individuals.
- Planned change to anticipate health service needs that correlate with changing national demographics.
- Steps to reduce health care costs include
  - Required usage of managed care in the public plan and encouraged in private plans.
  - Incentives for consumers and providers to utilize managed care arrangements.
  - Controlled growth of the health care system by planning and prudent resource allocation.
  - Incentives for consumers and providers to be cost efficient in exercising health care options.
  - Development of health care policies based on effectiveness and outcomes research.
  - Assurance of direct access to a full range of qualified providers.
  - Elimination of unnecessary bureaucratic controls and administrative procedures.
- Case management will be required for those with continuing health care needs. This will reduce the fragmentation of the present system, promote consumers' active participation in decisions about their health, and create an advocate on their behalf.
- Provisions for long-term care, which include
  - Public and private funding for services of short duration to prevent personal impoverishment.
  - Public funding for extended care if consumer resources are exhausted.
  - Emphasis on the consumers' responsibility to financially plan for their long-term care needs, including new personal financial alternatives and strengthened private insurance arrangements.
- Insurance reforms to improve access to coverage, including affordable premiums, reinsurance pools for catastrophic coverage, and steps to protect both insurers and individuals against excessive costs.
- Access to services assured by no payment at the point of service and elimination of balance billing in both public and private plans.
- Establishment of public/private sector review—operating under federal guidelines and including payers, providers, and consumers—to determine resource allocation, cost reduction approaches, allowable insurance premiums, and fair and consistent reimbursement levels for providers. This review would progress in a climate sensitive to ethical issues.

Source: American Nurses Association, *Nursing's Agenda for Health Care Reform* (Washington, DC: ANA, 1991). PR-3 220M 6/91. Reprinted with permission.

UNEVEN DISTRIBUTION OF HEALTH SERVICES

Serious problems in the distribution of health services exist in both the United States and Canada. Two facets of this problem are (a) uneven distribution and (b) increased specialization. Uneven distribution is evidenced by the relatively higher number of nurses per population in the New England states and lowest number in Louisiana and

Oklahoma. Physicians are also unevenly distributed: Mississippi, Kentucky, Tennessee, and Alabama have the lowest number of physicians per 100,000, whereas New England has the highest (Jonas 1992, p. 65).

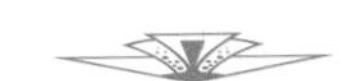

HEALTH CARE FOR THE 1990S

ANA RECOMMENDATIONS

In 1991, the American Nurses Association (ANA) published *Nursing's Agenda for Health Care Reform*, which sets forth the ANA's recommendations for health care reform. A central objective of this reform is to provide a basic "core" of essential health care services to everyone. The statement calls for a restructuring of the health care system to focus on consumers and their health needs. It also recommends that health care be delivered in such diverse settings as schools, workplaces, and homes and that the health care system shift its focus from illness and cure to wellness and care. See the box on page 74.

The American Organization of Nurse Executives (1992, p. 42) writes that effective health care must

1. Encourage consumer partnerships so that consumers can take an active role in their health and their care and in decisions about their care.
2. Allow all U.S. citizens and residents access to basic health care services.
3. Increase health care access by the use of physician and nonphysician providers.
4. Create incentives that promote health, wellness, and prevention; individuals with chronic illnesses will not be penalized.
5. Promote affordable, safe, and effective health care.
6. Make provisions for skilled and long-term care.
7. Make provisions for catastrophic care, with some limitation on extraordinary procedures.
8. Finance health care through a combination of public- and private-sector funding.

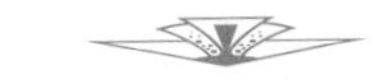

CRITICAL PATHWAYS

Critical pathways are multidisciplinary guidelines for client care. Critical pathways are also labeled as critical paths, multidisciplinary plans, anticipated recovery plans, multidisciplinary action plans, and action plans. Such pathways are developed for specific diagnoses, usually high volume, high risk, and high cost case types with the collaboration of members of the health care team. This type of client care management tool describes how resources will be utilized to achieve predetermined outcomes. These guidelines also provide the sequence of multidisciplinary interventions, incorporating education, discharge planning, consultations, nutrition, medications, activities, diagnostics, therapeutics, and treatments (Figure 4–1 on page 76).

The goals of critical pathways are as follows: to achieve realistic, expected client and family outcomes; to promote professional and collaborative practice and care; to ensure continuity of care; to guarantee appropriate use of resources; to reduce costs and length of stay; and to provide the framework for continuous quality improvement. Critical pathways generally emerge from case management models and quality improvement efforts. The overall goal is to improve the quality and proficiency of client care by designing pathways that facilitate a reproducible standard of care for specific client populations.

Variances from the critical pathways are recorded and studied by the nurses and case managers involved in the client's care. Variances are often grouped as either system, provider, or client variances. A typical system variance would be the unavailability of diagnostic testing. A provider variance may be related to a practitioner's level of experience. A client variance may result from an unexpected change in condition. The critical pathway can also be designed so that variances and interventions can be easily documented. A typical documentation system will include a check-off or initial line for interventions and a log for variances.

The process for developing a critical pathway is agency dependent. Information necessary for the development of any critical pathway includes literature reviews, chart reviews, expert opinion, and insurance reimbursements for the designated case type. A typical approach is to first identify high cost, high volume, and high risk case types for the agency. Next, a multidisciplinary team, including physicians, develops a consensus around the management of the case type and a critical pathway. The pathway is then piloted in a clinical setting and revised as indicated by the number and type of variances until it best meets the needs of clients in the practice setting.

In many agencies, critical pathways or similar models are replacing the traditional nursing care plans. The advantages of critical pathways are that they are outcome-driven and provide a time line to achieve their goals. Additionally, critical pathways encourage health care workers to collaborate to establish dynamic plans of care that reflect the totality of the client's needs. Although initially developed for acute hospitalizations, critical pathways are now being developed to manage clients in home health, outpatient, and long-term settings.

CRITICAL PATHWAY FOR CLIENT FOLLOWING LAPAROSCOPIC CHOLECYSTECTOMY

Expected length of stay: less than 24 hours

	DATE __________ PREOPERATIVE	DATE __________ 1st 24 hours following surgery
Daily outcomes	Client verbalizes understanding of preoperative teaching including: turning, coughing, deep breathing, incentive spirometer, mobilization, and pain management. Client verbalizes ability to cope.	Client is afebrile. Client has a dry, clean wound with edges well-approximated, healing by first intention. Client manages pain with non-pharmacologic measures or oral medications. Client is independent in self-care. Client is fully ambulatory. Client has resumed preadmission urine and bowel elimination pattern. Client verbalizes home care instructions. Client tolerates usual diet. Client verbalizes ability to cope with ongoing stressors.
Tests and treatments	CBC Urinalysis Baseline physical assessment: with a focus on respiratory status and gastrointestinal function Anesthesia consult	Vital signs and O_2 saturation, neurovascular assessment, dressing and wound drainage assessment q15 min x 4; q30 min x 4; q1h x 4 and then q4h if stable. Assess lung sounds and gastrointestinal function q4h and prn. Intake and output every shift. Assess voiding - if unable to void, try suggestive voiding techniques or cathetorize q8h or prn if unable to void.
Knowledge deficit	Orient to room and surroundings. Provide simple, brief instructions. Review preoperative preparation including hospital and surgical routines. Reinforce preoperative teaching regarding specific postoperative care: turning, coughing, deep breathing, incentive spirometer, mobilization, and pain management.	Reorient to room and postoperative routine. Review plan of care and importance of early mobilization. Begin discharge teaching regarding wound care/dressing change.
Psychosocial	Assess anxiety related to pending surgery. Assess fears of the unknown and surgery. Encourage verbalization of concerns. Provide information regarding surgical experience. Minimize external stimuli (eg, noise, movement).	Assess level of anxiety. Encourage verbalization of concerns. Provide information and ongoing support and encouragement.
Diet	NPO Baseline nutritional assessment	Advance to clear liquids, if tolerated advance to full liquids/soft diet morning following surgery.
Activity	OOB ad lib until premedicated for surgery.	Provide safety precautions. Bathroom privileges with assistance evening after surgery and begin progressive ambulation to tolerance the morning following surgery until fully ambulatory.
Medications	NPO except ordered medications.	IM or PO analgesics Antibiotics if ordered IV fluids until adequate PO intake then intermittent IV device Discontiue prior to discharge
Transfer/ discharge plans	Assess discharge plans and support system.	Probable discharge within 24 hours of surgery. Complete discharge home care teaching when fully awake and oriented and before discharge. Provide a written copy of discharge instructions.

Figure 4–1 Example of a critical pathway for a client who had a laparoscopic cholecystectomy. Courtesy of Susanne Beyea.

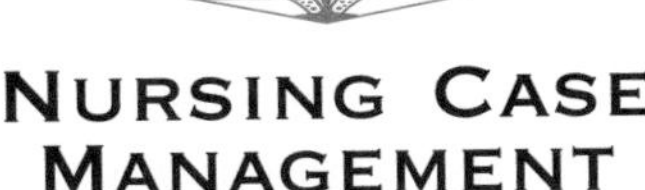

NURSING CASE MANAGEMENT

Nursing case management describes an innovative practice model utilized by a variety of health care agencies to ensure quality client care, reduce costs, and manage high volume and high risk cases. *Nursing case management* emerged when there were a number of changes in reimbursement programs and the need to manage clinical outcomes so as to limit costs. Two integral components of nursing care management are case management plans, such as critical pathways, and case managers.

Nurse case managers work with the multidisciplinary health care team to measure the effectiveness of the case management plan and monitor outcomes. Each agency or unit specifies the role of the nurse case manager. In some institutions, the case manager will work with primary/staff nurses to oversee the care of a specific caseload. In other agencies, the case manager will be the primary nurse or provide some level of direct care to the client and family. Insurance companies have also developed a number of roles for nurse case managers, and responsibilities may vary from managing acute hospitalizations to managing high cost clients or case types.

Nursing case management requires effective communication skills and a clinical background with clients of the specific case type. The nurse case manager in a hospital is responsible for developing case management plans with the health care team and then evaluating outcomes. Commonly used tools include critical pathways and variance analysis. **Critical pathways** are versions of the case management plan that clearly describe interventions and outcomes for a specific case type. **Variances** are departures from the expected pathway.

Regardless of the setting, case managers help ensure that care is oriented to the client, while at the same time controlling costs. Case managers may also be social workers, physicians, or paraprofessionals in any number of settings. Case managers are also in private practice, offering their services to families and individuals. With the ongoing need to limit costs and ensure quality, managed care and case management are increasingly important approaches to health care.

CHAPTER HIGHLIGHTS

- The health care delivery system is a large, complex organization comprising a variety of agencies and many health care professionals.
- Health care can be considered a right of all people.
- The idea that health is the responsibility of each individual in society is gaining greater acceptance.
- Health care delivery services can be categorized as primary, secondary, or tertiary, and generally, can also be grouped by the type of service: (1) health promotion and illness prevention, (2) diagnosis and treatment, and (3) rehabilitation.
- Various providers of health care coordinate their skills to assist a client. Their mutual goal is to restore a client's health and promote wellness.
- Hospitals provide a wide variety of services on an inpatient and outpatient basis. Hospitals can be categorized as for-profit or not-for-profit, public or private, acute care or long-term care.
- Outpatient services are expanding rapidly through hospitals, ambulatory care centers, and health maintenance organizations.
- In the United States, health care is financed largely through government agencies and private organizations that provide health care insurance, prepaid plans, and federally funded programs. Government-financed plans include Medicare and Medicaid. Private plans include Blue Cross and Blue Shield. Prepaid group plans include HMOs, PPOs, and PPAs.
- In Canada, health care is financed through a national health insurance plan.
- Current issues and problems impacting health care delivery include health care consumers, legislation, the women's movement, family characteristics, increasing number of elderly people, advances in knowledge and technology, economic factors, fragmentation of care, increased costs, health care of the homeless, and uneven distribution of health services.
- The ANA's *Nursing's Agenda for Health Care Reform* emphasizes a basic "core" of essential health care services for everyone and a restructuring of the health care system to focus on consumers and their health needs.

READINGS AND REFERENCES

SUGGESTED READINGS

Knollmueller, RN. October 1989. Case management: What's in a name? *Nursing Management* 20:38–40, 42.

In this article, Knollmueller provides several definitions of case management and describes a number of models. The author discusses the role of the case manager and points out that the value of case management will lie in the improved care that results.

Zander, K. September 1988. Nursing care management: Resolving the DRG paradox. *Nursing Clinics of North America* 23:503–19.

Zander describes the DRG paradox as cost-effective care versus quality care. The four components of nursing case management are designed to help resolve this paradox: (1) achievement of clinical and financial outcomes, (2) the caregiver as manager, (3) episode-based RN-MD group practice, and (4) active participation by clients and their support people in goal setting and evaluation. Zander further describes the New England Medical Center Hospital's model of case management.

RELATED RESEARCH

LeRoy, L. 1982. The cost-effectiveness of nurse practitioners. In Aiken, LH, editor. *Nursing in the 1980s: Crises, opportunities, challenges.* Philadelphia: Lippincott.

Neidig, JR, Megel, ME, and Koehler, KM. August 1992. The critical path: An evaluation of the applicability of nursing case management in the NICU. *Neonatal Network* 11:45–52.

SELECTED REFERENCES

American Hospital Association. 1992. A patient's bill of rights. Chicago: American Hospital Association.

American Nurses Association 1988. Case management: A challenge for nurses. Kansas City, MO: ANA.

———. 1991. *Nursing's Agenda for Health Care Reform.* Washington, DC: ANA.

American Organization of Nurse Executives. November 1992. Eight premises for a reformed American healthcare system. *Nursing Management* 23:42, 44.

Anspaugh, DJ, Hamrick, MH, and Rosato, FD. 1991. *Concepts and Applications: Wellness.* St Louis: Mosby Year Book.

Brecht, MC. January/February 1990. Nursing's role in assuring access to care. *Nursing Outlook* 38:6–7.

Commonwealth Department of Health, Housing and Community Services. 1993. *Medicare: The care you're entitled to. Your summary guide to Medicare.* Canberra, Australia.

Curtin, LL. May 1991. Rube Goldberg and the great American healthcare system. *Nursing Management* 22:9–11.

Curtin, LL and Zurlage, C. April 1991. Cornerstones of healthcare in the nineties: Forging a framework of excellence—a report of a landmark conference. *Nursing Management* 22:32–43, 46.

Deber, RB, Hastings, JE, and Thompson, GG. January 1991. Health care in Canada: Current trends and issues. *Journal of Public Health Policy* 12:72–82.

Del Togno-Armanasco, V, Olivas, GS, and Harter, S. October 1989. Developing an integrated nursing case management model. *Nursing Management* 20:26–29.

Dimond, M. March/April 1989. Health care and the aging population. *Nursing Outlook* 37:76–77.

Dougherty, CJ. 1988. *American Health Care: Realities, Rights, and Reforms.* New York: Oxford University Press.

Drew, JC. March 1990. Health maintenance organizations: History, evolution and survival. *Nursing Health Care* 11:144–49.

Faherty, B. July 1990. Case management: The latest buzzword: What it is and what it isn't. *Caring* 9:20–22.

Giuliano, KK and Poirier, CE. March 1991. Nursing case management: Critical pathways to desirable outcomes. *Nursing Management* 22:52–55.

Jonas, S. 1992. *An Introduction to the U.S. Health Care System.* 3d ed. New York: Springer Publishing.

Judd, V and Forgues, C. November 1989. Canada's homeless: Breaking down the barriers to health care. *Canadian Nurse* 85:18–19.

Knollmueller, RN. October 1989. Case management: What's in a name? *Nursing Management* 20:38–40, 42.

Kelly, M. September 1989. The Omnibus Budget Reconciliation Act of 1987: A policy analysis. *Nursing Clinics of North America* 24:791–94.

Lee, PR and Estes, CL, editors. 1990. *The Nations' Health.* Boston: Jones and Bartlett.

LeFort, SM. March 1993. Shaping health care policy. *Canadian Nurse* 89:23–27.

Lindsay, AM. March/April 1989. Health care for the homeless. *Nursing Outlook* 37:78–81.

McKenzie, CB, Torkelson, NG, and Holt, MA. October 1989. Care and cost: Nursing case management improves both. *Nursing Management* 20:30–34.

Mayer, D. November 1989. Accreditation panel to release hospital information to health care financing administration. *Medical Benefits* 6(11):12.

Mosher, C, Cronk, P, Kidd, A, McCormick, P, Stockton, S, and Sulla, C. January 1992. Upgrading practice with critical pathways. *American Journal of Nursing* 91:41–44.

Omachonu, VK and Nanda, R. April 1989. Measuring productivity: Outcome vs. output. *Nursing Management* 20:35–38, 40.

Sharp, N. March 1993. Healthcare reform—it ain't gonna be easy. *Nursing Management* 24:22–24.

Spasoff, R. 1987. *Health for All: Report of the Panel on Health Goals for Ontario.* Toronto: Ontario Ministry of Health.

Statistics Canada. 1991. *Population Projections for Canada, Provinces and Territories,* 1989–2011. Catalogue 91-520. Ottawa, Canada.

Thatcher, RM. September 1989. Community support: Promoting health and self-care. *Nursing Clinics of North America* 24:725–31.

U.S. Bureau of the Census. 1989. *Statistical Abstract of the United States.* 109th ed. Washington, DC: U.S. Government Printing Office.

U.S. Department of Health and Human Services. 1990. *Health United States.* Washington, DC: U.S. Government Printing Office.

———. 1991. *Health & People 2000: National Heath Promotion and Disease Prevention Objectives.* Washington, DC: U.S. Government Printing Office.

Zander, K. January 1988a. Managed care within acute care settings: Design and implementation via nursing case management. *Health Care Supervisor* 6:27–43.

———. April 1988b. Nursing case management: Strategic management of cost and quality outcomes. *Journal of Nursing Administration* 18:23–30.

———. September 1988c. Nursing case management: Resolving the DRG paradox. *Nursing Clinics of North America* 23:503–20.

———. May/June 1992. Focusing on patient outcome: Case management in the 90's. *Dimension of Critical Care Nursing* 11:127–29.

Zarle, NC. September 1989. Continuity of care: Balancing care of elders between health care settings. *Nursing Clinics of North America* 24:697–705.

The Nursing Process in Action

The nursing process is a systematic, rational method of planning and providing nursing care. Its goal is to identify a client's healthcare status, actual or potential health problems, to establish plans to meet the identified needs, and to deliver specific nursing interventions to address those needs. The nursing process is cyclical; that is, its components follow a logical sequence, but more than one component may be involved at one time. At the end of the first cycle, care may be terminated if goals are achieved, or the cycle may begin again with reassessment.

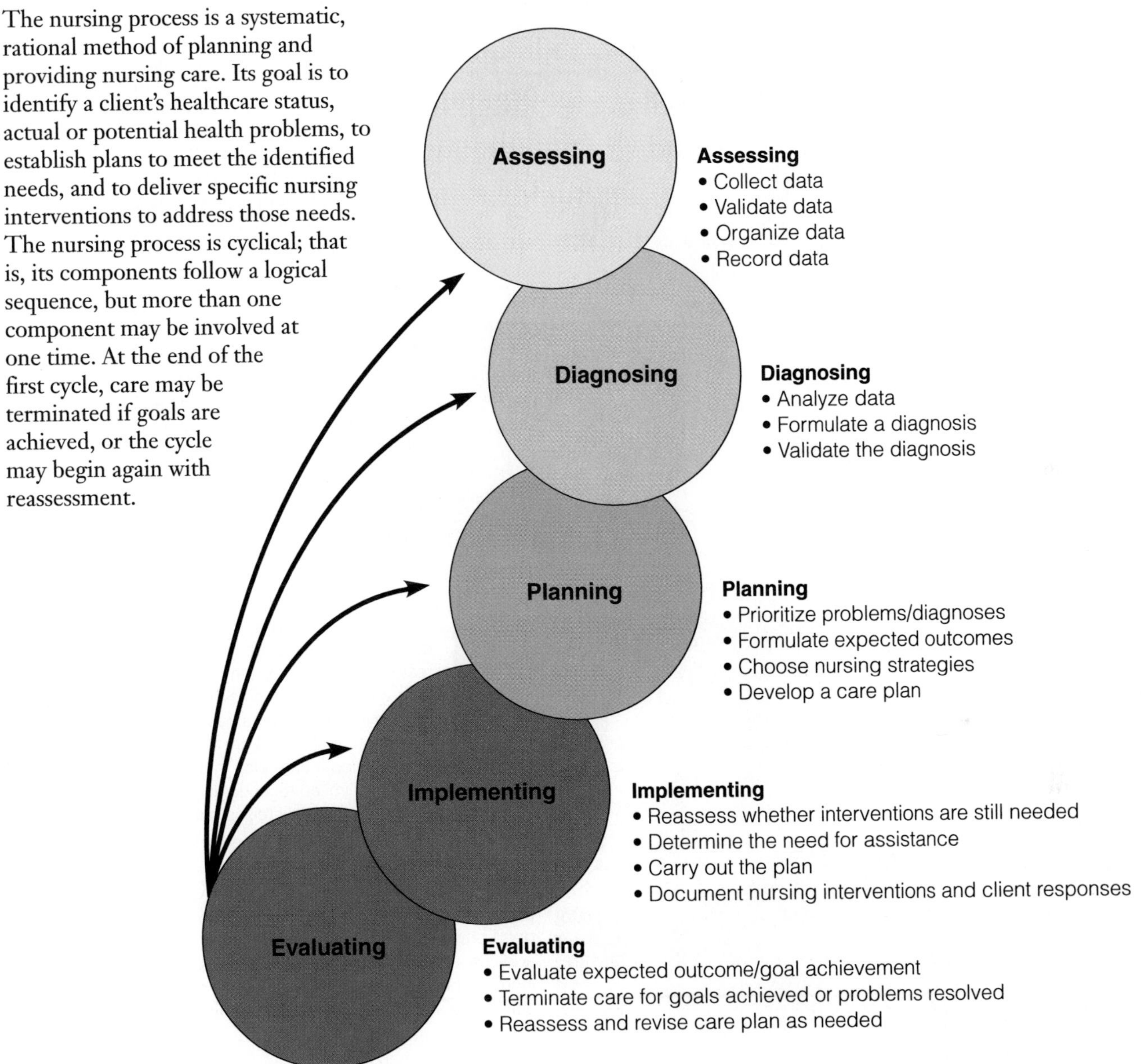

Assessing
Diagnosing
Planning
Implementing
Evaluating
Assessing
• Collect data
• Validate data
• Organize data
• Record data
Diagnosing
• Analyze data
• Formulate a diagnosis
• Validate the diagnosis
Planning
• Prioritize problems/diagnoses
• Formulate expected outcomes
• Choose nursing strategies
• Develop a care plan
Implementing
• Reassess whether interventions are still needed
• Determine the need for assistance
• Carry out the plan
• Document nursing interventions and client responses
Evaluating
• Evaluate expected outcome/goal achievement
• Terminate care for goals achieved or problems resolved
• Reassess and revise care plan as needed

The Nursing Process in Action

Luisa Sanchez, a 28-year-old married attorney, was admitted to the hospital with an elevated temperature, a productive cough, and rapid, labored respirations. In taking a nursing history, Mary Medina, RN, finds that Ms Sanchez has had a "chest cold" for two weeks, and has been experiencing shortness of breath upon exertion. Yesterday she developed an elevated temperature and began to experience "pain" in her "lungs."

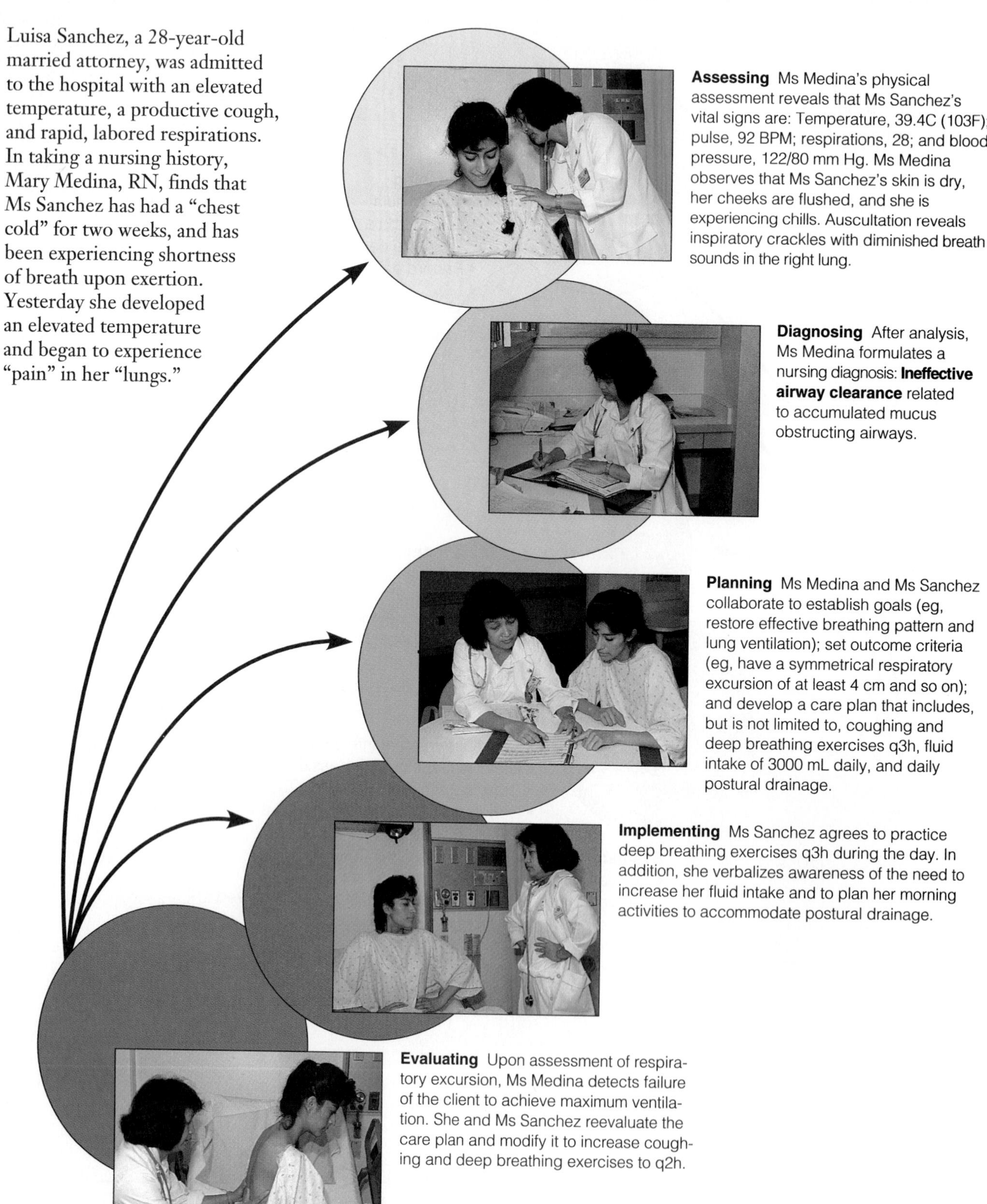

Assessing Ms Medina's physical assessment reveals that Ms Sanchez's vital signs are: Temperature, 39.4C (103F); pulse, 92 BPM; respirations, 28; and blood pressure, 122/80 mm Hg. Ms Medina observes that Ms Sanchez's skin is dry, her cheeks are flushed, and she is experiencing chills. Auscultation reveals inspiratory crackles with diminished breath sounds in the right lung.

Diagnosing After analysis, Ms Medina formulates a nursing diagnosis: **Ineffective airway clearance** related to accumulated mucus obstructing airways.

Planning Ms Medina and Ms Sanchez collaborate to establish goals (eg, restore effective breathing pattern and lung ventilation); set outcome criteria (eg, have a symmetrical respiratory excursion of at least 4 cm and so on); and develop a care plan that includes, but is not limited to, coughing and deep breathing exercises q3h, fluid intake of 3000 mL daily, and daily postural drainage.

Implementing Ms Sanchez agrees to practice deep breathing exercises q3h during the day. In addition, she verbalizes awareness of the need to increase her fluid intake and to plan her morning activities to accommodate postural drainage.

Evaluating Upon assessment of respiratory excursion, Ms Medina detects failure of the client to achieve maximum ventilation. She and Ms Sanchez reevaluate the care plan and modify it to increase coughing and deep breathing exercises to q2h.

UNIT 2

THE NURSING PROCESS

STUDENT PROFILE

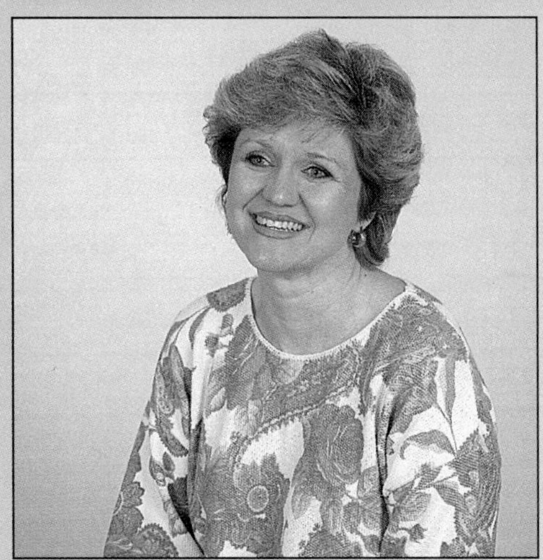

NAME	Christine Bartlett
SCHOOL OF NURSING	Lee College, Baytown, Texas
HOMETOWN	Liberty, Texas

WHY DID YOU ENTER THE FIELD OF NURSING?
I have always enjoyed helping people, especially children. My own children are in high school and I knew I would want to get into the job market, so I felt nursing was the career for me.

WHO OR WHAT INFLUENCED THAT DECISION?
A friend who was nearly killed in an auto accident about 5 years ago needed someone to help her after a 3-month hospital stay. She still needed some intensive care and they taught me how to care for her. It was a turning point in my career choice.

WHAT QUALITIES DO YOU THINK ARE NECESSARY TO BE A GOOD NURSE?
Compassion—always keep the feelings and fears of patients and their families in the front of all the care. Commitment—be on the floor to help people who need your knowledge and understanding to get them through the critical times.

WHAT HAS BEEN YOUR MOST GRATIFYING MOMENT AS A STUDENT NURSE?
The feeling of belonging and challenge the moment I walked into the neonatal unit was overwhelming.

WHAT ADVICE WOULD YOU GIVE A NEW STUDENT?
To know deep inside you that this is what you want to do. Nursing is not just a career, it is a lifestyle if you are ready to commit to the ideal of helping people, not just drawing a paycheck.

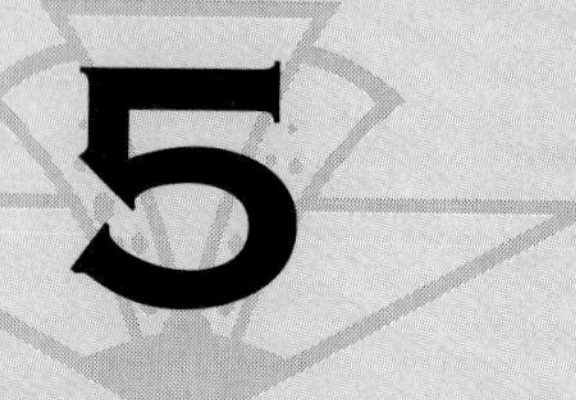

5 Assessing

Objectives

- Describe the components of the nursing process.
- Identify the contribution of selected nurses to the development of the nursing process.
- Identify essential characteristics of the nursing process.
- List benefits of the nursing process.
- Identify the four major activities associated with the assessment process.
- Identify the purpose of assessing.
- Differentiate objective and subjective data and primary and secondary data.
- Identify three methods of data collection, and give examples of how each is useful.
- Compare directive and nondirective approaches to interviewing.
- Compare closed and open-ended questions, providing examples and listing advantages and disadvantages of each.
- Describe important aspects of the interview setting.
- Contrast various frameworks used for nursing assessment.

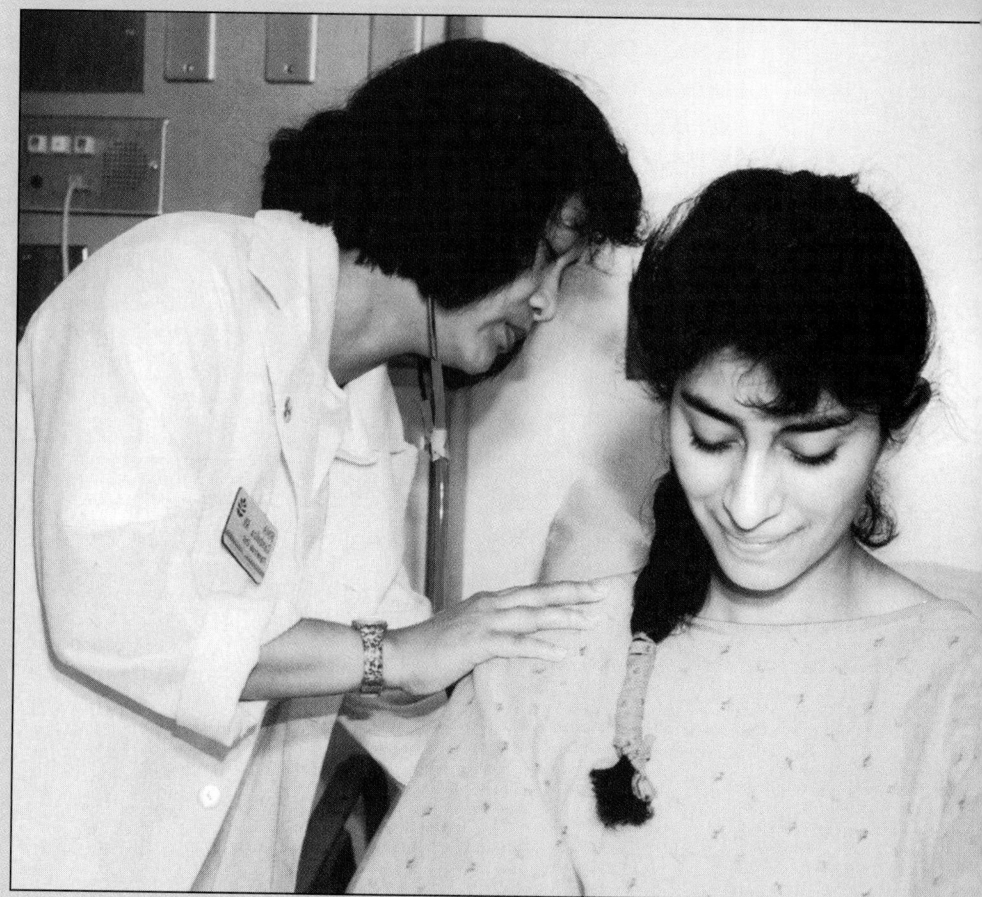

A **process** is a series of planned actions or operations directed toward a particular result or goal. The **nursing process** is a systematic, rational method of planning and providing individualized nursing care. Its purpose is to identify a client's health status, actual or potential health care problems or needs; to establish plans to meet the identified needs; and to deliver specific nursing interventions to meet those needs. The nursing process is cyclical; that is, the components of the nursing process follow a logical sequence, but more than one component may be involved at any one time (Figure 5–1).

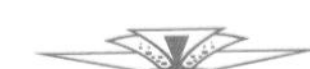

Overview of the Nursing Process

Components of the Nursing Process

The nursing process consists of a series of five components or phases: assessing, diagnosing, planning, implementing, and evaluating. Although nursing theorists may use different terms to describe these phases, the activities of the nurse using the process are similar. To avoid misunderstanding, nurses should be familiar with alternative terms that describe the phases. For example, *nursing diagnosis* may be called *analysis*, and *implementation (implementing)* may be called *intervention* or *intervening.*

An overview of the five-phase nursing process follows. See also Table 5–1 on page 84. Each of the five components of the nursing process is discussed in depth in this and subsequent chapters of this unit.

1. **Assessing** is collecting, organizing, validating, and recording data about a client's health status. Data are obtained from a variety of sources and are the basis for actions and decisions taken in subsequent phases. No conclusions about the data are drawn in this phase.
2. **Diagnosing** is a process which results in a diagnostic statement or nursing diagnosis. In this phase, the nurse sorts, clusters, and analyzes the data and asks, "What are the actual and potential health problems for which the client needs nursing assistance?" and "What factors contributed to this problem?" Responses to those questions establish the nursing diagnoses.
3. **Planning** involves a series of steps in which the nurse and the client set priorities and goals or expected outcomes to resolve or minimize the identified problems of the client. In collaboration with the client, the nurse develops specific interventions for each nursing diagnosis. The product of the planning phase is a written care plan used to coordinate the care provided by all the health team members.

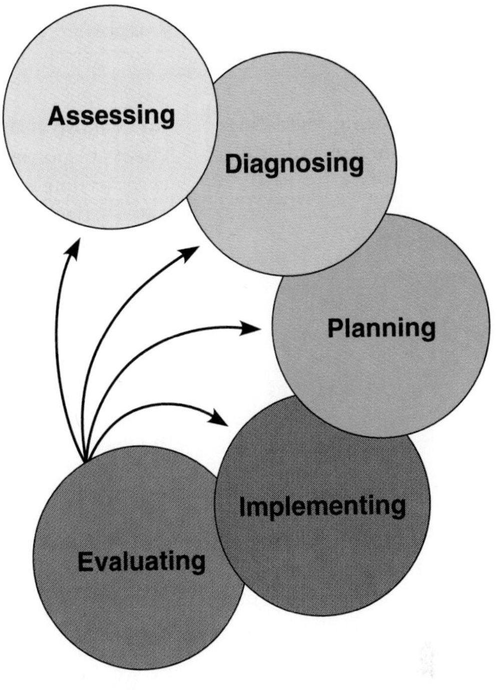

Figure 5–1 The five overlapping phases of the nursing process. Each phase depends on the accuracy of the preceding phase. Evaluating involves examination of all previous phases.

4. **Implementing** is putting the nursing care plan into action. During the implementation phase, the nurse carries out the prescribed nursing activities or delegates the care to an appropriate person, and validates the nursing care plan. This phase ends when the nurse records the care given and the client's responses to care in the client record (eg, the nursing progress notes).
5. **Evaluating** is assessing the client's response to nursing interventions and then comparing the response to the goals or outcome criteria written in the planning phase. The nurse determines the extent to which the outcomes/goals of care have been achieved. The care plan is reassessed in this phase, which may involve changes in any or all of the previous phases of the nursing process.

The five phases of the nursing process are not discrete entities but overlapping, continuing subprocesses. For example, assessing, the first phase of the nursing process, is often carried out during implementing and evaluating.

Each phase of the nursing process affects the others; they are closely interrelated. For example, if inadequate data are obtained during assessment, the nursing diagnoses will be incomplete or incorrect; this will be reflected

Table 5–1 Overview of the Purposes and Activities of the Nursing Process

Component and Description	Purpose	Activities
Assessing		
Collecting, organizing, validating, and communicating/recording client data	To establish a database about the client's response to health concerns or illness and the ability to manage health care needs	Establish a database ▪ Obtain health history ▪ Conduct physical assessment ▪ Review client records ▪ Review literature ▪ Consult support persons ▪ Consult health professionals Update data as needed Organize data Validate data Communicate/document data
Diagnosing		
Analyzing and synthesizing data	To identify client strengths and health problems that can be prevented or resolved by collaborative and independent nursing interventions To develop a list of nursing diagnoses and collaborative problems	Interpret and analyze data ▪ Compare data against standards ▪ Cluster or group data (generate tentative hypotheses) ▪ Identify gaps and inconsistencies Determine client's strengths, risks, and problems Formulate nursing diagnoses and collaborative problem statements
Planning		
Determining how to prevent, reduce, or resolve the identified client problems; how to support client strengths; and how to implement nursing interventions in an organized, individualized, and outcome/goal-directed manner	To develop an individualized care plan that specifies client goals/expected outcomes and related nursing interventions	Set priorities and goals/outcomes in collaboration with client Write goals/outcome criteria Select nursing strategies/interventions Consult other health professionals Write nursing orders and nursing care plan Communicate care plan to relevant health care providers
Implementing		
Carrying out the planned nursing interventions	To assist the client to meet desired goals/outcomes; promote health and wellness; prevent illness and disease; and facilitate coping with health problems	Reassess the client to update the database Determine need for nursing assistance Perform or delegate planned nursing interventions Communicate nursing actions implemented ▪ Document care and client responses to care ▪ Give verbal reports as necessary
Evaluating		
Measuring the degree to which goals/outcomes have been achieved and identifying factors that positively or negatively influence goal achievement	To determine the extent to which client goals/outcomes have been achieved and to determine whether to continue, modify, or terminate the plan of care	Collaborate with client and collect data related to expected outcomes Judge whether goals/outcomes have been achieved Relate nursing actions to client outcomes Make decisions about problem status Review and modify the care plan as indicated or terminate nursing care

in the planning, implementing, and evaluating phases. Incomplete or incorrect assessment necessarily means equivocal evaluation because the nurse will have incomplete or incorrect criteria against which to evaluate changes in the client and the effectiveness of intervention.

Historical Perspective of the Nursing Process

Before the nursing process was developed, nurses tended to provide care that was based on medical orders written by physicians and that focused on specific disease conditions rather than on the person being cared for. Nursing practice that was provided independently of the physician was often guided by intuition and experience rather than a scientific method.

The term *nursing process* and the framework it implies are relatively new. In 1955, Hall originated the term, and Johnson (1959), Orlando (1961), and Wiedenbach (1963) were among the first to use it to refer to a series of phases describing the process of nursing. Since then, various nurses have described the process of nursing and organized the phases in different ways. The five-phase process described earlier is currently accepted by most experts. Table 5–2, on page 86, summarizes the historical evolution of the nursing process.

The use of the nursing process in clinical practice gained additional legitimacy in 1973, when the American Nurses Association (ANA) published *Standards of Nursing Practice*, which describes the five phases of the nursing process: assessing, diagnosing, planning, intervention, and evaluation (ANA 1973). (See Table 2–2, page 30, for the most recently revised standards.) Most states have since revised their nurse practice acts to reflect these aspects of nursing.

Characteristics of the Nursing Process

The nursing process "provides the framework in which nurses use their knowledge and skills to express human caring" and to help clients meet their health needs (Wilkinson 1992, pp. 4–5). The nursing process is characterized by unique properties that enable it to respond to the changing health status of the client. Hence, the nursing process is *cyclic and dynamic* rather than static.

The nursing process is also *client centered.* The nurse organizes the plan of care according to client problems rather than nursing goals. In the assessment phase, the nurse collects data to determine the client's habits, routines, and needs, enabling the nurse to incorporate client routines into the care plan as much as possible.

The nursing process is *interpersonal and collaborative.* To ensure the delivery of quality nursing care, the nurse must share concerns and problems and participate in continuous evaluation of the care plan. This depends on open and meaningful communication and the development of rapport between the client and the nurse. To carry out the nursing process effectively and individualize approaches to each client's particular needs, the nurse must collaborate with each individual, family, group, or community as required.

Another characteristic of the nursing process is that it is *universally applicable.* It can be used with clients of any age at any point on the wellness–illness continuum. Furthermore, it is useful in a variety of settings (eg, schools, hospitals, clinics, home health) and across specialty areas (eg, orthopedic nursing, maternity nursing, surgical nursing).

The nursing process is an adaptation of *problem-solving techniques* (see Chapter 10) *and systems theory* (see Chapter 14). It can be viewed as parallel to but separate from the medical process. Table 5–3, page 87, offers a detailed comparison of the two processes. Both processes (a) begin with data gathering and analysis; (b) base action (intervention or treatment) on a problem statement (nursing diagnosis or medical diagnosis); and (c) include an evaluative component. Whereas the medical process focuses on the disease process, however, the nursing process is directed toward a client's *response* to disease and illness.

Nurses use a variety of interpersonal, technical, and intellectual skills in applying the nursing process. *Interpersonal skills* include communicating; listening; conveying interest, compassion, knowledge, and information; developing trust; and obtaining data in a manner that enhances the dignity of the client. *Technical skills* include using equipment and performing procedures. *Intellectual skills* include analyzing, problem solving, critical thinking, and making nursing judgments.

Decision making is involved in every component of the nursing process (Yura & Walsh 1988, p. 108). Nurses can be highly creative when using the nursing process. They are not bound by standard responses and may apply their repertoire of skills and knowledge to assist clients. See the box on page 88 for a summary of the characteristics of the nursing process.

Benefits of the Nursing Process

The nursing process benefits clients by improving the quality of care they receive. A high level of client participation, together with continuous evaluation, ensures an appropriate level of care designed to meet the client's unique needs. Because the nursing process provides for an organized, systematic approach, it enables nurses to use time and resources efficiently, to both their own and their clients' benefit.

Table 5–2 Evolution of the Nursing Process

Nurse	Selected Contributions
Peplau, H 1952	Identified four phases in an interpersonal relationship: orientation, identification, exploitation, and resolution. The phases are sequential and focus on interpersonal therapeutic interaction (George 1985, pp. 60–65).
Hall, L 1955	Originated the term *nursing process* (George 1985, p. 116).
Kreuter, FR 1957	Described steps in a nursing process as coordinating, planning, and evaluating nursing care and directing the family and the nursing auxiliary as they give nursing care. These were considered to promote the quality of professional practice (Kreuter 1957, p. 302).
Johnson, DE 1959	Saw the nursing process as assessing situations, arriving at decisions, implementing a course of action designed to resolve nursing problems, and evaluating (Johnson 1959, p. 200).
Orlando, IJ 1961	Saw the nursing process as interactive (Orlando, 1961, p. 29). Stated that the process included three phases: client's behavior, reaction of the nurse, and the nursing actions (George 1985, pp. 162–68).
Wiedenbach, E 1963, 1970	Introduced a three-step nursing process model: identify help needed, minister help, validate that help was given.
Henderson, V 1965	Stated that the nursing process was the same as the steps of the scientific method (Henderson 1965, pp. 3–10; 1980, p. 907).
Heidgerken, L 1965	Described steps of professional nursing care as evaluating behavior and situations; recognizing physical symptoms; diagnosing, planning, and meeting nursing needs; and coordinating the client's regimen through all stages of care (Heidgerken 1965, p. 95).
McCain, RA 1965	Was the first to use the term *assessment* in an article published in 1965. Used the functional abilities of the client as the framework for assessment. Collected and recorded objective and subjective data in assessment (McCain 1965, pp. 82–84).
Knowles, L 1967	Introduced a process model called the "five D's": discover, delve, decide, do, and discriminate. Stated that nurses collected data about the client's health during the first two stages.
Western Interstate Commission on Higher Education (WICHE) 1967	Listed the steps of the nursing process as perception and communication; interpretation; intervention; and discrimination.
Catholic University of America 1967	Proposed four components of the nursing process: assessment, planning, intervention, and evaluation (Yura & Walsh 1988, p. 22).
Orem, D 1971	Stated that there were three steps in nursing care: (a) initial and continuing determination of need for nursing care; (b) designing nursing actions for the client that will contribute to the client's achievement of health goals; and (c) the initiating, conducting, and control of assisting actions (Orem 1985, p. 224).
ANA Standards of Nursing Practice 1973	Referred to a five step process: assessing, diagnosing, planning, intervention, and evaluation.
Bloch, D 1974	Suggested a five-step nursing process that was similar to the four-step model: collection of data, definition of problem, planning of intervention, implementation of intervention, and evaluation of intervention (Bloch 1974, p. 693).
Gebbie, K and Lavin, MA 1975	Initiated first national conference on the classification of nursing diagnoses in 1973, which led to the use of a five-step nursing process model: assessment, nursing diagnosis, planning, intervention, and evaluation.
Roy, Sr C 1976	Used six-step nursing process: assessment of client behaviors and influencing factors, problem identification, goal setting, intervention, selection of approaches, and evaluation. Advocated the use of the term *nursing diagnosis* (Roy 1976, pp. 23–38).

Table 5–3 Comparison of the Nursing Process and the Medical Process

Nursing Process	Medical Process
1. Assessing Collection of data from a. Nursing history b. Health examination c. Review of records d. Consultation with other team members e. Review of literature	1. Assessing Collection of data from a. Medical history b. Physical examination c. Diagnostic tests d. Review of literature
2. Diagnosing a. Analysis and synthesis of data b. Identification of the health problems c. Formulation of nursing diagnosis	2. Medical diagnosis* a. Organization of data b. Analysis and interpretation of the data c. Formulation of a diagnosis
3. Planning a. Establishment of priorities b. Establishment of goals/expected outcomes c. Establishment of nursing interventions d. Written nursing care plan e. Delegation of nursing activities	3. Medical planning a. Establishment of priorities b. Establishment of goals for therapy c. Written plan of therapy
4. Implementing a. Preimplementation interventions b. Implementation c. Documentation of nursing interventions and client responses to care	4. Therapy a. Physician's orders b. Medical therapy c. Referrals
5. Evaluating a. Collection of data about the client's response b. Comparison of the data to the established goals/expected outcomes c. Determination of the effectiveness of the nursing plan d. Analysis of variables affecting the outcomes e. Review and modification of the care plan	5. Evaluating a. Establishment of the effectiveness of the medical therapy in terms of the goals b. Analysis of variables c. Revision of the plan of therapy as necessary

* Medical diagnosis has four or five phases:
1. Suspected diagnosis following the patient's initial complaint
2. Tentative diagnosis following the medical history
3. Provisional diagnosis following the physical examination
4. Definitive diagnosis following diagnostic tests
5. Anatomic diagnosis following a postmortem

Nurses benefit from knowing that they are delivering care that meets the expectations of health care consumers and the standards of their profession. The criteria developed by the ANA and set forth in *Standards of Clinical Nursing Practice* are based on the phases of the nursing process (ANA 1991). A portion of the Canadian Nurses Association's *Definition of Nursing Practice: Standards for Nursing Practice* (1987) also includes standards related to the nursing process. (See the boxes on pages 30 and 31.) In the United States, the Joint Commission on Accreditation of Healthcare Organizations (JCAHO) requires evidence that the nursing process phases are carried out for each hospitalized client (JCAHO 1992, *Nursing Care*, pp. 1–67). The nursing process, therefore, is a framework for nurses' accountability. It holds nurses both accountable and responsible for assessing, diagnosing, planning, implementing, and evaluating client care.

Because health team members work together to implement the care plan, the nursing process enhances collaboration, which in turn promotes a more positive work atmosphere. Finally, the nursing process can help nurses define their role to those outside the profession, clearly demonstrating nursing contributions to clients' health.

CHARACTERISTICS OF THE NURSING PROCESS

- The system is open and flexible to meet the unique needs of client, family, group, or community.
- It is cyclic and dynamic. Because all steps are interrelated, there is no absolute beginning or end.
- It is client centered; it individualizes the approach to each client's particular needs.
- It is interpersonal and collaborative. It requires the nurse to communicate directly and consistently with clients to meet their needs.
- It is planned.
- It is goal directed.
- It permits creativity for the nurse and client in devising ways to solve the stated health problem.
- It emphasizes feedback, which leads either to reassessment of the problem or to revision of the care plan.
- It is universally applicable. The nursing process is used as a framework for nursing care in all types of health care settings, with clients of all age groups.

ASSESSING

Assessing, the first phase of the nursing process, involves data collection, organization, and validation. It must take place before a nursing diagnosis can be made. "Assessment is part of each activity the nurse does for and with the patient" (Atkinson & Murray 1990, p. 7). The ANA's *Standards of Clinical Nursing Practice* (1991, p. 9) outlines nurses' accountability for collecting client data. See the box at the top of the next column.

In effect, assessing is a continuous process carried out during all phases of the nursing process. For example, in the evaluation phase, assessment is done to determine the outcomes of the nursing strategies and to evaluate goal achievement. All phases of the nursing process depend on the accurate and complete collection of **data** (information).

In *Nursing: A Social Policy Statement* (ANA 1980, p. 9), the American Nurses Association states that nursing is "the diagnosis and treatment of human responses to actual or potential health problems." Thus the purpose of assessment is to establish a database about a client's *response* to health concerns or illness in order to determine the client's nursing care needs. Clients' responses include

ANA STANDARDS

Standard I: Assessment

The nurse collects client health data.

Measurement Criteria

1. The priority of data collection is determined by the client's immediate condition or needs.
2. Pertinent data are collected using appropriate assessment techniques.
3. Data collection involves the client, significant others, and health care providers when appropriate.
4. The data collection process is systematic and ongoing.
5. Relevant data are documented in a retrievable form.

Source: Abstracted from American Nurses Association, *Standards of Clinical Nursing Practice* (Kansas City, MO: ANA, 1991), p. 9. Used with permission.

areas of daily living; health; and biophysical, emotional, socioeconomic, cultural, and spiritual concerns. In contrast to other health professionals, the nurse is concerned with human needs that affect the total person rather than one problem or segment of need fulfillment (Yura & Walsh 1988, p. 110).

There are four different types of assessment: initial assessment, focus assessment, emergency assessment, and time-lapsed assessment (Table 5–4). These types vary according to their purpose, timing, time available, and client status.

The Joint Commission on the Accreditation of Healthcare Organizations (1992) recommends that each client have a documented nursing admission assessment that follows institutional policies. This assessment is usually performed by a registered nurse, but parts of it (eg, measurement of height, weight, and body temperature) may be delegated to a nonprofessional. Delegation does not, however, absolve the registered nurse from the responsibility of ensuring the completeness and accuracy of the information. The status of the client may not allow a thorough admission assessment. In such cases, it is completed at a later time.

ASSESSMENT METHODS

The primary methods used to assess clients are observing, interviewing, and examining. Observation occurs when-

Table 5–4 Types of Assessment

Type	Time Performed	Purpose	Example
Initial assessment	Performed within specified time after admission to a health care agency	To establish a complete database for problem identification, reference, and future comparison	Nursing admission assessment (see Figure 5–2)
Focus or ongoing assessment	Ongoing process integrated with nursing care	To determine the status of a specific problem identified in an earlier assessment	Hourly assessment of the client's fluid intake and urinary output in an ICU
		To identify new or overlooked problems	Assessment of client's ability to perform self-care while assisting a client to bathe
Emergency assessment	During any physiologic or psychologic crisis of the client	To identify life-threatening problems	Rapid assessment of a person's airway, breathing status, and circulation during a cardiac arrest
			Assessment of suicidal tendencies or potential for violence
Time-lapsed assessment	Several months after initial assessment	To compare the client's current status to baseline data previously obtained	Reassessment of a client's functional health patterns in a home care or outpatient setting

ever the nurse is in contact with the client or support persons. The primary interviewing process used during assessment is taking the nursing health history. See Figure 5–2 on pages 95 and 96. Examining is the major method used in the physical health assessment.

In reality, the nurse uses all three methods simultaneously when assessing clients. For example, during the client interview, the nurse observes, listens, asks questions, and mentally retains information to explore in the physical examination.

OBSERVING

To **observe** is to gather data by using the five senses. Observation is a conscious, deliberate skill that is developed only through effort and with an organized approach. Although nurses observe mainly through sight, most of the senses are engaged during careful observations. Examples of client data observed through four senses are shown in Table 5–5 on page 90.

Observation has two aspects: (a) noticing the stimuli and (b) selecting, organizing, and interpreting the data (ie, perceiving them). A nurse who observes that a client's face is flushed must relate that observation to, for example, body temperature, activity, environmental temperature, and blood pressure. Because observation involves selecting, organizing, and interpreting data, errors can occur. For example, a nurse might not notice certain signs, either because they are unexpected or because they do not conform to preconceptions about a client's illness. Nurses often need to focus on specific stimuli in a clinical situation; otherwise, they may be overwhelmed by a multitude of stimuli. Observing, therefore, involves discriminating among stimuli, that is, distinguishing stimuli in a meaningful manner. For example, nurses caring for newborns learn to ignore the usual sounds of machines in the nursery but respond quickly to an infant's cry or movement.

The experienced nurse is often able to attend to an intervention (eg, giving a bed bath or monitoring an intravenous infusion) while at the same time making important observations (eg, noting a change in respiratory status or skin color). The beginning student must learn to make observations and complete tasks simultaneously.

Nursing observations must be organized so that nothing significant is missed. Most nurses develop a particular sequence for observing events, usually focusing on the client first. For example, a nurse walks into a client's room and observes, in the following order:

1. Clinical signs of client distress (eg, pallor or flushing, labored breathing, and behavior indicating pain or emotional distress)

Table 5–5 Observational Skills

Sense	Examples of Client Data
Vision	Overall appearance (body size, general weight, posture, grooming); signs of distress or discomfort; facial and body gestures; skin color and lesions; abnormalities of movement; nonverbal demeanor (eg, signs of anger or anxiety); religious or cultural artifacts (eg, books, icons, candles, beads)
Smell	Body or breath odors
Hearing	Breath and heart sounds; bowel sounds; ability to communicate; language spoken; ability to initiate conversation; ability to respond when spoken to; orientation to time, person, and place; thoughts and feelings about self, others, and health status
Touch	Skin temperature and moisture; muscle strength (eg, hand grip); pulse rate, rhythm, and volume; palpatory lesions (eg, lumps, masses, nodules)

2. Threats to the client's safety, real or anticipated (eg, a lowered side rail)
3. The presence and functioning of associated equipment (eg, intravenous equipment and oxygen)
4. The immediate environment, including the people in it

INTERVIEWING

An **interview** is a planned communication or a conversation with a purpose, for example, to give information, identify problems of mutual concern, evaluate change, teach, provide support, or provide counseling or therapy. Interviewing is a process that the nurse applies in most phases of the nursing process. During the assessment phase, however, the primary purpose of the interview is to gather data. One example of the interview is the nursing health history, which is a part of the nursing admission assessment. See Figure 5–2, pages 95 and 96. Components of the nursing history are discussed in Chapter 22.

There are two approaches to interviewing: directive and nondirective. The **directive interview** is highly structured and elicits specific information. The nurse establishes the purpose of the interview and controls the interview, at least at the outset, by asking closed questions (see the next section) that call for a specific amount of data. The client responds to questions but may not have an opportunity to ask questions or discuss concerns. Nurses frequently use directive interviews to gather and to give information in a limited amount of time (eg, in an emergency situation).

During a **nondirective interview,** or rapport-building interview, by contrast, the nurse allows the client to control the purpose, subject matter, and pacing. **Rapport** is an understanding between two or more people. The nurse encourages communication by asking open-ended questions (see the next section) and providing empathetic responses. Nurses use nondirective interviewing for problem solving, counseling, and performance appraisal (Stewart & Cash 1988, p. 7).

A combination of directive and nondirective approaches is usually appropriate during the information-gathering interview, the goals of which are to collect data and to begin to establish rapport. The nurse begins by asking open-ended questions to determine areas of concern for the client. If, for example, a client expresses worry about surgery, the nurse pauses to explore the client's worry and to provide support. Simply to note the worry, without dealing with it, can leave the impression that the nurse does not care about the client's concerns or dismisses them as unimportant. As the interview evolves, the nurse may use closed questions to obtain more specific data and to complete the nursing health history.

Kinds of Interview Questions Although there are many ways to categorize questions, in this book they are classified as open-ended or closed, and neutral or leading. **Closed questions,** used in the directive interview, are restrictive and generally require only short answers giving specific information. Thus the amount of information gained is generally limited. Closed questions often begin with "when," "where," "who," "what," "do (did, does)," "is (are, was)" and sometimes "how." Examples of closed questions are "What medication did you take?" "Are you having pain now? Show me where it is." "What is your occupation?" "How old are you?" "When did you fall?" The highly stressed person and the person who has difficulty communicating will find closed questions easier to answer than open-ended questions.

Open-ended questions, associated with the nondirective interview, are ones that lead or invite clients to discover and explore (elaborate, clarify, or illustrate) their thoughts or feelings. They allow clients the freedom to talk about what they wish. An open-ended question is broad, specifies only the topic to be discussed, and invites answers longer than one or two words. Such questions give clients the freedom to divulge only the information that they are ready to disclose. Responses may also convey clients' attitudes and beliefs. The open-ended question is useful at the beginning of an interview or to change topics.

Examples of open-ended questions are "How have you been feeling lately?" "What brought you to the hospital?" "How did you feel in that situation?" "Would you describe more about how you relate to your child?" "What would you like to talk about today?" These questions or

Table 5–6 Selected Advantages and Disadvantages of Open and Closed Questions

Open Questions: Advantages	Open Questions: Disadvantages	Closed Questions: Advantages	Closed Questions: Disadvantages
1. They let the interviewee do the talking.	1. They take more time.	1. Questions and answers can be controlled more effectively.	1. They may provide too little information and require follow-up questions.
2. The interviewer is able to listen and observe.	2. Only brief answers may be given.	2. They require less effort from the interviewee.	2. They may not reveal how the interviewee feels.
3. They are easy to answer and nonthreatening.	3. Valuable information may be withheld.	3. They may be less threatening, since they do not require explanations or justifications.	3. They do not allow the interviewee to volunteer possibly valuable information.
4. They reveal what the interviewee thinks is important.	4. They often elicit more information than necessary.	4. They take less time.	4. They may inhibit communication and convey lack of interest by the interviewee.
5. They may reveal the interviewee's lack of information, misunderstanding of words, frame of reference, prejudices, or stereotypes.	5. Responses are difficult to document and require skill in recording.	5. Information can be asked for before the information is volunteered.	5. The interviewer may dominate the interview with questions.
6. They can provide information the interviewer may not ask for.	6. The interviewer requires skill in controlling an open-ended interview.	6. Responses are easily documented.	
7. They can reveal the interviewee's degree of feeling about an issue.	7. Responses require psychologic insight and sensitivity from the interviewer.	7. They are easy to use and can be handled by unskilled interviewers.	
8. They can convey interest and trust because of the freedom they provide.			

Table constructed, with permission, from material on pp. 55–58 of Charles J Stewart and William B Cash, Jr, *Interviewing: Principles and Practices*, 6th ed. © 1991 WC Brown, Dubuque, IA. All rights reserved.

statements require more than a yes or no or other short response. Such questions usually begin with "what" or "how."

The type of question a nurse chooses depends on the needs of the client at the time. For example, the nurse asks closed questions in an emergency or other acute situation when information must be obtained quickly. The nurse often finds it necessary to use a combination of closed and open-ended questions throughout an interview to accomplish the goals of the interview and obtain needed information. See Table 5–6 for advantages and disadvantages of open and closed questions.

A **neutral question** is a question the client can answer without direction or pressure from the nurse. Examples are "How do you feel about that?" "Why do you think you had the operation?" A **leading question,** by contrast, directs the client's answer. The phrasing of the question suggests what answer is expected. Examples are "You're stressed about surgery tomorrow, aren't you?" "You will take your medicine, won't you?" The leading question does not give the client an opportunity to decide whether the answer is true or not. Leading questions create problems if the client, in an effort to please the nurse, gives inaccurate responses. This results in inaccurate data collection.

Planning the Interview and Setting Before beginning an interview, the nurse reviews what information is already available, for example, postoperative record, information about the current illness, or literature about the client's health problem. The nurse also reviews the data-collection form to make sure that the data to be collected are really needed and will serve some purpose related to the client's care. If a form is not available, most nurses prepare an interview guide to remember areas of information and determine what questions to ask. The guide includes a list of topics and subtopics rather than a series of questions.

Each interview and its setting is influenced by time, place, and seating arrangement.

PERSONAL SPACE VARIABLES

- North Americans and Asians tend to need more space than Arabs and Latin Americans.
- Men of all cultures usually require more space than women.
- Anxiety increases the need for space.
- Direct eye contact increases the need for space.

Source: A Arnold and K Boggs, *Interpersonal Relationships: Professional Communications Skills for Nurses* (Philadelphia: WB Saunders, 1989), 197–98.

Time Nurses need to schedule interviews with hospitalized clients for a time when the client is physically comfortable and free of pain, and when interruptions by friends, family, and other health professionals are absent or minimal. Nurses should schedule interviews with clients in their homes at a time selected by the client. In all instances, the client should be made to feel comfortable and unhurried.

Place The place of the interview must have adequate privacy to promote communication. A well-lighted, well-ventilated, moderate-sized room that is relatively free of noise, movements, and interruptions encourages communication. In addition, a place where others cannot overhear or see the client is desirable. Most people are inhibited when answering personal questions or expressing strong feelings in the sight or hearing of others.

Seating Arrangement A seating arrangement with the nurse behind a desk and the client seated across creates a formal setting that suggests a business meeting between a superior and a subordinate. In contrast, a seating arrangement in which the parties sit on two chairs placed at right angles to a desk or table or a few feet apart, with no table between, creates a less formal atmosphere, and the nurse and client tend to feel on equal terms. In groups, a horseshoe or circular chair arrangement can avoid a superior or head-of-the-table position.

When interviewing a client in bed, the nurse can sit at a 45-degree angle to the bed. This position is less formal than sitting behind a table in the room or standing at the foot of the bed. During an initial admission interview, a client may feel less confronted if there is an overbed table between the client and the nurse. Sitting on a client's bed hems the client in and makes staring difficult to avoid.

Distance The distance between the interviewer and interviewee should be neither too small nor too great, because people feel uncomfortable when talking to someone who is too close or too far away. Most people feel comfortable maintaining a distance of 3 to 4 feet during an interview. Communication at a distance greater than this tends to be more impersonal, and may suggest a lack of involvement on the part of the nurse. Some clients require more or less personal space, depending on their cultural and personal needs. See the box to the left.

Height also affects communication. By standing and looking down at a client, the nurse risks intimidating the client, who may perceive the nurse as having greater status. For additional information, see the discussion of personal space in Chapter 18.

Stages of an Interview An interview has three major stages: the opening or introduction, the body or development, and the closing.

The Opening The opening can be the most important part of the interview, because what is said and done at that time sets the tone for the remainder of the interview. The opening is a two-step process: establishing rapport and orienting the interviewee (Stewart & Cash 1988, p. 39). Either step can come first, depending on the situation, the relationship between the two parties, or the interviewer's choice. The rapport and orientation stages may occur at the same time and are often indistinguishable.

Establishing rapport is a process of creating good will and trust. It can begin with a greeting—"Good morning, John"—or a self-introduction—"Good morning. I'm Becky James, a nursing student"—accompanied by nonverbal gestures such as a smile, a handshake, and a friendly manner. The nurse continues to develop rapport by asking questions about the person and proceeding with some small talk about the weather, sports, families, and the like. The nurse must be careful not to overdo this stage; too much superficial talk can arouse anxiety about what is to follow and may appear insincere.

In the orientation step, the nurse explains the purpose and nature of the interview, for example, what information is needed, how long it will take, and what is expected of the client. The nurse usually states that the client has the right not to provide data and tells the client how the information will be used.

The following is an example of an interview introduction:

Step 1—Establish rapport

Nurse: Hello, Ms Goodwin, I'm Ms Fellows. I'm a nursing student, and I'll be assisting with your care here.
Client: Hi. Are you a student from the college?
Nurse: Yes, I'm in my final year. Are you familiar with the campus?
Client: Oh! yes! I'm an avid football fan. My nephew graduated in 1990, and I often attend football games with him.

Nurse: That's great! Sounds like fun.
Client: Yes, I enjoy it very much.

Step 2—Orientation

Nurse: May I sit down with you here for about 10 minutes to talk about how I can help you while you're here?
Client: All right. What do you want to know?
Nurse: Well, to plan your care after your operation, I'd like to get some information about your normal daily activities and what you expect here in the hospital. I'd like to make notes while we talk to get the important points and have them available to the other staff who will also look after you.
Client: OK. That's all right with me.
Nurse: If there is anything you don't want to talk about, please feel free to say so, and if there is anything you would rather I didn't write down, just tell me. Is this a good time for you?
Client: Sure, that will be fine.

The Body In the body of the interview, the client communicates what he or she thinks, feels, knows, and perceives in response to questions from the nurse. The nurse can make the transition from the opening stage to this stage by asking an open-ended question that is related to the stated purpose, is easy to answer, and does not embarrass or place stress on the person. For example: "What brought you to the hospital today?"

Effective development of the interview demands that the nurse use communication techniques that make both parties feel comfortable and serve the purpose of the interview. See communication techniques in Chapter 18. Brief guidelines for communicating during an interview are outlined in the accompanying box.

The Closing The nurse usually terminates the interview when the needed information has been obtained. In some cases, however, a client terminates it, for example, when deciding not to give any more information or when unable to offer more information for some other reason—fatigue, for example. The closing is important in maintaining the rapport and trust established during the interview and in facilitating future interactions. The following techniques are commonly used to close an interview (Stewart & Cash 1988, pp. 50–52):

1. Signal that the interview is coming to an end by offering to answer questions: "Do you have any questions?" "I would be glad to answer any questions you have." Be sure to allow time for the person to answer, or the offer will be regarded as insincere.
2. Declare completion of the purpose or task by saying "Well, that's about all I need to know for now" or "Well, those are all the questions I have for now." Preceding a remark with the word "well" generally signals that the end of the interaction is near.
3. State appreciation or satisfaction about what was accomplished: "I really enjoyed meeting you, and I think we accomplished a great deal." "Those are all the questions I have. Thank you for your time and help." "The questions you have answered will be helpful in planning your nursing care."
4. Express concern for the person's welfare and future: "Take care of yourself. I'll see you on Thursday." "I hope all goes well for you. If you run into additional problems, be sure to get in touch with me."
5. Plan for the next meeting, if there is to be one. Include the day, time, place, topic, and purpose: "Let's get together again here on the fifteenth at 9:00 AM to see how you are managing then."
6. Reveal what will happen next. For example: "Ms Goodwin, I will be responsible for giving you care three mornings per week while you are here. I will be in to see you each Monday, Tuesday, and Wednesday between eight o'clock and noon. At those times, we can adjust your care if we need to."
7. Signal that the time is up if a time limit was agreed on or explain why the interview must close at that time: "Well, I see our time is up; did it ever go quickly today." Or: "I'm sorry, but we're going to have to end

CLINICAL GUIDELINES

Communication During an Interview

- Listen attentively, using all your senses, and speak slowly and clearly.
- Use language the client understands, and clarify points that are not understood, for instance, by asking the person to describe what a word means to the person.
- Plan questions to follow a logical sequence.
- Ask only one question at a time. Double questions limit the client to one choice and may confuse both the nurse and the client.
- Allow the client the opportunity to look at things the way they appear to him or her and not the way they appear to the nurse or someone else.
- Do not impose your own values on the client.
- Avoid using personal examples, such as saying, "If I were you . . ."
- Nonverbally convey respect, concern, interest, and acceptance.
- Use and accept silence to help the client search for more thoughts or to organize them.
- Use eye contact and be calm, unhurried, and sympathetic.

our discussion; I have another appointment in 10 minutes."

8. Provide a summary to verify accuracy and agreement. Summarizing serves several purposes: It helps to terminate the interview, it reassures the client that the nurse has listened, it checks the accuracy of the nurse's perceptions, it clears the way for new ideas, and it helps the client to note progress and forward direction (Brammer 1993, pp. 82–83). Sometimes clients may spontaneously offer a summary; at other times, the nurse must initiate it or ask the client to do so. "Let's look at what has happened in this interview. What do you think has been accomplished?" Summaries are particularly helpful for clients who are anxious or who have difficulty staying with the topic. "Well, it seems to me that you are especially worried about your hospitalization and chest pain because your father died of a heart attack 5 years ago, your wife has multiple sclerosis and depends on you for support and care, and you don't want to ask for too much help from your children. Is that correct? . . . We'll do the best we can to help you with these concerns. I'll discuss this with you again tomorrow, and we'll decide what plans need to be made to help you."

EXAMINING

The **physical examination** is a systematic data-collection method that uses observational skills (ie, the senses of sight, hearing, smell, and touch) to detect health problems. To conduct the examination, the nurse uses techniques of inspection, auscultation, palpation, and percussion. These techniques are discussed in Chapter 22.

Developing the skills needed for physical assessment requires knowledge, practice, and time. However, the student nurse often begins by describing the general appearance of the client, assessing skin, range of motion, and mobility—often during morning care—and by monitoring vital signs.

The physical assessment is carried out systematically. It may be organized according to the examiner's preference, in a head-to-toe approach or as a body systems approach. Usually, the nurse first records a general impression about the client's overall appearance and health status, for example, age, body size, mental and nutritional status, speech, and behavior. Then, the nurse takes such measurements as vital signs, height, and weight. The nurse conducting a physical examination using the **cephalocaudal** (head-to-toe) approach begins the assessment at the head, progresses to the neck, thorax, abdomen, and extremities and ends at the toes. The nurse using a body systems approach investigates each system individually, that is, the respiratory system, the circulatory system, the nervous system, and so on. During the physical assessment, the nurse assesses all body parts and compares findings on each side of the body (eg, lungs). These techniques are discussed in detail in Chapters 21 and 22.

Instead of giving a complete examination, the nurse may focus on a specific problem area noted from the nursing assessment, such as the inability to urinate. On occasion, the nurse may find it necessary to resolve a client complaint or problem (eg, shortness of breath) prior to completing the examination. Alternatively, the nurse may perform a screening examination. A **screening examination,** also called a review of systems, is a brief review of essential functioning of various body parts or systems. An example of a screening examination is the nursing admission assessment form shown in Figure 5–2. Data obtained from this examination are measured against norms or standards, such as ideal height and weight standards or norms for body temperature or blood pressure levels.

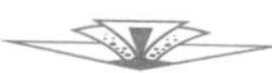

THE ASSESSMENT PROCESS

The assessment process involves four closely related activities:

- Collecting data
- Organizing data
- Validating data
- Recording data

COLLECTING DATA

Data collection is the process of gathering information about a client's health status. It must be both systematic and continuous to prevent the omission of significant data and reflect a client's changing health status.

A **database** (baseline data) is all the information about a client; it includes the nursing health history (Figure 5–2) and physical assessment, the physician's history and physical examination, results of laboratory and diagnostic tests, and material contributed by other health personnel.

Client data should include past history as well as current problems. For example, a history of an allergic reaction to penicillin is a vital piece of historical data. Past surgical procedures, folk healing practices, and chronic diseases are also examples of historical data. Current data relate to present circumstances, such as pain, nausea, sleep patterns, and religious practices. To collect data accurately, both the client and nurse must actively participate.

Types of Data Data can be subjective or objective. **Subjective data,** also referred to as **symptoms** or **covert data,** are apparent only to the person affected and can be described or verified only by that person. Itching, pain, and feelings of worry are examples of subjective data. Subjective data include the client's sensations, feelings, values,

ADMISSION DATA

Date 4-16-95 Time 3:15p.m. Primary Language English
Arrived Via: ☐ Wheelchair ☐ Stretcher ☑ Ambulatory
From: ☐ Admitting ☐ ER ☑ Home ☐ Nursing Home ☐ Other
Admitting M.D. R. Katz Time Notified 5 p.m.

ORIENTATION TO UNIT

	YES	NO		YES	NO
Arm Band Correct	☒	☐	Visiting Hours	☒	☐
Allergy Band	☒	☐	Smoking Policy	☒	☐
Telephone	☒	☐	TV, Lights, Bed Controls,		
Electrical Policy	☒	☐	Call Lights, Side Rails	☒	☐
Educational Mat'l	☒	☐	Nurses Station	☒	☐
(TV Brochure)	☒	☐			

Family M.D. R. Katz
Weight 125 lb. Height 5ft. 2in. BP:R — L 122/80
Temp. 103 F Pulse 92, weak Resp. 28, shallow
Source Providing Information ☑ Patient ☐ Other
Unable to Obtain History ☐
Reason for Admission (Onset, Duration, Pt.'s Perception) "Chest cold" X2 weeks S.O.B on exertion. "Lung pain, fever," "Dr. says I have pneumonia."

ALLERGIES & REACTIONS

Drugs Penicillin
Food/Other
Signs & Symptoms rash, nausea
Blood Reaction ☐ Yes ☑ No Dyes/Shellfish ☐ Yes ☑ No

MEDICATIONS

Current Meds	Dose/Freq.	Last Dose
Synthroid	0.1 mg. daily	4-16, 8 a.m.

Disposition of Meds: ☒ Home ☐ Pharmacy ☐ Safe *At Bedside

MEDICAL HISTORY

☑ No Major Problems ☐ Gastro
☐ Cardiac ☐ Arthritis
☐ Hyper/Hypotension ☐ Stroke
☐ Diabetes ☐ Seizures
☐ Cancer ☐ Glaucoma
☐ Respiratory ☑ Other Childbirth-1992

Surgery/Procedures	Date
Appendectomy	1978
Partial thyroidectomy	1991

SPECIAL ASSISTIVE DEVICES

☐ Wheelchair ☐ Contacts ☐ Venous Access Device ☐ Dentures ☐ Partial ☐ Upper ☐ Lower
☐ Braces ☐ Hearing Aid
☐ Cane/Crutches ☐ Prosthesis
☐ Walker ☐ Glasses ☐ Epidural Catheter
☐ Other None

VALUABLES

Patient informed Hospital not responsible for personal belongings.
Valuables Disposition: ☐ Patient ☐ Safe ☐ Given to
Patient/SO Signature None

PSYCHOSOCIAL HISTORY

Recent Stress None
Coping Mechanism Not assessed because of fatigue
Support System Husband, co-workers, friends
Calm: ☑ Yes ☐ No
Anxious: ☐ Yes ☐ No Facial muscles tense; trembling
Religion Catholic, Would want Last Rites
Tobacco Use: ☐ Yes ☑ No
Alcohol Use: ☐ Yes ☑ No
Drug Use: ☐ Yes ☑ No

NEUROLOGICAL

Oriented: ☑ Person ☑ Place ☑ Time ☐ Confused ☐ Sedated ☐ Alert ☐ Restless ☑ Lethargic ☐ Comatose
Pupils: ☑ Equal ☐ Unequal ☑ Reactive ☐ Sluggish ☐ Other 3mm.
Extremity Strength: ☑ Equal ☐ Unequal
Speech: ☑ Clear ☐ Slurred ☐ Other

MUSCULO-SKELETAL

Normal ROM of Extremities ☑ Yes ☐ No
☑ Weakness ☐ Paralysis ☐ Contractures ☐ Joint Swelling ☑ Pain
☐ Other ↓ related to fatigue when coughing

RESPIRATORY

Pattern: ☐ Even ☐ Uneven ☑ Shallow ☑ Dyspnea ☑ Other diminished breath sounds
Breathing Sounds: ☐ Clear ☑ Other inspiratory crackles
Secretions: ☐ None ☑ Other pink, thick sputum
Cough: ☐ None ☑ Productive ☐ Nonproductive

CARDIOVASCULAR

Pulses: Apical Rate 92-W ☑ Reg. ☐ Irregular ☐ Pacemaker
S = Strong W = Weak A = Absent D = Doppler
Radial R 92 L — Pedal R — L —
Edema: ☑ Absent ☐ Present Site
Perfusion: ☐ Warm ☐ Dry ☑ Diaphoretic ☐ Cool (Hot)

GASTROINTESTINAL

Oral Mucosa ☐ Normal ☑ Other pale and dry
Bowel Sounds: ☑ Normal ☐ Other Abd. soft
Wt. Change: ☐ ☑ N/V Stool Frequency/Character 1/day; soft
Last B/M 4-15-95 ☐ Ostomy (type)
Equip.

GENITOURINARY

Urine: Last Voided This morning
☐ Normal ☐ Anuria ☐ Hematuria ☐ Dysuri ☐ Incontinent
☒ Other ↓ amount & frequency since ill
☐ Catheter (type) Other
LMP 4-1-95 ☐ Vaginal/Penile Discharge
Other

SELF CARE

Need Assist with: ☐ Ambulating ☐ Elimination ☐ Meals ☒ Hygiene ☐ Dressing
while fatigued

ADDRESSOGRAPH PLATE

Luisa Sanchez. [F. age 28]
#4637651

NORTH BROWARD HOSPITAL DISTRICT
NURSING ADMINISTRATION ASSESSMENT

Figure 5–2 Assessment for Luisa Sanchez. Nursing assessment tool courtesy of North Broward Hospital District, Broward County, Florida. Reprinted with permission.

NUTRITION

General Appearance: ☑ Well Nourished ☐ Emaciated ☐ Other ______

Appetite: ☐ Good ☐ Fair ☑ Poor -x2 days

Diet Liquid Meal Pattern 3/day

☐ Feeds Self ☐ Assist ☐ Total Feed

SKIN ASSESSMENT

Color: ☐ Normal ☐ Flushed ☑ Pale ☐ Dusky ☐ Cyanotic ☐ Jaundiced ☑ Other Cheeks flushed, hot

General Description Surgical scars: RLQ abdomen; anterior neck

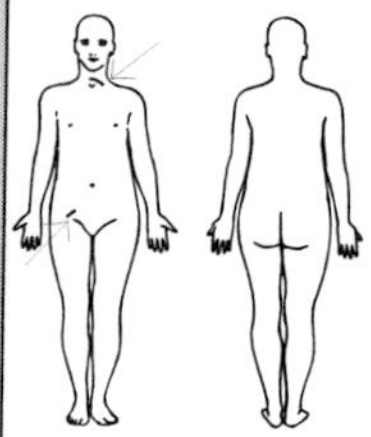

Note Cultures Obtained ______

PRESSURE SORE "AT RISK" SCREENING CRITERIA

OVERALL SKIN CONDITION

Grade		
	0	Turgor (elasticity adequate, skin warm and moist)
✓	1	Poor turgor, skin cold & dry
	2	Areas mottled, red or denuded
	3	Existing skin ulcer/lesions

BOWEL AND BLADDER CONTROL

Grade		
✓	0	Always able to ask for bedpan
	1	Incontinence of urine
	2	Incontinence of feces
	3	Totally incontinent Confined to bed

REHABILITATIVE STATE

Grade		
	0	Fully ambulatory
✓	1	Ambulated with assistance
	2	Chair to bed ambulation only
	3	Confined to bed
	4	Immobile in bed

NUTRITIONAL STATE

Grade		
	0	Eats all
✓	1	Eats very little
	2	Refuses food often
	3	Tube feeding
	4	Intravenous feeding

MENTAL STATE

Grade		
✓	0	Alert and clear
	1	Confused
	2	Disoriented/senile
	3	Stuporous
	4	Unconcious

CHRONIC DISEASE STATUS (i.e. COPD, ASCVD. Peripheral Vascular Disease, Diabetes, or Renal Disease, Cancer, Motor or Sensory Deficits, Elderly, Other)

Grade		
✓	0	Absent
	1	One Present
	2	Two Present
	3	Three or more Present

TOTAL ______ Refer to Skin Care Protocol

FALLS SCREENING

If one or more of the following are checked institute fall precautions/plan of care

☐ History of Falls ☐ Unsteady Gait ☐ Confusion/Disorientation ☐ Dizziness

If two or more of the following are checked institute fall precautions/plan of care

☐ Age over 80 ☐ Utilizes cane, walker, w/c ☐ Sleeplessness
☐ Impaired vision ☐ Urgency/frequency in elimination
☐ Multiple Diagnoses ☐ Impaired hearing
☐ Inability to understand or follow directions ☐ Medication/Sedative /Diuretic etc.

NURSE SIGNATURE/TITLE	DATE	TIME
Mary Medina, RN	4-16-95	3:30pm
NURSE SIGNATURE/TITLE	DATE	TIME

EDUACTION/DISCHARGE PLANNING

1. What do you know about your present illness? "Dr. says I have pneumonia." "I will have an I.V."
2. What information do you want or need about your illness? ______
3. Would you like family/SO involved in your care? Husband, Michael
4. How long do you expect to be in the hospital? "1-2 days"
5. What concerns do you have about leaving the hospital? ______

CHECK APPROPRIATE BOX

Will patient need post discharge assistance with ADLs/physical functioning? ☐ Yes ☑ No ☐ Unknown

Does patient have family capable of and willing to provide assistance post discharge?
☑ Yes ☐ No ☐ Unknown ☐ No family

Is assistance needed beyond that which family can provide?
☐ Yes ☑ No ☐ Unknown

Previous admission in the last six months?
☐ Yes ☑ No ☐ Unknown

Patient lives with Husband and 1 child

Planned discharge to Home

Comments: Fatigue and anxiety may have interfered with learning. Re-teach anything covered at admission, later.

Social Services Notified ☐ Yes ☑ No

NARRATIVE NOTES

S--c/O sharp chest pain when coughing and dyspnea on exertion. States unable to carry out regular daily exercise for past week. Coughing relieved "if I sit up and sit still." Nausea associated with coughing. Having occasional "chills." Occasionally becomes frightened, stating, "I can't breathe." Well groomed but "too tired to put on make-up."

O--Chest expansion < 3cm, no nasal flaring or use of accessory muscles. Breath sounds and insp. crackles in Ⓡ upper and lower chest.

Assesses own supports as "good" (eg, relationship c̄ husband). Is "worried" about daughter. States husband will be out of town until tomorrow. Left 3-year-old daughter with neighbor. Concerned too about her work (is attorney). "I'll never get caught up." Had water at noon—no food today. Informed of need to save urine for 24 hr. specimen. IV D_5W LR 1000 mL started in Ⓡarm, 100 mL/hr. Slow capillary refill. Keeping head of bed↑ to facilitate breathing.

NORTH BROWARD HOSPITAL DISTRICT
NURSING ADMINISTRATION ASSESSMENT

Figure 5–2 *continued*

EXAMPLES OF SUBJECTIVE AND OBJECTIVE DATA

Subjective	*Objective*
"I feel weak all over when I exert myself."	Blood pressure 90/50
	Apical pulse 104
	Skin pale and diaphoretic
Client states he has a cramping pain in his abdomen. States, "I feel sick to my stomach."	Vomited 100 mL green-tinged fluid
	Abdomen firm and slightly distended
	Active bowel sounds auscultated in all 4 quadrants
"I'm short of breath."	Lung sounds clear bilaterally; diminished in right lower lobe
"He doesn't seem so sad today." (Wife states.)	Cried during interview
"I would like to see the chaplain before surgery."	Holding open Bible
	Has small silver cross on bedside table

beliefs, attitudes, and perception of personal health status and life situation. Information supplied by family members, significant others, or other health professionals is also considered subjective, if it is based on opinion rather than fact.

Objective data, also referred to as **signs** or **overt data,** are detectable by an observer or can be tested against an accepted standard. They can be seen, heard, felt, or smelled, and they are obtained by observation or physical examination. For example, a discoloration of the skin or a blood pressure reading are objective data. During the physical examination, the nurse obtains the objective data needed to validate subjective data and to complete the assessment phase of the nursing process. A complete database of both subjective and objective data provides a baseline for comparing client's responses to nursing and medical interventions. Examples of subjective and objective data are shown in the box above.

Sources of Data Sources of data are *primary* or *secondary.* The client is the primary source of data. Family members or other support persons, other health professionals, records and reports, laboratory and diagnostic analyses, and relevant literature are secondary or indirect sources. Secondary sources provide data that supplement and validate data obtained from the client.

Client The best source of data is usually the client, unless the client is too ill, young, or confused to communicate clearly. The client can usually provide subjective data that no one else can offer. See Table 5–7 on page 98 for factors that may impede data collection from the client.

Support People Family members, friends, and caregivers who know the client well often can supplement or verify information provided by the client. They might convey information about the client's response to illness, the stresses the client was experiencing before the illness, family attitudes to illness and health, and the client's home environment.

Support people are an especially important source of data for a client who is very young, unconscious, or confused. In some cases—a client who is physically or emotionally abused, for example—the person giving information may wish to remain anonymous. Before eliciting data from support people, the nurse should ensure that the client, if mentally able, accepts such input. The nurse should also indicate on the nursing history that the data was obtained from a support person.

Client Records Client records include information documented by various health care professionals. Client records also contain data regarding the client's occupation, religion, and marital status. By reviewing such records before interviewing the client, the nurse can avoid asking questions for which answers have already been supplied. Repeated questioning can be stressful and annoying to clients and cause concern about the lack of communication among health professionals.

Medical records (eg, medical history, physical examination, progress notes, and consultations) are often a source of a client's present and past health and illness patterns. These records can provide nurses with information about the client's coping behaviors, health practices, previous illnesses, and allergies.

Records of therapies by other health professionals, such as social workers, nutritionists, dietitians, or physiotherapists, help the nurse obtain relevant data not expressed by the client. For example, a social agency's report on a

Table 5–7 Factors That May Impede Client Data Collection

Client Factor	Effect	Nursing Action
Language difficulty (eg, not fluent in English)	Unable to clearly communicate vital information	Use simple, clear language with client and obtain an interpreter.
High anxiety	Rapid, incoherent speech; distortion of information	Attempt to reduce anxiety by speaking slowly and quietly; emphasize importance of providing accurate information to get appropriate help.
Fear that illness is incapacitating or life-threatening	May deny certain symptoms or deliberately give misleading facts	Explore discrepancies between client statements and physical findings or data from other sources.
Acute illness and/or pain	Short responses; primary concern is intervention to alleviate the problem	Provide required intervention before obtaining data. Ask closed questions to obtain essential data.
Limited mental capacity	Possibility of inaccurate, unreliable information	Encourage client to provide as much information as able; then, use secondary sources.
Previous negative experience with health care professionals	Resists providing data; believes "it won't help me anyway. It didn't do any good before"	Acknowledge previous experience and the imperfection of health professionals. Request another chance to help. Convey competence. Respect client's thoughts and feelings.

client's living conditions or a home health care agency's report on a client's coping at home can also be helpful to the nurse conducting an assessment.

Laboratory records also provide pertinent health information. Laboratory tests are frequently ordered as part of the physician's initial examination to aid in a medical diagnosis or to monitor medical treatment. For example, the determination of blood glucose level allows health professionals to monitor the administration of oral hypoglycemic medications. In some cases, nurses can use the same laboratory test to monitor the client's response to nursing interventions. Any laboratory data about a client must be compared to established norms for that particular test and for the client's age, sex, and so on. Laboratory tests vary among agencies, and norms can therefore be different. Diagnostic studies commonly ordered for large numbers of clients are shown in the *Clinical Companion.*

The nurse must always consider the information in client records in light of the present situation. For example, if the most recent medical record is 10 years old, it is likely that the client's health practices and coping behaviors have changed. Stressors in an individual's life often change, for example, when an alcoholic husband leaves home or a sick infant recovers.

Health Care Professionals Because assessment is an ongoing process, verbal reports from other health care professionals serve as other potential sources of information about a client's health. Nurses, social workers, physicians, and physiotherapists, for example, may have information from either previous or current contact with the client. Sharing of information among professionals is especially important to ensure continuity of care when clients are transferred to and from home and health care agencies.

Literature The review of nursing and related literature, such as professional journals and reference texts, can provide additional information for the database. A literature review includes but is not limited to the following information:

- Standards or norms against which to compare findings (eg, height and weight tables, normal developmental tasks for an age group)
- Cultural and social health practices
- Spiritual beliefs
- Additional required assessment data
- Nursing interventions and evaluation criteria relative to a client's health problems
- Information about medical diagnoses, treatment, and prognoses

ORGANIZING DATA

To obtain data systematically, the nurse uses an organized assessment framework, often referred to as a *nursing health history* or *nursing assessment.* Data collected during the nursing health history are largely subjective. Components of a nursing history are discussed in Chapter 22, page 462.

GORDON'S TYPOLOGY OF 11 FUNCTIONAL HEALTH PATTERNS

- *Health-perception–health-management pattern.* Describes client's perceived pattern of health and well-being and how health is managed.
- *Nutritional-metabolic pattern.* Describes pattern of food and fluid consumption relative to metabolic need and pattern indicators of local nutrient supply.
- *Elimination pattern.* Describes patterns of excretory function (bowel, bladder, and skin).
- *Activity-exercise pattern.* Describes pattern of exercise, activity, leisure, and recreation.
- *Cognitive-perceptual pattern.* Describes sensory-perceptual and cognitive pattern.
- *Sleep-rest pattern.* Describes patterns of sleep, rest, and relaxation.
- *Self-perception–self-concept pattern.* Describes self-concept pattern and perceptions of self (eg, body comfort, body image, feeling state).
- *Role-relationship pattern.* Describes pattern of role-engagements and relationships.
- *Sexuality-reproductive pattern.* Describes client's patterns of satisfaction and dissatisfaction with sexuality; describes reproductive patterns.
- *Coping–stress-tolerance pattern.* Describes general coping pattern and effectiveness of the pattern in terms of stress tolerance.
- *Value-belief pattern.* Describes patterns of values, beliefs (including spiritual), or goals that guide choices or decisions.

Source: M. Gordon, *Nursing diagnosis: Process and application*, 2d ed. (Hightstown, NJ: McGraw-Hill, 1987), p. 93.

There are many frameworks available for the systematic collection and documentation of assessment data. The framework may be modified according to the client's physical status.

Nursing Conceptual Models Most schools of nursing and health care agencies have developed their own structured assessment tools. Many of these are based on selected nursing theories (see Chapter 3). Three examples are Gordon's functional health pattern framework, Orem's self-care model, and Roy's adaptation model (see the accompanying boxes).

Gordon (1987) established a framework of 11 functional health patterns. Gordon uses the word *pattern* to signify a sequence of behavior. The nurse collects data

OREM'S SELF-CARE MODEL

Universal Self-Care Requisites

1. The maintenance of a sufficient intake of air
2. The maintenance of a sufficient intake of water
3. The maintenance of a sufficient intake of food
4. The provision of care associated with elimination processes and excrements
5. The maintenance of a balance between activity and rest
6. The maintenance of a balance between solitude and social interaction
7. The prevention of hazards to human life, human functioning, and human well-being
8. The promotion of human functioning and development within social groups in accord with human potential, known human limitations, and human desire to be normal. (Normalcy is used in the sense of that which is essentially human and that which is in accord with the genetic and constitutional characteristics and the talents of individuals.)

Source: DE Orem, *Nursing: Concepts of Practice*, 4th ed. (St Louis: Mosby-Year Book, 1991), p. 126.

ROY'S ADAPTATION MODEL

Adaptive Modes

1. Physiologic needs
   - Activity and rest
   - Nutrition
   - Elimination
   - Fluid and electrolytes
   - Oxygenation
   - Protection
   - Regulation: temperature
   - Regulation: the senses
   - Regulation: endocrine system
2. Self-concept
   - Physical self
   - Personal self
3. Role function
4. Interdependence

Source: C Roy and HA Andrews, *The Roy Adaptation Model: The Definitive Statement* (Norwalk, CT: Appleton & Lange, 1991), pp. 15–17.

about dysfunctional as well as functional behavior. Thus, by using Gordon's framework to organize data, nurses are able to discern emerging patterns.

Orem (1991) delineates eight universal self-care requisites of humans. Roy (1984) outlines the data to be collected according to the Roy adaptation model and classifies observable behavior into four categories: physiologic, self-concept, role function, and interdependence.

The unitary person framework, created by the North American Nursing Diagnosis Association (NANDA 1989) characterizes each person by a unique organization of nine "human response patterns," which reflect the whole person in interaction with the environment. Note that this is not, strictly speaking, a nursing theory, but a framework for assessing and diagnosing. This framework for organizing nursing diagnoses is presented in the box on page 123.

Figure 5–2 is a concise data-collection tool that is organized according to body systems and specific nursing concerns (eg, screening for falls and allergies); it does not use one particular nursing model. In the box on page 101, the Luisa Sanchez data from Figure 5–2 is shown after being organized according to the 11 functional health patterns. Note how the categories in the box differ from those in Figure 5–2. As a rule, the nurse organizes the data using the same model on which the data-collection tool is based. However, different models are provided here to demonstrate differences in organizing frameworks, and to show that the nurse is not limited to the framework provided by the data-collection tool.

Wellness Models Nurses use wellness models to assist clients to identify health risks and to explore life-style habits and health behaviors, beliefs, values, and attitudes that influence levels of wellness. Such models generally include the following (see Chapter 13 for details):

- Health history
- Physical fitness evaluation
- Nutritional assessment
- Life-stress analysis
- Life-style and health habits
- Health beliefs
- Sexual health
- Spiritual health
- Relationships
- Health risk appraisal

Nonnursing Models Frameworks and models from other disciplines may also be helpful for organizing data. These frameworks are narrower than the model required in nursing; therefore, the nurse usually needs to combine these with other approaches to obtain a complete history.

Body Systems Model The body systems model of physicians focuses on abnormalities of the following systems:

- Integumentary system
- Respiratory system
- Cardiovascular system
- Nervous system
- Musculoskeletal system
- Gastrointestinal system
- Genitourinary system
- Reproductive system

Maslow's Hierarchy of Needs Maslow's hierarchy of needs clusters data pertaining to the following:

- Physiologic needs (survival needs)
- Safety and security needs
- Love and belonging needs
- Self-esteem needs
- Self-actualization needs

See Chapter 14, page 274, for detailed information.

Developmental Theories Several physical, psychosocial, cognitive, and moral developmental theories may be used by the nurse in specific situations. Examples include the following:

- Havighurst's age periods and developmental tasks
- Freud's five stages of development
- Erikson's eight stages of development
- Piaget's phases of cognitive development
- Kohlberg's stages of moral development

See Chapter 23, pages 570–579, for further information.

VALIDATING DATA

If the nursing process is to be a successful framework for nursing care, the information gathered during the assessment phase must be complete, factual, and accurate. **Validation** is the act of "double-checking" or verifying data (cues) to confirm that they are accurate and factual. Validating data helps the nurse

- Ensure that assessment information is complete.
- Ensure that objective and related subjective data agree.
- Obtain additional information that may have been overlooked.
- Differentiate between cues and inferences.
- Avoid jumping to conclusions and focusing in the wrong direction to identify problems.

Not all data require validation. For example, data such as height, weight, birth date, and most laboratory studies

DATA FOR LUISA SANCHEZ, ORGANIZED ACCORDING TO FUNCTIONAL HEALTH PATTERNS

Health Perception/Health Management

- Aware/understands medical diagnosis
- Gives thorough history of illnesses and surgeries
- Complies with Synthroid regimen
- Relates progression of illness in detail
- Expects to have antibiotic therapy and "Go home in a day or two"
- States usual eating pattern "3 meals a day"

Nutritional/Metabolic

- 158 cm (5 ft, 2 in) tall; weighs 56 kg (125 lb)
- Usual eating pattern "3 meals a day"
- "No appetite" since having "cold"
- Has not eaten today; last fluids at noon
- Nauseated
- Oral temp 39.4 C (103 F)
- Decreased skin turgor

Elimination

- Usually no problem
- Decreased urinary frequency and amount ×2 days
- Last bowel movement yesterday, formed, "normal"

Activity/Exercise

- No musculoskeletal impairment
- Difficulty sleeping because of cough
- "Can't breathe lying down"
- States, "I feel weak"
- Short of breath on exertion
- Exercises daily

Cognitive/Perceptual

- No sensory deficits
- Pupils 3 mm, equal, brisk reaction
- Oriented to time, place, and person
- Responsive, but fatigued
- Responds appropriately to verbal and physical stimuli
- Recent and remote memory intact
- "I can think OK. Just weak"
- States "short of breath" on exertion
- Reports "pain in lungs," especially when coughing
- Experiencing chills
- Reports nausea

Roles/Relationships

- Lives with husband and 3-year-old daughter
- Sexual relationship "satisfactory"
- Husband out of town; will be back tomorrow afternoon
- Child with neighbor until husband returns
- States "good" relationships with friends and co-workers
- Working mother, attorney
- Husband helps at home "some"

Self-Perception/Self-Concept

- Expresses "concern" and "worry" over leaving daughter with neighbors until husband returns
- Well-groomed; says, "Too tired to mess with hair and makeup"

Coping/Stress

- Anxious: "I can't breathe"
- Facial muscles tense; trembling
- "I can think OK. Just weak"
- Expresses concerns about work: "I'll never get caught up"

Value/Belief

- Catholic
- No special practices desired except last rites
- Middle-class, professional orientation
- No wish to see chaplain or priest at present

Medication/History

- Synthroid 0.1 mg per day
- Client has history of appendectomy, partial thyroidectomy

Nursing Physical Assessment

- 28 years old
- Height 158 cm (5 ft, 2 in); weight 56 kg (125 lb)
- TPR 39.4 C, 92, 28
- Radial pulses weak, regular
- Blood pressure 122/80 sitting
- Skin hot and pale, cheeks flushed
- Mucous membranes dry and pale
- Respirations shallow; chest expansion < 3cm
- Cough productive of small amounts of pale pink sputum
- Inspiratory crackles auscultated throughout right upper and lower chest
- Diminished breath sounds on right side
- Abdomen soft, not distended
- Old surgical scars: anterior neck, RLQ abdomen
- Diaphoretic

Table 5–8 Validating Assessment Data

Guidelines	Example
Compare subjective and objective data to verify the client's statements with your observations.	Client's perceptions of "feeling hot" need to be compared with measurement of the body temperature.
Clarify any ambiguous or vague statements.	*Client:* "I've felt sick on and off for 6 weeks." *Nurse:* "Describe what your sickness is like. Tell me what you mean by 'on and off'."
Be sure your data consists of cues and not inferences.	*Observation:* Dry skin and reduced tissue turgor *Inference:* Dehydration *Action:* Collect additional data that are needed to make the inference in the diagnosing phase. For example, determine the client's fluid intake, amount and appearance of urine, and blood pressure.
Double-check data that are extremely abnormal.	*Observation:* A resting pulse of 50 beats per minute or a blood pressure of 180/95 *Action:* Use another piece of equipment as needed to confirm abnormalities, or ask someone else to collect the same data.
Determine the presence of factors that may interfere with accurate measurement.	A crying infant will have an abnormal respiratory rate and will need quieting before accurate assessment can be made.
Use references (textbooks, journals, research reports) to explain phenomena.	A nurse considers tiny purple or bluish-black swollen areas under the tongue of an elderly client to be abnormal until reading about physical changes of aging. Such varicosities are not uncommon.

that can be measured with an accurate scale of measurement can be accepted as factual. As a rule, the nurse validates data when there are discrepancies between data obtained in the nursing interview (subjective data) and the physical examination (objective data), or when the client's statements differ at different times in the assessment. Guidelines for validating data are shown in Table 5–8.

Cues are subjective or objective data that can be directly observed by the nurse; that is, what the client says or what the nurse can see, hear, feel, smell, or measure. **Inferences** are the nurse's conclusions or interpretation of the cues (eg, a nurse observes the cues that an incision is red, hot, and swollen; the nurse makes the inference that the incision is infected).

To collect data accurately, nurses need to be aware of their own biases, values, and beliefs and to separate fact from inference, interpretation, and assumption (see Chapter 10). For example, a nurse seeing a man holding his arm to his chest might assume that he is experiencing chest pain, when in fact he has a painful hand.

The acceptance of assumptions as fact is called **premature closure.** To build an accurate database and avoid premature closure, nurses must validate assumptions regarding the client's physical or emotional behavior. In the previous example, the nurse should ask the client why he is holding his arm to his chest. The client's response may validate the nurse's assumptions or prompt further questioning. Figure 5–2 shows that the nurse auscultated Luisa Sanchez's heart and lungs to validate her statement that she had "pain" in her "lungs" and "shortness of breath" on exertion (see page 95). Failure to validate assumptions can lead to an inaccurate or incomplete nursing assessment.

RECORDING DATA

To complete the assessment phase, the nurse records data. Accurate documentation is essential and should include all data collected about the client's health status. Data are recorded in a factual manner and not interpreted by the nurse. For example, the nurse records the client's breakfast intake (objective data) as "coffee 240 mL, juice 120 mL, 1 egg, and 1 slice of toast," rather than as "appetite good" (a judgment). A judgment or a conclusion such as "appetite good" or "normal appetite" may have different meanings for different people. To increase accuracy, the nurse records subjective data in the client's own words. Restating in other words what someone says increases the chance of changing the original meaning. Details of recording are discussed in Chapter 9.

RESEARCH NOTE

How Can Valid Data Be Obtained from Elderly Clients?

While interviewing institutionalized elders in a study at a geriatric remotivation program, the researchers encountered difficulties that threatened the validity of their data. Using a qualitative approach, the researchers identified four clusters of elder characteristics that threaten validity by producing data that are "insufficient," "unclear," "nice," and "emotionally charged":

1. Physical characteristics, such as being in pain, being unable to see and hear, and urinary urgency
2. Cognitive characteristics, such as disorientation and memory deficits
3. Affective characteristics, such as the way in which the elders displayed their feelings (eg, blank faces, unexpressive eyes), depression, and sadness
4. Personal characteristics, such as socioeconomic and ethnic background, and differences in language usage

Implications As a result of their experience, the authors recommended the following strategies to increase the validity of research data. Some of these also have implications for assessment interviews conducted in nursing practice:

- Increase sample size. (This is a research technique.)
- Return to setting frequently. (It is common for elders to be confused at some times and alert and oriented at others. Gathering data at more than one time allows for comparison of answers and produces more accurate data.)
- Lengthen observation periods. (Elders may fall asleep, become disoriented, or cry during interviews. The nurse should plan enough time to deal with these eventualities.)
- Recognize the value of stories. (Rather than dismissing what may seem to be irrelevant "stories" the elderly often tell, the nurse should listen. Listening to these stories may provide insight and information and at the same time be therapeutic for the client.)
- Recognize the value of socializing. (Valuable data may be gained by chatting with the client during meals, while bathing, changing linen, and so forth.)
- Have elders view and respond to videotapes. (This may not be practical for bedside nurses.)
- Collect interview and observation data. (Validation is important because elders' words and actions are often hard to understand. Subjective and objective data together create a more interpretable picture of the client, because each provides a check on the other.)

Source: BL Rogers, Interviewing institutionalized elders: Threats to validity, *Image: Journal of Nursing Scholarship*, Fall 1991, 23:171–76.

CHAPTER HIGHLIGHTS

- The nursing process is a systematic, rational method of planning and providing individualized nursing care for individuals, families, groups, and communities.
- The goals of the nursing process are to identify a client's actual or potential health care needs, to establish plans to meet the identified needs, and to deliver and evaluate specific nursing interventions to meet those needs.
- The nursing process can be utilized in all health care settings; it is cyclic and dynamic, client centered, interpersonal and collaborative, and universally applicable. It provides a framework for nurses' accountability and responsibility.
- The nursing process is organized into five interrelated, interdependent phases: assessing, diagnosing, planning, implementing, and evaluating.
- Assessing involves collecting, organizing, verifying, and recording data.
- Diagnosing is the process of making a clinical judgment (nursing diagnosis) about a client's potential or actual health problems.
- Planning involves setting priorities, writing outcomes/goals, and establishing a written plan for nursing interventions.
- Implementing is carrying out or delegating the nursing interventions. It incorporates all of the

activities performed to promote health, prevent complications, treat present problems, and facilitate the client's coping with chronic alterations in health status.

- Evaluating is the process of comparing client responses to preselected outcomes to determine whether goals have been met. It includes review and modification of the care plan.
- Assessment involves active participation by the client and nurse in obtaining subjective and objective data about the client's health status.
- The client is the primary source of data. Secondary sources are families, friends, health team members, the health record, and pertinent literature.
- Subjective data are the client's personal perceptions, often gathered during the nursing health history.
- Objective data (eg, data collected during the physical examination) are detectable by an observer.
- The nursing assessment must be complete and accurate, because nursing diagnoses and interventions are based on this information.
- Data must be validated. Subjective data can be used to validate objective data, and vice versa. Primary and secondary data can also be used to validate each other.
- Skills required for data collection are communicating, interviewing, observing, and examining.
- Observation is a conscious, deliberate skill involving use of the senses.
- The nurse uses a combination of directive and nondirective interviewing (including closed and open-ended questions) to obtain the nursing health history.
- Nursing models provide frameworks for collecting and organizing client data.
- Data must be recorded in a factual manner, without interpretation or inferences.

READINGS AND REFERENCES

SUGGESTED READINGS

Brider, P. May 1991. Who killed the nursing care plan? *American Journal of Nursing* 91:34–38.

Clarifies the new Joint Commission on Accreditation of Healthcare Organizations standards for nursing care in hospitals. A handwritten care plan is no longer required by this agency. The nursing process, on the other hand, receives even more emphasis. Evidence of each phase of the nursing process must be found in each client's record.

Gehring, PE. November 1991. Physical assessment begins with a history. *RN* 54:26–33.

This is part of a series of 7 home-study articles. Each has a CEU test for 2 hours of continuing education credit. The articles cover basic assessment skills in a brief, easy-to-read manner.

RELATED RESEARCH

Ellis, A and Cavanagh, SJ. June 1992. Aspects of the neurosurgical assessment using the Glasgow Coma Scale. *Intensive and Critical Care Nursing* 8:94–99.

Steeves, RH. August 1992. A typology of data collected in naturalistic interviews. *Western Journal of Nursing Research* 14:532–36.

SELECTED REFERENCES

American Nurses Association. 1973. *Standards of Nursing Practice.* Kansas City, MO: ANA.

———. 1980. *Nursing: A Social Policy Statement.* Kansas City, MO: ANA.

———. 1991. *Standards of Clinical Nursing Practice.* Kansas City, MO: ANA.

Arnold, A and Boggs, K. 1989. *Interpersonal Relationships: Professional Communications Skills for Nurses.* Philadelphia: WB Saunders.

Atkinson, LD and Murray, ME. 1990. *Understanding the Nursing Process.* 4th ed. Elmsford, NY: Pergamon Press.

Benner, P and Tanner, C. January 1987. How expert nurses use intuition. *American Journal of Nursing* 87:23–31.

Bloch, D. November 1974. Some crucial terms in nursing: What do they really mean? *Nursing Outlook* 22:689–94.

Brammer, LM. 1993. *The Helping Relationship.* 5th ed. San Francisco: Jossey-Bass.

Brider, P. May 1991. Who killed the nursing care plan? *American Journal of Nursing* 91:34–38.

Brigdon, P and Todd, M. January 1990. In search of the perfect assessment. *Professional Nurse* 5:181–84.

Canadian Nurses Association. February 1987. *A Definition of Nursing Practice: Standards for Nursing Practice.* Ottawa: CNA.

Davis, D. 1993. Toward successful compliance with JCAHO standard NC.1. *Nursing Management* 24(4):50–51.

Gebbie, K and Lavin, M. 1975. *Classification of Nursing Diagnoses.* St Louis: Mosby.

George, JB, editor. 1985. *Nursing Theories: A Base for Professional Nursing.* 2d ed. Englewood Cliffs, NJ: Prentice Hall.

Hall, L. June 1955. Quality of nursing care. *Public Health News.* Newark, NJ: State Department of Health.

Heidgerken, LE. 1965. *Teaching and Learning in Schools of Nursing: Principles and Methods.* 3d ed. Philadelphia: Lippincott.

Henderson, V. January/February 1965. The nature of nursing. *International Nursing Review* 12:23–30.

———. 1966. *The Nature of Nursing.* Riverside, NJ: Macmillan.

———. May 22, 1980. Nursing: Yesterday and tomorrow. *Nursing Times* 76:905–07.

Hogstel, MO and Keen-Payne, R. 1993. *Practical Guide to Health Assessment Through the Lifespan.* Philadelphia: FA Davis.

Johnson, DE. April 1959. A philosophy of nursing. *Nursing Outlook* 7:198–200.

Joint Commission on Accreditation of Healthcare Organizations. 1994. *Accreditation Manual for Hospitals.* Chicago: JCAHO, Nursing Services.

Knowles, L. 1967. *Decision-Making in Nursing: A Necessity for Doing. ANA Clinical Sessions, 1966.* New York: Appleton-Century-Crofts.

Kreuter, FR. May 1957. What is good nursing care? *Nursing Outlook* 5:302–04.

McCain, RF. April 1965. Nursing by assessment—not intuition. *American Journal of Nursing* 65:82–84.

McGillan, PM. June 1990. Assessment and care planning increase autonomy of practice. *Provider* 16(6):37–38.

McHugh, M. April 1991. Does the nursing process reflect quality care? *Holistic Nursing Practice* 5:22–28.

Niziolek, C and Shaw, S. May/June 1991. Whose plan—whose care? *Journal of Professional Nursing* 7:145.

North American Nursing Diagnosis Association. 1989. *Classification of Nursing Diagnoses: Proceedings of the Eighth Conference.* Philadelphia: Lippincott.

Orem, D. 1985. *Nursing: Concepts of Practice.* 3d ed. St Louis: Mosby-Year Book.

Orlando, I. 1961. *The Dynamic Nurse-Patient Relationship.* New York: Putnam.

Reed, J and Bond, S. 1991. Nurses' assessment of elderly patients in hospital. *International Journal of Nursing Studies* 28:55–64.

Roy, C. 1976. *Introduction to Nursing: An Adaptation Model.* Englewood Cliffs, NJ: Prentice Hall.

———. 1984. *Introduction to Nursing: An Adaptation Model.* 2d ed. Englewood Cliffs, NJ: Prentice Hall.

Rundell, S. April 17–23, 1991. Care about care plans! *Nursing Times* 87:32.

Ryan-Wenger, NM. 1990. A nursing process methodology. *Nursing Outlook* 38:190–93.

Stewart, CJ and Cash, WG, Jr. 1991. *Interviewing: Principles and Practice.* 6th ed. Dubuque, IA: WC Brown.

———. 1988. *Interviewing: Principles and Practice.* 5th ed. Dubuque, IA: WC Brown.

Vessey, JA and Richardson, BL. 1993. A holistic approach to symptom assessment and intervention. *Holistic Nursing Practice* 7(2):13–21.

Western Interstate Commission on Higher Education. 1967. *Defining Clinical Content: Graduate Nursing Programs, Medical and Surgical Nursing.* Boulder, CO: Western Interstate Commission on Higher Education.

Wiedenbach, E. November 1963. The helping art of nursing. *American Journal of Nursing* 63:54.

———. May 1970. Nurses' wisdom in nursing theory. *American Journal of Nursing* 70:1057–62.

Wilkinson, J. 1992. *Nursing Process in Action: A Critical Thinking Approach.* Redwood City, CA: Addison-Wesley Nursing.

Wittert, DD and Lamb, KV. April 1992. Nursing admission form: Revision from the bottom up. *Nursing Management* 23:64–66.

Yura, H and Walsh, MB. 1988. *The Nursing Process: Assessing, Planning, Implementing, Evaluating.* 5th ed. Norwalk, CT: Appleton & Lange.

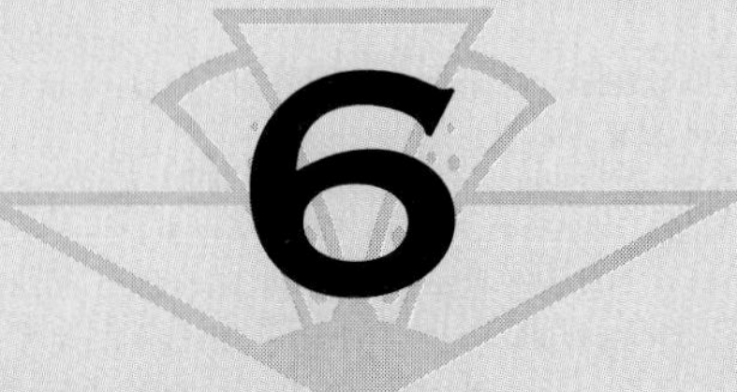

6 Diagnosing

Objectives

Differentiate various types of nursing diagnoses.

Identify the components of a nursing diagnosis.

Compare nursing diagnoses, medical diagnoses, and collaborative problems.

Identify basic steps in the diagnostic process.

Describe various formats for writing nursing diagnoses.

Describe the characteristics of a nursing diagnosis.

List common errors in writing diagnostic statements.

Describe the evolution of the nursing diagnoses movement.

List advantages of a taxonomy of nursing diagnoses.

Identify the challenges of the profession related to nursing diagnoses.

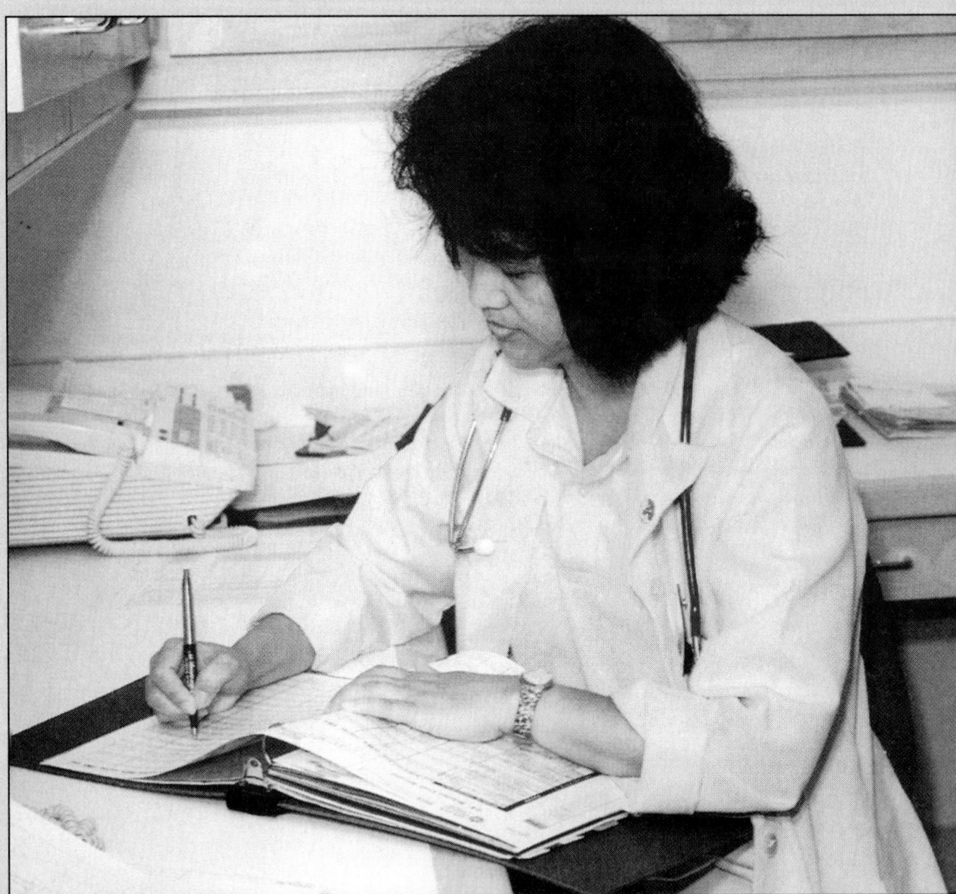

Diagnosing is the second phase of the nursing process. In this phase, nurses use critical-thinking skills to interpret assessment data and identify client strengths and problems. Diagnosing is a pivotal step in the nursing process. All activities preceding this phase are directed toward formulating the nursing diagnoses; all the care-planning activities following this phase are based on the nursing diagnoses (Figure 6–1).

The term *diagnosis* is often used to describe both a process and a product. Nurses use a reasoning process called *nursing diagnosis* to produce a statement of the client's health status; the product is also called a *nursing diagnosis.*

For clarity, this chapter uses the terms adapted from Carpenito (1995, p. 6). The term *diagnosis* refers to the reasoning process (diagnostic reasoning); the standardized North American Nursing Diagnosis Association (NANDA) terms (see inside back cover) are called *diagnostic labels;* and the product (problem statement) is called a *nursing diagnosis.*

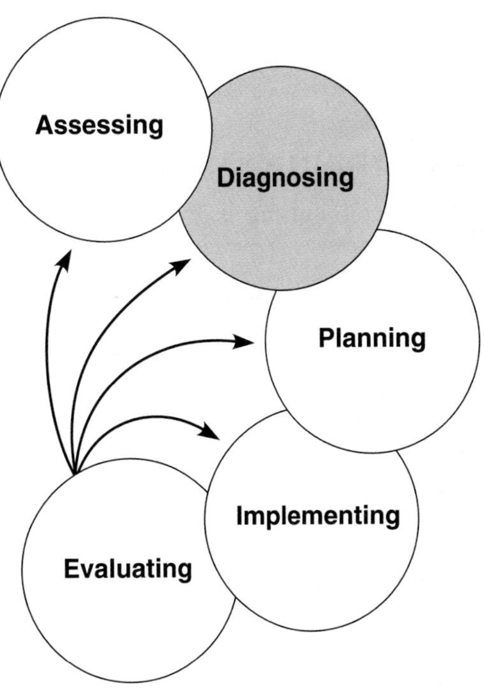

Figure 6–1 Diagnosing. The pivotal second phase of the nursing process in which the nurse interprets assessment data and identifies client strengths and problems amenable to nursing interventions.

DEFINITIONS

Several definitions of the term **nursing diagnosis** have been stated in the literature. Each has a different emphasis, but all are similar. In 1990, the North American Nursing Diagnosis Association (NANDA) adopted an official working definition of *nursing diagnosis,* shown in the box, below, as well as a definition of **wellness diagnosis.** These definitions imply the following:

1990 NANDA DEFINITIONS

Nursing Diagnosis

"Nursing diagnosis is a clinical judgment about individual, family, or community responses to actual and potential health problems/life processes. Nursing diagnoses provide the basis for selection of nursing interventions to achieve outcomes for which the nurse is accountable."

Wellness Diagnosis

"A wellness diagnosis is a clinical judgment about an individual, family, or community in transition from a specific level of wellness to a higher level of wellness" (1990). It describes "human responses to levels of wellness in an individual, family, or community that have a potential for enhancement to a higher state" (1994).

Source: North American Nursing Diagnosis Association, *Taxonomy I, Revised—1990* (St Louis: NANDA, 1990), pp. 114, 117, and *NANDA Nursing Diagnoses: Definitions and Classifications—1995–1996* by the North American Nursing Diagnosis Association, 1994, St Louis: NANDA.

- *Professional nurses (registered nurses) are responsible for making nursing diagnoses,* even though other nursing personnel may contribute data to the process of diagnosing and may implement specified nursing care. The American Nurses Association (ANA) *Standards of Clinical Nursing Practice* (1991, p. 9) reinforces that nurses are accountable for this phase of the nursing process (see the box on page 108). The Joint Commission for Accreditation of Healthcare Organizations (JCAHO) now requires evidence of nursing diagnosis in client's medical records as well (JCAHO 1992, p. 2).
- *Nursing diagnoses describe a continuum of health states:* (a) **actual health problems** (deviations from health), (b) **potential health problems** (presence of risk factors that predispose persons and families to health problems), and (c) healthy responses (areas of enriched personal growth).
- *The domain of nursing diagnosis includes only those health states that nurses are able and licensed to treat.* For example, nurses are not educated to diagnose or treat diseases such as diabetes mellitus; this task is defined legally as within the practice of medicine. Yet they can diagnose and treat **Knowledge deficit, Ineffective in-**

dividual coping, or **Altered nutrition**, all of which may accompany diabetes mellitus.

- *A nursing diagnosis is a judgment made only after thorough, systematic data collection.*

TYPES OF NURSING DIAGNOSES

There are various types of nursing diagnoses: actual, high risk, possible, and wellness.

1. An *actual diagnosis* is a judgment about a client's response to a health problem that is present at the time of the nursing assessment. An actual nursing diagnosis is based on the presence of associated signs and symptoms. Examples are **Ineffective breathing pattern** and **Anxiety.**
2. A *high risk nursing diagnosis*, as defined by NANDA, is a clinical judgment that a client is more vulnerable to develop the problem than others in the same or similar situation. For example, all people admitted to a hospital have some possibility of acquiring an infection; however, a client with diabetes or a compromised immune system is at higher risk than others. Therefore, the nurse would appropriately use the label **High risk for infection** to describe the client's health status.
3. A *possible nursing diagnosis* is one in which evidence about a health problem is unclear or the causative factors are unknown. A possible diagnosis requires more data either to support or to refute it. For example, an elderly widow who lives alone is admitted to the hospital. The nurse notices that she has no visitors and is pleased with attention and conversation from the nursing staff. Until more data are collected, the nurse may write a nursing diagnosis of **Possible social isolation** related to unknown etiology.
4. A *wellness diagnosis* is one indicating a healthy response of a client who desires a higher level of wellness. See the box on page 107.

ANA STANDARDS

Standard II: Diagnosis

The nurse analyzes the assessment data in determining diagnoses.

Measurement Criteria

1. Diagnoses are derived from the assessment data.
2. Diagnoses are validated with the client, significant others, and health care providers, when possible.
3. Diagnoses are documented in a manner that facilitates the determination of expected outcomes and plan of care.

Source: Abstracted from American Nurses Association, *Standards of Clinical Nursing Practice* (Washington, DC: ANA, 1991), p. 10. Used with permission.

COMPONENTS OF A NURSING DIAGNOSIS

A nursing diagnosis has three components: (1) the problem statement, (2) the etiology, and (3) the defining characteristics (Gordon 1987, pp. 15–18). Each component serves a specific purpose.

Problem Statement (Diagnostic Label) The problem statement, or diagnostic label, describes the client's health problem or response for which nursing therapy is given. It describes the client's health status clearly and concisely in a few words. See the inside back cover for a list of nursing diagnostic labels adopted by the Eleventh National Conference on Classification of Nursing Diagnoses in 1994. The purpose of the diagnostic label is to direct the formation of client goals and outcome criteria. It may also suggest some nursing interventions.

To be clinically useful, diagnostic labels need to be specific; when the word *specify* follows a label on this list, the nurse states the area in which the problem occurs, for example, **Knowledge deficit (medications)** or **Knowledge deficit (dietary adjustments).**

Qualifiers are words that have been added to some NANDA labels to give additional meaning to the diagnostic statement:

- **Altered** (a change from baseline)
- **Impaired** (made worse, weakened, damaged, reduced, deteriorated)
- **Decreased** (smaller in size, amount, or degree)
- **Ineffective** (not producing the desired effect)
- **Acute** (severe or of short duration)
- **Chronic** (lasting a long time, recurring, or constant)

Each diagnostic label approved by NANDA carries a definition that clarifies the characteristics of the human response under consideration. For example, the definition of the label **Activity intolerance** is shown in Table 6–1.

Etiology (Related Factors and Risk Factors) The etiology component of the diagnosis identifies one or more probable causes of the health problem, gives direction to the required nursing therapy, and enables the nurse to individualize the client's care. Etiology may include client behaviors, environmental factors, or interactions of the two. As shown in Table 6–1, the probable causes of **Activity intolerance** include sedentary life-

Table 6–1 Components of a Nursing Diagnostic Label

Diagnosis	Definition	Etiology/Related Factors	Defining Characteristics
Activity intolerance	A state in which an individual has insufficient psysiologic or psychologic energy to endure or complete required or desired daily activities	Sedentary life-style Generalized weakness Prolonged bedrest or immobility Sensory deficits Impaired motor function Fatigue Alterations in oxygen transport system Lack of motivation Obesity Acute or chronic pain	*Major (Must Be Present)* Altered response to activity (eg, dyspnea, shortness of breath, tachypnea, rapid shallow respirations) Weak, thready pulse, tachycardia, irregular pulse, failure to return to resting after 3 minutes, EKG changes during activity Failure of blood pressure to increase with activity, hypotension, increased diastolic pressure of 15 mm Hg Weakness and fatigue *Minor (May Be Present)* Pallor, cyanosis, vertigo, diaphoresis, confusion

Source: MJ Kim, GK McFarland, and AM McLane, editors, *Pocket Guide to Nursing Diagnosis,* 5th ed. (St Louis: Mosby, 1993), p. 2; LJ Carpenito, *Nursing Diagnosis: Application to Clinical Practice,* 5th ed. (Philadelphia: Lippincott, 1993), p. 101; JR Lederer, GL Marculescu, B Mocnik, and N Seaby, *Care Planning Pocket Guide: A Nursing Diagnosis Approach,* 5th ed. (Redwood City, CA: Addison-Wesley Nursing, 1993), p. 2.

Table 6–2 Examples of Nursing Interventions to Address Different Etiologies

Diagnostic Label (Problem)	Client	Etiology	Examples of Nursing Interventions
Colonic constipation	Ed Eilert	Long-term laxative use	Work with Mr Eilert to develop a plan for gradual withdrawal of the laxatives. Teach components of a high-fiber diet.
	Jerry Sims	Inactivity and insufficient fluid intake	Help Mr Sims develop an exercise regimen that he can follow at home. Obtain information about his daily schedule and type of fluids he likes. Help Mr Sims develop a plan for including sufficient amounts of fluids in his diet.
Ineffective breast-feeding	Ariel Dees	Breast engorgement	Teach Ms Dees to massage her breasts before feeding. Use hot packs or hot shower before nursing infant.
	June Biden	Inexperience and lack of knowledge	Teach to feed infant on demand. Show Ms Biden how to be sure infant is sucking and swallowing. Demonstrate different holding positions for feedings.

style, generalized weakness, prolonged inactivity, and so on. Differentiating among possible causes in the nursing diagnosis is essential, because each may require different nursing interventions. Refer to Table 6–2 for examples of health problems that have different etiologies and therefore require different interventions.

NANDA uses the term **related factor** to describe the etiology or likely cause of actual nursing diagnoses. The term **risk factor** is used to describe the etiology of **high risk** (potential) nursing diagnoses, because there are no subjective and objective signs present. Table 6–3 on page 110 compares related factors and risk factors.

Table 6–3 Comparison of Related Factors and Risk Factors

	Related Factors	Risk Factors
Definition	Factor that is causing or contributing to an actual problem	Factors present that place client at risk for developing a problem that has not yet occurred
Use as etiology of:	Actual problems	High risk (potential) problems
Use when signs and symptoms of problem are:	Present	Not present

Defining Characteristics Defining characteristics are the cluster of signs and symptoms that indicate the presence of a particular diagnostic label. For *actual* nursing diagnoses, the defining characteristics are the client's signs and symptoms. For *high risk* nursing diagnoses, the defining characteristics are the same as the etiology: the risk factors that cause the client to be more than "normally" vulnerable to the problem.

Nursing diagnosis labels are similar to medical diagnoses in that they are associated with a standard set of defining characteristics that are universally accepted. *Major* defining characteristics are those that *must* be present for the diagnosis to be valid. *Minor* characteristics may or may not be present. For example, for a nurse to make a diagnosis of **Activity intolerance,** the client would need to exhibit the defining characteristic of "altered response to activity," which might manifest as dyspnea, shortness of breath, tachypnea, or one of the other major symptoms listed in Table 6–1. For most nursing diagnoses, the list of defining characteristics is still being developed and refined. Partial listings have been published to assist nurses in developing and validating nursing diagnoses. Defining characteristics suggest criteria or client outcomes and may also suggest required nursing interventions.

RECOGNIZING CLIENT PROBLEMS

Because diagnosing involves problem identification, it is important to understand what a problem is and to be able to differentiate a problem from other phenomena such as symptoms or treatments. A **health problem** is recognized by the following characteristics (Wilkinson 1992, pp. 81–82):

- It is a human response to a life process, event, or stressor.
- It is a health-related condition that both the client and the nurse wish to change.
- It requires intervention in order to prevent or resolve illness, or to facilitate coping.
- It involves or results in ineffective coping/adaptation or daily living that is not satisfying to the client.
- It is an undesirable *client* state.

Clients have various kinds of problems. Some are nursing diagnoses, some are not. The nurse must be able to differentiate among different types of client problems.

DIFFERENTIATING NURSING DIAGNOSES FROM MEDICAL DIAGNOSES

Whereas a nursing diagnosis is a statement of nursing judgment and refers to a condition that nurses are licensed to treat, a **medical diagnosis** is made by a physician and refers to a condition that only a physician can treat. Medical diagnoses refer to disease processes—specific pathophysiologic responses that are fairly uniform from one client to another. In contrast, nursing diagnoses describe a client's physical, sociocultural, psychologic, and spiritual responses to an illness or a potential health problem. These responses vary among individuals. Whereas a client's medical diagnosis remains the same for as long as the disease process is present, nursing diagnoses change as the client's responses change, as in the following example:

> Seventy-year-old Mary Cain and 20-year-old Kristi Vidan both have rheumatoid arthritis. Their disease processes are much the same. X-ray studies show that, in both clients, the extent of inflammation and the number of joints involved are similar, and both clients experience almost constant pain. Ms Cain views her condition as part of the aging process and is responding with acceptance. Ms Vidan, however, is responding with anger and hostility, because she views her disease as a threat to her personal identity, role performance, and self-esteem.

Both medical and nursing diagnoses are client problems, and nurses have responsibilities related to both. Nurses are obligated to diagnose and prescribe within the

Table 6–4 Comparison of Nursing Diagnoses, Collaborative Problems, and Medical Diagnoses

Nursing Diagnoses	Collaborative Problems	Medical Diagnoses
Example: Activity intolerance related to decreased cardiac output	Example: Potential complication of myocardial infarction: congestive heart failure	Example: Myocardial infarction
Describes human responses to disease process or health problem	Involve human responses—mainly physiologic complications of disease, tests, or treatments	Describes disease and pathology; does not consider other human responses
Oriented to individual	Oriented to pathophysiology	Oriented to pathology
Nurses responsible for diagnosing	Nurses responsible for diagnosing	Physician responsible for diagnosing; diagnosis not within the scope of nursing practice
Nurse orders most interventions to prevent and treat	Nurse collaborates with physician and other health care professionals to prevent and treat (requires at least some medical orders)	Physician orders primary interventions to prevent and treat
Nursing focus: treat and prevent	Nursing focus: prevent and monitor for onset or status of condition	Nursing focus: implement medical orders for treatment and monitor status of condition
Independent nursing actions	Some independent actions, but primarily for monitoring and preventing	Dependent nursing actions, primarily
Can change frequently	Present when disease or situation is present	Remains the same while disease is present
Has no universally accepted classification system; such systems are in the process of development	Has no universally accepted classification system	Has a well-developed classification system accepted by the medical profession
Consists of a one-, two- or three-part statement, usually including problem and etiology	Consists of a two-part statement of situation/pathophysiology and the potential complication	Consists usually of not more than three words

limits of nurse practice acts. Nursing diagnoses relate to the nurse's **independent functions,** that is, the areas of health care that are unique to nursing and separate and distinct from medical management. With regard to medical diagnoses, nurses are obligated to carry out physician-prescribed therapies and treatments, that is, **dependent functions.**

Nurses may not prescribe *all* the care for a nursing diagnosis, but if the problem is a nursing diagnosis, the nurse can prescribe *most* of the interventions needed for prevention or resolution. For example, most clients with a nursing diagnosis of **Pain** have medical orders for analgesics, but there are also many independent nursing interventions for alleviating pain.

A nursing diagnosis may complement a medical diagnosis but is separate and distinct. A client who has one or more medical diagnoses and medical orders may also have one or more nursing diagnoses and nursing orders. See Table 6–4 for a comparison of nursing and medical diagnoses.

DIFFERENTIATING NURSING DIAGNOSES FROM COLLABORATIVE PROBLEMS

Like high risk nursing diagnoses, **collaborative problems** are a type of potential problem. However, independent nursing interventions for collaborative problems focus mainly on monitoring the client's condition and preventing development of the potential complication. Definitive treatment of the condition requires both medical and nursing interventions.

Because the number of physiologic complications for a given disease is limited, collaborative problems tend to be present any time a particular disease or treatment is present; that is, each disease or treatment has specific complications that are always associated with it. For example, Luisa Sanchez's collaborative problems might include "Potential complication of pneumonia: atelectasis, respiratory failure, pleural effusion, pericarditis, and meningitis" (see Chapter 5, page 95).

Nursing diagnoses, by contrast, involve human responses, which vary greatly from one person to the next. Therefore, the same set of nursing diagnoses cannot be expected to occur with a particular disease or condition; moreover, a single nursing diagnosis may occur as a response to any number of diseases. For example, all postpartum clients have similar collaborative problems (potential complications), such as "Potential complication of childbearing: postpartum hemorrhage" or "Potential complication of childbearing: thrombophlebitis." But not all new mothers have the same nursing diagnoses. Some might experience **Altered parenting (delayed bonding)**, but most will not; some might have a **Knowledge deficit** problem, whereas others will not. See Table 6–4 for a comparison of nursing diagnoses, collaborative problems, and medical problems.

THE DIAGNOSTIC PROCESS

The diagnosis process uses the critical-thinking skills of analysis and synthesis. **Analysis** is the separation into components, that is, breaking down the whole into its parts. **Synthesis** is the opposite, that is, putting together the parts into the whole. **Critical thinking** is a cognitive process during which a person reviews data and considers explanations before forming an opinion.

The diagnostic process is used continuously by most nurses. An experienced nurse may enter a client's room and immediately observe significant data about the client. The nurse is able to do this as a result of attaining knowledge, skill, and expertise in the practice setting.

Although experienced practitioners may seem to perform these mental processes automatically, the novice needs guidelines to understand and formulate nursing diagnoses. The diagnostic process has three steps:

- **Analyzing data**
  Compare data against standards
  Cluster data; generate tentative hypotheses
  Identify gaps and inconsistencies
- **Identifying health problems, risks, and strengths**
- **Formulating diagnostic statements**
  Nursing diagnoses
  Collaborative problems

ANALYZING DATA

In the diagnostic process, analyzing involves the following steps:

1. Compare data against standards (identify significant cues).
2. Cluster data (generate tentative hypotheses).
3. Identify gaps and inconsistencies.

These activities occur continuously rather than sequentially.

Comparing Data against Standards The nurse compares the client's data to a wide range of standards, such as normal health patterns, normal vital signs, laboratory values, basic food groups, growth, and development. The nurse also uses personal knowledge—for example, of physiology, psychology, and sociology—as well as past experience when comparing the data.

A **standard** or **norm** is a generally accepted rule, model, pattern, or measure. Standards must be both relevant and reliable. The nurse compares the client data against standards and norms to identify significant and relevant cues. A **cue** is any piece of information or data that influences decisions (Gordon 1987, p. 182). Refer to Table 6–5 for specific examples of client cues and norms to which they may be compared. A cue is considered significant if it does any of the following (Gordon 1987, p. 191):

1. **The cue points to change in a client's health status or pattern.** These may be positive or negative. For example, the client states: "I have recently experienced shortness of breath while climbing stairs," or "I have not smoked for 3 months."
2. **The cue varies from norms of the client population.** The client's pattern may fit within cultural norms but vary from norms of the general society. The client may consider a pattern—for example, eating very small meals and having a poor appetite—to be normal. This pattern, however, may not be productive and may require further exploration.
3. **The cue indicates a development delay.** Changes in health patterns occur as the person grows and develops. By age 9 months, the infant is usually able to sit alone without support and to stand while holding onto a support (Pillitteri 1992, pp. 864–65). The infant who has not accomplished these tasks needs further assessment for possible developmental delays. To identify significant cues, the nurse must be aware of normal patterns and changes.

Significant cues and data clusters for Luisa Sanchez, which were extracted from Figure 5–2 on pages 95 and 96 and the box on page 101 are shown in Table 6–6 on page 114.

Clustering Data Clustering or grouping data is a process of determining the relatedness of facts and finding

Table 6–5 Comparing Client Cues to Standards and Norms

Type of Cue	Client Cues	Standard/Norm
Deviation from population norms	Height is 158 cm (5 ft, 2 in.) tall. Woman with small frame. Weighs 109 kg (240 lbs).	Height and weight tables indicate that the "ideal" weight for a woman 158 cm (5 ft, 2 in.) tall with a small frame is 49–53 kg (108–121 lbs).
Developmental delay	Child is 18 months old. Parents state child has not yet attempted to speak. Child laughs aloud and makes cooing sounds.	Children usually speak their first word by 10 months to 1 year of age.
Changes in client's usual health status	States, "I'm just not hungry these days." Ate only 15% of food on breakfast tray. Has lost 13 kg (30 lbs) in past 3 months.	Client usually eats three balanced meals per day. Adults typically maintain stable weight.
Dysfunctional behavior	Amy's mother reports that Amy has not left her room for 2 days. Amy is age 16. Amy has stopped attending school and has withdrawn from social contact.	Adolescents usually like to be with their peers; social group very important. Functional behavior includes school attendance.
Changes in client's usual behavior	Mrs Stuart reports that lately her husband angers easily. "Yesterday he even yelled at the dog." "He just seems so tense."	Mr Stuart is usually relaxed and easygoing. He is friendly and kind to animals.

patterns in the facts. This is the beginning of synthesis. The nurse examines data to determine whether any patterns are present, whether the data represent isolated incidents, and whether the data are significant.

The nurse may cluster data *inductively* (as in Table 6–6) by combining data from different assessment areas to form a pattern, or the nurse may begin with a framework, such as Gordon's functional health patterns, and cluster the subjective and objective data into the appropriate categories (see the box in Chapter 5, page 101). The latter is a *deductive* approach to data clustering, or pattern formation.

Gordon (1987, p. 20) states that clustering information involves a search in the nurse's memory stores for previously learned meaningful groups of clinical cues that are associated with a diagnostic category. Gordon believes that clustering occurs in conjunction with data collection and interpretation, as evidenced in remarks or thoughts such as, "I'm getting a picture of" or "This cue doesn't fit the picture." The novice nurse does not have the knowledge base of the clinical experience that facilitates the recognition of cues related to diagnostic labels. Thus, the novice must take careful assessment notes, search data for abnormal cues, and use textbook resources for comparing the client's cues with the defining characteristics and etiologic factors of the accepted nursing diagnoses. After comparing the client cues against available resources, the novice can group data into clusters.

Data clustering involves making inferences about the data. An **inference** is the nurse's judgment or interpretation of cues. During data clustering, the nurse interprets the possible meaning of the cues and labels the cue clusters with tentative diagnostic hypotheses. Data clustering or grouping for Luisa Sanchez is illustrated in Table 6–6, in which data are clustered according to standardized diagnosis labels.

Identifying Gaps and Inconsistencies in Data Skillful assessment minimizes gaps and inconsistencies in data. However, data analysis should include a final check to ensure that data are complete and correct. *Gaps* are missing information needed to determine a data pattern. For example, information about a 15-month-old child's mobility may not specify whether the child crawls or walks. This information is essential for establishing the child's developmental stage.

Table 6–6 Formulating Nursing Diagnoses for Luisa Sanchez

Functional Health Pattern	Client Cue Clusters	Inferences (Tentative Identification of Problems)	Formulating Diagnostic Statements
Health perception/ Health management			No problem *Strength:* Shows healthy lifestyle, understanding of and compliance with treatment regimens
Nutritional/ Metabolic (includes hydration)	"No appetite" since having "cold" Has not eaten today; last fluids at noon today Nauseated ×2 days	**Altered nutrition: Less than body requirements**	**Altered nutrition: Less than body requirements** related to decreased appetite and nausea, and increased metabolism (secondary to disease process) *Strength:* Normal weight for height
	Last fluids at noon today Oral temp 39.4 C (103 F) Skin hot and pale, cheeks flushed Mucous membranes dry Poor skin turgor *Cues from elimination pattern:* Decreased urinary frequency and amount ×2 days	**Fluid volume deficit**	**Fluid volume deficit** related to intake insufficient to replace fluid loss secondary to fever and diaphoresis
Elimination	Decreased urinary frequency and amount ×2 days	Cues consist of elimination data but are actually symptoms of a fluid volume problem in the nutritional/metabolic functional health pattern	No elimination problem
Activity/Exercise	Difficulty sleeping because of cough "Can't breathe lying down" States, "I feel weak" Short of breath on exertion	**Sleep pattern disturbance**	**Sleep pattern disturbance** related to cough, pain, orthopnea, fever, and diaphoresis
	Cues from cognitive/perceptual pattern: Responsive but fatigued "I can think OK, just weak" *Cues from cardiovascular pattern:* Radial pulses weak, regular Pulse rate 92	**Activity intolerance** **Self-care deficit**	**Self-care deficit (level 2)** related to activity intolerance secondary to ineffective airway clearance and sleep pattern disturbance *Strength:* No musculoskeletal impairment. Normal energy level is satisfactory. Exercises regularly
Cognitive/ Perceptual	Reports pain in lungs," especially when coughing	**Chest pain**	**Chest pain** related to cough secondary to pneumonia
	Responsive but fatigued "I can think OK, just weak"	These are cognitive/perceptual data, but they reflect symptoms of problems in the activity/exercise pattern	*Strength:* No cognitive or sensory deficits
	Reports chills *Cue from nutritional/metabolic pattern:* Oral temp 39.4 C (103 F)	**Altered comfort: chills**	**Altered comfort: chills** related to fever and diaphoresis

Table 6–6 *continued*

Functional Health Pattern	Client Cue Clusters	Inferences (Tentative Identification of Problems)	Formulating Diagnostic Statements
Cognitive/Perceptual *(continued)*	*Cue from nursing physical assessment:* Diaphoretic		
Roles/Relationships	Husband out of town; will be back tomorrow afternoon Child with neighbor until husband returns	**Altered family processes** related to mother's illness and temporary unavailability of father to provide child care Cues also relate to a problem in the coping/stress pattern	**High risk for altered family processes** related to mother's illness and temporary unavailability of father to provide child care *Strength:* Husband supportive; neighbors available and willing to help
Self-Perception/ Self-Concept	Expresses "concern" and "worry" over leaving daughter with neighbors until husband returns	Cue is a symptom of a problem in the coping/stress pattern	No self-perception/self-concept problem
Coping/Stress	Anxious: "I can't breathe" Facial muscles tense; trembling Expresses concerns about work: "I'll never get caught up" *Cues from role/relationship pattern:* Husband out of town; will be back tomorrow afternoon Child with neighbor until husband returns *Cues from self-perception/self-concept patterns:* Expresses "concern" and "worry" over leaving daughter with neighbors	**Anxiety** related to difficulty breathing, inability to work, and childcare	**Anxiety** related to difficulty breathing and concerns over work and parenting roles
Medication/History	No significant cues	No problem	No problem
Physical Assessment			
Cardiovascular	Radial pulses weak, regular Pulse rate 92	Cues are symptoms only; symptoms of exercise/rest and oxygenation problems	No cardiovascular problem
Oxygenation	Skin hot and pale Respirations shallow; chest expansion < 3cm Cough productive of small amounts of pale pink sputum Inspiratory crackles auscultated throughout right upper and lower chest Diminished breath sounds on right side Mucous membranes pale	**Ineffective airway clearance** related to disease process	**Ineffective airway clearance** related to viscous secretions and shallow chest expansion secondary to pain, fluid volume deficit, and fatigue
Skin	Old surgical scars, anterior neck, RLQ abdomen	No problem now	Old problems; resolved

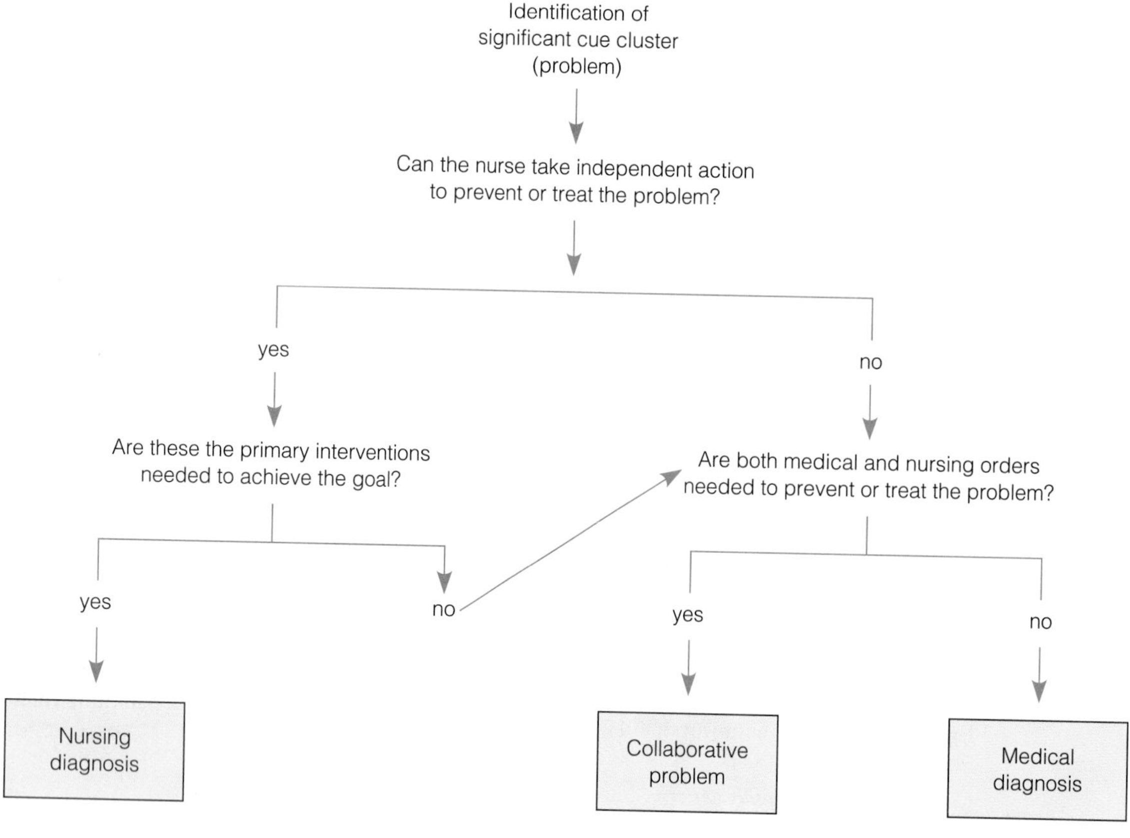

Figure 6–2 Decision tree for differentiating among nursing diagnoses, collaborative problems, and medical diagnoses.

Inconsistencies are conflicting data. Possible sources of conflicting data include measurement error, expectations, and conflicting or unreliable reports (Gordon 1987, p. 259). For example, if the client reports a history of high blood pressure but the nurse obtains a low reading, the nurse should check the equipment and procedure for possible error. In another situation, a nurse may learn from the nursing history that the client reports not having seen a doctor in 15 years, yet during the physical health examination he states, "My doctor takes my blood pressure every week." All inconsistencies must be clarified before a valid pattern can be established.

IDENTIFYING HEALTH PROBLEMS, RISKS, AND STRENGTHS

After data are analyzed, the nurse and client can together identify strengths and problems. This is primarily a decision-making process.

Health Problems and Risks During data analysis, the nurse groups the data and labels the clusters with tentative diagnoses. However, for health problems to have a successful outcome, the client must acknowledge that the problem exists. The nurse, by contrast, determines whether the client needs help dealing with the problem. Together they can make any of the following judgments:

1. *There is no problem* (eg, see Table 6–6, Elimination pattern).
2. *There is a potential problem.* The client has no signs and symptoms, but risk factors are present (eg, see Table 6–6, Role/Relationships pattern).
3. *There is a possible problem.* The nurse suspects a problem but needs more data to confirm it.
4. *There is an actual problem.* The client has signs and symptoms and needs help in resolving the problem (eg, see Table 6–6, Nutritional/Metabolic pattern).

When any kind of problem exists, the nurse must determine what type of problem it is. See Figure 6–2 for a decision tree to help differentiate nursing diagnoses, medical diagnoses, and collaborative problems. Also refer to Table 6–4.

Determining Etiologies After verifying problems with the client and determining the type of problem (ie, nursing diagnosis, medical diagnosis, or collaborative problem), the nurse examines the causal relationships between the problems and their related or risk factors. These are the problem **etiologies**—the physiologic, psychologic, sociologic, spiritual, or environmental factors believed to cause or contribute to the problem. As discussed on page 108 and shown in Table 6–2, the etiology gives direction to required nursing interventions. Therefore, if interventions are to be effective, the nurse must accurately identify the etiologies. When possible, the nurse should focus on etiologies that can be influenced by independent nursing actions.

Recall that early in data analysis, the nurse compares assessment data to standards and norms to identify significant cues. The nurse then interprets the cues in relation to other cues and hypothesizes possible problems. In the final level of data interpretation (determining etiologies), the nurse must apply knowledge and experience to the data to determine the exact nature of the cue relationships—that is, which cues represent problems and which are causes. The nurse must make inferences at this point, because the nurse cannot actually *observe* the link between problem and cause. For example, from Table 6–6, the following observations for Luisa Sanchez allow the nurse to conclude there is a problem of **Fluid volume deficit:**

Decreased urinary frequency and amount

Mucous membranes dry

Poor skin turgor

However, the nurse cannot *observe* that the cues "Last fluids at noon today" and "Oral temperature 39.4 C (103 F) are the cause of the fluid volume deficit. The nurse must use critical thinking and knowledge of fluid balance and the physiologic effects of fever and diaphoresis to infer this link between the problem and cause.

As illustrated in Table 6–6, the etiology is not necessarily found within the same pattern as the problem. In the Coping/Stress pattern, **Anxiety** was identified as a problem for Ms Sanchez. Note, however, that one of the causes of her anxiety (that a neighbor is keeping her child) is found in the Roles/Relationships pattern.

Different clients may have the same problem but different etiologies. For example, failure to comply with a medication regimen **(Noncompliance)** may be caused by denial of illness in Client A but by forgetfulness in Client B. Furthermore, a problem can have any number of etiologies. For example, Client C may fail to comply with the medication regimen *both* because he is denying his illness and because he is forgetful.

Strengths At this stage, the nurse and client also establish the client's strengths, resources, and abilities to cope. Generally, people have a clearer perception of their problems or weaknesses than of their strengths and assets, which they often take for granted. By taking an inventory of strengths, the client can develop a more well-rounded self-concept and self-image. Strengths can be an aid to mobilizing health and regenerative processes.

A client's strengths might be weight that is within the normal range for age and height, thus enabling the client to cope better with surgery. In another instance, a client's strengths might be absence of allergies and being a nonsmoker.

A client's strengths can be found in the nursing assessment record (health, home life, education, recreation, exercise, work, family and friends, religious beliefs, and sense of humor, for example), the health examination, and the client's records. See Table 6–6 for examples of Luisa Sanchez's strengths (eg, in the Health Perception/Health Management pattern).

ERRORS IN DIAGNOSTIC REASONING

Some error is inherent in any human undertaking, and diagnosis is no exception. However, it is important that nurses make nursing diagnoses with a high level of accuracy. Nurses can avoid some common errors of reasoning by recognizing them and applying the appropriate critical-thinking skills. Gordon (1987, p. 286) categorizes diagnostic errors as (a) errors of omission (ie, failure to diagnose a problem when one exists) and (b) errors of commission (ie, diagnosing a problem when no problem exists). Both kinds of error can occur at any point in the diagnostic process: data collection, data interpretation, and data clustering.

Data Collection Errors Correct, accurate diagnoses can be made only from a complete, accurate database. An organized assessment plan helps to prevent data collection errors. Missing data or large quantities of irrelevant data interfere with the nurse's ability to interpret the information. Interviewing skills and a good knowledge base help the nurse ask appropriate questions and thereby avoid collecting irrelevant data.

Data Interpretation Errors Data interpretation errors occur when the nurse misinterprets the meaning of cues. This is sometimes due to *premature data interpretation*, that is, making a judgment based on only one or two cues.

Example: The nurse observes that Mr Than repeatedly gets out of bed after the physician has ordered complete bed rest. The nurse interprets this as **Noncompliance.** However, Mr Than is actually experiencing diarrhea and is embarrassed to use the bedpan.

Biased interpretation is another source of error. *Personal bias*, the tendency to slant one's judgment in a particular way, is based on personal theories and stereotypes. Many of these ideas are based on life experience and may

RESEARCH NOTE

Can Clients Participate Meaningfully in the Diagnostic Process?

The researchers in this project were interested in determining chronically ill clients' perceptions of health and illness and the nursing diagnoses they considered relevant to themselves. To obtain this information, the researchers conducted interviews in the homes of 28 persons receiving home health care. They used open-ended questions to obtain clients' perceptions of illness and then asked subjects to identify their nursing diagnoses from the 1989 NANDA list of labels. Additionally, the subjects were asked if there were any diagnoses they wished to add to the list.

Subjects defined health in terms of their abilities to function independently (eg, being able to walk to the back door and sit on the porch). They defined illness in terms of their physical symptoms (eg, "I feel jittery").

Of the 166 nursing diagnoses selected by clients, the nurse-interviewer concurred with 164 (98.8%). However, the nurse identified 46 more diagnoses than the clients, for an overall rate of agreement of 78%. The difference was primarily the result of nurses' diagnoses of **Altered tissue perfusion** and **Knowledge deficit,** which clients may have lacked the knowledge to make.

Subjects identified four areas of concern that they believed were not covered by the NANDA list of diagnostic labels: (a) regimentation of eating, (b) frequency of urination, (c) disrupted relationships, and (d) medications. The researchers propose research and development of two new nursing diagnoses: (a) **Altered nutrition: regimentation,** and (b) **Adjustment to medication regimen.** They further recommend the development of wellness diagnoses.

Implications: The results of this study support the value of involving clients in every phase of the nursing process, including diagnosis.

Source: ME Loomis and D Conco, Patients' perceptions of health, chronic illness, and nursing diagnoses, *Nursing Diagnosis,* October/December 1991, 2(4):162–70.

or may not be accurate. For example, some people believe they will catch a cold if they get their feet wet or go outside with wet hair. Still others believe that illness is a punishment for wrongdoing. Such personal theories may affect the nurse's ability to interpret data for certain clients, for example, those with AIDS or other sexually transmitted diseases.

Nurses commonly and appropriately generalize from past experience when formulating tentative diagnoses. However, *relying too much on past experience* can lead to error. Although many clients behave similarly in similar situations, the nurse cannot assume that they all will.

> *Example:* Gwen Thomas, RN, has cared for several women who have had a hysterectomy. All of those clients did experience grief. Gwen is also familiar with the literature on the relationship between loss of a body part and grieving. Therefore, when she sees that Mrs Tracy is tearful, Gwen interprets this as grief, and writes a diagnosis of **Grieving** on the care plan.

Clients become upset for many reasons, and Nurse Thomas's inference is inaccurate for Mrs Tracy, who has just had an argument with her husband.

Another source of error in data interpretation is *overgeneralization* from one isolated observation of client behavior. For example, one episode of angry behavior does not mean that the client is hostile or lacking in coping skills.

Data Clustering Errors Incorrect clustering of data also leads to diagnostic error. For example, by clustering "decreased urinary frequency and amount," "oral temp 39.4 C (103 F)," and "experiencing chills," the nurse could erroneously diagnose a urinary problem for Luisa Sanchez (Table 6–6). However, clustering the urinary symptom and elevated temperature with "last fluids at noon," "dry mucous membranes," and "poor skin turgor," changes the diagnostic focus from a urinary problem to a problem of **Fluid volume deficit.**

Avoiding Errors Most sources of error are also legitimate sources of hypotheses about the meaning of client data. They cause error only when the nurse relies on these sources too heavily. The following suggestions should help to minimize diagnostic error:

- *Verify.* Hypothesize possible explanations of the data, but realize that all diagnoses are only tentative until they are verified. Begin and end the diagnostic process by talking with the client and family. When collecting data, ask them what their health problems are and what they believe the causes to be. At the end of the process, ask them to verify your diagnoses.
- *Build a good knowledge base, and acquire clinical experience.* Nurses must apply knowledge from many different areas to recognize significant cues and patterns and generate hypotheses about the data. To name only a few, principles from chemistry, anatomy, and pharmacology each help the nurse understand client data in a different way.
- *Have a working knowledge of what is normal.* Nurses need to know the norms (what is normal for most people) for vital signs, laboratory tests, speech development, breath sounds, and so on. In addition, nurses must determine what is normal for a particular person, taking

into account age, physical makeup, life-style, culture, and the person's own perception of what is normal. For example, normal blood pressure for adults is in the range of 110/60 to 140/80. However, a nurse might obtain a reading of 90/50 that is perfectly normal for a particular client. The nurse should compare findings to the client's baseline when possible.

- *Consult resources.* Both novices and experienced nurses should consult appropriate resources whenever in doubt about a diagnosis. Professional literature, agency policies, nursing colleagues, and other professionals are all appropriate resources. The nurse should use a nursing diagnosis handbook to ascertain that the client's signs and symptoms truly fit the NANDA label chosen.
- *Base diagnoses on patterns—that is, on behavior over time—rather than on an isolated incident.* For example, even though Luisa Sanchez is concerned today about needing to leave her child with a neighbor, it is likely that this concern will be resolved without intervention by the next day. Therefore, the admitting nurse should not diagnose **Altered family processes.**
- *Improve critical-thinking skills.* This helps the nurse to be aware of and avoid errors in thinking, such as overgeneralizing, stereotyping, making unwarranted assumptions, and so on. See Chapter 10.

FORMULATING DIAGNOSTIC STATEMENTS

The basic format for a diagnostic statement is **"Problem related to Etiology."** However, nurses must be able to write one-, two-, three-, and four-part diagnostic statements, as well as some variations of each. See Table 6–6 for nursing diagnoses formulated for Luisa Sanchez.

BASIC TWO-PART STATEMENTS

The basic two-part statement is used for actual, high risk, and possible nursing diagnoses. It includes the following:

1. Problem (P)—Statement of the client's response
2. Etiology (E)—Factors contributing to or probable causes of the responses

The two parts are joined by the words *related to* or *associated with* rather than *due to.* The phrase *due to* implies a cause-and-effect relationship; one clause causes or is responsible for the other clause. By contrast, the phrases *related to* and *associated with* merely imply a relationship. The phrase *related to* is most commonly used. If one part of the diagnostic statement changes, the other part may change as well. Some examples of two-part nursing diagnoses are shown in the box below. Some NANDA labels contain the word "Specify." For these, the nurse must add words to indicate the problem more specifically. The format is still a two-part statement, for example,

Noncompliance (specify)

Noncompliance (diabetic diet) related to denial of having disease

For ease in alphabetizing, many NANDA lists are arranged with qualifying words after the main word (eg, **Infection, high risk for**). Avoid writing diagnostic statement in that manner; instead, write them as they would be stated in normal conversation (eg, **High risk for infection**).

BASIC THREE-PART STATEMENTS

The basic three-part nursing diagnosis statement is called the **PES format** and includes

1. Problem (P)—Statement of the client's response
2. Etiology (E)—Factors contributing to or probable causes of the response
3. Signs and symptoms (S)—Defining characteristics manifested by the client

The three-part diagnostic statement includes the problem, the etiology, and the observed signs and symptoms (PES). Actual nursing diagnoses can be documented by using the three-part statement (using *related to* and *as manifested by,* or *as evidenced by*), because the signs and symptoms have been identified. This format cannot be used for high risk diagnoses, because the client does not have signs and symptoms of the diagnosis.

The PES format is especially recommended for beginning diagnosticians, because the signs and symptoms validate why the diagnosis was chosen and make the problem statement more descriptive. The box at the top of page 120 is an example of the PES format.

Problem	*Related to*	*Etiology*
Colonic constipation	related to	prolonged laxative use
Ineffective breastfeeding	related to	breast engorgement

Problem	*Related to*	*Etiology*	*As Manifested by*	*Signs and Symptoms*
Self-esteem disturbance	related to	rejection by husband	as manifested by	Hypersensitivity to criticism; states, "I don't know if I can manage by myself" and rejects positive feedback.

The disadvantage of this method is that it can create very long problem statements, thereby obscuring the problem and etiology. However, because the signs and symptoms can be helpful in planning nursing interventions, they should be easily accessible. To promote access without long problem statements, the nurse can record the signs and symptoms in the nursing progress notes instead of on the care plan. Another possibility, recommended for students, is to list the signs and symptoms on the care plan *below* the nursing diagnosis, grouping the subjective and objective data. The signs and symptoms are easily accessible, and the problem and etiology stand out clearly. For example:

Noncompliance (diabetic diet) related to unresolved anger about diagnosis
S—"I forget to take my pills."
"I can't live without sugar in my food."
O—Weight 98 kg (215 lbs) (gain of 4.5 kg [10 lbs])
Blood pressure 190/100

ONE-PART STATEMENTS

Some diagnostic statements, such as wellness diagnoses and syndrome nursing diagnoses, consist of a NANDA label only. As the diagnostic labels are refined, they tend to become more specific, so that nursing interventions can be derived from the label itself. Therefore, an etiology is not needed. For example, adding an etiology to the labels **Rape-trauma syndrome, Post-trauma response,** and **Defensive coping** does not make the label any more descriptive or useful.

For some nursing diagnoses, it is difficult to write an etiology other than a medical diagnosis, or writing the etiology is somewhat redundant. **Reflex incontinence,** for instance, is fully described by its NANDA definition ("The state in which an individual experiences an involuntary loss of urine, occurring at somewhat predictable intervals when a specific bladder volume is reached"). The etiology of **Reflex incontinence** is "neurologic impairment" (eg, spinal cord lesion that interferes with conduction of cerebral messages above the level of the reflex arc). This etiology does not suggest nursing actions, nor does it really add to the understanding of the problem label. Similarly, the nursing interventions for **Post-trauma response** would be much the same regardless of whether the etiology is "related to war experiences" or "related to earthquake."

There are currently four one-part NANDA labels reflecting healthy functioning: **Health-seeking behaviors, Family coping, Potential for growth, Effective breast-feeding,** and **Anticipatory grieving.** NANDA has specified that any new wellness diagnosis will be developed as a one-part statement beginning with the words "Potential for enhanced" followed by the desired higher-level wellness (for example, **Potential for enhanced parenting**).

VARIATIONS OF BASIC FORMATS

Variations of the basic one-, two-, and three-part statements include the following:

1. *Writing "unknown etiology"* when the defining characteristics are present but the nurse does not know the cause of contributing factors. One example is **Noncompliance (medication regimen)** related to unknown etiology.
2. *Using the phrase "complex factors"* when there are too many etiologic factors or when they are too complex to state in a brief phrase. The actual causes of **Decisional conflict** and **Chronic low self-esteem,** for instance, may be long-term and complex, as in the following nursing diagnoses: **Decisional conflict** and **Chronic low self-esteem** related to complex factors.
3. *Using the word "possible" to describe either the problem or the etiology.* When the nurse believes more data is needed about the client's response (problem) or the etiology, the word "possible" is inserted. Examples are ***Possible* low self-esteem** related to loss of job and rejection by family; **Altered thought processes *possibly*** related to unfamiliar surroundings; and ***Possible* low self-esteem** related to unknown etiology.
4. *Using "secondary to"* to divide the etiology into two parts, thereby making the statement more descriptive and useful. The part following "secondary to" is often a pathophysiologic or disease process, as in **High risk for impaired skin integrity** related to decreased peripheral circulation secondary to diabetes.
5. *Adding a second part to the general response or NANDA label to make it more precise.* For example, the diagnosis **Impaired physical mobility** does not indicate the degree of mobility impairment. To make this label more specific, the nurse can add a colon and descriptor, as in the box at the top of page 121.

Problem +	*Descriptor* →	*Related to* →	*Etiology*
Impaired physical mobility:	inability to walk	related to	knee joint stiffness and pain secondary to muscle atrophy
Pain:	severe headache	related to	fear of addiction to narcotics

6. **Four-part statements** are combinations of basic statements and variations 4 and 5, discussed above. For example, the nurse creates a four-part statement by using both variations 4 and 5 with a basic two-part statement, as in: (1) **High risk for impaired skin integrity:** (2) **pressure sores** related to (3) immobility (4) secondary to presence of casts and traction. A four-part statement is also created by using the basic three-part (PES) format and adding either variation 4 or 5; for example, (1) **Impaired skin integrity:** (2) **pressure sore on left heel** related to (3) immobility (4) as manifested by 2 cm × 2 cm red, excoriated area on the left heel and inability to move about in bed.

COLLABORATIVE PROBLEMS

Carpenito (1993, p. 31) suggests that all collaborative problems begin with the diagnostic label "Potential Complication" ("PC"). Student nurses should include in the diagnostic statement both the possible complication they are monitoring and the disease or treatment that is present to produce it. For example

Potential complication of head injury: increased intracranial pressure

When monitoring for a group of complications associated with a disease or pathology, the nurse states the disease and follows it with a list of the complications:

Potential complication of pregnancy-induced hypertension: seizures, fetal distress, pulmonary edema, hepatic/renal failure, premature labor, CNS hemorrhage

The PES format is not used for collaborative problems because they are potential problems. Therefore, the client has no signs and symptoms for the nurse to list.

There are some situations in which an etiology might be helpful in suggesting interventions, that is, when the complication is caused by something more specific than a disease process. Students should write the etiology, as in the following examples: (1) when it clarifies the problem statement, (2) when it can be concisely stated, and (3) when it helps to suggest nursing actions (Wilkinson 1992, p. 137). (See box below.)

EVALUATING THE QUALITY OF THE DIAGNOSTIC STATEMENT

In addition to using the correct format, nurses must consider the content of their diagnostic statements. The statements should, for example, be accurate, concise, descriptive, and specific. The nurse must always validate the diagnostic statements with the client and compare the client's signs and symptoms to the NANDA defining characteristics. For high risk problems, the nurse compares the client's risk factors to NANDA risk factors. After writing nursing diagnoses, the nurse checks them against the criteria in Table 6–7 on page 122.

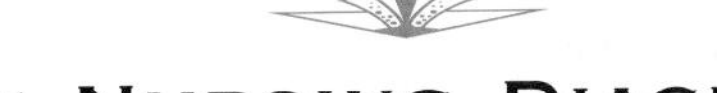

THE NURSING DIAGNOSIS MOVEMENT

Nursing diagnosis emerged in the 1970s and provided the profession with an appropriate focus on the content and diagnostic categories that were in the nursing domain.

HISTORICAL PERSPECTIVE

The earliest definition of nursing diagnosis was formulated by Abdellah (1957, p. 4), who stated that it was the "determination of the nature and extent of nursing problems presented by the individual patients or families receiving nursing care."

Disease/Situation	*Complication*	*Related to*	*Etiology*
Potential complication of childbirth:	hemorrhage	related to	1. uterine atony 2. retained placental fragments 3. bladder distention
Potential complication of diuretic therapy:	arrhythmias	related to	low serum potassium

Table 6–7 Guidelines for Writing a Nursing Diagnostic Statement

Guideline	Correct Statement	Incorrect and/or Ambiguous Statement
1. State in terms of a problem, not a need.	**Fluid volume deficit** (problem) related to fever	**Fluid replacement** (need) related to fever
2. State so that it is legally advisable.	**Impaired skin integrity** related to immobility (legally acceptable)	**Impaired skin integrity** related to improper positioning (implies legal liability)
3. Use nonjudgmental statements.	**Spiritual distress** related to inability to attend church services secondary to immobility (nonjudgmental)	**Spiritual distress** related to strict rules necessitating church attendance (judgmental)
4. Make sure that both elements of the statement do *not* say the same thing.	**High risk for impaired skin integrity** related to immobility	**Impaired skin integrity** related to ulceration of sacral area (response and probable cause are the same)
5. Make sure that the client's response precedes the contributing or causal factor.	**Noncompliance with diet** (response) related to lack of knowledge (contributing factor)	**Knowledge deficit** (contributing factor) related to noncompliance with diet (response)
6. Use statements that provide guidance for planning independent nursing interventions.	**Social isolation** related to loss of speech (loss of speech provides direction for planning alternative communication methods)	**Social isolation** related to laryngectomy (the nurse can do nothing about the laryngectomy)
7. Word diagnosis specifically and precisely to provide direction for planning nursing intervention.	**Altered oral mucous membrane** related to decreased salivation secondary to radiation of neck (specific)	**Altered oral mucous membrane** related to noxious agent (vague)
8. Use nursing terminology rather than medical terminology to describe the client's response.	**High risk for ineffective airway clearance** (nursing terminology)	**High risk for pneumonia** (medical terminology)
9. Use nursing terminology rather than medical terminology to describe the probable cause of the client's response.	**High risk for ineffective airway clearance** related to accumulation of secretions in lungs (nursing terminology)	**High risk for ineffective airway clearance** related to emphysema (medical terminology)
10. Do not start the nursing diagnosis with a nursing intervention.	**Altered nutrition: less than the body requirements** related to inadequate intake of protein (directs but does not state nursing intervention)	Provide high-protein diet because of **High risk for altered nutrition** (starts with nursing intervention)
11. Avoid using a symptom such as nausea as the problem. A symptom does not reflect a pattern and requires additional data collection.	Insufficient data for a diagnosis	**Nausea** related to medication
12. Use terminology generally understood by other professionals: do not use jargon or abbreviations.	**Self-care deficit: Toileting** related to inability to get out of bed without help	**Self-care deficit: Toileting** related to inability to get OOB w/o help
13. State the diagnosis concisely. (Using NANDA labels promotes conciseness.)	**Self-esteem disturbance** related to complex factors S—"I don't know if I can manage by myself" O—Hypersensitive to criticism, rejects positive feedback, no eye contact	**Self-esteem disturbance** related to long-standing feelings of failure aggravated by recently being rejected, as manifested by being hypersensitive to criticism, stating, "I don't know if I can manage by myself," rejecting positive feedback, and not making eye contact
14. Be sure that cause and effect are correctly stated (ie, the etiology causes the problem, or puts the client at risk for the problem).	**Pain: severe headache** related to fear of addiction to narcotics	**Pain** related to severe headache

The identification and development of nursing diagnoses began formally in 1973, when the National Conference Group for the Generation and Classification of Nursing Diagnoses was formed. This group originated through the efforts of two faculty members of Saint Louis University, Kristine Gebbie and Mary Ann Lavin, who perceived a need to identify their roles in an ambulatory care setting. The First National Conference held to identify nursing diagnoses was sponsored by the Saint Louis University School of Nursing and Allied Health Professions in 1973. Since that time, national conferences have been held in 1975, 1978, 1980, and every two years thereafter (Gebbie & Lavin 1975; Gebbie 1976; Kim & Moritz 1982; Kim et al 1984; Hurley 1986; McLane 1987). Through the efforts of these groups, much progress has been made in defining, classifying, and describing nursing diagnoses.

International recognition came with the First Canadian Conference, held in Toronto in 1977, and the International Nursing Conference held in May 1987 in Calgary, Alberta, Canada. In 1982, the conference group accepted the name North American Nursing Diagnosis Association (NANDA), thus recognizing the participation and contributions of nurses in the United States and Canada. The purpose of NANDA is to "define, refine and promote a taxonomy of nursing diagnostic terminology of general use to professional nurses" (Kim & Moritz 1982). The members of NANDA include staff nurses, clinical specialists, faculty, directors of nursing, deans, theorists, and researchers. In 1988, NANDA and the American Nurses Association (ANA) established a collaborative working agreement to "pursue development of the taxonomy" (Gordon 1988, p. 4). The group has currently approved more than 100 nursing diagnosis labels for clinical use and testing. See the list on the inside back cover.

APPROVAL OF NURSING DIAGNOSIS LABELS

Professional nurses wishing to submit a nursing diagnosis to NANDA do so through a review process developed by the Diagnosis Review Committee (DRC). After a diagnosis label is reviewed by clinical experts and the NANDA Board of Directors, it is voted on by the membership through a mail ballot. If the diagnosis is accepted, it is then included in the approved NANDA taxonomy. The approved labels are tentative and are modified and/or refined as necessary, according to clinical research data. At present these labels are considered the standard for use in the United States and Canada.

TAXONOMY OF NURSING DIAGNOSIS

A **taxonomy** is a classification system of groups, classes, or sets. The first taxonomy of nursing diagnoses was alphabetical. The nonhierarchic alphabetical ordering (see inside back cover) was considered unscientific by some, and a hierarchic structure was sought. In 1982, NANDA accepted the "nine patterns of unitary man" as an organizing principle. In 1984, NANDA renamed the "patterns of unitary man" as "human response patterns" (Kim et al 1984, p. 49). See the box above.

HUMAN RESPONSE PATTERNS

1. Exchanging: mutual giving and receiving
2. Communicating: sending messages
3. Relating: establishing bonds
4. Valuing: assigning relative worth
5. Choosing: selection of alternatives
6. Moving: activity
7. Perceiving: reception of information
8. Knowing: meaning associated with information
9. Feeling: subjective awareness of information

Having undergone refinements, revisions, and acceptance of new diagnoses, the taxonomy is now called *Taxonomy I, Revised* (NANDA 1990). All accepted nursing diagnoses now become subcategories of these nine human response patterns. For example, the human response pattern Feeling includes the following diagnostic labels:

- **Anxiety**
- **Fear**
- **Grieving (anticipatory, dysfunctional)**
- **Pain**
- **Chronic pain**
- **High risk for violence (self-directed or directed at others)**
- **Post-trauma response**
- **Rape-trauma syndrome (compound reaction, silent reaction)**

To prepare the taxonomy for possible inclusion in the World Health Organization's 10th revision of the *International Classification of Diseases (ICD 10)*, the NANDA Taxonomy Committee, in liaison with the ANA has modified the coding and made other revisions to conform to the ICD framework (Fitzpatrick et al 1989).

ADVANTAGES OF USING STANDARDIZED DIAGNOSTIC TERMINOLOGY

Diagnosing is now a standard by which professional care is measured. A uniform taxonomy of diagnostic labels can benefit both the nursing profession and health care consumers in the following ways:

- *Nursing diagnosis promotes professional accountability and autonomy by defining and describing the independent area of nursing practice.* According to Warren and Hoskins (1990, p. 162), "A profession must have a language that communicates its uniqueness and at the same time is understood by peers, other professionals, and consumers/clients." A nursing diagnosis, by definition, defines and describes problems for which the nurse can prescribe interventions (see the box on page 107).
- *Nursing diagnoses provide an effective vehicle for communication among nurses and other health care professionals.* Because a nursing diagnosis consolidates a great deal of information into concise statements and includes assessment parameters, it provides a shorthand method of communication. A nurse who knows a client's nursing diagnosis knows about the client's problem, the causal or contributing factors, and the necessary nursing actions.
- *Nursing diagnoses provide an organizing principle for the building of meaningful research.* The ability to access client data in relation to nursing diagnoses provides a framework for testing the validity of nursing interventions and feedback for further development of the unique body of nursing knowledge. In addition, the organization of data in this manner facilitates retrieval and analysis by computer-based information systems.
- *Nursing diagnoses facilitate individualized care.* Even though clients with identical medical conditions may need similar "routine" nursing interventions, the priorities of care may differ for each. In a health care system that is driven by cost considerations, there is ever-increasing emphasis on standardization of care as a way to promote efficiency and decrease cost. Nursing diagnoses can be used to focus on and promote attention to clients' unique needs, which may otherwise fail to be met.
- *Nursing diagnoses facilitate the delivery of quality care.* Nursing diagnoses facilitate comprehensive health care by identifying, validating, and responding to specific health problems (Risner 1986, p. 151). Because they identify the focus of a nursing activity, nursing diagnoses facilitate peer review of care and quality assurance within an agency. **Peer review** is the appraisal of a nurse's practice, education, or research by co-workers of equal status. **Quality assurance** is the evaluation of nursing services provided and the results achieved against an established standard. See discussion of evaluation in Chapter 8.
- *Nursing diagnoses facilitate continuity of care among nurses in an institution and when a client is transferred.* They guide the planning of nursing interventions from one shift to another in an acute care setting and when a client is transferred to a different unit (eg, from operating room to recovery room). They are also useful when a client moves from a hospital to a long-term care facility or is discharged from hospital to home but still requires nursing care.

CHALLENGES FOR THE FUTURE

The evolution of nursing diagnostic labels is in its early developmental stages, and the NANDA list is not to be considered a comprehensive guide for nursing practice. Although some nurses feel constrained by the existing list of diagnoses, it is well to remember that disciplines with well-established taxonomies, such as medicine, have taken many decades to develop. The usefulness of each diagnostic label must still be validated by appropriate research. **Validation** is the determination that the diagnosis accurately reflects the problem of the client, that the methods used for data gathering were valid, and that the conclusion or diagnosis is justified by the data. Many such studies have been done, and many more are in progress.

There is some concern that the use of nursing diagnoses may lead to stereotyping by the nurse and lessen the client's role in the decision-making process. Nurses must ensure that the client's perception of the problem is the focus of care. They need to be aware of the problems involved in professional labeling and make every effort to provide individualized client care.

The taxonomy has been criticized for the lack of focus on health promotion and health education. Nationally and internationally there is now an emphasis on consumer education and activities to promote a healthy life-style. The taxonomy is beginning to reflect these concerns. It now includes four wellness-oriented diagnostic labels: **Anticipatory grieving; Effective breastfeeding; Family coping: potential for growth;** and **Health-seeking behaviors.**

One of the major purposes of nursing diagnoses is to establish a method of validating independent nursing functions that would define nursing's unique role. A major task that is yet to be completed is the development of nursing interventions specific to each nursing diagnosis. Nurses will be accountable for these prescribed interventions. To date, a taxonomy of accepted clinical nursing interventions does not exist. However, lists of independent nursing functions are being developed. See Chapter 8 for further information.

CHAPTER HIGHLIGHTS

- Diagnosis is a reasoning process utilizing critical thinking.
- The critical-thinking skills used in diagnosing include analysis, synthesis, inductive reasoning, deductive reasoning, and decision making.
- The three phases of the diagnostic process are data analysis; identification of the client's health problems, health risks, and strengths; and formulation of nursing diagnoses.
- In data analysis and processing, the nurse compares data against standards to identify significant cues, clusters the data, and identifies gaps and inconsistencies.
- Significant cues are those that (a) point to change in a client's health status or pattern, (b) vary from norms of the client population, or (c) indicate a developmental delay.
- Professional standards of care hold that registered nurses are responsible for making nursing diagnoses, even though others may contribute data or implement care.
- The end product of the diagnostic process is a statement of client health status, called a nursing diagnosis.
- A nursing diagnosis is a clinical judgment about the client's responses to actual and potential health problems or life processes.
- A nursing diagnosis provides the basis for selecting independent nursing interventions to achieve outcomes for which the nurse is accountable.
- A wellness diagnosis is a clinical judgment about a client in transition from a specific level of wellness to a higher level of wellness.
- The basic format for a nursing diagnostic statement is "Problem related to etiology." However, there are several variations on this format.
- A nursing diagnosis should be clear, concise, client centered, related to only one problem, and based on reliable and relevant assessment data.
- Nursing diagnoses are complementary to but separate and distinct from a client's medical diagnoses.
- It is important to identify client strengths as well as problems.
- The client's perception of the nursing diagnoses must be validated.
- Diagnostic errors can be categorized as (a) errors of omission (ie, failure to diagnose a problem) and (b) errors of commission (ie, diagnosing a problem when no problem exists).
- Data interpretation errors occur when the nurse misinterprets the meaning of cues, makes a generalization based on an isolated cue, gathers incomplete data, or incorrectly clusters data.
- The purpose of the North American Nursing Diagnosis Association (NANDA) is to define, refine, and promote a taxonomy of nursing diagnostic terminology.
- The NANDA taxonomy of diagnostic labels is considered the standard for use in the United States and Canada.
- The organizing principle for the NANDA taxonomy is based on "human response patterns."
- A validated nursing diagnosis taxonomy would define the independent scope of practice, facilitate nursing research, and clarify communication among nurses and other health care professionals.
- The development of a taxonomy of nursing diagnosis labels is an ongoing process.

READINGS AND REFERENCES

SUGGESTED READINGS

Briody, ME, Carpenito, LJ, Jones, DA, and Fitzpatrick, JJ. July/September 1992. Toward further understanding of nursing diagnosis: An interpretation. *Nursing Diagnosis* 3(3):124–28.

This position article was presented to the NANDA Board of Directors and was intended to stimulate discussion about various interpretations of the term *nursing diagnosis* and surrounding issues. It asserts that nursing diagnoses are not reductionistic but holistic, and that the naming and classification of nursing's phenomena of concern will foster the growth of a nursing body of knowledge.

Whitley, GG. October/December 1992. Concept analysis of fear. *Nursing Diagnosis* 3(3):107–16.
The aim of this article was to clarify the meaning of the concept of Fear when used as a nursing diagnosis. The article is useful in helping nurses to differentiate between the closely related diagnoses of Anxiety and Fear.

RELATED RESEARCH

Kubsch, SM and Wichowski, HC. October/December 1992. Identification and validation of a new nursing diagnosis: "Sick role conflict." *Nursing Diagnosis* 3(4):141–47.

Lutjens, LRJ. 1993. The nature and use of nursing diagnosis in hospitals. *Nursing Diagnosis* 4: 107–13.

SELECTED REFERENCES

Abdellah, FG. June 1957. Methods of identifying covert aspects of nursing: A key to improved clinical teaching. *Nursing Research* 57:4–23.

American Nurses Association. 1991. *Standards of Clinical Nursing Practice.* Kansas City, MO: ANA.

Anderson, B and Hannah, KJ. 1993. A Canadian nursing data set: A major priority. *Canadian Journal of Nursing Administration* 6(2):7–13.

Avant, KD. April/June 1990. The art and science in nursing diagnosis development. *Nursing Diagnosis* 1(2):51–55.

Brackstone, A. 1993. Rekindling the nursing diagnosis flame. *The Canadian Nurse* 89(4):23–25.

Carnevali, DL and Thomas, MD. 1993. *Diagnostic Reasoning and Treatment Decision Making in Nursing.* Philadelphia: Lippincott.

Carpenito, LJ. 1995. *Nursing Diagnosis: Application to Clinical Practice.* 6th ed. Philadelphia: Lippincott.

Carroll-Johnson, RM, editor. 1991. *Classification of Nursing Diagnoses: Proceedings of the Ninth Conference.* Philadelphia: Lippincott.

Cox, HC et al. 1993. *Clinical Applications of Nursing Diagnosis: Adult, Child, Women's, Psychiatric, Gerontic and Home Health Considerations.* 2d ed. Philadelphia: FA Davis.

Dougherty, CM, Jankin, JJ, Lunney, MR, and Whitley, GG. 1993. Conceptual and research-based validation of nursing diagnoses: 1950–1993. *Nursing Diagnosis* 4(4):156–65.

Feild, L. 1991. Response of Feild to Leininger's nursing diagnosis article. *Journal of Transcultural Nursing* 3(1):25–29.

Fitzpatrick, J et al. 1989. Translating nursing diagnosis into ICD code. *American Journal of Nursing* 89:493–95.

Gebbie, KM. 1976. *Classification of Nursing Diagnoses: Summary of the Second National Conference.* St Louis: Mosby.

Gebbie, KM and Lavin MA, editors. 1975. *Classification of Nursing Diagnoses: Proceedings of the First National Conference.* St Louis: Mosby.

Gordon, M. 1987. *Nursing Diagnosis: Process and Application.* 2d ed. Hightstown, NJ: McGraw-Hill.

———. Summer 1988. President's column: North American Nursing Diagnosis Association. *Nursing Diagnosis Newsletter* 15:4–5.

Harvey, RM. 1993. Nursing diagnosis by computers: An application of neural networks. *Nursing Diagnosis* 4(1):26–34.

Hurley, ME, editor. 1986. *Classification of Nursing Diagnoses: Proceedings of the Sixth Conference, North American Nursing Diagnosis Association.* St Louis: Mosby.

Jones, JA. 1988. Clinical reasoning in nursing. *Journal of Advanced Nursing* 13:185–92.

Joint Commission on Accreditation of Healthcare Organizations. 1992. *Accreditation Manual for Hospitals.* Chicago: JCAHO, Nursing Services.

Kerr, M et al. 1993. Taxonomic validation: An overview. *Nursing Diagnosis* 4(1):6–14.

Kim, MJ, McFarland, GK, and McLane, AM. 1993. *Pocket Guide to Nursing Diagnoses.* 5th ed. St Louis: Mosby.

Kim, MJ, McFarland, GK, and McLane, AM, editors. 1984. *Classification of Nursing Diagnoses: Proceedings of the Fifth National Conference.* St Louis: Mosby.

Kim, MJ and Moritz, DA, editors. 1982. *Classification of the Third and Fourth National Conferences.* Highstown, NJ: McGraw-Hill.

Koch, B and McGovern, J. 1993. EXTEND: A prototype expert system for teaching nursing diagnosis. *Computers in Nursing* 11(1):35–41.

Kritek, PO. 1986. Development of a taxonomic structure for nursing diagnoses: A review and an update. In Hurley, ME, editor. *Classification of Nursing Diagnoses: Proceedings of the Sixth Conference, North American Nursing Diagnosis Association.* St Louis: Mosby.

Lederer, JR, Marculescu, GL, Mocnik, B, and Seaby, N. 1993. *Care Planning Pocket Guide: A Nursing Diagnosis Approach.* 5th ed. Redwood City, CA: Addison-Wesley Nursing.

McLane, AM, editor. 1987. *Classification of Nursing Diagnoses: Proceedings of the Seventh Conference.* St Louis: Mosby.

Mitchell, GJ. 1991. Nursing diagnoses: An ethical analysis. *Image: Journal of Nursing Scholarship* 23:99–103.

North American Nursing Diagnosis Association. 1990. *Taxonomy I, Revised—1990.* St Louis: NANDA.

———. 1994. *NANDA Nursing Diagnoses: Definitions and Classifications—1995–1996.* St Louis: NANDA.

Pillitteri, A. 1992. *Maternal and Child Nursing.* Philadelphia: Lippincott.

Pinkley, CL. January/March 1991. Exploring NANDA's definition of nursing diagnosis: Linking diagnostic judgments with the selection of outcomes and interventions. *Nursing Diagnosis* 2(1):26–32.

Popkess-Vawter, S. January/March 1991. Wellness nursing diagnosis: To be or not to be? *Nursing Diagnosis* 2(1):19–25.

Risner, PB. 1986. Analysis and synthesis. In Griffith, JW and Christensen, PJ, editors. pp. 124–50. *Nursing Process: Application of Theories, Frameworks, and Models.* St Louis: Mosby.

Thomas, RB, Barnard, KE, and Sumner, GA. 1993. In *The Nursing of Families: Theory/Research/Education/Practice. Selected Papers from the Second International Family Nursing Conference, Portland, OR, 1991.* Newbury Park, CA: Sage Publications.

Vincent, KG and Coler, MS. 1990. A unified nursing diagnostic model. *Image: Journal of Nursing Scholarship* 22:93–95.

Warren, J and Hoskins, L. 1990. The development of NANDA's nursing diagnosis taxonomy. *Nursing Diagnosis* 1(4):162–68.

Wilkinson, J. 1992. *Nursing Process in Action: A Critical Thinking Approach.* Redwood City, CA: Addison-Wesley Nursing.

Wooldridge, JB, Brown, DF, and Herman, J. Nursing diagnosis: The central theme in nursing knowledge. *Nursing Diagnosis* 4(2):50–55.

7 PLANNING

OBJECTIVES

- Describe the essential aspects of the planning phase of the nursing process.
- Identify five activities that occur in the planning phase.
- Identify factors that the nurse must consider when setting priorities.
- State the purposes of establishing client goals/expected outcomes.
- Describe the relationship of goals/expected outcomes to the nursing diagnoses.
- Identify guidelines for writing goals/expected outcomes.
- Describe the process of generating and choosing nursing strategies.
- List the five components of a nursing order.
- Identify major purposes of a written care plan.
- Identify essential guidelines for writing nursing care plans.
- Describe effective approaches to discharge planning.

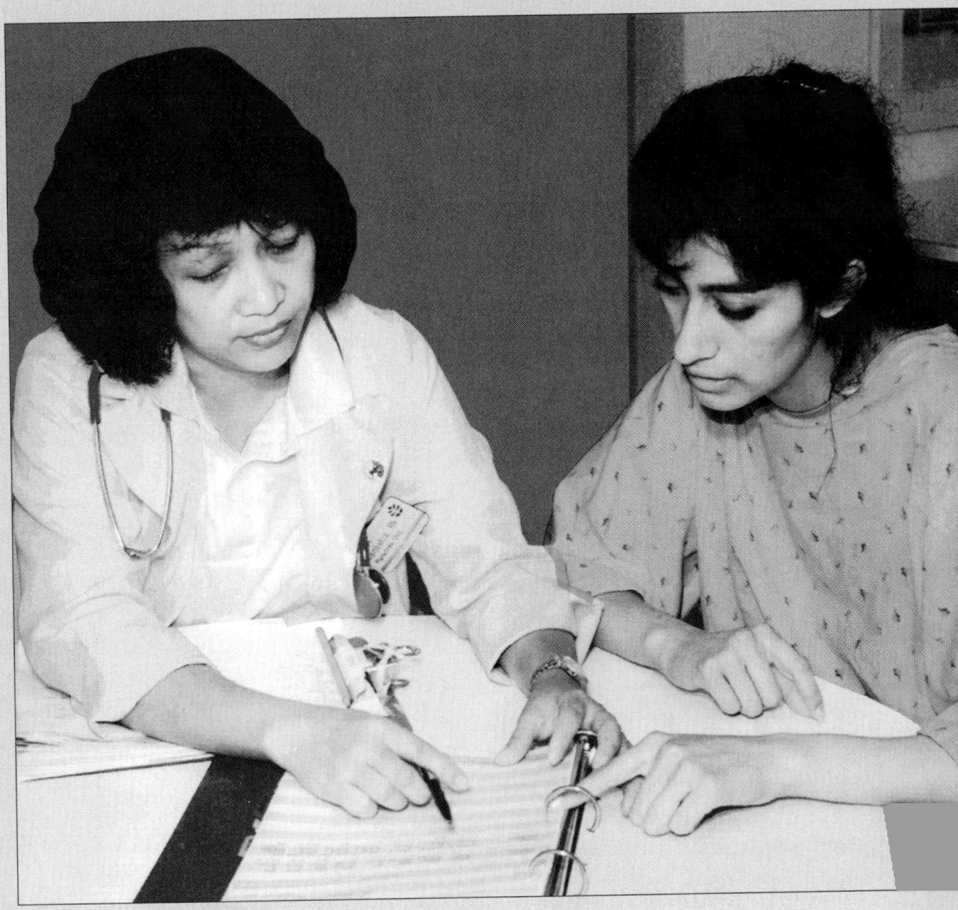

Planning is a deliberative, systematic phase of the nursing process that involves decision making and problem solving. In planning, the nurse refers to the client's assessment data and diagnostic statements for direction in formulating client goals and designing the nursing strategies required to prevent, reduce, or eliminate the client's health problems (Figure 7–1). The product of the planning phase is a client care plan. The box below describes the nurses' professional responsibilities for planning.

Although planning is basically the nurse's responsibility, input from the client and support persons is essential if a plan is to be effective. Nurses do not plan *for* the client, but encourage the client to participate actively to the extent possible. In a home setting, the client's support persons and/or caregivers are the ones who implement the plan of care; thus, its effectiveness depends largely on them. They can also provide information about problems the nurse might not otherwise discover.

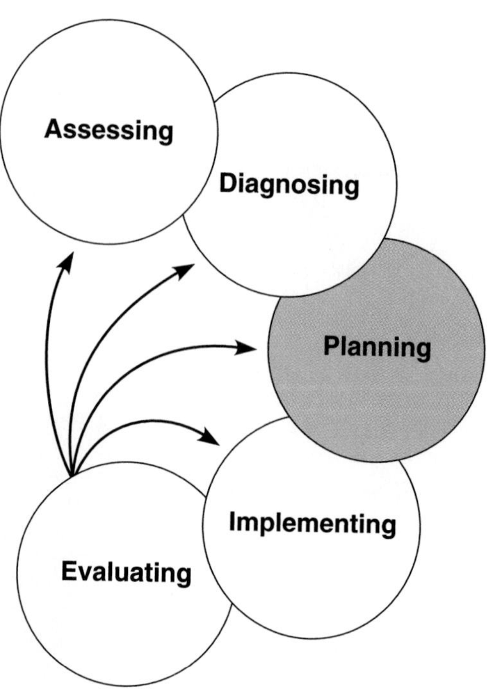

Figure 7–1 Planning. The third phase of the nursing process, in which the nurse and client develop client goals/outcomes and nursing strategies to prevent, reduce, or alleviate the client's health problems.

TYPES OF PLANNING

Planning begins with the first client contact and continues until the nurse-client relationship ends, usually when the client is discharged from the health care agency.

Initial Planning The nurse who performs the admission assessment usually develops the initial comprehensive plan of care. This nurse has the benefit of the client's body language as well as some intuitive kinds of information that are not available solely from the written database. Planning should be initiated as soon as possible after the initial assessment, especially because of the trend toward shorter hospital stays. Sometimes nurses use the available information to develop preliminary plans and refine them as the missing data become available.

> **ANA STANDARDS**
>
> ***Standard IV: Planning***
>
> The nurse develops a plan of care that prescribes interventions to attain expected outcomes.
>
> ***Measurement Criteria***
>
> 1. The plan is individualized to the client's condition or needs.
> 2. The plan is developed with the client, significant others, and health care providers, when appropriate.
> 3. The plan reflects current nursing practice.
> 4. The plan is documented.
> 5. The plan provides for continuity of care.
>
> **Source:** Abstracted from American Nurses Association, *Standards of Clinical Nursing Practice* (Washington, DC: ANA, 1991), pp. 11, 12. Used with permission.

Ongoing Planning Ongoing planning is done by all nurses who work with the client. As nurses obtain new information and evaluate the client's responses to care, they can individualize the initial care plan even more. Ongoing planning also occurs at the beginning of a shift as the nurse plans the care to be given that day. Using ongoing assessment data, the nurse carries out daily planning for the following purposes (Wilkinson 1992, pp. 165–66):

1. To determine whether the client's health status has changed
2. To set the priorities for the client's care during the shift
3. To decide which problems to focus on during the shift
4. To coordinate the nurse's activities so that more than one problem can be addressed at each client contact

STEPS IN THE CONSULTING PROCESS

1. *Identify the problem.* Have the problem clearly in mind, including the circumstances surrounding it.
2. *Collect all pertinent data.* When consulting another health professional who is unfamiliar with the client, collect all the data relevant to the problem.
3. *Select the consultant.* Consult a recognized health professional who has the skills or knowledge required.
4. *Communicate the problem and pertinent information.* The information often varies with each client and each problem. It is important to include information about the client's strengths and problems. Convey the information clearly and objectively, and make sure the data are factual and not interpretive.
5. *Discuss the recommendations with the consultant.* The consultant may provide recommendations at the time the nurse describes the problem, or a later meeting may be necessary. For example, an oncology nursing consultant may give immediate recommendations regarding activity, positioning, timing of medication, or the consultant might prefer to obtain further data before making recommendations.
6. *Include the recommendations in the client's nursing care plan.* The recommendations become part of the client's record. After implementing the recommendations, the nurse evaluates and records their effectiveness.

Discharge Planning Because the average client stay in acute care hospitals has become shorter, people are sometimes discharged still needing care. Although many clients are discharged to other agencies (eg, nursing homes), such care is increasingly being delivered in the home. **Discharge planning,** the process of anticipating and planning for needs after discharge, is becoming a crucial part of comprehensive health care. Effective discharge planning begins at the time of admission. Each client should be assessed for potential health needs, availability and ability of the client's support network to assist with these needs, and how the home environment supports the client. Client, family, and community resources should also be evaluated when considering discharge needs.

CONSULTING

Consulting, the process in which two people deliberate with one another, is frequently done in all phases of the nursing process, and in particular during planning. Nurses consult a variety of health professionals, including other nurses. Consulting implies that the nurse involved in the care seeks advice or clarification regarding client goals. Increasingly, nurses consult with other nurses within the agency about a variety of specialized nursing practice areas. Some agencies have a protocol to be followed by those consulting a health professional not currently involved in the client's care. For example, if a nurse wants to discuss a client's depression with an agency psychiatrist, the nurse may need to send a form to the psychiatrist requesting a consultation. However, many consultations take place on an informal basis. For example, the nurse may discuss a client's skin problem with the physician during the physician's rounds.

Nurses generally consult to verify findings, implement change, and obtain additional knowledge. They often ask other nurses to verify assessment data, such as extremely low blood pressure or exceptionally fast pulse, when their findings are unexpected or they are uncertain about them. Sometimes nurses discuss a client's care plan with another nurse, often to make sure the best possible plan has been arranged or to implement change in the plan. No nurse can know everything about nursing, and another nurse may have knowledge and experience about a particular problem. See the accompanying box for the six steps in the consulting process.

THE PLANNING PROCESS

The planning process includes the following activities:

- Setting priorities
- Establishing client goals/expected outcomes
- Selecting nursing strategies
- Developing nursing care plans

SETTING PRIORITIES

Priority setting is the process of establishing a preferential order for nursing strategies. The nurse and client begin planning by deciding which nursing diagnosis requires attention first, which second, and so on. Instead of rank-ordering diagnoses, nurses can group them as having high, medium, or low priority. Life-threatening problems, such as loss of respiratory or cardiac functioning, are designated as *high priority.* Health-threatening problems, such as acute illness and decreased coping ability, may result in delayed development or cause destructive physical or emotional changes; thus, they are usually assigned *medium priority.* A *low-priority* problem is one that arises from normal developmental needs or that requires only minimal nursing support.

Table 7–1 Assigning Priorities to Nursing Diagnoses for Luisa Sanchez

Nursing Diagnosis	Priority	Rationale
Ineffective airway clearance related to (1) viscous secretions secondary to fluid volume deficit and (2) shallow chest expansion secondary to pain and fatigue	High priority	Loss of respiratory functioning is a life-threatening problem. The nurse's primary concern must be to promote Ms Sanchez's oxygenation by addressing the etiologies of this problem.
Fluid volume deficit: intake insufficient to replace fluid loss related to fever and diaphoresis	High priority	Severe **Fluid volume deficit** is life-threatening. Although not that severe for Ms Sanchez, it is a high-priority problem because it is also a contributing factor for **Ineffective airway clearance.** Collaborative efforts to improve her hydration have already begun (intravenous fluids). The nurse must immediately and continuously assess and promote Ms Sanchez's hydration.
Anxiety related to (1) difficulty breathing and (2) concerns over work and parenting roles	Medium priority	Although Ms Sanchez is concerned about work and parenting roles, these are not a life threat. Also, treatment of her high-priority problem, **Ineffective airway clearance,** will relieve one of the etiologies of this problem (dyspnea). Meanwhile, the nurse must provide symptomatic relief of Ms Sanchez's anxiety during periods of dyspnea, because extreme anxiety could further compromise her oxygenation by causing her to breathe ineffectively and increasing the rate at which she uses oxygen.
Altered comfort: chills related to fever and diaphoresis	Medium priority	Although fever and diaphoresis will resolve with medical treatment, the nurse meanwhile must promote Ms Sanchez's comfort. Chills (and other discomfort) increase oxygen utilization and may contribute to **Anxiety** and **Sleep pattern disturbance.**
High risk for altered family processes related to mother's illness and temporary unavailability of father to provide child care	Low priority	Ms Sanchez's child is currently being cared for. If Mr Sanchez returns as planned, this potential problem will not develop into an actual problem. No interventions are needed at present, except for continued assessment and reassurance.
Altered nutrition: less than body requirements related to decreased appetite, nausea, and increased metabolism secondary to disease process	Low priority	This problem is not currently health-threatening, but it could be if it were to persist. It will almost certainly resolve in a day or two as the medical problem is treated. If the medical problem does not resolve quickly, this will change to a medium priority.
Self-care deficit (level 2) related to activity intolerance secondary to ineffective airway clearance and sleep pattern disturbance	Low priority	This problem is caused by other, higher-priority problems; therefore, it will resolve as they resolve. Meanwhile, the nurse merely needs to assist Ms Sanchez with bathing, and so on, to support and conserve her energy until she is strong enough to resume her own care. Because of the medical order for bed rest, few nursing actions are immediately required.
Sleep pattern disturbance related to cough, pain, orthopnea, fever, and diaphoresis	Low priority	Lack of sleep is health-threatening. But for the moment (until night) the nurse does not need to address this problem. **Sleep pattern disturbance** does contribute to Ms Sanchez's **Ineffective airway clearance,** but it is not the main cause. Therefore, measures to promote sleep will be low priority until evening. After the nurse has attended to Ms Sanchez's oxygenation and hydration needs, this problem priority will change.
Chest pain related to cough secondary to pneumonia	Not on care plan	The nurse did not write a **Pain** problem on the care plan because **Pain** is to be addressed as the etiology of **Sleep pattern disturbance** and **Ineffective airway clearance.** The pain etiologies (cough and pneumonia) will be treated by medications (collaborative interventions). Independent nursing actions would address the problem rather than the etiology and would be the same as the nursing actions for **Ineffective airway clearance.**

Using a framework makes priority setting easier. Although it is not, strictly speaking, a nursing framework, nurses frequently use Maslow's hierarchy of needs when setting priorities. See Figure 14–2 on page 274. In Maslow's hierarchy, physiologic needs, such as air, food, and water, are basic to life and receive higher priority than the need for security or activity. Growth needs, such as self-esteem, are not perceived as "basic" in this framework. Thus, when the nurse plans care for a client with unmet physiologic needs and unmet growth needs, the physiologic (basic) needs receive first priority.

Priority setting does not require that all the high-priority diagnoses be resolved before the nurse addresses any others. The nurse may partially address a high-priority diagnosis and then deal with a diagnosis of lesser priority. Furthermore, because clients usually have several problems, the nurse often addresses more than one diagnosis at a time. See Table 7–1 for priorities assigned to Luisa Sanchez's nursing diagnoses.

The priorities assigned to problems do not remain fixed; rather, they change as the client's responses, problems, and therapies change. The nurse assigns priorities on the basis of nursing judgment and, insofar as possible, client preference. The nurse must consider a variety of factors, for example, the client's values and priorities and the available resources.

Client's Health Values and Beliefs Values concerning health may be very important to the nurse but not to the client. For example, a client may believe being home for the children to be more urgent than a health problem. When there is such a difference of opinion, the client and nurse should discuss it openly to resolve any conflict. However, in a life-threatening situation, the nurse usually must take the initiative.

Client's Priorities Involving the client in prioritizing and care planning enhances cooperation between the nurse and client. Sometimes, however, the client's perception of what is important conflicts with the nurse's knowledge of potential problems or complications. For example, an elderly female may not regard ambulation or turning and repositioning in bed as important, preferring to be undisturbed. The nurse, however, aware of the potential complications of prolonged bed rest (eg, muscle weakness and decubitus ulcers), needs to inform the client and implement necessary interventions to prevent such debilitating effects.

Resources Available to the Nurse and Client If money, equipment, or personnel are scarce, then a health problem may be given a lower priority than usual. Nurses in a home setting, for example, do not have the resources of a hospital; therefore, if the resources needed for specific nursing strategies are not available, the solution of that problem might need to be postponed, or the client may need referral.

Client resources, such as finances or coping abilities, may also influence the setting of priorities. For example, a client who is unemployed may defer dental treatment; a client whose husband is terminally ill and dependent on her may consider nutritional guidance directed toward weight loss as too much to handle.

Urgency of the Health Problem Regardless of the framework used, life-threatening situations require that the nurse assign them high priority. This also applies to situations that affect the integrity of the client, that is, those that could have a negative or destructive effect on the client. Such health problems as drug abuse and radical alteration of self-concept due to amputation can be destructive not only to the individual but also to the family. For example, in Table 7–1, although Ms Sanchez is anxious about childcare, her **Ineffective airway clearance** has higher priority.

Medical Treatment Plan The priorities for treating health problems must be congruent with treatment by other health professionals. For example, a high priority for the client might be to become ambulatory; however, if the physician's therapeutic regimen calls for extended bed rest, then ambulation must assume a lower priority in the nursing care plan. The nurse can provide or teach exercises to facilitate ambulation later, provided the client's health permits. The diagnostic statement related to ambulation is not ignored; it is merely deferred.

ESTABLISHING CLIENT GOALS/EXPECTED OUTCOMES

After establishing priorities, the nurse sets goals for each nursing diagnosis. A **goal** is a desired outcome or change in client behavior. Goal attainment is the resolution of the problem specified in the nursing diagnosis. On a care plan, the goals describe, in terms of observable client responses, what the nurse hopes to achieve by implementing the nursing orders. The terms *goal* and *expected outcome* are sometimes used interchangeably. Some sources also use the terms *outcome criterion*, *objective*, and *predicted outcome*. The American Nurses Association (ANA) specifies outcome identification in *Standards of Clinical Nursing Practice*. See the box on page 132.

Some nursing literature differentiates by defining *goals* as broad statements about the effects of nursing interventions and *expected outcomes* as the more specific, measurable criteria used to evaluate whether the goal has been met. For example:

Goal (broad): Nutritional status will improve.

Expected outcome (specific): Will gain 5 lb by April 25.

ANA STANDARDS

Standard III: Outcome Identification

The nurse identifies expected outcomes individualized to the client.

Measurement Criteria

1. Outcomes are derived from the diagnoses.
2. Outcomes are documented as measurable goals.
3. Outcomes are mutually formulated with the client and health care providers, when possible.
4. Outcomes are realistic in relation to the client's present and potential capabilities.
5. Outcomes are attainable in relation to resources available to the client.
6. Outcomes include a time estimate for attainment.
7. Outcomes provide direction for continuity of care.

Source: Abstracted from American Nurses Association, *Standards of Clinical Nursing Practice* (Washington, DC: ANA, 1991), pp. 11, 12. Used with permission.

When goals are defined broadly, as in the above example, the client's care plan must include *both* goals and expected outcomes. In fact, they are sometimes combined into one statement linked by the words "as evidenced by," as follows:

> Nutritional status will improve, as evidenced by weight gain of 5 lb by April 25.

Writing the broad goal first may help students to think of the specific outcomes that are needed. But even though broad goals can be a starting point for planning, it is the specific, measurable outcomes that *must* be written on the care plan. Table 7–2 on page 133 shows that some of the expected outcomes are preceded by a broad goal.

Purpose of Goals/Expected Outcomes The purposes of goals/expected outcomes include the following:

1. Provide direction for planning nursing interventions that will achieve the desired changes in the client. Ideas for interventions come more easily if the goals state clearly and specifically what the nurse hopes to achieve.
2. Provide a time span for planned activities.
3. Serve as criteria for evaluation of client progress. Although developed in the planning step of the nursing process, the expected outcomes serve as criteria for judging nursing interventions and client progress in the evaluation step (see Chapter 8).
4. Enable the client and nurse to determine when the problem has been resolved.
5. Help motivate the client and nurse by providing a sense of achievement. As goals are met, both client and nurse can see that their efforts have been worthwhile. This provides motivation to continue following the plan, especially when difficult life-style changes need to be made.

Long-Term and Short-Term Goals Goals may be short term or long term. A short-term goal might be "Client will raise right arm to shoulder height by Friday." In the same context, a long-term goal might be "Client will regain full use of right arm in 6 weeks." In an acute care setting, much of the nurse's time is spent on the client's immediate needs, so most goals are short term. Short-term goals also enable the nurse to evaluate client progress more accurately.

Long-term goals are often used for clients who live at home and have chronic health problems and for clients in nursing homes, extended care facilities, and rehabilitation centers. Short-term goals are useful (a) for clients who require health care for a short time and (b) for those who are frustrated by long-term goals that seem difficult to attain and who need the satisfaction of achieving a short-term goal.

Relationship of Goals/Expected Outcomes to Nursing Diagnoses Goals/expected outcomes are derived from and relate to the client's nursing diagnoses—primarily from the first clause (problem). The problem clause contains the unhealthy response; it states what should change. Therefore, the *essential* client goals are derived from the problem clause. For example, if the nursing diagnosis is **High risk for fluid volume deficit** related to diarrhea and inadequate intake secondary to nausea, the *essential* goal statement might be "Client's fluid balance will be maintained, as evidenced by urinary and stool output in balance with fluid intake, normal skin turgor, and moist-mucous membranes." In this example, a general goal (fluid balance) is stated as the opposite of the problem **(Fluid volume deficit)** and then followed by a list of measurable expected outcomes. If achieved, the expected outcomes would be evidence that the problem, **Fluid volume deficit,** has been prevented. See Table 7–2 for additional expected outcomes from nursing diagnosis.

Goals may occasionally be derived from the second cause (etiology of the diagnosis), but they are different from those derived from the problem. Their achievement may help to resolve the problem, but they might also be achieved *without* resolving the problem. For example, in the diagnosis **High risk for fluid volume deficit** related to diarrhea and inadequate intake, the following expected outcome could be derived from the etiology: "Client will have daily fluid intake of 1500 mL." Note that drinking 1500 mL of fluid would help the client achieve fluid bal-

Table 7–2 Expected Outcomes from Nursing Diagnoses

Nursing Diagnosis	Problem Response	Opposite Healthy Response (Goals)	Expected Outcomes
Impaired physical mobility: inability to bear weight on left leg, related to inflammation of knee joint	**Impaired physical mobility: inability to bear weight on left leg**	Improved mobility	Client will ambulate with crutches by end of the week.
		Ability to bear weight on left leg	Client will be able to stand without assistance by end of the month.
Ineffective airway clearance related to poor cough effort, secondary to incision pain, and fear of damaging sutures	**Ineffective airway clearance**	Effective airway clearance	Lungs will be clear to auscultation during entire postoperative period.
			No skin pallor or cyanosis by 12 hours post op.
			*Within 24 hours after surgery, client will demonstrate good cough effort.

* Note that this outcome was derived from the etiology clause and that the client could achieve this outcome but still have the problem of **Ineffective airway clearance.**

ance; however, if the nurse discontinued the care plan on the basis of achieving this outcome, then the client's needs would not be met. The fact that the client's intake was 1500 mL does not "prove" that the problem was prevented. For example, continued diarrhea or a high fever that cause the client to lose more than 1500 mL of fluid could still create a problem of **Fluid volume deficit.**

Rule: For every nursing diagnosis, the nurse must write at least one outcome criterion that, when achieved, directly demonstrates resolution of the problem clause.

When developing outcome criteria, ask the following questions:

1. What is the problem clause?
2. What is the opposite, healthy response?
3. How will the client look or behave if the healthy response is achieved? (What will I be able to see, hear, palpate, smell, or otherwise observe with my senses?)
4. What must the client do and how well must the client do it to demonstrate problem resolution or to demonstrate the capability of resolving the problem?

The box on page 132 describes measurement criteria for expected outcomes.

EXAMPLES OF ACTION VERBS

Apply	Differentiate	Report
Arrange	Discuss	Select
Assemble	Drink	Share
Breathe	Explain	Show
Choose	Express	Sit
Communicate	Help	Sleep
Compare	Identify	State
Construct	Inject	Talk
Defend	Justify	Take
Define	List	Transfer
Demonstrate	Move	Turn
Describe	Name	Use
Design	Prepare	Verbalize
		Walk

Components of Goal/Expected Outcome Statements

Goal/expected outcome statements generally have the following four components:

1. *Subject.* The subject, a noun, is the client, any part of the client, or some attribute of the client, such as the client's pulse or urinary output. Often, the subject is omitted in nursing care plan goals; it is assumed that the subject is the client unless indicated otherwise.
2. *Verb.* The verb denotes an action the client is to perform, for example, what the client is to do, learn, or experience. Verbs that denote directly observable behaviors, such as *administer, demonstrate, show, walk,* and so on, are used. See the box above.

Table 7–3 Components of Goals/Expected Outcomes

Subject	Verb	Conditions/Modifiers	Criterion of Desired Performance
Client	drinks	2500 mL of fluid	daily (time)
Client	administers	correct insulin dose	using aseptic technique (quality standard)
Client	lists	three hazards of smoking (after reading literature)	(accuracy indicated by number of hazards)
Client	recalls	five symptoms of diabetes before discharge	(accuracy indicated by number of symptoms)
Client	walks	the length of the hall without a walker	by date of discharge (time)
Client's ankle	measures	less than 10 inches in circumference	in 48 hours (time)
Client	carries out	leg ROM exercises as taught	every 8 hours (time)
Client	identifies	foods high in salt from a prepared list	before discharge (time)
Client	states	the purposes of his medications	before discharge (time)

3. *Conditions or modifiers.* Conditions or modifiers may be added to the verb to explain the circumstances under which the behavior is to be performed. They explain what, where, when, or how. For example:

   Walks *with the help of a walker* (how).

   After attending two group diabetes classes, lists signs and symptoms of diabetes (when).

   When at home, maintains weight at existing level (where).

   Discusses *four food groups and recommended daily servings* (what).

   Conditions need not be included if the criterion of performance clearly indicates what is expected.

4. *Criterion of desired performance.* The criterion indicates the standard by which a performance is evaluated or the level at which the client will perform the specified behavior. These criteria may specify time or speed, accuracy, distance, and quality. To establish a time-achievement criterion, the nurse needs to ask, "How long?" To establish an accuracy criterion, the nurse asks, "How well?" Similarly, the nurse asks, "How far?" and "What is the expected standard?" to establish distance and quality criteria, respectively. Examples are:

   Weighs 75 kg *by April* (time).

   Lists *five out of six* signs of diabetes (accuracy).

   Walks *one block per day* (time and distance).

   Administers insulin *using aseptic technique* (quality).

See Tables 7–3 and 7–4 for other examples of expected outcomes. Table 7–3 illustrates the format that should be used to write outcomes, and Table 7–4 lists goals that were developed for Luisa Sanchez.

Guidelines for Writing Goals/Expected Outcomes

The following guidelines can help nurses write goals and expected outcomes.

1. Write goals and outcome criteria in terms of client behavior. Begin each goal and outcome criteria with "the client." This helps to focus on what the client will be able to do when the outcome criteria are achieved. Outcome criteria should focus on what the client will accomplish, *not what the nurse will do.* For example, a postoperative client may have the following goal. "The client will maintain clear, open airways, as evidenced by normal breath sounds, no wheezing or rales, normal rate of respirations, and absence of dyspnea and cyanosis.

   Avoid statements that start with *enable, facilitate, allow, let, permit,* or similar verbs followed by the word *client.* These verbs indicate what the nurse hopes to accomplish, not what the client will do. For example, the statement "Assist the client to deep breathe and cough every two hours" is a nursing action, not an observable client behavior.

2. Make sure the goal statement is appropriate for the nursing diagnosis. Validate the outcomes. If the outcomes are accomplished, will the client's nursing diagnosis be resolved?

3. Be sure that the outcomes are realistic for the client's capabilities, limitations, and designated time span, if it is indicated. *Limitations* refer to finances, equipment, family support, social services, physical and mental condition, and time. For example, the outcome "The client will walk with crutches on level surfaces and on stairs" may be unrealistic for an elderly woman with a heavy leg cast. "The client will walk with crutches from bed to bathroom with assistance" may be more realis-

Table 7–4 Expected Outcomes for Luisa Sanchez

Nursing Diagnosis*	Goal Statements (Expected Outcomes)
Ineffective airway clearance related to viscous secretions and shallow chest expansion secondary to fluid volume deficit, pain, and fatigue	Demonstrates adequate air exchange, as evidenced by ▪ Absence of pallor and cyanosis (skin and mucous membranes) ▪ Use of correct breathing/coughing technique after instruction ▪ Productive cough ▪ Demonstrating symmetric chest excursion of at least 4 cm ▪ Verbalizing chest pain of < 4 on a 1–10 scale within 30 min after receiving po analgesics Within 48–72 hours: ▪ Lungs clear to auscultation ▪ Respirations 12–22/min, pulse < 100 beats/min ▪ Inhales normal volume of air on incentive spirometer
Fluid volume deficit: intake insufficient to replace fluid loss related to vomiting, fever, and diaphoresis	Demonstrates fluid balance, as evidenced by ▪ Urine output greater than 30 mL/h ▪ Urine specific gravity 1.005–1.025 ▪ Good skin turgor ▪ Moist mucous membranes ▪ Relating the need for oral fluid intake ▪ Total fluid intake > output
Anxiety related to difficulty breathing and concerns about work and parenting roles	Demonstrates decreased anxiety, as evidenced by ▪ Listening to and following instructions for correct breathing and coughing technique, even during periods of dyspnea ▪ Verbalizing understanding of condition, diagnostic tests, and treatments ▪ Decrease in reports of fear and anxiety; none within 12 h ▪ Voice steady, not shaky ▪ Respiratory rate of 12–22/min ▪ Freely expressing concerns about work and parenting roles, but placing them in perspective in view of her illness
Altered comfort: chills related to fever and diaphoresis	Demonstrates relief from discomfort by ▪ Verbalizing relief ▪ Relaxed facial expression
High risk for altered family processes related to mother's illness and temporary unavailability of father to provide child care	Will not experience altered family processes, as evidenced by ▪ Husband returning tomorrow, as scheduled ▪ Report of satisfactory child care arrangements having been made ▪ Client and husband communicating effectively and working together to solve problems ▪ Family members expressing feelings and providing mutual support
Altered nutrition: Less than body requirements related to decreased appetite, nausea, and increased metabolism secondary to disease process	Demonstrates adequate nutritional intake to meet body needs, as evidenced by ▪ Eating at least 85% of each meal ▪ Maintaining present weight ▪ Verbalizing importance of adequate nutrition ▪ Verbalizing improved appetite
Self-care deficit (level 2) related to activity intolerance secondary to ineffective airway clearance and sleep pattern disturbance	▪ Feeds self unassisted† ▪ Ambulates to bathroom without dyspnea, fatigue, or shortness of breath ▪ Within 24 hours, bathes with assistance in bed; within 48 hours, bathes with assistance at sink; within 72 hours, bathes in shower without dyspnea ▪ Reports satisfaction and comfort with hygiene needs
Sleep pattern disturbance related to cough, pain, orthopnea, fever, and diaphoresis	▪ Observed sleeping at night rounds† ▪ Reports feeling rested ▪ Does not experience orthopnea

* The nursing diagnoses are listed in priority order.

† Note that these expected outcomes are written without using the broad statement of "opposite, healthy response to the problem."

CHARACTERISTICS OF WELL-STATED GOALS/EXPECTED OUTCOMES

- Expected outcomes are derived primarily from the first clause of the nursing diagnosis. Their achievement demonstrates problem resolution or prevention.
- The expected outcome is possible to achieve.
- The expected outcome is stated in terms of client responses rather than nursing activities.
- Each expected outcome is a statement of *one* specific client response or behavior.
- Each expected outcome is specific and concrete, to facilitate measurement.
- Each expected outcome is appraisable or measurable, that is, the outcome can be seen, heard, felt, or measured by another person.
- The goal/expected outcome is valued by the client and family.
- The goal/expected outcome is compatible with the therapies of other professionals.

tic. The outcome "Measures insulin accurately" may be unrealistic for a client who has poor vision due to cataracts.

4. Make sure the client considers the goals/outcomes important and values them. Some outcomes, such as those for problems related to self-esteem, parenting, and communication, involve choices that are best made by the client or in collaboration with the client.

   Some clients may know what they wish to accomplish with regard to their health problem. For instance, the client's goal may be "relief of pain." Other clients may not know all the outcome possibilities for their specific problem. The nurse must actively listen to the client to determine personal values, goals, and desired outcomes in relation to current health concerns. Then, discuss the nursing diagnosis and goals to determine whether the client agrees with the stated problem and goals. Clients are usually motivated and expend the necessary energy to reach goals they consider important.
5. Ensure that the goals and expected outcomes are compatible with the work and therapies of other professionals. The goal "Increase the client's activity tolerance" and the attending criterion "Will increase the time spent out of bed by 15 minutes each day" are not compatible with a physician's prescribed therapy of bed rest for 3 days.
6. Make sure that each goal is derived from only one nursing diagnosis. For example, the goal "The client will increase the amount of nutrients ingested and show progress in the ability to feed self" is derived from two nursing diagnoses: **Feeding self-care deficit** related to neuromuscular impairment and **Altered nutrition: less than body requirements** related to anorexia. Keeping the goal statement related to only one diagnosis facilitates evaluation of care by ensuring planned nursing interventions are clearly related to the diagnosis.
7. When writing expected outcomes, use observable, measurable terms; avoid words that are vague and require interpretation or judgment by the observer. For example, such phrases as "increase daily exercise," "increase participation in social activities," and "improve knowledge of nutrition" can mean different things to different people. If used in criteria, these phrases can lead to disagreements about whether the criterion was met. These phrases may be suitable for a broad client goal but are not sufficiently clear and specific for use in outcome criteria used to evaluate the client's response.

   Examples of expected outcomes associated with the diagnostic statements for Luisa Sanchez are shown in Table 7–4 on page 135. Note that the diagnostic statements have been reordered according to established priorities. Also see the box to the left for a summary of the characteristics of well-stated goals/outcomes.

SELECTING NURSING STRATEGIES

Nursing strategies or interventions are nursing activities relating to a specific nursing diagnosis that a nurse carries out to achieve client goals. The specific strategies chosen should focus on eliminating or reducing the etiology (cause) of the nursing diagnosis, which is the second clause of the diagnostic statement. Strategies for *potential* nursing diagnoses should focus on measures to reduce the client's risk factors and/or signs and symptoms, which are also found in the second clause.

Correct identification of the etiology during the diagnosing phase provides the framework for choosing successful nursing interventions. For example, **Activity intolerance** may have several etiologies—pain, weakness, sedentary life-style, anxiety, or cardiac arrhythmias, for example. The interventions will vary according to the cause of the problem.

Often, the nurse and the client can establish a number of nursing strategies for each problem statement. Too many alternatives can be confusing. Usually three to five alternative nursing strategies for each health problem are satisfactory.

A recent development is a set of 336 standardized nursing interventions (McCloskey & Bulechek 1992). They have yet to be reviewed by national nursing groups but have been put forth for clinical use and testing. Each broad intervention label includes a definition and a list of all the specific activities nurses perform to carry out the intervention. Not all the activities would be needed for every client, so the nurse chooses from the list those activities appropriate for the client, and individualizes them to fit the supplies, equipment, and so forth, available in the agency. See Table 7–5 for an example of one intervention label, definition, and a few of its specific activities.

Table 7–5 Example of a Standardized Nursing Intervention Label

Respiratory Monitoring

Definition: Collection and analysis of patient data to ensure airway patency and adequate gas exchange.

Activities (5 examples are given, from a list of 26):

- Monitor rate, rhythm, depth, and effort of respirations
- Monitor for noisy respirations such as crowing or snoring
- Percuss anterior and posterior thorax from apices to bases bilaterally
- Monitor for increased restlessness, anxiety, and air hunger
- Monitor patient's ability to cough effectively

Source: JC McCloskey and GM Bulechek, editors, *Nursing Interventions Classification (NIC)*. (St Louis: Mosby Year-Book, 1992), p. 409. Used with permission.

Considering the Consequences of Each Strategy

Once the nurse identifies a number of possible strategies to implement, the next step is to consider the risks and benefits of each action. Often, an action will have more than one consequence. For example, the strategy "Provide accurate information" could result in the following client behaviors:

- Increased anxiety
- Decreased anxiety
- Wish to talk with the physician
- Desire to leave hospital
- Relaxation

Determining the consequences of each strategy requires nursing knowledge and experience. The nurse's experience may suggest that providing information before the client's bedtime may increase the client's worry and tension, whereas maintaining the usual rituals before sleep is more effective. The nurse may consider implementing some alternative nursing actions during the day to facilitate sleep at night, for example, providing accurate information during the day and increasing daytime activity.

Criteria for Choosing Nursing Strategies After considering the consequences of the alternative nursing strategies, the nurse chooses one or more that are likely to be most effective. Although the nurse bases this decision on knowledge and experience, the client's input is very important. For example, a client may say: "I always have a sandwich and glass of milk before going to bed when I am home. I know I'll sleep if I can have that." Maintaining the client's routine may indeed help the client sleep, and this action might be the first choice as a nursing strategy.

The following criteria can help the nurse choose the best nursing strategy. The planned action must be

1. Safe and appropriate for the individual's age, health, and so on.
2. Achievable with the resources available (eg, in the previous example, sandwiches and milk must be available).
3. Congruent with the client's values and beliefs.
4. Congruent with other therapies (eg, if the client is not permitted food, the strategy of an evening snack must be deferred until health permits).
5. Based on nursing knowledge and experience or knowledge from relevant sciences (ie, based on a rationale). Example:

   Client's Diagnosis
   Potential impaired skin integrity related to immobility

   Nursing Strategies
   Assess skin integrity over bony prominences q2h.
   Turn and change position q30 min.
   Pad pressure points.
   Use egg crate mattress on bed.

   Rationale
   Continuous pressure on a body area compresses tissue, obstructs blood flow to and from an area, and can result in damaged tissue.
6. Within established standards of care as determined by state laws, professional associations (American Nurses Association, Canadian Nurses Association), and the policies of the institution.

   Each state has nurse practice acts that govern the scope of nursing practice. What nurses can do varies somewhat from state to state. Nurses should know the laws of the state where they practice and remain aware of current changes.

   Many agencies have policies to guide nursing activities and the activities of other health professionals. Policies are usually intended to safeguard clients. Rules for visiting hours and procedures to follow when a client has cardiac arrest are examples. If a policy does not benefit clients, nurses have a responsibility to bring this to the attention of the appropriate people.

Types of Nursing Strategies Nursing strategies (or interventions) are identified and written during the planning step of the nursing process; however, they are actually performed during the implementing step. A nursing intervention is any direct care treatment that a nurse performs on behalf of a client, whether nurse-initiated or physician-initiated (McCloskey & Bulechek 1992, p. xvii).

Independent interventions are those activities that nurses are licensed to initiate on the basis of their knowledge and skills. They include physical care, ongoing assessment, emotional support and comfort, teaching, counseling, environmental management, and making referrals to other health care professionals. Recall from Chapter 6 that nursing diagnoses are client problems that can be treated primarily by independent nursing interventions. McCloskey and Bulechek refer to these as *nurse-initiated treatments* (1992, p. xvii). Mundinger prefers the term *autonomous nursing practice.* She states, "Knowing why, when, and how to position clients and doing it skillfully makes the function an autonomous therapy" (1980, p. 4). In performing an autonomous activity, the nurse determines that the client requires certain nursing interventions, either carries these out or delegates them to other nursing personnel, and is accountable for the decision and the actions. To be **accountable** is to be answerable. An example of an independent action is planning and providing special mouth care to a client after diagnosing **Impaired oral mucous membranes.**

Dependent interventions are those activities carried out under the physician's orders or supervision, or according to specified routines. McCloskey and Bulechek call these *physician-initiated treatments* (1992, p. xvii). Medical orders commonly include orders for medications, intravenous therapy, diagnostic tests, treatments, diet, and activity. The nurse is responsible for explaining, assessing the need for, and administering the medical orders. Dependent interventions are usually directly related to the client's disease, and their importance should not be minimized. Nursing orders may be written to individualize the medical order, based on the client's status. For example, for a medical order of "Progressive ambulation, as tolerated," a nurse might write the following nursing orders:

1. Dangle for 5 min, 12 h post op.
2. Stand at bedside 24 h post op; observe for pallor, dizziness, and weakness.
3. Check pulse before and after ambulating. Do not progress if pulse > 110.

Collaborative interventions are actions the nurse carries out in collaboration with other health team members, such as physical therapists, social workers, dietitians, and physicians. Collaborative nursing activities reflect the overlapping responsibilities of, and collegial relationships between, health personnel. For example, the physician might order physical therapy to teach the patient crutch-walking. The nurse would be responsible for informing the physical therapy department and for coordinating the client's care to include the physical therapy sessions. When the client returns to the nursing unit, the nurse would assist with crutch-walking and collaborate with the physical therapist to evaluate the client's progress.

The ANA describes collaboration as "true partnership, in which the power on both sides is valued by both, with recognition and acceptance of separate and combined spheres of activity and responsibility, mutual safeguarding of legitimate interests of each party, and a commonality of goals that is recognized by both parties" (1980, p. 7). To achieve collaborative nursing practice, nurses must be clinically competent, feel confident in their knowledge and skills, and assume responsibility for their own actions.

The amount of time the nurse spends in an independent versus a collaborative or dependent role varies according to the clinical area, type of institution, and specific position of the nurse. Guzzetta (1987, p. 634) estimates that a critical care nurse spends only about 10% of the day functioning in the independent nursing role. In other settings, such as home health care, nurses may function independently 50% of the time. Clinical nurse specialists may work independently 100% of the time.

Writing Nursing Orders After choosing the appropriate nursing interventions, the nurse writes them on the care plan as nursing orders. **Nursing orders** are instructions for the specific activities the nurse performs to help the client meet established health care goals. The term *order* connotes a sense of accountability for the nurse who gives the order and for the nurse who carries it out. Carnevali and Thomas (1993, p. 132) use the term *nursing directives.* The degree of detail included in the nursing orders depends to some degree on the health personnel who will carry out the order. For the components of a nursing order, see Table 7–6.

Date Nursing orders are dated when they are written and reviewed regularly at intervals that depend on the individual's needs. If a client is acutely ill, in an intensive care unit, for example, the plan of care will be continually monitored and revised. In a community clinic, weekly or biweekly reviews may be indicated.

Action Verb The verb starts the order and needs to be precise. For example, "Explain (to the client) the actions of insulin" is a more precise statement than "Teach (the client) about insulin." "Measure and record ankle circumference daily at 0900 h" is more precise than "Assess edema of left ankle daily." Sometimes a modifier for the

Table 7–6 Components of Nursing Orders

Date	Action Verb	Content Area	Time Element	Signature
4/14/94	Monitor	for verbalization of interest in group activities	with each client contact	J. Jonas RN
4/14/94	Instruct	(client) to avoid drinking liquids with meals if nausea occurs	evening shift, 4/14/94	J. Jonas RN
4/14/94	Pad	side rails	during periods of restlessness and confusion	C. Van RN
4/14/94	Discuss	(with family) their need for help with client's care at home	on Friday	L. Taylor RN
4/14/94	Palpate	uterine fundus for firmness	hourly ×2, then q4h ×24 h	C. Patti RN

verb can make the nursing order more precise. For example, "Apply spiral bandage to left lower leg *firmly*" is more precise than "Apply spiral bandage to left leg."

Content Area The content is the where and the what of the order. In the above order, "spiral bandage" and "left leg" state the what and the where of the order. The nurse can also clarify in this example whether the foot or toes are to be left exposed.

Time Element The time element answers when, how long, or how often the nursing action is to occur. Examples are: "Assist client with tub bath *at 0700 daily*"; "Immerse client's left arm in sterile saline soak *for 1 h*"; or "Assist client to change position *every 2 h between 0700 and 2100 h*."

Signature The signature of the nurse prescribing the order shows the nurse's accountability and has legal significance.

Relationship of Nursing Orders to Problem Status

Depending on the type of client problem, the nurse writes orders for observation, prevention, treatment, and health promotion.

Observation orders include observations to determine whether a complication is developing, as well as observations of the client's responses to nursing and other therapies. The nurse should write observation orders for every problem type: actual, potential, and possible. Some examples are "Auscultate lungs q8h," "Observe for redness over sacrum q2h," and "Record intake and output hourly."

Prevention orders prescribe the care needed to prevent complications or reduce risk factors. They are used mainly for potential nursing diagnoses but may also be appropriate for actual nursing diagnoses. Examples of prevention orders are "Turn, cough, and deep-breathe q2h" (prevents respiratory complications) and "If fundus is boggy, massage until firm" (prevents postpartum hemorrhage).

Treatment orders include teaching, referrals, physical care, and other care needed to treat an actual nursing diagnosis. However, an order may accomplish either prevention or treatment functions, depending on the status of the problem. In the preceding examples, the order "Turn, cough, and deep-breathe q2h" can also be intended to treat an existing respiratory problem, and the order "If fundus is boggy, massage until firm" can also be intended to treat an actual postpartum hemorrhage.

Health promotion orders are appropriate when the client has no health problems or when the nurse makes a wellness nursing diagnosis. Such nursing interventions focus on helping the client identify areas for improvement that will lead to a higher level of wellness and actualize the client's overall health potential. Examples are "Discuss the importance of daily exercise" and "Explore infant-stimulation techniques" (Wilkinson 1992, pp. 186–87).

DEVELOPING NURSING PLANS

The **nursing care plan** (also referred to as the *client care plan*) is a written guide that organizes information about a client's care into a meaningful whole. It includes the actions nurses must take to address the client's nursing diagnoses and meet the stated goals. For example, the Care Planning Guide on pages 140–141 includes four of Luisa Sanchez's nursing diagnoses. The nurse starts the care plan as soon as the client is admitted to the health care agency and constantly updates it throughout the client's stay, in response to changes in the client's condition and evaluations of goal achievement.

CARE PLANNING GUIDE

CARE PLAN FOR LUISA SANCHEZ

NURSING DIAGNOSIS: Ineffective airway clearance

Outcome Criteria

Demonstrate adequate air exchange as evidenced by

- Absence of pallor and cyanosis (skin and mucous membranes).
- Using correct breathing/coughing technique after instruction.
- Productive cough.
- Demonstrating symmetric chest excursion of at least 4 cm.
- Verbalizing chest pain of < 4 on a 1-10 scale within 30 min after receiving oral analgesics.

Within 48–72 hours

- Lungs clear to auscultation.
- Respirations 12-22/min, pulse < 100 beats/min.
- Inhaling normal volume of air on incentive spirometer

Nursing Interventions	Rationale
Monitor respiratory status q4h: rate, depth, effort, skin color, mucous membranes, amount and color of sputum. Monitor results of blood gases, chest X-ray studies, and incentive spirometer volume as available. Monitor level of consciousness. Auscultate lungs q4h.	To identify progress toward or deviations from goal. **Ineffective airway clearance** leads to poor oxygenation, evidenced by pallor, cyanosis, lethargy, and drowsiness.
Vital signs q4h.	Inadequate oxygenation causes increased pulse rate. Respiratory rate may be decreased by narcotic analgesics. Shallow breathing further compromises oxygenation.
Instruct in breathing and coughing techniques. Remind to perform, and assist q3h.	To enable client to cough up secretions. May need encouragement and support because of fatigue and pain.
Administer prescribed expectorant; schedule for maximum effectiveness.	Helps loosen secretions so they can be coughed up and expelled.
Maintain Fowler's or semi-Fowler's position.	Gravity allows for fuller lung expansion by decreasing pressure of abdomen on diaphragm.
Administer prescribed analgesics. Notify physician if pain not relieved.	Controls pleuritic pain by blocking pain pathways and altering perception of pain, enabling client to increase thoracic expansion. Unrelieved pain may signal impending complication.
Administer oxygen as prescribed by nasal cannula. Provide portable oxygen if client goes off unit (eg, for X-ray examination).	Supplemental oxygen makes more oxygen available to the cells, even though less air is being moved by the client, thereby reducing the work of breathing.
Assist with postural drainage daily at 0930.	Gravity facilitates movement of secretions upward through the respiratory tree.
Administer prescribed antibiotic to maintain constant blood level. Observe for rash and GI or other side effects.	Resolves infection by schedule bacteriostatic or bactericidal effect, depending on type of antibiotic used. Constant level required to prevent pathogens from multiplying. Allergies to antibiotics are common.

NURSING DIAGNOSIS: Fluid volume deficit: intake insufficient to replace fluid loss (See standardized care plan for **Fluid volume deficit,** p. 143.)

NURSING DIAGNOSIS: Anxiety

Outcome Criteria	Nursing Interventions	Rationale
Demonstrates decreased anxiety, as evidenced by	When client is dyspneic, stay with her; reassure her you will stay.	Presence of a competent caregiver reduces fear of being unable to breathe. Control of anxiety will help client to maintain effective breathing pattern.
• Listening to and following instructions for correct breathing and coughing technique, even during periods of dyspnea.	Remain calm; appear confident	Reassures client that the nurse can help her.
• Verbalizing understanding of condition, diagnostic tests, and treatments (by end of day).	Encourage slow, deep breathing.	Focusing on breathing may help client to feel in control and decrease anxiety.
• Decrease in reports of fear and anxiety; none within 12 hours.	When client is dyspneic, give brief explanations of treatments and procedures. When acute episode is over, give detailed information about nature of condition, treatments, and tests.	Anxiety and pain interfere with learning. Knowing what to expect reduces anxiety.
• Voice steady, not shaky. • Respiratory rate of 12-22/min	As client can tolerate, encourage to express and expand on her concerns about her child and her work. Explore alternatives as needed.	Awareness of source of anxiety enables client to gain control over it.
• Freely expressing concerns about work and parenting roles, but placing them in perspective in view of her illness.	Note whether husband returns as scheduled. If not, institute care plan for actual Altered family processes.	Husband's continued absence would constitute defining characteristic for this nursing diagnosis.

NURSING DIAGNOSIS: Sleep pattern disturbance

Outcome Criteria	Nursing Interventions	Rationale
• Observed sleeping at night rounds (on day 1). • Reports feeling rested in the morning. • Does not experience orthopnea (by day 2).	Provide comfort measures, such as back rub, quiet environment, dim lights, dry linen when diaphoretic, and mouth care. Monitor and institute collaborative measures to control pain, fever, and dyspnea. Use flashlight when making night rounds.	These promote relaxation and remove stimuli that might prevent sleep.
	Use semi-Fowler's position if client cannot go to sleep in Fowler's.	Head of bed must be elevated somewhat for chest expansion. However, sleep is promoted by facilitating as much as possible the way she sleeps at home.
	Inquire daily if client feels rested.	Allows nurse to assess goal achievement.

RESEARCH NOTE

Registered Nurses' Attitudes Toward the Nursing Process and Written/Printed Nursing Care Plans

The use of the nursing process and the use of written or printed nursing care plans are being examined to determine their cost-effectiveness and usefulness in delivering quality care. Using a rating scale, the researchers surveyed 60 registered hospital nurses to determine their attitudes toward nursing care plans and the nursing process. The nurses had a more positive attitude toward the nursing process than toward nursing care plans. They indicated that they use the nursing process and that it facilitates delivery of their nursing care. However, most indicated that they do not use and do not need a written plan in order to give high-quality client care.

New graduates (employed for up to 1 year) valued both the nursing process and written care plans more than did nurses who were employed for 10 or more years. Possibly the nursing process and written care plans have been emphasized more in nursing education during recent years.

Implications: Nurses may view care plans as a learning tool and have less need for them after they have worked long enough to incorporate the necessary information into their knowledge base.

Source: TB Hildeman, Registered nurses' attitudes toward the nursing process and written/printed nursing care plans, *Journal of Nursing Administration,* October 1991, 21(10):20, 33, 45.

Purposes of a Written Care Plan The purposes of a written care plan are the following:

1. To provide direction for *individualized care* of the client. Because the plan flows from the client's list of nursing diagnoses (see Chapter 6), it is organized according to each client's unique needs. Standardized care plans are adapted and used in conjunction with handwritten plans as needed.
2. To provide for *continuity of care.* The written plan is a means of communicating and organizing the actions of a constantly changing nursing staff. The updated plan is often conveyed to all nursing staff at change-of-shift reports, nursing rounds, and client care conferences.
3. To provide *direction about what needs to be documented* on the client's progress notes. The care plan specifically outlines which observations to make, what nursing actions to carry out, and what instructions the client or family members require. This facilitates recording.
4. To serve as a *guide for assigning staff* to care for the client. Certain aspects of the client's care may need to be delegated to someone who can make necessary judgments about the client's responses.
5. To serve as a *guide for reimbursement* from medical insurance companies, often called third-party reimbursement. The medical record is used by the insurance companies to determine what they will pay in relation to the hospital care received by the client. If nursing care has not been documented precisely in the care plan, the nurse has no way to prove that it was done, and the insurers will not pay for care that is not documented.

Preprinted Care Plans A nursing care plan may be preplanned and preprinted, or it may be completely handwritten. Many agencies have devised preprinted, standardized guides for providing essential nursing care to specified groups of clients who have certain needs in common (eg, all clients with pneumonia, all clients with a nursing diagnosis of **Ineffective breastfeeding,** or all clients undergoing cardiac catheterization). Standardized care plans, standards of care, protocols, policies, and procedures are developed and accepted by the nursing staff in order to

1. Ensure that the minimally acceptable standards of care are provided.
2. Promote efficient use of nurses' time by making it unnecessary to hand-write common activities that are done over and over for all (or most) clients on a nursing unit.

Standards of care are "detailed guidelines that represent the predicted care indicated in a specific situation," such as a medical diagnosis, test, or treatment; a nursing diagnosis; or a collaborative problem (Carpenito 1991, p. 17). Standards of care describe nursing care for groups of clients rather than individuals, and they describe achievable rather than ideal nursing care. They define the interventions for which nurses are held accountable, and they do not contain medical orders. Standards of care are usually agency records and not part of the client's care plan, but they may be referred to in the plan (eg, a nurse might write, "See standards of care for cardiac catheterization"). Standards of care may or may not be organized according to problems or nursing diagnoses.

Standardized care plans (model care plans) are preplanned, preprinted guides for the nursing care of groups of clients with common needs (eg, a specific nursing diagnosis, or all the nursing diagnoses associated with a particular medical condition). However, they should not be confused with *standards of care.* Although the two have some similarities, they have important differences (see Figure 7–2 for a standardized care plan for **Fluid volume deficit**). The following are true of standardized care plans, but not of standards of care:

Standardized Care Plan for Nursing Diagnosis of FLUID VOLUME DEFICIT

Etiology	Expected Outcomes	Nursing Order (Identify Frequency)
√ Decreased oral intake √ Nausea __ Depression √ Fatigue, weakness __ Difficulty swallowing __ Other:______ √ Excess fluid loss √ Fever or increased metabolic rate √ Diaphoresis √ Vomiting __ Diarrhea __ Burns __ Other______ **Defining Characteristics** √ Insufficient intake √ Negative balance of intake and output √ Dry mucous membranes √ Poor skin turgor __ Concentrated urine __ Hypernatremia √ Rapid, weak pulse __ Falling B/P __ Weight loss	√ Urinary output > 30 mL/hr √ Urine specific gravity 1.005–1.025 √ Serum Na^+ normal √ Mucous membranes moist √ Skin turgor good √ No weight loss √ 8-hour intake = 400 mL oral Other:	√ Monitor intake and output q 1 h √ Weigh daily √ Monitor serum electrolyte levels X 1 or until normal √ Check skin turgor and mucous membranes q 8 h √ Monitor temperature q 4 h √ Administer prescribed IV therapy (Monitor according to protocol for "Intravenous Therapy") 1000 mL D5 LR at 100 mL/hr √ Offer oral liquids q 1 h Type clear, cold √ Instruct client regarding amount, type, and schedule of fluid intake. √ Assess understanding of type of fluid loss; teach accordingly √ Mouth care prn with mouthwash √ Institute measures to reduce fever (eg, lower room temperature, remove bed covers, offer cold liquids.) Other Nursing Orders:______ Monitor urine specific gravity q̄shift

Plan Initiated by: M. Medina RN **Date** 4-15-95

Plan/outcomes evaluated__________ **Date**______

Plan/outcomes evaluated__________ **Date**______

Client: Luisa Sanchez

Figure 7–2 A standardized care plan for nursing diagnosis of **Fluid volume deficit.**

1. Standardized care plans are kept with the client's active care plan on the nursing unit. When the client is discharged, they become part of the permanent medical record.
2. Standardized care plans provide more detailed instructions than standards of care and contain additions or deletions from the standards of care of the agency.
3. Standardized care plans typically take the usual nursing process format:

   Problem → Goals → Nursing Orders → Evaluation
4. Standardized care plans allow the nurse to add handwritten care plans. They frequently include checklists, blank lines, or empty spaces to allow the nurse to individualize goals and nursing orders (Wilkinson 1992, p. 299).

The use of standardized care plans is supported by the Joint Commission for the Accreditation of Healthcare Organization standards for nursing care (JCAHO 1992), which no longer require a handwritten care plan for every client.

Regardless of whether nursing orders are handwritten or chosen from a preprinted plan, nursing care must be individualized to fit the unique needs of each client. In practice, a care plan usually consists of both preprinted and handwritten sections. The nurse uses standardized care plans for predictable, commonly occurring problems and handwrites an individual plan for unusual problems or problems needing special attention. For example, a standardized care plan for all "clients with a medical diagnosis of pneumonia" would probably include a nursing diagnosis of **Fluid volume deficit** and direct the nurse to assess the client's hydration status. On a respiratory or medical unit, this would be a common nursing diagnosis; therefore, Luisa Sanchez's nurse was able to obtain a standardized plan directing care commonly needed by clients with **Fluid volume deficit.** However, the nursing diagnosis **High risk for altered family processes** would not be common to all clients with pneumonia; it is specific to Ms Sanchez. Therefore, the goals and nursing orders for that diagnosis were handwritten by the nurse. (See the Care Planning Guide on page 140 and Figure 7–2.)

Format for Care Plans Although formats differ from agency to agency, the plan is generally organized into four columns or categories: (a) nursing diagnoses or problem list, (b) goals and outcome criteria, (c) nursing orders, and (d) evaluation. Some agencies have a five-column plan that includes a column for assessment data before the nursing diagnoses column. Others use a three-column plan that subsumes the evaluation column under the goal column.

To help students learn to write care plans and apply their knowledge, educators often modify this plan by adding a column headed "Rationale" after the nursing intervention column. See Table 7–1 on page 130. A **rationale** is the scientific reason for selecting a specific nursing action. Students may also be required to cite supporting literature for this stated rationale. Many agencies use a nursing Kardex or Rand system for organizing and storing nursing care plans.

Like standards of care and standardized care plans, **protocols** are preprinted and preplanned to indicate the actions commonly required for a particular group of clients. For example, an agency may have a protocol for admitting a client to the intensive care unit, for administering magnesium sulfate to a client with preeclampsia, or for caring for a client receiving continuous epidural analgesia. Protocols may include both medical orders and nursing orders. Depending on the agency, protocols may or may not be included in the client's permanent record.

Policies and **procedures** are developed to govern the handling of frequently occurring situations. For example, a hospital may have a policy specifying the number of visitors a client may have. Some policies are similar to protocols and specify what is to be done, for example, in the case of cardiac arrest. If a policy covers a situation pertinent to client care, it is usually noted on the care plan (eg, "Make Social Service referral according to Unit Policy Manual"). Policies are institution records and do not become a part of the care plan or permanent record.

A **standing order** is a written document about policies, rules, regulations, or orders regarding client care. Standing orders give nurses the authority to carry out specific actions under certain circumstances, often when a physician is not immediately available. In a hospital critical care unit, a common example is the administration of emergency antiarrhythmic medications when a client's cardiac monitoring pattern changes.

In a home care setting, a physician may write a standing order for the administration of epinephrine for a client who becomes excessively dyspneic.

Computerized Care Plans Computers are increasingly being used to create and store nursing care plans. The computer can generate both standardized and individualized care plans. Nurses access the client's stored care plan from a centrally located terminal at the nurses' station or from terminals in client rooms. For an individualized plan, the nurse chooses the appropriate diagnoses from a menu suggested by the computer. The computer then lists possible goals and nursing interventions for those diagnoses; the nurse chooses those appropriate for the client and types in any additional goals and interventions not listed on the menu. The nurse can read the plan on the computer screen or print out an updated working copy each day. For further information, see Chapter 9, page 166.

Case Management Plans A case management plan (sometimes called a collaborative care plan, a critical pathway, or a care map) is a multidisciplinary care plan that sequences the care that needs to be given each day during the projected length of stay for a specific type of case (Zander 1992, p. 127). Like the traditional nursing care plan, a case management plan specifies goals and nursing orders to address client problems (including nursing diagnoses). However, it includes medical and other treatments as well. The care plan is usually organized with a column for each day, listing the interventions that should be carried out and the client goals that should be achieved on that day. In order for the case management plan to be effective, each member of the health team must agree on the plan and actively participate in the client's care in a timely manner. For further information, see Chapter 4, page 75.

Guidelines for Writing Nursing Care Plans In addition to following the earlier suggestions for writing nursing orders, the nurse can use the following guidelines when writing nursing care plans:

1. Date and sign the plan. The date the plan is written is essential for evaluation, review, and future planning. The nurse's signature demonstrates accountability to the client and to the nursing profession, since the effectiveness of nursing actions can be evaluated.
2. Use the category headings "Nursing Diagnoses," "Goals/Outcome Criteria," "Nursing Orders," and "Evaluation" and include a date for the evaluation of each goal.
3. Use standardized medical or English symbols and key words rather than complete sentences to communicate your ideas. For example, write "Turn and reposition q2h" rather than "Turn and reposition the client every two hours." Or write, "Clean decubitus ulcer c̄ H_2O_2 bid" rather than "Clean the client's decubitus ulcer with hydrogen peroxide twice a day, morning and evening."
4. Refer to procedure books or other sources of information rather than including all the steps on a written plan. For example, write: "See unit procedure book for tracheostomy care," or attach a standard nursing plan about such procedures as radiation-implantation care and preoperative or postoperative care.
5. Tailor the plan to the unique characteristics of the client by ensuring that the client's choices, such as preferences about the times of care and the methods used, are included. This reinforces the client's individuality and sense of control. For example, the written nursing order "Provide prune juice at breakfast rather than regular juice" indicates that the client was given a choice of beverages.
6. Ensure that the nursing plan incorporates *preventive* and health maintenance aspects as well as restorative. For example, carrying out the order "Provide active-assistance ROM exercises to affected limbs q2h" prevents joint contractures and maintains muscle strength and joint mobility.
7. Ensure that the plan contains orders for ongoing assessment of the client (eg, "Inspect incision q shift").
8. Include collaborative and coordination activities in the plan. For example, the nurse may write orders to ask a nutritionist or physical therapist about specific aspects of the client's care.
9. Include plans for the client's discharge and home care needs. It is often necessary to consult and make arrangements with the community health nurse, social worker, and specific agencies that supply client information and needed equipment.

CHAPTER HIGHLIGHTS

- Planning is the process of designing nursing strategies required to prevent, reduce, or eliminate a client's health problems.
- Planning involves the nurse, the client, support persons, and other caregivers.
- Nursing strategies are planned around a client's diagnostic statements and goals.
- Five activities of planning are setting priorities, establishing client goals, planning nursing strategies, writing nursing orders, and writing a nursing care plan.
- Nursing diagnoses are assigned high, medium, and low priorities in consultation with the client, if health permits.
- Client goals/outcome criteria are used to plan nursing strategies that will achieve anticipated changes in the client.
- Client goals/outcome criteria are derived from the *first* clause of the nursing diagnosis.
- Outcome criteria describe specific and measurable client responses and help the nurse evaluate the effectiveness of the nursing intervention.

- Goal statements and outcome criteria are written in terms of the client's behavior.
- Nursing strategies are focused on the etiology or *second* clause of the nursing diagnosis.
- Nursing strategies can be generated by brainstorming, hypothesizing, and extrapolating.
- Establishing the consequences of each nursing strategy requires nursing knowledge and experience.
- Nursing orders are the specific actions taken by the nurse to help the client meet established health care goals.
- Independent nursing interventions are those the nurse is licensed to prescribe or delegate.
- The nursing care plan provides direction for individualized care of the client.
- Preprinted, standardized care plans should be adapted and used with handwritten plans to meet individual client needs.
- The nurse consults with other nurses or health professionals to verify information, implement changes, or obtain additional knowledge to aid in client goals.
- Shorter acute care hospitalizations necessitate careful discharge planning.

READINGS AND REFERENCES

SUGGESTED READINGS

Tirk, JE. July 1992. Determining discharge priorities. *Nursing92* 22(7):55.

This one-page, "how-to" article has many useful tips for increasing the effectiveness of discharge planning for short-stay clients.

Tuazon, NC. April 1992. Discharge teaching: Use this MODEL. *RN* 55(4):19–22.

Presents a mnemonic device—the word MODEL—to facilitate recall of the basics of discharge planning.

RELATED RESEARCH

Ferrell-Torry, AT and Glock, OJ. 1993. The use of therapeutic massage as a nursing intervention to modify anxiety and the perception of cancer pain. *Cancer Nursing* 16(2):93–101.

Kitson, A, Harvey, G, Hyndman, S, and Yerrell, P. 1993. A comparison of expert- and practitioner-derived criteria for post-operative pain management. *Journal of Advanced Nursing* 18:218–32.

SELECTED REFERENCES

Allen, SK. March/April 1991. Selection and implementation of an automated care planning system for a health care institution. *Computers in Nursing* 9(2):61–68.

American Nurses Association. 1980. *Nursing: A Social Policy Statement.* Kansas City, MO: ANA.

———. 1991. *Standards of Clinical Nursing Practice.* Washington, DC: ANA.

Anderson, B and Hannah, KJ. 1993. A Canadian nursing minimum data set: A major priority. *Canadian Journal of Nursing Administration* 6(2):7–13.

Barriball, KL and Mackenzie, A. 1993. Measuring the impact of nursing interventions in the community: A selective review of the literature. *Journal of Advanced Nursing* 18(3):401–07.

Blaylock, A and Cason, CL. July 1992. Discharge planning: Predicting patients' needs. *Journal of Gerontological Nursing* 18(7):5–10, 37–38.

Brider, P. 1991. Who killed the nursing care plan? *American Journal of Nursing* 91(5):35–38.

Bulechek, GM and McCloskey, JC. May 1987. Nursing interventions: What they are and how to choose them. *Holistic Nursing Practice* 1:36–44.

———. 1990. Nursing intervention taxonomy development. In McCloskey, JC and Grace, HK, editors. pp. 23–28. *Current Issues in Nursing.* 3d ed. St Louis: Mosby.

———, editors. June 1992. Nursing interventions. *Nursing Clinics of North America* 27:289–602.

Carnevali, DL and Thomas, MD. 1993. *Diagnostic Reasoning and Treatment Decision Making in Nursing.* Philadelphia: Lippincott.

Carpenito. LJ. 1991. *Nursing Care Plans and Documentation.* Philadelphia: Lippincott.

Faherty, B. July 1990. Case management—The latest buzzword: What it is, and what it isn't. *Caring* 9(7):20–22.

Goodwin, DR. February 1992. Critical pathways in home healthcare. *Journal of Nursing Administration* 22(2):35–40.

Guzzetta, C. November 1987. Nursing diagnoses in nursing education: Effect on the profession. Part 1. *Heart and Lung* 16:629–35.

Haas, J. August 1993. Ethical considerations of goal setting for patient care in rehabilitation medicine. *American Journal of Physical Medicine and Rehabilitation* 72:228–32.

Handcock, M and Knight, D. February 12–18, 1992. Improving discharge planning standards. *Nursing Standard* 6(21):38–40.

Holdsworth, N. 1993. What are we about? . . . making a difference is far more important than the goals we may set for patients. RN 56(6):88.

Iowa Intervention Project. 1993. The NIC taxonomy structure. *Image: Journal of Nursing Scholarship 25*, 187–92.

Joint Commission on Accreditation of Healthcare Organizations. 1992. *Accreditation Manual for Hospitals.* Chicago: Joint Commission on Accreditation of Healthcare Organizations, Nursing Services.

Lekander, BJ, Lehmann, S, and Lindquist, R. 1993. Therapeutic listening: Key intervention for several nursing diagnoses. *Dimensions of Critical Care Nursing* 12:24–30.

McCloskey, JC and Bulechek, GM, editors. 1992. *Nursing Interventions Classification (NIC).* St Louis: Mosby-Year Book.

McFarland, GK and McFarlane, EA. 1993. *Nursing Diagnosis and Intervention.* 2d ed. St Louis: Mosby-Year Book.

McWilliams, G. March 1992. Care planning: A team effort. *Nursing Management* 23(3):67.

Matz, LB and Gary, B. 1993. Patient outcomes measure home health care accomplishments. *Nursing Management* 24(5): Long Term Care Ed: 96Y-Z, 96DD, 96FF.

Mundinger, MO. 1980. *Autonomy in Nursing.* Gaithersburg, MD: Aspen Systems.

Neufeld, KR, Degner, LF, and Dick, JAM. 1993. A nursing intervention strategy to foster patient involvement in treatment decisions. *Oncology Nursing Forum* 20:631–35.

Norris, J. 1992. Nursing intervention for self-esteem disturbances. *Nursing Diagnosis* 3(2):48–53.

Paquin-Cadotte, S, Rashotte, J, and Van-Volkingburgh, S. June 1990. The evolution and implementation of a P.I.C.U. standard nursing care plan: A nursing process. *Canadian Critical Care Nursing Journal* 7(2):14–18.

Pease, J and Guhde, B. Summer/Fall 1991. Implementing an automated care planning system. *Journal of Long-Term Care Administration* 19(2/3):17–19.

Petrucci, K et al. July/August 1992. Improving automated care planning with plan libraries. *Nursing Economics* 10:297–301.

Pinkley, CL. January/March 1991. Exploring NANDA's definition of nursing diagnosis: Linking diagnostic judgments with the selection of outcomes and interventions. *Nursing Diagnosis* 2(1):26–32.

Rundell, S. April 17–23 1991. Care about care plans! *Nursing Times* 87:32.

Schmidt, SM. February 1991. Goal-directed temporal plans of care. *Nursing Management* 23(2):60–62.

Stewart, BJ and Archbold, PG. 1993. Nursing intervention studies require outcome measures that are sensitive to change. Part 2. *Research in Nursing and Health* 16:77–81.

Taylor, D. 1989. Interventions. In ANA Pub no. NP-74-500. *Classification Systems for Describing Nursing Practice.* Kansas City, MO: ANA.

Wilkinson, JM. 1992. *Nursing Process in Action: A Critical Thinking Approach.* Redwood City, CA: Addison-Wesley Nursing.

Zander, K. January 1988a. Managed care within acute care settings: Design and implementation via nursing case management. *Health Care Supervisor* 6(2):27.

———. September 1988b. Nursing case management: Resolving the DRG paradox. *Nursing Clinics of North America* 23:503–20.

———. 1992. Focusing on patient outcome: Case management in the 90's. *Dimensions of Critical Care Nursing* 11(3):127–29.

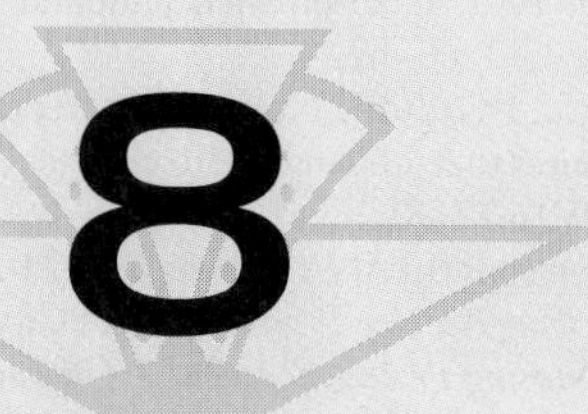

8 Implementing and Evaluating

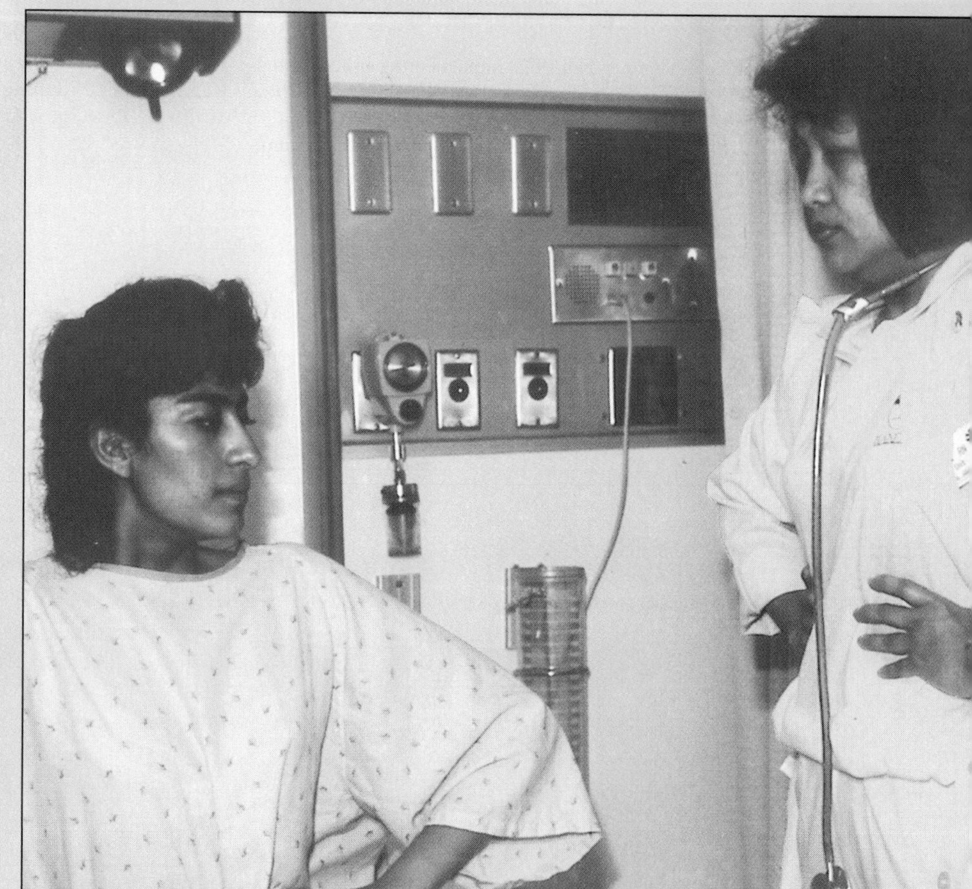

Objectives

Identify four activities of the implementing phase.

Explain how implementing relates to other phases of the nursing process.

Describe three categories of skills used to implement nursing strategies.

Identify essential guidelines for implementing nursing strategies.

Explain how evaluating relates to other phases of the nursing process.

Describe six components of the evaluation process.

Describe the steps involved in reexamining and modifying the client's care plan.

Name the two components of an evaluation statement.

Differentiate quality assessment from quality assurance.

Describe three approaches to quality evaluation.

Identify essential steps in developing tools to evaluate quality care.

The nursing process is action-oriented, client-centered, and goal-directed. After developing a plan of care based on the assessing and diagnosing phases, the nurse puts the plan into effect and evaluates the results. On the basis of this evaluation, the plan of care is either continued, modified, or terminated. As in all phases of the nursing process, clients and support persons are encouraged to participate as much as possible.

IMPLEMENTING

In the nursing process, implementing is the phase in which the nurse puts the nursing care plan into action. Broadly defined, implementing consists of doing, delegating, and recording. The nurse performs or delegates the nursing orders that were developed in the planning step and then concludes the implementing step by recording nursing activities and the resulting client responses. See the box at the right for professional standards describing nurses' accountability for implementing.

Although the nurse may act on the client's behalf (eg, referring the client to a community health nurse for home care), professional standards support client and family participation, as in all phases of the nursing process. The degree of participation depends on the client's health status. For example, an unconscious man is unable to participate in his care and therefore needs to have care given to him. By contrast, an ambulatory client may require very little care from the nurse and carry out health care activities independently.

Bulechek and McCloskey define nursing interventions as "any direct care treatment that a nurse performs on behalf of a client. These treatments include nurse-initiated treatments resulting from nursing diagnoses, physician-initiated treatments resulting from medical diagnoses and performance of the daily essential functions for the client who cannot do these" (1990, p. 26). Table 8–1 on page 150 shows 6 domains and 26 classes of nursing interventions developed by the Iowa Intervention Project. This is referrd to as the Nursing Interventions Classification (NIC) Taxonomy. While the nursing process enables nurses to emphasize their independent activities, "the full nursing role encompasses dependent and collaborative functions as well. Most nurses provide care for ill clients, whose comprehensive health needs include attention to their medical condition; therefore, during the implementing step, nurses implement both the nursing orders on the client's care plan and physicians' orders for the medical plan of care" (Wilkinson 1992, pp. 220–21). For further information about dependent and collaborative activities, see Chapter 7, page 138.

ANA Standards

Standard V: Implementation

The nurse implements the interventions identified in the plan of care.

Measurement Criteria

1. Interventions are consistent with the established plan of care.
2. Interventions are implemented in a safe and appropriate manner.
3. Interventions are documented.

Source: Abstracted from American Nurses Association, *Standards of Clinical Nursing Practice* (Washington, DC: ANA, 1991), p. 13. Used with permission.

RELATIONSHIP OF IMPLEMENTING TO OTHER NURSING PROCESS PHASES

Successful implementing depends, in part, on the quality of assessing, diagnosing, and planning that has been done. These first three nursing process phases provide the basis for the autonomous nursing actions performed during the implementing step. In turn, the implementing step provides the actual nursing activities and client responses that are evaluated in the final step (evaluating). The nursing process phases are interdependent and overlapping rather than separate and linear (see Chapter 5 and Figure 8–1 [on page 151]). Using data acquired during assessment, the nurse can individualize the care given in the implementing phase, tailoring the interventions to fit a specific client (eg, Luisa Sanchez) rather than applying them routinely to categories of clients (eg, all pneumonia clients).

Ongoing assessment occurs simultaneously with implementation. While implementing the nursing orders, the nurse continues to reassess the client at every contact, gathering data about the client's responses to the nursing actions and about any new problems that may develop. Reassessment is *not the same as* implementing; rather they occur concurrently. For example:

Implementation	*Assessment*
While bathing an elderly client,	the nurse observes a reddened area on the client's sacrum.
When emptying a catheter bag,	the nurse measures 200 mL of strong smelling urine.

Table 8–1 NIC Taxonomy

Level 1: Domains	Level 2: Classes (numbered for cross-referencing)
DOMAIN I **Physiological: Basic** Care that supports functional health status	1. **Activity and Exercise Enhancement:** Interventions to organize or assist with physical activity and energy expenditure 2. **Elimination Management:** Interventions to establish and maintain regular bowel and urinary elimination patterns and manage complications due to altered patterns 3. **Immobility Management:** Interventions to restrict body movement and manage the sequelae 4. **Nutrition Support:** Interventions to facilitate change in nutritional habit patterns or provide methods for nutritional intake 5. **Physical Comfort Promotion:** Interventions to promote comfort using physical techniques 6. **Self-Care Facilitation:** Interventions to provide, facilitate or assist with routines, basic activities of daily living
DOMAIN II **Physiological: Complex** Care that supports homeostatic regulation	7. **Electrolyte and Acid-Base Management:** Interventions to regulate electrolyte/acid-base balance and prevent complications 8. **Medication Management:** Interventions to facilitate desired effects of pharmacologic agents 9. **Neurologic Management:** Interventions to optimize neurologic function 10. **Perioperative Care:** Interventions to provide care prior to, during, and immediately after surgery 11. **Respiratory Management:** Interventions to promote airway patency and gas exchange 12. **Skin/Wound Management:** Interventions to maintain or restore tissue integrity 13. **Thermoregulation:** Interventions to maintain body temperature within a normal range 14. **Tissue Perfusion Management:** Interventions to optimize circulation of blood and fluids to the tissue
DOMAIN III **Behavioral** Care that supports psychological functioning and facilitates life style changes	15. **Behavior Therapy:** Interventions to reinforce or promote desirable behaviors or alter undesirable behaviors 16. **Cognitive Therapy:** Interventions to reinforce or promote desirable cognitive functioning or alter undesirable cognitive functioning 17. **Communication Enhancement:** Interventions to facilitate interaction with a patient who has difficulty delivering or receiving verbal or non-verbal messages 18. **Coping Assistance:** Interventions to assist another to build on own strengths to adapt to a change in function or achieve a higher level of function 19. **Patient Education:** Interventions to facilitate learning 20. **Psychological Comfort Promotion:** Interventions to promote comfort using pyschological techniques
DOMAIN IV **Family** Care that supports the family unit	21. **Childbearing Care:** Interventions to assist in understanding and coping with the psychological and physiological changes during the childbearing period 22. **Family Care:** Interventions to facilitate family unit functioning and promote the health and welfare of family members
DOMAIN V **Health System** Care that supports effective use of the health care delivery system	23. **Health System Management:** Interventions to enhance environmental support services for the delivery of care 24. **Health System Mediation:** Interventions to facilitate the interface between patient/family and the health care system
DOMAIN VI **Safety** Care that supports protection against harm	25. **Crisis Management:** Interventions to provide immediate, short term help in both psychological and physiological crises 26. **Risk Management:** Interventions to initiate risk reduction activities and continue monitoring risk over time

Source: Adapted from Iowa Intervention Project. McCloskey, J and Bulechek, G editors. Fall 1993. The NIC Taxonomy structure. *Image: Journal of Nursing Scholarship*. 25:190. Reprinted with permission.

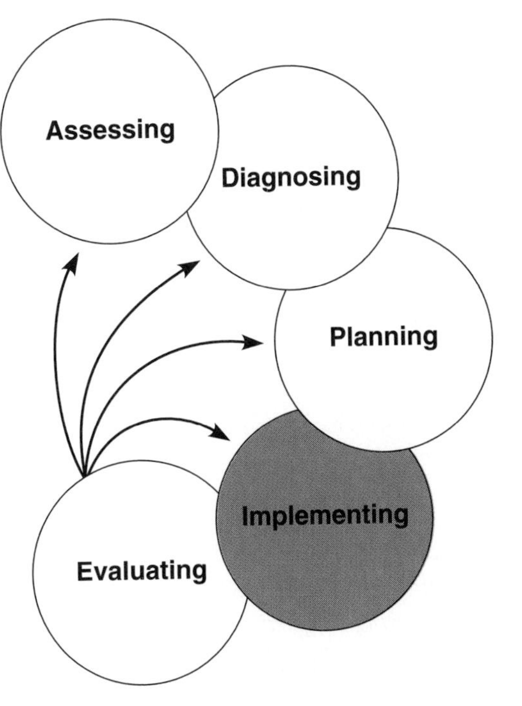

Figure 8–1 Implementing. The fourth phase of the nursing process, in which the nurse puts the nursing care plan into action, continues data collection, and documents care provided.

Finally, nurses implement nursing orders that specifically *direct* reassessment. For example, a nursing order on the client's care plan might read, "Auscultate lungs q4h." When performing this activity, the nurse is carrying out the nursing order (implementing) and performing the reassessment (Wilkinson 1992, p. 215).

IMPLEMENTING SKILLS

To implement the care plan successfully, nurses need good cognitive, interpersonal, and technical skills. The skills are distinct from one another; in practice, however, nurses use them in various combinations and with different emphasis, depending upon the activity. For instance, when inserting a urinary catheter, the nurse needs cognitive knowledge of the principles and steps of the procedure, technical skill in draping the client and manipulating the equipment, and interpersonal skills to inform and reassure the client.

The **cognitive skills** (intellectual skills) include problem solving, decision making, critical thinking, and creative thinking (see Chapter 10). They are crucial to safe, intelligent nursing care.

Interpersonal skills are all the activities people use when communicating directly with one another. They include verbal and nonverbal activities. The effectiveness of a nursing action often depends largely on the nurse's ability to communicate with others. Even when giving a medication to a client, the nurse needs to understand the client and in turn be understood. A nurse who is delegating a nursing action also needs to be understood.

Interpersonal skills are necessary for all nursing activities: caring, comforting, referring, counseling, and supporting are just a few. They include conveying knowledge, attitudes, feelings, interest, and appreciation of the client's cultural values and life-style. Before nurses can be highly skilled in interpersonal relations, they must have self-awareness and sensitivity to others. See Chapter 18 for more detailed explanations of interpersonal skills.

Technical skills are "hands-on" skills such as manipulating equipment, giving injections and bandaging, moving, lifting, and repositioning clients. These tasks are also called procedures or psychomotor skills. The term *psychomotor* includes the interpersonal component, for example, the need to communicate with the client.

Technical skills require knowledge and, frequently, manual dexterity. The number of technical skills expected of a nurse has increased greatly in recent years because of the increased use of technology, especially in acute care hospitals.

PROCESS OF IMPLEMENTING

The process of implementing normally includes

- Reassessing the client
- Determining the need for nursing assistance
- Implementing the nursing strategies
- Communicating the nursing actions

Reassessing the Client Assessing is carried out throughout the nursing process, whenever the nurse has contact with the client. Just before implementing, the nurse must reassess whether the intervention is still needed. Even though an order is written on the care plan, the situation or the client's condition may have changed. For example, Gayle Fischer has a nursing diagnosis of **Sleep pattern disturbance** related to anxiety and unfamiliar surroundings. During rounds, the nurse discovers that Gayle is sleeping; and, therefore, defers the back rub that had been planned as a relaxation strategy.

New data may, in the nurse's judgment, indicate a need to change the priorities of care or the nursing strategies. For example, a nurse begins to teach Ms Eves, who has diabetes, how to give herself insulin injections. Shortly after beginning the teaching, the nurse realizes that Ms Eves is not concentrating on the lesson. Subsequent discussion reveals that she is worried about her eyesight and fears she is going blind. The nurse ends the lesson because the client's level of stress is interfering with her learning

GUIDELINES FOR IMPLEMENTING NURSING STRATEGIES

- *Nursing actions should be based on scientific knowledge, nursing research, and professional standards of care.* The nurse must be aware of the scientific rationale for all interventions, as well as possible side effects or complications of the activities. When individualizing an action, the nurse takes care not to violate the scientific basis of the activity. For example, Ms Li prefers to take an oral medication after meals; however, this medication is not well absorbed in the presence of food. Therefore, the nurse will need to explain to Ms Li why this preference cannot be honored.
- *Nurses should understand clearly the orders to be implemented and question any that are not understood.* The nurse is responsible for intelligent implementation of medical and nursing plans of care. This requires knowledge of each intervention, its purpose in the client's plan of care, any contraindications (eg, allergies), and changes in the client's condition that may be applicable.
- *Nursing actions should be adapted to the individual client.* A client's beliefs, values, age, health status, and environment are factors that can affect the success of a nursing action. Although the nurse takes care not to violate the scientific basis of the activity, actions often need to be individualized. For example, Mr Ault cannot swallow pills, so his nurse consults with the physician to change the order to a liquid form of the medication.
- *Nursing actions should always be safe.* For example, when changing a sterile dressing, the nurse practices sterile technique to prevent infection; when giving a medication, the nurse takes care to administer the correct dosage by the ordered route.
- *Nursing actions often require teaching, support, and comfort.* These independent nursing activities can enhance the effectiveness of many nursing actions.
- *Nursing actions should be holistic.* The nurse must always view the client as a whole and consider the client's responses in that light.
- *Nursing actions should respect the dignity of the client and enhance the client's self-esteem.* Providing privacy and encouraging clients to make their own decisions are ways of respecting dignity and enhancing self-esteem.
- *Clients should be encouraged to participate actively in implementing the nursing actions.* Active participation enhances the client's sense of independence and control. However, clients vary in the degree of participation they desire. Some want total involvement in their care, whereas others prefer little involvement. The amount of desired involvement may be related to the severity of the illness; the number of stressors; or the client's energy, fear, understanding of the illness, and understanding of the intervention.

and makes arrangement for a physician to examine the client's eyes. The nurse also provides supportive communication to help alleviate the client's stress.

Determining the Need for Nursing Assistance

When implementing some nursing strategies, the nurse may require assistance for one of the following reasons:

1. The nurse is unable to implement the nursing strategies safely alone (eg, turning an obese client in bed).
2. It would reduce stress on the client (eg, turning a person who experiences acute pain when moved).
3. The nurse lacks the knowledge or skills to implement a particular nursing activity (eg, a nurse who is not familiar with a particular model of oxygen mask needs assistance the first time it is applied).

Implementing Nursing Strategies After reassessing the client and determining the need for assistance, the nurse implements the planned strategies. Nursing activities generally include caring, communicating, helping, teaching, counseling, acting as a client advocate and change agent, leading, and managing (see Chapter 2). In addition to performing nursing activities, nurses (a) assign and delegate care to other nursing personnel and (b) supervise and evaluate the nursing activities of others. Guidelines for implementing nursing strategies are shown in the box above.

Communicating Nursing Actions After carrying out the nursing orders, the nurse completes the implementing phase by recording the interventions, along with the client responses, in the nursing progress notes. These are a part of the agency's permanent record for the client. Nursing actions must not be recorded in advance, because the nurse may determine on reassessing the client that the action should not or cannot be implemented. For example, a nurse is authorized to inject 10 mg of morphine sulfate subcutaneously to a client, but the nurse finds that the client's respiratory rate is 4 breaths per minute. This finding contraindicates the administration of morphine (a respiratory depressant). The nurse withholds the morphine and reports the client's respiratory rate to the nurse in charge and/or physician. A nurse might also find that a

RESEARCH NOTE

Can an Independent Nursing Action Aid in Alleviating Symptoms and Controlling Pain of Terminally Ill People?

The purpose of this study was to explore the effectiveness of slow stroke back massage in promoting relaxation and helping terminally ill clients cope with pain and other stressors. Thirty adults were given this intervention on 2 succeeding days. Vital signs were measured before and after the intervention. The results revealed modest but statistically significant decreases in heart rate and blood pressure and an increase in skin temperature that were indicative of relaxation. Additionally, clients in the study appeared eager to participate and receive the intervention—reaffirming literature findings that human beings are often hungry for touch.

Implications: The technique of slow stroke back massage is cost-effective and relatively straightforward. Nurses do not need formal preparation in massage therapy to master the technique. It requires little time and minimal supplies and could easily be taught to family members. This study suggests that slow stroke back massage is an effective therapy and would be appropriate for nurses to add to their repertoire of independent interventions.

Source: S Meek, Effects of slow stroke back massage on relaxation in hospice clients, *Image: Journal of Nursing Scholarship,* Spring 1993, 25:17–21.

planned nursing action cannot be implemented (eg, the client objects; the client is too weak to ambulate; the nurse encounters an obstruction when inserting a rectal tube). Nursing activities, therefore, are always recorded after they are completed, when the nurse can accurately record exactly what occurred.

The nurse may record routine or recurring activities (eg, mouth care) at the end of a shift; in the meantime, the nurse maintains a personal record of these interventions. Many agencies have special forms for this type of recording.

In some instances, it is important to record a nursing action immediately after it is implemented. This is particularly true of the administration of medications and treatments because recorded data about a client must be up to date, accurate, and available to other nurses and health care professionals. Immediate recording helps safeguard the client, for example, from receiving a second dose of medication.

Nursing actions are communicated verbally as well as in writing. When a client's health is changing rapidly, the charge nurse and/or the physician may want to be kept up to date with verbal reports. Verbal reports are given to other nurses and other health professionals. Nurses also give verbal reports at a change of shift and on a client's discharge to another unit or health agency. For information on recording and reporting, see Chapter 9.

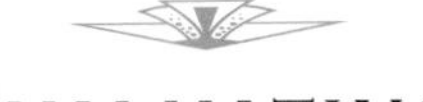

EVALUATING

To evaluate is to judge or to appraise. Evaluating is the fifth and last phase of the nursing process. In this context, **evaluating** is a planned, ongoing, purposeful activity, in which clients and health care professionals determine (1) the client's progress toward goal achievement and (2) the effectiveness of the nursing care plan. Evaluation is an exceedingly important aspect of the nursing process, because conclusions drawn from the evaluation determine whether the nursing interventions should be terminated, continued, or changed.

Evaluation may be ongoing, intermittent, or terminal. **Ongoing evaluation** is done while or immediately after implementing a nursing order; it enables the nurse to make on-the-spot modifications in an intervention. **Intermittent evaluation,** performed at specified intervals (eg, once a week), shows the extent of progress toward goal achievement and enables the nurse to correct any deficiencies and modify the care plan as needed. Evaluation continues (either ongoing or intermittently) until the client achieves the health goals and/or is discharged from nursing care. **Terminal evaluation** indicates the client's condition at the time of discharge. It includes the status of goal achievement and an evaluation of the client's self-care abilities with regard to follow-up care. Most agencies have a special discharge record for the terminal evaluation.

Through evaluating, nurses accept responsibility for their actions, indicate interest in the results of the nursing actions, and demonstrate a desire not to perpetuate ineffective actions but to adopt more effective ones. See the box on page 154 for professional standards describing the nurse's responsibility for evaluating.

RELATIONSHIP OF EVALUATING TO OTHER NURSING PROCESS PHASES

Evaluation depends on the effectiveness of the steps that precede it (Figure 8–2 on page 154). Assessment data must be accurate and complete so that the nurse can formulate appropriate expected outcomes in the planning step. The expected outcomes must be stated concretely in behavioral terms if they are to be useful for evaluating client responses. And finally, without the implementing

ANA STANDARDS

Standard VI: Evaluation

The nurse evaluates the client's progress toward attainment of outcomes.

Measurement Criteria

1. Evaluation is systematic and ongoing.
2. Client's responses to interventions are documented.
3. The effectiveness of interventions is evaluated in relation to outcomes.
4. Ongoing assessment data are used to revise diagnoses, outcomes, and the plan of care, as needed.
5. Revisions in diagnoses, outcomes, and the plan of care are documented.
6. The client, significant others, and health care providers are involved in the evaluation process, when appropriate.

Source: Abstracted from American Nurses Association, *Standards of Clinical Nursing Practice* (Washington, DC: ANA, 1991), p. 14. Used with permission.

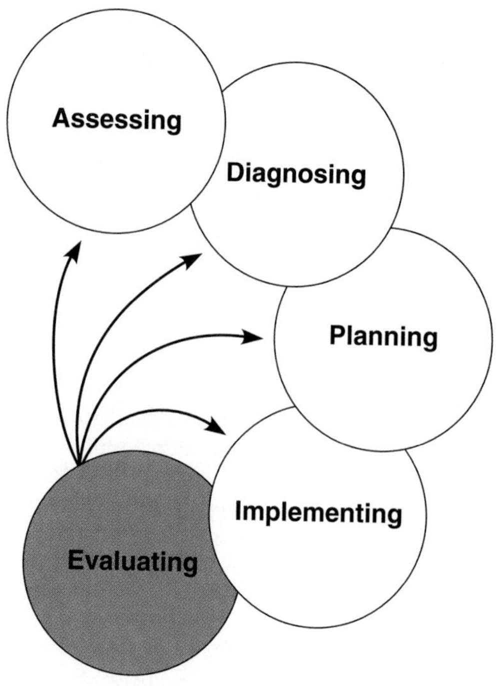

Figure 8–2 Evaluating. The final phase of the nursing process, in which the nurse determines the client's progress toward goal/outcome achievement and the effectiveness of the nursing care plan. The plan may be continued, modified, or terminated.

phase, in which the plan is put into action, there would be nothing to evaluate.

The evaluating and assessing phases overlap. As previously stated, assessment (data collection) is ongoing and continuous at every client contact. However, data are collected for different purposes at different points in the nursing process. During the assessing phase, the nurse collects data for the purpose of making diagnoses. During the evaluating step, the nurse collects data for the purpose of comparing it to preselected goals and judging the effectiveness of the nursing care. The *act* of assessing (data collection) is the same; the differences lie in (1) when the data are collected and (2) how the data are used.

EVALUATING CLIENT RESPONSES

The evaluation process has six components:

- Identifying the expected outcomes that the nurse will use to measure client goal achievement (This is done in the planning step.)
- Collecting data related to the expected outcomes
- Comparing the data with the expected outcomes and judging whether the goals have been achieved
- Relating nursing actions to client outcomes
- Drawing conclusions about problem status
- Reviewing and modifying the client's care plan

Identifying Expected Outcomes The expected outcomes formulated in the planning step (see Chapter 7) are the criteria used to evaluate the client's response to nursing care. Expected outcomes serve two purposes: They (1) establish the kind of evaluative data that need to be collected and (2) provide a standard against which the data are judged. For example, given the following expected outcomes, any nurse caring for the client would know what data to collect:

- Daily fluid intake will not be less than 2500 mL.
- Urinary output will balance with fluid intake.
- Residual urine will be less than 100 mL.

Collecting Data Using the clearly stated, precise, and measurable expected outcomes as a guide, the nurse collects data so that conclusions can be drawn about whether goals have been met. It is usually necessary to collect both objective and subjective data.

Some data may require interpretation. Examples of objective data requiring interpretation are the degree of tissue turgor of a dehydrated client or the degree of restlessness of a client with pain. When objective data need interpretation, the nurse may obtain the views of other nurses to substantiate changes. Examples of subjective data needing interpretation include complaints of nausea or pain by the client. When interpreting subjective data, the nurse must rely upon either (a) the client's statements (eg, "My pain is worse now than it was after breakfast") or (b) objective indicators of the subjective data, even though these indicators may require further interpretation (eg, decreased restlessness, decreased pulse and respiratory rates, and relaxed facial muscles as indicators of pain relief). Data must be recorded concisely and accurately to facilitate the third part of the evaluating process (see Chapter 9).

Judging Goal Achievement If the first two parts of the evaluation process have been carried out effectively, it is relatively simple to determine whether a goal has been met. Both the nurse and client play an active role in comparing the client's actual responses with the expected outcomes. Did the client drink 3000 mL of fluid in 24 hours? Did the client walk unassisted the specified distance per day? When determining whether a goal has been achieved, the nurse can draw one of three possible conclusions:

1. The goal was met; that is, the client response is the same as the expected outcome.
2. The goal was partially met; that is, either a short-term goal was achieved, but the long-term goal was not, or the expected outcome was only partially attained.
3. The goal was not met.

After determining whether a goal has been met, the nurse writes an evaluative statement (either on the care plan or in the nurse's notes). An **evaluation statement** consists of two parts: a conclusion and supporting data. The conclusion is a statement that the goal/expected outcome was met, partially met, or not met. The supporting data are the list of client responses that support the conclusion, for example:

> Goal met: Oral intake 300 mL more than output; skin turgor good; mucous membranes moist.

See Table 8–2 on page 156 for evaluation statements for Luisa Sanchez. Data in this table represent Ms Sanchez's responses to care as observed by the night nurse on the morning after her admission to the unit. In practice, care plans usually do not have a column for evaluation statements; rather, evaluation statements are recorded in the nurses' notes.

RELATING NURSING ACTIONS TO CLIENT OUTCOMES

The fourth aspect of the evaluating process is determining whether the nursing actions had any relation to the outcomes. It should never be assumed that a nursing action was the cause of or the only factor in meeting, partially meeting, or not meeting a goal. For example, Mrs Sophi Ringdale was obese and needed to lose 14 kg (30 lb). When the nurse and client drew up a care plan, one goal was "Lose 1.4 kg (3 lb) by 4/7/95." A nursing strategy in the care plan was "Explain how to plan and prepare a 900-calorie diet." On 4/7/95, the client weighed herself and had lost 1.8 kg (4 lb). The goal had been met—in fact, exceeded. It is easy to assume that the nursing strategy was highly effective. However, it is important to collect more data before drawing that conclusion. On questioning the client, the nurse might find any of the following: (a) the client planned a 900-calorie diet and prepared and ate the food; (b) the client planned a 900-calorie diet but did not prepare the correct food; (c) the client did not understand how to plan a 900-calorie diet, so she did not bother with it. If the first possibility is found to be true, the nurse can safely judge that the nursing strategy "Explain how to plan and prepare a 900-calorie diet" was effective in helping the client lose weight. However, if the nurse learns that either the second or third possibility actually happened, then it must be assumed that the nursing strategy did not affect the outcome. The next step for the nurse is to collect data about what the client actually did to lose weight. It is important to establish the relationship (or lack thereof) of the nursing actions to the client responses.

Drawing Conclusions about Problem Status The nurse uses the judgments about goal achievement (see preceding phase) to determine whether the care plan was effective in resolving, reducing, or preventing client problems. When goals have been met, the nurse can draw one of the following conclusions about the status of the client's problem:

- The actual problem stated in the nursing diagnosis has been resolved; or the potential problem is being prevented, and the risk factors no longer exist. In these instances, the nurse documents that the goals have been met and discontinues the care for the problem.
- The potential problem stated in the nursing diagnosis is being prevented, but the risk factors are still present. In this case, the nurse keeps the problem on the care plan.
- The actual problem still exists even though some goals are being met. For example, an expected outcome on Gina Suske's care plan is "Client will ingest 3000 mL of fluid daily." Even though the data show this outcome has been achieved, other data (dry oral mucous membranes) indicate that she still has **Fluid volume deficit.** Therefore, the nursing interventions must be continued even though this one goal was met.

When goals have been partially met or when goals have not been met, two conclusions may be drawn:

Text continued on page 158

Table 8–2 Modified Care Plan for Luisa Sanchez (Two problems only)*

Nursing Diagnosis	**Ineffective airway clearance** related to viscous secretions and shallow chest expansion secondary to fluid volume deficit, pain, and fatigue

Expected Outcomes	Evaluation Statements	Nursing Orders	Rationale
Demonstrates adequate air exchange, as evidenced by 1. Absence of pallor and cyanosis (skin and mucous membranes)	1. Goal partially met. Skin and mucous membranes not cyanotic, but still pale.	a. Monitor respiratory status q4h: rate, depth, effort, skin color, mucous membranes, amount and color of sputum. b. Monitor results of blood gases, chest x-ray studies, and incentive spirometer volume as available. c. Monitor level of consciousness d. Auscultate lungs q4h.	a, b, c, d. To identify progress toward or deviations from goal. **Ineffective airway clearance** leads to poor oxygenation, evidenced by pallor, cyanosis, lethargy, drowsiness. Shallow breathing further compromises oxygenation. *Retain nursing orders to continue to identify progress. Goal status indicates problem not resolved.*
2. Using correct breathing/coughing technique after instruction.	2. Goal partially met. Uses correct technique when pain well controlled by narcotic analgesics.	e. Vital signs q4h (TPR, B/P).	e. Inadequate oxygenation causes increased pulse rate. Respiratory rate may be decreased by narcotic analgesics or increased by dyspnea and anxiety.
3. Productive cough	3. Goal met. Cough productive of moderate amounts of thick, yellow, pink-tinged sputum.	f. ~~Instruct in breathing and coughing techniques.~~ *Remind to perform and assist q3h. Support, and encourage.* (4/17/95 JW)	f. *Does not need to be reinstructed as client demonstrates correct techniques. May still need support and encouragement because of fatigue and pain.*
4. Demonstrating symmetric chest excursion of at least 4 cm.	4. Goal not met. Chest excursion = 3cm.	g. Administer prescribed expectorant; schedule for maximum effectiveness	g. Helps loosen secretions so they can be coughed up and expelled.
5. Verbalizing chest pain of < 4 on a 1–10 scale within 30 min after receiving po analgesics.	5. Goal met. Tylenol #3 given at 0300. At 0330 stated, "Easier to breathe," rated pain at 3, and coughed effectively.	h. Maintain Fowler's or semi-Fowler's position. i. Administer prescribed analgesics. Notify physician if pain not relieved.	h. Gravity allows for fuller lung expansion by decreasing pressure of abdomen on diaphragm. i. Controls pleuritic pain by blocking pain pathways and altering perception of pain, enabling client to increase thoracic expansion. Unrelieved pain may signal impending complication.
6. Lungs clear to auscultation within 48–72 h.	6. Goal not met. Scattered inspiratory crackles auscultated throughout right anterior and posterior chest.	j. Administer oxygen as prescribed by nasal cannula. Provide portable oxygen if client goes off unit (eg, for X-ray examinations).	j. Supplemental oxygen makes more oxygen available to the cells, even though less air is being moved by the client, thereby reducing the work of breathing.
7. Respirations 12–22/min, pulse < 100 beats/min.	7. Goal partially met. Respirations 26/min, pulse 96.	k. Assist with postural drainage daily at 0930. *On 4/17 teach to continue prn at home.* (4/17/95, JW)	k. Gravity facilitates movement of secretions upward through the respiratory passage. *As soon as client is hydrated and fever is controlled, she will probably be discharged to self-care at home.*
8. Inhaling normal volume of air on incentive spirometer.	8. Goal not met. Tidal volume only 350 mL (Evaluated 4/17/95, JW)		

Table 8–2 ***continued***

Nursing Diagnosis — **Anxiety** related to difficulty breathing and concerns about work and parenting roles

Expected Outcomes	Evaluation Statements	Nursing Orders	Rationale
Demonstrates decreased anxiety, as evidenced by		a. When client is dyspneic, stay with her; reassure her you will stay.	a. Presence of a competent caregiver reduces fear of being unable to breathe. Control of anxiety will help client to maintain effective breathing pattern.
1. Listening to and following instructions for correct breathing and coughing technique, even during periods of dyspnea.	1. Goal met. Performed coughing techniques as instructed during periods of dyspnea.	b. Remain calm, appear confident. c. Encourage slow, deep breathing.	b. Reassures client the nurse can help her. c. Focusing on breathing may help client feel in control and decrease anxiety.
2. Verbalizing understanding of condition, diagnostic tests, and treatments (by end of day 1).	2. Goal met. See nurse's notes for 3–11 shift. Stated, "I know I need to try to breathe deeply even when it hurts." Demonstrated correct use of incentive spirometer and stated understanding of the need to use it. Understands IV is for hydration and antibiotics. *(Evaluated 4/17/95, JW)*	d. When client is dyspneic, give brief explanations of treatments and procedures. e. ~~When acute episode is over, give detailed information about nature of condition, treatments, and tests.~~ *Reassess whether client needs any information on condition, treatments, or tests. (4/17/95, JW)*	d. Anxiety and pain interfere with learning. Knowing what to expect reduces anxiety. e. *Detailed information has been given. Because client shows understanding, there is no need to repeat information.*
3. Decrease in reports of fear and anxiety; none within 12 h.	3. Goal met. States, "I know I can get enough air, but it still hurts to breathe."	f. As client can tolerate, encourage to express and expand on her concerns about her child and her work. Explore alternatives as needed.	f. Awareness of source of anxiety enables client to gain control over it.
4. Voice steady, not shaky. 5. Respiratory rate of 12–22/min.	4. Goal met. Speaks in steady voice. 5. Goal not met. Rate 26–36/min.	g. Note whether husband returns as scheduled. If he does not, institute care plan for actual **Altered family processes** *(do on 4/17, day shift) (4/17/95, JW)*	g. Husband's continued absence would constitute defining characteristic for this nursing diagnosis. *It is important that this assessment be made right away, so child care can be arranged if needed.*
6. Freely expressing concerns about work and parent but placing them in perspective in view of her illness.	6. Goal partially met. Discussed only briefly on 3–11 shift. Not done on 11–7 shift because of client's need to rest. *(Evaluated 4/17/95, JW)*		

* In this care plan, a line has been drawn through portions the nurse wished to delete; additions to the care plan are shown in italics.

Table 8–3 Evaluation Checklist

Assessing	Diagnosing	Planning	Implementing
___ Are data complete, accurate, and validated? ___ Do new data require changes in the care plan?	___ Are nursing diagnoses relevant and accurate? ___ Are nursing diagnoses supported by the data? ___ Has problem status changed (ie, potential, actual, possible)? ___ Are the diagnoses stated clearly and in correct format? ___ Have any nursing diagnoses been resolved?	***Expected Outcomes*** ___ Do new nursing diagnoses require new goals? ___ Are goals realistic? ___ Was enough time allowed for goal achievement? ___ Do the goals address all aspects of the problem? ___ Does the client still concur with the goals? ___ Have client priorities changed? ***Nursing Orders*** ___ Do nursing orders need to be written for new nursing diagnoses or new goals? ___ Do the nursing orders seem to be related to the stated goals? ___ Is there rationale to justify each nursing order? ___ Are the nursing orders clear, specific, and detailed? ___ Are new resources available? ___ Do the nursing orders address all aspects of the client's goals? ___ Were all nursing orders clearly effective?	___ Was client input obtained at each step of the nursing process? ___ Were goals and nursing interventions acceptable to the client? ___ Did the caregivers have the knowledge and skill to perform the interventions correctly? ___ Were explanations given to the client prior to implementing?

- The care plan may need to be revised, since the problem is only partially resolved. The revisions may need to occur during assessing, diagnosing, or planning phases, as well as interventions.
- The care plan does not need revision, because the client merely needs more time to achieve the previously established goal(s). In order to make this decision, the nurse must assess why the goals are being only partially achieved, including whether the evaluation was conducted too soon.

Reviewing and Modifying the Nursing Care Plan

After drawing conclusions about the status of the client's problems, the nurse modifies the care plan as indicated. Depending on the agency, modifications may be made by drawing a line through portions of the care plan, using a Hi-Liter pen, or writing "Discontinued (dc'd)" and the date.

Whether or not goals were met, there are a number of decisions to make about continuing, modifying, or terminating nursing care for each problem. Before making modifications, the nurse must first determine why the plan was not completely effective. This requires a review of the entire care plan and a critique of the nursing process steps involved in its development. See Table 8–3 for a checklist summary to use when reviewing a care plan.

Assessing An incomplete or incorrect database influences all subsequent steps of the nursing process and care plan. If data are incomplete, the nurse needs to reassess the client and record the new data. In some instances, new data may invalidate the database, necessitating new nursing diagnoses, new goals, and new nursing actions.

Diagnosing If the database is incomplete, new diagnostic statements may be required. If the database is complete, the nurse needs to analyze whether the problem was identified correctly and whether the nursing diagnoses are relevant to that database. After making judgments about problem status, the nurse revises or adds new diagnoses as needed to reflect the most recent client data.

Planning: Expected Outcomes If the nursing diagnosis is inaccurate, obviously the goal statement will need revision. If the nursing diagnosis is appropriate, the nurse then checks that the goals are realistic and attainable. Unrealistic goals require correction. The nurse should also determine whether priorities have changed and whether the client still agrees with the priorities. Goals must also be written for any new nursing diagnoses.

Planning: Nursing Orders The nurse investigates whether the nursing strategies were related to goal achievement and whether the best nursing strategies were selected. Even when diagnoses and goals are appropriate, the nursing strategies selected may not have been the best ones to achieve the goal. New nursing orders may reflect changes in the amount of nursing care the client needs, scheduling changes, or rearrangement of nursing activities to group similar activities or to permit longer rest or activity periods for the client. If new nursing diagnoses have been written, then new nursing orders will be necessary.

Implementing Even if all sections of the care plan appear to be satisfactory, the manner in which the plan was implemented may have interfered with goal achievement. Before selecting new interventions, the nurse should check whether the nursing orders were carried out. Other personnel may not have carried them out, either because the orders were unclear or because they were unreasonable in terms of external constraints such as money, staff, and equipment.

After making the necessary modifications to the care plan, the nurse implements the modified plan and begins the nursing process cycle again. Refer to Table 8–1 to see how the plan for Luisa Sanchez was modified after evaluation of goal achievement and review of the nursing process. A line has been drawn through portions the nurse wished to delete; additions to the care plan are shown in italics.

EVALUATING THE QUALITY OF NURSING CARE

Over the past 30 years, the quality of nursing care has undergone considerable evaluation to determine what good care is, whether the care nurses give is appropriate and effective, and whether the quality of care provided is good. Evaluating the quality of nursing care is an essential part of professional accountability. Other terms used for this measurement are quality assessment and quality assurance. **Quality assessment** is an examination of services only; **quality assurance** implies that efforts are made to evaluate *and* ensure quality health care.

Historical Perspective Evaluation of the quality of care is not a new concept. Florence Nightingale's *Notes on Hospitals*, published in 1859, included an evaluation of medical and nursing care. Since that time, evaluation has progressed through a number of stages. Initially, it focused on the environment, for example, whether equipment was available at the time it was needed. Later, organizational standards in agencies were developed. For example, the ratio of nurses to clients was studied and evaluated in terms of clients' needs. Since 1952, the Joint Commission on Accreditation of Hospitals (JCAH), a voluntary organization, has surveyed hospitals. Objective criteria were applied to evaluate a client's record after discharge from the hospital. This was called a **retrospective audit.** (*Retrospective* means relating to a past event, and *audit* means an examination or review of records.) A **nursing audit** is a review of clients' charts to evaluate nursing competence or performance. In 1972 and 1973, the JCAH (currently called the Joint Commission on Accreditation of Healthcare Organizations, or JCAHO) revised its standards to include the requirement that hospitals be subjected to medical and nursing audits before receiving accreditation.

In 1972, the United States government enacted legislation to control health care costs and evaluate the quality of health care services received by Medicare and Medicaid patients. Since that time, a national and statewide system of professional review organizations (PROs) has been developed (Gordon 1987). The purposes of the PROs include developing standards and monitoring the quality of, cost of, and access to care. The objective of these procedures is to ensure that the care given under federal programs was necessary and that the appropriate facilities were chosen to provide the care.

The PROs are based on the concept of peer review. A **peer review** is an encounter between two persons equal in education, abilities, and qualifications, during which one person critically reviews the practices that the other has documented in a client's record. These evaluative processes may be **concurrent audits,** that is, reviews of present practices.

Approaches to Quality Evaluation Three aspects of care—structure, process, and outcome—can be evaluated. Standards of care for each type of evaluation have been developed based on nursing and health-related research and expert opinion. A good evaluation needs to consider all three aspects of care.

The Structure in Which Client Care Takes Place **Structure evaluation** focuses on the organization of the client care system, for instance, administrative and financial procedures that direct the provision of care, staffing patterns, management styles, availability of equipment, and physical facilities. Information about these support structures can be obtained easily. Quality care cannot be delivered without adequate staff and resources. However, adequate staffing patterns and adequate facilities do not ensure quality care.

The Process of Care **Process evaluation** focuses on the activities of the nurse, that is, the performance of the caregiver in relation to the client's needs. The care given by the nurse is evaluated by talking with the client, auditing the client's record, and observing the nursing activities. Evaluators may seek answers to questions such as these: Are medications recorded correctly? Was client teaching documented? Is the care plan complete? This type of evaluation is time-consuming and requires the judgment of expert practitioners. The American Nurses Association (ANA) *Standards of Clinical Nursing Practice* (1991) are process standards that provide the nursing profession with a framework for the delivery and evaluation of care.

Outcomes of the Care The focus of **outcome evaluation** is the client's health status, welfare, and satisfaction, or the results of care in terms of changes in the client. Its advantage is that outcomes may be easily observed. However, in order for outcome evaluation to be successful, it is essential that nurses and other health care providers write measurable and objective criteria in their goal statements. Outcome evaluation may be concurrent or retrospective. It is usually accomplished by comparing the client's progress against the collaborative case management plan or care map. The Joint Commission on the Accreditation of Healthcare Organizations supports an interdisciplinary, collaborative approach to health care, and as of 1995 has begun to evaluate hospitals based on outcome criteria (Ignatavicius & Hausman 1995).

CHAPTER HIGHLIGHTS

- Implementing is putting planned nursing strategies into action.
- Reassessing occurs simultaneously with the implementing phase of the nursing process.
- Successful implementing and evaluating depend in part on the quality of the preceding phases of assessing, diagnosing, and planning.
- Implementing is action focused. Broadly stated, nursing activities in the implementing step include doing, delegating, and recording.
- More specifically, implementing activities include communicating, caring, teaching, counseling, leading, managing, and acting as a client advocate and change agent.
- Cognitive, interpersonal, and technical skills are used to implement nursing strategies.
- Prior to implementing a medical or nursing order, the nurse reassesses the client to be sure that the order is still appropriate.
- The nurse must determine whether assistance is needed to perform a nursing strategy knowledgeably, safely, and comfortably for the client.
- The implementing phase terminates with the documentation of the nursing activities and client responses.
- After the care plan has been implemented, the nurse evaluates the client's health status and the effectiveness of the care plan in achieving client goals.
- Evaluating is determining whether or to what degree the client goals have been met.
- Evaluating may be ongoing, intermittent, or terminal.
- Evaluating is purposeful and organized.
- The expected outcomes formulated during the planning phase serve as criteria for evaluating client progress and improved health status.
- The expected outcomes determine the data that must be collected to evaluate the client's health status.
- Reexamining the client care plan is a process of making decisions about problem status and critiquing each phase of the nursing process.
- Professional standards of care hold that nurses are responsible and accountable for implementing and evaluating the plan of care.
- Quality assurance evaluation includes consideration of the structures, processes, and outcomes of nursing care.

READINGS AND REFERENCES

SUGGESTED READINGS

Egan, E, Snyder, M, and Burns, K. July/August 1992. Intervention studies in nursing: Is the effect due to the independent variable? Nursing Outlook 40(4):187–90.

There is increased interest in and study of independent nursing interventions. This article raises a number of questions about the methodology used by many of the intervention studies that have been done. The authors believe that this explains the inconsistencies found in the effects of an intervention.

Hansten, R and Washburn, M. 1992. Tips for delegating to the right person. *American Journal of Nursing* 92(6):64–65.

Implementing is both doing and delegating. This article contains practical advice for those who are still unsure about delegating interventions to others.

RELATED RESEARCH

Richardson, M and O'Sullivan, S. March/May 1991. Preoperation interviews: A nursing intervention to reduce patients' anxiety. *Australian Journal of Advanced Nursing* 8:3–5.

White, P. 1993. Nurses' perceptions of quality assurance programs. *Journal of Nursing Care Quality* 7(4):44–55.

SELECTED REFERENCES

American Nurses Association. 1980. *Nursing: A Social Policy Statement.* Kansas City, MO: ANA.

______. 1991. *Standards of Clinical Nursing Practice.* Kansas City, MO: ANA.

Brennan, M. June 1992. Teaching tools for the Marker Model for standards development and the Umbrella Model for quality assurance. *Health Care Supervisor* 10(4):66–74.

Bulechek, GM and McCloskey, JC. 1990. Nursing intervention taxonomy development. In McCloskey, JC and Grace, HK, editors. pp. 23–28. *Current Issues in Nursing.* St Louis: Mosby.

Cesta, TG. 1993. The link between continuous quality improvement and case management. *Journal of Nursing Administration* 23(6):55–61.

Cox, DM. 1993. Keeping score: Triage tools for organized patient care and evaluation. *Emergency* 25(5):42–48.

Dickey, LL. 1993. Promoting preventive care with patient-held minirecords: A review. *Patient Education and Counseling* 20(1):37–47.

Finnegan, SA et al. 1993. Automated patient acuity: Linking nurse systems and quality measurement with patient outcomes. *Journal of Nursing Administration* 23(5):62–71.

Gordon, M. 1987. *Nursing Diagnosis: Process and Application.* 2d ed. Hightstown, NJ: McGraw-Hill.

Hodges, LC and Icenhour, ML. 1990. Measuring the quality of nursing care. In McCloskey, JC and Grace, HK, editors. pp. 242–48. *Current Issues in Nursing.* St Louis: Mosby.

Joint Commission on Accreditation of Healthcare Organizations. 1993. *Accreditation Manual for Hospitals.* Chicago: JCAHO, Nursing Services.

Katz, JM and Green, E. 1992. *Managing Quality: A Guide to Monitoring and Evaluating Nursing Services.* St Louis: Mosby-Year Book.

Koch, MW and Fairly, TM. 1992. *Integrated Quality Management: The Key to Improving Nursing Care Quality.* St Louis: Mosby-Year Book.

Lang, NM and Krejci, JW. 1991. Standards and holism: A reframing. *Holistic Nursing Practice* 5(3):14–21.

Ludwig-Beymer, P et al. 1993. Using patient perceptions to improve quality care. *Journal of Nursing Care Quality* 7(2):42–51.

McFarland, GK and McFarlane, EA. 1993. *Nursing Diagnosis and Intervention.* 2d ed. St Louis: Mosby-Year Book.

Marker, CGS. December 1991. Total quality management and the Marker Management System 1988: Part 1. An Overview. *Aspen's Advisor for Nurse Executives* 7(3):5–8.

Morison, MJ. April 1991. The Stirling model of nursing audit: Its relationship to standard setting and quality assurance. *Professional Nurse* 6:366, 368–70.

Mundinger, MO. 1980. *Autonomy in Nursing.* Gaithersburg, MD: Aspen Publishers.

Phaneuf, M. 1976. *The Nursing Audit: Self Regulation in Nursing Practice.* New York: Appleton-Century-Crofts.

Pike, AW et al. 1993. A new architecture for quality assurance: Nurse-physician collaboration. *Journal of Nursing Care Quality* 7(3):1–8.

Raynor, DK, Booth, TG, and Blenkinsopp, A. 1993. Effects of computer generated reminder charts on patients' compliance with drug regimens. *British Medical Journal* 306:1158–61.

Riley-Clark, A et al. 1993. How do you evaluate the effectiveness of your patient teaching? *Oncology Nursing Forum* 20:825–27.

Tucker, S, Canobbio, M, Paquette, E, and Wells, M. 1992. *Patient Care Standards: Nursing Process, Diagnosis and Outcome.* 5th ed. St Louis: Mosby.

Wilkinson, JM. 1992. *Nursing Process in Action: A Critical Thinking Approach.* Redwood City, CA: Addison-Wesley Nursing.

Wright, D. September 1984. An introduction to the evaluation of nursing care: A review of the literature. *Journal of Advanced Nursing* 9:457–67.

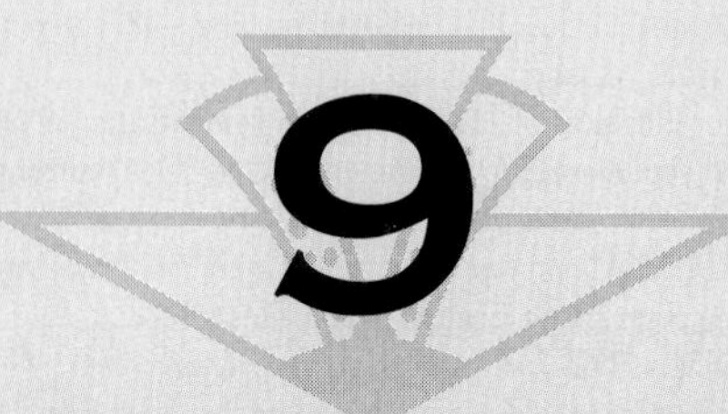

9 Documenting and Reporting

Objectives

Identify nine purposes of client records.

Describe the components of source-oriented clinical records and problem-oriented clinical records.

Describe three types of progress records.

Differentiate among narrative charting, SOAP charting, focus charting, and charting by exception.

Identify measures used to ensure that recording meets legal standards.

Identify abbreviations and symbols commonly used for charting.

Identify measures used to maintain the confidentiality of client records.

Describe the change-of-shift report.

Identify essential guidelines for reporting client data.

Compare the advantages and disadvantages of nursing care conferences and nursing care rounds.

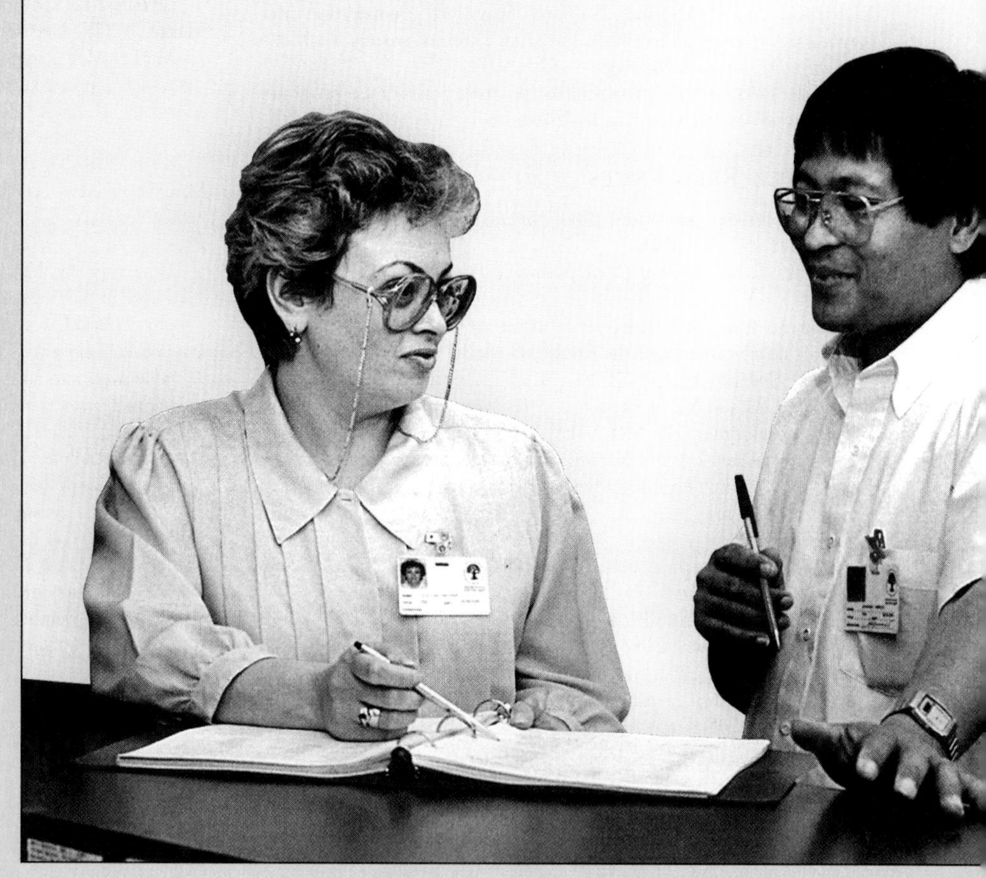

Written and verbal communication among health professionals is vital to the quality of client care. Generally, health personnel communicate through discussions, reports, and records. A **discussion** is an informal oral consideration of a subject by two or more health care personnel to identify a problem or establish strategies to resolve a problem. A **report** is oral, written, or computer-based communication intended to convey information to others. For instance, nurses always report on clients at the end of a hospital work shift. A **record** is always written; it is a formal, legal documentation of a client's progress. The process of making an entry on a client record is called **recording** or **charting.**

The Joint Commission on Accreditation of Healthcare Organizations (JCAHO) (1992) states that nursing data related to assessments, nursing diagnoses or client needs, nursing interventions, and client outcomes must be permanently filed in a client information system. Each health care organization has policies about recording and reporting client data, and each nurse is accountable for practicing according to these standards.

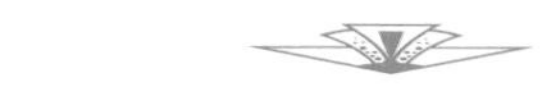

Purposes of Client Records

Client records are kept for a number of purposes.

Planning Client Care Each health professional uses data from the client's record to plan care for that client. A physician, for example, may order a specific antibiotic after establishing that the client's temperature is steadily rising and that laboratory tests reveal the presence of a certain microorganism. Nurses use baseline and ongoing data to evaluate the effectiveness of the nursing care plan. The social worker's data about the client's home environment can assist the nurse in developing an appropriate discharge teaching plan. Data from the physical therapist help the nurse to implement specific physical exercises for the client. Data from the dietitian helps the nurse reinforce necessary dietary adjustments.

Communication The record serves as the vehicle by which different health professionals who interact with a client communicate with each other. This prevents fragmentation, repetition, and delays in client care.

Legal Documentation The client's record is a legal document and is admissible in court as evidence. In some jurisdictions, however, the record is considered inadmissible as evidence when the client objects, because information the client gives to the physician is confidential. A record is usually considered the property of the agency, although there is increasing belief that the client has a right to the information in the record on request.

Research The information contained in a record can be a valuable source of data for research. The treatment plans for a number of clients with the same health problems can yield information helpful in treating a particular client.

Education Students in health disciplines often use client records as educational tools. A record can frequently provide a comprehensive view of the client, the illness, effective treatment strategies, and factors that affect the outcome of the illness.

Quality Assurance Monitoring The client's record is used to monitor the care the client is receiving and the competence of the people giving that care. During quality assurance monitoring of nursing, also referred to as a **nursing audit,** the nursing interventions are monitored and measured against established standards. Often an audit is a retrospective audit, in that the care has already been given.

A nursing audit carried out by other nurses is sometimes referred to as a **peer review.** Many agencies have committees that monitor the practice of individual and groups of nurses.

Statistics Statistical information from client records can help an agency anticipate and plan for people's future needs. For example, the number of births or kinds of illnesses can be obtained from records. Some statistics, such as records of births and deaths, are required by law. They are filed with a government agency and become a part of the local, national, and international statistics.

Accrediting and Licensing Organizations such as the Joint Commission on Accreditation of Healthcare Organizations (JCAHO), which accredits health care facilities, review clinical records of clients to ensure that the facility is meeting their standards.

Reimbursement Documentation also helps a facility receive reimbursement from the federal government. For a facility to obtain payment through Medicare, the client's clinical record must contain the correct diagnostic related group (DRG) codes and reveal that the appropriate care has been given.

Table 9–1 Components of the Source-Oriented Clinical Record

Form	Information
Admission (face) sheet	Legal name, birth date, age
	Social Security number
	Address
	Marital status; closest relatives or person to notify in case of emergency
	Date, time, and admitting diagnosis
	Food or drug allergies
	Name of admitting (attending) physician
	Insurance information
	Any assigned diagnostic related group (DRG)
Initial nursing assessment	Findings from the initial nursing assessment and physical health examination
Flowsheets	
▪ Graphic record (Figure 21–12, page 436)	Body temperature, pulse rate, respiratory rate, blood pressure, and weight
▪ Medication record	Name, dosage, route, time, date, site of regularly administered medications
▪ Activity flow record	Activity, diet, bathing, and elimination records; may also include restraints, isolation activities
▪ Special flowsheets	Examples: 24-hour fluid balance (Figure 38–8, page 1082), neurologic assessment
Nurse's notes (Figure 9–4, page 169)	Assessments, nursing diagnoses, nursing interventions, including client responses
Medical history and physical examination	Past and family medical history, present medical problems, differential or current diagnoses, findings of physical examination by the physician
Physician's order sheet	Medical orders for medications, treatments, and so on
Physician's progress notes	Medical observations, treatments, client progress, and so on
Consultation records	Reports by medical and clinical specialists
Diagnostic reports	Examples: laboratory reports, X-ray reports, CT scan reports
Consultation reports	Physical therapy, respiratory therapy
Client discharge plan and referral summary	Started on admission and completed upon discharge; includes nursing problems, general information and referral data

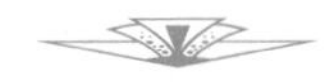

TYPES OF RECORDS

SOURCE-ORIENTED CLINICAL RECORDS

In the traditional client record, or source-oriented clinical record (formerly referred to as the *source-oriented medical record*), each person or department makes notations in a separate section or sections of the client's chart. For example, the admission department has an admission sheet; the physician has a doctor's order sheet, a doctor's history sheet, and progress notes; nurses use the nurse's notes; and other departments or personnel have their own records. In this type of record, information about a particular problem is distributed throughout the record. For example, if a client had left hemiplegia (paralysis of the left side of the body), data about this problem might be found in the physician's history sheet, on the physician's order sheet, in the nurse's notes, in the physical therapist's record, and in the social service record. See Table 9–1 for the components of a source-oriented clinical record.

PROBLEM-ORIENTED CLINICAL RECORDS

In a problem-oriented clinical record (POR), data about the client are recorded and arranged according to the problems the client has, rather than according to the source of the information. The record integrates all data about a problem, whether gathered by physicians, nurses, or others involved in the client's care. Plans for each active or potential problem are drawn up, and progress notes are recorded for each problem. Unlike the traditional record, which separates the medical data on a problem from the nursing data and other data into different sections of the record, the POR coordinates the care given by all health team members and focuses on the client and the client's health problems.

The POR has four basic components:

- Baseline data
- Problem list
- Initial list of orders or care plans
- Progress notes

Baseline Data Baseline data consist of all information known about the client when the client first enters the health care agency. It includes the nursing assessment, the physician's history, and the physical health examination. To these are added social and family data from other sources, such as the social worker, and baseline laboratory and roentgenographic data. In most agencies, a standardized form is used to help team members obtain a complete database. Data are constantly updated as the client's health status changes.

Problem List The problem list (Figure 9–1) is a list of problems that is carefully compiled once the database has been collected and analyzed. Some problems are obvious on initial contact with the client; others are established as additional data are gathered. In this context, a problem is essentially a need that the client is unable to meet without assistance from a health professional.

The initial problem list is usually made either by the first person to encounter the client or by the person who assumes primary responsibility for the client's care. Subsequent contributions are made by other health professionals.

To be complete, the problem list should include socioeconomic, demographic, psychologic, and physiologic data. The list is usually found at the front of the client's record. Each problem is labeled and numbered so that it can be identified throughout the record. This list has been likened to an index or table of contents. See Figure 9–1. Problems are usually categorized as active or inactive.

No.	Date Entered	Date Inactive	Client Problem	Related to
#1	Mar 9/93		Several CVAs resulting in Rt hemiplegia	
			and left-sided weakness. Redefined Feb 7/95	
#1A	Mar 9/93		Self-care deficit (hygiene, toileting,	
			grooming, feeding).	
#1B	Mar 9/93		Impaired physical mobility. Redefined Feb 7/95	
#1C	Mar 9/93		Total incontinence. Redefined Nov 17/94	
#1D	Mar 9/93		Progressive dysphasia.	
#2	Mar 9/93		Colonic constipation. Redefined Nov 10/93	
#3	Mar 9/93		History of depression.	
#4	Mar 9/93		Essential hypertension.	
#5	June 6/93	Nov 93	Pruritus.	
#2	Nov 10/93		Potential for constipation.	
#1C	Nov 17/94		Nocturnal urinary incontinence.	
#1	Feb 7/95		Cerebral vascular disease (multiple CVAs)	
			resulting in bilateral hemiplegia	
#1B	Feb 7/95		Needs major assistance to transfer/	
			unable to walk	

Figure 9–1 A client's problem list using the sublisting method to relate problems. Note that problems 1, 1B, 1C, and 2 were redefined on the dates indicated and listed subsequently.

Potential problems are entered on the progress notes rather than the problem list. Only when a problem actually becomes active is it added to the list.

Signs, symptoms, and abnormal diagnostic findings are considered temporary labels until diagnosis is established. With the development of nursing diagnoses, many nurses are now using the North American Nursing Diagnosis Association (NANDA) taxonomy of nursing diagnoses to state nursing problems. Problem statements should refer to one problem only, be written unambiguously (so that no interpretation is required) in behavioral terms, and should provide direction for client care.

When several problems have a common etiology or cause, two methods are used to relate the problems: sublisting and cross-referencing. A *sublist* is a group of all manifestations of a major problem that require separate management. Manifestations may be either behavioral or clinical indicators of the same problem. For example, consider the following segment of Figure 9–1:

No.	Client Problem
1	Several CVAs resulting in Rt hemiplegia and left-sided weakness
1A	Self-care deficit (hygiene, toileting, grooming, feeding)
1B	Impaired physical mobility
1C	Total incontinence
1D	Progressive dysphasia

The *cross-referencing method* lists all problems separately, using consecutive numbers. A "Related to" column to the right of the "Client Problem" column lists the number of the major problem to which the manifestations are related. For example, Figure 9–1 could also include the following:

No.	Client Problem	Related to
1	Multiple CVAs resulting in Rt hemiplegia and left-sided weakness	
2	Self-care deficit (hygiene, toileting, grooming, feeding)	#1
3	Impaired physical mobility	#1
4	Total incontinence	#1
5	Progressive dysphasia	#1

Major problems can also be cross-referenced to other major problems. An example of this would be the following:

No.	Client Problem	Related to
1	Cerebral vascular disease	#4
4	Essential hypertension	#1

"Redefinition" of problems is often necessary to reflect a change in the client's problem or to increase understanding of the problem. Redefining does *not* involve changing the stated nature of the problem; it involves changing the wording of the problem to reflect a change in its frequency or intensity, or increased knowledge. The problem retains the same number (eg, see Figure 9–1):

No.	Client Problem
1C	Total incontinence Redefined Nov 17/94
1C	Nocturnal urinary incontinence

Initial List of Orders or Care Plans The initial list of orders or care plans is made with reference to the active problems. Care plans or orders are generated by the person who lists the problems. Physicians write physician's orders or medical care plans; nurses write nursing orders or nursing care plans. The written plan in the record is listed under each problem in the progress notes (discussed next) and is not isolated as a separate list of orders.

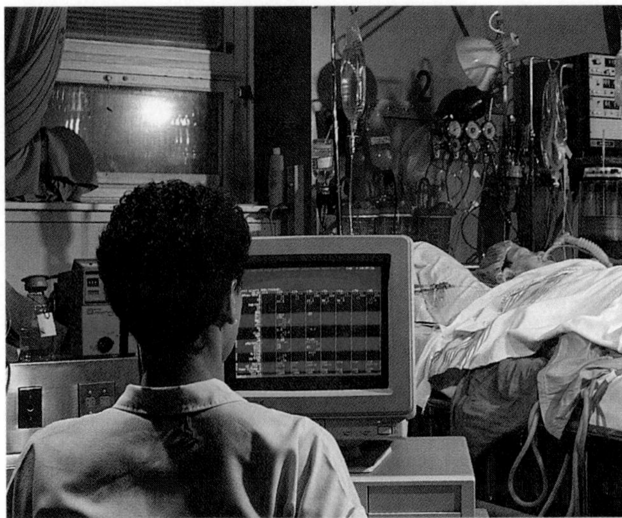

Figure 9–2 A bedside computer.

Progress Notes Progress notes in the POR are made by all health professionals involved in a client's care. All health personnel add progress notes on the same type of sheet. Progress notes are numbered to correspond to the problems on the problem list. See page 169 and Figure 9–5, later in this chapter.

COMPUTER RECORDS

In about 1968, a number of health institutions introduced computers. Initially, computers were installed primarily in hospital business offices. However, increasing numbers of computers are being used in health care planning and delivery as well as in laboratories and physicians' clinics. By the turn of the century, most nurses will use computers in many aspects of their practice. Already, "user-friendly" machines, often operated with a light-pen and simple keyboard, are of great help to the nurse in assessing, planning, implementing, recording, and evaluating nursing care. Bedside computers are becoming more common in hospitals (see Figure 9–2).

By using computerized systems, nursing staffs are able to create care plans easily, customize them for each client, type in additions as needed, evaluate and update information at any time, and retrieve data appropriate to a specific nursing diagnosis. Such systems can be programmed to provide work lists, as needed, directly from the com-

> **RESEARCH NOTE**
>
> ### Are There Advantages to Using Bedside Computers?
>
> These researchers investigated the acceptability, productivity, and return-on-investment (ROI) of bedside computers. The increased acuity of clients in hospitals and a shortage of nurses have prompted hospitals' increased use of bedside computers. All sites studied reported that bedside computers improved care by decreasing errors of omission; allowing greater accuracy and completeness of documentation; improving the standardization of charting quality; increasing nurses' accountability to charting and scheduling intravenous therapy; facilitating more timely responses to client needs, more accurate and up-to-date care plans, and greater timeliness of tests and procedures; and providing nurses with more time for client education.
>
> ***Implication:*** Bedside computers are a valuable adjunct to the provision of nursing care.
>
> **Source:** D Herring and R Rochman, A closer look at bedside terminals, *Nursing Management*, July 1990, 21:54–56, 60–61.

> ### SELECTED PROS AND CONS OF COMPUTER DOCUMENTATION
>
> ***Pros***
>
> - Storage and retrieval of information is fast and simple.
> - Links various sources of client information.
> - Client information, requests, and results are sent and received quickly.
> - Bedside terminals can synthesize information from monitoring equipment.
> - Facilitates client outcomes.
> - Information is legible.
> - Reinforces standards of care.
> - Standard terminology improves communication.
> - Bedside terminals eliminate need to take notes on a worksheet before recording
> - Bedside terminals permit the nurse to check an order immediately before administering a treatment or medication.
>
> ***Cons***
>
> - Client's privacy may be infringed on if security measures are not used.
> - Breakdowns make information temporarily unavailable.
> - System is expensive.

puter. In this way, lists generated for treatments, procedures, and medications can always be kept up-to-date. Such an application eliminates the need for multiple flowsheets, because all of the same information is available both in the computer and on computer-printed update forms. To record nursing actions, the nurse either enters data directly into the computerized records or completes the computer-generated flowsheet in the client's chart. Selected pros and cons of computer documentation are shown in the box above.

A well-designed database system can make the entry and retrieval of information a relatively easy task for the nurses who use it. Figure 9–3 on page 168 shows a client care plan using a computer-based information system.

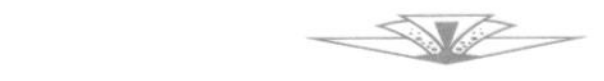

FORMATS FOR NURSING DOCUMENTATION

NURSING CARE PLANS

There are two types of nursing care plans: traditional and standardized. The **traditional care plan** is written for each client. The form varies from agency to agency according to the needs of the client and the department. Most forms have three columns: one for nursing diagnoses, a second for expected outcomes, and a third for nursing interventions. See Chapter 7, page 139, for additional information.

Standardized care plans have been developed to save documentation time. These plans may be based on an institution's standards of practice, thereby helping to provide a high quality of nursing care. For further information, see Chapter 7, page 142.

CRITICAL PATHWAYS

With the advent of managed care systems, tools such as critical paths and health care maps have been developed (Figure 4–1, page 76). The pathway includes interventions for a client with a specific diagnosis. For example, a critical pathway for a client who has undergone a knee replacement sets forth the essential care the client must receive on a day-to-day basis: physical activities, diet, medications, and so on.

All health professionals providing care to the client use the critical pathway as a monitoring and documenting tool.

Client name : Martha O'Brien Rm number 403

Admission date : 05/25/95

Sex : F Religion : Catholic

Age : 62 Date of birth : 03/13/33

Admitting physician : Dr. Raymond Atkins

Medical diagnosis : Diabetes

Primary nurse : Juana Briones, RN

Allergies : Penicillin Diet : 1500 c ADA

Risk factors : Hearing aid Vital signs : T.I.D.

Nursing diagnosis : Impaired skin integrity related to pruritus.

Long-term goals : Client will experience improved skin integrity within 48 hours.

Short-term goals	Nursing interventions	Evaluation
Given the prescribed care, client will experience decreased itching sensation.	1. Infrequent baths. 2. Use cool water. 3. Soap substitute. 4. Blot skin dry. DO NOT RUB! 5. Lubricate skin with lotion after bath.	
Client will understand and implement health teaching.	1. Explain phenomenon of itching. 2. Teach avoidance of excessive warmth. 3. Teach need for increased humidity.	

Figure 9–3 Computer-generated nursing care plan.

KARDEX

The Kardex is a widely used, concise method of organizing and recording data about a client, making information quickly accessible to all health professionals. The system consists of a series of cards kept in a portable index file. The card for a particular client can be quickly turned up to reveal specific data. Often Kardex data are recorded in pencil so that they can be changed and kept up to date.

The information on Kardexes may be organized into sections, for example:

- Pertinent information about the client, such as name, room number, age, religion, marital status, admission date, doctor's name, diagnosis, type of surgery and date, occupation, and next of kin
- List of medications, with the date of order and the times of administration for each

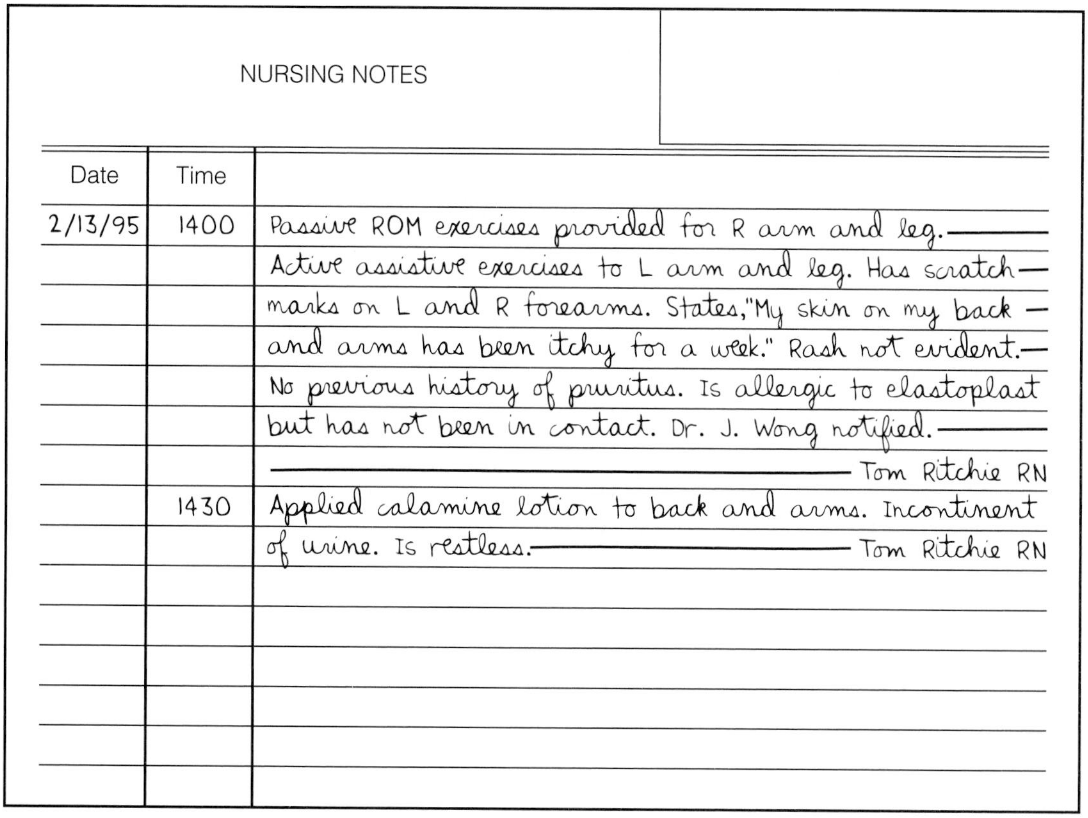

NURSING NOTES

Date	Time	
2/13/95	1400	Passive ROM exercises provided for R arm and leg.
		Active assistive exercises to L arm and leg. Has scratch-
		marks on L and R forearms. States, "My skin on my back
		and arms has been itchy for a week." Rash not evident.
		No previous history of pruritus. Is allergic to elastoplast
		but has not been in contact. Dr. J. Wong notified.
		Tom Ritchie RN
	1430	Applied calamine lotion to back and arms. Incontinent
		of urine. Is restless. Tom Ritchie RN

Figure 9–4 An example of narrative notes.

- List of intravenous fluids, with dates of infusions
- List of daily treatments and procedures, such as irrigations, dressing changes, postural drainage, or measurement of vital signs
- List of diagnostic procedures ordered, such as roentgenography or laboratory tests
- Allergies
- Specific data on how the client's physical needs are to be met, such as type of diet, assistance needed with feeding, elimination devices, activity, hygienic needs, and safety precautions (use of side rails, and so on)
- A problem list, stated goals, and a list of nursing approaches to meet the goals and relieve the problems

Although much of the information on the Kardex may be recorded by the nurse in charge or a delegate (eg, the ward clerk), any nurse who cares for the client plays a key role in initiating the record and keeping the data current.

PROGRESS NOTES

Six methods used to write progress notes are narrative charting, the SOAP format, the PIE format, use of flowsheets, focus charting, and charting by exception.

Narrative Charting Narrative charting is a description (narration) of information, and **chronologic charting** records data in sequence as time moves forward. Chronologic charting is commonly associated with source-oriented clinical records. Figure 9–4 is an example of narrative nurse's notes. The forms used for the nurse's notes may vary from place to place. Some agencies have separate columns for treatments, nursing observations, and comments. The major disadvantage of narrative charting is that it is difficult for a reader to find all the data about a specific problem without examining all of the recorded information. For this reason, specific flow records (discussed later) are often used.

SOAP Format SOAP is an acronym for subjective data, objective data, assessment, and planning. The SOAP format originated from the medical model with the POR but is used increasingly in many different types of records. The acronyms SOAPIE and SOAPIER refer to formats that add implementation, evaluation, and revision. Many agencies use only the SOAP format. A more recent format is the *APIE* (assessment, plan, implementation, and evaluation), which condenses the client data into fewer statements. In APIE, the assessment combines the subjective

SOAP Format

2/13/95 #5 Generalized pruritus
1400 S—"My skin is itchy on my back and arms, and it's been like this for a week."
O—Skin appears clear—no rash or irritations noted. Marks where client has scratched noted on left and right forearms. Allergic to elastoplast but has not been in contact.
A—No previous history of pruritus. Altered comfort (pruritus): cause unknown.
P—Instructed to not scratch skin.
—Applied calamine lotion to back and arms at 1430 h.
—Cut fingernails.
—Assess further to determine whether recurrence associated with specific drugs or foods.
—Refer to physician and pharmacist for assessment.

Tom Ritchie, RN

SOAPIER Format

2/13/95 #5 Generalized pruritus
1400 S—"My skin is itchy on my back and arms, and it's been like this for a week."
O—Skin appears clear—no rash or irritation noted. Marks where client has scratched noted on left and right forearms. Allergic to elastoplast but has not been in contact.
No previous history of pruritus.
A—Altered comfort.
P—Instruct to not scratch skin.
—Apply calamine lotion as necessary.
—Cut nails to avoid scratches.
—Assess further to determine whether recurrence associated with specific drugs or foods.
—Refer to physician and pharmacist for assessment.
I —Instructed not to scratch skin. Applied calamine lotion to back and arms at 1430 h. Assisted to cut fingernails. Notified physician and pharmcist of problem.
1600 E—States, "I'm still itchy. That lotion didn't help."
R—Remove calamine lotion and apply hydrocortisone ungt. as ordered.

Tom Ritchie, RN

APIE Format

2/13/95 #5 Generalized pruritus
1400 A—Altered comfort: cause unknown. States, "My skin is itchy on my back and arms, and it's been like this for a week." Skin appears clear.
—No rash or irritations noted. Marks where client has scratched noted on left and right forearms. Allergic to elastoplast but has not been in contact. No previous history of pruritus.
P—Instruct not to scratch skin.
—Apply calamine lotion as necessary.
—Cut nails to avoid scratches.
—Assess further to determine whether recurrence associated with specific drugs or foods.
—Refer to doctor and pharmacist for assessment.
I —Instructed not to scratch skin. Applied calamine lotion to back and arms at 1430 h. Assisted to cut fingernails. Notified physician and pharmacist of problem.
E—States, "I'm still itchy. That lotion didn't help."

Tom Ritchie, RN

Figure 9–5 Examples of nursing progress notes using SOAP, SOAPIER, and APIE formats.

and objective data; the plan combines the nursing actions with the expected outcomes; and the implementation and evaluation are the same. See Figure 9–5 for an example of a nurse's progress notes using the SOAP, SOAPIER, and APIE formats.

Subjective data report what the client perceives and the way the client expresses it. **Objective data** include measurements such as vital signs, observations made by health team members using their senses, laboratory and roentgenographic findings, and client responses to diagnostic and therapeutic measures such as medications. Examples of subjective and objective data are provided in Chapter 5.

In the *assessment* phase, the observer makes interpretations and draws conclusions from the subjective and objective data. Again, all health professionals have made assessments, using the knowledge in their possession. At this point, the nurse writes a nursing diagnostic statement in accordance with the guidelines discussed in Chapter 6. The *plan* is a plan for action based on the above data. The initial plan is written by the person who enters the problem into the record. All subsequent plans, including revisions, also are entered into the progress notes. Plans may include termination of certain activities if the problem is resolved, initiation of new actions if the problem is unchanged, and activities being done to resolve a particular problem.

Implementation, or *intervention*, is documentation of activities in the plan that were actually done for the client. These entries specify which plans were actually carried out. *Evaluation* is documentation of the client's response to the plan, stated in terms of client behavior (eg, what the client did or said). The question asked at this stage is "Does the client's behavior indicate that the plan was unsuccessful in lessening or alleviating the identified problem?" *Revision*, or *reassessment*, refers to changes that must be made in the initial or original plan. From the evaluation notes and decision, one may determine that the client's condition may have improved or deteriorated. New data may now be available.

PIE Charting The PIE charting model originated from the nursing process and is similar to the SOAP charting. PIE is an acronym for problems, interventions, and evaluation of nursing care. This system consists of a client care assessment flowsheet and progress notes. The flowsheet covers a 24-hour period and uses specific assessment criteria in a particular format, such as human needs or functional health patterns. After the assessment, the nurse establishes and records specific problems on the progress notes, often using NANDA diagnoses to word the problem. If there is no approved nursing diagnosis for a problem, the nurse develops a problem statement using NANDA's three-part format: human response, related factor, and "as evidenced by." See Chapter 6, page 119. The *problem statement* is labeled "P" and referred to by number (eg, P #6). The *interventions* employed to manage the problem are labeled "I" and numbered according to the problem (eg, I #6). The *evaluation* of the effectiveness of the interventions is also labeled and numbered according to the problem (eg, E #6).

Flowsheets When specific client variables such as pulse, blood pressure, medications, and progress in learning a new skill need to be recorded accurately, narrative notes are often too long. Instead, the **flowsheet,** a graphic record, is used as a quick way to reflect the client's condition. The time parameters for flowsheets can vary from minutes to months. In a hospital intensive care unit, a client's blood pressure may be monitored by the minute, whereas in an ambulatory clinic, a client's blood glucose level may be recorded once a month.

Flowsheets commonly used are the clinical record (also called the graphic chart or graphic observation record), the fluid intake and output record, the medication record, and daily nursing care records.

Clinical Record The clinical record (shown in Figure 21–12 on page 436) indicates body temperature, pulse rate, respiratory rate, blood pressure readings, and weight.

Some agencies also show special medications (such as dicumarol), central venous pressure (CVP), 24-hour fluid intake and output, bowel movement, glucose and acetone in the urine, and other significant clinical data.

24-Hour Fluid Balance Record A 24-hour fluid balance record is shown in Figure 38–8, page 1082. Before notations are made on a 24-hour fluid balance record, the nurse records the amount of the client's fluid intake and output on a form kept at the client's bedside. The client and support persons should be taught to use this record. It documents intake and output for the duration of one shift only (8 or 12 hours). The totals for each shift are then recorded on the 24-hour fluid balance record. In the sample shown in Figure 38–8, the totals for each 8-hour shift (days, evenings, and nights) are recorded, and then the 24-hour totals are calculated.

All routes of fluid intake and all routes of fluid loss or output must be measured and recorded. Information about ways to measure and record specific amounts of fluid intake and output are described in Chapter 38.

Medication Record Medication flowsheets usually include designated areas for the date of the medication order, the expiration date, the medication name and dose, the frequency of administration and route, and the nurse's signature. Some records also include a place to document the client's allergies.

Daily Nursing Care Record The daily nursing care is often recorded on a flowsheet such as the one in Figure 9–6 on pages 172 and 173.

Focus Charting Focus charting uses key words that describe what is happening to the client. Unlike problem-oriented charting, focus charting is *not* limited to clinical problems. The term *focus* was developed to encourage nurses to view the client's status from a positive perspective rather than the negative one that *problem* suggests. The term *focus* has a broad definition. It can denote any of the following:

- A current client concern or behavior (eg, decreased fluid intake)
- A significant change in the client status or behavior (eg, sudden loss of sensation in one extremity)
- A significant event in the client's therapy (eg, return from surgery)

In sum, a nursing focus outlines the occasions for and the activities of the *nursing care* the client is receiving. A focus is *not* a medical diagnosis, but it sometimes describes what is happening to the client as a result of the medical diagnosis. For example, some of the foci for a client with a medical diagnosis of myocardial infarction may include admission information, chest pain, anxiety about medical diagnosis, and education about cardiac medications.

The focus charting system often uses three columns:

Date/Hour	Focus	Progress Notes
2/11/95 0900	Neuro status	DATA: Unresponsive to verbal stimuli; responsive to painful stimuli. Pupils pinpoint and equal. Dr Ward visited. ACTION: Neuro assessment and vital signs q2h. RESPONSE: See flowsheets.

24-HOUR PATIENT CARE RECORD

Instructions: Document time of assessment in specified column. Document significant findings, interventions and outcomes in narrative as warranted.

Date: Time

PSYCHOSOCIAL	Calm						
	Anxious						
	Cooperates with care						
	Other						
NEURO-LOGICAL	Alert/Oriented X 3						
	Lethargic						
	Other						
MUSCULO-SKELETAL	CMS Intact						
	Proper alignment						
	Proper position						
	Other						
RESPIRATORY	Breath°° Clear						
	Sounds: Congested						
	Regular						
	Irregular						
	Unlabored						
	Labored						
	Caugh: Nonproductive						
	Productive						
	02 At ___						
	Via ___						
	Other ___						
	Other ___						
CARDIOVASCULAR	Skin Warm						
	Cool						
	Dry						
	Diaphoretic						
	Other ___						
	Apical: Regular						
	Irregular						
	Pedal: Present						
	Absent						
	Radial: Present						
	Absent						
	Edema						
	Antiembolic hose on						
	Other ___						
	Other ___						
GASTRO-INTESTINAL	Abd: Soft						
	Firm						
	Distended						
	Tender						
	Bowel Present						
	Sounds: Absent						
	Other ___						
	Other ___						

NORTH BROWARD HOSPITAL DISTRICT
24-HOUR PATIENT CARE RECORD

Time

GENITOURINARY	Clear Yellow Urine						
	Amber Urine						
	Dark Urine						
	Bloody Urine						
	Foley Patent/Secure						
	Incontinent						
	Other ___						
	Other ___						
WOUND/DECUBITUS	Site 1 ___						
	Site 2 ___						
	Site 3 ___						
	Clean/Dry/Intact						
	Open to air ___						
	Dressing ___						
	Sutures ___						
	Staples ___						
	Steristrips ___						
	Drain(s) 1. ___						
	2. ___						
	3. ___						
	Other ___						
	Other ___						
PARENTERAL	IV Site 1. ___						
	Site 2. ___						
	Patent Q ___						
	Site change						
	Tubing change						
	Central Venous Access						
	Site ___						
	Patent Q ___						
	Dressing change						
	Other ___						
	Other ___						

*IDENTIFY USE & SHIFT		11-7	7-3	3-11
EQUIPMENT	K-PAD			
	SPECIAL BED			
	Bio Gard			
	TRACTION/OHF			
	ORTHO DEVICE			
	FEEDING PUMP			
	SUCTION			
	IV PUMP			
	OTHER			
	OTHER			

ADDRESSOGRAPH

Figure 9–6 First two pages of 24-hour patient care record. **Source:** Courtesy of North BrowardHospital District, Florida. Used with permission.

** S = Self A = Assist T = Total **

	PATIENT CARE ACTIVITIES	11-7	7-3	3-11
DIET	Type:			
	Type:			
	% Taken			
	** S/A/T **			
HYGIENE	Shower			
	Bath ** S/A/T **			
	Mouthcare			
	Pericare			
	Antiembolic hose			
	P.M. Care			
	Other			
ACTIVITY	Asleep on Rounds q			
	Bedrest			
	BRP			
	Up w/assist			
	Up ad lib			
	ROM active/passive			
	OOB Chair			
	Amb. Hall **S/A**			
	Other			
OFF UNIT	To:	At	Via	Return
	To:	At	Via	Return
	To:	At	Via	Return
TEACHING	TOPIC:			
	Taught to: Patient			
	Family			
	S.O.			
	Teaching Method: discuss			
	slide			
	demo			
	video			
	handout			
	Level of Under-standing: good			
	fair			
	poor			
	reinforced			
	Eval. method: verbal			
	return demo			
	written			
	Comment:			

	PATIENT CARE ACTIVITIES	11-7	7-3	3-11
SPECIMEN	Type:			
	Type:			
	Type:			
SAFETY	Bed low position			
	Call light within reach			
	Siderails up			
	Fall precautions			
	Siezure precautions			
	Restraints:			
	Traction equipment ckd.			
	Isolation			
	Other			
	*Document Nursing Intervention/Outcome as Appropriate			
NURSING CARE ACTIVITIES	N/G irrigated			
	N/G suction			
	Decubitus care			
	Turned Q			
	Cough/deep breath			
	Suctioned			
	Trach care			
	Ostomy care			
	Dressing change			
	Foley care			
	Irrigation			
	CBI			
	Inc. Spirometer			
	Other:			
	NSG. CARE PLAN REVIEWED			
	DISCHARGE PLAN REVIEWED			

PROTOCOLS		
	1.	2.
	3.	4.
	5.	6.
	7.	8.

INITIAL	SIGNATURE/TITLE

Figure 9–6 *continued*

In the progress notes column, all entries are organized by DAR (data, action, response). *Data* include subjective and/or objective data. *Action* includes plans for action and immediate nursing interventions. *Response* includes the client's response to interventions (Lampe 1988, p. 23). This system is therefore compatible with use of the nursing process: the data component equates with assessment, action with planning and implementation, and response with evaluation.

Focus charting relies on an adequate database or assessment forms and the use of such flowsheets as vital signs records, neurologic checklists, intake and output flowsheets, and hygiene checklists. Agencies that use focus charting often provide a simple assessment checklist of key words that pertain to the special needs of clients in specific nursing units. For each key word, the checklist shows both normal and abnormal characteristics. Those applicable to the client can be circled. Normal characteristics may be underlined.

Charting by Exception Charting by exception (CBE) is a documentation system in which only significant findings or exceptions to norms are recorded. CBE incorporates three key components (Murphy & Burke 1990, p. 68):

1. Unique *flowsheets* that highlight significant findings and define assessment parameters and findings. These include the nursing/physician order flowsheet, the graphic record, the client teaching record, and the client discharge note.

2. Documentation by reference to *Standards of Nursing Practice*, which eliminates much of the repetitive charting of routine care. The *standards* must therefore be specific in describing actual nursing practice and apply to every nurse regardless of clinical area. Unit-specific standards may also be developed. Examples of standards related to hygiene patterns include: "The nurse shall ensure that the client has a complete linen change every three days and as needed," and "The nurse shall ensure that the client is offered oral care tid." Documentation of care according to these specified standards involves only a check mark in the routine standards box on the graphic record. If all of the standards are not implemented, an asterisk with reference to the nurse's notes is made. All exceptions to the standards should be clearly outlined in narrative form on the nurse's notes.

3. Bedside accessibility of documentation forms. In the CBE system, all flowsheets are kept at the client's bedside to allow immediate recording and to eliminate the need for transcribing data from the nurse's worksheet to the permanent record.

DISCHARGE NOTE AND REFERRAL SUMMARY

A discharge note and referral summary are completed when the client is being discharged and transferred to another institution or to a home setting where a visit by a community health nurse is required. See the discussion of discharge planning in Chapter 7, page 129. Discharge summaries usually include the following:

- Description of client's condition at discharge
- Current medications
- Treatments (eg, wound care, oxygen therapy)
- Diet
- Activity level
- Restrictions

Referral summaries usually include the following:

- Any active health problems
- Current medications
- Current treatments that are to be continued
- Eating and sleeping habits
- Self-care abilities
- Support networks
- Life-style patterns
- Religious preferences

This exchange of information ensures continuity of health care for the client.

DISCHARGING A CLIENT AGAINST MEDICAL AUTHORITY

Occasionally, clients leave an agency without the permission of the physician. These are *unauthorized discharges*, often referred to as *discharge against medical authority (AMA)*. The client is asked to sign a special form releasing the hospital from any responsibility after the departure (Figure 9–7).

It is important that the client understand that refusing a particular treatment or medication is not the same as refusing all treatments and desiring to leave the hospital. The AMA form is used in the latter instance, whereas refusing a particular aspect of care is the client's right and needs to be documented on the chart and reported to the nurse in charge.

When a client decides to leave a health care facility AMA, the following activities are indicated:

1. Ascertain why the person wants to leave the agency. Sometimes clients misunderstand information or have fears the nurse can resolve. As a result, the client may decide to stay in the agency.

EL CAMINO HOSPITAL

LEAVING HOSPITAL AGAINST ADVICE

Date

This is to certify that
a patient in the above named hospital, is leaving the hospital against the advice of the attending physician and the hospital administration. I acknowledge that I have been informed of the risk involved and hereby release the attending physician, and the hospital, from all responsibility and any ill effects which may result from this action.

Patient

Other Person Responsible

Relationship

Witness

Witness°

Figure 9–7 A discharge form for a client who is being released against medical authority.
Source: El Camino Hospital, Mountain View, California. Reprinted with permission.

2. Notify the physician of the client's decision.
3. Offer the client the appropriate form to complete.
4. If the client refuses to sign the form, document the fact on the form and have another health professional witness this.
5. Provide the client with the original of the signed form and place a copy in the record.
6. When the client leaves the agency, notify the physician, nurse in charge, and agency administration as appropriate.
7. Assist the client to leave as if this were a usual discharge from the agency. The agency is still responsible while the client is on the premises.

GUIDELINES FOR RECORDING

Because the client's record is a legal document and may be used to provide evidence in court, many factors are considered in recording. Health care personnel not only must maintain the confidentiality of the client's record but also meet legal standards in the process of recording. Elements of effective charting are summarized in the accompanying box.

ELEMENTS OF EFFECTIVE CHARTING

Timing	Appropriateness
Confidentiality	Completeness
Permanence	Standard Terminology
Signature	Brevity
Accuracy	Legal Awareness
Sequence	

Timing For *each* notation, documentation of the *date* and *time* of the recording and of the assessment or intervention is essential not only for legal reasons but also for client safety. Follow the agency's policy about the frequency of documenting, and adjust the frequency as a client's condition indicates; for example, a client whose blood pressure is changing requires more frequent documentation than a client whose blood pressure is constant.

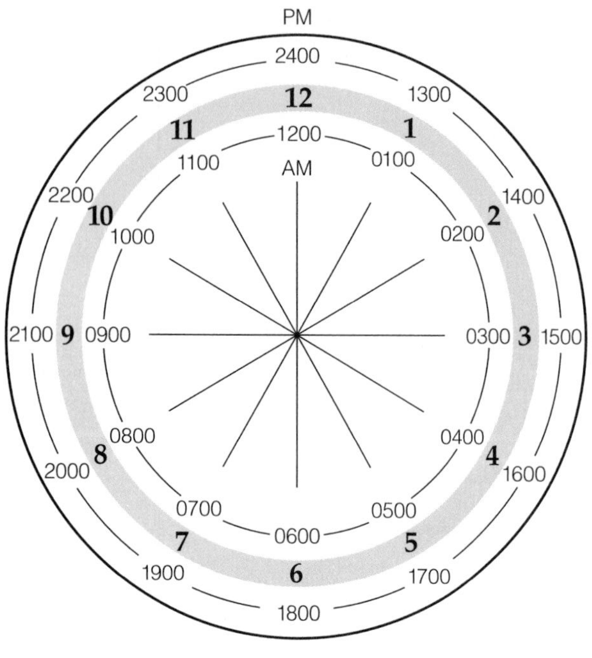

Figure 9–8 The 24-hour clock.

Documenting should also be done as soon as possible after an assessment or intervention.

No recording should be done *before* providing nursing care. For example, the time at which a narcotic was administered to a client needs to be determined before the next one can safely be given. Time can be recorded in the conventional manner (ie, 9:00 AM or 3:20 PM) or according to the 24-hour clock (military clock), which avoids confusion about whether a time was AM or PM (Figure 9–8).

Confidentiality The client's record is protected legally as a private record of the client's care. Thus, access to the record is restricted to health professionals involved in giving care to the client. Insurance companies, for example, have no legal right to demand access to medical records, even though they may be determining compensation to the client. However, a client who is making a claim for compensation may ask to have the medical history used as evidence. In this instance, the client must sign an authorization for review, copying, or release of information from the record. This form clearly indicates what information is to be released and to whom. In no instance may a nurse allow access to a client's record by significant others or any person other than a caregiver.

For purposes of education and research, most agencies allow student and graduate health professionals access to client records. The records are used in client conferences, clinics, rounds, and written papers or client studies. The student or graduate is bound by a strict ethical code to hold all information in confidence. Some agencies code medical records when they are filed, so that the names of clients are removed. This allows records to be used without identifying individuals. When this is not the practice, it is the responsibility of the student or health professional to protect the client's privacy by *not* using a name or any statements in the notations that would identify the client. Many agencies also require documentation from the student or health professional wishing to use medical records of discharged clients. A permission note from the student's instructor will confirm the person's status as a student at a particular school.

Permanence All entries on the client's record are made in dark-colored ink so that the record is permanent and changes can be identified. Dark-colored ink is generally required because it reproduces well on microfilm and in duplication processes. Entries need to be legible. Hand printing or easily understood handwriting is usually permissible. Nurses should follow the agency's policies about the type of pen and ink used for recording.

Signature Each recording on the nursing notes is signed by the nurse making it. The signature includes the *name* and *title*, for example, "Susan J. Green, RN." Nurses need to follow agency policy about how to sign their names. Some agencies permit initials rather than first name (eg, SJ Green). The following title abbreviations are often used, but nurses are advised to check the practice in their agencies.

RN registered nurse
LVN licensed vocational nurse
LPN licensed practical nurse
NA nursing assistant
NS nursing student
SN student nurse

Accuracy It is essential that notations on records be accurate and correct. Accurate notations consist of facts or exact observations, rather than opinions or interpretations of an observation. It is more accurate, for example, to write that the client "refused medication" (fact) than to write that the client "was uncooperative" (opinion); to write that a client "was crying" (observation) is preferable to noting that the client "was depressed" (interpretation). Opinions or interpretations may or may not be accurate. Similarly, when a client expresses worry about the diagnosis or problem, this should be quoted directly on the record: "Stated: 'I'm worried about my leg.'" Nurses should record what they hear as well as what they observe. When describing something, nurses should also avoid general words, such as *large*, *good*, or *normal*, which can be interpreted differently.

Table 9–2 Documentation for the Nursing Process

Step	Documentation Forms
Assessment	Initial assessment form, various flowsheets
Nursing diagnosis	Nursing care plan, protocols, critical path, progress notes, problem list
Planning	Nursing care plan, critical path, protocols
Intervention	Progress notes, flowsheets
Evaluation	Progress notes

Correct spelling is essential for accuracy in recording. If unsure how to spell a word, the nurse looks it up in a dictionary or other resource book. Most agency units have them available for this purpose. Two decidedly different medications may have similar spellings—for example, digitoxin and digoxin.

When the nurse makes a *recording error* in charting, the nurse draws a line through it and writes the word *error* above it, with the nurse's initials or name (depending on agency policy). Errors should not be erased or blotted out, so that there is no doubt about the nursing care given or the charting error made.

Sample Recording

Date: Dec 10/95	Time: 0100

error AJR
Pulse 180 beats/minute 108 beats/minute
__________ Abby J. Roberts NS

If the nature of the error is not clear, many attorneys feel it is helpful and legally acceptable for the nurse to indicate what the error was, to protect the client and the nurse. An example might be, "Charted for wrong client." The policy of the agency, however, needs to be checked.

If a *blank* appears in a notation, the nurse draws a line through the blank space so that no additional information can be recorded at any other time or by any other person, and signs the notation.

Sample Recording

Date: Nov 7/95	Time: 0730

Urine appears cloudy, light brown with dark flecks. No odor. ____ Lin I. Ma NS
C/o burning pain in pubic region prior to voiding. __________ Lin I. Ma NS

Sequence The nurse documents events in the order in which they occur; for example, the nurse records assessments, then the nursing interventions, and then the client's responses.

Appropriateness Only information that pertains to the client's health problems and care is recorded. Any other personal information that the client conveys to the nurse is inappropriate for the record. Recording irrelevant information may be considered an invasion of the client's privacy and/or libelous. A client's disclosure that she was addicted to heroin 20 years ago, for example, *would not* be recorded on the client's medical record unless it had a direct bearing on the client's health problem.

Completeness Not all data that a nurse obtains about a client can be recorded. However, the information that is recorded needs to be complete and helpful to the client and health care professionals. "The JCAHO specify that nurses' notes must reflect the nursing process" (Edelstein 1990, p. 40). See Table 9–2 for documentation for the nursing process.

Use of Standard Terminology The nurse needs to use only commonly accepted *abbreviations*, *symbols*, and *terms* that are specified by the agency. Then, if the record is used in court as evidence, other professionals responsible for interpreting the data can do so correctly. Many abbreviations are standard and used universally; others are used only in certain geographic areas. Some agencies supply a list of the abbreviations they accept. When in doubt about whether to use an abbreviation, the nurse writes the term out in full, until certain about the abbreviation. Abbreviations that are not official can lead to misunderstandings. For example, "D/c" may mean "discharge" or "discontinue"; "od" could mean "once a day" or "right eye." Table 9–3, page 178, lists some commonly used abbreviations (except those used for medications, which are described in Chapter 43). Table 9–4, page 179, indicates commonly accepted symbols.

Brevity Recordings need to be brief as well as complete, to save time in communication. The client's name and the word *client* are omitted. For example, the nurse may write "Perspiring profusely. Respirations shallow,

Table 9–3 Commonly Used Abbreviations

Abbreviation	Term	Abbreviation	Term
abd	abdomen	neg	negative
ABO	the main blood group system	nil (ō)	none
ac	before meals (*ante cibum*)	no. (#)	number
ADL	activities of daily living	NPO (NBM)	nothing by mouth (*per ora*)
ad lib	as desired (*ad libitum*)	NS (N/S)	normal saline
adm	admitted or admission	O_2	oxygen
AM	morning (*ante meridiem*)	od	daily (*omni die*)
amb	ambulatory	OD	right eye (*oculus dexter*); overdose
amt	amount	OOB	out of bed
approx	approximately (about)	os	mouth
bid	twice daily (*bis in die*)	OS	left eye (*oculus sinister*)
BM (bm)	bowel movement	pc	after meals (*post cibum*)
BP	blood pressure	PE (PX)	physical examination
BR	bed rest	per	by or through
BRP	bathroom privileges	PM	afternoon (*post meridiem*)
c̄ (C)	with	po	by mouth (*per os*)
C	Celsius (centigrade)	postop	postoperative(ly)
CBC	complete blood count	preop	preoperative(ly)
CBR	complete bed rest	prep	preparation
Cl	client	prn	when necessary (*pro re nata*)
c/o	complains of	pt	patient
DAT	diet as tolerated	q	every (*quaque*)
dc (disc)	discontinue	qd	every day (*quaque die*)
drsg	dressing	qh (q1h)	every hour (*quaque hora*)
Dx	diagnosis	q2h, q3h, and so on	every 2 hours, 3 hours, and so on
ECG (EKG)	electrocardiogram	qhs	every night at bedtime (*quaque hora somni*)
F	Fahrenheit	qid	four times a day (*quater in die*)
fld	fluid	req	requisition
GI	gastrointestinal	Rt (rt, R)	right
GP	general practitioner	S (s̄)	without (*sine*)
gtt	drops (*guttae*)	SI	seriously ill
h (hr)	hour (*hora*)	spec	specimen
H_2O	water	stat	at once, immediately (*statim*)
hs	at bedtime (*hora somni*)	tid	three times a day (*ter in die*)
I & O	intake and output	TL	team leader
IV	intravenous	TLC	tender loving care
Lab	laboratory	TPR	temperature, pulse, respirations
liq	liquid	Tr	tincture
LMP	last menstrual period	VO	verbal order
lt (L)	left	VS (vs)	vital signs
meds	medications	WNL	within normal limits
mL (ml)	milliliter	wt	weight
mod	moderate		

Table 9–4 Commonly Used Symbols

Symbol	Term	Symbol	Number
>	greater than	ō	0
<	less than	$\overline{ss}$	½
=	equal to	i̇	1
↑	increased	ii̇	2
↓	decreased	iii̇	3
♀	female	iv̇	4
♂	male	v̄	5
°	degree	vi̇	6
#	number; fracture	vii̇	7
ʒ	dram	viii̇	8
℥	ounce	ix̄	9
×	times	x̄	10
@	at		

wet, 28/min." Each thought or sentence is terminated with a period.

Legal Awareness Accurate, complete documentation should give legal protection to the nurse, the client's other caregivers, the health care facility, and the client. Admissible in court as a legal document, the clinical record provides proof of the quality of care given to a client.

For the best legal protection, the nurse should not only adhere to professional standards of nursing care but also follow agency policy and procedures for intervention and documentation in all situations—especially high-risk situations. For example:

> 1100 hours—Complained of feeling dizzy. Raised side rails and instructed to stay in bed and ring call bell if requiring assistance. 1130 hours—found beside bed on floor. Said, "I climbed over these rails all by myself." When asked about pain, replied, "I feel fine but a little dizzy." Helped into bed. BP 100/60 P90 R24 Dr RJ Naden notified. ________________ RS Woo RN

REPORTING

Reports can be either oral or written. The purpose of reporting, in general, is to communicate specific information to a person or group of people. A report should be concise. A good report includes pertinent information but no extraneous detail.

CHANGE-OF-SHIFT REPORTS

A *change-of-shift report* is an oral report given two or three times a day by nurses to all nurses on the next shift. Its purpose is to provide continuity of care for clients. Change-of-shift reports may be given either in a face-to-face exchange or by audiotape recording. Taped reports need to be taped near the end of the shift to make them as current as possible. The face-to-face report permits the listener to ask questions during the report. The tape-recorded report is often briefer and less time-consuming. Some agencies or units combine these methods of giving the change-of-shift report, following the taped report or a brief report to all oncoming staff with a more extensive individual report given by the nurse going off duty to the nurse who will be providing client care during the coming shift. This more detailed report is often given at the bedside, and clients as well as nurses may participate in the exchange of information. See the box on page 180 for key elements of a change-of-shift report.

TELEPHONE REPORTS

Health professionals frequently report on a client by telephone. Nurses inform physicians about a change in a client's condition; a radiologist reports the results of an X-ray study; a nurse may confer with a nurse on another unit about a transferred client.

To document a telephone report, the nurse receiving the information should include the date and time, the name of the person giving the information, what information was received, and the name of the person receiving the information. For example:

> June 6/95 10:35 AM GL Messina, laboratory technician, reported by telephone that Mrs Sara Ames's hematocrit was 39/100 mL. ____ Barbara Ireland RN

If there is any doubt about the information given over the telephone, the person receiving the information should repeat it back to the sender to ensure accuracy.

When giving a telephone report to a physician, it is important that the nurse be concise and accurate. Telephone reports usually include the client's name and medical diagnosis, changes in nursing assessment, vital signs related to baseline vital signs, significant laboratory data, and related nursing interventions. For example:

> Dorothy Mendes admitted 12 noon; burning abdominal pain upper right quadrant (URQ) BP 120/80, P100, R20 on admission. Demerol 100 mg IM on admission. At 3:15 PM BP 100/40, P120, R30. Pain unchanged. Color pale and perspiring. ____ RS Woo RN

The nurse should have the client's chart ready to give the physician any further information.

KEY ELEMENTS OF A CHANGE-OF-SHIFT REPORT

- Follow a particular order (eg, follow room numbers in a hospital).
- Provide basic identifying information for each client (eg, name, room number, bed designation).
- Provide the reason for admission of a new client or medical diagnosis (or diagnoses), surgery (date), diagnostic tests, and therapies in past 24 hours.
- Include significant recent changes in client's condition and present information in order (ie, assessment, nursing diagnoses [if appropriate], planning, intervention, and evaluation). For example, "Mr Ronald Oakes said he had an aching pain in his left calf at 1400 hours. Inspection revealed no other signs. Calf pain is related to altered blood circulation. Rest and elevation of his legs on a footstool for 30 minutes provided relief."
- Provide exact information, such as "Ms Jessie Jones received Demerol 100 mg intramuscularly at 2000 hours (8 PM)," *not* "Ms Jessie Jones received some Demerol during the evening."
- Report clients who may require special emotional support. For example, a client who has just learned that his biopsy results revealed malignancy and who is now scheduled for a laryngectomy needs time to discuss his feelings before the nurse commences preoperative teaching.
- Include current nurse-prescribed and physician-prescribed orders.
- Provide a summary of newly admitted clients, include diagnosis, age, general condition, plan of therapy, and significant information about significant others.
- Report clients that have been transferred or discharged from the unit.
- Clearly state priorities of care.

DOCUMENTATION WHEN A PHYSICIAN-ORDERED MEDICATION IS JUDGED INAPPROPRIATE

- The nurse must contact the physician and discuss why the nurse believes the medication or dosage is inappropriate.
- The nurse documents in notes the following: when the physician was notified, what was conveyed to the physician, and how the physician responded.
- If the nurse cannot reach the physician, the nurse documents all attempts to contact the physician and the reason for withholding the medication.
- If someone else gives the medication, the nurse documents data about the client's condition before and after the medication.
- If an incident report (see Chapter 12) is indicated, the nurse clearly documents factual information.

Source: Adapted from PW Iyer, Thirteen charting rules, *Nursing91*, June 1991, 21:42.

TELEPHONE ORDERS

Physicians often order a therapy (eg, a medication), for a client by telephone. Most agencies have specific policies about telephone orders. Many agencies allow only registered nurses to take telephone orders.

While the physician gives the order, the nurse should write it down and repeat it back to the physician to ensure accuracy. The nurse then transcribes the order onto the physician's order sheet, indicating it as a verbal order (VO) or telephone order (TO) (Figure 9–9).

The nurse should also question the physician about any order that is ambiguous, unusual (eg, an abnormally high dosage of a medication), or contraindicated by the client's condition.

Once the order is transcribed on the physician's order sheet, the order must be countersigned by the physician within a time period described by agency policy. Many acute care hospitals require that this be done within 24 hours. The box above provides the documentation required when the nurse judges a physician-ordered medication inappropriate.

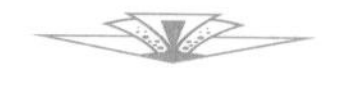

CONFERRING

To **confer** is to consult another person or persons for advice, information, ideas, or instructions. Nurses confer with colleagues and other health professionals about some

12/9/95 1800 h.	Demerol 100 mg I.M. stat Telephone order from— Dr CJ Emms. ———— ———— Betty Eng RN

Figure 9–9 Sample recording of a telephone order.

aspect of client care or to elicit or validate data needed to plan nursing care. Two ways nurses share information are through the nursing conference and nursing rounds.

NURSING CONFERENCE

A nursing care conference is a meeting of a group of nurses to discuss possible solutions to certain problems of a client, such as inability to cope with an event or lack of progress toward goal attainment. The nursing care conference allows each nurse an opportunity to offer an opinion about possible solutions to the problem. Other health professionals may be invited to attend the conference to offer their expertise; for example, a social worker may discuss the family problems of a severely burned child and his responses, or a dietitian may discuss the dietary problems of a client who has diabetes.

Nursing conferences are most effective when there is a climate of respect—that is, nonjudgmental acceptance of others even though their values, opinions, and beliefs may seem different. Nurses need to accept and respect each person's contributions, listening with an open mind to what others are saying even when there is disagreement. People can often learn new ways of approaching situations when they conscientiously listen to other perspectives.

NURSING ROUNDS

Nursing rounds are procedures in which a group of nurses visits all or selected clients at each client's bedside to

- Obtain information that will help plan nursing care.
- Provide clients the opportunity to discuss their care.
- Evaluate the nursing care the client has received.

During rounds, the nurse assigned to the client provides a brief summary of the client's nursing needs and the interventions being implemented. Nursing rounds offer advantages to both clients and nurses: Clients can participate in the discussions, and nurses can see the client being discussed and the equipment being used. To facilitate client participation in nursing rounds, nurses need to use terms that the client can understand. Medical terminology excludes the client from discussion.

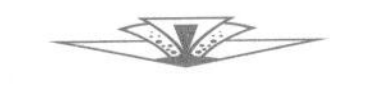

REFERRING

To *refer* is to send or direct a person to another person, or place for help or treatment. The process of sending or assisting the person for help is called referral. A client in a hospital may be referred on discharge to a community agency for home care or follow-up care. Departments within a hospital may also refer to another department. For example, nurses on a unit may refer a client to a social worker for financial assistance.

Most health agencies have policies about who can make referrals and how the process is carried out. The agency will likely require forms to be filled out as part of the referral process (Figure 9–10, page 182).

CHAPTER HIGHLIGHTS

- Nurses must accurately document each step of the nursing process on a client record.
- Client records are legal documents and are admissible as evidence in a court of law.
- In source-oriented clinical records, each health care professional group provides its own record. Recording is oriented around the source of the information.
- Source-oriented records generally have eight parts: admission (face) sheet, initial nursing assessment, flowsheets, physician's order sheet, medical history sheet, physician's progress notes, nurses' notes, and other special records, such as laboratory and consultation records.
- In problem-oriented clinical records, recording is oriented around client problems.
- The problem-oriented record (POR) has four basic components: a defined database, a complete problem list, an initial plan for each identified problem, and progress notes.
- Computer records have simplified nursing documentation. The use of computer terminals at the bedside allows immediate documentation of nursing actions.
- The Kardex record is used for quick access to current data about clients.
- Six methods are used to write progress notes: narrative notes, SOAP format, PIE format, flowsheets, focus charting, and charting by exception.
- Record entries should be brief, accurate, legible, chronologic, made on consecutive lines, and appropriately signed.

Chapter Highlights continued on page 183

Patient Name: Mr. Fabrizio D'Amico

Medical Record Number: 5447652001

(addressograph stamp)

INTER-AGENCY REFERRAL FORM
ALLIED HEALTH INFORMATION

Address Reply To:
STANFORD UNIVERSITY HOSPITAL
Discharge Planning Program
300 Pasteur Drive
Stanford, CA 94305-5232

Medicare No. 0721569702	Medi-Cal No.:
Admission Date: 7/15/95	Discharge Date: 8/1/95
Name and Address of Nearest Relative or Friend: KAY JONAS (neighbor) 14 MONTGOMERY ST., MENLO PARK, CA	

From (Ward or Clinic): 4 SOUTH (415) 723- 4499

Medications Administered Day of Discharge: COUMADIN 5 mg @ 0900 hrs.

NURSING EVALUATION

	GOOD	FAIR	POOR
Vision	✓		
Hearing		✓	
Speech			✓
Bladder Control			✓
Bowel Control		✓	
Date of last BM	7/31/95		

	MOBILITY
	Walks
	Cane
	Crutches
	Walker
A	Wheelchair
A	Bed/Chair
	Bedfast

	PERSONAL NEEDS
	Call Bell
A	Feeds Self
	Eating Device
A	Commode
	Bedpan
I	Urinal
A	Bathing
I	Wash Face
A	(Shave)/Make-Up
I	Comb Hair
A	Brush Teeth/(Dentures)

CODE:
I = Independent
A = Assist
D = Dependent

PATIENT USES:	YES	NO	COMMENTS
Glasses	✓		
Hearing Aide	✓		
Dentures	✓		
Catheter (condom)	✓		Type: Δ'd:
Tubes		✓	Type: Δ'd:
Prosthesis		✓	Type:
Colostomy		✓	Δ'd:

PATIENT IS:	YES	Describe Atypical Behavior
Alert/Appropriate		
Confused		
Combative		
Noisy		
Withdrawn	✓	DEPRESSED ABOUT DYSPHASIA
Wanderer		

SKIN (describe), DRESSING CHANGES, or TREATMENTS:
SKIN DRY BUT INTACT. SLING APPLIED TO (L) ARM

Myra Brown (SIGNATURE) RN (TITLE) 7/31/95 (DATE)

PHYSICAL AND OCUPATIONAL THERAPY:
ROM exercises To (L) arm and (L) leg daily. Quadriceps exercises To (R) leg.

Larry Chu (SIGNATURE) PT (TITLE) 7/31/95 (DATE)

DIET: NO RESTRICTIONS

TEACHING:

SIGNATURE TITLE DATE

SOCIAL (Current/future living arrangements; family composition, etc.)
AND OTHER PERTINENT INFORMATION:
THIS 86 YR. OLD WIDOWER LIVES ALONE. HAS ONE DAUGHTER (IN NEW YORK CITY) WHO IS EXPLORING LONG TERM CARE FACILITIES IN THIS AREA. CLIENT'S ATTEMPTS TO VERBALIZE NEED TO BE ENCOURAGED. HE UNDERSTANDS SLOW, DISTINCT SPEECH.

Myra Brown (SIGNATURE) RN (TITLE) 7/31/95 (DATE)

REPLY TO BE COMPLETED WITHIN 4 WEEKS:

SIGNATURE TITLE DATE

Figure 9–10 Sample referral form. **Source:** Stanford University Hospital, Stanford, California. Reprinted with permission.

Chapter Highlights *continued*

- Record entries are made *after* nursing assessments, interventions, and evaluations.
- Because the record is a legal document, nurses sign their legal names according to agency policy and use standard terms and abbreviations.
- Reports about clients need to be concise and pertinent and must include significant changes in the client's condition and therapy.
- Common methods of communication by nurses are reporting, conferring, and referring.

READINGS AND REFERENCES

SUGGESTED READINGS

Cohen, MR. July 1987. Play it safe: Don't use these abbreviations. *Nursing 87* 17:46–47.

Even though some abbreviations may be approved for use by staff, Cohen maintains that some abbreviations should never be used because they are so easily misunderstood. Alternatives are provided.

Iyer, PW. June 1991. Thirteen charting rules. *Nursing 91* 21:40–44.

Iyer presents 13 rules about charting that are designed to keep the nurse legally safe. Each rule is explained, and examples are provided.

RELATED RESEARCH

Edelstein, J. November 1990. A study on nursing documentation. *Nursing Management* 21:40–46.

Lower, MS and Navert, LB. July 1992. Charting: The impact of bedside computers. *Nursing Management* 23:40–42, 44.

SELECTED REFERENCES

Albarado, RS, McCall, V, and Thrane, JM. July 1990. Computerized nursing documentation. *Nursing Management* 21:64–65.

Bergerson, SR. April 1988. More about charting with a jury in mind. *Nursing88* 18:50–58.

Brown, BL and Brown, JW. January 1993. OSHA regulations demand strict documentation. *Provider* 19:37–38.

Buckley-Womack, C and Gidney, B. October 1987. A new dimension in documentations: The PIE method. *Journal of Neuroscience Nursing* 19:256–60.

Bunston, T, Elliott, M, and Rapuch, S. Spring 1993. A psychosocial summary flow sheet: Facilitating the coordination of care, enhancing the quality of care. *Journal of Palliative Care* 9:14–22.

Clinical Skillbuilders. 1992. *Better Documentation.* Springhouse, PA: Springhouse.

Comstock, LG and Moff, TE. July 1991. Cost-effective charting. *Nursing Management* 22:44–48.

Edelstein, J. November 1990. A study of nursing documentation. *Nursing Management* 21:40–43, 46.

Fischbach, F. 1991. *Documenting Care.* Philadelphia: FA Davis.

Fondiller, S. September 1991. The new look in nursing documentation. *American Journal of Nursing* 91:65–76.

Greve, P. July 1992. Documentation: Every word counts. *RN* 55:55–56, 59.

Iyer, PW. June 1991. Thirteen charting rules. *Nursing91* 21:40–44.

______. July 1991. Six more charting rules to keep you legally safe. *Nursing 91* 21:34–39.

Iyer, PW and Camp, NH. 1991. *Nursing Documentation: A Nursing Process Approach.* St Louis: Mosby-Year Book.

Joint Commission on Accreditation of Healthcare Organizations. 1994. *Accreditation Manual for Hospitals.* Chicago: JCAHO, Nursing Services.

Kettenbach, G. 1990. *Writing S.O.A.P. Notes.* Philadelphia: FA Davis.

Knapp-Spooner, C and Brett, J. March 1992. Less is more: A med/surg flow sheet. *RN* 55:36–39.

Lampe, SS. 1984. *Focus Charting.* Minneapolis: Creative Nursing Management.

______. July 1985. Focus charting: Streamlining documentation. *Nursing Management* 16:43–46.

______. 1988. *Focus Charting.* Minneapolis: Creative Nursing Management.

Meintz, SL and Shaha, SH. January 1992. Our hand-held computer beats them all. *RN* 55:52–55, 57.

Meyer, C. April 1992. Bedside computer charting: Inching toward tomorrow. *American Journal of Nursing* 92:38–42, 44.

Miller, P and Pastorino, C. November 1990. Daily nursing documentation can be quick and thorough! *Nursing Management* 21:47–49.

Murphy, J and Burke, LJ. May 1990. Charting by exception: A more efficient way to document. *Nursing90* 20:65, 68–69.

Rocerto, LR and Maleski, CM. July/August 1984. All about rights to medical records. *Nursing Life* 4:50–51.

Smith, CE. February 1986. Upgrade your shift reports with the three R's. *Nursing86* 16:63–64.

Weed, LL. 1971. *Medical Records, Medical Education and Patient Care: The Problem-Oriented Record as a Basic Tool.* Cleveland: Case Western Reserve University Press.

10

Critical Thinking, Problem Solving, and Decision Making

Objectives

- Differentiate critical thinking, problem solving, decision making, and creative thinking.
- Describe the importance of critical thinking for nurses.
- Discuss characteristics, skills, and attitudes of critical thinking.
- Differentiate trial-and-error, intuition, nursing process, scientific method, and modified scientific method as problem-solving methods.
- Compare the research process (scientific method) with the problem-solving process (modified scientific method).
- Describe the decision making process.
- Discuss the value of creativity in critical thinking and decision making.
- Discuss the relationship between nursing process, critical thinking, problem-solving process, and decision-making process.
- Evaluate your own critical-thinking skills.

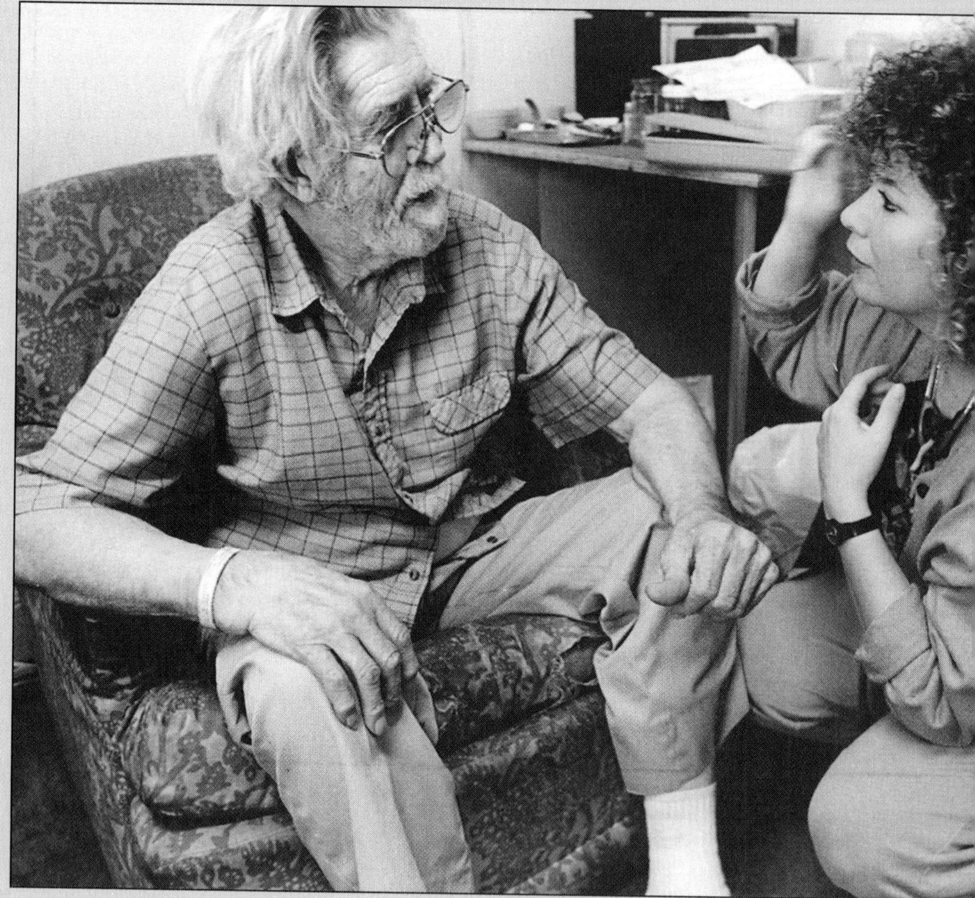

Nurses must be critical thinkers because of the nature of the discipline and the nature of their work. Nurses are expected to solve client problems by performing critical analysis of the factors associated with the problems. This critical analysis, or *critical thinking,* allows the nurse to make better decisions. Creativity in thinking, problem solving, and decision making can enhance the effectiveness of the solutions or decisions made. Thus critical thinking, problem solving, and decision making are interrelated processes, with creativity enhancing the result.

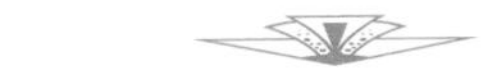

Critical Thinking

The thinking process that guides nursing practice must be organized, purposeful, and disciplined rather than random or undirected. This type of thinking is called critical thinking. **Critical thinking** is defined by Chaffee (1990, p. 37) as "making sense of our world by carefully examining the thinking process in order to clarify and improve our understanding." Paul (1988, pp. 2–3) describes critical thinking as "the art of thinking about thinking," that is, "the rational examination of ideas, inferences, assumptions, principles, arguments, conclusions, issues, statements, beliefs, and actions (Bandman & Bandman 1988, p. 5). Strader (1992, p. 226) describes critical thinking as "the process of examining underlying assumptions about current evidence and interpreting and evaluating arguments for the purpose of reaching a conclusion from a new perspective." The term *critical* means requiring careful judgment. The term *thinking* means to have an opinion, to reflect on (ponder), to call to mind (remember), to devise by thinking (devise a plan), to form a mental picture of (image), to reason. Therefore, critical thinking is a purposeful mental activity in which ideas are produced and evaluated, plans made, and desired conclusions determined. Strader (1992, p. 226) labels the conclusion reached as a **critical-thinking outcome.**

Critical Thinking in Nursing Practice

Because nursing decisions may profoundly affect the lives of clients and their families, nurses must think critically. But critical thinking is not limited to problem solving or decision making; professional nurses use critical thinking to make reliable observations, draw sound conclusions, create new information and ideas, evaluate lines of reasoning, and improve their self-knowledge. Critical thinking is considered so important to nursing that the National League for Nursing (NLN) has added it as a mandatory criterion for the accreditation of schools of nursing (NLN 1992). Nurses use their critical-thinking skills in a variety of ways:

- *Nurses use knowledge from other subjects and fields.* Using insight from one subject to shed light on another subject requires critical-thinking skills. Reilly and Oermann (1992, p. 217) state that "one cannot think critically about nursing without a basic knowledge of its concepts, theories, and content." Because nurses deal holistically with human responses, they must draw meaningful information from other subject areas in order to understand the meaning of client data and plan effective interventions. Nursing students are required to take courses in the biologic and social sciences and in the humanities so that they can acquire a strong foundation on which to build their nursing knowledge and skill. For example, the nurse might use knowledge from nutrition, physiology, and physics to promote wound healing and prevent further injury to a client with a decubitus ulcer.
- *Nurses deal with change in stressful environments.* Nurses work in rapidly changing situations. Treatments, medications, and technology change constantly, and a client's condition may change from minute to minute. Routine behaviors may therefore not be adequate to deal with the situation at hand. Familiarity with the routine for giving medications, for example, does not help the nurse deal with a client who is frightened of injections or with one who does not wish to take a medication. When unexpected situations arise, critical thinking enables the nurse to recognize important cues, respond quickly, and adapt interventions to meet specific client needs.
- *Nurses make important decisions.* During the course of a workday, nurses make vital decisions of many kinds. These decisions often determine the well-being of clients and even their very survival, so it is important that the decisions be sound. Nurses use critical-thinking skills to collect and interpret the information needed to make decisions. Nurses must, for example, use good judgment to decide which observations must be reported to the physician immediately and which can be noted in the client record for the physician to address later, during the routine visit with the client.

Characteristics of Critical Thinking

In addition to a strong knowledge base, other characteristics—summarized in Table 10–1 on page 187—are important for critical thinking.

RESEARCH NOTE

What Is the Nurse's Pattern of Personal Knowing in Clinical Decision Making?

A complex activity such as clinical decision making entails multiple patterns of knowing: empirical knowing, esthetic knowing, personal knowledge, and ethical knowing (see Chapter 1 for a discussion of nurses' ways of knowing). The authors interviewed nurses about their clinical decision making. These nurses stated that their success in making clinical decisions is highly dependent on the quality of interpersonal relationships with patients, peer nursing staff, and physicians. The dynamic of interpersonal relationships and the difficulties in establishing them are identified as important influencing factors in nurses' clinical decision making.

Implications: Nurses interact with clients, other nurses, physicians, and other health care providers when making clinical decisions. It is essential for nurses to establish relationships with these key players in order to gain the personal knowledge necessary for making clinical decisions.

Source: JM Jenks, The pattern of personal knowing in nurse clinical decision making, *Journal of Nursing Education,* November 1993, 32:399–405.

- *Critical thinking is reasonable and rational.* It is based on reason and logic rather than prejudice, preference, self-interest, or fear.
- *Critical thinking is reflective.* The person who thinks critically does not jump to conclusions or make a hurried decision; rather, the critical thinker takes the time to collect data and then think the matter through in a disciplined manner, weighing facts and evidence.
- *Critical thinking inspires an attitude of inquiry.* A critical thinker examines existing claims and statements to determine whether they are true or valid rather than blindly accepting them. Critical thinkers are constructively skeptical and ask questions. They ask, "Why?" and "How?" They want to know more. For example, the nurse who thinks critically wants to know how the body works and why it responds in the way it does to disease and to treatments and medications.
- *Critical thinking is autonomous thinking.* A critical thinker does not passively accept the beliefs of others but analyzes the issues and decides which authorities are credible. For example, the critical thinker examines beliefs acquired as a child, accepting them for rational reasons or rejecting those that have been held for the wrong reasons. Because they will neither accept nor reject a belief they do not understand, critical thinkers are not easily manipulated.
- *Critical thinking includes creative thinking.* Creative thinking is an intellectual process that creates original ideas by establishing relationships among or making connections between thoughts and concepts (Tappen 1989, p. 126). It involves the ability to transfer a concept to a new setting or apply it in a different way. Although it is more random than systematic, creative thinking is directed.
- *Critical thinking is fair thinking.* Critical thinkers attempt to remove bias and one-sidedness from their own thinking. They also attempt to recognize bias in the thinking of others and in accepted standards. Critical thinkers question suppositions and practices that are based on bias or prejudice. They examine reasons underlying choices and decisions. They are aware of their own values and feelings and are willing to examine the basis for them.
- *Critical thinking focuses on deciding what to believe or do.* Critical thinking is used to evaluate arguments and conclusions, relate new ideas or alternative courses of action, decide on a course of action, produce reliable observations, draw sound conclusions, and solve problems. Critical thinkers use accepted standards to examine their own views as well as the views of others. See the box on page 197 for suggested standards.

By using critical thinking, the nurse can differentiate facts, inferences, judgments, and opinions (Table 10–2 on page 188).

CRITICAL-THINKING ATTITUDES AND COGNITIVE SKILLS

Critical thinking is both an affective attitude and a cognitive reasoning process. To think critically, a person must not only have cognitive skills but also be disposed to use them. These **critical-thinking attitudes** (listed in the box on page 188) provide the motivation to use thinking skills carefully and fairly.

Critical-Thinking Attitudes Critical-thinking attitudes are interrelated and integrated, rather than used in isolation. For instance, it takes courage to acknowledge that one does not know something and to develop an inquiring attitude. Selected critical-thinking attitudes are discussed below.

Thinking Independently Critical thinking requires that individuals think for themselves. People acquire many beliefs as children, not because there are rational reasons for believing, but because there may be rewards for believing or because they do not question. As they mature and acquire knowledge, critical thinkers examine their beliefs,

Table 10–1 Characteristics of Critical Thinking

Characteristic	Explanation	Example
Is rational and reflective.	It is based on reasons and evidence rather than on preference or self-interest. Critical thinkers do not "jump to conclusions." They take the time to collect data, weigh the facts, and think the matter through.	Sarah decided to become a nurse after watching a film in which nurses were shown as attractive and heroic. Michelle, who thinks more critically, asked a counselor about the job opportunities available for nurses. She also talked to several nurses. After gathering and weighing her facts, Michelle decided to go to nursing school.
Involves healthy, constructive skepticism.	Critical thinkers do not accept or reject ideas unless they understand them. They do not mindlessly follow rules but seek to understand the rationale behind them, following those that make sense and working to improve those that do not.	When a salesperson insisted that a new intravenous tubing was better than that being used on Nurse Mackey's unit, Nurse Mackey asked, "What do you mean by 'better'? What information do you have to show that this is so?"
Is autonomous.	Critical thinkers are not easily manipulated. They think for themselves, rather than being led by their peer group.	No one in Lin's family had ever gone beyond high school. Although her sisters did not understand why she wanted to work so hard, Lin said, "I've thought it out, and this is what I want to do. I believe it will be worth the effort."
Includes creative thinking.	Critical thinkers create original ideas by finding connections among thoughts and concepts.	Nurse Wilson remembered a song his mother used to sing to him, and sang it to help comfort a frightened child in the hospital.
Is fair thinking.	Critical thinking is not biased or one-sided.	Nurse Maria Valdez, the unit manager, needed to make the schedule for the Christmas and New Year's holidays. Before responding to a nurse's request to be off for Christmas, she asked all staff members to submit their preference. Once she was able to determine that staffing was adequate for both holidays, she responded to the nurse's request.
Focuses on what to believe and do.	Critical thinking is used to decide on a course of action; make reliable observations; draw sound conclusions; solve problems; and evaluate policies, claims, and actions.	In the previous examples, Lin, Sarah, and Nurse Valdez decided what to do. Nurse Wilson creatively solved a problem. Nurse Mackey evaluated the salesperson's claim to decide what to believe and, ultimately, what to do.

holding those they can rationally support and rejecting those they cannot. Being an independent thinker does not mean ignoring what others think and acting on one's own; rather, following the ideas of others makes one dependent only if one accepts those ideas without question. Therefore, critical thinkers consider seriously a wide range of ideas, learn from them, and then make their own judgments about them. Nurses must be willing to challenge orders, activities, and rituals that have no rational support. For example, nurses traditionally have worn white, starched caps. Originally, nursing caps were head coverings or veils designed to cover the hair and to prevent hair or hair-borne contaminants from getting on patients and equipment. However, these head coverings evolved into small caps perched on the top or back of the head, no longer serving the original purpose. Eventually, most nurses and nursing institutions gave up the cap when they realized that there was no longer any functional reason for wearing them.

Humility Intellectual humility means having an awareness of the limits of one's own knowledge. Critical thinkers are willing to admit what they don't know; they are willing to seek new information and to rethink their con-

Table 10–2 Differentiating Types of Statements

Statement	Description	Example
Facts	Can be verified through investigation.	Blood pressure is affected by blood volume.
Inferences	Conclusions drawn from the facts. Go beyond facts to make a statement about something not currently known.	If blood volume is decreased (eg, in hemorrhagic shock), the blood pressure will drop.
Judgments	Evaluation of facts or information that reflect values or other criteria. A type of opinion.	It is harmful to the client's health if the blood pressure drops too low.
Opinions	Beliefs. Formed over time. Include judgments that may fit facts or be in error.	Nursing intervention can assist in maintaining the client's blood pressure within normal limits.

EXAMPLES OF CRITICAL-THINKING ATTITUDES AND COGNITIVE SKILLS

Attitudes

- Thinking independently
- Humility
- Courage
- Integrity
- Perseverance
- Empathy
- Fair-mindedness
- Exploring thoughts and feelings

Cognitive Skills

- Critical analysis
- Making valid inferences
- Differentiating fact from opinion
- Evaluating the credibility of information sources
- Reasoning inductively
- Reasoning deductively
- Clarifying concepts
- Recognizing assumptions

Source: Adapted from R Paul, *Critical Thinking* (Santa Rosa, CA: Foundation for Critical Thinking, 1993), pp. 129–30.

clusions in light of new knowledge. Critical thinking is impeded when one is unable to admit that one doesn't know. For example, a nurse working on a new unit may feel insecure and unsure about how to proceed. But as a critical thinker, the nurse would request a meeting with the nurse-manager to discuss professional strengths and areas of inexperience and to develop strategies for gaining the required new knowledge and skills. Admitting insecurity and requesting assistance when needed enables the nurse to obtain necessary support and to learn unit policies and procedures more rapidly. Admitting lack of knowledge or skill enables the nurse to gain new knowledge and skill and to grow professionally.

Courage With an attitude of courage, one is willing to consider and examine fairly one's own ideas or views, especially those to which one may have a strongly negative reaction. This type of courage comes from recognizing that beliefs are sometimes false or misleading. Values and beliefs are not always acquired "rationally." (Values are discussed in Chapter 11.) Rational beliefs are those which have been examined and found to be supported by solid reasons and data. After such examination, it is inevitable that some ideas previously held to be true are found to contain questionable elements and that some truth will emerge from ideas considered dangerous or false. Courage is needed to be true to new thinking in such cases, especially if social penalties for nonconformity are severe.

For example, Evelyn is a nurse in a community where there is a negative attitude toward homosexuality and acquired immune deficiency syndrome (AIDS). Her friends believe that the homosexual lifestyle is unacceptable and that AIDS is a punishment. In caring for clients with AIDS, Evelyn learns to view them as individuals rather than labels. Because some of her friends have difficulty accepting her view, Evelyn risks losing them. It requires courage for Evelyn to stand up for what she knows to be right.

Lack of courage can cause people to become resistant to change. Old beliefs can provide a sense of security. People may be resistant to new ideas because they produce discomfort. Chapter 20 describes strategies for dealing with resistance to change.

Integrity Intellectual integrity requires that individuals apply the same rigorous standards of proof to their own knowledge and beliefs as they apply to the knowledge and beliefs of others. Critical thinkers will question their own knowledge and beliefs as quickly and as thoroughly as they will challenge those of another. They are readily able to admit and evaluate inconsistencies within their own beliefs and between their own beliefs and those of another.

Perseverance Nurses who are critical thinkers show perseverance in finding effective solutions to client and nursing problems. This determination enables them to clarify concepts and sort out related issues, in spite of difficulties and frustrations. Confusion and frustration are uncomfortable, but critical thinkers resist the temptation to find a quick and easy answer. Important questions tend to be complex and confusing and therefore often require a great deal of thought and research.

Empathy *Empathy* is the ability to imagine oneself in the place of others in order to understand their actions and be sensitive to their feelings and beliefs. It is easy to misinterpret the words or actions of a person who is from a different cultural, religious, or socioeconomic background. It is also difficult to understand the beliefs or actions of a person experiencing a situation that one has never experienced. For example, it is difficult for a nurse to understand the feelings of a hospitalized client if the nurse has never been ill or hospitalized. Intellectual empathy is the ability to reason and understand from the other's perspective.

Fair-mindedness Critical thinkers are fair-minded, assessing all viewpoints with the same standards and not basing their judgments on personal or group bias or prejudice. Fair-mindedness helps one to consider opposing points of view and try to understand new ideas before rejecting or accepting them.

Exploring Thoughts and Feelings Although there is a distinct difference between thoughts and feelings, in reality they are inseparable. All feelings are based on some kind of thinking, and all thought creates some level of feeling. When confronted with someone else's feelings, critical thinkers consider what thoughts the person might have that contribute to those feelings. For example, when the critical thinker is dealing with an individual who is angry (feeling), they try to determine the reason (thought) for the anger. Critical thinkers ask similar questions about their own feelings. Critical thinkers try to identify whether their own feelings or the feelings of another are rational.

Critical Analysis Questions

- What is the central issue?
- What are the underlying assumptions?
- Is the evidence given valid?
  - Are stereotypes or clichés used?
  - Are emotional or biased arguments used?
  - Are the data adequate and verifiable?
  - Are important terms clearly defined?
  - Are the given data relevant?
  - Is the problem or issue correctly identified?
- Are the conclusions acceptable?
  - Is the conclusion accurate?
  - Is the conclusion applicable?
  - Is there any value conflict?

Source: RM Tappen, *Critical Thinking in Nursing Leadership and Management: Concepts and Practice*, 2d ed. (Philadelphia: FA Davis, 1989), p. 128. Used with permission.

Cognitive Skills Complex thinking processes such as critical analysis, problem solving, and decision making require the use of cognitive critical thinking skills. For example, when solving problems, nurses make inferences, differentiate facts from opinions, evaluate the credibility of information sources, and use a variety of other cognitive skills.

Decision making involves two types of reasoning: inductive and deductive. In **inductive reasoning,** generalizations are formed from a set of facts or observations. When viewed together, certain bits of information suggest a particular interpretation. For example, the nurse who observes that a client has dry skin, poor turgor, sunken eyes, and dark amber urine may make the generalization that the client is dehydrated. **Deductive reasoning,** by contrast, is reasoning from the general to the specific. The nurse starts with a conceptual framework—for example, Maslow's hierarchy of needs or a self-care framework—and makes descriptive interpretations of the client's condition in relation to that framework. For example, the nurse who uses the needs framework might categorize data and define the client's problems in terms of elimination, nutrition, or protection needs. In a more simplistic example, inductive reasoning is like looking at the piece of a jigsaw puzzle and attempting to describe the whole (without seeing a picture of the completed puzzle). As the puzzler puts more and more pieces together, the whole picture becomes clearer. In deductive reasoning, the puzzler sees the whole picture (from the box cover) and puts the puzzle together by organizing the pieces into border pieces, or colors, or some other grouping.

Critical thinking involves critical analysis. Tappen (1989, pp. 127–28) defines **critical analysis** as a set of questions one can apply to a particular situation or idea to determine essential information and ideas and discard superfluous information and ideas. The questions are not sequential steps; rather, they are a set of criteria for judging an idea. Not all questions will need to be applied to every situation, but one should be aware of all the questions in order to choose those questions appropriate to a given situation. The box at the top of the page lists critical analysis questions.

Critical thinking involves high-level cognitive processes that include problem solving, decision making, and creativity. Although the terms *problem solving* and *decision making* are sometimes used interchangeably, they are separate processes that are related in some situations. Solving a problem may require making a number of decisions, and making a decision may involve solving a number of problems. Effective solutions and decisions often require creative thinking.

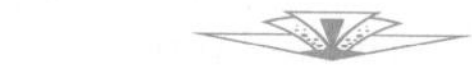

PROBLEM SOLVING

Nurses use critical thinking to rationally resolve problems related to direct client care. Nurse managers use critical thinking to resolve problems related to overall client care, unit administration, and staff interpersonal issues (see Chapter 20). Strader (1992, p. 228) defines problem solving as "the process used when a gap is perceived between an existing state (what *is* occurring) and a desired state (what *should be* occurring)." In problem solving, the nurse obtains information that clarifies the nature of the problem and suggests possible solutions. The nurse then carefully evaluates the possible solutions and chooses the best to implement. The situation is then carefully monitored over time to ensure its initial and continued effectiveness. The nurse does not discard the other solutions but holds them in reserve in the event that the first solution is not effective. The nurse may also encounter a similar problem in a different client situation where an alternative solution is determined to be the most effective. Therefore, problem solving for one situation contributes to the nurse's body of knowledge for problem solving in future similar situations.

PROBLEM-SOLVING METHODS

There are various approaches to problem solving. Five of the most commonly used are trial and error, intuition, the nursing process, the scientific method/research process, and the modified scientific method.

Trial and Error One way to solve problems is trial and error, in which a number of approaches are tried until a solution is found. However, without considering alternatives systematically, one cannot know why the solution works. Trial-and-error methods in nursing care can be dangerous because the client might suffer harm if an approach is inappropriate.

Intuition Intuition as a problem-solving method has not been considered either sound or legitimate. Rather, it has been viewed as a form of guessing and, as such, an inappropriate basis for nursing decisions. However, according to Benner and Tanner (1987), intuition appears to be an essential and legitimate aspect of clinical judgment acquired through knowledge and experience. Intuitive judgment in nursing is developed through clinical experience with similar types of situations. In other words, nurses develop expertise in a specialty area, such as cardiovascular nursing, through continuous and meaningful exposure to clients who have experienced cardiovascular problems.

Intuition is based on experience and knowledge. The nurse must first have the knowledge base necessary to practice in the clinical area then use that knowledge in clinical practice. Clinical experience allows the nurse to recognize cues and patterns and begin to make correct decisions.

The intuitive method of problem solving is gaining recognition as part of nursing practice. It is not a valid method of decision making for novices or students, however, because they usually lack the knowledge base and clinical experience on which to make a valid judgment.

Nursing Process The nursing process is the systematic method of planning, providing, and evaluating nursing care. It is the method used by nurses to solve clients' problems. See Chapters 5 through 8.

Scientific Method/Research Process The research process is a formalized, logical, systematic approach to solving problems. The classic scientific method is most useful when the researcher is working in a controlled situation. The steps in the research process are as follows:

1. *State a research question or problem.* The investigator's initial task is narrowing a broad area of interest to a circumscribed problem that specifies exactly the intent of the study.
2. *Define the purpose of or the rationale for the study.* The investigator indicates why the research question is important and what use the answer will serve.
3. *Review the related literature.* Before progressing with the development of the research design, the investigator finds out what is already known about the problem. A thorough review of the literature provides the foundation on which to build new knowledge. This also enables the investigator to develop a theoretical framework for the research. A theoretical framework is the way in which the investigator relates the existing knowledge of concepts, theories, and research findings to the study question and purpose.
4. *Formulate hypotheses and define variables.* **Hypotheses** are statements of the relationship between two or more concepts. In research, these concepts are called **variables,** because they can vary or take on different values (eg, temperature, blood pressure, weight). Some studies are intended to develop hypotheses, and others are intended to test hypotheses using statistical

procedures. Stating hypotheses requires not only sufficient knowledge about a topic to predict the outcome of the study but also definitions that specify the variables under investigation in measurable terms. Hypothesis generation is one example of a cognitive critical-thinking skill being used in a high-level thinking process.

5. *Select a plan or method to test the hypothesis (the research design).* A research design is a well-formulated, systematic, and controlled plan for finding answers to study questions. Everything from methods of data collection through methods of data analysis should be spelled out in the research design.
6. *Select the population, sample, and setting.* At this stage, the researcher chooses the study population, selects a sample, and decides on the setting where the sample can be located. The **population** includes all possible members of the group to be studied. The **sample** is that segment of the population from whom data will actually be collected.
7. *Conduct a pilot study.* A pilot study is sometimes done to help the researcher discover the strengths and weaknesses of the intended design, sample size, and data-collection instrument of the larger project.
8. *Collect the data.* The scientific method is characterized by a reliance on **empirical data,** that is, information collected from the observable world. These data are used to make statements or conclusions about what is observed. Data sources may be people, documents, or laboratory materials. Data-collection instruments include interviews, questionnaires, physiologic tests, and psychologic tests.
9. *Analyze the data.* In this step, the collected data are reorganized to relate them to the study question, research objectives, or stated hypotheses. The most important part of this step is to have a procedural plan in mind, have the requisite skills for analysis (such as knowledge of statistics), and realize that analysis provides the answers to the original research questions. Critical-thinking skills are essential for analyzing research data, as the investigator carefully studies the research outcomes to make valid conclusions.
10. *Communicate conclusions and implications.* Implicit in conducting research is the requirement to share the knowledge generated with others, either through publication in professional journals or by reporting results verbally at professional conferences. Communicating the conclusions, interpreting the meaning and implications of the findings, recognizing the study's limitations, and suggesting directions for further study culminate the research process.

Although the scientific method is used in nursing research, there are differences between conducting formal research in a controlled setting and solving clinical problems in the nurse's practice setting. Three of these differences are as follows:

- The nurse's time frame is often shorter than the researcher's. The researcher may take months or even years to carry out a study, whereas a nurse, for example, must give immediate help to a client in pain.
- The nurse's environment makes complete scientific control impossible, whereas the laboratory scientist strives to establish precise scientific controls in experiments. For example, a home care nurse striving to help regulate a client's diabetes through diet and insulin injections can outline a regimen and teach the client to administer insulin but has no control over whether the client will follow instructions later.
- The nurse deals with multiple, complex problems, especially because most clients have more than one problem when they are ill. The scientist often isolates and studies a single aspect of a problem.

The scientific method, therefore, must be adapted for nursing practice. The nurse requires a problem-solving system that is scientific, systematic, yet flexible enough to deal with the complex situations in the health care system.

Modified Scientific Method Health professionals require a modified approach of the scientific method for solving problems. This modified scientific problem solving method is used in the nursing process as well as the medical process. Strader (1992) describes seven steps in the problem solving process.

1. *Define the problem.* A problem is defined as the difference between what is occurring and what is desired. For example, when a client is experiencing pain (what is occurring), the nurse wants to assist the client by relieving the pain (what is desired).
2. *Gather information.* Problem solving begins with collecting relevant information or data. A part of information gathering is the search for additional facts that provide clues to the scope and solution of the problem. Sources of information available for nurses include clients and their families, other health professionals, textbooks, nursing and other professional journals, and other professional literature. If the information search is careful and thorough, the nurse will be more effective in accomplishing the goal and be better able to evaluate the effects of the solution. In the previous example, the information that the nurse needs includes the following:
   a. Location of the pain
   b. Description of the pain
   c. How long the client has had the pain
   d. Whether the pain is related to anything else (eg, surgery, exercise, injury)

e. Whether the client has found any specific type of pain relief to be effective in the past (Additional information nurses needed in assessing pain can be found in Chapter 36.)

3. *Analyze the information.* The information is first organized in an orderly fashion and then analyzed for its relevance to the situation. Strader suggests the following strategies for organizing data:
   a. Categorize information in order of reliability.
   b. List information from most important to least important.
   c. Organize information into a time sequence; for example, in the above situation, the nurse needs to know when the client first experienced the pain.
   d. Identify information in terms of cause and effect. Is A causing B, or vice versa? For example, in the above situation, what other associated factors were occurring either prior to or at the same time as the pain experience?
   e. Organize information into categories, such as nursing model formats, physiologic factors, psychosocial factors, or developmental factors.
4. *Develop solutions.* As the nurse analyzes the information, possible solutions will emerge. Depending on the nurse's knowledge and experience with the situation, various alternative strategies for resolving the problem will be suggested. Developing alternative solutions makes it possible to combine the best parts of several solutions into one best response. This also provides a back-up solution to try if the first cannot be implemented or is ineffective.
5. *Make a decision.* After identifying several possible solutions, the nurse must choose the one most appropriate to the situation. Factors that influence the decision include choosing the solution that has the fewest undesirable consequences. In the above example, the nurse knows that narcotic medications can depress respiratory function and are addictive. The nurse may request that the physician order a nonnarcotic pain medication for the client with chronic back pain who has a chronic respiratory disease. The nurse must be aware that solutions that require a change in behavior may be met with resistance. In such cases the nurse should encourage participation in the process to minimize resistance. Chapter 20 provides more information about the change process.
6. *Implement the decision.* The nurse implements the chosen solution.
7. *Evaluate the solution.* During and following implementation, the nurse must evaluate the response to the solution to determine its effectiveness. In evaluating, the nurse determines whether the desired outcome has been achieved. The nurse also observes for any unexpected negative outcomes. If the solution presents a problem, the nurse can review the alternative solutions previously identified.

Table 10–3 Comparison Between the Research Process and the Modified Scientific Method

Research Process (Scientific Method)	Modified Scientific Method
State a research question or problem.	Define the problem.
Define the purpose of or the rationale for the study.	
Review related literature.	Gather information.
Formulate hypotheses and defining variables.	Analyze the information.
Select method to test hypotheses.	Develop solutions.
Select population, sample, and setting.	
Conduct pilot study.	Make a decision.
Collect the data.	Implement the decision.
Analyze the data.	Evaluate the decision.
Communicate conclusions and implications.	

Table 10–3 compares the research process or scientific method with the modified scientific method. Critical thinking is important in all problem-solving processes as the nurse evaluates all potential solutions to a given problem and makes a decision to select the most appropriate solution for that situation.

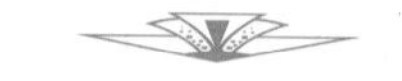

DECISION MAKING

Tschikota (1993, p. 389) states that "effective clinical decision making is critical to the future of professional nursing practice." Nurses make decisions in the course of solving problems, for example, in each step of the nursing process. Decision making, however, is also used in situations that do not involve problem solving. Nurses make value decisions (eg, to keep client information confidential); time management decisions (eg, taking clean linens to the client's room at the same time as the medication in order to save steps); scheduling decisions (eg, to bathe the client before visiting hours); and priority decisions (eg, which interventions are most urgent and which can be delegated).

Table 10–4 Elements of Decision Making

Element	Definition	Example
Cue	A piece of information or data	Vital signs, laboratory values, client history, signs and/or symptoms
Hypothesis	A projected or proposed possibility; may concern what is wrong with the client, what the nurse/doctor/client might do, think, or feel, or what possible doctor's orders or hospital policies might be used; often introduced by subjects with such words as *probably, might, if, could be, maybe, perhaps, sounds like,* or *looks like*	"Possible infection." "Possible allergic reaction." "Probable myocardial infarction." "If we change the intravenous flow rate, the blood pressure might change."
Knowledge base	Information, correct or incorrect, that is used as rationale or support for any statements made by the subject	"*Because the client has a fever,* he probably has an infection." "*When we increase the intravenous flow rate, we add to circulating volume;* therefore, the blood pressure should change."
Nursing intervention	Any proposed nursing action	"Increase the intravenous flow rate." "Administer prn acetominophen for fever."
Search	Indication of a desire for additional or supplementary information about the situation	"I think we need to know what the client's hemoglobin and hematocrit are." "Do we know what the client was doing prior to experiencing the pain?"
Assumption	A conclusion for which there is insufficient information; may lead to a search	"I believe the client is experiencing depression." (This could be based on observation of behavior without an adequate history to support the statement.)

Source: Adapted from S Tschikota, The clinical decision-making processes of student nurses, *Journal of Nursing Education,* November 1993, 32:393. Used with permission.

Decision making is a critical-thinking process for choosing the best actions to meet a desired goal. **Decision making** is defined by Strader (1992, p. 233) as "the process of establishing criteria by which alternative courses of action are developed and selected." Decisions must be made whenever there are several mutually exclusive choices. For example, the individual who wishes to become a nurse in the United States has several possible courses of action: a diploma program, an associate degree program, or a baccalaureate program. Prospective students must choose. Therefore, they must evaluate the different types of programs, as well as personal circumstances, to make a decision appropriate to their situation.

Nurses must make decisions and assist clients to make decisions. When faced with several client needs at the same time, the nurse must decide which client to assist first. When a client is trying to make a decision about what course of treatment to follow, the nurse may need to provide the client with information or resources to assist the client in making a decision. Nurses must make decisions in their own personal and professional lives. For example, the nurse must decide whether to work in a hospital or community setting, whether to join a professional association, and whether to carry professional liability insurance.

According to Schaefer (1974, p. 1852) three conditions must prevail in decision making: freedom, rationality, and voluntarity. *Freedom* means that the individual makes the decision without pressure from others and has the authority to make the decision. *Rationality* means that the best or optimal decision is made and that it is consistent with the decision maker's values and preferences. Rationality involves both deliberation and judgment. *Voluntarity* is making a choice voluntarily.

Tschikota (1993) states that clinical decision making is composed of six elements: cue, hypothesis, knowledge base, nursing intervention, search, and assumption (Table 10–4). Nurses use various combinations of these decision-making elements as part of their mental processing in making decisions.

Table 10–5 Comparison Between the Nursing Process, Decision-Making Process, Research Process, and Modified Scientific Method

Nursing Process	Decision-Making Process*	Research Process (Scientific Method)	Modified Scientific Method (Problem-Solving Method)
Assess	Identify the purpose	State a research question or problem	Define the problem
		Define the purpose of or the rationale for the study	
		Review related literature	Gather information
Diagnose		Formulate hypotheses and defining variables	Analyze the information
Plan	Set the criteria	Select method to test hypotheses	Develop solutions
	Weight the criteria	Select population, sample, and setting	Make a decision
	Seek alternatives	Conduct pilot study, if needed	
Implement	Test alternatives	Collect the data	Implement the decision
	Troubleshoot	Analyze the data	Evaluate the decision
Evaluate	Evaluate the action	Communicate conclusions and implications	

*The Decision-Making Process parallels each of the other processes but also is used during each step of the different processes.

Strader (1992) describes a seven-step decision making process:

1. *Identify the purpose.* In this step, the nurse identifies why a decision is needed and what needs to be determined.
2. *Set the criteria.* When the nurse sets the criteria for decision making, three questions must be answered: what needs to be achieved, what needs to be preserved, and what needs to be avoided. For example, in the previous example of a client with pain, the criteria would be as follows:
   a. What needs to be achieved? Relief of pain.
   b. What needs to be preserved? Physical functioning, cognitive functioning, psychologic functioning, client comfort.
   c. What needs to be avoided? Central nervous system depression, respiratory depression, nausea.
3. *Weight the criteria.* In this step, the decision maker sets priorities or ranks activities or services in order of importance from least important to most important as they relate to the specific situation. Because the weighting is specific to the situation, an activity may be ranked as most important in one situation and of less importance in another situation.
4. *Seek alternatives.* After establishing and weighting the criteria in the previous steps, the decision maker identifies all possible ways to meet the criterion. In clinical situations, the alternatives may be selected from a range of nursing interventions or client care strategies.
5. *Test alternatives.* The nurse analyzes the alternatives to ensure that there is an objective rationale in relation to the established criteria for choosing one strategy over another.
6. *Troubleshoot.* In troubleshooting, the nurse tries to determine what might go wrong as a result of a decision and develops plans to prevent, minimize, or overcome any problems.
7. *Evaluate the action.* In evaluating the strategies used, the nurse determines how effective they were and whether they achieved the initial purpose.

The research process, the problem-solving process, and the nursing process all share similarities. The nurse uses decision making in all of the steps of these processes. Table 10–5 compares the steps of these different processes.

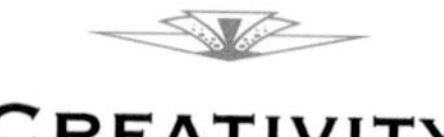

CREATIVITY

Creativity, or original thinking, is a major component of critical thinking. When nurses incorporate creativity into their thinking, they are able to find unique (one-of-a-kind) solutions to unique (one-of-a-kind) problems. **Creative thinking** is defined by Reilly and Oermann (1992, p. 217) as thinking that results in the development of new ideas and products. Creativity in problem solving and decision making is described by Strader (1992, p. 243) as the ability to develop and implement new and better solutions.

Strader (1992) describes four stages in the creative process: preparation, incubation, insight, and verification.

During the *preparation stage*, the creative thinker gathers information related to the problem or concern. During the *incubation phase*, the creative thinker unconsciously considers and works on possible solutions or decisions. All possibilities, both old and new, are considered during this phase. Old possibilities that are considered may include a creative application of an effective solution used in a previous situation that was similar in nature to the present situation. During the *insight stage*, appropriate solutions emerge and are developed, and the solution believed to be most appropriate is implemented. Finally, during the *verification stage*, the implemented solution is evaluated for its effectiveness.

During the first three stages, unconscious, intuitive, and creative thinking occurs that can result in a unique solution to the problem at hand. Creative thinking is required when the nurse encounters a new situation or a client situation where traditional interventions are not effective. For example, Nurse Ned Steele, a pediatric home health nurse, is caring for 9-year-old Pauline, who has ineffective respirations following abdominal surgery. The physician has ordered incentive spirometry (a treatment device that promotes alveolar expansion). Pauline is frightened by the equipment and tires quickly during the treatments. Ned offers Pauline a bottle of blow bubbles and a blowing wand. Pauline is delighted with blowing bubbles. He knows that the respiratory effort in blowing bubbles will promote alveolar expansion and suggests that Pauline blow bubbles between incentive spirometry treatments.

Creative thinkers must have knowledge of the problem. They must have assessed the present problem and be knowledgeable about the underlying facts and principles that apply. For example, in the previous situation, Ned knows the anatomy and physiology of respiratory function and is aware of the purpose of incentive spirometry. He also understands pediatric growth and development. In trying to assist Pauline, he builds on his knowledge and comes up with a creative solution (Figure 10–1). Strader (1992, p. 244) describes creative thinkers as

- Able to generate ideas rapidly.
- Flexible and spontaneous; that is, they are able to discard one viewpoint for another or change directions in thinking rapidly and easily.
- Able to provide original solutions to problems.
- Preferring complex thought processes to simple and easily understood ones.
- Independent and self-confident, even when under pressure.
- Exhibiting distinct individualism.

Brainstorming is a creative thinking technique used by groups for eliciting ideas, decisions, or solutions to problems. Brainstorming takes the form of concentrated, uninhibited discussion among a small group of knowledgeable persons. Creative thinkers ask questions such as "What if?" or "Why don't we try something different?" Often, the solutions proposed by creative thinkers seem wild and impossible. Brainstorming has been criticized as expensive, time-consuming, and superficial (Strader 1992, p. 245); however, the brainstorming outcomes can be filtered through critical thinking so that effective solutions are identified.

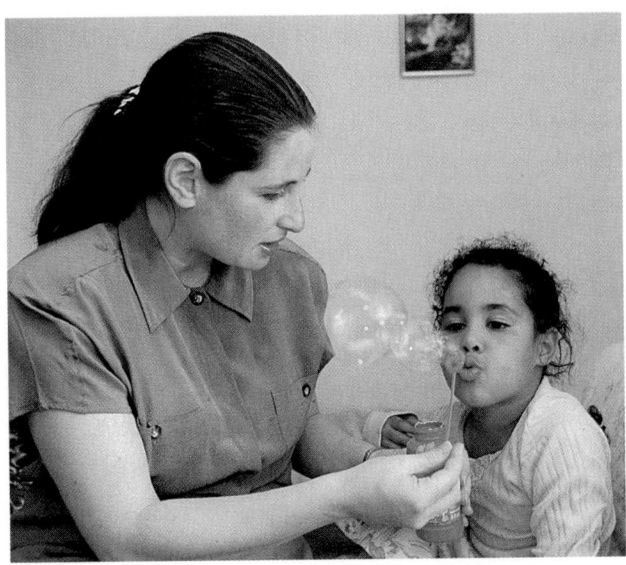

Figure 10–1 The nurse finds a creative solution to help a child improve lung expansion.

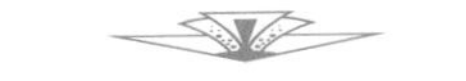

CRITICAL THINKING AND THE NURSING PROCESS

Nurses use a variety of critical thinking skills to carry out the nursing process (Chapters 5 through 8). The nursing process, however, does not necessarily require the nurse to use all the possible critical-thinking skills and attitudes. As discussed in Chapter 5, the nursing process is a problem-solving method. Table 10–6 on page 196 provides examples of critical thinking in the nursing process.

Assessing In the assessment phase of the nursing process, nurses gather data about the client and validate what the client says with what they observe. They must make reliable observations and distinguish relevant from irrelevant and important from unimportant data. These are basic critical-thinking skills. Assessing requires more complex thinking skills as well. For example, nurses organize and categorize relevant, important cues in some useful manner—usually according to a theory-based nursing framework (see Chapter 3).

Table 10–6 Examples of Critical Thinking in the Nursing Process

Nursing Process Activity	Critical-Thinking Skills
Assessing	Making reliable observations
	Distinguishing relevant from irrelevant data
	Distinguishing important from unimportant data
	Validating data
	Organizing data
	Categorizing data
Diagnosing	Finding patterns and relationships among cues
	Making inferences
	Stating the problem
	Suspending judgment
	Making interdisciplinary connections
Planning	Forming valid generalizations
	Transferring knowledge from one situation to another
	Making interdisciplinary connections
	Developing evaluative criteria
	Hypothesizing
Implementing	Applying knowledge and principles
	Testing hypotheses
Evaluating	Deciding whether hypotheses are correct
	Making criterion based evaluations

Source: Adapted from JM Wilkinson, *Nursing Process in Action: A Critical Thinking Approach* (Redwood City, CA: Addison-Wesley Nursing, 1991), p. 29. Used with permission.

Diagnosing When making nursing diagnoses, nurses examine the data they have organized to look for patterns and relationships among the various cues and make sound inferences about them. Nurses make inferences when they tentatively assign meaning to data they see, hear, or otherwise sense. For example, when the nurse observes that the client is grimacing and moving about restlessly in bed, the nurse's knowledge and previous experience suggest that these symptoms are associated with pain. This is only an inference and, until verified, not a fact.

Critical thinkers are careful to suspend judgment when they do not have enough data. This is what nurses do when they write a "possible" rather than an "actual" or "potential" nursing diagnosis. They weight the data and decide whether their conclusions are warranted, based on the data they have. In the preceding example, the nurse needs more data to be certain the inference is correct. The nurse should question the client to obtain further information about the client's behavior.

Critical thinking requires conceptualization. This skill is important in diagnosing, because each of the diagnostic statements in the North American Nursing Diagnosis Association (NANDA) taxonomy is actually a concept. **Concepts** are mental images of reality that enable one to make sense of the world by organizing it into patterns. **Conceptualization** is the intellectual process of forming a concept. People use concepts to distinguish one kind of thing from another, relate one kind of thing to another, and describe things to people who have the same understanding of the concept. When a nurse reports that a client has **Altered oral mucous membranes,** other nurses immediately have an idea of the cluster of symptoms associated with that NANDA diagnosis. Similarly, when observing that a client has a coated tongue, dry mouth, and oral lesions, the nurse would readily associate these signs with the concept of **Altered oral mucous membranes.**

Planning When planning care with clients, nurses use knowledge and reasoning to develop realistic client outcomes that are used to evaluate the effectiveness of their care. This is the same as developing and applying evaluative criteria, another skill in critical thinking, problem solving, and decision making. Another critical-thinking skill used during planning is forming valid generalizations, explanations, and predictions.

When planning nursing interventions and providing their rationales, nurses must make interdisciplinary connections. For example, nurses use their knowledge of physiology, psychology, and sociology to choose appropriate nursing orders and provide rationale for them. And finally, nurses use critical-thinking and problem-solving skills to hypothesize (research process) that particular nursing interventions will relieve the client's problem and help achieve the stated health goals.

Implementing In the implementation phase, nurses apply knowledge and principles from nursing and related courses to each specific client situation. The ability to apply, not simply memorize, principles is a mark of critical thinking. For example, when the obstetrics unit is short staffed, a float nurse, Ann Motta, is assigned there even though she has minimal experience in newborn care. Ann knows the principles that heat is lost through evaporation and that normal newborns are at risk for cold stress because of their physical characteristics. Although she has not bathed a newborn since nursing school and is not familiar with unit procedures, she knows to prevent cold stress by uncovering only the parts she is bathing and by drying the infant well.

Carrying out the nursing orders in the implementation step can also be compared to the skill of hypothesis testing that occurs in the scientific method. The nursing orders must be translated into action (or "tested") to determine whether they were successful.

Evaluating In the evaluation phase, nurses use new observations to determine whether the predetermined client outcomes have been met—that is, whether nursing orders were successful. Use of criterion-based evaluation is a critical-thinking skill. In the preceding example, Ann Motta realizes she must evaluate the results of her actions—that is, she must determine whether she has kept the infant warm enough. The obvious criterion to measure this is that the infant's body temperature will be at least 98 F. Though no one has told her to do so, Ann takes the infant's temperature to evaluate whether her goal of avoiding cold stress has been met. Even without knowing the unit's routine for obtaining vital signs, she realizes the importance of evaluating and maintaining the baby's body temperature.

STANDARDS FOR CRITICAL THINKERS?

Critical Thinkers

- Explore the thinking that underlies their emotions and feelings
- Suspend judgment when they lack sufficient data
- Develop criteria for evaluation and apply them fairly and accurately
- Evaluate the credibility of sources they use to justify their beliefs
- Make interdisciplinary connections and use insights from one subject or experience to illuminate and correct other subjects
- Differentiate facts from opinions
- Examine assumptions that underlie their thoughts and behavior
- Distinguish relevant from irrelevant data and important from trivial data
- Make plausible inferences and distinguish conclusions from the reasoning that supports them

Source: Adapted from R Paul, What, then, is critical thinking? From the Eighth Annual and Sixth International Conference on Critical Thinking and Educational Reform (Rohnert Park, CA: The Center for Critical Thinking and Moral Critique, Sonoma State University, 1988).

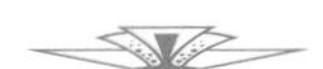

DEVELOPING SKILLS OF CRITICAL THINKING, PROBLEM SOLVING, AND DECISION MAKING

After gaining an idea of what it means to think critically, solve problems, and make decisions, nurses need to become aware of their own thinking style and abilities. Acquiring critical-thinking skills and a critical attitude then becomes a matter of practice. Critical thinking is not an "either-or" phenomenon; it exists on a continuum, along which people develop and use it more or less effectively. Some people make better evaluations than others; some people believe information from nearly any source; and still others seldom believe anything without carefully evaluating the credibility of the information. Critical thinking is not easy. (See the box above for standards that can help nurses evaluate and develop their critical-thinking skills and attitudes.) Solving problems and making decisions is risky. Sometimes the outcome is not what was desired. With effort, however, everyone can achieve some level of critical thinking to become effective problem solvers and decision makers.

CHAPTER HIGHLIGHTS

- Critical thinking is a purposeful mental activity in which ideas are produced and evaluated and judgments are made.
- Nurses use critical thinking as they apply knowledge from other subjects and fields to nursing practice, deal with change in stressful environments, and make important decisions related to client care.
- Critical thinking is reasonable, rational, reflective, autonomous, creative, and fair. Critical thinking inspires an attitude of inquiry that focuses on deciding what to believe or do.
- Critical thinkers have certain attitudes: autonomy, humility, courage, integrity, perseverance, empathy, and fair-mindedness.

- Critical thinking consists of high-level cognitive processes that include problem solving, decision making, and creativity.
- There are several problem solving methods: trial and error, intuition, the nursing process, the scientific method, and the modified scientific method. Nurses use the scientific method or research process when they participate in nursing and health research.
- The steps of the modified scientific method, when used as a problem-solving process, include defining the problem, gathering information related to the problem, analyzing the information, developing possible solutions, making a decision, implementing the decision, and evaluating the effectiveness of the solution.
- Decisions must be made whenever there are several mutually exclusive choices. Nurses must make decisions in both their personal and professional lives. The steps of the decision-making process include identifying the purpose of the decision, setting the criteria, weighting the criteria, seeking alternatives, testing alternatives, troubleshooting, and evaluating the action.
- Creativity is a major component of critical thinking that enables nurses to find unique (one-of-a-kind) solutions for unique (one-of-a-kind) problems.
- Nurses use critical thinking in applying the nursing process and achieving the purpose of nursing.
- Nursing process and critical thinking are interrelated and interdependent, but not identical. Both involve problem solving, decision making and creativity.
- Everyone has at least some level of critical thinking skill, and that skill can be developed with practice.

READINGS AND REFERENCES

SUGGESTED READINGS

Ruggiero, VR. 1989. *Critical Thinking.* Rapid City, SD: College Survival.
This small book presents the fundamentals of critical thinking in a combined text-workbook format. Chapters address such subjects as knowing one's attitudes and values, facts and opinions, errors of perception, unraveling arguments, and errors of judgment.

Wilkinson, J. 1992. *Nursing Process in Action: A Critical Thinking Approach.* Redwood City, CA: Addison-Wesley Nursing.
This interactive text provides exercises to develop the reader's critical-thinking skills in applying the nursing process to simulated and real client situations.

RELATED RESEARCH

Brooks, KL. March/April 1992. Professionalism vs. general critical thinking abilities of senior nursing students in four types of nursing curricula. *Journal of Professional Nursing* 8:87–95.

Saarmann, L, Freitas, L, Rapps, J, and Riegel, B. January/February 1992. The relationship of education to critical thinking ability and values among nurses: Socialization into professional nursing. *Journal of Professional Nursing* 8:26–34.

Tschikota, S. November, 1993. The clinical decision making processes of student nurses. *Journal of Nursing Education* 32:389–98.

SELECTED REFERENCES

Bandman, EL and Bandman, B. 1988. *Critical Thinking in Nursing.* Norwalk, CT: Appleton & Lange.

Benner, P and Tanner, C. January 1987. How expert nurses use intuition. *American Journal of Nursing* 87:23–31.

Chaffee, J. 1990. *Thinking Critically.* 3d ed. Boston: Houghton Mifflin.

Jenks, JM. November 1993. The pattern of personal knowing in nurse clinical decision making. *Journal of Nursing Education* 32:399–405.

Kramer, MK. November 1993. Concept clarification and critical thinking: Integrated processes. *Journal of Nursing Education* 32:406–14.

National League for Nursing. 1992. *Criteria for the Evaluation of Baccalaureate and Higher Degree Programs in Nursing.* 5th ed. New York: NLN.

Paul, R. 1988. What, then, is critical thinking? From the Eighth Annual and Sixth International Conference on Critical Thinking and Educational Reform. Rohnert Park, CA: The Center for Critical Thinking and Moral Critique, Sonoma State University.

Pless, BS and Clayton, GM. November 1993. Clarifying the concept of critical thinking in nursing. *Journal of Nursing Education* 32:425–28.

Polit, DF and Hungler, BP. 1989. *Essentials of Nursing Research: Methods, Appraisal, and Utilization.* 2d ed. Philadelphia: Lippincott.

Reilly, DE and Oermann, MH. 1992. Cognitive learning in the clinical setting. In *Clinical Teaching in Nursing Education.* 2d ed. pp. 207–46. New York: National League for Nursing.

Schaefer, J. October 1974. The interrelatedness of decision making and the nursing process. *American Journal of Nursing* 74:1852–55.

Strader, M. 1992. Critical thinking. In Sullivan, EJ and Decker, PJ. pp. 225–48. *Effective Management in Nursing.* 3d ed. Redwood City, CA: Addison-Wesley Nursing.

Tappen, RM. 1989. Critical thinking. In *Nursing Leadership and Management: Concepts and Practice.* 2d ed. pp. 124–33. Philadelphia: FA Davis.

Tschikota, S. November 1993. The clinical decision-making processes of student nurses. *Journal of Nursing Education* 32:389–98.

Wilkinson, JM. 1992. *Nursing Process in Action: A Critical Thinking Approach.* Redwood City, CA: Addison-Wesley Nursing.

Wilson, HS. 1989. *Research in Nursing.* 2d ed. Redwood City, CA: Addison-Wesley Nursing.

UNIT

3

PROFESSIONAL ACCOUNTABILITY AND ADVOCACY

STUDENT PROFILE

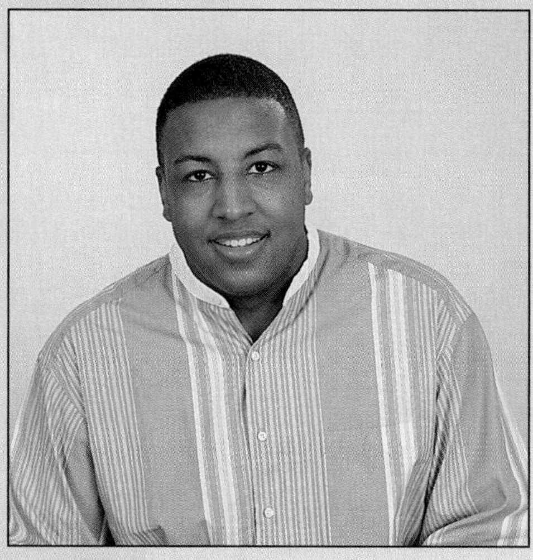

NAME	Brian McCain
SCHOOL OF NURSING	St Francis School of Nursing, Pittsburgh, Pennsylvania
HOMETOWN	Pittsburgh

WHY DID YOU ENTER THE FIELD OF NURSING?
I had planned to be an attorney, but I found that numbers bored me. My sister suggested I try nursing because I'm such a people person.

WHY DO YOU THINK THIS IS A GOOD TIME TO BE IN NURSING?
We will be the first group of nurses to have the opportunity to pioneer the new reform. Being part of the reform is really exciting. It makes you feel like what you are doing is really worthwhile.

WHAT QUALITIES DO YOU THINK ARE NECESSARY TO BE A GOOD NURSE?
Compassion, discipline, and organization.

WHAT HAS BEEN YOUR MOST GRATIFYING MOMENT AS A STUDENT NURSE?
I had a 21-year-old client with preeclampsia and cerebral hemorrhage, and she came back. It was really something. We didn't know whether or not she'd make it, and when she came back the joy was pretty intense.

WHAT ADVICE WOULD YOU GIVE A NEW STUDENT?
Stick with it!

11 Ethics and Values

Objectives

- Explain how to recognize a moral issue.
- Define the terms *ethics*, *bioethics*, and *nursing ethics*.
- Discuss sources of ethical problems in nursing.
- Explain the difference between decision-focused problems and action-focused problems.
- Differentiate the following moral frameworks: deontology, teleology, intuitionism, and the ethic of caring.
- When presented with an ethical situation, identify the moral principles involved.
- Explain the uses and limitations of professional codes of ethics.
- Explain how cognitive development, values, moral frameworks, and codes of ethics affect moral decisions.
- Explain how nurses acquire and clarify personal and professional values.
- Discuss the concept of an integrity-preserving compromise.
- Describe the elements of selected ethical issues nurses encounter.
- Discuss nursing roles and responsibilities with regard to ethics.

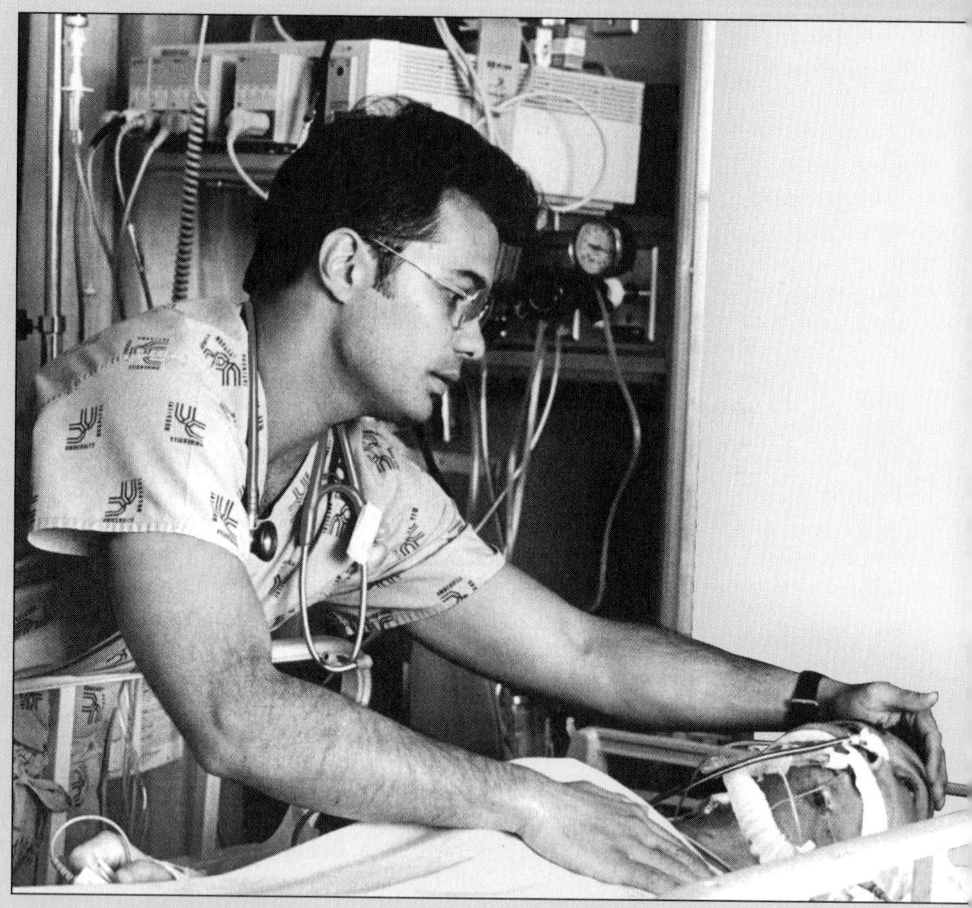

Because nurses deal with the most fundamental human events—birth, death, and suffering—they encounter many ethical issues surrounding these sensitive areas. Nurses must decide what their own moral actions ought to be in these situations, and because of the special nature of the nurse–client relationship, they must support and sustain clients and families who are facing hard moral choices. As client advocates and as continuously present caregivers, nurses must also support clients who are living out the consequences of choices made for and about them by others. Nurses can make better moral decisions by thinking in advance about their beliefs and values and about the kinds of problems they may encounter in caring for their clients.

Table 11–1 Comparison of Morals and Ethics

Morals	Principles and rules of right conduct
	Private, personal
	Commitment to principles and values are usually defended in daily life
Ethics	Formal reasoning process used to determine right conduct
	Professionally and publicly stated
	Inquiry or study of principles and values
	Process of questioning, and perhaps changing, one's morals

ETHICS, VALUES, AND MORALITY

The term **ethics** is derived from the Greek *ethos*, meaning custom or character. It has several meanings in common usage. First, it refers to a method of inquiry that assists people to understand the morality of human behavior (ie, it is the study of morality). When used in this sense, ethics is an activity; it is a way of looking at or investigating certain issues about human behavior. Second, ethics refers to the practices or beliefs of a certain group (ie, physicians' ethics, nursing ethics). Third, ethics refers to the expected standards of behavior of a particular group. These standards are described in the group's code of professional conduct. Nurses are expected to maintain certain ethical standards in their nursing practice. (See Codes of Ethics later in this chapter.) **Bioethics** is ethics as applied to life (ie, to life and death decision making). Nursing ethics refers to ethical issues involved in nursing practice.

Values are freely chosen, enduring beliefs or attitudes about the worth of a person, object, idea, or action. Freedom, courage, family, and dignity are examples of values, and form a basis for behavior; a person's real values are shown by consistent patterns of behavior. Once you are aware of your values, they become an internal control for behavior. "Values are significant in choice making" (Salladay & McDonnell 1989, p. 544). Each person has a small number of values.

Values exist in some relationship to one another within a person. A **value system** is the organization of a person's values along a continuum of relative importance. Values underlie **purposive behavior,** which refers to actions that are performed "on purpose" with the intention of reaching some goal or bringing about a certain result. Purposive behavior, then, is based on a person's decisions or choices, and these decisions or choices are based on underlying values.

Morals (or *morality*) is similar to ethics and many people use the two words interchangeably. **Morality** usually refers to *personal* standards of right and wrong. It denotes what is right and wrong in conduct, character, and attitude. Sometimes the first clue to the moral nature of a situation is an aroused conscience, or an awareness of feelings such as guilt, hope, or shame. The tendency to respond to the situation with words such as *ought*, *should*, *right*, *wrong*, *good*, and *bad*, is another indicator. And finally, moral issues are concerned with important social values and norms: they are not about trivial things. They may seem unusually complex or difficult in some undefined way, but this is not necessarily so. See Table 11–1 for a comparison of morals and ethics.

Nurses should distinguish between *morality* and *the law.* Laws frequently reflect the moral values of a society; however, an action can be legal but not moral. For example, an order for "full resuscitation" of a terminally ill client is legal; however, one could still question whether the act is moral. Conversely, an action can be moral but illegal. For example, if a child at home stops breathing, it is moral but not legal to exceed the speed limit en route to the hospital. Legal aspects of nursing practice are covered in Chapter 12.

Distinction can also be made between *morality* and *religion.* Morality and religion are often closely related. For example, many years ago in the United States, "witches" were burned because of the religious beliefs of their persecutors. The morality of that practice can be questioned today.

People learn moral reasoning during their **socialization,** the process by which individuals learn the knowledge, skills, and dispositions of their social group or society. Lawrence Kohlberg perceives six stages in the moral development of individuals. See Table 23–6, page 578, for Kohlberg's theory and page 577 for the theory of moral development as proposed by Gilligan.

VALUES

Each person, eg, nurse, client, and physician, has a personal set of values. A **value set** is the group of values a person holds. Individuals incorporate personal values into their lives as a result of observing the behavior and attitudes of parents and teachers and interacting with their cultural, religious, and social environments. Personal values also reflect experiences and a person's intelligence.

TYPES OF VALUES AND SELECTED MEANINGS

Religious:	Obtains strength from religious beliefs
Theoretical:	Holds truth, rationality, and empiricism in high esteem
Political:	Values power
Economic:	Values usefulness and practicality
Aesthetic:	Values beauty, harmony, and form
Social:	Values human interactions, is kind, sympathetic, and unselfish

TYPES OF VALUES

There are two general types of values: intrinsic and extrinsic. An **intrinsic value** relates to the maintenance of life, eg, food and water have intrinsic value. An **extrinsic value** originates outside the individual and is not necessary for the maintenance of life, eg, health, holism, and humanism (Steele & Harmon 1983, p. 2).

Values can be either positive or negative. A positive value is a view of what is desirable or how something *should be.* For example, some nurses value a holistic approach to nursing. Negative values, by contrast, are views of what is undesirable or how something *should not be.* For example, talking unkindly about clients is considered by many nurses to be undesirable. Therefore, being unkind is a negative value. The box above gives six categories of values.

VALUES TRANSMISSION

The origin of a person's values can be traced to culture, society, institutions, and personality. Values are learned and are greatly influenced by a person's sociocultural environment. For example, if a parent consistently demonstrates honesty in dealing with others, the child will probably begin to value honesty. Acquiring values is a gradual process, usually occurring at an unconscious level. Because values are learned through observation and experience, they are heavily influenced by a person's sociocultural environment. For example, some cultures value the treatment of a folk healer over that of a physician. For additional information about cultural values relative to health and illness, see Chapter 15.

Personal Values Most people derive some values from the society or subgroup of society in which they live. A person may internalize some or all of these values and perceive them as **personal values.** People need societal values to feel accepted, and they need personal values to individualize themselves. See the box on page 203 for selected personal and societal values.

Professional Values Professional values are often a reflection and expansion of personal values. They are acquired during socialization into nursing—from codes of ethics, nursing experiences, teachers, and peers. As members of a caring profession, nurses' values relate to both competence and compassion. Watson outlined four important values of nursing (1981, pp. 20–21).

1. *Strong commitment to service.* Nursing is a helping, humanistic service. Because they are responsible for assessing and promoting health, nurses should value the caring aspect of nursing as well as their contribution to the health and well-being of people.
2. *Belief in the dignity and worth of each person.* This value means that the nurse acts in the best interest of the client regardless of nationality, race, creed, color, age, sex, politics, social class, or health status.
3. *Commitment to education.* This reflects a societal value of lifelong learning. In nursing, continuing education is needed to maintain and expand the nurse's level of competence and to increase the body of professional knowledge.
4. *Autonomy.* Nurses need to become more assertive in promoting nursing care and developing the ability to assume independent functions.

In a sense, nurses should be "value-neutral." This does not mean that nurses can or should be divorced from their personal and professional values; it does mean that nurses should be aware of the client's values and not assume that their own are superior. This attitude permits a nurse to establish effective relationships with clients who have differing values. For information about health beliefs and values, see Chapter 13.

SELECTED SOCIETAL AND PERSONAL VALUES

Societal Values	*Personal Values*
▪ Human life	▪ Family unity
▪ Individual rights	▪ Self-worth
▪ Individual autonomy	▪ Worth of others
▪ Liberty	▪ Independence
▪ Democracy	▪ Religion
▪ Equal opportunity	▪ Honesty
▪ Power	▪ Fairness
▪ Health	▪ Love
▪ Wealth	▪ Sense of humor
▪ Youth	▪ Safety
▪ Vigor	▪ Peace
▪ Intelligence	▪ Financial security
▪ Imagination	▪ Material things
▪ Education	▪ Money
▪ Technology	▪ Property of self
▪ Conformity	▪ Property of others
▪ Friendship	▪ Leisure time
▪ Courage	▪ Work
▪ Compassion	▪ Travel
▪ Family	▪ Plants
	▪ Animals
	▪ Physical activity
	▪ Intellectual activity
	▪ Artistic activity
	▪ Neatness

VALUES CLARIFICATION

Values clarification is a process by which people identify, examine, and develop their own individual values. A principle of values clarification is that no one set of values is right for everyone. When people are able to identify their values, they can retain or change them and thus act on the basis of freely chosen, rather than unconscious, values. Values clarification promotes personal growth by fostering awareness, empathy, and insight.

A widely used theory of values clarification was developed in 1966 by Raths, Harmon, and Simon (cited in Fowler & Levine-Ariff 1987, p. 143). This "valuing process" includes cognitive, affective, and behavioral components, referred to as "choosing," "prizing," and "acting." See the box above.

VALUES CLARIFICATION

Choosing (cognitive)	Beliefs are chosen ▪ Freely, without outside pressure. ▪ From among alternatives. ▪ After reflecting and considering consequences.
Prizing (affective)	Chosen beliefs are prized and cherished.
Acting (behavioral)	Chosen beliefs are ▪ Affirmed to others. ▪ Incorporated into one's behavior. ▪ Repeated consistently in one's life.

Source: Adapted from L Raths, M Harmin, and S Simon, *Values and Teaching*, 2d ed. (Columbus, OH: Merrill, 1978), p. 47. Used with permission of authors.

Identifying Personal Values Nurses need to know specifically what values they hold about life, health, illness, and death. Nursing students should explore their own values and beliefs regarding

- Individual's right to make decisions for self
- Abortion
- Passive euthanasia
- Active euthanasia
- Blood transfusion
- Acquired immune deficiency syndrome (AIDS)
- Withholding fluids and nutrition
- Cultural differences
- Homelessness
- Spiritual/religious differences

One strategy for gaining awareness of personal values is to consider one's own attitudes about such issues as abortion and euthanasia. When considering these issues, the nurse should ask: "Can I accept this or live with this?" "Why does this bother me?" "What would I do or want done in this situation?" (Corey et al 1984, pp. 57–94).

Identifying Client Values Nurses need to identify clients' values as they influence and relate to a particular health problem. For example, a client with failing eyesight will probably place a high value on the ability to see, and

BEHAVIORS THAT MAY INDICATE UNCLEAR VALUES

Behavior	*Example*
Ignoring a health professional's advice	A client with heart disease who values hard work ignores advice to exercise regularly
Inconsistent communication or behavior	A pregnant woman says she wants a healthy baby but continues to drink alcohol and smoke tobacco
Numerous admissions to a health agency for the same problem	A middle-aged, obese woman repeatedly seeks help for back pain but does not lose weight
Confusion or uncertainty about which course of action to take	A woman wants to obtain a job to meet financial obligations but also wants to stay at home to care for an ailing husband

a client with chronic pain will value comfort. Normally, people take such things for granted. Values clarification can help clients whose unclear or conflicting values are detrimental to their health. Examples of behaviors that may indicate the need for values clarification are listed in the box above.

The following process may help clients clarify their values.

1. *List alternatives.* Make sure that the client is aware of all alternative actions and has thought about the consequences of each. Ask, "Are you considering other courses of action?"
2. *Examine possible consequences of choices.* Ask, "What do you think you will gain by doing that?" "What benefits do you foresee from doing that?"
3. *Choose freely.* To determine whether the client chose freely, ask: "Did you have any say in that decision?" "Did you have a choice?"
4. *Feel good about the choice.* To determine how the client feels, ask, "How do you feel about that decision (or action)?" Because some clients may not feel satisfied with their decision, a more sensitive question may be "Some people feel good after a decision is made; others feel bad. How do you feel?"
5. *Affirm the choice.* Ask, "What will you say to others (family, friends) about this?"
6. *Act on the choice.* To determine whether the client is prepared to act on the decision, ask, for example, "Will it be difficult to tell your wife about this?"
7. *Act with a pattern.* To determine whether the client consistently behaves in a pattern, ask, "How many times have you done that before?" or "Would you act that way again?"

When implementing these seven steps, the nurse assists the client to think each question through, never imposing personal values. When clarifying values, the nurse never offers an opinion (eg, "It would be better to do it this way") or offers a judgment (eg, "That's not the right thing to do"). The nurse offers an opinion only when the client asks the nurse for it and then only with care.

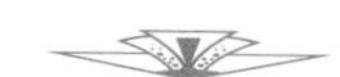

NURSING ETHICS

The growing awareness of nursing ethics is mainly a product of social and technologic change and of the nature of nursing itself.

Social Movements In the 1960s, the civil rights movement and a growing consumerism encouraged people to examine the morality of public institutions, exposing racial and economic discrimination in health care. The feminist movement linked oppression of nurses to discrimination against women in the health care setting and in the workplace, as well as in society as a whole. Currently, the large number of people without health insurance and the escalating cost of health care are raising issues of fairness and allocation of resources.

Technology Rapidly changing technologies create new issues that did not exist in earlier, simpler times. Before monitors, respirators, and parenteral feedings were available, there was no question about whether to "allow" an 800-gram premature infant to die. If the infant was very premature, there was no way to maintain life. The question has now become, *Should* we always do what we *can* do?

Nurses are accountable for their ethical conduct. In 1991 the American Nurses Association (ANA) published *Standards of Clinical Nursing Practice*, in which Standard V is ethics; see the box at the top left of page 205. Therefore, nurses need to understand their own values related to moral matters and to use ethical reasoning to determine and explain their moral positions. Sometimes nurses are aware of an ethical issue, but nurses also need moral principles and reasoning skills to explain their position. Otherwise they may give emotional responses, which often are not helpful.

ANA STANDARDS OF PROFESSIONAL PERFORMANCE

Standard V: Ethics

The nurse's decisions and actions on behalf of clients are determined in an ethical manner.

Measurement Criteria

1. The nurse's practice is guided by the *Code for Nurses.*
2. The nurse maintains client confidentiality.
3. The nurse acts as a client advocate.
4. The nurse delivers care in a nonjudgmental and nondiscriminatory manner that is sensitive to client diversity.
5. The nurse delivers care in a manner that preserves/protects client autonomy, dignity, and rights.
6. The nurse seeks available resources to help formulate ethical decisions.

Source: American Nurses Association, *Standards of Clinical Nursing Practice,* (Washington, DC: ANA, 1991), p. 15. Used by permission.

EXAMPLES OF NURSES' OBLIGATIONS IN ETHICAL DECISIONS

- Maximize the client's well-being.
- Balance the client's need for autonomy with family members' responsibilities for the client's well-being.
- Support each family member and enhance the family support system.
- Carry out hospital policies.
- Protect other clients' well-being.
- Protect the nurse's own standards of care.

FACTORS AFFECTING ETHICAL DECISIONS

Factors affecting ethical decision-making include nurses' perceptions of their roles and responsibilities, moral theories and frameworks, moral principles, the professional code of ethics, the level of cognitive development of the people involved, and the values, beliefs and attitudes of these people.

Perceptions of Roles and Responsibilities Nurses are responsible for determining their own actions and for supporting clients who are making ethical decisions or coping with the results of decisions made by others. A good decision is one that is in the client's best interest and at the same time preserves the integrity of all involved. Nurses have multiple obligations to balance in moral situations. See the box at the top of the next column for examples and Advocacy, on page 213.

Moral Theories and Frameworks There are four general approaches to moral theory: teleology, deontology, intuitionism, and the ethic of caring. **Teleology** looks to the consequences of an action in judging whether that action is right or wrong. Utilitarianism, one specific teleologic theory, is summarized in the ideas, "the greatest good for the greatest number" and "the end justifies the means."

Deontology proposes that the morality of a decision is not determined by its consequences. It emphasizes duty, rationality, and obedience to rules. For instance, a nurse might believe it is necessary to tell the truth no matter who is hurt. There are many deontologic theories; each justifies the rules of acceptable behavior differently. For example, some state that the rules are known by divine revelation; others refer to a natural law or social contract.

The difference between teleology and deontology can be seen when they are applied to the issue of abortion. A person taking a teleologic approach might consider that saving the mother's life (the end, or consequence) justifies the abortion (the means, or act). A person taking a deontologic approach might consider any termination of life as a violation of the rule, "Do not kill" and, therefore, would not abort the fetus regardless of the consequences to the mother. It is important to note that the approach, or framework, guides making the moral decision; it does not determine the outcome (eg, the person taking a teleologic approach might have considered that saving the life of the fetus justified the death of the mother).

A third framework is **intuitionism,** summarized as the notion that people inherently know what is right or wrong; determining what is right is not a matter of rational thought or learning. For example, a nurse inherently knows it is wrong to strike a client, this does not need to be taught or reasoned out.

Benner and Wrubel (1989) proposed **caring** as the central goal of nursing as well as a basis for nursing ethics. Unlike the preceding theories which are based on the concept of fairness (justice), an ethic of caring is based on relationships. Caring theories stress courage, generosity, commitment, and responsibility. Caring is a force for protecting and enhancing client dignity. Guided by this ethic,

CRITICAL THINKING CHALLENGE

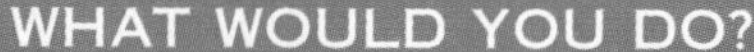

WHAT WOULD YOU DO?

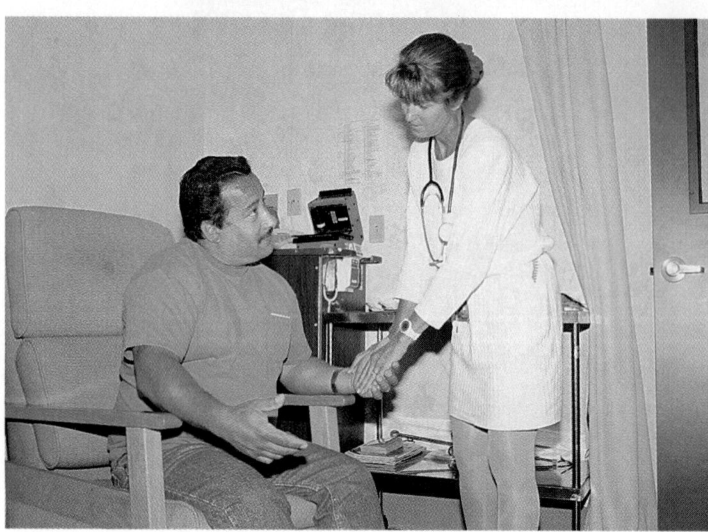

Jorge Zetina, a 47-year-old male, was admitted to your unit yesterday for diagnostic testing to confirm the diagnosis of stomach carcinoma. Mr Zetina's physician has told you that the tumor is malignant, with widespread metastases, but has not informed the patient of his poor prognosis. When you go into Mr Zetina's room, he seems worried and anxious, and then asks, "Did the doctor tell you things aren't going well?"

What would you do?

nurses use touch and truth-telling to affirm clients as persons rather than objects and to assist them to make choices and find meaning in their illness experiences.

Moral Principles Moral principles are statements about broad, general philosophic concepts such as autonomy and justice. They provide the foundation for **moral rules,** which are specific prescriptions for actions. For example, "People should not lie" (rule) is based on the moral principle of respect or autonomy for people. Principles are useful in ethical discussions because even people who do not agree on which action to take may be able to agree on the principles that apply. That agreement can serve as the basis for an acceptable solution. For example, most people would agree that nurses are obligated to respect their clients (a principle), even if they disagree about whether a nurse should deceive a client about the client's prognosis (action). **Autonomy** (respect for persons) refers to the right to make one's own decisions. Respect for autonomy means that nurses recognize the individual's uniqueness, the right to be what that person is, and the right to choose personal goals. People have "inward autonomy" if they have the faculty and ability to make choices. People have "outward autonomy" if their choices are not limited or imposed by others.

Nurses who follow the principle of autonomy respect a client's right to make decisions even when those choices seem not to be in the client's best interest. Respect for people also means treating others with consideration. In a health care setting, abuses of this principle occur when a nurse disregards clients' subjective accounts of their symptoms (ie, pain). Finally, respect for autonomy means that people should not be treated as "a means to an end" (eg, clients must provide an informed consent before tests and procedures are carried out). See Informed Consent in Chapter 12, page 228.

Nonmaleficence means the duty to do no harm. This principle is the basis of most codes of nursing ethics. Although this would seem to be a simple principle to follow in nursing practice, in reality it is complex. Harm can mean deliberate harm, risk of harm, and unintentional harm. In nursing, intentional harm is always unacceptable. However, the risk of harm is not so clear. A client may be at risk of harm during a nursing intervention that is intended to be helpful. For example, a client may react adversely to a medication. Sometimes, the degree to which a risk is morally permissible can be a conflict.

Beneficence means "doing good." Nurses are obligated to "do good," that is, to implement actions that benefit clients and their support persons. However, in an increasingly technologic health care system, "doing good" can also pose a risk of doing harm. For example, a nurse may advise a client about an intensive exercise program to improve general health but should not do so if the client is at risk of a heart attack.

Justice is often referred to as fairness. Nurses frequently face decisions in which a sense of justice should prevail. For example, a nurse is alone on a hospital unit,

Table 11–2 International Council of Nurses Code for Nurses

The fundamental responsibility of the nurse is fourfold: to promote health, to prevent illness, to restore health, and to alleviate suffering.

The need for nursing is universal. Inherent in nursing is respect for life, dignity, and rights of man. It is unrestricted by considerations of nationality, race, creed, color, age, sex, politics or social status.

Nurses render health services to the individual, the family, and the community and coordinate their services with those of related groups.

Nurses and People

The nurse's primary responsibility is to those people who require nursing care.

The nurse, in providing care, promotes an environment in which the values, customs and spiritual beliefs of the individual are respected.

The nurse holds in confidence personal information and uses judgment in sharing this information.

Nurses and Practice

The nurse carries responsibility for nursing practice and for maintaining competence by continual learning. The nurse maintains the highest standards of nursing care possible within the reality of a specific situation.

The nurse uses judgment in relation to individual competence when accepting and delegating responsibilities.

The nurse when acting in a professional capacity should at all times maintain standards of personal conduct which reflect credit upon the profession.

Nurses and Society

The nurse shares with other citizens the responsibility for initiating and supporting action to meet the health and social needs of the public.

Nurses and Coworkers

The nurse sustains a cooperative relationship with coworkers in nursing and other fields. The nurse takes appropriate action to safeguard the individual when his care is endangered by a coworker or any other person.

Nurses and the Profession

The nurse plays the major role in determining and implementing desirable standards of nursing practice and nursing education.

The nurse is active in developing a core of professional knowledge.

The nurse, acting through the professional organization, participates in establishing and maintaining equitable social and economic working conditions in nursing.

Source: International Council of Nurses, *ICN Code for Nurses: Ethical Concepts Applied to Nursing* (Geneva: Imprimeries Populaires, 1973). Reprinted with permission of the ICN.

and one client arrives to be admitted at the same time another client requires a medication for pain. Instead of running from one client to the other, weigh the facts in the situation and then act based on the principle of justice.

Fidelity means to be faithful to agreements and responsibilities one has undertaken. Nurses have responsibilities to clients, employers, government, society, and to themselves. Circumstances often affect which responsibilities take precedence at a particular time.

Veracity refers to telling the truth. Most children are taught to always tell the truth, but as adults the choices are often less clear. Does a nurse tell the truth when it is known that it will cause harm? Does a nurse tell a lie when it is known that the lie will relieve anxiety and fear? Bok (1978) concludes that lying to sick and dying people is rarely justified. The loss of trust in the nurse and the anxiety caused by not knowing the truth, for example, usually outweigh any benefits derived from lying.

Nursing Code of Ethics A **code of ethics** is a formal statement of a group's ideals and values. It is a set of ethical principles that is shared by members of the group, reflects their moral judgments over time, and serves as a standard for their professional actions. Codes of ethics are usually higher than legal standards, and they can never be less than the legal standards of the profession.

International, national, state, and provincial nursing associations have established codes of ethics. The International Council of Nurses (ICN) developed and adopted their first code of ethics in 1953. The ICN Code was revised in 1965 and again in 1973 (Table 11–2). The American Nurses Association (ANA) first adopted a code of ethics in 1950; it was revised in 1968, 1976, and 1985 (Table 11–3, p. 208). In 1980, the Canadian Nurses Association (CNA) adopted a code of ethics; it was revised in 1991 (Table 11–4, p. 208). Increasingly, professional nursing associations are taking an active part in improving

Table 11–3 American Nurses Association Code for Nurses

1. The nurse provides services with respect for human dignity and the uniqueness of the client unrestricted by considerations of social or economic status, personal attributes, or the nature of health problems.
2. The nurse safeguards the client's right to privacy by judiciously protecting information of a confidential nature.
3. The nurse acts to safeguard the client and the public when health care and safety are affected by the incompetent, unethical, or illegal practice of any person.
4. The nurse assumes responsibility and accountability for individual nursing judgments and actions.
5. The nurse maintains competence in nursing.
6. The nurse exercises informed judgment and uses individual competence and qualifications as criteria in seeking consultation, accepting responsibilities, and delegating nursing activities to others.
7. The nurse participates in activities that contribute to the ongoing development of the profession's body of knowledge.
8. The nurse participates in the profession's efforts to implement and improve standards of nursing.
9. The nurse participates in the profession's effort to establish and maintain conditions of employment conducive to high quality nursing care.
10. The nurse participates in the profession's effort to protect the public from misinformation and misrepresentation and to maintain the integrity of nursing.
11. The nurse collaborates with members of the health professions and other citizens in promoting community and national efforts to meet the health needs of the public.

Source: American Nurses Association, *Code for Nurses* (Kansas City, MO: ANA, 1985). Reprinted with permission.

and enforcing standards. Nurses are responsible for being familiar with the code that governs their practice.

Functions of Ethical Codes Nursing codes of ethics have the following purposes:

1. To inform the public about the minimum standards of the profession and to help them understand professional nursing conduct
2. To provide a sign of the profession's commitment to the public it serves
3. To outline the major ethical considerations of the profession
4. To provide general guidelines for professional behavior
5. To guide the profession in self-regulation

Table 11–4 Canadian Nurses Association Code of Ethics for Nursing*

Clients

I. A nurse treats clients with respect for their individual needs and values.

II. Based upon respect for clients and regard for their right to control their own care, nursing care reflects respect for the right of choice held by clients.

III. The nurse holds confidential all information about a client learned in the health care setting.

IV. The nurse is guided by consideration for the dignity of clients.

V. The nurse provides competent care to clients.

Nursing Roles and Relationships

VI. The nurse maintains trust in nurses and nursing.

VII. The nurse recognizes the contribution and expertise of colleagues from nursing and other disciplines as essential to excellent health care.

VIII. The nurse takes steps to ensure that the client receives competent and ethical care.

IX. Conditions of employment should contribute in a positive way to client care and the professional satisfaction of nurses.

X. Job action by nurses is directed toward securing conditions of employment that enable safe and appropriate care for clients and contribute to the professional satisfaction of nurses.

Nursing Ethics and Society

XI. The nurse advocates the interests of clients.

XII. The nurse represents the values and ethics of nursing before colleagues and others.

The Nursing Profession

XIII. Professional nursing organizations are responsible for clarifying, securing, and sustaining ethical nursing conduct. The fulfillment of these tasks requires that professional nurses' organizations remain responsive to the rights, needs, and legitimate interests of clients and nurses.

* This represents only one element of the code values. For each value noted the CNA Code of Ethics for Nursing provides obligations which provide more specific direction for conduct. In two instances, limitations are also listed which describe exceptional circumstances in which a value or obligation cannot be applied.

Source: Canadian Nurses Association. November 1991. *Code of Ethics for Nursing* (Ottawa: CNA). Reprinted with permission of the CNA.

6. To remind nurses of the special responsibility they assume when caring for the sick

Because the wording in a code of ethics is intentionally vague, such codes can serve as general guides. They do not give direction for actions to take in specific cases. For example, the first item in the ANA *Code for Nurses* refers to respect for human dignity and states that in caring for clients, nurses should be "unrestricted by considerations of the nature of health problems." Does this mean that it is wrong for a pregnant nurse to refuse to care for a client with active herpes? Or that it is wrong to refuse to care for a client who uses rude language? When making ethical decisions, nurses should consider their code of ethics together with a more unified ethical theory, ethical principles, and the relevant data about each situation.

Cognitive Moral Development Ethics problems require nurses to think and reason in making decisions, judgments, and choices. Reasoning is a cognitive function and is, therefore, developmental. See Chapter 23 for the cognitive moral development theories of Lawrence Kohlberg and Carol Gilligan.

In resolving ethics problems, one difficulty may be that the people involved in the situation operate at different levels of cognitive reasoning, as well as from different moral frameworks and different individual values. For example, when deciding whether it is right to resuscitate a dying client, a nurse reasoning "by the rules" would think, "According to policy, if there is no DNR (Do Not Resuscitate) order, we must resuscitate." A co-worker, reasoning on the basis of "not hurting others" might think, "Resuscitation will cause the client to suffer needlessly; therefore it is wrong." When trying to achieve consensus, nurses should keep these differences in mind and determine the reasoning of those involved (ie, the client and support persons), asking not only what they believe to be right, but also what process of reasoning led them to that belief.

Values, Beliefs, and Attitudes **Values** are an important aspect of decision making because they influence perceptions and motivation; therefore, it is important that nurses be consciously aware of their own values and the values of the others involved in a given situation. **Beliefs** (opinions) are interpretations or conclusions that we accept as true (Chaffee 1990, p. 187). Beliefs are based more on faith than on fact and may or may not be true.

Beliefs may or may not involve values. For example, the statement, "I believe if I study hard I will get good grades" expresses a belief that does not involve a value. By contrast the statement, "Good grades are really important to me. I believe I must study hard to obtain good grades" does involve a value.

Attitudes are mental positions or feelings made up of many different beliefs and are directed toward a person, object, or idea. They are often judged as good or bad, positive or negative, whereas beliefs are judged as correct or incorrect. The affective aspect of an attitude is the feelings associated with it. Because feelings vary so greatly among people, this may be the most important aspect of an attitude. For example, one client may feel very strongly about the sound from a television set in the next room, whereas another client may dismiss it as unimportant. The cognitive component of an attitude includes the beliefs and factual information associated with it (eg, the knowledge about effective and appropriate nurse-client communication). The behavioral component is the inclination to act as a result of one's attitude. For example, a nurse who disapproves of another nurse's behavior toward a client may think, "If she speaks that way to Mr B again, I shall talk to her."

TYPES OF ETHICS PROBLEMS

Nurses encounter two broad types of problems: decision-focused problems and action-focused problems. Each requires a different approach (Wilkinson 1993, p. 4).

In **decision-focused problems,** the difficulty lies in deciding what to do. The question is, What *should* I do? For example:

> Because Leon is committed to the sanctity of life, he wishes his client to have artificial nutrition and hydration. As a nurse, Leon also believes in relieving suffering, so when he sees that the tube-feedings are prolonging the client's pain, and even contributing to her discomfort, he wishes to have the feedings discontinued. He is not comfortable with either choice.

In this case, two principles clearly apply, so no matter what the nurse does, an important value must be sacrificed. This is the typical **moral dilemma** that people commonly equate with ethics, sometimes referred to as "being between a rock and a hard place." The nature of a dilemma dictates that there are no easy solutions. However, because the difficulty is personal and internal, nurses can address decision-focused problems by learning to make better decisions by, for example, reviewing their own personal value systems, taking advantage of staff development offerings, and attending ethics rounds.

In **action-focused problems,** the difficulty lies not in making the decision, but in implementing it. In these situations, nurses usually feel secure in their judgment about what is right but act on their judgment only at personal risk. The central question is, What *can* I do? or What risks am I willing to take to do what is right? **Moral distress,** one type of action-focused problem, occurs when the nurse knows the right course of action but cannot carry it out because of institutional policies or other constraints

(Jameton 1984, p. 6). This results in feelings of anger, guilt, and loss of integrity on the part of the nurse and can impact client care. For example:

> A resident physician has told the nurses to order complete blood count (CBC) and urinalysis on all clients and to get the results before calling him to the emergency room to examine the clients. The nurses believe this is unethical because it is wasteful and poses unnecessary discomfort and possible risks for clients. However, they do not have the authority or the access to decision-making channels needed to change the situation. So they order the tests, but they feel guilty and upset because they believe what they are doing is wrong.

Unlike decision-focused problems, action-focused problems cannot be resolved by improving one's decision-making skills. Even after a nurse decides what is *right* to do, the issue becomes what the nurse actually can do given the conditions of practice. Research indicates that nurses' actions are influenced by such constraints as verbal threats, fear of losing their jobs or their nursing licenses, fear of physicians, fear of the law or lawsuits, and lack of support from both peers and administrators (Wilkinson 1987/88, p. 21). Action-focused problems require knowledge, experience, communication, and the ability to make integrity-preserving compromises. To deal successfully with these problems, nurses must shift their attention away from "making the right decision" and focus on the factors that are preventing the "right action" (Wilkinson 1993, p. 5).

Conflicts Within Nursing Ethical conflicts also arise from nurses' unresolved questions about the nature and scope of their practice. High-technology and specialty roles (intensive care nurses, diabetes clinicians) have expanded the scope of nursing practice, often causing nursing and medical activities to overlap. This creates value conflicts for nurses. For example:

- Although nurses value health promotion and wellness, many still work in hospitals, and many are involved in high-tech treatment of illness.
- Although the profession values a humanistic, caring approach and emphasizes nurse-client relationships, many nurses spend much of their time attending to the client's machines.

Conflicting Loyalties and Obligations Because of their unique position in the health care system, nurses experience conflicting loyalties and obligations to clients, families, physicians, employing institutions, and licensing bodies. The client's needs may conflict with institutional policies, physician preferences, needs of the client's family, or even laws of the state. According to the nursing code of ethics, the nurse's first allegiance is to the client. However, it is not always easy to determine which action best serves the client's needs. For instance, a nurse may believe the client's interests require telling the client a truth that others have been withholding. But this might damage the client-physician relationship, in the long run causing harm to the client rather than the intended good.

RESOLVING ETHICAL PROBLEMS

Nurses need to be aware of ethical theories and principles, the nursing code of ethics, and their own hierarchy of values. These components enter into their decision-making process along with the facts of a specific situation. Good decision-making requires nurses to be "aware of the factors that contribute to and/or hinder one's ability to make a choice" (Thompson & Thompson 1990, p. 78). These factors include cultural values, societal expectations, degree of commitment, lack of time, lack of experience, ignorance or fear of the law, and conflicting loyalties.

Responsible ethical reasoning is rational thinking. It is also systematic and based upon principles. It should *not* be based upon emotions, intuition, fixed policies, or precedents. (A *precedent* is an earlier similar occurrence. For example, "We have always done it this way" is a statement using precedence.) However, intuition may actually improve the quality of one's ethical decisions, as shown by a study indicating that "individuals with high levels of intuitive ability make more effective decisions than individuals with low levels of intuitive ability" (Gearhart & Young 1990, p. 49).

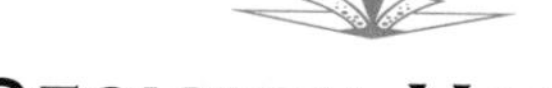

DECISION-MAKING MODELS

Various models including the decision-making models discussed in Chapter 10 can guide nurses in making ethical decisions. The following example utilizes a Bioethical Decision Model (Cassels & Redman 1989, pp. 465–66).

Situation:

> Mrs. LaVesque, a 67-year-old woman, is hospitalized with multiple fractures and lacerations caused by an automobile accident. Her husband, who was killed in the accident, was taken to the same hospital. Mrs. LaVesque, who was driving the automobile, constantly questions Kate Murillo, her primary nurse, about her husband. The surgeon, Dr. Mario Gonzales, has told the nurse not to tell Mrs. LaVesque about the death of her husband; however, he does not give the nurse any reason for these instructions. Ms. Murillo expresses concern to the charge nurse, who says the surgeon's

orders must be followed. Ms. Murillo is not comfortable with this and wonders what she should do.

1. *Identify the moral aspects of nursing care.* Not all problems have moral content. A decision to give Mrs. LaVesque prescribed prn analgesic requires scientific, not moral, judgment. The following criteria may be used to determine whether a moral situation exists (Fry 1989a, p. 491).
   a. There is a need to choose between alternative actions that conflict with human needs or the welfare of others. One conflict for the primary nurse is the need to be honest with Mrs. LaVesque without being disloyal to the surgeon and the charge nurse.
   b. The choice to be made is guided by universal moral principles or theories, which can be used to provide some kind of justification for the action.
   c. The choice is guided by a process of weighing reasons.
   d. The decision must be freely and consciously chosen.
   e. The choice is affected by personal feelings and by the particular context of the situation. For example, Kate's choice will probably be affected by her concern for Mrs. LaVesque and perhaps by the surgeon's incomplete communication with her.

2. *Gather relevant facts related to the issue.* Data should include information about the client's health problems. Determine who is involved, the nature of their involvement, and their motives for acting. In this case, the people involved are the client (who is concerned about her husband), the husband (who is deceased), the surgeon, the charge nurse, and the primary nurse. Motives are not known. Perhaps the nurse wishes to protect her therapeutic relationship with Mrs. LaVesque; possibly the physician believes he is protecting Mrs. LaVesque from psychologic trauma and consequent physical deterioration.

3. *Determine ownership of the decision.* In some cases, the most important question is *who* should make the decision. When the decision maker is the client, the nurse functions in a supportive role. Clients need knowledge about the probability and nature of consequences attending various courses of action. Nurses share their special knowledge and expertise with clients to enable them to make informed decisions. The following questions may be helpful in determining who owns a problem (Davis & Aroskar 1983, p. 218):
   a. For whom is the decision being made?
   b. Who should be involved in making the decision and why?
   c. What criteria (social, economic, psychologic, physiologic, or legal) should be used in deciding who makes the decision?
   d. What degree of consent is needed by the subject? In this case, the decision is being made for Mrs. LaVesque. The surgeon obviously believes that he should be the one to decide, and the charge nurse agrees. It would be helpful if caregivers agreed on criteria for deciding who the decision maker should be.

4. *Clarify and apply personal values.* We can infer from this situation that Mrs. LaVesque values her husband's welfare, the charge nurse values policy and procedure, and Ms. Murillo seems to value a client's right to have information. Ms. Murillo needs to clarify her own and the surgeon's values, as well as confirm the values of Mrs. LaVesque and the charge nurse.

5. *Identify ethical theories and principles.* For example, failing to tell Mrs. LaVesque the truth can negate her autonomy. The nurse would uphold the principle of honesty by telling Mrs. LaVesque. The principles of beneficence and nonmaleficence are also involved because of the possible effects of the alternative actions on Mrs. LaVesque's physical and psychologic well-being.

6. *Identify applicable laws or agency policies.* Because Dr. Gonzales simply "gave instructions" rather than an actual order, agency policies might not require Ms. Murillo to do as he says. She should clarify this with the charge nurse. She should also be familiar with the Nurse Practice Act in her state or province.

7. *Utilize competent interdisciplinary resources.* In this case, Kate might consult literature to find out if clients are harmed by receiving bad news when they are injured. She might also consult with the chaplain.

8. *Develop alternative actions and project their outcomes on the client and family.* Possibly because of the limited time available for ethical deliberations in the clinical setting, nurses tend to identify two opposing, either-or alternatives (eg, to tell or not to tell) instead of generating multiple options (DeWolf 1989, p. 80). This creates a dilemma even when none exists. Two alternative actions, with possible outcomes, include
   a. Follow the charge nurse's advice and do as the surgeon says. Possible outcomes: (a) Mrs. LaVesque might become increasingly anxious and angry when she finds out they have withheld information, or (b) by waiting until Mrs. LaVesque is stronger to give her the bad news, her health may not be affected.
   b. Discuss the situation further with the charge nurse and surgeon, pointing out Mrs. LaVesque's right to autonomy and information. Possible outcomes: (a) The surgeon acknowledges Mrs. LaVesque's right to be informed, or (b) he states that Mrs. LaVesque's health is at risk and insists that she not be informed until a later time.

Regardless of whether the action agrees with Ms. Murillo's personal value system, Mrs. LaVesque's best interests take precedence.

9. *Apply nursing codes of ethics to help guide actions.* Codes of nursing usually support client autonomy and nursing advocacy. If Ms. Murillo believes strongly that Mrs. LaVesque should hear the truth, then as a client advocate, she should choose to confer again with the charge nurse and surgeon.
10. *For each alternative action, identify the risk and seriousness of consequences for the nurse.* Nurses do not always have the autonomy to act on their moral/ethical decisions. If Ms. Murillo tells Mrs. LaVesque the truth without the agreement of the charge nurse and surgeon, she risks the surgeon's anger and a reprimand from the charge nurse. If Ms. Murillo follows the charge nurse's advice, she will receive approval from the charge nurse and surgeon; however, she risks being seen as unassertive, and she violates her personal value of truthfulness. If Ms. Murillo requests a conference she may gain respect for her assertiveness and professionalism, but she risks the surgeon's annoyance at having his instructions questioned.
11. *Participate actively in resolving the issue.* The appropriate degree of nursing input varies with the situation. Sometimes nurses participate in choosing what will be done; sometimes they merely support a client who is making the decision. If an action cannot be agreed on, Ms. Murillo must decide whether this issue is important enough to merit the personal risks involved.
12. *Implement the action.*
13. *Evaluate the action taken.* Begin by asking, "Did I do the right thing?" Involve the client, family, and other health members in the evaluation, if possible. Ms. Murillo can ask herself whether she would make the same decisions again if the situation were repeated. If she is not satisfied, review other alternatives, and work through the process again (Uustal 1990, p. 440).

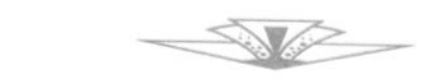

SPECIFIC ETHICAL ISSUES

Nurses encounter a variety of ethical issues. In a recent study, respondents reported being involved in issues of client's refusal of treatment, informed consent, discontinuation of life-saving treatment, withholding of information from clients, confidentiality, client competence, and allocation of scarce resources (Cassells & Redman 1989, pp. 467–69).

Acquired Immune Deficiency Syndrome (AIDS) Because of its association with homosexual and bisexual behavior, prostitution, illicit drug use, and inevitable physical decline and death, AIDS bears a social stigma. In a recent study, nurses caring for AIDS clients reported conflicting feelings of anger, fear, sympathy, fatigue, helplessness, and self-enhancement (Breault & Polifroni 1992). According to ANA, the moral obligation to care for an HIV-infected client cannot be set aside unless the risk exceeds the responsibility. "Not only must nursing care be readily available, . . . but nurses must also be advised of the risks and the responsibilities they face in providing care. . . . Accepting personal risk which exceeds the limits of duty is not morally obligatory; it is a moral option" (ANA 1988b, p. 31).

Abortion Abortion is a highly publicized issue about which many people, including nurses, feel very strongly. Debate continues, pitting the principle of sanctity of life against the principle of autonomy and the woman's right to control her own body. This is an especially volatile issue because no public consensus has yet been reached.

Most state and provincial laws have provisions known as *conscience clauses* that permit individual physicians and nurses, as well as institutions, to refuse to assist with an abortion if doing so violates their religious or moral principles. However, nurses have no right to impose their values on a client. Nursing codes of ethics support clients' rights to information and abortion counseling. For example, the CNA's *Code of Ethics for Nursing* 1991 says "Based upon respect for clients and regard for their right to control their own care, nursing care reflects respect for the right of choice held by clients."

Confidentiality In keeping with the principle of autonomy, nurses are obligated to respect clients' privacy and confidentiality. Clients must be able to trust that nurses will not reveal details of their situation inappropriately but will communicate the information necessary to provide for their health care. Computerized information management in acute care settings makes client data accessible to more people. Nurses should help develop security measures (eg, access codes) and policies to help ensure appropriate use of client data.

Withdrawing or Withholding Food and Fluids It is generally accepted that providing food and fluids is part of ordinary nursing practice and, therefore, a moral duty. A nurse is morally obligated, however, to withhold food and fluids when it is more harmful to administer than to withhold them (ANA 1988a, p. 2). In addition, "It is morally as well as legally permissible for nurses to honor the refusal of food and fluids by competent patients in their care" (ANA 1988a, p. 3). The *Code for Nurses* supports this statement through the nurse's role as a client advocate and through the moral principle of autonomy.

Termination of Life-Sustaining Treatment Antibiotics, organ transplants, and technologic advances (eg, ventilators) have helped prolong life. However, the ability to restore health has not kept pace with the capacity to prolong life. Clients may specify that they wish to have life-sustaining measures withdrawn, they may have advance directives on this matter, or they may specify a surrogate decision maker. When these decisions are made, the nurse, as the primary caregiver, must ensure that sensitive care and comfort measures are given as the client's illness progresses (Cassells & Redman 1989, pp. 467–68). A decision to withdraw treatment is not a decision to withdraw care.

Allocation of Health Resources Allocation of health care goods and services, such as organ transplants, artificial joints, and the services of specialists, has become an especially urgent issue as a result of cost-containment measures and the growing expense of medical care. For example, the number of office visits and the length of hospital stay are decisions that are increasingly being influenced by administrative policy.

ADVOCACY

An **advocate** is one who pleads the cause of another, and a **client advocate** is an advocate for clients' rights (see Chapter 1, page 20). The JCAHO *Standards Related to Ethics* states "3.2. Nursing staff members have a defined mechanism for addressing ethical issues in patient care." and "3.2.1. When the hospital has an ethics committee or other defined structures for addressing ethical issues in patient care, nursing staff members participate." (1992, p. 3.7.) Also see the box on page 205 for the ANA standard. The focus of the client advocacy role is to respect client decisions and enhance client autonomy.

According to Kohnke (1982, p. 5) the actions of an advocate are to *inform* and *support.* An advocate informs clients about their rights in a situation, and provides them with the information they need to make an informed decision. The first step in informing is to make sure the client agrees to receiving the information. In addition, an advocate must (a) either have the necessary information or know how to get it, (b) want the client to have the information, (c) present information in a way that is meaningful to the client, and (d) deal with the fact that there may be those who do not wish the client to be informed.

An advocate supports clients in their decisions. Support can involve action or nonaction. An advocate must know how to provide support in an objective manner, being careful not to convey approval or disapproval of the client's choices. Advocacy involves accepting and respecting the client's right to decide, even if the nurse believes the decision is wrong. As advocates, nurses do not make decisions for clients; clients must make their own decisions freely. For example: After being fully informed about the chemotherapy treatment, the alternative treatments, and the possible consequences of the available choices, Mr Rae decides against further chemotherapy for his malignancy. The client advocate supports Mr Rae in his decision. Underlying client advocacy are the beliefs that individuals have the following rights:

- the right to select values they deem necessary to sustain their lives
- the right to decide which course of action will best achieve the chosen values

RESEARCH NOTE

Do Nurses Have Ethical Experiences?

In response to a questionnaire sent to 1400 registered nurses, 200 nurses wrote a short description of an ethical situation that occurred in their practice. The most frequently cited dilemmas were those involving quality of life issues and life-sustaining treatment of the terminally ill. The remaining themes from their narratives were: (a) patient's right to know diagnosis and refuse treatment; (b) truth telling and informed consent; (c) difficulty in working with physicians; (d) standards of care; and (e) allocation of resources. Many nurses shared their frustration at not being able to do what they knew was right. Respondents described in great detail the pain endured by both the patient and themselves (eg, "I cried. I am crying now as I write this").

Implications: For nurses, ethical concerns are almost inseparable from concerns about the quality of patient care. Upon graduation from nursing school, nurses are expected to be competent in clinical skills and interpersonal communications, but competence in addressing ethical problems is usually left to on-the-job training or trial and error. Nurses' stories indicate that ethical problems affect them profoundly. More research is needed to help discover what nurses see as the solutions to moral problems in clinical nursing practice. This study supports the need for the nursing work environment to change to support nurses' participation in ethical decision making.

Source: AM Haddad, Problematic ethical experiences: Stories from nursing practice. *Bioethics Forum,* Fall 1993, 9:5–10.

- the right to dispose of values in a way they choose without coercion by others (Donahue 1985, p. 1037).

Nurses who function responsibly as advocates for themselves, their clients, and the community are in a position to effect change. A nurse functioning in this capacity must have an objective understanding of the ethical issues in health care as well as knowledge of the laws and regulations that affect nursing practice and public health (see Chapter 12).

ETHICS COMMITTEES

Because nurses have more contact with the client and family than other members of the health care team, they know the client better and have access to special kinds of information not available to other health care professionals (Mahon 1990, p. 266). Nurses offer unique perspectives that can greatly improve the quality of the ethical decisions made in health care settings. One important way for nurses to provide input is to serve on institutional ethics committees.

Ethics committees typically review cases, write guidelines and policies, and provide education and counseling. They ensure that relevant facts are brought out, provide a forum in which diverse views can be expressed, reduce stress for caregivers, and can reduce legal risks. These factors tend to produce better decisions than would otherwise be made (Hosford 1986, p. 15).

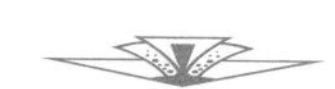

THE NURSE AS A MORAL AGENT

Nurses should develop the skills necessary to function as **moral agents**—that is to participate in ethical decision making. Cassells and Redman (1989, pp. 465–66) incorporated these skills as steps of their bioethical decision model. Professional nurses are responsible for acquiring these skills as a part of either their basic or continuing education.

Historically, nurses have looked on ethical decision making as the physician's responsibility. However, no one profession is responsible for an ethical decision, nor does expertise in one discipline (such as medicine or nursing) necessarily make a person an expert in ethics. As situations become more complex, multidisciplinary input becomes increasingly important.

Simply put, morality is the idea that people have choices and are responsible for their actions. Because professionals claim to use their expertise for social good, nurses need to be clear about the ethics of their work in order to conduct it well. Although nursing codes of ethics identify client advocacy as a part of the nursing role, many nurses work in settings that expect accountability but do not support nurses' authority or autonomy to act as advocates or moral agents. There are risks involved in putting advocacy into action (Parker 1990, p. 39). Some nurses have suggested that a viable nursing ethic must include an agenda of sociopolitical reform that empowers nurses to participate in ethical decision making.

CHAPTER HIGHLIGHTS

- Morality refers to what is right and wrong in conduct, character, or attitude.
- Nursing ethics refers to the moral problems that arise in nursing practice and to ethical decisions nurses make.
- Moral issues are those that arouse conscience, are concerned with important values and norms, and evoke words such as *good, bad, right, wrong, should,* and *ought.*
- Ethical problems are created as a result of changes in society, advances in technology, conflicts within the nursing role itself, and nurses' conflicting loyalties and obligations (ie, to clients, families, employers, physicians, and other nurses).
- Decision-focused problems are those in which it is difficult to arrive at a decision; they can be relieved by improving one's decision-making skills.
- Action-focused problems arise when nurses believe they know the right action but cannot act on their judgment without great personal risk; improved decision-making skills will not relieve the effects of these problems.
- Nurses' ethical decisions are influenced by their role perceptions, moral theories and principles, nursing codes of ethics, level of cognitive development, and personal and professional values.
- Four common moral frameworks (approaches) are teleology, deontology, intuitionism, and caring.

- Moral principles (eg, autonomy, beneficence, nonmaleficence, justice), fidelity, and veracity are broad, general philosophical concepts. Moral rules, by contrast, are specific prescriptions for actions.
- A professional code of ethics is a formal statement of a group's ideals and values that serves as a standard and guideline for the group's professional actions and informs the public of its commitment.
- Values give direction and meaning to life and guide a person's behavior.
- Values are freely chosen, prized and cherished, affirmed to others, and consistently incorporated into one's behavior.
- Values clarification is a process in which people identify, examine, and develop their own values.
- The goal of ethical reasoning, in the context of nursing, is to reach a mutual, peaceful agreement that is in the best interests of the client; reaching the agreement may require compromise.
- Integrity-preserving moral compromise requires shared moral language, a context of mutual respect, and acknowledgment of a situation's moral complexity.
- Nurses are responsible for determining their own actions and for supporting clients who are making moral decisions or for whom decisions are being made.
- Client advocacy involves concern for and defined actions on behalf of another person or organization in order to bring about change.
- The focus of the advocacy role is to inform and support.
- Ethics committees are multidisciplinary bodies that review cases, write guidelines and policies, and provide education and counseling.

READINGS AND REFERENCES

SUGGESTED READINGS

Barnett, T. January/March 1993. Are there employment risks to ethical decisions? *Nursing Forum* 28:17–21.

Describes a case in which a nurse was dismissed from her job after publicly protesting her employer's policy regarding withdrawal of food and fluids—a policy she believed was unethical, although legal. The article highlights that while nurses make ethical decisions, there may be a certain amount of risk in carrying them out.

Czerwinski, B. June 1990. An autopsy of an ethical dilemma. *Journal of Nursing Administration* 20:25–29.

Describes how an actual ethical dilemma involving a "No Code" order was resolved, and how nurses contributed to the creation of guidelines to use in similar situations.

RELATED RESEARCH

Breault, AJ and Polifroni, EC. January 1992. Caring for people with AIDS: Nurses' attitudes and feelings. *Journal of Advanced Nursing* 17:21–27.

Kelly, B. January 1992. Professional ethics as perceived by American nursing undergraduates . . . senior baccalaureate nursing students. *Journal of Advanced Nursing* 17:10–15.

SELECTED REFERENCES

American Nurses Association. 1985a. *Code for Nurses with Interpretive Statements.* Kansas City, MO: ANA.

______. 1985b. *Ethical Dilemmas Confronting Nurses.* Kansas City, MO: ANA.

______. 1988a. *Ethics in Nursing: Position Statements and Guidelines.* Kansas City, MO: ANA.

______. 1988b. *Nursing and the Human Immunodeficiency Virus: A Guide for Nursing's Response to AIDS.* Kansas City, MO: ANA.

______. 1991. *Standards of Clinical Nursing Practice.* Washington, DC: ANA.

Bandman, E. December 1979. Why ethics in nursing practice? *Imprint* 26:34–35, 58–59, 62 passim.

Bandman, EL. and Bandman, B. 1990. *Nursing Ethics Through the Life Span.* 2d ed. Norwalk, CT: Appleton & Lange.

Benner, P and Wrubel, J. 1989. *The Primacy of Caring.* Redwood City, CA: Addison-Wesley Nursing.

Bernal, EW. April 1985. Values clarification: A critique. *Journal of Nursing Education* 24:174–75.

Bishop, A and Scudder, J. April 1987. Nursing ethics in an age of controversy. *Advances in Nursing Science* 9:34–43.

Bok, S. 1978. *Moral choice in public and private life.* New York: Pantheon Books. As cited in Ellis, JR and Hartley, CL. 1992. *Nursing in today's world* 4th ed. Philadelphia: Lippincott.

Breault, AJ and Polifroni, EC. January 1992. Caring for people with AIDS: Nurses' attitudes and feelings. *Journal of Advanced Nursing* 17:21–27.

Canadian Nurses' Association. 1991. *Code of Ethics for Nursing.* Ottawa: CNA.

Cassells, J and Redman, B. June 1989. Preparing students to be moral agents in clinical nursing practice. *Nursing Clinics of North America* 24:463–73.

Chaffee, J. 1990. *Thinking Critically.* 3d ed. Boston: Houghton Mifflin.

College of Nurses of Ontario. 1985. *Guidelines for Ethical Behavior in Nursing.* Toronto: The College of Nurses.

Cooper, M. 1988. Covenantal relationships: Grounding for the nursing ethic. *Advances in Nursing Science* 10:48–59.

Corey, G, Corey, M, and Callahan, P. 1984. *Issues and Ethics in the Helping Professions.* 2d ed. Monterey, CA: Brooks/Cole.

Davis, A and Aroskar, M. 1983. *Ethical Dilemmas and Nursing Practice.* 2d ed. Norwalk, CT: Appleton-Century-Crofts.

DeWolf, M. May 1989. Ethical decision-making. *Seminars in Oncology Nursing* 5:77–81.

Donahue, MP. 1985. Viewpoints. Euthanasia: An ethical uncertainty. In McCloskey, JC and Grace, HK. *Current Issues in Nursing.* 2d ed. Cambridge, MA: Blackwell.

Fenton, M. October 1988. Moral distress in clinical practice: Implications for the nurse administrator. *Canadian Journal of Nursing Administration* 1:8–11.

Fowler, MD. January 1989a. Social advocacy. *Heart & Lung* 18:97–99.

———. December 1989b. Ethical decision making in clinical practice. *Nursing Clinics of North America* 24:955–65.

Fowler, MDM and Levine-Ariff, J. 1987. *Ethics at the Bedside.* Philadelphia: Lippincott.

Fry, S. June 1989a. Teaching ethics in nursing curricula. *Nursing Clinics of North America* 24:485–97.

———. May/June 1989b. The ethics of compromise. *Nursing Outlook* 37:152.

Gadow, S. 1990. Existential advocacy: Philosophical foundations of nursing. In Pence, T and Cantrall, J, editors. pp. 41–51. *Ethics in Nursing: An Anthology.* Pub. no. 20-2294. New York: National League for Nursing.

Gearhart, S and Young, S. April 1990. Intuition, ethical decision making, and the nurse manager. *Health Care Supervisor* 8:45–52.

Gilligan, C. 1982. In a different voice. Cambridge MA: Harvard University Press.

Grady, C. June 1989. Ethical issues in providing nursing care to human immunodeficiency virus-infected populations. *Nursing Clinics of North America* 24:523–34.

Haddad, AM. Fall 1993. Problematic ethical experiences: Stories from nursing practice. *Bioethics Forum* 9:5–10.

Hosford, B. 1986. *Bioethics Committees.* Rockville, MD: Aspen Publishers.

International Council of Nurses. 1973. *ICN Code for Nurses: Ethical Concepts Applied to Nursing.* Geneva: Imprimeries Populaires.

Jacobson, S. May/June 1978. Stressful situations for neonatal intensive care nurses. *American Journal of Maternal Child Nursing* 3:144–52.

Jameton, A. 1984. *Nursing Practice: The Ethical Issues.* Englewood Cliffs, NJ: Prentice Hall.

Joint Commission on Accreditation of Healthcare Organizations. 1992. *Accreditation Manual for Hospitals.* Oakbrook Terrace, IL: JCAHO.

Kohnke, MF. November 1980. The nurse as advocate. *American Journal of Nursing* 80:2038–40.

———. 1982. *Advocacy: Risk and Reality.* St Louis: Mosby.

Mahon, M. 1990. The nurse's role in treatment decisionmaking for the child with disabilities. *Issues in Law and Medicine* 6(3):247–68.

Murphy, C. 1990. Technological advances and ethical dilemmas. In McCloskey, J and Grace, H, editors. pp. 587–91. *Current Issues in Nursing.* St Louis: Mosby.

Noddings, N. 1984. *Caring: A Feminine Approach to Ethics and Moral Education.* Berkeley, CA: University of California Press.

Parker, RS. September 1990. Nurses' stories: The search for a relational ethic of care. *Advances in Nursing Science* 13:31–40.

Raths, L, Harmin, M, and Simon, S. 1978. *Values and Teaching.* 2d ed. Columbus, OH: Merrill.

Salladay, SA and McDonnell, MM. February 1992. Facing ethical conflicts. *Nursing92* 22:44–47.

Steele, SM and Harmon, VM. 1983. *Values Clarification in Nursing.* 2d ed. Norwalk, CT: Appleton-Century-Crofts.

Thompson, J and Thompson, H. June 1990. Moral development. *Neonatal Network* 8:77–78.

Uustal, D. September 1990. Enhancing your ethical reasoning. *Critical Care Nursing Clinics of North America* 2:437–42.

van Hooft, S. February 1990. Moral education for nursing decisions. *Journal of Advanced Nursing* 15:210–15.

Watson, J. Summer 1981. Socialization of the nursing student in a professional nursing education programme. *Nursing Papers* 13:19–24.

———. 1985. *Nursing: Human Science and Human Care.* Norwalk, CT: Appleton-Century-Crofts.

Wilkinson, J. 1987/88. Moral distress in nursing practice: Experience and effect. *Nursing Forum* 23:16–29.

———. January 1993. All ethics problems are not created equal. *The Kansas Nurse* 68(1):4–6.

Winslow, BJ and Winslow, GR. June 1991. Integrity and compromise in nursing ethics. *The Journal of Medicine and Philosophy* 16:307–23.

Yarling, R and McElmurry, B. January 1986. The moral foundation of nursing. *Advances in Nursing Science* 8:63–73.

12 Legal Aspects of Nursing Practice

Objectives

- Describe general legal concepts as they apply to nursing.
- Explain how nurse practice acts legally help the practicing nurse.
- Describe ways standards of care, agency policies, and nurse practice acts affect the scope of nursing practice.
- Identify essential types and elements of contracts.
- Identify rights and obligations associated with the nurse's legal roles.
- Describe collective bargaining with reference to nursing.
- Identify areas of potential liability for nurses.
- Differentiate crimes from torts, and give examples in nursing.
- Describe the purpose and essential elements of informed consent.
- List information that needs to be included in an incident report.
- Describe actions a nurse should take when a client is injured.
- Describe the purpose of the following legislated acts: Good Samaritan acts, Patient Self-Determination Act, Americans with Disabilities Act.
- Discuss the problem of sexual harassment in nursing.
- Discuss the problem of the chemically impaired nurse.
- Describe the purpose of professional liability insurance.
- Identify ways nursing students can minimize their chances of liability.

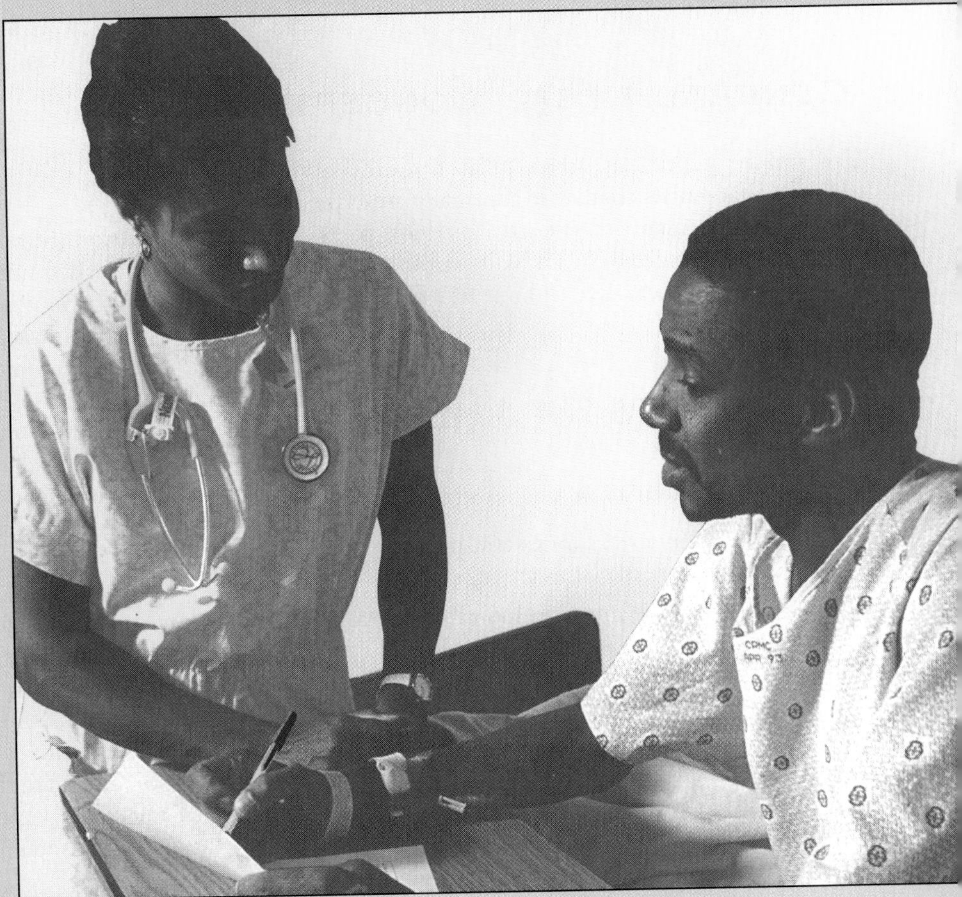

Nursing practice is governed by many legal concepts. It is important for nurses to know the basics of legal concepts, because nurses are accountable for their professional judgments and actions. Accountability is an essential concept of professional nursing practice and the law. Knowledge of laws that regulate and affect nursing practice is needed for two reasons:

1. To ensure that the nurse's decisions and actions are consistent with current legal principles
2. To protect the nurse from liability

General Legal Concepts

Law can be defined as "those rules made by humans which regulate social conduct in a formally prescribed and legally binding manner" (Bernzweig 1990, p. 3). Hall (1990, p. 35) states that laws prohibit extremes of behavior so that individuals can live without fear for their person or their property.

Functions of the Law in Nursing

The law serves a number of functions in nursing:

- It provides a framework for establishing which nursing actions in the care of clients are legal.
- It differentiates the nurse's responsibilities from those of other health professionals.
- It helps establish the boundaries of independent nursing action.
- It assists in maintaining a standard of nursing practice by making nurses accountable under the law.

Sources of Law

The legal systems in both the United States and Canada have their origins in the English common law system. Three primary sources of law are constitutions, statutes, and decisions of courts (common law).

Constitutions The Constitution of the United States and the Constitution of Canada are the supreme laws of their respective countries. They establish the general organization of the federal governments, grant certain powers to them, and place limits on what federal and state or provincial governments may do. Constitutions create legal rights and responsibilities and are the foundation for a system of justice.

Constitutions have due process and equal protection clauses. The due process clause applies to state or provincial and local agencies, including public hospitals, and to actions that deprive a person of life, liberty, or property. **Due process** has two primary elements (Black 1991, p. 346):

1. The procedural element, which guarantees a fair and orderly legal process.
2. The substantive element, which protects a person's property from unfair governmental interference or taking.

Black (1991, p. 371) defines **equal protection** as "a constitutional guarantee that no person or group of persons can be denied the same protection of the laws which is enjoyed by other persons or other classes in like circumstances."

Legislation (Statutes) Laws enacted by any legislative body are called **statutory laws.** When federal and state or provincial laws conflict, federal law supersedes. Likewise, state or provincial laws supersede local laws.

The regulation of nursing is a function of state or provincial law. State or provincial legislatures pass statutes that define and regulate nursing, that is, nurse practice acts. These acts, however, must be consistent with constitutional and federal provisions. Nurses practice acts, Good Samaritan laws, and adult or child abuse laws are examples of statutes that affect nurses.

Legislatures delegate responsibility and power to implement various laws to many administrative agencies who have the time and the expertise to address complex issues. State or provincial administrative agencies oversee the practice of the professions and regulate various aspects of commerce and public welfare. Examples pertinent to nurses are the state boards of nursing and provincial nursing associations, which implement and enforce nurse practice acts.

Common Law The body of principles that evolves from court decisions is referred to as **common law,** or decisional laws. Although courts are called on to interpret and apply constitutional or statutory law, they also are asked to resolve disputes between two parties. In such disputes, statutory and constitutional laws alone cannot support the case. Common law is continually being adapted and expanded. In deciding specific controversies, courts generally adhere to the doctrine of *stare decisis*—"to stand by things decided"—usually referred to as "following precedent." In other words, to arrive at a ruling in a particular case, the court applies the same rules and principles applied in previous, similar cases. Courts may depart

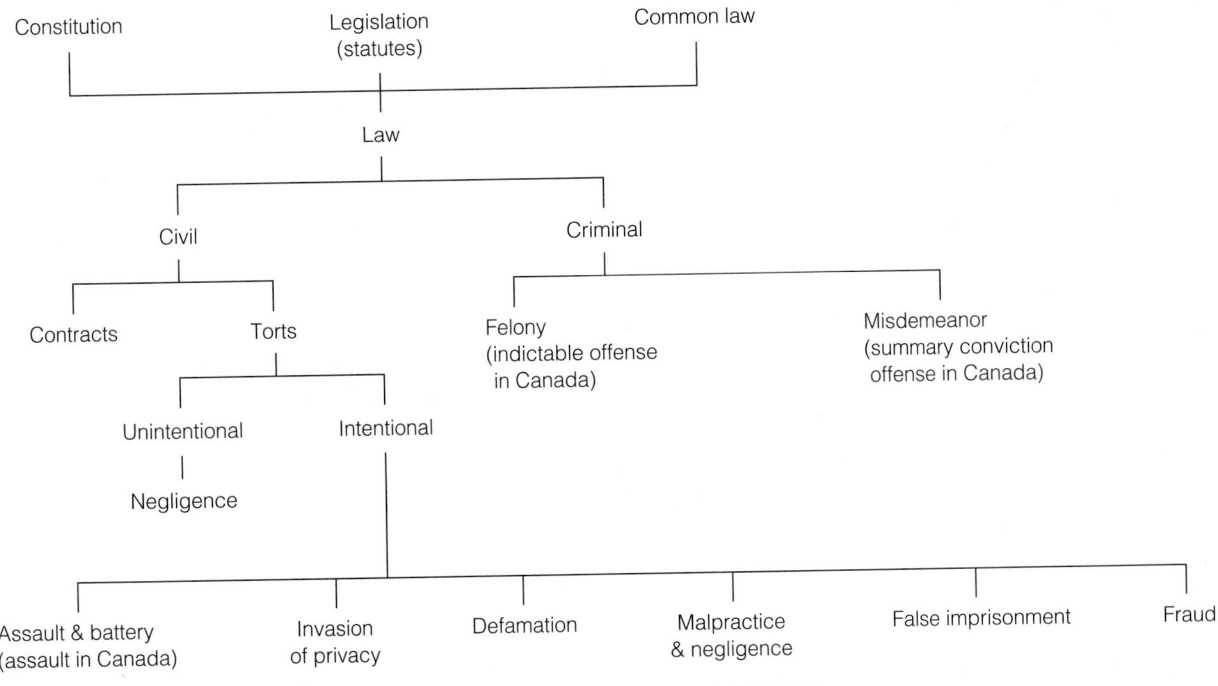

Figure 12–1 Categories of law pertinent to nursing.

from precedent when slight differences are noted between cases or when it is thought that a particular common law rule no longer applies to the needs of society.

TYPES OF LAWS

Laws govern the relationship of private individuals with government and with each other.

Public law refers to the body of law that deals with relationships between individuals and the government and governmental agencies. An important segment of public law is **criminal law,** which deals with actions against the safety and welfare of the public. Examples are homicide, manslaughter, and theft. In the United States, crimes are classified as felonies or misdemeanors; in Canada, as indictable offenses or summary conviction offenses. See the discussion of crimes and torts later in this chapter. Public law also includes numerous regulations designed to enhance societal objectives. Private individuals and organizations are required to follow specified courses of action in their activities. Noncompliance with these regulations can lead to criminal penalties.

Private law, or **civil law,** is the body of law that deals with relationships between private individuals. It is categorized as contract law and tort law. **Contract law** involves the enforcement of agreements among private individuals or the payment of compensation for failure to fulfill the agreements. **Tort law** defines and enforces duties and rights among private individuals that are not based on contractual agreements. The word *tort* comes from the Latin word *tortus,* meaning twisted. Loosely translated, it means "wrong" or "bad." Some examples of tort laws applicable to nurses are negligence and malpractice, invasion of privacy, and assault and battery. See Figure 12–1, above, and also Table 12–1, on page 220, for selected categories of law affecting nurses.

KINDS OF LEGAL ACTIONS

There are two kinds of legal actions: civil or private actions and criminal actions. **Civil actions** deal with the relationships between individuals in society; for example, a man may file a suit against a person who he believes cheated him. Civil actions that are of concern to nurses include the torts and contracts listed in Table 12–1, on page 220. Other civil actions that can concern nurses include those relating to wills and the estates of deceased persons. For example, nurses in long term care and home health may be called upon to attest to the validity of a client's will during **probate proceedings** if the nurse was witness to the signing of the will. **Criminal actions** deal with disputes between an individual and the society as a whole; for example, if a man shoots a person, society brings him to trial.

THE CIVIL JUDICIAL PROCESS

The judicial process primarily functions to settle disputes peacefully and in accordance with the law. A lawsuit has strict procedural rules. There are generally five steps:

Table 12–1 Selected Categories of Laws Affecting Nurses

Category	Examples
Constitutional	Due process
	Equal protection
Statutory (legislative)	Nurse practice acts
	Good Samaritan acts
	Child and adult abuse laws
	Living wills
	Sexual harassment laws
	Americans with Disabilities Act
Criminal (public)	Homicide, manslaughter
	Theft
	Arson
	Active euthanasia
	Sexual assault
	Illegal possession of controlled drugs
Contracts (private/civil)	Nurse and client
	Nurse and employer
	Nurse and insurance
	Client and agency
Torts (private/civil)	Negligence
	Libel and slander
	Invasion of privacy
	Assault and battery
	False imprisonment
	Abandonment

1. A document called a **complaint** is filed by a person referred to as the **plaintiff,** who claims that the person's legal rights have been infringed upon by one or more persons, referred to as **defendants.**
2. A written response, called an **answer,** is made by the defendants.
3. Both parties engage in pretrial activities, referred to as **discovery,** in an effort to gain all the facts of the situation.
4. In the **trial** of the case, all the relevant facts are presented to a jury or a judge.
5. The judge renders a **decision,** or the jury renders a **verdict.** If the outcome is not acceptable to one of the parties, an appeal can be made for another trial.

During a trial, a plaintiff must offer evidence of the defendant's wrongdoing. This duty of proving an assertion is called the **burden of proof.** An additional aspect of this burden of proof is that in order to prevail, the plaintiff must present a greater amount of convincing evidence than the defendant.

NURSES AS WITNESSES

A nurse may be called to testify in a legal action for a variety of reasons. The nurse may be a defendant in a malpractice or negligence action or may have been a member of the health team that provided care to the plaintiff. It is advisable that any nurse who is asked to testify in such a situation seek the advice of an attorney before providing testimony. In most cases, the attorney for the institution will provide support and counsel during the legal case. If the nurse is the defendant, however, it is advisable for the nurse to retain an attorney to protect the nurse's own interests.

A nurse may also be asked to provide testimony as an expert witness. An **expert witness** is one who has special training, experience, or skill in a relevant area and who is allowed by the court to offer an opinion on some issue within that nurse's area of expertise (Bernzweig 1990, p. 431). Such a witness is usually called to help a judge or jury understand evidence pertaining to the extent of damage and the standard of care.

When called into court as a witness, the nurse has a duty to assist justice as far as possible. The nurse should always respond directly and truthfully to the questions asked. The nurse is not expected to volunteer additional information, nor is the nurse expected to remember completely all the details of a situation that may have occurred months or even years prior to the legal action. The nurse may ask to refer to the client record or to personal notes related to the incident. If the nurse does not remember the details of the incident, it is advisable to say so rather than to report an inaccurate recollection. In any case, it is the nurse's professional responsibility to provide accurate testimony, both during the pretrial discovery phase and the trial phase of a legal action.

PRIVILEGED COMMUNICATION

A **privileged communication** is information given to a professional person who is forbidden by law from disclosing the information in a court without the consent of the person who provided it.

Legislation regarding privileged communications is highly complicated. A nurse would be unwise to encourage disclosures or advise a client about the subject. The privileged communication law is for the benefit of the client; a nurse who is given confidential information should be prepared to answer questions fully and honestly if required to testify in a court of law. Many states with statutes granting privileged communications between the client and various health care providers do not extend the privilege to nurse-client communication.

The American Nurses Association (ANA) refers to the matter of privileged communications in its *Code for Nurses* (1976). It advises the nurse to seek legal counsel in regard to a privileged communication and to become familiar with the rights and privileges of the client and the nurse.

In Canada, confidentiality of information is incorporated as an ethic in the legislation on nursing practice. Failure to maintain confidentiality can result in disciplinary action against the nurse.

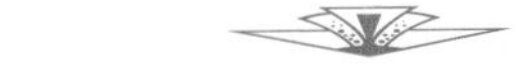

LEGAL ASPECTS OF NURSING

CREDENTIALING

Credentialing is the process of determining and maintaining competence in nursing practice. The credentialing process is one way in which the nursing profession maintains standards of practice and accountability for the educational preparation of its members. Credentialing includes licensure, registration, certification, and accreditation.

Licensure and Registration **Licenses** are legal permits a government agency grants to individuals to engage in the practice of a profession and to use a particular title. A particular jurisdiction or area is covered by the license. For a profession or occupation to obtain the right to license its members, it generally must meet three criteria:

1. There is a need to protect the public's safety or welfare.
2. The occupation is clearly delineated as a separate, distinct area of work.
3. There is a proper authority to assume the obligations of the licensing process, eg, in nursing, state and provincial boards of nursing.

Registration is the listing of an individual's name and other information on the official roster of a governmental or nongovernmental agency. Nurses who are registered are permitted to use the title "Registered Nurse."

In the United States, all registered nurses are licensed by the board of nursing of the state; in Canada, they are licensed or registered by the provincial nursing association or college of nursing. The requirements for licensure vary by state and province. In the United States, all nursing candidates write the National Council Licensure Examinations (NCLEX) for registered nursing or practical nursing.

Canada has a national comprehensive registered nurse examination, offered in both French and English. Nurses from other countries are granted registration by endorsement after successfully completing these examinations. Both licensure and registration must be renewed on an annual basis (in some states, every 2 years) to remain valid.

There are two types of licensure/registration: mandatory and permissive. Under *mandatory licensure/registration*, anyone who practices nursing must be licensed or registered. Under *permissive licensure/registration*, the title RN is reserved for licensed or, in Canada, registered practitioners, but the practice of nursing is not prohibited to others who are not licensed or registered. Registration is mandatory in most provinces of Canada. In the United States, nursing licensure is mandatory in all states. A strong movement is under way in Canada to make registration mandatory in all provinces.

In each state and province there is a mechanism by which licenses (or registration in Canada) can be revoked for just cause (eg, incompetent nursing practice, professional misconduct, conviction of a crime such as using illegal drugs or selling drugs illegally). In each situation, all the facts are generally reviewed by a committee at a hearing. Nurses are entitled to be represented by legal counsel at such a hearing. If the nurse's license is revoked as a result of the hearing, either the nurse can appeal the decision to a court of law, or, in some states, an agency is designated to review the decision before any court action is initiated.

Nurse Practice Acts Each state in the United States has a nurse practice act, and each province in Canada has a nurse practice act or an act for professional nursing practice. Nurse practice acts protect the nurse's professional capacity and legally control nursing practice through licensing. Nurse practice acts legally define and describe the scope of nursing practice, which the law seeks to regulate, thereby protecting the public as well. Because of the number of acts, there are many definitions and descriptions of nursing. In 1981, the ANA described nursing practice as including but not limited to "administration, teaching, counseling, supervision, delegation, and evaluation of practice and execution of the medical regimen, including the administration of medications and treatments prescribed by any person authorized by state law to prescribe" (ANA 1981, p. 6).

For advanced nursing practice, many states require a different license or have an additional clause that pertains to actions that may be performed only by nurses with advanced education. For example, an additional license may be required to practice as a nurse-midwife, nurse-anesthetist, or nurse-practitioner. The advanced practice nurse also requires a license to be able to prescribe medication or order treatments from physical therapists or other health professionals. There is some controversy about the requirement for additional licensure for advanced practice. The ANA's position is that it is the function of the professional association, not the law, to establish the scope of practice for advanced nursing practice and that the state boards of nursing can regulate advanced nursing practice within each state (ANA 1993b).

Certification Certification is the voluntary practice of validating that an individual nurse has met minimum standards of nursing competence in specialty areas, such as maternal-child health, pediatrics, mental health, gerontology, and school nursing. Certification programs are conducted by the ANA and by specialty nursing organizations. A certification program was established in Canada by the CNA in 1991. The CNA certification program for nurses includes seven specialized fields of nursing.

Accreditation/Approval of Basic Nursing Education Programs Accreditation is a process by which a voluntary organization, such as the National League for Nursing (NLN), or governmental agency, such as the state board of nursing, appraises and grants accredited status to institutions and/or programs or services that meet predetermined structure, process, and outcome criteria (ANA 1979). Minimum standards for basic nursing education programs are established in each state of the United States and in each province in Canada. State accreditation or provincial approval is granted to schools of nursing meeting the minimum criteria.

The purposes of NLN accreditation of programs in nursing are as follows (NLN 1991, p. vi; 1992, p. vi):

- To foster the continuous development and improvement in quality of educational programs in nursing throughout the United States and its territories
- To evaluate nursing programs in relation to their stated philosophy and outcomes and to the established criteria for accreditation
- To involve administrators of the governing institutions and the administrators, faculties, and students of nursing programs in the process of continuous self-study and improvement of their programs
- To bring together practitioners, administrators, faculty, and students in an activity directed toward improving educational preparation for nursing practice
- To provide an external peer review process

According to the NLN, "accreditation reflects a program that is flexible and progressive, meeting the changing needs of the society it serves through sound educational methods and a humanistic approach (NLN 1991, p. vii)." Unlike state approval or provincial accreditation, NLN accreditation is not a legal requirement. Some states, however, require NLN accreditation for any school wishing to maintain state accreditation.

STANDARDS OF PRACTICE

Another way the nursing profession attempts to ensure that its practitioners are competent and safe to practice is through the establishment of standards of practice (see Chapter 2). These standards are often used to evaluate the quality of care nurses provide. In addition to this basic set of standards, which are applicable in any practice setting, the ANA has developed standards of nursing practice for specific areas such as maternal-child, medical-surgical, geriatric, psychiatric, and community health nursing.

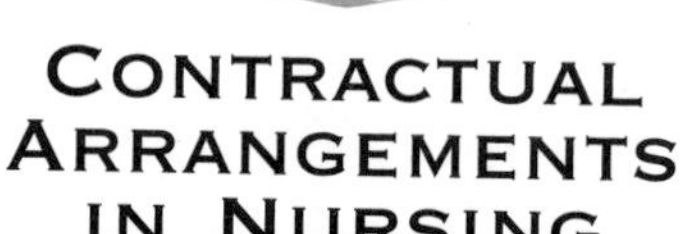

CONTRACTUAL ARRANGEMENTS IN NURSING

A contract is the basis of the relationship between a nurse and an employer—for example, a nurse and a hospital or a nurse and a physician. A **contract** is an agreement between two or more competent persons, on sufficient consideration (remuneration), to do or not to do some lawful act. A contract may be written or oral; however, a written contract cannot be changed legally by an oral agreement. If two people wish to change some aspect of a written contract, the change must be written into the contract, because one party cannot hold the other to an oral agreement that differs from the written one.

A contract is considered to be *expressed* when the two parties discuss and agree orally or in writing to its terms, for example, that a nurse will work at a hospital for a stated length of time and under stated conditions. An **implied contract** is one that has not been explicitly agreed to by the parties but that the law nevertheless considers to exist. In the contractual relationship between nurse and client, clients have the right to expect that nurses caring for them have the competence to meet their needs. This *implies* that the nurse has a responsibility to remain competent. The nurse has the associated right to expect the client to provide accurate information as required.

A lawful contract requires the following five elements (Creighton 1986, p. 25):

1. The consent of the parties or persons involved.
2. A valid consideration or something of value—in most cases, financial compensation for fulfilling the terms of the contract or agreement.
3. A lawful purpose; that is, the activity must be legal.
4. Competent parties or persons; that is, they are of legal age to enter into a contract and have the mental capacity to understand the requirements of the contract.
5. Completion of the appropriate documents required by the law.

A contract made by a client (with nurses, other health professionals, or health care institutions) is valid only if it meets these requirements. For example, a client contracts with a hospital to obtain health care, a legal activity. Clients who are minors are not usually admitted for care without consent from their parents or legal guardians. The parties agree to the terms of the contract when the client gives informed consent for care and the hospital offers care. The client promises to reimburse the hospital for its services through insurance coverage or other means.

LEGAL ROLES OF NURSES

Nurses have three separate, interdependent legal roles, each with rights and associated responsibilities: provider of service, employee or contractor for service, and citizen.

Provider of Service The nurse is expected to provide safe and competent care so that harm (physical, psychologic, or material) to the recipient of the service is prevented. Implicit in this role are several legal concepts: liability, standard of care, and contractual obligations.

Liability is the quality or state of being legally responsible to account for one's obligations and actions and to make financial restitution for wrongful acts. A nurse, for example, has an obligation to practice and direct the practice of others under the nurse's supervision so that harm or injury to the client is prevented and standards of care are maintained. Even when a nurse carries out treatments ordered by the physician, the responsibility for the nursing activity is the nurse's. When a nurse is asked to carry out an activity that the nurse believes will be injurious to the client, the nurse's responsibility is to refuse to carry out the order and report this to the nurse in charge.

The **standards of care** by which a nurse acts or fails to act are legally defined by nurse practice acts and by the rule of reasonable and prudent action—what a reasonable and prudent professional with similar preparation and experience would do in similar circumstances. **Contractual obligations** refer to the nurse's duty of care, that is, duty to render care, established by the presence of an expressed or implied contract discussed earlier.

Employee or Contractor for Service A nurse who is employed by a hospital works as an agent of the hospital, and the nurse's contract with clients is an implied one. However, a nurse who is employed directly by a client, for example, a private nurse, may have a written contract with that client in which the nurse agrees to provide professional services for a certain fee. If the client is dying, the nurse can be protected by a written contract that allows collection of the fee from the client's estate. A nurse might be prevented from carrying out the terms of the contract because of illness or death. However, personal inconvenience and personal problems, such as the nurse's car failure, are not legitimate reasons for failing to fulfill a contract.

Contractual relationships vary among practice settings. An independent nurse practitioner is a contractor for service whose contractual relationship with the client is an independent one. The nurse employed by a hospital functions within an employer–employee relationship, in which the nurse represents and acts for the hospital and therefore must function within the policies of the employing agency. This type of legal relationship creates the ancient legal doctrine known as **respondeat superior** ("let the master answer"). In other words, the master (employer) assumes responsibility for the conduct of the servant (employee) and can also be held responsible for malpractice by the employee. By virtue of the employee role, therefore, the nurse's conduct is the hospital's responsibility.

This doctrine does not imply that the nurse cannot be held liable as an individual. Nor does it imply that the doctrine will prevail if the employee's actions are extraordinarily inappropriate, that is, beyond those expected or foreseen by the employer. For example, if the nurse hits a client in the face, the employer could disclaim responsibility, because this behavior is beyond the bounds of expected behavior. Criminal acts, such as assisting with criminal abortions or taking tranquilizers from a client's supply for personal use, would also be considered extraordinarily inappropriate behavior. Nurses can be held liable for failure to act as well. For example, if a nurse sees another nurse hitting a client and fails to do anything to protect the client, the observer may also be considered negligent.

The nurse in the role of employee or contractor for service has obligations to the employer, the client, and other personnel. The nursing care provided must be within the limitations and terms specified. The nurse has an obligation to contract only for those responsibilities that the nurse is competent to discharge.

The nurse is expected to respect the rights and responsibilities of other health care participants. For example, although the nurse has responsibility to explain nursing activities to a client, the nurse does not have the right to comment on medical practice in a way that disturbs the client or denounces the physician. At the same time, the nurse has the right to expect reasonable and prudent conduct from other health professionals.

Citizen The rights and responsibilities of the nurse in the role of citizen are the same as those of any individual under the legal system. Rights of citizenship protect clients from harm and ensure consideration for their personal property rights, rights to privacy, confidentiality, and other rights discussed later in this chapter. These same rights apply to nurses.

Table 12–2 Nurses' Legal Roles, Rights, and Responsibilities

Role	Responsibilities	Rights
Provider of service	To provide safe and competent care commensurate with the nurse's preparation, experience, and circumstances	Right to adequate and qualified assistance as necessary
	To inform clients of the consequences of various alternatives and outcomes of care	Right to reasonable and prudent conduct from clients, eg, provision of accurate information as required
	To provide adequate supervision and evaluation of subordinates for whom the nurse is responsible	
	To remain competent	
Employee or contractor for service	To fulfill the obligations of contracted service with the employer	Right to adequate working conditions (eg, safe equipment and facilities)
	To respect the employer	Right to compensation for services rendered
	To respect the rights and responsibilities of other health care providers	Right to reasonable and prudent conduct by other health care providers
Citizen	To protect the rights of the recipients of care	Right to respect by others of the nurse's own rights and responsibilities
		Right to physical safety

Nurses move in and out of these roles when carrying out professional and personal responsibilities. An understanding of these roles and the rights and responsibilities associated with them promotes legally responsible conduct and practice by nurses. **Rights** are privileges or fundamental powers to which an individual is entitled unless they are revoked by law or given up voluntarily; **responsibilities** are the obligations associated with these rights. See Table 12–2 for examples of the responsibilities and rights associated with each role.

Collective Bargaining

Collective bargaining is the formalized decision-making process between representatives of management and representatives of labor to negotiate wages and conditions of employment, including work hours, working environment, and fringe benefits of employment (eg, vacation time, sick leave, and personal leave). Through a written agreement, both employer and employees legally commit themselves to observe the terms and conditions of employment. Collective bargaining is a controversial issue among nurses. Some nurses consider collective bargaining to be unprofessional and contrary to the altruistic nature of nursing. Others argue that collective bargaining is necessary to obtain control of nursing practice and economic security.

The collective bargaining process involves the recognition of a certified bargaining agent for the employees. This agent can be a union, a trade association, or a professional organization. The agent represents the employees in negotiating a contract with management. O'Connor and Gibson (1990, p. 454) reported that approximately 239,000, or 11%, of registered nurses in the United States were covered by collective bargaining agreements, and the majority were represented by their state constituents of the ANA.

When collective bargaining breaks down because an agreement cannot be reached, the employees usually call a strike. A **strike** is an organized work stoppage by a group of employees to express a grievance, enforce a demand for changes in conditions of employment or solve a dispute with management.

Because nursing practice is a service to people (often ill people), striking presents a moral dilemma to many nurses. Actions taken by nurses can affect the safety of people. When faced with a strike, each nurse must make an individual decision to cross or not to cross a picket line. Nursing students may also be faced with decisions about crossing picket lines in the event of a strike at a clinical agency used for learning experiences. The ANA supports striking as a means of achieving economic and general welfare.

Collective bargaining is more than the negotiation of salary terms and hours of work; it is a continuous process

Table 12–3 Categories and Examples of Grievances

Category	Examples
Contract violations	Shift or weekend work is assigned inequitably.
	A nurse is dismissed without cause.
Violations of federal and state law	A female nurse is paid less than a male nurse for the same work.
	Appropriate payment is not given for overtime work.
	Minority group nurses are not promoted.
Management responsibilities	Appropriate locker room facilities are not provided.
	Safe client care is jeopardized by inadequate staffing.
Violation of agency rules	Performance evaluations are conducted only at termination of employment, but the contract requires annual evaluations.
	A vacation period is assigned without the nurse's agreement, as required in personnel policies.

Source: American Nurses Association, *The Grievance Procedure* (Kansas City, MO: ANA, 1985), pp. 2–4. Used by permission.

in which day-to-day working problems and relationships can be handled in an orderly and democratic manner. Day-to-day difficulties or grievances are handled through the grievance procedure, a formal plan established in the contract that outlines the channels for handling and settling grievances through progressively higher levels of administration. A **grievance** is any dispute, difference, controversy, or disagreement arising out of the terms and conditions of employment. Grievances fall into four main categories, outlined in Table 12–3.

AREAS OF POTENTIAL LIABILITY IN NURSING

CRIMES AND TORTS

A **crime** is an act committed in violation of public (criminal) law and punishable by a fine and/or imprisonment. A crime does *not* have to be intended in order to be a crime. For example, a nurse may accidentally give a client an additional and lethal dose of a narcotic to relieve discomfort.

Crimes are classified as either felonies (or, in Canada, indictable offenses) or misdemeanors (or, in Canada, summary conviction offenses). A **felony** is a crime of a serious nature, such as murder, punishable by a term in prison. In some areas, second-degree murder is called **manslaughter.** A nurse who accidentally gives an additional and lethal dose of a narcotic can be accused of manslaughter. Other examples of felonies are arson and armed robbery.

Crimes are punished through criminal action by the state or province against an individual. A **misdemeanor** is an offense of a less serious nature and is usually punishable by a fine or short-term jail sentence, or both. A nurse who slaps a client's face could be charged with a misdemeanor.

A **tort** is a civil wrong committed against a person or a person's property. Torts are usually litigated in court by civil action between individuals. In other words, the person or persons claimed to be responsible for the tort are sued for damages. Tort liability almost always is based on fault, that is, something that was done incorrectly (an unreasonable act of commission) or something that should have been done was not done (act of omission).

Torts may be classified as intentional or unintentional. Intentional torts include fraud, invasion of privacy, libel and slander, assault and battery, and false imprisonment. **Fraud** is the false presentation of some fact with the intention that it will be acted upon by another person. For example, it is fraud for a nurse applying to a hospital for employment to fail to list two past employers for deceptive reasons when asked for five previous employers.

The right to privacy is the right of individuals to withhold themselves and their lives from public scrutiny. Invasion of privacy is a direct wrong of a personal nature. It injures the feelings of the person and does not take into account the effect of revealed information on the standing of the person in the community. The right to privacy can also be described as the right to be left alone. Liability can result if the nurse breaches confidentiality by passing along confidential client information to others or intrudes into the client's private domain.

In this context, there is a delicate balance between the need of a number of people to contribute to the diagnosis and treatment of a client and the client's right to confidentiality. In most situations, necessary discussion about a client's medical condition is considered appropriate, but unnecessary discussions and gossip are considered a breach of confidentiality. Necessary discussion involves only those engaged in the client's care.

Most jurisdictions of the country have a variety of statutes that impose a duty to report certain confidential client information. Four major categories are (a) vital statistics, such as births and deaths, (b) infections and communicable diseases, such as diphtheria, syphilis, and typhoid fever, (c) child or elder abuse, and (d) violent incidents, such as gunshot wounds and knife wounds.

Table 12–4 Elements of Negligence

Element	Definition	Example
Duty	The duties of the nurse to the client are described in standards of nursing practice, institutional policy and procedure manuals, and nursing literature.	The nurse has a duty to provide a safe environment for the client; for example, a client who is confused and disoriented should have side rails in place to prevent falls.
Breach of the duty	Failure to comply with the standard of care; may be an act of commission or omission.	The nurse inadvertently fails to put the side rails up.
Injury	An injury occurs to the client.	The client falls out of bed and suffers a fractured hip.
Causal relationship	A relationship between the breach of duty and the injury.	Because the nurse failed to put up the side rails, the client fell out of bed and suffered the injury.

Both libel and slander are wrongful actions that come under the heading of defamation. **Defamation** is communication that is false, or made with a careless disregard for the truth, and results in injury to the reputation of a person. **Libel** is defamation by means of print, writing, or pictures. Writing in the nurse's notes that a physician is incompetent because he didn't respond immediately to a call is an example of libel. **Slander** is defamation by the spoken word, stating unprivileged (not legally protected) or false words by which a reputation is damaged. An example of slander would be for the nurse to tell a client that another nurse is incompetent. A nurse has a qualified privilege to make statements that could be considered invasions of a client's privacy, both orally and in writing, but only as a part of nursing practice and only to a physician or another health team member caring directly for the client.

In the United States, the terms *assault* and *battery* are often heard together, but each has its own meaning. **Assault** can be described as an attempt or threat to touch another person unjustifiably. Assault precedes battery; it is the act that causes the person to believe a battery is about to occur. For example, the person who threatens someone by making a menacing gesture with a club or a closed fist is guilty of assault. In nursing, a nurse who threatened a client with an injection after the client refused to take the medication orally would be committing assault.

Battery is the willful touching of a person (or the person's clothes, or even something the person is carrying) that may or may not cause harm. To be actionable at law, however, the touching must be wrong in some way, for example, done without permission, embarrassing, or causing injury. In the previous example, if the nurse followed through on the threat and gave the injection without the client's consent, the nurse would be committing battery. Liability applies even though the physician ordered the medication or the activity and even if the client benefits from the nurse's action.

In Canada, the term *battery* is not used. Instead, assault is classified into three categories: assault with intention to injure (for example, threatening someone by making a menacing gesture with a knife), assault causing bodily injury, and sexual assault.

False imprisonment is the "unlawful restraint or detention of another person against his or her wishes." False imprisonment does not require force; the fear of force to restrain or detain the individual is sufficient (Bernzweig 1990, p. 228). False imprisonment accompanied by forceful restraint or threat of restraint is assault (Creighton 1986, p. 197).

Although nurses may suggest under certain circumstances that a client remain in the room or in bed, the client must not be detained against the client's will. The client has a right to insist upon leaving even though it may be detrimental to health. In this instance, the client can leave by signing an AWA (absence without authority) or AMA (against medical advice) form.

Negligence and malpractice are examples of unintentional torts that may occur in health care settings. **Negligence** is "failure to behave in a reasonably and prudent manner, whether as a layperson or a professional and whether engaged in the simplest or most complex type of activity" (Bernzweig 1990, p. 21). When harm or injury results from this failure, negligence is said to occur. **Malpractice** refers "to the negligent acts of persons engaged in professions or occupations in which highly technical or professional skills are employed" (Bernzweig 1990, p. 26). The elements of proof for nursing negligence and malpractice are (a) a duty of the nurse to the client, (b) a breach of the duty on the part of the nurse, (c) an injury to the client, and (d) a causal relationship between the breach of the duty and the client's subsequent injury.

BASIC NURSING CARE ERRORS RESULTING IN NEGLIGENCE

Assessment Errors

Failing to

- Gather and chart client information adequately
- Recognize the significance of certain information (eg, laboratory values, vital signs)

Planning Errors

Failing to

- Chart each identified problem
- Use language in the care plan that other care givers understand
- Ensure continuity of care by ignoring the care plan
- Give discharge instructions that the client understands

Intervention Errors

Failing to

- Interpret and carry out a doctor's orders
- Perform nursing tasks correctly
- Pursue the doctor if the doctor doesn't respond to calls or notify the nurse manager if the doctor is unavailable

Source: Adapted from BE Calfee, Protecting yourself—nursing negligence, *Nursing91*, December 1991, 21:34–40.

See Table 12–4. A nurse could be liable for malpractice if the nurse injured a client while performing a procedure differently from the way other nurses would have done it.

Nurses are responsible for their own actions, whether they are independent practitioners or employees of a health agency. The descriptions of negligence and malpractice do not mention good intentions; it is not pertinent that the nurse did not intend to be negligent. If a nurse administers an incorrect medication, even in good faith, the fact that the nurse failed to read the label correctly indicates malpractice if all of the elements of negligence are met. Negligence usually is the result of errors in basic nursing care. Calfee (1991, p. 35) describes three categories of nursing errors: assessment errors, planning errors, and intervention errors. The box above gives examples of each of these error types.

Another significant aspect of negligence and malpractice is that both omissions and commissions are included. That is, a nurse can be negligent by forgetting to give a medication as well as by giving the wrong medication. See Table 12–5 for a summary of the differences between intentional and unintentional torts.

Table 12–5 Comparison of Intentional and Unintentional Torts

Intentional	Unintentional (Negligence)
1. They involve the commission of a prohibited act.	1. They can result from either an act of commission or an act of omission.
2. The act in question is willful and deliberate (intentional).	2. The wrong results from failure to use due care.
3. They involve certain specific types of conduct listed as "wrong."	3. They are not spelled out in an all-inclusive list.

POTENTIAL MALPRACTICE SITUATIONS IN NURSING

To avoid charges of malpractice, nurses need to recognize those nursing situations in which negligent actions are most likely to occur and to take measures to prevent them. The most common situation is the *medication error*. Because of the large number of medications on the market today and the variety of methods of administration, these errors may be on the increase. Nursing errors include failing to read the medication label, misreading or incorrectly calculating the dosage, failing to identify the client correctly, preparing the wrong concentration, or administering a medication by the wrong route (eg, intravenously instead of intramuscularly). Some medication errors are very serious and can result in death. For example, administering dicumarol to a client recently returned from surgery could cause the client to have a hemorrhage. Nurses always need to check medications very carefully. Even after checking, the nurse is wise to recheck the medication order and the medication before administering it if the client states, for example, "I did not have a green pill before."

Sponges or other small items can be left inside a client during an operation because the nurse or surgical technician either failed to count them before the surgeon closed the incision or counted them incorrectly. In either case, the nurse responsible for the *sponge count* can be held liable for malpractice.

A relatively frequent malpractice action attributed to nurses is *burning a client.* Burns may be caused by hot water bottles, heating pads, and solutions that are too hot for application. Elderly, comatose, or diabetic people are

Guidelines for Reporting a Crime, Tort, or Unsafe Practice

- Write a clear description of the situation you believe you should report.
- Make sure that your statements are accurate.
- Make sure you are credible.
- Obtain support from at least one trustworthy person before filing the report.
- Report the matter starting at the lowest possible level in the agency hierarchy.
- Assume responsibility for reporting the individual by being open about it. Sign your name to the letter.
- See the problem through once you have reported it.

Source: DM Price and P Murphy, How—and when—to blow the whistle on unsafe practices, *Nursing Life*, January/February 1983, 3:50–54.

particularly vulnerable to burns because of their decreased sensitivity to pain and temperature. Hot objects can burn these people before they notice it. A nurse may also be held negligent for leaving a client without taking precautions (giving warnings or providing protections), for example, when using a steam vaporizer.

Clients often fall accidentally, sometimes with resultant injury. Some falls can be prevented by elevating the side rails on the cribs, beds, and stretchers of babies and small children and, when necessary, of adults. If a nurse leaves the rails down or leaves a baby unattended on a bath table, that nurse is guilty of malpractice if the *client falls* and is injured as a direct result. Most hospitals and nursing homes have policies regarding the use of safety devices such as side rails and restraints. The nurse needs to be familiar with these policies and to take indicated precautions to prevent accidents. Information about providing a safe environment for the client can be found in Chapter 28.

In some instances, ignoring a client's complaints can constitute malpractice. This type of malpractice is termed *failure to observe and take appropriate action.* The nurse who does not report a client's complaint of acute abdominal pain is negligent and may be found guilty of malpractice for ensuing appendix rupture and death. By failing to take the blood pressure and pulse and to check the dressing of a client who has just had abdominal surgery, a nurse omits important assessments. If the client hemorrhages and dies, the nurse may be held responsible for the death as a result of this malpractice.

Incorrectly identifying clients is a problem, particularly in busy hospital units. Unfortunate occurrences, such as removal of a healthy gallbladder from the wrong person, have resulted from nurses' preparing the wrong client for surgery. Cases of *mistaken identity* are costly to the client and render the nurse liable for malpractice.

Loss of Client Property

Client property, such as jewelry, money, eyeglasses, and dentures, is a constant concern to hospital personnel. Today, agencies are taking less responsibility for property and are generally requesting clients to sign a waiver on admission relieving the hospital and its employees of any responsibility for property. There are, however, situations in which the client cannot sign a waiver and the nursing staff must follow prescribed policies for safeguarding the client's property. In hospital units, dentures are often a major problem; they can be lost in bedding or left on a meal tray. Nurses are expected to take reasonable precautions to safeguard a client's property, and they can be held liable for its *loss or damage* if they do not exercise reasonable care.

Reporting Crimes, Torts, and Unsafe Practices

Nurses may need to report nursing colleagues or other health professionals for practices that endanger the health and safety of clients. For instance, alcohol and drug use, theft from a client or agency, and unsafe nursing practice should be reported. Reporting a colleague is not easy. The person reporting may feel disloyal, incur the disapproval of others, or endanger chances for promotion. When reporting an incident or series of incidents, the nurse must be careful to describe observed behavior only and not make inferences as to what might be happening. The box at the top of the page outlines guidelines for reporting a crime, tort, or unsafe practice. In cases of substance abuse, states such as California have established voluntary programs that allow nurses to receive help in resolving their problems without losing their licenses to practice. See additional information on the impaired nurse, later in this chapter.

Selected Legal Facets of Nursing Practice

Informed Consent

Informed consent is an agreement by a client to accept a course of treatment or a procedure after complete information, including the risks of treatment and facts relating to it, has been provided by the physician. Informed consent, then, is an exchange between a client and a physician. Usually the client signs a form provided by the agency. The form is a record of the informed consent, not the informed consent itself.

Obtaining informed consent for specific medical and surgical treatments is the responsibility of a physician (Bernzweig 1990, p. 194; Maher 1989, p. 38; Creighton 1986, p. 36). Although this responsibility is delegated to nurses in some agencies and there are no laws that prohibit the nurse from being part of the information-giving process, the practice nevertheless is highly undesirable (Maher 1989, p. 38). Often, the nurse's responsibility is to witness the giving of informed consent. This involves the following:

- Witnessing the exchange between the client and the physician
- Establishing that the client really did understand, that is, was really informed
- Witnessing the client's signature

If a nurse witnesses only the client's signature and not the exchange between the client and the physician, the nurse should write "witnessing signature only" on the form (Northrop 1984, p. 223). If the nurse finds that the client really does not understand the physician's explanation, then the physician must be be notified.

There are three major elements of informed consent:

1. The consent must be given voluntarily.
2. The consent must be given by an individual with the capacity and competence to understand.
3. The client must be given enough information to be the ultimate decision maker.

To give informed consent voluntarily, the client must not feel coerced. Sometimes fear of disapproval by a health professional can be the motivation for giving consent; such consent is not voluntarily given.

To give informed consent, the client must receive sufficient information to make a decision; otherwise, the client's right to decide has been usurped. Information needs to include benefits, risks, and alternative procedures. It is also important that the client understand. Technical words and language barriers can inhibit understanding. If a client cannot read, the consent form must be read to the client before it is signed. If the client does not speak the same language as the health professional who is providing the information, an interpreter must be acquired.

If given sufficient information, the client can make decisions regarding health. To do so, the client must be competent and an adult. A competent adult is a person over 18 years of age who is conscious and oriented. A person under 18 years who is considered "an emancipated minor" (ie, self-supporting or married) can also give consent. A client who is confused, disoriented, or sedated is not considered functionally competent at that time.

There are three groups of people who cannot provide consent. The *first* is minors. In most areas, a parent or guardian must give consent before minors can obtain treatment. The same is true of an adult who has the mental capacity of a child and who has an appointed guardian. In some states, however, minors are allowed to give consent for such procedures as blood donations, treatment for drug dependence and sexually transmitted disease, and procedures for obstetric care. The *second* group is persons who are unconscious or injured in such a way that they are unable to give consent. In these situations, consent is usually obtained from the closest adult relative if existing statutes permit. In a life threatening emergency, if consent cannot be obtained from the client or a relative, then the law generally agrees that consent is assumed. This is referred to as **implied consent.** The *third* group is mentally ill persons who have been judged to be incompetent. State and provincial mental health acts or similar statutes generally provide definitions of mental illness and specify the rights of the mentally ill under the law as well as the rights of the staff caring for such clients.

DEATH AND RELATED ISSUES

Legal issues surrounding death include issuing the death certificate, labeling of the deceased, autopsy, organ donation, and inquest. By law, a death certificate must be made out when a person dies. It is usually signed by the attending physician and filed with a local health or other government office. The family is usually given a copy to use for legal matters, such as insurance claims.

Nurses have a duty to handle the deceased with dignity and label the corpse appropriately. Mishandling can cause emotional distress to survivors. Mislabeling can create legal problems if the body is inappropriately identified and prepared incorrectly for burial or a funeral. Usually, the deceased's wrist identification tag is left on, and another tag is tied to the client's ankles, in case one of the tags becomes detached. Tags tied to the ankles are preferred, since any tissue damage they cause will be concealed by bed linen or clothing. A third tag is attached to the shroud. All identification tags should include the client's name, hospital number, and physician's name.

An **autopsy** or **postmortem examination** is an examination of the body after death. It is performed only in certain cases. The law describes under what circumstances an autopsy must be performed, for example, when death is sudden or occurs within 48 hours of admission to a hospital. The organs and tissues of the body are examined to establish the exact cause of death, to learn more about a disease, and to assist in the accumulation of statistical data.

It is the responsibility of the physician or, in some instances, of a designated person in the hospital to obtain consent for autopsy. Consent must be given by the decedent (before death) or by the next of kin. Laws in many states and provinces prioritize the family members who can provide consent as follows: surviving spouse, adult children, parents, siblings. After autopsy, hospitals cannot retain any tissues or organs without the permission of the person who consented to the autopsy.

Organ Donation Under the Uniform Anatomical Gift Act in the United States or the Human Tissue Act in Canada, any person 18 years or older and of sound mind may make a gift of all or any part of the body for the following purposes: for medical or dental education, research, advancement of medical or dental science, therapy, or transplantation. The donation can be made by a provision in a will or by signing a cardlike form in the presence of two witnesses. This card is usually carried at all times by the person who signed it. In most states and provinces, the gift can be revoked, either by destroying the card or by revoking the gift orally in the presence of two witnesses. Nurses may serve as witnesses for persons consenting to donate organs. In some states (eg, California), health care workers are required to ask survivors for consent to donate the deceased's organs.

Inquest An inquest is a legal inquiry into the cause or manner of a death. When a death is the result of an accident, for example, an inquest is held into the circumstances of the accident to determine any blame. The inquest is conducted under the jurisdiction of a coroner or medical examiner. A **coroner** is a public official, not necessarily a physician, appointed or elected to inquire into the causes of death, when appropriate. A **medical examiner** is a physician who usually has advanced education in pathology or forensic medicine. Agency policy dictates who is responsible for reporting deaths to the coroner or medical examiner.

EUTHANASIA

Euthanasia is the act of painlessly putting to death persons suffering from incurable or distressing disease. It is commonly referred to as "mercy killing." Because advanced technology has enabled the medical profession to sustain life almost indefinitely, people are increasingly considering the meaning of quality of life. For some people, the withholding of artificial life-support measures or even the withdrawal of life support is a desired and acceptable practice for clients who are terminally ill, in intractable pain, fear being a burden to family, or who are incurably disabled and believed unable to live their lives with some happiness and meaning.

Voluntary euthanasia refers to situations in which the dying individual desires some control over the time and manner of death. All forms of euthanasia are illegal except in states where right-to-die statutes and living wills exist. Currently, the legality of assisted suicide in the United States is being tested in the court of law. Right-to-die statutes legally recognize the client's right to refuse treatment. As society continues to contemplate the legality of euthanasia and assisted suicide, nurses must carefully evaluate their own beliefs and speak to the potential benefits and risks for clients.

PATIENT SELF-DETERMINATION ACT

The Patient Self-Determination Act of 1991 enables clients to participate in decisions about their care, including the right to refuse treatment, even if such treatment is necessary to preserve life. This act requires that hospitals and other health care organizations receiving payment through Medicare and Medicaid do the following:

- Tell clients that they have the right to declare their personal wishes regarding treatment decisions, including the right to refuse medical treatment.
- Inform the client regarding the hospital's policy on how advance directives are honored.
- Provide a written statement on the client's chart indicating whether the client has an advance directive. A copy of the advance directive should be included on the client's chart.
- Provide staff and community education on advance directives.

An **advanced medical directive** is a statement the client makes prior to receiving health care, specifying the client's wishes regarding health care decisions. There are three types of advance medical directives, the **living will,** the **health care proxy** or **surrogate,** and the **durable power of attorney for health care.** The living will (Figure 12–2) states what medical treatment the client chooses to omit or refuse in the event that the client is unable to make those decisions and is terminally ill. For example, the client can indicate a wish not to be kept alive by artificial means such as cardiopulmonary resuscitation (CPR), respiratory ventilation, or tube feeding. With a health care proxy (Figure 12–3, p. 232), the client appoints a proxy, usually a relative or trusted friend, to make medical decisions on the client's behalf in the event that the client is unable to do so. The health care proxy is not limited to terminal situations but can apply to any illness or injury in which the client is incapacitated. A durable power of attorney is a notarized statement appointing someone else to manage health care treatment decisions when the client is unable to do so.

The specific requirements of advance medical directives are directed by individual state legislation. In most states, advance directives must be witnessed by two people but do not require review by an attorney. Some states do not permit relatives, heirs, or physicians to witness advance directives.

LIVING WILL

Declaration made this______day of ________________, 19____ I, ____________________________
willfully and voluntarily make known my desire that my dying not be artificially prolonged under the circumstances set forth below, and I do hereby declare:

If at any time I have a terminal condition and if my attending or treating physician and another consulting physician have determined that there is no medical probability of my recovery from such condition, I direct that life-prolonging procedures be withheld or withdrawn when the application of such procedures would serve only to prolong artificially the process of dying, and that I be permitted to die naturally with only the administration of medication or the performance of any medical procedure deemed necessary to provide me with comfort care or to alleviate pain.

I do ( ), I do not ( ) desire that nutrition and hydration (food and water) be provided by either gastrointestinal or intravenous administration.

It is my intention that this declaration be honored by my family and physician as the final expression of my legal right to refuse medical or surgical treatment and to accept the consequences for such refusal.

In the event that I have been determined to be unable to provide express and informed consent regarding my witholding, withdrawal, or continuation of life-prolonging procedures, I wish to designate as my surrogate to carry out the provisions of this declaration:

Name: ____

Address: ____

Phone: ____

If my surrogate is unwilling or unable to perform his/her duties, I wish to designate as my alternate surrogate:

Name: ____

Address: ____

Phone: ____

I understand the full importance of this declaration, and I am emotionally and mentally competent to make this declaration.

Additional Instructions (Optional):

____

____

____
Signature of Declarant

____ ________________
Witness to Signature Relationship

____ ________________
Witness to Signature Relationship

Figure 12–2 A sample living will. **Source:** Pembroke Pines Hospital, Pembroke Pines, Florida. Reproduced with permission.

Pembroke Pines Hospital
DESIGNATION OF HEALTH CARE SURROGATE

NAME: ____________________

In the event that I have been determined to be incapacitated to provide informed consent for medical treatment and surgical and diagnostic procedures, I wish to designate as my surrogate for health care decisions:

Name: ____________________

Address: ____________________

Phone: ____________________

If my surrogate is unwilling or unable to perform his/her duties, I wish to designate as my alternate surrogate:

Name: ____________________

Address: ____________________

Phone: ____________________

I fully understand that this designation will permit my designee to make health care decisions and to provide, withhold, and withdraw consent on my behalf; to apply for public benefits to defray the cost of health care; and to authorize my admission to or transfer from a health care facility.

Additional Instructions (Optional):

____

____

I further affirm that this designation is not being made as a condition of treatment of admission to a health care facility.

I will notify and send a copy of this document to my surrogate and alternate, if any, and to the following persons other than my surrogate, so they may know who my surrogate is:

Name ____________________

Name: ____________________

Name: ____________________

____________________ ____________________
Signature of Declarant Date

____________________ ____________________
Witness to Signature Relationship

____________________ ____________________
Witness to Signature Relationship

Figure 12–3 A sample designation of health care surrogate/proxy. **Source:** Pembroke Pines Hospital, Pembroke Pines, Florida. Reproduced with permission.

The ANA (1991) supports the client's right to self-determination and believes that nurses must play a primary role in implementation of the law. The nurse is often the facilitator of discussions between clients and their families about health care and end-of-life decisions. The ANA recommends that the following questions be part of the nursing admission assessment regarding advance directives:

- Does the client have basic information about advance care directives, including living wills and durable power of attorney?

- Does the client wish to initiate an advance care directive?
- If the client has prepared an advance care directive, did the client bring it to the health care agency?
- Has the client discussed end-of-life choices with the family and/or designated surrogate, physician, or other health care team worker?

Nurses should learn the law regarding patient self-determination for the state in which they practice, as well as the policy and procedures for implementation in the institution where they work.

"Do Not Resuscitate" Orders

Physicians may order "no code" or **"do not resuscitate" (DNR)** for clients who are in a stage of terminal, irreversible illness or expected death. DNR orders require that no effort be made to resuscitate the client in the event of a respiratory or cardiac arrest. The ANA believes that "the appropriate use of DNR orders can prevent suffering for many clients who choose not to extend their lives after experiencing cardiac arrest (ANA 1992a, p. 2)." The ANA makes the following recommendations related to DNR orders:

- The competent client's values and choices should always be given highest priority, even when these wishes conflict with those of the family or health care providers.
- When the client is incompetent, an advance directive or the surrogate decision makers acting for the client should make health care treatment decisions.
- A DNR decision should always be the subject of explicit discussion between the client, family, any designated surrogate decision maker acting on the client's behalf, and the health care team.
- DNR orders must be clearly documented, reviewed, and updated periodically to reflect changes in the client's condition. Such documentation is required to meet standards of the Joint Commission on Accreditation of Healthcare Organizations (JCAHO 1992).
- A DNR order is separate from other aspects of a client's care and does not imply that other types of care should be withdrawn, for example, nursing care to ensure comfort or medical treatment for chronic but non-life-threatening illnesses.
- If it is contrary to the nurse's personal beliefs to carry out a DNR order, the nurse should consult the nurse-manager for a change in assignment.

The ANA also recommends that each health care organization put into place mechanisms to resolve conflicts between clients, their families, and health care professionals, or between different health care professionals. Institutional ethics committees usually deal with such conflicts. It is important that nurses be represented on these institutional ethics committees, so that nursing perspectives can be heard and nurses can be involved in developing DNR policies.

Wills

A **will** is a declaration by a person about how the person's property is to be disposed of after death. In order for a will to be valid the following conditions must be met:

- The person making the will must be of sound mind, that is, able to understand and retain mentally the general nature and extent of the person's property, the relationship of the beneficiaries and of relatives to whom none of the estate will be left, and the disposition being made of the property. A person, therefore, who is seriously ill and unable to carry out usual roles may be still able to direct preparation of a will.
- The person must not be unduly influenced by anyone else. Sometimes a client may be persuaded by someone who is close at that particular time to make that person a beneficiary. Clients sometimes are persuaded to leave their estates to persons looking after them rather than to their relatives. Frequently, the relatives contest the will in such situations and take the matter to court, claiming undue influence.

Nurses may be requested from time to time to witness a will, although most agencies have policies that nurses not do so. In most states and provinces, a will must be signed in the presence of two witnesses. In some situations, a mark can suffice if the person making the will cannot write a signature. When witnessing a will, the nurse (a) attests that the client signed a document that is stated to be the client's last will and (b) attests that the client appears to be mentally sound and appreciates the significance of their actions (Bernzweig 1990, p. 372).

If a nurse witnesses a will, the nurse should note on the client's chart the fact that a will was made and the nurse's perception of the physical and mental condition of the client. This record provides the nurse with accurate information if the nurse is called as a witness later. The record may also be helpful if the will is contested. If a nurse does not wish to act as a witness—for example, if in the nurse's opinion undue influence has been brought on the client—then it is the nurse's right to refuse to act in this capacity.

Abortions

Abortion laws provide specific guidelines for nurses about what is legally permissible. In 1973, when the *Roe v. Wade* and *Doe v. Bolton* cases were decided, the Supreme Court of the United States held that the constitutional rights of

INFORMATION TO INCLUDE IN AN INCIDENT REPORT

- Identify the client by name, initials, and hospital or identification number.
- Give the date, time, and place of the incident.
- Describe the facts of the incident. Avoid any conclusions or blame. Describe the incident as you saw it even if your impressions differ from those of others.
- Identify all witnesses to the incident.
- Identify any equipment by number and any medication by name and number.
- Document any circumstance surrounding the incident, for example, that another client was experiencing cardiac arrest.

privacy give a woman the right to control her own body to the extent that she can abort her fetus in the early stages of pregnancy. The state, however, has a legitimate interest in controlling abortion during later stages of pregnancy.

In 1989, the Supreme Court's decision in *Webster v. Reproductive Health Services* upheld a Missouri law banning the use of public funds or facilities for performing or assisting with abortions. The Supreme Court and state legislatures continue to struggle with the issue of abortion.

Many statutes also include conscience clauses, upheld by the Supreme Court, designed to protect nurses and hospitals. These clauses give hospitals the right to deny admission to abortion clients and give health care personnel, including nurses, the right to refuse to participate in abortions. When these rights are exercised, the statutes also protect the agency and employee from discrimination or retaliation.

In Canada, abortion is largely a matter between a woman and her physician. However, the law varies somewhat from province to province.

THE AMERICANS WITH DISABILITIES ACT

The Americans with Disabilities Act (ADA), passed by the United States Congress in 1990, prohibits discrimination on the basis of disability in employment, public services, and public accommodations. The purposes of the act are

- To provide a clear and comprehensive national mandate for eliminating discrimination against individuals with disabilities
- To provide clear, strong, consistent enforceable standards addressing discrimination against individuals with disabilities
- To ensure that the federal government plays a central role in enforcing standards established under the act

The ADA has "the potential to improve the lives of both clients and nurses with disabilities, and to change the nature of the nursing support that disabled people need" (Lippman 1991, p. 65). Nurses working in a variety of settings may be involved in educating disabled clients in accessing and using public transportation, communicating through telecommunications devices for the deaf, and patronizing grocery stores, restaurants, and theaters. Furthermore, an employer may not refuse to hire a nurse with disabilities if the nurse is able to fulfill the duties of the work role. The ADA also enables individuals of normal intelligence who have a physical or learning disability to pursue a nursing curriculum through alternative learning methods.

RECORD KEEPING

The client's medical record is a legal document and can be produced in court as evidence. Often, the record is used to remind a witness of events surrounding a lawsuit, because several months or years usually elapse before the suit goes to trial. The effectiveness of a witness's testimony can depend on the accuracy of such records. Nurses, therefore, need to keep accurate and complete records of nursing care provided to clients. Failure to keep proper records can constitute negligence and be the basis for tort liability. Insufficient or inaccurate assessments and documentation can hinder proper diagnosis and treatment and result in injury to the client. See Chapter 9 for types of records and facts about recording.

THE INCIDENT REPORT

An incident report is an agency record of an accident or incident. This report is used to make all the facts about an accident available to agency personnel, to contribute to statistical data about accidents or incidents, and to help health personnel prevent future accidents. All accidents are usually reported on incident forms. Some agencies also report other incidents, such as the occurrence of client infection or the loss of personal effects. The box above lists the information to be included in an incident report. The report should be completed as soon as possible, always within 24 hours of the incident, and filed according to agency policy. As incident reports are not part of the client's medical record, the facts of the incident should also be noted in the medical record.

Incident reports are often reviewed by an agency committee, which decides whether to investigate the incident further. The nurse may be required upon further investigation to answer such questions as what the nurse believes precipitated the accident, how it could have been prevented, and whether any equipment should be adjusted. Nurses who believe they may be dismissed or that suit may be brought should obtain legal advice. Even if the agency clears the nurse of responsibility, the client or the client's family may file suit. The plaintiff, however, bears the burden of proving that the accident occurred because reasonable care was not taken. Even if the accepted standard of care was not met, the plaintiff must prove that the accident was the direct result of failure to meet the acceptable standards of care and that the accident caused physical, emotional, or financial injury.

When an accident occurs, the nurse should first assess the client and intervene to prevent injury. If a client is injured, nurses must take steps to protect the client, themselves, and their employer. Most agencies have policies regarding accidents. It is important to follow these policies and not to assume one is negligent. Although negligence may be involved, accidents can and do happen even when every precaution has been taken to prevent them.

GOOD SAMARITAN ACTS

Good Samaritan acts are laws designed to protect health care providers who provide assistance at the scene of an emergency against claims of malpractice unless it can be shown that there was a gross departure from the normal standard of care or willful wrongdoing on their part. Gross negligence usually involves further injury or harm to the person. For example, an injured child left on the side of the road may be struck by an automobile when the nurse leaves to obtain help.

In the United States, most state statutes do not require citizens to render aid to people in distress. Such assistance is considered more of an *ethical* than a *legal* duty. A few states, however, have enacted legislation that requires people educated in health care to stop and aid the injured. To encourage citizens to be good Samaritans, most states have now enacted legislation releasing the good Samaritan from legal liability for injuries caused under such circumstances, even if the injuries resulted from negligence of the person offering emergency aid.

In Canada, some provinces specify in traffic acts that it is the responsibility of people to give aid at the scene of an accident. However, lawsuits against good Samaritans are rarely successful.

It is generally believed that a person who renders help in an emergency, at a level that would be provided by any reasonably prudent person under similar circumstances, cannot be held liable. The same reasoning applies to nurses, who are among the people best prepared to help at the scene of an accident. If the level of care a nurse provides is of the caliber that would have been provided by any other nurse, then the nurse will not be held liable.

PROFESSIONAL LIABILITY INSURANCE

Because of the increase in the number of malpractice lawsuits against health professionals, nurses are advised in many areas to carry their own liability insurance. Most hospitals have liability insurance that covers all employees, including all nurses. However, some smaller facilities, such as "walk-in" clinics, may not. Thus the nurse should always check with the employer at the time of hiring to see what coverage the facility provides. A physician or a hospital can be sued because of the negligent conduct of a nurse, and the nurse can also be sued and held liable for negligence or malpractice. Because hospitals have been known to countersue nurses when they have been found negligent and the hospital was required to pay, nurses are advised to provide their own insurance coverage and not rely on hospital-provided insurance.

Additionally, nurses often provide nursing services outside of employment-related activities, such as being available for first aid at children's sport or social activities or providing health screening and education at health fairs. Neighbors or friends may seek advice about illnesses or treatment for themselves or family members. In the latter situation, the nurse may be tempted to give advice; however, it is always advisable for the nurse to refer the friend or neighbor to the family physician. The nurse may be protected from liability under Good Samaritan acts when nursing service is volunteer; however, if the nurse receives any compensation or if there is a written or verbal agreement outlining the nurse's responsibility to the group, the nurse needs liability coverage to cover legal expenses in the event that the nurse is sued. Paxman (1993, p. 12) states that "it is the nurse's professional responsibility to be financially responsible in his or her practice. The public expects professionals to compensate harm caused by negligent practice, whether through an individual liability policy, an institutional policy, or through personal assets."

Liability insurance coverage usually defrays all costs of defending a nurse, including the costs of retaining an attorney. The insurance also covers all costs incurred by the nurse up to the face value of the policy, including a settlement made out of court. In return, the insurance company may have the right to make the decisions about the claim and the settlement.

Nursing faculty and nursing students are also vulnerable to lawsuits. In hospital nursing education programs, instructors and students are often specifically covered for liability by the hospital. An instructor, however, can still be sued by a hospital in cases of negligence and malpractice.

Students and teachers of nursing employed by community colleges and universities are less likely to be covered by the insurance carried by hospitals and health agencies. It is advisable for these people to check with their school about the coverage that applies to them. Increasingly, instructors are carrying their own malpractice insurance in both the United States and Canada. In the United States, insurance can be obtained through the ANA or private insurance companies; in Canada, it can usually be obtained through provincial nurses' associations. Nursing students in the United States can also obtain insurance through the National Student Nurses Association. In some states, hospitals do not allow nursing students to provide nursing care without liability insurance.

CONTROLLED SUBSTANCES

United States and Canadian laws regulate the distribution and use of controlled substances such as narcotics, depressants, stimulants, and hallucinogens. Misuse of controlled substances leads to criminal penalties. Controlled substances are kept in securely locked drawers or cupboards, and only authorized personnel have access to them. See Chapter 43 for the legal aspects of drug administration.

THE IMPAIRED NURSE

The impaired nurse refers to a nurse "whose practice has deteriorated because of chemical abuse, specifically the use of alcohol and drugs (Ellis & Hartley 1992, p. 234). Chemical dependence in health care workers has become a problem because of the high levels of stress involved in many health care settings and the easy access to addictive drugs. Sullivan et al (1988, pp. 16, 171–74) report that of disciplinary hearings held before 44 state boards of nursing in 1985, 67% were related to violations involving drug or alcohol abuse. They suggest that the percentage of chemically impaired nurses is probably equal to the percentage of chemically dependent people in the general population; that is, 10% of males and 5% of females abuse alcohol, and 1% to 2% of the total population abuse drugs.

In 1981, the ANA appointed a Task Force on Addiction and Psychological Disturbance to develop guidelines for identifying, treating, and assisting nurses impaired by alcohol or drug abuse or psychologic disturbance (AJN 1982, p. 242). Ellis and Hartley (1992, p. 236) cite two reasons for concern for the chemically impaired nurse: "the first concern is for the nurse whose illness may go undetected and untreated for years, the second concern is for the client, whose care may be jeopardized by the nurse whose judgment and skills are impaired." The box at the top of this page lists behaviors that may be seen in the impaired nurse. The guidelines presented in the box on page 228 can be used to report the nurse suspected of chemical impairment.

BEHAVIORAL INDICATORS OF CHEMICAL ABUSE

- Increasing isolation from colleagues, friends, and family
- Frequent reports of illness, minor accidents, and emergencies
- Complaints about poor work performance
- Inability to meet schedules and deadlines
- Tendency to avoid new and challenging assignments
- Mood swings, irritability, and depression
- Request for night shifts
- Social avoidance of staff
- Illogical and sloppy charting
- Excessive errors
- Increasing carelessness about personal appearance
- Medication "errors" that require many changes in charting
- Arriving on duty early or staying late for no reason
- Volunteering to administer client medications, especially pain medications

Source: Adapted from E Sullivan, L Bissell, and E Williams, *Chemical Dependency in Nursing: The Deadly Diversion* (Redwood City, CA: Addison-Wesley Nursing, 1988), pp. 30–32.

A variety of programs has been developed to assist impaired nurses to recovery. In many states, impaired nurses who enter an intervention program for treatment do not have their nursing license revoked, but their practice is closely supervised within the limitations placed by the intervention program.

SEXUAL HARASSMENT

Sexual harassment is a violation of the individual's rights and a form of discrimination. The Equal Employment Opportunity Commission (EEOC) defines sexual harassment as "unwelcome sexual advances, requests for sexual favors, and other verbal or physical conduct of a sexual nature" occurring in the following circumstances (EEOC 1980, sections 3950.10–3950.11):

- When submission to such conduct is considered, either explicitly or implicitly, a condition of an individual's employment
- When submission to or rejection of such conduct is used as the basis for employment decisions affecting the individual

RESEARCH NOTE

What Are the Effects of Sexual Harassment on Nursing Students?

This study investigated the frequency and type of sexual harassment experienced by nursing students. The 25-question Sexual Harassment of Nursing Students (SHONS) questionnaire was administered to 277 subjects to determine (a) the students' perceptions of the physical and emotional effects of these experiences on academic performance and (b) the resources the students used to cope with the experience. Twenty-one (8%) of the respondents reported sexual harassment experiences; 20 of these students were female, and one was male. Verbal abuse was the most common (48%) form of harassment. Other forms of harassment included sexist remarks about the student's clothing, body, or sexual activities; unnecessary touching, patting, or pinching of body parts; and leering or ogling. The majority (53%) of the students stated that the harassment had no initial effect on their academic performance; 43% stated that they were disturbed but did not consider dropping out of the nursing program; one student (5%) considered dropping out. Students discussed the experience with and received support from friends of the same sex, spouses, parents, and other faculty members. Most (90%) of the students did not file a formal report with administrators or faculty members in the school of nursing or the university. Fifty-one (20%) of the total sample reported sexual harassment in their clinical practice settings.

Implications: Nurses need to be aware of the types of harassment in the clinical practice setting, including verbal abuse and inappropriate touching, patting, or pinching by physicians, administrators, or other personnel.

Source: JJ Cholewinski and JM Burge, Sexual harassment of nursing students, *Image: Journal of Nursing Scholarship*, Summer 1990, 22:106–10.

- When such conduct interferes with an individual's work performance or creates an "intimidating, hostile, or offensive working environment"

In health care, both clients and health care professionals may experience sexual harassment. Because sexual harassment is generally related to a power imbalance, female nurses are more likely to experience sexual harassment from male physicians or administrators. Diaz and McMillin (1991, p. 100) reported that 30% of the nurses studied experienced sexual harassment in the form of having been "sexually propositioned," "suggestively touched," or "sexually insulted" by physicians during their career. Such behavior is considered sexual harassment and can negatively affect client care. For example, to avoid uncomfortable situations, the nurse may refuse to care for the clients of a particular offensive physician or work on a unit with an offensive administrator, or the nurse may avoid calling a physician to report changes in client status or to suggest changes to improve client care.

The victim or the harasser may be male or female. The victim does not have to be of the opposite sex. Moreover, the victim does not have to be the person harassed; anyone who is affected by the offensive conduct may be considered a victim (ANA 1992b, p. 2). Nurses must develop skills of assertiveness to deter sexual harassment in the workplace. See the box above.

STRATEGIES TO DETER SEXUAL HARASSMENT

- Confront the harasser, repeatedly if necessary, and clearly ask that the behavior stop.
- Report the harassment to authorities, using the "chain of command" and whatever formal complaint channels are available.
- Document the harassment, recording in detail the "who," "what," "where," and "when" of the situation and how you responded. Include witnesses if any.
- Seek support from others, such as friends, colleagues, relatives or an organized support group.

Source: Reprinted with permission from *Sexual Harassment: It's Against the Law*, © 1992 American Nurses Association, Washington, DC.

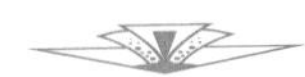

LEGAL RESPONSIBILITIES IN NURSING PRACTICE

CARRYING OUT A PHYSICIAN'S ORDERS

Nurses are expected to know basic information about procedures and medications ordered by the physician. It is the nurse's responsibility to seek clarification of ambiguous or seemingly erroneous orders from the prescribing physician. Clarification from any other source is unacceptable and regarded as a departure from competent nursing practice.

If the order is neither ambiguous nor apparently erroneous, the nurse is responsible for carrying it out. For example, if the physician orders oxygen to be administered at 4 liters per minute, the nurse must administer oxygen at that rate, and not at 2 or 6 liters per minute. If the orders state that the client is not to have solid food after a bowel resection, the nurse must ensure that no solid food is given to the client. Nurses also have a responsibility to check for changes in orders from previous shifts of duty.

Becker (1983, pp. 21–23) outlines four orders that nurses must question to protect themselves legally:

1. Question any order a client questions. For example, if a client who has been receiving an intramuscular injection tells the nurse that the doctor changed the order from an injectable to an oral medication, the nurse should recheck the order before giving the medication.
2. Question any order if the client's condition has changed. The nurse is considered responsible for notifying the physician of any significant changes in the client's condition, whether the physician requests notification or not. For example, if a client who is receiving an intravenous infusion suddenly develops a rapid pulse, chest pain, and a cough, the nurse must notify the physician immediately and question continuance of the ordered rate of infusion. If a client who is receiving morphine for pain develops severely depressed respirations, the nurse must withhold the medication and notify the physician.
3. Question and record verbal orders to avoid miscommunications. In addition to recording the time, the date, the physician's name, and the orders, the nurse documents the circumstances that occasioned the call to the physician, reads the orders back to the physician, and documents that the physician confirmed the orders as the nurse read them back.
4. Question standing orders, especially if the nurse is inexperienced. *Standing orders* give the nurse added responsibility to exercise appropriate judgment when implementing them. The nurse is delegated the authority to, for example, adjust the amount of a medication or other substances and make decisions about when a medication is needed. Nurses need to take the same precautions when implementing these orders as when implementing any other orders. In addition, the nurse who does not feel confident about exercising discretionary judgment should request specific guidelines from the physician or assistance from a more experienced nurse. In some states, standing orders are not allowed except in intensive care or coronary care units.

IMPLEMENTING DELEGATED AND INDEPENDENT NURSING INTERVENTIONS

Nurses implementing care need to take the following precautions:

- Know their job description. This enables nurses to function within the scope of the description and know what is and what is not expected. Job descriptions vary from agency to agency.
- Follow the policies and procedures of the agency in which they are working.
- Always identify clients, particularly before initiating major interventions (eg, surgical or other invasive procedures) or when administering blood transfusions.
- Make sure the correct medications are given in the correct dose, by the right route, at the scheduled time, and to the right client. See Chapter 43 for more detailed information about the administration of medications.
- Perform procedures appropriately. Negligent incidents during procedures generally relate to equipment failure, improper technique, and improper performance of the procedure. For instance, the nurse must know how to safeguard the client in the event that a respirator or other equipment fails.
- Promptly and accurately document all assessments and care given. Records must show that the nurse provided and supervised the client's care daily.
- Report all incidents involving clients. Prompt reports enable those responsible to attend to the client's well-being, to analyze why the incident occurred, and to prevent recurrences.
- Build and maintain good rapport with clients. Keeping clients informed about diagnostic and treatment plans, giving feedback on their progress, and showing concern for the outcome of their care prevent a sense of powerlessness and a buildup of hostility in the client.
- Maintain clinical competence in their area of practice. For students, this demands study and practice before caring for clients. For graduate nurses, it means continued study, including maintaining and updating clinical knowledge and skills.
- Know their own strengths and weaknesses. For example, nurses who recognize that they have difficulty calculating medication dosages should always ask someone to check the calculations before proceeding.
- When delegating nursing responsibilities, make sure that the person who is delegated a task understands what to do and that the person has the required knowledge and skill. The delegating nurse can be held liable for harm caused by the person to whom the care was delegated.
- Be alert when implementing nursing interventions and give each task their full attention and skill.

Ways nurses can protect themselves legally are summarized in the accompanying Clinical Guidelines box. Communication is an essential step in providing safe and effec-

CLINICAL GUIDELINES

Legal Precautions for Nurses

- Function within the scope of your education, job description, and area nurse practice act.
- Follow the procedures and policies of the employing agency.
- Observe and monitor the client accurately.
- Communicate and record significant changes in the client's condition to the physician.
- Check any orders that a client questions.
- Identify clients before initiating any interventions.
- Protect clients from falls and preventable injuries.
- Document all nursing assessments and interventions accurately.
- Ask for assistance and supervision in situations for which you feel inadequately prepared.
- Delegate tasks to persons with the knowledge and skill to carry them out.
- Build and maintain good rapport with clients.

Table 12–6 Communication Do's and Don'ts to Prevent Lawsuits

Do's	Don'ts
Approach every client with sincere concern.	Don't talk in a condescending manner.
Include the client in conversations—don't talk to other health care professionals or family members as if the client doesn't exist.	Don't make promises that can't be kept.
Admit when you don't know the answer to the client's question. Tell the client you will find out the answer and then follow through.	Don't guess or "create" information to make yourself look good.
Always respond professionally to clients and their families.	Don't complain to the client about working conditions, understaffing, or clashes with doctors or other staff members.
	Don't treat a difficult client any differently from a compliant client.

Source: BE Calfee, Protecting yourself—nursing negligence, *Nursing 91*, December 1991, 21:34–40.

tive client care and in protecting the nurse from negligence claims. Table 12–6 provides some communication guidelines that can help the nurse prevent negligence actions.

LEGAL RESPONSIBILITIES OF STUDENTS

Nursing students are responsible for their own actions and liable for their own acts of negligence committed during the course of clinical experiences. When they perform duties that are within the scope of professional nursing, such as administering an injection, they are legally held to the same standard of skill and competence as a registered professional nurse (Bernzweig 1990, p. 60). Lower standards are *not* applied to the actions of nursing students.

In cases arising from negligent acts by nursing students, the student has traditionally been treated as an employee of the hospital, which was held liable under the doctrine of *respondeat superior*. Today, associate degree and baccalaureate nursing students are not usually considered employees of the agencies in which they receive clinical experience, because these nursing programs contract with agencies to provide clinical experiences for students. In future cases of negligence involving such students, the hospital or agency (eg, public health agency) and the educational institution will be held potentially liable for negligent actions by students (Rhodes & Miller 1984, p. 164).

Students in clinical situations must be assigned activity within their capabilities and be given reasonable guidance and supervision. Nursing instructors are responsible for assigning students to the care of clients and for providing reasonable supervision. Failure to provide reasonable supervison and/or the assignment of a client to a student who is not prepared and competent can be a basis for liability.

To fulfill responsibilities to clients and to minimize chances for liability, nursing students need to

- Make sure they are prepared to carry out the necessary care for assigned clients.
- Ask for additional help or supervision in situations for which they feel inadequately prepared.
- Comply with the policies of the agency in which they obtain their clinical experience.
- Comply with the policies and definitions of responsibility supplied by the school of nursing.

Students who work as part-time or temporary nursing assistants or aides must also remember that *legally* they can perform only those tasks that appear in the job description of a nurse's aide or assistant. Even though a student may have received instruction and acquired competence in administering injections or suctioning a tracheostomy tube, the student cannot legally perform these tasks while employed as an aide or assistant.

CHAPTER HIGHLIGHTS

- Accountability is an essential concept of professional nursing practice under the law.
- Nurses need to understand laws that regulate and affect nursing practice to ensure that the nurses' actions are consistent with current legal principles and to protect the nurse from liability.
- Nurse practice acts legally define and describe the scope of nursing practice that the law seeks to regulate.
- Competence in nursing practice is determined and maintained by various credentialing methods, such as licensure, registration, certification, and accreditation, which protect the public's welfare and safety.
- Standards of practice published by national and state or provincial nursing associations and agency policies, procedures, and job descriptions further delineate the scope of a nurse's practice.
- The nurse has specific legal obligations and responsibilities to clients and employers. As a citizen, the nurse has the rights and responsibilities shared by all individuals in the society.
- Collective bargaining is one way nurses can improve their working conditions and economic welfare.
- Nurses can be held liable for intentional torts, such as fraud, invasion of privacy, defamation, assault and battery, and false imprisonment; and for unintentional torts, such as negligence and malpractice.
- Negligence or malpractice of nurses can be established when (a) the nurse (defendant) owed a duty to the client, (b) the nurse failed to carry out that duty, (c) the client (plaintiff) was injured, and (d) the client's injury was caused by the nurse's failure to carry out that duty.
- When a client is accidentally injured or involved in an unusual situation, the nurse's first responsibility is to take steps to protect the client and then to notify appropriate agency personnel.
- The nurse is responsible for ensuring that informed consents from clients (or from the closest relative in emergencies or from parents or guardians when the client is a minor) are in the medical record before treatment regimens and procedures begin.
- Informed consent implies that (a) the consent was given voluntarily; (b) the client was of age and had the capacity and competence to understand; and (c) the client was given enough information on which to make an informed decision.
- Nurses must be knowledgeable about their responsibilities in regard to legal issues surrounding death: ensuring completion of the death certificate, labeling of the deceased, autopsy, organ donation, and inquest.
- The Patient Self-Determination Act of 1991 enables clients to participate in decisions about their care, including the right to refuse treatment, even if such treatment is necessary to preserve life. Nurses need to familiarize themselves with implementation of the act within their work setting.
- Physicians may order "no code" or "do not resuscitate" (DNR) for clients who are in a stage of terminal, irreversible illness or expected death. Nurses need to know their responsibility to clients who have a DNR order.
- The Americans with Disabilities Act (ADA) prohibits discrimination on the basis of disability in employment, public services, and public accommodations. Nurses need to know how ADA affects nursing practice.
- Good Samaritan acts protect health professionals from claims of malpractice when they offer assistance at the scene of an emergency, provided that there is no willful wrongdoing or gross departure from normal standards of care.

- Practicing nurses who are not covered by liability insurance in their employing agency can obtain it through professional nursing associations.
- Chemical dependence in health care workers has become a problem because of the high levels of stress involved in many health care settings and the easy access to addictive drugs. Chemical impairment includes abuse of alcohol and addictive drugs. The nurse needs to know the proper reporting of nursing colleagues whose practice is chemically impaired.
- Sexual harassment is a violation of the individual's right and a form of discrimination. Sexual harassment can happen to both nurses and clients. The nurse needs to be aware of strategies to deter harassing behavior.
- Nursing students need to make certain that they are prepared to provide the necessary care to assigned clients and to ask for help or supervision in situations for which they feel inadequately prepared.

READINGS AND REFERENCES

SUGGESTED READINGS

Idemoto, BK et al. January 1993. Implementing the Patient Self-Determination Act. *American Journal of Nursing* 93:20–25.

The authors describe a multidisciplinary approach to the implementation of the Patient Self-Determination Act at a large university hospital. The implementation project included the education of nurses about the PSDA, an assessment of patient knowledge about advance directives, and admission education of patients about their right to make advance directives. The authors discuss unresolved issues related to the implementation project, but believe that nurses' "unique skills in talking to clients make them well suited to carry on such crucial conversations."

Powers, JL. 1993. Accepting and refusing assignments. *Nursing Management* 24(9):64–68.

Powers discusses legal guidelines for providing safe client care. She discusses reasons for which a nurse may feel compelled to refuse an assignment and then provides options available to both nursing managers and staff nurses to ensure safe practice and maintain staffing requirements.

RELATED RESEARCH

Diaz, AL and McMillin, FD. February 1991. A definition and description of nurse abuse. *Western Journal of Nursing Research* 13(1):97–109.

SELECTED REFERENCES

Alford, D. September/October 1987. How to avoid being a nurse defendant. *Nursing Life* 7:22–23.

American Heart Association. June 6, 1986. Standards and guidelines for cardiopulmonary resuscitation and emergency cardiac care. *Journal of the American Medical Association* 255:2841–3044.

American Nurses Association. 1961. *Legal Definition of Nursing.* Kansas City, MO: ANA.

———. 1976. *The Code for Nurses.* Kansas City, MO: ANA.

———. April 1979. Credentialing in nursing: A new approach. Report of the Committee for the Study of Credentialing in Nursing. *American Journal of Nursing* 79:674–83.

———. 1981. The Nursing Practice Act: Suggested state legislation. Kanas City, MO: ANA.

———. 1985. *The Grievance Procedure.* Kansas City, MO: ANA.

———. 1987. *Credentialing in Nursing: Contemporary Developments and Trends.* Kansas City, MO: ANA.

———. 1991. Position statement on nursing and the Patient Self-Determination Act. Washington, DC: ANA.

———. 1992a. Position statement on nursing care and do-not-resuscitate decisions. Washington, DC: ANA.

———. 1992b. Report to the Constituent Assembly on Sexual Harassment in the Workplace. Washington, DC: ANA.

———. 1993a. *Sexual Harassment: It's Against the Law.* Washington, DC: ANA.

———. 1993b. Regulation of advanced nursing practice. In *Summary of Proceedings, 1993 House of Delegates.* Washington, DC: ANA.

American Nurses Association, Cabinet on Economic and General Welfare. 1985. *The Nature and Scope of ANA's Economic and General Welfare Program.* Kansas City, MO: ANA.

Becker, M. January/February 1983. Five orders you must question to protect yourself legally. *Nursing Life* 3:21–23.

Bernzweig, EP. 1990. *The Nurse's Liability for Malpractice: A Programmed Course.* 5th ed. St Louis: Mosby.

Black, HC. 1991. Black's law dictionary. St Paul, MN: West Publishing Co.

Calfee, BE. December 1991. Protecting yourself—nursing negligence. *Nursing91* 21:34–39.

Creighton, H. 1986. *Law Every Nurse Should Know.* 5th ed. Philadelphia: WB Saunders.

Diaz, AL and McMillin, FD. February 1991. A definition and description of nurse abuse. *Western Journal of Nursing Research* 13:97–109.

Doe v Bolton, 1973. 410 US 179.

Ellis, JR and Hartley, CL. 1992. *Nursing in Today's World.* 4th ed. Philadelphia: Lippincott.

Equal Employment Opportunity Commission. 1980. Sex discrimination guideline. In *EEOC Rules and Regulations.* Chicago: Commerce Clearing House.

Fiesta, J. 1983, 1988. *The Law and Liability: A Guide for Nurses.* 2d ed. New York: Wiley.

Flanagen, L. 1983. *Collective Bargaining and the Nursing Profession.* Washington, DC: ANA.

Hall, JK. October 1990. Understanding the fine line between law and ethics. *Nursing90* 20:34–39.

Idemoto, BK et al. January 1993. Implementing the Patient Self-Determination Act. *American Journal of Nursing* 93:20–25.

Joint Commission on the Accreditation of Healthcare Organizations (JCAHO). 1992. *Nursing Care Standards: Accreditation Manual for Hospitals.* Oak Bluffs Terrace, IL: JCAHO.

Kemerer, AA. March/April 1989. Nurse practice acts. *A D Nurse* 4:29–33.

Labor-Management Relations Act. 1947. Section 8(d).

Lacombe, DC. June 1990. Avoiding a malpractice nightmare. *Nursing90* 20:42–43.

Lippman, H. April 1991. New rights for the disabled will affect you. *RN* 54:65–71.

Maher, VF. November 1989. Your legal guide to safe nursing practice. *Nursing89* 19:34–41.

Mezey, M and Latimer, B. January/February 1993. The Patient Self-Determination Act: An early look at implementation. *The Hastings Center Report* 23:16–20.

Moylan, LB. June 1988. Implications of the National Labor Relations Act. *Nursing Management* 19:80.

National League for Nursing. 1991. *Criteria and Guidelines for the Evaluation of Associate Degree Programs in Nursing.* New York: NLN.

———. 1992. *Criteria and Guidelines for the Evaluation of Baccalaureate and Higher Degree Programs in Nursing.* New York: NLN.

New ANA task force will seek answers for impaired RNs. *American Journal of Nursing* 82(2):242.

O'Connor, KS and Gibson, JF. 1990. Why are we seeing more unionization? In McCloskey, JC and Grace, HK, editors. *Current Issues in Nursing.* 3d ed. St Louis: Mosby.

Paxman, GF. September 27, 1993. Professional liability insurance. *Nursing Spectrum* 3:12–14.

———. 1990. Collective bargaining: Impact on nursing. In Chaska, NL, editor. *The Nursing Profession: Turning Points.* St Louis: Mosby.

Powers, JL. September, 1993. Accepting and refusing assignments. *Nursing Management* 24:64–68.

Roe v Wade. 1973. 410 US 113.

Rouse, F. September/October 1991. Patients, providers, and the PSDA. *Hastings Center Report* 21:S1–S3.

Rovner, J. July 1990. Provisions: Americans With Disabilities Act. Congressional Quarterly 48(30):2437–44.

Sabatino, CP. January/February 1993. Surely the wizard will help us, Toto? Implementing the Patient Self-Determination Act. *Hastings Center Report* 23:12–16.

Sullivan, E, Bissell, L, and Williams, E. 1988. *Chemical Dependency in Nursing: The Deadly Diversion.* Redwood City, CA: Addison-Wesley Nursing.

US Department of Labor. 1979. *Impact of the 1974 Health Care Amendments to the NLRA on Collective Bargaining in the Health Care Industry.* Washington, DC: US Government Printing Office.

Williams, RM. March/April 1984. Collective bargaining and political lobbying: Tools to accomplish professional nursing goals. *Michigan Nurse* 57:1.

UNIT 4

ELEMENTS OF HOLISTIC CARE

STUDENT PROFILE

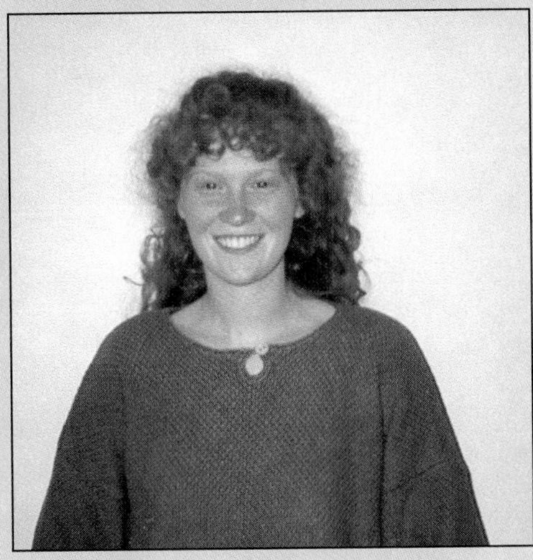

NAME Julie Moffat

SCHOOL OF NURSING Ryerson Polytechnical Institute, Toronto, Ontario, Canada

HOMETOWN Oakville, Ontario, Canada

WHY DID YOU ENTER THE FIELD OF NURSING?
Nursing is a very person-oriented profession, and I enjoy the close working relationships that are established between the client and nurse.

WHO OR WHAT INFLUENCED THAT DECISION?
The combination of volunteer work at two Toronto hospitals and my mom's enjoyment of the profession encouraged me to enter nursing.

WHY DO YOU THINK THIS IS A GOOD TIME TO BE IN NURSING?
The role of nursing is changing rapidly, for example, the expansion of community health care, and the role of nurse-practitioner. Nursing students can influence the growth of the profession by enhancing their skills to incorporate these changes.

WHAT QUALITIES DO YOU THINK ARE NECESSARY TO BE A GOOD NURSE?
Some of the most important qualities are intelligence, compassion, respect, and the ability to continually learn and adapt to a situation.

WHAT ADVICE WOULD YOU GIVE TO A NEW STUDENT?
Always practice in an intelligent and professional manner, making the client your first concern. If you are unsure of something, ask.

13

Wellness, Health, and Illness

Objectives

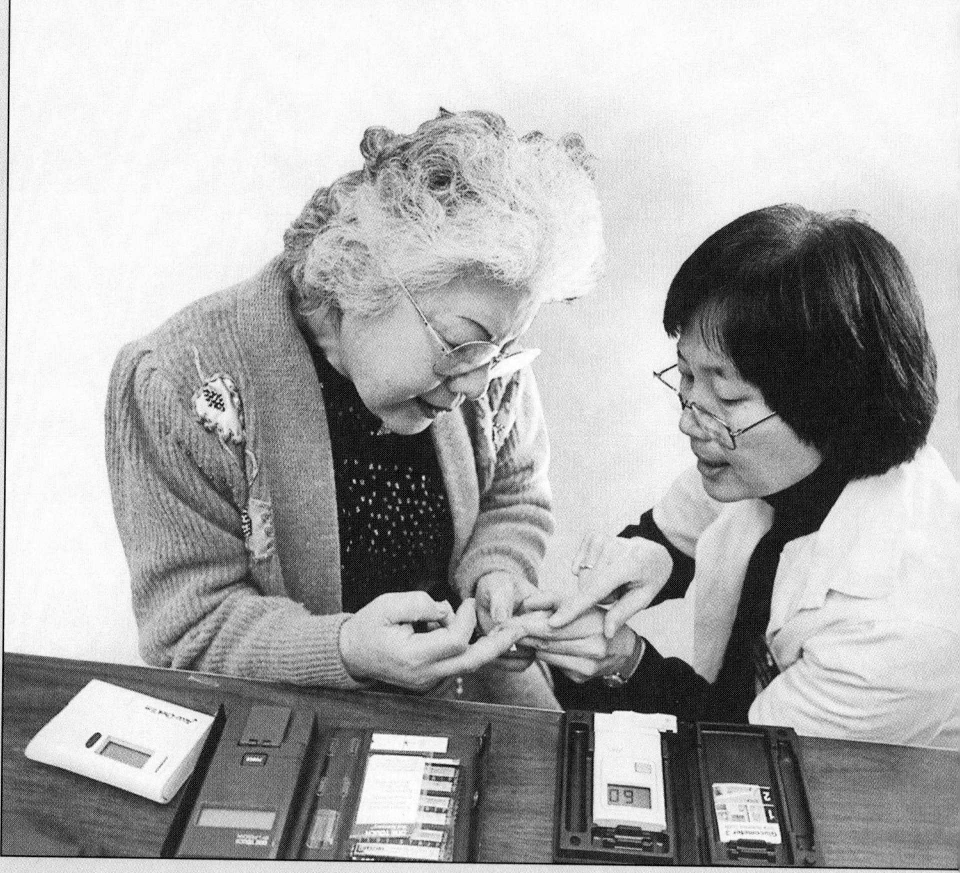

Differentiate health, wellness, and well-being.

Describe five dimensions of wellness.

Compare various models of health outlined in this chapter.

Identify factors affecting health status, beliefs, and practices.

Describe factors affecting health care compliance.

Identify nursing interventions to improve compliance.

Differentiate illness from disease and acute illness from chronic illness.

Explain Igun's stages of illness.

Identify Parsons' four aspects of the sick role.

Identify effects of hospitalization on clients.

Describe effects of illness on family members' roles and functions.

Identify changes in major causes of death, longevity, and morbidity during the latter part of this century.

Discuss three broad goals stated by the US Department of Health and Human Services to meet the health challenges of the 1990s.

Explain the essential facts about health promotion.

List the various types of health promotion programs.

Discuss the nurse's role in health promotion.

Explain the steps involved in health promotion, assessment, diagnosis, planning, and evaluation.

Discuss nursing strategies for enhancing behavior change.

Health is a changing, evolving concept that is basic to nursing. For centuries, the concept of disease was the yardstick by which health was measured. Until the late 19th century, the major concern of health professionals was the "how" of disease (pathogenesis). Now there is an increasing emphasis on health and wellness (salutogenesis).

Most people want to be healthy and feel a sense of loss when they are not. Today, many people actively seek ways to maintain or improve their health by exercising, attending health and fitness clubs, eating or dieting prudently, obtaining adequate sleep, stopping smoking, reducing alcohol intake, and by other means, such as purchasing products intended to enhance or restore health. Yet health, like happiness, is a quality of life that is difficult to define and impossible to measure.

Concepts of Health, Wellness, and Well-Being

Health

In 1947 the World Health Organization (WHO) proposed a broad definition of **health,** shown in the accompanying box. This definition was a notable departure from the traditional view of health, in which health was defined in terms of disease; that is, the state of people who were not sick or dying. Although the new definition is broad and has been criticized as meaningless, it takes a holistic view of health:

- It reflects concern for the individual as a total person functioning physically, psychologically, and socially. Mental processes determine people's relationship with their physical and social surroundings, their attitudes about life, and their interaction with others.
- It places health in the context of environment. People's lives, and therefore their health, are affected by everything they interact with—not only environmental influences such as climate and the availability of nutritious food, comfortable shelter, clean air to breathe, and pure water to drink but also other people, including family, lovers, employers, co-workers, friends, and associates of various kinds.
- It equates health with productive and creative living. It focuses on the living state rather than on categories of disease that may cause illness or death.

Some people, however, view the word "complete" in the definition as a major weakness. For example, a person who has a mild, chronic disease such as hayfever may not be regarded as healthy. In 1953 the (United States) President's Commission on Health Needs of the Nation made a statement about health, also shown in the accompanying box. This definition emphasizes health as an adaptive process rather than a state.

> **Definitions of Health**
>
> - "*Health* is a state of complete physical, mental, and social well-being, and not merely the absence of disease or infirmity" (WHO 1947, p. 1).
> - "*Health* is not a condition; it is an adjustment. It is not a state but a process. The process adapts the individual not only to our physical, but also our social environments" (President's Commission 1953, p. 4).

In the past few decades, a number of health professionals have provided definitions of health and wellness, including nurse theorists. See Table 3–1 on page 47.

Health is a highly individual perception. Consider the following examples of individuals who would probably say they are healthy even though they have physical impairments that some would consider an illness.

- Devon Dobrowski, a 15-year-old diabetic, takes injectable insulin each morning. He plays on the school soccer team and is editor of the high school newspaper.
- John Talbot, age 32, is paralyzed from the waist down and needs a wheelchair for mobility. He is taking accounting at a nearby college and uses a specially designed automobile for transportation.
- Susan Helmer, age 72, takes antihypertensive medications to treat high blood pressure. She bowls once a week, is a member of the neighborhood golf club, makes handicrafts for a local charity, and travels 2 months each year.

Most people define and describe health as the following:

- Being free from symptoms of disease and pain as much as possible
- Being able to be active and able to do what they want or must
- Being in good spirits most of the time

These characteristics indicate that health is not something that a person achieves suddenly at a specific time. It is an ongoing *process*—a way of life—through which a

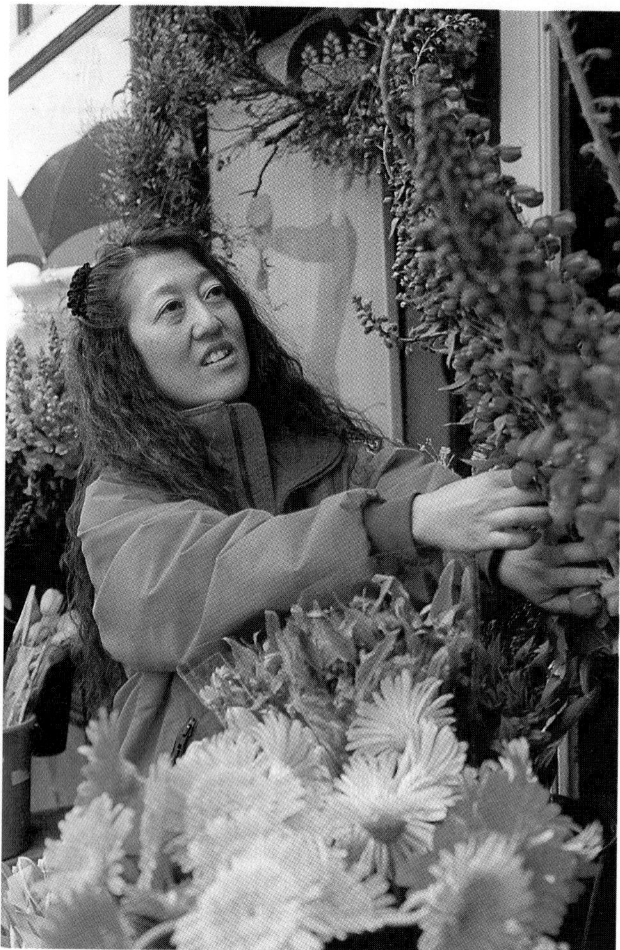

Figure 13–1 Satisfaction with work enhances a sense of well-being and contributes to wellness.

DEVELOPING A PERSONAL DEFINITION OF HEALTH

The following questions can help nurses develop a personal definition of health.

- Is a person more than a biophysiologic system?
- Is health more than the absence of disease symptoms?
- Is health the ability of an individual to perform work?
- Is health the ability of an individual to adapt to the environment?
- Is health a condition of a person's actualization?
- Is health a state or a process?
- Is health the effective functioning of self-care activities?
- Is health static or changing?
- Are health and wellness the same?
- Are disease and illness different?
- Are there levels of health?
- Are wellness, health, and illness separate entities or points along a continuum?
- Is health socially determined?
- How do you rate your health, and why?

person develops and encourages every aspect of the body, mind, and feelings to interrelate harmoniously as much as possible (Figure 13–1).

Many factors affect individual definitions of health. Definitions vary according to an individual's previous experiences, expectations of self, age, and sociocultural influences (see page 251).

Nurses should be aware of their own personal definitions of health and should appreciate that other people have their own individual definitions as well. The person's definition of health influences behavior related to health and illness. By understanding clients' perceptions of health and illness, nurses can provide more meaningful assistance to help clients regain or attain a state of health. To facilitate development of a personal definition of health, see the box above at the right.

WELLNESS AND WELL-BEING

Wellness is a state of well-being. It means engaging in attitudes and behaviors that enhance quality of life and maximize personal potential. (Anspaugh et al 1991, p. 2). Basic concepts of wellness include self-responsibility; an ultimate goal; a dynamic, growing process; daily decision-making in the areas of nutrition, stress management, physical fitness, preventive health care, emotional health, and other aspects of health; and, most importantly, the whole being of the individual.

Leddy and Pepper contend that people confuse the *process* of health with the *status* of well-being. **Well-being** is a *subjective* perception of balance, harmony, and vitality (Leddy & Pepper 1993, p. 221). It is a state that can be described objectively, occurs in levels, and can be plotted on a continuum.

Travis and Ryan (1988, p. xiv) state that wellness is a choice; a way of life; a process; efficient handling of energy; integration of body, mind, and spirit; and loving acceptance of self. See the box on page 247.

Anspaugh et al (1991, p. 3) propose five dimensions of wellness (Figure 13–2). To realize optimal health and wellness, people must deal with the factors within each dimension:

- *Physical.* The ability to carry out daily tasks, achieve fitness (eg, pulmonary, cardiovascular, gastrointestinal),

CONCEPTS OF WELLNESS

- Wellness is a choice—a decision you make to move toward optimal health.
- Wellness is a way of life—a life-style you design to achieve your highest potential for well-being.
- Wellness is a process—a developing awareness that there is no end point, but that health and happiness are possible in each moment, here and now.
- Wellness is an efficient channeling of energy—energy received from the environment, transformed within you, and sent on to affect the world outside.
- Wellness is the integration of body, mind, and spirit—the appreciation that everything you do, and think, and feel, and believe has an impact on your state of health.
- Wellness is the loving acceptance of yourself.

Source: Reprinted with permission, *Wellness Workbook*, Travis & Ryan, Ten Speed Press, Berkeley, CA. © 1981, 1988 by John W Travis, MD.

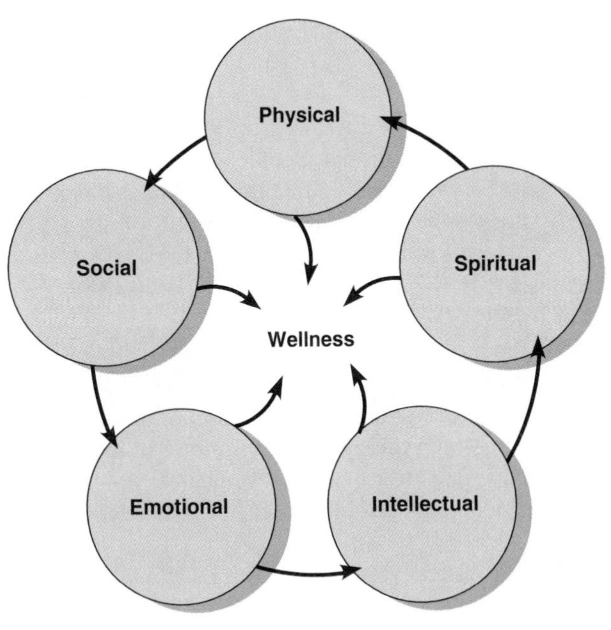

Figure 13–2 The dimensions of wellness.

maintain adequate nutrition and proper body fat, avoid abusing drugs and alcohol or using tobacco products, and generally to practice positive life-style habits.

- *Social.* The ability to interact successfully with people and within the environment of which each person is a part, to develop and maintain intimacy with significant others, and to develop respect and tolerance for those with different opinions and beliefs.
- *Emotional.* The ability to manage stress and to express emotions appropriately. Emotional wellness involves the ability to recognize, accept, and express feelings and to accept one's limitations.
- *Intellectual.* The ability to learn and use information effectively for personal, family, and career development. Intellectual wellness involves striving for continued growth and learning to deal with new challenges effectively.
- *Spiritual.* The belief in some force (nature, science, religion, or a higher power) that serves to unite human beings and provide meaning and purpose to life. It includes a person's own morals, values, and ethics.

Each of the five components overlap to some extent, and factors in one component often directly affect factors in another. For example, a person who learns to control daily stress levels from a physiologic perspective is also helping to maintain the emotional stamina needed to cope with a crisis. Wellness involves working on *all* aspects of the model.

MODELS OF HEALTH AND WELLNESS

Because health is such a complex concept, various researchers have developed models or paradigms to explain health and in some instances its relationship to illness or injury. Models can be helpful in assisting health professionals to meet the health and wellness needs of individuals. Nurses need to clarify their understanding of health, wellness, and illness for the following reasons:

- Nurses' definitions of health largely determine the scope and nature of nursing practice. For example, when health is defined narrowly as a physiologic phenomenon, nurses confine themselves to assisting clients regain normal physiologic functioning. When health is defined more broadly, the scope of nursing practice increases correspondingly.
- People's health beliefs influence their health practices. Thus, a nurse's health values and practices may differ from those of a client. Nurses need to ensure that plans of care developed for individuals relate to the client's conception of health. Otherwise, clients may fail to respond to a health care regimen.

SMITH'S MODELS OF HEALTH

Judith Smith (1981, p. 47) describes four models of health: (1) the clinical model, (2) the role performance model, (3) the adaptive model, and (4) the eudaemonistic model.

Clinical Model The narrowest interpretation of health occurs in the clinical model. People are viewed as physiologic systems with related functions, and health is identified by the absence of signs and symptoms of disease or injury. To laypersons, it is considered the state of not being "sick." In this model, the opposite of health is disease or injury.

Many medical practitioners use the clinical model. The focus of many medical practices is the relief of signs and symptoms of disease and the elimination of malfunctioning and pain. When the signs and symptoms of disease are no longer present in a person, the medical practitioner often considers that the individual's health is restored.

Role Performance Model Health is defined in terms of the individual's ability to fulfill societal roles, that is, to perform work. According to this model, people who can fulfill their roles are healthy even if they appear clinically ill. For example, a man who works all day at his job as expected is healthy even though an X-ray film of his lung indicates a tumor.

It is assumed in this model that sickness is the inability to perform one's work. A problem with this model is the assumption that a person's most important role is the work role. People usually fulfill several roles (eg, mother, daughter, friend), and certain individuals may consider nonwork roles paramount in their lives.

Adaptive Model The focus of the adaptive model is adaptation. In the adaptive model, health is a creative process; disease is a failure in adaptation, or *maladaptation.* The aim of treatment is to restore the ability of the person to adapt, that is, to cope. According to this model, extreme good health is flexible adaptation to the environment and interaction with the environment to maximum advantage (Smith 1981, p. 45). Sister Callista Roy's adaptation model of nursing (Roy & Andrews 1991) views the person as an adaptive system (see page 51). The focus of this model is stability, although there is also an element of growth and change.

Murry and Zentner (1989, p. 570) indicate this growth and change in their definition of health: "a state of well-being in which the person is able to use purposeful, adaptive responses and processes, physically, mentally, emotionally, spiritually, and socially, in response to internal and external stimuli (stressors) in order to maintain relative stability and comfort and to strive for personal objectives and cultural goals."

Eudaemonistic Model The eudaemonistic model incorporates the most comprehensive view of health (Smith 1981, p. 44). Health is seen as a condition of actualization or realization of a person's potential. Actualization is the apex of the fully developed personality. (Maslow presents this concept of health. See Chapter 14). In this model, the highest aspiration of people is fulfillment and complete development, i.e., actualization. Illness, in this model, is a condition that prevents self-actualization.

Pender includes stabilizing and actualizing tendencies in her definition of health: "Health is the actualization of inherent and acquired human potential through satisfying relationships with others while adjustments are made as needed to maintain structural integrity and harmony with the environment" (1987, p. 27).

LEAVELL AND CLARK'S AGENT-HOST-ENVIRONMENT MODEL

The *agent-host-environment model* of health and illness, also called the *ecologic model,* originated in the community health work of Leavell and Clark (1965) and has been expanded into a general theory of the multiple causes of disease. The model is used primarily in predicting illness rather than in promoting wellness, although identification of risk factors that result from the interaction of agent-host-environment are helpful in promoting and maintaining health.

The model has three dynamic interactive elements:

1. *Agent.* Any environmental factor or stressor (biologic, chemical, mechanical, physical, or psychosocial) that by its presence or absence (eg, lack of essential nutrients) can lead to illness or disease.
2. *Host.* Person(s) who may or may not be at risk of acquiring a disease. Family history, age, and life-style habits influence the host's reaction.
3. *Environment.* All factors external to the host that may or may not predispose the person to the development of disease. Physical environment includes climate, living conditions, sound (noise) levels, and economic level. Social environment includes interactions with others and life events, such as the death of a spouse.

Because each of the agent-host-environment factors constantly interacts with the others, health is an ever-changing state. When variables are in balance, health is maintained; when variables are not in balance, disease occurs.

HEALTH-ILLNESS CONTINUA

Health-illness continua (grids or graduated scales) can be used to measure a person's perceived level of wellness. Many continua have been developed; two, those of Dunn and Travis, are included here.

Dunn's High-Level Wellness Grid Dunn describes a health grid in which a health axis and an environmental axis intersect (1959a, p. 786). It demonstrates the interaction of the environment with the illness-wellness continuum. The health axis extends from peak wellness to death, and the environmental axis extends from very favorable to very unfavorable (Figure 13–3). The intersection of the two axes forms four health/wellness quadrants:

1. *High-level wellness in a favorable environment.* An example of this is a person who implements healthy life-style behaviors and has the biopsychosocial, spiritual, and economic resources to support this life-style.
2. *Emergent high-level wellness in an unfavorable environment.* An example of this is a woman who has the knowledge to implement healthy life-style practices but does not implement adequate self-care practices because of family responsibilities, job demands, or other factors.
3. *Protected poor health in a favorable environment.* An example of this is an ill person (eg, one with multiple fractures or severe hypertension) whose needs are met by the health care system and who has access to appropriate medications, diet, and health care instruction.
4. *Poor health in an unfavorable environment.* An example of this is a young child who is starving in a drought-stricken country.

In his book about high-level wellness in the individual, Dunn (1973) explores the concept of wellness as it relates to family, community, environment, and society. He believes that family wellness enhances wellness in individuals. In a well family that offers trust, love, and support, the individual does not have to expend energy to meet basic needs and can move forward on the wellness continuum. By providing effective sanitation and safe water, disposing of sewage safely, and preserving beauty and wildlife, the community enhances both family and individual wellness.

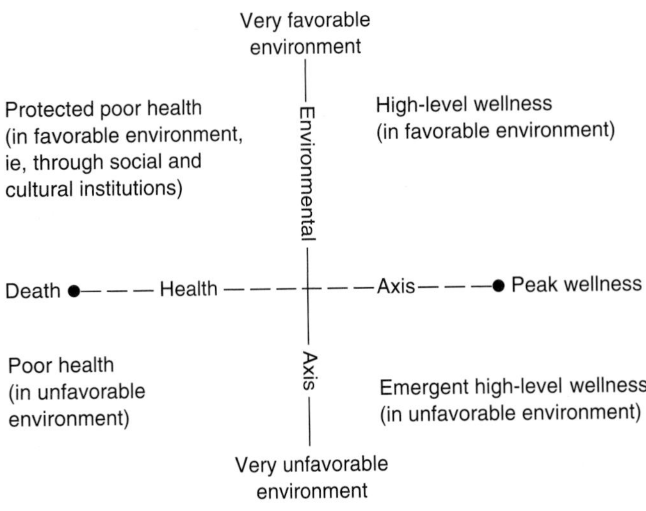

Figure 13–3 Dunn's health grid: its axes and quadrants. **Source:** HL Dunn, High-level wellness for man and society, *American Journal of Public Health.* June 1959, 49:788. Used with permission.

Environmental wellness is related to the premise that humans must be at peace with and guard the environment. Societal wellness is significant because the status of the larger social group affects the status of smaller groups. Dunn believes that social wellness must be considered on a worldwide basis.

Travis's Illness-Wellness Continuum The illness-wellness continuum, first developed by Travis in 1972 (Figure 13–4) ranges from high-level wellness to premature death (Travis & Ryan 1988, p. xvi). The model illustrates two arrows pointing in opposite directions and joined at a neutral point. Movement to the right of the neutral point indicates increasing levels of health and

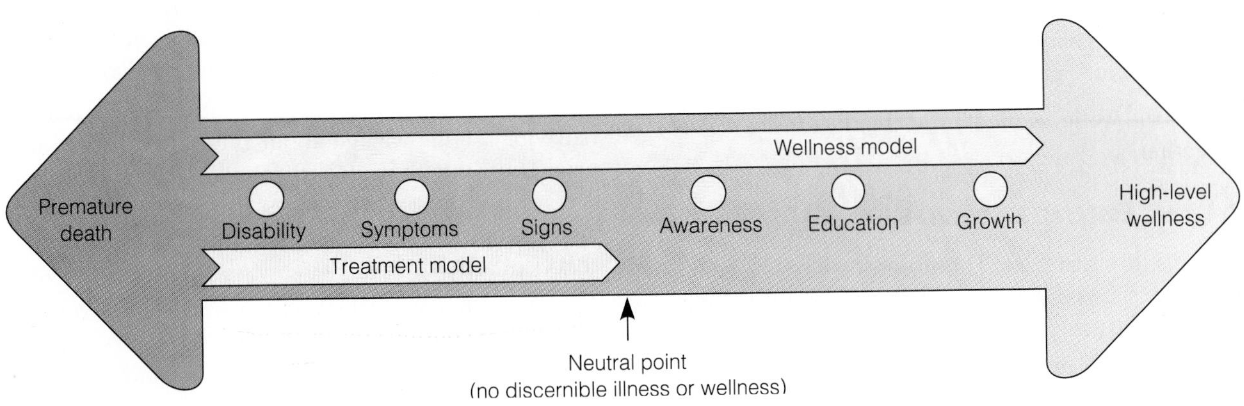

Figure 13–4 Illness-wellness continuum. **Source:** Reprinted with permission, *Wellness Workbook,* Travis & Ryan, Ten Speed Press, Berkeley, CA. © 1981, 1988 by John W Travis, MD.

well-being for an individual. This is achieved in three steps: (1) awareness, (2) education, (3) growth. In contrast, movement to the left of the neutral point indicates a progressively decreasing state of health.

Travis and Ryan believe it is possible to be physically ill and at the same time be oriented towards wellness, or physically healthy and at the same time be functioning from an illness mentality. Therefore, what matters most is not the point on the continuum the person might identify as the current state but *the direction on the pathway in which the person is facing*. For example, visualize a woman who is disabled, sick, or in pain yet takes responsibility for her life and has a genuinely optimistic or positive outlook. If only the physical dimension is considered, this woman would fall on the left side of the continuum. When the emotional, intellectual and spiritual dimensions are considered, however, this woman would be on the right side, facing the direction of high-level wellness.

The model also compares the traditional treatment model with the wellness model. The former can help an individual move from the left only to the neutral point, where symptoms of the illness are alleviated. For example, a man with hypertension who takes an antihypertensive medication to reduce blood pressure and relieve any associated symptoms moves to the neutral point. However, wellness-oriented measures such as reducing weight or ceasing to smoke are needed to move the person beyond the neutral point to a higher level of wellness.

Note that wellness interventions can be initiated at any point on the continuum. For example, a nurse treating the man with hypertension might incorporate the following measures:

1. Assess life stressors and emotional disturbances (awareness).
2. Instruct the client about nonpharmacologic approaches such as weight reduction; restriction of alcohol, sodium, and tobacco; exercise; and relaxation techniques (education).
3. Encourage the client to join support groups to control weight, smoking, and stress.

Thus, both the wellness model and treatment model can work together.

HEALTH BELIEF MODELS

In the 1950s, Rosenstock (1974) proposed a health belief model (HBM) intended to predict which individuals would or would not use such preventive measures as screening for early detection of cancer. Becker (1974) modified the health belief model to include these components: *individual perceptions*, *modifying factors*, and *variables likely to affect initiating action*.

The health belief model (Figure 13–5) is based on motivational theory. Rosenstock assumed that good health is an objective common to all people. Becker added "positive health motivation" as a consideration.

Individual Perceptions Individual perceptions include the following:

- *Perceived susceptibility*. A family history of a certain disorder, such as diabetes or heart disease, may make the individual feel at high risk.
- *Perceived seriousness*. The question here is: In the perception of the individual, does the illness cause death or have serious consequences? Concern about the spread of acquired immune deficiency syndrome (AIDS) reflects the general public's perception of the seriousness of this illness.
- *Perceived threat*. According to Becker, perceived susceptibility and perceived seriousness combine to determine the total perceived threat of an illness to a specific individual. For example, a person who perceives that many individuals in the community have AIDS may not necessarily perceive a threat of the disease; if the person is a drug addict or a homosexual, however, the perceived threat of illness is likely to increase because of the combined susceptibility and seriousness.

Modifying Factors Factors that modify a person's perceptions include the following:

- *Demographic variables*, such as age, sex, race, and ethnicity. An infant, for example, does not perceive the importance of a healthy diet; an adolescent may perceive peer approval as more important than family approval and participate as a consequence in hazardous activities or adopt unhealthy eating and sleeping patterns.
- *Sociopsychologic variables*. Social pressure or influence from peers or other reference groups (eg, self-help or vocational groups) may encourage preventive health behaviors even when individual motivation is low. Expectations of others may motivate people, for example, not to drive an automobile after drinking alcohol.
- *Structural variables* presumed to influence preventive behavior are knowledge about the target disease and prior contact with it. Becker found higher compliance rates with prescribed treatments among mothers whose children had frequent ear infections and occurrences of asthma.
- *Cues to action*. Cues can be either internal or external. Internal cues include feelings of fatigue, uncomfortable symptoms, or thoughts about the condition of an ill person who is close. External cues are listed in Figure 13–5.

Likelihood of Action The likelihood of a person's taking recommended preventive health action depends on

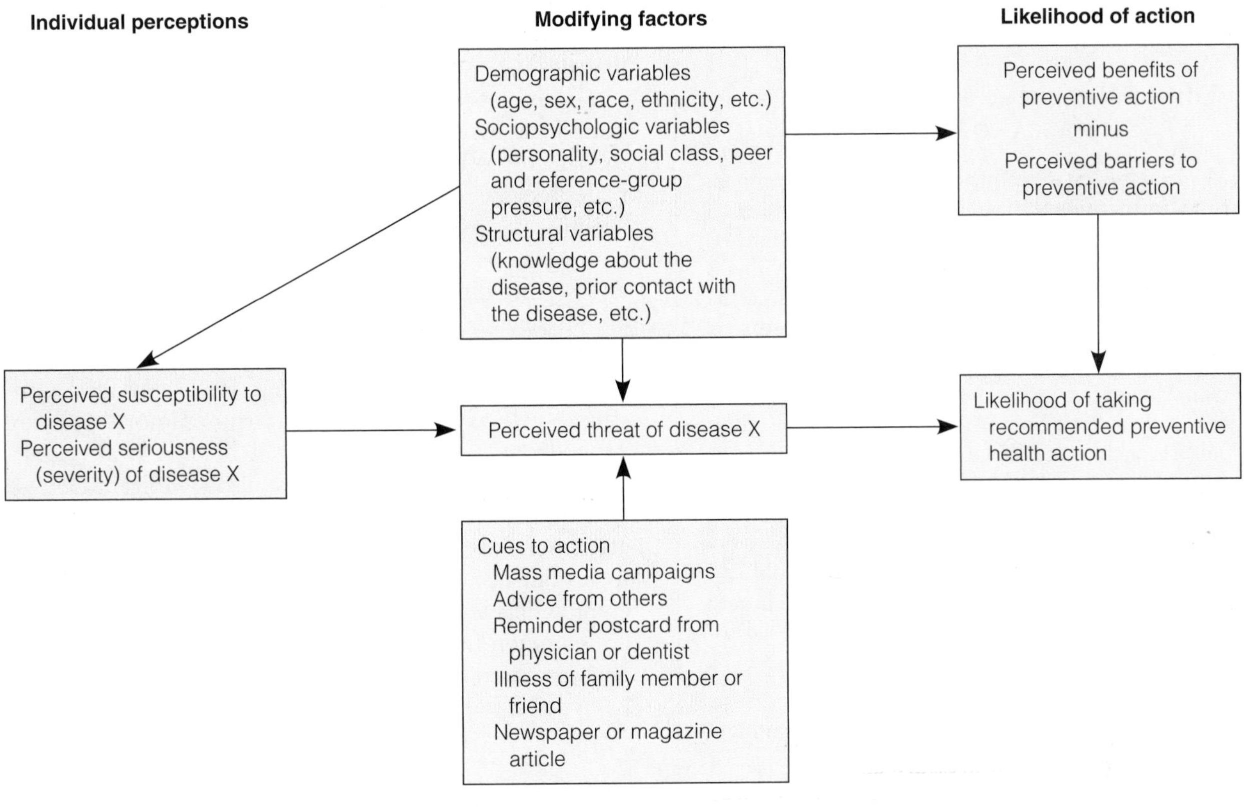

Figure 13–5 The health belief model. **Source:** MH Becker, DP Haefner, SV Kasi, et al, Selected psychosocial models and correlates of individual health-related behaviors, *Medical Care,* 1977. 15:27–46. Used with permission.

the perceived benefits of the action minus the perceived barriers to the action.

- *Perceived benefits of the action.* Examples include refraining from smoking to prevent lung cancer, and eating nutritious foods and avoiding snacks to maintain weight.
- *Perceived barriers to action* can include cost, inconvenience, unpleasantness, and life-style changes.

Pender (1987, p. 50) adds two further considerations: the importance of health as perceived by the individual and perceived control.

1. *The importance of health to the person.* Behavior indicating that health is perceived as something of value includes providing special foods and vitamins, having regular dental checkups, and participating in screening tests for cervical and testicular cancer, breast cancer, and cardiovascular disorders.
2. *Perceived control.* People who perceive that they have control over their own health are more likely to use preventive services than people who feel powerless. Control over health can relate to such behaviors as not smoking and using seat belts in automobiles.

Nurses play a major role in helping clients implement healthy behaviors. They help clients monitor health, supply anticipatory guidance, and impart knowledge about health. Nurses can also reduce barriers to action (eg, by minimizing inconvenience or discomfort) and can support positive actions.

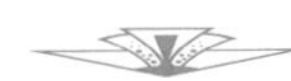

VARIABLES INFLUENCING HEALTH STATUS, BELIEFS, AND PRACTICES

Multiple variables influence a person's health status, beliefs, and behaviors or practices. The box on page 252 differentiates health status, health beliefs, and health behaviors. Some of the factors influencing health are internal to the person; others are external. They may or may not be under conscious control. People can usually control their health behaviors and can choose healthy or unhealthy activities. In contrast, people have little or no choice over their genetic makeup, age, sex, physical environments, culture, or areas of residence. To plan and provide holistic

DIFFERENTIATING HEALTH STATUS, BELIEFS, AND BEHAVIORS

- *Health status.* State of health of a person at a given time. In its general meaning, the term may refer to a problem-free state or to anxiety, depression, or acute illness and thus describes the individual's problem in general. Health status can also describe such specifics as pulse rate and body temperature.
- *Health beliefs.* Concepts about health that an individual believes true. Such beliefs may or may not be founded on fact. Some of these are influenced by culture, such as the "hot-cold" system of some Hispanic Americans. In this system, health is viewed as a balance of hot and cold qualities within a person. For example, a fever is said to be caused by an excess of "hot" foods. In this context, "hot" and "cold" do not denote temperature or spiciness but innate qualities of the food. Citrus fruits and some fowl are considered "cold" foods, and meats and bread are "hot" foods.
- *Health behavior.* The actions people take to understand their health state, maintain an optimal state of health, prevent illness and injury, and reach their maximum physical and mental potential. Behaviors such as eating wisely, exercising, paying attention to signs of illness, following treatment advice, and avoiding known health hazards such as smoking are all examples.

nursing care, nurses need to recognize how these factors affect people's health behavior. When preparing a plan of care with an individual, nurses need to consider the person's health beliefs before they attempt to change health behaviors.

INTERNAL FACTORS

Internal factors include biologic, psychologic, cognitive, and spiritual dimensions.

Biologic Dimension Genetic makeup, race, sex, age, and developmental level all significantly influence a person's health.

Genetic makeup influences biologic characteristics, innate temperament, activity level, and intellectual potential. It has been related to susceptibility to specific disease, such as diabetes and breast cancer.

Race is associated with predisposition to certain diseases. For example, blacks have a higher incidence of sickle-cell anemia and hypertension than the general population, and Native Americans have a higher rate of diabetes.

Sex influences the distribution of disease. Certain acquired and genetic diseases are more common in one sex than in the other. Disorders more common among females include osteoporosis, autoimmune diseases such as rheumatoid arthritis and systemic lupus erythematosus, anorexia nervosa and bulimia, gallbladder disease, obesity, and thyroid disease. Those more common among males are stomach ulcers, abdominal hernias, respiratory diseases, arteriosclerotic heart disease, hemorrhoids, and tuberculosis. Obviously, diseases that affect reproductive organs, such as testicular or uterine tumors, are sex dependent.

Age and developmental level are also significant factors. The distribution of disease varies with age. For example, arteriosclerotic heart disease is common in middle-aged males but occurs infrequently in younger persons; such communicable diseases as whooping cough and measles are common in children but rare in older persons, who have acquired immunity to them. Developmental level has a major impact on health status, for example:

- Infants lack physiologic and psychologic maturity. Defenses against disease are lower during the first years of life and again near the end of life.
- Toddlers who are learning to walk are more prone to falls and injury.
- Adolescents who have a need to conform with peers are more prone to risk-taking behavior and subsequent injury.
- Declining physical and sensory-perceptual abilities limit the ability of older adults to respond to environmental hazards and stressors.

Psychologic Dimension Psychologic (emotional) factors influencing health include mind-body interactions, self-concept, and job satisfaction.

Mind-body interactions can affect health status positively or negatively. Emotional responses to stress affect body function. For example, a student who is extremely anxious before a test may experience urinary frequency and diarrhea. A person worried about the outcome of surgery or about the behavior of a teenager may chain-smoke. Prolonged emotional distress may increase susceptibility to organic disease or precipitate it. Emotional distress may influence the immune system through central nervous system and endocrine alterations. Alterations in the immune system are related to the incidence of infections, cancer, and autoimmune diseases.

Increasing attention is being given to the mind's ability to direct the body's functioning. Relaxation, meditation, and biofeedback techniques are gaining wider recognition by individuals and health care professionals. For example, women often use relaxation techniques to decrease pain during childbirth. Other people may learn biofeedback skills to reduce hypertension.

Emotional reactions also occur in response to body conditions. For example, a person diagnosed with a terminal illness may experience fear and depression. *Self-concept* is how a person feels about self (self-esteem) and perceives the physical self (body image), needs, roles, and abilities. Self-concept affects how people view and handle situations. Such attitudes can affect health practices, responses to stress and illness, and the times when treatment is sought. An example is the anorexic woman who deprives herself of needed nutrients because she believes she is too fat even though she is well below an acceptable weight level. Self-concept is discussed in detail in Chapter 31. Self-perceptions are also associated with a person's definition of health. For example, a 75-year-old man who can no longer move large objects as he was accustomed to do may need to examine and redefine his concept of health in view of his age and abilities.

Cognitive Dimension Cognitive or intellectual factors influencing health include life-style choices and spiritual and religious beliefs.

Life-style choices include patterns of eating; exercise; use of tobacco, drugs, and alcohol; and methods of coping with stress. Overeating, getting insufficient exercise, and being overweight are closely related to the incidence of heart disease, arteriosclerosis, diabetes, and hypertension. Excessive sugar intake increases the risk of dental caries. Abuse of drugs and alcohol is physically and mentally debilitating. Excessive use of tobacco is clearly implicated in lung cancer, emphysema, and cardiovascular diseases.

Spiritual and religious beliefs can significantly affect health behavior. For example, Jehovah's Witnesses oppose blood transfusions; some fundamentalists believe that a serious illness is a punishment from God; some religious groups are strict vegetarians; and Orthodox Jews perform circumcision on the eighth day of a male baby's life. The influence of spirituality and religion is discussed further in Chapter 16.

EXTERNAL FACTORS

External factors influencing health status, beliefs, and practices include geography, physical environment, standards of living, family and cultural beliefs, and social support networks.

Geography Geography determines climate, and climate affects health. For instance, malaria and malaria-related conditions occur more frequently in tropical than temperate climates.

Environment People are becoming increasingly aware of their environment and how it affects their health and level of wellness. Pollution of the water, air, and soil can affect the support of life. Pollution can occur naturally (eg, lightening-caused fires produce smoke, which pollutes the air). Other substances in the environment, such as asbestos, are considered carcinogenic (ie, they cause cancer). Cigarette smoke is now considered "hazardous to one's health," with rates of all types of cancer higher among smokers.

Another environmental hazard is radiation. Two sources of radiation that can be hazardous to health are machines and drugs that emit radiation. The improper use of X rays, for example, can harm many of the body's organs. Another common source of radiation is the sun's ultraviolet rays. Light-skinned people are more susceptible to the harmful effects of the sun than are dark-skinned people.

The main component of acid rain is sulfur dioxide, produced by ore smelters and related industries. The other components are nitrogen oxides. These emissions are thought by scientists to damage forests, lakes, and rivers. As a result, fish and fish eggs are damaged by the increasingly acidic water.

Another environmental hazard that is receiving increasing attention is the "greenhouse effect." The glass roof of a greenhouse permits the sun's radiation to penetrate, but the resulting heat does not escape back through the glass. Carbon dioxide in the earth's atmosphere acts very much like the glass roof of a greenhouse, hence the surface temperature of the earth is increasing.

Other sources of environmental contamination are pesticides and chemicals used to control weeds and plant diseases. These contaminants can be found in some animals and plants that are subsequently ingested by people. In excessive levels, they are harmful to health.

Standards of Living An individual's standard of living (reflecting occupation, income, and education) is related to health, morbidity, and mortality. Hygiene, food habits, and the propensity to seek health care advice and follow health regimens vary among high-income and low-income groups. For example, preventing illness may not have as high a priority among the poor as generating and maintaining an income; even when prevention is a priority, the poor may not be able to afford regular medical examinations, housing, or nutritious foods that promote health.

Low-income families often define health in terms of work; if people can work they are healthy. They tend to be fatalistic and believe that illness is not preventable. Because their present problems are so great and all efforts are exerted toward survival, an orientation to the future may be lacking. Most low-income people do not have regular preventive medical checkups, because they cannot afford them. It is more important to them to work than to lose a day's pay visiting a physician. Reliance on public assistance and inability to afford health care insurance limit both the low-income person's access to health care and the type of care available.

The environmental conditions of poverty-stricken areas also have a bearing on overall health. Slum neighborhoods are overcrowded and in a state of deterioration. Neglect and disorder are common. Sanitation services tend to be inadequate. Many streets are strewn with garbage, and alleys are overrun by rats. Fires and crime are constant threats. Recreational facilities are almost nonexistent, forcing children to play in streets and alleys.

Occupational roles also predispose people to certain illnesses. For instance, some industrial workers may be exposed to carcinogenic agents. More affluent people may fulfill stressful social or occupational roles that predispose them to stress-related diseases. Such roles may also encourage overeating or social use of drugs or alcohol.

Family and Cultural Beliefs In addition to transmitting genetic predispositions, the family passes on patterns of daily living and life-styles to offspring. For example, a woman who was abused as a child may physically abuse her small son. Physical or emotional abuse may cause long-term health problems. Emotional health depends on a social environment that is free of excessive tension and does not isolate the person from others. A climate of open communication, sharing, and love fosters the fulfillment of the person's optimum potential.

Culture and social interactions also influence how a person perceives, experiences, and copes with health and illness. Each culture has ideas about health, and often these are transmitted from parents to children. For example, in some traditional Chinese families health is defined as a balance of energy (yin and yang). Yin is dark, cold, wet, negative, and female; yang is light, warm, dry, positive, and male. An imbalance of yin and yang results in disease. Ethnic and cultural influences on health are discussed in detail in Chapter 15.

People of certain cultures may perceive home remedies or tribal health customs as superior and more dependable than the health care practices of North American society. For example, a person of Asian origin may prefer to use herbal remedies and acupuncture to treat pain rather than analgesic medications. Cultural rules, values, and beliefs give people a sense of being stable and able to predict outcomes. The challenging of old beliefs and values by second-generation ethnic groups may give rise to conflict, instability, and insecurity, in turn contributing to illness.

Social Support Networks Social support networks are closely related to an individual's internal factors of self-concept, cognition, and psychologic make-up; these influence the person's motivation and ability to develop supportive networks. Having a support network (family, friends, or a confidant) and job satisfaction helps people avoid illness. Support people also help the person confirm that illness exists. Persons with inadequate support networks sometimes allow themselves to become increasingly ill before confirming the illness and seeking therapy. Support people also provide the stimulus for an ill person to become well again.

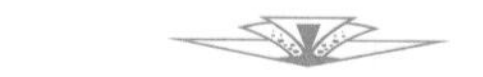

HEALTH CARE COMPLIANCE

Compliance, also referred to as adherence, is the extent to which an individual's behavior (for example, taking medications, following diets, or making life-style changes) coincides with medical or health advice. Degree of compliance may range from disregarding every aspect of the recommendations to following the total therapeutic plan. There are many reasons why some people comply and others do not. See the box at the top of page 255.

To enhance compliance, nurses need to ensure that the client is able to perform the prescribed therapy, understands the necessary instructions, is a willing participant in establishing goals of therapy, and values the planned outcomes of behavior changes.

When a nurse identifies noncompliance, it is important to find out why and, by taking the following steps, assist the client to comply:

- *Establish why the client is not following the regimen.* Where indicated, the nurse can, for example, provide information, correct misconceptions, attempt to decrease expense, or suggest counseling if psychologic problems are interfering with compliance. It is also essential that the nurse reevaluate the suitability of the health advice provided.
- *Demonstrate caring* by showing sincere concern about the client's problems and decisions and at the same time accepting the client's right to a course of action. For example, a nurse might tell a client who is not taking his heart medication, "I can appreciate how you feel about this, but I am very concerned about your heart."
- *Encourage healthy behaviors through positive reinforcement.* If the man who is not taking his heart medication is walking every day, the nurse might say, "You are really doing well with your walking."
- *Use aids to reinforce teaching.* For instance, the nurse can leave pamphlets for the client to read later or make a "pill calendar," a paper with the date and number of pills to be taken.

Factors Influencing Compliance

- Client motivation to become well
- Degree of life-style change necessary
- Perceived severity of the health care problem
- Value placed on reducing the threat of illness
- Difficulty in understanding and performing specific behaviors
- Degree of inconvenience of the illness itself or of the regimens
- Belief that the prescribed therapy or regimen will or will not help
- Complexity, side-effects, and duration of the proposed therapy
- Specific cultural heritage that may make compliance difficult
- Degree of satisfaction and quality and type of relationship with the health care providers
- Overall cost of prescribed therapy

- *Establish a therapeutic relationship of freedom, mutual understanding, and mutual responsibility with the client and support persons.* By providing knowledge, skills, and information, the nurse gives clients control over their health and establishes a cooperative relationship, which results in greater compliance.

Illness and Disease

People may view illness and disease as the same entity; however, health professionals generally view them as completely separate. Emotions are not believed to cause disease, but they may create an environment in which disease can develop through their effect upon the immune system. See the discussion of mind-body interactions on page 252.

Illness is a highly personal state in which the person feels unhealthy or ill. Illness may or may not be related to disease. An individual could have a disease, for example, a growth in the stomach, and not feel ill. By the same token, a person can feel ill, that is, feel uncomfortable, yet have no discernible disease. Illness is highly subjective; only the individual person can say he or she is ill.

Disease is a term that can be described as an alteration in body functions resulting in a reduction of capacities or a shortening of the normal life span. Traditionally, intervention by physicians has the goal of eliminating or ameliorating disease processes. Primitive people thought disease was caused by "forces" or spirits. Later, this belief was replaced by the single-causation theory. Today, multiple factors are considered to interact in causing disease and determining an individual's response to treatment.

Common Causes of Disease

- Biologic agents (eg, viruses, bacteria, rickettsia, fungi, protozoa, helminths [worms], and toxins)
- Inherited genetic defects
- Developmental defects resulting from exposure to environmental elements (eg, viruses or chemicals)
- Physical agents (eg, temperature extremes, radiation, and electricity)
- Chemical agents (eg, alcohol, strong acids and bases, many drugs, heavy metals, and industrial poisons)
- Tissue response to irritation or injury
- Faulty chemical or metabolic processes (eg, excessive or inadequate production of body secretions, such as hormones and enzymes)
- Emotional and physical reactions to stress

The causation of disease is called its **etiology.** A description of the etiology of a disease includes the identification of all causal factors that act together to bring about the particular disease. For example, the tubercle bacillus is designated as the biologic agent of tuberculosis. However, other etiologic factors, such as age, nutritional status, and even occupation, are involved in the development of tuberculosis and influence the course of infection. There are many diseases for which the cause is unknown (eg, multiple sclerosis). Common causes of disease are listed in the box above.

Traditionally, physicians have dealt with disease at a subsystem level. Subsystems are those aspects of the body subsumed in the larger system of the whole body. (See systems theory in Chapter 14, page 277.) A subsystem may be a cell, an organ, or an organ system. Only recently have physicians started looking at the person as an entity, or whole. Nurses, by contrast, have traditionally viewed the person as an entity, taking a holistic view of people. Nursing practice today is based on the multiple-causation theory of health problems. Unemployment, life-style, and stressful events, while not known to actually cause disease, may all contribute to it. These can be considered suprasystem problems, that is, problems stemming from systems in which the individual is a subsystem. Illness, then, is influenced by a person's family, social network, environ-

IGUN'S 11 STAGES OF HEALTH SEEKING

Stage 1 *Symptom experience.* Experiences symptoms and realizes there is a problem; often gives meaning to symptoms and labels them; responds emotionally.

Stage 2 *Self-treatment or self-medication.* Begins self-treatment; if believes symptoms are serious, moves to next state.

Stage 3 *Communication to others.* Communicates symptoms to significant others or a health professional.

Stage 4 *Assessment of symptoms.* Assesses symptoms to determine legitimacy and make tentative diagnosis.

Stage 5 *Sick-role assumption.* Assumes sick-role.

Stage 6 *Concern.* Significant others offer concern and support.

Stage 7 *Efficacy of treatment.* Assesses various treatments and sources of treatment.

Stage 8 *Selection of treatment.* Assesses various treatments and costs; may defer to health professional's advice.

Stage 9 *Treatment.* Implements treatment plan.

Stage 10 *Assessment of effectiveness of treatment.* If treatment not effective, may return to earlier stage.

Stage 11 *Recovery and rehabilitation.* Returns to earlier health status before illness or experiences temporary or permanent disability.

ment, and culture. It can be thought of as a result of interaction of the body, the mind, and the environment.

There are many ways to classify illness and disease; one of the most common is as acute or chronic. **Acute illness** is typically characterized by severe symptoms of relatively short duration. The symptoms often appear abruptly and subside quickly and, depending upon the cause, may or may not require intervention by a health care professional. Some acute illnesses are serious (for example, appendicitis may require surgical intervention) but many acute illnesses, such as colds, subside without medical intervention or with the help of over-the-counter medications. Following an acute illness, most people return to their normal level of wellness.

A **chronic illness** is one that lasts for an extended period of time, usually 6 months or longer, and often for the person's life. Often people who are chronically ill also have long-term disease processes (eg, osteoarthritis or multiple sclerosis). However, some people with chronic diseases do not regard themselves as ill. For example, an aging man who experiences physical changes from what was normal in earlier years may not consider himself ill.

Chronic illnesses usually have a slow onset and, often, periods of **remission,** when the symptoms disappear, and **exacerbation,** when the symptoms reappear.

Another distinction needs to be made between disease and deviance. **Deviance** is behavior that goes against social norms. Some deviant behaviors may be considered diseases according to the earlier definition of disease. For example, alcoholism can result in an alteration of body functioning, a reduction in capacities, and a shortening of the life span. Other deviant behavior can be considered disease, not because it alters the function of a body organ, but because it disrupts a family or a community. An example is drug addiction. However, differentiation between disease and deviance is not always clear and often depends on the perspective of the person observing the behavior.

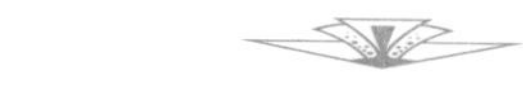

ILLNESS BEHAVIORS

By knowing stages of illness and the illness behaviors that accompany them, nurses can better understand their clients and determine ways to assist them. **Illness behavior** is "any activity undertaken by a person who feels ill, to define the state of his health and to discover a suitable remedy" (Igun 1979, p. 445).

Parsons (1972, pp. 436–37) describes four aspects of the sick role:

1. Clients are not held responsible for their condition.
2. Clients are excused from certain social roles and tasks.
3. Clients are obliged to try to get well as quickly as possible.
4. Clients or their families are obliged to seek competent help.

Igun (1979, pp. 445–46) describes 11 stages of illness or health seeking. See the box at the left above.

Bauman (1965, p. 208) found that people use three distinct criteria to determine if they are ill:

- The presence of symptoms (eg, elevated temperature or pain)
- The perception of how they feel (eg, well, tired, sick)
- Their ability to carry out daily activities (eg, work or schoolwork)

EFFECTS OF ILLNESS

When people are ill, there is usually a change in normal behavior. If the individual enters a health care agency (eg, a hospital), privacy is often affected. **Privacy** has been described as a comfortable feeling reflecting a deserved degree of social retreat *or* as freedom from unauthorized intrusion. Its dimensions and duration are controlled by the individual seeking the privacy. It is a personal internal state.

People need varying degrees of privacy and establish boundaries for privacy; when these boundaries are crossed, they feel invaded. For example, when clients are ill they are often asked to provide information they consider private, and their health is frequently discussed by a number of health professionals.

The boundaries of privacy are highly individual. A child from a large family may be accustomed to sharing activities such as bathing with others. It is important for nurses to ascertain what privacy means to the individual and try to support accustomed practices whenever possible. See also the discussion of territoriality in Chapter 18, page 363.

Ill people frequently give up much of their autonomy. Decisions about meals, hygienic practices, and sleeping are frequently adjusted for hospitalized clients. **Autonomy** is the state of being independent and self-directed without outside control. People vary in their sense of autonomy; some are accustomed to functioning independently in most of their life activities, whereas others are more accustomed to receiving direction.

Another effect of illness is the financial burden it places on clients and their families. Even people with health insurance may find that it does not cover all costs. In addition, many lose income during the illness. Nurses may be able to assist clients by facilitating referrals to social workers.

Illness also often necessitates a change in life-style. *Life-style* has been defined as "a general way of living based on the interplay between living conditions in the wide sense and individual patterns of behavior as determined by sociocultural factors and personal characteristics" (WHO, Health Education Unit 1986, p. 118). In addition to participating in treatments and taking medications, the ill person may need to change diet, activity and exercise, and rest and sleep patterns.

Nurses can help clients adjust their life-styles by

- Providing explanations about necessary adjustments.
- Making arrangements wherever possible to accommodate the client's life-style, such as providing a bath in the evening rather than in the morning.
- Encouraging other health professionals to become aware of the person's life-style practices and to support healthy aspects of that life-style.
- Reinforcing desirable changes in practices with a view to making them a permanent part of the client's life-style.

A person's illness affects not only the person who is ill but also the family or significant others. The kind of effect and its extent depend chiefly on three factors: (a) the member of the family who is ill, (b) the seriousness and length of the illness, and (c) the cultural and social customs the family follows.

The changes that can occur in the family include the following:

- Role changes
- Task reassignments and increased demands on time
- Increased stress due to anxiety about the outcome of the illness for the client and conflict about unaccustomed responsibilities
- Financial problems
- Loneliness as a result of separation and pending loss
- Change in social customs

See Chapter 14 for further information about the effects of illness on the family.

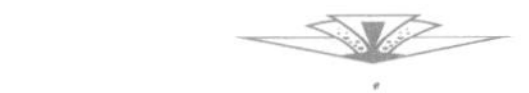

TRENDS IN HEALTH AND ILLNESS

Various data are obtained to measure the population's health. These include statistics on **mortality** (death rate), **longevity** (life expectancy), and **morbidity** (illness), and measures of people's sense of well-being or self-rated health status.

MORTALITY

Major causes of death (mortality) in the general population are shown in Figure 13–6 on page 258. In the past decades, much progress has been made in reducing the rates of death from three of the leading causes of death among Americans (US Department of Health and Human Services 1990, p. 3):

- Heart disease mortality has dropped more than 40% since 1970, reflecting notable increases in the detection and control of high blood pressure, a reduction in cigarette smoking, and an increasing awareness of the role of blood cholesterol and dietary fats.

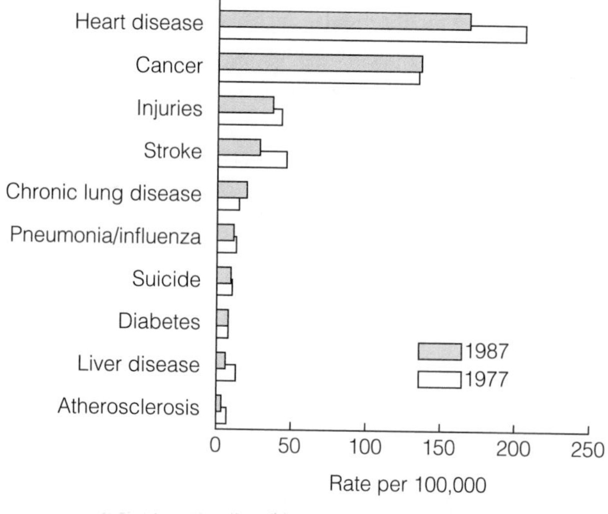

Figure 13–6 Changing incidence in the leading causes of death between 1977 and 1987. **Source:** National Center for Health Statistics, *Health United States 1989 and Preventive Profile,* DHHS Pub no. (PHS) 90-1232.

- Rates of death from stroke have dropped 50% in the same period. This decrease also reflects the gains in hypertension control and declines in smoking.
- Unintentional injuries have also declined. Traffic fatalities have dropped by one-third in the last few decades in part because of the increased use of seat belts, lower speed limits, and declines in alcohol use. Enhanced occupational safety standards have reduced fatal occupational injuries.

More progress is required, however, to reduce the death rate from diseases such as cancer, which have so far not declined. Although lung cancer deaths have increased since 1960, rates among men age 50 and younger showed improvement in the past decade due to changes in smoking patterns. Deaths from breast cancer remain high, but it is believed that early detection and treatment could reduce these deaths by as much as 30%. On the positive side, the widespread use of Papanicolaou tests has contributed to a 73% reduction in death rates from cervical cancer since 1950 (USDHHS 1990, p. 4).

In terms of children, progress has also been made. In 1990, the infant mortality rate reached a record low of 10.1 infant deaths per 1000 live births in the United States, representing a 65% decline since 1950 (National Center for Health Statistics 1990). However, this rate is still higher than in many other countries.

LONGEVITY

In this century, average life expectancy at birth has increased almost 60%, from 47 years in 1900 to 75 in 1987 (USDHHS 1990, p. 43). Since the eighteenth century, the health of infants and young children has been transformed. At that time, only about 3 of 10 newborn infants lived beyond the age of 25. Today in developed countries, fewer than 1 in 20 children die before they reach adulthood (McKeown 1990, p. 7).

The increased life expectancy is due primarily to a reduction of deaths from infectious diseases. Major factors responsible were the introduction of (a) antibiotics and vaccines; (b) basic hygienic measures such as water purification, efficient sewage disposal, and improved food hygiene, including the pasteurization of milk; (c) improved conditions in the home, workplace, and general environment; and (d) increased food supplies that led to better nutrition and increased resistance to infectious diseases (McKeown 1990, pp. 8–10).

MORBIDITY

The National Health Interview Survey (NHIS) provides annual reports about the United States population's health. Included are rates for incidence of acute conditions; restricted activity, bed disability, and absence from work (work loss) due to acute and chronic conditions; and limitations in activities due to chronic conditions.

Acute Conditions Compared to children and young adults, people aged 45 and older experience fewer acute conditions (eg, respiratory conditions, injuries, acute skin and musculoskeletal problems, genitourinary problems). Since the late 1950s, incidence rates for all acute conditions (with the exception of injuries for women) have declined for men and women over age 45. A lower incidence of respiratory conditions accounts for this decline. Injury rates have increased for women.

Disability Days for All Conditions Adults aged 65 and older have three times more restricted activity days per year and three times more bed-disability days than children under 17. This rise in disability with age reflects an increasing incidence of chronic conditions that is offset only minimally by a decreasing incidence in acute conditions.

Limitations Due to Chronic Conditions The percentage of people with major activity limitations rises with age. In 1981, it was 2% for children, 19% for middle-aged adults, and 39% for older adults. This indicates rising limitations since the late 1950s and may reflect rising chronic morbidity for adults or increased willingness to make role adjustments for chronic health problems.

"HEALTHY PEOPLE 2000" GOALS

Healthy People 2000, a report by the US Department of Health and Human Services (USDHHS 1990, p. 43) outlines three broad goals to meet the health challenge of the 1990s:

1. Increase the span of healthy life for Americans.
2. Reduce health disparities among Americans.
3. Achieve access to preventive services for all Americans.

A central purpose of *Healthy People 2000* is to increase the proportion of Americans who live long and healthy lives. Healthy life means a full range of functional capacity at each life stage. It extends into the final quarter of a person's life and focuses on freedom from chronic, disabling disease and conditions, from preventable infection, and from serious injury.

Health disparities occur among certain population groups in terms of life expectancy, infant mortality rate, years of healthy life, and potential years of life lost before age 65 (USDHHS 1990, pp. 46–48). For example

- Life expectancy for European Americans is 74.4 years but only 68 years for African Americans (1980).
- Years of healthy life for European Americans is 63 years compared to only 56 for African Americans and 62 for Hispanics (1990).
- Infant mortality rates are greater among African Americans than European Americans (17.9 deaths per 1000 live births compared to 8.6 in 1987).
- Compared to European-American males, African-American males have higher percentages of lost years of life before age 65: 55% higher for cancer, 180% higher for stroke, 100% higher for lung disease, and 630% higher for homicide (1987).
- Lost years of life before 65 were 134% higher among African-American women for heart disease, 166% higher for stroke, and 360% higher for homicide (1987).

Achievement of the second goal of *Healthy People 2000* depends on significant improvements in the health of populations (eg, African Americans) that are at the highest risk of disease, disability, and premature death.

Access to preventive services for all Americans means more than the availability of services. Preventive services must be integrated with basic primary health care. Approximately 18% of all Americans and 31% of those who lack private or public health insurance have no source of primary health care. Over the next decade, particular attention needs to be given to increasing the number of people who have a primary source of health care and who have adequate insurance coverage. Health care systems need to cover preventive services such as the following:

- Providing health care services that ensure the health of pregnant women and the birth of healthy babies
- Monitoring of child growth and development
- Immunizing children against childhood diseases and immunizing adults who are vulnerable to influenza and pneumonia
- Adequate screening to detect high blood pressure, high blood cholesterol, and cancer (eg, breast, cervical, oropharyngeal, and colorectal)
- Counseling on injury prevention, nutrition, and smoking cessation

These three goals can serve as basic values that underlie all health promotion, health protection, and disease prevention services.

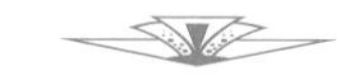

PROMOTING HEALTH AND WELLNESS

Health promotion is any activity undertaken for the purpose of achieving a higher level of health and well-being. It is directed toward improving well-being and actualizing the health potential of individuals, families, groups, and communities.

Health promotion is more than the avoidance or prevention of disease. It includes *primary* prevention activities (eg, immunization) as well as wellness-promotion activities not directed to specific diseases (eg, stress management and physical fitness). See Table 13–1 on page 260 for levels of prevention.

Health promotion can be offered to all clients regardless of their health and illness status or age. For example, weight-control measures can benefit both overweight clients without disease and clients with cardiac or joint disease. Age-specific health promotion activities are discussed in Chapters 24, 25, and 26. See the accompanying box for examples of health promotion topics for well or ill older adults.

HEALTH PROMOTION TOPICS FOR OLDER ADULTS

- Adequate sleep
- Appropriate use of alcohol
- Dental/oral health
- Drug managenment
- Exercise
- Foot health
- Health screening recommendations
- Hearing aid use
- Immunizations
- Medication instruction
- Nutrition
- Physical fitness
- Preventive health services
- Safety precautions
- Smoking cessation
- Stress management
- Weight control

Table 13-1 Levels of Prevention

Level/Description	Examples
Primary prevention. Generalized health promotion and specific protection against disease. It precedes disease or dysfunction and is applied to generally healthy individuals or groups.	▪ Health education about accident and poisoning prevention, standards of nutrition and growth and development for each stage of life, exercise requirements, stress management, protection against occupational hazards, and so on ▪ Immunizations ▪ Risk assessments for specific disease ▪ Family planning services and marriage counseling ▪ Environmental sanitation and provision of adequate housing, recreation, and work conditions
Secondary prevention. Emphasizes early detection of disease, prompt intervention, and health maintenance for individuals experiencing health problems. It includes prevention of complications and disabilities.	▪ Screening surveys and procedures of any type (eg, Denver Developmental Screening Test, hypertension screening) ▪ Encouraging regular medical and dental checkups ▪ Teaching self-examination for breast and testicular cancer ▪ Assessing the growth and development of children ▪ Nursing assessments and care provided in home, hospital, or other agency to prevent complications (eg, maintaining skin integrity; turning, positioning, and exercising clients; ensuring adequate rest, food, and fluid intake; promoting fecal and urinary elimination; administering medical therapies such as medications, and so on)
Tertiary prevention. Begins after an illness, when a defect or disability is fixed, stabilized, or irreversible. Its focus is to help rehabilitate individuals and restore them to an optimum level of functioning within the constraints of the disability.	▪ Referring a client who has had a colostomy to a support group ▪ Teaching a client who has diabetes to identify and prevent complications ▪ Referring a client with a spinal cord injury to a rehabilitation center to receive training that will maximize use of remaining abilities

Health promotion programs are found in many settings: work settings, schools, health care organizations, and other community agencies. A variety of individuals may provide instruction. For example, the fire department may disseminate fire-prevention information; the police may offer a bicycle safety program for children or safe-driving campaign for young adults; health care personnel may offer programs such as smoking cessation, exercise and fitness, time management, and women's health.

TYPES OF HEALTH PROMOTION PROGRAMS

A variety of programs can be used for the promotion of health, including (a) information dissemination, (b) health appraisal and wellness assessment, (c) life-style and behavior change, (d) worksite wellness programs, and (e) environmental control programs.

Information dissemination is the most basic type of health promotion program that raises the level of knowledge and awareness of individuals and groups about health habits. This method makes use of a variety of media to offer information to the public about the risk of particular life-style choices and personal behavior, as well as the benefits of changing that behavior and improving the quality of life. Billboards, posters, brochures, newspaper features, books, and health fairs all offer opportunities for the dissemination of health promotion information. Alcohol and drug abuse, driving under the influence of alcohol, good nutrition, hypertension, anorexia, and AIDS are some of the topics frequently discussed.

Health appraisal/wellness assessment programs are used to apprise individuals of the risk factors inherent in their lives in order to motivate them to reduce specific risks and develop positive health habits. Wellness assessment programs focus on more positive methods of enhancement, in contrast to the risk factor approach used in the health appraisal. A variety of tools are available to facilitate these assessments. Some of these tools are computer based and can therefore be offered to educational institutions and industries at a reasonable cost.

Life-style and behavior change programs require the participation of the individual and are geared toward enhancing the quality of life and extending the life span. Many programs are available to the public, both on a group and individual basis. These programs address stress management, nutrition awareness, weight control, smoking cessation, exercise, and similar topics.

Worksite wellness programs include programs that address air quality standards for the office, classroom, or plant; programs aimed at specific populations, such as accident prevention for the machine worker or back-saver programs for the individual involved in heavy lifting; programs to screen for high blood pressure; or health enhancement programs, such as fitness information and relaxation techniques.

Environmental control programs have been developed in response to the recent growth in the number of contaminants of human origin that have been introduced into our environment. The amount of contaminants already present in the air, food, and water will affect the health of our descendants for several generations. The most common concerns of community groups are toxic and nuclear wastes, nuclear power plants, air and water pollution, and herbicide and pesticide spraying.

THE NURSE'S ROLE IN HEALTH PROMOTION

- Model healthy life-style behaviors and attitudes.
- Facilitate client involvement in the assessment, implementation, and evaluation of health goals.
- Teach clients self-care strategies to enhance fitness, improve nutrition, manage stress, and enhance relationships.
- Assist individuals, families, and communities to increase their levels of health.
- Teach clients to be effective health care consumers.
- Assist clients, families, and communities to develop and choose health-promoting options.
- Guide the clients' development in effective problem solving and decision making.
- Reinforce the clients' personal and family health-promoting behaviors.
- Advocate in the community for changes that promote a healthy environment.

THE NURSE'S ROLE IN HEALTH PROMOTION

As a promoter of health, the nurse may act as advocate, consultant, teacher, or coordinator of services. For examples of the nurse's role in health promotion, see the accompanying box. In this role, the nurse may work with all age groups or be limited to a specific population (eg, new parents, school-age children, or senior citizens). In any case, the nursing process is a basic tool for the nurse in a health promotion role. Although the process is the same, the emphasis is on teaching the client self-care responsibility. The clients decide the goals, determine the health promotion plans, and take the responsibility for the success of the plans.

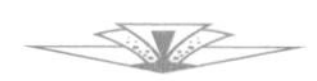

THE NURSING PROCESS AND HEALTH PROMOTION

ASSESSING

A thorough assessment of the client's health status is basic to health promotion. Components of this assessment are the health history and physical examination, physical-fitness assessment, nutrition assessment, health risk appraisal, life-style assessment, and life-stress review. To create a health promotion program that has relevance to clients, the nurse needs to first understand the clients' perspectives of their existing health status.

Health History and Physical Examination The health history and physical examination provide a means for detecting any existing problems. See Chapter 22 for detailed information about the health history and physical examination.

Physical Fitness Assessment During an evaluation of physical fitness, the nurse takes girth and skinfold measurements, administers the step test, and assesses strength and endurance of muscles and flexibility of joints. See Chapter 34, page 882.

Nutritional Assessment To assess nutritional status, the nurse compares the client's weight to body build and height (see Chapter 22), measures mid-upper arm circumference to determine muscle mass, observes for signs of malnutrition, and takes a dietary history. The latter three are discussed in Chapter 37.

Health Risk Appraisal A health risk appraisal (HRA) or health hazard appraisal (HHA) is an assessment and educational tool that indicates a client's risk of disease or injury. There are two objectives of the many HRA instruments available:

Health-Style: A Self-Test

All of us want good health. But many of us do not know how to be as healthy as possible. Health experts now describe *life-style* as one of the most important factors affecting health. In fact, it is estimated that as many as seven of the ten leading causes of death could be reduced through common-sense changes in life-style. That's what this brief test, developed by the Public Health Service, is all about. Its purpose is simply to tell you how well you are doing to stay healthy. The behaviors covered in the test are recommended for most Americans. Some of them may not apply to people with certain chronic diseases or disabilities, or to pregnant women. Such people may require special instructions from their physicians.

Cigarette Smoking

If you never smoke, enter a score of 10 for this section and go to the next section on *Alcohol and Drugs*.

	almost always	sometimes	almost never
1. I avoid smoking cigarettes.	2	1	0
2. I smoke only low tar and nicotine cigarettes *or* I smoke a pipe or cigars.	2	1	0

Smoking score: ____________

Alcohol and Drugs

	almost always	sometimes	almost never
1. I avoid drinking alcoholic beverages *or* I drink no more than one or two drinks a day.	4	1	0
2. I avoid using alcohol or other drugs (especially illegal drugs) as a way of handling stressful situations or the problems in my life.	2	1	0
3. I am careful not to drink alcohol when taking certain medicines (for example, medicine for sleeping, pain, colds, and allergies), or when pregnant.	2	1	0
4. I read and follow the label directions when using prescribed and over-the-counter drugs.	2	1	0

Alcohol and drugs score: ____________

Eating Habits

	almost always	sometimes	almost never
1. I eat a variety of foods each day, such as fruits and vegetables, whole grain breads and cereals, lean meats, dairy products, dry peas and beans, and nuts and seeds.	4	1	0
2. I limit the amount of fat, saturated fat, and cholesterol I eat (including fat on meats, eggs, butter, cream, shortenings, and organ meats such as liver).	2	1	0
3. I limit the amount of salt I eat by cooking with only small amounts, not adding salt at the table, and avoiding salty snacks.	2	1	0
4. I avoid eating too much sugar (especially frequent snacks of sticky candy or soft drinks).	2	1	0

Eating habits score: ____________

Exercise and Fitness

	almost always	sometimes	almost never
1. I maintain a desired weight, avoiding overweight and underweight.	2	1	0
2. I do vigorous exercises for 15 to 30 minutes at least three times a week (examples include running, swimming, brisk walking).	3	1	0
3. I do exercises that enhance my muscle tone for 15 to 30 minutes at least three times a week (examples include yoga and calisthenics).	2	1	0
4. I use part of my leisure time participating in individual, family, or team activities that increase my level of fitness (such as gardening, bowling, golf, and baseball).	2	1	0

Exercise/fitness score: ____________

Stress Control

	almost always	sometimes	almost never
1. I have a job or do other work that I enjoy.	2	1	0
2. I find it easy to relax and express my feelings freely.	2	1	0
3. I recognize early, and prepare for, events or situations likely to be stressful for me.	2	1	0
4. I have close friends, relatives, or others whom I can talk to about personal matters and call on for help when needed.	2	1	0
5. I participate in group activities (such as church and community organizations) or hobbies that I enjoy.	2	1	0

Stress control score: ____________

Safety

	almost always	sometimes	almost never
1. I wear a seat belt while riding in a car.	2	1	0
2. I avoid driving while under the influence of alcohol and other drugs.	2	1	0
3. I obey traffic rules and the speed limit when driving.	2	1	0
4. I am careful when using potentially harmful products or substances (such as household cleaners, poisons, and electrical devices.	2	1	0
5. I avoid smoking in bed.	2	1	0

Safety score: ____________

(continued)

Figure 13–7 Health style: A self-test. **Source:** National Health Information Clearinghouse. Reprinted with permission.

Health-Style: A Self-Test *(continued)*

What Your Scores Mean to You

Scores of 9 and 10
Excellent! Your answers show that you are aware of the importance of this area to your health. More important, you are putting your knowledge to work for you by practicing good health habits. As long as you continue to do so, this area should not pose a serious health risk. It's likely that you are setting an example for your family and friends to follow. Because you got a very high test score on this part of the test, you may want to consider other areas where your scores indicate room for improvement.

Scores of 6 to 8
Your health practices in this area are good, but there is room for improvement. Look again at the items you answered with "Sometimes" or "Almost never." What changes can you make to improve your score? Even a small change can often help you achieve better health.

Scores of 3 to 5
Your health risks are showing! Would you like more information about the risks you are facing and about why it is important for you to change these behaviors? Perhaps you need help in deciding how to successfully make the changes you desire. In either case, help is available.

Scores of 0 to 2
Obviously, you were concerned enough about your health to take the test, but your answers show that you may be taking serious and unnecessary risks with your health. Perhaps you are unaware of the risks and what to do about them. You can easily get the information and help you need to improve, if you wish. The next step is up to you.

Where Do You Go from Here

Start by asking youself a few frank questions: *Am I really doing all I can to be as healthy as possible? What steps can I take to feel better? Am I willing to begin now?* If you scored low in one or more sections of the test, decide what changes you want to make for improvement. You might pick that aspect of your life-style where you feel you have the best chance for success and tackle that one first. Once you have improved your score there, go on to other areas.

If you already have tried to change your health habits (to stop smoking or exercise regularly, for example), don't be discouraged if you haven't yet succeeded. The difficulty you have encountered may be due to influences you've never really thought about—such as advertising—or to a lack of support and encouragement. Understanding these influences is an important step toward changing the way they affect you.

There's help available. In addition to personal actions you can take on your own, there are community programs and groups (such as the YMCA or the local chapter of the American Heart Association) that can assist you and your family to make the changes you want to make. If you want to know more about these groups or about health risks, contact your local health department or the National Health Information Clearinghouse. There's a lot you can do to stay healthy or to improve your health—and there are organizations that can help you. Start a new "health-style" today!

For assistance in locating specific information on these and other health topics, write to the National Health Information Clearinghouse:

National Health Information Clearinghouse
P.O. Box 1133
Washington, DC 20013

1. To assess risk factors that may lead to health problems. A **risk factor** is a phenomenon (eg, age or life-style behavior) that increases a person's chance of acquiring a specific disease.
2. To change health behaviors that place the client at risk of developing an illness.

An HRA may have from 25 to 300 or more questions. Clients either score their responses themselves or send them to an organization for computer printouts. Scores are often tabulated according to an overall life-style profile, levels of health risk, and life expectancy.

Risk factors may be categorized according to (a) age, (b) genetic factors, (c) biologic characteristics, (d) personal health habits, (e) life-style, and (f) environment. Clients cannot control some of the risk factors appraised, such as age, sex, and family history; others, such as blood pressure, stress, and cigarette smoking, can be partially or totally controlled.

Life-Style Assessment Life-style assessment, which may or may not be part of the HRA, focuses on the personal life-style and habits of the client as they affect health. Categories of life-style generally assessed are physical activity, eating habits, safety practices, stress management, and such habits as smoking, alcohol consumption, and drug use. Other categories may be included.

Several tools are available to assess life-style ranging up to 100-item tools. A concise self-test life-style assessment form is shown in Figure 13–7.

The goals of life-style assessment tools are

1. To provide an opportunity for clients to assess the impact of their present life-style on their health.

2. To provide a basis for decisions related to desired behavior and life-style change.

Life-Stress Review There is abundant literature about the impact of stress on mental and physical well-being. Assessment of stressors, signs of anxiety, and stress is discussed in Chapter 32.

VALIDATION OF ASSESSMENT DATA

Following the collection of assessment data, the nurse and client need to review, validate, and summarize the information. This step is carried out jointly by the nurse and the client. During this process, the nurse verbally reviews the current practices and attitudes of the client. This allows validation of the information by the client and may increase awareness of the need to change behavior. The nurse and client need to consider:

- Any existing health problems
- The client's perceived degree of control over health status
- Level of physical fitness and nutritional status
- Illnesses for which the client is at risk
- Current positive health practices
- Ability to handle stress
- Information needed to enhance health care practices

DIAGNOSING

Nursing diagnoses accepted by NANDA (North American Nursing Diagnosis Association) have generally focused on altered health patterns or problems. There are, however, four NANDA wellness diagnoses that may be used for clients seeking a higher level of wellness. These are

- **Health seeking behavior** (specify)
- **Family coping: potential for growth**
- **Effective breast feeding**
- **Anticipatory grieving**

The diagnosis of **Health seeking behavior** needs to be specified (eg, physical fitness). In lieu of these diagnoses, the nurse may write wellness diagnoses by using the words "Potential for enhanced" followed by the wellness behavior, as follows:

- **Potential for enhanced nutritional status**
- **Potential for enhanced physical fitness**
- **Potential for enhanced family functioning**
- **Potential for enhanced coping patterns**
- **Potential for enhanced parenting skills**
- **Potential for enhanced use of safety precautions**
- **Potential for enhanced relationship with peers**

PLANNING

Health promotion plans need to be developed according to the needs, desires, and priorities of the client. The client decides on health promotion goals, the activities or interventions to achieve those goals, the frequency and duration of the activities, and the method of evaluation. During the planning process the nurse acts as a resource person rather than as an adviser or counselor. The nurse provides information when asked, emphasizes the importance of small steps to behavioral change, and reviews the client's goals and plans to make sure they are realistic, measurable, and acceptable to the client.

Steps in Planning Pender (1987, p. 214) outlines several steps in the process of health promotion planning, which are carried out jointly by the nurse and the client:

1. *Identify health care goals.* The client selects two or three top-priority goals or areas for improvement (eg, achieve desired weight).
2. *Identify possible behavior changes.* For each of the selected goals or areas in step 1, determine what specific behavioral changes are needed to bring about the desired outcome (eg, increase activity level and decrease fat in diet).
3. *Assign priorities to behavior changes.* Behavior must be acceptable to the client if it is to be adopted and integrated. From the list of behavior options in step 2, the clients select and assign priorities to those changes they are most willing to try.
4. *Make a commitment to change behavior.* Increasingly, a formal, written **behavioral contract** is being used to motivate the client to follow through with selected actions. Here is an example of a self-contract:

    I, Amy Martin, will exercise strenuously for 20 minutes three times per week for a period of 2 weeks and will then buy myself six yellow roses.

    Amy Martin
July 30, 1995

5. *Identify effective reinforcements and rewards.* Rewards tend to provide an incentive for behavior change, more so than individual willpower, provided the reward is meaningful to and selected by the client. Rewards can be objects, experiences, family activities, or praise.
6. *Determine barriers to change* such as lack of support from family members, cost of change, culture or peer pressure, lack of time, or inconvenience.
7. *Develop a schedule for implementing the behavior change.* Clients need to set up a time frame to make the behav-

ior changes required to meet each goal. Time frames may be several weeks or months. Scheduling short-term goals and rewards can offer the encouragement necessary to achieve long-term objectives. Clients may need help to be realistic and to deal with one behavior at a time.

Exploring Available Resources Another essential aspect of planning is identifying support resources available to the client. These may be community resources, such as a fitness program at a local gymnasium, or educational programs, such as stress management, breast self-examination, nutrition, smoking cessation, and health lectures. The nurse, too, may meet some of the client's educational needs. A major nursing role is to support the client. The nurse can contact the client or be available at specified intervals to review the contract and to assist with problem solving.

IMPLEMENTING

Implementing is the "doing" part of behavior change. Self-responsibility is emphasized for implementing the plan. Depending on the clients' needs, the nursing strategies may include supporting, teaching, consulting, coordinating, facilitating, counseling, and enhancing the behavior change.

Providing and Facilitating Support A vital component of life-style change is ongoing support that focuses on the desired behavior change and is provided in a nonjudgmental manner. Support can be offered by the nurse on an individual basis or in a group setting. The nurse can also facilitate the development of support networks for the client, such as family members and friends.

Individual Counseling Sessions Counseling sessions may be routinely scheduled as part of the plan or may be provided if the client encounters difficulty in carrying out interventions or meets insurmountable barriers to change. In a counseling relationship, the nurse and client share ideas. In this sharing relationship, the nurse acts as a facilitator, promoting the client's decision making regarding the health promotion plan.

Telephone Counseling Regular telephone sessions may be provided to the client to help in answering questions, reviewing goals and strategies, and reinforcing progress. The client may find that scheduling a weekly telephone session is helpful or may wish to initiate a call if a problem occurs. The client is asked, "Is your plan working?" If the plan is not working, the nurse asks, "What would you like to do?" The client may wish to continue or may wish to change the plan to a more realistic one. Telephone support is efficient for the busy client who may not have the time for regular, in-person sessions.

Group Support Group sessions provide an opportunity for participants to learn the experiences of others in changing behavior. Group contact gives individuals a renewed commitment to their goals. Groups can be scheduled at monthly or less frequent intervals for over a year.

Facilitating Social Support Social networks, such as families, friends, and community-based support groups such as Overeater's Anonymous can facilitate or impede the efforts directed toward health promotion and prevention. To provide the necessary support, families must communicate effectively, be aware of and support each other's needs and goals, and provide help and assistance to one another to achieve those goals. The client may wish the nurse to meet with the family or significant others and help in enlisting their understanding and support.

Providing Health Education Health education programs on a variety of topics can be provided to groups, individuals, or communities. Group programs need to be planned carefully before they are implemented. The decision to establish a health promotion program must be based on the assessed health needs of the people; also, specific health promotion goals must be set. After the program is implemented, program outcomes must be evaluated.

In the evaluation of health promotion programs, the client's understanding must be ascertained. Simply asking clients if they understand may be inappropriate. Using nondirective, open-ended questions (see Chapter 5, page 90), the nurse asks clients in their own words what they understand about the health promotion programs. This approach enables the nurse to ensure that the program is designed to meet the client's unique situation.

In some cases, the client may understand the information but may not be able to apply it or may have anxiety about doing a particular task. For instance, a new parent may understand all the principles of giving an infant a bed bath but have considerable anxiety about managing the procedure. Giving clients ample opportunity to demonstrate or practice routines and procedures, asking them to repeat important steps or information, and clarifying any unclear statements allow the nurse to evaluate the clients' knowledge and competence more fully.

Nurses may offer an abundance of information less formally. To do so, however, nurses need up-to-date knowledge, the ability to assess learning needs, and effective teaching skills. See Chapter 19 for detailed information. For example, nurses often disseminate information about parenting, breast and testicular self-examination, prevention of sexually transmitted disease, nutritional needs, and monitoring blood pressure and pulse rates.

Health fairs are a recent method being used to disseminate information to the public about health promotion and disease prevention and early detection. Nurses are

CLINICAL GUIDELINES

Enhancing Behavior Change

- Recognize that motivation is the basis of all behavior whether it is healthy or unhealthy, good or bad.
- Recognize that people are motivated by their needs.
- Avoid labeling people as unmotivated. The label simply means that the person does not comply with the wishes of the nurse who applies the label.
- Focus on the sources or factors that motivate the person's behavior rather than on the presence or absence of motivation.
- Remember that resistance is a normal part of change and a healthy response to a threat.
- Understand that a client may choose to keep unhealthy habits for many reasons.
  a. The habit may be a culturally learned response such as cigarette smoking and alcohol consumption. In North America, these habits were once associated with a glamorous or sophisticated life-style and a certain kind of satisfaction.
  b. The client may be directing all available energies to meet other needs. A person who is grieving the loss of a loved one, or a recently divorced person, for example, may not have the energy to follow a weight-loss diet.
  c. The conditions required to change may be absent. For example, clients need help first to "unlearn" or "unfreeze" old habits and recognize the benefits of new habits before they can consider or undertake action.
- Cast aside the idea that the client *must* change. This attitude is not conducive to a helping relationship with the client and does not convey respect for the client. The client who does not change is entitled to the nurse's interest and nonjudgmental response.
- Measure your competence in terms of how well you understand clients' needs and implement clients' care rather than by the extent to which clients change their behavior.

Source: MM Murphy. November/December 1982. Why won't they shape up? Resistance to the promotion of health. *Canadian Journal of Public Health* 73:427–30.

RESEARCH NOTE

What Are the Health Promotion Practices of Nursing Students?

Nursing students have the power to act as role models for classmates, family, friends, and clients. How well do they play this role? The purpose of this study was to identify the health practices of nursing students and to find out their overall opinion toward primary preventive practices. The sample for this study consisted of 1081 female nursing students from ten schools in the Buffalo, New York area. The ten schools included diploma, associate degree, and baccalaureate programs. The ages of the students ranged from 17 to 55 years, with a mean age of 24.

The results showed considerable variation in the extent to which students practiced health promotion and prevention. On the positive side, the majority of students obtained 6–8 hours of sleep per night, did not or had never smoked, brushed their teeth regularly, exercised regularly, had routine dental care, and had a yearly physical examination. However, fewer than half of the students ate breakfast daily, three-fourths of those surveyed ate between meals, and less than half limited fats, salt, and sugar in their diets. Breast self-examination was done by only one-third of the group; most did not wear seat belts; and 90% consumed alcoholic beverages.

These findings indicate that although nursing students, as future health care professionals, are expected to act as role models, their own health practices need improvement.

Implications: The authors suggest that faculty take a more active role in promoting positive health promotion behaviors by (a) increasing students' awareness regarding the information and resources that are available for facilitating behavior change, (b) increasing content related to health promotion and prevention within the core curriculum and in courses relating to health and life-styles, and (c) instituting no-smoking policies in classrooms and school buildings. In addition, nursing faculty members should be aware of their role in setting the appropriate example by practicing health promotion and prevention.

Source: S Dittmar, B Hoyghey, R O'Shea, and J Brasure, Health practices of nursing students, *Health Values*, March/April 1989, 13:24–31.

often the initiators of health fairs and may provide participants of all age groups with information, teaching, counseling, or screening. Health fairs are usually offered in convenient locations such as shopping malls, schools, hospitals, and business settings in order to encourage maximum participation.

Enhancing Behavior Change To help clients succeed in implementing behavior changes, the nurse needs to understand the process of change and the nature of the client's motivation or the client's current situation. An application of Lewin's stages of change (unfreezing, moving, and refreezing) can help the nurse recognize the client's needs. See Chapter 20 for additional information on Lewin's stages.

"*Stage 1 (unfreezing)* or 'unlearning' old habits is probably the most important stage of change but it is also the most difficult and challenging for the health promoter" (Murphy 1982, p. 428). The nurse can best help the client by emphasizing what that person values. Loss of an unhealthy behavior may then become tolerable. For example, a client may start to "unfreeze" a habit of eating excessive carbohydrates if emphasis is placed on maximizing energy potential through a balanced food intake rather than just on the components of a healthy diet. In *Stage 2 (moving)*, the client is ready to change and develop new responses. Many health promoters tend to focus their efforts on this stage of eliciting new desired responses. In *Stage 3 (refreezing)*, the client internalizes behavior changes and stabilizes a new level of functioning. Guidelines for assisting the client toward behavior change are offered in the box on page 266.

Modeling Modeling consists of observing the behavior of other people who have successfully achieved the goal that clients have set for themselves. Modeling is not imitating. Through observing a model, the client acquires ideas for behavior and coping strategies for specific problems. The client is not expected to mimic the sequence of actions or behavior patterns of the model.

The nurse and client should mutually select models with whom the client can identify, because the cultural and ethnic backgrounds of the nurse and client often differ. Models should be frequently available during the early learning and change stages of unfreezing and moving. Models should also be people the client respects.

Nurses should serve as models of wellness. To model effectively, nurses need to have a philosophy and life-style that demonstrate good health habits. They need to assess their own life-styles, develop a health promotion plan, and actually carry out the implementation strategies. Once nurses have had a firsthand experience with creating a health promotion plan and with the difficulties involved with behavior change, they will be able to work more effectively with peers and clients. Clients are more likely to respect and trust the nurse who can tell them what worked in the nurse's personal situation.

EVALUATING

Evaluation takes place on an ongoing basis, both during the attainment of short-term goals and after the completion of long-term goals. During evaluation, the client may decide to continue with the plan, reorder priorities, change strategies, or revise the health promotion contract.

CHAPTER HIGHLIGHTS

- The perspective from which health is viewed has changed; instead of absence of disease, health has come to mean a high level of wellness or the fulfillment of one's maximum potential for physical, psychosocial, and spiritual functioning.
- Wellness is an active, five-dimensional process of becoming aware of and making choices toward a higher level of well-being. The five dimensions of wellness are the physical, social, emotional, intellectual, and spiritual dimensions.
- Well-being is considered a subjective perception of balance, harmony, and vitality. It is a state rather than a process.
- Because notions of health are highly individual, the nurse must determine each client's perception of health to provide meaningful assistance. This involves well-developed communication skills. Nurses need to be aware of their own personal definitions of health.
- Most people describe health as freedom from symptoms of disease, the ability to be active, and a state of being in good spirits.
- Various models have been developed to explain health. These include Smith's clinical, role performance, adaptive, and eudaemonistic models; Leavell and Clark's agent-host-environment model; Dunn's high-level wellness grid; Travis's illness-wellness continuum; and Rosenstock's health belief model.
- Nurses need to clarify their understanding of health because nurse's definitions of health largely determine the scope and nature of nursing practice, and people's health beliefs influence their health practices.
- The health status of a person is affected by many internal and external variables over which the person has varying degrees of control.
- Internal variables include biologic, psychologic, and cognitive dimensions. The biologic dimension includes genetic makeup, race, sex, age, and developmental level. The psychologic dimension includes mind-body interactions and self-concept. The cognitive dimension includes life-style choices and spiritual and religious beliefs.

➤

- External variables influencing health are geography, physical environment, standards of living, family and cultural beliefs, and social support networks.
- A person's decision to implement health behaviors or to take action to improve health depends on such factors as the importance of health to the person, perceived threat of a particular disease or severity of the health care problems, perceived benefits of preventive or therapeutic actions, inconvenience and unpleasantness involved, degree of life-style change necessary, cultural ramifications, and cost.
- Nurses can enhance health care compliance by identifying the reasons for noncompliance if it occurs, demonstrating caring, using positive reinforcement to encourage healthy behaviors, using aids to reinforce teaching, and establishing a therapeutic relationship of freedom, mutual understanding, and mutual responsibility with the client and support persons.
- Illness is usually associated with disease but may occur independently of it. Illness is a highly personal state in which the person feels unhealthy or ill. Disease alters body functions and results in a reduction of capacities or a shortened life span.
- The single-causation theory of disease is being replaced by a multiple-causation theory. For many diseases, the cause is still unknown.
- Five categories of risk factors that predispose individuals to illness and disease are genetic factors, age, physiologic factors, life-style, and environment.
- One of the most common ways to classify illness and disease is by their acuteness or chronicity.
- Various theorists have described stages and aspects of illness. Igun describes 11 stages of illness or health-seeking behaviors. Parsons describes 4 aspects of the sick role. Bauman outlines 3 criteria people use to determine if they are ill.
- An individual's usual pattern of behavior changes with illness and hospitalization. Illness and hospitalization disrupt a person's privacy, autonomy, life-style, roles, and finances.
- Nurses need to be aware that the illness of one member of a family affects all other members.
- Various data are obtained to measure a population's health: mortality rates, longevity, and morbidity data.
- Health promotion activities are directed toward developing client resources that maintain or enhance well-being and raise the client's level of health.
- Health promotion programs can be categorized as information dissemination, health appraisal and wellness assessment, life-style and behavior change, worksite wellness, and environmental control programs.
- A thorough assessment of the client's health status is basic to health promotion.
- Health risk or hazard appraisals provide the data that often spur the client to adopt a healthier life-style.
- Life-style assessment tools give clients the opportunity to assess the impact of their present life-styles on their health and to make decisions about life-style changes.
- During planning, the client may wish to make a behavioral contract. A contract usually includes the client goal, activities to achieve the goals, and the methods of evaluation to measure goal achievement.
- To help clients change their life-styles or health behaviors, the nurse provides ongoing support, supplies additional information and education, explores the motivating sources of the client's behavior, and acts as a wellness role model.

READINGS AND REFERENCES

SUGGESTED READINGS

Alford, DM and Futrell, M. September/October 1992. Wellness and health promotion of the elderly. *Nursing Outlook* 40:221–26.
This paper presents the concepts that health should be restructured to include social and environmental aspects and disease should not characterize old age. Life-style changes such as exercising and eating a nutritious diet are to be encouraged. "Successful aging for most people means coping and adapting." This article presents a variety of health recommendations for the elderly.

McAllister, G and Farquhar, M. December 1992. Health beliefs: A cultural division? *Journal of Advanced Nursing* 17:1447–54.
The authors identify and compare the health beliefs of Asian women and white indigenous women living in London. The Asian women rated their health as poorer than did the white women. The article presents concepts of illness, health beliefs, and locus of control models. It also presents some specific recommendations to nurses regarding cultural sensitivity.

RELATED RESEARCH

Robertson, JF. June 1991. Promoting health among the institutionalized elderly. *Journal of Gerontological Nursing* 17:15–19.

Whetstone, WR and Reid, JC. November 1991. Health promotion of older adults: Perceived barriers. *Journal of Advanced Nursing* 16:1343–49.

SELECTED REFERENCES

Anspaugh, DJ, Hamrick, MH, and Rosata, FD. 1991. *Wellness: Concepts and Applications.* St Louis: Mosby-Year Book.

Bauman, B. 1965. Diversities in conceptions of health and physical fitness. In Skipper, JK, Jr and Leonard, RC, editors. *Social Interaction and Patient Care.* Philadelphia: Lippincott.

Becker, MH, editor. 1974. *The Health Belief Model and Personal Health Behavior.* Thorofare, NJ: Charles B. Slack.

Damrosch, S. December 1991. General strategies for motivating people to change their behavior. *Nursing Clinics of North America* 26:833–43.

Dubos, R. 1978. Health and creative adaptation. *Human Nature* 74(1):entire issue.

Dunn, HL. June 1959a. High-level wellness in man and society. *American Journal of Public Health* 49:786.

______. November 1959b. What high-level wellness means. *Canadian Journal of Public Health* 50:447.

______. 1973. *High-Level Wellness.* Arlington, VA: Beatty.

Edlin, G and Golanty, E. 1992. *Health and Wellness: A Holistic Approach.* 4th ed. Boston: Jones and Bartlett.

Igun, UA. 1979. Stages in health-seeking: A descriptive model. *Social Science and Medicine* 13A:445–56.

Jensen, L and Allen, M. Fall 1993. Wellness: The dialectic of illness. *Image: Journal of Nursing Scholarship* 25:220–23.

Leavell, HR and Clark, EG. 1965. *Preventive Medicine for the Doctor in His Community.* 3d ed. New York: McGraw-Hill.

Leddy, S and Pepper, JM. 1993. *Conceptual Bases of Professional Nursing.* 3d ed. Philadelphia: Lippincott.

Lee, PR and Estes, CL. 1990. *The Nation's Health.* 3d ed. Boston: Jones and Bartlett.

Lewin, K. 1951. *Field theory in social science.* New York: Harper and Row.

McCann/Flynn, JB and Heffron, PB. 1988. *Nursing: From Concept to Practice.* 2d ed. Norwalk, CT: Appleton & Lange.

McKeown, T. 1990. Determinants of health. In Lee, PR and Estes, CL. pp. 6–13. *The Nation's Health.* 3d ed. Boston: Jones and Bartlett.

Moll, JA. January 1982. High-level wellness and the nurse. *Topics in Clinical Nursing* 3:61–67.

Muhlenkamp, AF and Broerman, NA. May 1988. Health beliefs, health value, and positive health behaviors. *Western Journal of Nursing Research* 10:637–46.

Murphy, MM. November/December 1982. Why won't they shape up? Resistance to the promotion of health. *Canadian Journal of Public Health* 73:427–30.

Murray, RB and Zentner, JP. 1989. *Nursing Concepts for Health Promotion.* 4th ed. Norwalk, CT: Appleton & Lange.

National Center for Health Statistics. 1990. *Health United States 1989 and Preventive Profile.* DHHS Pub no. (PHS) 90-1232. Washington, DC: US Government Printing Office.

Palank, CL. December 1991. Determinants of health-promotive behavior: A review of current research. *Nursing Clinics of North America* 26:815–32.

Parsons, T. 1972. Definitions of health and illness in the light of American values and social structure. In Jaco, EG, editor. *Patients, Physicians and Illness.* 2d ed. New York: Free Press.

Pender, NJ. 1987. *Health Promotion in Nursing Practice.* 2d ed. Norwalk, CT: Appleton & Lange.

Rosenstock, IM. 1974. Historical origins of the health belief model. In Becker, MH, editor. *The Health Belief Model and Personal Health Behavior.* Thorofare, NJ: Charles B. Slack.

Rosenstock, IM, Strecher, VJ, and Becker, MH. Summer 1988. Social learning theory and the health belief model. *Health Education Quarterly* 15:175–83.

Roy, C and Andrews, HA. 1991. *The Roy Adaptation Model: The Definitive Statement.* Norwalk, CT: Appleton & Lange.

Smith, JA. April 1981. The idea of health: A philosophical inquiry. *Advanced Nursing Science* 3:43–50.

Spellbring, AM. December 1991. Nursing's role in health promotion: An overview. *Nursing Clinics of North America* 26:805–14.

Stoto, MA and Durch, JS. November 1991. National health objectives for the year 2000: The demographic impact of health promotion and disease prevention. *American Journal of Public Health* 81:1456–65.

Swinford, PA and Webster, JA, editors. 1989. *Promoting Wellness: A Nurse's Handbook.* Rockville, MD: Aspen Publishers.

Tanner, EKW. December 1991. Assessment of a health-promotion lifestyle. *Nursing Clinics of North America* 26:845–54.

Travis, JW and Ryan, RS. 1988. *Wellness Workbook.* 2d ed. Berkeley, CA: Ten Speed Press.

US Department of Health and Human Services, Public Health Service. 1990. *Healthy People 2000: National Health Promotion and Disease Prevention Objectives.* DHHS Pub no. (PHS) 91-50212. Washington, DC: US Government Printing Office.

Verbrugge, LM. 1990. Longer life but worsening health? Trends in health and mortality of middle-aged and older women. In Lee, PR and Estes, CL. pp. 14–34. *The Nation's Health.* 3d ed. Boston: Jones and Bartlett.

World Health Organization. 1947. *Constitution of the World Health Organization: Chronicle of the World Health Organization 1.* Geneva: WHO.

World Health Organization, Health Education Unit. 1986. Life-styles and health. *Social Science Medicine* 22:117–24.

14

Individuals and Families in the Home and Community

Objectives

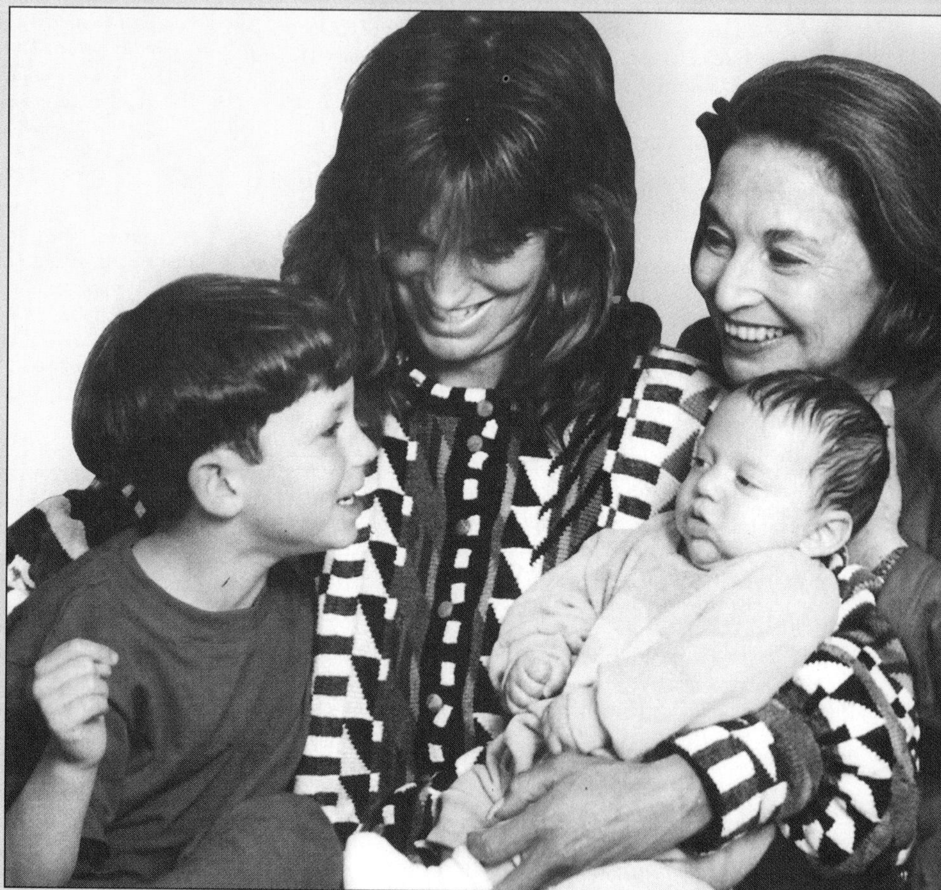

Explain the relationship of individuality and holism to nursing practice.

Give four main characteristics of homeostatic mechanisms.

Describe the components of individual health assessment.

Describe the roles and functions of the family.

Describe different types of families.

Identify the components of a family health assessment.

Identify common risk factors regarding family health.

Develop nursing diagnoses pertaining to family functioning.

Develop outcome criteria for specific nursing diagnoses related to family functioning.

Identify theoretical frameworks used in individual and family health promotion.

Identify Maslow's characteristics of the self-actualized person.

Identify various types of communities.

Describe six areas of community health practice.

Describe practice settings for community health nursing.

Describe the use of the nursing process in the community setting.

Identify advantages and disadvantages of caring for individuals and families in the home.

Describe the use of the nursing process in the home.

Discuss the interrelationship between the home health and community health nurse.

Nurses assess and plan health care for three types of clients: the individual, the family, and the community. Care of the individual is enhanced when the nurse understands the concepts of individuality, holism, homeostasis, human needs, and systems theory. The beliefs and values of each person and the support they receive come in large part from the family and are reinforced by the community. Thus an understanding of family dynamics and the context of the community assists the nurse in planning care. When a family is the client, the nurse determines the health status of the family and its individual members, the level of family functioning, family interaction patterns, and family strengths and weaknesses. When a community is the client, the nurse determines environmental problems, for example pollution, poor sanitation, waste disposal, incidence of crime, housing conditions, and so on, and intervenes to promote healthful living and prevent health problems.

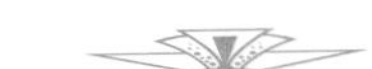

Individual Health

Concept of Individuality

To help clients attain, maintain, or regain an optimal level of health, nurses need to understand clients as individuals. Each individual is a unique being who is different from every other human being, with different genetic makeups, life experiences, and environmental interactions.

Dimensions of individuality include the person's total character, self-identity, and perceptions. The person's *total character* encompasses behaviors, emotional state, attitudes, values, motives, abilities, habits, and appearances. The person's *self-identity* encompasses perception of self as a separate and distinct entity alone and in interactions with others. The person's *perceptions* encompass the way the person interprets the environment or situation, directly affecting how the person thinks, feels, and acts in any given situation.

When providing health promotion care, nurses need to focus on the client within both a total care and an individualized care context. In the total care context, the nurse considers all the principles and areas that apply when taking care of any client of that age and condition. In the individualized care context, the nurse becomes acquainted with the client as an individual, referring to the total care principles and using those principles that apply to this person at this time. For example, a nurse who is advising the mother of a preschooler understands that the child's desire to explore his world is a developmental stage that all preschoolers experience. However, the preschooler diagnosed with attention deficit disorder with hyperactivity who is interacting with his environment may have an increased risk of accidents and injuries due to his impulsivity and poor self-control.

Concept of Holism

Nurses are concerned with the individual as a whole, complete, or holistic person, not as an assembly of parts and processes. The terms **holistic** and **holism** are derived from the Greek word meaning "whole." The term *holism* itself was coined by Jan Smuts, a South African statesman, in his book *Holism and Evolution* (1926). In holistic theory, all living organisms are seen as interacting, unified wholes that are more than the mere sums of their parts. Viewed in this light, any disturbance in one part is a disturbance of the whole system; in other words, the disturbance affects the whole being.

When applied to humans, the concept of holism emphasizes the fact that nurses must keep the whole person in mind and strive to understand how the area of client concern relates to the whole person. Therefore, when analyzing one part of an individual, the nurse must consider how that part relates to all others. The nurse must also consider the interaction and relationship of the individual to the external environment and to others. For example, in helping a man who is grieving over the death of his spouse, the nurse explores the impact of the loss on the whole person (ie, on the man's appetite, rest/sleep pattern, energy level, sense of well-being, mood, usual activities, family relationships, and relationships with others). Nursing interventions are directed toward restoring overall harmony and depend on the man's sense of purpose and meaning of his life.

The terms **holistic health** and **holistic health care** become popular during the 1960s, when people voiced dissatisfaction with the existing health care system. *Holistic health* involves the total person: the whole of the person's being and the overall quality of life-style. *Holistic health care* considers all the components of health: health promotion, health maintenance, health education and illness prevention, and restorative-rehabilitative care. Advocates of the holistic approach view all of these components with equal importance when identifying health needs, planning and implementing care, and evaluating the results.

Concept of Homeostasis

The concept of homeostasis was first introduced by WB Cannon (1939) to describe the relative constancy of the internal processes of the body, such as blood oxygen and carbon dioxide levels, blood pressure, body temperature, blood glucose, and fluid and electrolyte balance. To Canon, the word *homeostasis* did not imply something stagnant, set, or immobile; it meant a condition that might vary but remained relatively constant. Cannon viewed the human being as separate from the external environment and constantly endeavoring to maintain physiologic **equilibrium,** or balance, through adaptation to that environment. **Homeostasis,** then, is the tendency of the body to maintain a state of balance or equilibrium while continually changing.

Physiologic Homeostasis Physiologic homeostasis means that the internal environment of the body is relatively stable and constant. All cells of the body require a relatively constant environment to function; thus, the body's internal environment must be maintained within narrow limits. Homeostatic mechanisms have four main characteristics:

1. They are self-regulating.
2. They are compensatory.
3. They tend to be regulated by negative feedback systems.
4. They may require several feedback mechanisms to correct only one physiologic imbalance.

Self-regulation means that homeostatic mechanisms come into play automatically in the healthy person. However, if a person is ill, or if a respiratory organ such as a lung is injured, the homeostatic mechanisms may not be able to respond to the stimulus as they would normally. Homeostatic mechanisms are **compensatory** (counterbalancing), because they tend to counteract conditions that are abnormal for the person. An example is a sudden drop in temperature. The compensatory mechanisms are that the peripheral blood vessels constrict, thereby diverting most of the blood internally; and increased muscular activity and shivering occur to create heat. Through these mechanisms the body temperature remains stable despite the cold.

Feedback is the mechanism by which some of the output of a system is "fed back" into the system as input. This input influences the behavior of the system and its future output. **Negative feedback** inhibits change; **positive feedback** stimulates change. Most biologic systems are controlled by negative feedback to bring the system back to stability. This type of feedback system senses and counteracts any deviations from normal. The deviations may be greater or less than the normal level or range. Negative feedback is a common control mechanism for hormone levels. For example, an increase in the production of parathyroid hormone is stimulated by a drop in blood calcium, but, when parathyroid hormone is increased and raises the level of blood calcium, its production is then inhibited. Several negative feedback systems may be required to correct one physiologic imbalance. For example, with hypoxia (shortage of oxygen), the concentration of red blood cells increases and the heart rate becomes faster to transport the blood and available oxygen around the body adequately.

The two major homeostatic regulators are the autonomic nervous system and the endocrine system. In addition, the cardiovascular system, the renal system, the respiratory system, and the gastrointestinal system are important in maintaining homeostasis. See Figure 14–1.

Psychologic Homeostasis The term psychologic homeostasis refers to emotional or psychologic balance or a state of mental well-being. It is maintained by a variety of mechanisms. Each person has certain psychologic needs, such as the need for love, security, and self-esteem, that must be met to maintain psychologic homeostasis. When one or more of these needs is not met or is threatened, certain coping mechanisms are activated to protect the person and provide psychologic homeostasis.

Psychologic homeostasis is acquired or learned through the experience of living and interacting with others. In addition, societal norms and culture influence behavior. Some prerequisites for a person to develop psychologic homeostasis can be summarized as follows:

- A stable physical environment in which the person feels safe and secure. For example, the basic needs for food, shelter, and clothing must be met consistently from birth onward.
- A stable psychologic environment from infancy onward, so that feelings of trust and love develop. Growing children and adolescents also need kind but firm and consistent discipline, encouragement, and support to be their own unique selves.
- A social environment that includes adults who are healthy role models. Children learn the customs and values of society from these individuals.
- A life experience that provides satisfactions. Throughout life, people encounter many frustrations. People deal with these better if enough satisfying experiences have occurred to counterbalance the frustrating ones. See also unconscious ego defense mechanisms in Chapter 32, page 836.

ASSESSING THE HEALTH OF INDIVIDUALS

A thorough assessment of the individual's health status is basic to health promotion. Components of this assessment are the health history and physical examination, physical fitness assessment, life-style assessment, health risk appraisal, health beliefs review, and life stress review (Pender 1996).

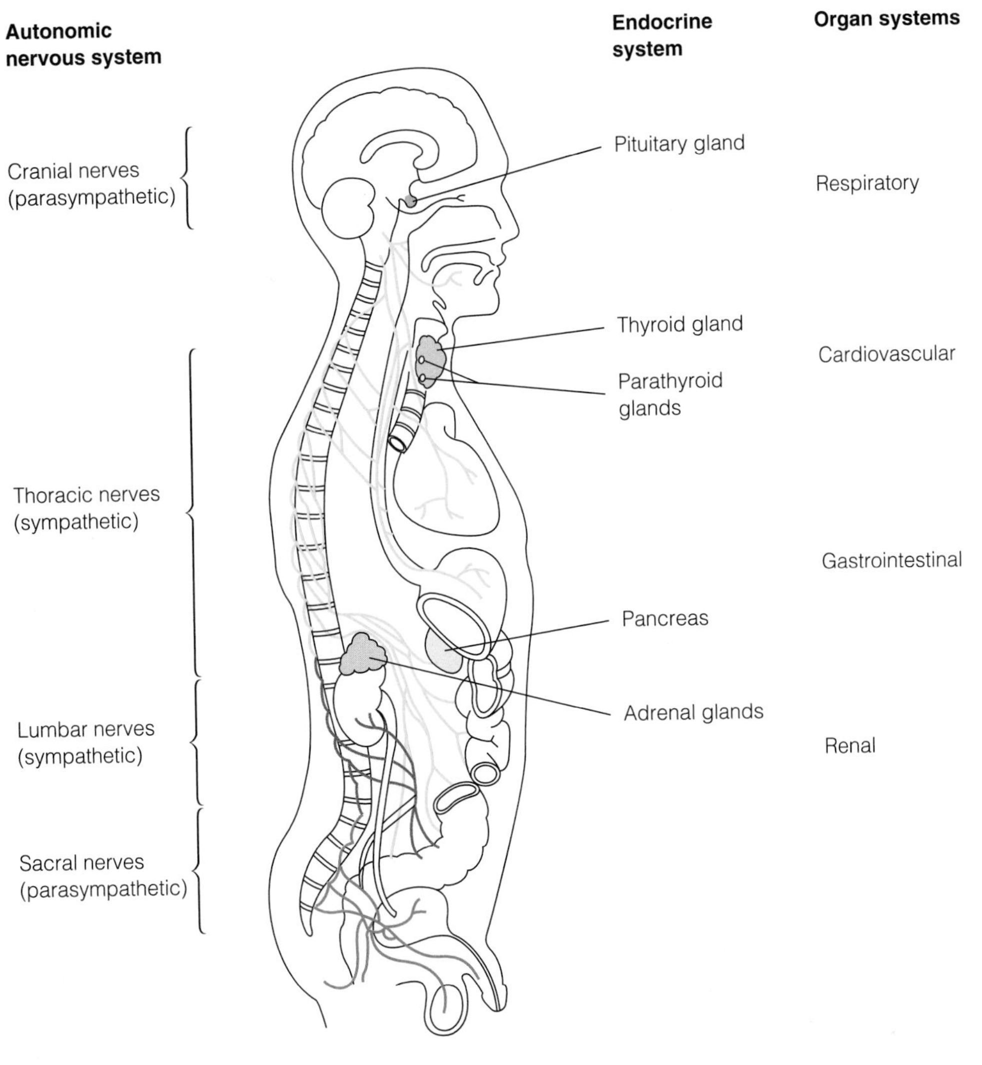

Figure 14–1 The homeostatic regulators of the body: autonomic nervous system, endocrine system, and specific organ systems.

The **health history and physical examination** provide a means for gathering data, detecting strengths, or identifying existing or potential problems. See Chapter 22 for a detailed discussion of history taking and physical examination.

During an evaluation of **physical fitness,** the nurse assesses several components of the body's physical functioning: muscle strength and endurance, joint flexibility, body composition, and cardiovascular endurance. Each of these components contributes to the calculation of overall fitness, a key aspect of health status.

Life-style assessment focuses on the personal life-style and habits of the client as they affect health. Categories of life-style generally assessed are physical activity, nutritional practices, stress management, and such habits as smoking, alcohol consumption, and drug use. The goals of life-style assessment are to provide an opportunity for clients to assess the impact of their life-style on their health and to provide a basis for decisions related to desired behavior and life-style change. Several tools are available to assess life-style.

A **health risk appraisal (HRA),** or health hazard appraisal, is an assessment and educational tool that indicates a client's risk for disease or injury over the next 10 years by comparing the client's health behavior and demographic data to behaviors of and data about a large national sample. Many HRAs that focus on the assessment of life-style factors, health behaviors, genetic and biologic characteristics, and environment are available today. The objectives of most HRAs are twofold: to assess risk factors that may lead to health problems, and to change health behaviors that place the client at risk of developing an illness.

Health care beliefs must also be clarified, particularly those beliefs that determine how clients perceive control of their own health care status. This assessment provides the nurse with an indication of how much the clients believe they can influence or control health through personal behaviors.

The **life stress review** is also an important component of health promotion assessment. There is abundant literature about the impact of stress on mental and physical well-being. A variety of instruments to assess stress levels are present in the literature. Studies have shown that a high score is associated with an increased possibility of illness in an individual.

FAMILY HEALTH

ROLES AND FUNCTIONS OF THE FAMILY

The **family** is a basic unit of society. There has been a resurgence of interest in the family unit and its impact on the health, values, and productivity of individual family members. In the nursing profession, this interest in the family as a unit has been expressed by the emergence of **family-centered nursing:** nursing that considers the health of the family as a unit in addition to the health of individual family members.

As the structure of the family has become more diverse, it has been necessary to define the family more broadly to encompass the wide variety of family forms seen in today's society.

To provide flexibility in the study of families, Mallinger (1989, p. 26) defines a family as "composed of one or more individuals closely related by blood, marriage, or friendship." A family of parents and their offspring is known as the **nuclear family.** The relatives of nuclear families, such as grandparents or aunts and uncles, comprise the **extended family.** In some families, members of the extended family live with the nuclear family. Although members of the extended family may live in different areas, they are a frequent source of support and companionship for the family.

The family's major roles are to protect and socialize its members. Among the many functions it serves, of prime importance is the role the family plays in providing emotional support and security to its members through love, acceptance, concern, and nurturing. This affective (emotional) component holds families together, gives family members a sense of belonging, and develops a sense of kinship.

In addition to providing an emotionally safe environment for members to thrive and grow, the family is also a basic unit of physical protection and safety. This is accomplished by meeting the basic needs of its members: food, clothing, and shelter. Provision of a physically safe environment requires knowledge, skills, and economic resources.

In modern society, the economic resources needed by the family are secured by adult members through employment or government programs. The family also protects the physical health of its members by providing adequate nutrition and health care services. Nutritional and life-style practices of the family not only influence the health of family members but also directly affect the developing health attitudes and life-style practices of the children.

In addition to providing an environment conducive to physical growth and health, the family creates an atmosphere that influences the cognitive and psychosocial growth of its members. Children and adults in healthy, functional families receive support, understanding, and encouragement as they progress through predictable developmental stages, as they move in or out of the family unit, and as they establish new family units. In families where members are physically and emotionally nurtured, individuals are challenged to achieve their potential in the family unit. As individual needs are met, family members are able to reach out to others in the family and the community, and to society.

The family is a major educator of its members. Parents are often called a child's first teachers. This early learning plays an influential part in the development of a child's attitudes about family, education, health, work, and recreation. These attitudes persist throughout their lives. In addition, families play a major role in the transmission of religious, cultural, and societal values. As the family socializes its new members to the expectations of home, community, and society, it provides a place of warmth, acceptance, and nurturing that insulates its members from the demands of society.

Families from different cultures are an integral part of North America's rich heritage. Each family has values and beliefs (*cultural heritage*) that are unique to their culture of origin and that shape the family's structure, methods of interaction, health care practices, and coping mechanisms. These factors interact to influence the health of families. Families from different cultures may cluster to form mutual support systems and to preserve their heritage; however, this practice may isolate them from the larger society.

Becoming acculturated is a slow, stressful process of learning the language and customs of a new country. Children in cultural clusters often have greater contact with the world around them than adults; through school, children become more proficient in language and more comfortable with new customs and behaviors. Sometimes children create conflict in the family when they bring home new ideas and values. For more information about cultural aspects of health of individuals and families, see Chapter 15.

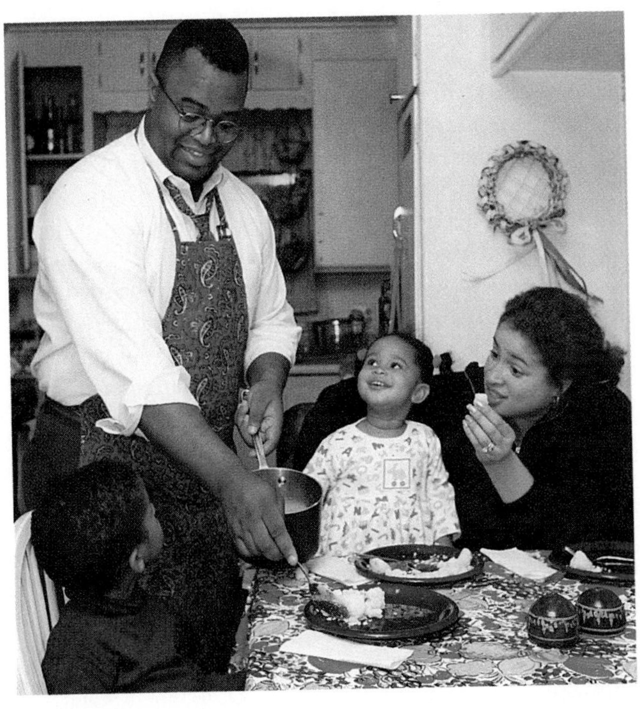

Figure 14–2 Role patterns within traditional families are changing.

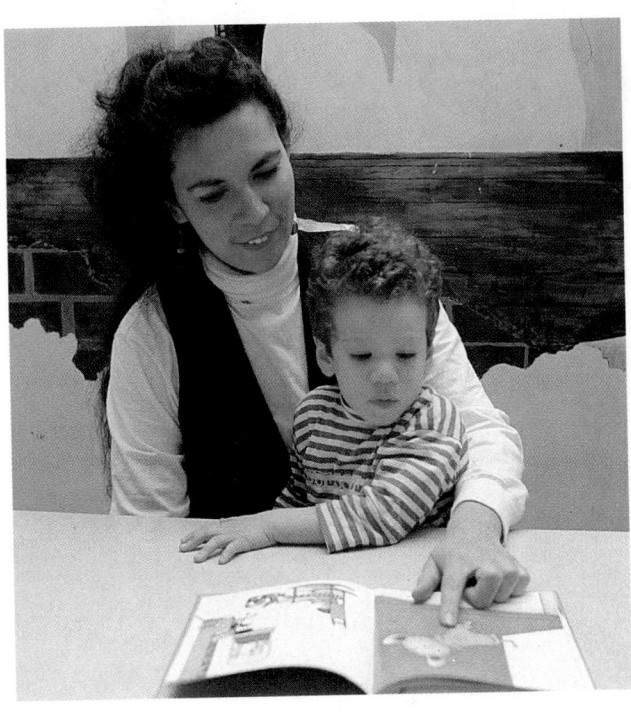

Figure 14–3 Single-parent families are prevalent in modern society.

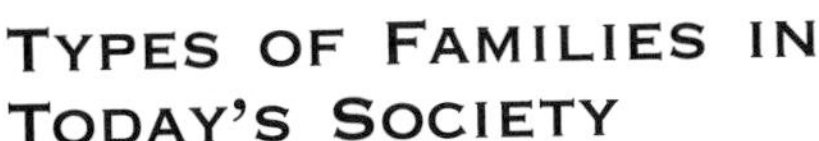

TYPES OF FAMILIES IN TODAY'S SOCIETY

Traditional Family The traditional family is viewed as an autonomous unit in which both parents reside in the home with their children, the mother assuming the nurturing role and the father providing the necessary economic resources. In today's society, both males and females are less bound to traditional role patterns. For example, fathers are more likely to be involved with the household chores, their children, and family life (Figure 14–2).

Two-Career Family In two-career (or dual career) families, both the husband and wife are employed. They may or may not have children. Two-career families have steadily increased since the 1960s because of increased career opportunities for women, a desire to increase their standard of living, and economic necessity. Finding quality, affordable child care is one of the greatest stresses faced by working parents.

Single-Parent Family Today it is estimated that over 50% of North American children live in a single-parent home. There are many reasons for single parenthood, including death of a spouse, separation, divorce, birth of a child to an unmarried woman, or adoption of a child by a single man or woman. Nearly 90% of single parent families are headed by a female (Figure 14–3). The stresses of single parenthood are many: child care concerns, adequate financial resources, role overload and fatigue in managing daily tasks, and social isolation.

Adolescent Family A growing proportion of infants are born each year to adolescent parents. These young parents are developmentally, physically, emotionally, and financially ill prepared to undertake the responsibility of parenthood. Adolescents pregnancies frequently interrupt or stop formal education. Children born to an adolescent are often at greater risk for health and social problems, and they have few role models to assist in breaking out of the cycle of poverty.

Blended Family Existing family units who join together to form new families are known as blended (or reconstituted) families. Families with children living with a birth and nonbirth parent are commonly called *step families.* Family integration requires time and effort. Stresses occur as blended families get acquainted with each other, respect differences, and establish new patterns of behavior.

Cohabiting Family Cohabiting (or communal) families consist of unrelated individuals or families who live under one roof. Reasons for cohabiting may be a need for companionship, a desire to achieve a sense of family, testing a relationship or commitment, or sharing expenses and household management. Cohabiting families

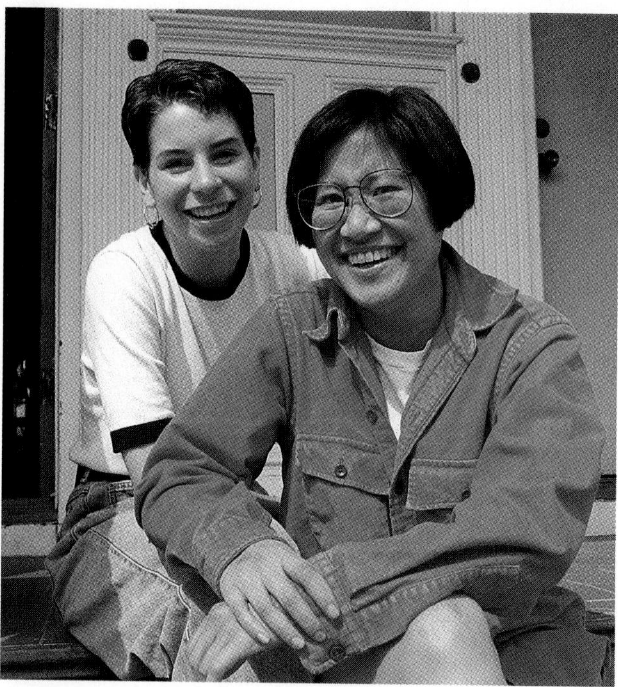

Figure 14–4 Many gay and lesbian relationships are based on long-term mutuality.

illustrate the flexibility and creativity of the family unit in adapting to individual challenges and changing societal needs.

Gay and Lesbian Family A number of homosexual adults in today's society have formed gay and lesbian families based on the same goals of caring and commitment seen in heterosexual relationships (Figure 14–4). Children raised in these family units develop sex role orientations and behaviors similar to children in the general population. The greater danger to children in these families is the prejudice and ridicule expressed by others in society.

Single Adults Living Alone Individuals who live by themselves represent a significant portion of today's society. Singles include young self-supporting adults who have recently left the nuclear family as well as the older adults living alone. Older adults find themselves single through divorce, separation, or the death of a spouse. Single adults frequently maintain contacts with other family members, such as parents, siblings, adult children, and grandchildren.

Assessing the Health of Families

The purpose of family assessment is to determine the level of family functioning, clarify family interaction patterns, identify family strengths and weaknesses, and describe the health status of the family and its individual members. Also important are family living patterns, including communication, child rearing, coping strategies, and health practices. An overall family assessment gives an overview of the family process and helps the nurse identify areas that need further assessment. Nurses carry out a more detailed assessment in specific target areas as they become more acquainted with the family and begin to understand family needs and strengths more fully. In planning interventions, nurses need to focus not only on problems but also on family strengths and resources as part of the nursing care plan. The box on the facing page provides a guide for a basic family assessment.

Risk assessment helps the nurse identify individuals and groups whose risk of developing specific health problems, such as stroke, diabetes, and lung cancer, is higher than that of the general population. The vulnerability of family units to health problems may be based on family developmental level, age of family members, heredity or genetic factors, sociologic factors, and life-style practices. The goal of the nurse is to promote optimal family health and functioning.

Developmental Factors Families at both ends of the age continuum are at risk of developing health problems. Newly formed families entering the childbearing and child-rearing phases of development experience many changes in roles, responsibilities, and expectations. These changes occur when adult family members are attempting to establish financial security. The many, often conflicting demands on the young family cause stress and fatigue, which may impede growth of family members and the functioning of the group as a unit.

Adolescent mothers, because of their developmental level and lack of knowledge about parenthood, and single-parent families, because of role overload experienced by the head of the household, are more likely to develop health problems. Moreover, the elderly are at risk of developing degenerative and chronic health problems. Because of the emphasis on youth in today's society, many elderly persons feel a lack of purpose and decreased self-esteem. These feelings in turn reduce their motivation to engage in health-promoting behaviors, such as exercise or community and family involvement.

Hereditary Factors Persons born into families with a history of certain diseases, such as diabetes or cardiovascular disease, are at greater risk of developing these conditions. A detailed family health history, including genetically transmitted disorders, is crucial to the identification of persons and families at risk. These data are used not only to monitor the health of individual family members but also to recommend modifications in health practices that potentially reduce the risk, minimize the conse-

FAMILY ASSESSMENT GUIDE

Family Structure

- Size and type: nuclear, extended, or other alternative family
- Age and sex of family members

Family Roles and Functions

- Persons working outside the home; type of work and satisfaction with it
- Household roles and responsibilities and how tasks are distributed
- Ways child-rearing responsibilities are shared
- Major decision maker and methods of decision making
- Family members' satisfaction with roles, the way tasks are divided, and the way decisions are made

Physical Health Status

- Current physical health status of each member
- Perceptions of own health and other family members' health
- Preventive health practices (eg, status of immunizations, oral hygiene practices, regularity and frequency of visits to the dentist, regularity of visual examinations)
- Routine health care; when and why physician last seen

Interaction Patterns

- Ways of expressing affection, love, sorrow, anger, and so on
- Most significant family member in person's life
- Openness of communication with all family members

Family Values

- Cultural/religious orientation; degree to which cultural practices are followed
- Use of leisure time and whether leisure time is shared with total family unit
- View of education, teachers, and the school system
- Health values: How much emphasis is put on exercise, diet, preventive health care

Coping Resources

- Degree of emotional support offered to one another
- Availability of support persons and affiliations outside the family (eg, friends, church memberships)
- Methods of handling stressful situations and conflicting family member goals
- Financial ability to meet current and future needs

quences, or postpone the development of genetically related conditions.

Life-Style Factors As the understanding of health and illness increases, it has become clear that many diseases are preventable and that life-style modification can minimize the effects of some diseases and delay the onset of others. Cancer, cardiovascular disease, adult-onset diabetes, and tooth decay are among the life-style diseases.

Sociologic Factors Poverty is a major problem that affects not only the family but also the community and society. A disproportionate number of today's poor belong to minority groups. Poverty is a real concern among the rising number of one-parent families headed by a female, and, as the number of these families increases, poverty will affect a large number of growing children.

Because many poor families do not possess the skills or support systems necessary to break out of the cycle of poverty, it is likely that poverty will continue to escalate rapidly in the future. When ill, the poor are likely to put off seeking services until the illness reaches an advanced state and requires longer or more complex treatment.

DIAGNOSING AND PLANNING

Data gathered during a family assessment may lead to the following nursing diagnoses: **Altered family processes,** the state in which a normally supportive family experiences a stressor that affects its functioning; **Family coping: potential for growth,** the state in which a family member exhibits a desire and readiness for enhanced health and growth; **Ineffective family coping: disabling,** the state in which a family demonstrates destructive behavior or adapts detrimentally to a stressor; **Ineffective family coping: compromised,** a state similar to **Altered family processes; Altered parenting,** the state in which one or more caregivers is unable to create an environment that promotes the optimal growth and development of a child or children; **Impaired home maintenance management,** the state in which an individual or family is unable to maintain independently a safe, growth-promoting immediate environment; **Caregiver role strain,** a caregiver's felt difficulty in performing the family caregiver role; and **High risk for caregiver role strain,** vulnerability for felt difficulty in performing the family caregiver role. Examples of contributing factors for selected diagnoses are shown below.

Altered family processes related to

- Illness of family member
- Loss of family member
- Gain of new family member
- Economic crises (eg, unemployment)
- Change in family role (eg, working mother)
- Retirement
- Divorce

Impaired home maintenance management related to

- Chronic debilitating disease
- Injury to family member
- Parent with cognitive, motor, or sensory deficit

Caregiver role strain related to

- Severity of illness of the care receiver
- Caregiver health impairment
- Lack of respite and recreation
- Inexperience with caregiving

Planned nursing interventions need to focus on assisting the family to plan realistic strategies that enhance family functioning, such as improving communication skills, identifying and utilizing support systems, developing and rehearsing parenting skills, and becoming involved in community activities. For families who are functioning well, anticipatory guidance may assist families in preparing for predictable developmental transitions that occur in the life of families (Denehy 1990, p. 53).

Examples of outcome criteria to evaluate the achievement of client goals and the effectiveness of nursing interventions are listed below.

The client or family

- Expresses feelings freely and appropriately.
- Participates in problem-solving process directed at appropriate solutions for the crisis.
- Participates in care of the ill family member.
- Encourages ill family member to handle situation in own way, progressing toward independence.
- Seeks appropriate external resources as needed.
- States an intent to use positive coping mechanisms and constructive stress management.
- Expresses more realistic understanding and acceptance of the family member demonstrating destructive or maladaptive behavior.
- Seeks assistance for abusive behavior.
- Verbalizes realistic expectations of parenting role.
- Demonstrates appropriate parenting behaviors (eg, attachment).
- Identifies own needs as well as strengths and resources to meet needs.
- Begins to verbalize positive feelings about infant.
- Identifies factors that restrict self-care and home management.
- Demonstrates ability to perform skills necessary for individual or home care.

The caregiver

- Verbalizes impact of situation on current life-style/role performance.
- Identifies personal strengths, social supports, and community resources.
- Ensures provision of appropriate level of care.

THE FAMILY EXPERIENCING A HEALTH CRISIS

Illness of a Family Member Illness of a family member is a crisis that affects the entire family system. See Chapter 13, page 257, for the effects of illness upon family members. The family is disrupted as members abandon their usual activities and focus the energy on restoring family equilibrium. Roles and responsibilities previously assumed by the ill person are delegated to other family members, or those functions may remain undone during the duration of the illness. The family experiences anxiety because members are concerned about the sick person and the resolution of the illness. This anxiety is compounded by additional responsibilities when there is less time or motivation to complete the normal tasks of daily living. See the accompanying box for examples of many of the factors that determine the impact of illness on the family unit.

The family's ability to deal with the stress of illness depends on the members' coping skills. Families with good communication skills are better able to discuss how they feel about the illness and how it affects family functioning. They can plan for the future and are flexible in adapting these plans as the situation changes. An established social support network provides strength, encouragement, and services to the family during the illness. During health crises, families need to realize that it is a strength, not a sign of weakness, to turn to others for support. Nurses can

FACTORS DETERMINING THE IMPACT OF ILLNESS ON THE FAMILY

- The nature of the illness, which can range from minor to life-threatening
- The duration of the illness, which ranges from short term to long term
- The residual effects of the illness, including none to permanent disability
- The meaning of the illness to the family and its significance to family systems
- The financial impact of the illness, which is influenced by factors such as insurance and ability of the ill member to return to work
- The effect of the illness on future family functioning (for instance, previous patterns may be restored or new patterns may be established)

be part of the support system for families, or they can identify other sources of support in the community.

During a crisis, families are often drawn together by a common purpose. In this time of closeness, family members have the opportunity to reaffirm personal and family values and their commitment to one another. Indeed, illness may provide a unique opportunity for family growth.

Intervening in Families Experiencing Illness Nurses committed to family-centered care involve both the ailing individual and the family in the nursing process. Through their interaction with families, nurses can give support and information. Nurses make sure that not only the individual but also each family member understands the disease, its management, and the effect of these two factors on family functioning. The nurse also assesses the family's readiness and ability to provide continued care and supervision at home when warranted. After carefully planned instruction and practice, families are given an opportunity to demonstrate their ability to provide care under the supportive guidance of the nurse. When the care indicated is beyond the capability of the family, nurses work with families to identify available resources that are socially and financially acceptable.

In helping families reintegrate the ill person into the home, nurses use data gathered during family assessment to identify family resources and deficits. By formulating mutually acceptable goals for reintegration, nurses help families cope with the realities of the illness and the changes it may have brought about, which may include new roles and functions of family members or the need to provide continued medical care to the ill or recovering person. Working together, nurses and families can create environments that restore or reorganize family functioning during illness and throughout the recovery process.

Death of a Family Member The death of a family member has a profound effect on the family. The structure of the family is altered, and this change may in turn affect how it functions as a unit. Individual members experience a sense of loss. They grieve for the lost person, and they grieve for the family that once was. (See Chapter 33 for a discussion of loss and grieving.) Some of the early stages of grief accompany family disorganization. However, as the family begins to recover, a new sense of normalcy develops, the family reintegrates its roles and functions, and it comes to grips with the reality of the situation. This painful blow takes time to heal. After the death of a member, families may need counseling to deal with their feelings and to talk about the person who died. They may also want to talk about their fears about and hopes for the future. At this time, families often derive comfort from their religious beliefs and their spiritual adviser. Support groups are also available for families experiencing the pain of death. It is often different for nurses to deal with grieving families because the nurses also feel the loss and feel inadequate in knowing what to say or do. By understanding the effect death has on families, nurses can help families resolve their grief and move ahead with life.

APPLYING THEORETICAL FRAMEWORKS TO INDIVIDUALS AND FAMILIES

A variety of theoretical frameworks provide the nurse with a holistic overview for health promotion of the individual and families across the life span. Major theoretical frameworks that nurses use in promoting the health of the *individual* are needs theories, developmental stage theories, and systems theories. Major theoretical frameworks that nurses use in promoting the health of the *family* are developmental stage theories, systems theories, and structural–functional theories.

NEEDS THEORIES

In needs theories, human needs are ranked on an ascending scale according to how essential the needs are for survival. Abraham Maslow, perhaps the most renowned needs theorist, ranks human needs on five levels. The five

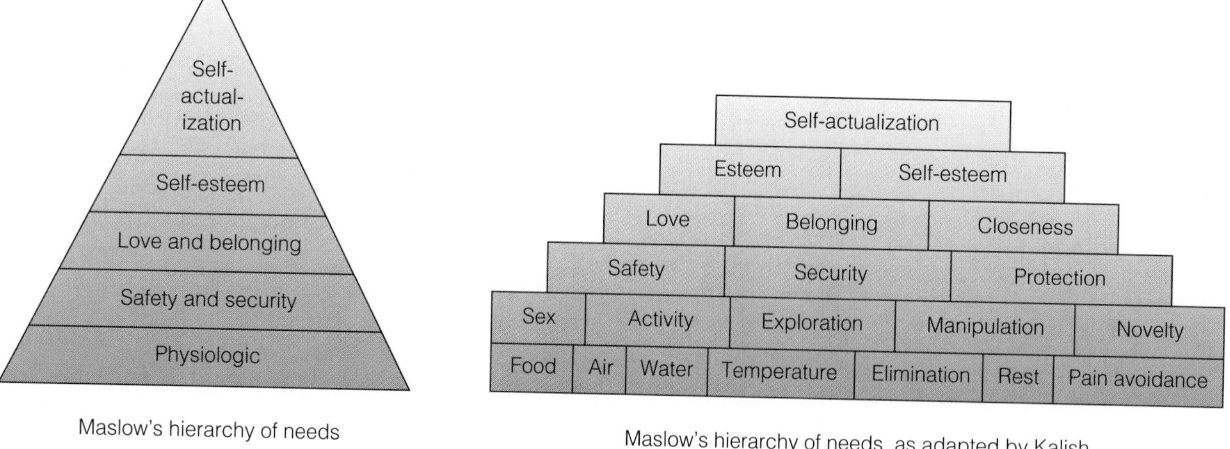

Figure 14–5 Maslow's needs. **Source:** RA Kalish. *The Psychology of Human Behavior,* 5th ed. Copyright 1983 by Wadsworth, Inc. Reprinted by permission of Brooks/Cole Publishing Company, Monterey, CA 93940.

levels in ascending order are physiologic needs, safety and security needs, love and belonging needs, self-esteem needs, and the need for self-actualization (1970, p. 37). See Figure 14–5 and the accompanying box.

- *Physiologic needs.* Needs such as air, food, water, shelter, rest, sleep, activity, and temperature maintenance, are crucial for survival.
- *Safety and security needs.* The need for safety has both physical and psychologic aspects. The person needs to feel safe, both in the physical environment and in relationships.
- *Love and belonging needs.* The third level of needs includes giving and receiving affection, attaining a place in a group, and maintaining the feeling of belonging.
- *Self-esteem needs.* The individual needs both self-esteem (ie, feelings of independence, competence, and self-respect) and esteem from others (ie, recognition, respect, and appreciation).
- *Self-actualization.* When the need for self-esteem is satisfied, the individual strives for self-actualization, the innate need to develop one's maximum potential and realize one's abilities and qualities.

Throughout their lifetimes, individuals strive to meet needs. A person's perception of a need and his or her response to satisfy a need may be influenced by ethnocultural standards, by external and internal stimuli (eg, hunger), and by self-determined priorities (eg, stopping smoking). Positive factors that affect the satisfying of needs are an individual's healthy position on the wellness–illness continuum, the presence of supportive relationships, a good self-concept, and the satisfactory achievement of developmental stages. For example, if an infant achieves the developmental task of learning to trust, then the basic needs of feeling loved and secure are readily resolved.

Knowledge of the theoretical bases of human needs assists nurses in responding therapeutically to a client's behaviors and in understanding themselves and their own responses to needs. Human needs serve as a framework for assessing behaviors, assigning priorities to outcome criteria, and planning nursing interventions. For example, an adult with poor self-esteem would have difficulty in accomplishing self-actualization. Therefore, nursing interventions would focus on increasing the client's self-esteem.

Developmental Stage Theories

Developmental stage theories related to individuals categorize a person's behaviors or tasks into approximate age ranges or in terms that describe the features of an age group. The age ranges of the stages do not take into account individual differences; however, the categories do describe characteristics associated with the majority of individuals at periods when distinctive developmental changes occur and with the specific tasks that must be accomplished. Because human development is highly complex and multifaceted, developmental stage theories describe only one aspect of development, such as cognitive, psychosexual, psychosocial, moral, and faith development. Stage theories emphasize a definite, predictable sequence of development that is orderly and continuous.

MASLOW'S CHARACTERISTICS OF A SELF-ACTUALIZED PERSON

- Is realistic, sees life clearly, and is objective about his or her observations.
- Judges people correctly.
- Has superior perception, is more decisive.
- Has clear notion of right and wrong.
- Is usually accurate in predicting future events.
- Understands art, music, politics, and philosophy.
- Possesses humility, listens to others carefully.
- Is dedicated to some work, task, duty, or vocation.
- Is highly creative, flexible, spontaneous, courageous, and willing to make mistakes.
- Is open to new ideas.
- Is self-confident and has self-respect.
- Has low degree of self-conflict; personality is integrated.
- Respects self, does not need fame, possesses a feeling of self-control.
- Is highly independent, desires privacy.
- Can appear remote and detached.
- Is friendly, loving, and governed more by inner directives than by society.
- Can make decisions contrary to popular opinion.
- Is problem centered rather than self-centered.
- Accepts the world for what it is.

Source: Based on Chapter 3, "The Study of Self-Actualization," from *The Third Force: The Psychology of Abraham Maslow*, by Frank Goble. Copyright © 1970 by Thomas Jefferson Research Center. Reprinted by permission of Viking Penguin, a division of Penguin Books U.S.A., Inc.

Each stage is affected by those stages preceding it and affects those stages that follow. For example, an adolescent who is unable to establish a stable sense of personal identity may have difficulty in later developmental stages with adult roles and career aspirations.

Developmental stage theories allow nurses to describe typical behaviors of an individual within a certain age group, explain the significance of those behaviors, predict behaviors that might occur in a given situation, and provide a rationale to control behavioral manifestations. Individuals can be compared with a representative group of people at the same point in time or compared at different points in time. During health promotion care, the nurse's knowledge of stage theories can be utilized in parental and client education, counseling, and anticipatory guidance.

Developmental stage theories view *families* as ever-changing and growing. Crucial, yet predictable, tasks occur at each level or stage of development. Achievement of tasks appropriate at one level is a prerequisite for successfully achieving the tasks expected at the next level. A major task of the family, from a developmental perspective, is to create an environment where the family can master critical developmental tasks. This ensures orderly progression through the stages of the family life cycle.

SYSTEMS THEORIES

Human systems theories assert that the individual is an open system in constant interaction with a changing environment. The human being is a complex system with multiple subsystems. Because individuals are biopsychosocial beings, their physiologic, psychologic, social, and ethnocultural, developmental, and spiritual components can be regarded as systems with hierarchic subsystems. All parts of human systems are interrelated, and the whole system responds to changes in one of its subsystems. This interrelatedness is the basis for nursing's holistic view of individuals. For example, a person under stress may exhibit both physiologic and psychologic symptoms, such as changes in cardiac function and reacting with anger to a work situation.

Open systems function through the quality and quantity of input (information, material, energy coming into the system), throughput (processing of that information, material, energy), and output (information, material, energy given out). Persons interact with the environment by adjusting themselves to it or adjusting it to themselves. Constant input into the system and feedback to it maintains the system in a state of dynamic equilibrium (homeostasis). This premise directs the nurse to look at environmental factors influencing the system and to plan nursing interventions to help the client maintain homeostasis. For example, the individual who is experiencing severe anxiety may be taught a variety of stress management techniques.

The family unit can also be viewed as a system. Its members are interdependent, working toward specific purposes and goals. Many families are described as *open systems*, for they are continually interacting and influenced by other systems in the community. Boundaries regulate the input from other systems that interact with the family system; they also regulate output from the family system to the community or to society. Boundaries protect the family from the demands and influences of other systems. Open families are likely to welcome input from without, encouraging individual members to adapt beliefs and practices to meet the changing demands of society. Such families are more likely to seek out health care information and use community resources. These families are adaptable and therefore better prepared to cope with changes in life-style needed to restore, maintain, or promote health.

Family systems also can be described as *closed systems*. Closed families are self-contained units resistant to outside interaction or influence. Such families may be suspicious of others and are content with the status quo. They are less likely to change values and practices; they tend to exert more control over the lives of their members and distrust recommendations made by nonfamily members. It is more difficult for closed family systems to use community resources that may be helpful in dealing with a family health crisis or to incorporate new behaviors that may promote a healthier family. The boundaries of most families, however, are permeable and flexible, regulating input and output according to family needs, values, and developmental stage.

STRUCTURAL–FUNCTIONAL THEORIES

The structural–functional theory, as the name implies, focuses on family structure and function. The structural component of the theory addresses the membership of the family and the relationships among family members. Intrafamily relationships are complex because of the numerous relationships that exist within the family structure—mother–daughter, brother–sister, husband–wife, and so on. These relationships are constantly evolving as children mature and leave the family nest and adults age and become more dependent on others to meet their daily needs.

The functional aspect of the theory examines the effects of intrafamily relationships on the family system, as well as their effects on other systems. Some of the main functions of the family include developing a sense of family purpose and affiliation, adding and socializing new members, and providing and distributing care and services to members. A healthy family organizes its members and resources in meeting family goals; it functions in harmony, working toward shared goals.

Nurses generally use a combination of theoretical frameworks in promoting the health of individuals and families. For example, the nurse may provide education for the mother of a toddler who is struggling to accomplish Erikson's (1963) developmental stage of autonomy. Simultaneously, the nurse may also provide guidance for the toddler's family who is undergoing a stressful "transition period" between developmental stages (described by Duvall & Miller 1985) as their older school-age child becomes an adolescent.

COMMUNITY HEALTH

DEFINITIONS OF A COMMUNITY AND COMMUNITY NURSING

To understand community health nursing one must first define the word community and other terms associated with community health. A **community** is a collection of people who share some attribute of their lives. It may be that they live in the same locale, attend a particular church, or even share a particular interest, such as painting. Groups that constitute a community because of common member interests are often referred to as a *community of interest* (eg, religious and ethnic groups). A community can also be defined as a *social system* in which the members interact formally or informally and form networks that operate for the benefit of all people in the community. Five of the functions of the community are described in the lefthand box on page 283. In community health, the community may be viewed as having a common health problem, for example, populations where there is a high incidence of infant mortality or communicable disease, such as tuberculosis or HIV infection. See the righthand box on page 283 for characteristics of a healthy community.

Stanhope and Lancaster (1996, p. 1086) define **community health nursing** as "the synthesis of nursing and public health practice applied to promoting and preserving the health of populations. The practice is general and comprehensive, with the dominant responsibility being to the population as a whole." For many, this definition is more appropriately used to describe the practice of public health nursing, and the term community health nursing "refers more broadly to nursing in the community" (Spradley & Allender 1996, p. 77). Spradley and Allender (1996, p. 77) suggest that the "distinction between the two terms might be that community health nursing is the beginning level of specialization and public health nursing is an advanced level of practice."

ELEMENTS OF COMMUNITY HEALTH NURSING PRACTICE

There are six basic elements of community health practice: (1) promotion of healthful living, (2) prevention of health problems, (3) remedial care for health problems, (4) rehabilitation, (5) evaluation, and (6) research (Spradley & Allender 1996, p. 13).

Promotion of Healthful Living The promotion of the health of individuals and groups has long been recognized as an important aspect of community health nursing. Health promotion programs are provided to raise the lev-

FIVE FUNCTIONS OF A COMMUNITY

1. *Production, distribution, and consumption of goods and services.* These are the means by which the community provides for the economic needs of its members. This function includes not only the supplying of food and clothing but also the provision of water, electricity, and police and fire protection and the disposal of refuse.
2. *Socialization.* Socialization refers to the process of transmitting values, knowledge, culture, and skills to others. Communities usually contain a number of established institutions for socialization: families, churches, schools, media, voluntary and social organizations, and so on.
3. *Social control.* Social control refers to the way in which order is maintained in a community. Laws are enforced by the police; public health regulations are implemented to protect people from certain diseases. Social control is also exerted through the family, church, and schools.
4. *Social interparticipation.* Social interparticipation refers to community activities that are designed to meet people's needs for companionship. Families and churches have traditionally met this need; however, many public and private organizations also serve this function.
5. *Mutual support.* Mutual support refers to its ability to provide resources at a time of illness or disaster. Although the family is usually relied on to fulfill this function, health and social services may be necessary to augment the family's assistance if help is required over an extended period.

TEN CHARACTERISTICS OF A HEALTHY COMMUNITY

A healthy community:

- Is one in which members have a high degree of awareness that "we are a community."
- Uses its natural resources while taking steps to conserve them for future generations.
- Openly recognizes the existence of subgroups and welcomes their participation in community affairs.
- Is prepared to meet crises.
- Is a problem-solving community; it identifies, analyzes, and organizes to meet its own needs.
- Possesses open channels of communication that allow information to flow among all subgroups of citizens in all directions.
- Seeks to make each of its systems' resources available to all members.
- Has legitimate and effective ways to settle disputes that arise within the community.
- Encourages maximum citizen participation in decision making.
- Promotes a high level of wellness among all its members.

els of wellness of individuals, families, groups, and the entire community. At the individual level, programs may include smoking cessation, reduction of alcohol and drug abuse, exercise and fitness, and stress management. At the family level, preventive health services such as family planning, pregnancy and infant care, immunizations, and information about sexually transmitted diseases may be offered. At the group level, occupational safety and health, and accidental injury may be considered. At the community level, toxic agent control, fluoridation of water supplies, and infectious agent control are of significance.

Prevention of Health Problems Health protection activities are highly varied. They may include the prevention of nutritional deficiency, accidents at work and at home, communicable diseases, cardiovascular disease, lung cancer, child abuse, poisoning, pollution, and so on.

Remedial Care for Health Problems Community health care nurses provide direct and indirect services to individuals with chronic health problems. A variety of health care services provide **direct services,** such as home visits for the assessment and monitoring of health problems, dietary planning, administration of injections, personal care, homemaking services, and information about equipment resources (eg, bath seats, wheelchairs, canes, walkers, syringes, dressing materials, and so on). **Indirect services** focus on assisting people with health problems to obtain treatment. For example, a community health nurse may assist a person to get a physician's appointment after eliciting data about an elevated blood pressure, a persistent cough, or vaginal bleeding. In other instances, the nurse may refer an individual or family to other agencies that provide information and/or therapy such as (a) a family therapy and counseling program, (b) a self-help group or association, or (c) a chemical dependency counseling and treatment center.

On a community level, individual community members and health workers may lobby for the development of programs to remedy unhealthy situations or to initiate services that are lacking. Examples of unhealthy situations are an inadequate school lunch program, inhumane conditions in a nursing home, and excessive pollution of water supplies from industrial wastes. Examples of new initiatives are increased shelters for abused women, low-cost housing for the elderly, the establishment of nursing services on the streets, and provision of health care to the homeless.

Rehabilitation **Rehabilitation** services that focus on reducing disability and/or restoring function are provided at the individual, family, and community level. At the individual level, a community health nurse in conjunction with other allied health workers (eg, physical and occupational therapists) may assist physically disabled persons (eg, those with cerebrovascular accidents, heart conditions, amputations, or paralysis) regain some degree of lost function, prevent further disability, and develop new skills that enable them to assume an appropriate vocation or degree of independence. Many rehabilitative community groups are available to assist families and individuals with chronic health problems. Examples are colostomy clubs, postmastectomy groups, halfway houses for the discharged mentally ill, and Alcoholics Anonymous. The community health nurse can be instrumental in informing clients of available services.

Evaluation Ongoing evaluation of health and health care services at the individual, national, and international levels is an essential component of community health practices. Its aim is to (a) determine the effectiveness of current activities, (b) determine needs, and (c) develop improved services. For example, evaluation of services available for rape victims may reveal a need for more comprehensive counseling programs.

Research Research, a critical component of community health care practice, provide the means to identify problems and examine improved methods of providing health services. Research occurs at all levels—from federal agencies such as the US Public Health Service to state and municipal groups. Researchers may investigate (a) patterns of illness and health, (b) possible causes and means of preventing specific problems such as child abuse, suicide, homicide, trauma, and substance abuse, (c) deficiencies in services such as day care centers or services for the elderly, (d) the effectiveness of treatment programs such as weight reduction, stress management, or substance abuse programs, (e) the effect of societal and environmental changes on existing services, and (f) utilization of existing health services.

SETTINGS FOR COMMUNITY HEALTH NURSING PRACTICE

Community health nursing is practiced in diverse settings, including community centers, schools, and the workplace, among others.

Community Centers Community health nurses utilize a variety of community sites for practice. In community centers, the client is usually a group of individuals with common needs or interests. Nurses may provide health-related education and influenza immunizations for older adults in an adult day-care center, offer blood pressure screenings and nutritional counseling at a community health fair, lead a discussion in stress management at a local church, and teach cardiopulmonary resuscitation (CPR) in a school. Community health nurses also staff stationary or mobile clinics that provide primary care and health screening services for the medically indigent or disadvantaged. Using clinics increases nurse efficiency and decreases nurse travel time. Community health nurses may also collaborate with other community professionals, such as environmental health professionals who regulate day-care facilities. This collaboration provides opportunities for the nurse to educate day-care staff on managing ill children, identifying children who are neglected or abused, preventing injuries, and promoting normal growth and development (Stanhope & Lancaster 1996, p. 614).

Schools Community schools reflect the society they are part of. Today, school systems are encountering increasingly complex health-related morbidities in children, such as substance abuse and pregnancies; dealing with major environmental risks, such as violence and poverty; and accommodating children with significant physical and psychosocial impairments. The core components of a **school health** program are health services, health education, and a healthy environment (Stanhope & Lancaster 1996, p. 884). Nursing services are in integral part of the school health program. School nurses provide direct care in school clinics, manage immunization programs, provide health education in classrooms, offer health-related expertise during student conferences, coordinate student health services, promote safety, and advocate for student health programs at the local and state level. Although the health needs of today's children have increased, many school systems have cut support for school health programs in order to cut costs. Other school systems recognize that providing health services today is an investment in children's future, and they directly or indirectly support health services at school sites by, for example, maintaining primary care clinics. Nurses who wish to pursue a specialty and certification in school nursing will find a variety of graduate programs that provide advanced degrees in this field.

Occupational Health **Occupational health** nurses consider an organization's needs as well as workers' needs (Stanhope & Lancaster 1996, p. 908). The primary functions of the occupational nurse are to provide emergency treatment and promote worker health and safety; however, rapid changes in technology, the health care system, and societal expectations have expanded the nurse's role and made it increasingly complex. Occupational health nurses may now develop and carry out health promotion, health maintenance, and risk management programs and consult with their employers in reducing health-related costs. They may offer direct care to employees, manage program evaluation, and analyze work-related injuries and illnesses. In companies where management positions have been pared, the occupational health nurse may assume expanded responsibilities in job analysis, safety, and benefits management. Specialization in the field is often a requirement for additional responsibilities. Nurses who wish to pursue specialization and certification in occupational health will find a number of graduate programs that offer advanced education in this field.

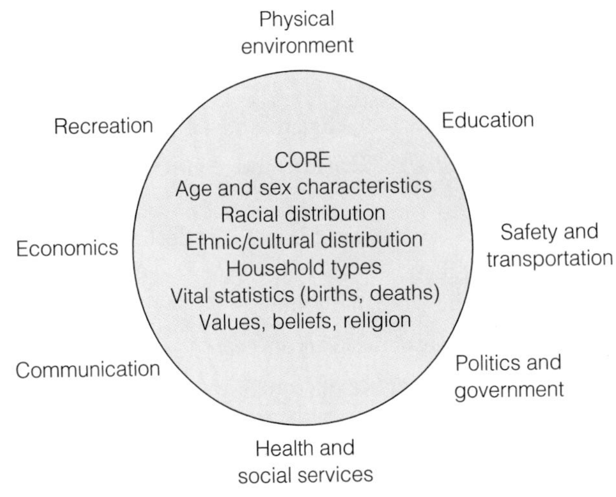

Figure 14–6 Community assessment wheel. **Source:** Adapted from ET Anderson and JM McFarlane. 1988. *Community as Client: Application of the Nursing Process* (Philadelphia: Lippincott), p. 170.

ASSESSING COMMUNITY HEALTH

Several community assessment frameworks have been devised. In one, Anderson and McFarlane (1988, p. 171) identify eight subsystems of the community for analysis. The subsystems are illustrated around a "core," which consists of the people, their characteristics, values, history, and beliefs. The first stage in assessment is to learn about the people in the community. Figure 14–6 shows some of the major components of the community core. Surrounding the core are the eight subsystems. The boxes on pages 286 and 287 provide questions to focus on in a community assessment and sources of data.

DIAGNOSING

After assessing, validating, and summarizing data, the nurse identifies nursing diagnoses for the community. NANDA diagnoses have largely focused on individual and family responses. McCloskey and Bulechek (1996) identify three community-focused NANDA nursing diagnoses:

- **Ineffective community coping:** a pattern of community activities for adaptation and problem solving that is unsatisfactory for meeting the demands or needs of the community (McCloskey & Bulechek 1996, p. 618).
- **Potential for enhanced community coping:** a pattern of community activities for adaptation and problem solving that is satisfactory for meeting the demands or needs of the community but can be improved for management of current and future problems/stressors (McCloskey & Bulechek 1996, p. 619).
- **Ineffective community management of therapeutic regimen:** a pattern of regulating and integrating into the community processes programs for treatment of illness and the sequelae of illness that are unsatisfactory for meeting health-related goals (McCloskey & Bulechek 1996, p. 619).

PLANNING AND IMPLEMENTING

Planning community health may be oriented toward improved crisis management, disease prevention, health maintenance, or health promotion. The responsibility for planning at the community level is usually broadly based. The exact resources and skills of members of the community will often be dependent on the size of the community. A broadly based planning group is most likely to create a plan that is acceptable to members of the community. Also, people who are involved in planning become educated about the problems, the resources, and the interrelationships within the system relative to health and problems.

When setting priorities, health planners must work with consumers, interest groups, or other involved persons to prioritize health problems. It is important to take into consideration the values and interests of community members, the severity of the problems, and the resources available in order to identify and act on the problems. Because any plan will probably result in change, members of the planning group should be cognizant of and employ planned change theory (see Chapter 20).

Establishing goals also requires consumer participation. The goals should reflect a desirable state—for example, to reduce infant mortality 15%. National statistics and/or *Healthy People 2000* goals may be helpful in keeping goals realistic (see Chapter 13). Among the many other factors that must be considered are the traditions of people in the community, vested interests, current organizations, and resources, all of which may be barriers to change. An example of a goal of a community would be to reduce the incidence of infectious disease in a school.

Aspects of Community Assessment

Physical Environment

- What are the terrain, climate, and natural boundaries?
- What is the size, density, and composition of the community?
- Is the area experiencing growth or decline in population?
- What are the types of dwellings?
- Are there signs of decay or poverty?
- What is the incidence of crime, vandalism, gang activity, and drug addiction in the community?

Education

- What educational facilities are in the community?
- How many residents attend school?
- Do people go outside the community to school?
- What are the existing school health facilities, services, and personnel?
- What type and amount of health services are handled by the school nurses?
- Is there a nutritious lunch program available in the schools?
- What additional services are available (eg, extracurricular sports, libraries, and counseling services)?
- What services or personnel are available for students with physical, mental, or learning challenges?
- Are continuing education or extended education programs available?
- What is the extent of parental involvement in the schools?

Safety and Transportation

- What are the fire, police, and sanitation services?
- What are the sources of water and its treatment?
- What is the quality of the air?
- How is garbage disposed of?
- Is safe public transportation available 24 hours per day?
- Are ambulance services available?

Politics and Government

- What kind of government does the community have?
- What organizations are active in the community?
- Who are the influential people in the community?
- What issues have recently appeared on local ballots?
- What is the average election turnout?

Health and Social Services

- What hospitals, health care facilities, and health care services exist in the community?
- What are the number, type, and routine caseloads of the health professionals in the community?
- Is there geographic, economic, and cultural accessibility to health care services?
- What are the sources of health information in the community?
- What is the level of immunization among children in the community?
- What is the life expectancy of members of the community?
- Are home health care and long term care services available?
- What services are provided by the public health system?
- Is there transportation service available to all major health facilities?

Communication

- What newspapers are available to the community?
- Are there radio and TV stations, postal services, and telephone services?
- Are public forums held?
- Are there informal bulletin boards?

Economics

- What are the main industries and occupations in the community?
- What percentage of the population is employed or attending school?
- What are the income levels and quality and type of housing?
- Are there occupational health programs?
- Who are the major employers in the community?
- What services are available to the community?

Recreation

- What recreational facilities are available in the community? Outside the community?
- Are there theaters and movie houses?
- What is the number and utilization of playgrounds, pools, parks, and sports facilities?
- Are there family-centered programs?
- What are the number and types of church and religious services available?
- What is the level of participation in various church programs?
- Do any churches provide recreational activities or facilities?
- What are the number and type of social committees, organizations, and clubs available?

SOURCES OF COMMUNITY ASSESSMENT DATA

- City maps to locate community boundaries, roads, churches, schools, parks, hospitals, and so on.
- State or provincial census data for population composition and characteristics.
- Chamber of Commerce for employment statistics, major industries, and primary occupations.
- Municipal, state, or provincial health departments for location of health facilities, occupational health programs, numbers of health professionals, numbers of welfare recipients, and so on.
- City or regional health planning boards for health needs and practices.
- Telephone book for location of social, recreational, and health organizations, committees, and facilities.
- Public and university libraries for district social and cultural research reports.
- Health facility administrators for information about employee caseloads, prevalent types of problems, and dominant needs.
- Recreational directors for programs provided and participation levels.
- Police department for incidence of crime, vandalism, and drug addiction.
- Teachers and school nurses for incidence of children's health problems and information on facilities and services to maintain and promote health.
- Local newspapers for community activities related to health and wellness, such as health lectures or health fairs.
- On-line computer services that may provide access to public documents related to community health.

Outcome criteria or objectives are specific, measurable targets. An example of such an objective is an increase in immunization levels by 20%, to be achieved by September 1999.

Implementing nursing strategies in community health is generally a collaborative action. According to Spradley (1990), nurses are also frequently catalysts and facilitators in implementation of plans. The primary goal in community health nursing is to help people help themselves.

McCloskey and Bulechek (1996), through the Nursing Intervention Classification (NIC) Project, describe three specific interventions appropriate to the management of community health problems: **environmental management: community, health policy monitoring,** and **health education.** In implementing health education (NIC 5510) as an intervention, the nurse "develops and provides instruction and learning experiences to facilitate voluntary adaptation of behavior conducive to health in individuals, families, groups, or communities." In promoting community environmental management (NIC 6486), the nurse "monitors and influences the physical, social, cultural, economic, and political conditions that affect the health of groups and communities" through the following activities (McCloskey & Bulechek 1996, p. 258):

- Initiating screening for health risks from the environment.
- Participating in multidisciplinary teams to identify threats to safety in the community.
- Monitoring the status of known health risks.
- Participating in community programs to deal with known risks.
- Collaborating in the development of community action programs.
- Promoting governmental policy to reduce specified risks.
- Encouraging neighborhoods to become active participants in community safety.
- Coordinating services to at-risk groups and communities.
- Conducting educational programs for targeted risk groups.
- Working with environmental groups to secure appropriate governmental regulations.

McCloskey and Bulechek also describe the nurse's role in political advocacy in the nursing intervention health policy monitoring (NIC 7970), which is defined as the "surveillance and influence of government and organization regulations, rules, and standards that affect nursing systems and practices to ensure quality care of patients." The nurse does this by carrying out the following activities (McCloskey & Bulechek 1996, p. 310):

1. Reviewing proposed policies and standards in organizational, professional, and governmental literature, and in the popular media.
2. Assessing implications and requirements of proposed policies and standards for quality client care.

3. Comparing requirement of policies and standards with current practices.
4. Assessing negative and positive effects of health policies and standards on nursing practice, client, and cost outcomes.
5. Identifying and resolving discrepancies between health policies and standards and current nursing practice.
6. Acquainting policy makers with implications of current and proposed policies and standards for client welfare.
7. Lobbying policy makers to make changes in health policies and standards to benefit clients.
8. Testifying in organizational, professional, and public forums to influence the formulation of health policies and standards that benefit clients.
9. Assisting consumers of health care to be informed of current and proposed changes in health policies and standards and the implications for health outcomes.

EVALUATING

In community health, evaluation determines whether the planned interventions have led to the achievement of the established goals and objectives; for example, was the immunization rate of preschool children improved. Because community health is usually a collaborative process between health providers, including nurses, community leaders, politicians, and consumers, all may be involved in the evaluation process. Often the community health nurse is the agent of evaluation in collecting and assessing the data that determines the effectiveness of implemented programs. Evaluation data may include community statistics related to changes in disease incidence rates, mortality and morbidity rates, the costs to provide programs and the availability of required financial and other resources, and citizen program utilization and satisfaction rates. Leaders must decide whether the benefits of a program merit the costs in money, time, and other resources. Based on such evaluation, effective programs may be continued, ineffective programs may be discontinued, existing programs may be modified, or new programs might be implemented.

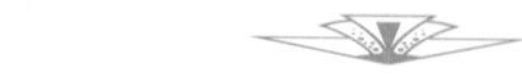

HOME HEALTH NURSING

DEFINITIONS AND PERSPECTIVES OF HOME HEALTH NURSING

The delivery of nursing services in the home has been called by a variety of terms, including home health nursing, home care nursing, and visiting nursing. Spradley and Allender (1996, p. 484) define home health care as "all the services and products provided to clients in their homes to maintain, restore, or promote their physical, mental, and emotional health." Stanhope and Lancaster (1996, p. 806) add that "home health care cannot simply be defined as 'care at home' but includes an arrangement of disease prevention, health promotion, and episodic illness–related services provided to people in their places of residence." This suggests that home health nursing services might be provided in long-term care facilities, residential hospices, residential shelters for abused women and children and the homeless, and adult congregate living facilities (ACLFs). According to the American Nurses Association (1992), home health nursing is a "synthesis of community health nursing and selected technical skills from other nursing specialties," including medical-surgical nursing, psychiatric–mental health nursing, gerontologic nursing, parent–child nursing, and community health nursing. The Department of Health and Human Services presented a more comprehensive definition of home health care in 1980 (Warhola 1980). The USDHHS states that

> home health care is that component of a continuum of comprehensive health care whereby health services are provided to individuals and families in their places of residence for the purposes of promoting, maintaining or restoring health, or of maximizing the level of independence while minimizing the effects of disability and illness, including terminal illness. Services appropriate to the needs of the individual patient and family are planned, coordinated, and made available by providers organized for the delivery of home care through the use of employed staff, contractual arrangements, or a combination of the two patterns.

The focus, then, of home health care nursing is individuals and their families. This differs somewhat from the focus of community health nursing, which focuses on the health of the community as a whole.

Home health care nurses have identified significant advantages in caring for individuals and families in the home. The home setting is intimate; this intimacy fosters familiarity, sharing, connections, and caring between clients, families, and their nurse. Behaviors are more natural, cultural beliefs and practices are more visible, and multigenerational interactions tend to be displayed. Home health care nurses become realistic about what they can remedy and learn how to provide various supports and use creative interventions for what they cannot remedy (Stulginsky 1993b, pp. 477–480).

Home health care nurses have also identified issues that negatively impact care in the home. More than any other care providers, these nurses have first-hand knowledge and experience about the burden of caregiving. In the interest of cutting health care costs, policy makers, third-party payors, and medical providers are placing increasingly complex responsibilities on clients' families and significant other(s). Caregiving demands may go on for months or years, placing the caregivers themselves (many of whom are older adults) at risk for physiologic and psychosocial problems. Additionally, nurses enter homes where the living conditions and support systems may be inadequate. When additional support or improved caregiving cannot be obtained for the client, home health care nurses face difficult decisions (Stulginsky 1993a, p. 406).

Hospice nursing is often considered a subspecialty of home health nursing as hospice services are frequently delivered to terminally ill clients in their residence.

APPLYING THE NURSING PROCESS IN THE HOME

The application of the nursing process is focused on the needs of individual clients and their caregivers. According to the American Nurses Credentialing Center (1995, p. 12), "the framework of home health practice is care management, which includes: the use of the nursing process to assess, diagnose, plan, and evaluate care; performing nursing interventions, including teaching; coordinating and using referrals and resources; providing and monitoring all levels of technical care; collaborating with other disciplines and providers; identifying clinical problems and using research knowledge; supervising ancillary personnel; and advocating for the client's right to self-determination."

Assessing McFarland and McFarlane (1993, pp. 308–317) state that the nurse "must assess not only the health care demands of the patient and family but also the home and community environment." The home health nurse obtains a health history from the client, reviews documents from the referral agency, examines the client, observes the client and caregiver relationship, and assesses the home and community environment. Parameters of assessment of the home environment include client and caregiver mobility, client ability to perform self-care, the cleanliness of the environment, the availability of caregiver support, safety, food preparation, financial supports, and emotional status of the client and caregiver.

Diagnosing In addition to nursing diagnoses specific to the client's health needs, nursing diagnoses related to the home environment may be identified. An example of a nursing diagnosis appropriate for home care is **Impaired home maintenance management,** which is defined by Carpenito (1992, p. 479) as the "state in which an individual or family experiences or is at risk to experience a difficulty in maintaining self or family in a home environment." Impaired home maintenance management may be related to impaired cognition, immobility, fatigue, or financial constraints (McFarland & McFarlane 1993, p. 313).

Planning and Intervention Planning and intervention, done in collaboration with the client and caregivers, focuses on establishing a realistic plan for home health management, teaching the client and family the techniques of home care, and identifying appropriate resources to assist the client and family in maintaining self-sufficiency.

Evaluating Evaluation can be done by the nurse on subsequent home visits by observing the same parameters assessed on the initial home visit. The nurse can also teach caregivers parameters of evaluation so that they can obtain professional intervention if needed.

INTEGRATION OF HOME AND COMMUNITY NURSING

"Home care has been an organized system of care in the United States for approximately 100 years. Home care was developed in response to (a) the needs and preferences of families to care for ill and infirm members at home and (b) limitations and costs of institutional care" (Barkauskas 1990, p. 394). The focus of home nursing has always been on individual clients and their families. Community nursing has an equally prestigious history as nurses focused on the health needs of the community as a whole. In many ways the roles and practice settings of the home health care nurse and the community health nurse are separate and distinct. For example, the home health care nurse works exclusively in the client's residence. Community nurses may work in the home but are more frequently found in clinics, immigrant and refugee centers, public health centers, community nursing centers, and other community-based providers of care outside the home or hospital. The home health care nurse is usually providing care to a client who is recovering from illness or injury; the community health nurse is usually working in areas of health promotion and illness prevention.

The home health care nurse is the care provider, teacher, and advocate for clients and their families. The nurse may intervene to mobilize the resources of the community or the hospital to meet the client's identified needs, but the focus remains the client and family. The community nurse may work with individual clients and their families but often must subjugate the needs of the individual to the needs of the community. For example, clients with a highly communicable disease may have their freedom of movement restricted in order to protect the community, or clients diagnosed with a sexually transmitted disease may have to defer their right of confidentiality for the identification and treatment of their contacts.

Some consider home health nursing an aspect of community nursing as the client's residence is within his or her community and the strengths and weaknesses of the community impact on the client's ability to stay well or recover from illness in the home. While the issue of whether home health nursing is community nursing may be debated, it is more important that nurses recognize the wide range of professional opportunities for nurses to influence the health of individuals, families, and communities.

CHAPTER HIGHLIGHTS

- Nursing involves viewing the client as an individual and in a holistic way.
- To ensure holistic health care, the nurse considers all the components of health (health promotion, health maintenance, health education and illness prevention, and restorative-rehabilitative care) and recognizes that disturbance in one part of a person affects the whole being.
- Homeostasis is the tendency of the body to maintain a state of relative balance or constancy in response to a changing internal and external environment.
- Physiologic homeostasis is maintained by coordinated functioning of the autonomic nervous, endocrine, respiratory, cardiovascular, renal, and gastrointestinal systems.
- Homeostatic mechanisms regulate hormone secretion, fluid and electrolyte levels, the functions of body viscera, and metabolic processes that provide energy for the body.
- Psychologic homeostasis, or emotional well-being, is acquired or learned through the experience of living and interacting with others.
- Although each individual has unique characteristics, certain needs are common to all people.
- The family is the basic unit of society.
- The family plays an important role in forming the health beliefs and practices of its members.
- Family-centered nursing addresses the health of the family as a unit, as well as the health of family members.
- In today's society, many types of families exist: traditional, two-career, single-parent, those headed by one or more adolescent parent, blended, cohabiting, gay and lesbian, and families from different cultures. In addition, many single adults live alone.
- The purpose of family assessment is to determine the level of family functioning, to clarify family interaction patterns, to identify family strengths and weaknesses, and to describe the health status of the family and its individual members.
- An overall family assessment gives an overview of the family process and helps the nurse identify areas that need further assessment. Nurses carry out a more detailed assessment in specific target areas as they become more acquainted with the family and begin to understand family needs and strengths more fully.
- Families at risk for health problems may be considered on the basis of family developmental level and age of family members, presence of hereditary factors, life-style practices, and sociologic factors, such as poverty.
- Nursing diagnoses that relate to family health needs and problems include **Family coping: potential for growth; Ineffective family coping: disabling** or **compromised; Altered family processes; Altered parenting; Impaired home maintenance management; Caregiver role strain;** and **High risk for caregiver role strain.**
- Nurses must examine their own values about family, health, illness, and death to be effective in supporting families in crisis.
- There are a variety of social, psychologic, and nursing theoretical frameworks that provide the nurse with a holistic overview of health promotion of individuals and families across the lifespan.
- Maslow's hierarchy of human needs consists of five categories: physiologic (survival) needs,

safety needs, love and belonging needs, self-esteem needs, and self-actualization needs.

- People vary in how they rank their needs at any given moment.
- Needs satisfaction can be altered by illness, significant relationships, self-concept, and developmental levels.
- A community is a collection of people who share some attribute of their lives.
- Six elements of community nursing practices are promotion of healthful living, prevention of health problems, development of health programs, rehabilitation, evaluation, and research.
- For community assessment, eight subsystems proposed by Anderson and McFarlane can be used: physical environment, education, safety and transportation, politics and government, health and social services, communication, economics, and recreation.
- The focus of home health care nursing is individuals and their families. This differs somewhat from the focus of community health, which focuses on the health of the community as a whole.
- Hospice nursing is often considered a subspecialty of home health nursing as hospice services are frequently delivered to terminally ill clients in their residence.
- In many ways the roles and practice settings of the home health care nurse and the community health nurse are separate and distinct.

READINGS AND REFERENCES

SUGGESTED READINGS

Anderson, KH and Tomlinson, PS. Spring 1992. The family health system as an emerging paradigmatic view for nursing. *Image: Journal of Nursing Scholarship* 24:57–63.

This paper explores family health from a nursing perspective. The authors propose a holistic definition of family health that incorporates wellness and illness, and focuses on five realms of family experience that direct nursing practice: the interactive processes, the developmental processes, the coping processes, the integrity processes, and the health processes of the family.

Dea, LW. October 1994. The effectiveness of community health nursing interventions: A literature review. *Public Health Nursing* 11(5):315–323.

In this era of increasingly limited health care resources, it is imperative that community health nurses document the effectiveness of their interventions. This article describes a variety of interventions community health nurses provide in response to needs of high-risk families, specific geographical communities, and other vulnerable population groups. The effectiveness of these interventions is based on available literature. Descriptive analyses and outcome evaluation studies are used to support the effectiveness of home-based and community-centered nursing interventions and to provide a basis for eliciting local, state, and national support.

Fugate Woods, N, Yates, BC, and Primomo, J. Spring 1989. Supporting families during chronic illness. *Image: Journal of Nursing Scholarship* 21:46–50.

This article summarizes what is known about support for individuals and families in which an adult member is living with a chronic illness such as cancer, heart disease, or diabetes. It discusses types, sources, timing, and outcomes of support helpful to the family.

Spradley, BW. 1991. *Readings in Community Health Nursing.* 4th ed. Philadelphia: Lippincott.

This anthology of reprinted articles is designed to provide insights into the nature of community health nursing in today's world. The articles present important contemporary aspects of health care and community health nursing in an interesting and meaningful manner. The book discusses topics related to community health nursing: the issues, trends, and mission; assessment and health planning; tool utilization; nursing populations, groups, and families; cultural dimensions; and ethical and political influences.

RELATED RESEARCH

Quayhagen, MP and Roth, PA. May/June 1989. From models to measures in assessment of mature families. *Journal of Professional Nursing* 5:144–51.

Lundeen, SP. 1992. Health needs of a suburban community: A nursing assessment approach. *Journal of Community Nursing* 9:235–44.

SELECTED REFERENCES

American Nurses Association. 1992. *A Statement on the Scope of Home Health Nursing Practice.* Washington, DC: ANA.

American Nurses Credentialing Center. 1995. *1995 Certification Catalog.* Washington, DC: ANCC.

Anderson, ET and McFarlane, JM. 1988. *Community as Client: Application of the Nursing Process.* Philadelphia: Lippincott.

Anderson, KH and Tomlinson, PS. Spring 1992. The family health system as an emerging paradigmatic view for nursing. *Image: Journal of Nursing Scholarship* 24:57–63.

Barkauskas, VH. 1990. Home health care: Responding to need, growth, and cost containment. In Chaska, NL, editor. Pp. 394–405. *The Nursing Profession: Turning Points.* St Louis: Mosby.

Bull, MJ. December 1990. Factors affecting family care-giver burden and health. *Western Journal of Nursing Research* 12:775–76.

Cannon, WB. 1939. *The Wisdom of the Body.* 2d ed. New York: Norton.

Carpenito, LJ. 1992. *Nursing Diagnosis: Application to Clinical Practice.* 4th ed. Philadelphia: Lippincott.

Cetinski, G and Milne, R. January 1991. Family caregivers. *Canadian Nurse* 87:33–34.

Danielson, CB, Hamel-Bissel, BP, and Winstead-Fry, PW. 1992. *Families, Health, and Illness: Perspectives on Coping and Interventions.* St Louis: Mosby-Year Book.

Deheny, JA. 1990. Anticipatory guidance. In Craft, MJ and Deheny, JA. editors. Pp. 53–67. *Nursing Interventions for Infants and Children.* Philadelphia: Saunders.

Duval, EM. 1977. *Marriage and Family Development.* 5th ed. Philadelphia: Lippincott.

Duvall, E and Miller, B. 1985. *Marriage and Family Development.* 6th ed. New York: Harper & Row.

Erikson, E. 1963. *Childhood and Society.* 2d ed. New York: Norton.

Friedman, M. 1992. *Family Nursing: Theory and Assessment.* 3d ed. Norwalk, CT: Appleton & Lange.

Gaynor, SE. Winter 1990. The long haul: The effects of home care on caregivers. *Image: Journal of Nursing Scholarship* 22:208–12.

Goble, FG. 1970. *The Third Force: The Psychology of Abraham Maslow.* Richmond Hill, Ontario: Simon & Schuster.

Hegyvary, ST. January/February 1990. Education: Redefining community. *Journal of Professional Nursing* 6:7.

Johnson, DE. 1980. The behavioral system model for nursing. In Riehl, JP and Roy, C, editors. Pp. 207–16. *Conceptual Models for Nursing Practice.* 2d ed. New York: Appleton-Century-Crofts.

Jourard, S. 1963. *Personality Adjustment.* 2d ed. New York: Macmillan.

Kalish, RA. 1983. *The Psychology of Human Behavior.* 5th ed. Monterey, CA: Brooks/Cole.

Kim, MJ, McFarland, GK, and McLane, AM. 1993. *Pocket Guide to Nursing Diagnoses.* 5th ed. St Louis: Mosby-Year Book.

Leahey, M, Stout, L, and Myrak, I. February 1991. Family systems nursing: How do you practice it in an active community hospital? *Canadian Nurse* 87:31–33.

Lederer, JR, Marculescu, GL, Mocnik, B, and Seaby, N. 1993. *Care Planning Pocket Guide: A Nursing Diagnosis Approach.* 5th ed. Redwood City, CA: Addison-Wesley Nursing.

Mallinger, KM. 1989. The American family: History and development. In Bomar, PJ, editor. *Nurses and Family Health Promotion: Concepts, Assessment, and Interventions.* Baltimore: Williams and Wilkins.

Maslow, AH. 1968. *Toward a Psychology of Being.* 2d ed. New York: Van Nostrand Reinhold.

______. 1970. *Motivation and Personality.* 2d ed. New York: Harper & Row.

______. 1971. *The Farther Reaches of Human Nature.* New York: Penguin Books.

McClelland, E, Kelly, K, and Buckwalter, K. 1985. *Continuity of Care: Advancing the Concept of Discharge Planning.* Orlando: Grune & Stratton.

McCloskey, JC and Bulechek, GM. 1996. *Iowa Intervention Project: Nursing Interventions Classification (NIC).* 2d ed. St Louis: Mosby.

McFarland, GK and McFarlane, EA. 1993. *Nursing Diagnosis and Intervention: Planning for Patient Care.* 2d ed. St Louis: Mosby.

Neuman, B. 1989. *The Neuman Systems Model.* 2d ed. Norwalk, CT: Appleton & Lange.

Pender, NJ. 1996. *Health Promotion in Nursing Practice.* 3d ed. Norwalk, CT: Appleton & Lange.

Ross, B and Cobb, KL. 1990. *Family Nursing: A Nursing Process Approach.* Redwood City, CA: Addison-Wesley Nursing.

Shamansky, SL and Clausen, CE. February 1980. Levels of prevention: Examination of the concept. *Nursing Outlook* 28:104–08.

Smuts, J. 1926. *Holism and Evolution.* New York: Macmillan.

Spradley, BW. 1990. *Community Health Nursing: Concepts and Practice.* 3d ed. Glenview, IL: Scott, Foresman.

Spradley, BW 1991. *Readings in Community Health Nursing.* 4th ed. Philadelphia: Lippincott.

Spradley, JW, and Allender, A. 1996. *Community Health Nursing: Concepts and Practice.* 4th ed. Philadelphis: Lippincott.

Stanhope, M and Lancaster, J. 1996. *Community Health Nursing: Promoting Health of Aggregates, Families, and Individuals.* 4th ed. St. Louis: Mosby.

Stulginsky, MM. October 1993a. Nurses' home health experience. Part 1: The practice setting. *Nursing & Health Care* 14(8):402–7.

Stulginsky, MM. November 1993b. Nurses' home health experience. Part 2: The unique demands of home visits. *Nursing & Health Care* 14(9): 476–85.

von Bertalanffy, L. 1969. *General System Theory.* New York: George Braziller.

Warhola, C. August 1980. *Planning for Home Health Services: A Resource Handbook.* (Pub No. HRA 80–14017). Washington, DC: USDHHS, Public Health Service.

Woods, NF, Yates, BC, and Primomo, J. Spring 1989. Supporting families during chronic illnesses. *Image: Journal of Nursing Scholarship* 21:46–50.

Wright, LM and Leahey, M. February 1990. Trends in nursing of families. *Journal of Advanced Nursing* 15:148–54.

Zinn, MB and Eitzen, DS. 1990. *Diversity in American Families.* 2d ed. New York: Harper & Row.

15

Ethnicity and Culture

Objectives

- Describe the concept of culture.
- Identify concepts pertaining to cultural diversity in nursing.
- Differentiate cultural awareness, cultural sensitivity, and cultural competence.
- Discuss components of culture pertinent to nursing care.
- Identify components of Leininger's Sunrise Model.
- Identify guidelines to foster culturally sensitive health care.
- Describe the different health views of culturally diverse clients: magico-religious, biomedical, and holistic.
- Differentiate folk healing from biomedical care.
- Identify factors related to communication with culturally diverse clients and colleagues.
- Assess clients from a cultural perspective and plan culturally competent client care.

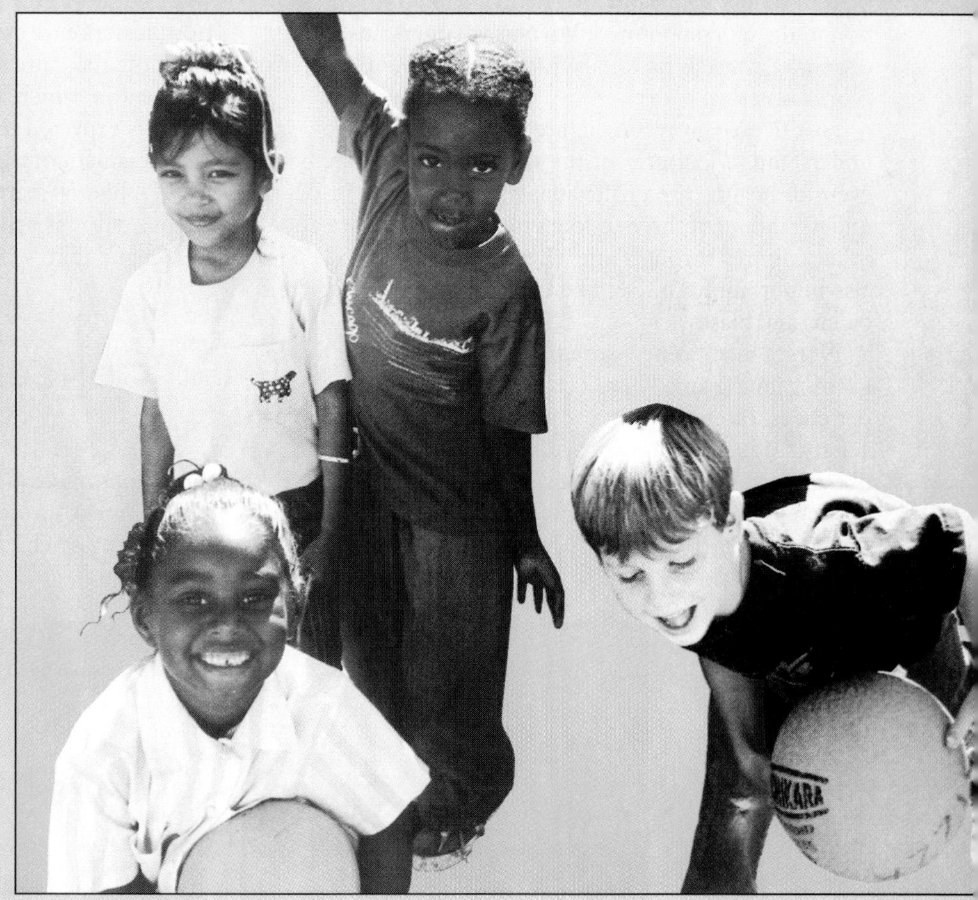

Nurses need to become informed about and sensitive to culturally diverse subjective meanings of health, illness, caring, and healing practices. A transcultural care perspective is now considered essential for nurses and other health care professionals to deliver quality health care to all clients.

North America is a continent of many cultural groups. It has been called a "melting pot" of peoples: however, the term "cultural mosaic" may be a more accurate description of the way in which many people of different cultures maintain the cultural values, beliefs, traditions, and practices of their "homeland" for many generations. In addition to the indigenous peoples (Native Americans and Aboriginals), there is much diversity in immigrant groups in North America.

Health care professionals are not expected to know and understand *all* cultures of the world; it is possible, however, for health care professionals to develop an in-depth understanding of three or four cultures and to learn about other cultures through time (Leininger 1993, p. 32). It is also important for nurses to understand their own cultural beliefs and biases.

Nurses need to be aware that although people from a given ethnic group share certain beliefs, values, and experiences, often there is also widespread intra-ethnic diversity. Major differences within ethnic groups may be due to such factors as age, sex, level of education, socioeconomic status, religious affiliation, and area of origin in the home country (rural or urban). Such factors influence the client's beliefs about health and illness, health and illness practices, help-seeking behaviors, and expectations of health professionals (Anderson, Waxler-Morrison et al 1990, p. 246). For these reasons, nurses should make special effort to avoid ethnic stereotyping.

In 1991, the American Nurses Association (ANA) stated that "culture is one of the organizing concepts upon which nursing is based and defined" (ANA 1991, p. 1). Nurses need to understand how cultural groups understand life processes, how cultural groups define health and illness, what cultural groups do to maintain wellness, what cultural groups believe to be the causes of illness, how healers cure and care for members of cultural groups, and how the cultural background of the nurse influences the way in which the nurse provides care. Because the nurse is expected to provide individualized care based on an assessment of the client's physiologic, psychologic, and developmental status, the nurse must understand how the client's cultural beliefs and practices can affect the client's health and illness (ANA 1991, p. 1).

Concepts Related to Culture

All groups of people face similar issues in adapting to their environment: providing nutrition and shelter, caring for and educating children, division of labor, social organiza-

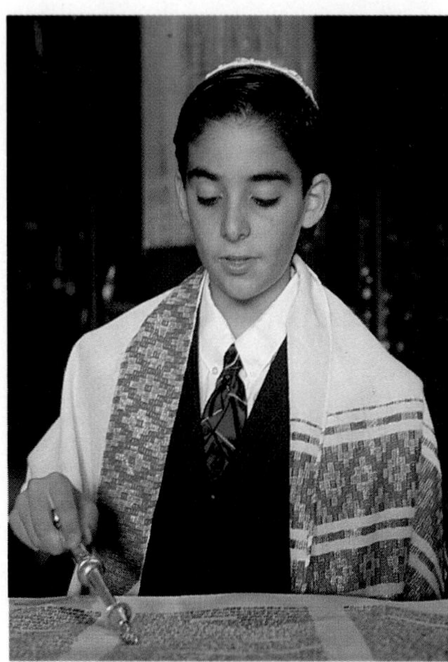

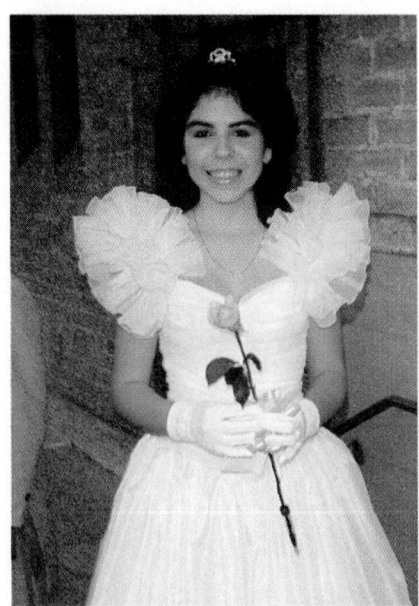

Figure 15–1 Celebrations of the passage to adulthood: the Jewish bar mitzvah and the Latino or Hispanic "quince" or "quinceañero" party.

tion, controlling disease, and maintaining health. Humans adapt to varying environments by developing cultural solutions to meet these needs. An understanding of the cultural dimension of people is the focus of the field of anthropology. Cultural anthropologists attempt to understand culture by studying both similarities and differences among human groups. Nurses use the cultural information gained by cultural anthropologists to understand and help clients (individuals, their families, or groups) to achieve optimum health.

Culture is a universal experience, but no two cultures are exactly alike. Two important terms identify the differences and similarities among peoples of different cultures. **Culture-universals** are the commonalities of values, norms of behavior, and life patterns that are similar among different cultures. **Culture-specifics** are those values, beliefs, and patterns of behavior that tend to be unique to a designated culture and do not tend to be shared with members of other cultures. For example, most cultures have ceremonies to celebrate the passage from childhood to adulthood; this practice is a culture-universal. However, different cultural groups celebrate this important life event in very different ways (Figure 15–1). In Latin or Hispanic cultures, the "quince" or "quinceañero" party, which celebrates a girl's fifteenth birthday, signifies that the young girl has now become a woman. In the Jewish tradition, the bar mitzvah (for boys) and the bat mitzvah (for girls) are celebrations of the passage to adulthood.

Anthropologists have also traditionally divided culture into material and nonmaterial culture. **Material culture** refers to objects (such as dress, art, religious artifacts, or eating utensils) and ways these are used. **Nonmaterial culture** refers to beliefs, customs, languages, and social institutions.

The terms *culture*, *diversity*, *ethnicity*, and *race* are often used interchangeably, but they are not synonymous. **Culture** is defined as "the learned, shared, and transmitted values, beliefs, norms, and lifeway practices of a particular group that guide thinking, decisions, and actions in patterned ways" (Leininger 1988, p. 158).

Because cultural patterns are learned, it is important for nurses to note that members of a particular group may not share identical cultural experiences. Thus, each member of a cultural group will be somewhat different from his or her own cultural counterparts (Waxler-Morrison et al 1990, p. 6). For example, white Roman Catholics will have cultural patterns and beliefs different from those of white Seventh-Day Adventists. Third-generation Japanese Americans, or *Sansei*, will differ in cultural understandings from first-generation Japanese, or *Issei*.

Large cultural groups often have cultural subgroups or subsystems. A **subculture** is usually composed of people who have a distinct identity and yet are also related to a larger cultural group. A subcultural group generally shares ethnic origin, occupation, or physical characteristics with the larger cultural group. Examples of cultural subgroups include occupational groups (eg, nurses), societal groups (eg, feminists), and ethnic groups (eg, Cajuns, who are descendants of French Acadians).

Bicultural is used to describe a person who crosses two cultures, life-styles, and sets of values (Giger & Davidhizar 1991, p. 51). For example, a young man whose father is Cherokee and whose mother is European American may maintain his traditional Cherokee heritage while also being influenced by his mother's cultural values.

Diversity refers to the "fact or state of being different" (Steinmetz & Braham 1993, p. 141). Many factors account for differences: race, gender, sexual orientation, culture, ethnicity, socioeconomic status, educational attainment, religious affiliation, and so on. Diversity therefore occurs not only between cultural groups but also within a cultural group.

The term **ethnic** refers to a group of people who share a common and distinctive culture and who are members of a specific group. The **ethnic group** shares a common social and cultural heritage that is passed on to successive generations (Giger & Davidhizar 1991, p. 51). The characteristics of the group give an individual a sense of **cultural identity. Ethnicity** has been defined as "a consciousness of belonging to a group that is differentiated from others by symbolic markers (culture, biology, territory). It is rooted in bonds of a shared past and perceived ethnic interest" (Sprott 1993, p. 190). Other factors that help to define ethnicity are religion and geographic background of the family.

Race is the classification of people according to shared biologic characteristics, genetic markers, or features. They have common characteristics such as skin color, bone structure, facial features, hair texture, and blood type. Different ethnic groups can belong to the same race, and different cultures can be found within the same ethnic group. For example, the term *Causasian* and *European American* describe the race of people whose origins are in Europe. Whereas British Americans are a subgroup of European Americans, Scottish Americans (an ethnic subgroup of British Americans) may share different cultural practices than other British Americans. It is important to understand that not all people of the same race have the same culture. Culture should not be confused with either race or ethnic group.

It is helpful to differentiate the terms *acculturation* and *ethnic identity*. **Acculturation** is often defined in terms of such observable factors as dress, food, language, and values. Individuals who are acculturated may no longer eat foods associated with their culture or always wear traditional dress (Lynam 1992, p. 151). **Ethnic identity,** in contrast, refers to a subjective perspective of the person's heritage and to a sense of belonging to a group that is distinguishable from other groups. Thus, people may be visibly acculturated to the mainstream culture but may retain an identity that differs from the mainstream.

The cultural beliefs and practices regarding the health and illness of North America's many different ethnic and cultural groups are important considerations for nurses in planning nursing care. Nursing ethnoscientists study the health beliefs of cultures so that nurses can provide culturally competent care to clients of different cultures. Madeleine Leininger, a nurse anthropologist, described **transcultural nursing** as the study of different cultures and subcultures with respect to nursing and health illness caring practices, beliefs, and values (1978, p. 493). The goal of transcultural nursing is to provide culture-specific and culture-universal nursing care. Cultural awareness and cultural sensitivity are prerequisite to the provision of culturally competent nursing care. **Cultural awareness** is the conscious and informed recognition of the differences and similarities between different cultural or ethnic groups. Cultural awareness is not knowledge derived solely from myths and stereotypes. **Cultural sensitivity** is the respect and appreciation for cultural behaviors based on an understanding of the other person's perspective. **Cultural competence** is "knowing, utilizing, and appreciating the culture of another in assisting with the resolution of a problem" (DeSantis & Lowe 1992, p. 1). The culturally competent nurse, therefore, works within the cultural belief system of the client to resolve health problems. To provide culturally competent care, nurses need data about the client's personal and cultural views regarding health and illness. To make valid assessments, nurses need to try to see and hear the world as their clients do. When developing care plans, nurses need to consider the client's world and daily experiences. Although a client's needs and behaviors can be better understand when particular cultural health norms are identified, nurses must take care to avoid stereotyping clients by culture norms. This allows for individualized care.

Culture shock can occur when members of one culture are abruptly moved to another culture or setting. **Culture shock** is the state of being disoriented or unable to respond to a different cultural environment because of its sudden strangeness, unfamiliarity, and incompatibility to the stranger's perceptions and expectations (Leininger 1978, p. 490). For example, when immigrants first enter the United States or Canada, language and behavior differences may initially cause them difficulty in carrying out normal activities. People can also experience culture shock when they are abruptly thrust into the health care subculture. Nursing students, for example, may experience culture shock when they enter nursing school and must learn medical terminology (a new language) and provide care for clients in clinical environments with which they are unfamiliar. Expressions of culture shock can range from silence and immobility to agitation.

Not uncommonly, people of a minority group assume the attitudes, values, beliefs, and practices of the dominant or host society, resulting in a new blended cultural pattern. This process is referred to as cultural **assimilation** or **acculturation.**

CHARACTERISTICS OF CULTURE

Culture exhibits several characteristics.

- *Culture is learned.* It is neither instinctive nor innate. It is learned through life experiences from birth.
- *Culture is taught.* It is transmitted from parents to children over successive generations. All animals can learn, but only humans can pass along culture. Verbal and nonverbal communication patterns are the transmitters of culture.
- *Culture is social.* It originates and develops through the interactions of people: families, groups, and communities.
- *Culture is adaptive.* Customs, beliefs, and practices change as people adapt to the social environment and as biologic and psychologic needs of people change. Some traditional forms in a culture may cease to provide satisfaction and are eliminated. For example, in many cultures it is customary for family members of different generations to live together (extended family); however, education and employment considerations may require children to leave their parents and move to other parts of the country. In such cases, the extended family norm may change.
- *Culture is satisfying.* Cultural habits persist only as long as they satisfy people's needs. Gratification strengthens habits and beliefs. Once they no longer bring gratification, they may disappear.
- *Culture is difficult to articulate.* Members of a specific cultural group often find it different to articulate their own culture. Many of the values and behaviors are habitual and are carried out subconsciously.
- *Culture exists at many levels.* Culture is most easily identified at the material level. For example, art, tools, and clothes usually reveal aspects of a culture relatively readily. More abstract concepts, such as values, beliefs, and traditions, are often more difficult to find out about. Nurses may need to ask culture-sensitive questions of the client or support persons to obtain this information.

COMPONENTS OF CULTURE

Cultures are very complex. They consist of facets that relate to all aspects of life: language, art, music, values systems (beliefs, morals, rules), religion, philosophy, family interaction, patterns of behavior, childrearing practices, rituals or ceremonies, recreation and leisure activities, fes-

PROVIDING CULTURALLY COMPETENT CARE TO FAMILIES

- Learn the rituals, customs, and practices of the major cultural groups with whom you come into contact. Learn to appreciate the richness of diversity as an asset rather than a hindrance in your practice.
- Identify personal biases, attitudes, prejudices, and stereotypes.
- Include cultural assessment of the client and family as part of overall assessment.
- Recognize that it is the client's (or family's) right to make their own health care choices.
- Convey respect and cooperate with traditional helpers and caregivers.

tivals and holidays, nutrition, food preferences, and health practices. Many facets of culture (eg, health and illness practices, attitudes about touch, territory and privacy, childbirth, and death and dying practices) have an impact on nursing practice.

Religious values are part of the cultural values of groups that have one dominant religion. For example, the roles of men and women in Islamic cultures is clearly defined by the Koran. The tenets of Roman Catholicism dictate the value for life and family and influence both laws and customs in many Roman Catholic cultures around the world. Culture and religion are deeply intertwined among many Jews, most notably in the nation of Israel, which is founded on Jewish beliefs and traditions.

Religions values associated with any culture influence many facets of life, including dietary restrictions, family planning, use of blood transfusions, and death-related practices, such as autopsy, organ donation, cremation, and prolonging life.

CULTURE AND HEALTH CARE

Two transcultural health care systems generally exist side by side with limited awareness by practitioners of both systems: an indigenous health care system and a professional health care system (Leininger 1993, p. 36). The *indigenous health care system* refers to traditional folk health care methods, such as folk medicines and other home treatments. The modern *professional health care system* refers to a structured system maintained by individuals who have engaged in a formal program of study. The indigenous system is the older system and has often provided health care long before a professional system enters the culture. According to Leininger, few professional health care workers are knowledgeable about the indigenous health care system or its practitioners. Some professionals regard the indigenous system as unscientific or "primitive," or even as "quackery." Leininger emphasizes that the goal of health care should be to use the best of both systems and that health professionals need to consider ways to interface with the two systems for the benefit of the people served. "Every culture has health, caring, and caring processes, techniques, and practices viewed as important to the people" (1993, p. 38).

LEININGER'S SUNRISE MODEL

Leininger produced the Sunrise Model to depict her theory of cultural care diversity and universality (Figure 15–2). This model emphasizes that health and care are influenced by elements of the social structure, such as technology, religious and philosophical factors, kinship and social systems, cultural values, political and legal factors, economic factors, and educational factors. These social factors are addressed within environmental contexts, language expressions, and ethnohistory. Each of these systems is part of the social structure of any society; health care expressions, patterns, and practices are also integral parts of these aspects of social structure (Leininger 1993, p. 35).

Technologic factors, such as the availability of technical and electrical equipment, greatly determine what health equipment will be used. For example, many European Americans regard resuscitative equipment as essential. The *economic* system determines the quality of health care within a culture, for example, the availability of funds for health care services materially affects the health of the culture's infants and aged. The *political* system is a major determinant of what health programs will be available and which health practitioners may provide health services. *Legal* aspects govern the roles, functions, and standards of health professionals within cultures. *Kinship* and the *social system* often influence who will or will not receive health care and how promptly it will be provided. For example, in some cultures a person of high status (eg, tribal leader, CEO, or king) may receive prompt care; a person of lower status (eg, a peasant, housewife, or child) may experience a considerable waiting period for care. Because of male dominance in many cultures, men may receive care before a wife or female child. *Cultural, educational, religious,* and *philosophical* factors are closely related. They influence the type, quality, and quantity of health care considered desirable, appropriate, or acceptable to the culture. *Environmental* and *demographic* factors relate to the health needs of the culture and which strategies of care can be used in the setting.

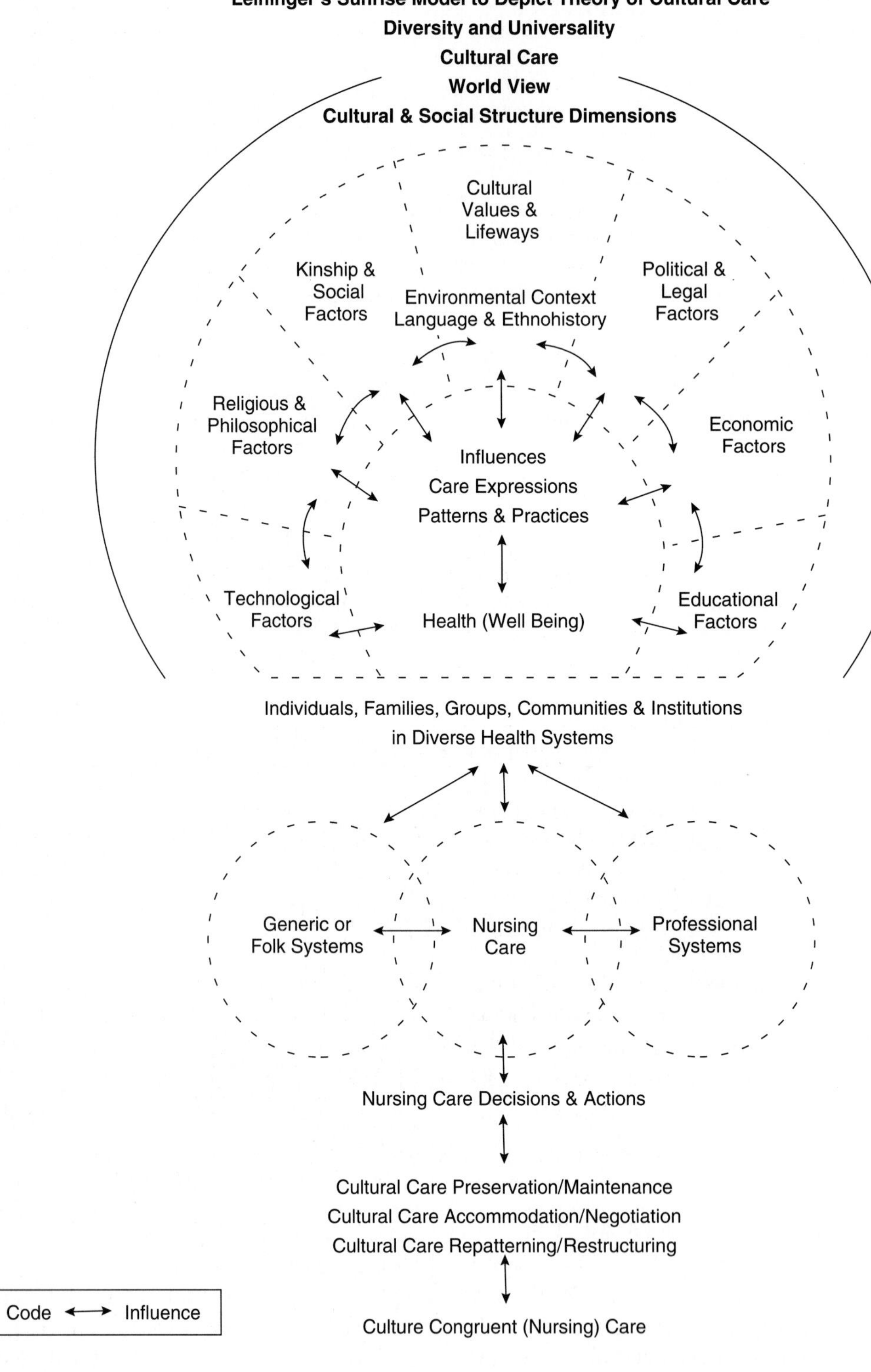

Figure 15–2 Leininger's Sunrise Model. **Source:** *Culture Care Diversity and Universality: A Theory of Nursing* by M. Leininger, 1991, New York: National League for Nursing Pub. No. 15-2402, p. 43. Reprinted with permission.

CULTURALLY SENSITIVE CARE

Kittler and Sucher (1990) suggest a four-step process to improve cultural sensitivity:

1. *Become aware of one's own cultural heritage.* Nurses should identify their own cultural values and beliefs. For example, does the nurse value stoic behavior in relation to pain? Are the rights of the individual valued over and above the rights of the family? Only by knowing one's own culture (values, practices, and beliefs) can a person be ready to learn about another's.
2. *Become aware of the client's culture as described by the client.* It is important to avoid assuming that all people of the same ethnic background have the same culture. When the nurse has a knowledge of the client's culture, mutual respect between client and nurse is more likely to develop.
3. *Become aware from the client of adaptations made to live in a North American culture.* During this interview, a nurse can also identify the client's preferences in health practices, diet, hygiene, and so on.
4. *Form a nursing care plan with the client that incorporates his or her culture.* In this way, cultural values, practices, and beliefs can be incorporated with care and judgment.

BARRIERS TO CULTURAL SENSITIVITY

Many factors can be barriers to providing culturally sensitive or culturally congruent care to clients and their support persons. These factors can also affect communication and working relationships with other health care personnel. Ethnocentricism, stereotyping, prejudice, and discrimination are some of these factors.

Ethnocentrism refers to an individual's belief that his or her culture's beliefs and values are superior to those of other cultures. In the health care area, ethnocentrism means that the only valid health care beliefs and practices are those held by the health care culture. Nurses who take a transcultural view, however, value their own beliefs and practices while respecting the belief and practices of others. It is important for nurses to realize that although many people of differing racial and religious backgrounds have combined their traditional health practices with Western health practices, other people may be unable to do so.

Most people are gradually exposed to the cultural beliefs, values, and practices over a period of years starting at birth. Ethnocentricism is thought to result from lack of exposure or knowledge of cultures other than one's own. **Ethnorelativity** is the ability to appreciate and respect other viewpoints different from one's own.

Stereotyping is assuming that all members of a culture or ethnic group are alike. For example, a nurse may assume that all Italians express pain volubly or that all Chinese people like rice. Stereotyping may be based on generalizations founded in research, or it may be unrelated to reality. For example, research indicates that Italians are likely to express pain verbally; however, an Italian client may not verbalize pain. Stereotyping that is unrelated to reality may be either positive or negative and is frequently an outcome of racism or discrimination.

It is important for nurses to realize that not all people of a specific group will have the same health beliefs, practices, and values. It is therefore essential to identify a specific client's beliefs, needs, and values rather than assuming they are the same as those attributable to the larger group.

Prejudice is strongly held opinion about some topic or group of people. A prejudice may be positive or negative. A positive prejudice often stems from a strong sense of ethnocentrism (Eliason 1993, p. 226), that is, beliefs that one's cultural group are vastly superior to the beliefs held by others. One example is that American nursing education is superior to European nursing education. Prejudice may also derive from ignorance, misinformation, past experience, or fear. Other types of negative prejudice are ageism, which includes negative attitudes toward older adults; sexism, meaning negative attitudes toward women; and homophobia, which is negativism toward lesbians and gay men.

Banks and Banks (1989, p. 37) define **discrimination** as "the differential treatment of individuals or groups based on categories such as race, ethnicity, gender, social class, or exceptionality." For example, a nurse takes a child who is waiting in an emergency department ahead of another child. The child taken ahead appears clean, is neatly dressed, and is smiling; the other child appears dirty, is wearing worn clothes, and is angry. **Racism** is a form of discrimination related to ethnocentrism where a person believes that race is the primary determinant of human traits and capacities and that racial differences produce an inherent superiority of a particular race.

CONVEYING CULTURAL SENSITIVITY

It is important for nurses to be culturally sensitive and to convey this sensitivity to clients, support persons, and other health care personnel. Some of the ways to do so follow.

- Always address clients by their last names (eg, Mrs Aylia, Dr Rush) until they give you permission to use other names. In some cultures, the more formal style of address is a sign of respect, whereas the informal use of first names may be considered disrespect. It is important to ask clients how they wish to be addressed.

- When meeting a person for the first time, introduce yourself by name, and, when appropriate, explain your position. This helps establish a relationship and provides an opportunity for both clients and nurses to clarify pronunciation of one another's names, and so on.
- Be authentic with people, and share your lack of knowledge about their culture.
- Use language that is culturally sensitive; for example, say "gay," "lesbian," or "bisexual" rather than "homosexual"; do not use "man" or "mankind" when referring to a woman; "African American" and "Latino" are currently preferred over "black" or "Hispanic." "Asian" is more acceptable than "Oriental" (Eliason 1993, p. 228). However, nurses need to keep up with language changes.
- Find out what the client knows about his or her health problems, illness, and treatments. Assess whether this information is congruent with the dominant health care culture. If the beliefs and practices are incongruent, establish whether this will have a negative effect on the client's health.
- Do not make any assumptions about the client, and always ask about anything you don't understand.
- Respect the client's values, beliefs, and practices, even if they differ from your own or from those of the dominant culture. If you don't agree with them, it is important to respect the client's right to hold these beliefs.
- Show respect for the client's support people. In some cultures males in the family make decisions affecting the client, while in other cultures females make the decisions.
- Make a concerted effort to obtain the client's trust, but do not be surprised if it develops slowly or not at all.

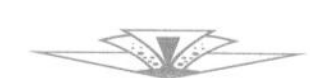

SELECTED CULTURAL PARAMETERS FOR NURSING

This section outlines selected cultural and ethnic phenomena of significance to nursing.

HEALTH BELIEFS AND PRACTICES

Andrews and Boyle (1995, pp. 22–29) describe three health belief views: magico-religious, scientific, and holistic. In the **magico-religious health belief view,** health and illness are controlled by supernatural forces. The client may believe that illness is the result of "being bad" or opposing God's will. Getting well is also viewed as dependent on God's will. The client may make statements such as, "If it is God's will, I will recover," or "What did I do wrong to be punished with cancer?" Some cultures believe that magic can cause illness. A sorcerer or witch may put a spell or hex on the client. Some people view illness as possession by an evil spirit. Although these beliefs are not supported by empirical evidence, clients who believe that such things can cause illness may, in fact, become ill as a result. Such illnesses may require magical treatments in addition to scientific treatments. For example, a man who experiences gastric distress, headaches, and hypertension after being told that a spell has been placed on him may recover only if the spell is removed by the culture's healer.

The **scientific** or **biomedical health belief view** is based on the belief that life and life processes are controlled by physical and biochemical processes that can be manipulated by humans (Andrews & Boyle 1995, p. 23). The client with this view will believe that illness is caused by germs, viruses, bacteria, or a breakdown of the human machine, the body. This client will expect a pill, or treatment, or a surgery to cure health problems.

The **holistic health belief view** holds that the forces of nature must be maintained in balance or harmony. Human life is one aspect of nature that must be in harmony with the rest of nature. When the natural balance or harmony is disturbed, illness results. The Medicine Wheel is an ancient symbol used by Native Americans of North and South American to express many concepts. Related to health and wellness, the Medicine Wheel teaches the four aspects of the individual's nature: the physical, the mental, the emotional, and the spiritual. Each of the dimensions must be in balance to be healthy. The Medicine Wheel can also be used to express the individual's relationship with the environment as a dimension of wellness. The concept of yin and yang in the Chinese culture and the hot/cold theory of illness in many Spanish cultures are examples of holistic health beliefs. When the client has a yin illness or a "cold" illness, the treatment will need to include a yang or "hot" food. For example, a Chinese client who has been diagnosed with cancer, a yin disease, will want to eat cultural foods that have yang properties. What is considered as hot or cold varies considerably across cultures. In many cultures, the mother who has just delivered a baby should be offered warm or hot foods and kept warm with blankets, because childbirth is seen as a "cold" condition. Conventional scientific thought recommends cooling the body to reduce a fever. The physician may order liquids for the client and cool compresses to be applied to the forehead, the axillae, or the groin. Galanti (1991, p. 97) states that many cultures believe that the best way to treat a fever is to "sweat it out." Clients from these cultures may want to cover up with several blankets, take hot baths, and drink hot beverages. Giger and Davidhizar (1995, p. 84) state that the nurse must keep in mind that a treatment strategy that is consistent with the client's beliefs may have a better chance of being successful. For example, the Mexican-American client who avoids "hot" foods when he has a stomach disturbance such as an ulcer may be eating foods consistent with the bland diet that is normally prescribed by physicians for clients with ulcers.

Sociocultural forces, such as politics, economics, geography, religion, and the predominant health care system, can influence the client's health status and health care behavior. For example, people who have limited access to scientific health care may turn to folk medicine or folk healing. **Folk medicine** is defined as those beliefs and practices relating to illness prevention and healing which derive from cultural traditions rather than from modern medicine's scientific base. The student may recall special teas or "cures" that were used by older family members to prevent or treat colds, fevers, indigestion, and other common health problems. For example, many people continue to use chicken soup as a treatment for "flu."

Why do individuals use these nontraditional folk healing methods? Folk medicine, in contrast to biomedical health care, is thought to be more humanistic. The consultation and treatment takes place in the community of the recipient, frequently in the home of the healer. It is less expensive than scientific or biomedical care, because the health problem is identified primarily through conversation with the client and the family. The healer often prepares the treatments, for example, teas to be ingested, poultices to be applied, or charms or amulets to be worn. A frequent component of treatment is some ritual practice on the part of the healer or the client to cause healing to occur. Because folk healing is more culturally based, it is often more comfortable and less frightening for the client.

It is important for the nurse to obtain information about folk or family healing practices that may have been used prior to the client's seeking Western medical treatment. Often clients are reluctant to share home remedies with health care professionals for fear of being laughed at or rebuked. The nurse should remember that treatments once considered to be folk treatments, including acupuncture, therapeutic touch, and message are now being investigated for their therapeutic effect.

FAMILY PATTERNS

The family is the basic unit of society. Cultural values can determine communication within the family group, the norm for family size, and the roles of specific family members. In some families the man is usually the provider and decision maker. The woman may need to consult her husband prior to making decisions about her medical treatment or the treatment of her children (Galanti 1991, p. 63). Some families are matriarchal; that is, the mother or grandmother is viewed as the leader of the family and is usually the decision maker. The nurse needs to identify who has the "authority" to make decisions in a client's family. If the decision maker is someone other than the client, the nurse needs to include that person in health care discussions.

The value placed on children and elderly within a society is culturally derived. In some cultures, children are not disciplined by spanking or other forms of physical punishment. Rather, children are allowed to interact with their environment while caregivers provide subtle direction to prevent harm or injury. In other cultures, the elderly are considered the holders of the culture's wisdom and are therefore highly respected. Responsibility for caring for elder relatives is determined by cultural practices. In many cultures, older relatives who cannot live independently often live with a married daughter and her family.

Cultural sex-role behavior may also affect nurse-client interaction. In some countries, the male dominates and women have little status. The male client from these countries may not accept instruction from a female nurse or physician but be receptive to the same instruction given by a male physician or nurse (Galanti 1991, pp. 66–78). In some cultures, there is a prevailing concept of machismo, or male superiority. The positive aspects of machismo require that the adult male provide for and protect his family, including extended family members. The woman is expected to maintain the home and raise the children.

Cultural family values may also dictate the extent of the family's involvement in the hospitalized client's care. In some cultures, the nuclear and the extended family will want to visit for long periods of time and participate in care. In other cultures, the entire clan may want to visit and participate in the client's care (Galanti 1991, p. 55). This can cause concern on nursing units with strict visiting policies. The nurse should evaluate the positive benefits of family participation in the client's care and modify visiting policies as appropriate.

Cultures that value the needs of the extended family as much as those of the individual may hold the belief that personal and family information must stay within the family. Some cultural groups are very reluctant to disclose family information to outsiders, including health care professionals. This attitude can present difficulties for health care professionals who require knowledge of family interaction patterns to help clients with emotional problems.

In many cultures naming systems differ from those in North America. In some cultures (eg, Japanese and Vietnamese) the family name comes first and the given name second. One or two names may or may not be added between the family and given names. Other nomenclature may be used to delineate sexual, child, or adult status. For example, in traditional Japanese culture, adults address other adults by their surname followed by *san*, meaning *Mr, Mrs*, or *Miss*. An example is Murakami san. The children are referred to by their first names followed by *kun* for boys and *chan* for girls. Sikhs and Hindus traditionally have three names. Hindus have a personal name, a complimentary name, and then a family name. Sikhs have a personal name, then the title *Singh* for men and *Kaur* for women, and lastly the family name. Names by marriage also vary. In Central America, a woman who marries retains her father's name and takes her husband's. For example, if Louisa Viccario marries Carlos Gonzales she becomes Louisa Viccario de Gonzales. The connecting *de* means "belonging to." A male child will be Pedro Gonzales Viccario. Nurses need to become familiar with appropriate ways to address clients. In many cultures, using a client's first name is considered patronizing.

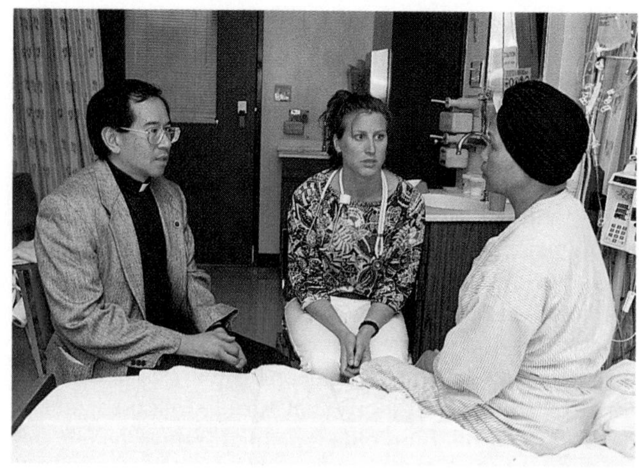

Figure 15–3 Group leaders such as clergy can often help bridge the gap between cultures, including the health care culture.

COMMUNICATION STYLE

Communication and culture are closely interconnected. Through communication, the culture is transmitted from one generation to the next, and knowledge about the culture is transmitted within the group and to those outside the group. Communicating with clients of various ethnic and cultural backgrounds is critical to providing culturally competent nursing care. There can be cultural variations in both verbal and nonverbal communication.

Verbal Communication The most obvious cultural difference is in verbal communication: vocabulary, grammatical structure, voice qualities, intonation, rhythm, speed, pronunciation, and silence (Giger & Davidhizar 1995, p. 23). In North America, the dominant language is English; however, immigrant groups who speak English still encounter language differences, because English words can have different meanings in different English-speaking cultures. For example, in the United States a boot is a type of footwear that comes to the ankle or higher; in England, a boot can also be the trunk of a car. Spanish is spoken by people in several regions of the world: Spain, South America, Central America, Mexico, the Caribbean, and the Philippines. It is the second most commonly spoken language in the United States. Nevertheless, each cultural group that speaks Spanish may use different vocabulary, apply rules of grammar differently, and use different pronunciation, so that often two people of different Latino cultures, speaking Spanish together, may not completely understand each other.

Initiating verbal communication may be influenced by cultural values. The busy nurse may want to complete nursing admission assessments quickly. The client, however, may be offended when the nurse immediately asks personal questions. In some cultures, it is believed that social courtesies should be established before business or personal topics are discussed. Discussing general topics can convey that the nurse is interested in the client and has time for the client. This enables the nurse to develop a rapport with the client before progressing to more personal discussion.

Verbal communication becomes even more difficult when an interaction involves people who speak different languages. Both clients and health professionals experience frustration when they are unable to communicate verbally with each other. For clients who have limited knowledge of English, the nurse should avoid slang words, medical terminology, and abbreviations. Augmenting spoken conversation with gestures or pictures can increase the client's understanding. The nurse should speak slowly, in a respectful manner, and at a normal volume. Speaking loudly does not help the client understand and may be offensive. The nurse must also frequently validate the client's understanding of what is being communicated. The nurse must be wary of interpreting a client's broad smiling and head nodding to mean that the client understands; the client may only be trying to please the nurse and not understand what is being said.

For the client who speaks a different language, a translator may be necessary. Galanti (1991, p. 16) states that cultural rules often dictate who can discuss what with whom. Guidelines for using an interpreter are shown in the accompanying box.

Translators should be objective individuals who can provide accurate translation of the client's information and of the health professional's questions, information, and instruction. Many institutions that are located in culturally diverse communities have translators available on staff or maintain a list of employees who are fluent in other languages. Embassies, consulates, ethnic churches (eg, Russian Orthodox, Greek Orthodox), ethnic clubs (eg, Polish-American Club, Italian-American Club) or telephone communication companies may also be able to provide translating services. Nursing and other health personnel can use pictures and gestures to augment verbal communication. Some schools of nursing and health care institutions do not permit nursing students to translate for a procedure consent because a lack of knowledge about the procedure may lead the student to give inaccurate information. The student should check the institution's policy prior to agreeing to translate for institutional staff and physicians.

Nurses and other health care providers must remember that clients for whom English is a second language may lose command of their English when they are in stressful situations. It is not uncommon for clients who have used English comfortably for years in social and business communication to forget and revert back to their primary language when they are ill or distressed. It is important for the nurse to assure the client that this is normal and to promote behaviors to facilitate verbal communication.

Using an Interpreter

- Avoid asking a member of the client's family, especially a child or spouse, to act as interpreter. The client, not wishing family members to know about his or her problem, may not provide complete or accurate information.
- Be aware of gender and age differences; it is preferable to use an interpreter of the same sex as the client to avoid embarrassment and faulty translation of sexual matters.
- Avoid an interpreter who is politically or socially incompatible with the client. For example, a Bosnian Serb may not be the best interpreter for a Muslim, even if he speaks the language.
- Address the questions to the client, **not** to the interpreter.
- Ask the interpreter to translate as closely as possible to the words used by the nurse.
- Speak slowly and distinctly. Do **not** use metaphors, for example, "Does it swell like a grapefruit?" or "Is the pain stabbing like a knife?"
- Observe the facial expressions and body language that the client assumes when listening and talking to the interpreter.

Nonverbal Communication

To communicate effectively with culturally diverse clients, the nurse needs to be aware of two aspects of nonverbal communication behaviors: what nonverbal behaviors mean to the client and what specific nonverbal behaviors mean in the client's culture. It is not required that the nurse be knowledgeable about the nonverbal behavior patterns of all cultures; however, before the nurse assigns meaning to nonverbal behavior, the nurse must consider the possibility that the behavior may have a different meaning for the client and the family. Furthermore, to provide safe and effective care, nurses who work with specific cultural groups should learn more about cultural behavior and communication patterns within these cultures.

Nonverbal communication can include the use of silence, touch, eye movement, facial expressions, and body posture. Some cultures are quite comfortable with long periods of silence, whereas others consider it appropriate to speak before the other person has finished talking. Many persons value silence and view it as essential to understanding a person's needs or use silence to preserve privacy. Some cultures view silence as a sign of respect, whereas to other persons silence may indicate agreement (Giger & Davidhizar 1995, p. 28).

Touch and touching is a learned behavior that can have both positive and negative meanings. In the American culture, a firm handshake is a recognized form of greeting that conveys character and strength (Giger & Davidhizar 1995, p. 28). In some European cultures, greetings may include a kiss on one or both cheeks along with the handshake. In some societies, touch is considered magical and because of the belief that the soul can leave the body on physical contact, casual touching is forbidden. In the Hmong culture, only certain elders are permitted to touch the head of others, and children are never patted on the head. Nurses should therefore touch a client's head only with permission (Rairdan & Higgs 1992, p. 55). The sex of the person touching and being touched often has cultural significance. Galanti (1991, p. 82) describes a situation in which an Orthodox Jewish husband could not touch his wife during labor and delivery; to Orthodox Jews, the blood of both menstruation and birth render a woman unclean, and her husband is forbidden to touch her during those times.

Cultures also dictate what forms of touch are appropriate for individuals of the same sex and opposite sex. In many cultures, for example, a kiss is not appropriate for a public greeting between persons of the opposite sex, even those who are family members; however, a kiss on the cheek is acceptable as a greeting among individuals of the same sex. The nurse should watch interaction among clients and families for cues to the appropriate degree of touch in that culture. The nurse can also assess the client's response to touch when providing nursing care, for example, by noting the client's reaction to the physical examination or the bath.

Facial expression can also vary between cultures. Giger and Davidhizar (1995, p. 31) state that Italian, Jewish, African-American, and Spanish-speaking persons are more likely to smile readily and use facial expression to communicate feelings, whereas Irish, English, and northern European persons tend to have less facial expression and are less open in their response, especially to strangers. Facial expressions can also convey the opposite meaning of what is felt or understood. For example, clients who have difficulty understanding English may smile and nod their heads as though they understood what is being said, when, in fact, they do not understand at all, but do not want to displease the caregiver.

Eye movement during communication has cultural foundations. In Western cultures, direct eye contact is regarded as important and generally shows that the other is attentive and listening. It conveys self-confidence, openness, interest, and honesty. Lack of eye contact may be interpreted as secretiveness, shyness, guilt, lack of interest, or even a sign of mental illness. Other cultures may view eye contact as impolite or an invasion of privacy. In the Hmong culture, continuous direct eye contact is considered rude, but intermittent eye contact is acceptable (Rairdan & Higgs 1992, p. 53). The nurse should not misinterpret the character of the client who avoids eye contact.

Body posture and gesture are also culturally learned. Finger pointing, the "V" sign with the index and middle fingers, and the "thumbs up" sign may have different meanings. For example, the "V" sign means victory in some cultures, while it may be an offensive gesture in other cultures (Galanti 1991, p. 22). In the Hmong culture, bowing the head slightly when entering the room where an elder is present or using both hands to give something to someone are considered signs of respect (Rairdan & Higgs 1992, p. 52).

Communication is an essential part of establishing a relationship with a client and their family. It is also important for developing effective working relationships with health care colleagues. To enhance their practice, nurses can observe the communication patterns of clients and colleagues and be aware of their own communication behaviors. A variety of strategies for communicating with clients from different cultures are presented in several references listed at the end of this chapter. The same strategies can be used in communication with professional colleagues.

SPACE ORIENTATION

Space is a relative concept that includes the individual, the body, the surrounding environment, and objects within that environment. The relationship between the individual's own body and objects and persons within space is learned and is influenced by culture. For example, in nomadic societies space is not owned; it is occupied temporarily until the tribe moves on. In Western societies people tend to be more territorial, as reflected in phrases such as "This is my space" or "Get out of my space." In Western cultures, spatial distances are defined as the intimate zone, the personal zone, and the social and public zones. The intimate zone is the smallest area of space around the individual, the public zone the largest area. The size of these areas may vary with the specific culture. Nurses move through all three zones as they provide care for clients. The nurse needs to be aware of the client's response to movement toward the client. The client may physically withdraw or back away if the nurse is perceived as being too close. The nurse will need to explain to the client why there is a need to be close to the client. To assess the lungs with a stethoscope, for example, the nurse needs to move into the client's intimate space. The nurse should first explain the procedure and await permission to continue.

Clients who reside in long-term care facilities, or are hospitalized for an extended time, may want to personalize their space. They may want to arrange their space differently and control the placement of objects on their bedside cabinet or over-bed table. The nurse should be responsive to clients' needs to have some control over their space. When there are no medical contraindications, clients should be permitted and encouraged to wear their own clothing and have objects of personal significance. Wearing cultural dress or having personal and cultural items in one's environment can increase self-esteem by promoting not only one's individuality but also one's cultural identity. Of course, the nurse should caution the client about responsibility for loss of personal items.

TIME ORIENTATION

Time orientation refers to an individual's focus on the past, the present, or the future (Galanti 1991, p. 29). Most cultures combine all three time orientations, but one orientation is more likely to dominate. The American focus on time tends to be directed to the future, emphasizing time and schedules (Smith 1992, p. 27). Nursing students know what times they "must" be in class or clinical. They know what courses they will take in future semesters. European Americans often plan for next week, their vacation, or their retirement. Other cultures may have a different concept of time. Leininger (1987, pp. 256, 262) describes the Navajo emphasis as "on the flow of life within the natural environment without specific time boundaries." For example, a Navajo mother may not become upset if her child does not achieve a specific developmental milestone, such as walking or toileting, on schedule.

The culture of nursing and health care values time. Appointments are scheduled, and treatments are prescribed with time parameters (eg, changing a dressing once a day). Medication orders include how often the medicine is to be taken and when (eg, digoxin 0.25 mg, once a day, in the morning). Nurses need to be aware of the meaning of time for clients. Giger and Davidhizar (1995, p. 109) state that when caring for clients who are "present-oriented," it is important to avoid fixed schedules. The nurse can offer a time range for activities and treatments. For example, instead of telling the client to take digoxin every day at 10:00 AM, the nurse might tell the client to take it every day in the morning, or every day after getting out of bed.

NUTRITIONAL PATTERNS

Most cultures have staple foods, that is, foods that are plentiful or readily accessible in the environment. For example, the staple food for Asians is rice; of Italians, pasta; and of Eastern Europeans, wheat. Even clients who have been in the United States or Canada for several generations often continue to eat the foods of their cultural homeland.

The way food is prepared and served is also related to cultural practices. For example, in the United States, a traditional food served for the Thanksgiving holiday is stuffed turkey; however, in different regions of the country the contents of the stuffing may vary. In Southern states, the stuffing may be made of cornbread; in New England, of seasoned bread and chestnuts.

The ways in which staple foods are prepared also varies. For example, some Asian cultures prefer steamed rice; others prefer boiled rice. Southern Asians from India prepare unleavened bread from wheat flour rather than the leavened bread of Anglo-Americans.

Food-related cultural behaviors can include whether to breastfeed or bottle feed infants, and when to introduce solid foods to them. Food can also be considered part of the remedy for illness. Foods classified as "hot" foods or foods that are hot in temperature may be used to treat illnesses that are classified as "cold" illnesses. For example, corn meal (a "hot" food) may be used to treat arthritis (a "cold" illness). Each culture group defines what it considers to be hot and cold entities.

Religious practice associated with specific cultures also affects diet. Some Roman Catholics avoid meat on certain days, such as Ash Wednesday and Good Friday, and some Protestant faiths prohibit meat, tea, coffee, or alcohol. Both Orthodox Judaism and Islam prohibit the ingestion of pork or pork products. Orthodox Jews observe Kosher customs, eating certain foods only if they are inspected by a rabbi and prepared according to dietary laws. For example, the eating of milk products and meat products at the same meal is prohibited. Some Buddhists, Hindus, and Sikhs are strict vegetarians. The nurse must be sensitive to such religious dietary practices.

PAIN RESPONSES

It has been demonstrated that beliefs about and responses to pain vary among ethnic/racial groups. Cultural response to pain must be viewed in relation both to the actual perception of pain and to the meaning or significance of pain to the client and family. In some cultures, pain may be considered a punishment for bad deeds; the individual is, therefore, to tolerate pain without complaint in order to atone for sins. In other cultures, self-infliction of pain is a sign of mourning or grief. In other groups, pain may be anticipated as a part of the ritualistic practices of passage ceremonies, and therefore tolerance of pain signifies strength and endurance. In yet other cultures, the expression of pain elicits attention and sympathy, while in other cultures, boys especially are taught "to take pain like a man" and "big boys don't cry."

Cavillo and Flaskerud (1991, p. 16) found that nurses and clients assess pain differently. In a study of Mexican-American clients with pain, they found that nurses and physicians tend to underestimate and undertreat their client's pain in relation to the client's expression of pain. Client responses to pain should be assessed within the context of their culture. If the client does not complain of pain, it should not be assumed that the client is not experiencing pain. The nurse must be aware of what conditions are likely to cause pain and offer clients pain relief as appropriate.

Treatment for pain may also vary with culture. In European-American cultures, medication is typically used for pain relief. In other cultures, heat, cold, relaxation, or other techniques and treatments may be used.

DEATH AND DYING PRACTICES

Death is a universal experience, and people want to die with dignity. Various cultural and religious traditions and practices associated with death, dying, and grieving process help people cope with these experiences. Nurses are often present through the dying process and at the moment of death, especially when it occurs in a health care facility. Knowledge of the client's religious and cultural heritage helps nurses provide individualized care to clients and their families, even though they may not participate in the rituals associated with death.

Dying in solitude is generally unacceptable in most cultures. In many cultures, people prefer a peaceful death at home rather than in the hospital. Some ethnic groups may request that health professionals not reveal the prognosis to dying clients. They believe the person's last day should be free of worry and pain. People in other cultures prefer that a family member (preferably a male in some cultures) be told the diagnosis so that the client can be tactfully informed by a family member in gradual stages or not be told at all. Nurses also need to determine whom to call, and when, as the impending death draws near.

Beliefs and attitudes about death, its cause, and the soul also vary amongst cultures. Unnatural deaths, or "bad deaths," are sometimes distinguished from "good deaths." The death of a person who has behaved well in life is considered less threatening because that person will be reincarnated into a good life next time.

Beliefs about preparation of the body, autopsy, organ donation, cremation, and prolonging life are closely allied to the person's religion. *Autopsy*, for example, may be prohibited, opposed, or discouraged by Eastern Orthodox religions, Muslims, Jehovah's Witnesses, and Orthodox Jews. Some religions prohibit the removal of body parts and dictate that all body parts be given appropriate burial. *Organ donation* is prohibited by Jehovah's Witnesses and Muslims, whereas Buddhists in America consider it an act of mercy and encourage it. *Cremation* is discouraged, opposed, or prohibited by the Mormon, Eastern Orthodox, Islamic, and Jewish faiths. Hindus, in contrast, prefer cremation and cast the ashes in a holy river. *Prolongation of life* is generally encouraged; however, some religions, such as Christian Science, are unlikely to use medical means to prolong life, and the Jewish faith generally opposes prolonging life after irreversible brain damage. In hopeless illness, Buddhists may permit euthanasia.

Nurses also need to be knowledgeable about the client's death-related rituals, such as last rites and administration of Holy Communion, chanting at the bedside, and other rituals, such as special procedures for washing, dressing, positioning, and shrouding the dead. For example, certain immigrants may wish to retain their native customs, in which family members of the same sex wash and prepare the body for burial and cremation. Muslims also customarily turn the body toward Mecca. Nurses need to ask family members about their preference and verify who will carry out these activities. Burial clothes and other cultural or religious items are often important symbols for the funeral. For example, faithful Mormons are often dressed in their "temple clothes." Some Native Americans may be dressed in elaborate apparel and jewelry and wrapped in new blankets with money. The nurse must ensure that any ritual items present in the health care agency be given to the family or to the funeral home.

CHILDBIRTH AND PERINATAL CARE

Prenatal Care In North America, emphasis is placed on regular prenatal medical visits, dental care, prenatal classes for both parents, and avoidance of communicable disease. These practices are accepted in varying degrees by people of other cultures. To some for example, regular medical checkups are often avoided because they are equated with problems or abnormalities. Traditionally, these women will see a physician only if there is a problem. Many immigrants may also prefer not to attend prenatal classes for a variety of reasons. Some of these relate to language problems or discomfort and embarrassment about doing exercises in front of others, discussing sexual matters, or seeing movies about childbirth.

Because in many cultures pregnancy and childbirth are considered the exclusive realm of women, some women prefer to have a female friend or relative attend prenatal classes and the birth rather than the husband. Nurses need to respect this choice. However, some new immigrant husbands, in the absence of a mother, mother-in-law or other female, may indicate interest in attending prenatal classes and the birth, if only to act as interpreters for their wives.

Prenatal practices vary in regard to safeguarding the health of the fetus and mother. People in several cultures (eg, Mexican-Americans, Asians, Chinese) emphasize the equilibrium model of health—that is, balancing yin and yang or hot and cold—during pregnancy. Pregnant women therefore avoid too much "hot" or "cold" food as determined by their culture. Some women believe that hot foods during the first trimester of pregnancy can cause miscarriage or a premature delivery; as a result, they emphasize the ingestion of cool foods, such as some fruit, coconut, buttermilk, and yogurt, and the avoidance of hot foods, such as meat, nuts, and eggs, during this period (Waxler-Morrison et al 1990, p. 168).

Labor and Delivery In some cultures, pregnant women traditionally return to their parents' home for the delivery of the first child and, sometimes, subsequent births. Births in the home are usually managed by a midwife, with the assistance of the woman's mother, mother-in-law, or married sister. Traditionally, the husband is not present. In other cultures, childbirth takes place in homes, hospitals, and clinics and is attended by physicians and certified nurse-midwives.

Positions used for delivery vary from the standard lithotomy position of North Americans. For example, squatting, kneeling, sitting, or standing may be preferred.

Responses to labor pain vary. Some women of certain cultures tolerate considerable pain and stoically accept pain for many reasons. They may, for example, want to avoid showing weakness or calling undue attention to themselves for fear of shaming themselves and their families, or they may act accordingly simply because it is expected behavior within their culture. In other cultures, women express pain and anguish more freely. For example, screaming and sobbing are acceptable and expected responses. It is important for the nurse to know that the absence of crying and moaning does not necessarily mean that pain is absent, nor does the presence of crying and moaning necessarily mean that pain relief is desired at that moment. With clients from some cultures, nurses may use touching and the support of others (husband, female relative, or friend) to decrease pain during labor. Various other cultures may or may not value the same comfort measures. Pain relief medications may also be used, but some clients are hesitant to request it.

Postpartum Care Most cultures emphasize certain postpartal routines or rituals for mother and baby. These are frequently designed to restore harmony or the hot-cold balance of the body. In many cultures, the mother's health status is classified as cold due to stress and the loss of blood. Thus, people take care to warm the body and to avoid cold after birth. This prohibition includes cold air and wind, as well as designated foods and fluids. Showers, tub baths, and shampoos are restricted, often until the lochia stops or longer, to avoid chilling. Sponge baths may be taken using warm water and/or special products that have medicinal properties. Foods considered "hot" by the specific culture are provided, whereas foods considered "cold" are avoided. Some women may wear binders around the abdomen and perineum not only to protect the body from cold but also to aid the uterus to return to its normal size. Mexican Americans may also cover the head, body, and feet to avoid cold air, infection, and other problems, such as sterility.

Confinement periods also vary and in many cultures are considerably longer than that of the health care system of North America. For example, traditional Chinese practice a "sitting in" period for 1 month to avoid cold winds. This confinement also applies to the newborn. New Mexican-American mothers may remain in bed for 3 days following delivery, begin to walk inside the home after 1 week and may go outside after 2 weeks.

For most cultures, the extended family frequently plays an essential role during the postnatal period. A grandmother, mother, mother-in-law, aunt, or married sister may be the primary helper for the mother and newborn. This gives the new mother time to rest as well as access to someone who can help with problems and concerns as they arise.

The Newborn Breast-feeding is the traditional feeding method in most cultures. However, bottle feeding is becoming more common among women who are employed. The current emphasis in North America on breast-feeding is confusing to some new immigrants because effective advertising campaigns have convinced women of the superiority of bottle feeding; they believe babies grow faster on the formulas. Nurses need to provide additional encouragement and clear explanations for these women.

In some cultures, newborn babies may have a coin placed on the umbilicus or their waist tied with a belly band to prevent a protruding umbilicus or hernia (Waxler-Morrison et al 1990, p. 60). Islamic practice requires a family member to pray in the newborn's ear as soon as possible after birth. Circumcision is mandatory according to some religious doctrines and cultural practices. However, in many cultures, circumcision is not performed.

It is important to remember that younger members of a specific culture group may have been acculturated to the dominant culture and no longer follow traditional practices. In other instances, they follow some practices but not others. Sensitive nurses can work toward a blending of old and new behaviors to meet the goals of all concerned.

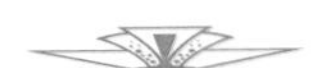

Providing Culturally Competent Care

All phases of the nursing process are affected by the client's and the nurse's cultural values, beliefs, and behaviors. As the client's culture and the nurse's culture come together in the nurse-client relationship, a unique cultural environment is created that can improve or impair the client's outcome. Self-awareness of personal biases can enable nurses to develop modifying behaviors or (if they are unable to do so) to remove themselves from situations where care may be compromised. Nurses can become more aware of their own culture through a values clarification (see Chapter 5). The nurse must also consider the cultural values of the health care setting because they, too, may influence the client's outcome.

To obtain cultural assessment data, the nurse uses broad statements and open-ended questions that encourage clients to express themselves fully. The important principle to remember when conducting an assessment is that "the client is the teacher and expert regarding his or her culture, and the nurse is the learner" (Rosenbaum 1995, p. 188). At this stage, the nurse makes no conclusions but obtains information from the client.

There are many cultural assessment tools available. The nurse needs to use a tool appropriate to the situation and adapt it as required. For example, a nurse in an emergency department of an urban hospital may need a different format than a nurse working in a home care setting. Tripp-Reimer, Brink, and Saunders (1984, p. 78) note that it is unnecessary to complete a total cultural assessment for every client. Instead, nurses need to collect enough basic cultural data to identify patterns of behavior that may either facilitate or interfere with a nursing strategy or treatment plan.

Anderson et al (1990, pp. 256–262) emphasize the following points relevant to cultural assessment.

- A cultural assessment takes time and usually needs to extend over several time periods.

- Recognition of one's own ethnicity and social background is essential. Even when the nurse and client share the same ethnic background, the nurse should expect differences in beliefs and values.
- The *process* of assessment is important. How and when questions are asked requires sensitivity and clinical judgment.
- The timing and phrasing of questions needs to be adapted to the individual. Timing is important in introducing questions. Sensitivity is needed in phrasing questions.
- Trust needs to be established before clients can be expected to volunteer and share sensitive information. The nurse therefore needs to spend time with the clients, introduce some social conversation, and convey a genuine desire to understand their values and beliefs.

Before a cultural assessment begins, the nurse determines what language the client speaks and the client's degree of fluency in the English language. The nurse can also learn about the client's communications patterns and space orientation by observing both verbal and nonverbal communication. For example, does the client speak for self or defer to another? What nonverbal communication behaviors does the client exhibit (eg, touching, eye contact)? What significance do these behaviors have for the nurse-client interaction? What is the client's proximity to other people and objects within the environment? How does the client react to the nurse's movement toward the client? What cultural objects within the environment have importance for health promotion/health maintenance?

For the initial cultural assessment, regardless of the approach used, nurses should ask themselves the following questions (Grant 1994, pp. 180–181):

- What does the client think about the nature of the illness? What does the client believe to be its cause? How does the client usually deal with the problem? How can others help?
- What support systems are available to the client? Is support from family, religious, community, or ethnic groups available to the client during and after treatment? Does the client need assistance contacting these individuals?
- What treatments is the client using to maintain health and fight illness? Are nontraditional healers involved? What remedies or treatments are ongoing or under consideration? What assistance will be needed from the health care institution or staff to accommodate a combined approach to the problem?
- What biologic and social factors should the nurse consider when planning client care? What health care risks and individual needs characterize the client's culture? What communication problems might occur?
- What does the client want from traditional medicine? What problems are foreseeable? What decisions can be anticipated? How might any legal or ethical problems be addressed?

As the client answers these questions, the sensitive nurse will identify other concerns and issues that can be queried.

To provide *culturally congruent care* the benefits, satisfies, and is meaningful to the people nurses serve, Leininger (1991, pp. 41–42) conceptualizes three major modes to guide nursing judgments, decisions, and actions:

1. *Cultural care preservation and/or maintenance.* The nurse accepts and complies with the client's cultural beliefs. For example, the nurse provides herbal tea to ease a "nervous stomach," a practice the client says has worked well in the past.
2. *Cultural care accommodation and/or negotiation.* The nurse plans, negotiates, and accommodates the client's culturally specific food preferences, religious practices, kinship needs, child care practices, and treatment practices.
3. *Cultural care repatterning or restructuring.* The nurse is knowledgeable about culture care and develops ways to repattern or restructure nursing care.

Cultural care preservation may involve, for example, encouraging the use of cultural health care practices, such as ingesting herbal tea, chicken soup, or "hot foods" to the ill client. Accommodating the client's viewpoint and negotiating appropriate care require expert communication skills, such as responding empathetically, validating information, and effectively summarizing content. Negotiation is a collaborative process. It acknowledges that the nurse–client relationship is reciprocal and that differences exist between the nurse and client about notions of health, illness, and treatment. The nurse attempts to bridge the gap between the nurse's (scientific) and the client's (cultural) perspectives. During the negotiation process, the nurse first elicits the client's views and acknowledges these views and then, if appropriate, provides relevant scientific information. If the client's views reveal that certain behaviors would not affect the client's condition adversely, then the nurse incorporates these views in planning care. If the client's views can lead to harmful behaviors, then the nurse attempts to shift the client's perspectives to the scientific view. Negotiation therefore occurs when cultural treatment practices conflict with those of the health care system and when the cultural practices are considered harmful to the client's well-being. The nurse must determine precisely how the client is managing the illness, what practices could be harmful, and which practices can be safely combined with Western medicine. For example, reducing dosages of an antihypertensive medication or replacing insulin therapy with herbal measures may be detrimental. In situations where harm may occur, the nurse needs to inform the client about possible outcomes. When a client chooses to follow only cultural practices and refuses all prescribed medical or nursing interventions, the nurse needs to adjust the client's goals. Anderson et al (1990, p. 264) point out that monitoring the client's condition to identify changes in health state and to recognize impending crises before they become irreversible may be all that is realistically achievable. At a time of crisis, the nurse may then have the opportunity to renegotiate the original care approach.

Transcultural nursing care is challenging. It requires discovery of the meaning of the client's behavior, flexibility, creativity, and knowledge to adapt nursing interventions. For example, a culturally sensitive nurse knows that a Chinese woman who has just given birth and refuses to eat fruit and vegetables, refuses to drink the cold water at her bedside, stays in bed, and refuses to take sitz baths, baths, or showers needs to increase the return of yang forces. The nurse will make plans to adapt nursing interventions accordingly.

Nurses also need to identify community resources that are available to assist clients of different cultures. Nurses should try to learn from each transcultural nursing situation they encounter to improve the delivery of culture-specific care to future clients. The box on page 297 offers suggestions for providing culturally competent nursing care.

CHAPTER HIGHLIGHTS

- North Americans come from a variety of ethnic and cultural backgrounds, and many North Americans retain at least some of their traditional values, beliefs, and practices.
- Many groups in North America are bicultural; that is, they embrace two cultures: their original ethnic culture and a North American culture.
- An individual's ethnic and cultural background can influence beliefs, values, and practices.
- Through acculturation, most ethnic and cultural groups in North America modify some of their traditional cultural characteristics.
- Personal characteristics also modify an individual's cultural values, beliefs, and practices.
- Health beliefs and practices, family patterns, communication style, space and time orientation, nutritional patterns, pain response, death and dying practices, childbirth and perinatal care, and ethnic-related health problems influence the relationship between the nurse and the client who have different cultural backgrounds.
- When assessing a client, the nurse considers the client's cultural values, beliefs, and practices related to health and health care.

READINGS AND REFERENCES

SUGGESTED READINGS

Bell, R. May 1994. Prominence of women in Navajo healing beliefs and values. *Nursing and Health Care* 15:232–240.
This nurse describes her experiences in the Indian Health Service of the U.S. Public Health Service in Arizona, where she grew to understand that "the Navajo views of health are closely related to traditional beliefs and values in a harmonious relationship with all living things."

Candle, P. December 1993. Providing culturally sensitive health care to Hispanic clients. *Nurse Practitioner* 18:40–51.
It is projected that Hispanics will constitute the largest minority in the United States by the year 2000. She discusses prevalent health problems, lack of care resources for Hispanics, and the implications for nursing practice.

Giger, JN and Davidhizar, R. Fall 1990. Developing communication skills for use with black patients. *The ABNF Journal* 1:3–35.
These authors believe that the nurse who works with African-American clients must develop sensitivity to communication variances that exist between and within various ethnic and cultural groups. To help nurses communicate better with African-American clients, the authors delineate the conceptual and historical development of Black English and describe the variations in its pronunciation.

O'Hara, EM and Zhan, L. October 1994. Cultural and pharmacologic considerations when caring for Chinese elders: Knowledge of traditional Chinese medicine is necessary. *Journal of Gerontological Nursing* 20:11–16.
These authors state that to provide effective care for Chinese elders, nurses should be familiar with the philosophical perspectives of Confucianism and with traditional Chinese medicine, including herbal treatments, diet therapy, and the use of animal secretions and organs. The authors also describe the effects of some common Chinese herbal medicines and other nursing implications of caring for this group of clients.

Wilson, S and Billones, H. August 1994. The Filipino elder: Implications for nursing practice—knowledge of heritage essential. *Journal of Gerontological Nursing* 20:31–36.
This article provides information about five significant Filipino cultural values influencing health behaviors: bahala, na, pakikisamu, hiya, amor propio, and utang na loob. The authors also discuss the immigration experience, changes in life-style patterns of immigrants, and nursing implications.

AFRICAN-AMERICAN LITERATURE

Angelou, M. 1969. *I Know Why the Caged Bird Sings.* New York: Bantam Books.

Ellison, R. 1947. *Invisible Man.* New York: Vintage.

Walker, A. 1982. *The Color Purple.* New York: Washington Square Press.

ASIAN LITERATURE

Buck, P. 1931. *The Good Earth.* New York: Washington Square Press.

Tan, A. 1989. *The Joy Luck Club.* New York: Vintage.

HISPANIC LITERATURE

Marquez, GG. 1967. *One Hundred Years of Solitude.* New York: Avon Books.

Marquez, GG. 1985. *Love in the Time of Cholera.* New York: Penguin Books.

RELATED RESEARCH

Calvillo, ER and Flaskerud, JH. Winter 1991. Review of literature on culture and pain of adults with focus on Mexican Americans. *Journal of Transcultural Nursing* 2:16–23.

Rooda, LA. May 1993. Knowledge and attitudes of nurses toward culturally different patients: Implications for nursing education. *Journal of Nursing Education* 32:209–13.

SELECTED REFERENCES

American Nurses Association. 1991. *Position statement on cultural diversity in nursing practice.* Washington, DC: ANA.

Anderson, JM. May/June 1990. Health care across the cultures. *Nursing Outlook* 38:136–139.

Anderson, JM, Waxler-Morrison, N, Richardson, E, Herbert, C, and Murphy, M. 1990. Delivering culturally-sensitive health care. In Waxler-Morrison, N, Anderson, J, and Richardson, E. pp. 245–267. *Cross Cultural Caring: A Handbook for Health Professionals in Western Canada.* Vancouver, BC: UBC Press.

Andrews, MM and Boyle, JS. 1995. *Transcultural Concepts in Nursing.* 2d ed. Philadelphia: Lippincott.

Banks, J and Banks, C. 1989. *Multicultural Education and Perspectives.* Boston: Allyn & Bacon.

Baye, AL. Summer/Fall 1995. A lesson in culture. *Minority Nurse* pp. 35–38.

Bernal, H. December 1993. A model for delivering culture-relevant care in the community. *Public Health Journal* 10:228–232.

Bushy, A. April 1992. Cultural considerations for primary health care: Where do self-care and folk medicine fit? *Holistic Nursing Practice* 6:10–18.

Calvillo, ER and Flaskerud, JH. Winter 1991. Review of literature on culture and pain of adults with focus on Mexican Americans. *Journal of Transcultural Nursing* 2:16–23.

DeSantis, L and Lowe, J. 1992. Moving from cultural sensitivity to cultural competence in nursing practice: Pitfalls and progress. *Paper presented at the 18th Annual Transcultural Nursing Society Conference, Miami, FL, October* 22–24, 1992.

DeSantis, L and Thomas, JT. Summer 1990. The immigrant Haitian mother: Transcultural nursing perspective on preventive health care for children. *Journal of Transcultural Nursing* 2:2–15.

Diaz-Gilbert, M. October 1993. Caring for culturally diverse patients. *Nursing93,* 23:44–45.

Eliason, MJ. September/October 1993. Ethics and transcultural nursing care. *Nursing Outlook* 4:225–228.

Galanti, G. 1991. *Caring for Patients from Different Cultures.* Philadelphia: University of Pennsylvania Press.

Giger, JN and Davidhizar, R. January/February 1990. Transcultural nursing assessment: A method for advancing nursing practice. *International Nursing Review* 37:199–202.

Giger, JN and Davidhizar, R. 1995. *Transcultural Nursing: Assessment and Interventions.* 2d ed. St Louis: Mosby-Year Book.

Grant, AB. 1994. *The Professional Nurse: Issues and Actions.* Springhouse, PA: Springhouse.

Grossman, D and Taylor, R. February 1995. Working with people: Cultural diversity on the unit. *American Journal of Nursing* 95:64, 65–67.

Kavanaugh, KH and Kennedy PH. 1992. *Promoting Cultural Diversity.* Newbury Park: Sage Publications.

Kittler, PG and Sucher, KP. March/April 1990. Diet counseling in a multicultural society. *Diabetes Educator* 16:127–134.

Lea, A. August 1994. Nursing in today's multicultural society: A transcultural perspective. *Journal of Advanced Nursing* 20:307–313.

Leininger, MM. 1978. *Transcultural Nursing: Concepts, Theories, and Practices.* New York: Wiley.

Leininger, MM. November 1988. Leininger's theory of nursing: Cultural care diversity and universality. *Nursing Science Quarterly* 14:152–160.

Leininger, MM. editor. 1991. *Culture Care Diversity and Universality: A Theory of Nursing.* New York: National League for Nursing Press. Pub. No. 15–2402.

Leininger, MM. Winter 1993. Towards conceptualization of transcultural health care systems: Concepts and a model. *Journal of Transcultural Nursing* 4:32–40.

Lynam, MJ. February 1992. Towards the goal of providing culturally sensitive care: Principles upon which to build nursing curricula. *Journal of Advanced Nursing* 17:149–157.

Outlaw, FH. April 1994. A reformulation of the meaning of culture and ethnicity for nurses delivering care. *Medical-Surgical Nursing* 3:108–111.

Price, JL and Cordell, B. July/August 1994. Cultural diversity and patient teaching. *Journal of Continuing Education in Nursing* 25:163–166.

Rairdan, B and Higgs, ZR. March 1992. When your patient is a Hmong refugee. *American Journal of Nursing* 92:52–55.

Rosenbaum, JN. April 1991. A cultural assessment guide: Learning cultural sensitivity. *Canadian Nurse* 88:32–33.

Rosenbaum, JN. April 1995. Teaching cultural sensitivity. *Journal of Nursing Education* 34:188–189.

Smith, S. 1992. *Communications in Nursing.* 2d ed. St Louis: Mosby-Year Book.

Spector, RE. 1991. *Cultural Diversity in Health and Illness.* 3d ed. Norwalk, CT: Appleton-Century-Crofts.

Sprott, J. 1993. The black box in family assessments: Cultural diversity. In Feetham, S, Meister, S, Bell, J, and Gilliss, C. pp. 189–199. *The Nursing of Families: Theory, Research, Education, Practice.* Beverly Hills, CA: Sage Publications.

Steinmetz, S and Braham, CG. editors. 1993. *Random House Webster's Dictionary.* New York: Ballantine Reference Library.

Stringfellow, I. 1978. The Vietnamese. In Clark, AL. editor. *Culture, Childbearing, Health Professionals.* Philadelphia: FA Davis.

Thiederman, SB. September 1986. Health care issues: Ethnocentrism: A barrier to effective health care. *Nurse Practitioner* 11:52–54, 59.

Tripp-Reimer, T, Brink, PJ, and Saunders, JM. March/April 1984. Cultural assessment: Content and process. *Nursing Outlook* 32:78–82.

Waxler-Morrison, N, Anderson, J, and Richardson, E. editors. 1990. *Cross Cultural Caring: A Handbook for Health Professionals in Western Canada.* Vancouver, BC: UBC Press.

Wenger, AFZ. January 1993. Cultural meaning of symptoms. *Holistic Nursing Practice* 7:22–23.

16

Spirituality and Religion

Objectives

Compare and contrast the concepts of spirituality, faith, and religion.

Describe the spiritual development of the individual across the life span.

Discuss Fowler's stages of spiritual development.

Discuss Westerhoff's stages of faith.

Describe characteristics of spirituality.

Assess the spiritual needs of clients.

Plan nursing care to assist the client with spiritual needs.

Describe nursing interventions to support client's spiritual beliefs and religious practices.

State outcome criteria for evaluating the client's spiritual well-being.

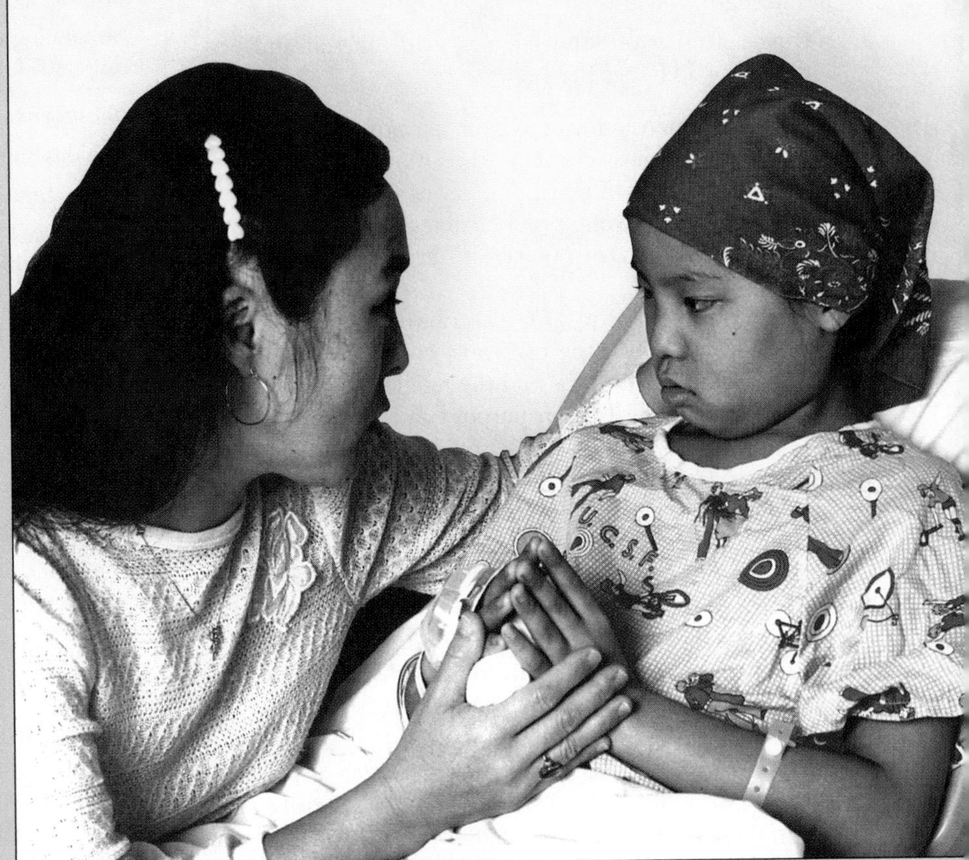

Spirituality, faith, and religion are separate entities, yet some people use the words interchangeably. **Spirituality** or spiritual belief is a belief in or relationship with some higher power, creative force, divine being, or infinite source of energy. For example, a person may believe in "God," in "Allah," the "Creator," or in a "Higher Power." Spirituality includes the following aspects (Burkhardt 1993, p. 12):

- Dealing with the unknown or uncertainties in life.
- Finding meaning and purpose in life.
- Being aware of and able to draw upon inner resources and strength.
- Having a feeling of connectedness with oneself and with God or a Higher Being.

"The spiritual dimension tries to be in harmony with the universe, strives for answers about the infinite and especially comes into focus or sustaining power when the person faces emotional stress, physical illness, or death. It goes outside a person's own power" (Murray & Zentner 1993, p. 86).

Mickley et al (1992, p. 267) describe spirituality as being multidimensional; the two most commonly cited dimensions are the existential and the religious. The existential dimension focuses on purpose and meaning in life; the religious dimension focuses on one's relationship with God or a Higher Power.

Stoll (1989, p. 7) describes spirituality as a two-dimensional concept: the vertical dimension is the relationship with the transcendent/God or whatever supreme values guide the person's life; the horizontal dimension is the person's relationship with self, others, and the environment. There is a continuous interrelationship between and among the two dimensions. Characteristics of spirituality are listed in the box at the right.

Spiritual needs are described by Carson (1989, p. 17) as "the need for a forgiving, loving, trusting relationship with a God (as defined by the individual) and meaningfully lived out in the love, forgiveness, hope, and trust of oneself and others."

It is often the nurse who identifies a need for spiritual assistance and obtains the desired help. According to Shelly and Fish, certain spiritual needs underlie all religions: (a) the need for meaning and purpose, (b) the need for love and relatedness, and (c) the need for forgiveness (1988, pp. 40–53). Some people believe that these needs are common to all humanity.

Faith, according to Fowler and Keen (1985, p. 18), is a universal—a feature of living, acting, and self-understanding. To have faith is to believe in or be committed to something or someone. In a general sense, religion or spiritual beliefs are one's attempt to understand one's place in the universe, that is, how one sees the self in relation to the total environment.

Religion is an organized system of worship. Religions have central beliefs, rituals, and practices usually related to death, marriage, and salvation. They also often have rules of conduct applicable to daily life. Many people satisfy their spiritual needs through a specific religion or religious framework. The most common religions in North America are listed in Table 16–1.

Characteristics of Spirituality

Relationship with Self

Inner strength/self-reliance

- Self knowledge (who one is, what one can do)
- Attitudes (trust in self, trust in life/future, peace of mind, harmony with self)

Relationship with Nature

Harmony

- Knowing about plants, trees, wildlife, weather
- Communing with nature (gardening, walking, being outside); preserving nature

Relationship with Others

Harmonious/supportive

- Sharing time, knowledge, and resources; reciprocating
- Caring for children, elderly, sick
- Reaffirming the living and the dead (visiting, photos, cemetery meetings)

Nonharmonious

- Conflict with others
- Resolution leading to harmony or long-term disharmony with friction and limited association

Relationship with Deity

Religious or non-religious

- Prayer/meditation
- Religious articles
- Being in nature
- Church participation

Source: M Burkhardt, Characteristics of spirituality in the lives of women in a rural Appalachian community, *Journal of Transcultural Nursing,* Winter 1993, 4:12–18. Used with permission.

Table 16–1 Religions of North America, 1991

Religion	Numbers of Believers (Millions)
Christianity	96.3 Roman Catholic 95.6 Protestant 7.2 Anglican 38.0 Other Christian
Judaism	7.0
Islam	2.6
Hinduism	1.3
Buddhism	0.6
Baha'i	0.4
Sikh	0.3
Nonreligious (no religion, nonbelievers, agnostics, freethinkers, and dereligionized secularists indifferent to all religion)	25.2
Atheists	1.3

Source: *Statistical Abstract of the United States*, 112th ed. (Washington, DC: US Department of Commerce, 1992).

Religious development of an individual refers to the acceptance of specific beliefs, values, rules of conduct, and rituals. Religious development may or may not parallel spiritual development. For example, a person may follow certain religious practices and yet not internalize the symbolic meaning behind the practices. An **agnostic** is a person who doubts the existence of God or a supreme being or believes the existence of God has not been proved. An **atheist** denies the existence of God. **Monotheism** is the belief in the existence of one God who created and rules the universe. **Polytheism** is the belief in more than one God. The moral and ethical codes of agnostics and atheists are not derived from theistic beliefs.

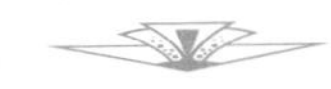

SPIRITUAL DEVELOPMENT

Faith is defined as the acceptance of a truth that cannot be demonstrated or proved by logical thought. Fowler (1974), Aden (1976), and Westerhoff (1976) have studied the development of faith. Each has described several stages in the development of faith in the individual. Fowler (Table 16–2, p. 314) builds on the moral development theory of Kohlberg and the developmental theories of Piaget and Erikson (see Chapter 23). He describes faith as being present in both religious and nonreligious individuals. Faith gives life meaning for the individual, providing the individual with strength in times of difficulty. Aden, who has also been influenced by Erikson, describes faith as a gift from a higher power. He describes eight stages of faith, starting during infancy, when faith is manifested as trust in caregivers, and developing across life's stages, as faith evolves into courage, obedience, assent, identity, self-surrender, unconditional caring, and unconditional acceptance as one's physical abilities decline in older years. Westerhoff (Table 16–3, p. 314) describes faith as a way of being and behaving that evolves from an experienced faith guided by parents and others during a person's infancy and childhood to an owned faith that is internalized in adulthood and serves as a directive for personal action. For the client who is ill, faith—whether in a higher authority (eg, God, Allah, Jehovah), the client's own self, in the health care team, or in a combination of all—provides strength and trust.

Hope is a concept that also has a spiritual dimension. **Hope** is defined as a confident expectation that a desire will be fulfilled. Hope is necessary for the individual to survive illness or other difficult times. Grimm (1991, p. 511) states that hope "is an interpersonal process that is created through trust and is nurtured by trusting relationships with others, including God." Whereas faith is the belief in someone or something, hope is the belief that things will get better. Stotland (1969, p. 1) states that "without hope, the individual is often dull, listless, and moribund." In the absence of hope, the client gives up, and illness—especially terminal illness—may progress more rapidly. Table 16–4 on page 315 summarizes spiritual and religious behaviors during different life stages.

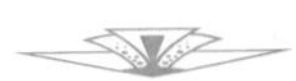

RELIGION AND ILLNESS

Spiritual and religious beliefs are important in many people's lives. They can influence life-style, attitudes, and feelings about illness and death. Some organized religions

Table 16–2 Fowler's Stages of Spiritual Development

Stage	Age	Description
0. Undifferentiated	0 to 3 years	Infant unable to formulate concepts about self or the environment
1. Intuitive-projective	4 to 6 years	A combination of images and beliefs given by trusted others, mixed with the child's own experience and imagination
2. Mythic-literal	7 to 12 years	Private world of fantasy and wonder; symbols refer to something specific; dramatic stories and myths used to communicate spiritual meanings
3. Synthetic-conventional	Adolescent or adult	World and ultimate environment structured by the expectations and judgments of others; interpersonal focus
4. Individuating-reflexive	After 18 years	Constructing one's own explicit system; high degree of self-consciousness
5. Paradoxical-consolidative	After 30 years	Awareness of truth from a variety of viewpoints.
6. Universalizing	Maybe never	Becoming an incarnation of the principles of love and justice

Source: Adapted from J Fowler and S Keen, *Life Maps: Conversations in the Journey of Faith* (Waco, TX: Word Books, 1985) and A Hollander, *How to Help Your Child Have a Spiritual Life: A Parents' Guide to Inner Development* (New York: A and W Publishers, 1980). Used by permission.

specify practices about diet, birth control, appropriate medical therapy, and proper care of the dying or dead. Some religious groups condemn modern science because of "false teachings," such as evolution. Other groups support medical therapy in general but object to specific practices; for example, Christian Science urges members to avoid all drugs unless they are exceedingly ill.

Spiritual beliefs may assume greater importance at a time of illness than at any other time in a person's life, helping some people accept illness and explaining illness for others. Some clients may look upon illness as a test of faith; that is, they believe that if their faith is great enough, they will get well. Viewed from this perspective, illness is usually accepted by the client and the client's support persons and does not shake their religious beliefs.

Other people may look on illness as punishment and think, "What have I done to deserve this?" These people associate disease with immoral behavior and believe their illness is punishment for past sins. They may believe that through prayer, promises, and perhaps penance, the cause of the disease will disappear. Such people may believe that health professionals treat only the symptoms of disease and that they will become well if they are forgiven. If such an individual does not get well, then the support persons either accept the "punishment" or view the "punishment" as unfair.

Usually, spiritual beliefs help people to accept illness and to plan for the future. Religion can help people prepare for death and strengthen them during life. It can provide a meaning to life and to death; a haven of strength, serenity, and faith at a time of crisis; a sense of security; and a tangible network of social support.

Certain spiritual beliefs are in conflict with accepted medical practice. When a person's faith leads the person

Table 16–3 Westerhoff's Four Stages of Faith

Stage	Age	Behavior
Experience faith	Infancy/early adolescence	Experiences faith through interaction with others who are living a particular faith tradition
Affiliative faith	Late adolescence	Actively participates in activities that characterize a particular faith tradition; experiences awe and wonderment; feels a sense of belonging
Searching faith	Young adulthood	Through a process of questioning and doubting own faith, acquires a cognitive as well as an affective faith
Owned faith	Middle adulthood/old age	Puts faith into personal and social action and is willing to stand up for what the individual believes even against the nurturing community

Source: Adapted from J Westerhoff, *Will Our Children Have Faith?* (New York: Seabury Press, 1976), pp. 79–103.

Table 16–4 Summary of Spiritual Development

Developmental Stage	Characteristics
Infants and toddlers	Both infants and toddlers have no sense of right or wrong, spiritual beliefs, or convictions to guide activities. Toddlers may follow rituals (eg, saying prayers at bedtime) in imitation of their parents. Toddlers may attend a church nursery school, but emphasis is on enhancing their positive self-image.
Preschoolers	Parental attitudes toward moral codes and religion convey to children what is considered good and bad. Preschoolers copy what they see rather than what they are told. If what they see and what they are told are contradictory, problems arise. They often ask questions about morality and religion (eg, "Why is [some action or word] wrong?" and "What is heaven?"). They believe that their parents, like God, are omnipotent. Two methods of spiritual education are used with preschool children: indoctrinating them and letting them choose their own way. Preschoolers follow a religion not because they understand it but because it is part of daily life. Five-year-olds often make up prayers themselves. They believe that God or human beings are responsible for such natural events as rain and wind. They may reason, "The rain is God crying; the wind is God blowing air out of His mouth." Many go to church school and participate in religious holidays. They ask many questions about the meaning of the holidays and need explanations about them. However, they are more occupied with such rituals as Santa Claus coming at Christmas than with the reason behind the holiday. When children begin to question such myths as the Easter Bunny, they are ready for a more sophisticated explanation about Easter or Passover.
School-age children	Young school-age children expect that their prayers will be answered, good rewarded, and bad punished. During the prepuberty stage, children become aware of spiritual disappointments. They realize that their prayers are not always answered on their own terms, and they begin to reason rather than accept a faith blindly. Some children drop or modify certain religious practices (eg, praying for tangible benefits); others continue to follow religious practices because of dependence on their parents. During adolescence, children compare the standards of their parents with others and determine which ones they want to incorporate into their own behavior. Adolescents also compare the scientific viewpoint with the religious viewpoint and try to bring the two together. By 16 years, many adolescents have decided whether to accept the family religion. They may experience personal religious awakenings, such as being saved or converted, either suddenly or gradually. Adolescents with parents of different faiths may choose one faith over the other or no faith. For some, a firm faith provides strength during these turbulent years.
Adults	Young adults who need to answer the religious questions of their own children may find that the teaching of their own early childhood are more acceptable to them now than during adolescence. During the middle years, adults often find that they have more time for religious activities because their children are older. Older adults who have developed religious values often endeavor to broaden them and to understand the newer values of younger people. Elderly adults who do not have mature religious beliefs may experience a feeling of deprivation as they become less active (eg, because of retirement). During later years, people face death (their own, their spouses', and their friends'). This recognition may make them despondent. The development of a mature religious philosophy can often help older people face reality, participate in life, have feelings of self-worth, and accept death as inevitable.

CRITICAL THINKING CHALLENGE

WHAT WOULD YOU DO?

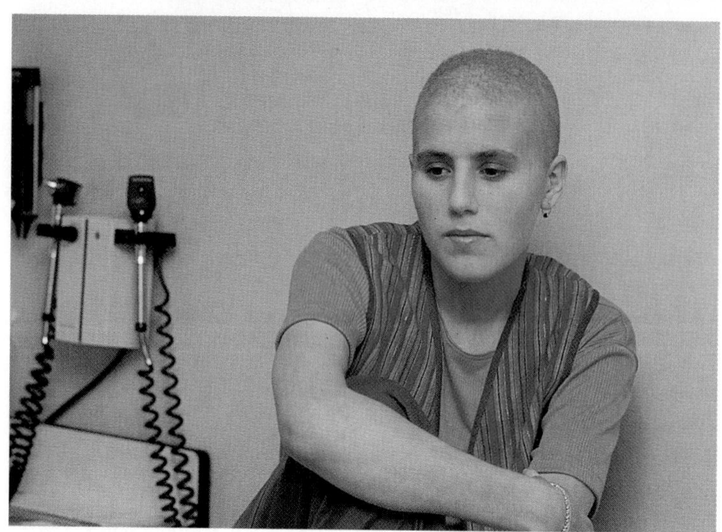

Bettina Clark, a 23-year-old female, has been receiving chemotherapy agents for the treatment of leukemia. After her treatment she asks, "Why is God punishing me? I've tried to be a good person all of my life."

What would you do?

to reject certain medical treatment, life may be threatened. For example, many practicing Jehovah's Witnesses will not accept blood transfusions because their religious doctrine forbids the treatment.

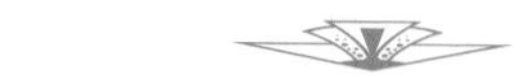

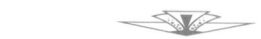

Religious Beliefs Related to Health Care

Meeting the spiritual needs of clients and their support persons is part of the function of nurses as well as designated chaplains and other clergy. The term **clergy** refers to priests, rabbis, ministers, church elders, deacons, and other spiritual advisers. Some religious groups, such as the Church of Latter Day Saints and the Christian Scientists, do not have ordained clergy; they usually do have people whose role it is to minister to the ill, and these people must be recognized by nurses as having appropriate functions. In Christian Science, the role of ministering to the sick is carried out by a practitioner (reader).

Although nurses cannot expect to be well versed about the practices of all the religious groups in North America, it is important to be familiar with the major religious groups of the community. Watson (1985, p. 92) states that the "nurse's acknowledgment, appreciation, and respect for the spiritual meaning in a person's life can be comforting to the person. Spiritual and religious awareness is one of the nurse's responsibilities." Representatives of a religion usually give nurses information required in the care of clients. Table 16–5 (page 318) identifies holy days and sacraments and discusses the beliefs related to health care of selected major religions of North America.

Protestantism is a major religious group in North America. There are more than 50 Protestant denominations in North America, for example, Episcopalians, Methodists, Lutherans, Presbyterians, and Baptists. Some Protestant denominations are further divided; for example, the Baptists comprise American Baptists, Southern Baptists, and National Baptists. These denominations share some doctrines, but each denomination has its own interpretation of scripture and its own religious practices that may affect health care practices. The following are major common tenets of Protestant beliefs (Carson 1989, pp. 88–89):

- The Bible (Old and New Testaments) is the source of authority.
- God is revealed through the Bible, the life of Jesus, and the presence of the Holy Spirit (Holy Ghost).
- The Holy Trinity consists of God the Father, God the Son (Jesus Christ), and God the Holy Spirit. All are one God.
- Jesus initiated baptism and holy communion. These are the only sacraments practiced.
- Sin requires forgiveness from God and is obtained through a personal relationship with God through Jesus Christ.
- One is able to communicate with God through prayer.
- Holy remembrance and celebration of events in the life of Jesus, such as his birth (Christmas), death (Holy

SPIRITUAL WELL-BEING

Religious Component

I believe that God loves me and cares about me.

I have a personal and meaningful relationship with God.

I believe God is concerned about my problem.

My relationship with God helps me not to feel lonely.

I feel most fulfilled when I am in close communion with God.

My relationship with God contributes to my sense of well-being.

Meaning and Purpose in Life

I feel that life is a positive experience.

I feel very fulfilled and satisfied with life.

I feel a sense of well-being about the direction my life is headed in.

I feel good about my future.

I believe there is some real purpose in life.

Source: Sample statements from a scale on religious meaning and purpose of life. © Spiritual Well-Being Scale. 1982 by Craig W. Ellison and Raymond F. Paloutzian. All rights reserved. Used with permission.

ASSESSMENT INTERVIEW

Spirituality

- Are any particular religious practices important to you? If so, could you please tell me about them?
- Will being here interfere with your religious practices?
- Do you feel your faith is helpful to you? In what ways is it important to you right now?
- In what ways can I help you carry out your faith? For example, would you like me to read your prayer book to you?
- Would you like a visit from your spiritual counselor or the hospital chaplain?
- What are your hopes and your sources of strength right now?

Week, Maundy Thursday, Good Friday) and resurrection (Easter).

- The organized church is responsible for carrying out the teachings of Jesus Christ.
- There is life after death, and that afterlife is determined by one's relationship with God.

When the client demonstrates a need for or requests spiritual assistance, the nurse must determine the individual client's specific spiritual requirements.

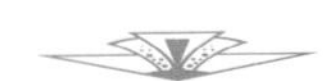

SPIRITUAL HEALTH AND THE NURSING PROCESS

ASSESSING

Spiritual health, or **spiritual well-being,** is a feeling of being "generally alive, purposeful, and fulfilled" (Ellison 1983, p. 332). According to Pilch (1988, p. 31), spiritual wellness is "a way of living, a lifestyle that views and lives life as purposeful and pleasurable, that seeks out life-sustaining and life-enriching options to be chosen freely at every opportunity, and that sinks its roots deeply into spiritual values and/or specific religious beliefs."

Ellison and Paloutzian (1982) designed a spiritual well-being scale that includes specific questions for a client (see the box at the left for sample statements). They found that people who scored high on the scale tended to be less lonely, more socially skilled, and higher in self-esteem; furthermore, their religious commitment was more intrinsic to their personalities.

Nursing History Nurses may elicit data about a client's spiritual beliefs as part of the general history. Often the information elicited is limited to the client's religious affiliation. Nurses should never assume, however, that a client follows all the practices of the client's stated religion.

Stoll (1979, p. 1574) suggests a spiritual history guide to elicit information in four areas: (a) the person's concept of God or deity, (b) the person's source of hope and strength, (c) the significance of religious practices and rituals to the person, and (d) the relationship the person perceives between the individual's spiritual beliefs and state of health. Stoll further cautions that all people have a right to their own values and beliefs and that they have a right not to discuss or reveal these beliefs to others. The spiritual assessment is best taken at the end of the assessment process or following the psychosocial assessment, once the nurse has developed a relationship with the client and/or support person and feels that it is appropriate to discuss spiritual matters. The questions provided in the box above may be suitable.

Text continued on page 320

Table 16–5 Religious Beliefs of Selected Religions

Religion	Holy Days	Sacraments
Baha'i International Community	March 21: Naw-Ruz (Baha'i New Year); April 21: Ridvan (12 days, commemorates the declaration of Baha'u'llah); July 9: Martyrdom of the Bab; October 20: Birth of the Bab; November 12: Baha'u'llah Birthday. All holy days begin at sunset of the previous day.	No sacraments as understood by Christians. Obligatory prayers, holy days, and the Nineteen-Day Fast.
Buddhist Churches of America	February 15: Death of Buddha; March 21: Higan-e (First Day of Spring); April 8: Hanamatsuri (Birth of Buddha); July 15: Obon-e (Memorial Day); September 23: Higan-e (First Day of Fall); December 8: Bodhi Day (Enlightenment).	No sacraments. A ritual that symbolizes one's entry into the Buddhist faith is the Three Treasures (Buddha, Dharma, and Sangha).
Christian Science	Sundays (day of worship); Wednesdays are considered gathering times for testimony meetings. Traditional Christian holidays may be observed on an individual basis.	Baptism, which is the daily purification and spiritualization of thought. Communion, which is the finding of one's conscious unity with God through prayer.
Hinduism	Are based on the lunar calendar and include Purnima (full moon), Janamasthtimi (birthday of Lord Krishna), Ramnavmi (birthday of Rama), Shivratri (birth of Lord Shiva), Dusserah (Good over Evil), Vasant Panchami (Advent of Spring), Diwali, (Festival of Lights).	No sacraments.
Islam	Are based on the lunar calendar and include Ramadan (30 days of fasting, from sunup to sundown, to honor the first revelations to the Prophet (Muhammad); Idul-Fitr (the end of Ramadan); Idul-Adha (Day of Sacrifice); Maulid An-Nabi (Prophet Muhammad's Birthday).	No sacraments.
Judaism	Sabbath (Friday at sunset until after sunset on Saturday); Rosh Hashanah (Jewish New Year); Yom Kippur (Day of Atonement); Sukkot (Feast of Tabernacles); Chanukah (Festival of Lights); Shavuot (Festival of Weeks). All holy days begin at sunset of the previous day.	Circumcision is performed on the 8th day following birth (may be done by a ritual circumciser, *mohel*).
Protestantism Over 50 denominations	All Sundays December 25; Christmas; Good Friday (date varies); Easter Sunday (date varies).	Baptism Communion Confirmation is a holy day in some denominations.
Roman Catholicism	All Sundays. December 25: Christmas; January 1: Solemnity of Mary, Mother of God; Ash Wednesday (date varies); Good Friday (date varies); Easter Day (date varies); Ascension (date varies, always on a Thursday); August 15: Feast of the Assumption; November 1: All Saints' Day; December 8: Feast of the Immaculate Conception.	Baptism, Reconciliation (Confession), Holy Communion, Confirmation, Matrimony, Holy Orders, Anointing of the Sick.

Sources: MM Andrews and PA Hanson. Religious beliefs: Implications for nursing practice, in JS Boyle and MM Andrews, *Transcultural Concepts in Nursing Care.* (Philadelphia: Lippincott, 1989); and *A Calendar of Religious Holidays and Ethnic Festivals* (New York: National Conference of Christians and Jews, 1992).

Religion and Healing	Dietary and Medication Beliefs	Treatment Procedures
Believe there is a harmony between religion and science; therefore, they seek out competent medical care and pray for health.	Alcoholic beverages are prohibited. Tobacco use is discouraged. Narcotic drugs are prohibited except by prescription.	Permanent sterilization is prohibited. Abortion is discouraged. Forbids monastic celibacy.
Spiritual peace and liberation from anxiety by adherence to and achievement of awakening to Buddha's wisdom can be important factors in promoting healing and the recovery process.	No special beliefs. Medications should be used in accordance with the nature of the illness and the capacity of the individual.	Treatments such as amputations, organ transplants, biopsies, or amniocentesis that prolong life and allow individual to attain Enlightenment are encouraged.
Human imperfection, including physical illness, reflects a fundamental misunderstanding of creation; therefore, healing is through prayer and spiritual regeneration. Christian Science operates facilities where nursing care can be provided if needed.	No dietary restrictions; however, members usually abstain from alcoholic beverages. Some abstain from tea and coffee. Medications are not used. Immunizations and vaccines are acceptable only when required by law.	Blood and blood products are avoided. Organ transplantation, either donor or recipient, rare.
Some believe illness is God's punishment for sin. May believe in faith healing.	The eating of meat is forbidden. No medication restrictions.	No restrictions.
Pregnant women, nursing mothers, elderly, and ill need not fast for Ramadan. Any attempt to shorten one's life or terminate it is prohibited. Ritual cleansing and preparation of the dead for burial by a Muslim are required.	Eating pork and drinking intoxicating beverages are forbidden. No medication restrictions. Medications containing alcohol are permitted if prescribed as medicine.	No restrictions.
According to Jewish law, medical care from a physician is expected when ill. Autopsy is permitted only in special circumstances, and all body parts must be returned for burial.	For Orthodox Jews, dietary laws are strict and forbid eating of pork, predatory fowl, and shellfish. Milk dishes and meat dishes are not to be mixed. Only fish with fins and scales are permitted. Food must be Kosher, (ie, animals ritually killed). Conservative and Reform Jews may modify these dietary restrictions. No medication restrictions.	Abortion is permitted if the mother's health is in jeopardy. Abortion on demand is not considered acceptable.
Religious practices vary with different denominational beliefs; may include prayer, "laying on of hands," and anointing.	Beliefs vary; some denominations may prohibit alcoholic beverages, whereas others do not. No medication restrictions.	No restrictions.
At the client or family's request, a priest should be called to administer the Sacrament of the Sick, which includes anointing of the sick, communion, if possible, and a blessing. The nurse may baptize a critically ill newborn when a priest is not available.	Use food in moderation and in such a way that it is not injurious to health. Fasting is viewed as a valued discipline. Days of fast include Ash Wednesday and Good Friday; days of abstinence include all Fridays in Lent. Fasting is not required when ill. Medications are allowed as long as they are used for the good of the whole person.	Abortion is considered morally wrong. Only natural means of birth control are accepted: abstinence, rhythm method, and temperature method. Permanent sterilization is forbidden.

NURSING DIAGNOSES

CLIENTS WITH SPIRITUAL DISTRESS

NURSING DIAGNOSIS: Spiritual distress (distress of the human spirit): The state in which the individual or group experiences or is at risk of experiencing a disturbance in the belief or value system that provides strength, hope and meaning to life

Defining Characteristics

Major

- Disturbance in belief or value system that provides emotional strength and hope and gives life meaning

Minor

- Requests spiritual assistance
- Expresses doubt in belief system
- Expresses doubt over the meaning of life
- Expresses concern over death and afterlife
- Expresses despair
- Expresses anger toward God or Higher Authority
- Verbalizes that illness is a punishment
- Questions the treatment plan because of spiritual beliefs
- Is unable or refuses to perform spiritual rituals
- Exhibits behaviors associated with mood alterations, such as crying, withdrawal, anxiety, anger, or hostility
- Physical complaints, including loss of appetite, sleep disturbance, headaches, tension

Related Factors

Illness or threat to well-being, including loss of body part or function, terminal illness, debilitating disease, pain, trauma, or stillbirth/miscarriage; loss of meaningful roles related to divorce, the illness or death of a significant other, or childbirth; separation from religious, cultural, or family ties; belief and value system that is challenged or questioned by others, including social, familial, institutional, or medical opposition to practicing spiritual rituals.

Sources: LJ Carpenito. *Nursing Diagnosis: Application to Clinical Practice*, 4th ed. (Philadelphia: Lippincott, 1992, pp. 802–23); M Gordon. *Manual of Nursing Diagnosis, 1993–1994.* (St Louis: Mosby, 1993, p. 381); GK McFarland and EA McFarlane. *Nursing Diagnosis & Intervention: Planning for Patient Care*, 2d ed. (St Louis: Mosby, 1993, pp. 747–54); NANDA. *Nursing Diagnoses: Definitions and Classifications 1992–1993.* (Philadelphia: NANDA, 1992, p. 46).

Clinical Assessment **Spiritual distress** may be revealed by one or more of the following:

1. *Affect and attitude.* Does the client appear lonely, depressed, angry, anxious, agitated, apathetic, or preoccupied?
2. *Behavior.* Does the client appear to pray before meals or at other times or read religious literature? Does the client complain frequently, need unusually high doses of sedation, pace the halls at night, joke inappropriately, have nightmares and sleep disturbances, or express anger at religious representatives or a deity?
3. *Verbalization.* Does the client mention God, prayer, faith, the church, or religious topics (even briefly)? Does the client ask about a visit from the clergy? Does the client express fear of death, concern with the meaning of life, inner conflict about religious beliefs, concern about a relationship with the deity, questions about the meaning of existence, the meaning of suffering, or the moral/ethical implications of therapy?
4. *Interpersonal relationships.* Who visits? How does the client respond to visitors. Does a minister come? How does the client relate to other clients and nursing personnel?
5. *Environment.* Does the client have a Bible, prayer book, devotional literature, religious medals, a rosary, or religious get-well cards in the room? Does a church send altar flowers or Sunday bulletins? (Shelley & Fish 1988, pp. 61–62).

DIAGNOSING

The nursing diagnosis that relates to problems with spirituality is **Spiritual distress** or **Distress of the human spirit** (NANDA 1992, p. 46). This diagnosis, with its definition, contributing factors, and defining characteristics, is shown in the special Nursing Diagnoses box above. Clinical applications of this diagnosis are shown in Table 16–6.

Table 16–6 Clinical Application: Assessment Data Clusters and Related Nursing Diagnoses for Clients with Spiritual Distress

Data Cluster	Nursing Diagnosis
Marilyn Eckhardt, 72 years old, is crying, fingering her rosary, and verbalizing concern that she has not seen her priest for confession since being admitted to the hospital. She states that "she is afraid to die without confessing her sins." She also states that she does not want to see the hospital chaplain, but rather her own priest, whose parish is about 30 miles away. The hospital record indicates that Ms Eckhardt is Roman Catholic.	**Spiritual distress** related to inability to practice spiritual ritual (confession with parish priest)
John Ames, 42 years old, is in a terminal state with an AIDS-related condition. He has become withdrawn but states to the nurse, "What have I done that God has punished me so?" The nurse observes religious literature on his bedside cabinet.	**Spiritual distress** related to crisis of illness and impending death

O'Brien (1982, p. 81) subcategorizes spiritual distress as follows:

- Spiritual *pain:* difficulty accepting the loss of a loved one or intense suffering (physical or emotional)
- Spiritual *alienation:* separation from religious or faith community
- Spiritual *anxiety:* challenge to beliefs and value systems (eg, by moral/ethical nature of therapy, such as abortion, blood transfusion, or surgery)
- Spiritual *guilt:* failure to abide by religious rules
- Spiritual *anger:* difficulty accepting illness, loss, or suffering
- Spiritual *loss:* difficulty finding comfort in religion
- Spiritual *despair:* feeling that no one cares

The following alternative diagnoses may be related to the client's spiritual state:

- **Hopelessness** (see Chapter 33 for more information)
- **Powerlessness**
- **Fear**
- **Dysfunctional grieving** (see Chapter 33 for more information)
- **Ineffective coping**
- **Self-esteem disturbance** (see Chapter 31 for more information)
- **Sleep pattern disturbance** (see Chapter 35 for more information)
- **Decisional conflict** related to conflict between treatment plan and spiritual beliefs

PLANNING

In the planning phase, the nurse identifies interventions to help the client achieve the overall goals of spiritual strength, serenity, and satisfaction.

Planning in relation to **Spiritual distress** should be designed to meet one or more of the following needs:

- To help the client fulfill religious obligations
- To help the client draw on and use inner resources more effectively to meet the present situation
- To help the client maintain or establish a dynamic, personal relationship with a supreme being in the face of unpleasant circumstances.
- To help the client find meaning in existence and the present situation
- To promote a sense of hope
- To provide spiritual resources otherwise unavailable.

Sometimes clients ask directly for a visit from the hospital chaplain or their own clergyman. Others may discuss their concerns with the nurse and ask about the nurse's beliefs as a way of seeking an empathic listener. Some people are embarrassed to ask for spiritual counsel but may hint at their concern in such statements as, "I've been wondering what will happen to me when I die," or "Do you go to a church?"

Any client or support person may desire spiritual assistance. The client facing death may have accepted it, but the family and support persons may not. Often relatives are grateful for spiritual support by a nurse or pastor. Assisting them may indirectly assist the client. Among those who may desire spiritual assistance are

- Clients who appear lonely and have few visitors.
- Clients who express fear and anxiety.
- Clients about to have surgery.
- Clients whose illness is related to the emotions or whose illness has religious or social implications.
- Clients who must change their life-style as a result of illness or injury.

RESEARCH NOTE

What Feelings of Spiritual Well-Being, Religiousness, and Hope Do Women with Breast Cancer Experience?

This study explored the spiritual health of 175 women diagnosed with varying stages of breast cancer. Participants were asked to complete the Spiritual Well-Being Scale (Ellison 1983), Feagin's Intrinsic/Extrinsic Religiousness Scale (Feagin 1964), and the Nowotny Hope Scale (Nowotny 1989). Findings demonstrated that the well-being scores of intrinsically religious women were higher than those of extrinsically religious women. The women with an intrinsic religious orientation endeavored to internalize a religious creed and follow it fully. Those with an extrinsic religious orientation tended to regard religion in a utilitarian manner, that is, as a means to obtain security or to interact socially. Findings also indicated a positive relationship between spiritual well-being and hope, primarily related to existential well-being, which focuses on life purpose and satisfaction. The authors suggest that spiritual well-being may be important to the client's ability to cope with illness but found no difference between the hope scores of intrinsically religious women and extrinsically religious women.

Implications: As a result of this study, the investigators suggest the following nursing interventions: (a) assist the client to maintain social support networks and religious beliefs; (b) structure the environment to allow visits from church members or group prayer; (c) be available to listen, accept, and explore client questions about existential concerns; and (d) be able to address secular aspects of promoting hope in clients.

Source: JR Mickley, K Soeken, and A Belcher, Spiritual well-being, religiousness, and hope among women with breast cancer, *Image: Journal of Nursing Scholarship*, Winter 1992, 24:267–72.

- Clients preoccupied about the relationship of their religion and health.
- Clients whose pastor is unable to visit.

It is important that the nurse ask the client before obtaining assistance. Some people profess no religious beliefs and may be angered if the nurse makes arrangements for a chaplain to visit. The nurse needs to respect the client's wishes and not make a judgment of right or wrong, good or bad. Planning also involves establishing particular outcome criteria.

IMPLEMENTING

Once **Spiritual distress** has been identified as a relevant nursing diagnosis and specific strategies have been planned, the nurse is ready to implement the plan. To be effective when intervening, nurses should have already examined and clarified their own spiritual beliefs and values (see Chapter 11). A nurse who feels uncomfortable assisting the client spiritually (eg, reading devotional material or praying with the client on request) should verbalize this discomfort and offer to obtain assistance for the client. It is important to respect the client's beliefs and maintain a supportive relationship. It is equally important for nurses not to feel guilty about their discomfort.

To decrease spiritual distress, nurses should focus attention on the client's perceived spiritual needs rather than on the practices or beliefs of the client's religious affiliation. Individual spiritual beliefs may vary greatly among members of a given religion. People join religious groups for many reasons (eg, to have a place of worship; to find an avenue for social action, such as helping the poor or homeless; to gain friends for recreational purposes; or to have a place for important life events such as weddings and funerals). Nurses should not assume that a client has no spiritual needs because the record states no religious affiliation or specifies atheist or agnostic.

To further individualize care, the nurse determines the meaning the client attaches to the situation. Such meanings can influence the client's response to an illness or condition and may either hinder nursing intervention or provide hope, courage, and strength. For example, a person who believes that illness is God's punishment may feel powerless and demonstrate little interest in therapy designed to prevent illness.

When orienting clients to the nursing unit, the nurse can provide information about hospital services to help clients meet spiritual needs and arrange for clients to participate in these as they are able. Many large hospitals have full-time chaplains who assist clients, support persons, and staff with spiritual needs. For smaller hospitals that do not have chaplains, clergy in the community usually provide this service. Many nursing units have a list of clergy who are on call when needed.

Some agencies have a chapel where religious services are regularly held for clients, support persons, and staff. Most hospitals also have quiet rooms that can be used for meditation, counsel, and even worship services. Sometimes a client prefers to meet the chaplain in a quiet, private room, particularly when the client shares a hospital room. A hospital may hold nondenominational religious services or several services for different denominations. If a client expresses a desire to attend services, the nurse needs to help organize the client's care so that attendance is possible if health permits.

The nurse sometimes determines that there is a true conflict between spiritual beliefs and medical therapy. In this case, the nurse encourages the client and physician to discuss the conflict and consider alternative methods of therapy. The nurse always supports the client's right to make an informed decision. If the beliefs of the nurse and client conflict, the nurse should discuss this conflict with the nurse in charge and the nurse's own spiritual leader. It may be preferable for the client to receive care from a nurse with compatible views. The nurse may also wish to discuss feelings with other health professionals, such as nurses on the team.

EVALUATING

To evaluate whether the client achieved the goals established during the planning phase, the nurse collects data pertaining to the outcome criteria established. Skill in observation, helping relationships, and communication are required. The nurse needs to observe the client when alone and when interacting with others and listen to what the client says and does not say. The accompanying box lists characteristics indicative of spiritual well-being.

CHARACTERISTICS INDICATIVE OF SPIRITUAL WELL-BEING

Sense of inner peace
Compassion for others
Reverence for life
Gratitude
Appreciation of both unity and diversity
Humor
Wisdom
Generosity
Ability to transcend the self
Capacity for unconditional love

Source: VB Carson, *Spiritual Dimensions of Nursing Practice* (Philadelphia: WB Saunders, 1989).

CHAPTER HIGHLIGHTS

- The spiritual needs of clients and support persons often come into focus at a time of illness.
- Nurses must respect the rights of people to hold their own spiritual beliefs and to communicate or not communicate these to others.
- Spiritual beliefs and practices are highly personal.
- Spiritual and religious beliefs influence life-style, attitudes, and feelings about illness and death.
- Spiritual beliefs often help people accept illness and plan for the future.
- A spiritual assessment is best obtained after the nurse has developed a relationship with the client. Information about a client's concept of God or deity, the client's source of hope and strength, the significance of religious practices and rituals, and the relationship the client perceives between health and spiritual beliefs should be obtained.
- Spiritual distress may be reflected in a number of behaviors, including depression, anxiety, and verbalizations of fear of death.
- Nurses should be aware of their own spiritual beliefs in order to be comfortable assisting others.
- Nurses and clergy may intervene directly to help clients and support persons meet spiritual needs.

READINGS AND REFERENCES

SUGGESTED READINGS

Andrews, MM and Hanson, PA. 1989. Religious beliefs: Implications for nursing practice. In Boyle, JS and Andrews, MM. *Transcultural Concepts in Nursing Care*. Philadelphia: Lippincott.
The authors discuss the beliefs and religious practices, holy days, sacraments, religious beliefs related to healing, and religious beliefs about diet, medications, medical treatment and surgical procedures of major world religions. Health issues that may be controversial within the religious group, the religious support system for ill believers, and religion specific issues related to death and dying are also discussed.

Carson, VB. 1989. *Spiritual Dimensions of Nursing Practice.* Philadelphia: WB Saunders.

Carson lays the foundation for the nurse's spiritual care for the client by first discussing spirituality and the nursing profession. She then describes the influence of major religious belief systems on clients' responses to medical treatment plans. Spirituality and the nursing process is described.

RELATED RESEARCH

Boutell, KA and Bozett, RW. July/August 1990. Nurses' assessment of patients' spirituality: Continuing education implications. *Journal of Continuing Education in Nursing* 21:172–76.

Highfield, MF. February 1992. Spiritual health of oncology patients: Nurse and patient perspectives. *Cancer Nursing* 15:1–8.

SELECTED REFERENCES

Aden, L. 1976. Faith and the developmental cycle. *Pastoral Psychology.* 24(2):215–30.

Andrews, MM and Hanson, PA. 1989. Religious beliefs: Implications for nursing practice. In Boyle, JS and Andrews, MM. *Transcultural Concepts in Nursing Care.* Philadelphia: Lippincott.

Arnold, E and Boggs, K. 1989. *Interpersonal Relationships: Professional Communication Skills for Nurses.* Philadelphia: WB Saunders.

Brooke, V. July/August 1987. The spiritual well-being of the elderly. *Geriatric Nursing* 8:194–95.

Burkhardt, M. Winter 1993. Characteristics of spirituality in the lives of women in a rural Appalachian community. *Journal of Transcultural Nursing* 4:12–18.

Burkhardt, MA and Nagai-Jacobson, MG. April 1985. Dealing with spiritual concerns of clients in the community. *Journal of Community Health Nursing* 2:191–98.

Burnard, P. May 1987. Spiritual distress and the nursing response: Theoretical considerations and counselling skills. *Journal of Advanced Nursing* 12:377–82.

Carpenito, LJ. 1992. *Nursing Diagnosis: Application to Clinical Practice.* 4th ed. Philadelphia: Lippincott.

Carson, VB. 1989. *Spiritual Dimensions of Nursing Practice.* Philadelphia: WB Saunders.

Danielson, CB, Hamel-Bissell, B, and Winstead-Fry, P. 1993. *Families, Health and Illness: Perspectives on Coping and Intervention.* St Louis: Mosby-Year Book.

Ellison, CW. April 1983. Spiritual well-being: Conceptualization and measurement. *Journal of Psychology and Theology* 11:330–40.

Feagin, JR. 1964. Prejudice and religious types: A focused study of Southern fundamentalists. *Journal for the Scientific Study of Religion.* 4:3–13.

Forbis, PA. May/June 1988. Meeting patients' spiritual needs: Helping patients to fulfill their spiritual needs is part of the nursing process. *Geriatric Nursing* 9:158–59.

Fowler, JW. 1974. Toward a developmental perspective on faith. *Religious Education* 69(2):207–19.

Fowler, J and Keen, S. 1978. *Life Maps: Conversations in the Journey of Faith.* Waco, TX: Word Books.

———. *Life Maps: Conversations on the Journey of Faith.* Waco, TX: Word Books.

Giger, JN and Davidhizar, RE. 1991. *Transcultural Nursing: Assessment and Intervention.* St Louis: Mosby-Year Book.

Gordon, M. 1993. *Manual of Nursing Diagnosis, 1993–1994.* St Louis: Mosby-Year Book.

Grimm, PM. 1991. Hope. In Creasia, JL and Parker, B. *Conceptual Foundations of Professional Nursing Practice.* St Louis: Mosby-Year Book.

Harmon, Y. May/June 1985. The relationship between religiosity and health. *Health Values* 9:23–25.

Highfield, MF and Cason, C. June 1983. Spiritual needs of patients: Are they recognized? *Cancer Nursing* 6:187–92.

Hollander, A. 1980. *How to Help Your Child Have a Spiritual Life: A Parent's Guide to Inner Development.* New York: A and W Publishers.

Labun, E. May 1988. Spiritual care: An element in nursing care planning. *Journal of Advanced Nursing* 13:314–20.

Lyon, JL and Nelson, S. May/June 1988. Mormon health. *Health Values* 12:37–44.

McFarland, GK and McFarlane, EA. 1993. *Nursing Diagnosis and Intervention: Planning for Patient Care.* 2d ed. St Louis: Mosby-Year Book.

Mealey, AR, Richardson, H, and Dimico, G. 1989. Family stress management. In Bomar, PJ, editor. *Nurses and Family Health Promotion: Concepts, Assessment, and Interventions.* Philadelphia: WB Saunders.

Mickley, JR, Soeken, K, and Belcher, A. Winter 1992. Spiritual well-being, religiousness, and hope among women with breast cancer. *Image: Journal of Nursing Scholarship* 24:267–72.

Murray, RB and Zentner, JB. 1993. *Nursing Assessment and Health Promotion Strategies Through the Life Span.* 5th ed. Norwalk, CT: Appleton & Lange.

Nagai-Jacobson, MG and Burkhardt, MA. May 1989. Spirituality: Cornerstone of holistic nursing practice. *Holistic Nursing Practice* 3:18–26.

National Conference of Christians and Jews. 1992. *A Calendar of Religious Holidays and Ethnic Festivals.* New York: National Conference of Christians and Jews.

North American Nursing Diagnosis Association. 1992. *Nursing Diagnoses: Definitions and Classifications 1992–1993.* Philadelphia: NANDA.

Nowotny, ML. 1989. Assessment of hope in patients with cancer: Development of an instrument. *Oncology Nursing Forum* 16(1):57–61.

O'Brien, ME. 1982. The need for spiritual integrity. In Yura, H and Walsh, M, editors. pp. 81–115. *Human Needs and the Nursing Process.* Norwalk, CT: Appleton-Century-Crofts.

Paloutzian, RT and Ellison, CW. 1982. Loneliness, spiritual well-being, and the quality of life. In Peplau, LA and Perlman, D, editors. *Loneliness: A Sourcebook of Current Theory, Research and Therapy.* New York: Wiley.

Pilch, JJ. May/June 1988. Wellness spirituality. *Health Values* 12:28–31.

Shelly, JA and Fish, S. 1988. *Spiritual Care: The Nurse's Role.* 3d ed. Downers Grove, IL: Inter Varsity Press.

Stoll, RT. September 1979. Guidelines for spiritual assessment. *American Journal of Nursing* 79:1574–77.

———. 1989. The essence of spirituality. In Carson, VB, editor. *Spiritual Dimensions of Nursing Practice.* Philadelphia: WB Saunders.

Stotland, E. 1969. *The Psychology of Hope.* San Francisco: Jossey-Bass.

US Department of Commerce. 1992. *Statistical Abstract of the United States.* 112th ed. Washington, DC: US Department of Commerce.

Watson, J. 1985. *Nursing: The Philosophy and Science of Caring.* Boulder, CO: Colorado Associated University Press.

Westerhoff, J. 1976. *Will Our Children Have Faith?* New York: Seabury Press.

17 SEXUALITY

OBJECTIVES

- Describe selected aspects of sexuality.
- Compare selected physical and psychologic sexual stimulation patterns.
- Identify physiologic changes occurring in males and females during each phase of the sexual response as described by Masters and Johnson.
- List factors that affect an individual's sexual attitudes and behaviors.
- Describe nursing skills for working with clients' sexual needs.
- Give examples of how to obtain data about sexual functioning when conducting a health history.
- Identify factors contributing to sexual dysfunction.
- List factors that increase and decrease sexual motivation.
- Describe common problems of genital sexuality and possible causes.
- Identify common illnesses affecting sexuality.
- Compare selected intervention models for sexual counseling.
- Identify essential aspects about selected contraceptive methods to include in health teaching.
- Describe guidelines for the prevention of sexually transmitted diseases (STDs).
- Identify interventions for the client who demonstrates inappropriate sexual behavior.
- Describe essential outcome criteria that permit evaluation of client progress toward meeting planned goals.

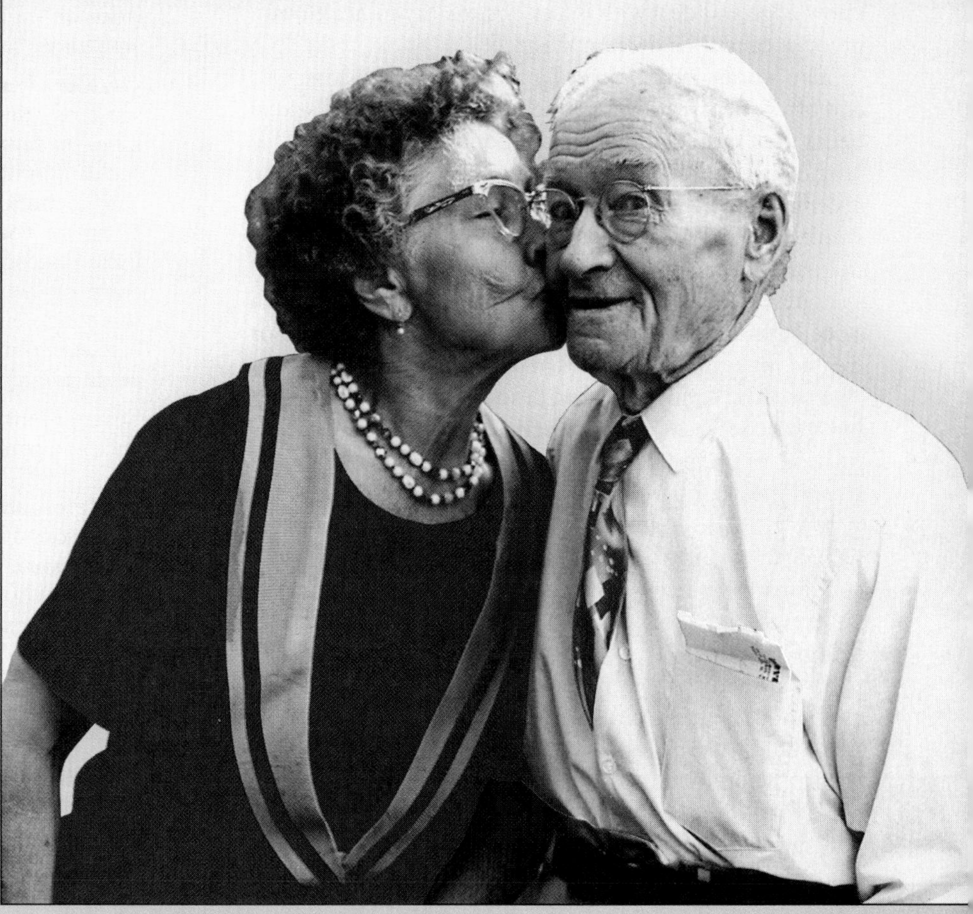

Sexuality is an integral characteristic of every human being. We are all born with the capacity to function as sexual beings. Clients do not leave their sexuality behind when they enter the health care system—their sexuality comes along as part of the whole person. Professional nurses, as health care providers focusing on the holistic nature of care, have a responsibility to provide effective sexual health care for their clients.

A holistic approach to client health care needs indicates that all aspects of being interact. Thus, sexuality influences and is influenced by the biologic, psychologic, sociologic, and spiritual aspects of being. The need to acknowledge and deal with issues of sexuality in health care practice cannot be overemphasized.

The words *sex* and *sexuality* are used interchangeably, and often incorrectly, to define different aspects of sexual being. **Sex** is the term most commonly used to denote biologic male or female status, but it is also used to describe specific sexual behavior, such as sexual intercourse. Examples of such usage include the labeled boxes on questionnaire forms to indicate male or female (M☐, F☐) and the question "How many partners have you had sex with since your last visit?" asked of a person being assessed or treated for sexually transmitted disease.

The more appropriate and descriptive term when dealing with sexual issues is **sexuality.** Girts makes this distinction between sex and sexuality: "Sex is defined as something we do, while sexuality is something we are" (1990, p. 205). "As human beings we express ourselves sexually from birth to death. Aging, chronic and disabling conditions may necessitate certain adaptations in the way we express our sexuality, but we do not cease to be sexual beings" (Parke 1991, p. 40). Sexuality is a crucial part of people's identity. It reflects our human character, not solely our genital nature.

Although sexuality is an integral part of the whole human being, it can also be categorized and studied according to three separate aspects: (a) biologic sex, (b) gender identity, and (c) gender role. See the accompanying box.

Terms Relative to Sexuality

- **Sexuality** includes all of those aspects of the human being that relate specifically to being boy or girl, woman or man. It is subject to lifelong dynamic change. As a function of the total personality, it is concerned with the biologic, psychologic, sociologic, spiritual, and cultural variables of life.
- **Biologic sex** includes all of the human being's genetically determined anatomy and physiology, which is also influenced by intrauterine conditions. The result of genetic plus other prenatal factors usually is clearly developed primary sex characteristics or variations of these characteristics, called ambiguous sex.
- **Gender identity** is the individual's persisting inner sense of being male or female, masculine or feminine. Its development is based on biologic sex and sociocultural reinforcement, which beings at birth with identification of the baby as male or female. Ultimate congruence between biologic sex and learned sense of sexual self is the most common outcome of this developmental process. Variations of this congruence are common, principally at periods of significant change in the life span (eg, adolescence, menopause, climacteric, old age).
- **Sexual identity** or sexual orientation is the preference of a person for one sex or the other. Examples are:
  - **Heterosexual:** one who is sexually attracted to persons of the opposite sex ("straight")
  - **Bisexual:** one who is sexually attracted to persons of both sexes ("bi")
  - **Homosexual:** one who is sexually attracted to persons of the same sex ("gay" [both sexes], lesbian [women])
  - **Transsexual:** one's belief that one is not the sex of one's physical body but of the opposite sex (trapped in the wrong body; sex-change surgery may be desired and undertaken)
- **Gender-role behavior** is the way a person acts as female or male, including the expression of what is perceived as gender-appropriate behavior.

Characteristics of Sexual Health

Sexual health includes biologic, psychologic, sociocultural, and spiritual components. Characteristics of sexually healthy people are shown in the box on page 327. These characteristics reflect the integral, holistic nature of sexuality as part of the human experience, and they provide a useful guide for measuring sexual health. Sexual health is possible for many people who have a variety of health problems and disabilities.

Because sexuality and sexual functioning are aspects of health and well-being, they are a part of nursing care. Nurses may need to assess sexuality and sexual function nonjudgmentally. They should encourage clients to discuss their concerns and offer suggestions to assist the return of intimacy and sexual function.

CHARACTERISTICS OF SEXUAL HEALTH

- Expression of a positive body image
- Cognitive knowledge about human sexuality
- Congruence between biologic sex, gender identity, and gender-role behavior
- Behavior consistent with self-concept
- Awareness of own sexual feelings and attributes
- Capacity for physical and psychosexual responsiveness, which is enhancing to self and others
- Comfort with a range of sexual behavior and lifestyles
- Acceptance of responsibility for pleasure, reproduction, and physical safety
- Ability to create effective interpersonal relationships with both sexes
- Value system that is developing and usable

Source: Adapted from EM Lion (editor), *Human Sexuality in Nursing Process* (New York: Wiley) 1982, pp. 9–10.

Research indicates that clients prefer health care professionals to initiate a discussion about sexual concerns, while many nurses expect clients to do this (Waterhouse & Metcalfe 1991, p. 1048). When no one introduces the topic of sexuality, the client is often left to resolve sexual concerns alone.

Nurses require four basic skills to help clients in the area of sexuality:

1. Self-knowledge and comfort with their own sexuality.
2. Acceptance of sexuality as an important area for nursing intervention and a willingness to work with clients expressing their sexuality in a variety of ways.
3. Knowledge of basic sexuality, including how certain health problems and treatments may affect sexuality and sexual function and which interventions facilitate sexual expressions and functioning.
4. Communication skills.

RESEARCH NOTE

Nurses Discussing Sexual Concerns: What Do Clients Think?

The purposes of this study were (a) to investigate the attitudes of healthy people toward nurses' discussing sexual concerns with their clients and (b) to identify factors that may influence people's attitudes toward nurses' discussing sexual issues. The factors investigated for possible influence on clients' attitudes included: age, sex, race, marital status, occupation, education, current importance of sexual activity, frequency of discussing sexual relationship with partner, and the number of others with whom sexual concerns are discussed. The primary question asked was "Do you believe that nurses should discuss sexual concerns with their patients?" The sample included 88 people between the ages of 25 and 75 years.

The results indicated that most people (92%) believe it is appropriate for nurses to provide sexual counseling for clients at some times. Only two factors were significant predictors of attitudes: race and the number of others with whom sexual concerns were discussed.

Implications: Nurses can generally expect clients to react favorably to a discussion of sexual concerns, and the nurse should initiate these discussions. Because clients' attitudes about discussing sexuality concerns with the nurse is not influenced by age, marital status, or education, nurses need to be careful not to limit sexual concerns to certain categories of clients.

Source: J Waterhouse and M Metcalfe, Attitudes toward nurses discussing sexual concerns with patients, *Journal of Advanced Nursing*, September 1991, 16:1048–54.

FACTORS INFLUENCING SEXUALITY

Many factors influence a person's sexuality: developmental level, culture, religious values, personal ethics, disease processes, and medications.

DEVELOPMENTAL LEVEL

The development of sexuality begins with conception and changes throughout the life span. Every society develops expectations about acceptable forms of sexual expression. Table 17–1 on page 328 outlines characteristics of sexual development throughout life, with nursing interventions and teaching guidelines for each developmental stage.

CULTURE

All cultural groups have their own practices and values relating to sexuality. Many North Americans have strong negative attitudes about homosexuality; in a number of subcultures, however, homosexual behavior is tolerated, and in some instances it has become an integral part of rituals such as coming of age.

Table 17–1 Sexual Development Through Life

Stage	Characteristics	Nursing Interventions and Teaching Guidelines
Infancy: Birth to 18 Months	Given gender assignment of male or female. Differentiates self from others gradually. External genitals are sensitive to touch. Male infants have penile erections; females, vaginal lubrication. Dress and toys are gender oriented.	Self-manipulation of the genitals is normal, not "bad."
Toddler: 1–3 Years	Continues to develop gender identity. Develops control over bladder and bowels. Able to identify own gender.	Permit toddler to indicate readiness for toilet training. Rigid measures may result in compulsive behavior. Body exploration and genital fondling is normal. Use correct names for body parts. Children from single-parent homes should have contact with adults of both sexes.
Preschooler: 4 and 5 Years	Becomes increasingly aware of self. Explores own and playmates' body parts. Learns correct names for body parts. Learns to control feelings and behavior. Focuses love on parent of the opposite sex.	Answer questions about "where babies come from" honestly and simply. Parental overreaction to exploration of genitals and masturbation can lead to feelings that sex is "bad."
School age: 6–12 Years	Tends to have friends of the same sex. Has increasing awareness of self. Continues self-stimulating behavior.	Provide explanations of places, times, and relationships for sexual expression within the religious and cultural values of the family.
Adolescence: Early: 12–13 Years; Middle: 14–16 Years; Late: 17–18 or 20 Years	Primary and secondary sex characteristics develop. Menarche takes place. Develops relationships with the opposite sex.	Requires information about body changes. Peer groups have great importance at this time and assist in forming sexual roles. Dating helps adolescents prepare for adult roles.

Different groups hold diverse attitudes about husband/wife roles, childhood sexuality, nudity, and appropriate sexual behavior. Because clients (and, often, colleagues) may differ in their approaches to sexuality, nurses must be aware of and consider cultural factors when approaching sexual issues in health care. As simple a practice as giving a bed bath can have sexual implications, depending on the cultural traditions of the client and/or nurse. See Chapter 15 for additional information about culture.

RELIGIOUS VALUES

Religion influences sexual expression. It provides guidelines for sexual behavior and acceptable circumstances for the behavior, as well as prohibited sexual behavior and the consequences of breaking the sexual rules. The guidelines or rules may be detailed and rigid or broad and flexible. For example, some religions view forms of sexual expression other than male-female intercourse as unnatural and hold virginity before marriage to be the rule.

Many religious values conflict with the more flexible values of society that have developed over the last few decades (often labeled the "sexual revolution"), such as the acceptance of premarital sex, unwed motherhood, homosexuality, and abortion. These conflicts create marked anxiety and potential sexual dysfunctions in some individuals. See Chapter 16 for additional information about religious values.

PERSONAL ETHICS

Although ethics is integral to religion, ethical thought and ethical approaches to sexuality can be viewed separately. Many individuals and groups have developed written or

Table 17–1 *continued*

Stage	Characteristics	Nursing Interventions and Teaching Guidelines
Adolescence *continued*	Masturbation is common. May participate in sexual activity.	Parents share values and beliefs regarding behavior. Teenagers require information about contraceptive measures and precautions to take in regard to sexually transmitted disaeases (STDs).
Young Adulthood: 20–40 Years	Sexual activity before marriage is common. Many prefer cohabitation instead of marriage; however, many marry and start families by age 30. Establishes own life-style and values. Many couples share financial obligations and tasks around the home.	Young adults often require information about measures to prevent unwanted pregnanacies (ie, abstinence or contraceptive devices). Require information to prevent STDs. Regular communication is required to understand partner's sexual needs and to work through problems and stresses.
Middle Adulthood: 40–65 Years	Men and women experience decreased hormone production. The menopause occurs in women, usually anywhere between 40 and 55 years. The climacteric occurs gradually in men. Quality rather than the number of sexual experiences becomes important. Divorce is common. Individuals establish independent moral and ethical standards.	Women and men may need help adjusting to new roles. People may require counseling to help them reevaluate and direct their energies. Encourage couples to look at the positive aspects of this time of life.
Late Adulthood: Young-Old: 65–74 Years; Middle-Old: 75–84 Years; Old-Old: 85 Years and Older	Interest in sexual activity may continue. Sexual activity becomes less frequent. Women's vaginal secretions diminish, and breasts atrophy. Men produce fewer sperm.	Elderly people can continue sexual activity. Couples may require counseling about adapting their affection and sexual needs to physical limitations.

unwritten codes of conduct based on ethical principles. What one person views as bizarre, perverted, or wrong may be completely natural and right to another. Examples include masturbation, oral or anal intercourse, and cross-dressing. Many people accept sexual expression of various forms if it is performed by consenting adults, is practiced in privacy, and is not harmful.

HEALTH STATUS

Healthy minds, bodies, and emotions are necessary for sexual wellness. Many factors can interfere with a person's expression of sexuality.

Heart Disease Heart disease frequently influences sexual expression. Clients experiencing or at risk for myocardial infarction are often anxious about their sexuality and sexual activity. Concerns about the effect of sexual activity on the heart may cause people to restrict or avoid sexual activity.

Diabetes Mellitus Many men with long-term diabetes mellitus develop erectile dysfunction related to neurologic changes associated with the disease process. Women who have diabetes may experience orgasmic dysfunction (loss of ability for orgasm), difficulty experiencing arousal, loss of vaginal lubrication, and painful intercourse related to a *Monilia* infection of the vagina. The latter commonly occurs with diabetes.

Spinal Cord Injury Because the level of the injury to the spinal cord determines the effect on sexual functioning, individuals may be capable of erection and ejaculation

EFFECTS ON SEXUAL FUNCTION BY SELECTED TYPES OF DRUGS

- Loss of sexual desire: antianxiety medications, antidepressants, antihypertensives, diuretics, hormonal preparations
- Diminution or erectile dysfunction: antiarrhythmics, anticholinergics, antipsychotic medications
- Orgasmic or ejaculatory dysfunction: antidepressants, antihypertensives, antianxiety medications

and be fertile, may have psychogenic or reflexogenic genital arousal, or may have no physiologic genital responses.

Surgical Procedures Any surgical procedure has the potential to alter a person's body image, especially when the surgery involves mutilating, removing, or altering parts of the body. Examples include amputation of a leg, radical neck surgery, excision of large portions of the lower jaw, and ostomies. Impact is even greater when the surgery alters or removes body parts linked directly with sexual functioning, for instance, mastectomy, hysterectomy, and vaginal excision in women; orchiectomy (removal of the testicles) and penectomy in men. Feelings of ugliness and loss of masculinity or femininity are common after these surgeries.

Many men fear that prostatectomy can cause impotence and may delay seeking medical advice and treatment. Most surgical approaches for prostatectomy, however, do *not* result in impotence. Because of anatomic changes in the posterior urethra following a prostatectomy, retrograde ejaculation sometimes results; after ejaculation the seminal fluid enters the bladder and is excreted in the urine. This affects fertility. In most instances, the man may resume sexual activity in 6 to 8 weeks. The client needs to know that ejaculate will be decreased or absent and the urine is often cloudy.

Some radical prostatectomies (eg, radical perineal prostatectomy) performed for cancer of the prostate may cause impotence because of damage to the nerves responsible for producing erections. However, surgeons are now performing nerve-sparing radical prostatectomies that maintain sexual function in certain clients (Moore et al 1992, p. 59).

Joint Disease Joint disease may indirectly affect sexual function because of pain, stiffness, loss of joint motion, and fatigue. Such symptoms influence sexual motivation, and sexual positioning and methods.

Chronic Pain Chronic pain that accompanies many chronic illnesses often decreases sexual motivation. Altered positions for coitus may be necessary, and alternative ways to express sexual stimulation and warmth may need to be emphasized.

Sexually Transmitted Disease (STD) There are numerous sexually transmitted diseases (STDs), including acquired immune deficiency syndrome (AIDS), gonorrhea, syphilis, chlamydial urethritis (nongonococcal urethritis [NGU]), herpes genitalis, trichomoniasis, and genital warts. For clinical signs of these diseases, see Table 17–7, later in this chapter. The presence of an STD in one partner induces fear of transmission in the other, often resulting in abstinence of sexual contact. In some situations, the presence of an STD is unknown and transmission occurs.

Many STDs can be treated quickly and effectively. Others may have serious consequences. For example, women may develop pelvic inflammatory disease (PID) resulting in damage to the reproductive structures and possible infertility. AIDS has no effective treatment. The anxiety about AIDS transmission has caused many individuals to alter their sexual behavior, such as using a condom during intercourse.

Mental Disorders Because the mind and thought processes are involved in sexual functioning, any impairment of the mind may affect sexual expression. For example, depression lowers libido and can affect both the depressed and nondepressed partner. Some clients with mental disorders may behave in an inappropriate sexual manner, such as touching their genitals or removing their clothing. Other clients, such as those with Alzheimer's disease, may not remember any previous sexual contact with their partners.

Medications Many medications prescribed by physicians and essential for therapy have side effects that affect sexual functioning. The box above lists common side effects of selected medications. Some people also take drugs to enhance sexual motivation. See page 336.

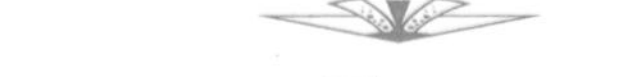

SEXUAL EXPRESSION

Sexual expression varies greatly among people. The nurse's personal sexual preference of sexual expression may not be that of the client. Some people may be involved sexually with one or more long-term partners; others have concurrent relationships with several partners.

The manner of sexual expression (eg, sexual stimulation and sexual positions) also varies. In addition, the frequency of sexual expression and the kind of foreplay (activity before intercourse) also vary. Forms of sexual expression include gender-role behavior, sexual stimulation, and sexual intercourse.

Gender-Role Behavior

Gender-role behavior is the outward expression of a person's sense of maleness or femaleness as well as the expression of what is perceived as gender-appropriate behavior. Even newborns are influenced by expectations regarding gender-appropriate role behavior, and this influence continues throughout life. Each society or culture establishes boundaries for acceptable gender-role behavior. Congruence between an individual's gender identity and expression of role behavior is the ideal, but this ideal is not always easy to achieve.

Physical structure, variations in the internal sense of what is male or female, family values, and cultural values all influence gender-role behavior. As a result, the limits of appropriate gender-role behavior are fairly flexible in North America. Expected adult male roles include breadwinner, heterosexual lover, father, and athlete. Expected male behaviors include wearing trousers, demonstrating physical strength, and expressing feelings in a controlled fashion. Women are expected to express their emotions more freely and to be more gentle in their physical responses; they also have a broader choice of clothing than men.

These descriptions represent the kinds of gender-role behaviors that are reinforced in our society. However, many individuals today express themselves with gender-role behaviors that do not conform to these stereotypes. This stretching of the boundaries can create stress for the individual and for society. Though there has been more variation in gender roles and gender-role behavior in recent years, these variations frequently are still portrayed as aberrant, humorous, or wrong.

In actuality, however, many people are challenging these stereotypes. Men sport long hair, earrings, and cosmetics. Women wear construction boots, jeans, and men's suits. Men make loving and sensitive single fathers. Women are capably functioning as competitive and assertive executives and world leaders. Openly gay male and lesbian relationships are on the increase. Sexual activity in older adults is common. Such gender-role behaviors are legitimate expressions of the self as a sexual being. All individuals need sanction of and support for those gender-role behaviors that validate their sense of self. Labeling these behaviors as aberrant and intervening for change should rightly occur only when the behaviors create significant problems for individuals and their relationship with the world.

Sexual Stimulation

The sexually functional human is capable of responding to a wide variety of physical and psychologic stimuli. These sexually arousing stimuli, often called **erotic,** may be real or symbolic. In the right circumstances, imagination, sight, hearing, smell, and touch can all invoke sexual arousal.

Physical Stimulation Physical stimulation involves touch and/or pressure to parts of the body and may be applied by one's self, by another's body contact or by inanimate objects. Examples include kissing, stroking, hugging, squeezing, breast stimulation, manual stimulation of the genitals, oral-genital stimulation, and anal stimulation. Any of these may be engaged in for sexual pleasure on their own or as a prelude to genital intercourse. Physical stimulation used as a prelude to intercourse is called **foreplay** or **precoital stimulation.** Physical stimulation used for sexual pleasure is called **sex play.** Wide variations exist in the amount and types of physical stimulation used.

Certain parts of the body are richly supplied with nerve endings and give sexual pleasure when stimulated. These areas are called **erogenous zones.** There is also a psychologic component that involves the linking of particular stimuli to a sexual context. The most common erogenous zones are, of course, the genitals of both sexes. Other areas include the breasts, the mouth, thighs, buttocks, earlobes, neck, and anus; however, stimulation of any body area can become sexually arousing. Erogenous zones adapt rapidly to continuous stimulation by becoming decreasingly responsive. Because touch and pressure receptors respond better to *changes* in stimulation, sexual arousal can be increased by alternating sites of stimulation rather than stimulating one or two areas continuously.

Kissing, which involves the senses of touch, taste, and smell, is unique to humans as a source of erotic stimulation. This type of sexual stimulation ranges from lip-to-lip kissing to deep tongue kissing. Stroking, hugging, and squeezing are behaviors that vary according to the preferences of the individuals involved, extending from light, gentle hugging and stroking, through firm, energetic hugging and stroking, to hard squeezing, pinching, biting, and scratching. These last examples involve some pain, which can be erotically stimulating when engaged in *voluntarily* by sexual partners.

Oral or manual stimulation of the female breasts can produce sexual pleasure. Stimulation of the breasts causes the release of the pituitary hormone oxytocin, which stimulates milk secretion and may cause smooth muscle contractions in the uterus and related structures. Breast stimulation thus can produce pleasurable contractions in the pelvic region. These sensations can be a source of sexual satisfaction on their own and may lead to orgasm, or breast stimulation may be used as an adjunct to other sexual interaction. Breast-feeding mothers may also experience these contractions and the release of milk during sexual stimulation. They should be reassured that this is a healthy phenomenon. Stimulation of men's nipples may also produce erotic responses.

Manual stimulation of the genitals may be used to produce **orgasm** (climax of sexual excitement) or as a prelude to sexual intercourse. Manual self-stimulation is called **masturbation.** Reciprocal manual stimulation is called **mutual masturbation.** Stimulation of the penis generally produces a more erotic response than stimulation of the scrotum. The most common form of male masturbation is firm gripping and stroking of the shaft and glans of the penis. Light rubbing or tugging at the **frenulum** (the fold of tissue that connects the lower surface of the glans to the prepuce) can also produce sexual excitement. Whatever method is used, as sexual excitement increases, manipulation often becomes more rapid and intense, until **ejaculation** (expulsion of seminal fluid and sperm) occurs. After ejaculation, the glans penis is often hypersensitive to touch.

Stimulation of the **clitoris** is usually a major erotic focus for females. This highly sensitive area rarely requires direct stimulation. Rubbing pressure on the **mons pubis (mons veneris),** pulling or rubbing the clitoral hood (prepuce), or pulling on the labia stimulate the clitoral shaft and produce intensely erotic responses. Some women use external manipulation as well as insertion of fingers into the vagina to produce sexual excitement.

Masturbation in itself is neither physically nor mentally harmful. It is very common in preschool children and is often associated with comfort and pleasure. Most men begin to masturbate earlier in life (often before the age of 20 years) than women. Some individuals use sexual implements when masturbating, including vibrators, artificial penises, and other genital substitutes.

There are three forms of oral-genital stimulation: cunnilingus, fellatio, and soixante-neuf. **Cunnilingus** is oral stimulation (kissing, licking, or sucking) of the female genitals, including the mons pubis, vulva, clitoris, labia, and vagina. **Fellatio** is oral stimulation of the penis by licking and sucking. **Soixante-neuf** ("69") is simultaneous oral-genital stimulation by two persons. These practices, like other physical stimulation, may be engaged in for the pleasure they give, including orgasm, or as a prelude to genital intercourse. As with masturbation, there is no evidence that oral-genital contact is harmful. However, some people hold strong negative feelings about these behaviors.

Anal stimulation can be a source of sexual pleasure, because the anus is richly innervated. Oral-anal stimulation is called **anilingus.** Stimulation may also be applied by hands or by sex aids such as vibrators. Because the anus is associated with feces, many people do not include anal stimulation in their sexual repertoire.

Psychologic Sexual Stimulation Although the excitatory process involves physiology, erotic stimulation through smell, taste, hearing, sight, or fantasy is considered psychologic because the responses relate to thought processes and feelings. The stimuli evoke pleasant past experiences or hopes and desires. Certain odors (eg, body odors, perfumes, leather, flowers) can produce erotic responses in sexual situations.

Because of their specific associations, certain sights can also produce erotic responses. The more obvious sights include naked bodies and pictures of naked bodies and sexual acts. Other less obvious sights include romantic photographs, decor, lighting, and colors.

Sexual excitement is often enhanced by sound. The spoken word and music are frequent adjuncts to sexual activity. "Whispering sweet nothings" and "talking dirty" are examples. Music is frequently associated with specific sexual situations.

Most people engage in **sexual fantasy.** The fantasizing usually involves idealized sexual situations but may also include so-called forbidden fantasies: mental imagery of unusual or risqué activities that are out of bounds in real life. People engage in fantasy both during masturbation and when with a partner.

Sexual Intercourse

Physiologic responses to sexual stimulation are basically the same for all individuals, male or female. However, such responses are highly variable, with differences occurring between males and females, among members of the same sex, and in the same person at different times. The most common form of sexual activity with a partner is heterosexual **genital intercourse,** also known as **coitus** or **copulation.** Penile-vaginal intercourse can be both physically and emotionally satisfying. There are a variety of positions for this kind of intercourse; the most common is lying face to face (with female or male on top). Side-lying, standing, sitting, and rear-entry positions are also used. Side-lying, female-on-top, and rear-entry positions facilitate clitoral stimulation, either by penile contact or manual contact. The choice of intercourse positions and activities depends on physical comfort and beliefs, values, and attitudes about different practices.

The other form of genital intercourse is **anal intercourse,** during which the penis is inserted into the anus and rectum of the partner. Anal intercourse is most commonly practiced by gay men, but some heterosexual couples engage in it as well. Positions for anal intercourse are similar to those for penile-vaginal intercourse, with minor differences due to the position of the anus.

Current practice dictates the use of a condom in both forms of intercourse to prevent the transmission of disease. Because anorectal tissue is not self-lubricating, a lubricant must be used on the condom. Also, since normal bacterial flora from the bowel can produce infection in other parts of the body, the used condom should be removed and another applied before inserting the penis into other body orifices. (Condoms are used for contraception as well as for preventing sexually transmitted diseases. See the discussion of sexual health teaching, later in this chapter.)

Lesbians and gay men engage in a variety of sexual activities that collectively can be labeled intercourse. Oral sex, manual sex, frottage (body rubbing), and the use of sex aids are among these. There is no evidence that this type of sexual interaction is less satisfying than heterosexual penile-vaginal intercourse.

VARIANT FORMS OF SEXUAL EXPRESSION

Variant forms of sexual expression, some of which are illegal and harmful to others, include **transvestism** (cross-dressing, or adopting the dress and, often, the behavior of the opposite sex); **sadomasochism bondage** (heterosexual or homosexual activities that involve inflicting pain or experiencing pain during sexual stimulation; can involve being tied up, hitting, whipping, pinching, scratching, and other activities); and **pedophilia** (sexual acts with children).

Nurses may also care for clients who act out sexually or who are sexually aggressive toward or harass other clients or the nurse. Such behaviors infringe on the rights of others or are harmful to others. Nurses need to recognize this behavior as unacceptable but also recognize it as a possible expression of a sexual concern or problem that the client may be experiencing.

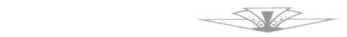

SEXUAL RESPONSE CYCLE

Two primary physiologic changes occur during sexual arousal: **Vasocongestion** (congestion of the blood vessels in the genital area) and **myotonia** (increased muscle tension). Physiologic changes have been identified in one model of physiologic response that fall into four phases: excitement, plateau, orgasm, and resolution (Masters & Johnson 1966, p. 4). Table 17–2 on page 334 summarizes the physiologic changes associated with each of the phases of the sexual response cycle in both males and females. It is important to remember that many individual variations in this cycle fall within the norm.

During the **excitement phase,** erotic stimuli cause a gradual increase in the level of sexual arousal. This phase may last minutes to hours. The **plateau phase,** the period during which sexual tension increases to levels nearing orgasm, may last from 30 seconds to 3 minutes. The **orgasmic phase** is the involuntary climax of sexual tension, accompanied by physiologic and psychologic release. This phase is considered the measurable peak of the sexual experience. Although the entire body is involved, the major focus of the orgasm is felt in the pelvic region. The orgasmic phase is short, lasting 3 to 10 seconds. The **resolution phase,** the period of return to the unaroused state, may last 10 to 15 minutes after orgasm, or longer if there is no orgasm.

ALTERED SEXUAL FUNCTION

The ability to engage in genital intercourse is of great importance to most people. Many people experience transient problems with their ability to respond to sexual stimulation or to maintain the response. Problems are classified as primary or secondary. **Primary sexual dysfunction** results from a problem that has always been present or is longstanding. **Secondary sexual dysfunction** is a new occurrence in a previously asymptomatic individual. It is often the outcome of other health problems or treatments. Nurses are involved in the initial assessment of both types of dysfunctions.

MALE DYSFUNCTION

Common concerns for the male are the ability to achieve and maintain an erection and to develop orgasmic timing with the partner. For women, common concerns relate to their ability to become and stay aroused and to achieve orgasm.

The inability to achieve or maintain an erection sufficient for sexual satisfaction for the self and/or partner is called **erectile dysfunction.** Many believe that the term **impotence,** also commonly used, is inappropriate, because for many clients it has negative connotations. All men have transient interferences with the ability to attain and maintain erection.

Erectile dysfunction becomes a problem when it interferes significantly with the client's ability to satisfy himself or his partner. Such interference may occur consistently in all sexual situations, with or without a partner, or it may occur only in certain situations, such as with one partner but not with others, or with masturbation. A man with primary erectile dysfunction has never been able to achieve an erection sufficient for intercourse. A man with secondary erectile dysfunction has functioned adequately for some time before developing erectile dysfunction. Both types of erectile dysfunction can be caused by physiologic or psychologic factors, but primary erectile dysfunction is more often associated with psychologic factors. Physiologic factors include the following:

- Neurologic disorders created by spinal cord injuries, injury to the genitals or perineal nerves, extensive surgery such as abdominal-perineal bowel resections, radical perineal prostatectomy, diabetes mellitus, multiple sclerosis, and Parkinson's disease

Table 17–2 Physiologic Changes Associated with the Sexual Response Cycle

Phase of the Sexual Response Cycle	Signs Present in Both Sexes	Signs Present in Males Only	Signs Present in Females Only
Excitement	Increased muscle tension Moderate increase in heart rate, respirations, and blood pressure Sex flush (less prevalent in men than in women; present in 75% of women) Nipple erection (60% of men and most women)	Penile erection Tensing, thickening, and elevation of the scrotum Partial elevation and increase in size of testicles	Enlargement of the clitoral glans Vaginal lubrication Widening and lengthening of vaginal barrel Separation and flattening of the labia majora Reddening of the labia minora and vaginal wall Breast tumescence (enlargement) and enlarged areolae
Plateau	Increased voluntary and involuntary myotonia Abdominal, intercostal, anal, and facial muscle contraction Accelerated heart rate and respiratory rate, and increased blood pressure Sex flush (appearance in some men late in the phase; spread over the entire body in women)	Increase in penile circumference, at the coronal ridge, and deepening of color 50% increase in testicular size, and elevation close to the perineum Appearance of a few drops of mucoid secretions from the bulbourethral glands at tip of penis; may contain sperm	Retraction of the clitoris under the hood Appearance of the orgasmic platform, increase in the size of the outer one-third of the vagina and the labia minora Slight increase in the width and depth of the inner two-thirds of the vagina Further reddening of the labia minora Appearance of a few drops of mucoid secretion from the Bartholin's glands to lubricate inner labia Further increase in breast size and areolar enlargement
Orgasmic	Involuntary spasms of muscle groups throughout the body	Rhythmic, expulsive contractions of the penis at 0.8-second intervals	Approximately 5–12 contractions in the orgasmic platform at 0.8-second intervals

- Prolonged use of drugs, such as alcohol, sedatives, heroin, antidepressants, and antipsychotics (phenothiazines)
- Vascular diseases, such as sickle-cell anemia and leukemia
- Endocrine disorders, such as hypothyroidism and Addison's disease.

Psychologic factors are often signaled by a sudden rather than a gradual onset. They may include the following:

- Doubts about one's ability to perform or about one's masculinity
- Fatigue, anger, or stress caused by problems at work, in the family, or in interpersonal relationships
- Traumatic early sexual experiences (eg, rejection)
- Pain, fear, or guilt associated with erection
- Boredom associated with a specific partner

The treatment for erectile dysfunction depends largely on the cause. Penile implants have been used to treat physiologic erectile dysfunction. Erectile dysfunction of psychologic origin often requires a change in both partners' views of sexuality. Awareness of the cause of the condition and exercises designed to increase sensations are also used.

Table 17–2 *continued*

Phase of the Sexual Response Cycle	Signs Present in Both Sexes	Signs Present in Males Only	Signs Present in Females Only
Orgasmic *continued*	Diminished sensory awareness Involuntary contractions of the anal sphincter Peak heart rate 110–180 b/min), respiratory rate (40/min or greater), and blood pressure (systolic 30–80 mm Hg and diastolic 20–50 mm Hg above normal)	Emission of seminal fluid into the prostatic urethra from contraction of the vas deferens and accessory organs (stage 1 of the expulsive process) Closing of the internal bladder sphincter just before ejaculation to prevent retrograde ejaculation into bladder Orgasm may occur without ejaculation Ejaculation of semen through the penile urethra and expulsion from the urethral meatus. The force of ejaculation varies from man to man and at different times but diminishes after the first two to three contractions (stage 2 of the expulsive process)	Contraction of the muscles of the pelvic floor and the uterine muscles Varied pattern of orgasms, including minor surges and contractions, multiple orgasms, or a simple intense orgasm similar to that of the male
Resolution	Reversal of vasocongestion in 10–30 min; disappearance of all signs of myotonia within 5 min Genitals and breasts return to their preexcitement states Sex flush disappears in reverse order of appearance Heart rate, respiratory rate, and blood pressure return to normal Other reactions include sleepiness, relaxation, and emotional outbursts such as crying or laughing	A **refractory period** during which the body will not respond to sexual stimulation; varies, depending on age and other factors, from a few moments to hours or days	

Premature ejaculation occurs when a man is unable to delay ejaculation long enough to satisfy his partner. This usually means that ejaculation occurs after only very limited stimulation of the penis. Often the ejaculation occurs either during penetration (of the vagina, mouth, or anus) or immediately following. The condition may develop when the need for rapid orgasm or performance demands continue over time. To address the problem of premature ejaculation, many sex therapists advise couples to increase sexual communication and responsiveness and to decrease performance demands. The couple together practice sensate exercises (learning to enjoy the sensation of touch without attempting intercourse) and then work together to establish satisfying coitus.

Retarded ejaculation, or **ejaculatory incompetence,** is either the inability to ejaculate into the vagina or a delayed ejaculation. Like erectile dysfunction, retarded ejaculation may have physical or psychologic origins.

FEMALE DYSFUNCTION

Orgasmic dysfunction is the inability of a woman to achieve orgasm. A woman with primary orgasmic dysfunction has never been able to achieve orgasm. A woman with secondary dysfunction has experienced at least one orgasm but is currently nonorgasmic. Orgasmic dysfunction can be caused by drugs, alcohol, aging, and anatomic abnormalities of the genitals. However, most cases have psychologic causes, including hostility between partners, fear or guilt about enjoying the sexual act, and concern about performance. Therapy usually involves helping both partners to establish new attitudes about sex. Pelvic muscle exercises (Kegel's exercises) can also increase the woman's capacity to achieve orgasm by increasing the strength of the pubococcygeal muscle.

Vaginismus is the irregular and involuntary contraction of the muscles around the outer third of the vagina when coitus is attempted—that is, the vagina closes before penetration. Its causes can be severe sexual inhibition, often associated with early learning. Other causes can be rape, incest, and painful intercourse.

Treatment often involves sensate focus exercises and therapy to bring about psychologic changes. In some instances graduated vaginal dilators are used.

Dyspareunia describes the pain experienced by a woman during intercourse, a result of inadequate lubrication, scarring, vaginal infection, or hormonal imbalance. Treatment—such as supplying additional lubrication before intercourse—corrects the underlying cause.

CHANGES IN SEXUAL MOTIVATION

The urge or desire for sexual ativity is called **libido** (sexual motivation, sex drive). Libido fluctuates within each person and varies from person to person. The range of fluctuation in each individual is broad and is considered a problem only when the client (or those interacting with the client) identifies it as interfering with the ability to have satisfying sexual interactions.

DECREASED MOTIVATION

Factors that may contribute to *decreased* sexual motivation include the following:

- *Drugs.* The following decrease sexual drive: all central nervous system depressants (eg, alcohol, barbiturates, sedatives, morphine, heroin, and methadone), estrogens and adrenal steroids in large doses, certain psychotropic drugs, and some antihypertensive agents (eg, reserpine [Serpasil] and methyldopa [Aldomet]).
- *Depression.* This condition slows all body functions and lowers libido. It can affect both the depressed and nondepressed partner.
- *Disease.* Libido diminishes with general ill health and chronic diseases that cause debility or pain. Any disorder that causes dyspareunia (eg, vaginitis, genital herpes, and **imperforate hymen**) also lowers libido.
- *Pregnancy.* Pregnancy affects sexuality if it is associated with physical discomfort, fear of injury to the fetus, or perceived loss of attractiveness. For about 4 weeks following delivery, libido is often reduced due to decreased vaginal lubrication, thinner vaginal walls, pain or fear of pain after an episiotomy, and a slower response to stimulation.
- *Aging.* Older people vary greatly in their sexual motivation. Psychosocial factors, such as beliefs and attitudes about sexual functioning, play an important role in this variation. Physical factors, such as energy levels, pain, and immobility, also have an effect. See the box on page 337 on sexuality and the elderly client.

INCREASED MOTIVATION

Sexual motivation may also be enhanced by a number of various conditions and circumstances. This may or may not be a problem for the individual. Factors contributing to *increased* sexual motivation include the following:

- *Puberty and adolescence.* Both males and females experience increased sexual motivation during puberty and adolescence as a result of hormonal and body changes. This population is at risk of pregnancy and sexually transmitted disease if they do not receive appropriate sex education.
- *Drugs.* Amphetamines and cocaine enhance sexual motivation for some people for short periods. Lysergic acid diethylamide (LSD) and marijuana increase libido in some but inhibit it in others.

ASSESSING SEXUAL HEALTH

Information about a client's sexual health status should always be an integral part of a nursing assessment. The amount and kind of data collected depend on the context of the assessment, that is, the client's reason for seeking health care and how the client's sexuality interacts with other problems. The nurse's professional preparation is another factor that influences the level of sexual health assessment.

Watts (1979, p. 1570) outlines four levels of sexual assessment, each of which requires varying degrees of professional competence:

Level 1 focuses on screening for sexual function and dysfunction. It is conducted by the professional nurse during a health history.

Level 2 is a sexual history conducted by a professional nurse who has postgraduate education in sex education and counseling.

Sexuality Considerations for the Elderly Client

Men

- Erectile dysfunction is not a normal outcome of the aging process.
- Interest in sexual activity is not lost as men age.
- More time is needed to achieve an erection and to ejaculate.
- More direct genital stimulation is required to achieve an erection.
- Volume of ejaculated fluid decreases.
- Intensity of contractions with orgasm may decrease.
- Refractory period after orgasm is longer.
- Testes may decrease in size.
- Performance anxiety may occur with normal changes associated with aging or with medical problems or surgical procedures.
- Possibility of erectile dysfunction (impotence) related to disease, surgery, treatments, and medications increases with age.

Women

- Remain capable of multiple orgasm and may, in fact, experience an increase in sexual desire after the menopause.
- Vaginal lubrication and elasticity decrease with menopause and decreased estrogen.
- Breast tissue loses fat, affecting the shape and size of the breast.
- Phases of the sexual response cycle may require longer to occur.
- Possibility of pain during sexual activity and intercourse (dyspareunia) related to vaginal dryness or chronic health conditions (eg, diabetes or arthritis) increases.

Men and Women

- Many define sexuality far more broadly and include in their definition such things as touching, hugging, romantic gestures (eg, getting roses), comfort, warmth, dressing up, joy, spirituality, and beauty.
- Medications may interfere with sexual functioning and libido. The effects may be dose related; decreasing the dose may reduce or eliminate troubling symptoms.
- Voluntary termination of sexual activity may occur because the person may consider it inappropriate for age or may no longer feel sexually attractive or desirable.
- Loss of partner from illness or death is not uncommon.
- Lack of privacy may be a concern if the person lives with family or in a rehabilitation or nursing home facility.

Sources: C Kain, N Reilly, and E Schultz, The older adult—a comparative assessment, *Nursing Clinics of North America*, December 1990, 25:845; R. Nay, Sexuality and aged women in nursing homes, *Geriatric Nursing*, December 1992, 313–14; F Parke, Sexuality in later life, *Nursing Times*, December 11–17, 1991, 87:40–41; and K Payling, A safe way to reduce the symptoms? Advising women on hormone replacement therapy, *Professional Nurse*, October 1992, 7:37.

Level 3 is a sexual problem history conducted by qualified sex therapists.

Level 4 is a psychiatric and psychosexual history conducted by professionals who are specialized in sex therapy.

Generally, the nurse conducts a sexual history on the following categories of clients:

- Those receiving care for pregnancy, infertility, contraception or STD
- Those whose illness or therapy will affect sexual functioning (eg, diabetes, gynecologic problem, heart disease)
- Those currently experiencing a sexual problem (eg, erectile dysfunction)

Nursing History

Many aspects of sexuality are integrated into the nursing history. For example, the need to collect data about erectile dysfunction in a male who has diabetes may be indicated in the review of the cardiovascular, neurologic, and genitourinary systems. Baldness (integumentary system) may also be important to note as a physiologic influence on sexual self-image.

Collecting such physiologic data for the nursing history does not require extensive or detailed questioning. The screening process of the systems review allows the nurse and client to identify problem areas. For example, answers to the question "Do you have any concerns about the amount or regularity of your menstrual flow?" can give clues to the presence of problems not otherwise

ASSESSMENT INTERVIEW

Sexual Health History

Women

- When did your menstrual periods first begin, and when did you have your last menstrual period?
- What is the usual length of your period in days and usual amount of bleeding?
- Do you have any concerns about the amount or regularity of your menstrual flow?
- If periods are irregular, problematic, or have stopped: Have you been evaluated for this change or done anything yourself to deal with it?
- Are you having any burning with urination, any vaginal itching or discharge, midcycle spotting, pain with intercourse, or any other problems?
- Have you ever been pregnant? (Explore number and outcome of pregnanacies, including miscarriages and induced abortions.)
- How often do you do breast self-examination?
- Is there a history of breast or ovarian cancer in your family?
- When did you have your last Pap smear and mammogram?

Men

- Are you having any difficulty with initiating urination, urinary frequency, or frequent urination at night?
- Are you having any itching or discharge from your penis?
- How often do you do testicular self-examination?
- Is there a history of testicular cancer in your family?

Men and Women

- Are you currently sexually active?
- What type of birth control do you use? Do you have any questions about this method or other methods?
- What do you do to protect yourself from infection when you are sexually active?
- Have you ever had a sexually transmitted disease?
- Has any disease, injury, surgery, medication, or other situation affected your sexual health and happiness or your feelings about yourself as a woman or wife (man or husband)?
- Do you have any questions about your sexual health or functioning, or is there anything else we have discussed that you would like clarified or explained?

identified. Also, questions asked about the functioning of systems directly related to sexuality often provide clients with an opportunity to give clues to sexual concerns or problems. The thoroughness of the sexual assessment is directly related to the potential impact of sexuality on the health problem, or vice versa.

Important psychosexual influences include development, culture, religion, attitudes, and values. Again, specific, detailed questions about psychosexual issues are not necessary in the usual nursing history unless there are clues that potential or actual problems exist. A useful approach to psychosexual assessment is a review of sexual self-concept. Manner of dress, tone of voice, and comments about self and relationships with others can all give the nurse opportunities to explore issues of sexual self-concept more fully. Because illnesses and other health concerns can have a strong influence on sexual concept, assessment of these areas often provides the first clues to client concerns.

The accompanying Assessment Interview box provides questions that the nurse can ask as part of the health history. Notice that lead-in questions are asked before the questions about sexuality.

PHYSICAL EXAMINATION

Physical examination of the female genitals and reproductive tract and the male genitals is part of a routine physical examination in some agencies. Check agency protocol. (See Chapter 22, page 553). If the client has not been examined within 1 year or when data from the recent nursing history indicate a need, the nurse performs a physical examination. Nursing history data indicating the need for a physical examination include the following:

- Suspicion of infertility, pregnancy, or an STD
- Reports of discharge, presence of a lump, or change in color, size, and shape of a genital organ
- Changes in urinary function
- Need for Papanicolaou smear
- Request for birth control

IDENTIFYING CLIENTS AT RISK

Clients at risk for altered sexual patterns include those experiencing

- Altered body structure or function due to disease or trauma, pregnancy, recent childbirth, or anatomic abnormalities of the genitals. Common diseases affecting sexuality are discussed earlier on page 329.
- Physical, psychosocial or sexual abuse; sexual assault.

NURSING DIAGNOSES
CLIENTS WITH SEXUAL/SEXUALITY PROBLEMS

NURSING DIAGNOSIS: Altered sexuality patterns (includes sexual identity, sexuality, and sexual function): The state in which one expresses concern regarding one's sexuality

Related Factors

Impaired relationship with partner; fear of pregnancy, of acquiring an STD, or of coitus following a heart attack; lack of significant other; lack of privacy; body image disturbance; self-esteem disturbance; knowledge/skill deficit about altered body function, illness, medical therapy, or alternative responses to health-related changes.

Defining Characteristics

- Reported difficulties, limitations, or changes in sexual activities or behaviors

---

NURSING DIAGNOSIS: Sexual dysfunction: The state in which an individual experiences an unsatisfactory, unrewarding, or inadequate change in sexual function

Related Factors

Altered body structure or function secondary to disease process, trauma, medical therapy (eg, surgery, radiation); pregnancy; recent childbirth; drugs.

Defining Characteristics

- Verbalization of problem
- Inability to achieve sexual satisfaction
- Values conflict
- Change in sexual motivation
- Change of interest in self and others
- Altered relationship with significant other
- Seeking confirmation of desirability
- Actual or perceived limitation imposed by disease and/or therapy

Sources: LJ Carpenito, *Nursing Diagnosis: Application to Clinical Practice*, 4th ed. (Philadelphia: Lippincott, 1992), pp. 750–72; MJ Kim, GK McFarland, and AM McLane, *Pocket Guide to Nursing Diagnoses*, 5th ed. (St Louis: Mosby-Year Book, 1993), pp. 53–54; GK McFarland and EA McFarlane, *Nursing Diagnosis and Intervention: Planning for Patient Care* (St Louis: Mosby, 1989), pp. 799–813; North American Nursing Diagnosis Association, *NANDA Nursing Diagnoses: Definitions and Classification 1992–1993*, (Philadelphia: NANDA, 1992), pp. 40–41, 45; and JR Lederer, GL Marculescu, B Mocnik, and N Seaby, *Care Planning Pocket Guide: A Nursing Diagnosis Approach*, 5th ed. (Redwood City, CA: Addison-Wesley Nursing, 1993), pp. 178–81.

- Disfiguring conditions, such as burns, skin conditions, birthmarks, scars (eg, mastectomy), and ostomies.
- Specific medication therapy that decreases sexual drive or causes erectile or ejaculatory dysfunction (see the box on page 330).
- Temporary or long-term impaired physical ability to perform grooming and maintain sexual attractiveness.
- Value conflicts between personal beliefs and religious doctrine.
- Loss of a partner.
- Lack of knowledge or misinformation about sexual functioning and expression.

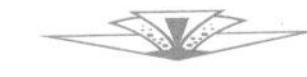

DIAGNOSING

The nursing diagnoses identified by the North American Nursing Diagnosis Association (NANDA 1992, pp. 40–41, 45) relating specifically to sexuality include the following:

- **Altered sexuality patterns**
- **Sexual dysfunction**

These diagnoses, with definitions, contributing factors, and defining characteristics, are shown in the box above. Clinical applications of these diagnoses are shown in Table 17–3 on page 340.

Table 17–3 Clinical Application: Assessment Data Clusters and Related Nursing Diagnoses for Clients with Sexuality Problems

Data Cluster	Nursing Diagnosis
Marsha Ogilvy, 55 years old, reports vaginal burning and pain whenever she and her husband make love. Her last menses was 14 months ago. She says her husband is concerned about the lack of her usual response to lovemaking.	**Sexual dysfunction** related to painful intercourse from inadequate vaginal lubrication
Georgina Honey, 49 years old, had a total mastectomy 2 weeks ago. She says, "I'm sure not going to be sexually appealing to my husband anymore. How on earth will he ever want to make love to me again? I feel like a lopsided oddity."	**Altered sexuality pattern** related to body image disturbance secondary to mastectomy
Larry Stogryn, 52 years old, has a history of hypertension for which he has been taking an antihypertensive (reserpine [Serpasil]). He says he has lost interest in sex in the past few months, and when he does have sex, he has trouble keeping an erection.	**Altered sexuality pattern** related to altered body function secondary to use of antihypertensive medication

Frequently, the nurse makes a high-risk diagnosis of one of the above diagnoses because of risk factors in the client's database or because the client's illness, surgery, or therapies are associated with a high incidence of sexual concerns and problems.

Altered sexuality patterns and **Sexual dysfunction** can also be the etiology of other diagnoses, including the following:

- **Knowledge deficit** (eg, about conception, STDs, contraception, or normal age-related sexual changes) related to misinformation and sexual myths
- **Pain** related to inadequate vaginal lubrication or effects of genital surgery
- **Anxiety** related to loss of sexual desire or functioning
- **Fear** related to history of sexual abuse or dyspareunia
- **Body image disturbance** (mastectomy) related to perceived feelings of rejection by spouse.

PLANNING

The overall client goal for persons with sexual problems is to maintain, restore, or improve sexual health. Some suggested evaluation outcome criteria follow:

- Verbalizes concerns about altered pattern of sexuality:
  a. Body image
  b. Sex role
  c. Desirability as sexual partner
  d. Sexual orientation
  e. Sexual responses
- Verbalizes understanding of
  a. Sexual anatomy and function
  b. Ways to avoid STD
  c. Physiologic changes of pregnancy
  d. Chosen contraceptive device
  e. Factors related to altered sexuality pattern or dysfunction
  f. Alternative modes of dealing with sexual expression
- Verbalizes satisfaction with
  a. Proposed changes in modes of sexual expression
  b. Current sexual practices and responses
  c. Body image
  d. Sex role/relationships
  e. Sexual orientation

See also the Care Planning Guide on page 341 for clients with sexual problems.

IMPLEMENTING

Interventions to meet sexuality needs include one or more of the following activities:

- Teaching (see "Limited Information," on page 342)
- Discussing fears and concerns
- Providing support and encouragement
- Enhancing the client's body image and self-esteem (see Chapter 31)
- Maintaining the client's sexuality by
  a. Providing privacy during intimate body care
  b. Involving the client's partner in physical care
  c. Giving attention to the client's appearance and dress.
  d. Conveying the attitude that people are sexual beings from birth to death
  e. Giving clients privacy to meet their sexual needs alone or with a partner within the context of what is physically safe at this point in recovery

CARE PLANNING GUIDE

CLIENTS WITH SEXUAL/SEXUALITY PROBLEMS

NURSING DIAGNOSIS: Altered sexuality patterns

Outcome Criteria	Nursing Interventions	Rationale
The client		
▪ Verbalizes concerns about altered pattern of sexuality	Provide the client with caregivers who are comfortable discussing sexual concerns and have developed rapport with the client.	Discomfort with sexual topics will be communicated to the client and hinder open expression of thoughts and feelings.
	Offer privacy, and allow sufficient time for client to express concerns.	Clients are more comfortable discussing guilt-ridden, embarrassing, or intimate matters in privacy and need time to verbalize them.
	Allow partner to be involved in discussion *only* if the client wishes.	Client may feel uncomfortable discussing some concerns with the partner present (eg, anxiety about death during coitus or extramarital sex)
	Listen actively.	Assists in validating that the client's message has been understood correctly.
▪ Verbalizes understanding of factors related to altered pattern of sexuality and alternative ways of dealing with sexual expression	Assess client's understanding of reasons for change in sexual functioning or sexual desire.	Enables nurse to identify misinformation and focus on information the client requires.
	Establish a teaching plant that provides appropriate information (eg, need for limitations in sexual activity, altered position or method of sexual activity, effects of prescribed medications on sexual functioning).	Plan ensures that all necessary information is provided.
▪ Verbalizes satisfaction with proposed changes in modes of sexual expression	Encourage open communication between the client and partner.	Helps them verbalize satisfaction or dissatisfaction with plan of care.
	Explore client's and partner's feelings about alternative methods of sexual activity (eg, positioning, oral-genital stimulation, and mutual masturbation).	Adverse feelings about specific alternative methods dictate changes that are inappropriate for these particular people.
	Provide referrals when indicated (eg, to clinical specialist, enterostomal therapist, psychologist).	Unresolved sexuality difficulties require interventions that lie beyond the scope of nursing practice.

SELECTING APPROPRIATE INTERVENTIONS

The interventions the nurse selects are based on the data obtained from the client and the identified nursing diagnoses. Many interventions are directed at preventing high-risk problems and providing knowledge about changes and adaptations to those changes.

The **PLISSIT model of intervention** was developed by Annon (1974) for helping clients with sexual problems. There are four progressive levels of this model represented by the acronym PLISSIT:

P Permission giving
LI Limited information
SS Specific suggestions
IT Intensive therapy

At each level, the nurse provides additional guidance and information to the client and therefore requires more specialized and specific knowledge and skill.

All professional nurses should be able to function at the first two levels.

Permission Giving Clients may feel that they need permission to be sexual beings, to ask questions, to show affection, and express themselves sexually. Giving permission means that the nurse by attitude or word lets the client know that sexual thoughts, fantasies, and behaviors between informed consenting adults are allowed. Giving permission begins when the nurse acknowledges the client's verbal and nonverbal sexual concerns. For example, an older male client with a reduced libido may feel that he cannot discuss sex with the nurse unless the nurse broaches the subject. Other clients may need acknowledgment to feel comfortable about virginity, homosexual activities, oral-genital sex, or masturbation. Often, the nurse can alleviate many sexual concerns by giving the client permission to engage or not to engage in certain sexual behaviors. The nurse conveys the attitude that sexual concerns and needs are important to health and recovery.

Limited Information Clients need accurate but concise information. The nurse might explain what is normal; how some medical conditions, treatments, injuries, or surgeries may affect sexuality and functioning; or how aging may affect sexuality and functioning. The nurse may give the following types of information:

1. General information about sexuality, including
   a. Anatomy and physiology of sexual organs
   b. Stages of sexual development
   c. Breast and testicular self-examination
   d. Sexual response cycles
   e. Coital positions
2. Information specific to the client's needs, such as
   a. Alterations in sexuality made necessary by certain disease processes, medications, surgery, or therapies
   b. Alternative modes of sexual expression
   c. Contraception
   d. STDs and prevention of infection
   e. Pregnancy
   f. Abortion
   g. Infertility

The combination of the first two levels of the PLISSIT model is generally effective in dealing with many sex-related concerns and problems. The nurse requires basic and specific knowledge on sexuality and functioning and how health problems can affect sexual functioning.

Specific Suggestions At this level the nurse requires specialized knowledge and skill about how sexuality and functioning may be affected by a disease process or therapy and what interventions might be effective. The nurse offers suggestions to help the client adapt sexual activity to promote optimal functioning, such as what measures might be used to alleviate vaginal dryness, safe positions for intercourse following a total hip replacement, and safe and unsafe sexual practices following a heart attack. Similarly, nurses on a cardiac unit need specialized knowledge about sexual readjustment during cardiac rehabilitation, and nurses working with clients with spinal cord injuries need information about the sexual consequences of spinal injuries at various levels. For the client with the nursing diagnosis of **Sexual dysfunction** related to neurologic changes secondary to insulin-dependent diabetes mellitus, implementation might involve teaching about etiology, supportive counseling related to self-image, teaching about continued ability to ejaculate, and providing information about options that address erectile dysfunction such as vacuum devices or penile implants.

Intensive Therapy Intensive therapy, provided by a clinical nurse-specialist or sex therapist, is used when the first three levels of counseling are ineffective. It may involve such issues as sexual motivation, marriage, or self-concept.

CLIENT TEACHING

Preventing AIDS and HIV Transmission

- Avoid sexual contact with persons *known* to or *suspected* to have AIDS or HIV infection.
- Practice "safe sex" (no exchanges of body fluids, including semen, urine, feces, or blood; no contact of body fluids with mucous membranes).
- Wear a condom during intercourse, regardless of birth control method being used, unless you have a monogamous partner who you know is not infected.
- Avoid unnecessary transfusions of blood or blood products.
- Encourage autologous transfusions (donation of own blood before surgery) for elective surgery whenever possible.
- Screen all potential blood donors carefully.
- Advise intravenous drug users to use only clean, disposable needles and syringes and not to share drug equipment.
- Provide educational programs on AIDS for the public and school children.
- Use appropriate blood/body fluid precautions with all clients.

Table 17–4 Clinical Signs of Sexually Transmitted Diseases

Disease	Male	Female
Gonorrhea	Painful urination; urethritis with watery white discharge, which may become purulent.	May be asymptomatic; or, vaginal discharge, pain, and urinary frequency may be present.
Syphilis	Chancre, usually on glans penis, which is painless and heals in 4–6 weeks; secondary symptoms—skin eruptions, low-grade fever, inflammation of lymph glands—in 6 weeks to 6 months after chancre heals.	Chancre on cervix or other genital areas, which heals in 4–6 weeks; symptoms same as for male.
Genital warts (condyloma acuminatum)	Single lesions or clusters of lesions growing beneath or on the foreskin, at external meatus, or on the glans penis. On dry skin areas, lesions are hard and yellow-gray. On moist areas, lesions are pink or red and soft with a cauliflowerlike appearance.	Lesions appear at the bottom part of the vaginal opening, on the perineum, the vaginal lips, inner walls of the vagina, and the cervix.
Herpes genitalis (Herpes simplex of the genitals)	Primary herpes involves the presence of painful sores or large, discrete vesicles that last for weeks; vesicles rupture. Recurrent herpes is itchy rather than painful; it lasts for a few hours to 10 days.	Same as for males.
Chlamydial urethritis	Urinary frequency; watery, mucoid urethral discharge.	Commonly a carrier; vaginal discharge, dysuria, urinary frequency.
Trichomoniasis	Slight itching; moisture on tip of penis; slight, early morning urethral discharge. Many males are asymptomatic.	Itching and redness of vulva and skin inside thighs; copious watery, frothy vaginal discharge.
Candidiasis	Itching, irritation, discharge, plaque of cheesy material under foreskin.	Red and excoriated vulva; intense itching of vaginal and vulvar tissues; thick, white, cheesy or curdlike discharge.
Acquired immune deficiency syndrome (AIDS)	Symptoms can appear anytime from several months to several years after acquiring the virus. The person has reduced immunity to other diseases. Symptoms include any of the following for which there is no other explanation: persistent heavy night sweats; extreme fatigue; severe weight loss; enlarged lymph glands in neck, axillae, or groin; persistent diarrhea; skin rashes; blurred vision or chronic headache; harsh, dry cough; thick gray-white coating on tongue or throat.	

PROVIDING SEXUAL HEALTH TEACHING

Providing education for sexual health is an important component of nursing implementation. Many sexual problems exist as a result of sexual ignorance; many others can be prevented with effective sexual health teaching. Examples of important areas of teaching include breast and testicular self-examination (see Chapter 22), prevention of STDs, and contraception.

Preventing Sexually Transmitted Diseases (STDs)

Human immunodeficiency virus (HIV) infection, or acquired immune deficiency syndrome (AIDS), is a health problem of increasing severity. This growing health problem has implications for nurses in health teaching as well as in providing direct care to individuals with AIDS and related conditions. Important issues noted earlier in this chapter, such as nonjudgmental attitudes and the need for accurate information, are vital to the proper understanding and care of individuals with HIV infection. AIDS is an extremely complex and sensitive issue. Information about the specifics of AIDS is available in and best sought from specialty publications, many of which are written specifically for nurses. Specific strategies to prevent AIDS are shown in the box on page 342.

Other STDs are shown in Table 17–4. Note that *Trichomonas* and *Candida* infections can also be acquired nonsexually. Increases in these diseases are due to two factors: (a) changing sexual mores that permit increased sexual activity, and (b) an increase in the number of sexual partners. Because the term *sexually transmitted disease* elicits feelings of guilt, shame, and fear, people frequently do not seek medical help as early as they should. Clients need education about these diseases, preventive measures, and early treatment. Table 17–4 lists common signs of STDs

CLIENT TEACHING

Decreasing Exposure to STDs

- Limit the number of sexual partners.
- Use condoms for protection.
- Abstain from sexual activity with a partner who has symptoms of an STD.
- Report to a health care facility for examination whenever in doubt about possible exposure or when signs of an STD are evident.
- When an STD is diagnosed, notify all partners, and encourage them to seek treatment.

for which people should seek medical care. Ways to decrease exposure to STDs are described in the box above.

Contraception Contraception is the voluntary prevention of conception or **impregnation** (fertilizing or making pregnant). Contraceptive methods include fertility awareness, mechanical and chemical contraception, and surgical procedures. Most people use several methods during their lives, so they need to be familiar with the various methods available. Increasingly, people are choosing methods that do not employ the use of artificial substances within the body. So-called natural methods have long been preferred by people whose religious beliefs conflict with artificial birth-control methods.

Fertility awareness methods depend on identifying the days of the month when conception could take place and abstaining during that time. The nurse providing instruction describes the signs of ovulation (see the box below right) to the client and explains that because conception is possible when a woman is ovulating, she should abstain from heterosexual genital intercourse during that time.

Coitus interruptus is another method that does not employ chemical or mechanical barriers. The man withdraws his penis from his partner's vagina prior to ejaculation. While this is one of the oldest methods of birth control, it has certain disadvantages: It requires considerable self-control; the required constraint may decrease sexual gratification; and some semen may escape into the vagina prior to ejaculation.

Mechanical contraceptive methods (using a condom, diaphragm, or sponge) are also current popular choices. The **intrauterine device** (IUD), a preferred mechanical contraceptive method of the 1970s, is now used less frequently because of complications associated with its use and numerous lawsuits against its manufacturers. The **condom** is a covering sheath placed over the penis prior to intercourse. Since the ejaculate is deposited in the condom rather than in the vagina, the condom should be inspected for holes prior to application. The man or his partner places the condom on the erect penis, leaving a small space at the end of the condom for the ejaculate and rolling down the sheath from the tip to the end of the shaft. For maximum effectiveness, the penis should be carefully withdrawn after intercourse while still erect, with the rim of the condom held to prevent spillage. Should the penis become flaccid, the man should hold the edge of the condom while withdrawing from the vagina to prevent the condom from slipping off and spilling semen.

The **vaginal diaphragm** is a round rubber cup inserted into the vagina and placed over the cervix. It offers greater contraceptive protection than condoms, especially when used with **spermicides** (substances, usually incorporated into jellies or creams, that kill sperm). However, the diaphragm requires proper fitting (including refitting after the birth of a child or a change in body weight of 20 pounds) by trained personnel and yearly replacement. The diaphragm can be inserted by the women or her partner up to 2 hours before intercourse. Longer time spans require additional application of spermicides. For maximum effectiveness, the diaphragm should be left in place for 6 hours following intercourse to ensure that the spermicide has killed all sperm in the vaginal folds. The nurse should instruct the client to hold the diaphragm up to a light periodically and inspect it for holes.

To insert the diaphragm, the woman is instructed to

1. Apply a tablespoon of spermicidal jelly into the cup of the diaphragm and around the rim that will face the cervix.
2. Cup the diaphragm between the thumb and fingers and insert it, cream side up, into the vagina, over the cervix.

FERTILITY AWARENESS: SIGNS OF OVULATION

- Changes in vaginal mucus: when a woman is not ovulating, her mucus is thick and yellow, and sometimes cloudy; it becomes clearer and thinner near the time of ovulation.
- Breast tenderness.
- Tenderness at either side of the lower abdomen.
- Midcycle spotting of blood.
- Changes in basal body temperature: temperature upon arising in the morning drops slightly for 1 to 2 days before ovulation and rises above normal for 1 to 2 days after ovulation.

Table 17–5 Using Oral Contraceptives

Minor Side Effects	Major Side Effects	Contraindications for Use
Nausea	Severe headaches	Cardiovascular disorders (eg, hypertension)
Weight gain	Severe abdominal pain	Severe migraine headaches
Breast tenderness	Blurred vision	Liver disease
Headaches	Chest pain	Diabetes mellitus
Decreased menstrual flow	Thrombophlebitis	Known or increased risk of breast cancer
Spotting	Hypertension	Smoker, over age 40 years
Missed periods		Pregnancy
Vaginal itching		History of thrombophlebitis
Yeast infections		Hyperlipidemia
Transient depression		
Decreased libido		

3. Push the anterior rim of the diaphragm up under the symphysis pubis. (Some women report a popping sensation.)
4. Check its placement by touching the diaphragm with the index finger and feeling the cervix beneath. The **cervix** is a small rounded structure that feels somewhat like the tip of the nose. The diaphragm should be centered over the cervix.

The **vaginal sponge** is a modification of the diaphragm, easier to use and requiring no professional fitting, but less effective as a contraceptive device. It is shaped like a mushroom cap, is saturated with spermicide, and fits into the upper vagina. It is moistened with water and inserted so that the concave surface is over the cervix. Some people maintain that using a diaphragm or sponge inhibits the spontaneity of intercourse; others report finding the genital manipulation necessary for insertion and removal offensive. Many people are successful in incorporating this procedure into their lovemaking experience.

Chemical contraception includes the use of synthetic **estrogen** and **progesterone** (birth control pills, or *oral contraceptives*) and inserting spermicidal foams, jellies, creams, or suppositories into the vagina prior to intercourse. The effectiveness of *spermicides* increases substantially when combined with the use of a condom or diaphragm. *Douching* after intercourse is *not* an effective contraceptive. The client who reports using douching for contraception should be informed that she may actually be increasing her chances for impregnation, as douching may assist the sperm in moving up toward the uterus (Olds et al 1992, p. 177).

Oral contraceptives are preferred by many North American women. The increased estrogen levels suppress ovulation, and increased progesterone levels change the characteristics of the cervical mucus, interfering with the passage of sperm through the cervix. The woman choosing to use birth control pills should be instructed to follow the specific instructions included with her prescription. The nurse should also inform the woman of possible side effects and indications for contacting the primary care provider (ie, the prescribing nurse-practitioner or physician). Table 17–5 lists minor and major side effects of oral contraceptives, as well as conditions contraindicating the use of oral contraceptives. Women using oral contraceptives should be instructed to contact the primary care provider if minor side effects persist. Major side effects are warnings of potentially serious problems and require a physician's immediate attention.

A new hormonal contraceptive, **Norplant,** consists of several subdermal implants of synthetic progestin. Physicians and nurse-practitioners implant the silicone capsules containing the same hormone as in birth control pills, levonorgestrel. It diffuses slowly over time and lasts for up to 5 years (Runner 1992, p. 44). Six capsules are implanted with a special tool in the woman's upper arm, on the inner aspect. The protective contraceptive effect begins 24 hours after implantation. Norplant's initial effectiveness rate of 99.95% decreases to 96% in the fifth year. Women who are not candidates for birth control pills are also not candidates for Norplant, because it contains the same hormone. The implants need to be removed by the physician or nurse-practitioner when the client wishes to become fertile again or when the hormone has been used up. Norplant offers no protection against STDs, so condoms are still necessary. Norplant is the most expensive form of birth control other than surgical sterilization (Runner 1992, p. 47).

COMMON SEXUAL MISCONCEPTIONS

Misconception	*Fact*
Nearly all men over 70 years are impotent.	Sexual desire and ability decrease very little after middle age.
Masturbation causes certain mental instability.	Masturbation is totally harmless.
Sexual activity weakens a person.	There is no evidence that sexual activity weakens a person.
Women who have experienced orgasm are more likely to become pregnant.	Conceiving is not related to experiencing orgasm.
A large penis provides greater sexual satisfaction to a woman than a small penis.	There is no evidence that a large penis provides greater satisfaction.
Alcohol is a sexual stimulant.	Alcohol is a relaxant and central nervous system depressant. Chronic alcoholism is associated with impotence.

Surgical contraceptive methods include tubal ligation and vasectomy. Although other surgical procedures involving reproductive organs (eg, hysterectomy or bilateral orchiectomy) produce infertility, they are not performed for contraceptive purposes. A **tubal ligation** is the tying of a woman's fallopian tubes to interrupt tubal continuity. A small abdominal incision is made below the umbilicus under local or general anesthesia.

A **vasectomy** is the ligation and cutting of the man's vas deferens on either side of the scrotum. The procedure is usually performed under local anesthesia. Sperm are not cleared from the genitourinary system for 4 to 6 weeks (approximately 6 to 36 ejaculations) after a vasectomy. The client should be instructed to use other contraceptive methods during that time span.

CORRECTING SEXUAL MYTHS AND MISCONCEPTIONS

There is an increasing awareness today of sexuality and sexual functioning. Nevertheless, some people still hold certain myths and misconceptions about sexuality. Many of these are handed down in families and are part of the beliefs associated within a particular culture. It is highly important that nurses learn about the beliefs clients hold and that they provide up-to-date information in this regard. Otherwise, misconceptions can negate health teaching and even have an adverse affect on the client's health. See the box above for some common sexual myths and misconceptions.

PROMOTING SAFE SEXUAL EXPRESSION

Clients recuperating from childbirth, for example, or specific illness or disease (eg, heart attack) need instruction about safe sexual activities and the effects that therapy may have on sexual functioning. The following topics need to be considered:

- When sexual activity is safe
- Specific sexual activities that are unsafe, and why
- Adaptations needed for resuming a satisfactory sexual life
- The side effects of prescribed medications on sexual functioning, and the need to notify the physician for possible dose or medication adjustment should problems develop
- Ways to handle ostomy appliances, Foley catheters, casts, or other devices (eg, prostheses) during sexual activity

To promote safe sexual activity, the nurse uses a process of assessing, sharing information, and discussing client concerns.

The *assessment phase* involves asking the client questions and evaluating the answers. For example, the nurse might ask a client recuperating from a heart attack the following questions:

> "Now that you're recuperating and you've had some time to sort out your feelings, have you thought about how your heart attack might alter your sex life?"
>
> "Have you and your partner discussed how you both feel about it?"

Information sharing and discussion should follow each question. In this example, *sharing information* means the nurse informs the client about how his heart attack might affect his sex life, including the following:

WHAT WOULD YOU DO?

CRITICAL THINKING CHALLENGE

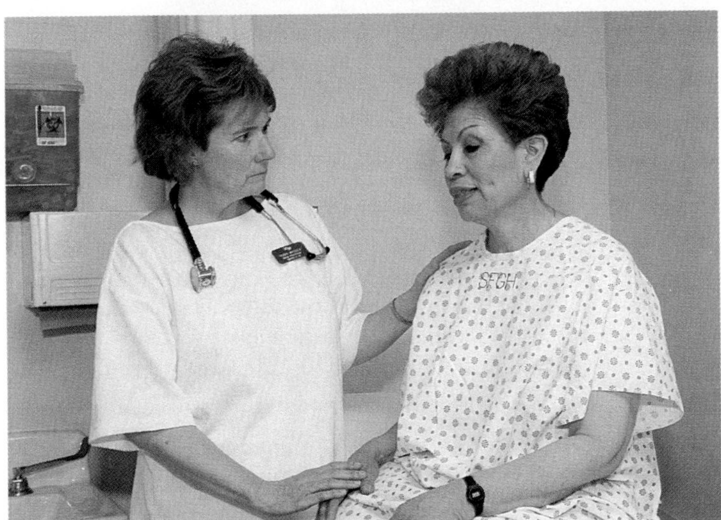

Geri Williams, a 46-year-old female, had a total mastectomy and returns to your clinic for a follow-up examination. When you enter the examination room, Mrs Williams says, "I feel like my husband doesn't want to be close to me."

What would you do?

> "Your heart attack will not alter your capacity for sexual response. Most people can resume intercourse in 4 to 6 weeks, but this should be confirmed by your doctor."
>
> "Many postcoronary clients fear sexual intercourse because of increased heart and respiratory rates associated with it. However, your prescribed program of progressive physical activity will also increase your tolerance for sexual activity."

After sharing information, the nurse should encourage *discussion.* If the nurse cannot answer the client's questions, the nurse refers the client to someone who can. The nurse may offer helpful suggestions during discussion, for example:

> "Many people express concern about the stress of certain positions for intercourse, but you may use whatever position is comfortable for you and your partner, or try side-lying or partner-on-top positions."

DEALING WITH INAPPROPRIATE SEXUAL BEHAVIOR

Nurses may encounter a variety of sexually inappropriate behaviors for a variety of reasons. The behavior may be either aggressive or nonaggressive. Clients may act out sexually by

- Exposing themselves.
- Asking the nurse to provide intimate physical care, such as bathing genital areas, when they are capable of doing this themselves.
- Touching or grabbing the nurse (eg, on the breasts or bottom); trying to pull the nurse into bed.
- Making blatant sexual statements to the nurse.
- Offering the nurse sex.
- Whistling; making comments about the nurse's attractiveness or desirability.
- Making sexual comments to another client in the same room or to visitors about the "sexy" nurse or what they would like to do sexually with the nurse.

Possible reasons for this inappropriate behavior are:

- Fear or anxiety over future ability to function sexually.
- Unmet need for intimacy and sexual closeness because of hospitalization, injury, illness, treatment, lack of a partner, lack of privacy.
- Misinterpretation of the nurse's behavior as sexual or provocative.
- Need for reassurance that they are still sexual beings and still sexually attractive.
- Need for attention.
- Confusion: Neurologic impairment or trauma can lead clients to use profane sexual language, engage in masturbation, expose themselves, or inappropriately touch or grab at the nurse.
- Need to control; clients may be experiencing loss of control over their lives because of hospitalization, injury, or illness.
- Need for power.

NURSING STRATEGIES FOR INAPPROPRIATE SEXUAL BEHAVIOR

- Communicate that the behavior is not acceptable by saying, for example, "I really do not like the things you are saying," or "I see you are not dressed. I will be back in 10 minutes and will help you with breakfast when you get your clothes on."
- Tell the client how the behavior makes you feel: "When you act like that toward me, I don't even want to come into your room. It embarrasses me and makes it hard for me to give you the kind of nursing care you need."
- Identify the behavior you expect: "Please call me by my name, not 'honey'," or "I expect you to keep yourself covered when I am in the room. If you are feeling hot or something is uncomfortable, let me know, and I will try to make you more comfortable."
- Set firm limits: Take the client's hand and move it away, use direct eye contact, and say, "Don't do that!"
- Try to refocus clients from the inappropriate behavior to their real concerns and fears; offer to discuss sexuality concerns: "All morning you have been making very personal sexual comments about yourself. Sometimes people talk like that when they are concerned about the sexual part of their life and how their illness will affect them. Are there things that you have questions about or would like to talk about?"
- Report the incident to your nursing instructor, charge nurse, or nursing clinical specialist. Discuss the incident, your feelings, and possible inter-ventions.
- Assign a nurse who will confront the behavior and relate to the client in a consistent manner.
- Clarify the consequences of continued inappropriate behavior (avoidance, withdrawal of services, no chance to help resolve underlying concerns of client).

- Belief that flirtatious behavior is expected due to influence of media portrayal of nurses as sexy, available, and experienced.

Before implementing any nursing interventions, the nurse should first ensure that the behavior *is* inappropriate and not an attempt to communicate a physical need. For example, clients may expose themselves if they are febrile, pull at the penis if a catheter is uncomfortable or irritating, or reach for the nurse if unable to communicate verbally. Nursing strategies to deal with inappropriate sexual behavior are shown in the box above.

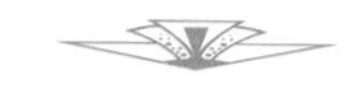

EVALUATING

The nurse uses data collected during care (eg, during health teaching about sexuality or contraception, or correcting myths or misconceptions held by the client) to establish whether client outcomes have been achieved. If any outcomes have *not* been achieved, the nurse should explore the reasons, which may include the following:

- Were risk factors correctly identified?
- Did the client convey all significant fears and concerns about sexuality?
- Was the client more comfortable following discussions about sexual matters?
- Did the client understand the nurse's teaching?
- Was the health teaching compatible with the client's culture and religious values?
- Was the client ready to deal with sexuality problems?

See also Evaluation Checklist on page 158.

CHAPTER HIGHLIGHTS

- Sexuality is important in developing self-identity, interpersonal relationships, intimacy, and love.
- In its broad sense, sexuality involves physical, emotional, social, and ethical aspects of being and behaving.
- An understanding of the structure and function of the male and female genitals is essential for nurses.

- The components that contribute to the development of sexuality are numerous; both biologic and psychologic components exist at all ages.
- In adults many secondary sexual problems are related to illnesses, injuries, and medical therapies.
- During the middle and later years, the genitals undergo physical changes. However, the desire and ability to maintain satisfying sexual relationships can remain.
- Assessing actual or high risk for sexual problems is part of the initial nursing assessment. Assessment should also be carried out when clients or support persons present cues that problems exist or when they have an illness that could cause sexual problems.
- Nurses assess attitudes toward sexuality, including factors that affect attitudes and behaviors.
- An understanding of sexual stimuli and response patterns can help individuals have satisfying sexual relationships. This understanding is also vital for nurses wishing to help clients with psychologic problems, such as feelings of inadequacy, or medical problems, such as spinal cord injuries or myocardial infarctions.
- Common sexual problems of healthy adults are changes in libido, erectile dysfunction, premature ejaculation, retarded ejaculation, orgasmic dysfunction, vaginismus, and dyspareunia.
- Illnesses that commonly affect sexuality include myocardial infarction and diabetes mellitus. Many surgical procedures, including mastectomy, hysterectomy, orchiectomy, and enterostomy, also affect sexual abilities and sexual self-image.
- Nursing diagnoses for clients with sexual problems are related to many contributing factors, including altered body structure or function, lack of knowledge or misinformation about sexual matters, physical or psychologic abuse, value conflicts, and loss or lack of a partner.
- Before assisting clients with sexual problems, nurses must acquire accurate information about sexuality, identify and accept their own sexual values and behaviors as well as those of others, and be comfortable acquiring and disseminating information about sexuality.
- Nursing interventions include helping clients develop awareness of sexuality, giving permission, giving information, and offering suggestions.

READINGS AND REFERENCES

SUGGESTED READINGS

King, J. March/April 1992. Helping patients choose an appropriate method of birth control. *The American Journal of Maternal/Child Nursing* 17(2):91–95.

This article gives suggestions about appropriate birth control measures based on consideration of effectiveness, acceptability, and medical safety for the individual.

Stampfer, M, Colditz, G, Willett, W, Manson, J, Rosner, B, Speizer, F, and Hennekens, C. September 1991. Postmenopausal estrogen therapy and cardiovascular disease. *The New England Journal of Medicine* 325(11):756–62.

This article examines the risks and benefits related to estrogen replacement for menopausal women. The conclusion is that the use of estrogen decreases mortality and morbidity in post-menopausal women and should be considered unless contraindicated.

RELATED RESEARCH

Cleary, P, Van Devanter, N, Rogers, T, Singer, E, Shipton-Levy, R, Steilen, M, Stuart, A, Avorn, J, and Pindyck, J. December 1991. Behavior changes after notification of HIV infection. *American Journal of Public Health* 81:1586–90.

Nay, R. December 1992. Sexuality and aged women in nursing homes. *Geriatric Nursing* 13:312–14.

SELECTED REFERENCES

Andrist, LC. December 1988. Taking a sex history and educating clients about safe sex. *Nursing Clinics of North America* 23:959–73.

Annon, J. 1974. *The Behavioral Treatment of Sexual Problems.* Vol. 1. *Brief Therapy.* New York: Harper & Row.

Carpenito, LJ. 1992. *Nursing Diagnosis: Application to Clinical Practice.* 4th ed. Philadelphia: Lippincott.

Finnis, S and Robbins, I. November 25–December 1, 1992. Tip of the iceberg? *Nursing Times* 88:29–31.

Flaskerud, JD. 1989. *AIDS/HIV Infection: A Resource Guide for Nursing Professionals.* Philadelphia: WB Saunders.

Girts, C. 1990. Nursing attitudes about sexuality needs of spinal cord injury patients. *Rehabilitation Nursing* 15:205–6.

Heinrich, K. March/April 1987. Effective responses to sexual harassment. *Nursing Outlook* 35:70–72.

Kain, C, Reilly, N, and Schultz, E. December 1990. The older adult—a comparative assessment. *Nursing Clinics of North America* 25:833–48.

Kim, MJ, McFarland, GK, and McLane, AM. 1993. *Pocket Guide to Nursing Diagnoses.* 5th ed. St Louis: Mosby-Year Book.

King, J. March/April 1992. Helping patients choose an appropriate method of birth control. *The American Journal of Maternal/Child Nursing* 17:91–95.

Lederer, JR, Marculescu, GL, Mocnik, B, and Seaby, N. 1993. *Care Planning Pocket Guide: A Nursing Diagnosis Approach.* 5th ed. Redwood City, CA: Addison-Wesley Nursing.

Lion, EM, editor. 1982. *Human Sexuality in Nursing Process.* New York: Wiley.

McAndrew, T. January 1990. Elderly sexuality examined. *Pennsylvania Nurse* 45:16.

McCann, M. September 1989. Sexual healing after heart attack. *American Journal of Nursing* 89:1133–38.

McCracken, A. October 1988. Sexual practice by elders: The forgotten aspect of functional health. *Journal of Gerontological Nursing* 14:13–17.

McFarland, GK and McFarlane, EA. 1989. *Nursing Diagnosis and Intervention: Planning for Patient Care.* St Louis: Mosby.

McKenzie, F. May 18–24, 1988. Sexuality after total pelvic exenteration. *Nursing Times* 84:27–30.

Martin, F. March 1990. When the solution is a prosthesis. *RN* 53:32–35.

Masters, WH and Johnson, VE. 1966. *Human Sexual Response.* Boston: Little, Brown.

Moore, S, Kubrik, M, Shea, L, and Kubrik, N. April 1992. Nerve-sparing prostatectomy. *American Journal of Nursing* 92:59–64.

Nay, R. December 1992. Sexuality and aged women in nursing homes. *Geriatric Nursing* 13:312–14.

North American Nursing Diagnosis Association. 1992. *NANDA Nursing Diagnoses: Definitions and Classification 1992–1993.* Philadelphia: NANDA.

Olds, S, London, M, and Ladewig, P. 1992. *Maternal-Newborn Nursing.* 4th ed. Redwood City, CA: Addison-Wesley Nursing.

Parke, F. December 11–17, 1991. Sexuality in later life. *Nursing Times* 87:40–42.

Payling, K. October 1992. A safe way to reduce the symptoms? Advising women on hormone replacement therapy. *Professional Nurse* 7:37–40.

Redefining AIDS. May 1993. *Aliveness Newsletter* 3:1, 5.

Reznichek, C and Reznichek, R. March 1990. The problem most men won't talk about. *RN* 53:28–32.

Rothman, B and Sebastian, H. May 1990. Intimacy and cognitively impaired elders. *Canadian Nurse* 86:32, 34.

Runner, J. June 1992. If you're asking about Norplant. *RN* 55:44–47.

Stockard, S. November 1991. Caring for the sexually aggressive patient. *Nursing91* 21:72–73.

Talashek, M, Tichy, A, and Epping, H. April 1990. Sexually transmitted diseases in the elderly—issues and recommendations. *Journal of Gerontological Nursing* 16:33–40.

Wall-Hass, C. November/December 1991. Nurses' attitudes toward sexuality in adolescent patients. *Pediatric Nursing* 17:549–55.

Waterhouse, J and Metcalfe, M. 1991. Attitudes toward nurses discussing sexual concerns with patients. *Journal of Advanced Nursing* 16:1048–54.

Watts, R. September 1979. Dimensions of sexual health. *American Journal of Nursing* 79:1568–72.

Williamson, M. January/February 1992. Sexual adjustment after hysterectomy. *Journal of Obstetric, Gynecologic, and Neonatal Nursing* 21:42–47.

UNIT

5

Integral Components of Client Care

STUDENT PROFILE

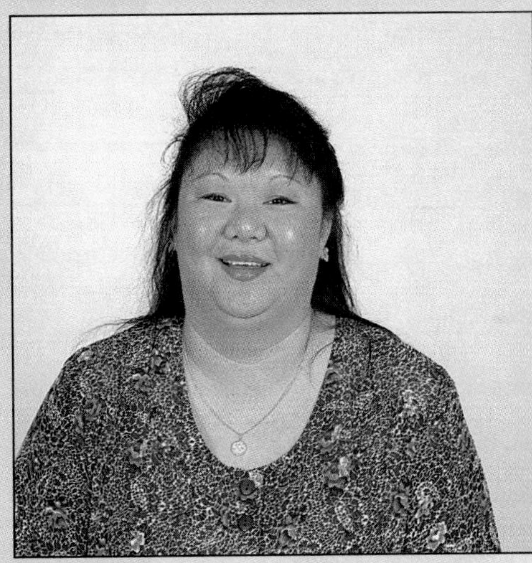

NAME	Margie Sologuren
SCHOOL OF NURSING	Central Florida Community College Ocala, Florida
HOMETOWN	Ocala

WHY DID YOU ENTER THE FIELD OF NURSING?
Nineteen years ago I worked as a nursing assistant while putting my husband through school. After raising three children, I've returned to the medical field.

WHO OR WHAT INFLUENCED THAT DECISION?
My father is a physician and my mother an RN, and I love to care for people. I also want to be independent and self-supporting.

WHAT QUALITIES DO YOU THINK ARE NECESSARY TO BE A GOOD NURSE?
Humility, compassion, self-awareness, and belief in yourself.

WHAT HAS BEEN YOUR MOST GRATIFYING MOMENT AS A STUDENT NURSE?
The daughter of an elderly woman got into a confrontation with her mother's doctor. I was there to comfort both the client, who was upset with the loud verbal exchange, and the daughter, who had a lot to work through.

WHAT ADVICE WOULD YOU GIVE A NEW STUDENT?
Try to focus on nursing as a whole picture, from the micro to the macro (local, state, national, worldwide). Don't be too hard on yourself or pump yourself up above everyone else; be willing to adapt and change.

18 Helping and Communicating

Objectives

Describe four phases of the helping relationship.

Describe essential aspects of communication and the communication process.

Explain the four elements of the communication process outlined in this chapter.

Identify ways in which selected factors influence the communication process.

Differentiate verbal, nonverbal communication.

Give guidelines for assessing problems in communication.

List examples of nursing diagnoses pertaining to communication.

Describe strategies for planning to resolve communication problems.

Describe effective and ineffective methods used by nurses when communicating with clients.

List outcome criteria that can be used to evaluate whether communication problems have been resolved.

Identify features of effective groups.

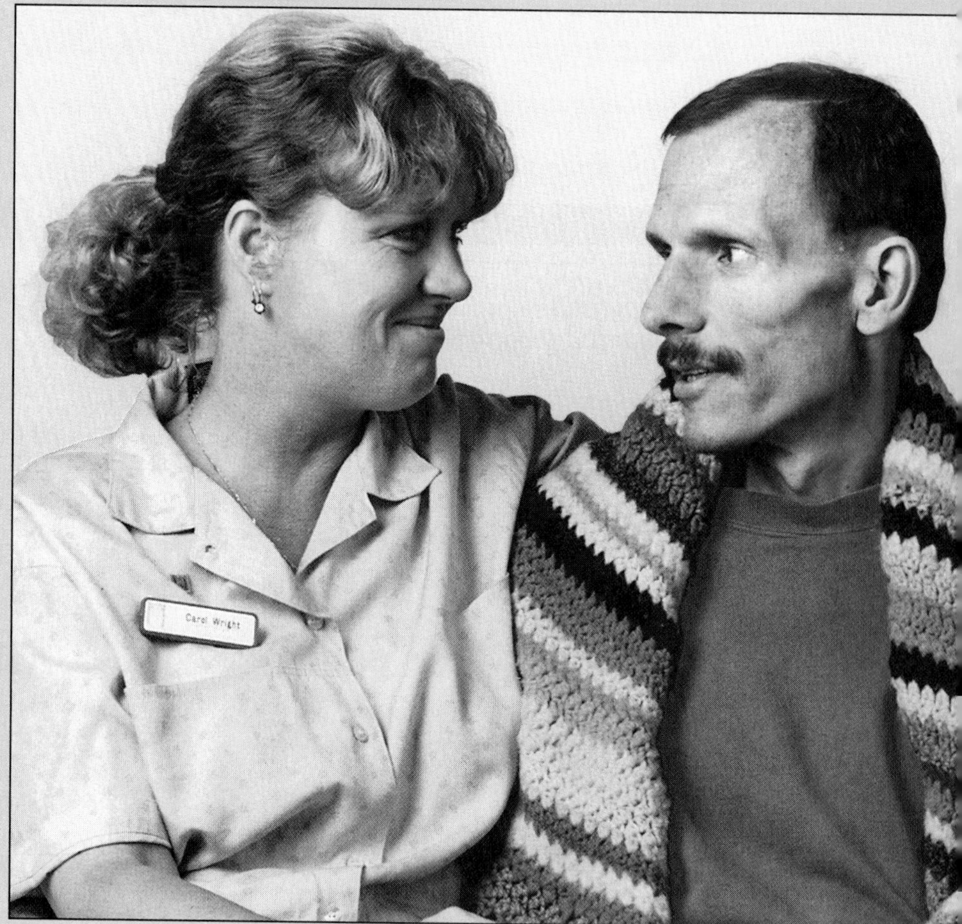

Nurse-client relationships are referred to by some as **interpersonal relationships,** by others as *therapeutic relationships* and by still others as *helping relationships.* Helping is a growth-facilitating process in which one person assists another to solve problems and to face crises in the direction the assisted person chooses (Brammer 1988, p. 5). This **helping (therapeutic) relationship** forms the basis for the caring, which is the hallmark of nursing practice (Thobaben 1991, p. 46). See Chapter 3, page 53, for a detailed discussion of caring. The helping relationship is a dynamic, ever-changing relationship with another human being whose welfare is the focus of the interaction. The nurse helps individuals, caregivers, families, and groups. A helping relationship may develop over weeks of working with a client, or over minutes. The keys to the helping relationship are (a) the development of trust and acceptance between the nurse and the client, and (b) an underlying belief that the nurse cares about and wants to help the client.

The helping relationship is influenced by the personal and professional characteristics of the nurse and the client. Age, sex, appearance, diagnosis, education, values, ethnic and cultural background, personality, expectations, and setting can all affect the development of the nurse-client relationship. Consideration of all these factors, combined with good communication skills and sincere interest in the client's welfare, will enable the nurse to create a helping relationship.

Characteristics of helping relationships are shown in the accompanying box.

Characteristics of a Helping Relationship

A helping relationship

- Is an intellectual and emotional bond between the nurse and the client and is focused on the client.
- Respects the client as an individual:
  - maximizes client's abilities to participate in decision making and treatments.
  - considers ethnic and cultural aspects.
  - considers family relationships and values.
- Respects client confidentiality.
- Focuses on the client's well-being.
- Is based on mutual trust, respect, and acceptance.

Phases of a Helping Relationship

The helping relationship process can be described in terms of four sequential phases, each of which is characterized by identifiable tasks and skills. The relationship must progress through the stages in succession, because each builds on the one before. Nurses can identify the progress of a relationship by understanding these phases: preinteraction phase, introductory phase, working (maintaining) phase, and termination phase. Table 18–1 on page 354 summarizes the tasks and skills required.

Preinteraction Phase

The preinteraction phase is similar to the planning stage before an interview. In most situations, the nurse has information about the client before the first face-to-face meeting. Such information may include the client's name, address, age, medical history, and/or social history. Planning for the initial visit may generate some anxious feelings in the nurse. If the nurse recognizes these feelings and identifies specific information to be discussed, positive outcomes will evolve.

Introductory Phase

The introductory phase, also referred to as the *orientation phase* or the *prehelping phase*, is important because it sets the tone for the rest of the relationship. During this initial encounter, the client and the nurse closely observe each other and form judgments about the other's behavior. The three stages of this introductory phase are opening the relationship, clarifying the problem, and structuring and formulating the contract (Brammer 1988, p. 51). Other important tasks of the introductory phase include getting to know each other and developing a degree of trust.

After introductions, the nurse may initially engage in some social interaction to put the client at ease. For example, the nurse and client may talk about what a nice day it is and what they would like to do if at home.

During the initial parts of the introductory phase, the client may display some resistive behaviors and some testing behaviors. *Resistive behaviors* are those that inhibit involvement, cooperation, or change. They may be due to difficulty in acknowledging the need for help and thus a dependent role, fear of exposing and facing feelings, anxiety about the discomfort involved in changing problem-causing behavior patterns, and fear or anxiety in response to the nurse's approach, which may, in the client's opinion, be inappropriate.

Testing behaviors are those that examine the nurse's interest and sincerity. For example, to test whether the

Table 18–1 Tasks and Skills for Each Phase of the Helping Relationship

Phase	Tasks	Skills
Preinteraction phase	The nurse reviews pertinent knowledge, considers potential areas of concern, and develops plans for interaction.	Recognizing limitations and seeking assistance as required.
Introductory phase		
1. Opening the relationship	Both client and nurse identify each other by name. When the nurse initiates the relationship, it is important to explain the nurse's role to give the client an idea of what to expect. When the client initiates the relationship, the nurse needs to help the client express concerns and reasons for seeking help. Vague, open-ended questions, such as "What's on your mind today?" are helpful at this stage.	A relaxed attending attitude to put the client at ease. It is not easy for all clients to receive help.
2. Clarifying the problem	Because the client initially may not see the problem clearly, the nurse's major task is to help clarify the problem.	Attentive listening, paraphrasing, clarifying, and other effective communication techniques discussed in this chapter. A common error at this stage is to ask too many questions of the client.
3. Structuring and formulating the contract (obligations to be met by both the nurse and client)	Nurse and client develop a degree of trust and verbally agree about: (a) location, frequency, and length of meetings, (b) overall purpose of the relationship, (c) how confidential material will be handled, (d) tasks to be accomplished, and (e) duration and indications for termination of the relationship.	Communication skills listed above and ability to overcome resistive and/or testing behaviors if they occur.
Working phase	Nurse and client accomplish the tasks outlined in the introductory phase, enhance trust and rapport, and develop caring.	
1. Exploring and understanding thoughts and feelings	The nurse assists the client to explore thoughts and feelings and acquires an understanding of the client. The client explores thoughts and feelings associated with problems, develops the skill of listening, and gains insight into personal behavior.	Listening and attending skills, empathy, respect, genuineness, concreteness, self-disclosure, and confrontation. Skills acquired by the client are non-defensive listening and self-understanding.
2. Facilitating and taking action	The nurse plans programs within the client's capabilities and considers long- and short-term goals. The client needs to learn to take risks (ie, accept that either failure or success may be the outcome). The nurse needs to reinforce successes and help the client recognize failures realistically.	Decision-making and goal-setting skills. In addition: For the nurse: reinforcement skills. For the client: risk-taking.
Termination phase	Nurse and client accept feelings of loss. The client accepts the end of the relationship without feelings of anxiety or dependence.	For the nurse: summarizing skills. For the client: abilities to handle problems independently.

nurse will stay for a certain period of time, a client may refuse to talk.

Resistive and testing behaviors can be overcome by conveying a caring attitude, genuine interest in the client, and competency. These behaviors of the nurse also foster the development of trust in the relationship. **Trust** can be described as a reliance on someone without doubt or question, or the belief that the other person is capable of assisting in times of distress and, in all likelihood, will do so. To trust another person involves risk; clients become vulnerable when they share thoughts, feelings, and attitudes with the nurse. Trust, however, enables the client to express thoughts and feelings openly.

By the end of the introductory phase, clients should be begin to

- Develop trust in the nurse.
- View the nurse as a competent professional capable of helping.
- View the nurse as honest, open, and concerned about their welfare.
- Believe the nurse will try to understand and respect their cultural values and beliefs.
- Believe the nurse will respect client confidentiality.
- Feel comfortable talking with the nurse about feelings and other sensitive issues.
- Understand the purpose of the relationship and the roles.
- Feel that they are active participants in developing a mutually agreeable plan of care.

RESEARCH NOTE

Client Teaching: Effective or Not?

Client teaching has long been considered a key role for nurses. Previous research has demonstrated that clients who are well informed experience less pain and report less stress and greater satisfaction than clients who have not received teaching. This study evaluated the quality of client teaching to inpatients in acute care hospitals.

Over the course of one year, the study surveyed 1903 clients who were discharged from medical/surgical wards of an acute care hospital after at least a one-day stay. Within two weeks of discharge, clients were asked to respond to a questionnaire focused on the teaching they received while hospitalized. Approximately 81% (1544 clients) responded. Clients reported general satisfaction with teaching, especially in the areas of medical and surgical treatments; however, they reported low levels of satisfaction with the level of information provided about bedrest, discharge instructions (especially regarding medications), side effects, and what to report to health care providers for follow-up.

Implications: The authors conclude that deficits exist in current client teaching practice. As health care increasingly moves into the community, deficits in discharge teaching may assume greater importance.

Source: J Cortis and A Lacey, Measuring the quality and quantity of information-giving to inpatients, *Journal of Advanced Nursing*, October 1996, 24(4):674–681.

WORKING PHASE

During the working phase of a helping relationship, the nurse and the client begin to view each other as unique individuals. They begin to appreciate this uniqueness and care about each other. *Caring* is sharing deep and genuine concern about the welfare of another person. Once caring develops, the potential for empathy increases.

The working phase has two major stages: *exploring and understanding thoughts and feelings*, and *facilitating and taking action*. The nurse helps the client to explore thoughts, feelings, and actions and helps the client plan a program of action to meet pre-established goals.

Exploring and Understanding Thoughts and Feelings The nurse requires the following skills for this phase of the helping relationship:

- *Empathy* Nurses must communicate (respond) in ways that indicate they have listened to what was said and understand how the client feels. The nurse responds to content or feelings or both, as appropriate. The nurse's nonverbal behaviors are also important. Nonverbal behaviors indicating empathy include moderate head nodding, a steady gaze, moderate gesturing, and little activity or body movement. Two models of empathy may operate: therapeutic and emotional. **Therapeutic empathy** is a learned, conscious way of responding in which the nurse uses various communications techniques to convey understanding of the client's reality. Therapeutic empathy focuses on learned communication skills and problem-solving skills. **Emotional empathy** is the nurse's spontaneous response to the client's condition of distress or need: "the caregiver's intuitive sensing and response to the other's plight" (Morse et al 1992, p. 810).

This model of communication and helping relationships (also referred to as **emotive engagement** or **embodiment**) is seen as the essence of the nurse-client relationship (Morse et al 1992, p. 819). The client's suffering is the trigger that "engages" the nurse who then

COMPONENTS OF GENUINENESS

- The genuine helper does not take refuge in or overemphasize the role of counselor.
- The genuine person is spontaneous.
- The genuine person is nondefensive.
- The genuine person displays few discrepancies—that is, the person is consistent and does not think or feel one thing but say another.
- The genuine person is capable of deep self-disclosure (self-sharing) when it is appropriate.

"embodies" the client's suffering; that is, the nurse actually "feels" the client's distress at some level. Suffering thus becomes a shared experience at both a cognitive and an emotional level. Emotional empathy or bonding requires energy and strength on the part of the nurse. The result is comforting and caring for the client and a helping, healing relationship.

- *Respect* The nurse must show respect for the client's willingness to be available, and desire to work with the client.
- *Genuineness* Personal statements can be helpful in solidifying the rapport between the nurse and the client. The nurse might offer such comments as "I recall when I was in (a similar situation), and I felt angry about being put down." Egan (1982, p. 128) refers to this quality as *genuineness* and outlines five behaviors that are components of it. See the box above. Nurses need to exercise caution when making references about themselves. These statements must be used with discretion. The extreme of matching each of the client's problems with a better story of the nurse's own is of little value to the client.
- *Concreteness* The nurse must assist the client to be concrete and specific rather than to speak in generalities. When the client says, "I'm stupid and clumsy," the nurse narrows the topic to the specific by pointing out, "You tripped on the scatter rug."

During this first stage of the working phase, the intensity of interaction increases, and feelings such as anger, shame, or self-consciousness may be expressed. If the nurse is skilled in this stage and if the client is willing to pursue self-exploration, the outcome is a beginning understanding on the part of the client about behavior and feelings.

- *Self-disclosure* The nurse willingly but discreetly shares personal experiences.
- *Confrontation* The nurse points out discrepancies between thoughts, feelings, and actions that inhibit the client's self-understanding or exploration of specific areas. This is done empathetically, not judgmentally.

Facilitating and Taking Action Ultimately the client must make decisions and take action to become more effective. The responsibility for action belongs to the client. The nurse, however, collaborates in these decisions, provides support, and may offer options or information.

TERMINATION PHASE

The termination phase of the relationship is often expected to be difficult and filled with ambivalence. However, if the previous phases have evolved effectively, the client generally has a positive outlook and feels able to handle problems independently. However, because caring attitudes have developed, it is natural to expect some feelings of loss, and each person needs to develop a way of saying goodbye.

Many methods can be used to terminate relationships. Summarizing or reviewing the process can produce a sense of accomplishment. This may include sharing reminiscences of how things were at the beginning of the relationship and comparing them to how they are now. It is also helpful for both the nurse and the client to express their feelings about termination openly and honestly. Thus termination discussions need to start in advance of the termination interview. This allows time for the client to adjust to independence. In some situations referrals are necessary, or it may be appropriate to offer an occasional standby meeting to give support as needed. Follow-up phone calls are another intervention that eases the client's transition to independence.

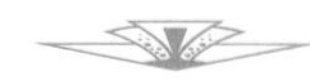

DEVELOPING HELPING RELATIONSHIPS

Whatever the practice setting, the nurse establishes some type of helping relationship in which mutual goals (outcomes) are set with the client or, if the client is unable to participate, with support persons. Although special training in counseling techniques is advantageous, there are many ways of helping clients that do not require special training.

- *Listen actively* (See the discussion of attentive listening, later in this chapter.)
- *Help to identify what the person is feeling* Often clients who are troubled are unable to identify or to label their feelings and consequently have difficulty working them out or talking about them. Responses such as "You

CRITICAL THINKING CHALLENGE

WHAT WOULD YOU DO?

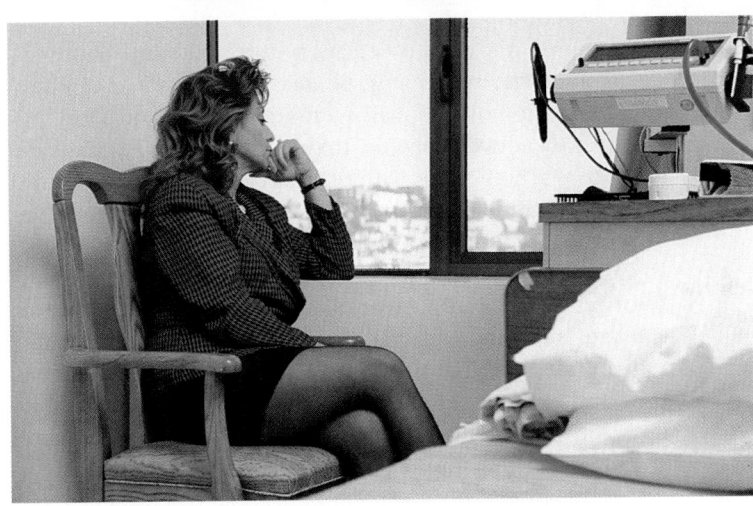

Anna San Luis, a 38-year-old female, has been admitted to the nursing unit for removal of multiple gallstones. When you enter her room to assess her status, you find her looking out the window and crying. When you ask, "Do you need someone to talk to?" Ms San Luis answers, "My boyfriend just dropped me off at the hospital and didn't even come in. I don't think he cares about me or what happens to me."

What would you do?

---

seem angry about taking orders from your boss" or "You sound as if you've been lonely since your wife died" can help clients recognize what they are feeling and talk about it.

- *Put yourself in the other person's shoes (ie, empathize)* Communicate to the client in a way that shows an understanding of the client's *feelings* and the *behavior* and *experience* underlying these feelings.
- *Be honest* In effective relationships nurses honestly recognize any lack of knowledge by saying, "I don't know the answer to that right now"; openly discuss their own discomfort by saying, for example, "I feel uncomfortable about this discussion"; and admit tactfully that problems do exist, for instance, when a client says "I'm a mess, aren't I?"
- *Do not tell a person not to feel* Feelings expressed by clients often make nurses uncomfortable. Common examples are a client's expressions of anger or worry or a client's crying. A nurse who feels this discomfort often responds by saying, "Don't worry about it, everything will be fine," or "Please don't cry." Such responses inhibit the client's expression of feelings. Unless feelings are extremely inappropriate, it is best to encourage the client to ventilate (voice) them. This allows the client to express feelings in words and examine them objectively. Indirectly, such an attitude conveys this message: "Your feelings are not that awful, since I am not bothered by them."
- *Do not tell a person what to feel* Statements that tell clients how they should feel, rather than how they actually do feel, in essence deny their true feelings and suggest that these feelings are inappropriate. Examples are "You shouldn't complain about pain; many others have gone through this same experience stoically," and "You should be glad that you are alive and not worry about the loss of your arm."
- *Do not make excuses for the other person* When a person reacts with an intense feeling such as anger or grief and seems to have lost control of behavior to the astonishment or discomfort of others, a common error is to explain the behavior by offering excuses. Examples are "Well, Mr Brown, you're upset about not finishing your lunch, but the dietitian and I gave you too much." This response discourages and diverts the person from discussing feelings of anger or inadequacy. The nurse has made assumptions about the reasons for the client's behavior and therefore inhibits exploration of what the client is really experiencing and feeling. Instead the nurse can reflect the feeling back to the client and ask for clarification: "You seem very angry. Did something happen today that upset you?"
- *Be genuine* Clients will sense whether or not the nurse is truly concerned.
- *Use your ingenuity* There are always many courses of action to consider in handling problems. Whatever course is chosen needs to further the achievement of the client's goals (outcomes), be compatible with the client's value system, and offer the probability of success. The client needs to choose the ways to achieve goals (outcomes); however, the nurse can assist in identifying options. For example, a client has asked for help because he is depressed and anxious about retirement. The nurse knows he loves animals, young children, and story telling. In this case, the nurse might direct his thoughts toward exploring a hobby or volunteer position related to these interests.

- *Be aware of cultural differences* that may affect meaning and understanding. See the section on Communication related to culture in Chapter 15, page 295. To facilitate nurse-client interaction, recognize the language(s) and/or dialect(s) the client uses. Provide a bilingual interpreter as needed for clients limited in the English language.
- *Maintain client confidentiality* To maintain the client's right to privacy, share information only with other health care professionals as needed for effective care and treatment.
- *Use communication techniques* that enable you to identify the client's perception of health, illness, treatments, and desired outcomes. Avoid closed questions that can be answered with "yes" or "no." (See Chapter 5, page 90 and Table 5–6.) Make verbal and nonverbal messages congruent. Be aware of your body language and what it conveys.
- *Focus on information needed to formulate an individualized plan of care* Include the client in formulating any plan of care.
- *Know your role and your limitations* Every person has unique strengths and problems. When you feel unble to handle some problems, the client should be informed and referred to the appropriate health professional. Clarify functions and roles, specifically what is expected of the client, the nurse, and the physician. This is especially important for clients who are unfamiliar with the health care system. Be honest about your limitations.

The ease with which nurses establish a helping relationship varies. Clients who are very young, who are unable to speak or to understand, whose mental abilities are impaired, or who have a different cultural background all pose challenges for the nurse. The nurse should approach every client with the belief that a helping relationship is possible, no matter how little feedback or participation the client is capable of at the time of initiation. For example, talking with a comatose client may seem ineffective, but the nurse who believes that the client hears and relates on some level to voice and touch can establish a helping relationship.

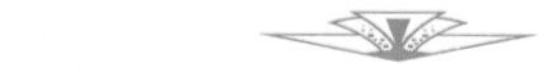

COMMUNICATION IN NURSING

The term **communication** has various meanings, depending on the context in which it is used. To some, communication is the interchange of information between two or more people; in other words, the exchange of ideas or thoughts. This kind of communication uses methods such as talking and listening or writing and reading. However, painting, dancing, and storytelling are also methods of communication. Thoughts are conveyed to others not only by spoken or written words but also by gestures or body actions.

Communication may have a more personal connotation than the interchange of ideas or thoughts. It can be a transmission of feelings, or a more personal and social interaction between people. In this context, communication often is synonymous with relating. Frequently, one member of a couple comments that the other is not communicating. Some teenagers complain about a generation gap—being unable to communicate with understanding or feeling to a parent or authority figure. Sometimes a nurse is said to be efficient but lacking in something called *bedside manner*. For the purpose of this text, *communication* is any means of exchanging information or feelings between two or more people. It is a basic component of human relationships.

The intent of any communication is to elicit a response. Thus, communication is a process. It includes all the techniques by which an individual affects another. It has two main purposes: to influence others and to obtain information. Communication can be described as helpful or unhelpful. The former encourages a sharing of information, thoughts, or feelings between two or more people. The latter hinders or blocks the transfer of information and feelings.

Nurses who communicate effectively are better able to initiate change that promotes health, establish a trusting relationship with a client and support persons, and prevent legal problems associated with nursing practice. Effective communication is essential for the establishment of the nurse-client relationship.

MODES OF COMMUNICATION

Communication is generally carried out in two different modes: verbal and nonverbal. **Verbal communication** uses the spoken or written word; **nonverbal communication** uses other forms, such as gestures or facial expressions, and touch. Although both kinds of communication occur concurrently, the majority of communication (some say 80% to 90%) is nonverbal. Learning about nonverbal communication is thus an important consideration for nurses in developing effective communication patterns and relationships with clients.

VERBAL COMMUNICATION

Verbal communication is largely conscious, because people choose the words they use. The words used vary among individuals according to culture, socioeconomic background, age, and education. As a result, countless possibilities exist in the way ideas are exchanged. An abundance of words can be used to form messages. In addition, a wide variety of feelings can be conveyed when people talk. The intonation of the voice can express animation, enthusiasm, sadness, annoyance, or amusement. The pacing or rhythm of a person's communication is another variable. Monotonous rhythms or very rapid rhythms can be products of lack of energy or interest, anxiety, or fear.

When choosing words to say or to write, nurses need to consider (a) simplicity, (b) clarity, (c) timing and relevance, (d) adaptability, and (e) credibility.

Simplicity Simplicity includes the use of commonly understood words, brevity, and completeness. Many complex technical terms become natural to nurses. However, laypersons often misunderstand these terms. Words such as *vasoconstriction* or *cholecystectomy* are meaningful to the nurse and easy to use but are ill-advised when communicating with clients. Nurses need to learn to select simple words intentionally even though effort is required to do so. For example, instead of saying to a client, "The nurse will be catheterizing you tomorrow for a urine specimen," it is better to say, "Tomorrow we need a sample of urine and we will collect it by putting a tube into your bladder." The latter statement is likely to produce a response from the client about why it is needed and whether it will hurt or be uncomfortable. The former statement may simply make the client wonder what the nurse means.

Another aspect of simplicity is brevity. By using short sentences and avoiding unnecessary material, the speaker or writer can achieve brevity. Brevity is of particular importance in writing, for example, in nurse's notes (see Chapter 9). Reports or memos need to be concise and should be condensed into a single paragraph or page, if possible.

The opposite of overcommunicating is undercommunicating. Shortcuts for the sake of simplicity can lead to incomplete or unclear communication. For example, initials or abbreviations such as "bid" (twice a day) or "ICU" (intensive care unit) should be avoided unless the nurse is certain that the client will understand them. At the first use, terms should be expressed in full; they can be shortened once the nurse is sure that the client or reader knows the meanings.

Clarity *Clarity* means saying exactly what is meant. It also is aligned with meaning what is said. The latter involves a blending of the speaker's behavior (nonverbal communication) with the words that are spoken. When the words and the behavior blend together or are unified, the communication is regarded as consistent or congruent.

The goal of clarity is to communicate so that people know the what, how, why (if necessary), when, who, and where of any specific event. Without knowing these facts, people are left to make assumptions. To ensure clarity in communication, the nurse also needs to speak slowly and enunciate words well. It may be helpful to repeat the message and to reduce distractions such as surrounding noises.

Some common pitfalls that can produce unclear communications are ambiguous statements, generalizations, and opinions. For example, "Men are stronger than women" is both a generalization and an opinion, and the word *stronger* is open to several interpretations. Another example is a nurse's statement to a client, "Mrs Smith, you need to keep busy today." The specific actions Mrs Smith is expected to carry out and the reasons for them are open to many interpretations.

Timing and Relevance No matter how clearly or simply words are stated or written, the timing needs to be appropriate to ensure that words are heard. Moreover, the messages need to relate to the person or to the person's interests and concerns.

Nurses need to be aware of both relevance and timing when communicating with clients. This involves being sensitive to the client's needs and concerns. For example, a client who is enmeshed in fear of cancer may not hear the nurse's explanations about the expected procedures before and after gallbladder surgery. In this situation it is better for the nurse first to encourage the client to express concerns, and to then deal with those concerns. The necessary explanations can be provided at another time.

Asking several questions at once bombards and confuses the client. For example, a nurse enters a client's room and says in one breath, "Good morning, Mrs Brody. How are you this morning? Did you sleep well last night? Your husband is coming to see you before your surgery, isn't he?" The client no doubt wonders which question to answer first, if any. A related pattern of poor timing is to ask a question and then not wait for an answer before making another comment.

Adaptability Spoken messages need to be altered in accordance with behavioral cues from the receiver. This adjustment is referred to as *adaptability.* Moods and behavior may change minute by minute, hour by hour, or from day to day. What the nurse says and how it is said must be individualized and carefully considered. This requires astute assessment and sensitivity on the part of the nurse. For example, a nurse who usually smiles, appears cheerful, and greets her client every afternoon with an enthusiastic "Hi, Mr Brown!" notices that he is not smiling and appears distressed when she appears. In response to the client's cues, the nurse adapts her usual greeting and tones down her cheery manner. She may say "Hi" in a much softer and caring manner and express concern in her facial expression while she moves toward him.

Credibility *Credibility* means worthiness of belief, trustworthiness, reliability. Credibility may be the most important criterion of effective communication. A nurse's credibility to clients depends in part on the opinion of others. If other health professionals and clients regard the nurse as trustworthy, then the client also is likely to.

To become credible, the nurse needs to be knowledgeable about the subject matter being discussed and to have accurate information. Nurses also need to convey confidence and certainty in what they are saying. This is often referred to as *positivism.* People tend to perceive confidence, which is dynamic and emphatic, as more credible than hesitance or uncertainty, which is less forceful and less active. However, the nurse should not sound overconfident or authoritarian. To avoid this perception by the client, the nurse states messages in a constructive way and focuses on being helpful to clients.

Nurses foster credibility by being consistent, dependable, and honest. People value the nurse who acknowledges limitations and can say, "I don't know the answer to that, but I'll find someone who does."

NONVERBAL COMMUNICATION

Nonverbal communication is sometimes called *body language.* It includes gestures, body movements, use of touch, and physical appearance, including adornment. Nonverbal communication often tells others more about what a person is *feeling* than what is actually said, because nonverbal behavior is controlled less consciously than verbal behavior. Nonverbal communication either reinforces or contradicts what is said verbally. For example, if a nurse says to a client, "I'd be happy to sit here and talk to you for a while," yet glances nervously at a watch every few seconds, the actions contradict the verbal message. The client is more likely to believe the nonverbal behavior, which conveys "I am very busy."

Observers cannot always be sure of the correct interpretation of the feelings expressed nonverbally. On the one hand, the same feeling can be expressed nonverbally in more than one way. For example, anger may be communicated by aggressive or excessive body motion, or it may be communicated by a frozen stillness. In some cultures, a smile may be used to conceal anger. On the other hand, a variety of feelings, such as embarrassment, pleasure, or anger, can be expressed by a single nonverbal cue, such as blushing.

Observing and interpreting the client's nonverbal behavior are essential skills for nurses. Interpreting the observations requires validation with the client. For example, the nurse might say "You look like you have been crying. Is something upsetting you?"

The nurse's own nonverbal behavior is under constant scrutiny by clients. It is therefore necessary for nurses to gain awareness of their actions and to learn to convey understanding, respect, and acceptance to clients.

To observe nonverbal behavior efficiently requires a systematic approach. As part of an initial assessment, the nurse should observe the person's overall physical appearance, including adornments, posture, and gait, and then assesses specific parts of the body, such as the face and the hands, for nonverbal cues. The person's overall appearance includes physical characteristics and manner of dress. Whatever is observed, the nurse needs to exercise caution in interpretation. For example, pale skin may be normal for a particular client. Nails may be short because they were bitten nervously or because they were broken by hard manual labor. For additional information regarding appearance, see Chapter 22, page 472.

Clothing and adornments are sometimes rich sources of information about a person. Choice of apparel is highly personal. Clothing may convey social and financial status, culture, religion, group association, and self-concept. Adornments such as jewelry, perfume, and cosmetics reveal additional information.

How a person dresses is often an indicator of how the person feels. People who are tired or ill may not have the energy or the desire to maintain their normal grooming. The nurse also needs to be alert to sudden changes in a person's dress. When a person known for immaculate grooming becomes lax about appearance, the nurse may suspect a loss of self-esteem or a physical illness. The nurse validates these observed nonverbal data by, for example, asking the client, "You look different to me today. When we met last week, your hair was fixed, you had makeup on, and you were smiling. Today you didn't fix yourself up, and you look kind of sad. Is anything wrong?"

For clients in acute general hospital settings, a change in grooming habits or personal adornment often signals that the client is feeling better. A male client may request a shave, or a female client may request a mirror and her lipstick.

Posture and Gait The ways people walk and carry themselves are often reliable indicators of self-concept, current mood, and health. Erect posture and an active, purposeful stride suggest a feeling of well-being. Slouched posture and a slow, shuffling gait suggest dejection or physical discomfort. Tense posture and a rapid, determined gait suggest anxiety or anger. Likewise, the sitting or lying postures of clients can communicate feelings. Again, the nurse clarifies the meaning of the observed behavior by describing to the client what the nurse sees and then asking what it means or whether the nurse's interpretation is correct. For example, "You look like it really hurts you to move. I'm wondering how your pain is and if you might need something to make you more comfortable?"

Facial Expression No part of the body is as expressive as the face (Figure 18–1). Feelings of joy, sadness, fear, surprise, anger, and disgust can be conveyed by facial expressions. The muscles around the eyes and the mouth are particularly expressive. Although actors learn to control these muscles to convey emotions to audiences, facial expressions generally are not consciously controlled.

Clients are quick to notice the nurse's facial expression, particularly when they feel unsure or uncomfortable. The client who questions the nurse about a feared diagnostic result will watch the nurse to see whether the nurse maintains eye contact or looks away when answering. The client who has had disfiguring surgery will examine the nurse's face for signs of disgust. Nurses, like actors, need to be aware of their facial expressions and what they are communicating to others. Although it is impossible to control all facial expressions, the nurse must learn to control feelings such as fear and disgust in certain situations.

Many facial expressions generally convey a universal meaning. The smile conveys happiness. Contempt is conveyed by the mouth turned down, the head tilted back, and the eyes directed down the nose. No single expression can be interpreted accurately, however, without considering (a) other reinforcing physical cues, (b) the setting in which it occurs, (c) the expression of others in the same setting, and (d) the cultural background of the client.

Eye contact is another essential element of facial communication. See Chapter 15, page 299. In many cultures, mutual eye contact acknowledges recognition of the other person and a willingness to maintain communication. Often a person initiates contact with another person with a glance, capturing the person's attention prior to communicating. A person who feels weak or defenseless often averts the eyes or avoids eye contact; the communication received may be too embarrassing or too dominating. Animals are known to succumb to dominance first by averting their eyes and then by moving away.

Hand Movements and Gestures Like faces, hands are expressive. They can communicate feelings at any given moment. An anxious person, for instance a man awaiting word about his daughter in surgery, may wring his hands or pick his nails; relaxed persons may interlock their fingers over their laps or allow their hands to fall over the ends of armrests. Hands also communicate by touch: slapping someone's face or caressing another's head communicates obvious feelings.

Hands are frequently involved in gestures. The handshake, the victory sign, the wave good-bye, the hand motion to ask a visitor to sit down are gestures that have relatively universal meanings. Some gestures, however, are culture-specific. European women walk together holding hands as a sign of friendship; in North American society, this gesture may be regarded as unacceptable. Even the same gesture can have different meanings in different cultures. The North American gesture meaning "shoo" or "go away" means "come here" or "come back" in some Asian cultures.

Hands are also very expressive in illustrating or stylizing verbal communication. The French and Italians are noted for using their hands in this manner. When describing the shape and size of an object, a French person uses the hands to reinforce the verbal message.

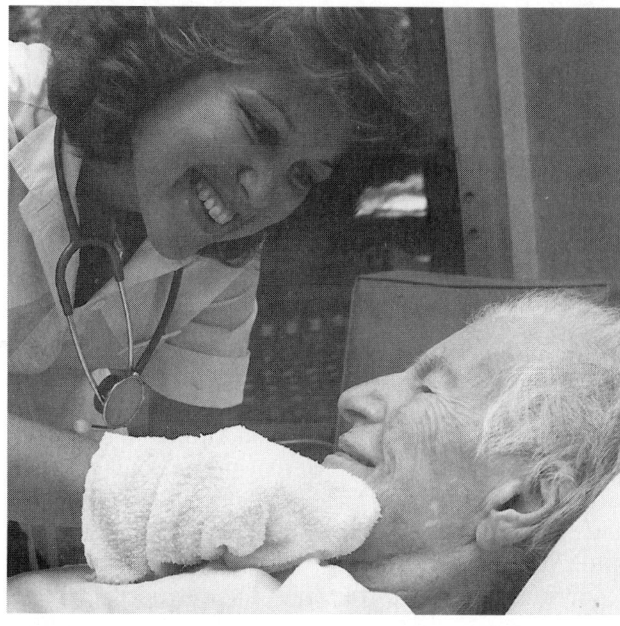

Figure 18–1 The nurse's facial expression communicates warmth and caring.

For people with special communication problems, such as the deaf, the hands are invaluable in communication. Many deaf people learn sign language. Ill persons who are unable to reply verbally can similarly devise a unique communication system using the hands. The client may be able to raise an index finger once for "yes" and twice for "no." Other signals can often be devised by the client and the nurse to denote other meanings.

THE COMMUNICATION PROCESS

In face-to-face communication there is a sender, a message, a receiver, and a response, or feedback (Figure 18–2, p. 362). In its simplest form, communication is a two-way process involving the sending and the receiving of a message. Because the intent of communication is to elicit a response, the process is ongoing; the receiver of the message then becomes the sender of a response, and the original sender then becomes the receiver.

Sender The sender, a person or group who wishes to convey a message to another, is sometimes called the *source-encoder*. This term suggests that the person or group sending the message must have an idea or reason for communicating (source) and must put the idea or feeling into a form that can be transmitted. **Encoding** involves the selection of specific signs or symbols (codes) to transmit the

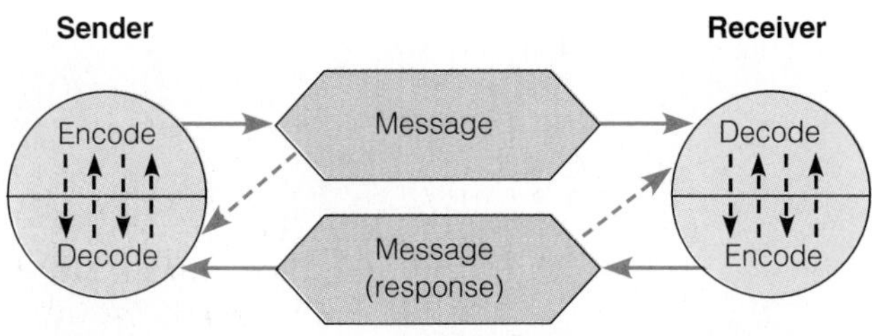

Figure 18–2 The communication process. The dashed arrows indicate intrapersonal communication (self-talk). The solid lines indicate interpersonal communication.

message, such as which language and words to use, how to arrange the words, and what tone of voice and gestures to use. For example, if the receiver speaks English, the sender usually selects English words. If the message is "No, Mr Johnson, smoking is not permitted in patient rooms in this hospital!" the tone of voice selected will be one of firmness, and a shake of the head or a pointing index finger can reinforce it. The nurse must not only deal with dialects and foreign languages but also must cope with two language levels—the layperson's and the health professional's.

Message The second component of the communication process is the **message** itself—what is actually said or written, the body language that accompanies the words, and how the message is transmitted. Various channels can be used to convey messages, and frequently combinations are used. It is important that the channel be appropriate for the message and make the intent of the message clear.

Talking face-to-face with a person may be more effective in some instances than telephoning or writing a message. Recording messages on tape or communicating by radio or television may be more appropriate for larger audiences. Written communication is often appropriate for long explanations or for a communication that needs to be preserved. The nonverbal channel of touch is often highly effective (Figure 18–3, p. 363).

Receiver The receiver, the third component of the communication process, is the listener, who must listen, observe, and attend. This person, sometimes called the *decoder*, must perceive what the sender intended (sensation) and then analyze the information received (interpretation). Perception involves use of all the senses to receive all verbal and nonverbal messages. To **decode** means to relate the message perceived to the receiver's storehouse of knowledge and experience and to sort out the meaning of the message. Whether the message is decoded accurately by the receiver, according to the sender's intent, depends largely on their similarities in knowledge and experience. For example, Mr Johnson may perceive the message accurately—"No smoking is allowed in my room." However, if experience has taught him that he can smoke in his room if a certain nurse is on duty, he will interpret the intent of the message differently.

Response The fourth component of the communication process, the response, is the message that the receiver returns to the sender. It is also called **feedback.** Feedback can be either verbal, nonverbal, or both. Nonverbal examples are a nod of the head or a yawn. Either way, feedback allows the sender to correct or reword a message. In the case of Mr Johnson, the receiver may appear irritated or say, "Well—the nurse on evening shift lets me smoke." The sender then knows the message was interpreted accurately. However, now the original sender becomes the receiver, who is required to decode and respond.

INTRAPERSONAL COMMUNICATION

Intrapersonal communication is the communication that you have with yourself; another name is *self-talk*. Both the sender and the receiver of a message usually engage in this type of communication. It involves thinking about the message before it is sent, while it is being sent, and after it is sent, and it occurs constantly (Farley 1992, p. 481). Consequently, intrapersonal communication can interfere with a person's ability to hear a message as the sender intended. It also tends to be evaluative, especially when the emotions of the receiver are involved. Nurses can facilitate communication by controlling self-talk and delaying any evaluation of the message or sender.

FACTORS INFLUENCING THE COMMUNICATION PROCESS

In addition to factors such as a person's sociocultural background, language, age, and education, and the limitations and attributes of nonverbal communication, the following factors affect the communication process: ability of the communicator; perceptions; personal space; territoriality; roles and relationships; time; environment; attitudes; and emotions and self-esteem.

Ability of the Communicator The person's abilities to speak, hear, see, and comprehend stimuli influence the communication process. People who are hard of hearing may require messages that are short, loud, and clear. Those who are unable to read will be unable to comprehend written information. Some, because of disease processes, are unable to see or to speak, and individual methods for communication need to be devised with them.

The receiver of a message also needs to be able to interpret the message. Mental faculties can be impaired for such reasons as brain damage or use of sedative drugs or alcohol. Even if a client is free of physical impairments, the nurse needs to determine how many stimuli the client is capable of receiving in a given time frame. Frequently the receiver is expected to assimilate too much information. The nurse must be careful not to talk too quickly or present too many ideas at once, particularly when offering health instruction.

Perceptions Because each person has unique personality traits, values, and life experiences, each will perceive and interpret messages differently. For example, the nurse may draw the curtains around a crying woman and leave her alone. The woman may interpret this as "The nurse thinks that I will upset others in the room and that I shouldn't cry" or "The nurse doesn't like crying" or "The nurse respects my need to be alone." It is important in many situations to validate or correct the perceptions of the receiver.

Personal Space Personal space is the distance people prefer in interactions with others. **Proxemics** is the study of distance between people in their interactions. Middle-class North Americans use definite distances in various interpersonal relationships, along with specific voice tones and body language. Communication thus alters in accordance with four distances, each with a close and a far phase, that have been described by Hall (1969, p. 45):

1. Intimate: Physical contact to 1½ feet
2. Personal: 1½ to 4 feet
3. Social: 4 to 12 feet
4. Public: 12 feet and beyond

Intimate distance communication is characterized by body contact, heightened sensations of body heat and smell, and vocalizations that are low. Vision is intense, restricted to a small body part, and may be distorted. Intimate distance is frequently used by nurses. Examples occur in cuddling a baby, touching the sightless client, positioning clients, observing an incision, and restraining a toddler for an injection. It is a natural protective instinct for people to maintain a certain amount of space immediately around them, and the amount varies with individuals and cultures. When someone who wants to communicate steps too close, the receiver automatically steps back a pace or two. In their therapeutic roles, nurses often are required to violate this personal space. However, it is important for them to be aware when this will occur and to forewarn the client. In many instances, the nurse can respect (not come as close as) a person's intimate distance. In other instances, the nurse may come within intimate distance to communicate warmth and caring.

Personal distance is less overwhelming than intimate distance. Voice tones are moderate, and body heat and smell are noticed less. Physical contact such as a handshake or touching a shoulder is possible. More of the person is perceived at a personal distance, so that nonverbal behaviors such as body stance or full facial expressions are seen with less distortion. Much communication between nurses and clients occurs at this distance. Examples occur when nurses are sitting with a client, giving medications, or establishing an intravenous infusion. Communication at a close personal distance can convey involvement by facilitating the sharing of thoughts and feelings. At the outer extreme of 4 ft, however, less involvement is conveyed. Bantering and some social conversations are usual at this distance.

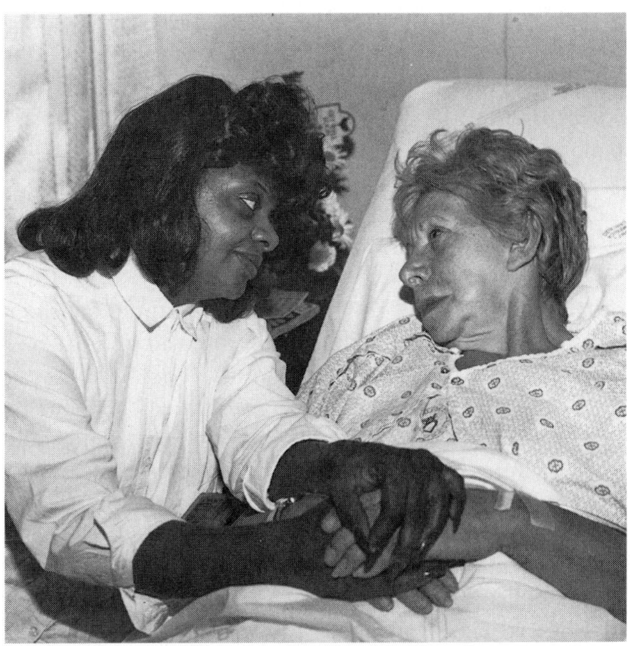

Figure 18–3 Appropriate forms of touch can communicate caring.

Social distance is characterized by a clear visual perception of the whole person. Body heat and odor are imperceptible, eye contact is increased, and vocalizations are loud enough to be overheard by others. Communication is therefore more formal and is limited to seeing and hearing. The person is protected and out of reach for touch or personal sharing of thoughts or feelings. Social distance allows more activity and movement back and forth. It is expedient in communicating with several people at the same time or within a short time. Examples occur when nurses make rounds or wave a greeting to someone. Social distance is important in accomplishing the business of the day. However, it is frequently misused. For example, the nurse who stands in the doorway and asks a client "How are you today?" will receive a more noncommittal reply than the nurse who moves to personal distance to inquire.

Public distance requires loud, clear vocalizations with careful enunciation. Although the faces and forms of people are seen at public distance, individuality is lost. Instead, a general notion is perceived about a group of people or a community.

Territoriality Territoriality is a concept of the space and things that an individual considers as belonging to the self. Territories marked off by people may be visible to others. For example, clients in a hospital often consider their territory as bounded by the curtains around the bed unit or by the walls of a private room. This human tendency to claim territory must be recognized by all health care workers. Clients often feel the need to defend their territory when it is invaded by others; for example, when a visitor or nurse removes a chair to use at another bed, the visitor has inadvertently violated the territoriality of the client whose chair was moved. Nurses need to obtain permission from clients to remove, rearrange, or borrow objects in their hospital area.

Roles and Relationships The roles and the relationship between sender and receiver affect the communication process. Roles such as nursing student and instructor, client and physician, or parent and child affect the content and responses in the communication process. Choice of words, sentence structure, and tone of voice vary considerably from role to role. In addition, the specific relationship between the communicators is significant. The nurse who meets with a client for the first time communicates differently from the nurse who has previously developed a relationship with that client.

Time The time factor in communication includes the events that precede and follow the interaction. The hospitalized client who is anticipating surgery or who has just received news that a spouse has lost a job will not be very receptive to information. A client who has had to wait for some time to express needs may respond quite differently from one who has endured no waiting period. The setting also influences communication. If the room lacks privacy or is hot, noisy, or crowded, the communication process can break down.

Nurses' use of time can facilitate or inhibit a client's communication. The nurse who tells a client, "I'll be back in a moment" while delivering medications is likely to convey "I haven't time now" or "I've got work to do." This inhibits client communications. However, by saying to the client, "Would you tell me now what your concern is about, and then when I've finished delivering medications I'll come back and help you with it," the nurse facilitates the communication process.

Environment People usually communicate most effectively in a comfortable environment. Temperature extremes, excessive noise, and a poorly ventilated environment can all interfere with communication. Also, lack of privacy may interfere with a client's communication about matters the client considers private. For example, a client who is worried about the ability of his wife to care for him after discharge from hospital may not wish to discuss this concern with a nurse within the hearing of other clients in the room. Environmental distraction can impair and distort communication.

Attitudes Attitudes convey beliefs, thoughts, and feelings about people and events. Attitudes are communicated convincingly and rapidly to others. Attitudes such as caring, warmth, respect, and acceptance facilitate communication, whereas condescension, lack of interest, and coldness inhibit communication.

Caring and *warmth* convey a feeling of emotional closeness, in contrast to impersonal distance. Caring is more enduring and intense than warmth. It conveys deep and genuine concern for the person, whereas warmth conveys friendliness and consideration, shown by acts of smiling and attention to physical comforts (Brammer 1988, p. 37). Caring involves giving feelings, thoughts, skill, and knowledge. It requires psychologic energy and poses the risk of gaining little in return, yet by caring, people usually reap the benefits of greater communication and understanding.

Respect is an attitude that emphasizes the other person's worth and individuality. It conveys that the person's hopes and feelings are special and unique even though similar to others in many ways. People have a need to be different from—and at the same time similar to—others. Being too different can be isolating and threatening. A nurse conveys respect by listening open-mindedly to what the other person is saying, even if the nurse disagrees. Nurses can learn new ways of approaching situations when they conscientiously listen to another person's perspective.

Acceptance emphasizes neither approval nor disapproval. The nurse willingly receives the client's honest feelings and actions without judgment. An accepting attitude allows clients to express personal feelings freely and to be themselves. The nurse may need to restrict acceptance in situations where clients' actions are harmful to themselves or to others.

In contrast, *condescension* is an attitude that conveys superiority over the other person. Clients who feel helpless often perceive nurses to be in a superior position because of their knowledge and skill. In these instances, the nurse may convey condenscension by an air of superiority and intellectualism. One common condescending act by nurses is to call clients "honey" or "dear." This casts the nurse in the role of the superior mother and the client in the role of the inferior child. Another condescending act is patting an elderly client on the head.

Lack of interest also inhibits communication by indicating a lack of concern or a belief that what the person is saying is not important. The nurse conveys lack of interest by forgetting part of the client's conversation or not concentrating on it sufficiently to respond. Being tired near the end of a long day's work or in a hurry to complete tasks may contribute to giving the appearance of not being interested in the client.

Coldness is the opposite of caring and warmth. Nurses convey this attitude to clients by appearing more interested in the technical and procedural aspects of nursing than in the concerns of the person receiving the therapy. For example, the nurse can convey coldness by appearing more concerned about the neatness of the client's bed than about the client's restlessness or more interested in the efficient functioning of a cardiac monitor than in the client's anxiety. A rigid body posture and aloof tone of voice also convey a nurse's lack of genuine concern for the client.

Emotions and Self-Esteem Most people have experienced overwhelming joy or sorrow that is difficult to express in words. Anger may produce loud, profane vocalizations or controlled speechlessness. Fright may produce screams of terror or paralyzed silence.

Emotions also affect a person's ability to interpret messages. Large parts of a message may not be heard, or the message may be misinterpreted when the receiver is experiencing strong emotion. This situation occurs frequently in nursing. For example, the client feeling great fear may not remember all the preoperative instructions offered by a nurse.

Self-esteem also influences communication patterns. People whose self-esteem is high communicate honestly, with confidence, and with **congruence** (agreement or coinciding) between verbal and nonverbal messages. For example, a nurse explaining the importance of preoperative exercises would present a sincere and serious facial expression. Those with low self-esteem or under high stress tend to give double messages; that is, their verbal and nonverbal messages are incongruent (lack consistency). For example, while a client explains about his colostomy to his family he laughs.

ASSESSING COMMUNICATION ABILITIES

To assess the client's communication abilities, the nurse determines communication impairments or barriers and communication style. Remember that culture may influence when and how a client speaks. Obviously, language varies according to age and development. With children, the nurse observes sounds, gestures, and vocabulary.

BARRIERS TO COMMUNICATION

Various barriers may alter a client's ability to send, receive, or comprehend messages. These include language deficits, sensory deficits, cognitive impairments, structural deficits, and paralysis. The nurse must assess each to determine their presence.

Language Deficits Determine the client's primary language for communicating and whether or not a fluent interpreter is required. Some clients who use English as a second language may have language skills that are adequate to meet their needs.

Sensory Deficits The ability to hear, see, feel, and smell are important adjuncts to communication. Deafness can significantly alter the message the client receives; impaired vision alters the ability to observe nonverbal behavior, such as a smile or a gesture; inability to feel and smell can impair the client's capabilities to report injuries or detect the smoke from a fire. For clients with severe hearing impairments, follow these steps:

- Look for a *Medic Alert* indicating hearing loss
- Determine whether the client wears a hearing aid and it's functioning
- Observe whether the client is attempting to see your face to read lips
- Observe whether the client is attempting to use hands to communicate with sign language

Cognitive Impairments Any disorder that impairs cognitive functioning (eg, cerebrovascular disease, Alzheimer's disease, and brain tumors or injuries) may affect a client's ability to use and understand language. These clients may develop total loss of speech, impaired articulation, or the inability to find or name words. Certain medications such as sedatives, antidepressants, and neuroleptics may also impair speech, causing the client to use incomplete sentences or to slur words.

The nurse assesses whether these clients respond when asked a question and if so: Is the client's speech fluent or hesitant? Does the client use words correctly? Can the client comprehend instructions as evidenced by following directions? Can the client name objects or familiar people? Can the client repeat words or phrases? In addition, the nurse assesses the client's ability to understand written words: Can the client follow written directions? Can the client respond correctly by pointing to a written word? Can the client read aloud? Can the client recognize words or letters if unable to read whole sentences? The nurse uses large, clearly written words when trying to establish abilities in this area.

When the client is unconscious, the nurse looks for any indication that suggests comprehension of what is communicated (eg, tries to arouse the client verbally and through touch). Ask a closed question like "Can you hear me?" and watch for a nonverbal response such as a nod of the head for yes or a shake for no; a hand squeeze once for yes or twice for no; one blink of the eye for yes or two blinks for no.

Structural Deficits Structural deficits of the oral and nasal cavities and respiratory system can alter a person's ability to speak clearly and spontaneously. Examples include cleft palate, artificial airways such as an endotracheal tube or tracheostomy, and laryngectomy (removal of the larynx). Extreme dyspnea (shortness of breath) can also impair speech patterns.

Paralysis If paralysis of the upper extremities impairs the client's ability to write, the nurse should determine whether the client can point, nod, shrug, blink, or squeeze a hand. Any of these could be used to devise a beginning communication system.

STYLE OF COMMUNICATION

In assessing communication style, the nurse considers both verbal and nonverbal communication. In addition to physical barriers, some psychologic illnesses (eg, depression or psychosis) influence the ability to communicate. The client may demonstrate constant verbalization of the same words or phrases, a loose association of ideas, or flight of ideas.

Verbal Communication When assessing verbal communication, the nurse focuses on three areas: the content of the message, the themes, and verbalized emotions. In addition, the nurse considers the following:

- Whether the communication pattern is slow, rapid, quiet, spontaneous, hesitant, evasive, and so on.
- The vocabulary of the individual, particularly any changes from the vocabulary normally used. For example, a person who normally never swears may indicate increased stress or illness by an uncharacteristic use of profanity.
- The presence of hostility, aggression, assertiveness, reticence, hesitance, anxiety, or loquaciousness (incessant verbalization) in communication.
- Difficulties with verbal communication, such as slurring, stuttering, inability to pronounce a particular sound, lack of clarity in enunciation, inability to speak in sentences, loose association of ideas, flight of ideas, or the inability to find or name words or identify objects.
- Refusal or inability to speak.

Nonverbal Communication Consider nonverbal communication in relation to the client's culture. Pay particular attention to facial expression, gestures, body movements, affect, tone of voice, posture, and eye contact.

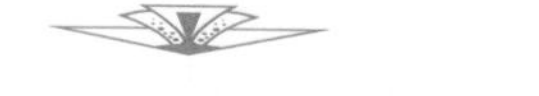

DIAGNOSING COMMUNICATION PROBLEMS

Impaired verbal communication is the NANDA nursing diagnosis given to clients with communication problems. As implied in the diagnostic label, this diagnosis focuses on *verbal* communication. The definition, defining characteristics, and contributing factors are shown in the accompanying box.

Other nursing diagnoses used for clients experiencing communication problems that involve impaired verbal communication as the etiology include the following:

- **Anxiety** related to impaired verbal communication
- **Powerlessness** related to impaired verbal communication
- **Self-esteem disturbance** related to impaired verbal communication
- **Social isolation** related to impaired verbal communication

PLANNING FOR EFFECTIVE COMMUNICATION

When problems in communication have been identified, the nurse and client set goals (outcomes) and begin planning ways to promote effective communication. The overall client goal (outcome) for persons with **Impaired verbal communication** is to reduce or resolve the impaired communication. Specific nursing interventions are planned from the stated etiology.

Examples of outcome criteria to evaluate the achievement of client goals and the effectiveness of nursing interventions follow.

The client

- Communicates that needs are being met
- Begins to establish a method of communication:
  a. Signals yes/no to direct questions using words, eye blinks, hand squeezes, word boards, or head movements
  b. Uses verbal or nonverbal techniques to indicate needs

NURSING DIAGNOSES

CLIENTS WITH COMMUNICATION PROBLEMS

NURSING DIAGNOSIS: Impaired verbal communication: The state in which an individual experiences a decreased or absent ability to use or understand language in human interaction

Defining Characteristics

- Difficulty speaking or verbalizing
- Absence of speech or inability to speak
- Inability to speak dominant language*
- Stuttering or slurring of words
- Difficulty finding or naming words or forming sentences
- Difficulty expressing thoughts verbally
- Inappropriate verbalizations
- Dyspnea
- Disorientation

Related Factors

Physical barriers such as cleft palate, brain injury, and tracheostomy; psychologic barriers such as psychosis and depression; developmental or age-related disability; cultural differences.

* Some nurses question the appropriateness of this defining characteristic because it does not relate to a health problem or wellness.

- Perceives the message accurately, as evidenced by appropriate verbal and/or nonverbal responses
- Uses resources appropriately
- Regains maximum communication abilities
- Expresses minimum fear, anxiety, frustration, and depression
- Communicates effectively:
  a. Uses dominant language
  b. Uses a word board or picture board
  c. Uses translator
  d. Uses sign language
  e. Uses a computer

IMPLEMENTING

THERAPEUTIC COMMUNICATION

Therapeutic communication promotes understanding by both the sender and the receiver. A number of techniques can help establish a constructive relationship between the nurse and the client, although the use of the techniques is no guarantee of effective communication. So many factors are involved in communication that the nurse is ill-advised to rely on any one technique or even several techniques. Not all people feel comfortable with all techniques, and skill in using them appropriately is essential. The nurse must be comfortable with the technique used and convey sincerity to the client. A phony or false response is usually quickly identified by clients and hinders the development of an effective relationship.

Nurses can learn by examining and becoming aware of their own reactions (feelings) and responses. Although it is difficult for nurses to see their own nonverbal communication other than by videotape feedback, a great deal can be learned by reflecting on what was heard, what the nurse said, and when and how it was said. Methods such as role playing, process recordings, and audiotapes can be useful.

Nurses need to respond not only to the content of a client's verbal message but also to the feelings expressed. It is important to understand how the client views the situation and feels about it before responding. The content of the client's communication is the words or thoughts, as distinct from the feelings. Sometimes people can convey a thought in words while their emotions contradict the words; that is, words and feelings are incongruent. For example, a client says, "I am glad he has left me; he was very cruel." However, the nurse observes that the client has tears in her eyes as she says this. To respond to the client's *words*, the nurse might simply rephrase, saying "You are pleased that he has left you." To respond to the client's *feelings*, the nurse would need to acknowledge the tears in the client's eyes, saying, for example, "You seem saddened by all this." Such a response helps the client to focus on her feelings. In some instances, the nurse may need to know more about the client and her resources for coping with these feelings.

Sometimes clients need time to deal with their feelings. Strong emotions are often draining. People usually need to deal with feelings before they can cope with other matters, such as learning new skills or planning for the future. This is most evident in hospitals when clients learn that they have a terminal illness. Some require hours, days, or even weeks before they are ready to start other tasks. Some need only time to themselves, others need someone to listen, others need assistance identifying and verbalizing feelings, and others need assistance making decisions about future courses of action.

Attentive Listening Attentive listening is listening actively, using all the senses, as opposed to listening passively with just the ear. It is probably the most important technique in nursing and is basic to all other techniques. Attentive listening is an active process that requires energy and concentration. It involves paying attention to the total message, both verbal messages and nonverbal messages, and noting whether these communications are congruent. Attentive listening means absorbing both the content and the feeling the person is conveying, without selectivity. The listener does not select or listen solely to what the listener wants to hear; the nurse focuses not on the nurse's own needs but rather on the client's needs. Attentive listening conveys an attitude of caring and interest, thereby encouraging the client to talk.

Attentive listening also involves listening for key themes in the communication. The nurse must be careful not to react quickly to the message. The speaker should not be interrupted and the nurse (the responder) should take time to think about the message before responding. As a listener, the nurse also should ask questions either to obtain additional information or to clarify.

Nurses need to be aware of their own biases. A message that reflects different values or beliefs should not be discredited for that reason. Rondeau (1992, p. 80) suggests that the message sender (ie, the client) should decide when to close a conversation. When the nurse closes the conversation the client may assume that the nurse considers the message unimportant.

In summary, attentive listening is a highly developed skill, but fortunately it can be learned with practice. A nurse can convey attentiveness in listening to clients in various ways. Common responses are nodding the head, uttering "uh huh" or "mmm," repeating the words that the client has used, or saying "I see what you mean." Each nurse has characteristic ways of responding, and the nurse must take care not to sound insincere or phony.

Physical Attending Egan (1982, pp. 60–61) has outlined five specific ways to convey physical attending, which he defines as the manner of being present to another or being with another. Listening, in his frame of reference, is what a person does while attending. The five actions of physical attending, which convey a "posture of involvement," are shown in the box above.

ACTIONS OF PHYSICAL ATTENDING

- *Face the other person squarely.* This position says, "I am available to you." Moving to the side lessens the degree of involvement.
- *Maintain good eye contact.* Mutual eye contact, preferably at the same level, recognizes the other person and denotes a willingness to maintain communication. Eye contact neither glares at nor stares down another but is natural.
- *Lean toward the person.* People move naturally toward one another when they want to say or hear something—by moving to the front of a class, by moving a chair nearer a friend, or by leaning across a table with arms propped in front. The nurse conveys involvement by leaning forward, closer to the client.
- *Maintain an open posture.* The nondefensive position is one in which neither arms nor legs are crossed. It conveys that the person wishes to encourage the passage of communication, as the open door of a home or an office does.
- *Remain relatively relaxed.* Total relaxation is not feasible when the nurse is listening with intensity, but the nurse can show relaxation by taking time in responding, allowing pauses as needed, balancing periods of tension with relaxation, and using gestures that are natural. See Figure 18–4.

These five attending postures need to be adapted to the specific needs of clients in a given situation. For example, leaning forward may not be appropriate at the beginning of an interview. It may be reserved until a closer relationship grows between the nurse and the client. The same applies to eye contact, which is generally uninterrupted when the communicators are very involved in the interaction.

Therapeutic communication techniques facilitate communication and focus on the client's concerns (Table 18–2 on pages 370 and 371). Techniques that specifically focus on comforting a client are shown in Table 18–3 on page 372.

NONTHERAPEUTIC COMMUNICATION

Nurses need to recognize nontherapeutic techniques that interfere with effective communication. See Table 18–4 on page 372. Failure to listen, improperly decoding the client's intended message, and placing the nurse's needs above the client's needs are major barriers to communication.

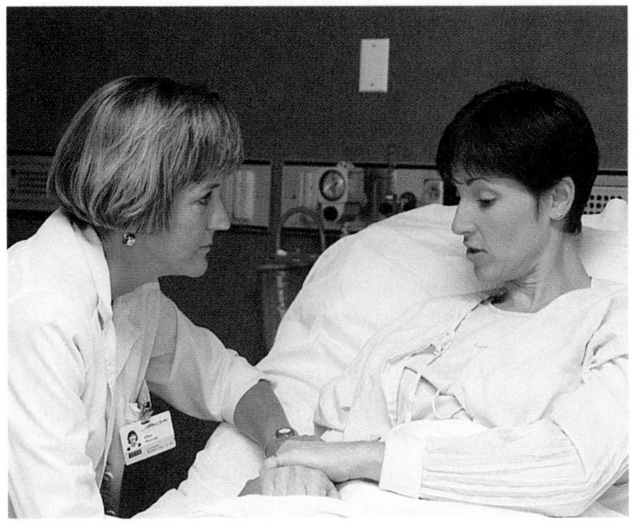

Figure 18–4 The nurse conveys attentive listening through a posture of involvement.

HELPING CLIENTS WHO HAVE COMMUNICATION PROBLEMS

When nurses interact with clients who have problems with speech or language, Boss (1992, pp. 992–95) suggests four categories of nursing interventions to facilitate communication.

Manipulate the Environment Initially, the nurse needs to provide a calm, relaxed environment, which will help reduce any anxiety the client might have. It should be remembered that impaired speech often creates feelings of frustration, anxiety, depression, or hostility in the client. In addition, some clients feel isolated and confused. Communication normally contributes to a client's sense of security and feelings that he or she is not alone. To further reduce these emotions, the nurse should acknowledge and praise the client's attempts at communication. For the hearing impaired, there should be sufficient light so the client can clearly see the nurse for lip reading.

Provide Support The nurse should convey encouragement to the client and provide nonverbal reassurance, perhaps by touch, if this is appropriate. If the nurse does not understand the client, tell the client, but continue the conversation so that the client can try other words or another way of communicating. When speaking with a client who has difficulty understanding, it is preferable to behave as if the client understands until lack of understanding is apparent. When providing care, anticipate the client's needs and ask about them. The nurse's body language (eg, gestures, posture, facial expression, and eye contact) should convey acceptance and approval.

Employ Measures to Enhance Communication
Ways to help communication include keeping words simple and concrete and discussing topics of interest to the client. It is often helpful to use alternative communication strategies such as word boards, pictures, and paper and pencil. Often interpreters can assist a client and nurse to communicate. Some hospitals have a list of interpreters for a variety of languages who will come to the bedside. In some instances, these interpreters are employed at the facility. In addition, the client's support persons often can provide this assistance.

Educate the Client and Support Persons Sometimes clients and support persons can be prepared in advance about communication problems, for example before an intubation or throat surgery. By explaining anticipated problems, the client is often less anxious when problems arise.

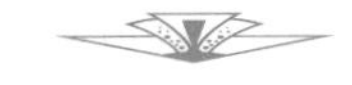

EVALUATING COMMUNICATION

Evaluating involves client and nurse communication. To establish whether client goals have been met, it is important to listen actively, to communicate verbally, and to observe nonverbal communication. Examples of evaluative statements indicating goal (outcome) achievement are "Using slateboard effectively to indicate needs x 1 week" or "The client stated, 'I listened more closely to my daughter yesterday and found out how she feels about our divorce.' "

For nurses to evaluate the effectiveness of their own communications with clients, process recordings are frequently used. A **process recording** is a verbatim (word-for-word) account of a conversation. It can be taped or written, and it includes all verbal and nonverbal interactions.

One method of writing a process recording is to make two columns on a page. The first column lists what the nurse and the client said and did, and the second contains interpretive comments about the nurse's responses. See an example in Table 18–5 on page 374.

Once a process recording his been completed, it should be analyzed in terms of (a) the direction and development of the interaction (process), and (b) the content. The nurse's interaction can be analyzed for process according to a number of questions:

1. Was the client's verbal and nonverbal behavior really heard and seen?
2. Were any cues missed?
3. Were the nurse's verbal responses and behavior congruent?

Text continued on page 376

Table 18–2 Therapeutic Communication Techniques

Technique	Description	Examples
Using silence	Accepting pauses or silences that may extend for several seconds or minutes without interjecting any verbal response.	Sitting quietly (or walking with the client) and waiting attentively until the client is able to put thoughts and feelings into words.
Providing general leads	Using statements or questions that (a) encourage the client to verbalize; (b) choose a topic of conversation; and (c) facilitate continued verbalization.	"Perhaps you would like to talk about . . ." "Would it help to discuss your feelings?" "Where would you like to begin?" "And then . . . what?" "I follow what you are saying."
Being specific and tentative	Making statements that are specific rather than general, and tentative rather than absolute.	"You scratched my arm." (specific statement) "You are as clumsy as an ox." (general statement) "You seem unconcerned about Mary." (tentative statement) "You don't give a damn about Mary and you never will." (absolute statement)
Using open-ended questions	Asking broad questions that lead or invite the client to explore (elaborate, clarify, describe, compare, or illustrate) thoughts or feelings. Open-ended questions specify only the topic to be discussed and invite answers that are longer than one or two words.	"I'd like to hear more about that." "Tell me about . . ." "How have you been feeling lately?" "What brought you to the hospital?" "What is your opinion?" "You said you were frightened yesterday. How do you feel now?"
Using touch	Providing appropriate forms of touch to reinforce caring feelings. Because tactile contacts vary considerably among individuals, families, and cultures, the nurse must be sensitive to the differences in attitudes and practices of clients and self.	Putting an arm over the client's shoulder. Placing the hand over the client's hand.
Restating or paraphrasing	Actively listening for the client's basic message and then repeating those thoughts and/or feelings in similar words. This conveys that the nurse has listened and understood the client's basic message and also offers clients a clearer idea of what they have said.	Client: "I couldn't manage to eat any dinner last night—not even the dessert." Nurse: "You had difficulty eating yesterday." Client: "Yes, I was very upset after my family left." Client: "I have trouble talking to strangers." Nurse: "You find it difficult talking to people you do not know?"
Seeking clarification	A method of making the client's *broad overall* meaning of the message more understandable. It is used when paraphrasing is difficult or when the communication is rambling or garbled. To clarify the message, the nurse can restate the basic message or confess confusion and ask the client to repeat or restate the message.	"I'm puzzled." "I'm not sure I understand that." "Would you please say that again?" "Would you tell me more?"
	Nurses can also clarify their own message with statements.	"I meant this rather than that." "I guess I didn't make that clear—I'll go over it again."
Perception checking or seeking consensual validation	A method similar to clarifying that verifies the meaning of *specific words* rather than the overall meaning of a message.	Client: "My husband *never* gives me any presents." Nurse: "You mean he has *never* given you a present for your birthday or Christmas?" Client: "Well—not *never*. He does get me something for my birthday and Christmas, but he never thinks of giving me anything at any other time."

Table 18–2 *continued*

Technique	Description	Examples
Offering self	Suggesting one's presence, interest, or wish to understand the client without making any demands or attaching conditions that would make the client comply to the suggestion to receive the nurse's attention.	"I'll stay with you until your daughter arrives." "We can sit here quietly for a while; we don't need to talk unless you would like to." "I'll help you to dress to go home."
Giving information	Providing, in a simple and direct manner, specific factual information the client may or may not request. When information is not known, the nurse states this and indicates who has it or when the nurse will obtain it.	"Your surgery is scheduled for 11 AM tomorrow." "You will feel a 'pulling' sensation when the tube is removed from your abdomen." "I do not know the answer to that, but I will find out from Mrs King, the nurse in charge."
Acknowledging	Giving recognition, in a nonjudgmental way, of a change in behavior, an effort the client has made, or a contribution to a communication. Acknowledgment may be with or without understanding, verbal or nonverbal.	"You trimmed your beard and mustache and washed your hair." "I notice you keep squinting your eyes. Are you having difficulty seeing?" "You walked twice as far today with your walker."
Clarifying time or sequence	Helping the client clarify an event, situation, or happening in relationship to time.	Client: "I vomited this morning." Nurse: "Was that after breakfast?" Client: "I feel that I have been asleep for weeks." Nurse: "You had your operation Monday, and today is Tuesday."
Presenting reality	Helping the client to differentiate the real from the unreal.	"That telephone ring came from the program on television." "That's not a dead mouse in the corner; it is a discarded washcloth." "Your magazine is here in the drawer. It has not been stolen."
Focusing	Helping the client expand on and develop a topic of importance. It is important for the nurse to wait until the clients think they have talked about the main concerns before attempting to focus. The focus may be an idea or a feeling; however, the nurse often emphasizes a feeling to help the client recognize an emotion disguised behind words.	Client: "My wife says she will look after me, but I don't think she can, what with the children to take care of, and they're always after her about something—clothes, homework, what's for dinner that night." Nurse: "You are worried about how well she can manage."
Reflecting	Directing ideas, feelings, questions, or content back to clients to enable them to explore their own ideas and feelings about a situation.	Client: "What can I do?" Nurse: "What do you think would be helpful?" Client: "Do you think I should tell my husband?" Nurse: "You seem unsure about telling your husband."
Summarizing and planning	Stating the main points of a discussion to clarify the relevant points discussed. This technique is useful at the end of an interview or to review a health-teaching session. It often acts as an introduction to future care planning.	"During the past half hour we have talked about . . ." "Tomorrow afternoon we may explore this further." "In a few days I'll review what you have learned about the actions and effects of your insulin."

Table 18–3 Communication Strategies Providing Comfort

Characteristic	Description	Examples of the Nurse's Verbal Reponse
Pity	An expression of regret or sorrow *for* a client who is suffering, distressed, or unhappy; confirms the sufferer's state; facilitates acceptance of reality.	"I don't know how you can deal with all this." "This must be really awful for you." "This is the worst kind of grief—losing a baby."
Sympathy	An expression of the nurse's *own* sorrow for the client's condition or situation; has an "I am sorry" focus; shows acceptance of the client's state, thereby providing comfort.	"I feel sad for you." "I'm so sorry about the results of the biopsy."
Compassion	Expresses a strong emotional response to the client's distress; leads to sharing of the suffering; shows acceptance of the client's problem; strengthens and comforts; nurse experiences the client's pain.	"It could have happened to any of us; it's nothing you did." "It's so unfair! How can this be happening?" "If you want to talk, I'm here to listen."
Consolation	Involves soothing and encouraging to ease discomfort and pain; may offer support and hope; expresses feelings of concern in nurse; can alter focus to the positive without negating crisis.	***To a family member*** "She's holding her own; she's still very sick but she's stable; this has been difficult for her." ***To a client:*** "You've done very well so far."
Commiseration	Used commonly in support groups or when the nurse has experienced the client's problem in some form; nurse and client have mutual response to a common experience; the nurse sincerely communicates agreement and understanding.	"I can truly understand some of what you're going through. I had a mastectomy 2 years ago." "I was really scared, too, the first time I saw a baby on a respirator; I was afraid to touch anything."
Reflexive reassurance	Spontaneous reaction by the nurse to try to calm the client who feels anxiety and distress over some circumstance. The nurse's response is intended to balance the client's feelings.	"You're going to be fine" (when you know the client will be). "No, I don't think you're being silly, but you know they will make sure the spinal is working before they begin the surgery."

Source: Adapted from JM Morse, J Bottorff, G Anderson, B O'Brien, and S Solberg, Beyond empathy: Expanding expressions of caring, *Journal of Advanced Nursing*, July 1992, 17:809–21.

Table 18–4 Nontherapeutic Responses

Technique	Description	Examples
Stereotyping	Offering generalized and oversimplified beliefs about groups of people that are based on experiences too limited to be valid. These responses categorize clients and negate their uniqueness as individuals.	"Two-year olds are brats." "Women are complainers." "Men don't cry." "Most people don't have any pain after this type of surgery."
Agreeing and disagreeing	Akin to judgmental responses, agreeing and disagreeing imply that the client is either right or wrong and that the nurse is in a position to judge this. These responses deter clients from thinking through their position and may cause a client to become defensive.	Client: "I don't think Dr Broad is a very good doctor. He doesn't seem interested in his patients." Nurse: "Dr Broad is head of the Department of Surgery and is an excellent surgeon."

Table 18–4 *continued*

Technique	Description	Examples
Being defensive	Attempting to protect a person or health care services from negative comments. These responses prevent the client from expressing true concerns. The nurse is saying, "You have no right to complain." Defensive responses protect the nurse from admitting weaknesses in the health care services, including personal weaknesses.	Client: "Those night nurses must just sit around and talk all night. They didn't answer my light for over an hour." Nurse: "I'll have you know we literally run around on nights. You're not the only client, you know."
Challenging	Giving a response that makes clients prove their statement or point of view. These responses indicate that the nurse is failing to consider the client's feelings, making the client feel it necessary to defend a position.	Client: "I felt nauseated after that red pill." Nurse: "Surely you don't think I gave you the wrong pill?" Client: "I feel as if I am dying." Nurse: "How can you feel that way when your pulse is 60?" Client: "I believe my husband doesn't love me." Nurse: "You can't say that; why, he visits you every day."
Probing	Asking for information chiefly out of curiosity rather than with the intent to assist the client. These responses are considered prying and violate the client's privacy. Often asking "why" is probing and places the client in a defensive position.	Client: "I was speeding along the street and didn't see the stop sign." Nurse: "Why were you speeding?" Client: "I didn't ask the doctor when he was here." Nurse: "Why didn't you?"
Testing	Asking questions that make the client admit to something. These responses permit the client only limited answers and often meet the nurse's need rather than the client's.	"Who do you think you are?" (enforces people to admit their status is only that of client) "Do you think I am not busy?" (forces the client to admit that the nurse really *is* busy)
Rejecting	Refusing to discuss certain topics with the client. These responses often make clients feel that the nurse is rejecting not only their communication but also the clients themselves.	"I don't want to discuss that. Let's talk about . . ." "Let's discuss other areas of interest to you rather than the two problems you keep mentioning." "I can't talk now. I'm on my way for coffee break."
Changing topics and subjects	Directing the communication into areas of self-interest rather than considering the client's concerns often arises as a self-protecting response to anxiety-causing topics. These responses imply that what the nurse considers important will be discussed and that clients are not capable of helping themselves.	Client: "I'm separated from my wife. Do you think I should have sexual relations with another woman?" Nurse: "I see that you're 36 and that you like gardening. This sunshine is good for my roses. I have a beautiful rose garden."
Unwarranted reassurance	Using cliches or comforting statements of advice as a means to reassure the client. These responses block the fears, feelings, and other thoughts of the client.	"You'll feel better soon." "I'm sure everything will turn out all right." "Don't worry."
Passing judgment	Giving opinions and approving or disapproving responses, moralizing, or implying one's own values. These responses imply that the client *must* think as the nurse thinks, fostering client dependence.	"That's good (bad)." "You shouldn't do that." "That's not good enough." "What you did was wrong (right)."
Giving common advice	Telling the client what do to. These responses deny the client's right to be an equal partner. Note that giving *expert* rather than common advice is therapeutic.	Client: "Should I move from my home to a nursing home?" Nurse: "If I were you, I'd go to a nursing home, where you'll get your meals cooked for you."

Table 18–5 Sample Process Recording

Mary Jane Adams, a nursing aide, reports to Irene Olsen, the staff nurse, that Sandra Barrett, the client in room 815, had finished only her orange juice when Ms Adams collected the breakfast trays. Mrs Barrett had been admitted 2 days earlier for diagnostic studies. Concerned about her client, Ms Olsen walks down the corridor to room 815, knocks, and enters. Mrs Barrett turns away from the window, tears in her eyes, as Ms Olsen enters.

Nurse/Client Dialog	Comments
NURSE: Good morning, Mrs Barrett.	Acknowledging.
CLIENT: Hello.	
NURSE: I understand you didn't eat your breakfast.	Making a specific statement, but ignoring the nonverbal.
CLIENT: I wasn't hungry.	
NURSE: Is something wrong?	Asking a closed-ended question that fails to facilitate exploration.
CLIENT: No. (Eyes fill with tears.)	
NURSE: You look sad; as if you're about to cry.	Giving feedback.
CLIENT: (Cries)	
NURSE: I'll sit here a while with you. (Sits down.)	Offering self.
CLIENT: (Continues to cry.)	
NURSE: (After a 30-second pause): Sometimes it's hard to share the things you're concerned about with someone you don't know well. I'd like to be able to help.	Empathizing. Supporting. Offering self.
CLIENT: (Angrily): You can help me by telling me the truth.	
NURSE: (Leans forward and maintains eye contact.)	Actively listening and demonstrating interest.
CLIENT: Everyone beats around the bush when I ask them what's wrong with me. The head nurse said, "What do *you* think is wrong?" That kind of put-off drives me up the wall!	
NURSE: You're angry because you're not getting any answers. It seems as if the staff knows something about your condition and they're keeping it from you.	Paraphrasing.
CLIENT: They all seem to be in cahoots. Nobody tells me anything. (Pause.) (Softly): If the news was good, they wouldn't beat around the bush.	
NURSE: I'm wondering if you're worried that because people haven't answered your question it means that you have a serious illness?	Paraphrasing.
CLIENT: Good news is always easy to give.	
NURSE: Yes, people do seem to be able to deliver good news easier and faster. I also know that we don't have any news—good or bad—to give you, because none of the laboratory or X-ray results are back yet. I know that doesn't help answer your questions, but I hope it relieves you a bit from worrying that there is some bad news that's being withheld.	Giving information. Supporting.

Table 18–5 ***continued***

Nurse/Client Dialog	Comments
CLIENT: Well, when my father-in-law had surgery for a bleeding ulcer, the X-ray and laboratory results were available immediately.	
NURSE: When there's a question of emergency surgery being needed, then tests results are asked for immediately. Usually, though, it's preferable to wait for an accurate reading and a thorough written report.	Giving information.
CLIENT: Are you absolutely sure?	
NURSE: You don't sound convinced.	Acknowledging the implied.
CLIENT: Listen, I don't mean to give you a hard time. It's just that . . . it may not seem like an emergency to my doctor or the lab people, but it sure is to me. I can't stand not knowing. I don't know the results of the tests I had yesterday. I don't know how many more tests I have to have. Will I have to have surgery? When can I go home?	
NURSE: The problem you need help with now is finding out the answers to four questions: What are the results of yesterday's tests? Is your doctor considering any other tests for you, and if so what are they? Is surgery being planned? And when can you go home? Let's try to figure out how you can get the answers to these questions.	Summarizing. Encouraging problem solving.
CLIENT: Well, I can't call my doctor on the phone. All his receptionist will do is take the message. And, anyway, I'm afraid that he'll be offended if he thinks I'm complaining about him. You won't tell him, will you?	
NURSE: No, not unless you and I decide together that it would be the best solution.	Encouraging collaboration.
CLIENT: I suppose I could try to forget about it and be patient, just like everyone tells me to.	
NURSE: You've tried that, but you're still worried, fearful, and angry. Let's think of some other possibilities.	Encouraging further exploration.
CLIENT: Maybe you could call his office for me! Since you're a nurse, they'll probably put your call right through.	
NURSE: So far there are three possible solutions—calling his office yourself, waiting until he comes to visit you later this afternoon, or having me call his office. Are there any other possible solutions that we haven't considered?	Focusing on solutions.
CLIENT: I can't think of any others.	
NURSE: Okay, then, which do you think would be best?	Demonstrating respect for the client.
CLIENT: I guess I'd feel better if you called his office. I just don't want him to think that I'm criticizing him.	
NURSE: You're concerned about what he might think of you because of this phone call. Let's discuss how I should handle the call and what I should say.	Paraphrasing. Encouraging collaboration and problem solving.

After a few minutes they develop a plan for calling Mrs Barrett's physician, and Ms Olsen makes the call. The physician has decided to call both the laboratory and the X-ray department for the results of Mrs Barrett's tests and promises to phone her as soon as he learns the results. They will discuss further possible tests and treatment plans that afternoon when he makes his hospital rounds. Mrs Barrett asks Ms Olsen to stay with her while she receives the physician's telephone call about the test.

Source: Adapted from material by Carol Ren Kneisl, President and Educational Director, Nursing Transitions, Williamsville, New York.

4. Did the client respond to the nurse or independently of the nurse?
5. Did the communication process flow smoothly?
6. Were the nurse's responses consistent with what the nurse observed and heard? Or were they unrelated, exaggerated, or underresponsive?
7. Were the nurse's responses therapeutic or nontherapeutic? See the previous sections on responding therapeutically or nontherapeutically.

Each response can also be analyzed for content in terms of facilitating or inhibiting communication.

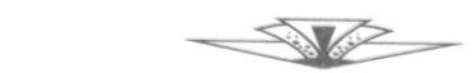

GROUP INTERACTION

People are born into a group (ie, a family) and interact with others at all stages of their lives in various groups: peer groups, work groups, recreational groups, religious groups, and so on. A **group** is defined as two or more persons who have shared needs and goals, who take each other into account in their actions, and who thus are held together and set apart from others by virtue of their interactions. Groups exist to help people achieve goals (outcomes) that would be unattainable by individual effort alone. For example, groups can often solve problems more effectively than one person by pooling the ideas and expertise of several individuals; in addition, information can be disseminated to groups more quickly than to individuals. The overall effectiveness of groups in attaining goals depends on many factors, discussed on page 378.

TYPES OF HEALTH CARE GROUPS

Much of a nurse's professional life is spent in a wide variety of groups, ranging from **dyads** (two-person groups) to large professional organizations. As a participant in a group, the nurse may be required to fulfill different roles: member or leader, teacher or learner, adviser or advisee, and so on.

Common types of health care groups include task groups, teaching groups, self-help groups, self-awareness/growth groups, therapy groups, and work-related social support groups. There are similarities and differences among the characteristics of these various types of groups and the nurse's role.

Task Groups The task group is one of the most common types of work-related groups to which nurses belong. Examples are health care planning committees, nursing service committees, nursing team meetings, nursing care conference groups, and hospital staff meetings. The focus of such groups is the completion of a specific task, and the format is defined at the outset by the leader and/or members. The methods used to perform the task vary according to the task to be performed.

The leader of a task group, usually called the *chairperson,* must be accepted by the members as an appropriate leader and therefore should be an expert in the area of task emphasis. The chairperson's role is to identify the specific task, clarify communication, and assist in expressing opinions and offering solutions. *Committee members* are generally selected in terms of their individual functional role and employment status, rather than in terms of their personal characteristics. Member participation is determined by the task. A target date for termination of the group is usually set in advance.

Teaching Groups The major purpose of teaching groups is to impart information to the participants. Examples of teaching groups include group continuing education and client health care groups. Numerous subjects are often handled via the group teaching format: childbirth techniques, birth control methods, effective parenting, nutrition, management of chronic illness such as diabetes, exercise for middle-aged and older adults, and instructions to family members about follow-up care for discharged clients. A nurse who leads a group in which the primary purpose is to teach or learn must be skilled in the teaching-learning process discussed in Chapter 19.

Self-Help Groups A self-help group is a small, voluntary organization composed of individuals who share a similar health, social, or daily living problem (Rollins 1987, p. 403). These groups are based on the helper-ther-

POSITIVE ASPECTS OF SELF-HELP GROUPS

- Members can experience almost instant kinship, because the essence of the group is the idea that "you are not alone."
- Members can talk about their feelings and listen to the concerns of others, knowing they all share this experience.
- The group atmosphere is generally one of acceptance, support, encouragement, and caring.
- Many members act as role models for newer members and can inspire them to attempt tasks they might consider impossible.
- The group provides the opportunity for people to help as well as to *be* helped—a critical component in restoring self-esteem.

Source: VJ Gilbey. Self-help. *Canadian Nurse* April 1987, 83:25.

Table 18–6 Comparative Features of Effective and Ineffective Groups

Factor	Effective Groups	Ineffective Groups
Atmosphere	Informal, comfortable, and relaxed. It is a working atmosphere in which people demonstrate their interest and involvement.	Obviously tense. Signs of boredom may appear.
Goal setting	Goals, tasks, and objectives are clarified, understood, and modified so that members of the group can commit themselves to cooperatively structured goals.	Unclear, misunderstood, or imposed goals may be accepted by members. The goals are competitively structured.
Leadership and member participation	Shift from time to time, depending on the circumstances. Different members assume leadership at various times, because of their knowledge or experience.	Delegated and based on authority. The chairperson may dominate the group, or the members may defer unduly. Member participation is unequal, with high-authority members dominating. One or more functions may not be emphasized.
Communication	Open and two-way. Ideas and feelings are encouraged, both about the problem and about the group's operation.	Closed or one-way. Only the production of ideas is encouraged. Feelings are ignored or taboo. Members may be tentative or reluctant to be open and may have "hidden agendas" (personal goals at cross-purposes with group goals).
Decision making	By consensus, although various decision-making procedures appropriate to the situation may be instituted.	By the highest authority in the group, with minimal involvement by members; or an inflexible style is imposed.
Cohesion	Facilitated through high levels of inclusion, trust, liking, and support.	Either ignored or used as a means of controlling members, thus promoting rigid conformity.
Conflict tolerance	High. The reasons for disagreements or conflicts are carefully examined, and the group seeks to resolve them. The group accepts unresolvable basic disagreements and lives with them.	Low. Attempts may be made to ignore, deny, avoid, suppress, or override controversy by premature group action.
Power	Determined by the members' abilities and the information they possess. Power is shared. The issue is how to get the job done.	Determined by position in the group. Obedience to authority is strong. The issue is who controls.
Problem solving	High. Constructive criticism is frequent, frank, relatively comfortable, and oriented toward removing an obstacle to problem solving.	Low. Criticism may be destructive, taking the form of either overt or covert personal attacks. It prevents the group from getting the job done.
Self-evaluation as a group	Frequent. All members participate in evaluation and decisions about how to improve the group's functioning.	Minimal. What little evaluation there is may be done by the highest authority in the group rather than by the membership as a whole.
Creativity	Encouraged. There is room within the group for members to become self-actualized and interpersonally effective.	Discouraged. People are afraid of appearing foolish if they put forth a creative thought.

Source: HS Wilson and CR Kneisl, *Psychiatric Nursing*, 4th ed. (Redwood City, CA: Addison-Wesley Nursing, 1992), p. 695. Used by permission.

apy principle: those who help are helped most. One of the central beliefs of the self-help movement is that persons who experience a particular social or health problem have an understanding of that condition which those without it do not.

There are many self-help groups available for a range of problems (eg, stillbirth, parenting, pregnant adolescents, divorce, drug abuse, cancer, menopause, mental illness, diabetes, AIDS, women's health, caregivers of elderly people, and grief). Alcoholics Anonymous was the first self-help group established. Positive aspects of self-help groups are outlined in the box on page 376.

The major functions of the nurse's role in self-help groups include the following:

1. Helping clients form such groups by identifying key people who can act as facilitators.
2. Sharing expertise with clients and helping them gain appropriate knowledge and skills.
3. Informing clients and support persons about existing self-help groups available to them.
4. Participating as a member of a self-help group when this is appropriate. The nurse's role is that of a resource person, that is, being "on tap, but not on top."
5. Helping out in times of crisis.

Self-Awareness/Growth Groups The purpose of self-awareness/growth groups is to develop or use interpersonal strengths. The overall aim is to improve the person's functioning in the group to which they return, whether job, family, or community. From the beginning, broad goals are usually apparent, for example, to study communication patterns, group process, or problem solving. Because the focus of these groups is interpersonal concerns around current situations, the work of the group is oriented to reality testing with a here-and-now emphasis. Members are responsible for correcting inefficient patterns of relating and communicating with each other. They learn group process through participation and involvement and guided exercises.

Therapy Groups Therapy groups work toward self-understanding, more satisfactory ways of relating or handling stress, and changing patterns of behavior toward health.

Members of the therapy group are referred to as clients or, in some settings, as patients. They are selected by health professionals after extensive selection interviews that consider the pattern of personalities, behaviors, needs, and identification of group therapy as the treatment of choice. Duration of therapy groups is not usually set. A termination date is usually mutually determined by the therapist and members.

Work-Related Social Support Groups Many nurses experience some of the high levels of vocational stress, for example, hospice, emergency, and critical care nurses. Social support groups can help reduce stress for such nurses if various types of support are provided to buffer the stress. Group members who know about the work of others can encourage and challenge members to be more creative and enthusiastic about their work and to achieve more. For example, a nurse may help another team member consider alternative strategies for intervention. Members also can share the joys of success and the frustration of failure through active listening without giving advice or making judgments. This type of social support is best given *outside* of the work-related support group.

FEATURES OF EFFECTIVE GROUPS

To be effective, a group must achieve three main functions:

1. Accomplish its goals
2. Maintain its **cohesion** (degree of group unity or oneness; sense of members being "we")
3. Develop and modify its structure to improve its effectiveness

Characteristics of an effectively functioning group are shown in Table 18–6 on page 377.

CHAPTER HIGHLIGHTS

- The effective nurse-client relationship is a helping relationship that facilitates growth and provides support, comfort, and hope.
- Four phases of the helping relationship include the preinteraction phase, the introductory phase, the working phase, and the termination phase; each has a specific purpose or goal and requires specific skills of the nurse.
- Communication incorporates exchanging information between two or more people and is a basic component of human relationships and nurse-client relationships.
- Communication is usually categorized as verbal or nonverbal.
- Verbal communication is effective when the criteria of simplicity, clarity, timing, relevance, adaptability, and credibility are met.
- Nonverbal communication often reveals more about a person's thoughts and feelings than verbal communication; it includes physical appearance, posture and gait, facial expressions, hand movements, use of touch, and other gestures.

- When assessing verbal and nonverbal behaviors, the nurse needs to consider cultural influences and be aware that a variety of feelings can be expressed by a single nonverbal expression and that words can have various meanings.
- When communication is effective, verbal and nonverbal expressions are congruent.
- Communication is a two-way interpersonal process involving the sender of the message and the receiver of the message. It also involves intrapersonal messages, or self-talk, which can affect the message, the interpretation of the message, and the response.
- Because the sender must encode the message and determine the appropriate channels for conveying it, and because the receiver must perceive the message, decode it, and then respond, the communication process includes four elements: sender, message, receiver, and feedback.
- Many factors influence the communication process: the ability of the communicator, perceptions, personal space (intimate, personal, social, and public distance), territoriality, roles and relationships, purposes, time and setting, attitudes, emotions, and self-esteem.
- To assess a client's communication abilities, the nurse determines (a) the presence of communication barriers such as a language deficit, sensory deficits, cognitive impairments, and structural deficits, and (b) the style of verbal and nonverbal communication.
- The NANDA nursing diagnosis used for clients with communication problems is **Impaired verbal communication.**
- Many techniques facilitate therapeutic communication: attentive listening; paraphrasing; clarifying; using open questions and statements; focusing; being specific; using touch and silence; clarifying reality, time, or sequence; providing general leads; and summarizing.
- Communication techniques specifically used to provide comfort to a distressed client include honest and sincere expression of pity, sympathy, compassion, commiseration, consolation, and reflexive reassurance.
- Techniques that inhibit communication include offering unvalidated reassurance, stating approval or disapproval, giving common (not expert) advice, stereotyping, and being defensive.
- To help clients with communication problems the nurse manipulates the environment, provides support, employs measures to enhance communication, and educates the client and support persons.
- Process recordings are frequently made by nurses to evaluate their own communication. With them, nurses can analyze both the process and the content of the communication.
- Nurses interact with groups of clients and colleagues in a wide variety of settings. To use groups rationally and effectively, nurses must understand the features of effective groups.
- Effective groups produce outstanding results, succeed in spite of difficulties, and have members who feel responsible for the output of the group. They accomplish their goals (outcomes), maintain cohesion, and develop and modify their structure in ways that improve effectiveness.

READINGS AND REFERENCES

SUGGESTED READINGS

Boss, BJ. December 1991. Managing communication disorders in stroke. *Nursing Clinics of North America* 26:985–96.

Boss describes the various communication problems a person may have following a stroke. The author also discusses assessments that help the nurse identify the client's specific communication problems and any abilities remaining intact. Finally, the author addresses nursing interventions that may be helpful to the client and to the family in restoring some form of communication and maximizing return of function.

Peplau, HE. July 1960. Talking with patients. *American Journal of Nursing* 60:964–66.

This classic article differentiates nursing communication with a client from that of a layperson. It offers a beginning nursing student helpful suggestions for meaningful communication with clients.

RELATED RESEARCH

Frees, C, Thomas, S, Lynch, J, Stein, R, and Friedman, E. January1989. Blood pressure, heart rate, and heart rhythm changes in patients with heart disease during talking. *Heart and Lung* 18:17–21.

Harrison, TM, Pistolessi, TV, and Stephen, TD. February 1989. Assessing nurses' communication: A cross-sectional study. *Western Journal of Nursing Research* 11:75–91.

SELECTED REFERENCES

Boss, BJ. December 1991. Managing communication disorders in stroke. *Nursing Clinics of North America* 26:985–96.

Bradley, S. August 1991. The signs of silence. *Journal of Emergency Medical Services* 16:26–32.

Brammer, LM. 1988. *The Helping Relationship: Process and Skills.* 4th ed. Englewood Cliffs, NJ: Prentice Hall.

Brown, KC. June 1991. Strategies for effective communication. *AAOHN Journal* 39:292–93.

Burnard, P. May 1992. Viewpoint communication: Born to be mild. *Nursing Standard* 6:53–54.

Carpenito, LJ. 1992. *Nursing Diagnosis: Application to Clinical Practice.* 4th ed. Philadelphia: Lippincott.

Farley, MJ. September 1992. Thought and talk: The intrapersonal component of human communication. *AORN Journal* 56:481–84.

Gordon, M. 1993. *Manual of Nursing Diagnosis 1993–1994.* 6th ed. St Louis: Mosby-Year Book.

Giger, JN and Davidhizar, R. Fall 1990a. Developing communication skills for use with black patients. *Association of Black Nursing Faculty Journal* 1:33–35.

———. November/December 1990b. Culture and space. *Advancing Clinical Care* 5:8–11.

———. 1991. *Transcultural Nursing.* St Louis: Mosby.

Hall, ET. 1969. *The hidden dimension.* Garden City, NY: Doubleday.

Kasch, CR. January 1984. Interpersonal competence and communication in the delivery of nursing care. *Advances in Nursing Science* 6:71–88.

Kim, MJ, McFarland, GK, and McLane, AM. 1993. *Pocket Guide to Nursing Diagnoses.* 5th ed. St Louis: Mosby-Year Book.

Kneisl, CR. 1992. Group process. In Wilson, HS and Kneisl, CR. pp. 270–89. *Psychiatric Nursing.* 4th ed. Redwood City, CA: Addison-Wesley Nursing.

Kozier, B, Erb, G, Blais, K, Johnson, JY, and Temple, JS. 1993. *Techniques in Clinical Nursing.* 4th ed. Redwood City, CA: Addison-Wesley Nursing.

Lederer, JR, Marculescu, GL, Mocnik, B, and Seaby, N. 1993. *Care Planning Pocket Guide: A Nursing Diagnosis Approach.* 5th ed. Redwood City, CA: Addison-Wesley Nursing.

Meadows, JL. 1991. Multicultural communication. *Physical & Occupational Therapy in Pediatrics* 11(4):31–42.

McFarland, GK and McFarlane, EA. 1993. *Nursing Diagnosis and Intervention: Planning for Patient Care.* 2d ed. St Louis: Mosby.

Morse, JM, Bottoroff, J, Anderson, G, O'Brien, B, and Solberg, S. July 1992. Beyond empathy: Expanding expressions of caring. *Journal of Advanced Nursing* 17:809–21.

North American Nursing Diagnosis Association. 1992. *NANDA Nursing Diagnoses: Definitions and Classification 1992–1993.* Philadelphia: NANDA.

Northouse, PG and Northouse, LL. 1992. *Health Communication: Strategies for Health Professionals.* 2d ed. Norwalk, CT: Appleton & Lange.

Puterbaugh, S. January 1991. Communication when the patient cannot speak English. *Today's OR Nurse* 13:31.

Raudsepp, E. April 1990. Seven ways to cure communication breakdowns. *Nursing90* 20:132, 134, 137–38.

Rollins, JA. November/December 1987. Self-help groups for parents. *Pediatric Nursing* 13:403–9.

Rondeau, KV. 1992. Effective communication means really listening. *Canadian Journal of Medical Technology* 54:78–80

Sundeen, SJ, Stuart, GW, Rankin, EAD, and Cohen, SA. 1989. *Nurse-Client Interaction.* 4th ed. St Louis: Mosby.

Thobaben, M. May/June 1991. Evaluation of the therapeutic nurse-patient relationship. *Home Healthcare Nurse* 9:46–47.

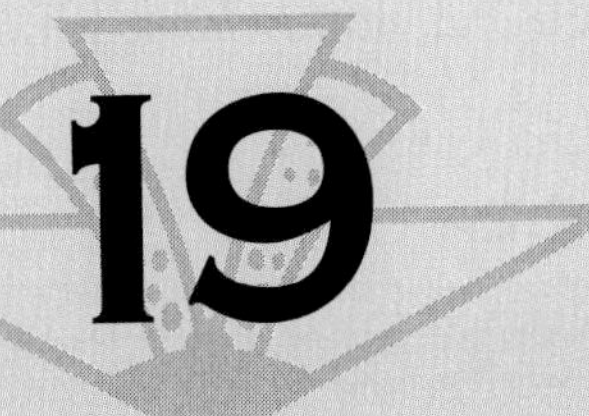

19 Teaching and Learning

Objectives

Explain how andragogy can guide client teaching.

Discuss factors that facilitate learning throughout the life span.

Identify factors that interfere with learning.

Explain the three domains, or areas, of learning.

Contrast the nursing process and the teaching process.

Identify client data nurses need to make a **Knowledge deficit** diagnosis and to plan appropriate teaching.

Describe guidelines for effective teaching.

Describe the essential aspects of a teaching plan.

Explain how client learning is evaluated.

Identify eight guidelines that help nurses implement the teaching plan.

Describe barriers to teaching clients of different cultures and possible ways to reduce or eliminate the barriers.

Describe different teaching strategies and situations in which they might be most effective.

Identify characteristics of effective written information for client education.

Describe how to adapt teaching to throughout the life span.

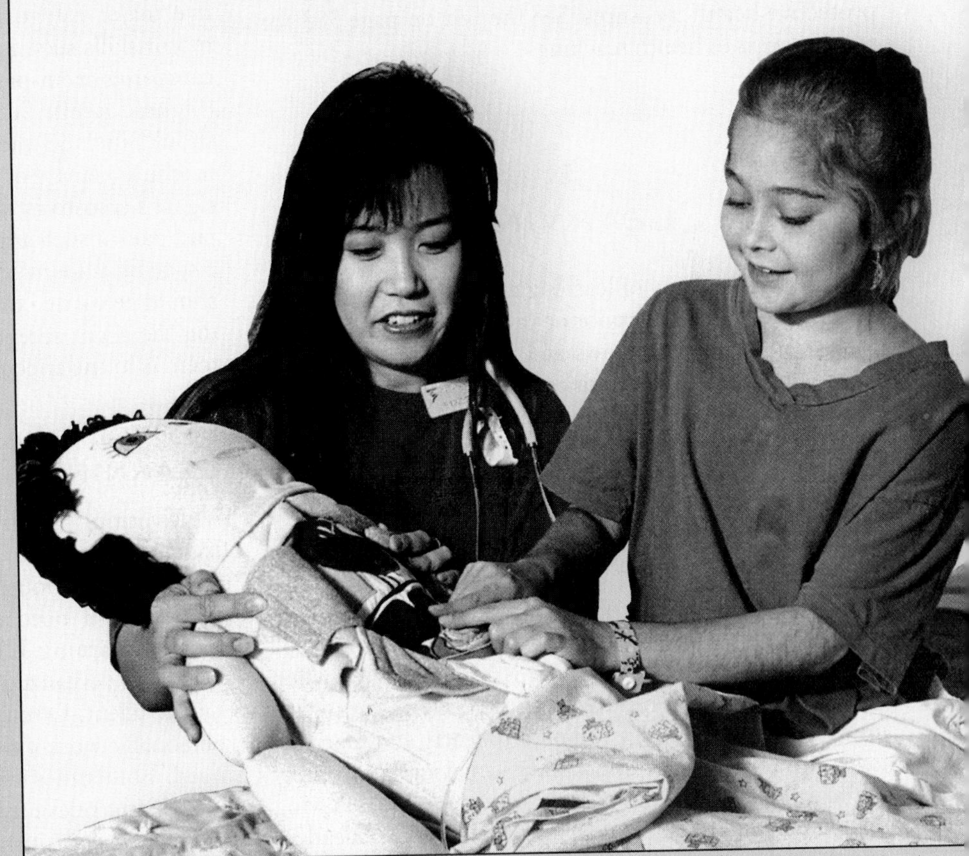

Client education is a major aspect of nursing practice and an important independent nursing function. In 1992, the American Hospital Association passed the Patients' Bill of Rights mandating client education as a right of all clients. In addition, legislation relating to nursing frequently has included client teaching as a function of nursing, thereby making teaching a legal and professional responsibility.

Client education is multifaceted, involving promoting, protecting, and maintaining health. It involves teaching about reducing health risk factors, increasing a person's level of wellness, and providing information about specific protective health measures. See the box on page 383 for specific areas of health teaching.

LEARNING

Clients have a variety of learning needs. A **learning need** is a need to change behavior or "a gap between the information an individual knows and the information necessary to perform a function or care for self" (Gessner 1989, p. 593). **Learning** is a change in human disposition or capability that persists over a period of time and that cannot be solely accounted for by growth. Learning is represented by a change in behavior. An important aspect of learning is the individual's desire to learn and to act on the learning. This is referred to as **compliance.** In the health care context compliance is "the extent to which a person's behavior coincides with medical or health advice" (Haynes 1979, p. 1). Compliance is best illustrated when the person recognizes and accepts the need to learn, willingly expends the energy required to learn, and then follows through with the appropriate behaviors that reflect the learning. For example, a person diagnosed as having diabetes willingly learns about the special diet needed, and then plans and follows the learned diet.

Andragogy is "the art and science of helping adults learn" (Knowles 1980, p. 43) in contrast to **pedagogy,** the discipline concerned with helping children learn. Nurses can use the following andragogic concepts about learners as a guide for client teaching (Knowles 1984):

- As people mature, they move from dependence to independence.
- An adult's previous experiences can be used as a resource for learning.
- An adult's readiness to learn is often related to a developmental task or social role.
- An adult is more oriented to learning when the material is immediately useful, not useful sometime in the future.

DOMAINS OF LEARNING

Bloom (1956) has identified three domains, or areas of learning: cognitive, affective, and psychomotor. The *cognitive domain* includes six intellectual skills such as knowing, comprehending and applying in an order from simple to complex. The *affective domain* includes feelings, emotions, interests, attitudes, and appreciations. It involves five major categories. The *psychomotor domain* includes motor skills such as giving an injection. It includes seven categories from perception (lowest level) to origination (highest level). See Table 19–1 on page 384. Nurses should include each of these three domains in client teaching plans. For example, teaching a client how to irrigate a colostomy is the psychomotor domain. An important part of such a teaching plan is to teach the client why a specific amount of fluid is used and when the irrigation should be carried out; this is the cognitive domain. Helping the client accept the colostomy and maintain self-esteem is in the affective domain.

FACTORS FACILITATING LEARNING

Motivation Motivation to learn is the desire to learn. It greatly influences how quickly and how much a person learns. Motivation is generally greatest when a person recognizes a need and believes the need will be met through learning. It is not enough for the need to be identified and verbalized by the nurse; it must be experienced by the client. Often the nurse's task is to help the client personally work through the problem and identify the need. Sometimes clients or support persons need help identifying relevant situational elements before they can see a need. For instance, clients with heart disease may need to know the effects of smoking before they recognize the need to stop smoking. Or adolescents may need to know the consequences of an untreated sexually transmitted disease before they see the need for treatment.

Readiness Readiness to learn is the behavior that reflects motivation at a specific time. Readiness reflects a client's willingness and ability to learn. The nurse's role is often to encourage the development of readiness.

Active Involvement Active involvement in the process makes learning more meaningful. If the learner actively participates in planning and discussion, learning is faster

AREAS FOR CLIENT EDUCATION

Promotion of Health

- Increasing a person's level of wellness
- Growth and development topics
- Fertility control
- Hygiene
- Nutrition
- Exercise
- Stress management
- Lifestyle modification
- Resources within community

Prevention of Illness/Injury

- Health screening (eg, blood glucose levels, blood pressure, blood cholesterol, Pap test, mammograms, vision, hearing, routine physical examinations)
- Reducing health risk factors (eg, lowering cholesterol level)
- Specific protective health measures (eg, immunizations, use of condoms, use of sunscreen, use of medication, umbilical cord care)
- First aid
- Safety (eg, using seat belts, helmets, walkers)

Restoration of Health

- Information about tests, diagnosis, treatment, medications
- Self-care skills or skills needed to care for family member
- Resources within health care setting and community

Adapting to Altered Health and Function

- Adaptations in life-style
- Problem-solving skills
- Adaptation to changing health status
- Strategies to deal with current problems (eg, home IV skills, medications, diet, activity limits, prostheses)
- Strategies to deal with future problems (eg, fear of pain with terminal cancer, future surgeries, or treatments)
- Information about prognosis, treatments, and likely outcomes
- Referrals to other health care facilities or services
- Facilitation of strong self-image
- Grief and bereavement counseling

and retention is better. See Figure 19–1 on page 385. Passive learning, such as listening to a lecture or watching a film, does not foster optimal learning.

Once learners have succeeded in accomplishing a task or understanding a concept, they gain self-confidence in their ability to learn. This reduces their anxiety about failure and can motivate greater learning. Successful learners have increased confidence with which to accept failure. People learn best when they believe they are accepted and will not be judged. The person who expects to be judged as a "poor" or "good" client will not learn as well as the person who feels no such threat.

Feedback Feedback is information relating a person's performance to a desired goal. It has to be meaningful to the learner. Feedback that accompanies practice of psychomotor skills helps the person to learn those skills. Support or desired behavior through praise, positively worded corrections, and suggestions of alternative methods are ways of providing positive feedback. Negative feedback such as ridicule, anger, or sarcasm can lead people to withdraw from learning. Such feedback, viewed as a type of punishment, may cause the client to avoid the teacher in order to avoid punishment.

Simple to Complex Learning is facilitated by material that is logically organized and proceeds from the *simple to the complex*. Such organization enables the learner to comprehend new information, assimilate it with previous learning, and form new understandings. Of course, simple and complex are relative terms, depending on the level at which the person is learning. What is simple for one person may be complex for another.

Repetition Repetition of key concepts and facts facilitates retention of newly learned material. Practice of psychomotor skills, particularly with feedback from the nurse, improves performance of those skills and facilitates their transfer to another setting. Also when a person appreciates the relevance of specific material, learning is facilitated.

Table 19–1 Major Categories in Each Learning Domain

Category/Description	Example
Cognitive Domain	
Knowledge Remembers previously learned material	A client learns the side effects of a medication and describes them two days later.
Comprehension Understands the meaning of learned material	A client describes how the side effects of a medication can be recognized and what to do about them.
Application Applies newly learned material in new concrete situations	A client learns to take the medication after meals to minimize side effects.
Analysis Breaks learned material into component parts and separates important from unimportant material	A client describes which side effects are serious and when the physician is to be notified.
Synthesis Takes parts of learned material and puts them together to form new material	A client learns to take steps to prevent side effects of a medication.
Evaluation Judges the value of the learned material	A client describes how the knowledge of new material can help prevent accidents at work.
Affective Domain	
Receiving Willingness to attend to particular stimuli	A female client is willing to listen to a nurse's description of the preparation for breast surgery.
Responding Actively participates by listening and responding	The female client asks questions about the preparation for the scheduled surgery.
Valuing Attaches a value or worth to a particular object, phenomenon, or behavior	The female client refuses to look at the incision following her breast removal.
Organization Develops a value system by bringing together different values and resolving conflicts	The client accepts changes brought about by the breast surgery.
Characterization Acts according to a value system	After surgery, the client returns to a life-style consistent with her value system.
Psychomotor Domain	
Perception Uses the senses to obtain cues to guide motor activity	A male client immediately calls a nurse when he sees another client fall from his bed.
Set Refers to readiness to take immediate action: includes mental, physical, and emotional sets	The client becomes ready to act when he sees the client who fell from his bed preparing to get out of his chair.
Guided Response Performs an act under the guidance of a nurse	A client moves himself from his bed to a wheelchair with a nurse's guidance.
Mechanism Performs a learned activity with confidence and proficiency	The client moves himself between his bed and a wheelchair quickly and competently.
Complex Overt Response Performs a motor skill competently, accurately, and smoothly	The client moves between the bed and the wheelchair at the same time adjusting his intravenous line and his catheter.
Adaption Performs skills and adapts them to special circumstances	The client stops transferring to the wheelchair and adjusts his intravenous line when it stops dripping
Origination Creates new movement patterns to suit a particular problem	The client transfers from his bed to the wheelchair in a different way to avoid pull on the intravenous line.

Sources: Adapted from NE Gronlund, *Stating Objectives for Classroom Instruction*, 3d ed. (New York: Macmillan, 1985), pp. 34–40; and BS Bloom, editor, *Taxonomy of Educational Objectives. Vol 1: Cognitive Domain*, (New York: David McKay Company Inc, 1956), pp. 18–24.

Timing People retain information and psychomotor skills best when the *time between learning and use is short*; the longer the time interval, the more is forgotten. For example, a woman who is taught how to administer her own insulin but is not permitted to do so until discharge from hospital is unlikely to remember much of what she learned. However, if she is allowed to give her own injections while in hospital, her learning will be enhanced.

Environment An *optimal learning environment* facilitates learning by reducing distraction and providing physical and psychological comfort. It has adequate lighting that is free from glare, a comfortable room temperature, and good ventilation. Most students know what it is like to try to learn in a hot, stuffy room; the subsequent drowsiness interferes with concentration. Noise can also distract the student and interfere with listening and thinking. To facilitate learning in a hospital setting, nurses should choose a time when there are no visitors present and interruptions are unlikely. Privacy is essential for some learning. For example, when a client is learning to irrigate a colostomy, the presence of others can be embarrassing and thus interfere with learning. When a client is particularly anxious, having support persons present often gives the client confidence.

FACTORS INHIBITING LEARNING

Many factors inhibit learning. Some of the most common are described below and in Table 19–2 on page 386.

Emotions A greatly *elevated anxiety* level can impede learning. Clients or families who are very worried may not hear spoken words or may retain only part of the communication. Extreme anxiety might be reduced by medications or by information that relieves uncertainty. By contrast, clients who appear disinterested and unconcerned may need to be cautioned about potential problems to enhance their motivation to learn.

Physiologic Events Learning can be inhibited by *physiologic events* such as a critical illness, pain, or impaired hearing. Because the client cannot concentrate and apply energy to learning, the learning itself is impaired. The nurse should try to reduce the physiologic barriers to learning as much as possible before teaching. Providing analgesics and rest before teaching is often helpful.

Cultural Barriers There are also *cultural barriers* to learning, such as language or values. Obviously the client who does not understand the nurse's language will learn little. Western medicine may conflict with cultural healing beliefs and practices. Nurses must deal directly with this conflict to be effective, otherwise the client may be partially or totally noncompliant with recommended treatments. In addition, another impediment to learning is *differing values* held by the client and the health team.

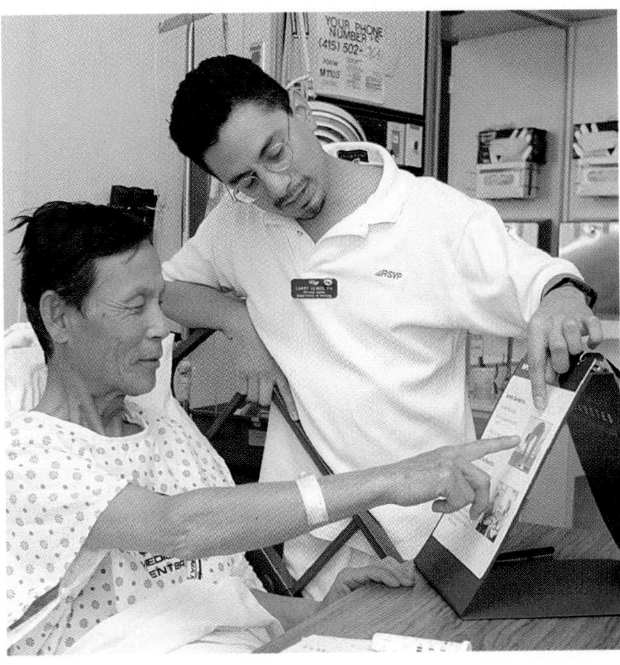

Figure 19–1 Learning is facilitated when the client is interested and actively involved.

For example, a client who does not value being thin may have difficultly learning about a reducing diet.

DEVELOPMENTAL AND HEALTH FACTORS AFFECTING LEARNING

Cognitive Ability The intellectual development of the individual is an important factor to consider when planning teaching. Piaget's theory of intellectual development explains how people normally learn to think, reason, and use language. See Chapter 23, page 575 and Table 23–5 for Piaget's stages of intellectual development and significant behavior at these various stages of development. Age may or may not reflect cognitive development. Although most people develop cognitively along predictable lines, there are also wide variations in the population. In addition, some people are never able to read or write and others are unable to do simple mathematical calculations. For example, a 27-year-old male client who has not developed intellectually beyond a 4-year-old level will be unable to read instructions about wound care. However, a 30-year-old female client who is a university graduate will probably be able to understand complex instructions regarding her self-care.

It is important that the nurse know the clients' knowledge level and intellectual abilities.

Psychomotor Ability Psychomotor development involves strength, coordination, energy, and sensory acuity. Havighurst describes the developmental tasks (motor

Table 19–2 Barriers to Learning

Barrier	Explanation	Nursing Implications
Acute illness	Client requires all resources and energy to cope with illness.	Defer teaching until client is less ill.
Pain	Pain decreases ability to concentrate.	Deal with pain before teaching.
Age	Vision, hearing, and motor control can be impaired in the elderly.	Consider sensory and motor defects in teaching plan.
Prognosis	Client can be preoccupied with illness and unable to concentrate on new information.	Defer teaching to a better time.
Biorhythms	Mental and physical performances have a circadian rhythm.	Adapt time of teaching to suit client.
Emotion (eg, anxiety, denial, depression, grief)	Emotions require energy and distract from learning.	Deal with emotions first and possible misinformation.
Language and ethnic background	Client may not be fluent in the nurse's language.	Obtain services of an interpreter or nurse with appropriate language skills.
Iatrogenic barriers	The nurse may set up barriers by appearing condescending or hurried, ignoring client cues, or appearing incompetent or unsure.	Establish a helping relationship and be sensitive to the client's needs. Plan and prepare for teaching ahead of time with current information appropriate for the learner.

skills) that occur throughout life. See Table 23–2 and page 570. It is important that the nurse be aware of a client's psychomotor skills when planning teaching. Psychomotor skills can be affected by health. For example, an elderly male client who has severe osteoarthritis of the hands may not be able to tie a bandage. The following physical abilities are important for learning psychomotor skills:

1. *Muscle strength.* For example, an elderly female client who cannot rise from a chair because of insufficient leg and muscle strength, cannot be expected to learn to lift herself out of a bathtub.
2. *Motor coordination.* Gross motor coordination is required for movements such as walking and fine motor coordination is needed when using utensils such as a fork for eating. For example, a female client who has advanced amyotrophic lateral sclerosis (ALS) involving the lower limbs will probably be unable to use a walker.
3. *Energy.* Energy is required for most psychomotor skills, and learning these skills uses more energy. Often when people are ill or elderly, energy resources are limited; learning and carrying out these skills must be timed for when the client's energy sources are not depleted.
4. *Sensory acuity.* Sight is used for most learning (ie, walking with crutches, changing a dressing, drawing a medication into a syringe). Clients who are visually impaired often need the assistance of support persons to carry out such tasks.

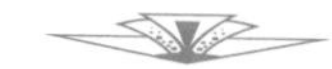

TEACHING

Teaching is a system of activities intended to produce learning. The teaching process is intentionally designed to produce specific learning.

The teaching/learning process involves dynamic interaction between teacher and learner. Each participant in the process communicates information, emotions, perceptions, and attitudes to the other. The teaching process and the nursing process are very much alike. See Table 19–3.

The relationship between the teacher and the learner is essentially one of trust and respect. The client trusts that the nurse has the knowledge and skill to teach, and the nurse respects the client's ability to attain the recognized goals. Once a nurse starts to instruct a client and/or support persons, it is important that the teaching process continue until the participants reach the learning goals, change the goals, or decide that the goals cannot be met.

LEARNING/TEACHING GUIDELINES

The following guidelines for effective learning/teaching may be helpful to nursing students:

- Teaching activities should help the client meet individual learning objectives. These objectives should be determined by the client (learner) and the nurse

Table 19–3 Comparison of the Teaching Process and the Nursing Process

Step	Teaching Process	Nursing Process
1	Collect data; analyze client's learning strengths and deficits.	Collect data; analyze client's strengths and deficits.
2	Make educational diagnoses.	Make nursing diagnoses.
3	Prepare teaching plan: ▪ Write learning objectives. ▪ Select content and time frame. ▪ Select teaching strategies.	Plan nursing goals/outcomes, and select interventions.
4	Implement teaching plan.	Implement nursing strategies.
5	Evaluate client learning based on achievement of learning objectives.	Evaluate client outcomes based on achievement of outcome criteria.

(teacher). If certain activities do not assist the learner, these need to be reassessed; perhaps other activities can replace them. For example, explanation alone may not be able to teach a client to handle a syringe. Actually handling the syringe may be more effective (Figure 19–2).

- Rapport between teacher and learner is essential. A relationship that is both accepting and constructive will best assist learning. The nurse should take time to establish rapport before teaching.
- The teacher who uses the client's previous learning in the present situation encourages the client and facilitates learning new skills. For example, a person who already knows how to cook can use this knowledge when learning to prepare food for a special diet.
- The nurse-teacher must be able to communicate clearly and concisely. The words the nurse uses need to have the same meaning to the learner as to the teacher. For example, a client who is taught not to put water on an area of the skin may think a wet washcloth is permissible for washing the area. In effect, the nurse needs to explain that no water or moisture should touch the area.
- Nurses often need to communicate effectively with individuals and small groups, and sometimes with large groups.
- A knowledge of the clients and the factors that affect their learning should be established before planning the teaching.

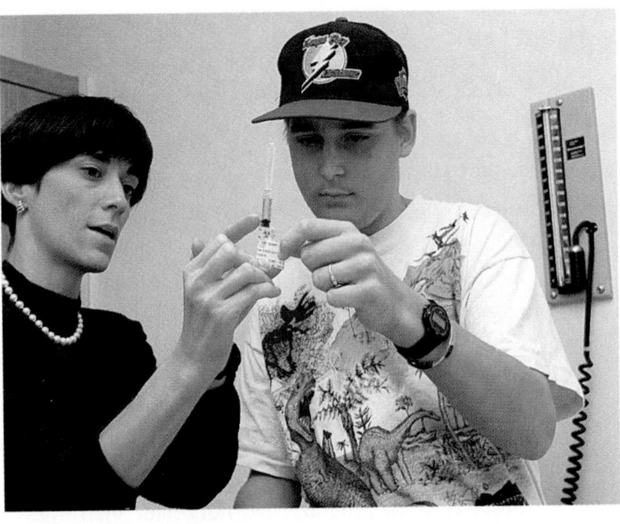

Figure 19–2 Teaching activities may need to include hands-on client participation.

- When a client is involved in planning, learning is often enhanced.
- Teaching that involves a number of the client's senses often enhances learning. For example, when learning about changing a surgical dressing, the nurse can tell the client about the procedure (hearing), show how to change the dressing (sight), and show how to manipulate the equipment (touch).
- The anticipated behavioral changes that indicate that learning has taken place must always be within the context of the client's life-style and resources. For example, it would probably not be reasonable to expect a woman to soak in a tub of hot water four times a day if she did not have a bathtub and had to heat water on a stove.

See the box on page 388 for the characteristics of effective teaching.

ASSESSING

A comprehensive assessment of learning needs incorporates data from the nursing history and physical assessment and addresses the client's support system. It also considers client characteristics that may influence the learning process: readiness to learn, motivation to learn, and reading and comprehension level, for example. Nurses also make many informal observations of clients' abilities and needs. For example, the nurse may identify a learning need by observing the client perform a procedure incorrectly. Clients themselves may express learning needs by asking the nurse to give them specific information or by stating their lack of knowledge or skill in a particular area.

CHARACTERISTICS OF EFFECTIVE TEACHING

- Holds the learner's interest.
- Fosters a positive self-concept in the learner; learner believes learning is possible and probable.
- Supports the learner with positive reinforcement.
- Makes partners of the learner and the teacher.
- Is accurate and current.
- Is appropriate for the learner's age, condition, and abilities.
- Is optimistic, positive, and nonthreatening.
- Is directed at helping the learner meet learning objectives.
- Uses several methods of teaching to accommodate a variety of learning styles; provides learning opportunities through hearing, seeing, and doing.
- Is cost-effective (the cost of the nurse's time spent teaching is less than the cost of treating health problems occurring when clients do not follow recommended treatments, fail to take medications correctly, or do not adapt life-style to changing health needs).

The nurse's own knowledge of common learning needs required by clients experiencing similar health problems is another source of information. The first time clients undergo a procedure, treatment, or surgery, they need to know what is to be done, why it is to be done, what it will feel like, and what the outcome will be. For example, clients scheduled for hip replacement are often brought in for teaching about the surgery itself and what to do beforehand to promote recovery and functioning. After surgery, clients need to learn how to perform leg exercises in bed, how to get out of bed safely, how to walk, and how to manage the pain. The nurse anticipates these learning needs. Learning needs change as the client's health status changes, so nurses must constantly reasses them.

NURSING HISTORY

Several elements in the nursing history provide clues to learning needs. These elements include, (a) age, (b) the client's understanding and perceptions of the health problem, (c) health beliefs and practices, (d) cultural factors, (e) economic factors, (f) learning style, and (g) client's support system. Examples of interview questions to elicit this information are shown in the box on page 389.

Age Age provides information on the person's developmental status that may indicate distinctive health teaching content and teaching approaches. Simple questions to school-age children and adolescents will elicit information on what they know. Observing children in play provides information about their motor and intellectual development as well as relationships with other children. For the elderly person, conversation and questioning may reveal slow recall or limited psychomotor skills and learning difficulties. For additional information, see the discussion of special teaching strategies, later in this chapter.

Client's Understanding of Current Health Problem Clients' perceptions of their current health problems and concerns may indicate knowledge deficits and/or misinformation. In addition, the effects of the problem on the client's usual activities can alert the nurse to other areas requiring instruction. For example, persons who cannot arrange self-care at home often need information about community resources and services.

Health Beliefs and Practices A client's health beliefs and practices are important to consider in any teaching plan. The health belief model described in Chapter 13, page 250, provides a predictor of preventive health behavior. However, even if a nurse is convinced that a client's health beliefs should be changed, doing so may not be possible because so many factors are involved in a person's health beliefs.

Cultural Factors Many cultural groups have their own beliefs and practices, a number of them related to diet, health, illness, and life-style. It is therefore important to know how the practices and values held by clients impinge on their learning needs. Although a nurse may be inclined to assume that because a client belongs to a specific ethnic or cultural group the client will follow the norms of the group, this is not always the case. Thus, nurses should avoid stereotyping and should determine the relevant beliefs and values of each client. For example, although the diet of some Jews excludes pork, other Jews have no objection to eating pork.

Folk beliefs of certain groups may also affect learning. Although the client may readily understand the health care information being taught, this learning may not be implemented in the home, where folk medical practices prevail. For additional information, see Chapter 15 and the section on transcultural teaching later in this chapter.

Economic Factors Economic factors can also affect a client's learning. For example, a client who cannot afford to obtain a new sterile syringe for each injection of insulin may find it difficult to learn to administer the insulin when the nurse teaches that a new syringe should be used each time.

Learning Style Considerable research has been done on people's learning styles. The best way to learn varies with the individual. Some people are visual learners and learn best by watching. Other people do not visualize an

ASSESSMENT INTERVIEW

Learning Needs and Characteristics

Primary Health Problem

- Tell me what you know about your current health problem. What do you think caused it?
- What concerns do you have about it?
- How has the problem affected what you can or cannot do during your usual activities (eg, work, recreation, shopping, housework)?
- What do you or did you do at home to relieve the problem? How helpful was it?
- How have the treatments you have started helped your problem?
- What, if any, difficulties have the treatments caused you (eg, inconvenience, cost, discomfort)?
- Tell me about the tests (surgery, treatments) you are going to have.

Health Beliefs

- How would you describe your health generally?
- What things do you usually do to keep healthy?
- What health problems do you think you may be at risk for because of family history, age, diet, occupation, inadequate exercise, or other habits, such as smoking?
- What changes would you be willing to make to decrease your risk for these problems or to improve your health?

Cultural Factors

- What language do you use most often when speaking and writing?
- Do you seek the advice of another health practitioner?
- Do you use herbs or other medicines or treatments commonly used by persons in your cultural group?
- Does your current doctor know about these?
- What advice or treatments given previously by your doctor conflicted with values or beliefs you consider important?
- When a conflict arose, what did you do?

Learning Style

- Note the client's age and development level.
- What level of education have you achieved?
- Do you like to read?
- How do you best learn new things:
  - By reading about them?
  - By talking about them?
  - By watching a movie or demonstration?
  - By computer?
  - By listening to the teacher?
  - By first being shown how something works and then doing it?
  - On your own or in a group?

Client Support System

- Would you like a family member or friend to help you learn about things you need to do to take care of yourself?
- Who do you think would be interested in learning with you?

activity well; they learn best by actually manipulating equipment and discovering how it works. Other people can learn well from reading things presented in an orderly fashion. Still other people learn best in groups relating to other people. For some, stressing the thinking part of a skill and the logic of something will promote learning. For other people, stressing the feeling part or interpersonal aspect motivates and promotes learning.

The nurse seldom has the time or skills to assess each learner, identify the person's particular learning style, and then adapt teaching accordingly; what the nurse can do, however, is to ask clients how they have learned things best in the past or how they like to learn. Many people know what helps them learn, and the nurse can use this information in planning the teaching. Using a variety of teaching techniques and varying activities during teaching are good ways to match learners with learning styles. One technique will be most effective for some clients, whereas other techniques will be suited to clients with different learning styles.

Client Support System The nurse explores the client's support system to determine the extent to which others may enhance learning and offer support. Family members or a close friend may help the client perform required skills at home and maintain required life-style changes. (Figure 19–3, p. 390).

PHYSICAL EXAMINATION

The general survey part of the physical examination provides useful clues to the client's learning needs, such as mental status, energy level, and nutritional status. Other

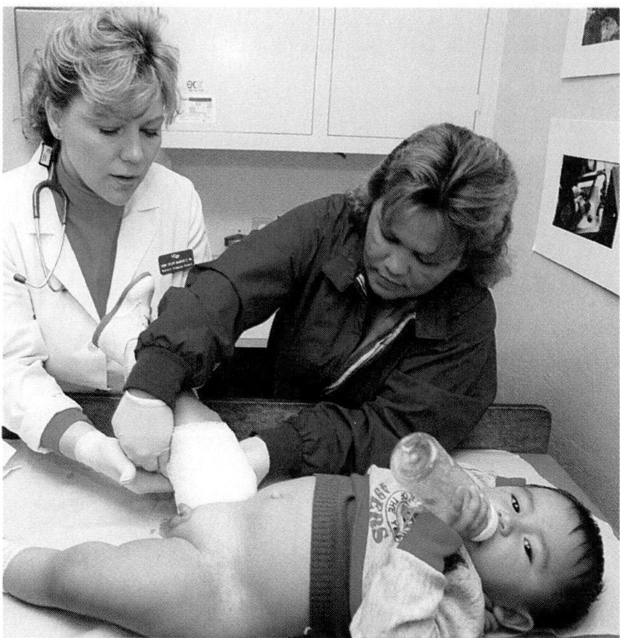

Figure 19–3 Members of the client's support system are an important part of the learning process.

parts of the physical examination reveal data about the client's physical capacity to learn and to perform self-care activities. Visual ability and hearing ability affect the selection of content and approaches to teaching. Musculoskeletal function affects the performance of psychomotor skills and self-care abilities. Activity tolerance, too, can alter a client's capacity to perform certain activities.

READINESS TO LEARN

Clients who are ready to learn often behave differently from those who are not. A client who is ready may search out information, for instance, by asking questions, reading books or articles, talking to others, and generally showing interest. The person unready to learn is more likely to avoid the subject or situation. In addition, the unready client may change the subject when it is brought up by the nurse. For example, the nurse might say, "I was wondering about a good time to show you how to change your dressing," and the client responds, "Oh, my wife will take care of everything." Furthermore, somatic symptoms (such as headaches, upset stomach, or gas pains experienced by clients having surgery) may make it difficult for clients to focus on anything but their physical discomforts. Until their discomfort is reduced, these clients are not ready to learn.

The nurse assesses for

- *Physical readiness.* Is the client able to focus on things other than physical status, or are pain, fatigue, and immobility using up all of the client's time and energy?
- *Emotional readiness.* Is the client emotionally ready to learn self-care activities? Clients who are extremely anxious, depressed, or grieving over their health status are not ready.
- *Cognitive readiness.* Can the client think clearly at this point? Are the effects of anesthesia and analgesia altering the client's level of consciousness?

Nurses can promote readiness to learn by providing physical and emotional support during the critical stage of recovery. As the client stablizes physically and emotionally, the nurse can provide opportunities to learn and encouragement.

MOTIVATION

As discussed earlier, motivation relates to whether the client wants to learn and is usually greatest when the client is ready, the learning need is recognized, and the information being offered is meaningful to the client.

Assessment of motivation to learn is often part of a general health assessment or of a more specific problem assessment. A nurse assessing motivation and a client's present abilities must have a full understanding of the subject to be learned. For example, a man who has had diabetes for several years may already understand how to test his urine for sugar, but he may not know how to inject insulin because he has always taken medication by mouth.

Nurses can increase a client's motivation in several ways:

- By relating the learning to something the client values and helping the client see the relevance of the learning
- By helping the client make the learning situation pleasant and nonthreatening
- By encouraging self-direction and independence
- By demonstrating a positive attitude about the client's ability to learn
- By offering continuing support and encouragement as the client attempts to learn (ie, positive reinforcement)
- By creating a learning stituation where the client is likely to succeed (succeeding in small tasks motivates the client to continue learning)

READING LEVEL

The nurse should not assume that a client's reading level is equal to the highest grade or level of formal education the client has completed. An eighth-grade reading level or lower is recommended for health education material designed for the general client population (Estey 1991, p. 290). The nurse can use the SMOG index to assess the reading levels of client educational material and thereby determine its appropriateness for the population who will be reading it. See the box on the next page.

DETERMINING READABILITY LEVEL OF WRITTEN MATERIALS USING THE SMOG INDEX

To determine the reading level of learning materials for clients, choose 30 sentences in the reading. Pick 10 from the beginning, 10 from the middle, and 10 from the end of the reading. Count all the words with 3 or more syllables; total these. Find the number in the list below, and read across to find the reading grade level.

Number of Words with 3 or More Syllables	*Reading Grade Level*
0–2	4
3–6	5
7–12	6
13–20	7
21–30	8
31–42	9
43–56	10
57–72	11
73–90	12

To decrease the reading level of and simplify the client educational material,

- Use smaller words.
- Avoid words with several syllables.
- Write shorter sentences.
- Explain terms that must be used.
- Use easy, common words.

Sources: ST Stephens, Patient educational materials: Are they readable? *Oncology Nursing Forum*, January/February 1992, 19:84; M Wong, Self-care instructions: Do patients understand educational materials? *Focus on Critical Care*, February 1992, 19:47–49.

DIAGNOSING

Nursing diagnoses pertinent to a client's learning needs are all grouped under the diagnostic category of **Knowledge deficit** (specify). This diagnosis, with its definition, defining characteristics, and related factors, is shown in the box on page 392. Knowledge deficit diagnosis can be written in a number of ways. In all situations, the nurse specifies which deficit the client has.

Examples using the NANDA label as the client response include the following:

- **Knowledge deficit: low-calorie diet** related to inexperience with newly ordered therapy
- **Knowledge deficit: diabetic diet** related to unfamiliarity with prescribed treatment
- **Knowledge deficit: preoperative care** related to inexperience with impending surgical procedure
- **Knowledge deficit: effects of medications** related to language differences and misinterpretation of information
- **Knowledge deficit: home safety hazards** related to denial of declining health and lack of interest in learning
- **Knowledge deficit: substance abuse** related to lack of interest in learning information

Another way to deal with identified learning needs of clients is to write the knowledge deficit as the etiology, or second part, of the diagnosis statement. Such nursing diagnoses are written in the following format:

- **High risk for** (specify) related to knowledge deficit (or lack of skill)

Examples include the following:

- **High risk for altered parenting** related to knowledge deficit: skills in infant care and feeding
- **High risk for infection** related to knowledge deficit: sexually transmitted diseases and their prevention
- **High risk for injury** related to incorrect crutch walking technique
- **High risk for Altered health maintenance** related to incorrect technique of home blood glucose monitoring

Other nursing diagnoses in which **Knowledge deficit** can be the etiology include:

- **Ineffective breast-feeding**
- **Impaired adjustment**
- **Ineffective individual coping**
- **Altered health maintenance**
- **Health-seeking behaviors**
- **Noncompliance (specify)**
- **Ineffective individual management of therapeutic regimens**

Clinical applications of this diagnosis are shown in Table 19–4 on page 392.

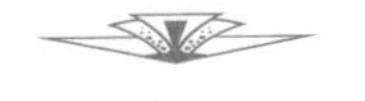

PLANNING

Developing a teaching plan (see a sample teaching plan for wound care on page 396) is accomplished in a series of steps. Involving the client at this time promotes the formation of a meaningful plan and stimulates client motivation. The client who helps formulate the teaching plan is more likely to achieve the desired outcomes.

NURSING DIAGNOSES

CLIENTS WITH KNOWLEDGE DEFICITS

NURSING DIAGNOSIS: Knowledge deficit: The state in which an individual or family does not comprehend, learn, or demonstrate knowledge of health care measures necessary to maintain health

Defining Characteristics

- Verbalization of the problem
- Inaccurate follow-through of instructions
- Inaccurate performance on a test
- Inappropriate or exaggerated behaviors (eg, hysteria, hostility, agitation, apathy)

Related Factors

Lack of exposure; lack of recall; information misinterpretation; cognitive limits; lack of interest in learning; unfamiliarity with information resources.

Sources: B Ackley and G Ladwig, *Nursing Diagnosis Handbook—A Guide to Planning Care* (St Louis: Mosby, 1993), p. 222; North American Nursing Diagnosis Association, *NANDA Nursing Diagnoses: Definitions and Classifications 1992–1993* (Philadelphia: NANDA, 1992), p. 70; JR Lederer, GL Marculescu, B Mocnik, and N Seaby, *Care Planning Pocket Guide: A Nursing Approach*, 5th ed. (Redwood City, CA: Addison-Wesley Nursing, 1993), p. 110; and LJ Carpenito, *Nursing Diagnoses: Application to Clinical Practice*, 4th ed. (Philadelphia: Lippincott, 1992), p. 558.

Table 19–4 Clinical Application: Assessment Data Clusters and Related Nursing Diagnoses

Data Cluster	Nursing Diagnosis
Mr Jack Bond is a retired 65-year-old man who will be having hip replacement surgery next week. He is in a preoperative joint teaching class, as requested by his physician. He states no knowledge of postoperative activities to prevent respiratory complications. States he has heard the new hip can become dislocated and asks what can prevent that. He asks how painful the recovery will be. He states he is really worried about the pain because a friend had this surgery and said the pain was almost unbearable.	**Knowledge deficit: postoperative activities to reduce risk of complications** related to unfamiliarity with hip replacement surgery and recovery **Fear** of postoperative pain related to knowledge deficit of pain control available
Mrs Mangiafuoco is learning new baby care after her delivery. She watches the nurse take the baby's temperature and states she has never done that to a baby. She was unable to read the thermometer when requested to by the nurse. Asks, "Will I ever have to do that? What is normal? When should I call the doctor?"	**Knowledge deficit: infant temperature taking** related to lack of exposure to information
The nurse brings Mr Steinberg the first dose of a medication ordered by his physician. The nurse asks whether anyone has explained what this medication is and why he is taking it. He says no.	**Knowledge deficit: medication information** related to lack of exposure to newly prescribed medication
Ms Kodo is a new postoperative client. She has her call light on. The nurse finds her crying quitely. She states her pain is really terrible and wants something for it. She states, "I waited as long as I could before asking for my pain shot, but I just can't bear it any longer. I don't want to get hooked on any of those drugs like my brother did."	**Fear** of addiction related to knowledge deficit: action and effects of analgesics given for pain

DETERMINING TEACHING PRIORITIES

The client's learning needs must be ranked according to priority. The client and the nurse should do this together, with the client's priorities always being considered. Once a client's priorities have been addressed, the client is generally more motivated to concentrate on other identified learning needs. For example, a man who wants to know all about coronary artery disease may not be ready to learn how to change his life-style until he meets his own need to learn more about the disease. Nurses can also use theoretical frameworks, such as Maslow's hierarchy of needs, to establish priorities. See Chapter 14.

SETTING LEARNING OBJECTIVES/OUTCOMES

Learning objectives can be considered the same as outcome criteria for other nursing diagnoses. They are written in the same way, but outcome criteria for learning needs are traditionally called *learning objectives*. Like client outcomes, learning objectives

- State the client (learner) behavior or performance, not nurse behavior. For example, "Will write his own diets as instructed" (client behavior), not "To teach the client about his diet" (nurse behavior).
- Reflect an observable, measurable activity. The performance may be visible (eg, walking) or invisible (eg, adding a column of figures). However, it is necessary to be able to deduce whether an unobservable activity has been mastered from some performance that represents the activity. Therefore, the performance of an objective might be written: "Writes the total for a column of figures in the indicated space" (observable), not "Adds a column of figures" (unobservable). Selected measurable verbs used for learning objectives are shown in the box at the right. Avoid using words such as knows, understands, believes, and appreciates; these are neither observable nor measurable.
- May add conditions/modifiers as required to clarify what, where, when, or how the behavior will be performed. Examples are "Walks to the end of the hall and back *without crutches*" (condition), "Irrigates his colostomy *independently* (condition) as taught," or "States *three* (condition) factors that affect blood sugar level."
- Include criteria specifying the time by which learning should have occurred. For example, "The client will state three things that affect blood sugar level *by end of second diabetic class*," "The client will demonstrate correct technique for crutch walking *before discharge on third postoperative day*," or "The client will safely inject own insulin dose *before discharge*."

SELECTED VERBS FOR LEARNING OBJECTIVES

Cognitive Domain	Affective Domain	Psychomotor Domain
compares	alters	adapts
contrasts	answers	arranges
defines	attends	assembles
describes	chooses	begins
draws	complies	calculates
differentiates	conforms	calibrates
explains	completes	changes
identifies	defends	constructs
labels	differentiates	creates
lists	discusses	demonstrates
matches	displays	dismantles
names	follows	manipulates
prepares	helps	measures
plans	initiates	moves
recites	joins	organizes
restates	justifies	proceeds
selects	modifies	rearranges
solves	participates	reacts
sorts	responds	shows
states	revises	starts
summarizes	shares	works
underlines	uses	
writes	verifies	

Source: Adapted from NE Gronlund, *Stating Objectives for Classroom Instruction*, 3d ed. (Toronto: Collier Macmillan, 1985), pp. 37–40.

CHOOSING CONTENT

The content, or what is to be taught, is determined by learning objectives. For instance, "Identify appropriate sites for insulin injection" means the nurse must include content about the body sites suitable for insulin injections. Nurses can select among many sources of information. The knowledge they have acquired through their own education, books, nursing journals, and other nurses and physicians are all good resources. Whatever sources the nurse chooses, content should be

- Accurate
- Current
- Based on learning objectives
- Adjusted for the learner's age, culture, and ability
- Consistent with information the nurse is teaching
- Selected with consideration for how much time and resources are available for teaching

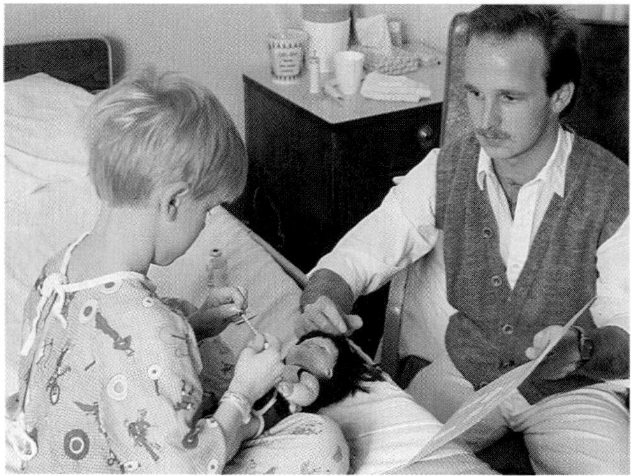

Figure 19–4 Teaching materials and strategies should be suited to the client's age and learning abilities.

> **CHARACTERISTICS OF EFFECTIVE READING MATERIALS**
>
> - Visual appeal: features colorful illustrations.
> - Current and accurate.
> - Reading level appropriate for the learners.
> - Key points emphasized with bold or enlarged print and underlining.
> - Print size appropriate for reader's visual acuity.
>
> **Source:** Adapted from A Estey, Evaluating educational materials for patients, *Journal of Nursing Staff Development,* November/December 1991, 7:290–91.

SELECTING TEACHING STRATEGIES

The method of teaching the nurse chooses should be suited to the individual, to the material to be learned, and to the teacher (Figure 19-4). For example, the person who cannot read needs material presented in other ways; a discussion is usually not the best strategy for teaching to give an injection; and a teacher using group discussion for teaching should be a competent group leader. As stated earlier, some people are visually oriented and learn best through seeing; others learn best through hearing and having the skill explained. See Table 19–5 for selected teaching strategies. Characteristics of effective reading materials are shown in the box above right.

ORDERING LEARNING EXPERIENCES

To save nurses time in constructing their own teaching guides, some health agencies have developed teaching guides for teaching sessions that nurses commonly give. These guides standardize content and teaching methods and make it easier for the nurse to plan and implement client teaching. Whether the nurse is implementing a plan devised by another or developing an individualized teaching plan, some guidelines can help the nurse order the learning experience.

- Start with something the learner is concerned about; for example, before learning how to administer insulin to himself, an adolescent wants to know how he can adjust his life-style and still play football.
- Begin with what the learner knows, and proceed to the unknown. This gives the learner confidence. Sometimes you will not know the client's knowledge or skill base and will need to elicit this information, either by asking questions or by having the client fill out a form, such as a pretest.
- Address first any area that is causing the client anxiety. A high level of anxiety can impair concentration in other areas. For example, a woman highly anxious about turning her husband in bed might not be able to learn about bathing him until she has successfully learned to turn him.
- Teach the basics first, then proceed to the variations or adjustments. It is very confusing to learners to have to consider possible adjustments and variations before they master the basic concepts. For example, when teaching a female client how to insert a retention catheter, it is best to teach the basic procedure before teaching any adjustments that might be needed if the catheter stops draining after insertion.
- Schedule time for review of content and questions the learner(s) may have to clarify information.

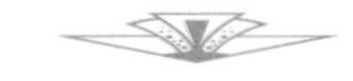

IMPLEMENTING

The nurse needs to be flexible in implementing any teaching plan, because the plan may need revising. The client may tire sooner than anticipated, or be faced with too much information too quickly; the client's needs may change; or external factors may intervene. For instance, the nurse and the client, Mr Brown, have planned to irrigate his colostomy at 10 AM but when the time comes, Mr Brown wants additional information before actually doing it himself.

In this case, the nurse alters the teaching plan and discusses the desired information, provides written information, and defers teaching the psychomotor skill until

Text continued on page 397

Table 19–5 Selected Teaching Strategies

Strategy	Major Type of Learning	Characteristics
Explanation or description (eg, lecture)	Cognitive	Teacher controls content and pace. Learner is passive; therefore retains less information than when a participant. Feedback is determined by teacher. May be given to individual or group.
One-to-one discussion	Affective, cognitive	Encourages participation by learner. Permits reinforcement and repetition at learner's level. Permits introduction of sensitive subjects.
Answering questions	Cognitive	Teacher controls most of content and pace. Teacher must understand question and what it means to learner. Learner may need to overcome cultural perception that asking questions is impolite and may embarrass the teacher. Can be used with individuals and groups. Teacher sometimes needs to confirm whether question has been answered by asking learner, for example, "Does that answer your question?"
Demonstration	Psychomotor	Often used with explanation. Can be used with individuals, small or large groups. Does not permit use of equipment by learners; learner is passive.
Discovery	Cognitive, affective	Teacher guides problem-solving situation. Learner is active participant; therefore retention of information is high.
Group discussion	Affective, cognitive	Learner can obtain assistance from supportive group. Group members learn from one another. Teacher needs to keep the discussion focused and prevent monopolization by one or two learners.
Practice	Psychomotor	Allows repetition and immediate feedback. Permits "hands-on" experience.
Printed and audiovisual materials	Cognitive	Forms include books, pamphlets, films, programmed instruction, and computer learning. Learners can proceed at their own speed. Nurse can act as resource person, need not be present during learning. Potentially ineffective if reading level is too high. Teacher needs to select language that meets learner needs if English is a second language.
Role playing	Affective, cognitive	Permits expression of attitudes, values, and emotions. Can assist in development of communication skills. Involves active participation by learner. Teacher must create supportive, safe environment for learners to minimize anxiety.
Modeling	Affective, psychomotor	Nurse sets example by attitude, psychomotor skill.
Computer-assisted learning programs	All types of learning	Learner is active. Learner controls pace. Provides immediate reinforcement and review. Use with individuals or groups.

TEACHING PLAN WOUND CARE

Assessment of Learner: A 24-year-old male college student suffered a 2.5 inch (7 cm) laceration on the left lower anterior leg during a hockey game. The laceration was cleansed, sutured, and bandaged. The client was given an appointment to return to the health clinic in ten days for suture removal. Client states that he lives in the college dormitory and is able to care for wound if given instructions. Client is able to understand and read English.

Nursing Diagnosis: **Knowledge deficit** related to care of sutured wound.

Long-term Goal: Client's wound will heal completely without infection, loss of function, or other complication.

Intermediate Goal: At clinic appointment, client's wound will be healing without signs of infection, loss of function, or other complication.

Short-term Goal: Client will respond to questions regarding wound care and perform return demonstration of wound cleansing and bandaging.

Behavioral Objectives	*Content Outline*	*Teaching Methods*
Upon completion of the instructional session, the client will:		
1. Describe normal wound healing	I. Normal wound healing	Describe normal wound healing with the use of audiovisuals.
2. Describe signs and symptoms of wound infection	II. Infection Signs and symptoms include wound warm to touch, malalignment of wound edges, and purulent wound drainage. Signs of systemic infection include fever and malaise.	Discuss the mechanism of wound infection. Use audiovisuals to demonstrate infected wound appearance. Provide handout describing signs and symptoms of wound infection.
3. Identify equipment needed for wound care	III. Wound care equipment a. Cleansing solution as prescribed by physician (eg, clear water, mild soap and water, antimicrobial solution, or hydrogen peroxide). b. Bandaging material: telfa, gauze wrap, adhesive tape.	Demonstrate equipment needed for cleansing and bandaging wound. Provide handout listing equipment needed.
4. Demonstrate wound cleansing and bandaging	IV. Demonstration of wound cleansing and bandaging on the client's wound or a mannikin	Demonstrate wound cleansing and bandaging on the client's wound or a mannikin. Provide handout describing procedure for cleansing and bandaging wound.
5. Describe appropriate action if questions or complications arise	V. Resources available for client questions include health clinic, emergency department.	Discuss available resources. Provide handout listing available resources, and follow-up treatment plan.
6. Identify date, time and location of follow-up appointment for suture removal	VI. Follow-up treatment plan; where and when	Provide written instructions.

Evaluation: The client will

1. Respond to questions regarding self care of wound
2. Return demonstration of wound cleansing and bandaging
3. State contact person and telephone number to obtain assistance
4. State date, time, and location of follow-up appointment

the next day. It is also important for nurses to use teaching techniques that enhance learning and reduce or eliminate any barriers to learning. See Table 19–2, earlier, for barriers to learning.

GUIDELINES FOR TEACHING

When implementing a teaching plan, the nurse may find the following eight guidelines helpful.

1. The optimal time for each session depends largely on the learner. Some people, for example, learn best at the beginning of the day, when they are most rested; others prefer late afternoon, when no other activities are scheduled. Whenever possible, ask the client for help to choose the best time.
2. The pace of each teaching session also affects learning. Nurses should be sensitive to any signs that the pace is too fast or too slow. A client who appears confused or does not comprehend material when questioned may be finding the pace too fast. When the client appears bored and loses interest, the pace may be too slow, the learning period may be too long, or the client may be tired.
3. An environment can detract from or assist learning; for example, noise or interruptions usually interfere with concentration, whereas a comfortable environment promotes learning.
4. Teaching aids can foster learning and help focus a learner's attention. To ensure the transfer of learning, the nurse should use the type of supplies or equipment that the client will eventually use. Before the teaching session, the nurse needs to assemble all equipment and visual aids and ensure that all audiovisual equipment is functioning effectively.
5. Learning is more effective when the learners discover the content for themselves. Ways to increase learning include stimulating motivation and stimulating self-direction, for example, by providing specific, realistic, achievable objectives, giving feedback, and helping the learner derive satisfaction from learning. The nurse may also encourage self-directed independent learning by encouraging the client to explore sources of information required.
6. Repetition—for example, summarizing content, rephrasing (using other words), and approaching the material from another point of view—reinforces learning. For instance, after discussing the kinds of foods that can be included in a diet, the nurse describes the foods again, but in the context of the three meals eaten during one day.
7. It is helpful to employ "organizers" to introduce material to be learned. Advanced organizers provide a means of connecting unknown material to known material and generating logical relationships. For example: "You understand how urine flows down a catheter from the bladder. Now I will show you how to inject fluid so that it flows up the catheter into the bladder." The details that follow such an introduction are then seen within its framework, and the details have added meaning.
8. Using a layperson's vocabulary enhances communication. Often nurses use terms and abbreviations that have meaning to other health professionals but make little sense to clients. Even words such as *urine* or *feces* may be unfamiliar to clients, and abbreviations such as "RR" (recovery room) or "PAR" (postanesthesia room) are often misunderstood.

TEACHING AND LEARNING THROUGHOUT THE LIFE SPAN

Learning occurs throughout a person's life, and teaching is required at various times during that life.

Infants Infants rely primarily upon their primary caregiver (ie, parents) for their basic needs. Learning best takes place through consistent routines in an atmosphere of love and security. The infant uses mostly the sensory organs to explore and to learn.

Toddlers Toddlers like to explore and handle equipment. They are continually learning to understand words and to express feelings verbally. Toddlers like to handle equipment (eg, an anesthetic mask). When a parent is present, the toddler's anxiety is often allayed and learning is facilitated. When toddlers feel overwhelmed, they frequently say "no" and it is best to delay teaching until another time.

Preschoolers Most preschoolers want to learn. They often use language fluently, although much of it is used without understanding the meaning. They tend to express their feelings through actions rather than words. Preschoolers ask questions but the nurse's answers need to be brief, using a vocabulary the child understands. Preschoolers usually respond well to rewards (eg, stickers) for participating in learning activities.

School-Age Children School-age children begin to relate events to mental concepts and to express themselves verbally and symbolically. For example, a child can learn to apply ointment to the face at specific times of the day.

Children of this age need to be encouraged to express their emotions, including fear. School-age children like to do things "right" and often will not accept any changes that they consider "not right." See the box on page 398 describing teaching tools for children.

TEACHING TOOLS FOR CHILDREN

- *Visits.* Visiting the hospital and treatment rooms; seeing people dressed in uniforms, scrub suits, protective gear.
- *Dress-up.* Touching and dressing up in the clothing they will see and wear.
- *Coloring books.* Using coloring books to prepare for treatments, surgery, or hospitalization; shows what rooms, people, and equipment will look like.
- *Story books.* Story books describe how the child will feel, what will be done, and what places will look like. Parents can read these stories to children several times before the experience. Younger children like this repetition.
- *Dolls.* Practicing procedures on dolls or teddy-bears that they will later experience; gives a sense of mastery of the situation. Custom dolls are often available for inserting tubes and giving injections, for example.
- *Puppet play.* Puppets can be used in role-play situations to provide information and show the child what the experience will be like; they help the child express emotions.
- *Health fairs.* Health fairs can educate children about their bodies and ways to stay healthy. Fairs can focus on high-risk problems children face, such as accident prevention, poison control, and other topics identified in the community as a concern.

Adolescents Adolescents may prefer to learn in the absence of their parents. Because adolescents tend to identify with peers, learning is often facilitated in a peer group. Although they do have knowledge about their bodies, some of it may be incorrect. Adolescents learn best when they see immediate benefit to themselves. For example, an adolescent who understands that taking his medicine regularly will permit him to continue playing football is more likely to follow through than if he is told the medication will prevent heart problems when he is in his forties.

Young and Middle-Aged Adults Young adults often take health for granted ("It won't happen to me"), and they may not be interested in learning about other people's problems. However, when young adults understand how something affects them, learning is facilitated. Young adults not living at home may find it unacceptable to be dependent on parents for health matters, and they may prefer a friend or the nurse to help them through a health problem.

Middle-aged adults are usually aware of the problems that can result from unhealthy life-styles. This is the period when changes in life-style are often indicated. Some middle-aged people change despite difficulty, and others still believe "it won't happen to me."

Elderly Adults Healthy elderly adults can learn new techniques and procedures and usually desire to do so if it will promote their continued health and independence. Recent research has shown that there is no general decline in intelligence with age.

Teaching methods should be geared to the older person's memory. Those who, for example, have difficulty with recent memory should be taught by methods that take this into consideration. In addition, like people of other ages, elderly people must be motivated to learn. People who have always assumed responsibility for their own health will probably be better motivated to change life-style and learn skills designed to improve health than will people who have had others assume this responsibility. Also, elderly people who prefer dependence may find it difficult to learn health practices that promote independence.

Elderly clients often have more complex health problems than younger adults. For example, many take several medications each day. The elderly client may have the added problems of reduced vision and hearing, increased time needed to learn, decreased short-term memory and attention span, and decreased ability to think abstractly (Weinrich & Boyd 1992, p. 16). It may also be challenging for the elderly client to learn a new psychomotor skill: decreased manual dexterity, decreased sense of touch, and the presence of chronic conditions (eg, arthritis) may make manipulation of small objects difficult and painful.

SPECIAL TEACHING STRATEGIES

There are a number of special teaching strategies that nurses can use: client contracting, group teaching, computer-assisted instruction, discovery/problem-solving, and behavior modification. Any strategy the nurse selects must be appropriate for the client and the learning objectives.

Client Contracting Client contracting involves establishing a contract with a client that specifies certain objectives and when they are to be met. The contract, drawn up and signed by the client and the nurse, specifies not only the learning objectives but also the responsibilities of the client and the nurse, and the teaching plan. The agreement allows for freedom, mutual respect, and mutual responsibility. For additional information about client contracting see Chapter 13, page 264.

Group Teaching Group instruction is economical, and it provides members with an opportunity to share with and learn from others. A small group allows for discussion in which everyone can participate. A large group often necessitates a lecture technique or use of films, videos, slides, or role-playing by teachers.

It is important that all members involved in group instruction have a need in common (eg, prenatal health or preoperative instruction). It is also important that sociocultural factors be considered in the formation of a group. Whereas middle-class Americans may value sharing experiences with others, people from a culture such as Japan may consider it inappropriate to reveal their thoughts and feelings.

Computer-Assisted Instruction (CAI) Computer-assisted instruction (CAI) is becoming more popular. Initially, cognitive learning of facts was the primary use of computer educational materials. Now, however, computers can also be used to teach the following:

- Complex problem-solving skills
- Application of information
- Psychomotor skills

Programs can be used for

- Individual clients using one computer.
- Families or small groups of three to five clients gathered around one computer taking turns running the program and answering questions together.
- Large groups, with the computer display screen projected onto a overhead screen and a teacher or one learner using the keyboard.

Individual clients using a computer are able to set the pace that meets their individual learning needs. Small groups are less able to do this, and large groups progress through the program at a pace that may be too slow for some learners and too fast for others. It is therefore helpful to group learners of similar needs and abilities together. Whether using the computer alone or in large groups, learners read and view informational material, answer questions, and receive immediate feedback. The correct answer is usually indicated by the use of colors, flashing signs, or written praise. When the learner selects an incorrect answer, the computer responds with an explanation of why that was not the best answer and encouragement to try again. Many programs ask learners whether they want to review material on which the question and answer were based. Some computer programs feature simulated situations that allow learners to manipulate objects on the screen to learn psychomotor skills. When used to teach such skills, CAI must be followed up with practice on actual equipment supervised by the teacher.

Some clients may have a negative attitude about computers that could act as a barrier to learning. The nurse helps these clients by explaining the steps to start and run the program, to turn the computer on and off, and where and when to insert the computer disk so that the client can use the program when the nurse is not present. Most media catalogs, professional journals, and health care libraries contain information about computer programs available to the nurse for client education. The media specialist or librarian in a health care facility or college is an excellent resource to help the nurse locate appropriate computer programs. Computer educational material is also available for clients with different language needs, for clients with special visual needs, and for clients at different growth and development levels.

Discovery/Problem-Solving In using the discovery/problem-solving technique, the nurse presents some initial information and then asks the learners a question or presents a situation related to the information. The learner applies the new information to the situation and decides what to do. Learners can work alone or in groups. This technique is well suited to family learning. The teacher guides the learners through the thinking process necessary to reach the best solution to the question or the best action to take in the situation. This may also be referred to as anticipatory problem solving. For example, the nurse-educator might present information on diabetes and blood glucose management. Then, the nurse might ask the learners how they think their insulin and/or diet should be adjusted if their morning glucose level was too low. In this way, clients learn what critical components they need to consider to reach the best solution to the problem.

Behavior Modification The behavior modification system for changing behavior has as its basic assumptions (a) that human behaviors are learned and can be selectively strengthened, weakened, eliminated, or replaced and (b) that a person's behavior is under conscious control. Under this system, desirable behavior is rewarded and undesirable behavior is ignored. The client's response is the key to behavior change. For example, clients trying to quit smoking are not criticized when they smoke, but they are praised or rewarded when they go without a cigarette for a certain period of time. For some people a learning contract is combined with behavior modification.

Pertinent features of behavior modification include the following:

- Positive reinforcement (eg, praise) is used.
- The client participates in the development of the learning plan.
- Undesirable behavior is ignored, not criticized.
- The expectation of the client and the nurse is that the task will be mastered (ie, the behavior will change).
- Success is maximized through positive reinforcement; failure and the threat of failure are minimized.

CRITICAL THINKING CHALLENGE

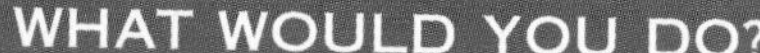

WHAT WOULD YOU DO?

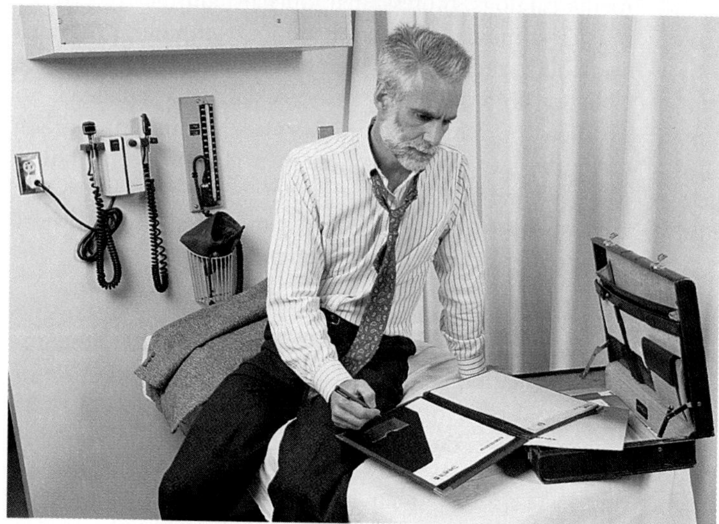

Stuart Spellman, a 52-year-old male, is being admitted for chest pains. When you enter the room, Mr Spellman is working, and exclaims, "I can't wait to get out of here. I've got so much work to catch up on."

What would you do?

TRANSCULTURAL CLIENT TEACHING

The nurse and clients of different cultural and ethnic backgrounds have additional barriers to overcome in the teaching-learning process. These barriers include language and communication problems, differing concepts of time, conflicting cultural healing practices, beliefs that may positively or negatively influence compliance with health teaching, and unique high-risk or high-frequency health problems needing health promotion instruction. See Chapter 15 for detailed information. Nurses should consider the following guidelines when teaching clients from various ethnic backgrounds:

- Obtain teaching materials, pamphlets, and instructions in languages used by clients in the health care setting. Nurses who are unable to read the foreign language material for themselves can have the translator read the material to them. The nurse can then evaluate the quality of the information and update it with the translator's help as needed.
- Use visual aids, such as pictures, charts or diagrams, to communicate meaning. Audiovisual material may be helpful if the English language is spoken clearly and slowly. Even if understanding the verbal message is a problem for the client, seeing a skill or procedure may be helpful. In some instances, a translator can be asked to clarify the video. Alternatively the video may be available in several languages, and the nurse can request the necessary version from the company.
- Use concrete rather than abstract words. Use simple language (short sentences, short words), and present only one idea at a time.
- Allow time for questions. This helps the client mentally separate one idea or skill from another.
- Avoid the use of medical terminology or health care language such as "taking your vital signs" or "apical pulse." Rather, nurses should say they are going to take a blood pressure or listen to the client's heart.
- If understanding another's pronunciation is a problem, validate brief information in writing. For example, during assessments, write down numbers, words, or phrases, and have the client read them to verify accuracy.
- Use humor very cautiously; meaning can change in the translation process.
- Do not use slang words or colloquialisms; these may be interpreted literally.
- Do not assume that a client who nods, uses eye contact or smiles is indicating an understanding of what is being taught. These responses may simply be the client's way of indicating respect. The client may feel that asking the nurse questions or stating a lack of understanding is inappropriate because it might embarrass the nurse or cause the nurse to "lose face."
- Invite and encourage questions during teaching. Let clients know they are urged to ask questions and be involved in making information more clear. When asking questions to evaluate client understanding, avoid

asking negative questions. These can be interpreted differently by people for whom English is a second language. "Do you understand how far you can bend your hip after surgery?" is better than the negative question "You don't understand how far you can bend your hip after surgery, do you?" With particularly difficult information or skills teaching, the nurse might say, "Most people have some trouble with this. May I please help you go through this one more time?" In some cultures, expressing a need is not appropriate, and expressing confusion or asking to be shown something again is considered rude.

- When explaining procedures or functioning related to personal areas of the body, it may be appropriate to have a nurse of the same sex do the teaching. Because of modesty concerns in many cultures and beliefs about what is considered appropriate and inappropriate male-female interaction, it is wise to have a female nurse teach a female client about personal care, birth control, sexually transmitted diseases (STDs), and other potentially sensitive areas. If a translator is needed during explanation of procedures or teaching, the translator should also be female.

- Include the family in planning and teaching. This promotes trust and mutual respect. Identify the authoritative family member and incorporate that person into the planning and teaching to promote compliance and support of health teaching. In some cultures, the male head of household is the critical family member to include in health teaching; in other cultures, it is the eldest female member.

- Consider the client's time orientation. The client may be oriented to the past, present, future, or a combination of all three. The client may be more oriented to the present than the nurse is. Cultures with a predominant orientation to the present include Mexican Americans, Navajo Native Americans, Appalachians, Eskimos, and Filipino Americans. For such clients, preventing future problems may be less significant, and teaching them how to do so may be more difficult. For example, teaching a client why and when to take medications may be more difficult if the client is oriented to the present. In such instances, the nurse can emphasize preventing short-term problems rather than long-term problems. Failure to keep clinic appointments or to arrive on time is common in clients who have a presenttime orientation. The nurse can help by arranging transportation and by accommodating these clients when they do come rather than rescheduling an appointment that they probably will not keep.

  Schedules may be very flexible in present-oriented societies, with sleeping and eating patterns varying greatly. Teaching clients to take medications at bedtime or with a meal does not necessarily mean that these activities will occur at the same time each day. For this reason, the nurse should assess the client's daily routine before teaching the client to pair a treatment or medication with an event the nurse assumes occurs at the same time every day. When teaching a client when to take medication, the nurse should determine whether a clock or watch is available to the client and whether the client can tell time.

- Identify cultural health practices and beliefs. Noncompliance with health teaching may be related to conflict with folk medicine beliefs. Noncompliance may also be related to lack of understanding or a fatalism, a belief system in which life events are held to be predestined or fixed in advance and the individual is powerless to change them. To encourage compliance, the nurse may need to involve the client in learning about the causes and preventability of certain health problems.

  The nurse should treat the client's cultural healing beliefs with respect and try to identify whether any are in agreement or in conflict with what is being taught. The nurse can then focus on the ones in agreement to promote the integration of new learning with familiar health practices. The client will need an explanation of why certain folk healing practices are harmful and must be stopped and how the recommended health practices will help improve health.

  The nurse might begin assessment by assuming that the client has already tried culturally accepted remedies for the health problem and that because these have not worked, the client is now seeking help from the health care system. The nurse should identify what folk remedies were tried and whether any are still being used. Some practices may put the client at risk. Self-medication is common in some cultures, such as migrant Hispanic workers (Foulk et al 1991, p. 284) and should be assessed. These medications can include not only herbal remedies and over-the-counter drugs but also injectable drugs, such as antibiotics or vitamins, which in some countries can be obtained without a doctor's perscription.

Evaluating

Evaluating Client Learning

Evaluating is both an ongoing and a final process in which the client, the nurse, and, often, the support persons determine what has been learned. This process is the same as evaluating client achievement of goals and outcomes for other nursing diagnoses. Learning is measured against the predetermined learning objectives that were selected in the planning phase of the teaching process. Thus,

RESEARCH NOTE

How Accurately Do Clients Perform Home Urine Glucose Monitoring?

Nurse-educators investigated diabetic clients' techniques in home urine glucose monitoring. One hundred clients participated in the study, all of whom had been diagnosed with diabetes and were doing home urine glucose monitoring. The client population had tested their urine at home for a minimum of 6 months up to 20 years. The results showed that in testing their urine, 61% of the clients displayed errors that would result in inaccurate results. Errors were caused by the following factors:

- Impaired vision resulted in incorrect number of drops of urine and water when using Clinitest tablets.
- Arthritis caused difficulty for some clients in using the dropper correctly.
- Incorrect timing of the reaction or incorrect timing before reading results: inability to read the second hand of a clock; test timed according to directions that were specified for another product and were incorrect for the current product; estimated the time rather than timing the test accurately.
- Inability to see small print led to errors in reading the glucose value.
- Inability to read the product directions (print too small, client unable to speak English, client's literacy level too low).

Implications: The researchers concluded that nurses need to reevaluate a client's skills periodically, even for clients who have been performing the skill for years; a client's report of ability to perform a skill is not always accurate. Nurses also need to assess the client's physical limitations, reading skills, and equipment available at home, such as clocks, to help determine the best product for the clients. Clients should be taught to ask for products by name, because a substitute product may have different directions and lead to errors.

Source: J Smolowitz and A Zaldivar. Evaluation of diabetic patients' home urine glucose testing techniques and ability to interpret results, *Diabetes Educator* May/June 1992, 18:207–10.

the objectives serve not only to direct the teaching plan but also to provide outcome criteria for evaluation. For example, the objective "Selects foods that are low in carbohydrates" can be evaluated by asking the client to name such foods or to select low-carbohydrate foods from a list.

The best method for evaluating depends on the type of learning. In *cognitive learning*, the client demonstrates acquisition of knowledge. Examples of the evaluation tools for cognitive learning include the following:

- Direct observation of behavior (eg, observing the client selecting the solution to a problem using the new knowledge).
- Written measurements (eg, tests).
- Oral questioning (eg, asking the client to restate information or correct verbal responses to questions).
- Self-reports and self-monitoring. These can be useful during follow-up phone calls and home visits. Evaluating individual self-paced learning, as might occur with computer-assisted instruction, often incorporates self-monitoring.

The acquisition of *psychomotor skills* is best evaluated by observing how well the client carries out a procedure such as changing a dressing or carrying out a urinary self-catheterization.

Affective learning is more difficult to evaluate. Whether attitudes or values have been learned may be inferred by listening to the client's responses to questions, noting how the client speaks about relevant subjects, and by observing clients behavior that expresses feelings and values. For example, have parents learned to value health sufficiently to have their children immunized? Do clients who state that they value health actually use condoms every time they have sex with a new partner?

Following evaluation, the nurse may find it necessary to modify or repeat the teaching plan if the objectives have not been met or have been met only partially. For the hospitalized client, follow-up teaching in the home or by phone may be needed.

Behavior change does not always take place immediately after learning. Often individuals accept change intellectually first and then change their behavior only periodically (for example, Mrs Green, who knows that she must lose weight, diets and exercises off and on). If the new behavior is to replace the old behavior, it must emerge gradually; otherwise, the old behavior may prevail. The nurse can assist clients with behavior change by allowing for client vacillation and by providing encouragement.

EVALUATING TEACHING

It is important for nurses to evaluate their own teaching. This is the same as evaluating the effectiveness of nursing interventions for other nursing diagnoses. Evaluation should include a consideration of all factors—the timing, the teaching strategies, the amount of information, whether the teaching was helpful, and so on. The nurse may find, for example, that the client was overwhelmed with too much information, was bored, or was motivated to learn more.

Both the client and the nurse should evaluate the learning experience. The client may tell the nurse what was helpful, interesting, and so on. Feedback questionnaires and videotapes of the learning sessions can also be helpful.

The nurse should not feel ineffective as a teacher if the client forgets some of what is taught. Forgetting is normal and should be anticipated. Having the client write down information, repeating it during teaching, giving handouts on the information and having the client be active in the learning process all promote retention.

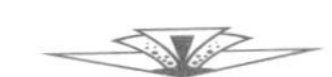

DOCUMENTING

Documentation of the teaching process is essential, because it provides a legal record that the teaching took place and communicates the teaching to other health professionals. If teaching is not documented, legally it did not occur. It is also important to document the responses of the client and support persons. What did the client or support person say or do to indicate that learning occurred? The nurse records this in the client's chart as evidence of learning. The parts of the teaching process that should be documented in the client's chart include the following:

- Diagnosed learning needs
- Learning objectives
- Topics taught
- Client outcomes
- Need for additional teaching
- Resources provided

The written teaching plan that the nurse uses as a resource to guide future teaching sessions might also include these elements:

- Actual information and skills taught
- Teaching stategies used
- Time framework and content for each class

CHAPTER HIGHLIGHTS

- Teaching clients and families about their health needs is a major role of the nurse.
- Learning is represented by a change in behavior.
- Bloom has identified three learning domains: cognitive, affective, and psychomotor.
- A number of factors facilitate learning, including motivation, readiness, active involvement, success at learning feedback, and moving from simple to complex.
- Factors such as extreme anxiety, certain physiologic processes, and cultural barriers impede learning.
- Teaching is a system of activities intended to produce learning. Rapport between the teacher and the learner is essential for effective teaching.
- Teaching, like the nursing process, consists of five activities: assessing the learner, diagnosing learning needs, developing a teaching plan, implementing the plan, and evaluating learning outcomes and teaching effectiveness.
- Learning objectives guide the content of the teaching plan and are written in terms of client behavior.
- Teaching strategies should be suited to the client, the material to be learned, and the teacher. It should be adjusted to the client's developmental level and health status.
- A teaching plan is a written plan consisting of learning objectives, content to teach, a time frame for teaching, and strategies to use in teaching the content. The plan must be revised when the client's needs change or the teaching strategies prove ineffective.
- Adaptations in teaching will facilitate learning for clients who are illiterate, elderly, or from non-Western cultural and ethnic backgrounds.
- Barriers to overcome transcultural teaching include language and communication problems, different concepts of time, and cultural beliefs and practices that conflict with those of Western medicine.
- Evaluation of the teaching/learning process is both an ongoing and a final process.
- Documentation of client teaching is essential to communicate the teaching to other health professionals and to provide a record for legal purposes.

READINGS AND REFERENCES

SUGGESTED READINGS

Weinrich, SP and Boyd, M. January 1992. Education in the elderly—adapting and evaluating teaching tools. *Journal of Gerontological Nursing* 18:15–20.

The elderly population is increasing, and their education needs are complex because of their multiple health problems, coupled with physical and psychosocial changes related to aging. The article gives specific guidelines for selecting written and audiovisual material for educating the elderly client. A case example and clinical implications are included.

Wong, M. February 1992. Self-care instructions: Do patients understand educational materials? *Focus on Critical Care* 19:47–49.

Wong contends that up to 50% of clients are unable to read and comprehend the health education materials designed for them. The author offers suggestions to help the nurse evaluate or develop health education literature for clients. Wong also contrasts examples of material presented at 9th-grade level to that at 4th-grade level.

RELATED RESEARCH

Baldwin, D, Hill, P, and Hanson, G. October 1991. Performance of psychomotor skills: A comparison of two teaching strategies. *Journal of Nursing Education* 30:367–70.

Estey, A, Musseau, A, and Keehn, L. October 1991. Comprehension levels of patients reading health information. *Patient Education and Counseling* 18:165–69.

SELECTED REFERENCES

American Hospital Association. 1992. A patient's *Bill of Rights*. Chicago: American Hospital Association.

American Nurses Association. 1991. *Standards of Clinical Nursing Practice*. Washington, DC: ANA.

Armstrong, ML. September 1989. Orchestrating the process of patient education: Methods and approaches. *Nursing Clinics of North America* 24:597–604.

Barnes, LP. May/June 1992. The illiterate client: Strategies in patient teaching. *Journal of Maternal-Child Nursing* 17:127.

Bloom, BS, editor. 1956. *Taxonomy of Education Objectives*. Book 1, *Cognitive Domain*. New York: Longman.

Carroll, P. December 1991. Using multiple teaching techniques in a continuing education program. *Focus on Critical Care* 18:502–5.

Chally, PS. March 1992. Empowerment through teaching. *Journal of Nursing Education* 31:117–20.

Clement, SC and Gay, N. May/June 1992. Tool chest: A better method for demonstrating the relationship between factors affecting glycemic control. *Diabetes Educator* 18:243-45.

Cordell, B and Smith-Blair, N. January 1994. Streamlined charting for patient education. *Nursing94* 24:57–59.

Estey, A. November/December 1991. Evaluating educational materials for patients. *Journal of Nursing Staff Development* 7:290–91.

Estey, A, Musseau, A, and Keehn, L. October 1991. Comprehension levels of patients reading health information. *Patient Education and Counseling* 18:165–69.

Forbes, K. Spring 1992. The complexity of teaching. *Clinical Nurse Specialist* 6:40.

Foulk, D, Lafferty, J, and Ryan, R. September/October 1991. Developing culturally sensitive materials for AIDS education specifically targeted to migrant farm workers. *Journal of Health Education* 22:283–86.

Gessner, BA. September 1989. Adult education: The cornerstone of patient teaching. *Nursing Clinics of North America* 24:589–95.

Giger, JN and Davidhizar, RE. 1991. *Transcultural Nursing*. St. Louis: Mosby.

Gronlund, NE. 1985. *Stating Objectives for Classroom Instruction*. 3d ed. New York: Macmillan Publishing Co.

Harrison, M. Winter 1992. Toward effective intercultural teaching. *Nursing Administration Quarterly* 16:29–34.

Joint Commission on Accreditation of Heathcare Organizations. 1993. *Accreditation Manual for Hospitals*. Chicago IL: JCAHO.

Kick, E. September 1989. Patient teaching for elders. *Nursing Clinics of North America* 24:681–86.

Knowles, MS. 1980. *The Modern Practice of Adult Education: From Pedagogy to Andragogy*. Chicago: Follet.

———. 1984. *Andragogy in Action*. San Francisco: Jossey-Bass.

Lederer, JR, Marculescu, GL, Mocnik, B, and Seaby, N. 1993. *Care Planning Pocket Guide: A Nursing Diagnosis Approach*. 5th ed. Redwood City, CA: Addison-Wesley Nursing.

Locke, JA. June 1992. Establishing an education program for non-English speaking families. *Journal of Pediatric Nursing* 7:227–28.

Logan, J and Boss, M. March 1993. Nurses' learning patterns. *Canadian Nurse* 89:18–22.

North American Nursing Diagnosis Association. 1992. *NANDA Nursing Diagnoses: Definitions and Classification 1992–1993*. Philadelphia: NANDA.

Miller, PH. 1989. *Theories of Developmental Psychology*. 2d ed. New York: Freeman.

Redman, BK. 1992. *The Process of Patient Education*. 7th ed. St. Louis: Mosby.

Rodriguez, L. September/October 1991a. Teaching tips: Using visualization as a teaching technique. *Journal of Continuing Education in Nursing* 22:222–23.

———. November/December 1991b. Teaching tips: Of crocodiles and research concepts. *Journal of Continuing Education in Nursing* 22:267–68.

Smolowitz, JL and Zaldivar, A. May/June 1992. Evaluation of diabetic patients' home urine glucose testing technique and ability to interpret results. *Diabetes Educator* 18:207–10.

Stephens, ST. January/February 1992. Patient education materials: Are they readable? *Oncology Nursing Forum* 19:83–85.

Thurlow, JG. Spring 1990. Tools for patient education. *Gastroenterological Nursing* 12:286–88.

Weinrich, SP and Boyd, M. January 1992. Education in the elderly—adapting and evaluating teaching tools. *Journal of Gerontological Nursing* 18:15–20.

Wong, M. February 1992. Self-care instructions: Do patients understand educational materials? *Focus on Critical Care* 19:47–49.

20

Leading, Managing, and Influencing Change

Objectives

- Differentiate formal from informal leaders.
- Compare and contrast the following leadership styles: charismatic, authoritarian, democratic, laissez-faire, situational, and transformational.
- Identify characteristics of an effective leader.
- Describe the management concepts of authority, accountability, and delegation.
- Compare and contrast the following nursing delivery models: case method, functional method, team nursing, primary nursing, case management, managed care, differentiated practice, and shared governance.
- Describe the roles of mentors and preceptors.
- Describe networking and its value for nursing professionals.
- Describe the role of the nurse as a change agent and characteristics of an effective change agent.
- Discuss the various types of change.
- Compare and contrast the change theories of Lewin, Lippitt, Havelock, and Rogers.
- Identify strategies for dealing with resistance to change.
- Discuss the seven steps in the change process as identified by Sullivan and Decker.

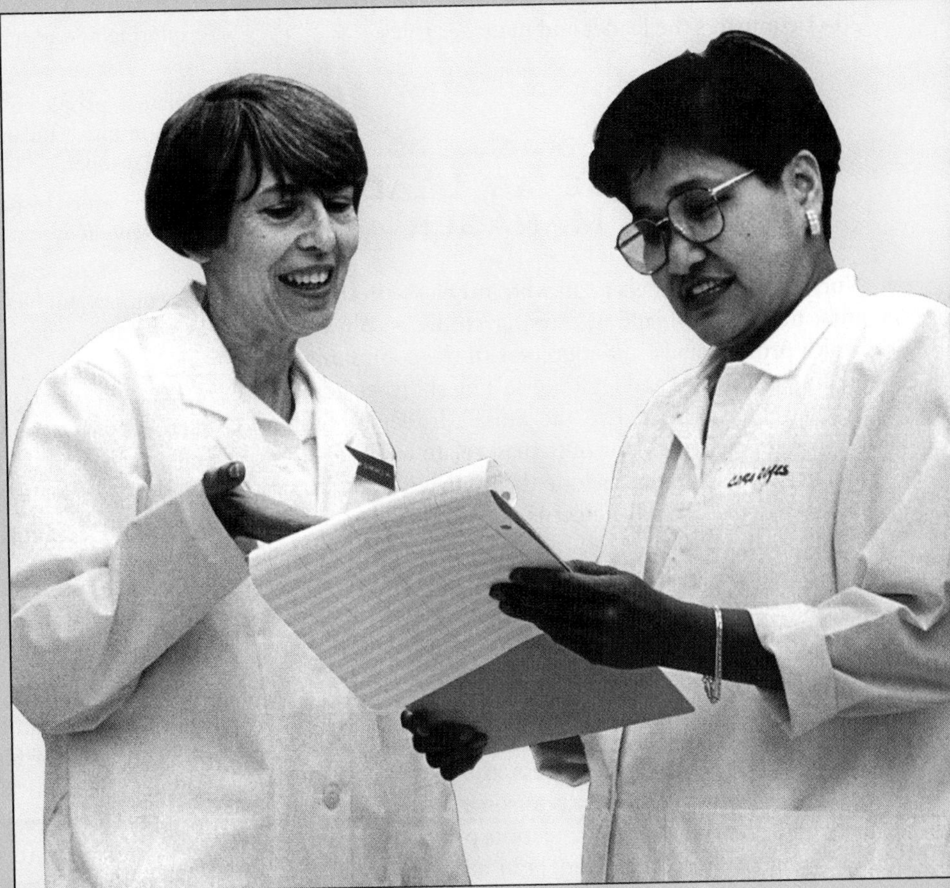

The professional nurse frequently assumes the roles of leader and manager. These two roles are often linked; that is, managers must have leadership abilities, and leaders often manage, but the two roles are uniquely different. Tappen (1989, p. 57) describes a **leader** as one who is successful in influencing others to work together in a productive and satisfying manner. Douglass (1992, p. 2) defines **nursing leadership** as "the process whereby a nurse influences one or more persons to achieve specific goals in the provision of nursing care for one or more clients." A **manager** is the person who has been appointed to a particular position in an organization and therefore has the power to implement the process of guiding and directing the work of others according to predetermined policies (Douglass 1992, p. 6). Table 20–1 compares the leader and manager roles.

Table 20–1 Comparison of Leader and Manager Roles

Leaders	Managers
May or may not have official appointment to the position.	Are appointed officially to the position.
Have power and authority to enforce decisions only so long as followers are willing to be led.	Have power and authority to enforce decisions.
Influence others toward goal setting, either formally or informally.	Carry out predetermined policies, rules, and regulations.
Interested in risk taking and exploring new ideas.	Maintain an orderly, controlled, rational, and equitable structure.
Relate to people personally in an intuitive and empathetic manner.	Relate to people according to their roles.
Feed rewarded by personal achievements.	Feel rewarded when fulfilling organizational mission or goals.
May or may not be successful as managers.	Are managers as long as the appointment holds.

Source: LM Douglass, *The Effective Nurse: Leader and Manager*, 4th ed. (St Louis: Mosby Year-Book, 1992), p. 6. Used with permission.

The Nurse as Leader and Manager

Nurses are role models to all who interact with them: clients; nursing colleagues; nursing students; physicians; health professionals; and members of the community, including politicians and legislators. The ability to advocate for the client is linked to the nurse's leadership ability. Leadership activities not only may relate to professional practice, but also may include the application of nursing knowledge to personal concerns. As members of the community, nurses provide leadership in matters related to health because of their special knowledge of risk factors and health-promotion behaviors. This leadership behavior is exemplified in nursing involvement in such organizations as Mothers Against Drunk Drivers (MADD), the American Cancer Society, the American Heart Association, and so on. Nurses also demonstrate leadership activity in programs for the homeless, the elderly, victims of acquired immune deficiency syndrome (AIDS), child welfare, and environmental protection programs. Most recently, nurses have been leaders in advocating and planning for a reformed health care system that will provide quality health care at an affordable cost to all residents of the United States.

The nurse assumes management functions in several ways. As manager and provider of client care, the nurse coordinates the various health professionals who provide service to the client, including those in the radiology department, pharmacy, respiratory therapy, physical therapy, social work, or occupational therapy. The nurse may also assume a formal role of manager as the head nurse or nursing supervisor. In this management role, the nurse directs and evaluates the nursing and nonnursing staff members.

The nurse can be a leader in the care of the individual client, the client family, groups of clients, professional colleagues, or the larger community (see Chapter 1). The purposes of nursing leadership vary according to the level of application and include (a) improving the health status of individuals or families, (b) increasing the effectiveness and level of satisfaction among professional colleagues who provide care, and (c) improving the attitudes of citizens and legislators toward the nursing profession and their expectations of it (Leddy & Pepper 1993, p. 383). Additionally, nurses as leaders promote the concept of caring in society by advocating for changes that promote physical, psychologic, and social wellness in the society as a whole.

Leadership

Douglass (1992, p. 3) describes two types of leaders: formal and informal. The **formal leader,** or appointed

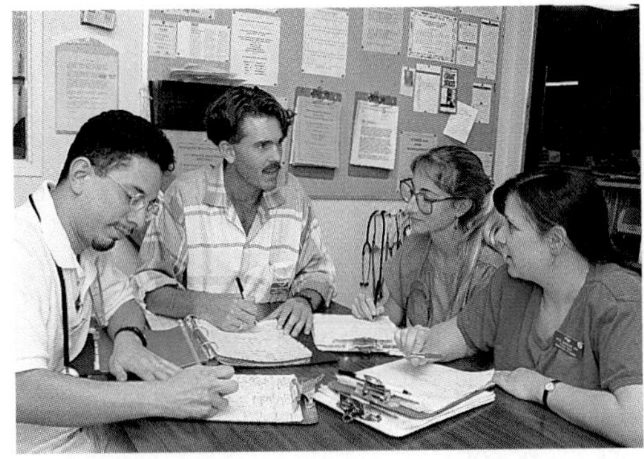

A

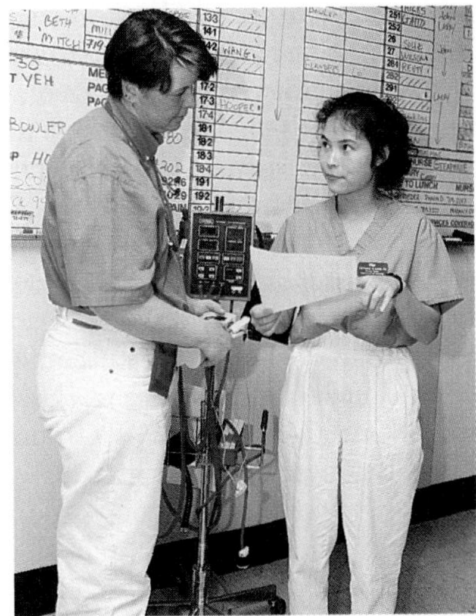

B

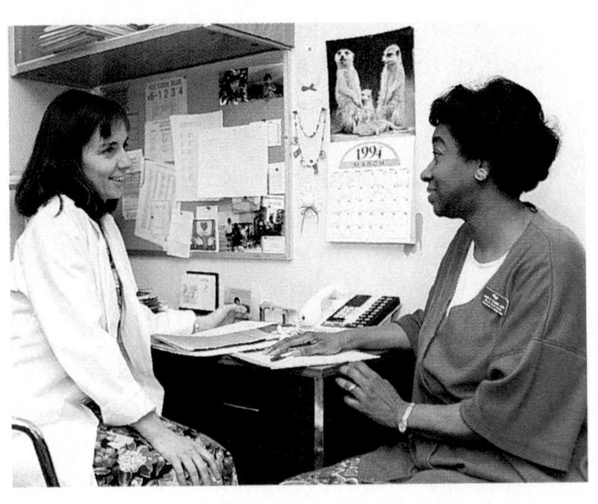

C

Figure 20–1 Nurses as leaders and managers: *A,* The nurse-manager discusses work assignments during change-of-shift report; *B,* The nurse delegates basic client care activities to the nursing assistant; *C,* The nurse consults the social worker during discharge planning.

leader, is selected by administrations and given official authority to make decisions and act. An **informal leader** does not have an appointed position to direct the activities of others but can play an important role in influencing colleagues, co-workers, or other group members to achieve goals. An informal leader is chosen by the group itself. Informal leaders usually become leaders because of seniority, age, special abilities, or a charismatic personality.

LEADERSHIP STYLE THEORY

Leadership style refers to "the individual's pattern of relating to others or how the leader gets along with members of the work group" (Wywialowski 1993, p. 127). Several leadership styles have been described: charismatic leadership, authoritarian or directive leadership, democratic or participative leadership, laissez-faire or nondirective leadership, situational leadership, and transformational leadership.

Charismatic leadership is characterized by an emotional relationship between the leader and the group members in which the leader "inspires others by obtaining an emotional commitment from followers and by arousing strong feelings of loyalty and enthusiasm" (Marriner-Tomey 1992, p. 261). A charismatic relationship exists when the leader can communicate a plan for change and the followers adhere to the plan because of their faith and belief in the abilities of the leader (Marriner-Tomey 1993, pp. 19–20). The followers of a charismatic leader may be able to overcome extreme hardship to achieve the goal because of their faith in the leader.

In **authoritarian leadership,** or **directive leadership,** the leader makes the decisions for the group. This style of leadership, which has also been referred to as **autocratic leadership,** is likened to dictatorship and presupposes that the group is incapable of making its own decisions. The leader determines policies and gives orders and directions to the members. Authoritarian leadership generally has negative connotations and often makes group members dissatisfied. There are times, however, when authoritarian leadership may be most effective. When decisions are necessary in an urgent situation (eg, a cardiac arrest, a unit fire, or a mass casualty event), one person must assume the responsibility to make decisions without being challenged by other team members. When group members are unable or do not wish to participate in making a decision, the authoritarian style effects resolution of the problem and enables the individual or group to move on. This style can also be effective when a project must be completed quickly and efficiently.

In **democratic leadership,** or **participative leadership,** the leader participates as a facilitator, encouraging group discussion and decision making. This leadership style is also referred to as **consultative leadership.** The leader focuses on the human aspects of the work relationship and tries to build effective work groups. Group members participate in decision making through collaboration and cooperation. This style increases group productivity and satisfaction. It presupposes that group members are capable of making decisions, are motivated to do so, and value independence. The participatory process permits each member to identify with the work setting by establishing challenging goals and providing opportunities to change or improve work methods. The participatory process enables group members to pursue professional and personal growth and learn about each other's achievement and contribution to the work effort (Douglass 1992, p. 23). Democratic leadership is based on the following principles (Tappen 1989, p. 34):

- Every group member should participate in decision making.
- Freedom of belief and action is allowed within reasonable bounds that are set by society and by the group.
- Each individual is responsible for himself or herself and for the welfare of the group.
- There should be concern and consideration for each group member as a unique individual.

In **laissez faire leadership,** or **nondirective leadership,** the leader participates minimally and often only on request of the members. This leadership style is also referred to as *permissive* or *ultraliberalism* (Douglass 1992, p. 21). This style is described as a "hands-off" approach. It recognizes the group's need for autonomy and self-regulation. Tappen (1989, p. 37) states, however, that in a laissez-faire group, members may act independently of each other and at cross-purposes because of a lack of cooperation or coordination. A laissez-faire style is most effective for groups whose members have both personal and professional maturity, so that once the group has made a decision, the members become committed to it and have the required expertise to implement it. Individual group members then perform tasks in their area of expertise. The leader acts as a resource person.

Situational leadership theory encourages managers to consider the environment or context in which management decisions are made. Douglass (1992, p. 24) states that situational leadership theorists share a basic assumption that successful leadership occurs when the leader's style matches the situation. Situational leadership theory predicts the most appropriate leadership style from the maturity level of the followers (Marriner-Tomey 1992, p. 266).

Nurse-managers assess their own management styles, the experience and ability of each group member, and the goals of the situation to determine appropriate leadership techniques. One factor influencing situational leadership is the personal and professional maturity of the group members. In groups whose members have a high level of maturity, little structure is required for the accomplishment of tasks; however, in groups whose members are novices and have little professional and/or personal maturity, increased structure and direction is needed.

Also important in situational leadership is the value given to the accomplishment of tasks and the concern given to the interpersonal relationships between leader and group members and among group members. For example, the nurse-manager encourages input from staff members when planning daily work assignments so that both staff needs and client needs are met. The nurse-manager may solicit input from staff members when doing both short-range and long-range planning for the unit. However, when a new staff member is being oriented to the unit, the nurse-manager may be more directive in making assignments until the staff member develops experience and professional maturity. In emergency situations or situations in which the task needs to be completed quickly, the nurse-manager may be more authoritative in directing the actions of all staff members.

Transformational leadership is a style in which the leader motivates others through values, vision, and empowerment (Marriner-Tomey 1992, p. 267). The leader envisions a clear, attractive, and attainable goal and enlists others to participate in attaining the goal. Through shared values, honesty, trust, and continuous learning, the leader empowers the group to share in goal attainment. Cottingham (1988) suggests that through transformational leadership, "followers are converted into leaders and leaders are converted into change agents." Marriner-Tomey (1992, p. 268) cites the following behaviors involved in situational leadership as applicable to transformational leadership:

- Challenging the process by searching for opportunities, experimenting, and taking risks

CHARACTERISTICS OF EFFECTIVE LEADERS

- Use a leadership style that is natural to them.
- Use a leadership style appropriate to the task and the members.
- Assess the effects of their behavior on others and the effects of others' behavior on themselves.
- Are sensitive to forces acting for and against change.
- Express an optimistic view about human nature.
- Are energetic.
- Are open and encourage openness, so that real issues are confronted.
- Facilitate personal relationships.
- Plan and organize activities of the group.
- Are consistent in behavior toward group members.
- Delegate tasks and responsibilities to develop members' abilities, not merely to get tasks performed.
- Involve members in all decisions.
- Value and use group members' contributions.
- Encourage creativity.
- Encourage feedback about their leadership style.

- Inspiring a shared vision by envisioning the future and enlisting others
- Enabling others to act by fostering collaboration and strengthening others
- Modeling the way by setting an example and planning small victories
- Building morale by recognizing individual contributions and celebrating accomplishments

EFFECTIVE LEADERSHIP

Effective leadership is a learned process requiring an understanding of the needs and goals that motivate people, the knowledge to apply the leadership skills, and the interpersonal skills to influence others. Much has been written about effective leadership and style; some descriptive statements about effective leaders are listed in the box above. Glennon (1992, p. 41) encourages humanistic leadership as a means of creating an environment "that is stimulating, motivating, and empowering to the professional nurse." Strategies for humanistic leadership are identified in the box to the right, above.

STRATEGIES FOR PUTTING HUMANISTIC LEADERSHIP INTO ACTION

- Praise or positively recognize staff and colleagues.
- Always think good thoughts about yourself and others.
- Always give before you get—give colleagues and staff a reason for doing whatever it is that you are asking of them.
- Smile often—it generates enthusiasm and goodwill.
- Remember the names of the people you work with.
- Think, act, and look successful.
- Always greet others with a positive, affirmative statement.
- Write informal appreciation notes; this shows appreciation and reinforces positive performance.
- Get out of the nurse's station or office; make a point of circulating among those who work in your circle of influence.
- Talk less and listen more; encourage communication and the sharing of ideas and information.
- Don't condemn, criticize or complain; instead, work on ways to improve the situation or solve the problem.

Source: Adapted from: TK Glennon. Empowering nurses through enlightened leadership, *Revolution: The Journal of Nurse Empowerment*, Spring 1992, 2:40–44.

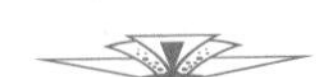

MANAGEMENT PRACTICES

Nurses function differently in various types of organizations. An organization may be autocratic, with one person having primary knowledge and power while other persons are subordinate. Bureaucratic organizations control through policy, structured jobs, and compartmentalized actions. Other organizations decentralize control and emphasize self-direction and self-discipline of members. Another organization may be a component of a system that interacts interdependently and adapts dynamically to change. This organization is particularly useful for the nurse who manages the care of individuals, families, and communities. On a larger scale, the nurse-manager must work in the organizational framework of the employing agency.

Authority is defined as the official power given by the organization to direct the work of others (Marquis & Huston 1994, p. 125). It is an integral component of managing. Authority is conveyed through leadership actions; it is determined largely by the situation, and it is always associated with responsibility and accountability.

Accountability is the ability and willingness to assume responsibility for one's actions and to accept the consequences of one's behavior. Accountability can be viewed within a hierarchic systems framework, starting at the individual level, through the institutional/professional level, and then to the societal level. At the individual or client level, accountability is reflected in the nurse's ethical integrity. At the institutional level, it is reflected in the statement of philosophy and objectives of the nursing department and nursing audits. At the professional level, it is reflected in standards of practice developed by national or provincial nursing associations. At the societal level, it is reflected in legislated nurse practice acts.

Delegation is the process by which responsibility and authority for performing tasks is assigned to individuals (Sullivan & Decker 1992, p. 216). Because it is often impossible to provide all of the nursing care needed by a group of clients, the nurse-delegator must assign aspects of the client's care to other nursing personnel. It may also be necessary to delegate work to the unit secretary, dietitian, housekeeping department, auxiliary nursing personnel, or other support departments (Tappen 1989, p. 241).

Delegation is a major tool in making the most efficient use of time. Delegation is a high-level implementation skill. The nurse-delegator must have the following information: (a) needs of the client and family, (b) goals of the client, (c) nursing activity that can help the client meet the goals, and (d) skills and knowledge of various nursing and support personnel.

The nurse-delegator must also determine how many and what type of personnel are needed. This information may be indicated on the client's records. Other sources of this information are the client, the charge nurse, other nursing personnel, and the nurse-delegator's own judgment. Nurses may require assistance to give client care quickly in certain situations. Assistance may also be necessary to ensure client safety.

After establishing that assistance is required, the nurse-delegator must identify what type of help is needed, how long help is required, when it is required, and what assistance is available. The nurse must arrange for assistance, usually by asking the appropriate person on the unit, before beginning the nursing activity. Delegation does not require that the nurse-delegator have the personal knowledge and expertise to perform a specific nursing activity, but rather that the nurse-delegator know who does have the knowledge and expertise and delegate responsibility to that person to provide the required care. For example, the nurse-delegator may call the dietitian to assist a client in making menu decisions or a social worker to assist a client who needs financial assistance and homemaker services after discharge.

An important aspect of delegation is the development of the potential of nursing and support personnel. By knowing the background, experience, knowledge, skills, and strengths of each person, a nurse can delegate responsibilities that help develop each person's competence. Nursing personnel to whom aspects of care have been delegated need to be supervised and evaluated. The amount of supervision required is highly variable, depending on the knowledge and skills of each person. As the person who assigns the activity and observes the performance, the nurse-delegator contributes to the evaluation process. Because individual motivation varies, the nurse-delegator needs to realize that not all persons perform equally. Thus, standards of performance must be evaluated against written job descriptions, rather than by comparing one person to another. It is essential, too, for the nurse-delegator to realize that people require ongoing feedback about their performance. Feedback should be given in an objective manner and include both positive and negative input.

Characteristics of effective nurse managers as described by Sullivan and Decker (1988, p. 576) are listed in the box on page 411.

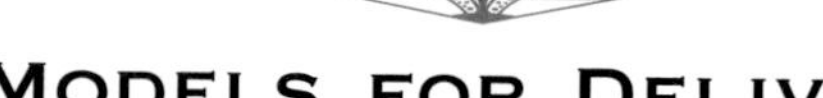

MODELS FOR DELIVERY OF NURSING

Common configurations for the delivery of nursing care include the case method, the functional method, team nursing, primary nursing, case management, managed care, differentiated practice, and shared governance.

Case Method The case method, also referred to as total care, is one of the earliest models developed. This method was used by private-duty nurses in providing total care to the client (Wywialowski 1993, pp. 40–41). This method is client centered. One nurse is assigned to and is responsible for the comprehensive care of a group of clients during an 8- or 12-hour shift. For each client, the nurse assesses needs, makes nursing plans, formulates diagnoses, implements care, and evaluates the effectiveness of care. In this method, a client has consistent contact with one nurse during a shift but may have different nurses on other shifts. The case method, considered the precursor of primary nursing, continues to be used in a variety of practice settings such as intensive care nursing. With the shortage of nursing personnel during World

CHARACTERISTICS OF EFFECTIVE NURSE-MANAGERS

- Have a face; that is, they join committees and groups and "work the crowd."
- Prepare themselves by pursuing educational programs that are directed toward their goals.
- Present a positive image; that is, they know the unwritten dress code and follow it, and their carriage and energy proclaim confidence.
- Demonstrate an above-average grasp of written and oral communication skills, expressing themselves clearly, concisely, and with impact.
- Network effectively. They have a circle of people internally and externally from whom to draw information and support. They carry business cards so as to be ready to validate new liaisons.
- Have mentors and sponsors and a clear awareness of the responsibilities and obligations inherent in these types of relationships.
- Know their organization's values (ie, where their organization is headed and why).
- Do not wound the lion or lioness; that is, they know the "hot buttons" and do not push them and never publicly make moves that discredit themselves or others.
- Mobilize resources. Know who or what can be of help in given situations and how to mobilize these resources.
- Have a vision of what may or could be and assume leadership in moving toward those goals.

Source: EJ Sullivan and PJ Decker. *Effective Management in Nursing*, 2d ed. (Redwood City, CA: Addison-Wesley Nursing, 1988), pp. 576–77. Reprinted with permission.

War II, the case method could no longer be the chief mode of care for clients. To meet staff shortages, managers hired personnel with less educational preparation than the professional nurse and developed on-the-job training programs for auxiliary helpers. The total care method became unfeasible in such situations, and the functional method was developed in response.

Functional Method The functional nursing method, which evolved from concepts of scientific management used in the field of business administration, focuses on the jobs to be completed. In this task-oriented approach, personnel with less preparation than the professional nurse perform less complex care requirements. It is based on a production and efficiency model that gives authority and responsibility to the person assigning the work, for example, the head nurse. Clearly defined job descriptions, procedures, policies, and lines of communication are required. The functional approach to nursing is economical and efficient and permits centralized direction and control. Its disadvantages are fragmentation of care and the possibility that nonquantifiable aspects of care, such as meeting the client's emotional needs, may be overlooked.

Team Nursing In the early 1950s, Eleanor Lambertson (1953) and her colleagues proposed a system of team nursing to overcome the fragmentation of care resulting from the task-oriented functional approach and to meet increasing demands for professional nurses created by advances in technologic aspects of care. **Team nursing** is the delivery of individualized nursing care to clients by a nursing team led by a professional nurse. A nursing team consists of registered nurses, licensed practical nurses, and often nurses' aides. This team is responsible for providing coordinated nursing care to a group of clients during an 8- or 12-hour shift.

With the advent of managed care, team nursing is experiencing a resurgence. In this revisited form of team nursing, licensed nursing personnel (RNs and LPNs) are frequently paired with an unlicensed assistive person (UAP). The licensed nurse retains responsibility and authority for client care but delegates appropriate tasks to the UAP. Contemporary proponents of this model believe the team approach increases the efficiency of the licensed nurse. Opponents state that the high acuity of inpatients leaves little to be delegated.

Primary Nursing Primary nursing, a system in which one nurse is responsible for total care of a number of clients 24 hours a day, 7 days a week, was introduced at the Loeb Center for Nursing and Rehabilitation, the Bronx, New York, under the leadership of Lydia Hall (1963). It is a method of providing comprehensive, individualized, and consistent care.

Primary nursing uses the nurse's technical knowledge and management skills. The primary nurse assesses and prioritizes each client's needs, identifies nursing diagnoses, develops a plan of care with the client, and evaluates the effectiveness of care. Associates provide some care, but the primary nurse coordinates it and communicates information about the client's health to other nurses and other health professionals. Primary nursing encompasses all aspects of the professional role, including teaching, advocacy, decision making, and continuity of care. The primary nurse is the first-line manager of the client's care with all its inherent accountabilities and responsibilities.

Case Management Case management is a more recent nursing care delivery method, in which case managers are responsible for a case load of clients across the health care continuum that is; case managers track the client's health progress from home, to hospital, to clinic or other agency, and back home. Case management is used in a variety of settings. Initially, public health and psychiatric-mental health nurses served as case managers. Today, case management is used in insurance-based programs, employer-based health programs, workers' compensation programs, maternal-child health settings, mental health settings and hospital-based nursing practice. Many case managers work with broad client populations, whereas others deliver care to specific populations. Clients may be grouped by diagnosis, age, nursing diagnosis, physician, insurance payer, or within the acute-chronic continuum (Bower 1992, p. 9).

For example, Mary Ellis, a 49-year-old obese female, is admitted to the hospital with severe hypertension and diabetes. During her hospital stay, she is met by a nurse who is a case manager for Ms Ellis's health insurance provider. This nurse not only consults with the hospital nursing staff to plan Ms Ellis's care but also plans for home care services that Ms Ellis may need after discharge. When Ms Ellis is discharged, the same nurse follows up on her status with either home visits, telephone communication, or clinic follow-up. This nurse ensures that treatment plans are followed and makes referrals, if they are needed, for social assistance, diabetic instruction, nutrition counseling, physician's follow-up, or other needed services. The case manager actually follows up on Ms Ellis's needs both during her hospital stay and after discharge.

According to Bower (1992, p. 25) the American Nurses Association (ANA) recommends that case managers have a minimum educational preparation of a baccalaureate in nursing and 3 years of clinical experience.

Managed Care Managed care is a heterogeneous array of cost containment strategies that attempts to balance cost and quality by altering the organization of health care, reimbursement for care, and the relationship between providers and insurers throughout the continuum of care.

Case management may be used as a cost-containment strategy in managed care. Both case management and managed care systems use **critical pathways** to track the client's progress. Critical pathways are treatment plans all health team members use to plan the sequence of client care based on medical diagnosis and projected length of stay. For additional information, see Chapter 4, page 75. Managed care can be used with primary, team, functional, and alternative nursing care delivery systems (Cohen & Cesta 1993, p. 33).

Managed care has gained popularity with the health care reform movement in the United States. The ANA (1991a) suggests that managed care will reduce health care costs and ensure consumer access to the most effective treatments. Although managed care has been embraced as a model for health care reform, many question the application of this business approach to a commodity as precious as health.

Differentiated Practice According to the National League for Nursing (NLN), differentiated practice "is an approach to assure quality care through the most appropriate utilization of nursing resources" (NLN 1991). As with managed care and case management, differentiated nursing practice seeks to provide quality care at an affordable cost. The model is developed within each health care institution by the nurses employed there. The institution must first identify the nursing competencies required by the clients within the specific practice environment. This model further requires the delineation of roles among both licensed nursing personnel and nursing support personnel. This enables nurses to progress and assume roles and responsibilities appropriate to their level of experience, capability, and education.

Shared Governance The shared governance model can be used in concert with other models of nursing delivery. Marrelli (1993, p. 97) describes shared governance as "an organizational model that gives staff the authority for decisions, autonomy to make those decisions, and control over the implementation and outcomes of the decisions." The focus of this model is to encourage participation of nurses in decision making at all levels of the organization. Individuals may participate either at their own request or as part of their job role criteria. More commonly, nurses participate through serving in decision-making groups, such as committees and task forces. The decisions made may address employment conditions, cost-effectiveness, long-range planning, productivity, and wages and benefits. The underlying principle of shared governance is that employees will be more committed to the organizational goals if they have had input into planning and decision making.

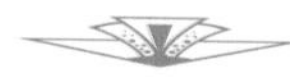

MENTORS AND PRECEPTORS

The term **mentor** is defined by Ardery (1990) as "an experienced guide, adviser, or advocate who assumes responsibility for promoting the growth and professional advancement of a less experienced individual—the protege." Most nursing literature describes the nurse-mentor relationship as important for career development in nursing administration or nursing education. The concept of mentoring should also be encouraged to assist the nurse's professional growth from new graduate to experienced nurse. The nurse then, in turn, may choose to mentor those who follow. Marriner-Tomey (1992, p. 210) describes three phases to the mentoring process:

1. *The invitational stage.* In this stage, the mentor must be willing to use time and energy to nurture an individual who is goal directed, willing to learn, and respectfully trusting of the mentor. The nurse-mentor invites the relationship with a young nurse to share knowledge, skill, and personal experiences of professional growth.
2. *The questioning stage.* In this stage, the novice experiences self-doubt and fears being unable to meet the goals. The mentor helps the protege clarify the goals and the strategies for achieving the goals, shares personal experiences, and serves as a sounding board and a source of support during times of doubt.
3. *The transitional stage.* In this stage, the mentor assists the protege to become aware of the protege's own strengths and uniqueness. The protege now is able to mentor someone else.

In the clinical area, the term **preceptor** is used to describe mentoring relationships in which the experienced nurse assists the "new" nurse in improving clinical nursing skill and judgment. The preceptor also instills understanding of the routines, policies, and procedures of the institution and the unit.

Mentors provide support. Often, the mentor relationship is one of teacher-learner: The mentor instructs the protege in the expected role, introduces the protege to those who are important to the achievement of goals, listens to and helps the protege evaluate ideas in light of institutional policy, and challenges the protege to advance the protege's professional practice. Marriner-Tomey (1992, p. 210) describes a mentor as "a confidante who becomes a role model and a sounding board for decision making."

Nurses who wish to improve and advance their professional practice, whether in education, administration, or clinical practice, should seek mentors to assist them. Mentors are usually of the same sex, 8 to 15 years older, and have a position of authority in the organization. Most are knowledgeable individuals who are willing to share their knowledge and experience. Mentors often choose proteges because of their leadership and/or managerial qualities.

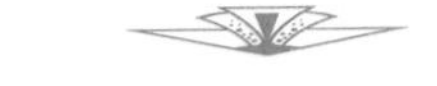

NETWORKING

To function effectively in all nursing roles, but especially in leadership and management roles, the nurse needs to network with other professionals. Marriner-Tomey (1993, p. 175) describes **networking** as a process in which people communicate, share ideas and information, and offer support and direction to each other. Network development builds linkages with people throughout the profession, both within and outside the work environment. Getting to know people helps build a trust relationship that can facilitate the achievement of professional goals. It is easier to access people one knows than it is to access strangers. This provides for the exchange of ideas, knowledge, and information. Tappen (1989, p. 73) states "the sharing of information and opportunities with fellow professionals can have a synergistic effect: The nurse can increase her energy, supply of information, and influence by sharing it."

Nurses can develop networks by (a) attending local, regional, and national conferences, (b) taking classes for continuing education or toward an academic degree, (c) joining the alumni association and attending alumni meetings, (d) joining and participating in professional organizations, (e) keeping in touch with former teachers and co-workers, and (f) socializing with professional colleagues (O'Leary et al 1986, pp. 14–15). Keeping an updated card file of colleagues and keeping in touch socially can keep the network fresh.

CHANGE

Change is all around. It is a dynamic process and a normal part of people's lives. It is a means by which people grow, develop, and adapt. Throughout the previous sections of this chapter, the word *change* has appeared numerous times in relation to the leading and managing roles of the nurse. Change is an integral aspect of nursing. To be effective and influential in today's world, nurses need to understand change theory and apply its precepts in the workplace, in government and professional organizations, and in the community. Planning and implementing change are professional responsibilities as well as largely unrealized power sources that are vital to the practice of nursing. In *Standards of Professional Performance* (1991b, p. 13), the ANA identifies measurement criteria for the nurse's role in change: Nurses use "the results of quality of care activities to initiate changes in practice" and "to initiate changes throughout the health care delivery system." Some synonyms for change are *alter, transform, modify, convert,* and *vary.* All these terms suggest that a fundamental difference or substitution is the outcome of change.

Change can be positive or negative, planned or unplanned. Change can involve gaining new knowledge or adapting what is currently known in the light of new information. Change can also involve obtaining new skills. Change can be especially difficult when it presents challenges to one's values and beliefs, ways of thinking, or

CHARACTERISTICS OF EFFECTIVE CHANGE AGENTS

- Have excellent communication and interpersonal skills with individuals, groups, administration, and all levels of the organization involved in change.
- Project expertise.
- Have knowledge of available resources and how to use them: people, time, money, facilities, information.
- Are skilled in problem solving.
- Are skilled in teaching.
- Are respected by those involved in the change.
- Have ability to encourage and nurture those going through change.
- Are self-confident, are able to take risks, and can inspire trust in themselves and in others.
- Are able to make decisions.
- Have a broad base of knowledge.
- Have a good sense of timing.

ways of relating. Change can involve individual clients, families, communities, organizations, nursing as a profession, and the entire health care delivery system.

CHANGE AGENT

A change agent is one who works to bring about a change (Sullivan & Decker 1992, p. 429). The change agent is the person or group who initiates, motivates, and implements the change. Change agents are leaders. The nurse uses the nursing process, critical thinking (see Chapter 10) and knowledge of change theory to be an effective change agent in a variety of health care settings.

An effective change agent must be highly skilled. As the nurse moves through the process of change with clients, families, groups, communities, or institutions, the nurse assumes a variety of roles, depending on the type of change and the needs of the individuals involved in the change. Some of these roles may include "investigator, collaborator, consultant, facilitator, evaluator, teacher, observer, organizer, and manager" (Kaplan 1991, p. 422). It is also important for the change agent to be accessible to all people involved in the change process. The change agent should be honest and straightforward about goals and problems. The box above describes characteristics of effective change agents.

A key element in the change process is trust. The change agent must trust the participants in the change, and they in turn must trust the change agent. One of the greatest risks of change is that it can disrupt the system or even render it nonfunctional. For example, changing the method of nurse assignments could result in gaps and missed care for some clients. To avoid this problem, the change agent must closely observe the situation during the change process.

A change agent may be formally or informally designated. A *formally designated change agent* is one who has the role and responsibility for change, such as a clinical nurse-specialist expected to make changes beneficial to specified clients. This person has the authority to plan and implement change. An *informally designated change agent* does not have the authority to make change by virtue of a position but does have the leadership skills and respect of others and therefore can serve an important function in the change process. A change agent who has formal status carries authority, whereas an informal change agent can operate only through persuasion (Ehrenfeld et al 1992, p. 23).

Change agents may also be internal or external. An *internal change agent* is a person who is part of the situation or system, for example, a charge nurse on a hospital unit or a public health nurse providing school health services to a specific school or within a school system. Internal change agents are familiar with the situation and the organization. However, they may have vested interests in the present system as well as biases. An *external change agent* comes to the situation from the "outside," for example, a nursing administrator from another hospital, a nurse-specialist from another health care facility, or a nurse-educator from a local college. External change agents are able to view the problem and the situation objectively and usually have no biases; they are often viewed as experts and are called consultants. However, they may not have personal knowledge of the situation and the problems. They may not be viewed as openly as an "insider"; therefore, they must develop a cooperative working relationship with the people involved in the change. A third option is to pair the external expert with the internal person to serve together as change agents. If this course is taken, it is critical that the two have similar philosophies about change and agree on the goals and process of the change (Kaplan 1991, p. 420). There are advantages and disadvantages to each of these options, and it is important for any change agent to be aware of both in each situation.

TYPES OF CHANGE

There are many types of change; in fact, change can occur without effort on anyone's part. Change of this type is referred to as "drift." It occurs as individuals and groups respond to the environment and is usually recognized retrospectively. For example, after the birth of a baby, changes may take place in the parents' life-style. They may go out socially less frequently. They may become aware of this change only after a period of time, when they realize they have not seen old friends as often as they had been accustomed.

Change is frequently differentiated as planned or unplanned. **Unplanned change** is usually haphazard, and the results can be unpredictable. "Drift" is a type of unplanned change. *Situational change* or *natural change* may be considered unplanned and occurs without any control by a person or group. An example is the change that occurs as a result of a war or a natural disaster. However, not all situational changes are negative; for example, Nurse Smith may be unexpectedly offered a position that she had considered a future goal but had not applied for at the present. According to Lippitt (1973), **planned change** is an intended, purposive attempt by an individual, group, organization, or larger social system to influence the status quo of itself, another organism, or a situation. Problem-solving skills, decision-making skills, and interpersonal skills are important factors in planned change.

Change may also be considered covert or overt. A *covert change* is hidden or occurs without the individual's awareness. For example, a person can become increasingly deaf without being aware of this fact. *Overt change* is change about which a person is aware, for example, the development of abdominal pain or shortness of breath while walking up stairs. People who experience overt change may also experience anxiety. Overt change often necessitates behavioral changes that are at variance with the person's needs or goals. An example is a client's diagnosis of cancer and the subsequent need for therapy even though it interferes with the person's work and family life.

Another type of change is *developmental change,* which refers to the physiopsychosocial changes that occur during the life cycle (see Chapters 23 through 26). This type of change is normally gradual and often not consciously planned. An example is the decreasing physical capability of an elderly person. This kind of change is slow and generally permits the individual time to adapt. The individual does not plan the physical changes of aging; they just happen. However, the individual may make plans for dealing with the physical changes (eg, moving to a smaller, one-floor residence which is easier to care for and in which it is easier to move around).

Marriner-Tomey (1992, pp. 161–62) states that three variables are differentiating factors in the change process: (a) mutual goal setting, (b) the power ratio between the change agent and the client system, and (c) the deliberativeness of changes. She cites the following types of change and describes the relationship between these three variables as they affect change:

- *Coercive change* is characterized by nonmutual goal setting, imbalanced power ratio, and one-sided deliberativeness.
- *Emulative change* is fostered through identification with and emulation of those perceived to have power.
- *Indoctrination* uses mutual goal setting, has an imbalanced power ratio, and is deliberative. Subordinates are instructed in and are expected to assume the beliefs of the power sources.
- *Interactional change* is characterized by mutual goal setting and fairly equal power, but no deliberativeness. Parties may be unconsciously committed to changing one another.
- *Socialization change* has a direct relationship with interactional change. One conforms to the needs of a social group. When there is greater deliberativeness on the power side, change becomes indoctrination.
- *Technocratic change* is brought about by collecting and interpreting data. A technocrat merely reports the findings of the analysis to bring about change.
- *Planned change,* by contrast, involves mutual goal setting, an equal power ratio, and deliberateness.

THEORIES OF PLANNED CHANGE

There are a number of theories of planned change. They all have in common an emphasis less on knowledge than on collaboration among the people involved. Of particular value to nurses are four theories about change, proposed by Lewin, Lippitt, Havelock, and Rogers. See Table 20–2 on page 416.

Kurt Lewin (1948) originated change theory. He saw change as having three basic stages: unfreezing, moving, and refreezing. During the *unfreezing* stage, the motivation to establish some sort of change occurs. The individual becomes aware of the need for change. This stage is a cognitive process in which the person becomes aware of a problem or of a better method of accomplishing a task and hence of the need for change. Having identified this need, the individual must also identify restraining and driving forces. The restraining forces are those that inhibit change, and the driving forces are those that support change. For example, a nurse who is instructing an adolescent client and his mother in dietary management of type I (juvenile-onset) diabetes may see the client's mother as a driving force, and the client's father and siblings, who don't want to change their sugar-loaded diet, as restraining forces.

In the second stage, *moving,* the actual change is planned in detail and then started. Information about the problem is gathered from one or several sources. At this stage, it is important that the people involved agree that the status quo is undesirable. In the above example, the

Table 20–2 Theories of Change

Lewin (1948)	Lippitt (1958)	Havelock (1973)	Rogers (1983)
1. Unfreezing 2. Moving 3. Refreezing	1. Diagnosing the problem 2. Assessing the motivation and the capacity for change 3. Assessing the change agent's motivation and resources 4. Selecting progressive change objectives 5. Choosing an appropriate role for the change agent 6. Maintaining the change once it has been initiated 7. Terminating the helping relationship	1. Building a relationship 2. Diagnosing the problem 3. Acquiring relevant resources 4. Choosing the solution 5. Gaining acceptance 6. Stabilization and generating self-renewal	1. *Knowledge.* The individual, called the decision-making unit, is introduced to change and begins to comprehend it. 2. *Persuasion:* The individual develops an attitude toward the change that may be favorable or unfavorable. 3. *Decision.* The person makes a choice to adopt or not to adopt the change. 4. *Implementation.* The person acts on the choice. At this time, alterations may take place. 5. *Confirmation.* The individual looks for confirmation that the choice was right. If the person encounters mixed messages, the choice may be changed.

Sources: K Lewin, *Field Theory in Social Science* (New York: Harper and Row, 1951); R Havelock, *The Change Agent's Guide to Innovations in Education* (Englewood Cliffs, NJ: Educational Technology Publications, 1973); E Rogers, *Diffusion of Innovations*, 3d ed. (New York: Free Press, 1983); R Lippitt, J Watson, and B Westley, *The Dynamics of Planned Change* (New York. Harcourt Brace, 1958).

nurse needs to help the family understand the importance of dietary management for diabetics and to enlist the family members' support for the client. The nurse could ask the dietitian to meet with the client and his family to demonstrate how a diabetic diet can be nutritious and tasty. The nurse might also provide printed food exchange lists, sample menus, and recipes, as well as resources for diabetic information. As change agent, the nurse should work with the family to create an environment that is conducive to the change, including, perhaps, rewards to reinforce desired behaviors. An environment that fosters change should be supportive, nonthreatening, and educational (Olson 1979).

In the third stage, *refreezing*, the changes are integrated and stabilized. According to Welch (1979), the individuals involved in the change integrate the idea into their own value system. Thus, in the above example, the client and his family would come to value the importance of family involvement in dietary management of their diabetic son and sibling. The family may develop their own strategies for assisting their loved one to comply with the plan.

Gordon Lippitt (1958) described planned change as having seven phases. See Table 20–2. For a detailed discussion of each of these seven stages, see Welch (1979).

Ronald Havelock (1973) modified Lewin's theory regarding planned change. See Table 20–2. His theory emphasizes planning the change process, which he believed takes the most time and involves the most significant changes (Welch 1979).

Everett Rogers (1983) viewed people's backgrounds and the environment as important in the process of change. He described change as a five-step process, which he called the *innovation-decision process* (Rogers 1983). See Table 20–2. The individual who undergoes change can also reject the change at a later time. Rogers thus introduced the idea that an adopted change is not necessarily permanent but may be reversed in the future. Rogers emphasized that for change to succeed, the people involved must be interested in the change and committed to implementing it.

ACCEPTANCE OF CHANGE

Important aspects of planning change are establishing the likelihood of the acceptance of the change and then determining the criteria by which that acceptance can be identified. Accepting change often takes time, particularly when it does not fit into a person's attitudinal frame of

Stages in the Acceptance of Change

The individual

1. Becomes aware of the new idea, system, or practice.
2. Seeks more information about the change.
3. Evaluates the information and relates it to the present situation.
4. Mentally tries out the proposed change.
5. Actually tries out the change, on a small scale if possible.
6. Adopts and integrates the change into the present system.

When introducing a change, the nearer the people involved in the change are to the process, the easier the implementation of the change. These stages of acceptance can then naturally evolve.

Source: B. Stevens, Effecting change, *Journal of Nursing Administration*, February 1975, 5:25. Used with permission.

reference; in such a case, change may not occur at all. For example, to stop smoking may not be accepted as a desirable behavior change by a person who values smoking and does not believe it is harmful. Optimally, this belief changes before the person tries to change the behavior. Stages in the acceptance of change are shown in the box above. Some characteristics and beliefs that can help people survive the stress of change include the following (Brown 1990, pp. 586–87):

- *Hardiness*—the ability to endure and grow in spite of difficult conditions
- *Positive outlook*—the ability to view change as an opportunity
- *Commitment*—the belief in the value of the change and the desire to work actively to promote the change
- *Control*—the sense that one can influence events; a sense of empowerment
- *Social support*—the feeling of support from and assistance of others involved in the change; the feeling that one is not alone
- *Stress management*—the ability to use stress management strategies (see Chapter 32) to cope effectively with stressors associated with the change process
- *Timing*—the ability to determine the appropriate time to introduce change, to provide time for everyone to participate in all steps of the change process, and to pace the implementation of change so as not to overwhelm those affected by it

Resistance to Change

Resistance to change is not merely lack of acceptance but rather behavior intended to maintain the status quo—that is, to prevent the change. The change agent should anticipate some resistance to change, no matter how beneficial the change may seem (Sullivan & Decker 1992, p. 443). When resistance is encountered, it is important to determine whether the resistance should be overcome. Sometimes the change is inadvisable, for example, when there are insufficient resources for making the change. Resistance to change is often greatest when the idea is not concurrent with existing trends, such as trying to change from primary nursing to functional nursing when primary nursing is currently popular. Resistance is also usually great when the proposed change would alter a situation with which people are comfortable.

Robinson (1991, p. 823) suggests that some degree of resistance to change is a natural response and should not be viewed negatively. Resistance may help people adapt to the proposed change as they try to understand the meaning on a personal level, establish a thread of continuity, and then accept and grow with the change. Sometimes change is opposed for valid, logical reasons.

Reasons for Resistance According to New and Couillard (1981), people resist change for one or more of the following reasons: (a) threatened self-interest, (b) inaccurate perceptions, (c) objective disagreement with the change, (d) psychologic reactance, and (e) low tolerance for change.

Threatened self-interest as a reason for resistance to change often involves people's perception that the personal costs will be greater than any gains. These may be costs in time, money, or status, for example. Opposition to a change may be based on *incorrect perceptions* of the change itself. Incomplete or inaccurate information may cause apprehension about the change, resulting in resistance on the part of the people involved. *Objective disagreement* can also cause resistance to a change. In some instances, people may have information that leads them to believe the change will not attain stated objectives. Sometimes others have more experience or information than the change agent, and their resistance can cause a planned change to be reconsidered, perhaps benefiting the people involved. *Psychologic reactance* is a reaction motivated by a perceived loss of freedom to engage in particular behaviors. According to New and Couillard (1981), psychologic reactance is manifested when threatened or eliminated behaviors suddenly assume greater importance than they did previously and the person attempts to reestablish eliminated behaviors.

Finally, some people simply have a *low tolerance* for change. Although they may intellectually understand the

Table 20–3 Balancing Resistive and Motivating Forces

Resisting Change	Motivating Change
No ownership	Involvement in assessing, planning, implementing, and evaluating the change
No time or energy	Reassigning other responsibilities; discussing/planning change activities when people are rested
No recognition of problem	Involvement in assessment and diagnosis; education; communication and update
Threat to job security, self-esteem	Active listening to concerns; redefining job or roles in a positive light; ensuring support; reducing anxiety; acknowledging feelings of loss
Narrow focus; failure to see big picture	Clarifying outcomes of change; communicating vision of changed future

Source: Adapted from J Reis, Computers in the OR—Using change dynamics to implement a new software system in the OR, *AORN Journal*, April 1991, 53:1052.

change, they are unable to accept it emotionally. This may be due to feelings of low self-esteem, fear of risk, or minimal tolerance for uncertainty.

Dealing with Resistance Sullivan and Decker (1992, pp. 444–45) give the following guidelines for dealing with resistance:

- Communicate with those who oppose the change. Get to the root of their reasons for opposition.
- Clarify information, and provide accurate feedback.
- Be open to revisions but clear about what must remain.
- Present the negative consequences of resistance (in client care situations, increased disability or death; in organizational situations, compromised client care, threat to organizational survival, decreased client satisfaction).
- Emphasize the positive consequences of the change and how the individual will benefit.
- Keep resisters involved in face-to-face contact with supporters. Recognize valid objections, and relieve unnecessary fears.
- Maintain a climate of trust, support, and confidence.
- Redirect resistance by diverting attention to a "more important" problem inside or outside the system. Sometimes when participants perceive a greater external threat, they unify internally.

Table 20–3 offers strategies for balancing resistive and motivating forces during the change process.

STEPS IN THE CHANGE PROCESS

Sullivan and Decker (1992) outline seven steps to planned change:

1. *Identify the problem or the opportunity.* Both problems and new opportunities require change. Douglass (1992, p. 224) states that one must "perceive the need for change."
2. *Collect data.* Once the problem or opportunity has been clearly defined, the change agent collects data internal and external to the proposed change. This enables the nurse to identify the driving forces and restraining forces. The nurse may review the professional literature related to the problem and identify solutions tried by others.
3. *Analyze data.* Explore alternative solutions in terms of their risks, benefits, driving and restraining forces, advantages, disadvantages, and probable outcomes. (One effective technique used by change agents is brainstorming; see Chapter 10.)
4. *Plan the change strategy.* Plan the who, how, and when of the change. Steps in planning the change include the following (Spradley 1980):
   a. Write measurable objectives.
   b. Determine a timetable.
   c. Plan a budget.
   d. Recruit individuals to carry out each aspect of the plan.
   e. Ensure the change agent's ability to work with the client system.
   f. Evaluate resources (driving forces) and resistance (restraining forces), and plan strategies to manage both. See Table 20–3.
   g. Design a plan to evaluate the outcomes of the change effort.
   h. Identify measures to refreeze or establish the change within the client system.
5. *Implement the change.* Interventions are designed to gain the necessary compliance. The change agent creates a supportive environment, acts as energizer, obtains and provides feedback, and overcomes resistance. (Pilot-testing a new idea affords one the opportunity to evaluate it on a small scale and then "sell" it to the larger client system.)
6. *Evaluate effectiveness.* Evaluate the outcome(s) on the basis of the measurable objectives, and make appropriate adjustments.

7. *Stabilize the change.* Refreeze the client system so that the changes are seen as standard operating procedures and the system is once again stable.

APPLYING THE CHANGE PROCESS TO CLIENT CARE

During the assessment phase, the nurse establishes trust and identifies the client's health status and motivation for change. In the diagnosis phase, problems are specified. In the planning phase, objectives or goals for change are mutually established. In the implementation phase, the nurse implements and maintains the change strategies. In the evaluation phase, the nurse determines whether the change process has been successful and what support or strategies will continue to be needed to maintain or enhance the change.

The nurse as change agent in direct care situations uses many strategies to help clients and families make changes for improved levels of health and well-being. Providing information and teaching new skills is the most obvious change behavior of nurses. Equally important interventions to promote change involve communicating with, supporting, encouraging, and empowering the client and family so that they believe they are capable of making the change through their own efforts. On a larger scale, the nurse can be instrumental in promoting change at the institutional, professional, or societal levels.

The following examples outline changes initiated by nurses who have identified a need to "do something" in each of four spheres of influence: the workplace, organizations, government, and the community.

The Workplace At each of three shift meetings, Mrs Hawkins, Head Nurse, listened to nurses complain about problems with getting clients' laboratory work done and reported to the unit in a timely manner. She conferred with other head nurses and with the attending and resident physicians on her unit. It appeared that similar complaints were widespread.

At the next head nurse meeting, Mrs Hawkins described the problem. The group appointed a task force, with Mrs Hawkins as chair, and asked it to present a plan to solve the problem at the next meeting. After gathering more data, the task force invited representatives from the attending and resident staff and the laboratory director to meet with them to review the data, consider alternative solutions, and select a plan to solve the problem.

By the next head nurse meeting, a preliminary plan to alter the system of laboratory reporting had been devised, and all concerned were working cooperatively to implement the plan.

The Professional Organization Nurses on the Education Committee of a district nurses' association recognized the need to make a public policy statement concerning the care of clients with AIDS. Because the board of directors had recently expressed interest in promulgating such policy statements, the committee sensed the timing was right and that the board would welcome its draft despite the controversial subject matter.

Members of the committee researched and drafted a statement. The full committee offered a critique and selected an articulate spokesperson to present the statement to the association president and seek support before asking to have the statement presented to the board. Once the president had approved the statement, it was placed on the agenda for the next board meeting.

After making minor additions, the board approved it for distribution to the lay and nursing press and asked the Education Committee to suggest a nurse to present the statement at a local hearing of the City Council Health Committee.

The Government While the pressure to contain health care costs escalated through the 1980s, a coalition representing the shared interests of the ANA, the NLN, and the American Association of Colleges of Nursing (AACN) mounted a campaign to convince Congress of the cost-effectiveness of a center for nursing research within the National Institutes of Health (NIH). Despite incredible odds, including a presidential veto and opposition from the American Medical Association, the American Association of Medical Colleges, and the NIH administrations, the proposal was passed by Congress in the fall of 1985, and in 1993 the center became an institute with equal standing with other components of NIH. The success of this effort demonstrates the effectiveness of carefully planned change including the collaboration of nursing organizations. It also illustrates the clout organized nurses can wield on any level and in any sphere.

The Community Every nurse plays several roles besides that of registered nurse. Each resides in a community, and many are parents. Some serve on school boards, belong to the League of Women Voters, or participate in religious, club, or scouting activities. There are numerous opportunities for nurses to contribute to the health and welfare of the communities in which they live. For example, a group of nursing students recognized a health problem within their community and developed a plan to intervene. Many of the students were parents of children in local elementary schools where a high percentage of children were being sent home daily with head lice. Because of previously enacted budget cuts, the district's school nurses were each responsible for between three and five schools. The students volunteered to work with the district nurses to provide screening and health teaching at each of the elementary schools, thereby helping to resolve the community's problem.

All nurses are affected by change; nobody can avoid it. Knowledgeable nurses make rational plans to deal with both opportunities to initiate and guide needed change as well as to respond to change that affects them in the workplace, government, organizations, and the community. To recognize these opportunities for change and respond to the factors that influence nursing from without, it is helpful to consider the history of nursing, current trends in nursing, and present political, social, technologic, and economic issues.

CHAPTER HIGHLIGHTS

- The professional nurse frequently assumes the roles of leader and manager.
- Several leadership styles have been described, including charismatic, authoritarian, democratic, laissez-faire, situational, and transformational. These styles are often blended to fit the situation. Nurses should know which style is most consistent with their behavior and learn to incorporate aspects of other styles into their practice.
- Nurse-managers work in the organizational framework of the employing agency. Principles of management include authority, accountability, and delegation.
- Nursing delivery systems that have been or are currently being used to provide client care include case method, functional method, team nursing, primary nursing, case management, managed care, and differentiated practice.
- Mentors and preceptors are important in the support and professional development of beginning nurses. Nurses should seek out mentoring relationships to enhance career growth.
- Networking is the establishment of professional linkages to obtain information, share ideas, and facilitate the accomplishment of professional goals. Nurses can develop professional networks throughout their careers in a variety of settings, including school, work, professional organizations, and social groups.
- To be effective and influential in current and future health care delivery systems, nurses need to understand and apply change theory.
- Planned change requires problem-solving skills, decision-making skills, and interpersonal competence.
- Nurses frequently act as formal or informal change agents in relation to clients, families, work settings, and communities.
- Change is stressful, and the individual experiencing change needs to be supported and empowered.
- Resistance to change can have a number of causes, including threatened self-interest, inaccurate perceptions, objective disagreement, psychologic reactance, and low tolerance for change.
- Nurses who assume a change agent role can plan and implement change using a nursing process framework.
- Nurses have been effective in promoting change in the workplace through professional organizations, in the legislative arena, and in the community.

READINGS AND REFERENCES

SUGGESTED READINGS

Cauthorne-Lindstrom, C and Tracy, T. July/August 1992. Organizational change from the "mom and pop" prespective. *Journal of Nursing Administration* 22:61–64.

This article describes elements for being successful with large scale changes. The elements discussed include *vision*, a clear picture of what the change will look like; a *culture* of trust and communication; *championship*, or enthusiasm for the change; and *involvement* of all those affected by the change.

RELATED RESEARCH

Davis, PS. January 1991. The meaning of change to individuals within a college of nurse education. *Journal of Advanced Nursing* 16:108–15.

SELECTED REFERENCES

American Nurses Association. 1991a. *Nursing's Agenda for Health Care Reform.* Washington, DC: ANA.

———.1991b. *Standards of Clinical Nursing Practice.* Washington, DC: ANA.

Ardery, G. 1990. Mentors and protégés: From ideology to knowledge. In McCloskey, JC and Grace, HK, editors. *Current Issues in Nursing.* 3d ed. St Louis: Mosby.

Benner, P. 1984. *From Novice to Expert: Excellence and Power in Clinical Nursing Practice.* Redwood City, CA: Addison-Wesley Nursing.

Bennis, WG, Benne, KD, and Chin, R, editors. 1985. *The Planning of Change.* 4th ed. New York: Holt, Rinehart & Winston.

Bolton, LB, Aydin, C, Popolow, G, and Ramseyer, J. June 1992. Ten steps for managing organizational change. *Journal of Nursing Administration* 22:14–20.

Bower, KA. 1992. *Case Management by Nurses.* Washington, DC: ANA.

Brown, K. December 1990. Managing change. *AAOHN Journal* 38:586–87.

Cauthorne-Lindstrom, C and Tracy, T. July/August 1992. Organizational change from the "mom and pop" perspective. *Journal of Nursing Administration* 22:61–64.

Cohen, EL and Cesta, TG. 1993. *Nursing Case Management: From Concept to Evaluation.* St Louis: Mosby-Year Book.

Cohen, LB. March 1992. Power and change in health care: Challenge for nursing. *Journal of Nursing Education* 31:113–16.

Cottingham, C. June 1988. Transformational leadership: A strategy for nursing. *Today's OR Nurse* 10:24–27.

Davis, PS. January 1991. The meaning of change to individuals within a college of nurse education. *Journal of Advanced Nursing* 16:108–15.

Del Togno-Armanasco, V, Hopkin, LA, and Harter, S. 1993. *Collaborative Nursing Case Management: A Handbook for Development and Implementation.* New York: Springer.

Douglass, LM. 1992. *The Effective Nurse: Leader and Manager.* St Louis: Mosby-Year Book.

Ehrenfeld, M, Bergman, R and Ziv, L. January/February 1992. Academia—a stimulus for change. *International Nursing Review* 39:23–26.

Glennon TK. Spring 1992. Empowering nurses through enlightened leadership. *Revolution: The Journal of Nurse Empowerment* 2:40–44.

Hall, L. November 1963. A center for nursing. *Nursing Outlook* 11:805–6.

Havelock, R. 1973. The change agent's guide to innovations in education. Englewood Cliffs, NJ: Educational Technology Publications.

Haynes, S. July 1992. Let the change come from within: The process of change in nursing. *Professional Nurse* 7:635–38.

Huston, CJ and Marquis, B. Summer 1988. Ten attitudes and behaviors necessary to overcome powerlessness. Nursing Connections 1:39–47.

Huxley, E. 1975. *Florence Nightingale.* New York: Putnam.

Kaplan, SM. December 1991. The nurse as change agent. *Dermatology Nursing* 3:419–22.

Koernier, JG, Bunkers, SS, and Nelson, J. Fall 1991. Change: A professional challenge. *Nursing Administrative Quarterly* 16:15–21.

Lambertson, E. 1953. *Nursing Team Organization and Functioning.* New York: Teachers College Press.

Leddy, S and Pepper, JM. 1993. *Conceptual Bases of Professional Nursing.* 3d ed. Philadelphia: Lippincott.

Lewin, K. 1948. *Resolving Social Conflicts.* New York: Harper and Brothers.

———. 1951. *Field Theory in Social Science.* New York: Harper and Row.

Lippitt, GL. 1973. *Visualizing Change: Model Building and the Change Process.* La Jolla, CA: University Associates.

Lippitt, R, Watson, J, and Westley, B. 1958. *The Dynamics of Planned Change.* New York: Harcourt Brace.

Marquis, BL and Huston, CJ. 1994. *Management Decision Making for Nurses.* 2d ed. Philadelphia: Lippincott.

Marrelli, TM. 1993. *The Nurse Manager's Survival Guide: Practical Answers to Everyday Problems.* St Louis: Mosby-Year Book.

Marriner-Tomey, A. 1992. *Guide to Nursing Management.* 4th ed. St Louis: Mosby-Year Book.

———. 1993. *Transformational Leadership in Nursing.* St Louis: Mosby-Year Book.

Mason, DJ. 1985. The politics of patient care. In Mason, DJ and Talbott, SW, editors. *Political Action Handbook for Nurses.* Redwood City, CA: Addison-Wesley Nursing.

Mason, DJ, Talbott, SW, and Leavitt, JK. 1993. *Policy and Politics for Nurses.* 2d ed. Philadelphia: WB Saunders.

National League for Nursing. 1991. *Differentiated Nursing Practice: Position Statement.* New York: NLN.

New, JR and Couillard, NA. March 1981. Guidelines for introducing change. *Journal of Nursing Administration* 11:17–21.

O'Leary, JG, Wendelgass, ST, and Zimmerman, HE. 1986. *Winning Strategies for Nursing Managers.* Philadelphia: Lippincott.

Olson, EM. June 1979. Strategies and techniques for the nurse change agent. *Nursing Clinics of North America* 14:323–36.

Reis, J. April 1991. Computers in the OR—Using change dynamics to implement a new software system in the OR. *AORN Journal* 53:1052.

Richards, MB. November 1987. Developing "participative leaders." *Nursing Management* 18:113–15.

Robinson, J. July 1991. Project 2000: The role of resistance in the process of professional growth. *Journal of Advanced Nursing* 16:820–24.

Rogers, E. 1983. *Diffusion of Innovations.* 3d ed. New York: Free Press.

Spradley, BW. 1980. Making change creatively. *Journal of Nursing Administration* 10:32–37.

Stevens, B. February 1975. Effecting change. *Journal of Nursing Administration* 5:23–25.

———. November 1980. Power and politics for the nurse executive. *Nursing and Health Care* 1:208–10.

Strudthoff, M. July 1991. Orchestrating change in nursing service. *Nursing Management* 22:96, 98.

Sullivan, EJ, and Decker, PJ. 1988. *Effective Management in Nursing.* 2d ed. Redwood City, CA: Addison-Wesley Nursing.

———.1992. *Effective Management in Nursing.* 3d ed. Redwood City, CA: Addison-Wesley Nursing.

Tappen, RM. 1989. *Nursing Leadership and Management: Concepts and Practice.* 2d ed. Philadelphia: FA Davis.

Teasley, D. November 1987. Situational leadership for nurses. *Nursing Management* 18:112–13.

Vance, C, Talbott, SW, McBride, AB, and Mason, DJ. November/December 1985. An uneasy alliance: Nursing and the women's movement. *Nursing Outlook* 33:281–85.

Welch, LB. June 1979. Planned change in nursing: The theory. *Nursing Clinics of North America* 14:307–21.

Wywialowski, E. 1993. *Managing Client Care.* St Louis: Mosby-Year

UNIT 6

ASSESSING HEALTH

STUDENT PROFILE

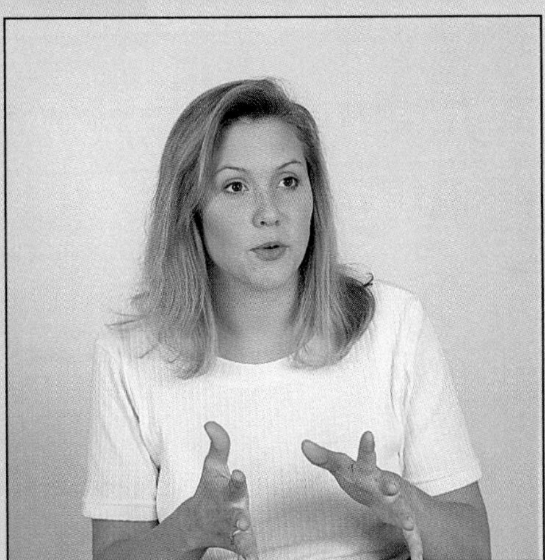

NAME	Melissa Joncas
SCHOOL OF NURSING	University of New Hampshire, Durham, New Hampshire
HOMETOWN	Londonderry, New Hampshire

WHY DID YOU ENTER THE FIELD OF NURSING?
When I was in junior high, I often visited my nana in the hospital, and observed the nurses who cared for her. Although she was quite sick, she always seemed comforted by these nurses, and I knew that someday I would like to have this kind of impact.

WHY DO YOU THINK THIS IS A GOOD TIME TO BE IN NURSING?
Nurses are taking an active role in health care reform. I like to see nurses taking a leadership role and promoting their perspectives.

WHAT QUALITIES DO YOU THINK ARE NECESSARY TO BE A GOOD NURSE?
I think the most important quality is passion—an excitement for what you're doing. To that I would add empathy, compassion, a caring nature.

WHAT HAS BEEN YOUR MOST GRATIFYING MOMENT AS A STUDENT NURSE?
I assisted in a birth last semester. Later I met the couple and their baby at a childbirth class I was observing, and they made a big point of telling everyone how helpful I was and that they should have a student present at their birthing experience, too. It felt great.

WHAT ADVICE WOULD YOU GIVE A NEW STUDENT?
Get involved!

21

Assessing Vital Signs

Objectives

- Describe factors that affect the vital signs and accurate measurement of them.
- Identify the normal ranges for each vital sign.
- Identify the variations in normal body temperature, pulse, respirations, and blood pressure that occur from infancy to old age.
- Describe five factors influencing the body's heat production.
- Identify four ways in which the body loses heat.
- Describe the body's temperature-regulating system.
- Compare oral, rectal, and axillary methods of measuring body temperature.
- Describe advantages and disadvantages of using each body temperature site.
- Identify indications and contraindications for using oral, rectal, and axillary body temperature sites.
- Describe selected alterations of body temperature and appropriate nursing care for these alterations.
- Identify nine pulse sites commonly used to assess the pulse and state the reasons for their use.
- List the characteristics that should be included when assessing pulses.
- Explain how to measure the apical pulse and apical-radial pulse.
- Describe the mechanics of breathing and the mechanisms that control respirations.
- Identify the characteristics that should be included in a respiratory assessment.
- Differentiate systolic from diastolic blood pressure.
- Describe five phases of Korotkoff's sounds.
- Describe various methods and sites used to measure blood pressure.

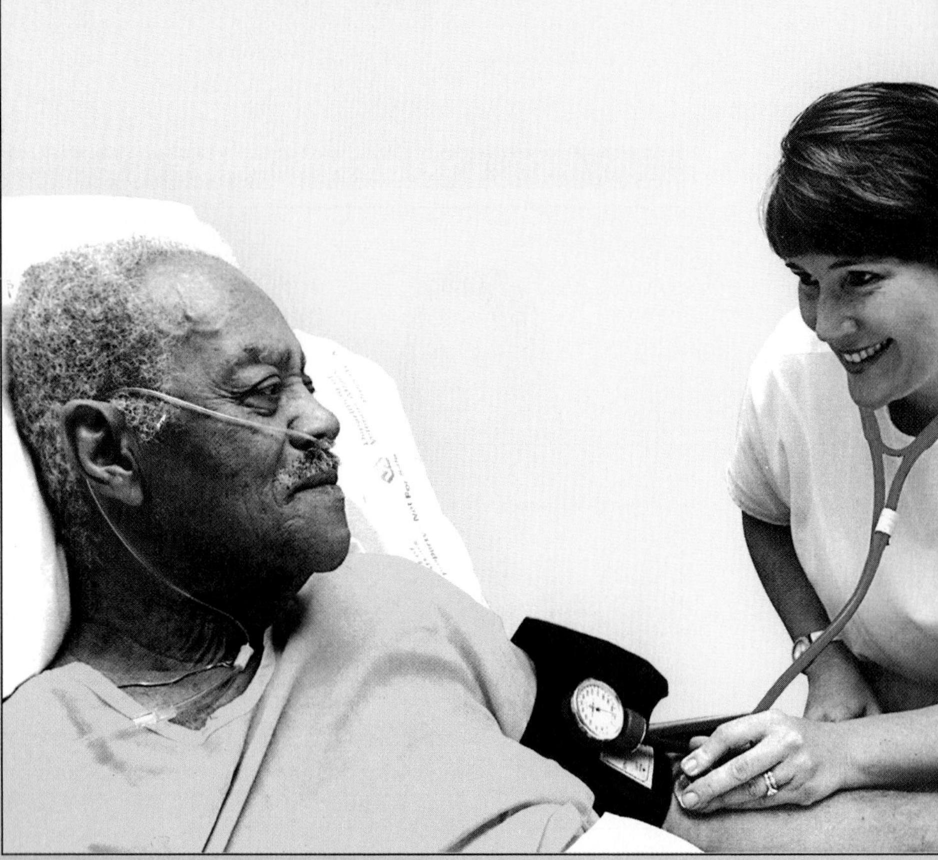

The **vital** or **cardinal signs** are body temperature, pulse, respirations, and blood pressure. These signs, which should be looked at in total, are determined to monitor the functions of the body. The signs reflect changes in function that otherwise might not be observed. Monitoring a client's vital signs should not be an automatic or routine procedure; it should be a thoughtful, scientific assessment. Vital signs, which should be evaluated with reference to the client's present and prior health status, are compared to accepted normal standards.

When and how often to assess a specific client's vital signs are chiefly nursing judgments, depending on the client's health status. Some agencies have policies about taking clients' vital signs, and physicians may specifically order a vital sign (eg, "Blood pressure q2h"). Ordered assessments, however, should be considered the minimum; a nurse should measure vital signs more often if the client's health status requires it. Examples of times to assess vital signs are listed in the accompanying box.

Times to Assess Vital Signs

- On admission to a health care agency to obtain baseline data
- When a client has a change in health status or reports symptoms such as chest pain or feeling faint
- According to a nursing or medical order
- Before and after surgery or an invasive diagnostic procedure
- Before and/or after the administration of a medication that could affect the respiratory or cardiovascular systems, for example, before giving a digitalis preparation
- Before and after any nursing intervention that could affect the vital signs (eg, ambulating a client who has been on bed rest)

Body Temperature

Body temperature is the balance between the heat produced by the body and the heat lost from the body. In other words, it is the heat of the body measured in heat units, called *degrees.* There are two kinds of body temperature: core temperature and surface temperature. **Core temperature** is the temperature of the deep tissues of the body, such as the cranium, thorax, abdominal cavity, and pelvic cavity. It remains relatively constant (37 C, 98.6 F). Accurate measurement is usually done using a pulmonary catheter. The **surface temperature** is the temperature of the skin, the subcutaneous tissue, and fat. It, by contrast, rises and falls in response to the environment. It can vary from 20 C (68 F) to 40 C (104 F).

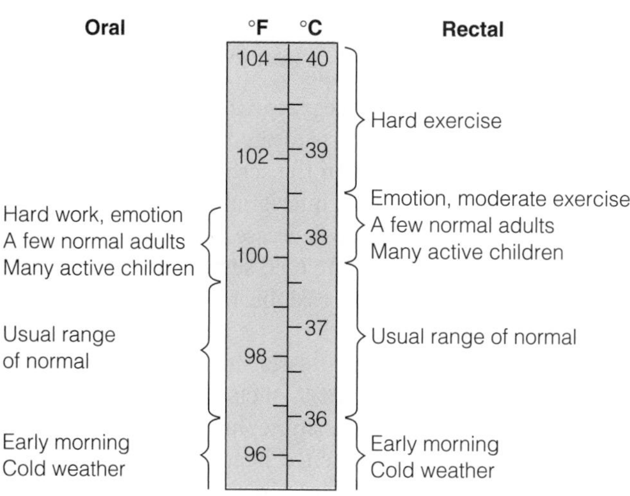

Figure 21–1 Estimated ranges of body temperatures in normal persons. **Source:** EF DuBois, *Fever and the Regulation of Body Temperature* (Springfield, IL: Charles C Thomas, 1948). Courtesy of Charles C Thomas, Publisher.

The sites nurses commonly use to measure body temperature reflect or estimate core temperature. When measured orally, the average body temperature of an adult is between 36.7 C (98 F) and 37 C (98.6 F). See Figure 21–1 for the normal ranges of body temperature.

The body continually produces heat as a by-product of metabolism. Carbohydrates, fats, and proteins are used to synthesize large quantities of adenosine triphosphate (ATP), which in turn is used as a source of energy by body cells. However, about 35% of the energy in food becomes heat rather than ATP, and further heat is produced as the food is changed to ATP (Guyton 1991, p. 792). When the amount of heat produced by the body exactly equals the amount of heat lost, the person is in **heat balance** (Figure 21–2, p. 426).

A number of factors affect the body's heat production. The most important are these five:

1. *Basal metabolic rate (BMR).* The **basal metabolic rate (BMR)** is the rate of energy utilization in the body required to maintain essential activities such as breathing. Metabolic rates decrease with age. In general, the younger the person, the higher the BMR (Marieb 1992, p. 862).

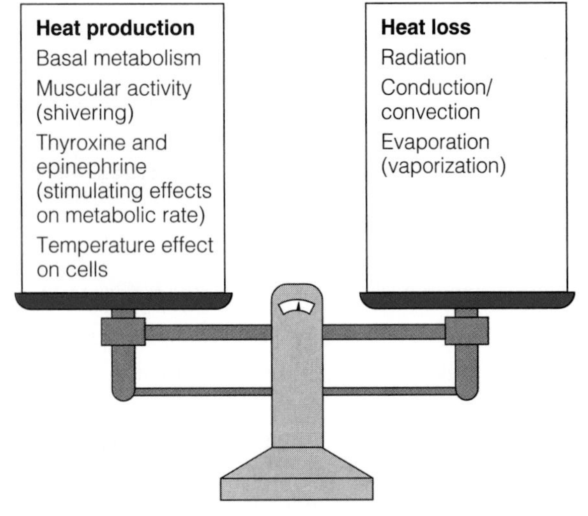

Figure 21–2 As long as heat production and heat loss are properly balanced, body temperature remains constant. Factors contributing to heat production (and temperature rise) are shown on the left side of the scale; those contributing to heat loss (and temperature fall) are shown on the right side of the scale. **Source:** Adapted from EN Marieb, *Human Anatomy and Physiology,* 2d ed. (Redwood City, CA: Benjamin/Cummings, 1992) p. 863. Adapted with permission.

2. *Muscle activity.* Muscle activity, including shivering, increases the metabolic rate.
3. *Thyroxine output.* Increased thyroxine output increases the rate of cellular metabolism throughout the body. This effect is called **chemical thermogenesis,** the stimulation of heat production in the body through increased cellular metabolism.
4. *Epinephrine, norepinephrine, and sympathetic stimulation.* These hormones immediately increase the rate of cellular metabolism in many body tissues, thereby increasing cell metabolism. Epinephrine and norepinephrine directly affect liver and muscle cells, thereby increasing cellular activity.
5. *Fever.* Fever increases the cellular metabolic rate and thus increases the body's temperature further.

Heat is lost from the body through radiation, conduction, convection, and vaporization. **Radiation** is the transfer of heat from the surface of one object to the surface of another without contact between the two objects, mostly in the form of infrared rays. For example, radiation accounts for 60% of the heat lost by a nude person standing in a room at normal room temperature (Guyton 1991, p. 799).

Conduction is the transfer of heat from one molecule to another. Again, a temperature gradient is implied. The heat transfers to a molecule of lower temperature. Conductive transfer cannot take place without contact between the molecules and normally accounts for minimal heat loss except, for example, when a body is immersed in ice water. The amount of heat transferred depends on the temperature difference and the amount and duration of the contact.

Convection is the dispersion of heat by air currents. There is usually a small amount of warm air adjacent to the body. This warm air rises and is replaced by cooler air, and so people always lose a small amount of heat through convection. **Vaporization** (evaporation) is continuous evaporation of moisture from the respiratory tract and from the mucosa of the mouth and from the skin. This continuous and unnoticed water loss is called insensible water loss, and the accompanying heat loss is called **insensible heat loss.** Insensible heat loss accounts for about 10% of basal heat production. When the body temperature increases, vaporization accounts for greater heat loss.

REGULATION OF BODY TEMPERATURE

The system that regulates body temperature has three main parts: sensors in the shell and in the core, an integrator in the hypothalamus, and an effector system that adjusts the production and loss of heat. Most *sensors* or *sensory receptors* are in the skin, which is a major part of the shell. The skin has more receptors for cold than warmth. Therefore, skin sensors detect cold more efficiently than warmth.

When the skin becomes chilled over the entire body, three physiologic processes to increase the body temperature take place:

1. Shivering increases heat production.
2. Sweating is inhibited to decrease heat loss.
3. Vasoconstriction decreases heat loss.

The **hypothalamic integrator,** the center that controls the core temperature, is located in the preoptic area of the hypothalamus. When the sensors in the hypothalamus detect heat, they send out signals intended to reduce the temperature, that is, to decrease heat production and increase heat loss. When the cold sensors are stimulated, signals are sent out to increase heat production and decrease heat loss.

The signals from the cold-sensitive receptors of the hypothalamus initiate *effectors,* such as vasoconstriction, shivering, and the release of epinephrine, which increases cellular metabolism and hence heat production. When the warmth-sensitive receptors in the hypothalamus are stimulated, the effector system sends out signals that initiate sweating and peripheral vasodilation. Also, when this system is stimulated, the person consciously makes appropriate adjustments, such as putting on additional clothing in response to cold or turning on a fan in response to heat.

Table 21–1 Variations in Body Temperatures by Age

Age	Average Temperature		
Newborn	Axillary:	36.1–37.7 C	(97.0–100 F)
1 year	Oral:	37.7 C	(99.7 F)
3 years	Oral:	37.2 C	(99.0 F)
5 years	Oral:	37.0 C	(98.6 F)
Adult	Oral:	37.0 C	(98.6 F)
	Axillary:	36.4 C	(97.6 F)
	Rectal:	37.6 C	(99.6 F)
	Forehead:	34.4 C	(94.0 F)
	Tympanic:	37.7 C	(99.9 F)
Elderly (over 70 yr)	Oral:	36.0 C	(96.8 F)

FACTORS AFFECTING BODY TEMPERATURE

Nurses should be aware of the factors that can affect a client's body temperature so that they can recognize normal temperature variations and understand the significance of body temperature measurements that deviate from normal. Among the factors that affect body temperature are the following:

1. *Age.* The infant is greatly influenced by the temperature of the environment and must be protected from extreme changes. Children's temperatures continue to be more labile than those of adults until puberty. Many elderly people, particularly those over 75 years, are at risk of hypothermia (temperatures below 36 C, or 96.8 F) for a variety of reasons, such as lack of central heating, inadequate diet, loss of subcutaneous fat, lack of activity, and reduced thermoregulatory efficiency. Elderly people are also particularly sensitive to extremes in the environmental temperature due to decreased thermoregulatory controls. Table 21–1 provides a summary of the variations in body temperatures by age.
2. *Diurnal variations (circadian rhythms).* Body temperatures normally change throughout the day, varying as much as 1.0 C (1.8 F) between the early morning and the late afternoon. The point of highest body temperature is usually reached between 2000 and 2400 hours (8:00 PM and midnight), and the lowest point is reached during sleep between 0400 and 0600 hours (4:00 and 6:00 AM). See Figure 21–3.
3. *Exercise.* Hard work or strenuous exercise can increase body temperature to as high as 38.3 to 40 C (101 to 104 F) measured rectally.

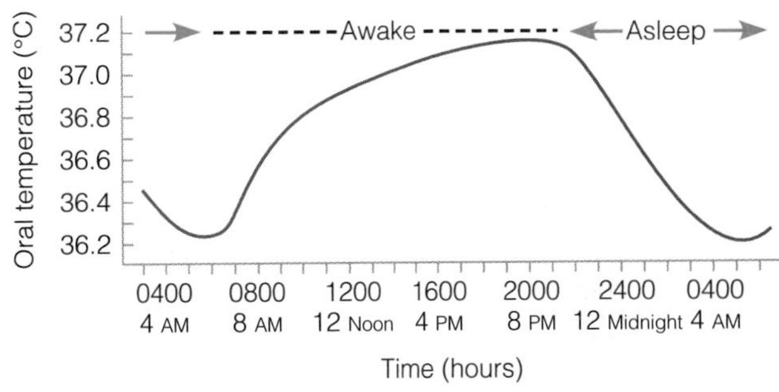

Figure 21–3 Range of oral temperatures during 24 hours for a healthy young adult.

4. *Hormones.* Women usually experience more hormone fluctuations than men. In women, progesterone secretion at the time of ovulation raises body temperature by about 0.3 C to 0.6 C (0.5 F to 1.0 F) above basal temperature (Olds et al 1992, p. 114).
5. *Stress.* Stimulation of the sympathetic nervous system can increase the production of epinephrine and norepinephrine, thereby increasing metabolic activity and heat production. Nurses may anticipate that a highly stressed or anxious client could have an elevated body temperature for that reason.
6. *Environment.* Extremes in environmental temperatures can affect a person's temperature regulatory systems. If the temperature is assessed in a very warm room and the body temperature cannot be modified by convection, conduction, or radiation, the temperature will be elevated. Similarly, if the client has been outside in an extremely cold weather without suitable clothing, the body temperature may be low.

ALTERATIONS IN BODY TEMPERATURE

Pyrexia A body temperature above the usual range is called **pyrexia, hyperthermia,** or (in lay terms) **fever.** A very high fever, such as 41 C (105.8 F) is called **hyperpyrexia** (Figure 21–4, p. 428). The client who has a fever is referred to as **febrile;** the one who has not is **afebrile.**

Four common types of fevers are intermittent, remittent, relapsing, and constant. During an **intermittent fever,** the body temperature alternates at regular intervals between periods of fever and periods of normal or subnormal temperatures. During a **remittent fever,** a wide range of temperature fluctuations (more than 2 C [3.6 F]) occurs over the 24-hour period, all of which are *above* normal. In a **relapsing fever,** short febrile periods of a few days are interspersed with periods of 1 or 2 days of normal temperature. During a **constant fever,** the body temperature fluctuates minimally but always remains above normal.

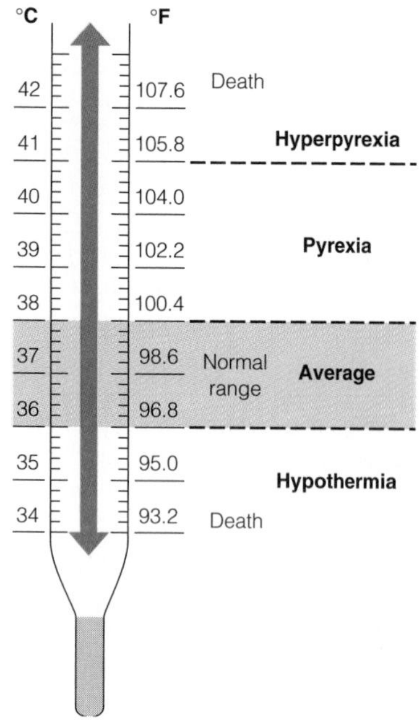

Figure 21–4 Terms used to describe alterations in body temperature (oral measurements).

The clinical signs of fever vary with the onset, course, and abatement stages of the fever (see the accompanying box). These signs occur as a result of changes in the *set-point* of the temperature control mechanism regulated by the hypothalamus. Whenever the core temperature rises above 37 C (98.6 F), the rate of heat loss is greater than heat production, resulting in a fall in temperature toward the set-point level. Conversely, when the core temperature falls below 37 C (98.6 F), the rate of heat production is greater than heat loss, resulting in a rise in temperature toward the set-point.

In a fever, however, the set-point of the hypothalamic thermostat changes suddenly from the normal level to a higher than normal value (eg, 39.5 C, 103.1 F) as a result of the effects of tissue destruction, pyrogenic substances, or dehydration on the hypothalamus. Although the set-point changes rapidly, the core body temperature (ie, the blood temperature) reaches this new set-point only after several hours. During this interval, the usual heat production responses that cause elevation of the body temperature occur: chills, feeling of coldness, cold skin due to vasoconstriction, and shivering.

When the core temperature reaches the new set-point, the person feels neither cold nor hot and no longer experiences chills. Depending on the degree of temperature elevation, various other signs (shown in the accompanying box) may occur at this stage. Very high temperatures, such as 41 to 42 C (106 to 108 F), damage the parenchyma of cells throughout the body, particularly in the brain, where destruction of neuronal cells is irreversible. Damage to the liver, kidneys, and other body organs can also be great enough to disrupt functioning and eventually cause death.

When the cause of the high temperature is suddenly removed, the set-point of the hypothalamic thermostat is suddenly reduced to a lower value, perhaps even back to the original normal level. In this instance, the hypothalamus now attempts to lower the temperature to 37 C (98.6 F), and the usual heat loss responses causing a reduction of the body temperature occur: excessive sweating and a hot, flushed skin due to sudden vasodilation. This sudden change of events is known as the *crisis* or the *flush* or the *defervescent stage* of a pyrexic condition. A more gradual return of the body temperature to normal is referred to as resolution of pyrexia by *lysis.*

CLINICAL SIGNS OF FEVER

Onset (cold or chill stage)

- Increased heart rate
- Increased respiratory rate and depth
- Shivering due to increased skeletal muscle tension and contractions
- Pallid, cold skin due to vasoconstriction
- Complaints of feeling cold
- Cyanotic nail beds due to vasoconstriction
- "Gooseflesh" appearance of the skin due to contraction of the arrectores pilorum muscles
- Cessation of sweating
- Rise in body temperature

Course

- Absence of chills
- Skin that feels warm
- Feelings of being neither hot nor cold
- Increased pulse and respiratory rates
- Increased thirst
- Mild to severe dehydration
- Simple drowsiness, restlessness, or delirium and convulsions due to irritation of the nerve cells
- Herpetic lesions of the mouth
- Loss of appetite (if the fever is prolonged)
- Malaise, weakness, and aching muscles due to protein catabolism

Defervescence (fever abatement)

- Skin that appears flushed and feels warm
- Sweating
- Decreased shivering
- Possible dehydration

NURSING INTERVENTIONS FOR CLIENTS WITH FEVER

- Monitor vital signs.
- Assess skin color and temperature.
- Monitor white blood cell count, hematocrit value, and other pertinent laboratory records.
- Remove excess blankets when the client feels warm, but provide extra warmth when the client feels chilled.
- Provide adequate food and fluids (eg, 2500–3000 mL per day) to meet the increased metabolic demands and prevent dehydration, if health permits. Clients who sweat profusely can become dehydrated.
- Measure intake and output.
- Maintain prescribed intravenous fluids.
- Reduce physical activity to limit heat production, especially during the flush stage.
- Administer antipyretics (drugs that reduce the level of fever) as ordered.
- Provide oral hygiene to keep the mucous membranes moist. They can become dry and cracked as a result of excessive fluid loss.
- Provide a tepid sponge bath to increase heat loss through conduction (physician's order often required).
- Provide dry clothing and bed linens to increase heat loss through conduction.

Nursing interventions for a client who has a fever are designed to support the body's normal physiologic processes, provide comfort, and prevent complications. During the course of fever, the nurse needs to monitor the client's vital signs closely.

Nursing measures during the chill phase are designed to help the client decrease heat loss. At this time, the body's physiologic processes are attempting to raise the core temperature to the new set-point temperature. During the flush or crisis phase, the body processes are attempting to lower the core temperature to the reduced or normal temperature set-point. At this time, the nurse takes measures to increase heat loss and decrease heat production. Nursing interventions for a client with fever are shown in the box above.

Hypothermia Hypothermia is a core body temperature below the lower limit of normal. The three physiologic mechanisms of hypothermia are (a) excessive heat loss, (b) inadequate heat production to counteract the heat loss, and (c) impaired hypothalamic thermoregula-

CLINICAL SIGNS OF HYPOTHERMIA

- Decreased body temperature
- Severe shivering (initially)
  Feelings of cold and chills
- Pale, cool, waxy skin
- Hypotension
- Decreased urinary output
- Lack of muscle coordination
- Disorientation
- Drowsiness progressing to coma

tion. The clinical signs of hypothermia are given in the box at the top of this column.

Hypothermia may be accidental or induced. *Accidental hypothermia* can occur as a result of exposure to a cold environment, (ie, below 16 C [60.8 F]) or from immersion in cold water. In elderly people, the problem can be compounded by a decreased metabolic rate and the use of sedatives, which depress the metabolic rate further. See the box directly below for clients at risk for hypothermia and

CLIENTS AT RISK FOR HYPOTHERMIA AND HYPERTHERMIA

People at risk for hypothermia:

- People who participate in cold-weather sports (eg, skiing and mountain climbing)
- Infants and children whose thermoregulatory systems are immature
- Elderly people who have insufficient food, clothing, or fuel
- People who have neurologic deficits and are unable to identify or respond to cold
- Alcoholics who have extreme heat loss secondary to vasodilation
- "Street people" who lack adequate clothing and shelter

People at risk for hyperthermia:

- People who have an infection
- Debilitated clients who are vulnerable to infection
- People with disease processes of the central nervous system that may impair thermoregulation
- People who have head trauma causing increased intracranial pressure
- Neonates who have ineffective thermoregulation

Table 21–2 Advantages and Disadvantages of Four Sites for Body Temperature Measurement

Site	Advantages	Disadvantages
Oral	Most accessible and convenient	Mercury-in-glass thermometers can break if bitten, therefore, they are contraindicated for children under 6 years and clients who are confused or who have convulsive disorders.
		Inaccurate if client has just eaten very hot or cold food or fluid or smoked.
		Inaccurate if client breathes through the mouth, therefore contraindicated for clients who have nasal surgery.
		Could injure the mouth following oral surgery.
Rectal	Most reliable measurement	Inconvenient and more unpleasant for clients; difficult for client who cannot turn to the side.
		Could injure the rectum following rectal sugery.
		Placement of the thermometer at different sites within the rectum yields different temperatures, yet placement at the same site each time is difficult.
		A rectal thermometer does not respond to changes in arterial temperatures as quickly as an oral thermometer, a fact that may be potentially dangerous for febrile clients, because misleading information may be acquired.
		Presence of stool may interfere with thermometer placement. If the stool is soft, the thermometer may be embedded in stool rather than against the wall of the rectum. If the stool is impacted, the depth of the thermometer insertion may be insufficient.
		In newborns and infants, insertion of the rectal thermometer has resulted in ulcerations and rectal perforations. *Many agencies advise against using rectal thermometers on neonates.*
Axillary	Safest and most noninvasive	The thermometer must be left in place a long time to obtain an accurate measurement.
Tympanic membrane	Readily accessible; reflects the core temperature	Equipment is expensive. Can be uncomfortable and involves risk of injuring the membrane if the probe is inserted too far.

hyperthermia. Managing the hypothermia involves removing the client from the cold and rewarming the client's body. For the client with mild hypothermia, the body is rewarmed by applying blankets; for the client with severe hypothermia, a hyperthermia blanket (an electronically controlled blanket that provides a specified temperature) is applied, and warm intravenous fluids are given. Wet clothing, which increases heat loss because of the high conductivity of water, should be replaced with dry clothing.

Induced hypothermia is the deliberate lowering of the body temperature to decrease the need for oxygen by the body tissues. Induced hypothermia can involve the whole body or a body part. It is sometimes indicated prior to surgery (eg, cardiac and brain surgery).

ASSESSING BODY TEMPERATURE

There are a number of sites for measuring body temperature. The three most common are oral, rectal, and axillary. In recent years, the tympanic membrane site has also been used. Each of the sites has advantages and disadvantages (Table 21–2). In a resting adult, rectal temperature is slightly higher than the temperature of the arterial blood, about the same as the temperature of the liver, and slightly lower than that of the brain. When measured in the axilla or orally (by mouth), the temperature is about 0.65 C (1 F) less than the rectal temperature.

The body temperature is usually measured *orally.* This method reflects changing body temperature more quickly than the rectal method. Traditionally, the oral method was not used for clients receiving oxygen, because the accuracy of the measurement was considered questionable. Recent evidence, however, suggests that oral readings are accurate in clients who receive oxygen by nasal cannula or face mask and clients who have nasogastric tubes and nasal endotracheal tubes, provided that the client can breathe through the nose (Heinz 1985, p. 128; Lukasiewicz 1986, p. 72). If a client has been taking cold or hot food or fluids or smoking, the nurse should wait 30 minutes before taking the temperature orally to ensure that the temperature of the mouth is not affected by the temperature of the food, fluid, or warm smoke.

RESEARCH NOTE

Are Chemical Dot Thermometers Accurate?

The chemical dot thermometer is widely used by clients of all ages in numerous community sites (eg, homes, schools, and day care centers). Despite its widespread use, the clinical accuracy of this convenient tool has not been well documented.

Erickson, Meyer, and Woo conducted a study to determine the accuracy of this community health tool. Chemical dot temperatures were compared with temperatures taken with an electronic thermometer at the oral site in 27 adults and at the axillary site in 44 adults and 34 young children in critical care units.

Chemical dot thermometers were found to provide a rough estimate of temperature and to perform differently at each of the sites and in the two age groups. In the adult subsample, mean readings with chemical dot thermometers were 0.4C lower than those taken at the oral site with an electronic thermometer. In contrast, mean readings with chemical dot thermometers were 0.4C higher in those adults measured at the axillary site with an electronic thermometer. No significant difference was found between axillary temperature readings with either method among the children's subsample group, although individual differences of ± 0.4C were common.

Implications: Chemical dot thermometers provide a rough estimate of temperature among children and adults; however, when accuracy is required, electronic thermometers should be used. Clients should be informed that chemical dot thermometers may be useful for tracking temperature trends, but they are not as accurate as electronic or glass thermometers.

Source: RS Erickson, LT Meyer, and TM Woo, Accuracy of chemical dot thermometers in critically ill adults and young children, *Image: Journal of Nursing Scholarship*, Spring 1996, 28:23–28.

Rectal temperature readings are considered to be the most accurate. In some agencies, taking temperatures rectally is contraindicated for clients with myocardial infarction. It is believed that inserting a rectal thermometer can produce vagal stimulation, which in turn can cause myocardial damage. However, not all authorities share this belief. Rectal temperatures are usually contraindicated for clients who are undergoing rectal surgery or have diarrhea or diseases of the rectum.

The axilla was the preferred site for measuring temperature in newborns because it was accessible and because there was no possibility of rectal perforation. However, newer research indicates that the axillary method is inaccurate when assessing a fever and that rectal perforation during temperature measurement is relatively rare (11 reported cases in the past 30 years) (Morley 1992, p. 28). Nursing students should check agency protocol when taking the temperature of newborns, infants, toddlers, and children. Clients for whom the axillary method of temperature assessment is appropriate include adult clients with oral inflammation or wired jaws, clients recovering from oral surgery, clients who are breathing through their mouths (eg, following nasal surgery), irrational clients, and clients for whom oral and rectal temperatures are contraindicated.

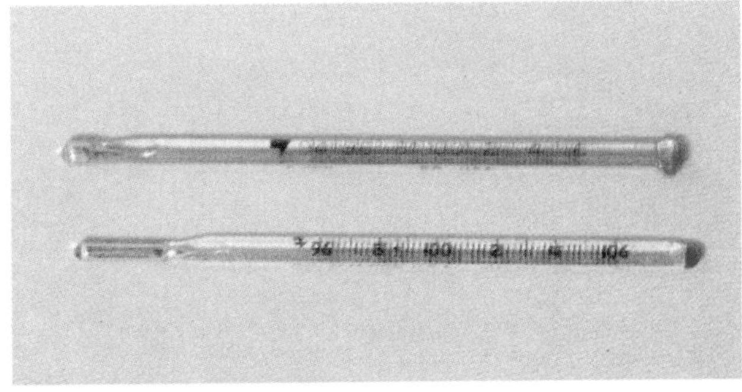

Figure 21–5 Two types of thermometer tips.

The *tympanic membrane*, or nearby tissue in the ear canal, is another core body temperature site. Tympanic membrane temperature readings average 1.1 to 1.5 F higher than oral temperature readings (Erickson & Yount 1991, p. 92). Like the sublingual oral site, the tympanic membrane has an abundant arterial blood supply, primarily from branches of the external carotid artery. Because temperature sensors applied directly to the tympanic membrane can be uncomfortable and involve risk of membrane injury or perforation, noninvasive *infrared thermometers* are now used.

Types of Thermometers Traditionally, body temperatures have been measured using *mercury-in-glass thermometers*. Oral thermometers may have long, slender tips or short, rounded tips (Figure 21–5). The rounded thermometer can be used at the rectal as well as other sites. In some agencies, thermometers may be color coded; for example, blue-colored or red-colored thermometers may be used for rectal temperatures and silver-colored ones for oral and axillary temperatures. *Disposable thermometers* are also manufactured; these are used only once.

Electronic thermometers offer another method of assessing body temperatures. They can provide a reading in only 2 to 60 seconds, depending on the model. The

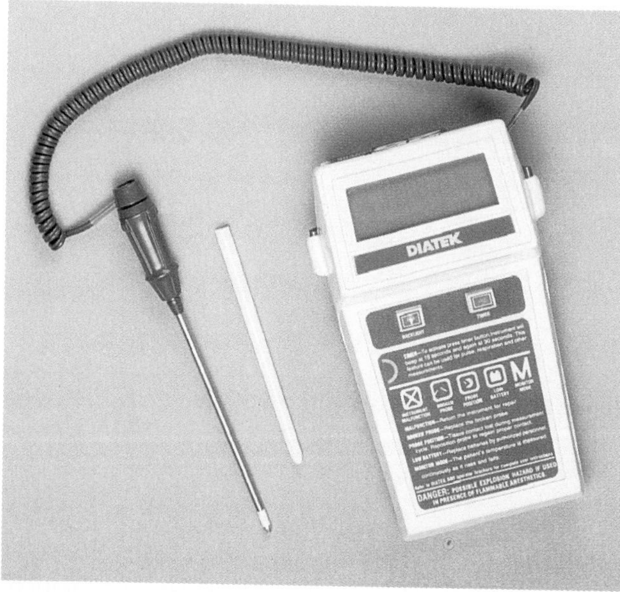

Figure 21–6 An electronic thermometer. Note the probe and probe cover.

equipment consists of a battery-operated portable electronic unit, a probe that the nurse attaches to the unit, and a probe cover, which is usually disposable (Figure 21–6). Some models have a different circuit for each method of measurement, and the nurse needs to make sure that the correct circuit is switched on before taking the temperature.

Chemical disposable thermometers are also used to measure body temperatures. They come in individual cases and are discarded after use. One type has small chemical dots at one end that respond to body heat by changing color, thereby providing a reading of the body temperature. The thermometer comes in a plastic case. To activate the chemicals, nurses hold the thermometer with the handle toward themselves, move the handle up and down, and then pull the plastic straight off the thermometer. The thermometer is inserted under the client's tongue, in the same way as a glass thermometer, and left in place for the time recommended by the manufacturer (eg, 45 seconds). After removing the thermometer, the nurse observes the dots for a change in color. To read the temperature, the nurse notes the highest reading among the dots that have changed color (Figure 21–7). The chemical thermometer is discarded after use.

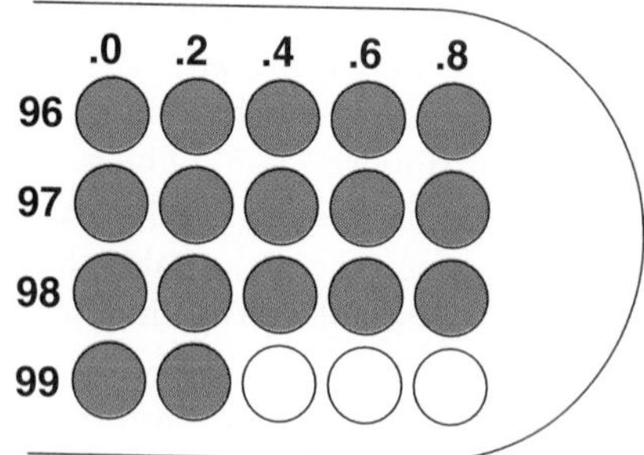

Figure 21–7 A chemical thermometer showing a reading of 99.2 F.

Temperature-sensitive tape may also be used to obtain a general indication of body surface temperature. It does not indicate the core temperature. When applied to the skin, usually of the forehead or abdomen, the tape responds by changing color. The skin area should be dry. After the length of time specified by the manufacturer (eg, 15 seconds), a color appears on the tape. The tape is removed and discarded after the color has been compared to the scale provided by the manufacturer. This method is particularly useful at home and for infants whose temperatures are to be monitored for any reason.

Infrared thermometers sense body heat in the form of infrared energy given off by a heat source, which in the ear canal is primarily the tympanic membrane (Erickson & Yount 1991, p. 91). See Figure 21–8. Because the infrared thermometer makes no contact with the tympanic membrane or moist mucous membrane, the risk of spreading infection is reduced. The ear canal has no mucous membrane and is normally dry.

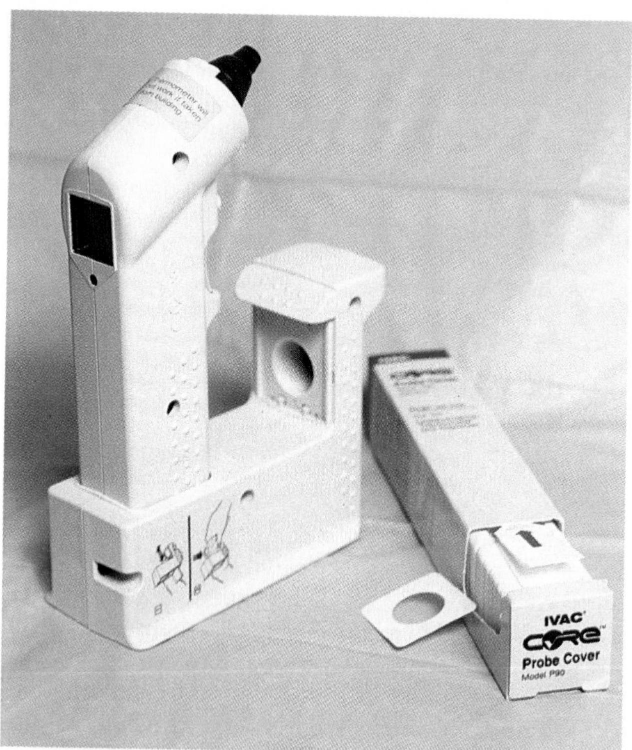

Figure 21–8 An infrared (tympanic) thermometer used to measure the tympanic membrane temperature.

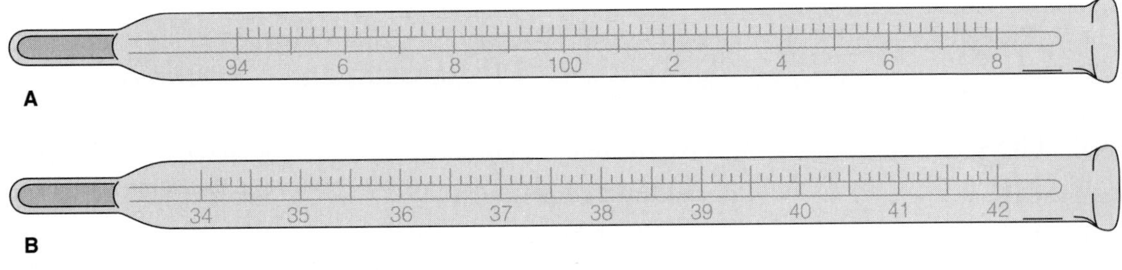

Figure 21–9 Glass thermometers. The upper one shows the Fahrenheit scale; the lower one shows the Celsius (centigrade) scale.

Temperature Scales The body temperature is measured in degrees on two scales: Celsius (centigrade) and Fahrenheit. A common type of thermometer is a glass tube with a column of mercury inside it. Heat expands the mercury, thus expanding the column along the tube, where it can be measured against marked calibrations. The Celsius scale normally extends from 34.0 to 42.0 C; the Fahrenheit scale usually extends from 94 to 108 F (Figure 21–9). Body temperatures rarely extend beyond these scales.

Sometimes a nurse needs to convert a Celsius reading to Fahrenheit, or vice versa. To convert from Fahrenheit to Celsius, deduct 32 from the Fahrenheit reading and then multiply by the fraction 5/9; that is:

$$C = (\text{Fahrenheit temperature} - 32) \times 5/9$$

For example, when the Fahrenheit reading is 100:

$$\begin{aligned} C &= (100 - 32) \times 5/9 \\ &= (68) \times 5/9 \\ &= 37.7 \end{aligned}$$

To convert from Celsius to Fahrenheit, multiply the Celsius reading by the fraction 9/5 and then add 32; that is:

$$F = (\text{Celsius temperature} \times 9/5) + 32$$

For example, when the Celsius reading is 40:

$$\begin{aligned} F &= (40 \times 9/5) + 32 \\ &= (72) + 32 \\ &= 104 \end{aligned}$$

Procedure 21–1 explains how to measure body temperature.

Text continued on page 437

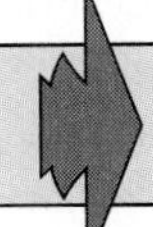

PROCEDURE 21–1 ASSESSING BODY TEMPERATURE USING A MERCURY THERMOMETER

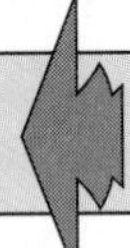

PURPOSES

- To establish baseline data for subsequent evaluation
- To identify whether the body temperature is within normal range
- To determine changes in the body temperature in response to specific therapies (eg, antipyretic administration, immunosuppressive therapy, invasive procedure)
- To monitor clients at risk for alterations in temperature (eg, clients at risk for infection or diagnosis of infection; those who have been exposed to temperature extremes; those with a leukocyte count below 5000 or above 12,000)

ASSESSMENT FOCUS

Clinical signs of fever (see page 428); clinical signs of hypothermia (see page 429); site most appropriate for measurement (see pages 430–431); factors that may alter core body temperature (see page 427).

EQUIPMENT

- ☐ Oral, rectal, axillary, or tympanic thermometer
- ☐ Lubricant and tissue, if the rectal site is used
- ☐ Towel, if the axillary site is used
- ☐ Disposable gloves, if the rectal site is used

➤

PROCEDURE 21–1 ASSESSING BODY TEMPERATURE USING A MERCURY THERMOMETER *continued*

INTERVENTION

1. Prepare the client.

- Ascertain which method of taking the temperature is appropriate for the client.

For an Oral Temperature

- Determine the time the client last took hot or cold food or fluids or smoked. *To obtain an accurate oral temperature reading, allow the amount of time according to agency protocol to elapse between a client's intake or smoking and the measurement.*

For a Rectal Temperature

- Assist the client to assume a lateral position. Place newborn in a lateral or prone position. Place a young child in a lateral position with knees flexed, or prone across the lap.
- Provide privacy before folding the bedclothes back to expose the buttocks. *Privacy is essential, because exposure of the buttocks embarrasses most people.*

For an Axillary Temperature

- Expose the client's axilla. If the axilla is moist, dry it with the towel, using a patting motion. *Friction created by rubbing can raise the temperature of the axilla.*

2. Prepare the equipment.

- Remove the thermometer from its package, and check the temperature reading on the thermometer.
- Shake down the mercury (if necessary) by holding the thermometer between the thumb and forefinger at the end farthest from the bulb. Snap the wrist downward.
- Repeat until the mercury is below 35 C (95 F).

3. Take the temperature.

For an Oral Temperature

- Place the thermometer or probe at the base of the tongue to the right or left of the frenulum, the posterior sublingual pocket (Figure 21–10). *The thermometer needs to reflect the core temperature of the blood in the larger blood vessels of the posterior pocket.*

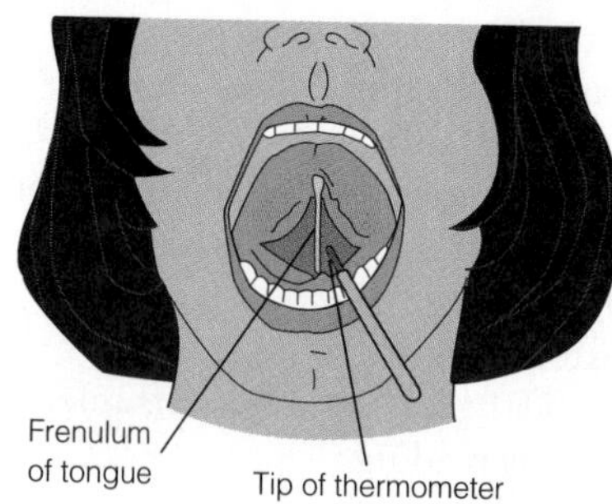

Figure 21–10 The tip of the oral thermometer is placed beside the frenulum below the tongue.

- Ask the client to close the lips, not the teeth, around the thermometer. *A client who bites the thermometer can break it and injure the mouth.*
- Leave the thermometer in place a sufficient time for the temperature to register or for the length of time recommended by the agency. The recommended time is generally either 2 minutes (Baker et al 1984, p. 111) or 3 minutes (Graves & Markarian 1980, p. 323). If an electronic oral thermometer is used, the client holds the thermometer under the tongue 10 to 20 seconds or until it completes registering.

For a Rectal Temperature

- Place some lubricant on a piece of tissue. Then apply lubricant to the thermometer about 2.5 cm (1 in) above the bulb. *The lubricant facilitates insertion of the thermometer without irritating the mucous membrane.*
- Wear disposable gloves on both hands. With the nondominant hand, raise the client's upper buttock to expose the anus.
- Ask the client to take a deep breath, and insert the thermometer into the anus anywhere from 1.5 to 4 cm (0.5 to 1.5 in), depending on the age and size of the client (for example, 1.5 cm [0.5 in] for an infant, 2.5 cm [0.9 in] for a child, and 3.7 cm [1.5 in] for an adult). *Taking a deep breath often relaxes the external sphincter muscle, thus easing insertion.*
- Do not *force* insertion of the thermometer. *Inability to insert the thermometer into a newborn could indicate the rectum is not patent.*
- Hold the thermometer in place for 2 minutes (Nichols 1972, p. 1093) or for the length of time recommended by the agency. For neonates hold the thermometer in place for 5 minutes or according to agency protocol (Schiffman 1982, p. 276). Hold the young child firmly while the probe is in the rectum. *The thermometer may become displaced inside or outside the anus if not held in place.*

For an Axillary Temperature

- Place the thermometer in the client's axilla (Figure 21–11).
- Assist the client to place the arm tightly across the chest to keep the thermometer in place.
- Leave the thermometer in place for 9 minutes or according to agency protocol (Nichols et al 1966, p. 310). For infants and children, leave the thermometer

PROCEDURE 21-1 *continued*

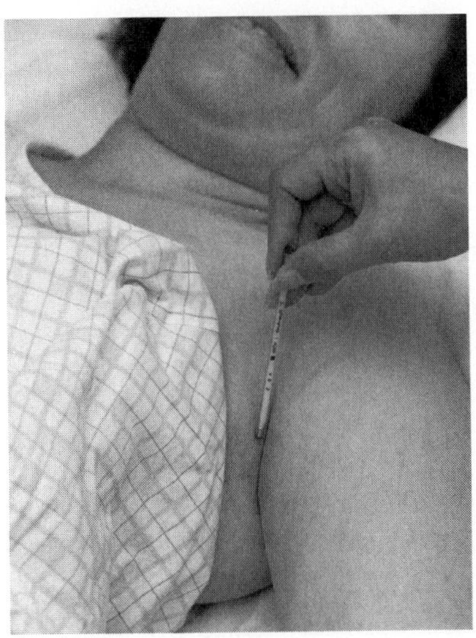

Figure 21–11 The bulb of the thermometer is placed in the center of the axilla.

in place 5 minutes (Eoff and Joyce 1981, p. 1011).

- Remain with the client, and hold the thermometer in place if the client is irrational or very young.

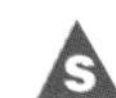

4. **Remove the thermometer.**
- Remove the plastic sheath, or wipe the thermometer with a tissue. Wipe in a rotating manner toward the bulb. *The thermometer is wiped from the area of least contamination to that of greatest contamination.*
- Discard the tissue in a receptacle used for contaminated items.

5. **Read the temperature.**
- Hold the thermometer at eye level, and rotate it until the mercury column is clearly visible. The upper end of the mercury column registers the client's body temperature. On the Fahrenheit thermometer, each long line reflects 1 degree, and each short line 0.2 degree. On the Celsius (centigrade) thermometer, each long line reflects 0.5 degree, and each short line 0.1 degree.

6. **Clean and shake down the thermometer.**
- Wash the thermometer in tepid, soapy water. Organic material, such as mucus, must be removed before the thermometer can be stored. *Organic materials on the thermometer can harbor microorganisms.*
- Rinse the thermometer in *cold* water, dry it, and store it dry. *Hot water expands the mercury and may break the thermometer.*
- Shake down the thermometer, and return it to its container or discard it. Some agencies also have special equipment for spinning down the mercury levels.
- If the thermometer is to be disinfected before storage, use recommended agency disinfectant.
- Return an electronic thermometer to the battery base for recharging.

7. **Document the temperature.**
- Record the temperature to the nearest indicated tenth (for example, 98.4 F, 37.1 C) on a flowsheet or in a notebook. See Figure 21–12 on page 436. *Recording the temperature immediately ensures it is not forgotten.*

Variation: Using an Electronic Thermometer

- Remove the electronic unit from the battery charging area.
- Remove the temperature probe from the unit. If the probe is not attached, attach it to the appropriate circuit (oral, rectal, or axillary) in models that have separate circuits for each.
- Place a disposable cover securely on the probe.
- Warm up the machine by switching it on if removal of the probe does not automatically prepare the machine for functioning.
- Take the temperature as indicated above in Step 3.
- Listen for a sound indicating that the maximum measurement has been reached, and read the temperature on the dial or readout.
- Remove the thermometer.
- Remove and discard the probe cover.

Variation: Using an Infrared Thermometer

- Apply a disposable sheath to the probe. There are sheaths that fit adults and infants. They can be applied without being touched.
- Place the probe tip into the outer position of the ear canal just at the opening. The probe tip seals the opening of the canal.
- Press the button on the electronic thermometer.
- Read the temperature on the screen. In 1 to 2 seconds, the temperature is digitized by computer onto the screen.
- Remove the thermometer.
- Remove and discard the probe cover. Covers can be ejected without being touched.

EVALUATION FOCUS

The temperature measurement in relation to baseline data or normal range for age of client; time of day and any other influencing factors; relationship to other vital signs.

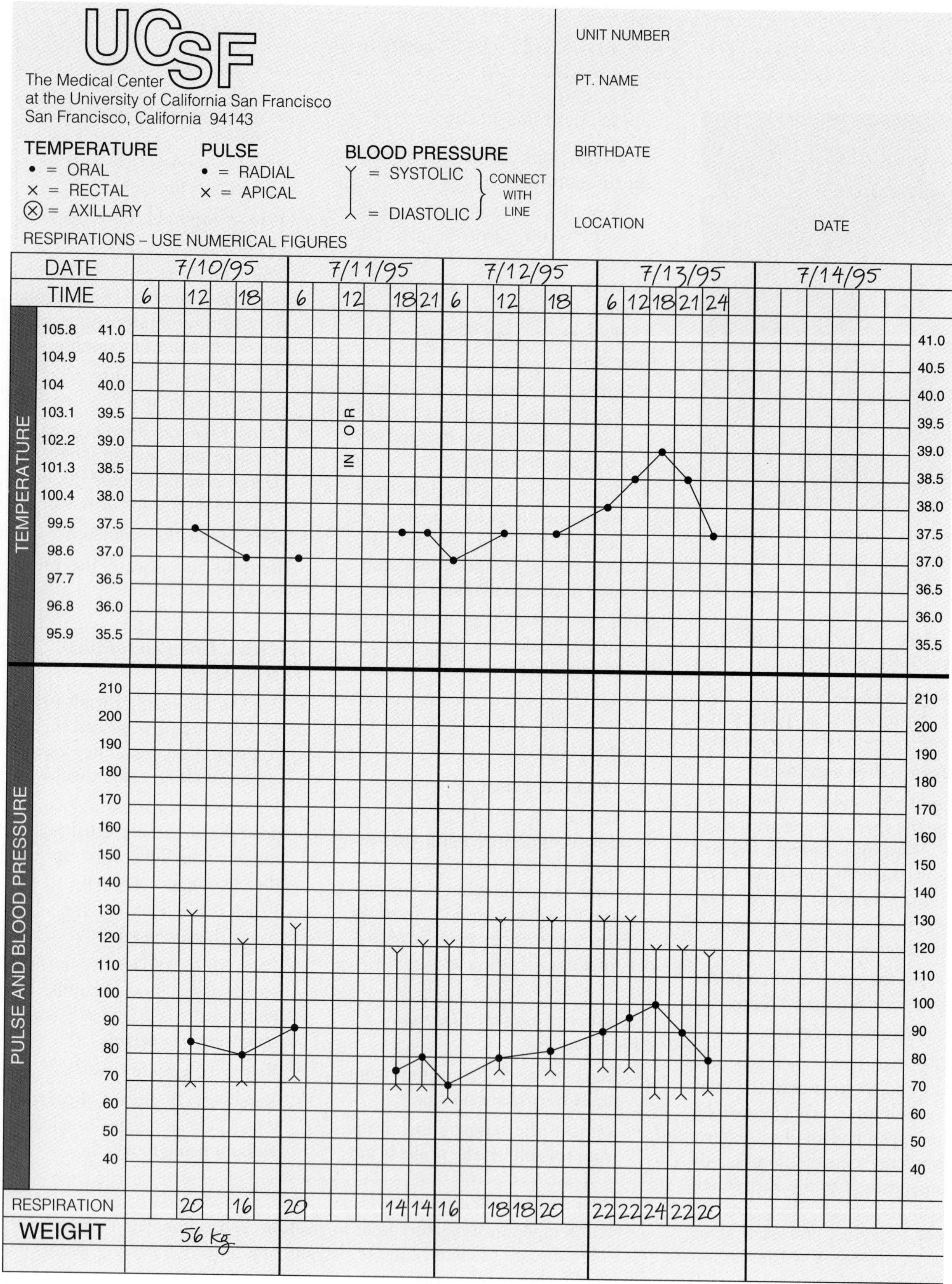

Figure 21–12 A clinical graph record. **Source:** Courtesy of the Department of Nursing, The Medical Center at the University of California, San Francisco. Reprinted with permission.

IDENTIFYING CLIENTS AT RISK FOR ALTERED BODY TEMPERATURE

The nursing assessment should include identifying individuals at risk for alterations in body temperature (see the box on page 429) as well as the clinical signs of specific conditions and the defining characteristics of possible nursing diagnoses.

RELATED NURSING DIAGNOSES

There are currently four accepted NANDA diagnostic categories concerning body temperature that reflect clients' actual and potential health problems. These are **High risk for altered body temperature, Hyperthermia, Hypothermia,** and **Ineffective thermoregulation. High risk for altered body temperature** is the state in which an individual is at risk for failure to maintain body temperature within normal range (Kim et al 1993, p. 6) due to internal factors such as the effects of disease and/or injury to the individual. Although modifying the causative factors is a medical responsibility (eg, the physician orders antibiotics to treat the infection causing the alteration in body temperature), the nurse is responsible for maintaining comfort, hydration, and nutrition appropriate for the individual client (Carpenito 1992, p. 157).

The remaining three nursing diagnoses reflect changes in body temperature in response to external factors such as the environment. **Hyperthermia** is the state in which body temperature is elevated above the individual's normal range, that is, greater than 37.8 C (100 F) orally or 38 C (100.5 F) rectally. **Hypothermia** is the state in which body temperature is reduced below the individual's normal range but not below a rectal temperature of 35.6 C (96 F) in adults and children and 36.4 C (97.5 F) in newborns (Kim et al 1993, p. 30). **Ineffective thermoregulation** exists when the client's temperature fluctuates between hyperthermia and hypothermia (Kim et al 1993, p. 60). The major nursing responsibility to clients with any of these three diagnoses related to external factors is modifying or controlling the causative factor or factors. Both hyperthermia and hypothermia, if not treated promptly, can result in medical emergencies; therefore, the nursing focus is often on prevention of these conditions in clients known to be at risk. The diagnoses are often recorded on the nursing care plan as **High risk for hyperthermia** or **High risk for hypothermia** (Carpenito 1992, p. 157).

The accepted NANDA nursing diagnoses, along with their related factors, are summarized below:

High risk for altered body temperature related to

- Illness or trauma affecting temperature regulation
- Medication causing vasoconstriction, vasodilation, altered metabolic state, or sedation
- Inactivity or vigorous activity

Hyperthermia related to

- Exposure to excessively hot environment
- Increased metabolic rate
- Dehydration

Hypothermia related to

- Exposure to excessively cool environment
- Debilitating illness or trauma
- Lack of adequate clothing and shelter

Ineffective thermoregulation related to

- Decreased basal metabolism secondary to aging
- Trauma or illness

Examples of assessment data clusters and related nursing diagnoses are shown in Table 21–3.

Table 21–3 Assessment Data Clusters and Related Nursing Diagnoses

Data Cluster	Nursing Diagnosis
Lakisha Jones, aged 3, was admitted to hospital with pyrexia of unknown origin. T, 39.8 C (104 F); P, 118; and R, 24. Skin is dry, flushed, and warm to touch. Mother reports she has been vomiting, has not been able to tolerate food or fluids for 48 hours, has become increasingly listless, and has had all required immunizations.	**Hyperthermia** related to illness not yet diagnosed and to dehydration.
Shelby Finn, aged 71, was brought to a homeless shelter by two other street people. T, 35.8 C (96.7 F); P, 122; and R, 20 and shallow; skin is pale and cool; nail beds are cyanotic. Friends state he is an alcoholic who sleeps under a viaduct but has little warm clothing or bedding for this cold winter climate.	**Hypothermia** related to exposure to cold environment and consumption of alcohol.

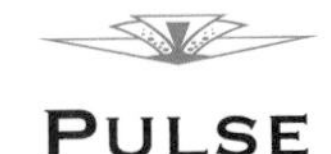

PULSE

The **pulse** is a wave of blood created by contraction of the left ventricle of the heart. The heart is a pulsating pump, and the blood enters the arteries with each heartbeat, causing pressure pulses or pulse waves. Generally, the pulse wave represents the stroke volume output and the compliance of the arteries. **Stroke volume output** is the amount of blood that enters the arteries with each ventricular contraction. Normally the heart empties about 70% of its volume with each contraction, that is, about 70 mL of blood in a healthy adult (Guyton 1991, p. 103). **Compliance** of the arteries is their ability to contract and expand. When a person's arteries lose their distensibility, as can happen in old age, greater pressure is required to pump the blood into the arteries.

When an adult is resting, the heart pumps 4 to 6 liters of blood each minute. This volume is called the **cardiac output.** The cardiac output (CO) is the result of the stroke volume (SV) times the heart rate (HR) per minute:

$$CO = SV \times HR$$

In a healthy person, the pulse reflects the heartbeat; that is, the pulse rate is the same as the rate of the ventricular contractions of the heart. However, in some types of cardiovascular disease the heartbeat and pulse rates can differ. For example, a client's heart may produce very weak or small pulse waves that are not detectable in a peripheral pulse far from the heart. In these instances, the nurse should assess the heartbeat *and* the peripheral pulse. See the section on assessing the apical pulse, later in this chapter. A **peripheral pulse** is a pulse located in the periphery of the body, for example, in the foot, hand, or neck. The **apical pulse,** in contrast, is a central pulse; that is, it is located at the apex of the heart.

The pulse rate is regulated by the autonomic nervous system (ANS). Impulses pass through the parasympathetic branch to the sinoatrial node (SA node), which is the pacemaker of the heart. These impulses decrease the heart rate. When body demands indicate a need for an increased heart rate, the impulses of the parasympathetic system are inhibited and the impulses of the sympathetic system increase.

FACTORS AFFECTING PULSE RATE

The rate of the pulse is expressed in beats per minute (BPM). A pulse rate varies according to a number of factors. The nurse should consider each of the following factors when assessing a client's pulse:

- *Age.* As age increases, the pulse rate gradually decreases. See Table 21–4 for specific variations in pulse rates from birth to adulthood.
- *Sex.* After puberty, the average male's pulse rate is slightly lower than the female's.
- *Exercise.* The pulse rate normally increases with activity. The rate of increase in the professional athlete is often less than in the average person because of greater cardiac size, strength, and efficiency.
- *Fever.* The pulse rate increases (a) in response to the lowered blood pressure that results from peripheral vasodilation associated with elevated body temperature and (b) because of the increased metabolic rate.
- *Medications.* Some medications decrease the pulse rate, and others increase it. For example, cardiotonics (eg, digitalis preparations) decrease the heart rate, whereas epinephrine increases it.
- *Hemorrhage.* Loss of blood from the vascular system (hemorrhage) normally increases pulse rate. The loss of a small amount of blood (eg, 500 mL, the amount lost after a blood donation) results in a temporary adjustment of the heart rate as the body compensates for the lost blood volume. An adult has about 5 liters of blood in the system and can usually lose up to 10% without adverse effects.
- *Stress.* In response to stress, sympathetic nervous stimulation increases the overall activity of the heart. Stress increases the rate as well as the force of the heartbeat. Fear and anxiety as well as the perception of severe pain stimulate the sympathetic system.
- *Position changes.* When a person assumes a sitting or standing position, blood usually pools in dependent vessels of the venous system. Pooling results in a transient decrease in the venous blood return to the heart and a subsequent reduction in blood pressure and increase in heart rate.

Table 21–4 Variations in Pulse Rate by Age

Age	Pulse Rate/Minute	
	Average	Range
Newborn to 1 month	130	80–180
1 year	120	80–140
2 years	110	80–130
6 years	100	75–120
10 years	70	50–90
Adult	80	60–100

PULSE SITES

Nine of the sites where a pulse is commonly taken (Figure 21–13) are the following:

1. *Temporal,* where the temporal artery passes over the temporal bone of the head. The site is superior (above) and lateral to (away from the midline of) the eye.
2. *Carotid,* at the side of the neck below the lobe of the ear, where the carotid artery runs between the trachea and the sternocleidomastoid muscle.
3. *Apical,* at the apex of the heart. In an adult this is located on the left side of the chest, no more than 8 cm

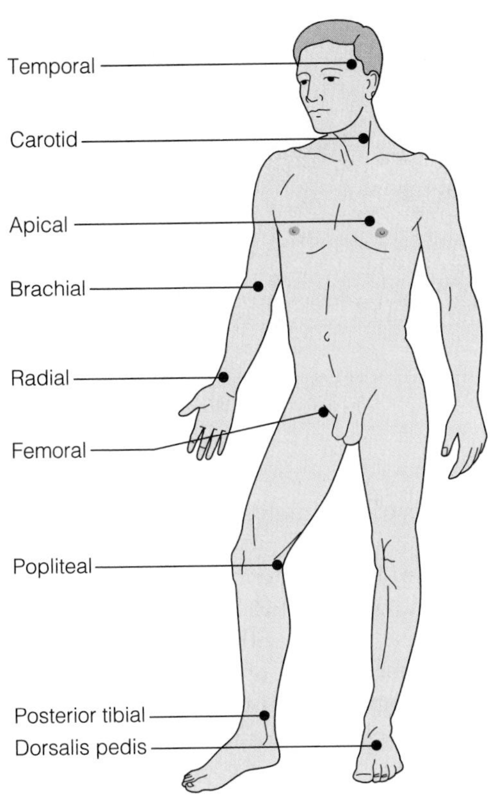

Figure 21–13 Nine sites commonly used for assessing a pulse.

(3 in) to the left of the sternum (breastbone) and under the fourth, fifth, or sixth intercostal space (area between the ribs). For a child 7 to 9 years of age, the apical pulse is located between the fourth and fifth intercostal spaces. Before 4 years of age it is left of the midclavicular line (MCL); between 4 and 6 years, it is at the MCL. See Figure 21–14.

4. *Brachial*, at the inner aspect of the biceps muscle of the arm (especially in infants) or medially in the antecubital space (elbow crease).
5. *Radial*, where the radial artery runs along the radial bone, on the thumb side of the inner aspect of the wrist.
6. *Femoral*, where the femoral artery passes alongside the inguinal ligament.
7. *Popliteal*, where the popliteal artery passes behind the knee. This point is difficult to find, but it can be palpated if the client flexes the knee slightly. See also Figure 21–25, later in this chapter.
8. *Posterior tibial*, on the medial surface of the ankle where the posterior tibial artery passes behind the medial malleolus.
9. *Pedal (dorsalis pedis)*, where the dorsalis pedis artery passes over the bones of the foot. This artery can be

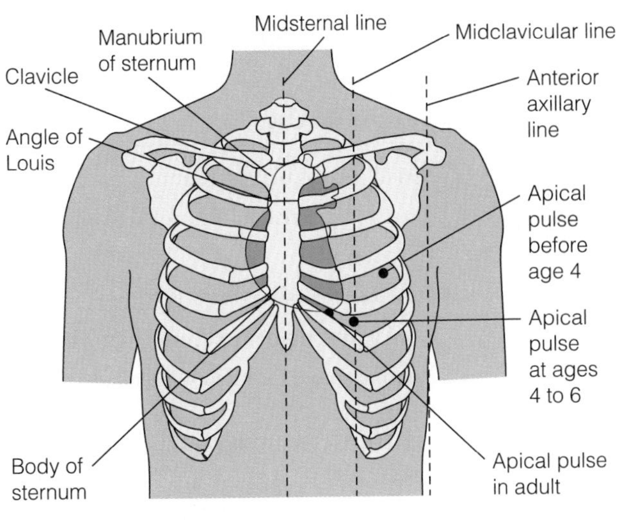

Figure 21–14 Location of the apical pulse for a child under 4 years, a child 4 to 6 years, and an adult.

palpated by feeling the dorsum (upper surface) of the foot on an imaginary line drawn from the middle of the ankle to the space between the big and second toes.

The radial site is most commonly used. It is easily found in most people and readily accessible. The reasons for use of each site are given in Table 21–5 on page 440.

ASSESSING THE PULSE

A pulse is commonly assessed by palpation (feeling) or auscultation (hearing). The middle three fingertips are used for palpating all pulse sites except the apex of the heart. A stethoscope is used for assessing apical pulses and fetal heart tones. Increasingly, a Doppler ultrasound stethoscope (DUS; see Figure 21–15, p. 440) is being used for pulses that are difficult to assess. The DUS headset has earpieces similar to standard stethoscope earpieces, but it has a long cord attached to a volume-controlled audio unit and an ultrasound transducer. The DUS detects movement of red blood cells through a blood vessel. In contrast to the conventional stethoscope, it excludes environmental sounds. It cannot detect blood flow in deep vessels or in those underlying bone, such as the vessels in the abdomen, thorax, or skull. The DUS is battery operated, and batteries must be replaced about every 6 months.

The cardiac monitoring machine is another device for assessing the apical pulse. It indicates the rate on a screen or readout graph.

A pulse is normally palpated by applying moderate pressure with the three middle fingers of the hand. The pads on the most distal aspects of the finger are the most sensitive areas for detecting a pulse. With excessive pressure, one can obliterate a pulse, whereas with too little

Table 21–5 Reasons for Using Specific Pulse Site

Pulse Site	Reasons for Use
Radial	Readily accessible and routinely used
Temporal	Used when radial pulse is not accessible
Carotid	Used for infants
	Used in cases of cardiac arrest
	Used to determine circulation to the brain
Apical	Routinely used for infants and children up to 3 years of age
	Used to determine discrepancies with radial pulse
	Used in conjunction with some medications
Brachial	Used to measure blood pressure
	Used during cardiac arrest for infants
Femoral	Used in cases of cardiac arrest
	Used for infants and children
	Used to determine circulation to a leg
Popliteal	Used to determine circulation to the lower leg
	Used to determine leg blood pressure
Posterial tibial	Used to determine circulation to the foot
Pedal	Used to determine circulation to the foot

pressure, one may not be able to detect it. Before the nurse assesses the *resting* pulse, the client should assume a comfortable position. The nurse should also be aware of the following:

- Any medication that could affect the heart rate.
- Whether the client has been physically active. If so, wait 10 to 15 minutes until the client has rested and the pulse has slowed to its usual rate.
- Any baseline data about the normal heart rate for the client. For example, a physically fit athlete may have a heart rate below 60 beats per minute.
- Whether the client should assume a particular position (eg, sitting). In some clients, the rate changes with the position because of changes in blood flow volume and autonomic nervous system activity.

When assessing the pulse, the nurse collects the following data: the rate, rhythm, volume, arterial wall elasticity, and presence or absence of bilateral equality. The *normal pulse rates* are shown in Table 21–4. An excessively fast heart rate (eg, over 100 beats per minute in an adult) is referred to as **tachycardia.** A heart rate in an adult of 60 beats per minute or less is called **bradycardia.** If a client has either tachycardia or bradycardia, the apical pulse should be assessed.

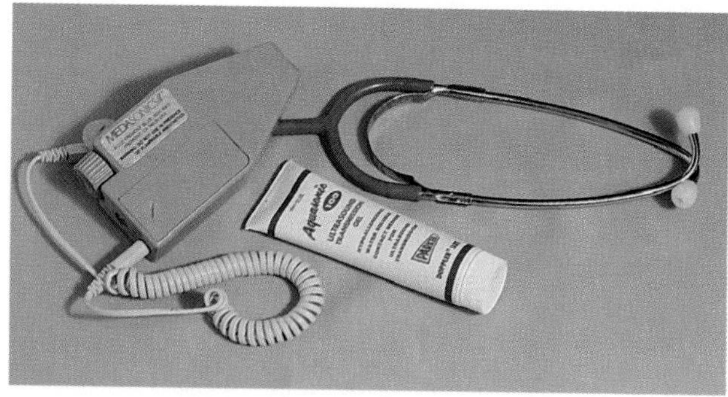

Figure 21–15 An ultrasound (Doppler) stethoscope.

The **pulse rhythm** is the pattern of the beats and the intervals between the beats. Equal time elapses between beats of a normal pulse. A pulse with an irregular rhythm is referred to as a **dysrhythmia** or **arrhythmia.** It may consist of random, irregular beats or a predictable pattern of irregular beats. When a dysrhythmia is detected, the apical pulse should be assessed. An electrocardiogram (ECG or EKG) is necessary to define the dysrhythmia further.

Pulse volume, also called the pulse strength or amplitude, refers to the force of blood with each beat. Usually, the pulse volume is the same with each beat. It can range from absent to bounding. A normal pulse can be felt with moderate pressure of the fingers and can be obliterated with greater pressure. A forceful or full blood volume that is obliterated only with difficulty is called a *full* or *bounding* pulse. A pulse that is readily obliterated with pressure from the fingers is referred to as *weak, feeble,* or *thready.* A pulse volume is usually measured on a scale of 0 to 3 (Table 21–6).

The **elasticity of the arterial wall** reflects its expansibility or its deformities. A healthy, normal artery feels straight, smooth, soft, and pliable. Elderly people often have inelastic arteries that feel twisted (tortuous) and irregular upon palpation. The elasticity of the arteries may

Table 21–6 Scale for Measuring Pulse Volume

Scale	Description of Pulse
0	Absent, not discernible
1	Thready or weak, difficult to feel
2	Normal, detected readily, obliterated by strong pressure
3	Bounding, difficult to obliterate

not affect the pulse rate, rhythm, or volume, but it does reflect the status of the client's vascular system.

When assessing a peripheral pulse to determine the adequacy of blood flow to a particular area of the body, the nurse should also assess the corresponding pulse on the other side of the body. The second assessment gives the nurse data with which to compare the pulses. For example, when assessing the blood flow to the right foot, the nurse assesses the right dorsalis pedis pulse and then the left dorsalis pedis pulse. If the client's right and left pulses are the same, the client's dorsalis pedis pulses are *bilaterally equal.*

PERIPHERAL PULSE ASSESSMENT

A peripheral pulse, usually the radial pulse, is assessed by palpation in all individuals *except:*

- Newborns and children up to 2 or 3 years. Apical pulses are assessed in these clients.
- Very obese or elderly clients, whose radial pulse may be difficult to palpate. Doppler equipment may be used for these clients, or the apical pulse is assessed.
- Individuals with a heart disease, who require apical pulse assessment.
- Individuals in whom the circulation to a specific body part must be assessed; for example, following leg surgery, the pedal (dorsalis pedis) pulse is assessed.

Procedure 21–2 provides guidelines for assessing peripheral pulses.

APICAL PULSE ASSESSMENT

Assessment of the apical pulse is indicated for clients whose peripheral pulse is irregular as well as for clients with known cardiovascular, pulmonary, and renal diseases. It is commonly assessed prior to administering medications that affect heart rate. The apical site is also used to

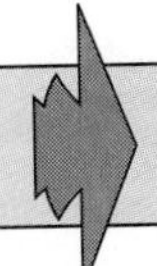

PROCEDURE 21–2 ASSESSING A PERIPHERAL PULSE

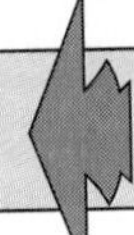

PURPOSES

- To establish baseline data for subsequent evaluation
- To identify whether the pulse rate is within normal range
- To determine whether the pulse rhythm is regular and the pulse volume is appropriate
- To compare the equality of corresponding peripheral pulses on each side of the body
- To monitor and assess changes in the client's health status
- To monitor clients at risk for pulse alterations (eg, those with a history of heart disease or experiencing cardiac arrhythmias, hemorrhage, acute pain, infusion of large volumes of fluids, fever)

ASSESSMENT FOCUS

Clinical signs of cardiovascular alterations, other than pulse rate, rhythm, or volume (eg, dyspnea [difficult respirations], fatigue, pallor, cyanosis [bluish discoloration of skin and mucous membranes], palpitations, syncope [fainting], impaired peripheral tissue perfusion as evidenced by skin discoloration and cool temperature); factors that may alter pulse rate (eg, emotional status and activity level); site most appropriate for assessment.

EQUIPMENT

- ☐ Watch with a second hand or indicator
- ☐ If using Doppler ultrasound stethoscope, the transducer in the DUS probe, a stethoscope headset, and transmission gel

INTERVENTION

1. Prepare the client.

- Select the pulse point. Normally, the radial pulse is taken, unless it cannot be exposed or circulation to another body area is to be assessed.
- Assist the client to a comfortable resting position. When the radial pulse is assessed, the client's arm can rest alongside the body, the palm facing downward. Or, the forearm can rest at a 90-degree angle across the chest with the ➤

Procedure 21–2 Assessing a Peripheral Pulse *continued*

palm downward. For the client who can sit, the forearm can rest across the thigh, with the palm of the hand facing downward or inward. Position a child comfortably in the parent's arms, or have the parent remain close by. *This may decrease anxiety and yield more accurate results.*

2. Palpate and count the pulse.

- Place two or three middle fingertips lightly and squarely over the pulse point (Figure 21–16). *Using the thumb is contraindicated because the thumb has a pulse that the nurse could mistake for the client's pulse.*
- If the pulse is regular, count for 30 seconds and multiply by 2. If it is irregular, count for 1 minute. If taking a client's pulse for the first time or when obtaining baseline data, count the pulse for a full minute. *An irregular pulse requires a full minute's count for a correct assessment.*

3. Assess the pulse rhythm and volume.

- Assess the pulse rhythm by noting the pattern of the intervals between the beats. A normal pulse has equal time periods between beats. If this is an initial assessment, assess for 1 minute.
- Asses the pulse volume. A normal pulse can be felt with moderate pressure, and the pressure is equal with each beat. A forceful pulse volume is full; an easily obliterated pulse is weak.

4. Assess the arterial wall.

- Compress the artery firmly, and run a finger distal to the heart along the artery (Figure 21–17). A normal arterial wall is smooth and straight.

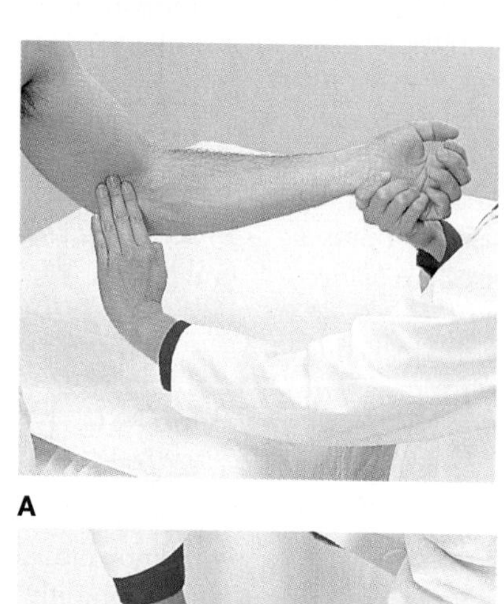

A

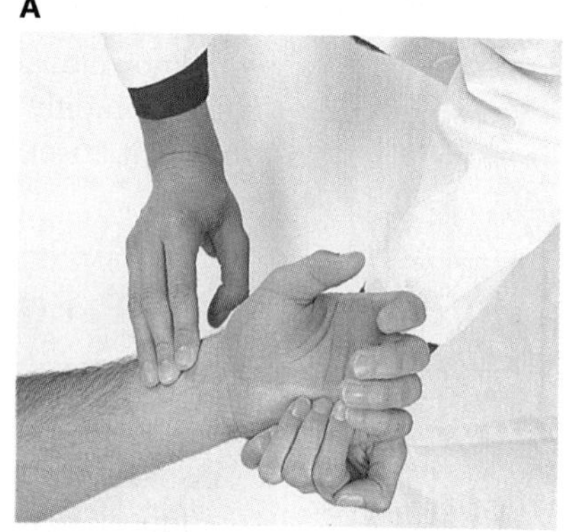

B

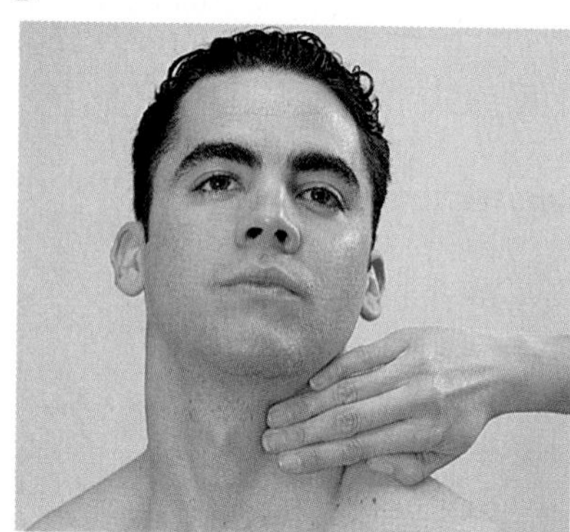

C

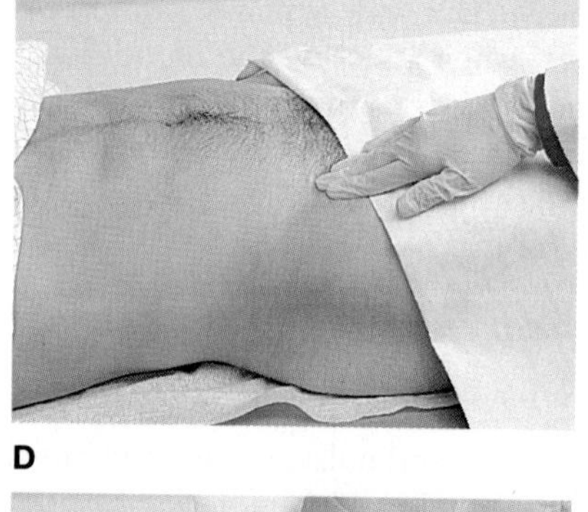

D

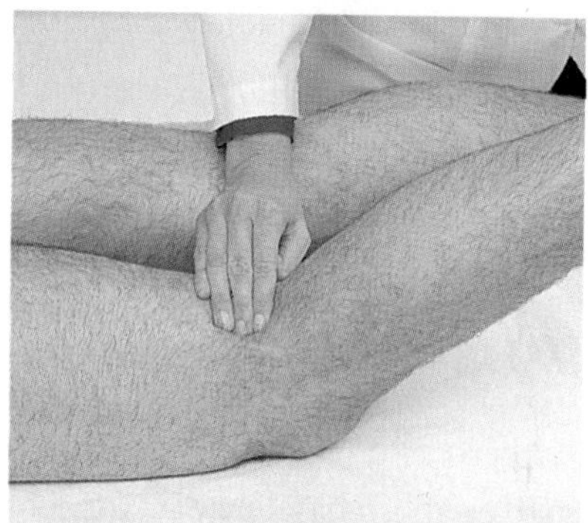

E

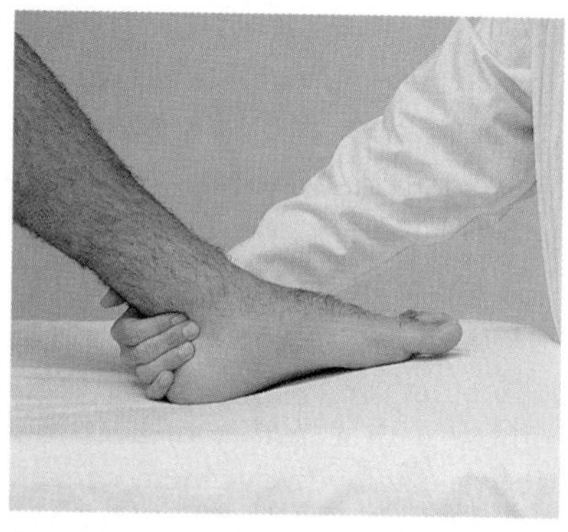

F

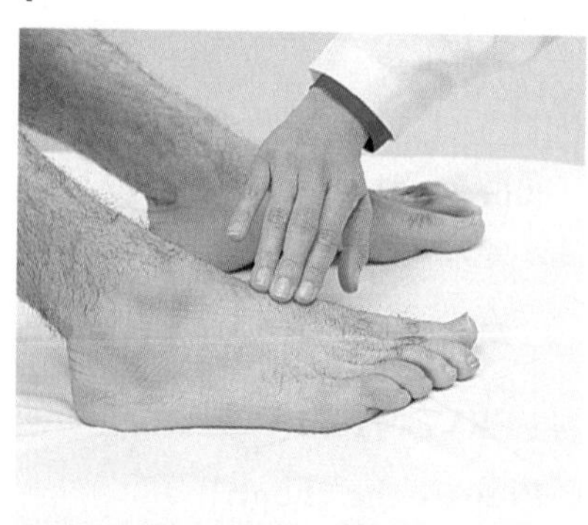

G

Figure 21–16 Assessing the pulses: *A*, brachial; *B*, radial; *C*, carotid; *D*, femoral; *E*, popliteal; *F*, posterior tibial; and *G*, pedal.

PROCEDURE 21–2 *continued*

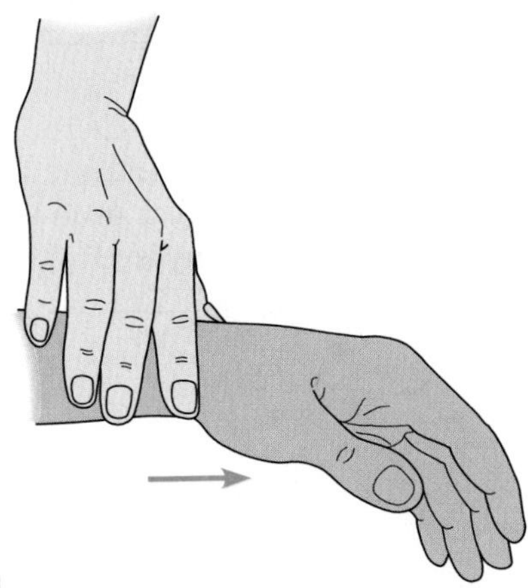

Figure 21–17 Assessing the status of the arterial wall.

5. Document and report pertinent assessment data.

- Record the pulse rate, rhythm, and volume, and the condition of the arterial wall.
- Report to the nurse in charge pertinent data such as (a) pale skin color and cool skin temperature, (b) a pulse rate faster or slower than normal for the client, (c) a full, bounding, or weak pulse volume, (d) an irregular pulse rhythm, and (e) a tortuous arterial wall.

Variation: Using a DUS

- Plug the stethoscope headset into one of the two output jacks located next to the volume control. DUS units have jacks for two headpieces and accessory loudspeakers so that a second person can listen to the signals.
- Apply transmission gel either to the probe (a device resembling a small transistor radio), at the narrow end of the plastic case housing the transducer, or to the client's skin. *Ultrasound beams do not travel well through air. The gel makes an airtight seal, which then promotes optimal ultrasound wave transmission.*
- Press the "on" button.
- Hold the probe at a 45-degree angle against the skin over the pulse site. Use a light pressure, and keep the probe in contact with the skin. *Too much pressure can stop the blood flow and obliterate the signal.*
- Distinguish artery sounds from vein sounds. The artery sound (signal) is distinctively pulsating and has a pumping quality. The venous sound is like the wind, is intermittent, and varies with respirations. *Both artery and vein sounds are heard simultaneously through the DUS, because major arteries and veins are situated close together throughout the body.*
- If arterial sounds cannot be easily heard, then reposition the probe.
- After assessing the pulse, remove all the gel from the probe to prevent damage to its surface. Clean the transducer with aqueous solutions. *Alcohol or other disinfectants may damage the face of the transducer.* Remove all gel from the client.

EVALUATION FOCUS

The pulse rate in relation to baseline data or normal range for age of client; relationship of pulse rate and volume to other vital signs; pulse rhythm and volume in relationship to baseline data and health status; if assessing peripheral pulses, equality, rate, and volume in corresponding extremities.

assess the pulse for newborns, infants, and children up to 2 to 3 years old. Procedure 21–3 on page 444 presents guidelines for assessing the apical pulse.

APICAL-RADIAL PULSE ASSESSMENT

An **apical-radial pulse** may need to be assessed for clients with certain cardiovascular disorders. Normally, the apical and radial rates are identical. An apical pulse rate greater than a radial pulse rate can indicate that the thrust of the blood from the heart is too feeble for the wave to be felt at the peripheral pulse site, or it can indicate that vascular disease is preventing impulses from being transmitted. Any discrepancy between the two pulse rates needs to be reported promptly. In no instance is the radial pulse greater than the apical pulse.

An apical-radial pulse can be taken by two nurses or one nurse, although the two-nurse technique may be more accurate. Procedure 21–4 on page 446 outlines the steps for assessing an apical-radial pulse.

RESPIRATIONS

Respiration is the act of breathing; it includes the intake of oxygen and the output of carbon dioxide. **External**

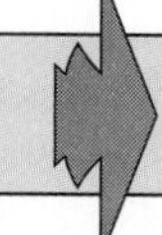

PROCEDURE 21–3 ASSESSING AN APICAL PULSE

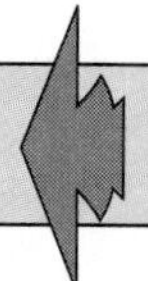

PURPOSES

- To obtain the heart rate of newborns, infants, and children 2 to 3 years old or of an adult with an irregular peripheral pulse
- To establish baseline data for subsequent evaluation
- To determine whether the cardiac rate is within normal range and the rhythm is regular
- To monitor clients with cardiac disease and those receiving medications to improve heart action

ASSESSMENT FOCUS
Clinical signs of cardiovascular alterations, other than pulse rate, rhythm, or volume (eg, dyspnea, fatigue, pallor, cyanosis, syncope); factors that may alter pulse rate (eg, emotional status, activity level).

EQUIPMENT

- ☐ Watch with a second hand or indicator
- ☐ Stethoscope with a bell-shaped or flat-disc diaphragm
- ☐ Antiseptic wipes
- ☐ If using ultrasound, a DUS, probe (transducer), and transmission gel

INTERVENTION

1. Position the client appropriately.

- Assist an adult or young child to a comfortable supine position with the head of the bed elevated, or to a sitting position on a chair, the edge of the bed, or the examination table.
- Place a baby in a supine position, and offer a pacifier if the baby is crying or restless. *Crying and physical activity will increase the pulse rate.* For this reason, take the apical pulse rate of infants and small children before assessing body temperature.
- Demonstrate the procedure to the child using a stuffed animal or doll, and allow the child to handle the stethoscope before beginning the procedure. *This will decrease anxiety and promote cooperation.*
- Expose the area of the chest over the apex of the heart.

2. Locate the apical impulse.

- This is the point over the apex of the heart where the apical pulse can be most clearly heard. It is also referred to as the point of maximal impulse (PMI). In 50% of the adult population, the apical impulse can be palpated (Malasanos et al 1990, p. 337).
- Palpate the angle of Louis (the angle between the manubrium, the top of the sternum, and the body of the sternum). It is palpated just below the suprasternal notch and is felt as a prominence (Figure 21–14, earlier).
- Place your index finger just to the left of the client's sternum, and palpate the second intercostal space.
- Place your middle or next finger in the third intercostal space, and continue palpating downward until you locate the apical impulse, usually about the fifth intercostal space, if the client is an adult or a child 7 years or older. If the client is a young child, palpate downward to the fourth intercostal space. *The apex of the heart is normally located in the fifth intercostal space in individuals who are 7 years of age and over; it is in the fourth intercostal space in young children, and one or two spaces above the adult apex during infancy (Malasanos et al 1990, p. 627).*
- Palpate the apical impulse. If the client is an adult, move your index finger laterally along the fifth intercostal space to the MCL. Normally, the apical impulse is palpable at or just medial to the MCL. For a young child, move your finger along the fourth intercostal space to a position between the MCL and the anterior axillary line (Figure 21–14, earlier).

3. Auscultate and count heartbeats.

- Use antiseptic wipes to clean the earpieces and diaphragm of the stethoscope (Figure 21–18) if their cleanliness is in doubt. *The diaphragm needs to be cleaned and disinfected if soiled with body substances.*
- Warm the diaphragm of the stethoscope by holding it in the palm of the hand for a moment. *The metal of the diaphragm is usually cold and can startle the client*

PROCEDURE 21–3 *continued*

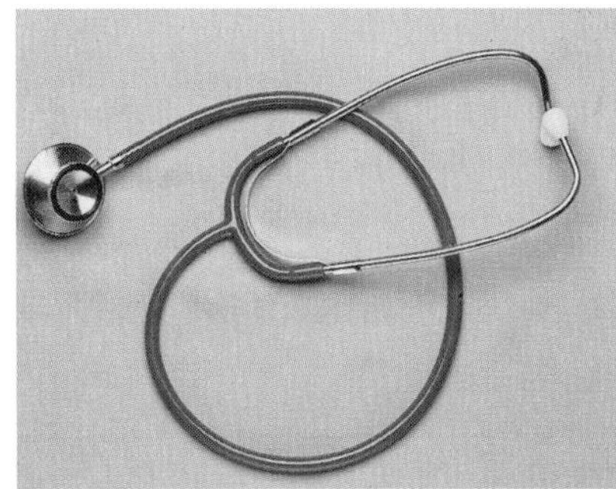

Figure 21–18 A stethoscope with both bell-shaped and flat-disc diaphragms.

when placed immediately on the chest.

- Insert the earpieces of the stethoscope into your ears. The earpieces may be straight or bent. If they are bent, place them in the direction of the ear canals, or slightly forward, to facilitate hearing.
- Place the diaphragm of the stethoscope over the apical impulse and listen for the normal S_1 and S_2 heart sounds, which are heard as "lub dub." Each lub dub is counted as one heartbeat. *The heartbeat is normally loudest over the apex of the heart. The two heart sounds are produced by closure of the valves of the heart.* The S_1 heart sound (lub) occurs when the atrioventricular valves close after the ventricles have been sufficiently filled. The S_2 heart sound (dub) occurs when the semilunar valves close after the ventricles empty.
- Count the heartbeats for 30 seconds and multiply by 2 if the rhythm is regular; count the beats for 60 seconds if the rhythm is irregular or if the apical impulse is being taken on an infant or child. *A 60-second count provides a more accurate assessment of an irregular pulse than a 30-second count.*

4. Assess the rhythm and the strength of the heartbeat.

- Assess the rhythm of the heartbeat by noting the pattern of intervals between the beats. A normal pulse has equal time periods between beats.
- Assess the strength (volume) of the heartbeat. Normally, the heartbeats are equal in strength and can be described as strong or weak.

5. Document and report pertinent assessment data.

- Record the pulse site and rate, rhythm, and volume.
- Report to the nurse in charge any pertinent data such as pallor, cyanosis, dyspnea, tachycardia, bradycardia, irregular rhythm, and reduced strength of the heartbeat.

EVALUATION FOCUS

The apical rate in relation to baseline data or normal range for the age of the client; relationship to other vital signs; apical pulse rhythm and volume in relationship to baseline data and health status.

respiration refers to the interchange of oxygen and carbon dioxide between the alveoli of the lungs and the pulmonary blood. **Internal respiration,** by contrast, takes place throughout the body; it is the interchange of these same gases between the circulating blood and the cells of the body tissues.

The term **inhalation** or **inspiration** refers to the intake of air into the lungs. **Exhalation** or **expiration** refers to breathing out or the movement of gases from the lungs to the atmosphere. **Ventilation** is another word that is used to refer to the movement of air in and out of the lungs. **Hyperventilation** refers to very deep, rapid respirations; **hypoventilation** refers to very shallow respirations.

There are basically two types of breathing that nurses observe, **costal (thoracic) breathing** and **diaphragmatic (abdominal) breathing.** Costal breathing involves chiefly the external intercostal muscles and other accessory muscles, such as the sternocleidomastoid muscles. It can be observed by the movement of the chest upward and outward. By contrast, diaphragmatic breathing chiefly involves the contraction and relaxation of the diaphragm, and it is observed by the movement of the abdomen, which occurs as a result of the diaphragm's contraction and downward movement.

MECHANICS AND CONTROL OF BREATHING

During *inhalation*, the following processes normally occur (Figure 21–19, p. 447): The diaphragm contracts (flattens), the ribs move upward and outward, and the sternum moves outward, thus enlarging the thorax and permitting the lungs to expand. During *exhalation* (Figure 21–20,

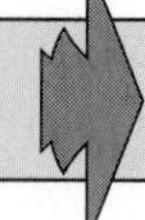

PROCEDURE 21–4 ASSESSING AN APICAL–RADIAL PULSE

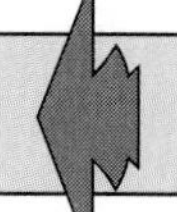

PURPOSE

- To determine adequacy of peripheral circulation or presence of pulse deficit

ASSESSMENT FOCUS
Clinical signs of hypovolemic shock (hypotension, pallor, cyanosis, and cold, clammy skin).

EQUIPMENT

- ☐ Watch with a second hand
- ☐ Stethoscope
- ☐ Antiseptic wipes

INTERVENTION

1. Position the client appropriately.

- Assist the client to assume the position described for taking the apical pulse. See Procedure 21–3, Step 1.
- If previous measurements were taken, determine what position the client assumed, and use the same position. *This ensures an accurate comparative measurement.*

2. Locate the apical and radial pulse sites.

- In the two-nurse technique, one nurse locates the apical impulse by palpation or with the stethoscope while the other nurse palpates the radial pulse site. See Procedures 21–2 and 21–3.

3. Count the apical and radial pulse rates.

Two-Nurse Technique

- Place the watch where both nurses can see it. The nurse who is taking the radial pulse may hold the watch.
- Decide on a time to begin counting. A time when the second hand is on 12, 3, 6, or 9 is usually selected. The nurse taking the radial pulse says "Start" at the designated time. *This ensures that simultaneous counts are taken.*
- Each nurse counts the pulse rate for 60 seconds. Both nurses end the count when the nurse taking the radial pulse says "Stop." *A full 60-second count is necessary for accurate assessment of any discrepancies between the two pulse sites.*
- The nurse who assesses the apical rate also assesses the apical pulse rhythm and volume (ie, whether the heartbeat is strong or weak). If the pulse is irregular, note whether the irregular beats come at random or at predictable times. The latter situation creates a regular irregularity.
- The nurse assessing the radial pulse rate also assesses the radial pulse rhythm and volume.

One-Nurse Technique

- Assess the apical pulse for 60 seconds.
- Assess the radial pulse for 60 seconds.

4. Document and report pertinent assessment data.

- Promptly report to the nurse in charge any notable changes from previous measurements or any discrepancy between the two pulses.
- Document the apical and radial (AR) pulse rates, rhythm, volume, and any pulse deficit.
- Record any other pertinent observations, such as pallor, cyanosis, or dyspnea.
- Check the physician's orders for any directions related to a discrepancy in the AR pulse rates.

EVALUATION FOCUS
Equality of apical and radial pulse rates; relationship to other vital signs, in particular respiratory rate and blood pressure; skin color and temperature.

p. 447), the diaphragm relaxes (its curvature increases), the ribs move downward and inward, and the sternum moves inward, thus decreasing the size of the thorax as the lungs are compressed. Normally breathing is carried out automatically and effortlessly. An inspiration lasts 1 to 1.5 seconds, and an expiration lasts 2 to 3 seconds.

Respiration is controlled by (a) respiratory centers in the medulla oblongata and the pons of the brain and (b) by chemoreceptors located centrally in the medulla and peripherally in the carotid and aortic bodies. These centers and receptors respond to changes in the concentrations of oxygen (O_2), carbon dioxide (CO_2) and hydrogen

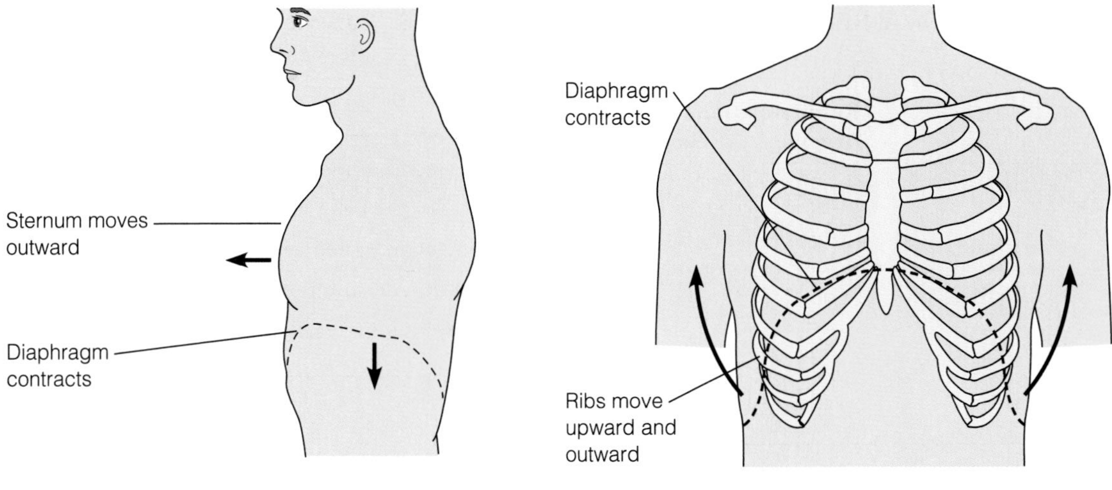

Figure 21–19 Respiratory inhalation: anterior and lateral views.

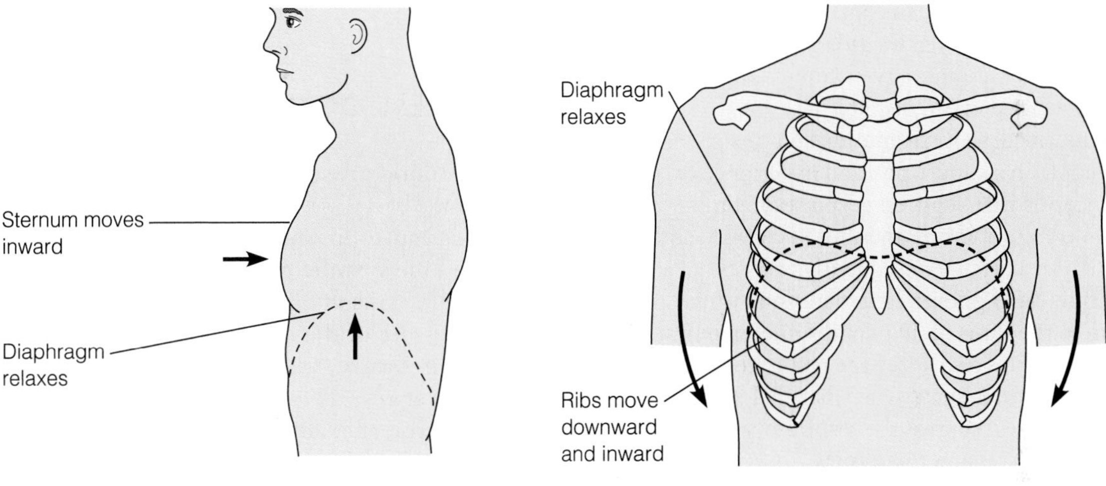

Figure 21–20 Respiratory exhalation: anterior and lateral views.

(H^+) in the arterial blood. See Chapter 39, page 1133, for details.

ASSESSING RESPIRATIONS

Resting respirations should be assessed when the client is at rest because exercise affects respirations, increasing their rate and depth. Anxiety is likely to affect respiratory rate and depth as well. Respirations may also need to be assessed after exercise to identify the client's tolerance to activity. Before assessing a client's respirations, a nurse should be aware of

- The client's normal breathing pattern
- The influence of the client's health problems on respirations
- Any medications or therapies that might affect respirations
- The relationship of the client's respirations to cardiovascular function

The rate, depth, rhythm, and special characteristics of respirations should be assessed.

The *respiratory rate* is normally described in breaths per minute. A healthy adult normally takes between 15 and 20 breaths per minute. Breathing that is normal in rate and depth is called **eupnea.** Abnormally slow respirations are referred to as **bradypnea,** and abnormally fast respirations are called **tachypnea** or **polypnea.** For the respiratory rates for different age groups, see Table 21–7 on page 448. Several factors influence respiratory rate; some are listed in Table 21–8 on page 448.

The *depth* of a person's respirations can be established by watching the movement of the chest. Respiratory depth is generally described as normal, deep, or shallow. *Deep respirations* are those in which a large volume of air is

Table 21–7 Variations in Respiratory Rate by Age

Age	Respiratory Rate/Minute Average	Range
Newborn	35	30–80
1 year	30	20–40
2 years	25	20–30
8 years	20	15–25
16 years	18	15–20
Adult	16	12–20

Table 21–8 Major Factors Influencing Respiratory Rate

Factor	Influence
Excercise: increases metabolism	Increase
Stress: readies the body for "fight or flight"	Increase
Environment: increased temperature	Increase
Increased altitude: lower oxygen concentration	Increase
Certain medications (eg, narcotic, analgesic)	Decrease

inhaled and exhaled, inflating most of the lungs. *Shallow respirations* involve the exchange of a small volume of air and often the minimal use of lung tissue. During a normal inspiration and expiration, an adult takes in about 500 mL of air. This volume is called the **tidal volume.** For further information about pulmonary volumes and pulmonary capacities, see Chapter 39, page 1130.

Body position also affects the amount of air that can be inhaled. People in a supine position experience two physiologic processes that suppress respiration: an increase in the volume of blood inside the thoracic cavity and compression of the chest. Consequently, clients in a back-lying position have poorer lung aeration, which predisposes them to the stasis of fluids and subsequent infection. Certain medications also affect the respiratory depth. For example, barbiturates such as secobarbital sodium, when taken in large doses, depress the respiratory centers in the brain, thereby depressing the respiratory rate and depth.

Respiratory rhythm or **pattern** refers to the regularity of the expirations and the inspirations. Normally, respirations are evenly spaced. Respiratory rhythm can be described as *regular* or *irregular*. An infant's respiratory rhythm may be less regular than an adult's. See Chapter 39, page 1135, for details about abnormal respiratory rhythms.

Respiratory quality or **character** refers to those aspects of breathing that are different from normal, effortless breathing. Two of these are the amount of effort a client must exert to breathe and the sound of breathing. Usually, breathing does not require noticeable effort; some clients, however, breathe only with decided effort.

The *sound* of breathing is also significant. Normal breathing is silent, but a number of abnormal sounds such as a wheeze are obvious to the nurse's ear. Many sounds occur as a result of the presence of fluid in the lungs and are most clearly heard with a stethoscope. See Chapter 22, page 515, for auscultation and percussion methods used to assess lung sounds. For details about altered breathing patterns and terms used to describe various patterns and sounds, see the box at the right. Procedure 21–5, on page 450, provides guidelines for assessing respirations.

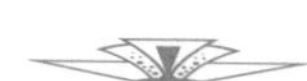

BLOOD PRESSURE

Arterial blood pressure is a measure of the pressure exerted by the blood as it flows through the arteries. Because the blood moves in waves, there are two blood pressure measures: the **systolic pressure,** which is the pressure of the blood as a result of contraction of the ventricles, that is, the pressure of the height of the blood wave; and the **diastolic pressure,** which is the pressure when the ventricles are at rest. Diastolic pressure, then, is the lower pressure, present at all times within the arteries. The difference between the diastolic and the systolic pressures is called the **pulse pressure.**

Blood pressure is measured in millimeters of mercury (mm Hg) and recorded as a fraction. The systolic pressure is written over the diastolic pressure. The average blood pressure of a healthy adult is 120/80 mm Hg. A number of conditions are reflected by changes in blood pressure. The most common is **hypertension,** an abnormally high blood pressure over 140 mm Hg systolic and/or 90 mm Hg diastolic when these are confirmed during a minimum of two consecutive visits by a client. See Table 21–9 on page 451 for classifications of hypertension and recommendations for follow-up care. **Hypotension** is an abnormally low blood pressure below 100 mm Hg systolic.

Because blood pressure can vary considerably among individuals, it is important for the nurse to know a specific client's baseline blood pressure. For example, if a client's usual blood pressure is 180/100 mm Hg and it is assessed following surgery to be 120/80 mm Hg, this drop in pressure must be reported to the charge nurse or physician. Many conditions influence blood pressure. Some of these are listed in Table 21–10 on page 451.

BREATHING PATTERNS AND SOUNDS

Breathing Patterns

Rate

- *Eupnea*—normal respiration that is quiet, rhythmic, and effortless
- *Tachypnea*—rapid respiration marked by quick, shallow breaths
- *Bradypnea*—abnormally slow breathing
- *Apnea*—cessation of breathing

Volume

- *Hyperventilation*—an increase in the amount of air in the lungs, characterized by prolonged and deep breaths; may be associated with anxiety
- *Hypoventilation*—a reduction in the amount of air in the lungs; characterized by shallow respirations

Rhythm

- *Cheyne-Stokes breathing*—rhythmic waxing and waning of respirations, from very deep to very shallow breathing and temporary apnea; often associated with cardiac failure, increased intracranial pressure, or brain damage

Ease or effort

- *Dyspnea*—difficult and labored breathing during which the individual has a persistent, unsatisfied need for air and feels distressed
- *Orthopnea*—ability to breath only in upright sitting or standing positions

Breath Sounds

Audible without amplification

- *Stridor*—a shrill, harsh sound heard during inspiration with laryngeal obstruction
- *Stertor*—snoring or sonorous respiration, usually due to a partial obstruction of the upper airway
- *Wheeze*—continuous, high-pitched musical squeak or whistling sound occurring on expiration and sometimes on inspiration when air moves through a narrowed or partially obstructed airway
- *Bubbling*—gurgling sounds heard as air passes through moist secretions in the respiratory tract

Audible by stethoscope

- *Crackles* (formerly called *rales*)—dry or wet crackling sounds simulated by rolling a lock of hair near the ear. Generally heard on inspiration as air moves through accumulated moist secretions. *Fine-to-medium* crackles occur when air passes through moisture in small air passages and alveoli. *Medium-to-coarse* crackles occur when air passes through moisture in brochioles, bronchi, and the trachea.
- *Gurgles* (formerly called *rhonchi*)—coarse, dry, wheezy, or whistling sound more audible during expiration as the air moves through tenacious mucus or narrowed bronchi
- *Pleural friction rub*—coarse, leathery, or grating sound produced by the rubbing together of inflamed pleura

Chest Movements

- *Intercostal retraction*—indrawing between the ribs
- *Substernal retraction*—indrawing beneath the breastbone
- *Suprasternal retraction*—indrawing above the clavicles
- *Tracheal tug*—indrawing and downward pull of the trachea during inspiration
- *Flail chest*—the ballooning out of the chest wall through injured rib spaces; results in *paradoxical breathing*, during which the chest wall balloons on expiration but is depressed or sucked inward on inspiration

Secretions and Coughing

- *Hemoptysis*—the presence of blood in the sputum
- *Productive cough*—a cough accompanied by expectorated secretions
- *Nonproductive cough*—a dry, harsh cough without secretions

PHYSIOLOGY OF ARTERIAL BLOOD PRESSURE

Arterial blood pressure is the result of several factors: the pumping action of the heart, the peripheral vascular resistance (the resistance supplied by the blood vessels through which the blood flows) and the blood volume and viscosity.

Pumping Action of the Heart *Cardiac output* is the volume of blood pumped into the arteries by the heart. When the pumping action of the heart is weak, less blood is pumped into arteries, and the blood pressure decreases. When the heart's pumping action is strong and the volume of blood pumped into the circulation increases, the blood pressure increases. Cardiac output increases with

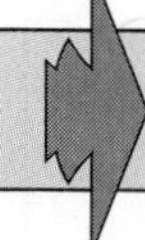

PROCEDURE 21–5 ASSESSING RESPIRATIONS

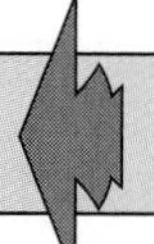

PURPOSES

- To acquire baseline data against which future measurements can be compared
- To monitor abnormal respirations and identify changes
- To assess respirations before the administration of a medication such as morphine (an abnormally slow respiratory rate may warrant withholding the medication)
- To monitor respirations following the administration of a general anesthetic or any medication that influences respirations
- To monitor clients at risk for respiratory alterations (eg, those with fever, pain, acute anxiety, chronic obstructive pulmonary disease, respiratory infection, pulmonary edema or emboli, chest trauma or constriction, brain stem injury)

ASSESSMENT FOCUS

Skin and mucous membrane color (eg, cyanosis or pallor); position assumed for breathing (eg, use of orthopneic position); signs of cerebral anoxia (eg, irritability, restlessness, drowsiness, or loss of consciousness); chest movements (eg, retractions between the ribs or above or below the sternum); activity tolerance; chest pain; dyspnea; medications affecting respiratory rate.

EQUIPMENT

☐ Watch with a second hand or indicator

INTERVENTION

1. Determine the client's activity schedule.

- Choose a suitable time to monitor the respirations. *A client who has been exercising will need to rest for a few minutes to permit the accelerated respiratory rate to return to normal. An infant or child who is crying will have an abnormal respiratory rate and will need quieting before respirations can be accurately assessed.*

2. Observe or palpate and count the respiratory rate.

- Place a hand against the client's chest to feel the client's chest movements, or place the client's arm across the chest and observe the chest movements, while supposedly taking the radial pulse. Because young children are diaphragmatic breathers, observe the rise and fall of the abdomen. *Awareness of respiratory rate assessment could cause the client voluntarily to alter the respiratory pattern.*
- Count the respiratory rate for 30 seconds if the respirations are regular. Count for 60 seconds if they are irregular. An inhalation and an exhalation count as one respiration.

3. Observe the depth, rhythm, and character of respirations.

- Observe the respirations for depth by watching the movement of the chest. During deep respirations a large volume of air is exchanged; during shallow respirations a small volume is exchanged.
- Observe the respirations for regular or irregular rhythm. Normally, respirations are evenly spaced.
- Observe the character of respirations—the sound they produce and the effort they require. Normally, respirations are silent and effortless.

4. Document and report pertinent assessment data.

- Document the respiratory rate, depth, rhythm, and character on the appropriate record.
- Report to the nurse in charge:
  a. Respiratory rate significantly above or below the normal range and any notable change in respirations from previous assessments
  b. Irregular respiratory rhythm
  c. Inadequate respiratory depth
  d. Abnormal character of breathing—orthopnea, wheezing, stridor, rales (crackles), or rhonchi (gurgles)
  e. Any complaints of dyspnea

EVALUATION FOCUS

The respiratory rate in relation to baseline data or normal range for age; relationship to other vital signs; respiratory depth, rhythm, and character in relation to baseline data and health status.

Table 21–9 Classification of Hypertension in Adults 18 Years or Older and Recommended Follow-Up

Blood Pressure Findings	Follow-Up
Diastolic Blood Pressure	
< 85 Normal	Recheck within 2 years.
85–90 High-normal	Recheck within 1 year.
90–104 Mild hypertension	Confirm within 2 months.
105–114 Moderate hypertension	Evaluate or refer promptly to source of care within 2 weeks.
> 115 Severe hypertension	Refer immediately to source of care.
Systolic Blood Pressure When Diastolic is Less than 90	
< 140 Normal	Recheck within 2 years.
140–159 Borderline isolated systolic hypertension	Confirm within 2 months.
> 160 Isolated systolic hypertension	If below 200, confirm within 2 months. If above 200, refer promptly for care within 2 weeks.

Source: US Department of Health and Human Services, Public Health Service, National Institutes of Health, *The 1988 Report of the Joint National Committee on Detection, Evaluation, and Treatment of High Blood Pressure,* May 1988, NIH Pub. no. 88–1088, pp. 3, 6.

fever and exercise, and the systolic pressure may increase as a result.

Peripheral Vascular Resistance *Peripheral resistance* can increase blood pressure. The diastolic pressure especially is affected. Some factors that create resistance in the arterial system are the size of the arterioles and capillaries, the compliance of the arteries, and the viscosity of the blood.

The *size* of the arterioles and the capillaries determines in great part the peripheral resistance to the blood in the body. A *lumen* is a channel within a tube: the smaller the lumen of a vessel, the greater the resistance. Normally, the arterioles are in a state of partial constriction. Increased vasoconstriction raises the blood pressure, whereas decreased vasoconstriction lowers the blood pressure.

The arteries contain smooth muscles that permit them to contract, thus decreasing their compliance (distensibility). The arteries account for most of the peripheral resistance. The major factor reducing arterial compliance is pathologic change affecting the arterial walls. The elastic and muscular tissues of the arteries are replaced with fibrous tissue; thus, the arteries lose much of their compliance. The condition, most common in middle-aged and elderly adults, is known as **arteriosclerosis.**

Table 21–10 Selected Conditions Affecting Blood Pressure

Condition	Effect	Cause
Fever	Increase	Increases metabolic rate
Stress	Increase	Increases cardiac output
Arteriosclerosis	Increase	Decreases artery compliance
Obesity	Increase	Increases peripheral resistance
Hemorrhage	Decrease	Decreases blood volume
Low hematocrit	Decrease	Decreases blood viscosity
External heat	Decrease	Increases vasodilation and thus decreases peripheral vascular resistance
Exposure to cold	Increase	Causes vasoconstriction and thus increases peripheral vascular resistance

Blood Volume When the blood volume decreases (for example, as a result of a hemorrhage or dehydration), the blood pressure decreases because of decreased fluid in the arteries. Conversely, when the volume increases (for example, as result of an intravenous infusion), the blood pressure increases because of the greater fluid volume within the circulatory system.

Blood Viscosity Viscosity is a physical property that results from friction of molecules in a fluid. In a viscous (or "thick") fluid, there is a great deal of friction among the molecules as they slide by each other. The blood pressure is higher when the blood is highly viscous, that is, when the proportion of red blood cells to the blood plasma is high. This ratio is referred to as the **hematocrit.** The viscosity increases markedly when the hematocrit is more than 60% to 65%.

FACTORS AFFECTING BLOOD PRESSURE

Among the factors influencing blood pressure are age, exercise, stress, race, obesity, sex, medications, and diurnal variations.

- *Age.* Newborns have a mean systolic pressure of 78 mm Hg. The pressure rises with age, reaching a peak at the onset of puberty, and then tends to decline somewhat. One quick way to determine the normal systolic blood

Table 21–11 Variations in Blood Pressure by Age

Age	Mean Blood Pressure (mm Hg)
Newborn	73/55
1 year	90/55
6 years	95/57
10 years	102/62
14 years	120/80
Adult	120/80
Elderly (over 70 years)	Diastolic pressure may increase

pressure of a child is to use the following formula:

Normal systolic BP = 80 + (2 × child's age in years)

In elderly people, elasticity of the arteries is decreased—the arteries are more rigid and less yielding to the pressure of the blood. This produces an elevated systolic pressure. Because the walls no longer retract as flexibly with decreased pressure, the diastolic pressure is also higher. Several baseline blood pressure readings should be taken in the elderly person who has an elevated blood pressure. See age variations in Table 21–11.

- *Exercise.* Physical activity increases both the cardiac output and hence the blood pressure; thus, a rest of 20 to 30 minutes following exercise is indicated before the blood pressure can be reliably assessed, unless the blood pressure is being assessed during or after exercise.
- *Stress.* Stimulation of the sympathetic nervous system increases cardiac output and vasoconstriction of the arterioles, thus increasing the blood pressure reading; however, severe pain can decrease blood pressure greatly and cause shock by inhibiting the vasomotor center and producing vasodilation.
- *Race.* African-American males over 35 years have higher blood pressures than European-American males of the same age.
- *Obesity.* Pressure is generally higher in some overweight and obese people than in people of normal weight.
- *Sex.* After puberty, females usually have lower blood pressures than males of the same age; this difference is thought to be due to hormonal variations. After menopause, women generally have higher blood pressures than before.
- *Medications.* Many medications may increase or decrease the blood pressure; nurses should be aware of the specific medications a client is receiving and consider their possible impact when interpreting blood pressure readings.
- *Diurnal variations.* Pressure is usually lowest early in the morning, when the metabolic rate is lowest, then rises throughout the day and peaks in the late afternoon or early evening.
- *Disease process.* Any condition affecting the cardiac output, blood viscosity, and/or compliance of the arteries has a direct effect on the blood pressure. See the discussion in the previous section.

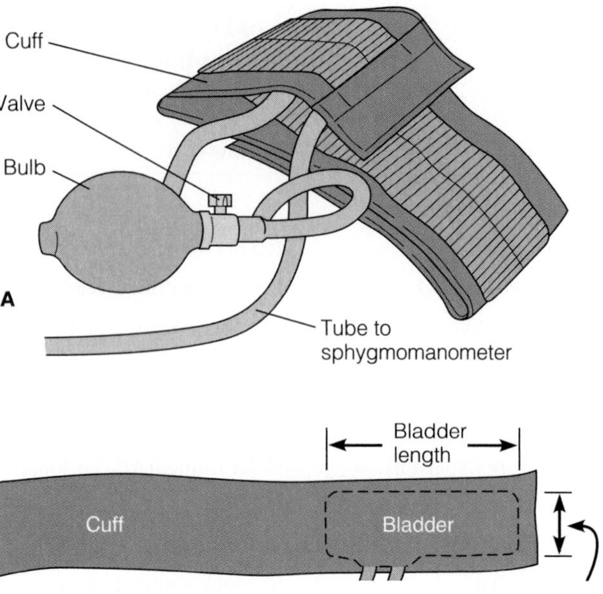

Figure 21–21 *A,* A blood pressure cuff and bulb; *B,* the bladder inside the cuff.

ASSESSING BLOOD PRESSURE

Equipment Blood pressure is measured with a *blood pressure cuff,* a *sphygmomanometer,* and a *stethoscope.* The blood pressure cuff consists of a rubber bag that can be inflated with air. It is called the *bladder* (Figure 21–21). It is usually covered with cloth and has two tubes attached to it. One tube connects to a rubber bulb that inflates the bladder. When turned counterclockwise, a small valve on the side of this bulb releases the air in the bladder. When the valve is tightened (turned clockwise), air pumped into the bladder remains there. The other tube is attached to a sphygmomanometer.

The sphygmomanometer indicates the pressure of the air within the bladder. There are two types of sphygmomanometers: *aneroid* and *mercury* (Figure 21–22). The aneroid sphygmomanometer is a calibrated dial with a

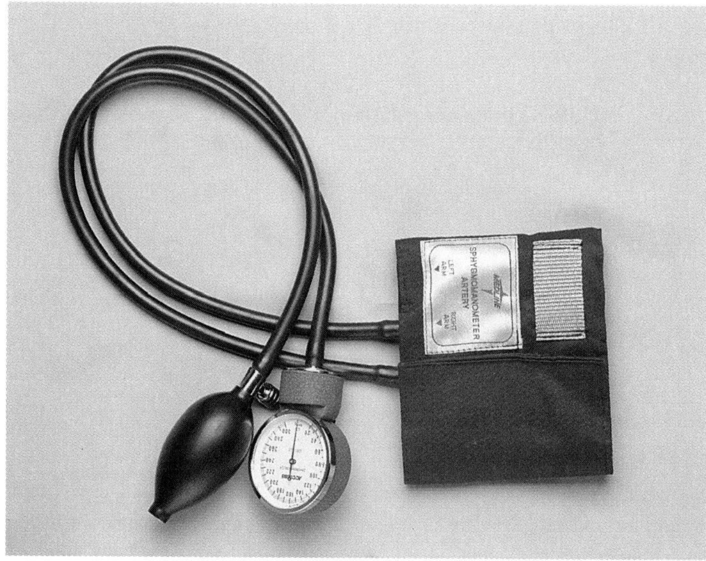

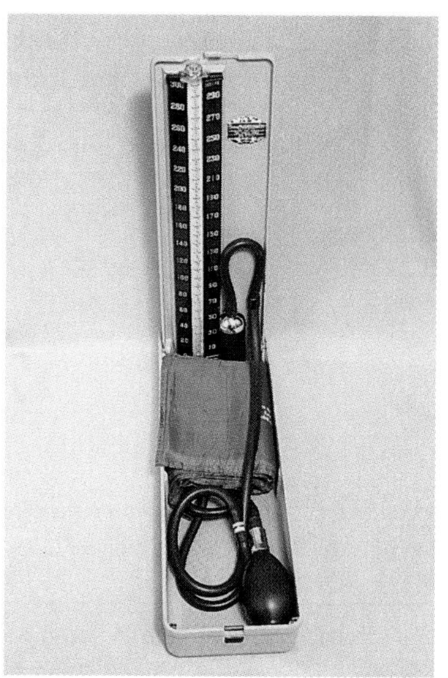

Figure 21–22 Blood pressure equipment: *A,* an aneroid manometer and cuff; *B,* a mercury manometer and cuff.

needle that points to the calibrations. The mercury sphygmomanometer is a calibrated cylinder filled with mercury. The pressure is indicated at the point to which the base of the *meniscus* of the mercury rises, that is, the point where the meniscus touches the sides of the glass tube (American Heart Association 1987, p. 12).

Some agencies use electronic sphygmomanometers, which eliminate the need to listen to the sounds of the client's systolic and diastolic blood pressures through a stethoscope. With some electronic sphygmomanometers, as the pressure in the cuff is lowered, a light flashes to indicate the systolic and diastolic pressures.

Ultrasound (Doppler) stethoscopes are also used to assess blood pressure. See Figure 21–15, earlier. These are of particular value when blood pressure sounds are difficult to hear, such as in infants, obese clients, and clients in shock. The nurse applies transmission gel to a transducer probe, places the probe over the pulse point, and measures the blood pressure. A systolic blood pressure assessed with a Doppler stethoscope is recorded with a large D, for example, 85D. Systolic pressure may be the only blood pressure obtainable with some ultrasound models.

Blood pressure cuffs come in various sizes, because the bladder must be the correct width and length for the client's arm. If the bladder is too narrow, the blood pressure reading will be erroneously elevated; if it is too wide, the reading will be erroneously low. The width should be 40% of the circumference, or 20% wider than the diameter of the midpoint of the limb on which it is used (American Heart Association 1987, p. 4). The bladder dimensions by arm circumference are shown in Table 21–12 on page 454; the arm circumference, not the age of the client, should always be used to determine bladder size. The nurse can also determine whether the width of a blood pressure cuff is appropriate: Lay the cuff lengthwise at the midpoint of the upper arm, and hold the outermost side of the bladder edge laterally on the arm. With the other hand, wrap the width of the cuff around the arm, and ensure that the width is 40% of the arm circumference (Figure 21–23, p. 454).

The length of the bladder also affects the accuracy of measurement. The bladder should be sufficiently long almost to encircle the limb and to cover at least two-thirds of its circumference.

Blood pressure cuffs are made of nondistensible material so that an even pressure is exerted around the limb. Most cuffs are held in place by hooks, snaps, or Velcro. Others have a cloth bandage that is long enough to encircle the limb several times; this type is closed by tucking the end of the bandage into one of the bandage folds.

Sites The blood pressure is usually assessed in the client's arm using the brachial artery and a standard stethoscope. If the arm is very large or grossly misshapen and the conventional cuff cannot be properly applied, leg or forearm measurements can be taken. To obtain a *leg blood pressure,* a standard-sized cuff is applied over the lower leg with the distal border of the cuff at the malleoli. Auscultate blood pressure sounds over the posterior tibial or dorsalis pedis arteries. To obtain a *thigh blood pressure,* apply an appropriate-sized cuff to the thigh, and auscultate the pulsations of the blood over the popliteal artery. To obtain a *forearm blood pressure,* apply an appropriate-sized cuff to the forearm 13 cm (5 in) below the elbow. Blood pressure sounds then can be heard over the radial artery.

Table 21-12 Recommended Bladder Sizes of Blood Pressure Cuffs for People with Different Arm Circumferences

Client	Arm Circumference at Midpoint (cm)*	Cuff Bladder Length (cm)	Cuff Bladder Width (cm)
Newborn	5–7.5	5	3
Infant	7.5–13	8	5
Child	13–20	13	8
Adult	24–32	24	13
Large adult	32–42	32	17
Thigh	42–50†	42	20

* The midpoint is half the distance between the acromion process and the olecranon process.

† In people with very large limbs, the indirect blood pressure should be measured in the leg or forearm.

Source: Reproduced with permission. © "Recommendations for Human Blood Pressure Determination by Sphygmomanometers," 1967, 1980, 1987. Copyright American Heart Association.

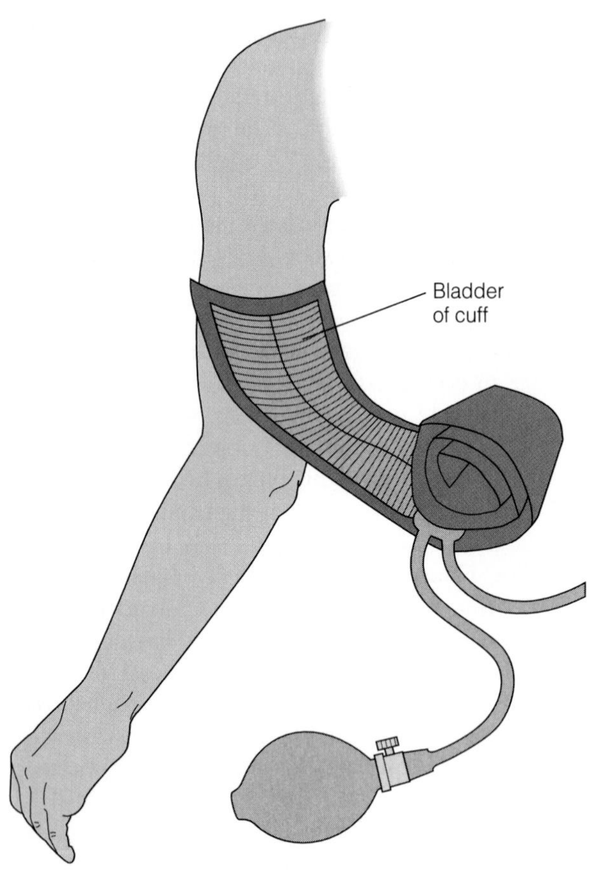

Figure 21-23 Determining that the bladder of a blood pressure cuff is 40% of the arm circumference or 20% wider than the diameter of the midpoint of the limb.

Assessing the blood pressure on a client's thigh is usually indicated in these situations:

- The blood pressure cannot be measured on either arm, (eg, because of burns or other trauma).
- The blood pressure in one thigh is to be compared with the blood pressure in the other thigh.

Blood pressure is *not* measured on a client's arm or thigh in the following situations:

- The shoulder, arm, or hand (or the hip, knee, or ankle) is injured or diseased.
- There is a cast or bulky bandage on any part of the limb.
- The client has had breast or axilla (or hip) surgery on that side.
- The client has an intravenous infusion or a blood transfusion running.
- The client has an arteriovenous fistula (eg, for renal dialysis).

Methods Blood pressure can be assessed directly or indirectly. *Direct (invasive monitoring) measurement* involves the insertion of a catheter into the brachial, radial, or femoral artery. Arterial pressure is represented as wavelike forms displayed on an oscilloscope. Generally, physicians insert the catheters, and nurses monitor the pressure readings. With correct placement, this pressure reading is highly accurate.

There are three *noninvasive indirect methods* of measuring blood pressure: the auscultatory, palpatory, and flush methods. The *auscultatory method* is most commonly used in hospitals, clinics, and homes. Required equipment is a sphygmomanometer, cuff, and a stethoscope. External pressure is applied to a superficial artery, and the nurse reads the pressure from the sphygmomanometer when the blood flow is first heard through a stethoscope. When carried out correctly, the auscultatory method is relatively accurate.

When taking a blood pressure using a stethoscope, the nurse identifies five phases in the series of sounds called **Korotkoff's sounds.** First, the nurse pumps the cuff up to about 30 mm Hg above the point where the last sound is heard; that is the point when the blood flow in the artery is stopped. Then the pressure is released slowly (2 to 3 mm Hg per sound), while the nurse observes the pressure readings on the manometer and relates them to the sounds heard through the stethoscope. Five phases occur (American Heart Association 1987, p. 4):

Phase 1 The pressure level at which the first faint clear tapping sounds are heard. These sounds gradually become more intense. To ensure that they are not extraneous sounds, the nurse should identify at least two consecutive tapping sounds.

Phase 2 The period during deflation when the sounds have a swishing quality.

Phase 3 The period during which the sounds are crisper and more intense.

Phase 4 The time when the sounds become muffled and have a soft, blowing quality.

Phase 5 The pressure level when the sounds disappear.

The American Heart Association (AHA) recommends that the systolic pressure be considered the point where the first tapping sound is heard during deflation of the cuff (phase 1). In adults, the diastolic pressure is the point where the last audible sound is heard (phase 5). In children, however, the AHA recommends that the onset of phase 4, where the sounds become muffled, be considered the diastolic pressure. In agencies where the fourth phase is considered the diastolic pressure of adults, three measures are recommended (systolic pressure, diastolic pressure, and phase 5). These may be referred to as systolic, first diastolic, and second diastolic pressures. The phase 5 (second diastolic pressure) reading may be zero; that is, the muffled sounds are heard even when there is no air pressure in the blood pressure cuff. In some instances, muffled sounds are never heard, in which case a dash is inserted where the reading would normally be recorded (eg, 190/—/110).

The *palpatory method* is sometimes used when Korotkoff's sounds cannot be heard and electronic equipment to amplify the sounds is not available, or when an auscultatory gap occurs. An **auscultatory gap,** which occurs particularly in hypertensive clients, is the temporary disappearance of sounds normally heard over the brachial artery when the cuff pressure is high and the reappearance of the sounds at a lower level. This temporary disappearance of sounds occurs in the latter part of phase 1 and phase 2 and may cover a range of 40 mm Hg. Instead of listening for the blood flow sounds, the nurse palpates the pulsations of the artery as the pressure in the cuff is released. The systolic pressure is read from the sphygmomanometer when the first pulsation is felt. A single whiplike vibration, felt in addition to the pulsations, identifies the point at which the pressure in the cuff nears the diastolic pressure. This vibration is no longer felt when the cuff pressure is below the diastolic pressure. To palpate the diastolic pressure, the nurse applies light to moderate pressure over the pulse point.

The *flush method* for determining blood pressure is another method used when Korotkoff's sounds cannot be heard by auscultation and electronic equipment is not available. The measurement is determined by a change in skin color when blood flow to an extremity resumes, that is, when the extremity is no longer extremely pale but becomes reddened (vascular flush). This method is less reliable in clients with peripheral vascular disease or a circulatory problem of varied origin. The cuff is applied to the client's arm and the limb is wrapped in a bandage distally to proximally to force venous blood out of and restrict arterial flow into the extremity. The cuff is then inflated and the bandage is removed. The cuff pressure is released, and the nurse reads the pressure from the sphygmomanometer when the extremity flushes. This reading is the **mean blood pressure,** the midway point between the systolic and diastolic pressures. Procedure 21–6 on page 456 gives guidelines for assessing blood pressure.

Common Errors in Assessing Blood Pressure

The importance of the accuracy of blood pressure assessments cannot be overemphasized. Many judgments about a client's health are made on the basis of blood pressure. It is an important indicator of the client's condition and is used extensively as a basis for nursing interventions. Two possible reasons for blood pressure errors are haste on the part of the nurse and subconscious bias. For example, a nurse may be influenced by the client's previous blood pressure measurements or diagnosis and "hear" a value consonant with the practitioner's expectations. An example of such a bias is "digit preference," a predilection for pressures ending with zero (eg, 130 systolic, 70 diastolic) more often than would be expected (AHA 1987, p. 14). Some reasons for erroneous blood pressure readings are given in Table 21–13 on page 458.

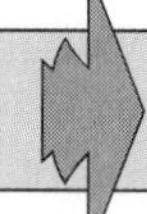

PROCEDURE 21–6 ASSESSING BLOOD PRESSURE (ARM)

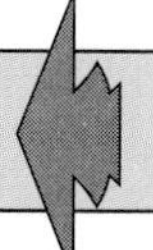

PURPOSES

- To obtain a baseline measure of arterial blood pressure for subsequent evaluation
- To determine the client's hemodynamic status (eg, stroke volume of the heart and blood vessel resistance)
- To identify and monitor changes in blood pressure resulting from a disease process and medical therapy (eg, presence or history of cardiovascular disease, renal disease, circulatory shock, or acute pain; rapid infusion of fluids or blood products)

ASSESSMENT FOCUS

Signs and symptoms of hypertension (eg, headache, ringing in the ears, flushing of face, nosebleeds, fatigue); signs and symptoms of hypotension (eg, tachycardia, dizziness, mental confusion, restlessness, cool and clammy skin, pale or cyanotic skin); factors affecting blood pressure (eg, activity, emotional stress, pain, and time the client last smoked or ingested caffeine).

EQUIPMENT

- ☐ Stethoscope or DUS
- ☐ Blood pressure cuff of the appropriate size (newborn, infant, child, small adult, adult, large adult, thigh)
- ☐ Sphygmomanometer

INTERVENTION

1. Prepare and position the client appropriately.

- Make sure that the client has not smoked or ingested caffeine within 30 minutes prior to measurement (US Department of Health 1988, p. 5).
- Make sure that the bladder of the cuff encircles at least two-thirds of the arm and that the width of the cuff is appropriate.
- Position the client in a sitting position unless otherwise specified. The arm should be slightly flexed with the palm of the hand facing up and the forearm supported at heart level. Readings in any other position should be specified. *The blood pressure is normally similar in sitting, standing, and lying positions, but it can vary significantly by position in certain persons and may need to be measured in all three positions. The blood pressure increases when the arm is below heart level and decreases when the arm is above heart level.*
- Expose the upper arm.

2. Wrap the deflated cuff evenly around the upper arm.

- Apply the center of the bladder directly over the medial aspect of the arm. *The bladder inside the cuff must be directly over the artery to be compressed if the reading is to be accurate.*
- For an adult, place the lower border of the cuff approximately 2.5 cm (1 in) above the antecubital space. The lower edge can be closer to the antecubital space of an infant.

3. If this is the client's initial examination, perform a preliminary palpatory determination of systolic pressure. The initial estimate tells the nurse the maximal pressure to which the manometer needs to be elevated in subsequent determinations. It also prevents underestimation of the systolic pressure or overestimation of the diastolic pressure should an auscultatory gap occur.

- Palpate the brachial artery with the fingertips. The brachial artery is normally found medially in the antecubital space (Figure 21–24).
- Close the valve on the pump by turning the knob clockwise.
- Pump up the cuff until you no longer feel the brachial pulse. *At that pressure the blood cannot flow through the artery.*
- Note the pressure on the sphygmomanometer at which the pulse is no longer felt. *This gives an estimate of the maximum pressure required to measure the systolic pressure.*
- Release the pressure completely in the cuff, and wait 1 to 2 minutes before making further measurements. *A waiting period gives the blood trapped in the veins time to be released.*

4. Position the stethoscope appropriately.

- Insert the ear attachments of the stethoscope in your ears so that

Procedure 21–6 *continued*

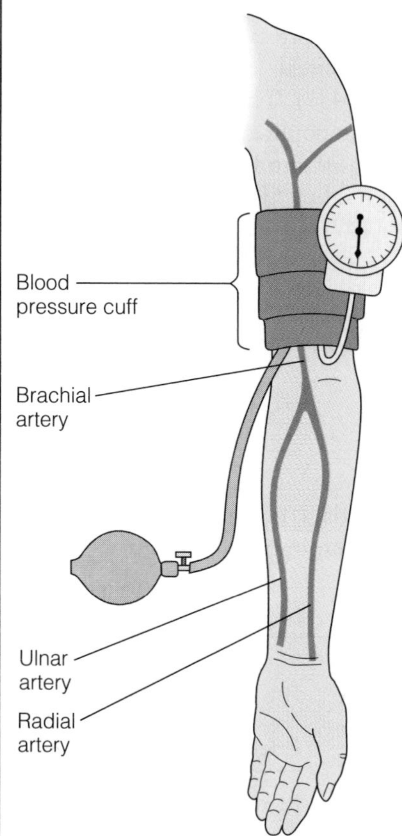

Figure 21–24 Location of the brachial artery.

they tilt slightly forward. *Sounds are heard more clearly when the ear attachments follow the direction of the ear canal.*

- Ensure that the stethoscope hangs freely from the ears to the diaphragm. *Rubbing the stethoscope against an object can obliterate the sounds of the blood within an artery.*
- Place the diaphragm of the stethoscope over the brachial pulse. Use the bell-shaped diaphragm (Figure 21–18, earlier). *Because the blood pressure is a low-frequency sound, it is best heard with the bell-shaped diaphragm* (Hill & Grim 1991, p. 38). Hold the diaphragm with the thumb and index finger.

5. Auscultate the client's blood pressure.

- Pump up the cuff until the sphygmomanometer registers about 30 mm Hg above the point where the brachial pulse disappeared.
- Release the valve on the cuff carefully so that the pressure decreases at the rate of 2 to 3 mm Hg per second. *If the rate is faster or slower, an error in measurement may occur.*
- As the pressure falls, identify the manometer reading at each of the five phases.
- Deflate the cuff rapidly and completely.
- Wait 1 to 2 minutes before making further determinations. *This permits blood trapped in the veins to be released.*
- Repeat the above steps once or twice as necessary to confirm the accuracy of the reading.

6. Remove the cuff from the client's arm.

7. If this is the client's initial examination, repeat the procedure on the client's other arm.

- There should be a difference of no more than 5 to 10 mm Hg between the arms.
- The arm found to have the higher pressure should be used for subsequent examinations.

8. Document and report pertinent assessment data.

- Document the blood pressure according to agency policy. Record two pressures in the form "130/80" where "130" is the systolic (phase 1) and "80" is the diastolic (phase 5) pressure. Record three pressures in the form "130/110/90," where "130" is the systolic, "110" is the first diastolic (phase 4), and "90" is the second diastolic (phase 5) pressure. Use the abbreviations *RA* for right arm *LA* for left arm. Record a difference of greater than 10 mm Hg in the arms.
- Report any significant change in the client's blood pressure to the nurse in charge. Also report these findings:
  a. Systolic blood pressure (of an adult) above 140 mm Hg

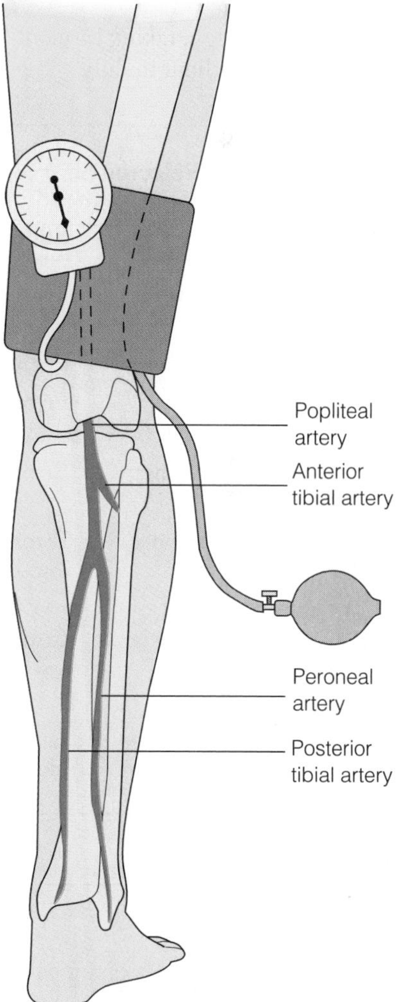

Figure 21–25 Location of the popliteal artery.

PROCEDURE 21–6 ASSESSING BLOOD PRESSURE (ARM) *continued*

b. Diastolic blood pressure (of an adult) above 90 mm Hg
c. Systolic blood pressure (of an adult) below 100 mm Hg

Variation: Taking a Thigh Blood Pressure

- Help the client to assume a prone position. If the client cannot assume this position, measure the blood pressure while the client is in a supine position with the knee slightly flexed. *Slight flexing of the knee will facilitate placing the stethoscope on the popliteal space.*
- Expose the thigh, taking care not to expose the client unduly.
- Wrap the cuff evenly around the midthigh with the compression bladder over the posterior aspect of the thigh and the bottom edge above the knee. *The bladder must be directly over the posterior popliteal artery if the reading is to be accurate.*
- If this is the client's initial examination, perform a preliminary palpatory determination of systolic pressure by palpating the popliteal artery (Figure 21–25, p. 457). The systolic pressure in the popliteal artery is usually 20 to 30 mm Hg higher than that in the brachial artery (Hill & Grim 1991, p. 42) because of use of a larger bladder; the diastolic pressure is usually the same.
- Auscultate the pressure as above.

EVALUATION FOCUS

The blood pressure in relation to baseline data, normal range for age, and health status; relationship to pulse and respirations.

Table 21–13 Selected Sources of Error in Blood Pressure Assessment

Error	Effect	Error	Effect
Bladder cuff too narrow	Erroneously high	Deflating cuff too slowly	Erroneously high diastolic reading
Bladder cuff too wide	Erroneously low		
Arm unsupported	Erroneously high	Failure to use the same arm consistently	Inconsistent measurements
Insufficient rest before the assessment	Erroneously high	Arm above level of the heart	Erroneously low
Repeating assessment too quickly	Erroneously high systolic or low diastolic readings	Assessing immediately after a meal or while client smokes or has pain	Erroneously high
Cuff wrapped too loosely or unevenly	Erroneously high	Failure to identify auscultatory gap	Erroneously low systolic pressure and erroneously low diastolic pressure
Deflating cuff too quickly	Erroneously low systolic and high diastolic readings		

CHAPTER HIGHLIGHTS

- Vital signs reflect changes in body function that otherwise might not be observed.
- Various sites and methods can be used to assess vital signs. The nurse selects the site and method that is safe for the client and that will provide the most accurate measurement possible.
- The most accurate values are obtained when the client is at rest and comfortable.

- Changes in one vital sign can trigger changes in other vital signs.
- Vital signs are assessed when a client is admitted to a health care agency to establish baseline data and when there is a change or possibility of a change in the client's condition.
- Data obtained from measurements of vital signs are used to plan and implement appropriate nursing interventions.
- Measurements of vital signs are also used to evaluate a client's response to nursing interventions or prescribed medical therapy.
- Knowledge of the normal ranges of vital signs and of the factors that regulate and influence vital signs helps the nurse interpret the measurements that deviate from normal.
- Body temperature is the balance between heat produced by the body and heat lost from the body.
- Heat is produced by the body's metabolic processes, which can be accelerated by muscle activity, thyroxine output, stimulation of the sympathetic nervous system, and fever.
- Knowledge of factors affecting heat production and heat loss helps the nurse to implement appropriate interventions when the client has a fever or hypothermia.
- The system that regulates body temperature has three parts: sensory receptors, primarily in the skin; the hypothalamic integrator, which controls the core temperature; and an effector system, which initates responses that either prevent heat loss and increase heat production (eg, peripheral vasoconstriction, shivering, and release of epinephrine, which increases metabolism) or increase heat loss through sweating and peripheral vasodilation.
- Factors affecting body temperature include age, diurnal variations, exercise, hormones, stress, and environmental temperatures.
- Pyrexia (fever) is a common sign of disease. Four common types of fever are intermittent, remittent, relapsing, and constant. Clinical signs of fever vary during the onset, course, and abatement stages.
- During a fever, the set-point of the hypothalamic thermostat changes suddenly from the normal level to a higher than normal level, but several hours elapse before the core temperature reaches the new set-point.
- Hypothermia involves three mechanisms: excessive heat loss, inadequate heat production by body cells, and increasing impairment of hypothalamic thermoregulation.
- Body temperature can be measured orally, rectally, or by axilla. The nurse selects the most appropriate site according to the client's age and condition.
- An important nursing function is to identify clients at risk for altered body temperature.
- Four NANDA nursing diagnoses are associated with body temperature: **High risk for altered body temperature, Hyperthermia, Hypothermia,** and **Ineffective thermoregulation.** Each has specific defining characteristics and contributing factors.
- Pulse rate and volume reflect the stroke volume output, the compliance of the client's arteries, and the adequacy of blood flow.
- Normally, a peripheral pulse reflects the client's heartbeat, but it may differ from the heartbeat in clients with certain cardiovascular diseases; in these instances, the nurse takes an apical pulse and compares it to the peripheral pulse.
- Many factors affect a person's pulse rate: age, sex, exercise, presence of fever, certain medications, hemorrhage, stress, and (in some situations) position changes.
- Although the radial pulse is the site most commonly used, eight other sites may be used in certain situations.
- Respirations are normally quiet, effortless and automatic and are assessed by observing respiratory rate, depth, rhythm, and sound.
- Blood pressure reflects cardiac output, peripheral vascular resistance, blood volume, and blood viscosity; peripheral vascular resistance varies according to the size of the arterioles and capillaries, and compliance of the arteries.

READINGS AND REFERENCES

SUGGESTED READINGS

Phoenix, J. November 1990. Low blood pressure: How to investigate this ominous sign. *Nursing* 20:34–40.

A sudden drop in a client's blood pressure requires rapid assessment to ensure effective intervention. This article includes blood pressure basics, risk factors, and emergency assessment tips. Two case studies are provided to assist nurses in appropriate assessment and intervention.

Trottier, D and Kochar, MS. November 1992. Around-the-clock blood pressure monitoring: How to get good results. *Nursing* 22:66–68, 70.

Ambulatory blood pressure (ABP) monitoring measures and records a client's blood pressure at preset intervals while the client performs routine activities. Throughout the day ABP is used to help diagnose hypertension more accurately in some clients. This article describes the monitoring device, how to apply it, how to obtain good results, and some of its disadvantages.

RELATED RESEARCH

Erickson, RS and Yount, ST. March/April 1991. Comparison of tympanic and oral temperatures in surgical patients. *Nursing Research* 40:90–93.

Norman, E, Gadaleta, D, and Griffin, CC. March/April 1991. An evaluation of three blood pressure methods in a stabilized acute trauma population. *Nursing Research* 40:86–89.

SELECTED REFERENCES

American Heart Association. 1967, 1980, 1987. *Recommendations for Human Blood Pressure Determination by Sphygmomanometers.* Pub no. 701005. American Heart Association.

Baker, NC, Cerone, SB, Gaze, N, and Knapp, TR. March/April 1984. The effect of thermometer and length of time inserted on oral temperature measurements of afebrile subjects. *Nursing Research* 33:109–11.

Carpenito, LJ. 1992. *Nursing Diagnosis: Application to Clinical Practice.* 4th ed. Philadelphia: Lippincott.

Cooper, KM. April 1992. Measuring blood pressure the right way. *Nursing* 22:75.

Eoff, MJ and Joyce, B. May 1981. Temperature measurement in children. *American Journal of Nursing* 81:1010–11.

Erickson, RS and Yount, ST. March/April 1991. Comparison of tympanic and oral temperatures in surgical patients. *Nursing Research* 40:90–93.

Feury, D and Nash, D. November 1990. Hypertension: The nurse's role. *RN* 53:54–60.

Graves, RD and Markarian, MF. September/October 1980. Three-minute intervals when using an oral mercury-in-glass thermometer without J-temperature sheaths. *Nursing Research* 29:323–24.

Giuffre, M, Heidenreich, T, Carney-Gersten, P, Dorsch, JA, and Heidenreich, E. May 1990. The relationship between axillary and core body temperature measurements. *Applied Nursing Research* 3:52–55.

Guyton, AC. 1991. *Textbook of Medical Physiology.* 8th ed. Philadelphia: WB Saunders.

Heinz, J. March 1985. Validation of sublingual temperatures in patients with nasogastric tubes. *Heart and Lung* 14:128–30.

Hill, MN and Grim, CM. February 1991. How to take a precise blood pressure. *American Journal of Nursing* 91:38–42.

Hollerbach, AD and Sneed, NV. May 1990. Accuracy of radial pulse assessment by length of counting interval. *Heart and Lung* 19:258–64.

Jolly, A. April 10–16, 1991. Taking blood pressure: *Nursing Times* 87:40–43.

Kennedy, WC, Jr. May 1990. Vital signs: Reading the essentials. *Journal of Emergency Medical Services* 15:26–30, 34, 36–39.

Kim, MJ, McFarland, GK, and McLane, AM 1993. *Pocket Guide to Nursing Diagnoses.* 5th ed. St Louis: Mosby.

Lukasiewicz, P. January/February 1986. Rectal temperatures are as accurate as oral temperatures in patients receiving oxygen therapy . . . fact or fantasy. *Critical Care Nurse* 6:72–73.

Malasanos, L, Barkauskas, V, Moss, M, and Stoltenberg-Allen, K. 1990. *Health Assessment.* 4th ed. St Louis: Mosby.

Marieb, EN. 1992. *Human Anatomy and Physiology.* Redwood City, CA: Benjamin/Cummings.

Morley, CJ. February 1992. Measuring infants' temperatures. *Midwives Chronicle* 105:26–29.

Nichols, GA, Ruskin, MM, Glor, BAK, and Kelly, WH. Fall 1966. Oral, axillary, and rectal determinations and relationships. *Nursing Research* 15:307–16.

North American Nursing Diagnosis Association. 1992. *NANDA Nursing Diagnoses: Definitions and Classification 1992–1993.* St Louis: NANDA.

Olds, SB, London, ML, and Ladewig, PA. 1992. *Maternal-Newborn Nursing: A Family-Centered Approach.* 4th ed. Redwood City, CA: Addison-Wesley Nursing.

Scharff, K. June 1991. Vital signs revisted: What you may be missing. *Nursing* 21:59.

Stone, S. February 1986. A new concept in routine vital signs measurement. *Nursing Management* 17:28–29.

Temperature taking—getting it right. December 1990. *Nursing Standard* 5:4–5.

US Department of Health and Human Services, Public Health Service, National Institutes of Health. May 1988. *The 1988 Report of the Joint National Committee on Detection, Evaluation, and Treatment of High Blood Pressure.* NIH Pub. no. 88–1088.

Wells, D. October 1990. A case for accuracy—monitoring pressure. *Professional Nurse* 30:30, 32.

Whaley, LF, and Wong, DL. 1991. *Nursing Care of Infants and Children.* 4th ed. St Louis: Mosby.

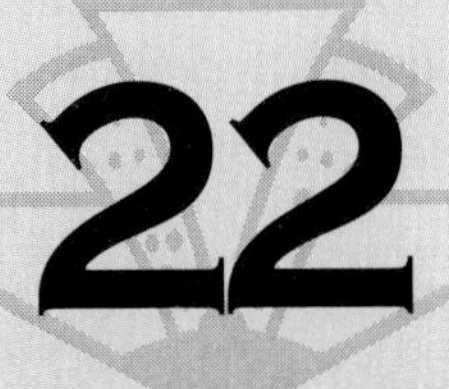

22 Assessing Adult Health

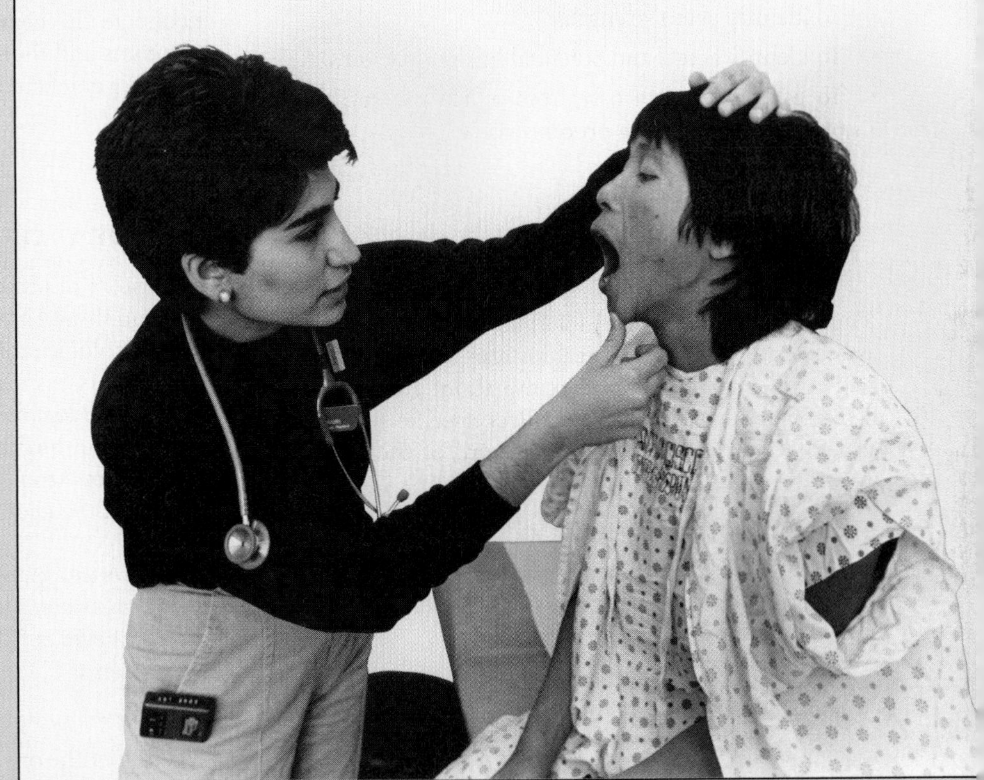

Objectives

- Define terms associated with health assessment.
- Describe ten components of a nursing health history.
- Identify purposes of physical health examination.
- Explain the four methods of examining.
- Explain the significance of selected physical findings.
- Identify expected outcomes of health assessment.
- Identify the various steps in selected assessment procedures.
- Describe suggested sequencing to conduct a physical health assessment in an orderly fashion.

Assessing a client's health status (ie, **nursing assessment**) is a major component of nursing care and has two aspects: (1) the health history and (2) a physical health examination. A nursing assessment can be any of three types: (a) a complete assessment (eg, when a client is admitted to a health care agency); (b) assessment of a body system (eg, the cardiovascular system); (c) assessment of a body part (eg, the lungs, when difficulty breathing is observed).

The purposes of a health assessment are

- To establish the client-nurse relationship.
- To obtain information about the client's health, including physiologic, psychologic, sociocultural, cognitive, developmental, and spiritual aspects.
- To identify client strengths.
- To identify actual and potential health problems.
- To establish a data base from which the subsequent phases of the nursing process evolve.

NURSING HEALTH HISTORY

The nursing health history interview is the first part of the assessment of the client's health status and is usually carried out before the physical examination. This is a structured interview designed to collect specific health data and to obtain a detailed health record of the client. Its purposes are

- To elicit information about all the variables that may affect the client's health status.
- To obtain data that help the nurse understand and appreciate the client's life experiences.
- To initiate a nonjudgmental, trusting interpersonal relationship with the client.

Data obtained are then used in collaboration with the client to develop nursing diagnoses and subsequent plans for individualized care. Skill in interviewing is essential when obtaining a health history (see Chapter 5, page 90).

Detailed nursing histories are discussed in each chapter in Unit 9 (Promoting Psychosocial Health) and Unit 10 (Promoting Physiologic Health). Many health history forms are designed as checklists that the client fills out independently. The nurse then reviews the information with the client and clarifies or amplifies the data as needed. Components of the nursing history include (a) biographic data, (b) chief complaint or reason for visit, (c) history of present illness (current health status), (d) past history, (e) family history of illness, (f) review of systems, (g) life-style, (h) social data, (i) psychologic data, and (i) patterns of health care.

BIOGRAPHIC DATA

Biographic data obtained include the client's name, address, age, sex, race, marital status, occupation, religious orientation, health care financing, and usual source of medical care.

CHIEF COMPLAINT OR REASON FOR VISIT

The chief complaint (CC) is the answer given to the question "What is troubling you?" or "What brought you to the hospital or clinic?" The chief complaint should be recorded in the client's own words. If the client states, "I have heart trouble," or "I have cancer," the nurse should encourage the client to elaborate by discussing specific symptoms and their duration. Further investigation may produce a chief complaint, such as "I've had chest pain for the past 2 hours," or "I've lost 45 pounds in the past month."

HISTORY OF PRESENT ILLNESS

The history of present illness (HPI) is sequentially developed and should include four parts: (a) usual health status, (b) chronologic story, (c) relevant family history, and (d) disability assessment. To obtain a description of the client's *usual health status*, ask the client, "How would you describe your health up until this time?" Answers such as "terrible" or "good" need to be clarified further. For example, ask the client, "What do you mean by terrible (or good)?"

The *chronologic story* is a narrative section where the client's chief complaint is documented in the proper sequence of events. The chronologic story includes the following items:

- When the symptoms started
- Whether the onset of symptoms was sudden or gradual
- If available, specific dates when the problem was experienced
- How often the problem occurs
- Exact location of the distress
- Character of the complaint (eg, intensity of pain or quality of sputum, emesis, or discharge)
- Amount of discharge, mucus, blood, stool, or urine or the size of a lesion
- Activity in which the client was involved when the problem occurred
- Phenomena or symptoms associated with the chief complaint
- Factors that aggravate or alleviate the problem

In the third part of the HPI, the *relevant family history*, the nurse asks the client about related problems of family members. If the client's chief complaint is chest pain, for example, the nurse may ask the client whether there is any family history of heart disease. If so, the specific problem of each affected family member is documented.

In the last part of the HPI, the *disability assessment*, the nurse explores how the problem has interfered with the client's daily life in terms of work or school and family resources and relationships. This part of the HPI provides the nurse with information about the severity of the problem from the client's perspective.

PAST HISTORY

Included in the past history are all previous immunizations and experiences with illness, including the following:

- *Childhood illnesses*, such as chickenpox, mumps, measles, rubella (German measles), rubeola (red measles), streptococcal infections, scarlet fever, rheumatic fever, and other significant illnesses
- *Childhood immunizations* and the date of the last tetanus shot
- *Allergies* to drugs, animals, insects, or other environmental agents and the type of reaction that occurs
- *Accidents and injuries:* how, when, and where the incident occurred, type of injury, treatment received, and any complications
- *Hospitalization* for serious illnesses: reasons for the hospitalization, dates, location of the hospital, name of the physician, surgery performed, course of recovery, and any complications
- *Medications:* all currently used prescription and over-the-counter medications, such as aspirin, nasal spray, vitamins, or laxatives

FAMILY HISTORY OF ILLNESS

The family history reveals risk factors for certain diseases. This information should include the ages of siblings, parents, and grandparents and their current state of health or (if they are deceased) the cause of death. Particular attention should be given to disorders such as heart disease, cancer, diabetes, hypertension, obesity, allergies, arthritis, tuberculosis, jaundice, bleeding, ulcers, migraine, and alcoholism.

REVIEW OF SYSTEMS (ROS)

The review of systems (ROS) is a review of all health problems by body system. Its purpose is to prevent the omission of data related to the present illness and to discover any other problems that might have been missed. It is a review of the past and present status of each system. Generally, a head-to-toe approach is used, and agency checklists are often available. A head-to-toe approach is also used in the physical examination, but the data obtained in this part of the history focus on *subjective data* given by the client. An example of a client checklist for the review of systems is shown in the box on page 464. The client is asked to circle or underline any symptoms experienced. The nurse then explores in depth with the client any symptoms that have not previously been mentioned. An alternative frame of reference for the ROS is the *functional health pattern* approach. See the box in Chapter 5, page 99.

Assessment of specific functional health patterns are shown throughout this book. See assessment interviews in each chapter in Units 8, 9, and 10.

LIFE-STYLE

Investigation of the client's life-style provides data about factors that can be used for planning health promotion, maintenance, and restoration. The nurse obtains data about personal habits, diet, sleep/rest patterns, activities of daily living, and recreation/hobbies.

- *Personal habits.* The nurse documents the frequency of all substance abuse, including the use of tobacco, alcohol, coffee, cola, tea, and illicit or recreational drugs. The type of tobacco (cigarette, cigar, or pipe) and the number of packs or smokes per day should be described. The nurse also notes the number of years the client has smoked. The type of alcohol (eg, beer, wine, or hard liquor), number of bottles or glasses per day, and pattern of drinking (morning, evenings, or weekends) should also be specified. The same descriptive data apply to the consumption of coffee, tea, and cola. When asking about the use of illicit or recreational drugs, the nurse focuses on drugs used extensively in the past, frequency and duration of use, and the good and bad effects.
- *Diet.* Dietary data may include the description of a typical diet on a normal day or of any prescribed special diet, number of meals and snacks per day, who cooks and shops for food, ethnically distinct food patterns, methods used for food preparation, and food likes, dislikes, and allergies. A more detailed nutritional history is provided in Chapter 37, page 1033.
- *Sleep/rest patterns.* Sleep and rest clearly affect the total well-being of the client. The nurse notes the usual daily sleep/wake times, difficulties sleeping, and remedies used for difficulties. A detailed sleep/rest history is provided in Chapter 35, page 960.
- *Activities of daily living (ADLs).* The nurse collects data about the client's perception of any difficulties experienced in the basic activities of eating, grooming, dressing, elimination, and locomotion.

EXAMPLE OF CLIENT CHECKLIST FOR REVIEW OF SYSTEMS

- *General health.* Weight loss, weakness, feelings of fatigue, mood changes, night sweats, or bleeding tendencies?
- *Skin.* Skin diseases such as eczema, psoriasis, acne; change in pigmentation; tendency toward bruising; excessive dryness or moisture; jaundice; itching, rashes, hives; change in color or size of moles; or open sores that are slow to heal?
- *Hair.* Itchy scalp, loss of hair, excessive body hair? Do you wear a wig?
- *Nails.* Color changes, biting, clubbing, splitting?
- *Head.* Frequent or severe headaches, fainting, dizziness, fall or accident resulting in unconsciousness?
- *Eyes.* Difficulty seeing, eye infection, eye pain, excessive tearing, double vision, blurring, sensitivity to light, cataracts, itching, spots in front of eyes? Do you wear glasses (for near or far vision) or contact lenses? When was your last eye examination?
- *Ears.* Any infection, loss of hearing, pain, discharge, ringing in the ears? Do you wear a hearing aid?
- *Nose.* Frequent colds, nosebleeds, allergies, pain, tenderness, postnasal drip?
- *Mouth and throat.* Sore gums; bleeding gums; sores, lumps or white spots on mouth, lips, or tongue; toothaches, cavities, difficulty swallowing; voice change or hoarseness? Do you wear dentures (upper, lower, partial)? When was your last dental appointment?
- *Neck.* Pain, swelling, stiffness, limited movement, swollen glands?
- *Breasts.* Nipple discharge, scaling or cracks around nipples, dimples, lumps, pattern of breast self-examination? When did you last have a mammogram?
- *Respiratory system.* Chest pain; cough; shortness of breath; wheezing; coughing up blood; lung disease such as tuberculosis, emphysema, asthma, bronchitis? Have you ever had a chest X ray? When? Results?
- *Cardiovascular system.* Heart disease, palpitations, heart murmur, high blood pressure, anemia, varicose veins, leg swelling or ulcer?
- *Gastrointestinal system.* Nausea, vomiting, loss of appetite, indigestion, heartburn, bright blood in stools, tarry-black stools, diarrhea, constipation, abdominal pain, excessive gas, hemorrhoids, rectal pain, colostomy, ileostomy?
- *Genitourinary system.* Frequency, dribbling, urgency, urination at night, difficulty starting stream, blood in urine, incontinence, pain or burning upon urination, urinary tract infection, ureterostomy, sexually transmitted disease such as gonorrhea ("clap" or "morning drip") or syphilis ("bad blood")?
  Females: Age of menarche, last menstrual period (LMP), duration, amount of flow, regularity of cycle? Any problem with painful menstruation, bleeding between periods, pain during intercourse, vaginal discharge, vaginal itching, vaginal infection?
  Males: Penile discharge, swelling, masses or lesions, difficulty in sexual functioning?
- *Musculoskeletal system.* Muscular pain, swelling, or weakness; joint swelling, soreness, or stiffness; leg cramps; bone defects?
- *Neurologic system.* Difficulty walking; unconsciousness; seizures; tremors; paralysis; numbness, tingling, or burning sensations in any body part; weakness on one side of body; speech problems; loss of memory; disorientation; forgetfulness; unclear thinking; changes in emotional state?
- *Endocrine system.* History of goiter; heat or cold intolerance; diabetes; excessive thirst; excessive eating?

- *Recreation/hobbies.* The client's exercise activity and tolerance, hobbies and other interests, vacations, and time spent with family and friends are discussed.

SOCIAL DATA

Social assessment includes family relationships and friendships, ethnic affiliation, educational history, occupational history, economic status, and home and neighborhood conditions.

Family Relationships/Friendships Because of the many different types of family arrangements and relationships in society today (eg, single parents, unmarried couples, homosexual couples), the nurse must obtain such data with care. The nurse needs to keep in mind the purposes of eliciting such data, which are to determine (a) whether the client has a support system in times of stress, (b) what effect the client's illness has on the family, and (c) whether any family problems are affecting the client. The nurse may ask these questions: "Do you live alone? Who helps you in times of need? What person would you like us to contact in case of an emergency? What person do you feel close to in your family? What effect has your illness on family members or friends? Are the other members of your family healthy?" If problems are suspected, the nurse may need to explore the quality of support relationships. To explore specific relationships, the nurse may ask, for example, "How would you describe your father? How would your father describe you?" Open-ended statements, such as "Tell me more about it," also encourage elaboration by the client. See also the discussion of family assessment in Chapter 14.

Ethnic Affiliation Data about ethnic affiliation help the nurse understand the client's customs and beliefs. Ethnic data may be obtained by indirect assessment of the client's language, manner of dress, and food preferences or by direct questions such as these: "What country are you and your parents and grandparents from? Do you identify with a particular ethnic group? What cultural practices should we know about that may affect your health care and recovery?"

Educational History Data about the client's highest level of education attained and any past difficulties with learning can help the nurse make appropriate adjustments in plans for client teaching.

Occupational History The occupational history should focus on all jobs the client has held, the client's current employment status, the number of days missed from work because of illness, any history of accidents on the job, any occupational hazards with a potential for future disease or accident, the client's need to change jobs because of past illness, the employment status of both spouses or partners and the way child care is handled, and the client's overall satisfaction with the work.

Economic Status Financial status is another sensitive area of inquiry that is best handled initially by an open-ended question, such as "How would you describe your financial status?" The nurse obtains information about how the client is paying for medical care (including what kind of medical and hospitalization coverage the client has), whether the client feels the family income is sufficient to meet the family's basic needs, and whether the client's illness presents financial concerns.

Home and Neighborhood Conditions Information about the client's home environment reveals conditions that may or may not be conducive to health. Much of these data may already be surmised from economic, employment, and financial data. The client's physical and mental status and age are especially important in the nurse's review of home safety measures and adjustments in physical facilities that may be required to help the client manage a physical disability, activity intolerance, and activities of daily living. The nurse also inquires about the availability of neighborhood and community services to meet the client's needs.

Psychologic Data

The general survey of appearance and behavior (a component of the physical assessment) reveals much information about the client's emotional state. When a further psychologic assessment is indicated, the nurse notes the client's major stressors, usual coping pattern, communication style, self-concept, and mood.

- *Major stressors.* The nurse determines major stressors the client has experienced in the past year and the client's perception of them.
- *Usual coping pattern.* The nurse asks what the client normally does to cope with a serious problem or a high level of stress. See the section on assessing client coping in Chapter 32, page 841.
- *Communication style.* The nurse observes the client's nonverbal communication and ability to verbalize appropriate emotion. Nonverbal communication—such as eye movements, gestures, use of touch, and posture—and the client's interactions with support persons can reveal anxiety, suspicion, withdrawal, anger, or other feelings. The nurse should note particularly the congruence of nonverbal behavior and verbal expression. Examples of incongruent expression are being overly cheerful in response to bad news, laughing while discussing a serious topic, or crying when talking about a pleasant topic.
- *Self-concept.* See questions in Chapter 31 on page 810.
- *Mood.* The nurse may need to ask about mood if the client appears underactive (flat or unresponsive). The nurse may ask whether the client sleeps well at night, gets discouraged, feels down, or cries frequently. The client's answers help the nurse determine whether the client is depressed. The nurse can then ask other questions to probe the depth of a depression. For example, a nurse may ask whether the client ever feels life is not worth living or whether things are getting too bad for the client to cope. Affirmative answers to these questions warrant other questions: "Have you ever thought of killing yourself or tried to kill yourself?" "How did you do it or how did you plan to do it?" By gradually leading up to questions of suicide, the nurse can gauge the depth of depression.

Patterns of Health Care

The nurse needs to note all health care resources the client is currently using and has used in the past. These include the family physician, specialists (eg, ophthalmologist or gynecologist), dentist, folk practitioners (eg, herbalist or curandero), health clinic, or health center. In addition, the nurse should determine whether the client considers the care being provided adequate and whether access to health care is a problem.

PHYSICAL HEALTH EXAMINATION

A complete health assessment is generally conducted from the head to the toes; however, the procedure can vary according to the age of the individual, the severity of the illness, the preferences of the nurse, and the agency's priorities and procedures. The order of head-to-toe assessment is given in the box below. Regardless of what procedure is used, the client's energy and time need to be considered. The health assessment is therefore conducted in a systematic and efficient manner that requires the fewest position changes for the client.

Frequently, nurses assess a specific body area instead of the entire body. These specific assessments are made in relation to client complaints, the nurse's own observation of problems, the client's presenting problem, nursing interventions provided, and medical therapies. Examples of these situations and assessments are provided in Table 22–1.

These are some of the purposes of the physical health examination:

- To obtain baseline data about the client's functional abilities
- To supplement, confirm, or refute data obtained in the nursing history
- To obtain data that will help the nurse establish nursing diagnoses and plan the client's care
- To evaluate the physiologic outcomes of health care and thus the progress of a client's health problem
- To screen for the presence of cancer (see the American Cancer Society's guidelines in the box on page 467)

HEAD-TO-TOE ORDER OF EXAMINATION AREAS

- Skin
- Hair
- Nails
- Head
- Face
- Ears
- Eyes
- Nose
- Sinuses
- Mouth
- Throat
- Neck
- Breasts and axillae
- Thorax/back
- Heart and peripheral vessels
- Upper extremities
- Abdomen
- Anus and rectum
- Genitals
- Lower extremities

Table 22–1 Nursing Assessments Addressing Specific Client Situations

Situation	Physical Assessment
Client complains of abdominal pain.	Inspect, palpate, and auscultate the abdomen; assess vital signs.
Client is admitted with a head injury.	Assess level of consciousness using Glasgow Coma Scale; assess pupils for reaction to light and accommodation; assess vital signs.
The nurse administers a cardiotonic drug to a client.	Assess apical pulse and compare with baseline data.
The nurse administers postural drainage.	Auscultate lungs before and after the procedure.
The client has just had a cast applied to the lower leg.	Assess peripheral perfusion of toes, capillary blanch test, pedal pulse if able, and vital signs.
The client's fluid intake is minimal.	Assess tissue turgor, fluid intake and output, and vital signs.

PREPARING THE CLIENT

Most people need an explanation of the physical health examination. The nurse should explain when and where the examination will take place, why it is necessary, who will conduct it, and what will happen during the examination. The nurse should also inform the client of any special circumstances—for instance, the need to go to a different room or assume a special position—and tell the adult client that appropriate draping will be provided so that the body will not be unnecessarily exposed.

Most clients should empty their bladders before the examination. Doing so helps them feel more relaxed and facilitates palpation of the abdomen and pubic area. Since an empty rectum facilitates rectal examination, the client should be encouraged to defecate before a complete physical examination. If a urinalysis is required, the urine should be collected in a container for that purpose. Clients must often assume special positions during the health examination. See Table 22–2 on page 468.

Dorsal and Horizontal Recumbent and Supine Positions The appropriate drapes for a client in these positions usually include (a) a hospital gown or bath towel for the chest and (b) a bath blanket or sheet to cover the remainder of the body from the waist to the toes. The nurse places the bath towel across the chest, and the bath blanket or sheet diagonally over the person. If the client's

CANCER SCREENING GUIDELINES FOR ASYMPTOMATIC PEOPLE

Colorectal Cancer (Males and Females)

- Digital rectal examination annually beginning at age 40
- Fecal occult blood test annually beginning at age 50
- Sigmoidoscopy every 3 to 5 years beginning at age 50

Breast Cancer (Females)

- Monthly breast self-examination beginning at age 20
- Breast examination by a physician every 3 years beginning at age 20 to age 40, and then annually beginning at age 40
- Mammogram every 1 to 2 years beginning at age 40 up to age 49, and then annually at age 50 and over

Uterine Cancer (Females)

- Papanicolaou (Pap) smear annually for all women who are or who have been sexually active or have reached age 18 (After a woman has had three or more consecutive satisfactory normal annual examinations, the Pap test may be performed less frequently at the discretion of her physician.)
- Pelvic examination every 1 to 3 years with Pap test beginning at age 18 to age 40, and annually for women over 40
- Endometrial tissue sample at menopause if at high risk and thereafter at the discretion of the physician

Prostate Cancer (Males)

- Prostate examination annually

Health Counseling and Cancer Checkup (Males and Females)

- Examination for cancers of the thyroid, testicles, ovaries, lymph nodes, oral region, and skin every 3 years over age 20 and annually over age 40

Source: *Summary of American Cancer Society Recommendations for Early Detection of Cancer in Asymptomatic People*, (Atlanta: American Cancer Society, Inc, January 1, 1994).

perineal area is to be examined, opposite corners of the sheet are wrapped around the feet to cover the legs. The corner between the client's legs can be raised to expose the perineum at the appropriate time.

Sitting Position This position is frequently assumed during examinations of the chest, neck, and head. The client requires a gown.

Lithotomy Position The lithotomy position is frequently used for examinations of the vagina and sometimes for urinary catheterizations in women.

The drapes usually used are (a) a gown for the upper body (optional), (b) a rectangular sheet or a **fenestrated drape** (with an opening in its center), and (c) socks (optional). The socks are put on the client before the feet are placed in the stirrups. The sheet is placed diagonally so that the top part covers the client's chest and abdomen. The side corners are wrapped around the client's legs and feet. If the client is wearing socks, the drape need not cover the feet. The corner between the client's legs is lifted to expose the perineal area. A fenestrated drape is placed the same way as a rectangular sheet but with the opening directly over the area to be examined.

Genupectoral (Knee-Chest) Position The genupectoral position is a kneeling position in which the head is turned to one side and the arms are held above the head. Special tables, provided in many agencies, support clients in this position.

The drapes required are (a) a hospital gown to cover the upper body, (b) socks to cover the feet and lower legs (optional), and (c) a fenestrated drape to cover the client's back, buttocks, and thighs. The hole in the drape exposes only the area to be examined. A rectangular drape can be used instead. The two lateral corners are tucked around the client's thighs. The corner between the thighs can then be lifted up to expose the area to be examined, for example, the anus.

Sims' Position In Sims' position, the lower arm is behind the client, and the upper arm is flexed at both the shoulder and the elbow. Both legs are also flexed, the upper one more so at the hip and the knee than the lower one.

The drape is usually one rectangular sheet, placed diagonally on the client. At the time of examination, the corner is folded back to expose the area. Because this position can be difficult for some clients to assume, particularly the elderly and the obese, it is normally not assumed until immediately before the examination.

Prone Position A client in the **prone position** usually turns the head to the side. A sheet to cover the client is required.

METHODS OF EXAMINING

Four primary techniques are used in the physical examination: inspection, palpation, percussion, and auscultation. These are discussed throughout this chapter as they apply to each body system.

Inspection Inspection is the visual examination, that is, assessing by using the sense of sight. The nurse inspects with the naked eye and with a lighted instrument such as

Table 22–2 Client Positions and Body Areas Examined

Position	Description	Areas Examined	Cautions
Dorsal recumbent 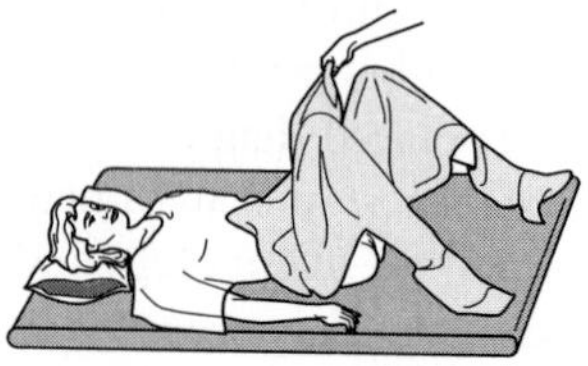	Back-lying position with knees flexed and hips externally rotated; small pillow under the head	Head and neck, axillae, anterior thorax, lungs, breasts, heart, abdomen, extremities, peripheral pulses, vital signs, and vagina	May be difficult for clients who have cardiopulmonary problems to assume
Horizontal recumbent 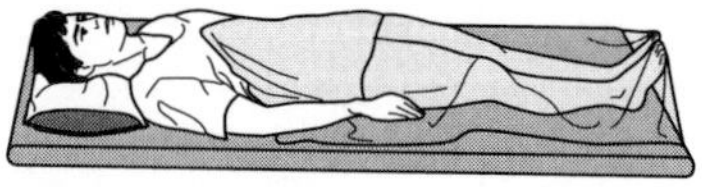	Back-lying position with legs extended; small pillow under the head	Head, neck, axillae, anterior thorax, lungs, breasts, heart, extremities, peripheral pulses	Not used for abdominal assessment because of the increased tension of abdominal muscles
Dorsal (supine) 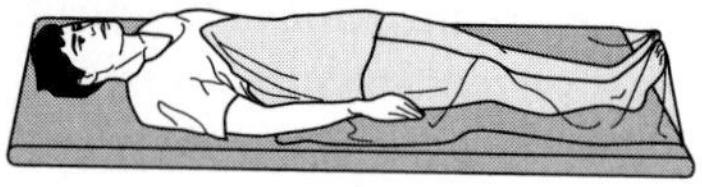	Back-lying position without a pillow	As for horizontal recumbent	Tolerated poorly by clients with cardiovascular and respiratory problems
Sitting 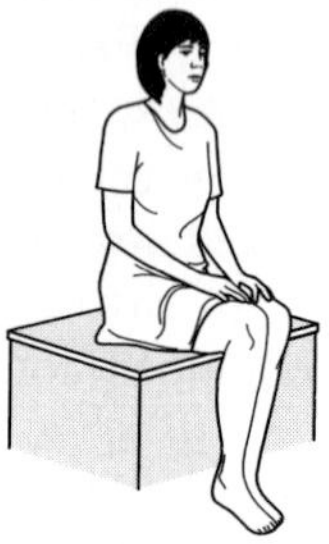	A seated position, back unsupported and legs hanging freely	Head, neck, posterior and anterior thorax, lungs, breasts, axillae, heart, vital signs, upper and lower extremities, reflexes	Elderly and weak clients may require support
Lithotomy 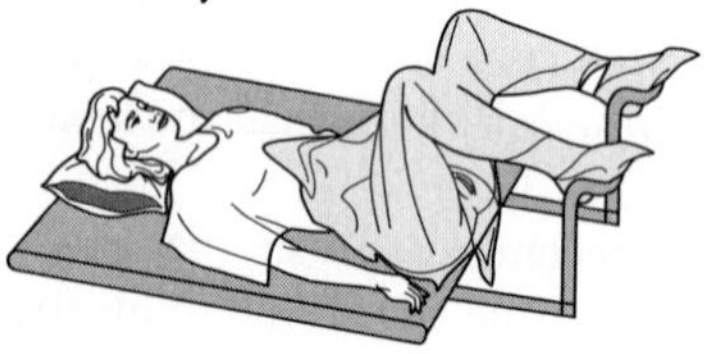	Back-lying position with feet supported in stirrups; the hips should be in line with the edge of the table	Female genitals, rectum, and female reproductive tract	May be difficult and tiring for elderly people
Genupectoral (knee-chest) 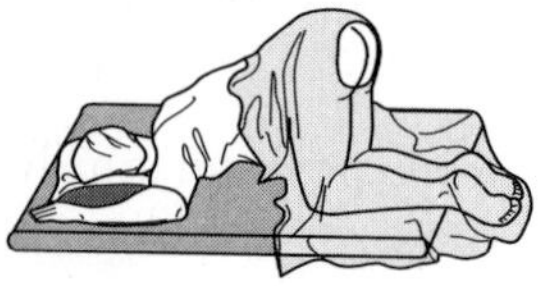	Kneeling position with torso at a 90-degree angle to hips	Rectum	Uncomfortable position, tolerated poorly by clients who have respiratory problems
Sims' 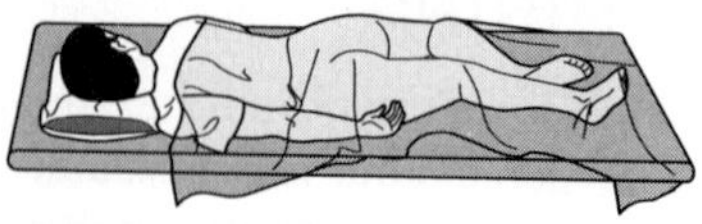	Side-lying position with lowermost arm behind the body and uppermost leg flexed	Rectum, vagina	Difficult for the elderly and people with limited joint movement
Prone 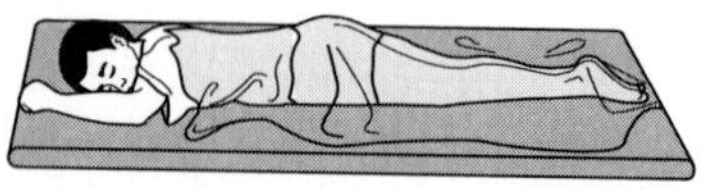	Face-lying position, with or without a small pillow	Posterior thorax, hip movement	Often not tolerated by the elderly and people with cardiovascular and respiratory problems

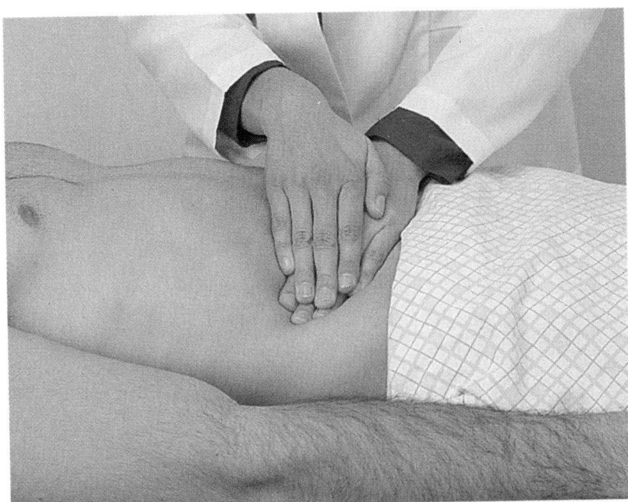

Figure 22–1 The position of the hands for deep bimanual palpation.

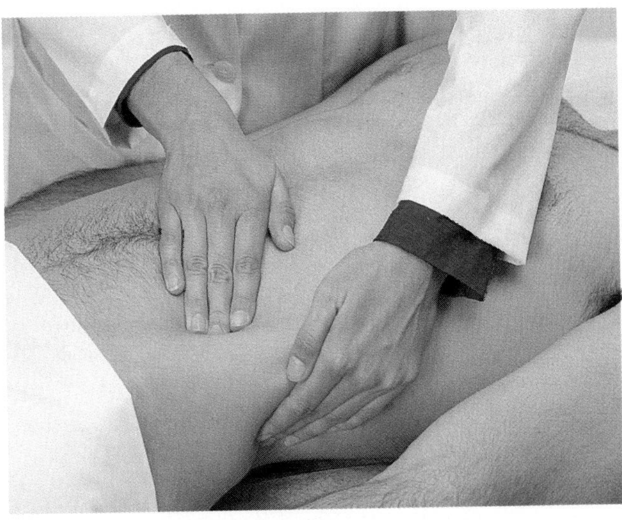

Figure 22–2 Deep palpation using the lower hand to support the body while the upper hand palpates the organ.

an otoscope (used to view the ear). Some authors consider the use of the senses of hearing and smell as part of the inspection (Malasanos et al 1990, p. 138). Nurses frequently use this technique to assess color, rashes, scars, body shape, facial expressions that may reflect emotions, and body structures (eg, the inner eye). Inspection is an active process, not a passive one. The nurse must know what to look for and where. Inspection should be systematic, so that nothing is missed. Lighting must be sufficient; either natural or artificial light can be used.

Palpation Palpation is the examination of the body using the sense of touch. The pads of the fingers are used because their concentration of nerve endings makes them highly sensitive to tactile discrimination. Palpation is used to determine (a) texture (eg, of the hair); (b) temperature (eg, of a skin area); (c) vibration (eg, of a joint); (d) position, size, consistency, and mobility of organs or masses; (e) distention (eg, of the urinary bladder); (f) presence and rate of peripheral pulses; and (g) tenderness or pain.

There are two types of palpation: light and deep. *Light* (superficial) *palpation* should always precede *deep palpation*, because heavy pressure on the fingertips can dull the sense of touch. For light palpation, the nurse extends dominant hand fingers parallel to the skin surface and presses gently while moving the hand in a circle. If it is necessary to determine the details of a mass, the nurse presses lightly several times rather than holding the pressure.

Deep palpation is done with two hands (bimanually) or one hand. In deep bimanual palpation, the nurse extends the dominant hand as for light palpation, then places the fingerpads of the nondominant hand on the dorsal surfaces of the distal interphalangeal joint of the middle three fingers of the dominant hand (Figure 22–1). The top hand applies pressure while the lower hand remains relaxed to perceive the tactile sensations. For deep palpation using one hand, the fingerpads of the dominant hand press over the area to be palpated. Often the other hand is used to support a mass or organ from below (Figure 22–2). *Deep palpation is a technique used more commonly by nurse practitioners and clinical specialists than by nurses in general practice.*

The effectiveness of palpation depends largely on the client's relaxation. Nurses can assist a client to relax by (a) gowning and/or draping the client appropriately; (b) positioning the client comfortably; (c) ensuring that their own hands are warm before beginning, for example, by running them under warm water if they are cold; and (d) commencing palpation with areas that are not painful. During palpation, the nurse should be sensitive to the client's verbal and facial expressions indicating discomfort.

Percussion Percussion is an assessment method in which the body surface is struck to elicit sounds that can be heard or vibrations that can be felt. There are two types of percussion: direct, or immediate, percussion and indirect, or mediate, percussion. In *direct percussion*, the nurse strikes the area to be percussed directly with the pads of two, three, or four fingers or with the pad of the middle finger. The strikes are rapid, and the movement is from the wrist. This technique is not generally used to percuss the thorax but is useful in percussing an adult's sinuses.

The second type, *indirect percussion*, is the striking of an object (eg, a finger) held against the body area to be examined. In this technique, the middle finger of the nondominant hand, referred to as the **pleximeter,** is placed firmly on the client's skin. Only the distal phalanx and joint of this finger should be in contact with the skin.

Table 22–3 Percussion Sounds and Tones

Sound	Intensity	Pitch	Duration	Quality	Example of Location
Flatness	Soft	High	Short	Extremely dull	Muscle, bone
Dullness	Medium	Medium	Moderate	Thudlike	Liver, heart
Resonance	Loud	Low	Long	Hollow	Lung
Hyperresonance	Very loud	Very low	Very long	Booming	Emphysematous lung
Tympany	Loud	High (distinguished mainly by musical timbre)	Moderate	Musical	Stomach filled with gas (air)

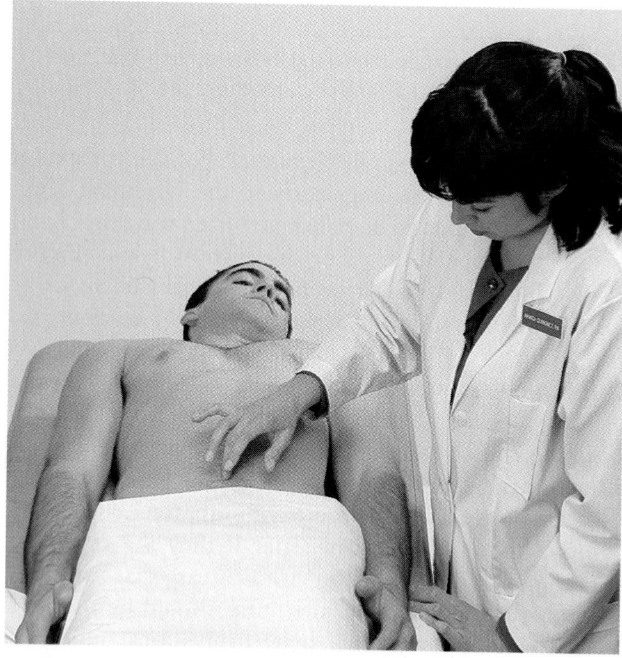

Figure 22–3 The position of the fingers for direct percussion. Only the middle finger of the nondominant hand is firmly in contact with the client's skin.

Using the tip of the flexed middle finger of the other hand, called the **plexor,** the nurse strikes the pleximeter, usually at the distal interphalangeal joint (Figure 22–3). Some nurses may find a point between the distal and proximal joints to be a more comfortable pleximeter point. The motion comes from the wrist; the forearm remains stationary. The angle between the plexor and the pleximeter should be 90 degrees, and the blows must be firm, rapid, and short to obtain a clear sound.

Percussion is used to determine the size and shape of internal organs by establishing their borders. It indicates whether tissue is fluid-filled, air-filled, or solid. Percussion elicits five types of sound: flatness, dullness, resonance, hyperresonance, and tympany. **Flatness** is an extremely dull sound produced by very dense tissue, such as muscle or bone. **Dullness** is a thudlike sound produced by dense tissue such as the liver, spleen, or heart. **Resonance** is a hollow sound such as that produced by lungs filled with air. **Hyperresonance** is not produced in the normal body. It is described as booming and can be heard over an emphysematous lung. **Tympany** is a musical or drumlike sound produced from an air-filled stomach. On a continuum, flatness reflects the most dense tissue (the least amount of air) and tympany the least dense tissue (the most amount of air). A percussion sound is described according to its intensity, pitch, duration, and quality. See Table 22–3.

Auscultation Auscultation is the process of listening to sounds produced within the body. Auscultation may be direct or indirect. *Direct auscultation* is the use of the unaided ear, for example, to listen to a respiration wheeze or the grating of a moving joint. *Indirect auscultation* is the use of a stethoscope, which amplifies the sounds and conveys them to the nurse's ears. A stethoscope is used primarily to listen to sounds from within the body, such as bowel sounds or valve sounds of the heart.

The stethoscope should be 30 to 25 cm (12 to 14 in) long, with an internal diameter of about 0.3 cm (1/8 in). It should have both a flat-disc and a bell-shaped diaphragm. See Figure 21–18 on page 445. The flat-disc diaphragm best transmits high-pitched sounds (eg, bronchial sounds) and the bell-shaped diaphragm best transmits low-pitched sounds, such as some heart sounds. The earpieces of the stethoscope should fit comfortably into the nurse's ears. The diaphragm of the stethoscope is placed firmly but lightly against the client's skin. If a client is very hairy, it may be necessary to dampen the hairs with a moist cloth so that they will lie flat against the skin and not cause scratching sounds.

Auscultated sounds are described according to their pitch, intensity, duration, and quality. The **pitch** is the frequency of the vibrations (the number of vibrations per

Table 22–4 Equipment and Supplies Used for a Health Examination

Instruments and Supplies	Purpose
Flashlight or penlight	To assist viewing of the pharynx and cervix or to determine the reactions of the pupils of the eye
Head mirror	To direct light to a specific body area (eg, the pharynx)
Laryngeal or dental mirror	To observe the pharynx and oral cavity
Nasal speculum	To permit visualization of the lower and middle turbinates; usually a penlight is used for illumination
Neurologic hammer	To test reflexes; often has a soft brush and needle in the handle that come out when it is unscrewed
Ophthalmoscope	A lighted instrument to visualize the interior of the eye
Otoscope	A lighted instrument to visualize the eardrum and external auditory canal (a nasal speculum may be attached to the otoscope to inspect the nasal cavities)
Percussion (reflex) hammer	An instrument with a rubber head to test reflexes
Smells (1 or 2 vials)	To test the sense of smell
Sphygmomanometer and cuff (see Figure 21–22, p. 453)	To measure the blood pressure
Stethoscope (see Figure 21–18, p. 445)	To auscultate body sounds (eg, blood pressure, chest, bowel sounds)

second). Low-pitched sounds, such as some heart sounds, have fewer vibrations per second than high-pitched sounds, such as bronchial sounds. The **intensity** (amplitude) refers to the loudness or softness of a sound. Some body sounds are loud, for example, bronchial sounds heard over the trachea; others are soft, for example, normal breath sounds heard in the lungs. The **duration** of a sound is its length (long or short). The **quality** of sound is a subjective description of a sound, for example, whistling, gurgling, or snapping.

INSTRUMENTATION

Photographs of various equipment are shown in Table 22–4. All equipment required for the health examination should be clean, in good working order, and readily accessible. Equipment is frequently set up on trays, ready for use.

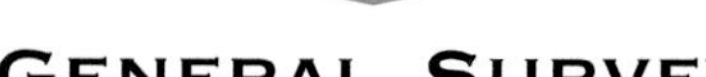

GENERAL SURVEY

The nurse assesses many components of the general survey while taking the health history. Other data obtained as part of the survey include appearance and mental status, vital signs, and height and weight.

Mental status and the level of consciousness or state of awareness are often determined at the beginning of the

Table 22–4 ***continued***

Instruments and Supplies	Purpose
Thermometer (see Figures 21–6, 21–7, 21–8, and 21–9 on pp. 432 and 433)	To measure body temperature
Tuning fork	A two-pronged metal instrument used to test hearing acuity and vibratory sense
Vaginal speculum (various sizes) (see Figure 22–77, p. 557)	To assess the cervix and the vagina
Ayre spatula (see Figure 22–78, p. 557)	To obtain a cervical scrape
Assorted containers and slides	For specimens
Cotton applicators	To obtain specimens
Disposable pads	To absorb liquid
Drapes	To cover the client
Gauze dressings	To cover wounds
Gloves (sterile and unsterile)	To protect the nurse
Lubricant 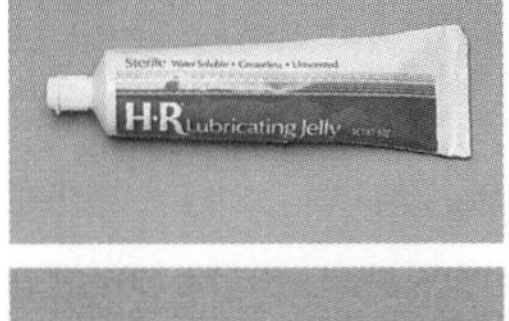	To ease insertion of instruments (eg, vaginal speculum)
Sterile safety pins	To test sensory function
Tongue blades (depressors)	To depress the tongue during assessment of the mouth and pharynx

physical examination. Ask the client to state name, the day or date, present location, and the reason for hospitalization or for seeking assistance. Record the client's ability to provide this information. For clients who are unable to speak, describe their specific responses to verbal and physical stimuli. See the discussion of the neurologic assessment, later in this chapter.

APPEARANCE AND MENTAL STATUS

The general appearance and behavior of an individual must be assessed in terms of culture, educational level, socioeconomic status, and current circumstances. For example, an individual who has recently experienced a personal loss may appropriately appear depressed. Also, the client's age, sex, and race are useful factors in interpreting findings that suggest increased risk for known conditions. Procedure 22–1 describes how to assess general appearance and mental status.

VITAL SIGNS

Vital signs are measured (a) to establish baseline data against which to compare future measurements and (b) to detect actual and future health problems. See Chapter 21 for measurements of temperature, pulse, respirations, and blood pressure.

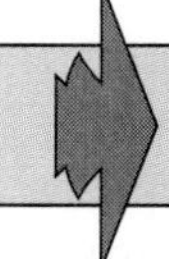

PROCEDURE 22-1 ASSESSING GENERAL APPEARANCE AND MENTAL STATUS

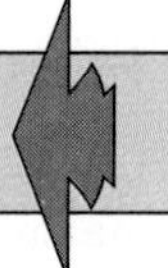

NURSING HISTORY FOCUS

Chronologic age, race, cultural background, and general health status; achievement of developmental tasks; body image concerns; self-esteem; educational level, thought processes; general health history; stressors (past and present); changes in personality, behavior, or memory; life-long problems (eg, poor job history, alcoholism, drug abuse, disciplinary problems).

ASSESSMENT	NORMAL FINDINGS	DEVIATIONS FROM NORMAL
General Appearance		
Observe body build, height, and weight in relation to the client's age, life-style, and health.	Varies with life-style	Excessively thin or obese
Observe the client's posture and gait, standing, sitting, and walking. See Chapter 34, pages 898 and 900.	Relaxed, erect posture; coordinated movement	Tense, slouched, bent posture; uncoordinated movement; tremors
Observe the client's overall hygiene and grooming. Relate these to the person's activities prior to the assessment.	Clean, neat	Dirty, unkempt
Note body and breath odor in relation to activity level.	No body odor or minor body odor relative to work or exercise; no breath odor	Foul body odor; ammonia odor; acetone breath odor; foul breath
Observe for signs of distress in posture (eg, bending over because of abdominal pain) **or facial expression** (eg, wincing or labored breathing).		
Note obvious signs of health or illness (eg, in skin color or breathing).	Healthy appearance	Pallor; weakness; obvious illness
Mental Status		
Assess the client's attitude.	Cooperative	Negative, hostile, withdrawn
Note the client's affect/mood; assess the appropriateness of the client's responses.	Appropriate to situation	Inappropriate to situation
Listen for quantity of speech (amount and pace), **quality** (loudness, clarity, inflection), **and organization** (coherence of thought, overgeneralization, vagueness).	Understandable, moderate pace Exhibits thought association	Rapid or slow pace Use generalizations; lacks association; exhibits confabulation (ie, tells stories that are untrue)
Listen for relevance and organization of thoughts.	Logical sequence Makes sense; has sense of reality	Illogical sequence Flight of ideas; confusion

HEIGHT AND WEIGHT

In adults, the ratio of weight to height provides a general measure of health. By asking clients about their height and weight before actually measuring them, the nurse obtains some idea of the person's self-image. Excessive discrepancies between the client's responses and the measurements may provide clues to actual or potential problems in self-concept. It is also important that the nurse and client be aware of any weight gains or losses over a specific time period.

The nurse measures height with a measuring stick attached to weight scales or to a wall. The client removes the shoes and stands erect, with heels together, buttocks and head against the measuring stick, and eyes looking straight ahead. The nurse raises the L-shaped sliding arm on the weight scale until it rests on top of the client's head, or places a small flat object, such as a ruler or book, on the client's head. The edge of the ruler should abut the measuring guide. More accurate results can be obtained with a right-angled instrument.

Weight is usually measured when a client is admitted to a health agency and often regularly, for example, each morning before breakfast. When accuracy is essential, the nurse should use the same scale each time (because every scale weighs differently), take the measurements at the same time each day, and make sure the client wears the same kind of clothing and no shoes. The client stands on a platform, and the weight is read from a digital display panel or a balancing arm. Clients who cannot stand are weighed on bed and chair scales. The bed scales have canvas straps or a stretcherlike apparatus. A machine lifts the client above the bed, and the weight is reflected either on a digital display panel or on a balance arm like that of a standing scale.

Standardized charts reflect average heights and weights of children and adults. It is important to remember that standardized charts reflect average heights and weights and provide only general guidelines for assessing growth, development, and nutritional status.

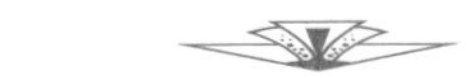

THE INTEGUMENT

The integument includes the skin, hair, and nails. The examination begins with a generalized inspection using a good source of lighting, preferably indirect natural daylight.

SKIN

Assessment of the skin involves inspection and palpation. In some instances, the nurse may also need to use the olfactory sense to detect unusual skin odors; these are usually most evident in the skinfolds or in the axillae. Pungent body odor is frequently related to poor hygiene, **hyperhidrosis** (excessive perspiration), or **bromhidrosis** (foul-smelling perspiration). The entire skin surface may be assessed at one time or as each aspect of the body is assessed.

Pallor may be difficult to determine in clients with dark skin. It is usually characterized by the absence of underlying red tones in the skin and may be most readily seen in the buccal mucosa. In brown-skinned clients, pallor may appear as a yellowish brown tinge; in black-skinned clients, the skin may appear ashen gray. Pallor in people with light skins may also be evident in the face, the conjunctiva of the eyes, and the nails. **Cyanosis** (a bluish tinge) is most evident in the nail beds, lips, and buccal mucosa. In dark-skinned clients, close inspection of the palpebral conjunctiva (the lining of the eyelids) and palms and soles may also show evidence of cyanosis. **Jaundice** (a yellowish tinge) may first be evident in the sclera of the eyes and then in the mucous membranes and the skin. Nurses should take care not to confuse jaundice with the normal yellow pigmentation in the sclera of a dark-skinned or black client. In these clients, the best place to inspect is the part of the sclera that is observable when the eye is open. If jaundice is suspected, the posterior part of the hard palate should also be inspected for a yellowish color tone. **Erythema** is a redness associated with a variety of rashes.

Dark-skinned clients have areas of lighter pigmentation, such as the palms, lips, and nail beds. Localized areas of hyperpigmentation (increased pigmentation) and hypopigmentation (decreased pigmentation) may also occur as a result of changes in the distribution of **melanin** (the dark pigment) or in the function of the melanocytes in the epidermis. An example of hyperpigmentation in a defined area is a birthmark; an example of hypopigmentation is vitiligo. **Vitiligo,** seen as patches of hypopigmented skin, is caused by the destruction of melanocytes in the area. *Albinism* is the complete or partial lack of melanin in the skin, hair, and eyes. Other localized color changes may indicate a problem such as edema or a localized infection. **Edema** is the presence of excess interstitial fluid. An area of edema appears swollen, shiny, and taut and tends to blanch the skin color. Edema is most often an indication of impaired venous circulation and in some cases reflects cardiac dysfunction or vein abnormalities.

A skin lesion is a traumatic or pathologic interruption of the skin. There are many kinds of lesions. Nurses must observe the location (eg, face), distribution (ie, body region or location), configuration (the arrangement or position of several lesions) as well as color, shape, size, firmness, texture, and characteristics of individual lesions. See Table 22–5 for the different types of skin lesions. Procedure 22–2 describes how to assess the skin.

GUIDE TO

Selected Skin Lesions

Nurses are responsible for describing skin lesions accurately, as shown below. Medical diagnoses are given in parentheses. See also Table 22–5 on page 475.

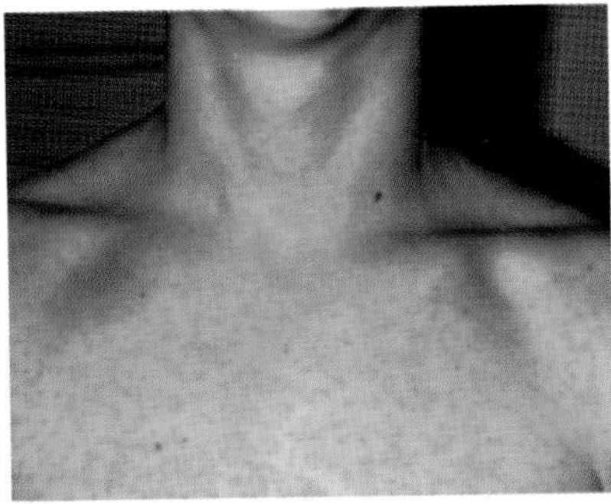

Diffuse discreet erythematous macules (rubella)

Diffuse varying-sized, confluent maculo-papular lesions (rubeola)

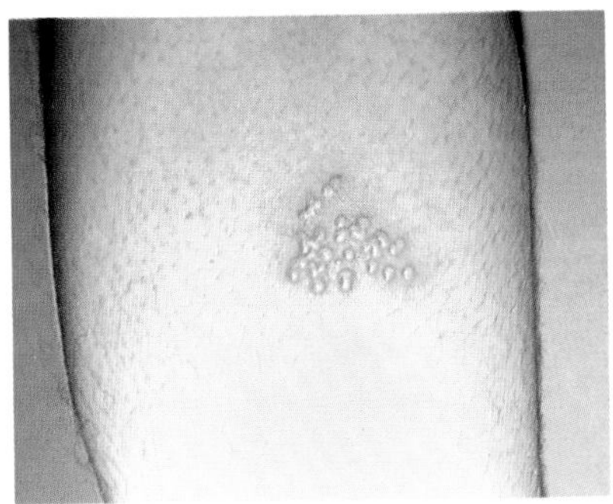

Clustered vesicles on an erythematous base (herpes simplex)

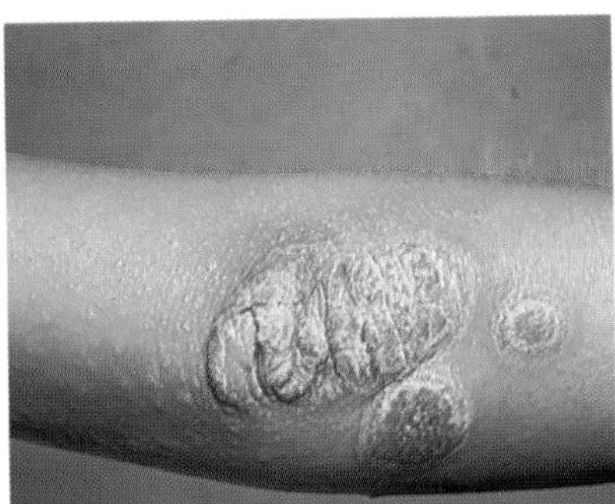

Grouped thick, silvery, scaly plaques (psoriasis)

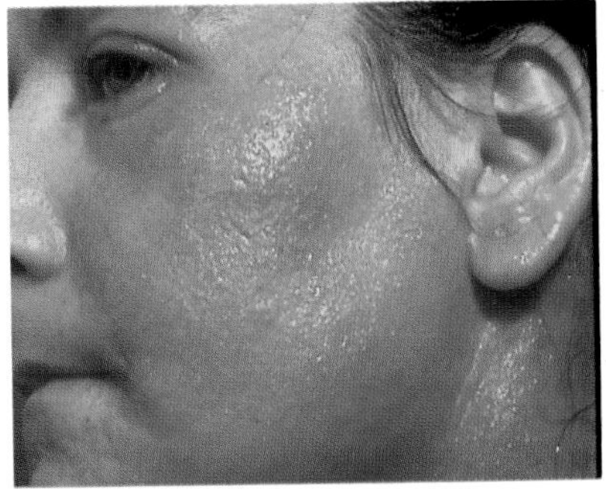

Diffuse edematous, bright erythema (contact dermatitis)

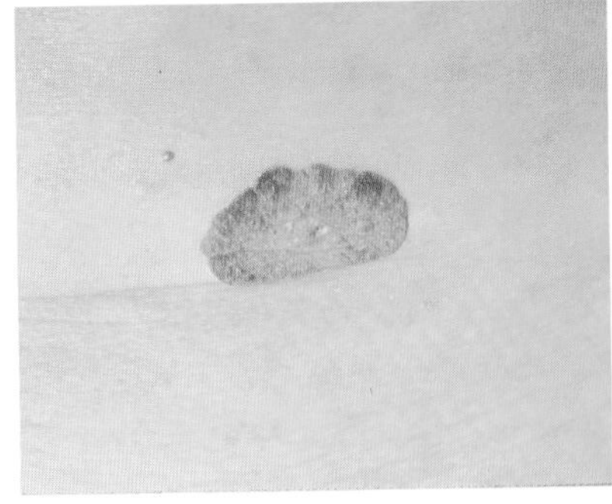

Circumscribed, oval, mottled, brown, slightly elevated lesion (sebborheic keratosis)

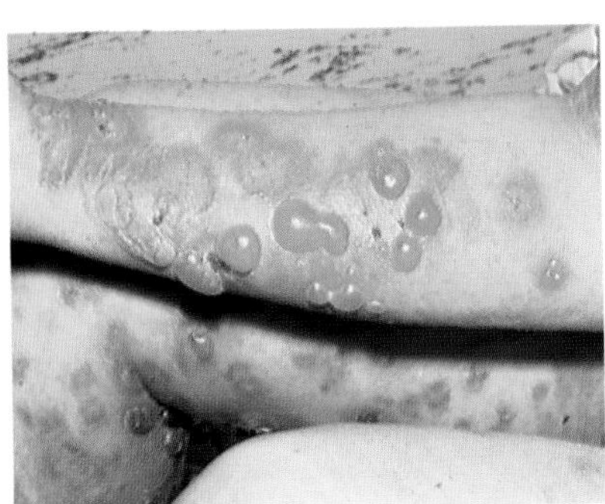

Grouped giant blisters on non-erythematous base (bullous pemphigoid)

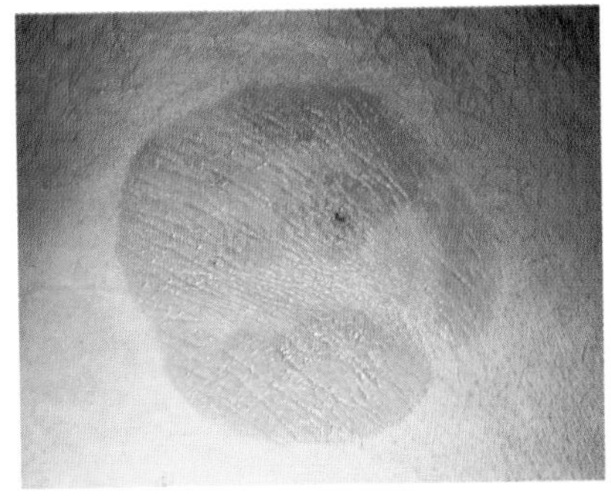

Coin-like, circumscribed, slightly elevated erythematous lesion (mycosis fungoides)

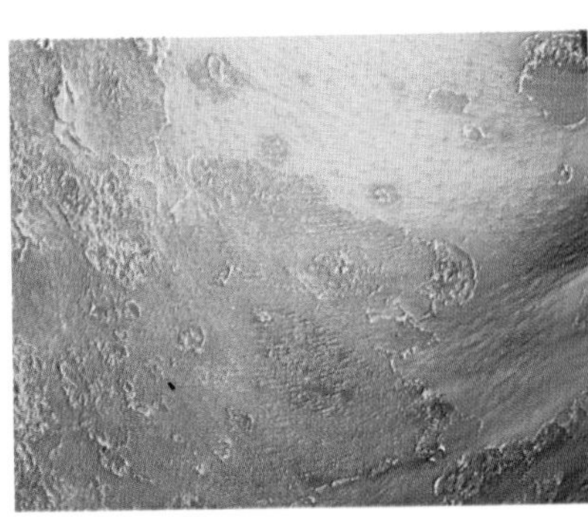

Irregular, varying-sized, pale erythematous patches with superficial fine scaling (pemphigus foliaceus)

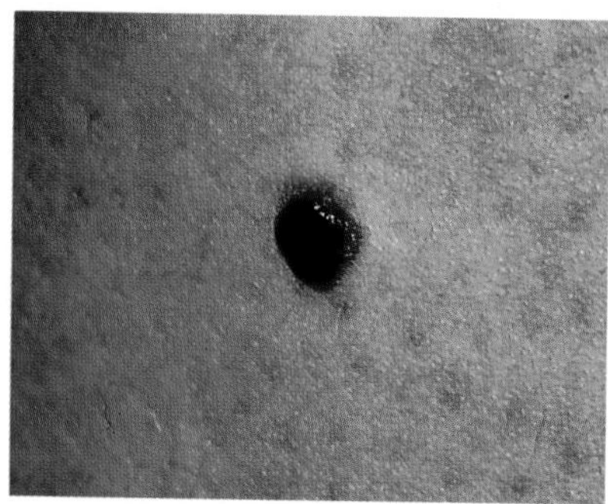

Solitary, deep brown, one-half inch nodule exhibiting a pale halo (malignant melanoma)

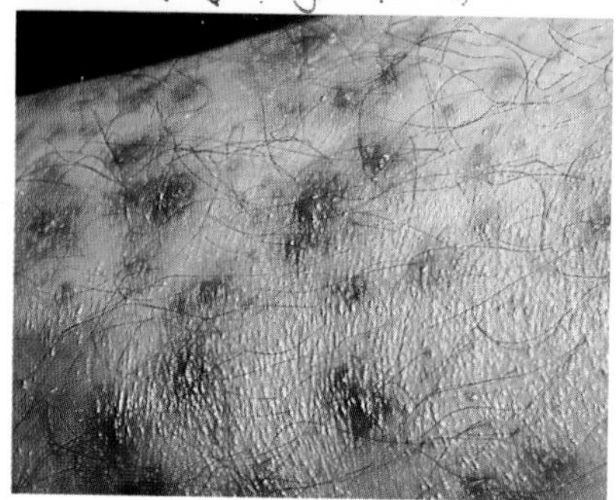

Purple discoloration with petechiae and ecchymoses (Henoch-Schönlein purpura)

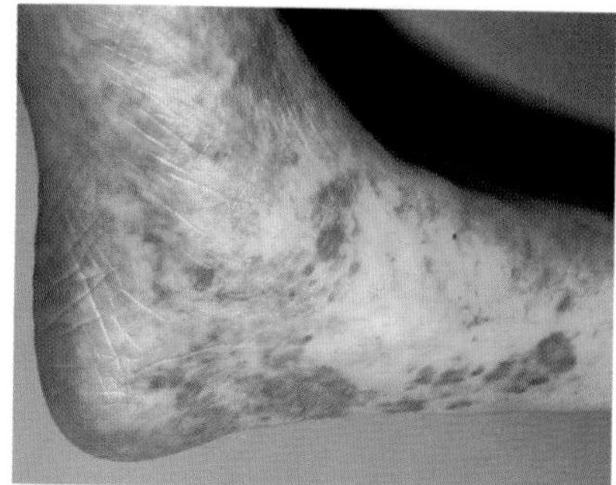

Extensive erythematous patches with small hemorrhagic nodules (Kaposi's sarcoma)

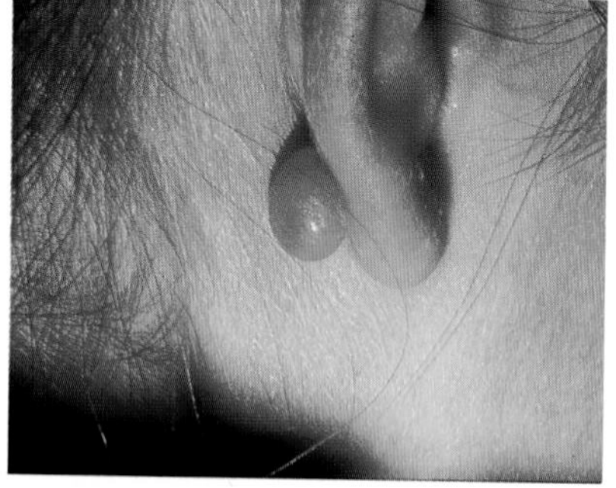

Solitary circumscribed, smooth, lentil-like papilloma (keloid)

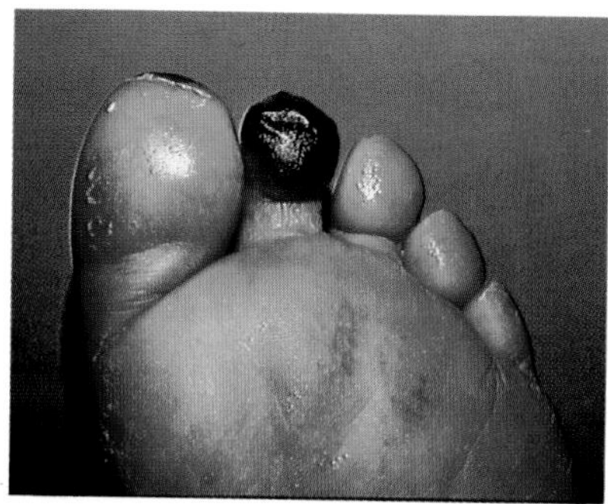

Distal half of toe exhibiting gangrene

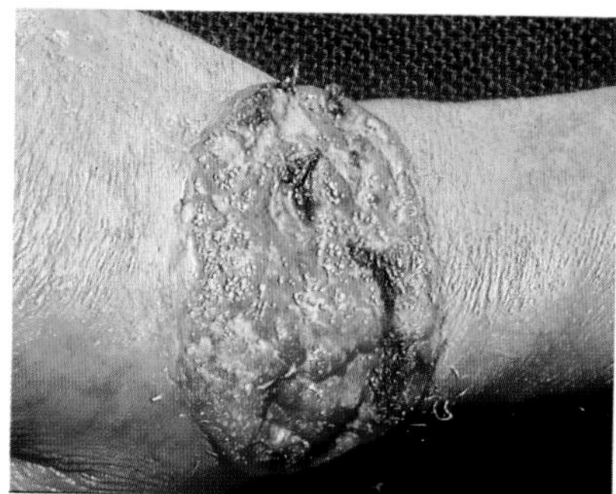

Fungating, ulcerating tumor exhibiting suppuration and necrosis (squamous cell carcinoma)

Decubitus Ulcers

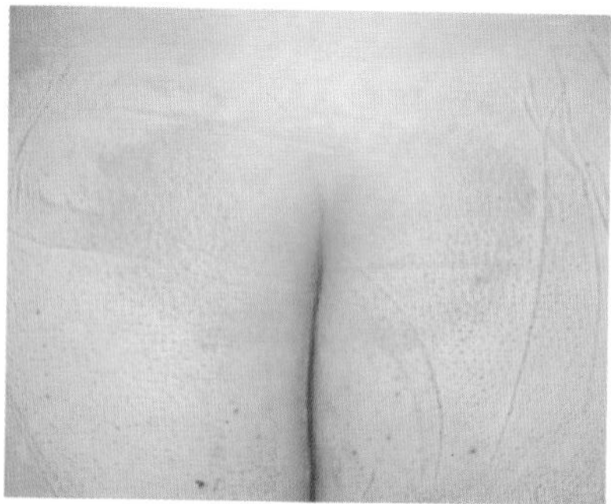

Stage I Non-blanchable erythema signalling potential ulceration

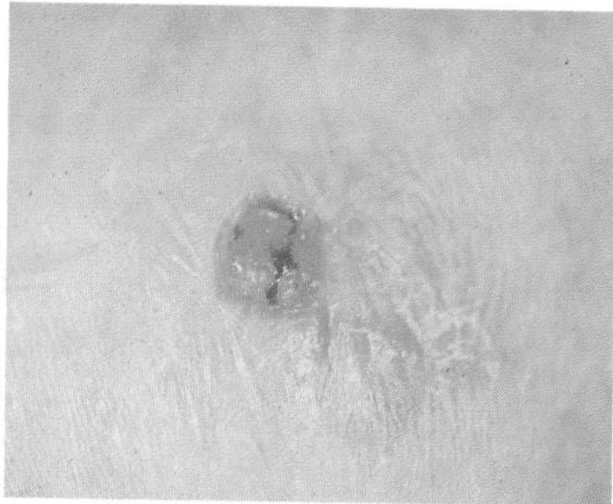

Stage II Abrasion, blister, or shallow crater involving the epidermis and possibly the dermis

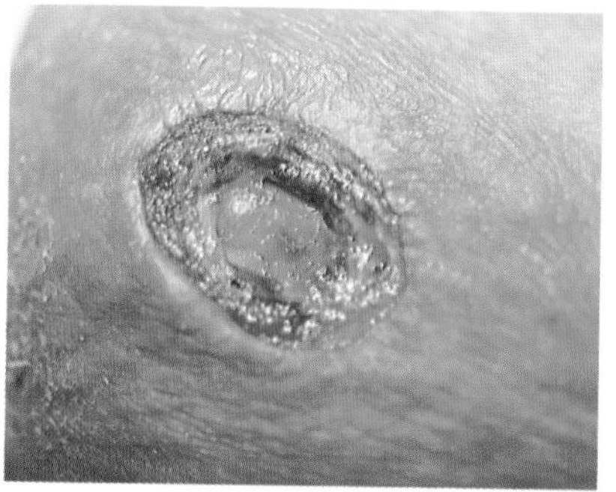

Stage III Deep ulcer exhibiting necrotic tissue and extending through the subcutaneous layer

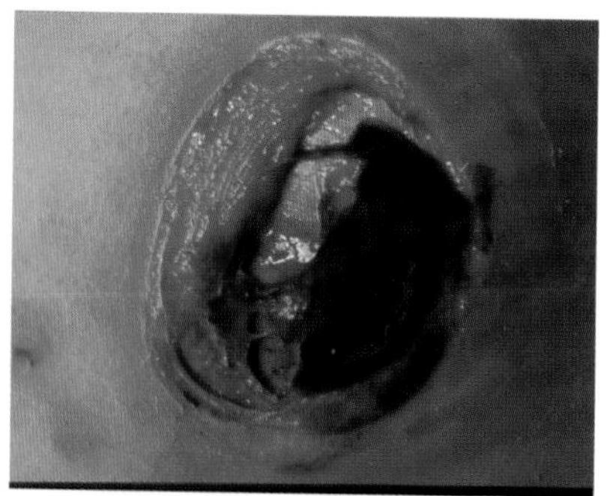

Stage IV Tissue necrosis and damage involving muscle, bone, or supporting structures

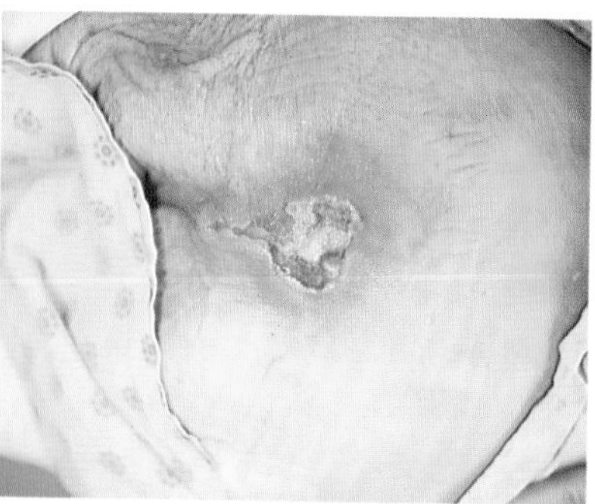

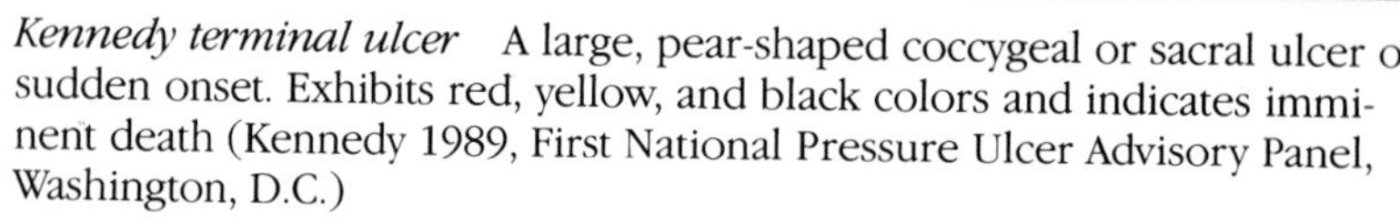

Kennedy terminal ulcer A large, pear-shaped coccygeal or sacral ulcer of sudden onset. Exhibits red, yellow, and black colors and indicates imminent death (Kennedy 1989, First National Pressure Ulcer Advisory Panel, Washington, D.C.)

Table 22–5 Skin Lesions

Type of Lesion	Description	Examples
Primary		
Macule	A flat, circumscribed area of color with no elevation of its surface; 1 mm to 1 cm	Freckles, flat nevi (moles)
Patch	Same as macule, but larger than 1 cm	Port wine birthmark
Papule	A circumscribed, solid elevation of skin; less than 1 cm	Warts, acne, pimples
Plaque	Same as papule, but larger than 1 cm	Eczema
Nodule	A solid mass that extends deeper into the dermis than does a papule	Pigmented nevi
Tumor	A solid mass larger than a nodule	Epitheliomas
Vesicle	A circumscribed elevation containing serous fluid or blood; less than 1 cm	Blister, chickenpox
Bulla	A larger fluid-filled vesicle	Blister, second-degree burns
Pustule	A vesicle or bulla filled with pus	Acne vulgaris, impetigo
Wheal	A relatively reddened, elevated, localized collection of edema fluid; irregular in shape	Mosquito bites, hives
Telangiectasia	Dilated capillary; fine red lines	Seen chiefly in pregnancy and cirrhosis of the liver
Petechiae	Pinpoint red spots	May indicate a problem in blood-clotting mechanisms
Secondary		
Scale	Thickened epidermal cells that flake off	Dandruff, psoriasis
Crust	Dried serum or pus on the skin surface	Impetigo, scab on abrasion
Fissure	A linear crack	Athlete's foot
Erosion	Loss of all or part of the epidermis	Chickenpox and smallpox following rupture
Excoriation	Linear or hollowed out crusted area exposing dermis	Scratch, abrasion
Atrophy	A decrease in the volume of epidermis	Striae, aged skin
Scar	A formation of connective tissue	Healed wound
Ulcer	An excavation extending into the dermis or below	Stasis ulcer

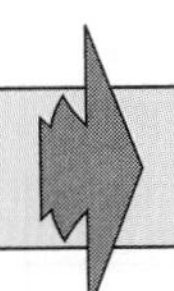

PROCEDURE 22–2 ASSESSING THE SKIN

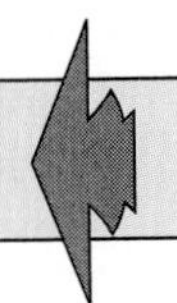

NURSING HISTORY FOCUS

Pain or itching; presence and spread of any lesions, bruises, abrasions, pigmented spots; previous experience with skin problems; associated clinical signs; family history; presence of problems in other family members; related systemic conditions; use of medications, lotions, home remedies; excessively dry or moist feel to the skin; tendency to bruise easily; any association of the problem to season of year, stress, occupation, medications, recent travel, housing, personal contact, and so on; any recent contact with allergens (eg, metal paint).

ASSESSMENT	NORMAL FINDINGS	DEVIATIONS FROM NORMAL
Inspect skin color (best assessed under natural light and on areas not exposed to the sun).	Varies from light to deep brown; from ruddy pink to light pink; from yellow overtones to olive	Pallor, cyanosis, jaundice, erythema

➤

PROCEDURE 22–2 ASSESSING THE SKIN *continued*

ASSESSMENT	NORMAL FINDINGS	DEVIATIONS FROM NORMAL
Inspect uniformity of skin color.	Generally uniform except in areas exposed to the sun; areas of lighter pigmentation (palms, lips, nail beds) in dark-skinned people	Areas of either hyperpigmentation or hypopigmentation (eg, vitiligo, albinism, edema)
Assess edema, if present (ie, location, color, temperature, shape, and the degree to which the skin remains indented or pitted when pressed by a finger).	**Scale for Describing Edema** 1+ Barely detectable 2+ Indentation of less than 5 mm 3+ Indentation of 5 to 10 mm 4+ Indentation of more than 10 mm	
Inspect, palpate, and describe skin lesions (see Table 22–5). Palpate lesions to determine shape and texture. Describe lesions according to type or structure, color, distribution, and configuration.	Freckles, some birthmarks, some flat and raised nevi (moles); no abrasions or other lesions	Various interruptions in skin integrity

Describing Skin Lesions

- *Type or structure.* Skin lesions are classified as *primary* (those that appear initially in response to some change in the external or internal environment of the skin) and *secondary* (those that do not appear initially but result from modifications such as chronicity, trauma, or infection of the primary lesion). For example, a vesicle (primary lesion) may rupture and cause an erosion (secondary lesion).
- *Color.* There may be no discoloration, one discrete color (eg, red, brown, or black), or several colors, as with *ecchymosis* (a bruise), in which an initial dark red or blue color fades to a yellow color. When color changes are limited to the edges of a lesion, they are described as *circumscribed;* when spread over a large area, they are described as *diffuse.*
- *Distribution.* Distribution is described according to the location of the lesions on the body and symmetry or asymmetry of findings in comparable body areas.
- *Configuration.* Configuration refers to the arrangement of lesions in relation to each other. Configurations of lesions may be annular (arranged in a circle); clustered together or grouped; linear (arranged in a line); arc- or bow-shaped; merged together, or indiscrete; follow the course of cutaneous nerves; or meshed in the form of a network.

ASSESSMENT	NORMAL FINDINGS	DEVIATIONS FROM NORMAL
Observe and palpate skin moisture.	Moisture in skinfolds and the axillae (varies with environmental temperature and humidity, body temperature, and activity)	Excessive moisture (eg, in hyperthermia); excessive dryness (eg, in dehydration)
Palpate skin temperature. Compare the two feet and the two hands, using the backs of your fingers.	Uniform; within normal range	Generalized hyperthermia (eg, in fever); generalized hypothermia (eg, in shock); localized hyperthermia (eg, in infection); localized hypothermia (eg, in arteriosclerosis)

PROCEDURE 22–2 *continued*

ASSESSMENT	NORMAL FINDINGS	DEVIATIONS FROM NORMAL
Note skin turgor (fullness or elasticity) by lifting and pinching the skin on an extremity.	When pinched, skin springs back to previous state	Skins stays pinched or tented or moves back slowly (eg, in dehydration)

THE ELDERLY: PHYSICAL CHANGES OF THE SKIN

- Aging changes of the skin result from many factors: enzymatic changes in connective and epithelial tissues, heredity, inadequate nutrition from vascular changes, endocrine changes, and environmental factors (eg, exposure to the elements).
- The skin loses its elasticity and wrinkles. Wrinkles first appear on the skin of the face and neck, which are abundant in collagen and elastic fibers.
- The skin appears thin and translucent because of loss of dermis and subcutaneous fat. Atrophy of the epidermal structures results from degeneration of collagen and elastin.
- The skin is dry and flaky because sebaceous and sweat glands are less active. Dry skin is more prominent over the extremities, where circulation is not as efficient.
- The skin takes longer to return to its natural shape after being pinched between the thumb and finger. Because there is loss of skin turgor over the extremities, the skin of the forehead is recommended for the pinch-fold test for dehydration.
- Flat tan to brown-colored macules, referred to as *senile lentigines* or *melanotic freckles,* may appear on skin areas that are exposed to the sun. These macules may be as large as 1 to 2 centimeters. They occur because cells lose their ability to spread out melanin.
- Warty lesions (*seborrheic keratosis*) with irregularly shaped borders and a scaly surface often occur on the face, shoulders, and trunk.
- Vitiligo tends to increase with age and is thought to result from an autoimmune response.
- Cutaneous tags (*acrochordons*) are most commonly seen in the neck and axillary regions. These skin lesions vary in size and are soft, often flesh colored, and pedicled.
- Visible, bright red, fine dilated blood vessels (*telangiectasias*) commonly occur as a result of the thinning of the dermis and the loss of support for the blood vessel walls.
- Pink to slightly red lesions with indistinct borders (*actinic keratoses*) may appear at about age 50, often on the face, ears, backs of the hands, and arms. They often become malignant.

HAIR

Assessing a client's hair includes inspecting the hair, considering developmental changes, and determining the individual's hair care practices and the factors influencing them. Much of the information about hair can be obtained by questioning the client.

Normal hair is resilient and evenly distributed. In people with severe protein deficiency (kwashiorkor), the hair color is faded and appears reddish or bleached, and the texture is coarse and dry. Some therapies for cancer cause **alopecia** (hair loss), and some disease conditions affect the coarseness of hair. Procedure 22–3 describes how to assess the hair.

NAILS

Parts of the nail are shown in Figure 22–4 on page 478. Nails are inspected for nail plate shape, angle between the nail and the nail bed, nail texture, nail bed color, and the intactness of the tissues around the nails.

The nail plate is normally colorless and a convex curve. The angle between the nail and the nail bed is normally 160 degrees (Figure 22–5, *A*, on page 479). One nail abnormality is the spoon shape. Here, the nail curves upward from the nail bed (Figure 22–5, *B*). This condition, called **koilonychia,** may be seen in clients with iron deficiency anemia. **Clubbing** is a condition in which the angle between the nail and the nail bed is 180 degrees or greater (Figure 22–5, *C* and *D*). Clubbing may be caused by long-term oxygen lack and is seen in the elderly.

Nail texture is normally smooth. Excessively thick nails can appear in the elderly or in the presence of poor circulation; excessively thin nails or the presence of grooves

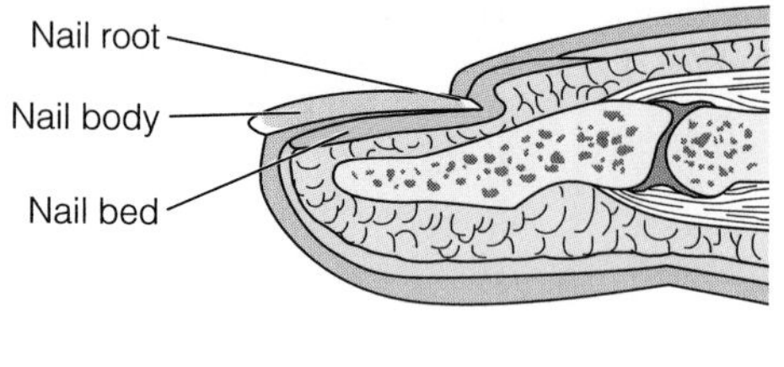

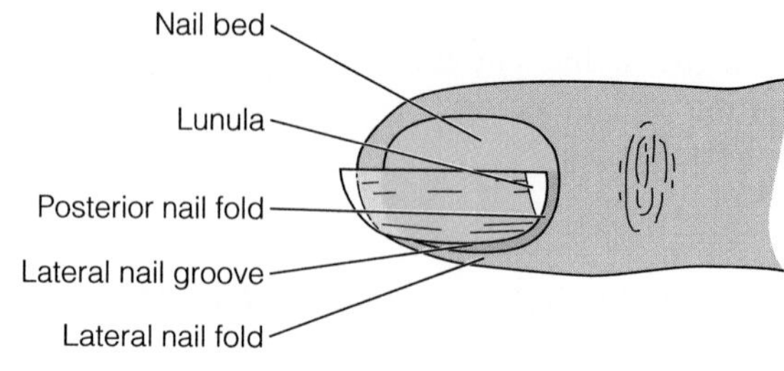

Figure 22–4 The parts of a nail.

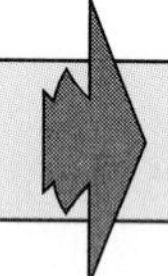

PROCEDURE 22–3 ASSESSING THE HAIR

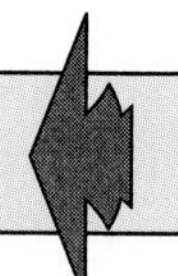

NURSING HISTORY FOCUS

Recent use of hair dyes, rinses, or curling or straightening preparations; recent chemotherapy (if alopecia is present); presence of disease, such as hypothyroidism, which can be associated with dry, brittle hair.

ASSESSMENT	NORMAL FINDINGS	DEVIATIONS FROM NORMAL
Inspect the evenness of growth over the scalp.	Evenly distributed hair	Patches of hair loss (ie, alopecia)
Inspect hair thickness or thinness.	Thick hair	Very thin hair (eg, in hypothyroidism)
Inspect hair texture and oiliness.	Silky, resilient hair	Brittle hair (eg, in hypothyroidism); excessively oily or dry hair
Note presence of infections or infestations by parting the hair in several areas.	No infection or infestation	Flaking, sores, lice, nits (louse eggs), and ringworm
Inspect amount of body hair.	Variable	**Hirsutism** (excessive hairiness) in women and children

THE ELDERLY: PHYSICAL CHANGES OF THE HAIR

- The age at which the scalp hair grays is influenced largely by genetic factors.
- There is loss of scalp, pubic, and axillary hair.
- In women, the hair of the eyebrows and some facial hair become coarse.
- Hairs of the eyebrows, ears, and nostrils become bristlelike and coarse.

or furrows can reflect prolonged iron-deficiency anemia. *Beau's lines* are horizontal depressions in the nail that can result from injury or severe illness (Figure 22–5, *E*).

The nail bed is highly vascular, a characteristic that accounts for its pink color in white people. In blacks, brown or black pigmentation in longitudinal streaks or along the edge of the nail bed may normally be present. A bluish or purplish tint to the nail bed may reflect cyanosis, and pallor may reflect poor arterial circulation.

The tissue surrounding the nails is normally intact epidermis. **Paronychia** is an inflammation of the tissues surrounding a nail. The tissues appear inflamed and swollen, and tenderness is usually present.

A **blanch test** can be carried out to test the capillary refill, that is, peripheral circulation. Normal nail bed capillaries blanch when pressed but quickly turn pink (in light-skinned people) or their usual color when pressure is released. In dark-skinned people, the rate of return of nail bed color may be more significant than the color. A slow rate of capillary refill may indicate circulatory problems. Procedure 22–4 describes how to assess the nails.

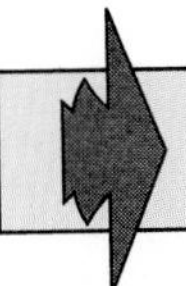

PROCEDURE 22–4 ASSESSING THE NAILS

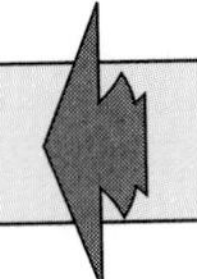

NURSING HISTORY FOCUS

Presence of diabetes mellitus, peripheral circulatory disease, previous injury, or severe illness.

ASSESSMENT	NORMAL FINDINGS	DEVIATIONS FROM NORMAL
Inspect nail plate shape to determine its curvature and angle.	Convex curvature; angle between nail and nail bed of about 160 degrees (Figure 22–5, *A*)	Spoon nail (Figure 22–5, *B*); clubbing (180 degrees or greater) (Figure 22–5, *C* and *D*)
Inspect nail texture.	Smooth texture	Excessive thickness (eg, result of poor circulation, iron deficiency anemia); excessive thinness or presence of grooves or furrows (eg, in iron deficiency anemia); Beau's lines (transverse white lines or grooves; Figure 22–5, *E*)

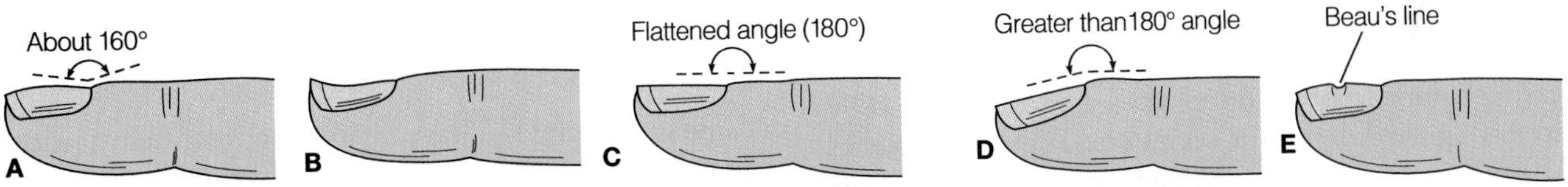

Figure 22–5 *A,* A normal nail, showing the convex shape and the nail plate angle of about 160 degrees; *B,* a spoon-shaped nail, which may be seen in clients with iron deficiency anemia; *C,* early clubbing; *D,* late clubbing (may be caused by long-term oxygen lack); *E,* Beau's line on nail (may result from severe injury or illness).

ASSESSMENT	NORMAL FINDINGS	DEVIATIONS FROM NORMAL
Inspect nail bed color.	Highly vascular and pink in light-skinned clients; dark-skinned clients may have brown or black pigmentation in longitudinal streaks	Bluish or purplish tint (may reflect cyanosis); pallor (may reflect poor arterial circulation)
Inspect tissues surrounding nails.	Intact epidermis	Hangnails; paronychia (inflammation)
Perform blanch test to test capillary refill. Press two or more nails between your thumb and index finger; look for blanching and return of usual color to nail bed.	Prompt return of pink or usual color	Delayed return of pink or usual color (may indicate circulatory impairment)

PROCEDURE 22–4 ASSESSING THE NAILS *continued*

THE ELDERLY: PHYSICAL CHANGES OF THE NAILS

- The nails grow more slowly and thicken.
- Longitudinal bands commonly develop, and the nails tend to split.
- Bands across the nails may indicate protein deficiency; white spots, zinc deficiency; and spoon shaped nails, iron deficiency.

HEAD

During an examination of the head, the nurse often inspects and palpates simultaneously, as well as auscultating. The nurse examines the skull, face, eyes, ears, nose, sinuses, mouth, and pharynx.

THE SKULL AND FACE

There is a large range of normal shapes of skulls. A normal head size is referred to as **normocephalic.** Names of areas of the head are derived from names of the underlying bones: frontal, parietal, occipital, mastoid process, mandible, maxilla, and zygomatic (Figure 22–6).

In adults, a large head may result from osteitis deformans or from acromegaly. **Osteitis deformans (Paget's disease)** is a disorder in which bony thickness increases. The skull, spine, pelvis, and femur are the usual sites of involvement. When the skull is involved, it appears enlarged, with prominent superficial veins, and often the hearing is impaired. **Acromegaly** is a disorder caused by excessive growth hormone secretion. The skull becomes thickened and enlarged, mandible length increases, the nose and forehead become more prominent, and the facial features look coarsened.

Many disorders cause a change in facial shape or condition. Kidney or cardiac disease can cause edema of the eyelids. Thyroid overactivity (hyperthyroidism) can cause **exophthalmus,** a protrusion of the eyeballs with elevation of the upper eyelids, resulting in a startled or staring expression. Thyroid underactivity (hypothyroidism, or **myxedema**) can cause a dry, puffy face with dry skin and coarse features, referred to as **myxedema facies,** and thinning of scalp hair and eyebrows. **Cushing's syndrome,** a disorder in which there is increased adrenal hormone production, can cause a round face with reddened cheeks, referred to as **moon face,** and excessive hair growth on the upper lips, chin, and sideburn areas. Intake of synthetic adrenal hormones also produces these changes. Prolonged illness, starvation, and dehydration can result in sunken eyes, cheeks, and temples.

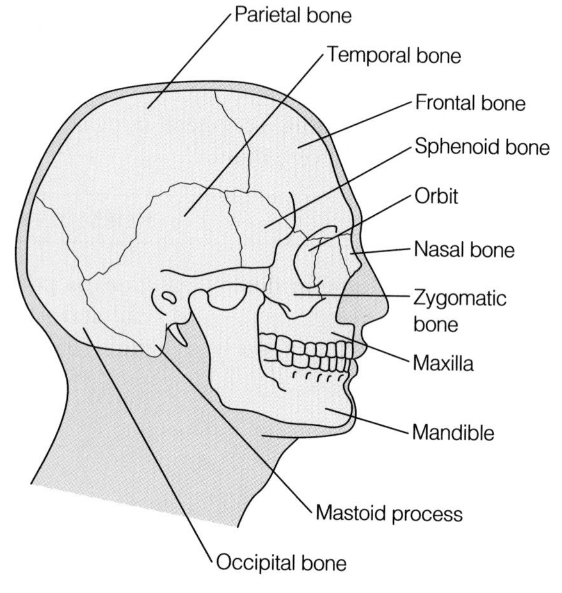

Figure 22–6 The bones of the head.

Procedure 22–5 describes how to assess the skull and face.

THE EYES AND VISION

Many people consider vision the most important sense because it allows them to interact freely with their environment and enjoy the beauty of life around them. To maintain optimum vision, people need to have their eyes examined throughout life. It is recommended that people under age 40 have their eyes tested every 3 to 5 years, or more frequently if there is a family history of diabetes, hypertension, blood dyscrasia, or eye disease (eg, glaucoma). After age 40, an eye examination is recommended every 2 years to rule out the possibility of glaucoma.

An eye assessment should be carried out as part of the client's initial physical examination; periodic reassess-

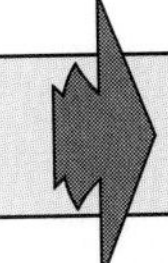

PROCEDURE 22–5 ASSESSING THE SKULL AND FACE

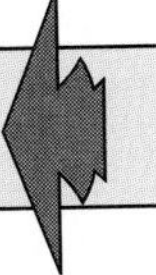

NURSING HISTORY FOCUS

Any past problems with lumps or bumps, itching, scaling, or dandruff; any history of loss of consciousness, dizziness, seizures, headache, facial pain, or injury; when and how any lumps occurred; length of time any other problem existed; any known cause of problem; associated symptoms, treatment, and recurrences.

ASSESSMENT	NORMAL FINDINGS	DEVIATIONS FROM NORMAL
Inspect the skull for size, shape, and symmetry. If skull is of abnormal size, measure its circumference just above the eyebrows.	Rounded (normocephalic and symmetric, with frontal, parietal, and occipital prominences); smooth skull contour	Lack of symmetry; increased skull size with more prominent nose and forehead; longer mandible (may indicate excessive growth hormone or increased bone thickness)
Palpate the skull for nodules or masses and depressions. Use a gentle rotating motion with the fingertips. Begin at the front and palpate down the midline, then palpate each side of the head.	Smooth, uniform consistency; absence of nodules or masses	Sebaceous cysts; local deformities from trauma
Inspect the facial features (eg, symmetry of structures and of the distribution of hair).	Symmetric or slightly asymmetric facial features; palpebral fissures equal in size; symmetric nasolabial folds	Increased facial hair; thinning of eyebrows; asymmetric features; exophthalmus; myxedema facies; moon face
Inspect the eyes for edema and hollowness.		Periorbital edema; sunken eyes
Note symmetry of facial movements. Ask the client to elevate the eyebrows, frown, or lower the eyebrows, close the eyes tightly, puff the cheeks, and smile and show the teeth. See Table 22–13 on page 545.	Symmetric facial movements	Asymmetric facial movements (eg, eye on affected side cannot close completely); drooping of lower eyelid and mouth; involuntary facial movements (ie, tics or tremors)

ments need to be made for long-term care clients. Examination of the eyes includes assessment of **visual acuity** (the degree of detail the eye can discern in an image), ocular movement, **visual fields** (the area an individual can see when looking straight ahead), and external structures. Most eye assessment procedures involve inspection. Consideration is also given to developmental changes and to individual hygienic practices, if the client wears contact lenses or an artificial eye. For the anatomic structures of the eye, see Figures 22–7 and 22–8 on page 482.

Many people wear eyeglasses or contact lenses to correct common refractive errors of the lens of the eye. These errors include **myopia** (nearsightedness), **hyperopia** (farsightedness), and **presbyopia** (loss of elasticity of the lens and thus loss of ability to see close objects). Presbyopia begins at about 45 years of age. People notice that they have difficulty reading newsprint. Often two corrective lenses (bifocals) are required—one for near vision or reading, the other for far vision. **Astigmatism,** an uneven curvature of the cornea that prevents horizontal and vertical rays from focusing on the retina, is a common problem that may occur in conjunction with myopia and hyperopia.

Three types of eye charts are available to test visual acuity (Figure 22–9, p. 482). The child acquires normal 20/20 vision by 6 years of age. Persons with denominators of 40 or more on the Snellen chart with or without corrective lenses need to be referred to an opthalmologist.

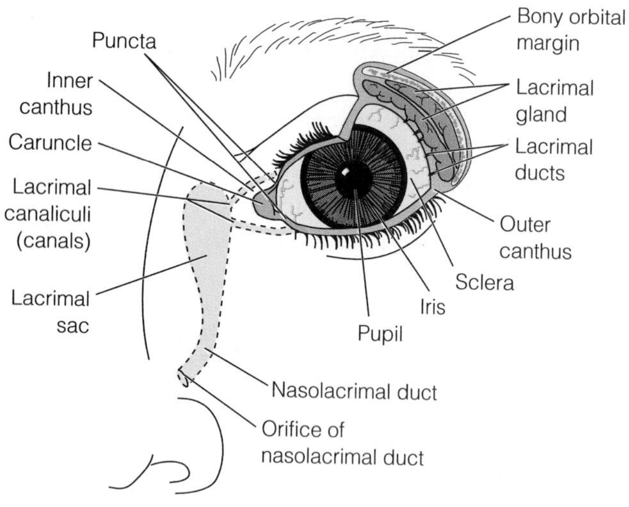

Figure 22–7 The external structures and lacrimal apparatus of the left eye.

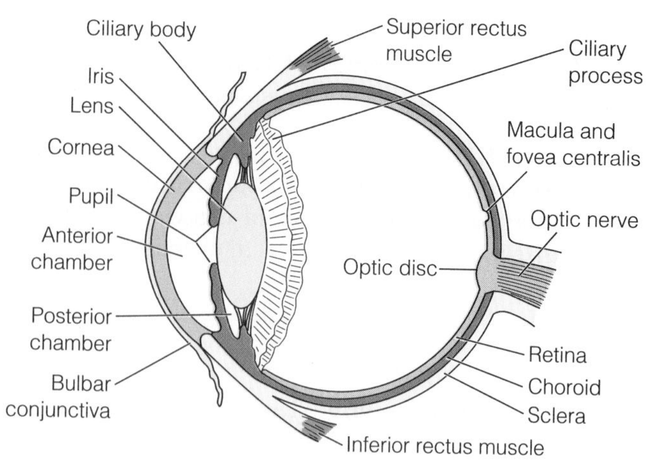

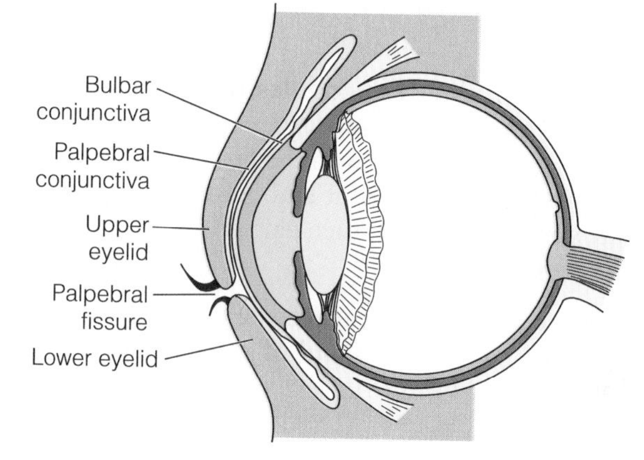

Figure 22–8 Anatomic structures of the right eye, lateral view.

Common inflammatory visual problems that nurses may encounter in clients include conjunctivitis, dacryocystitis, hordeolum, iritis, and contusions or hematomas of the eyelids and surrounding structures. **Conjunctivitis** (inflammation of the bulbar and palpebral conjunctiva) may result from foreign bodies, chemicals, allergenic agents, bacteria, or viruses. Redness, itching, tearing, and mucopurulent discharge occur. During sleep, the eyelids may become encrusted and matted together. **Dacryocystitis** (inflammation of the lacrimal sac) is manifested by tearing and a discharge from the nasolacrimal duct. **Hordeolum** (sty) is a redness, swelling, and tenderness of the hair follicle and glands that empty at the edge of the eyelids. **Iritis** (inflammation of the iris) may be caused by local or systemic infections and results in pain, tearing, and **photophobia** (sensitivity to light). **Contusions** or **hematomas** are "black eyes" resulting from injury.

Cataracts tend to occur in those over 65 years old. This opacity of the lens or its capsule, which blocks light rays, is frequently corrected by surgery. Cataracts may also occur in infants due to a malformation of the lens if the mother contracted rubella in the first trimester of pregnancy. **Glaucoma** (a disturbance in the circulation of aqueous fluid, which causes an increase in intraocular pressure) is the most frequent cause of blindness in people over 40. It can be controlled if diagnosed early. Danger signs of glaucoma include blurred or foggy vision, loss of peripheral vision, difficulty focusing on close objects, difficulty adjusting to dark rooms, and seeing rainbow-colored rings around lights.

Eyelids that lie at or below the pupil margin are referred to as **ptosis** and are usually associated with aging, edema from drug allergy or systemic disease (eg, kidney

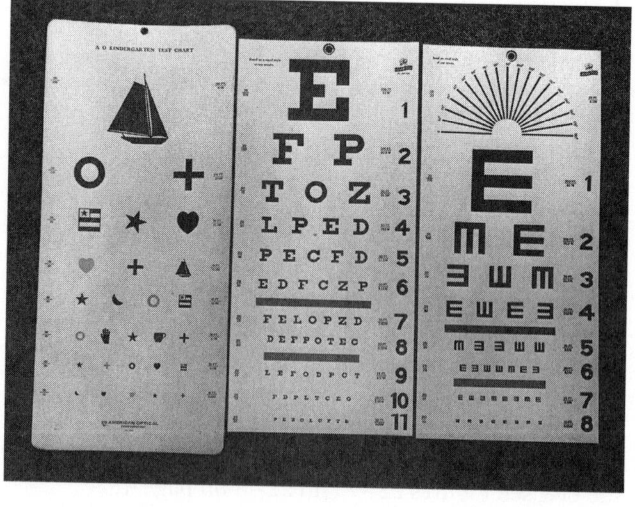

Figure 22–9 Three types of eye charts: the preschool children's chart (left), Snellen standard chart (center), and the Snellen E chart for clients unable to read (right).

disease), congenital lid muscle dysfunction, neuromuscular disease (eg, myasthenia gravis), and third cranial nerve impairment. Eversion, an outturning of the eyelid, is called **ectropion;** inversion, an inturning of the lid, is called **entropion.** These abnormalities are often associated with scarring injuries or the aging process.

Pupils are normally black, are equal in size (about 3 to 7 mm in diameter), and have round, smooth borders. Cloudy pupils are often indicative of cataracts. Enlarged pupils **(mydriasis)** may indicate injury or glaucoma, or result from certain drugs (eg, atropine). Constricted pupils **(miosis)** may indicate an inflammation of the iris or result from such drugs as morphine or pilocarpine. It is also an age-related change in older adults. Unequal pupils **(anisocoria)** may result from a central nervous system disorder; however, slight variations may be normal. The iris is normally flat and round. A bulging toward the cornea can indicate increased intraocular pressure. Procedure 22–6 describes how to assess a client's eye structures and visual acuity.

Text continued on page 491

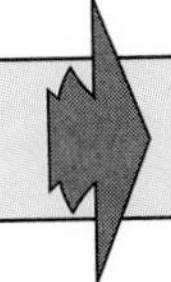

PROCEDURE 22–6 ASSESSING THE EYE STRUCTURES AND VISUAL ACUITY

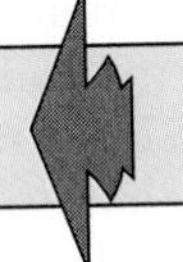

NURSING HISTORY FOCUS

Family history of diabetes, hypertension, blood dyscrasia, or eye disease, injury, or surgery; client's last visit to an ophthalmologist; current use of eye medications; use of contact lenses or eyeglasses; hygienic practices for corrective lenses; current symptoms of eye problems (eg, changes in visual acuity, blurring of vision, tearing, spots, photophobia, itching, or pain).

ASSESSMENT	NORMAL FINDINGS	DEVIATIONS FROM NORMAL
External Eye Structures		
Inspect the eyebrows for hair distribution and alignment and skin quality and movement. (Ask client to raise and lower the eyebrows.)	Hair evenly distributed; skin intact Eyebrows symmetrically aligned; equal movement	Loss of hair; scaling and flakiness of skin Unequal alignment and movement of eyebrows
Inspect the eyelashes for evenness of distribution and direction of curl.	Equally distributed; curled slightly outward	Turned inward (see box on page 484)
Inspect the eyelids for surface characteristics (eg, skin quality and texture), **position in relation to the cornea, ability to blink, and frequency of blinking.** For proper visual examination of the upper eyelids, elevate the eyebrows with your thumb and index fingers, and have the client close the eyes (Figure 22–10). Inspect the lower eyelids while the client's eyes are closed.	Skin intact; no discharge; no discoloration Lids close symmetrically Approximately 15 to 20 involuntary blinks per minute; bilateral blinking When lids open, no visible sclera above corneas, and upper and lower borders of cornea are slightly covered	Redness, swelling, flaking, crusting, plaques, discharge, nodules, lesions Lids close asymmetrically, incompletely, or painfully Rapid, monocular, absent, or infrequent blinking Ptosis, ectropion, or entropion; rim of sclera visible between lid and iris (possible hyperthyroidism)

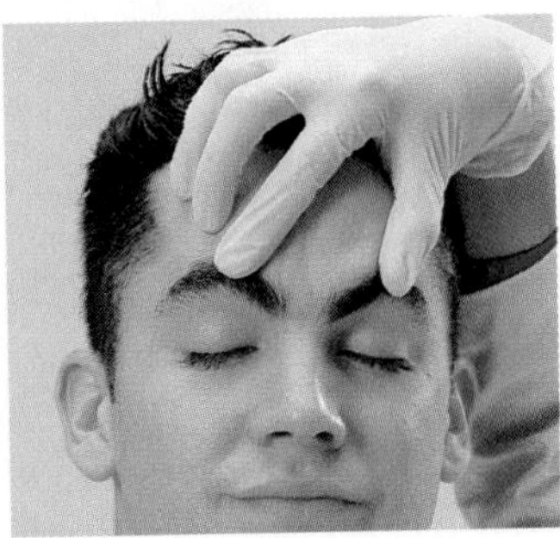

Figure 22–10 Inspecting the upper eyelids.

PROCEDURE 22–6 ASSESSING THE EYE STRUCTURES AND VISUAL ACUITY *continued*

ASSESSMENT	NORMAL FINDINGS	DEVIATIONS FROM NORMAL
External Eye Structures *continued*		
Inspect the bulbar conjunctiva (lying over the sclera) **for color, texture, and the presence of lesions.** Retract the eyelids with your thumb and index finger, exerting pressure over the upper and lower bony orbits, and ask the client to look up, down, and from side to side.	Transparent; capillaries sometimes evident; sclera appears white (yellowish in dark-skinned clients)	Jaundiced sclera (eg, in liver disease); excessively pale sclera (eg, in anemia); reddened sclera; lesions or nodules (may indicate damage by mechanical, chemical, allergenic, or bacterial agents)
Inspect the palpebral conjunctiva (lining the eyelids) **by everting the lids. Note color, texture, and the presence of lesions.** Evert both lower lids, and ask the client to look up. Then gently retract the lower lids with the index fingers.	Shiny, smooth, and pink or red	Extremely pale (possible anemia); extremely red (inflammation); nodules or other lesions
Evert the upper lids if a problem (eg, a foreign body) **is suspected.** See the box below.		

Everting the Upper Eyelid

- Ask the client to look down while keeping the eyes slightly open. *Closing the eyelids contracts the orbicular muscle, which prevents lid eversion.*
- Gently grasp the client's eyelashes with the thumb and index finger. Pull the lashes gently downward. *Upward or outward pulling on the eyelashes causes muscle contraction.*
- Place a cotton-tipped applicator stick about 1 cm above the lid margin, and push it gently downward while holding the eyelashes (Figure 22–11). These actions evert the lid, that is, flip the lower part of the lid over on top of itself.
- Hold the margin of the everted lid or the eyelashes against the ridge of the upper bony orbit with the applicator stick or the thumb (Figure 22–12).
- Inspect the conjunctiva for color, texture, lesions, and foreign bodies.
- To return the lid to its normal position, gently pull the lashes forward, and ask the client to look up and blink.

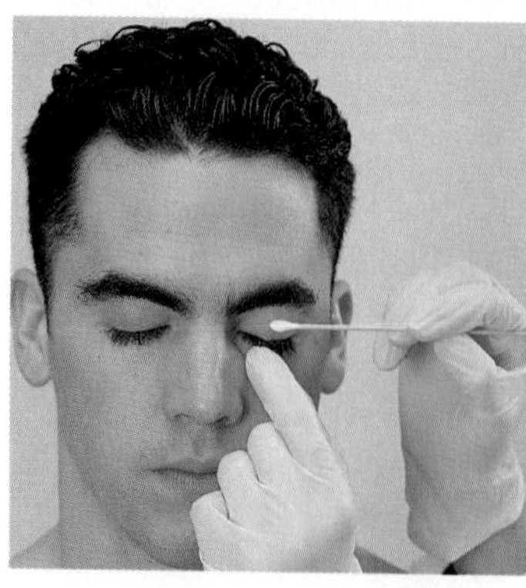

Figure 22–11 Everting the upper eyelid.

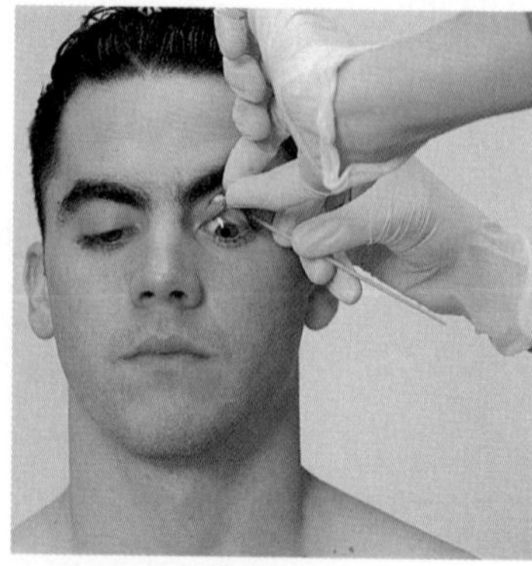

Figure 22–12 Holding the margin of the everted upper eyelid.

PROCEDURE 22-6 *continued*

ASSESSMENT	NORMAL FINDINGS	DEVIATIONS FROM NORMAL
Inspect and palpate the lacrimal gland. See the accompanying box.	No edema or tenderness over lacrimal gland	Swelling or tenderness over lacrimal gland
Inspect and palpate the lacrimal sac and nasolacrimal duct.	**No edema or tearing**	Evidence of increased tearing; regurgitation of fluid on palpation of lacrimal sac

Palpating the Lacrimal Gland, Lacrimal Sac, and Nasolacrimal Duct

- Using the tip of your index finger, palpate the lacrimal gland (Figure 22-13).
- Observe for edema between the lower lid and the nose.
- Observe for evidence of increased tearing.
- Using the tip of your index finger, palpate inside the lower orbital rim near the inner canthus (Figure 22-14).

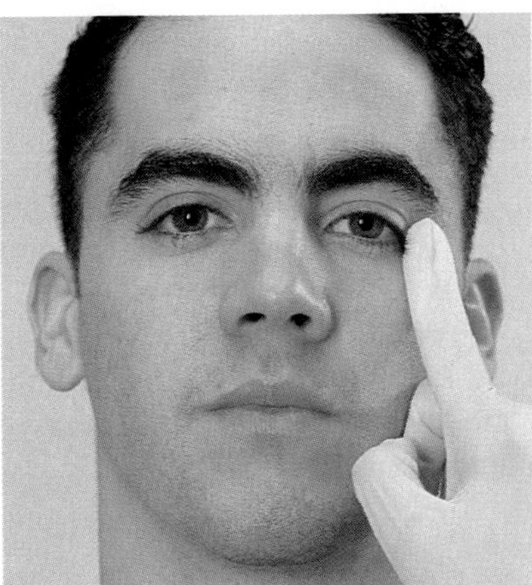

Figure 22-13 Palpating the lacrimal gland.

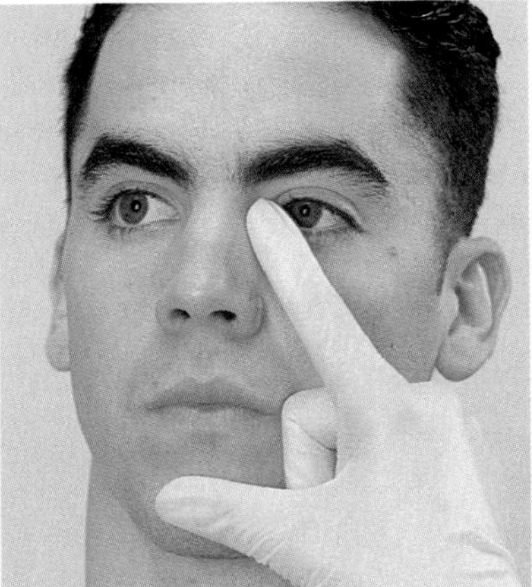

Figure 22-14 Palpating the lacrimal sac and nasolacrimal duct.

ASSESSMENT	NORMAL FINDINGS	DEVIATIONS FROM NORMAL
Inspect the cornea for clarity and texture. Ask the client to look straight ahead. Hold a penlight at an oblique angle to the eye, and move the light slowly across the corneal surface.	Transparent, shiny and smooth; details of the iris are visible In older people, a thin, grayish white ring around the margin, called arcus senilis, may be evident	Opaque; surface not smooth (may be the result of trauma or abrasion) Arcus senilis in clients under age 40 is abnormal
Perform the corneal sensitivity (reflex) test to determine the function of the fifth (trigeminal) cranial nerve. Ask the client to keep both eyes open and look straight ahead. With a wisp of cotton, approach from behind and beside the client, and lightly touch the cornea with the cotton wisp.	Client blinks when the cornea is touched, indicating that the trigeminal nerve is intact	One or both eyelids fail to respond

Procedure 22–6 Assessing the Eye Structures and Visual Acuity *continued*

ASSESSMENT	NORMAL FINDINGS	DEVIATIONS FROM NORMAL
Inspect the anterior chamber for transparency and depth. Use the same oblique lighting as used to test the cornea.	Transparent No shadows of light on iris Depth of about 3 mm	Cloudy Crescent-shaped shadows on far side of iris Shallow chamber (possible glaucoma)
Inspect the pupils for color, shape, and symmetry of size. Pupil charts are available in some agencies. See Figure 22–15 for variations in pupil diameters.	Black in color; equal in size; normally 3 to 7 mm in diameter; round, smooth border, iris flat and round	Cloudiness, mydriasis, miosis, anisocoria; bulging of iris toward cornea

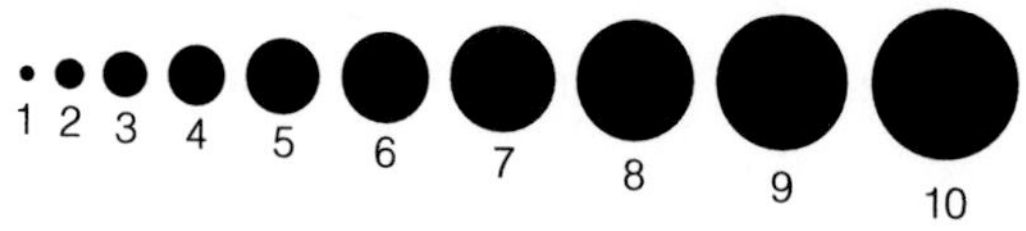

1 2 3 4 5 6 7 8 9 10

Figure 22–15 Variations in pupil diameters in millimeters.

ASSESSMENT	NORMAL FINDINGS	DEVIATIONS FROM NORMAL
Assess each pupil's direct and consensual reaction to light to determine the function of the third (oculomotor) and fourth (trochlear) cranial nerves. See the box below.	Illuminated pupil constricts (direct response) Nonilluminated pupil constricts (consensual response)	Neither pupil constricts Unequal responses Absent responses
Assess each pupil's reaction to accommodation.	Pupils constrict when looking at near object; pupils dilate when looking at far object; pupils converge when near object is moved toward nose	One or both pupils fail to constrict, dilate, or converge

Assessing Pupil Reactions

Direct and Consensual Reaction to Light

- Partially darken the room.
- Ask the client to look straight ahead.
- Using a penlight or flashlight and approaching from the side, shine a light on the pupil.
- Observe the response of the illuminated pupil. It should constrict (direct response).
- Again shine the light on the pupil, and observe the response of the other pupil. It should also constrict (consensual response).

Reaction to Accommodation

- Hold an object (a penlight or pencil) about 10 cm (4 in) from the bridge of the client's nose.
- Ask the client to look first at the top of the object and then at a distant object (eg, the far wall) behind the penlight. Alternate the gaze from the near to the far object.
- Observe the pupil response. The pupils should constrict when looking at the near object and dilate when looking at the far object.
- Next, move the penlight or pencil toward the client's nose. The pupils should converge.

To record normal assessment of the pupils, use the abbreviation PERRLA (pupils equally round and react to light and accommodation).

Procedure 22–6 *continued*

ASSESSMENT	NORMAL FINDINGS	DEVIATIONS FROM NORMAL
Visual Fields		
Assess peripheral visual fields to determine function of the retina and neuronal visual pathways to the brain and second (optic) cranial nerve.	When looking straight ahead, client can see objects in the periphery	Visual field smaller than normal (possible glaucoma); one-half vision in one or both eyes (indicates nerve damage)

Assessing Peripheral Visual Fields

- Have the client sit directly facing you at a distance of 60 to 90 cm (2 to 3 ft).
- Ask the client to cover the right eye with a card and look directly at your nose.
- Cover or close your eye directly opposite the client's covered eye (ie, your left eye), and look directly at the client's nose.
- Hold an object (eg, a penlight or pencil) in your fingers, extend your arm, and move the object into the visual field from various points in the periphery (Figure 22–16). The object should be at an equal distance from the client and yourself. Ask the client to tell you when the moving object is first spotted.
  - **a.** To test the *temporal field* of the left eye, extend and move your right arm in from the client's right periphery. Temporally, peripheral objects can be seen at right angles (90 degrees) to the central point of vision.
  - **b.** To test the *upward field* of the left eye, extend and move the right arm down from the upward periphery. The upward field of vision is normally 50 degrees because the orbital ridge is in the way.
  - **c.** To test the *downward field* of the left eye, extend and move the right arm up from the lower periphery. The downward field of vision is normally 70 degrees because the cheekbone is in the way.
  - **d.** To test the *nasal field* of the left eye, extend and move your left arm in from the periphery. The nasal field of vision is normally 50 degrees away from the central point of vision because the nose is in the way.
- Repeat the above steps for the right eye, reversing the process.

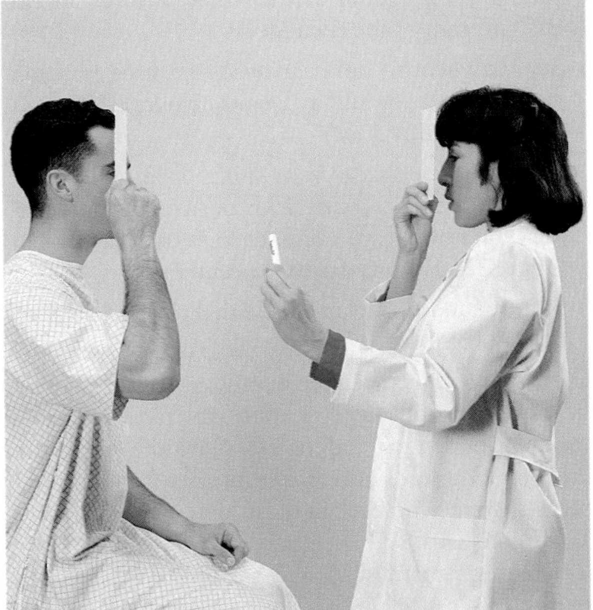

Figure 22–16 Assessing the client's left peripheral visual field.

ASSESSMENT	NORMAL FINDINGS	DEVIATIONS FROM NORMAL
Extraocular Muscle Tests		
Assess six ocular movements to determine eye alignment and coordination. These can be performed on clients over 6 months of age. See the box on page 488.	Both eyes coordinated, move in unison, with parallel alignment	Eye movements not coordinated or parallel; one or both eyes fail to follow a penlight in specific directions, such as **strabismus** (cross-eye or squint)

PROCEDURE 22–6 ASSESSING THE EYE STRUCTURES AND VISUAL ACUITY *continued*

ASSESSMENT	NORMAL FINDINGS	DEVIATIONS FROM NORMAL
	End-point **nystagmus** (rapid involuntary movement of the eyeball on the extreme lateral gaze)	Nystagmus other than end-point (may indicate neurologic impairment)

Assessing the Six Ocular Movements

- Stand directly in front of the client, and hold the penlight at a comfortable distance, such as 30 cm (1 ft) in front of the client's eyes.
- Ask the client to hold the head in a fixed position facing you and to follow the movements of the penlight with the eyes *only.*
- Move the penlight in a slow, orderly manner through the six cardinal fields of gaze, that is, from the center of the eye along the lines of the arrows in Figure 22–17 and back to the center.
- Stop the movement of the penlight periodically so that nystagmus can be detected.

These six positions are used because six muscles guide the movements of each eye. Four *rectus* muscles (superior, inferior, lateral, and medial) move the eye in the direction indicated. Two *oblique* muscles (superior and inferior) rotate the eyeball on its axis. Cranial nerves III (oculomotor), IV (trochlear), and VI (abducens) innervate these muscles. Moving the object through the six positions can identify a nonfunctioning muscle or associated cranial nerve.

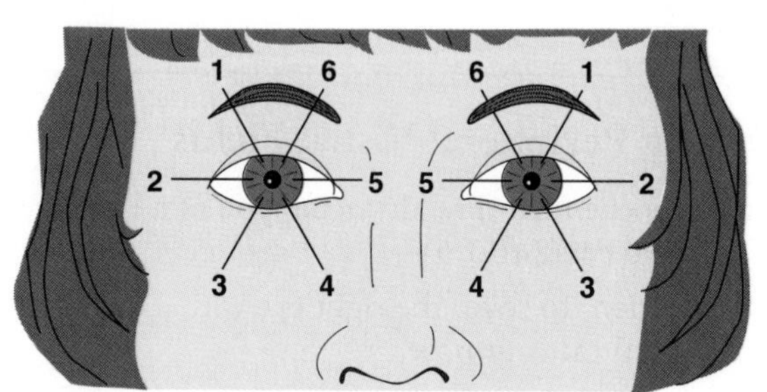

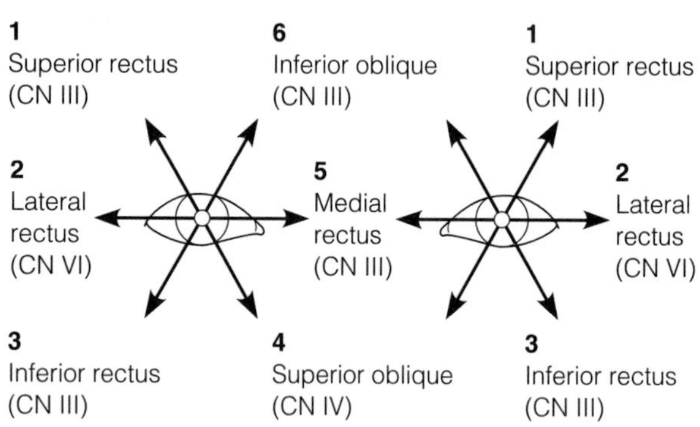

Figure 22–17 The six muscles that govern eye movement.

ASSESSMENT	NORMAL FINDINGS	DEVIATIONS FROM NORMAL
Perform the cover-uncover patch test to determine eye alignment. See the box on page 489.	Uncovered eye does not move from fixed point when other eye is covered	Uncovered eye moves to focus on fixed point, indicating it was *not* well aligned before other eye was covered; it is shifting from a lateral to central gaze
	Newly uncovered eye, if well aligned, does not move when index card is removed	Newly uncovered eye moves to focus on fixed point, indicating it was *not* well aligned when covered; muscle weakness is apparent when eye turns outward while covered; as eye is uncovered, it quickly moves inward to bring itself back in alignment
Perform the corneal light reflex test to determine eye alignment. See the box on page 489.	Light reflection appears at symmetric spots in both eyes	Light reflection appears at different spots in each eye (asymmetric)

PROCEDURE 22–6 *continued*

Testing Eye Alignment

Cover-Uncover Patch Test

- Ask the client to stare straight ahead at a fixed point, for example, at a penlight held 15 cm (6 in) in front of the eyes.
- Cover one of the client's eyes with an eye cover or index card while observing the uncovered eye.
- Remove the eye cover, and observe the newly uncovered eye for movement.
- Repeat the above steps for the other eye.
- Test each eye several times to confirm findings.

Corneal Light Reflex Test

- Darken the room.
- Ask the client to stare straight ahead.
- Shine a penlight on the bridge of the nose.
- Observe the light reflection in both corneas.

ASSESSMENT	NORMAL FINDINGS	DEVIATIONS FROM NORMAL
Visual Acuity		
Assess near vision by providing adequate lighting and asking the client to read from a magazine or newspaper held at a distance of 36 cm (14 in). If the client normally wears corrective lenses, the glasses or lenses should be worn during the test.	Able to read newsprint	Difficult reading newsprint unless due to aging process
Assess distance vision by asking the client to wear corrective lenses, unless they are used for reading only, that is, for distances of only 36 cm (12 to 14 in).	20/20 vision on Snellen chart from age 6 onward	Denominator of 40 or more on Snellen chart with corrective lenses

Assessing Distance Vision

- Ask the client to stand or sit 6 m (20 ft) from a Snellen chart, cover the eye not being tested, and identify the letters on the Snellen chart.
- Take three readings: right eye, left eye, both eyes.
- Record the readings of each eye and both eyes, that is, the smallest line from which the person is able to read one-half or more of the letters.

At the end of each line of the Snellen chart are standardized numbers (fractions). The top line is 20/200. The numerator (top number) is always 20, the distance the person stands from the chart. The denominator (bottom number) is the distance from which the normal eye can read the chart. Therefore, a person who has 20/40 vision, can see at 20 feet from the chart what a normal-sighted person can see at 40 feet from the chart. Visual acuity is recorded as "s̄c" (without correction), or "c̄c" (with correction). Also indicate how many letters were misread in the line, for example, "visual acuity 20/40–2c̄c" indicates that two letters were misread in the 20/40 line by a client wearing corrective lenses.

PROCEDURE 22–6 ASSESSING THE EYE STRUCTURES AND VISUAL ACUITY *continued*

ASSESSMENT	NORMAL FINDINGS	DEVIATIONS FROM NORMAL
Perform functional vision tests if the client is unable to see the top line (20/200) of the Snellen chart.		Functional vision only (eg, light perception, hand movements, counting fingers at 1 ft)

Performing Functional Vision Tests

Light Perception

Shine a penlight into the client's eye from a lateral position, and then turn the light off. Ask the client to tell you when the light is on or off. If the client knows when the light is on or off, the client has light perception, and the vision is recorded as "LP."

Hand Movements (H/M)

Hold your hand 30 cm (1 ft) from the client's face, and move it slowly back and forth, stopping it periodically. Ask the client to tell you when your hand stops moving. If the client knows when your hand stops moving, record the vision as "H/M 1 ft."

Counting Fingers (C/F)

Hold up some of your fingers 30 cm (1 ft) from the client's face, and ask the client to count your fingers. If the client can do so, note on the vision record "C/F 1 ft."

THE ELDERLY: PHYSICAL CHANGES OF THE EYES AND VISION

Visual Acuity

- Visual acuity decreases as the lens ages and becomes more opaque and loses elasticity (presbyopia).
- The ability of the iris to accommodate to darkness and dim light diminishes.
- Peripheral vision diminishes.
- The adaptation to light (glare) and dark decreases.
- Accommodation to far objects often improves, but accommodation to near objects decreases.
- Color vision declines; older people are less able to perceive purple colors and to discriminate pastel colors.
- Many older people wear corrective lenses; they are most likely to have hyperopia. Visual changes are due to loss of elasticity (presbyopia) and transparency of the lens.
- The number of vitreous floaters increases with age.

External Eye Structures

- The skin around the orbit of the eye may darken.
- The eyes may appear dry and lusterless because of the decrease in tear production from the lacrimal glands.
- The eyeball may appear sunken because of the decrease in orbital fat.
- Skinfolds of the upper lids may seem more prominent, and the lower lids may sag.
- A thin, grayish white arc or ring (*arcus senilis*) appears around part or all of the cornea. It results from an accumulation of a lipid substance on the cornea. The cornea tends to cloud with age.
- The iris may appear pale with brown discolorations as a result of pigment degeneration.
- The conjunctiva of the eye may appear paler than that of younger adults and may take on a slightly yellow appearance because of the deposition of fat.
- Pupil reaction to light and accommodation is normally symmetrically equal but may be less brisk.
- The pupils can appear smaller in size, unequal, and irregular in shape because of sclerotic changes in the iris.

Internal Eye Structures

- The fundus may appear yellower and lack luster.
- The blood vessels narrow slightly.
- The macula and fovea are less bright.

The Ears and Hearing

Assessment of the ear includes direct inspection and palpation of the external ear, inspection of the remaining parts of the ear by an **otoscope,** and determination of auditory acuity. The ear is usually assessed during an initial physical examination; periodic reassessments may be necessary for long-term clients or those with hearing problems.

The ear is divided into three parts: external ear, middle ear, and inner ear. Most of the structures mentioned below are illustrated in Figure 22–18. The external ear includes the **auricle** or **pinna,** the external auditory canal, and the **tympanic membrane,** or eardrum. Landmarks of the auricle include the **lobule** (earlobe), **helix** (the posterior curve of the auricle's upper aspect), **anthelix** (the anterior curve of the auricle's upper aspect), **tragus** (the cartilaginous protrusion at the entrance to the ear canal), **triangular fossa** (a depression of the antihelix), and **external auditory meatus** (the entrance to the ear canal). Although not part of the ear, the **mastoid,** a bony prominence behind the ear, is another important landmark. The external ear canal is curved, is about 2.5 cm (1 in) long in the adult, and ends at the tympanic membrane. It is covered with skin that has many fine hairs, glands, and nerve endings. The glands secrete **cerumen** (earwax), which lubricates and protects the canal.

The middle ear is an air-filled cavity that starts at the tympanic membrane and contains three **ossicles** (bones of sound transmission): the **malleus** (hammer), which is the most easily seen, the **incus** (anvil), and the **stapes** (stirrups) (Figure 22–18). The **eustachian tube,** another part of the middle ear, connects the middle ear to the nasopharynx. The tube stabilizes the air pressure between the external atmosphere and the middle ear, thus preventing rupture of the tympanic membrane and discomfort produced by marked pressure differences.

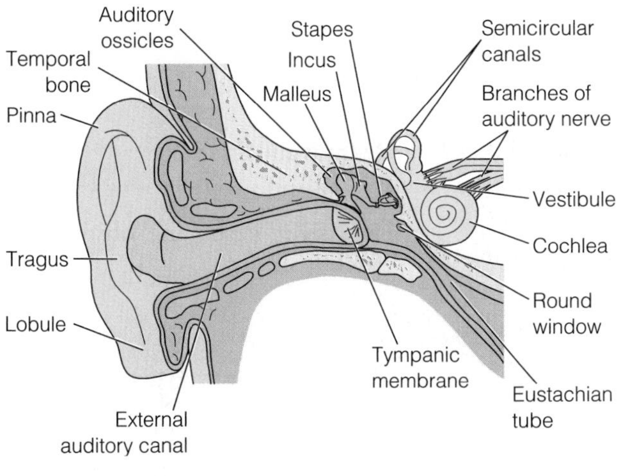

Figure 22–18 Anatomic structures of the external, middle, and inner ear.

The inner ear contains the **cochlea,** a seashell-shaped structure essential for sound transmission and hearing, and the **vestibule** and **semicircular canals,** which contain the organs of equilibrium (Figure 22–18).

Sound transmission and hearing are complex processes. In brief, sound can be transmitted by air conduction or bone conduction. Air-conducted transmission occurs by this process:

1. A sound stimulus enters the external canal and reaches the tympanic membrane.
2. The sound waves cross the tympanic membrane and reach the ossicles.
3. The sound waves travel from the ossicles to the opening in the inner ear (oval window).
4. The cochlea receives the sound vibrations.
5. The stimulus travels to the auditory nerve (the eighth cranial nerve) and the cerebral cortex.

Bone-conducted sound transmission occurs when skull bones transport the sound directly to the auditory nerve.

The curvature of the external ear canal differs with age. In the infant and toddler, the canal has an upward curvature. By age 3, the ear canal assumes the more downward curvature of adulthood.

Audiometric evaluations, which measure hearing at various decibels, are recommended for the elderly. A common hearing deficit with age is loss of ability to hear high-frequency sounds, such as *f, s, sh,* and *ph.* This neurosensory hearing deficit does not respond well to use of a hearing aid.

To inspect the external ear canal and tympanic membrane, the nurse inserts an otoscope (see page 493) into the external auditory canal.

In some practice settings, the nurse does not perform otoscopic examinations. In others, the nurse's examination is limited to inspection of the external ear canal and the color of the tympanic membrane.

Advanced practitioners use tuning fork tests to assess whether the client's hearing loss is a conduction, sensorineural, or mixed problem. **Conduction hearing loss** is the result of interrupted transmission of sound waves through the outer and middle ear structures. Possible causes are a tear in the tympanic membrane or an obstruction, due to swelling or other causes, in the auditory canal. **Sensorineural hearing loss** is the result of damage to the inner ear, the auditory nerve, or the hearing center in the brain. **Mixed hearing loss** is a combination of conduction and sensorineural loss. Procedure 22–7 describes how to assess the ears and hearing.

Text continued on page 496

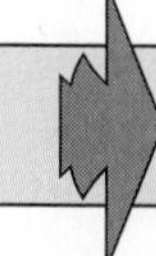

PROCEDURE 22–7 ASSESSING THE EARS AND HEARING

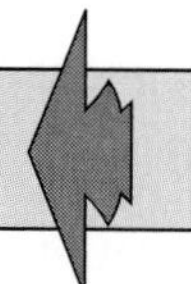

NURSING HISTORY FOCUS

Family history of hearing problems or loss; presence of any ear problems; medication history, especially if there are complaints of ringing in ears; any hearing difficulty: its onset, factors contributing to it, and how it interferes with activities of daily living; use of a corrective hearing device: when and from whom it was obtained.

ASSESSMENT	NORMAL FINDINGS	DEVIATIONS FROM NORMAL
Auricles		
Inspect the auricles for color, symmetry of size, and position. To inspect position, note the level at which the superior aspect of the auricle attaches to the head in relation to the eye.	Color same as facial skin	Bluish color of earlobes (eg, cyanosis); pallor (eg, frostbite); excessive redness (inflammation or fever)
	Symmetric position. Line drawn from lateral angle of eye to point where top part of auricle joins head is horizontal; imaginary line drawn from the top to the bottom of the ear varies no more than 10 degrees from the vertical.	Low-set ears (associated with a congenital abnormality, such as Down syndrome)
Palpate the auricles for texture, elasticity, and areas of tenderness. ▪ Pull the auricle upward, downward, and backward. ▪ Fold the pinna forward (it should recoil). ▪ Push in on the tragus. ▪ Apply pressure to the mastoid process.	Mobile, firm, and not tender; pinna recoils after it is folded	Lesions (eg, cysts); flaky, scaly skin (eg, seborrhea); tenderness when moved or pressed (may indicate inflammation or infection of external ear)
External Ear Canal and Tympanic Membrane		
Using an otoscope, inspect the external ear canal for cerumen, skin lesions, pus, and blood and the tympanic membrane for color. See the box on page 493.	Distal third contains hair follicles and glands Dry cerumen, grayish-tan color; or sticky, wet cerumen in various shades of brown	Redness and discharge Scaling Excessive cerumen obstructing canal
Inspect the tympanic membrane for color and gloss.	Pearly gray color, semitransparent	Pink to red, some opacity Yellow-amber White Blue or deep red Dull surface

PROCEDURE 22–7 *continued*

Inspecting the External Ear Canal with an Otoscope

- Attach a speculum to the otoscope. Use the largest diameter that will fit the ear canal without causing discomfort. *This achieves maximum vision of the entire ear canal and tympanic membrane.*
- Tip the client's head away from you, and straighten the ear canal. For an adult, straighten the ear canal by pulling the pinna up and back (Figure 22–19). *Straightening the ear canal facilitates vision of the ear canal and the tympanic membrane.*
- Hold the otoscope either (a) right side up, with your fingers between the otoscope handle and the client's head, or (b) upside down, with your fingers and the ulnar surface of your hand against the client's head (Figure 22–20). *This stabilizes the head and protects the eardrum and canal from injury if a quick head movement occurs.*
- Gently insert the tip of the otoscope into the ear canal, avoiding pressure by the speculum against either side of the ear canal. *The inner two-thirds of the ear canal is bony; if the speculum is pressed against either side, the client will experience discomfort.*

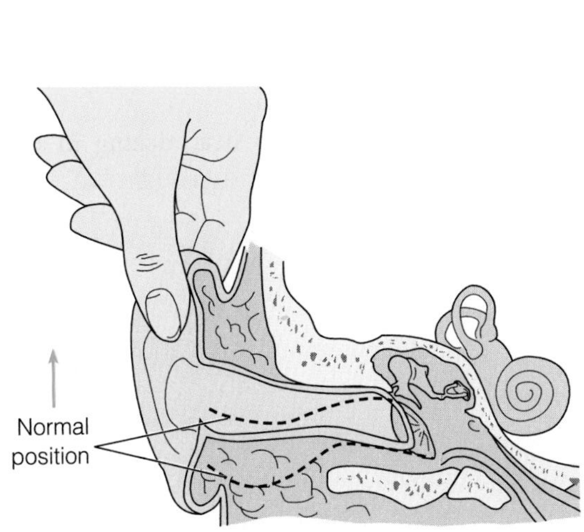

Figure 22–19 Straightening the ear canal of an adult by pulling the pinna up and back.

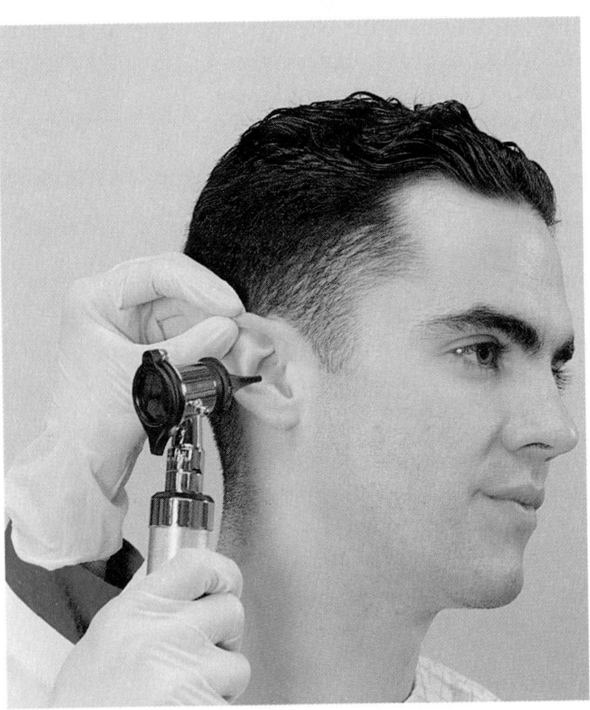

Figure 22–20 Inserting an otoscope.

ASSESSMENT	NORMAL FINDINGS	DEVIATIONS FROM NORMAL
Gross Hearing Acuity Tests **Assess client's response to normal voice tones.** If client has difficulty hearing the normal voice, proceed with the following tests.	Normal voice tones audible	Normal voice tones not audible (eg, requests nurse to repeat words or statements, leans toward the speaker, turns the head, cups the ears, or speaks in loud tone of voice)

PROCEDURE 22–7 ASSESSING THE EARS AND HEARING *continued*

ASSESSMENT	NORMAL FINDINGS	DEVIATIONS FROM NORMAL
Assess client's response to whispered voice. This test is used for screening purposes only, because maintaining consistency in the whispered voice is difficult.		
▪ Stand 30 to 60 cm (1 to 2 ft) from the client in a position where the client cannot read your lips. Ask the client to occlude one ear by putting a finger in it.		
▪ Whisper some nonconsecutive numbers and have the client tell you what was heard. Increase the loudness of the whisper until the client can identfy at least 50% of the numbers. Repeat the process with the other ear. *Nonconsecutive numbers are used so that the client cannot anticipate what number will follow.*	Able to repeat nonconsecutive numbers	Unable to repeat 50% of numbers whispered
Perform the watch tick test. The ticking of a watch has a higher pitch than the human voice.	Able to hear ticking in both ears	Unable to hear ticking in one or both ears
▪ Have the client occlude one ear. Out of the client's sight, place a ticking watch 2 to 3 cm (1 to 2 in) from the unoccluded ear.		
▪ Ask whether the client can hear it. Repeat with the other ear.		
Tuning Fork Tests		
Perform Weber's test to assess bone conduction. See the upper box on page 495. Note findings as Weber positive and indicate whether right or left ear.	Sound is heard in both ears or is localized at the center of the head (Weber negative)	Sound is heard better in impaired ear, indicating a bone-conductive hearing loss (eg, due to obstruction of ossicles), *or* sound is heard better in ear without a problem, indicating a sensorineural disturbance (nerve or inner ear damage)
Conduct the Rinne test to compare air conduction to bone conduction. See the upper box on page 495.	Air-conducted (AC) hearing is greater than bone-conducted (BC) hearing, that is, AC > BC (positive Rinne)	Bone conduction time is equal to or longer than the air conduction time, that is, BC > AC or BC = AC (negative Rinne; indicates a conductive hearing loss)

PROCEDURE 22–7 *continued*

Performing Tuning Fork Tests

Weber's Test

This test assesses bone conduction by testing the lateralization (sideward transmission) of sounds

- Hold the tuning fork at its base. Activate it by tapping the fork gently against the back of your hand near the knuckles or by stroking the fork between your thumb and index fingers. It should be made to ring softly.
- Place the base of the vibrating fork on top of the client's head (Figure 22–21) and ask where the client hears the noise.

Rinne Test

This test compares air conduction to bone conduction.

- Ask the client to block the hearing in one ear intermittently by moving a fingertip in and out of the ear canal.
- Hold the handle of the activated tuning fork on the mastoid process of one ear (Figure 22–22) until the client states that the vibration can no longer be heard.
- Immediately hold the still vibrating fork prongs in front of the client's ear canal (Figure 22–23). Push aside the client's hair if necessary. Ask whether the client now hears the sound. Sound conducted by air is heard more readily than sound conducted by bone. The tuning fork vibrations conducted by air are normally heard longer.

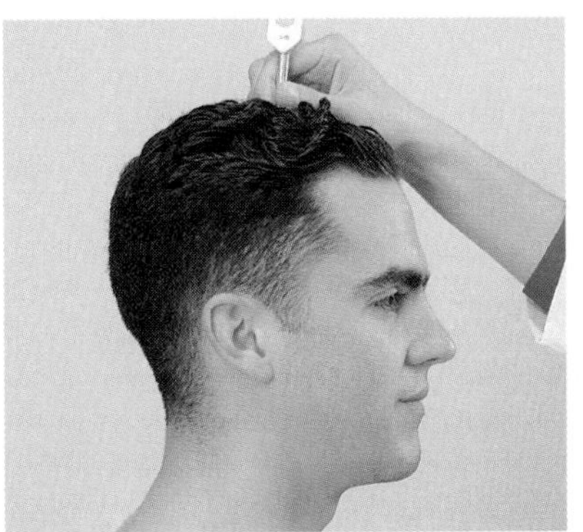

Figure 22–21 Placing the base of the tuning fork on the client's skull (Weber's test).

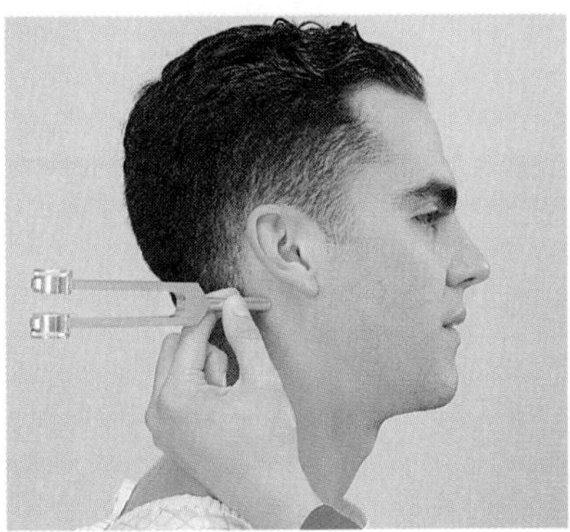

Figure 22–22 Placing the base of the tuning fork on the mastoid process (Rinne test).

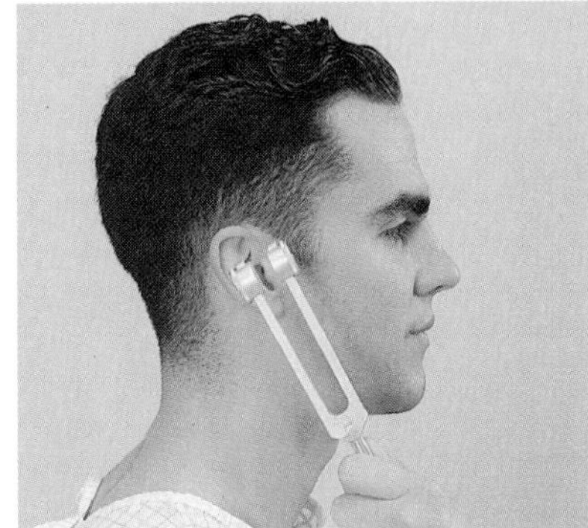

Figure 22–23 Placing the tuning fork prongs in front of the client's ear canal (Rinne test).

THE ELDERLY: PHYSICAL CHANGES OF THE EARS AND HEARING

- The skin of the ear may appear dry and be less resilient because of the loss of connective tissue.
- Increased coarse and wirelike hair growth occurs along the pinna, anthelix, and tragus. See Figure 22–18 on page 491.
- The tympanic membrane is more translucent and less flexible. The intensity of the light reflex may diminish slightly.
- Earwax is drier.
- The pinna increases in both width and length, and the earlobe elongates.
- Sensorineural hearing loss occurs.
- Generalized hearing loss (*presbycusis*) occurs in all frequencies, although the first symptom is the loss of high-frequency sounds: the *f*, *s*, *sh*, and *ph* sounds. To such persons, conversation can be distorted and result in what appears to be inappropriate or confused behavior.

THE NOSE AND SINUSES

A nurse can inspect the nasal passages very simply with a flashlight. However, a nasal *speculum*, which is a lighted instrument, facilitates examination of the nasal chambers.

Assessment of the nose includes inspection and palpation of the external nose (the upper third of the nose is bone; the remainder is cartilage); patency of the nasal cavities; and inspection of the nasal cavities. Major structures of the nose are shown in Figure 22–24. The nasal turbinates increase the surface of the mucous membrane in the nares. The clefts between the turbinates are called meati. Each meatus is named for the adjacent turbinate; for example, the inferior meatus is near the inferior turbinate. The nurse also inspects and palpates the facial sinuses (Figure 22–25). Advanced practitioners may perform transillumination of the sinuses. Procedure 22–8 describes how to assess the nose and sinuses.

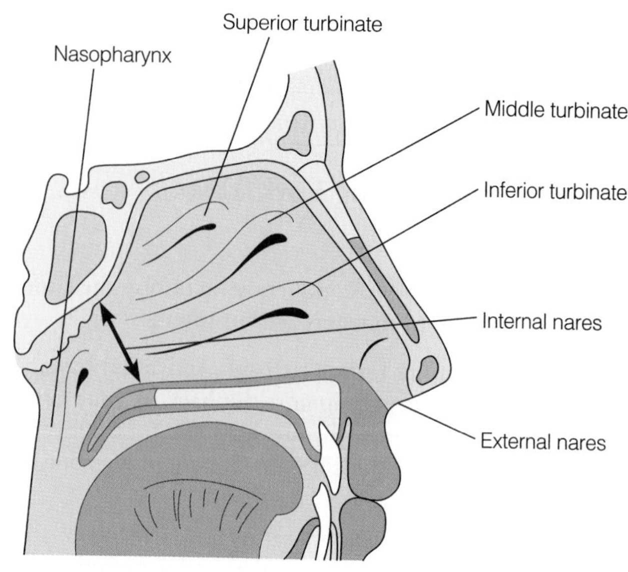

Figure 22–24 Major structures of the nose.

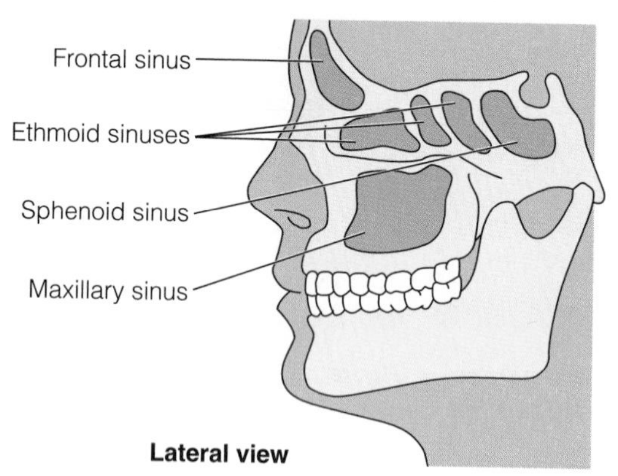

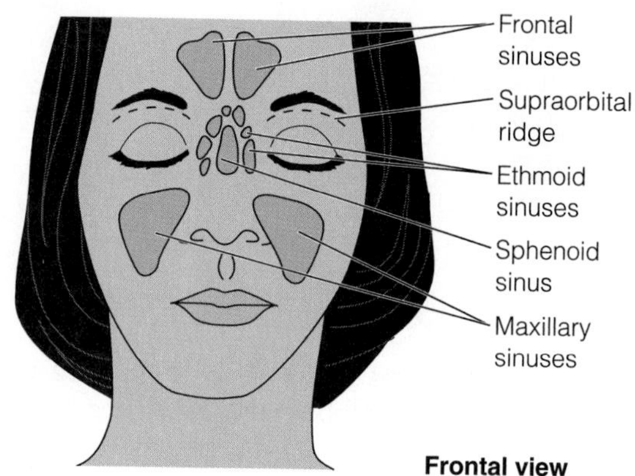

Figure 22–25 The facial sinuses.

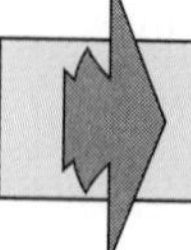

PROCEDURE 22–8 ASSESSING THE NOSE AND SINUSES

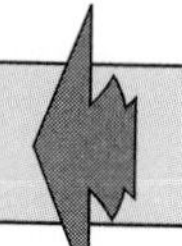

NURSING HISTORY FOCUS

History of allergies, difficult breathing through the nose, sinus infections, injuries to nose or face, nosebleeds; any medications taken; any changes in sense of smell.

PROCEDURE 22–8 *continued*

ASSESSMENT	NORMAL FINDINGS	DEVIATIONS FROM NORMAL
Nose		
Inspect the external nose for any deviations in shape, size, or color and flaring or discharge from the nares.	Symmetric and straight No discharge or flaring Uniform color	Asymmetric Discharge from nares Localized areas of redness or presence of skin lesions
Lightly palpate the external nose to determine any areas of tenderness, masses, and displacements of bone and cartilage.	Not tender; no lesions	Tenderness on palpation; presence of lesions
Determine patency of both nasal cavities. Ask the client to close the mouth, exert pressure on one naris, and breathe through the opposite naris. Repeat the procedure to assess patency of the opposite naris.	Air moves freely as the client breathes through the nares	Air movement is restricted in one or both nares
Inspect the nasal cavities using a flashlight or a nasal speculum:		
▪ Tip the client's head back.		
▪ If using a speculum, hold it in your nondominant hand, and place your index finger on the side of the nose to stabilize its position. Use your dominant hand to position the head and hold the light.		
▪ Inspect the lining of the nares (mucosa) and the coarse hairs that filter the air. Observe for the presence of redness, swelling, growths, and discharge.	Mucosa pink Clear, watery discharge No lesions	Mucosa red, edematous Abnormal discharge (eg, purulent) Presence of lesions (eg, polyps)
▪ Inspect the position of the nasal septum between the nasal chambers, noting in particular any deviation to right or left.	Nasal septum intact and in midline	Septum deviated
Facial Sinuses		
Palpate the maxillary and frontal sinuses for tenderness.	Not tender	Tenderness in one or more sinuses
Transilluminate the frontal sinuses by placing a penlight against the inner aspect of the supraorbital ridge of the frontal bone (see Figure 22–25). This is best done in a darkened room.	Sinuses are well outlined, contain air, and light up equally	Fluid in sinuses appears darker on transillumination

➤

PROCEDURE 22-8 ASSESSING THE NOSE AND SINUSES *continued*

ASSESSMENT	NORMAL FINDINGS	DEVIATIONS FROM NORMAL
Transilluminate the maxillary sinuses by placing a penlight in the mouth and shining it to the left and to the right.	As above	As above

THE ELDERLY: PHYSICAL CHANGES OF THE NOSE AND SENSE OF SMELL

- The sense of smell markedly diminishes because of a decrease in the number of olfactory nerve fibers and atrophy of the remaining fibers. Older persons are less able to identify and discriminate odors.
- Nosebleeds may result from hypertensive disease or other arterial vessel changes.

THE MOUTH AND OROPHARYNX

The mouth and pharynx are composed of a number of structures: lips, inner and buccal mucosa, the tongue and floor of the mouth, teeth and gums, hard and soft palate, uvula, salivary glands, tonsillar pillars, and tonsils. Anatomic structures of the mouth are shown in Figure 22–26.

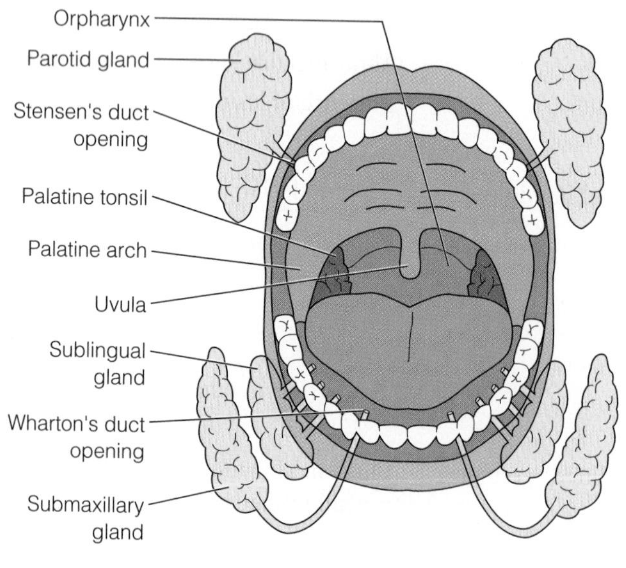

Figure 22–26 Anatomic structures of the mouth.

By age 25, most people have all their permanent teeth. For information about structures of the teeth, see Chapter 29, page 750.

Normally, three pairs of salivary glands empty into the oral cavity: the parotid, submandibular, and sublingual glands (Figure 22–26). The *parotid gland* is the largest and empties through the Stensen's duct opposite the second molar. The *submandibular gland* empties through Wharton's duct, which is situated at the side of the frenulum on the floor of the mouth. The *sublingual salivary gland* lies in the floor of the mouth and has numerous openings.

Dental **caries** (cavities) and **peridontal disease (pyorrhea)** are two problems that most frequently affect the teeth. Both problems are commonly associated with plaque and tartar deposits. **Plaque** is an *invisible* soft film that adheres to the enamel surface of teeth; it consists of bacteria, molecules of saliva, and remnants of epithelial cells and leukocytes. When plaque is unchecked, tartar (dental calculus) forms. **Tartar** is a visible, hard deposit of plaque and dead bacteria that forms at the gum lines. Tartar buildup can alter the fibers that attach the teeth to the gum and eventually disrupt bone tissue. Periodontal disease is characterized by **gingivitis** (red, swollen *gingiva,* ie, gum) bleeding, receding gum lines, and the formation of pockets between the teeth and gums. In advanced periodontal disease, the teeth are loose, and pus is evident when the gums are pressed.

Other problems nurses may see are **glossitis** (inflammation of the tongue), **stomatitis** (inflammation of the oral mucosa), and **parotitis** (inflammation of the parotid salivary gland). The accumulation of foul matter (food, microorganisms, and epithelial elements) on the teeth and gums is referred to as **sordes.**

Physical examination of the mouth includes inspection and palpation techiques. The CDC recommends that the nurse wear gloves when in contact with the buccal mucosa. Equipment needed for assessment of the mouth and pharynx includes tongue blade, gauze squares (2 × 2), a penlight or flashlight, and disposable gloves. See Procedure 22–9.

Text continued on page 503

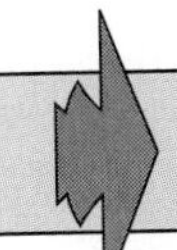

PROCEDURE 22–9 ASSESSING THE MOUTH AND OROPHARYNX

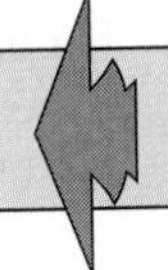

NURSING HISTORY FOCUS

Routine pattern of dental care, last visit to dentist; length of time ulcers or other lesions have been present; any denture discomfort; any medications client is receiving.

ASSESSMENT	NORMAL FINDINGS	DEVIATIONS FROM NORMAL
Lips and Buccal Mucosa		
Inspect the outer lips for symmetry of contour, color, and texture. Ask the client to purse the lips as if to whistle.	Uniform pink color (darker, eg, bluish hue, in Mediterranean groups and dark-skinned clients)	Pallor; cyanosis
	Soft, moist, smooth texture	Blisters; generalized or localized swelling; fissures, crusts, or scales (may result from excessive moisture, nutritional deficiency, or fluid deficit)
	Symmetry of contour	
	Ability to purse lips	Inability to purse lips (indicative of facial nerve damage)
Inspect and palpate the inner lips and buccal mucosa for color, moisture, texture, and the presence of lesions. See the box on page 500.	Uniform pink color (freckled brown pigmentation in dark-skinned clients)	Pallor; white patches (leukoplakia)
	Moist, smooth, soft, glistening, and elastic texture (drier oral mucosa in elderly due to decreased salivation)	Excessive dryness Mucosal cysts; irritations from dentures; abrasions, ulcerations; nodules
Teeth and Gums		
Inspect the teeth and gums while examining the inner lips and buccal mucosa. See the box on page 500.	32 adult teeth	Missing teeth Ill-fitting dentures
	Smooth, white, shiny tooth enamel	Brown or black discoloration of the enamel (may indicate staining or the presence of caries)
	Pink gums (bluish or dark patches in dark-skinned clients)	Excessively red gums
	Moist, firm texture to gums	Spongy texture; bleeding; tenderness (may indicate periodontal disease)
	No retraction of gums (pulling away from the teeth)	Receding, atrophied gums; swelling that partially covers the teeth

PROCEDURE 22–9 ASSESSING THE MOUTH AND OROPHARYNX *continued*

Inspecting and Palpating the Inner Lip, Buccal Mucosa, Teeth, and Gums

Inner Lip and Front Teeth

- Ask the client to relax the mouth, and, for better visualization, pull the lip outward away from the teeth.
- Grasp the lip on each side between the thumb and index finger (Figure 22–27).
- Palpate any lesions for size, tenderness, and consistency.
- Inspect the front teeth and gums.

Buccal Mucosa and Back Teeth

- Ask the client to open the mouth. Using a tongue blade, retract the cheek (Figure 22–28). View the surface buccal mucosa from top to bottom and back to front. A flashlight or penlight will help illuminate the surface. Repeat the procedure for the other side.
- Ask the client to open the mouth again. Using a fingercot (or gloves) and a penlight, move a finger along the inside cheek. Another finger may be moved outside the cheek.
- Examine the back teeth. For proper vision of the molars, use the index fingers of both hands to retract the cheek (Figure 22–29). Ask the client to relax the lips and first close, then open, the jaw. Closing the jaw assists in observation of tooth alignment and loss of teeth; opening the jaw assists in observation of dental fillings and caries. Observe the number of teeth, tooth color, the state of fillings, dental caries, and tartar along the base of the teeth. Note the presence and fit of partial or complete dentures.

Gums

- Inspect the gums around the molars. Observe for bleeding, color, retraction (pulling away from the teeth), edema, and lesions.
- Assess the texture of the gums by gently pressing the gum tissue with a tongue blade.

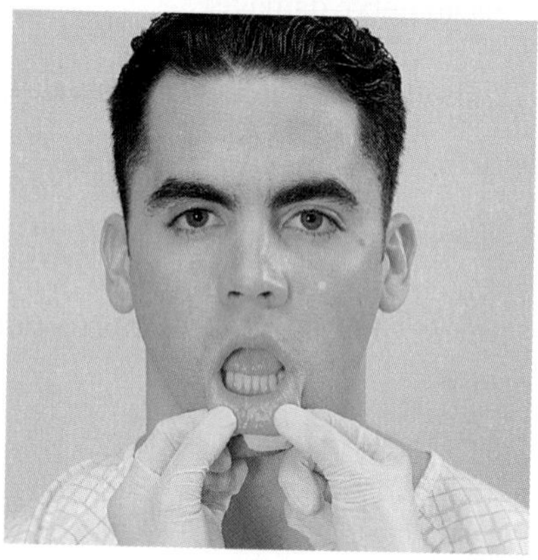

Figure 22–27 Inspecting the mucosa of the lower lip.

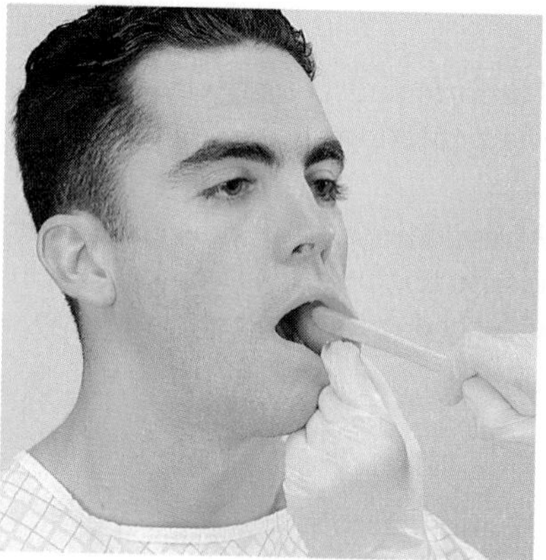

Figure 22–28 Inspecting the buccal mucosa using a tongue blade.

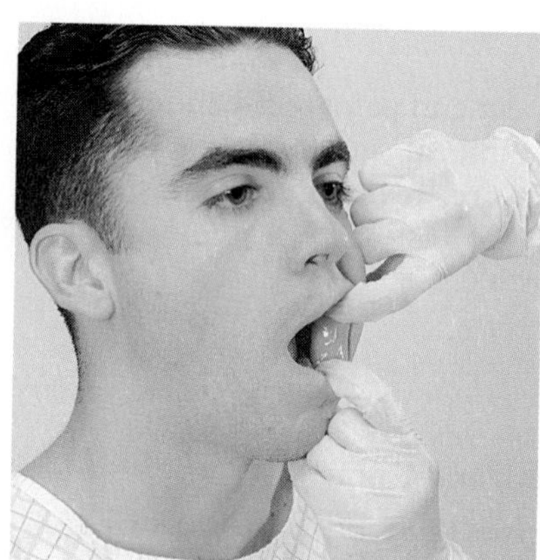

Figure 22–29 Inspecting the back teeth.

ASSESSMENT	NORMAL FINDINGS	DEVIATIONS FROM NORMAL
Inspect the dentures. Ask the client to remove complete or partial dentures. Inspect their condition, noting in particular broken or worn areas.	Smooth, intact dentures	Ill-fitting dentures; irritated and excoriated area under dentures

PROCEDURE 22–9 *continued*

ASSESSMENT	NORMAL FINDINGS	DEVIATIONS FROM NORMAL
Tongue/Floor of the Mouth		
Inspect the surface of the tongue for position, color, and texture. Ask the client to protrude the tongue.	Central position	Deviated from center (may indicate damage to hypoglossal [twelfth cranial] nerve)
	Pink color (some brown pigmentation on tongue borders in dark-skinned clients); moist; slightly rough; thin whitish coating	Smooth red tongue (may indicate iron, vitamin B_{12}, or vitamin B_3 deficiency)
		Dry, furry tongue (associated with fluid deficit)
	Smooth, lateral margins; no lesions	Nodes, ulcerations, discolorations (white or red areas); areas of tenderness
Inspect tongue movement. Ask the client to roll the tongue upward and move it from side to side.	Moves freely; no tenderness	Restricted mobility
Inspect the base of the tongue, the mouth floor, and the frenulum. Ask the client to place the tip of the tongue against the roof of the mouth.	Smooth tongue base with prominent veins Varicosities (tiny bluish-black or purple swollen areas) in elderly people	Swelling, ulceration
Palpate the tongue and floor of the mouth for any nodules, lumps, or excoriated areas. To palpate the tongue, use a piece of gauze to grasp its tip (stabilizes it), and with the index finger of your other hand, palpate the back of the tongue, its borders, and its base (Figure 22–30). To assess function of the glossopharyngeal and hypoglossal nerves, see the neurologic assessment, later in this chapter.	Smooth with no palpable nodules	Swelling, nodules

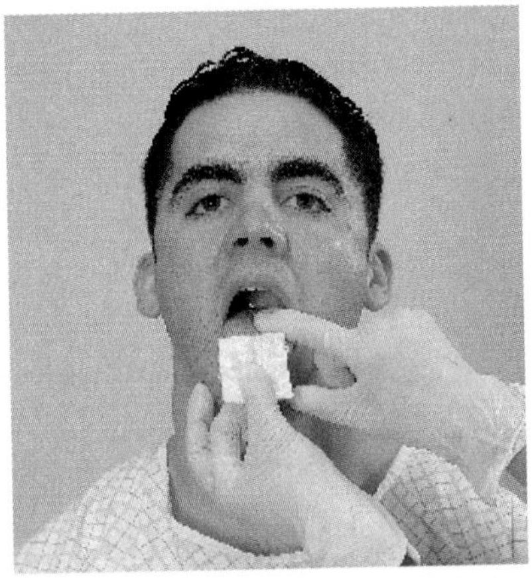

Figure 22–30 Palpating the tongue.

ASSESSMENT	NORMAL FINDINGS	DEVIATIONS FROM NORMAL
Salivary Glands		
Inspect salivary duct openings for any swelling or redness. See the discussion of salivary glands, page 498.	Same as color of buccal mucosa and floor of mouth	Inflammation (redness and swelling)

➤

Procedure 22–9 Assessing the Mouth and Oropharynx *continued*

ASSESSMENT	NORMAL FINDINGS	DEVIATIONS FROM NORMAL
Palates and Uvula		
Inspect the hard and soft palate for color, shape, texture, and the presence of bony prominences. Ask the client to open the mouth wide and tilt the head backward. Then, depress tongue with a tongue blade as necessary, and use a penhlight for appropriate visualization.	Light pink, smooth, soft palate Lighter pink hard palate, more irregular texture	Discoloration (eg, jaundice or pallor) Palates the same color Irritations Bony growths (exostoses) growing from the hard palate
Inspect the uvula for position and mobility while examining the palates. To observe the uvula, ask the client to say "ah" so that the soft palate rises.	Positioned in midline of soft palate	Deviation to one side from tumor or trauma; immobility (may indicate damage to trigeminal (fifth cranial) nerve or vagus (tenth cranial) nerve
Oropharynx and Tonsils		
Inspect the oropharynx for color and texture. Inspect one side at a time to avoid eliciting the gag reflex. To expose one side of the oropharynx, press a tongue blade against the tongue on the same side about halfway back while the client tilts the head back and opens the mouth wide. Use a penlight for illumination, if needed.	Pink and smooth posterior wall	Reddened or edematous; presence of lesions, plaques, or exudate
Inspect the tonsils (behind the fauces) **for color, discharge, and size.**	Pink and smooth No discharge Of normal size (see the accompanying box for a grading system to describe the size of tonsils)	Inflamed Presence of discharge Swollen
Elicit the gag reflex by pressing the posterior tongue with a tongue depressor.	Present	Absent (may indicate problems with glossopharyngeal or vagus nerves)

Grading System to Describe Size of Tonsils

- Grade 1 (normal): The tonsils are behind the tonsillar pillars, (the soft structures supporting the soft palate).
- Grade 2: The tonsils are between the pillars and the uvula.
- Grade 3: The tonsils touch the uvula.
- Grade 4: One or both tonsils extend to the midline of the oropharynx.

PROCEDURE 22–9 *continued*

THE ELDERLY: PHYSICAL CHANGES OF THE MOUTH AND SENSE OF TASTE

- The oral mucosa may be drier than that of younger persons because of decreased salivary gland acitivity. Decreased salivation occurs only in elderly people taking prescribed medications such as antidepressants, antihistamines, decongestants, diuretics, antihypertensives, tranquilizers, antispasmodics, and antineoplastics. Extreme dryness is associated with dehydration.
- Some receding of the gums occurs, giving an appearance of increased toothiness.
- There may be a brownish pigmentation to the gums, especially in black persons.
- Taste sensations diminish. Sweet and salty tastes are lost first. Elderly persons may add more salt and sugar to food than they did when they were younger. Diminished taste sensation is due to atrophy of the taste buds and a decreased sense of smell. It indicates diminished function of the fifth and seventh cranial nerves.
- Tiny purple or bluish black swollen areas (varicosities) under the tongue, known as *caviar* spots, are not uncommon.
- The teeth may show signs of staining, erosion, chipping, and abrasions due to loss of dentin. Tooth loss occurs as a result of gum disease but is preventable with good dental hygiene.
- The gag reflex may be slightly sluggish.

THE NECK

Examination of the neck includes the muscles, lymph nodes, trachea, thyroid gland, carotid arteries, and jugular veins. Areas of the neck are defined by the sternocleidomastoid muscles, which divide each side of the neck into two triangles: the anterior and posterior (Figure 22–31). The trachea, thyroid gland, anterior cervical nodes, and carotid artery lie within the anterior triangle (Figure 22–32, p. 504); the carotid artery runs parallel and anterior to the sternocleidomastoid muscle. The posterior lymph nodes lie within the posterior triangle (Figure 22–33, p. 504).

Each sternocleidomastoid muscle extends from the upper sternum and the medial third of the clavicle to the mastoid process of the temporal bone behind the ear (Figure 22–31). These muscles turn and laterally flex the head. Each trapezius muscle extends from the occipital bone of the skull to the lateral third of the clavicle. These muscles draw the head to the side and back, elevate the chin, and elevate the shoulders to shrug them.

Lymph nodes in the neck that collect lymph from the head and neck structures are grouped serially and referred to as *chains*. See Figure 22–33 and Table 22–6, both on page 504. The deep cervical chain is not shown in Figure 22–33 because it lies beneath the sternocleidomastoid muscle.

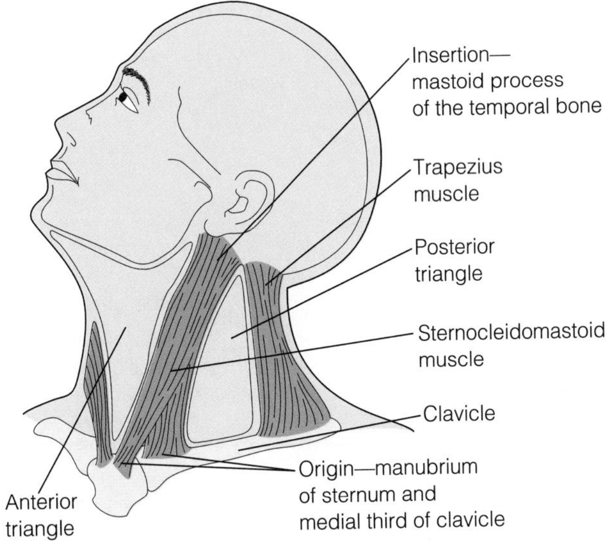

Figure 22–31 Major muscles of the neck.

Procedure 22–10 describes how to assess the neck.

Text continued on page 508

Table 22–6 Lymph Nodes of the Head and Neck

Node Center	Location	Area Drained
Head		
Occipital	At the posterior base of the skull	The occipital region of the scalp and the deep structures of the back of the neck
Postauricular (mastoid)	Behind the auricle of the ear over or in front of the mastoid process	The parietal region of the head and part of the ear
Preauricular	In front of the tragus of the ear	The forehead and upper face
Floor of Mouth		
Submandibular (submaxillary)	Along the medial border of the lower jaw, halfway between the angle of the jaw and the chin	The chin, upper lip, cheek, nose, teeth, eyelids, part of the tongue and of the floor of the mouth
Submental	Behind the tip of the mandible, in the midline, under the chin	The anterior third of the tongue, gums, and floor or the mouth
Neck		
Superficial (anterior) cervical chain	Along and anterior to the sternocleidomastoid muscle	The skin and neck
Posterior cervical chain	Along the anterior aspect of the trapezius muscle	The posterior and lateral regions of the neck, occiput, and mastoid
Deep cervical chain	Under the sternocleidomastoid muscle	The larynx, thyroid gland, trachea, and upper part of the esophagus
Supraclavicular	Above the clavicle, in the angle between the clavicle and the sternocleidomastoid muscle	The lateral regions of the neck and lungs

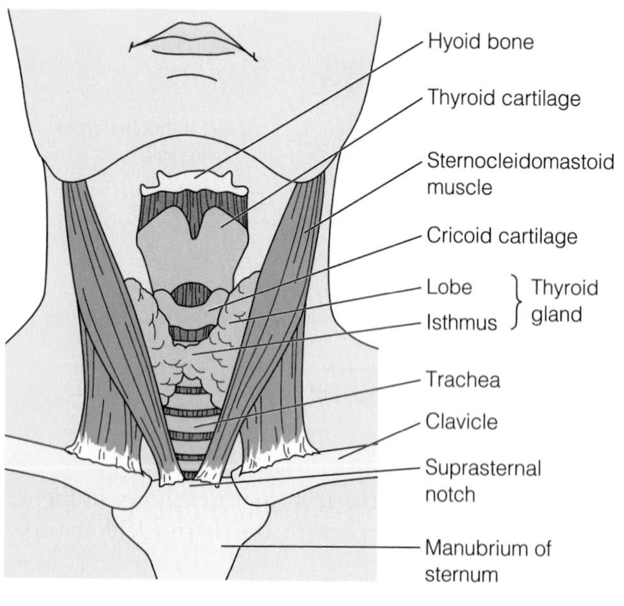

Figure 22–32 Structures of the neck.

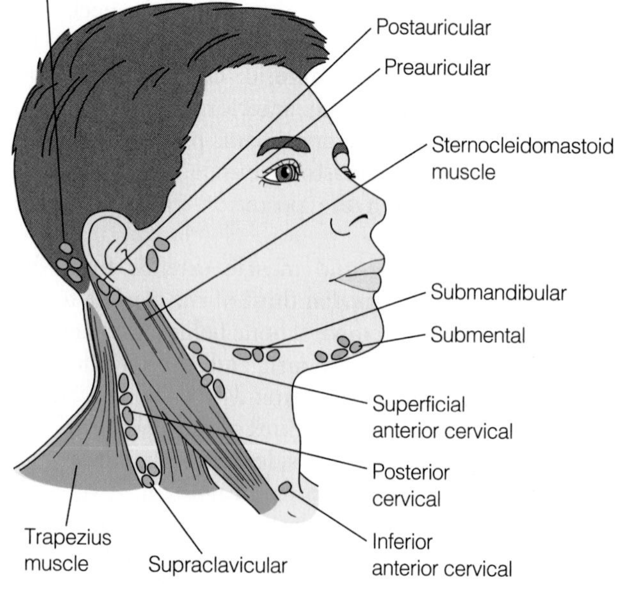

Figure 22–33 Lymph nodes of the neck.

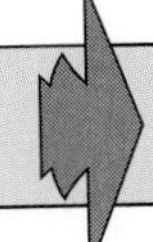

Procedure 22–10 Assessing the Neck

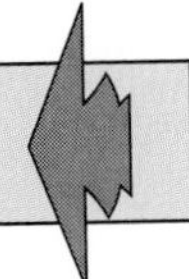

Nursing History Focus

Any problems with neck lumps; neck pain or stiffness; when and how any lumps occurred; any previous diagnoses of thyroid problems: over- or underfunction of the thyroid; tests taken, test results, medications ordered, former and current dosages, and any other treatments provided (eg, surgery, radiation).

ASSESSMENT	NORMAL FINDINGS	DEVIATIONS FROM NORMAL
Neck Muscles		
Inspect the neck muscles (sternocleidomastoid and trapezius) for abnormal swellings or masses. Ask the client to hold the head erect.	Muscles equal in size; head centered	Unilateral neck swelling; head tilted to one side (indicates presence of masses, injury, muscle weakness, shortening of sternocleidomastoid muscle, scars)
Observe head movement. Ask client to	Coordinated, smooth movements with no discomfort	Muscle tremor, spasm, or stiffness
▪ Move the chin to the chest (determines function of the sternocleidomastoid muscle).	Head flexes 45 degrees	Limited range of motion; painful movements; involuntary movements (eg, up-and-down nodding movements associated with Parkinson's disease)
▪ Move the head back so that the chin points upward (determines function of the trapezius muscle).	Head hyperextends 60 degrees	Head hyperextends less than 60 degrees
▪ Move the head so that the ear is moved toward the shoulder on each side (determines function of the sternocleidomastoid muscle).	Head laterally flexes 40 degrees	Head laterally flexes less than 40 degrees
▪ Turn the head to the right and to the left (determines function of the sternocleidomastoid muscle).	Head laterally rotates 70 degrees	Head laterally rotates less than 70 degrees
Assess muscle strength. Ask client to		
▪ Turn the head to one side against the resistance of your hand. Repeat with the other side (determines the strength of the sternocleidomastoid muscle).	Equal strength	Unequal strength
▪ Shrug the shoulders against the resistance of your hands (determines the strength of the trapezius muscles).	As above	As above
Lymph Nodes		
Palpate the entire neck for enlarged lymph nodes, using the guidelines shown in the box on the following page.	Not palpable	Enlarged, palpable, possibly tender (associated with infection and tumors)

➤

PROCEDURE 22–10 ASSESSING THE NECK *continued*

Palpating Neck Lymph Nodes

- Face the client, and bend the client's head forward slightly or toward the side being examined to relax the soft tissue and muscles.
- Palpate the nodes using the pads of the fingers. Move the fingertips in a gentle rotating motion.
- When examining the submental and submandibular nodes, place the fingertips under the mandible on the side nearest the palpating hand, and pull the skin and subcutaneous tissue laterally over the mandibular surface so that the tissue rolls over the nodes.
- When palpating the supraclavicular nodes, have the client bend the head forward to relax the tissues of the anterior neck and to relax the shoulders so that the clavicles drop. Use your hand nearest the side to be examined when facing the client (ie, use your left hand to palpate the client's right nodes). Use your free hand to flex the client's head forward if necessary. Hook your index and third fingers over the clavicle lateral to the sternocleidomastoid muscle (Figure 22–34).
- When palpating the anterior cervical nodes and posterior cervical nodes, move your fingertips slowly in a forward circular motion against the sternocleidomastoid and trapezius muscles, respectively.
- To palpate the deep cervical nodes, bend or hook your fingers around the sternocleidomastoid muscle.

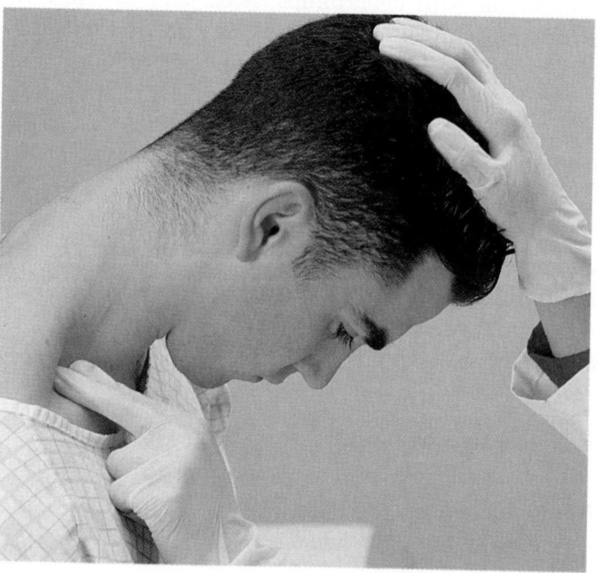

Figure 22–34 Palpating the supraclavicular lymph nodes.

ASSESSMENT	NORMAL FINDINGS	DEVIATIONS FROM NORMAL
Trachea		
Palpate the trachea for lateral deviation. Place your fingertip or thumb on the trachea in the suprasternal notch (Figure 22–32, earlier), and then move your finger laterally to the left and the right in spaces bordered by the clavicle, the anterior aspect of the sternocleidomastoid muscle, and the trachea.	Central placement in midline of neck; spaces are equal on both sides	Deviation to one side, indicating possible neck tumor; thyroid enlargement; enlarged lymph nodes
Thyroid Gland		
Inspect the thyroid gland.		
▪ Stand in front of the client.		
▪ Observe the lower half of the neck overlying the thyroid gland for symmetry and visible masses.	Not visible on inspection	Visible diffuseness or local enlargement

PROCEDURE 22–10 *continued*

ASSESSMENT	NORMAL FINDINGS	DEVIATIONS FROM NORMAL
▪ Ask the client to hyperextend the head and swallow. If necessary, offer a glass of water to make it easier for the client to swallow. This action determines how the thyroid and cricoid cartilages move and whether swallowing causes a bulging of the gland.	Gland ascends during swallowing but is not visible	Gland is not fully movable with swallowing
Palpate the thyroid gland for smoothness. Note any areas of enlargement, masses, or nodules. See the box below for palpation methods.	Lobes may not be palpated If palpated, lobes are small, smooth, centrally located, painless, and rise freely with swallowing	Solitary nodules
If enlargement of the gland is suspected, auscultate over the thyroid area for a bruit (a soft rushing sound created by turbulent blood flow). Use the bell-shaped diaphragm of the stethoscope.	Absence of bruit	Presence of bruit (see page 522 for further discussion of bruits)

Palpating the Thyroid Gland

Stand in front of or behind the client, and ask the client to lower the chin slightly. *Lowering the chin relaxes the neck muscles, facilitating palpation.*

Posterior Approach

- Place your hands around the client's neck, with your fingertips on the lower half of the neck over the trachea (Figure 22–35).
- Ask the client to swallow (taking a sip of water, if necessary), and feel for any enlargement of the *thyroid isthmus* as it rises. The isthmus lies across the trachea, below the cricoid cartilege. See Figure 22–32, earlier.
- To examine the right thyroid lobe, have the client lower the chin slightly and turn the head slightly to the right (the side being examined). With your left fingers, displace the trachea slightly to the right. With your right fingers, palpate the right thyroid lobe. Have the client swallow while you are palpating.
- Repeat the last step, in reverse, to examine the left thyroid lobe.

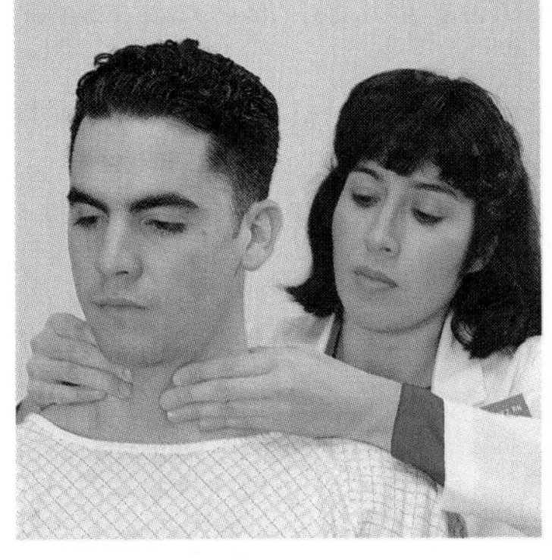

Figure 22–35 Placement of fingertips over the trachea to begin palpation of the thyroid gland (posterior approach).

Anterior Approach

- Place the tips of your index and middle fingers over the trachea, and palpate the thyroid isthmus as the client swallows.
- To examine the right thyroid lobe, have the client lower the chin slightly and turn the head slightly to the right. With your right fingers, displace the trachea slightly to the client's right (your left). With your left fingers, palpate the right thyroid lobe.
- To examine the left thyroid lobe, repeat the above step in reverse.

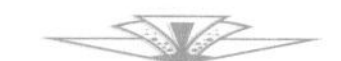

THE THORAX AND LUNGS

Assessing the thorax and lungs is frequently critical to assessing the client's aeration status. Changes in the respiratory system can come about slowly or quickly. In clients with chronic obstructive pulmonary disease (COPD), such as chronic bronchitis, emphysema, and asthma, changes are frequently gradual; however, in clients who are acutely ill, such as those who have a **pneumothorax** (accumulation of gas or fluid in the pleural cavity), changes occur quickly, and death can result if immediate action is not taken.

The client's posture is important to note. Some people with chronic respiratory problems tend to bend forward or even prop their arms on a support to elevate their clavicles. This posture is an attempt to expand the chest fully and thus breathe with less effort.

CHEST LANDMARKS

Before beginning the assessment, the nurse must be familiar with a series of imaginary lines on the chest wall and be able to locate the position of each rib and some spinous processes. These landmarks help the nurse to identify the position of underlying organs (eg, lobes of the lung) and to record abnormal assessment findings. Figure 22–36 shows the anterior, lateral, and posterior series of lines. The *midsternal line* is a vertical line running through the center of the sternum. The *midclavicular lines* (right and left) are vertical lines from the midpoints of the clavicles. The *anterior axillary lines* (right and left) are vertical lines from the anterior axillary folds (Figure 22–36, *A*). Figure 22–36, *B* shows the three imaginary lines of the lateral chest. The *posterior axillary line* is a vertical line from the posterior axillary fold. The *midaxillary line* is a vertical line from the apex of the axilla. The anterior axillary line is described above. Figure 22–36, *C* shows the posterior chest landmarks. The *vertebral line* is a vertical line along the spinous processes. The *scapular lines* (right and left) are vertical lines from the inferior angles of the scapulae.

Locating the position of each rib and certain spinous processes is essential for identifying underlying lobes of the lung. Figure 22–37, *A*, shows an anterior view of the chest and underlying lungs; Figure 22–37, *B*, a posterior view; and Figure 22–37, *C*, right and left lateral views. Each lung is first divided into the upper and lower lobes by an oblique fissure that runs from the level of the spinous process of the third thoracic vertebra (T-3) to the level of the sixth rib at the midclavicular line (Figure 22–37, *A*). The right upper lobe is abbreviated RUL; the right lower lobe, RLL. Similarly, the left upper lobe is abbreviated LUL; the left lower lobe, LLL. The right lung is further divided by a minor fissure into the right upper lobe and right middle lobe (RML). This fissure runs anteriorly from the right midaxillary line at the level of the fifth rib to the level of the fourth rib.

These specific landmarks, that is, T-3 and the fourth, fifth, and sixth ribs, are located as follows. The starting

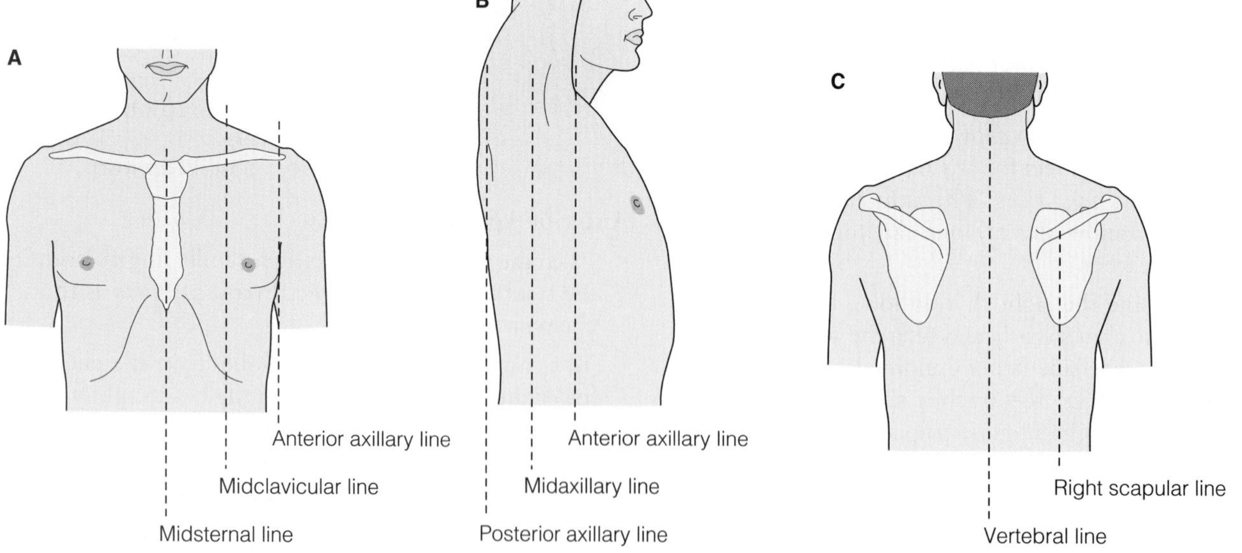

Figure 22–36 Chest wall landmarks: *A*, anterior chest; *B*, lateral chest; *C*, posterior chest.

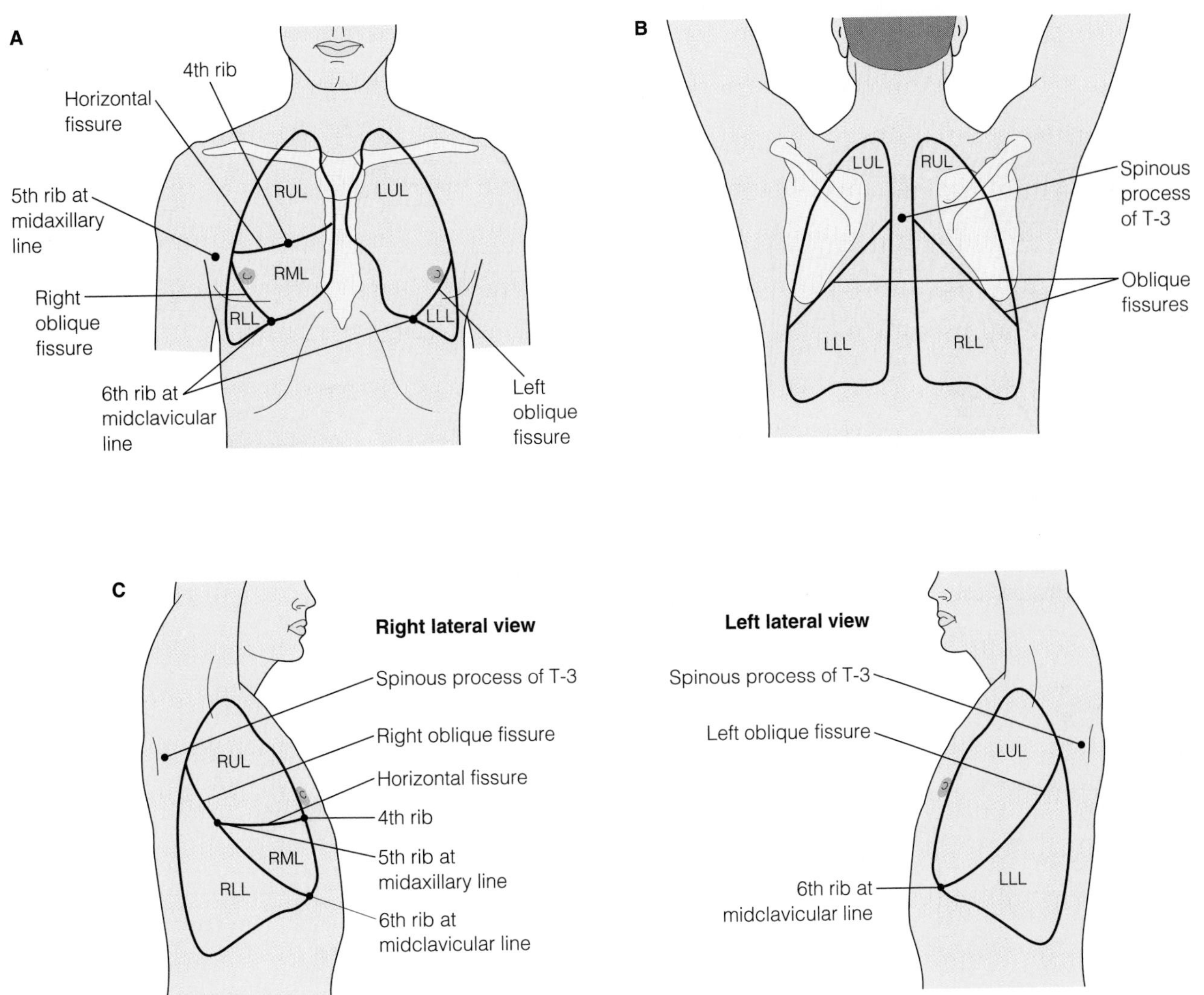

Figure 22–37 Chest landmarks: *A,* anterior chest landmarks and underlying lungs; *B,* posterior chest landmarks and underlying lungs; *C,* lateral chest landmarks and underlying lungs.

point for locating the ribs anteriorly is the **angle of Louis,** the junction between the body of the **sternum** (breastbone) and the **manubrium** (the handelike superior part of the sternum that joins with the clavicles). The superior border of the second rib attaches to the sternum at this manubriosternal junction (Figure 22–38, p. 510). The nurse can identify the manubrium by first palpating the clavicle and following its course to its attachment at the manubrium. The nurse then palpates and counts distal ribs and intercostal spaces (ICS) from the second rib. It is important to note that an ICS is numbered according to the number of the rib immediately *above* the space. When palpating for rib identification, the nurse should palpate along the midclavicular line rather than the sternal border, because the rib cartilages are very close at the sternum. Only the first seven ribs attach directly to the sternum.

The counting of ribs is more difficult on the posterior than on the anterior thorax. For identifying underlying lung lobes, the pertinent landmark is T-3. The starting point for locating T-3 is the spinous process of the seventh cervical vertebra (C-7), also referred to as the *vertebra prominens* (Figure 22–39, p. 510). When the neck is flexed anteriorly, a prominent process can be observed and palpated. This is the spinous process of the seventh cervical vertebra. If two spinous processes are observed,

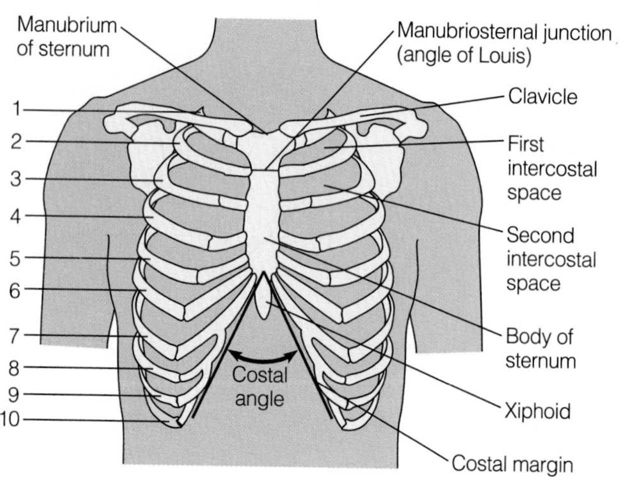

Figure 22–38 Location of the anterior ribs in relation to the angle of Louis and the sternum.

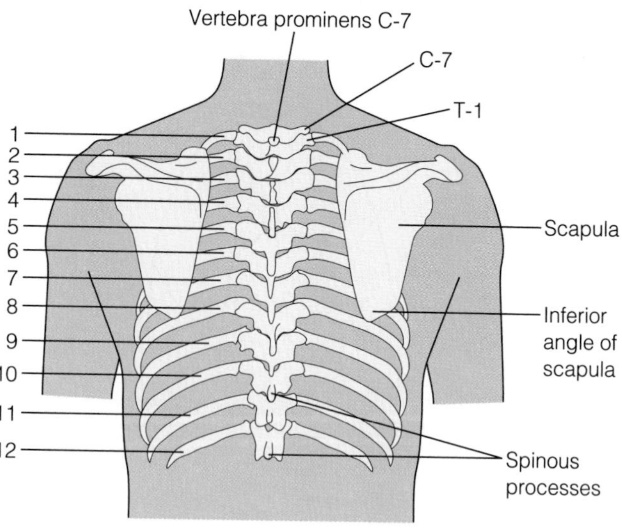

Figure 22–39 Location of the posterior ribs in relation to the spinous processes of the vertebrae.

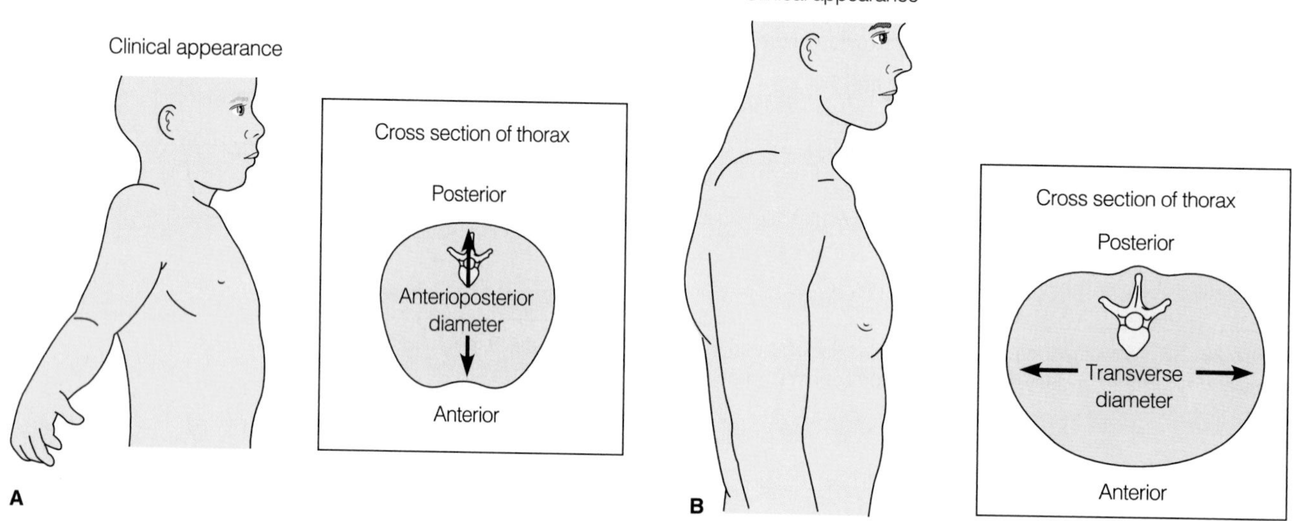

Figure 22–40 Configurations of the thorax showing anteroposterior diameter and transverse diameter: *A*, infant; *B*, adult.

the superior one is C-7, and the inferior one is the spinous process of the first thoracic vertebra (T-1). The nurse then palpates and counts the spinous processes from C-7 to T-3. Each spinous process up to T-4 is adjacent to the corresponding rib number; for example, T-3 is adjacent to the third rib. After T-4, however, the spinous processes project obliquely, causing the spinous process of the vertebra to lie, not over its correspondingly numbered rib, but over the rib below. Thus, the spinous process of T-5 lies over the body of T-6 and is adjacent to the sixth rib.

Chest Shape and Size

In the infant, the thorax is rounded; that is, the diameter from the front to the back (anteroposterior) is equal to the transverse diameter. It is also cylindrical, having a nearly

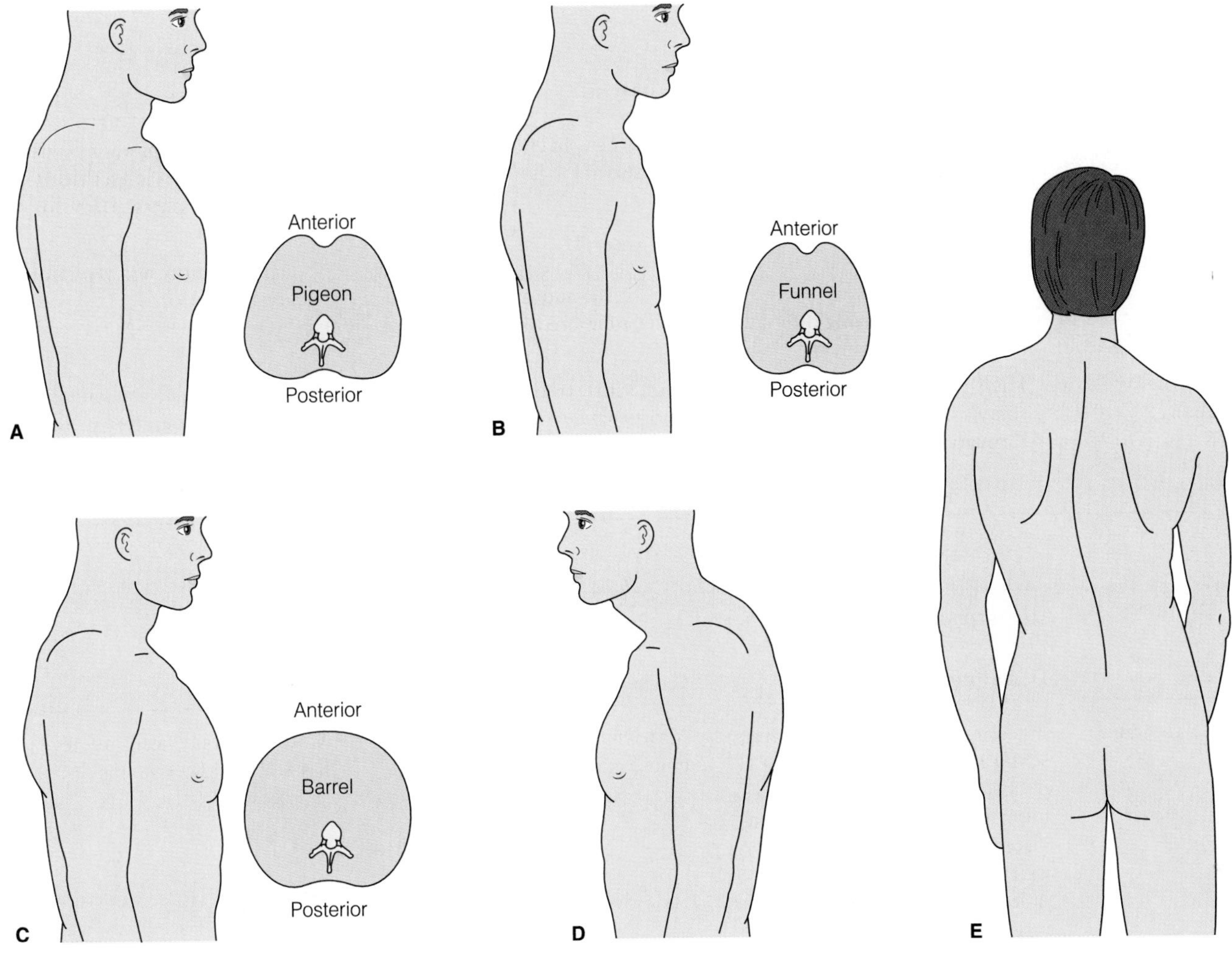

Figure 22–41 Chest deformities: *A,* pigeon chest; *B,* funnel chest; *C,* barrel chest; *D,* kyphosis; *E,* scoliosis.

equal diameter at the top and the base. When a child reaches 6 years, the anteroposterior diameter has decreased in proportion to the transverse one. In adults, the thorax is oval. Its anteroposterior diameter is two times smaller than its transverse diameter (Figure 22–40). The overall shape of the thorax is elliptical; that is, its diameter is smaller at the top than at the base. In the elderly, kyphosis and osteoporosis alter the size of the chest cavity as the ribs move downward and forward.

There are several deformities of the chest (Figure 22–41). **Pigeon chest (pectus carinatum),** a permanent deformity, may be caused by rickets. Pigeon chest is characterized by a narrow transverse diameter, an increased anteroposterior diameter, and a protruding sternum. A **funnel chest (pectus excavatum),** a congenital defect, is the opposite of pigeon chest in that the sternum is depressed, narrowing the anteroposterior diameter. Because the sternum points posteriorly in clients with a funnel chest, abnormal pressure on the heart may result in altered function. A **barrel chest,** in which the ratio of the anteroposterior to lateral diameter is 1 to 1, is seen in clients with thoracic **kyphosis** (excessive convex curvature of the thoracic spine) and **emphysema** (chronic pulmonary condition in which the air sacs, or alveoli, are dilated and distended). **Scoliosis** is a lateral deviation of the spine.

BREATH SOUNDS

Abnormal breath sounds, called **adventitious breath sounds,** occur when air passes through narrowed airways or airways filled with fluid or mucus, or when pleural linings are inflamed. See Table 22–7 on page 512 for normal breath sounds. Adventitious sounds are often superimposed over normal sounds. The three types of adventitious sounds—crackles (referred to as rales or **crepitations**), gurgles, and pleural friction rub—are described in the box in Chapter 21 on page 449, and in Table 22–8.

Table 22–7 Normal Breath Sounds

Type	Description	Location	Characteristics
Vesicular	Soft-intensity, low-pitched, "gentle sighing" sounds created by air moving through smaller airways (bronchioles and alveoli)	Over peripheral lung; best heard at base of lungs	Best heard on inspiration, which is about 2.5 times longer than the expiratory phase (5:2 ratio)
Bronchovesicular	Moderate-intensity and moderate-pitched "blowing" sounds created by air moving through larger airways (bronchi)	Between the scapulae and lateral to the sternum at the first and second intercostal spaces	Equal inspiratory and expiratory phases (1:1 ratio)
Bronchial (tubular)	High-pitched, loud, "harsh" sounds created by air moving through the trachea	Anteriorly over the trachea; not normally heard over lung tissue	Louder than vesicular sounds; have a short inspiratory phase and long expiratory phase (1:2 ratio)

Table 22–8 Adventitious Breath Sounds

Name	Description	Cause	Location
Crackles (rales)	Fine, short, interrupted crackling sounds; alveolar rales are high-pitched; bronchial rales are lower-pitched. Sound can be simulated by rolling a lock of hair near the ear. Best heard on inspiration but can be heard on both inspiration and expiration. May not be cleared by coughing.	Air passing through fluid or mucus in any air passage	Most commonly heard in the bases of the lower lung lobes.
Gurgles (rhonchi)	Continuous, low-pitched, coarse, gurgling, harsh, louder sounds with a moaning or snoring quality. Best heard on expiration but can be heard on both inspiration and expiration. May be altered by coughing.	Air passing through narrowed air passages as a result of secretions, swelling, tumors	Loud sounds can be heard over most lung areas but predominate over the trachea and bronchi.
Friction rub	Superficial grating or creaking sounds heard during inspiration and expiration. Not relieved by coughing.	Rubbing together of inflamed pleural surfaces	Heard most often in areas of greatest thoracic expansion (eg, lower anterior and lateral chest).
Wheeze	Continuous, high-pitched, squeaky musical sounds. Best heard on expiration. Not usually altered by coughing.	Air passing through a constricted bronchi as a result of secretions, swelling, tumors	Heard over all lung fields.

Absence of breath sounds over some lung areas is also a significant finding that is associated with collapsed and surgically removed lobes.

Assessment of the lungs and thorax includes all methods of examination: inspection, palpation, percussion, and auscultation. The following are needed for the examination: (a) stethoscope, (b) a marking pencil, and (c) a centimeter ruler. For efficiency, the nurse usually examines the posterior chest first, then the anterior chest. For posterior and lateral chest examinations, the client is uncovered to the waist and in a sitting position. A sitting or lying position may be used for anterior chest examination. The sitting position is preferred because it maximizes chest expansion. Good lighting is essential, especially for chest inspection. See Procedure 21–11.

Text continued on page 518

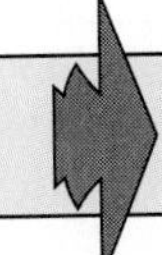

PROCEDURE 22–11 ASSESSING THE THORAX AND LUNGS

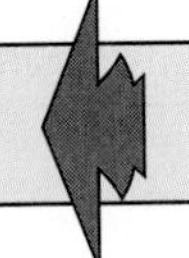

NURSING HISTORY FOCUS

Family history of illness (eg, cancer, allergies, tuberculosis); life-style (eg, smoking and occupational hazards like inhaling fumes); any medications being taken; current problems, (eg, swellings, coughs, wheezing, pain).

ASSESSMENT	NORMAL FINDINGS	DEVIATIONS FROM NORMAL
Posterior Thorax		
Inspect the shape and symmetry of the thorax from posterior and lateral views. Compare the anteroposterior diameter to the lateral diameter.	Anteroposterior to lateral diameter in ratio of 1:2 Chest symmetric	Barrel chest; increased anteroposterior to lateral diameter Chest asymmetric
Inspect the spinal alignment for deformities. Have the client stand. From a lateral position, observe the three normal curvatures: (cervical, thoracic, and lumbar). From the posterior, drop a plumb line from the occiput of the skull to the gluteal cleft.	Spine vertically aligned	Exaggerated spinal curvatures (kyphosis, lordosis); lateral deviation of spine (scoliosis)
Palpate the posterior thorax.		
▪ For clients who have no respiratory complaints, rapidly assess the temperature and integrity of all chest skin.	Skin intact; uniform temperature	Skin lesions; areas of hyperthermia
▪ For clients who do have respiratory complaints, palpate all chest areas for bulges, tenderness, or abnormal movements. Avoid deep palpation for painful areas, especially if a fractured rib is suspected. *In such a case, deep palpation could lead to displacement of the bone fragment against the lungs.*	Chest wall intact; no tenderness; no masses	Lumps, bulges; depressions; areas of tenderness; movable structures (eg, rib)
Palpate the posterior chest for respiratory excursion (thoracic expansion). Place the palms of both your hands over the lower thorax with your thumbs adjacent to the spine and your fingers stretched laterally (Figure 22–42, p. 514). Ask the client to take a deep breath while you observe the movement of your hands and any lag in movement.	Full and symmetric chest expansion (ie, when the client takes a deep breath, your thumbs should move apart an equal distance and at the same time; normally the thumbs separate 3 to 5 cm [1½ to 2 in] during deep inspiration)	Asymmetric and/or decreased chest expansion

Procedure 22–11 Assessing the Thorax and Lungs *continued*

ASSESSMENT	NORMAL FINDINGS	DEVIATIONS FROM NORMAL

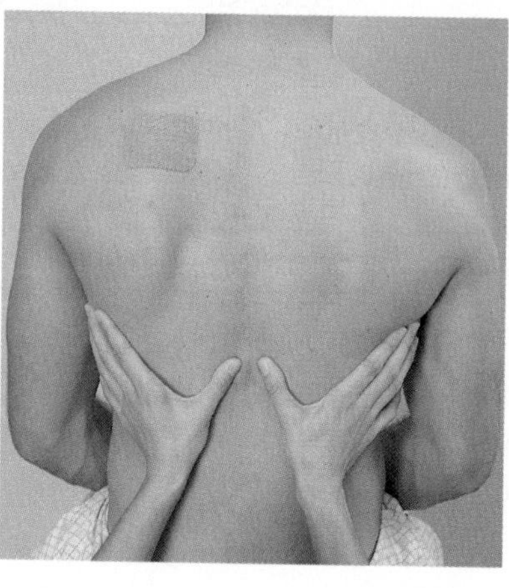

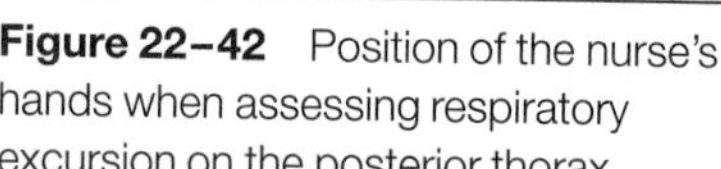

Figure 22–42 Position of the nurse's hands when assessing respiratory excursion on the posterior thorax.

Palpate the chest for vocal (tactile) fremitus, the faintly perceptible vibration felt through the chest wall when the client speaks.

- Place the palmar surfaces of your fingertips or the ulnar aspect of your hand or closed fist on the posterior chest, starting near the apex of the lungs (Figure 22–43, position A).
- Ask the client to repeat such words as "blue moon" or "one, two, three."
- Repeat the two steps, moving your hands sequentially to the base of the lungs, through positions B through E in Figure 22–43.
- Compare the fremitus on both lungs and between the apex and the base of each lung, using either one hand and moving it from one side of the client to the corresponding area on the other side

  or

  using two hands that are placed simultaneously on the corresponding areas of each side of the chest.

Normal findings:

Bilateral symmetry of vocal fremitus

Fremitus is heard most clearly at the apex of the lungs

Low-pitched voices of males are more readily palpated than higher-pitched voices of females

Deviations from normal:

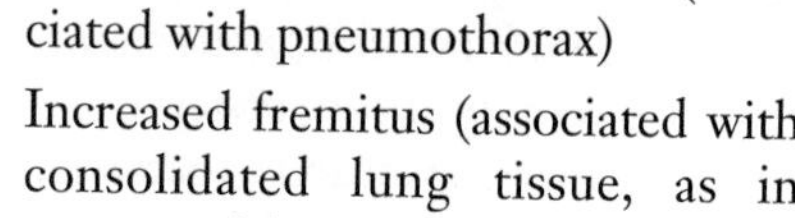

Decreased or absent fremitus (associated with pneumothorax)

Increased fremitus (associated with consolidated lung tissue, as in pneumonia)

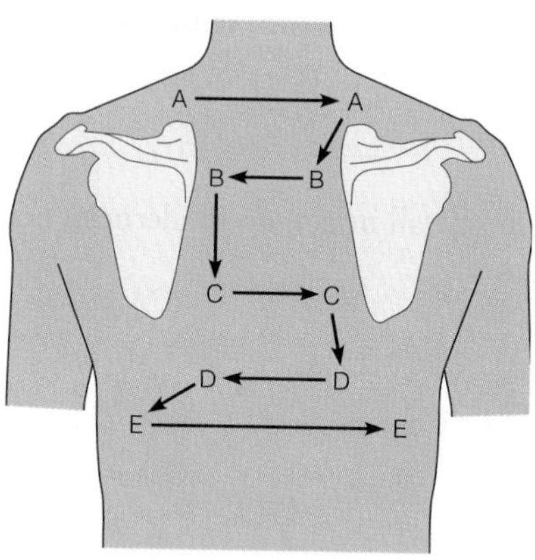

Figure 22–43 Areas and sequence for palpating tactile fremitus on the posterior chest.

Percuss the thorax. See the box on page 515.

Normal findings: Percussion notes resonate, except over scapula

Deviations from normal: Asymmetry in percussion

PROCEDURE 22–11 *continued*

ASSESSMENT	NORMAL FINDINGS	DEVIATIONS FROM NORMAL
	Lowest point of resonance is at the diaphragm (ie, at the level of the eighth to tenth rib posteriorly) *Note:* percussion on a rib normally elicits dullness	Areas of dullness or flatness over lung tissue (associated with consolidation of lung tissue or a mass)
Percuss for diaphragmatic excursion (movement of the diaphragm during maximal inspiration and expiration).	Excursion is 3 to 5 cm (1½ to 2 in) bilaterally in females and 5 to 6 cm (2 to 3 in) in males Diaphragm is usually slightly higher on the right side	Restricted excursion (associated with lung disorder)

Percussing the Thorax

Percussing for Normal Thorax Sounds

Percussion of the thorax is performed to determine whether underlying lung tissue is filled with air, liquid, or solid material and to determine the positions and boundaries of certain organs. Because percussion penetrates to a depth of 5 to 7 cm (2 to 3 in), it detects superficial rather than deep lesions. Percussion sounds and tones are described in Table 22–3, page 470.

- Ask the client to bend the head and fold the arms forward across the chest. *This separates the scapula and exposes more lung tissue to percussion.*
- Percuss in the intercostal spaces at about 5 cm (2 in) intervals in a systematic sequence (Figure 22–44). Figure 22–45 shows normal percussion sounds in the posterior chest.
- Compare one side of the lung with the other.
- Percuss the lateral thorax every few inches, starting at the axilla and working down to the eighth rib.

Percussing for Diaphragmatic Excursion

- Ask the client to take a deep breath and hold it while you percuss downward along the scapular line until dullness is produced at the level of the diaphragm. Mark this point with a marking pencil, and repeat the procedure on the other side of the chest.
- Ask the client to take a few normal breaths and then expel the last breath completely and hold it. Meanwhile, percuss upward from the marked point to assess and mark the diaphragmatic excursion during deep expiration on each side.
- Measure the distance between the two marks.

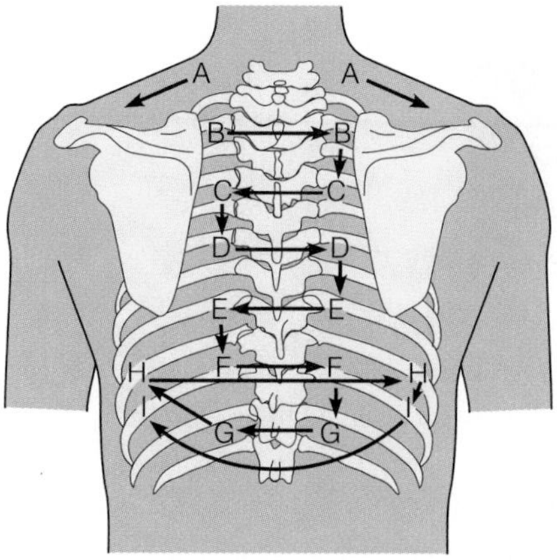

Figure 22–44 Sequence for posterior chest percussion.

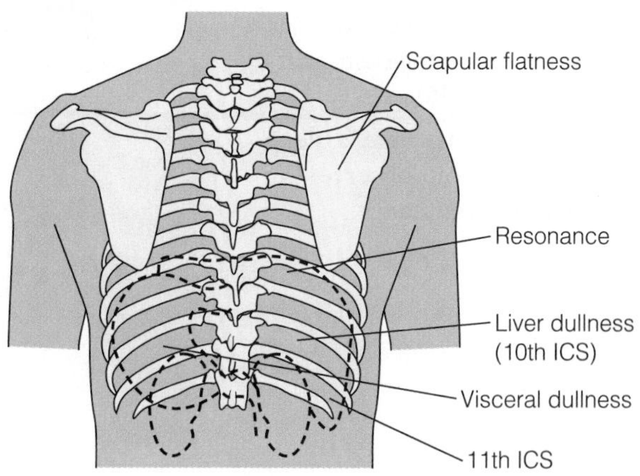

Figure 22–45 Normal percussion sounds on the posterior chest.

Procedure 22–11 Assessing the Thorax and Lungs *continued*

ASSESSMENT	NORMAL FINDINGS	DEVIATIONS FROM NORMAL
Auscultate the chest using the flat-disc diaphragm of the stethoscope (best for transmitting the high-pitched breath sounds). ▪ Use the systematic zigzag procedure used in percussion (Figure 22–44, p. 515) ▪ Ask the client to take slow, deep breaths through the mouth. Listen at each point to the breath sounds during a complete inspiration and expiration. ▪ Compare findings at each point with the corresponding point on the opposite side of the chest.	Vesicular and bronchovesicular breath sounds (see Table 22–7, p. 512)	Adventitious breath sounds (eg, crackles, rhonchi, wheeze, friction rub; see Table 22–8, p. 512) Absence of breath sounds (associated with collapsed and surgically removed lung lobes)
Anterior Thorax		
Inspect breathing patterns (eg, respiratory rate and rhythm).	See Chapter 21, page 447	See Chapters 21, page 449, and 39, page 1135, for abnormal breathing patterns and sounds
Inspect the costal angle (angle formed by the intersection of the costal margins) **and the angle at which the ribs enter the spine.**	Costal angle is less than 90 degrees, and the ribs insert into the spine at approximately a 45-degree angle (Figure 22–38, p. 510)	Costal angle is widened (associated with chronic obstructive pulmonary disease)
Palpate the anterior chest (see posterior chest palpation).		
Palpate the anterior chest for respiratory excursion. ▪ Place the palms of both hands on the lower thorax, with fingers laterally along the lower rib cage and thumbs along the costal margins (Figure 22–46). ▪ Ask the client to take a deep breath while you observe the movement of your hands.	Full symmetric excursion; thumbs normally separate 3 to 5 cm (1½ to 2 in) 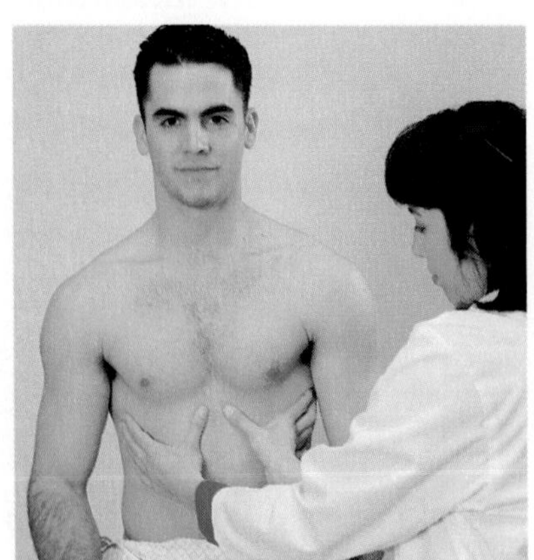 **Figure 22–46** Position of nurse's hands when assessing respiratory excursion on the anterior thorax.	Asymmetric and/or decreased respiratory excursion

PROCEDURE 22–11 *continued*

ASSESSMENT	NORMAL FINDINGS	DEVIATIONS FROM NORMAL
Palpate tactile fremitus in the same manner as for the posterior chest and using the sequence shown in Figure 22–47. If the breasts are large and cannot be retracted adequately for palpation, this part of the examination is usually omitted.	Same as posterior vocal fremitus Fremitus is normally decreased over heart and breast tissue	Same as posterior fremitus

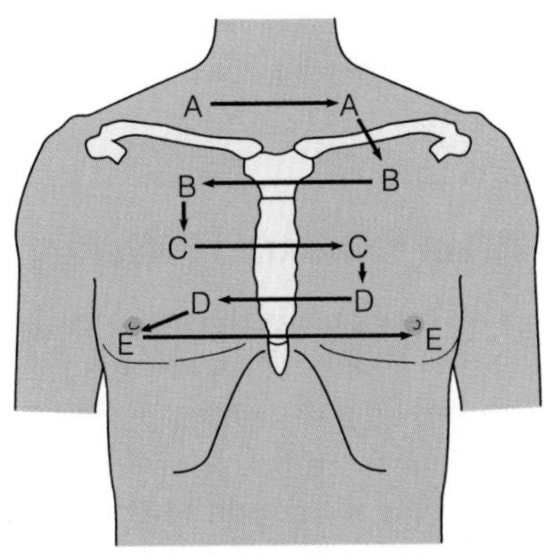

Figure 22–47 Areas and sequence for palpating tactile fremitus on the anterior chest.

ASSESSMENT	NORMAL FINDINGS	DEVIATIONS FROM NORMAL
Percuss the anterior chest systematically. ▪ Begin above the clavicles in the supraclavicular space, and proceed downward to the diaphragm (Figure 22–48). ▪ Compare one side of the lung to the other. ▪ Displace female breasts for proper examination.	Percussion notes resonate down to the sixth rib at the level of the diaphragm but are flat over areas of heavy muscle and bone, dull on areas over the heart and the liver, and tympanic over the underlying stomach (Figure 22–49)	Asymmetry in percussion notes Areas of dullness or flatness over lung tissue

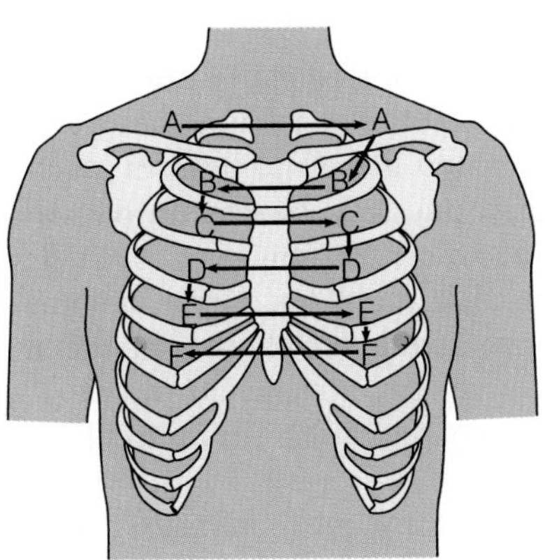

Figure 22–48 Sequence for anterior chest percussion.

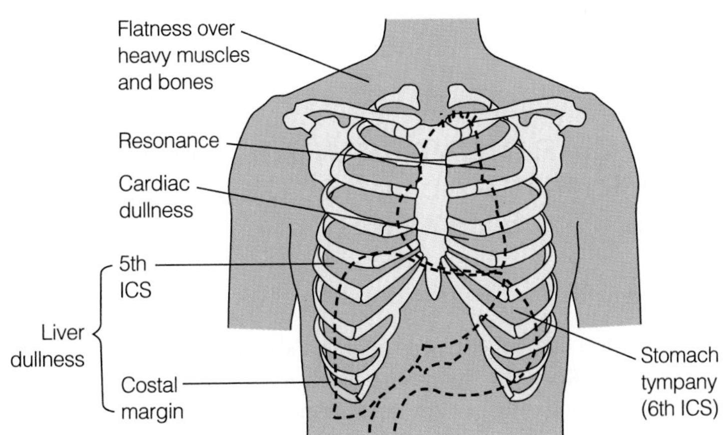

Figure 22–49 Normal percussion sounds on the anterior chest.

ASSESSMENT	NORMAL FINDINGS	DEVIATIONS FROM NORMAL
Auscultate the trachea.	Bronchial and tubular breath sounds (see Table 22–7, p. 512)	Adventitious breath sounds (see Table 22–8, p. 512)

➤

PROCEDURE 22–11 ASSESSING THE THORAX AND LUNGS *continued*

ASSESSMENT	NORMAL FINDINGS	DEVIATIONS FROM NORMAL
Auscultate the anterior chest. Use the sequence used in percussion (Figure 22–48, p. 517), beginning over the bronchi between the sternum and the clavicles.	Bronchovesicular and vesicular breath sounds (see Table 22–7, p. 512)	Adventitious breath sounds (see Table 22–8, p. 512)

THE ELDERLY: PHYSICAL CHANGES OF THE THORAX AND BREATHING PATTERNS

- The thoracic curvature may be accentuated (kyphosis) because of osteoporosis and changes in cartilage, resulting in collapse of the vertebrae.
- The anteroposterior diameter of the chest widens, giving the person a barrel-chested appearance. This is due to loss of skeletal muscle strength in the thorax and diaphragm and constant lung inflation from excessive expiratory pressure on the alveoli.
- Breathing rate and rhythm are unchanged at rest; the rate normally increases with exercise but may take longer to return to the preexercise rate.
- Inspiratory muscles become less powerful, and the inspiration reserve volume decreases. A decrease in depth of respiration is therefore apparent.
- Expiration may require the use of accessory muscles. The expiratory reserve volume significantly increases because of the increased amount of air remaining in the lungs at the end of a normal breath.
- Deflation of the lung is incomplete.
- Small airways lose their cartilaginous support and elastic recoil; as a result, they tend to close, particularly in basal or dependent portions of the lung.
- Elastic tissue of the alveoli loses its stretchability and changes to fibrous tissue. This thicker alveolar membrane decreases the pulmonary diffusion capacity. As a result, arterial oxyhemoglobin saturation and PaO_2 are slightly lower than those of young adults. Exertional capacity also decreases.
- Cilia in the airways decrease in number and are less effective in removing mucus; elderly clients are therefore at greater risk for pulmonary infections.

THE CARDIOVASCULAR AND PERIPHERAL VASCULAR SYSTEMS

HEART

Heart function can be assessed to a large degree by findings in the history, by symptoms such as shortness of breath, by the client's general appearance (eg, cyanosis and edema of the legs suggest impaired function), and by pulse rate, rhythm, and quality. Direct examination of the heart, however, offers more specific information, including the heart sounds, the heart size, and such findings as lifts, heaves, or **murmurs** (more prolonged sounds during systole and diastole). Nurses assess heart functions through observations (inspection), palpation, and auscultation, in that sequence. Auscultation is more meaningful when other data are obtained first. The heart is usually assessed during an initial physical assessment; periodic reassessments may be necessary for long-term or at-risk clients or those with cardiac problems. Heart examinations are usually performed while the client is in a semi-reclined position. The practitioner stands at the client's right side, where palpation of the cardiac area is facilitated and optimal inspection allowed.

To assess the client's heart, the nurse must first determine its exact location. In the average adult, most of the heart lies behind and to the left of the sternum. A small portion (the right atrium) extends to the right of the sternum. The upper portion of the heart (both atria), referred to as its **base,** lies toward the back. The lower portion (the ventricles), referred to as its **apex,** points forward. The

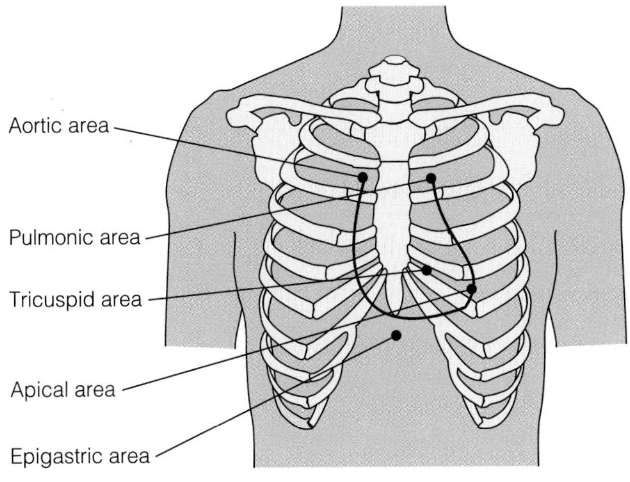

Figure 22–50 Anatomic sites of the precordium.

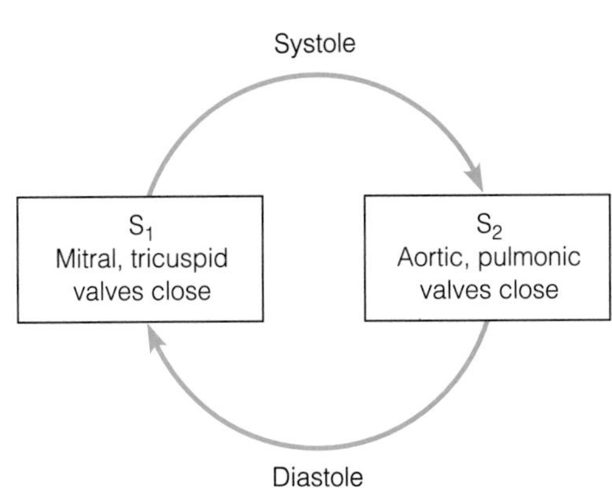

Figure 22–51 Relationship of heart sounds to systole and diastole.

apex of the left ventricle actually touches the anterior chest wall at or medial to the left midclavicular line (MCL) and at or near the fifth left intercostal space (LICS), which is slightly below the left nipple. See Figure 21–14 on page 439. This point where the apex touches the anterior chest wall is known as the **point of maximal impulse (PMI).**

The **precordium,** the area of the chest overlying the heart, is inspected and palpated simultaneously for the presence of abnormal pulsations or lifts or heaves. The terms **lift** and **heave,** often used interchangeably, refer to a rising along the sternal border with each heartbeat. A lift occurs when cardiac action is very forceful (overactive). It should be confirmed by palpation with the palm of the hand. Enlargement or overactivity of the left ventricle produces a heave lateral to the apex, whereas enlargement of the right ventricle produces a heave at or near the sternum.

Several heart sounds can be heard by auscultation. Only the first and second heart sounds (S_1 and S_2) will be emphasized in this book. The normal first two heart sounds are produced by closure of the valves of the heart. The first heart sound, $\mathbf{S_1}$, occurs when the atrioventricular (A-V) valves close. These valves close when the ventricles have been sufficiently filled. Although the right and left A-V valves do not close simultaneously, the closures occur closely enough to be heard as one sound (S_1), a dull, lowpitched sound described as "lub." After the ventricles empty their blood into the aorta and pulmonary arteries, the semilunar valves close, producing the second heart sound, $\mathbf{S_2}$, described as "dub." S_2 has a higher pitch than S_1 and is also shorter. These two sounds, S_1 and S_2 ("lub-dub"), occur within 1 second or less, depending on the heart rate.

The two heart sounds are audible anywhere on the precordial area, but they are best heard over the aortic, pulmonic, tricuspid, and apical areas (Figure 22–50). Each area is associated with the closure of heart valves: the aortic area with the aortic valve (inside the aorta as it arises from the left ventricle); the pulmonic area with the pulmonic valve (inside the pulmonary artery as it arises from the right ventricle); the tricuspid area with the tricuspid valve (between the right atrium and ventricle); and the apical (mitral) area with the mitral valve (between the left atrium and ventricle).

Associated with these sounds are systole and diastole. **Systole** is the period in which the ventricles contract. It begins with the first heart sound and ends at the second heart sound. Systole is normally shorter than diastole. **Diastole** is the period in which the ventricles relax. It starts with the second sound and ends at the subsequent first sound. Normally no sounds are audible during these periods (Figure 22–51). The experienced nurse, however, may perceive extra heart sounds (S_3 and S_4) during diastole. Both sounds are low in pitch and heard best at the apical site, with the bell of the stethoscope, and with the client lying on the left side. S_3 occurs early in diastole right after S_2 and sounds like "lub-dub-*ee*" (S_1, S_2, S_3) or "Kentuc-*ky*." It often disappears when the client sits up. S_3 is normal in children and young adults. In older adults, it may indicate heart failure. S_4 is rarely heard in healthy clients. It occurs near the very end of diastole just before S_1 and creates the sound of "*dee*-lub-dub" (S_4, S_1, S_2) or "*Ten*-nessee." S_4 may be heard in many elderly clients and can be a sign of hypertension.

Normal heart sounds are summarized in Table 22–9 on page 520. Procedure 22–12 describes how to assess the cardiovascular system.

Text continued on page 522

Table 22–9 Normal Heart Sounds

Sound or Phase	Description	Area: Aortic	Pulmonic	Tricuspid	Apical
S_1	Dull, low-pitched, and longer than S_2; sounds like "lub"	Less intensity than S_2	Less intensity than S_2	Louder than or equal to S_2	Louder than or equal to S_2
S_2	High-pitched, snappy, and shorter than S_1; creates sound of "dub"	Louder than S_1	Louder than S_1; abnormal if louder than the aortic S_2 in adults over 40	Less intensity than or equal to S_1	Less intensity than or equal to S_1
Systole	Normally silent interval between S_1 and S_2				
Diastole	Normally silent interval between S_2 and next S_1				

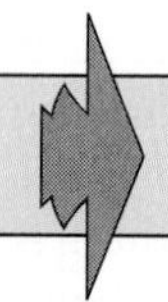

PROCEDURE 22–12 ASSESSING THE CARDIOVASCULAR SYSTEM

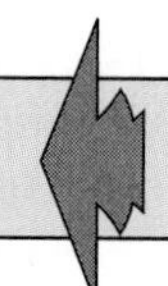

NURSING HISTORY FOCUS

Family history of incidence and age of heart disease, high cholesterol levels, high blood pressure, stroke, obesity, congenital heart disease, and rheumatic fever; client's past history of rheumatic fever, heart murmur, heart attack, or heart failure; present symptoms indicative of heart disease (eg, fatigue, dyspnea, orthopnea, edema, cough, chest pain, palpitations, syncope, hypertension, wheezing, hemoptysis); presence of diseases that affect heart (eg, obesity, diabetes, lung disease, endocrine disorders); life-style habits that are risk factors for cardiac disease (eg, smoking, alcohol intake, eating and exercise patterns, areas and degree of stress perceived).

ASSESSMENT	NORMAL FINDINGS	DEVIATIONS FROM NORMAL
Simultaneously inspect and palpate the precordium for the presence of abnormal pulsations, lifts, or heaves. To locate the valve areas of the heart, see the box on page 521.		
▪ Inspect and palpate the aortic and pulmonic areas, observing them at an angle and to the side, to note the presence or absence of pulsations. *Observing these areas at an angle increases the likelihood of seeing pulsations.*	No pulsations, although some people have aortic pulsations	Pulsations

PROCEDURE 22–12 *continued*

ASSESSMENT	NORMAL FINDINGS	DEVIATIONS FROM NORMAL
▪ Inspect and palpate the tricuspid area for pulsations and heaves or lifts.	No pulsations No lift or heave	Pulsations Diffuse lift or heave, indicating enlarged or overactive right ventricle
▪ Inspect and palpate the apical area for pulsation, noting its specific location (it may be displaced laterally or lower) and diameter. If displaced laterally, record the distance between the apex and the MCL in centimeters.	Pulsations visible in 50% of adults and palpable in most PMI in fifth LICS at or medial to MCL Diameter of 1 to 2 cm (⅓ to ½ in) No lift or heave	PMI displaced laterally or lower (indicates enlarged heart) Diameter over 2 cm (indicates enlarged heart or aneurysm) Diffuse lift or heave lateral to apex (indicates enlargement or overactivity of left ventricle)
▪ Inspect and palpate the epigastric area at the base of the sternum for abdominal aortic pulsations.	Aortic pulsations	Bounding abdominal pulsations (eg, aortic aneurysm)

Locating the Aortic, Pulmonic, Tricuspid, and Apical Areas of the Precordium

- Locate the angle of Louis (the point of tracheal bifurcation). It is felt as a prominence on the sternum.
- Move your fingertips down each side of the angle until you can feel the second intercostal spaces. The client's right second intercostal space is the *aortic area*, and the left second intercostal space is the *pulmonic area.*
- From the pulmonic area, move your fingertips down three left intercostal spaces along the side of the sternum. The left fifth intercostal space close to the sternum is the *tricuspid* or *right ventricular area.*
- From the tricuspid area, move your fingertips laterally 5 to 7 cm (2 to 3 in) to the left midclavicular line (LMCL). This is the *apical* or *mitral area*, or point of maximal impulse (PMI). If you have difficulty locating the PMI, have the client roll onto the left side to move the apex closer to the chest wall.

ASSESSMENT	NORMAL FINDINGS	DEVIATIONS FROM NORMAL
Auscultate the heart in all four anatomic sites: aortic, pulmonic, tricuspid, and apical (mitral). Auscultation need not be limited to these areas; however, the nurse may need to move the stethoscope to find the most audible sounds for each client. The upper box on page 522 describes the steps involved in auscultating the heart.	S_1: Usually heard at all sites Usually louder at apical area	Increased or decreased intensity Varying intensity with different beats
	S_2: Usually heard at all sites Usually louder at base of heart	Increased intensity at aortic area Increased intensity at pulmonic area
	Systole: Silent interval Slightly shorter duration than diastole at normal heart rate (60 to 90 beats/min)	Sharp-sounding ejection clicks
	Diastole: silent interval Slightly longer duration than systole at normal heart rates	S_3 in older adults
	S_3 in children and young adults	
	S_4 in many older adults	S_4 may be a sign of hypertension

PROCEDURE 22–12 ASSESSING THE CARDIOVASCULAR SYSTEM *continued*

Auscultating the Heart

- Eliminate all sources of room noise. *Heart sounds are of low intensity, and other noise hinders the nurse's ability to hear them.*
- Keep the client in a supine position with head elevated 30 to 45 degrees.
- Use both the flat-disc diaphragm and the bell-shaped diaphragm to listen to all areas.
- In every area of auscultation, distinguish both S_1 and S_2 sounds.
- When auscultating, concentrate on one particular sound at a time in each area: the first heart sound, followed by systole, then the second heart sound, then diastole. Systole and diastole are normally silent intervals.
- Later, reexamine the heart while the client is in the upright sitting position. *Certain sounds are more audible in certain positions.*

THE ELDERLY: PHYSICAL CHANGES OF THE HEART

- If no disease is present, heart size remains the same size throughout life.
- Cardiac output and strength of contraction decrease, thus lessening the older person's activity tolerance.
- The heart rate returns to its resting rate more slowly after exertion than it did when the individual was younger.
- S_4 heart sound is considered normal in older adults.
- Extra systoles commonly occur. Ten or more systoles per minute are considered abnormal.
- Sudden emotional and physical stresses may result in cardiac arrhythmias and heart failure.

PERIPHERAL VASCULAR SYSTEM

Assessing the peripheral vascular system includes measuring the blood pressure; palpating peripheral pulses; inspecting, palpating, and auscultating the carotid pulse; inspecting the jugular and peripheral veins; and inspecting the skin and tissues to determine **perfusion** (passage of blood constituents through the vessels) to the extremities. Certain aspects of peripheral vascular assessment are often incorporated into other parts of the assessment procedure. For example, blood pressure is usually measured at the beginning of the physical examination (see the section on assessing blood pressure in Chapter 21).

Pulse sites and pulse assessments are described in Chapter 21. Figures 21–13 and 21–16 illustrate the sites for palpating the peripheral pulses.

The *carotid arteries* supply oxygenated blood to the head and neck (Figure 22–52). Because they are the only source of blood to the brain, prolonged occlusion of one of these arteries can result in serious brain damage. The carotid pulses correlate with central aortic pressure, thus reflecting cardiac function better than the peripheral pulses. When cardiac output is diminished, the peripheral pulses may be difficult or impossible to feel, but the carotid pulse should be felt easily.

The carotid is also auscultated for a bruit, and if a bruit is found, the carotid artery is then palpated for a thrill. A **bruit** (a blowing or swishing sound) is created by turbulence of blood flow due either to a narrowed arterial lumen (a common development in older people) or to a condition, such as anemia or hyperthyroidism, that elevates cardiac output. A **thrill,** which frequently accompanies a bruit, is a vibrating sensation like the purring of a cat or water running through a hose. It, too, indicates turbulent blood flow due to arterial obstruction.

The *jugular veins* drain blood from the head and neck directly into the superior vena cava and right side of the heart (Figure 22–52). The external jugular veins are superficial and may be visible above the clavicle. The internal jugular veins lie deeper along the carotid artery and may transmit pulsations onto the skin of the neck. Normally, external neck veins are distended and visible when a person lies down; they are flat and not as visible when a person stands up, because gravity encourages venous drainage. By inspecting the jugular veins for pulsations and distention, the nurse can assess the adequacy of function of the right side of the heart and venous pressure. Bilateral jugular vein distention (JVD) may indicate right-sided heart failure.

Procedure 22–13 describes how to assess the peripheral vascular system.

Text continued on page 527

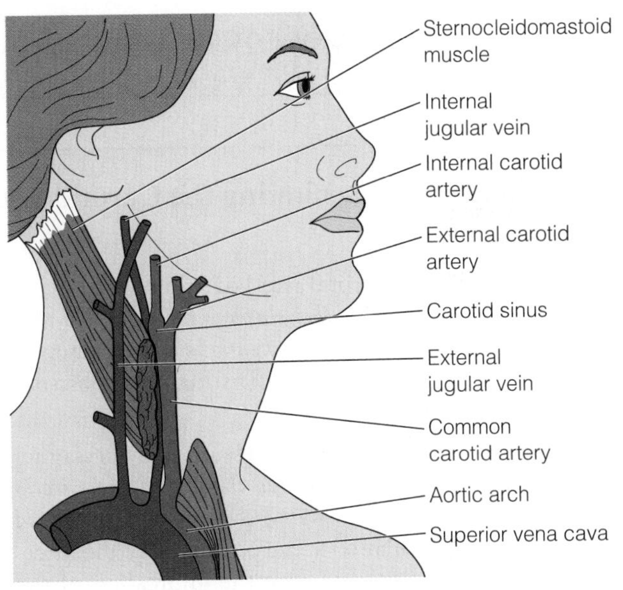

Figure 22–52 Arteries and veins of the right side of the neck.

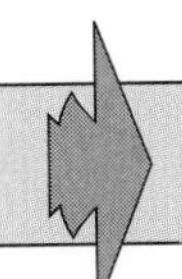

PROCEDURE 22–13 ASSESSING THE PERIPHERAL VASCULAR SYSTEM

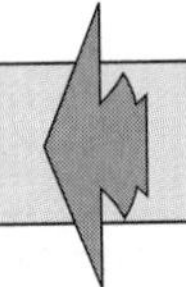

NURSING HISTORY FOCUS

Past history of heart disorders, varicosities, arterial disease, and hypertension; life-style, specifically exercise patterns, activity patterns and tolerance, smoking habits, and use of alcohol.

ASSESSMENT	NORMAL FINDINGS	DEVIATIONS FROM NORMAL
Peripheral Pulses		
Palpate the peripheral pulses (except the carotid pulse) **on both sides of the client's body simultaneously and systematically to determine the symmetry of pulse volume.** If it is difficult to palpate some of the peripheral pulses, use a Doppler ultrasound probe.	Symmetric pulse volumes	Asymmetric volumes (indicate impaired circulation)
	Full pulsations	Absence of pulsation (indicates arterial spasm or occlusion)
		Decreased, weak, thready pulsations (indicate impaired cardiac output)
		Increased pulse volume (may indicate hypertension, high cardiac output, or circulatory overload)
Carotid Arteries		
Palpate the carotid artery, using extreme caution. See the box on page 524.	Symmetric pulse volumes	Asymmetric volumes (possible stenosis or thrombosis)
	Full pulsations, thrusting quality	Decreased pulsations (may indicate impaired left cardiac output)
	Quality remains same when client breathes, turns head, and changes from sitting to supine position	Increased pulsations

PROCEDURE 22–13 ASSESSING THE PERIPHERAL VASCULAR SYSTEM *continued*

Palpating and Auscultating the Carotid Artery

Palpation

- Palpate only one carotid artery at a time. *This ensures adequate cerebral blood flow through the other and thus prevents possible ischemia. Ischemia* is a deficiency of blood in a body part due to constriction or obstruction of a blood vessel.
- Avoid exerting too much pressure and massaging the area. *Pressure can occlude the artery and carotid sinus massage can precipitate bradycardia.* The *carotid sinus* is a small dilation at the beginning of the internal carotid artery just above the bifurcation of the common carotid artery, in the upper third of the neck.
- Ask the client to turn the head slightly toward the side being examined. *This makes the carotid artery more accessible.*

Auscultation

- Turn the client's head slightly away from the side being examined. *This facilitates the placement of the stethoscope.*
- Auscultate the carotid artery on one side and then the other.
- Listen for the presence of a bruit.
- If you hear a bruit, gently palpate the artery to determine the presence of a thrill.

ASSESSMENT	NORMAL FINDINGS	DEVIATIONS FROM NORMAL
	Elastic arterial wall	Thickening, hard, rigid, beaded, inelastic walls (indicate arteriosclerosis)
Auscultate the carotid artery to determine the presence of a bruit. See the accompanying box.	No sound heard on auscultation	Presence of bruit in one or both arteries (suggests occlusive artery disease)
Jugular Veins		
Inspect the jugular veins for distention while the client is placed in a semi-Fowler's position (30- to 45-degree angle), with the head supported on a small pillow.	Veins not visible (indicating right side of heart is functioning normally)	Veins visibly distended (indicating advanced cardiopulmonary disease) Bilateral measurements above 3 cm are considered elevated (may indicate right-sided heart failure) Unilateral distention (may be caused by local obstruction)
If jugular distention is present, assess the jugular venous pressure (JVP). ▪ Locate the highest visible point of distention of the internal jugular vein. Although either the internal or the external jugular vein can be used, the internal jugular vein is more reliable. *The external jugular vein is more easily affected by obstruction or kinking at the base of the neck.*		

PROCEDURE 22–13 *continued*

ASSESSMENT	NORMAL FINDINGS	DEVIATIONS FROM NORMAL
▪ Measure the vertical height of this point in centimeters from the sternal angle (the point at which the clavicles meet; Figure 22–53). ▪ Repeat the steps above on the other side.		

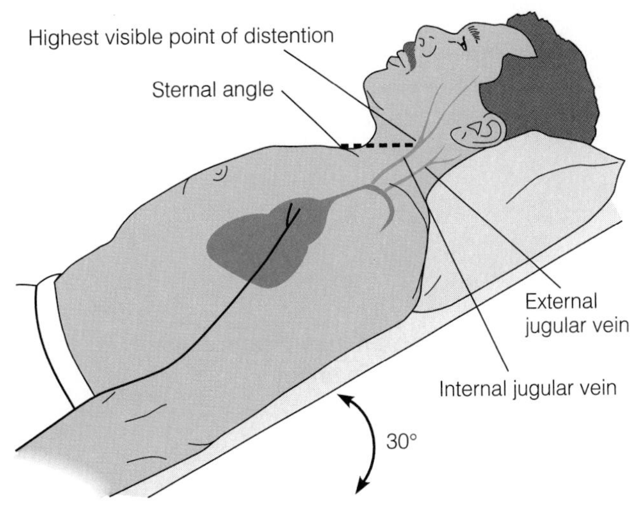

Figure 22–53 Assessing the highest point of distention of the internal jugular vein.

ASSESSMENT	NORMAL FINDINGS	DEVIATIONS FROM NORMAL
Peripheral Veins **Inspect the peripheral veins in the arms and legs for the presence and/or appearance of superficial veins** when limbs are dependent and when limbs are elevated.	In dependent position, distention and nodular bulges at calves are present When limbs are elevated, veins collapse (veins may appear tortuous or distended in older people)	Distended veins in the anteromedial part of thigh and/or lower leg or on posterolateral part of calf from knee to ankle
Assess the peripheral leg veins for signs of phlebitis.	Limbs not tender Symmetric in size	Tenderness on palpation Pain in calf muscles with forceful dorsiflexion of the foot **(Homans' sign)** Warmth and redness over vein Swelling of one calf or leg

Assessing Peripheral Leg Veins for Signs of Phlebitis

- Inspect the calves for redness and swelling over vein sites.
- Palpate the calves for firmness or tension of the muscles, the presence of edema over the dorsum of the foot, and areas of localized warmth. *Palpation augments inspection findings, particularly in more highly pigmented people, in whom redness may not be visible.*
- Push the calves from side to side to test for tenderness.
- Firmly dorsiflex the client's foot while supporting the entire leg in extension (Homans' sign), or have the person stand or walk.

PROCEDURE 22–13 ASSESSING THE PERIPHERAL VASCULAR SYSTEM *continued*

ASSESSMENT	NORMAL FINDINGS	DEVIATIONS FROM NORMAL
Peripheral Perfusion		
Inspect the skin of the hands and feet for color, temperature, edema, and skin changes.	Skin color pink	Cyanotic (venous insufficiency) Pallor that increases with limb elevation Dusky red color when limb is lowered (arterial insufficiency) Brown pigmentation around ankles (arterial or chronic venous insufficiency)
	Skin temperature not excessively warm or cold	Skin cool (arterial insufficiency)
	No edema	Marked edema (venous insufficiency) Mild edema (arterial insufficiency)
	Skin texture resilient and moist	Skin thin and shiny or thick, waxy, shiny, and fragile, with reduced hair and ulceration (venous or arterial insufficiency)
Assess the adequacy of arterial flow if arterial insufficiency is suspected.	**Buerger's test:** Original color returns in 10 seconds; veins in feet or hands fill in about 15 seconds	Delayed color return or mottled appearance; delayed venous filling; marked redness of arms or legs (indicates arterial insufficiency)
	Capillary refill test: Immediate return of color	Delayed return of color (arterial insufficiency)

Assessing the Adequacy of Arterial Blood Flow

Buerger's Test (Arterial Adequacy Test)

- Assist the client to a supine position. Ask the client to raise one leg or one arm about 30 cm (1 ft) above heart level, move the foot or hand briskly up and down for about 1 minute, and then sit up and dangle the leg or arm.
- Observe the time elapsed until return of original color and vein filling. Original color normally returns in 10 seconds, and the veins fill in about 15 seconds.

Capillary Refill Test

- Squeeze the client's fingernail and toenail between your fingers sufficiently to cause blanching.
- Release the pressure, and observe how quickly normal color returns. Color normally returns immediately.

Other Assessments

- Inspect the fingernails for changes indicative of circulatory impairment. See the section on assessment of nails, earlier in this chapter.
- See also peripheral pulse assessment, earlier.

PROCEDURE 22–13 *continued*

THE ELDERLY: PHYSICAL CHANGES IN THE PERIPHERAL VASCULAR SYSTEM

- The overall effectiveness of blood vessels decreases as smooth muscle cells are replaced by connective tissue. The lower extremities are more likely to show signs of arterial and venous impairment because of the more distal and dependent position.
- Proximal arteries become thinner and dilate.
- Peripheral arteries become thicker and dilate less effectively because of arteriosclerotic changes in the vessel walls.
- Blood vessels lengthen and become more tortuous and prominent. Varicosities occur more frequently.
- In some instances, arteries may be palpated more easily because of the loss of supportive surrounding tissues. Often, however, the most distal pulses of the lower extremities are more difficult to palpate because of decreased arterial perfusion.
- Systolic and diastolic blood pressures increase, but the increase in the systolic pressure is greater. As a result, the pulse pressure widens. Any client with a blood pressure reading above 140/90 should be referred for follow-up assessments.
- Peripheral edema is frequently observed and is most commonly the result of chronic venous insufficiency or low protein levels in the blood (hypoproteinemia).
- Carotid artery assessment is an essential aspect of peripheral vascular examination in the older adult.

THE BREASTS AND AXILLAE

The breasts of men and women need to be inspected and palpated. Men have some glandular tissue beneath each nipple, a potential site for malignancy, whereas mature women have glandular tissue throughout the breast. During adolescence, asymmetric development is not unusual, because one breast may develop more rapidly than the other. Boys may have some breast development in early adolescence. Stages of breast development are shown in the box below. In females, the largest portion of glandular breast tissue is located in the upper outer quadrant of each breast. From this quadrant there is a projection of breast tissue into the axilla, called the **axillary tail of Spence** (Figure 22–54). The majority of breast tumors are located

FIVE STAGES OF BREAST DEVELOPMENT*

Stage 1 Elevation of the nipple

Stage 2 Enlargement of the areola

Stage 3 Enlargement of the breast

Stage 4 Projection of the areola and nipple

Stage 5 Recession of the areola by about age 14 or 15, leaving only the nipple projecting

*The 2-year transient breast growth that occurs in males reaches only the second stage.

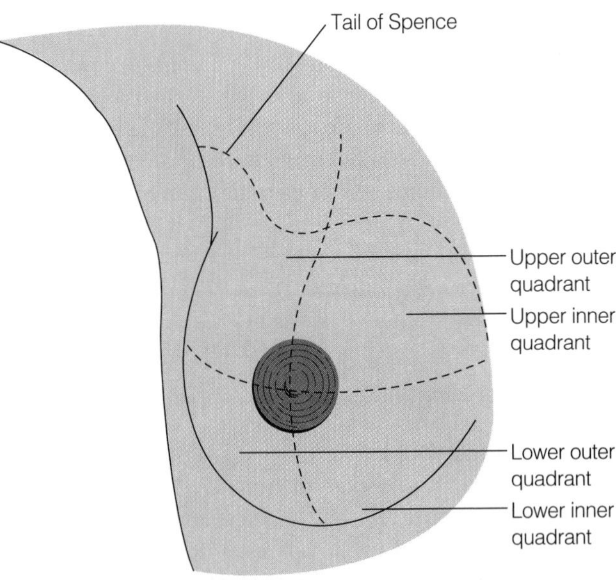

Figure 22–54 Four breast quadrants and the axillary tail of Spence.

CLIENT TEACHING

Breast Palpation

Instruct the woman to

- Examine the right breast by placing a pillow or folded towel under the right shoulder and the right hand behind the head. This position distributes breast tissue more evenly on the breast.
- With the left hand:
  a. Press the palmar surfaces of the middle three fingers on the skin surface, starting in the upper lateral quadrant, that is, the outermost top of the breast.
  b. Use a gentle rotating motion to press the breast tissue against the chest wall.
  c. Palpate from the periphery to the areola.
  d. Move the peripheral starting point around the breast clockwise.
  e. Finally, squeeze the nipple of each breast gently between the thumb and index finger. Note any clear or bloody discharge.
- Repeat the above for the left breast with a pillow under the left shoulder and the left hand behind the head.
- Report a lump or nipple discharge to the physician immediately. A ridge of firm tissue in the curve of each breast is normal.

in this upper outer breast quadrant and in the tail of Spence. During assessment, the nurse can localize specific findings by using this division of the breast into quadrants and the axillary tail.

Breast self-examination (BSE) should be conducted once a month. A regular time is best—such as immediately following menstruation, when breast tenderness and fullness caused by fluid retention have subsided, or on the first day of the month. Women who examine themselves regularly become familiar with the shape and texture of their breasts. Any changes must be reported immediately to a physician for accurate diagnosis. Before beginning to teach BSE to a client, the nurse needs to identify the client's attitudes toward this procedure. Some women are reluctant to conduct BSE because they fear what they might find. The nurse needs to explore these fears with the client. Women often offer these reasons for avoiding BSE: "I don't have time" and "I just don't think of doing it." The nurse also needs to explore these reasons with the client with particular reference to her self-esteem (see Chapter 31) and her need to spend time on herself.

BSE includes inspection as well as palpation. The nurse should instruct the client to inspect the breasts while standing in front of a mirror, placing the arms in four positions:

- Arms at the sides, at rest
- Hands on the hips and pressed into the hips (Figure 22–57)
- Hands over the head
- Torso leaning forward

Each breast is observed in each position for the following:

- Lumps or thickening
- Indentations, rippling, puckering, or dimpling
- Asymmetry of the nipples (eg, a nipple pulled to one side)
- Discoloration
- Discharge from the nipple
- Any change in the size or shape of the breasts

Palpation can be carried out in the bath or shower or in a supine position. The latter is recommended because it is preferable for larger breasts and for palpation of the axilla. For palpation techniques, see the Client Teaching box.

Procedure 22–14 describes a nursing assessment of the breasts and axillae.

Text continued on page 533

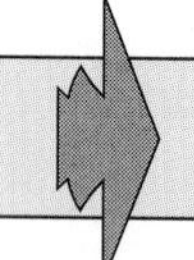

PROCEDURE 22–14 ASSESSING THE BREASTS AND AXILLAE

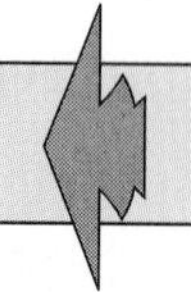

NURSING HISTORY FOCUS

History of breast self-examination; technique used and when performed in relation to the menstrual cycle; history of breast masses and what was done about them; any pain or tenderness in the breasts and relation to menstrual cycle; any discharge from the nipple; medication history (some medications, like oral contraceptives, steroids, digitalis, and diuretics, may cause nipple discharge; exogenous estrogens and phenothiazine are associated with developing cysts or cancer, respectively); risk factors for breast cancer (eg, mother, sister, aunt, or grandmother with breast cancer; menarche before age 13; menopause after age 50; age 35 or more at first pregnancy).

PROCEDURE 22–14 *continued*

ASSESSMENT	NORMAL FINDINGS	DEVIATIONS FROM NORMAL
Inspect the breasts for size, symmetry, and contour or shape while the client is in a sitting position.	Females: Rounded shape; slightly unequal in size; generally symmetric Males: Breasts even with the chest wall; if obese, may be similar in shape to female breasts	Recent change in breast size; swellings; marked asymmetry
Inspect the skin of the breast for localized discolorations or hyperpigmentation, retraction or dimpling, localized hypervascular areas, swelling or edema (Figure 22–55).	Skin uniform in color (same in appearance as skin of abdomen or back)	Localized discolorations or hyperpigmentation
	Skin smooth and intact	Retraction or dimpling (result of scar tissue or an invasive tumor)
	Diffuse symmetric horizontal or vertical vascular pattern in light-skinned people	Unilateral, localized hypervascular areas (associated with increased blood flow)
	Striae (stretch marks); moles and nevi	Swelling or edema appearing as pig skin or orange peel due to exaggeration of the pores

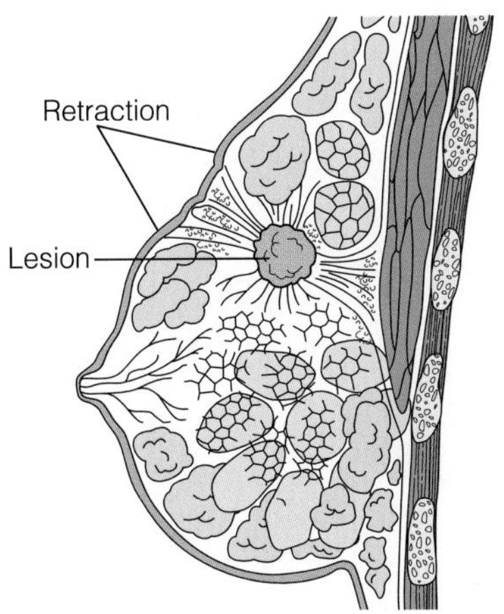

Figure 22–55 A lesion causing retraction of the skin.

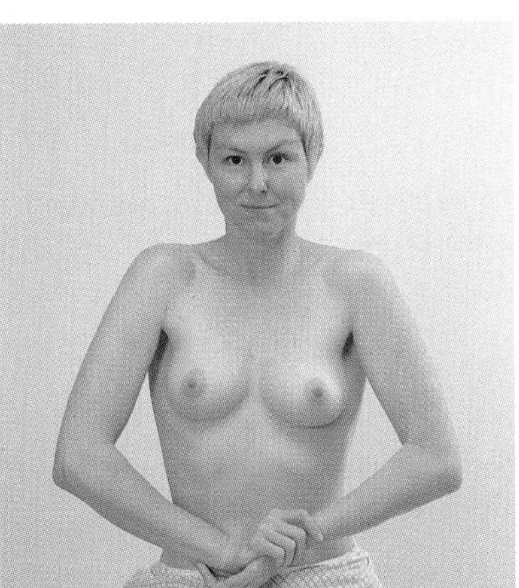

Figure 22–56 Pushing the hands together to accentuate retraction of breast tissues.

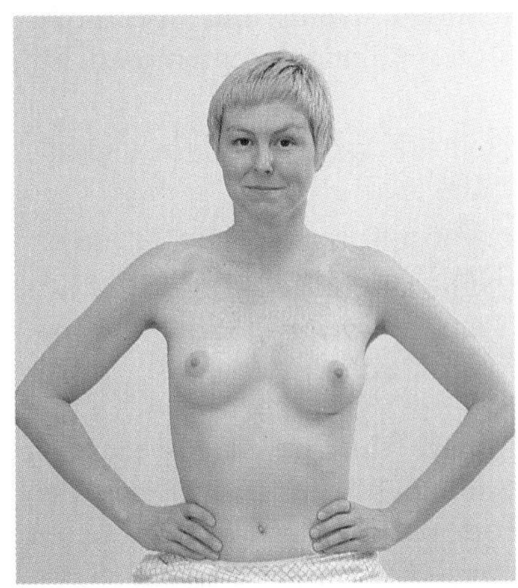

Figure 22–57 Pressing the hands down on the hips to accentuate retraction of breast tissue.

ASSESSMENT	NORMAL FINDINGS	DEVIATIONS FROM NORMAL
Accentuate any retraction by having the client ▪ Raise the arms above the head. ▪ Push the hands together, with elbows flexed (Figure 22–56). ▪ Press the hands down on the hips (Figure 22–57).		
Inspect the areola area for size, shape, symmetry, color, surface characteristics, and any masses or lesions.	Round or oval and bilaterally the same Color varies widely, from light pink to dark brown Irregular placement of sebaceous glands on the surface of the areola (Montgomery's tubercles)	Any asymmetry, mass, or lesion

➤

PROCEDURE 22–14 ASSESSING THE BREASTS AND AXILLAE *continued*

ASSESSMENT	NORMAL FINDINGS	DEVIATIONS FROM NORMAL
Inspect the nipples for size, shape, position, color, discharge, lesions.	Round, everted, and equal in size; similar in color; soft and smooth; both nipples point in same direction	Asymmetrical size and color
	No discharge, except for colostrum in pregnant females	Presence of discharge, crusts, or cracks
	Inversion of one or both nipples that is present from puberty	Recent inversion of one or both nipples
Palpate the axillary, subclavicular, and supraclavicular lymph nodes (Figure 22–58) while the client sits with the arms abducted and supported on the nurse's forearm. For palpation of clavicular lymph nodes, see page 506. Use the palmar surfaces of all fingertips to palpate the four areas of the axilla: ▪ The edge of the greater pectoral muscle (musculus pectoralis major) along the anterior axillary line ▪ The thoracic wall in the midaxillary area ▪ The upper part of the humerus ▪ The anterior edge of the latissimus dorsi muscle along the posterior axillary line	No tenderness, masses, or nodules	Tenderness, masses, or nodules
Palpate the breast for masses, tenderness, and any discharge from the nipples. See the box on page 531 for palpation methods.	No tenderness, masses, nodules, or nipple discharge	Tenderness, masses, nodules, or nipple discharge
Palpate the areola and the nipples for masses. Compress each nipple to determine the presence of any discharge. If discharge is present, milk the breast along its radii to identify the discharge producing lobe. Assess any discharge for amount, color, consistency, and odor. Note also any tenderness on palpation.	No tenderness, masses, nodules, or nipple discharge	Tenderness, masses, nodules, or nipple discharge
Palpate the male breasts and the axillary lymph nodes when the client is supine.	As above for female client	As above for female client

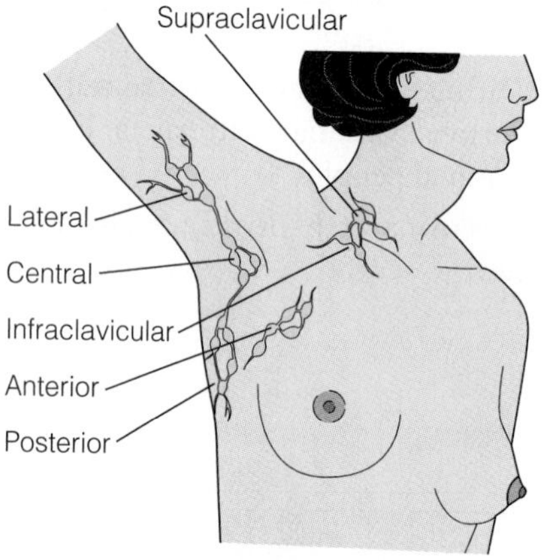

Figure 22–58 Lymph nodes that drain the breast tissues.

PROCEDURE 22–14 *continued*

Palpating a Client's Breast

Palpation of the breast may be performed while the client is supine or sitting. For clients who have a past history of breast masses, who are at high risk for breast cancer, or who have pendulous breasts, examination in both positions is recommended (Malasanos et al 1990, p. 289).

Bimanual Palpation

A bimanual technique is often preferred, particularly if the breasts are large. The nondominant hand is placed under the breast, and the dominant hand palpates the breast. This bimanual technique can be most effective in detecting small deep masses. The client is in the *sitting* position. The bimanual technique is performed as follows:

- If the client reports a breast lump, start with the "normal" breast to obtain baseline data that will serve as a comparison to the reportedly involved breast.
- Press the palmar surface of the middle three fingertips (held together) on the skin surface, starting at the periphery of the breast (Figure 22–59).
- Use a smooth rotary motion or back-and-forth technique to press the breast tissue against the other hand.
- Palpate from the periphery to the areola.
- Move from the peripheral starting point around the breast systematically until all breast surfaces are thoroughly surveyed.
- Pay particular attention to the upper outer quadrant area and the tail of Spence, where about 50% of breast cancers develop.

One-Handed Palpation

This technique is often performed after bimanual palpation, with the client in the *supine* position. *In the supine position, the breasts flatten evenly against the chest wall, facilitating palpation.* It is performed as follows:

- To enhance flattening of the breast, instruct the client to abduct the arm and place her hand behind her head. Then place a small pillow or rolled towel under the client's shoulder.
- Use the fingertips of one hand, and visualize the breast as a clock (Figure 22–60).
- Palpate the breast tissue along the hands of the clock, moving from the periphery toward the areola.
- Choose any starting point for palpation, but start and end at a fixed point to ensure that all breast surfaces are assessed.
- If you detect a mass, record the following data:
  - **a.** *Location:* the exact location relative to the clock (as in Figure 22–60) and the distance from the nipple in centimeters.
  - **b.** *Client's position:* whether the arms were raised or lowered and whether the client was sitting or supine. The position can change the perceived location of the mass.

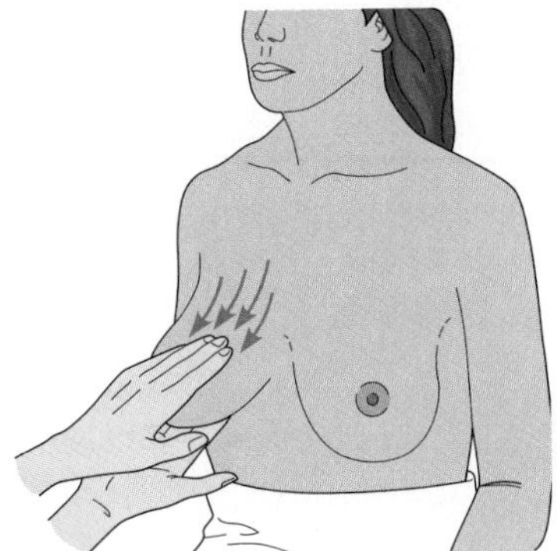

Figure 22–59 Bimanual breast palpation with the client in a sitting position.

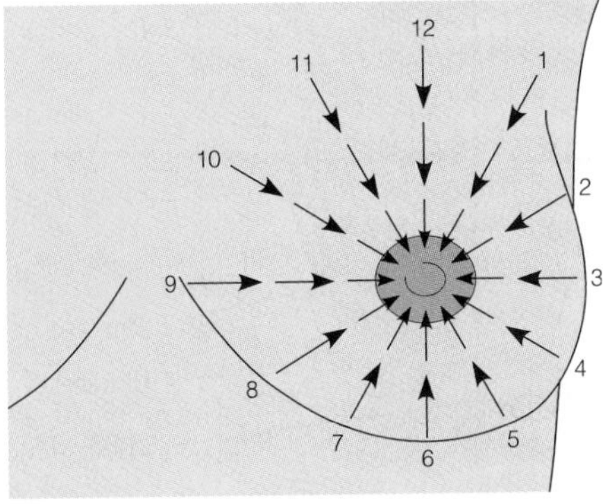

Figure 22–60 Pattern for palpating a breast, using the clock to describe the location of any masses.

Procedure 22–14 Assessing the Breasts and Axillae *continued*

Palpating a Client's Breast *continued*

c. *Size:* the length, width, and thickness of the mass in centimeters. If you are unable to determine the discrete edges, record this fact.
d. *Mobility:* whether the mass is movable or fixed. If it is fixed, determine whether it is firmly or moderately fixed, if possible.
e. *Consistency:* whether the mass is hard or soft.
f. *Surface:* whether the surface is smooth or irregular.
g. *Tenderness:* whether palpation is painful.
h. *Shape:* whether the mass is round, discoid, regular, or irregular.

The Elderly: Physical Changes of the Breasts

- In the postmenopausal female, breasts change in shape and often appear pendulous or flaccid; they lack the firmness they had in younger years.
- The presence of breast lesions may be detected more readily because of the decrease in connective tissue.
- General breast size remains the same. Although glandular tissue atrophies, the amount of fat in breasts (predominantly in the lower quadrants) increases in most women.

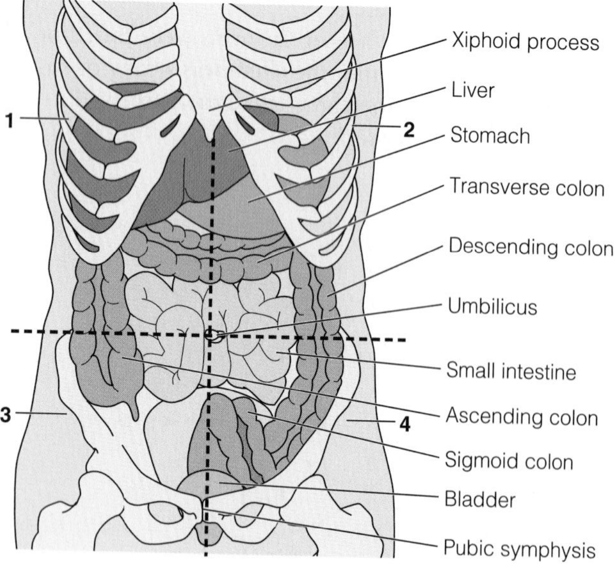

Figure 22–61 The four abdominal quadrants and the underlying organs: *1,* right upper quadrant; *2,* left upper quadrant; *3,* right lower quadrant; *4,* left lower quadrant.

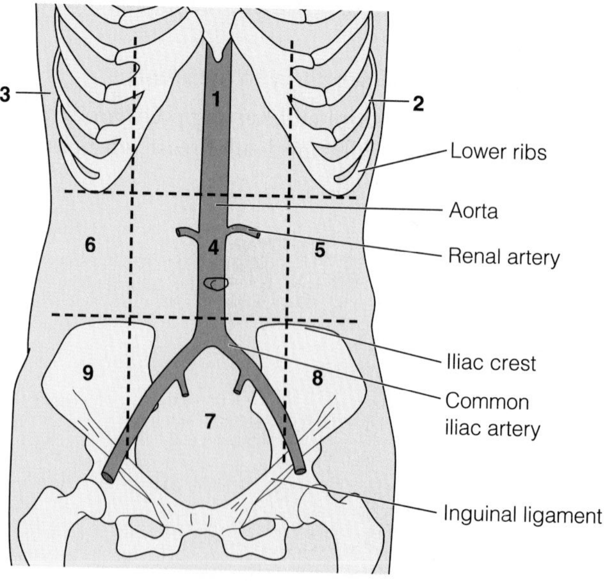

Figure 22–62 The nine abdominal regions: *1,* epigastric; *2, 3,* left and right hypochondriac; *4,* umbilical; *5, 6,* left and right lumbar; *7,* suprapubic and hypogastric; *8, 9,* left and right inguinal or iliac.

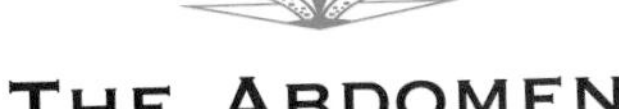

THE ABDOMEN

The nurse locates and describes abdominal findings in a client by using two common methods of subdividing the abdomen: quadrants and nine regions. To divide the abdomen into quadrants, the nurse imagines two lines: a vertical line from the xiphoid process to the pubic symphysis, and a horizontal line across the umbilicus (Figure 22–61). These quadrants are labeled right upper quadrant *(1)*, left upper quadrant *(2)*, right lower quadrant *(3)*, and left lower quadrant *(4)*. Using the second method, division into nine regions, the nurse imagines two vertical lines that extend superiorly from the midpoints of the inguinal ligaments, and two horizontal lines, one at the level of the edge of the lower ribs and the other at the level of the iliac crests (Figure 22–62). Specific organs or parts of organs lie in each abdominal region. See Tables 22–10 and 22–11.

In addition, practitioners often use certain landmarks to locate abdominal signs and symptoms. These are the xiphoid process of the sternum, the costal margins, the midline (a line drawn from the tip of the sternum through the umbilicus to the pubic symphysis), the anterosuperior iliac spine, the inguinal ligaments (Poupart's ligaments), and the superior margin of the pubic symphysis (Figure 22–63, p. 534).

Assessment of the abdomen involves all four methods of examination (inspection, auscultation, palpation, and percussion). Of these, beginning practitioners usually perform only inspection and auscultation. In some agencies, the nurse also performs palpation. Check agency protocol.

When assessing the abdomen, the nurse performs inspection first, followed by auscultation, palpation, and/or percussion. *Auscultation is done before palpation and percussion, because palpation and percussion cause movement or stimulation of the bowel, which can increase bowel motility and thus heighten bowel sounds, creating false results.*

Table 22–10 Organs in the Four Abdominal Quadrants

Right Upper Quadrant	*Left Upper Quadrant*
Liver	Left lobe of liver
Gallbladder	Stomach
Duodenum	Spleen
Head of pancreas	Upper lobe of left kidney
Right adrenal gland	Pancreas
Upper lobe of right kidney	Left adrenal gland
Hepatic flexure of colon	Splenic flexure of colon
Section of ascending colon	Section of transverse colon
Section of transverse colon	Section of descending colon
Right Lower Quadrant	***Left Lower Quandrant***
Lower lobe of right kidney	Lower lobe of left kidney
Cecum	Sigmoid colon
Appendix	Section of descending colon
Section of ascending colon	Left ovary
Right ovary	Left fallopian tube
Right fallopian tube	Left ureter
Right ureter	Left spermatic cord
Right spermatic cord	Part of uterus
Part of uterus	

Table 22–11 Organs in the Nine Abdominal Regions

Right Hypochondriac	*Epigastric*	*Left Hypochondriac*
Right lobe of liver	Aorta	Stomach
Gallbladder	Pyloric end of stomach	Spleen
Part of duodenum	Part of duodenum	Tail of pancreas
Hepatic flexure of colon	Pancreas	Splenic flexure of colon
Upper half of right kidney	Part of liver	Upper half of left kidney
Suprarenal gland		Suprarenal gland
Right Lumbar	***Umbilical***	***Left Lumbar***
Ascending colon	Omentum	Descending colon
Lower half of right kidney	Mesentery	Lower half of left kidney
Part of duodenum and jejunum	Lower part of duodenum	Part of jejunum and ileum
	Part of jejunum and ileum	
Right Inguinal	***Hypogastric (Pubic)***	***Left Inguinal***
Cecum	Ileum	Sigmoid colon
Appendix	Bladder	Left ureter
Lower end of ileum	Uterus	Left spermatic cord
Right ureter		Left ovary
Right spermatic cord		
Right ovary		

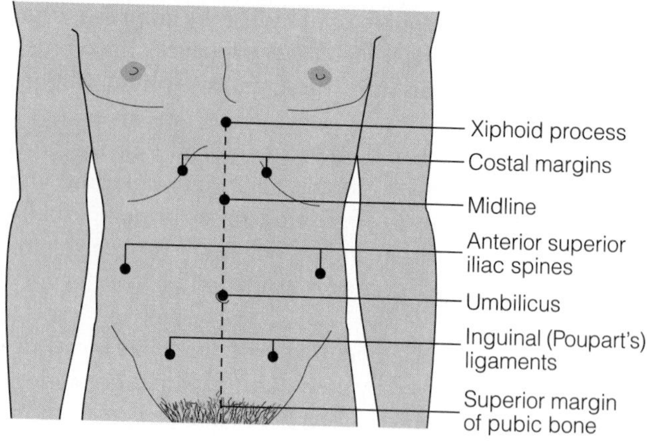

Figure 22–63 Landmarks commonly used to identify abdominal areas.

To facilitate validity of observations and enhance client comfort, the nurse asks the client to urinate before beginning the assessment and assists the client to a supine position, with the arms placed comfortably at the sides. The nurse also places small pillows beneath the knees and the head. This position and an empty bladder prevent tension in the abdominal muscles. By contrast, the abdominal muscles tense when the client is sitting or supine with knees and arms extended and with hands clasped behind the head.

The nurse should ensure that the room is warm and expose only the client's abdomen from chest line to the pubic area to avoid chilling and shivering, which can tense the abdominal muscles. An examining light, a tape measure (metal or unstretchable cloth), a water-soluble skin-marking pencil, and a stethoscope are necessary for the examination. Procedure 22–15 describes how to assess the abdomen.

Text continued on page 540

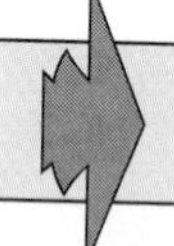

PROCEDURE 22–15 ASSESSING THE ABDOMEN

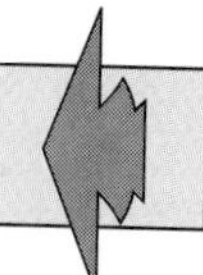

NURSING HISTORY FOCUS

Incidence of abdominal pain: its location, onset, sequence, and chronology; its quality (description); its frequency; associated symptoms (eg, nausea, vomiting, diarrhea); bowel habits; incidence of constipation or diarrhea (have client describe what client means by these terms); change in appetite, food intolerances, and foods ingested in last 24 hours; specific signs and symptoms (eg, heartburn, flatulence and/or belching, difficulty swallowing, hematemesis, blood or mucus in stools, and aggravating and alleviating factors); previous problems and treatment (eg, stomach ulcer, gallbladder surgery, history of jaundice).

ASSESSMENT	NORMAL FINDINGS	DEVIATIONS FROM NORMAL
Inspection of the Abdomen		
Inspect the abdomen for skin integrity (refer to the discussion about skin assessment, earlier in this chapter).	Unblemished skin Uniform color	Presence of rash or other lesions Tense, glistening skin (may indicate ascites, edema)
	Silver-white striae or surgical scars	Purple striae (associated with Cushing's disease)
Inspect the abdomen for contour and symmetry.		
▪ Observe the abdominal contour (profile line frm the rib margin to the pubic bone) while standing at the client's side when the client is supine.	Flat, rounded (convex), or scaphoid (concave)	Distended
▪ Ask the client to take a deep breath and to hold it (makes an enlarged liver or spleen more obvious).	No evidence of enlargement of liver or spleen	Evidence of enlargement of liver or spleen

PROCEDURE 22–15 *continued*

ASSESSMENT	NORMAL FINDINGS	DEVIATIONS FROM NORMAL
▪ Assess the symmetry of contour while standing at the foot of the bed.	Symmetric contour	Asymmetric contour, such as localized protrusions around umbilicus, inguinal ligaments, or scars (possible hernia or tumor)
▪ If a hernia is suspected, ask the client to raise the head and shoulders from the pillow without using the arms for support (increases intra-abdominal pressure and may cause upward protrusion of the hernia).	No appearance of bulges or marked ridges	Bulges or masses appear
▪ If distention is present, measure the abdominal girth by placing a tape around the abdomen at the level of the umbilicus (Figure 22–64).	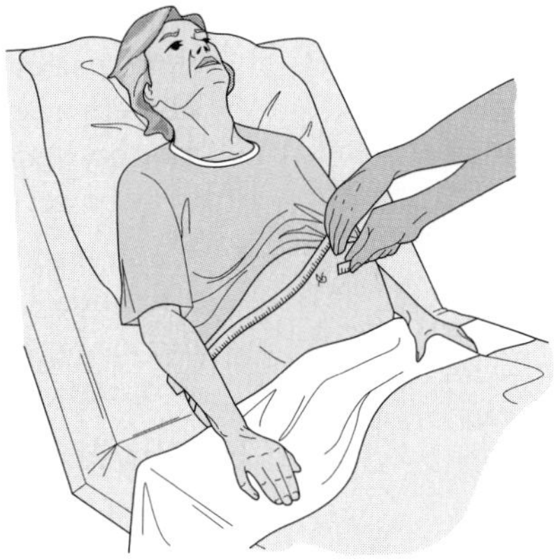	
Observe abdominal movements associated with respiration, peristalsis, or aortic pulsations.	Symmetric movements caused by respiration Visible peristalsis in very lean people Aortic pulsations in thin persons at epigastric area	Limited movement due to pain or disease process Visible peristalsis in nonlean clients (with bowel obstruciton) Marked aortic pulsations
Auscultation of the Abdomen **Auscultate the abdomen for bowel sounds, vascular sounds, and peritoneal friction rubs.** The auscultation procedure is shown in the box on page 536.	Audible bowel sounds Absence of arterial bruits Absence of friction rub	Absent or hypoactive bowel sounds Hyperactive bowel sounds Loud bruit over aortic area (possible aneurysm) Bruit over renal or iliac arteries Friction rub
Palpation of the Abdomen **Perform light palpation first to detect areas of tenderness and/or muscle guarding.** Systematically explore all four quadrants. See the box on page 537.	No tenderness; relaxed abdomen with smooth, consistent tension	Tenderness and hypersensitivity Superficial masses Localized areas of increased tension
Perform deep palpation over all four quadrants. See the box on page 537.	Tenderness may be present near xiphoid process, over cecum, and over sigmoid colon	Generalized or localized areas of tenderness Mobile or fixed masses

Figure 22–64 Measuring the abdominal girth at the level of the umbilicus.

PROCEDURE 22–15 ASSESSING THE ABDOMEN *continued*

Auscultating the Abdomen

Warm the hands and the stethoscope diaphragms. *Cold hands and a cold stethoscope may cause the client to contract the abdominal muscles, and these contractions may be heard during auscultation.*

For Bowel Sounds

- Use the flat-disc diaphragm. *Intestinal sounds are relatively high-pitched and best accentuated by the flat-disc diaphragm.* Light pressure with the stethoscope is adequate to detect sounds.
- Ask when the client last ate. *The frequency of sounds relates to the state of digestion or the presence of food in the gastrointestinal tract. Shortly after or long after eating, bowel sounds may normally increase. They are loudest when a meal is long overdue. Four to 7 hours after a meal, bowel sounds may be heard continuously over the ileocecal valve area while the digestive contents from the small intestine empty through the valve into the large intestine.*
- Place the flat-disc diaphragm of the stethoscope in each of the four quadrants of the abdomen over all the auscultation sites shown in Figure 22–65. Many nurses begin in the lower right quadrant in the area of the cecum.

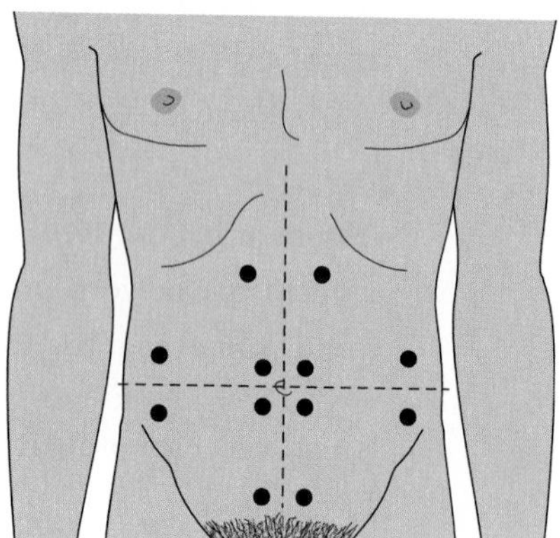

Figure 22–65 Auscultation sites of the abdomen.

- Listen for active bowel sounds—irregular gurgling noises occurring about every 5 to 20 seconds. The duration of a single sound may range from less than a second to more than several seconds.
- Normal bowel sounds are described as *audible*. Alterations in sounds are described as *absent* or *hypoactive*, that is, extremely soft and infrequent (eg, one per minute), and *hyperactive* or *increased*, that is, high-pitched, loud, rushing sounds that occur frequently (eg, every 3 seconds) also known as **borborygmi.** Absence of sounds indicates a cessation of intestinal motility. Hypoactive sounds indicate decreased motility and are usually associated with manipulation of the bowel during surgery, inflammation, paralytic ileus, or late bowel obstruction. Hyperactive sounds indicate increased intestinal motility and are usually associated with diarrhea, an early bowel obstruction, or the use of laxatives.
- If bowel sounds appear to be absent, listen for 3 to 5 minutes before concluding that they are absent. *Because bowel sounds are so irregular, a longer time and more sites are used to confirm absence of sounds.*

For Vascular Sounds

Use the bell of the stethoscope over the aorta, renal arteries, and iliac arteries as follows, and listen for bruits.

- Auscultate the aorta superior to the umbilicus.
- Auscultate the renal arteries at or to the left and right of the upper abdominal midline or farther toward the flank.
- Auscultate the iliac arteries to the left and right of the abdominal midline below the umbilicus. See Figure 22–62, page 532, to locate these areas.

Peritoneal Friction Rubs

Peritoneal friction rubs sound like two pieces of leather rubbing together. Friction rubs may be caused by infectious or abnormal growth processes, including metastases. Listen for peritoneal friction rubs at the various auscultating sites, especially above the liver and spleen. *The liver and spleen have large surface areas in contact with the peritoneum; thus they are most frequently the begining sites for friction rubs.*

- To auscultate the splenic site, place the stethoscope over the left lower rib cage in the anterior axillary line, and ask the client to take a deep breath. *A deep breath may accentuate the sound of a friction rub area.*
- To auscultate the liver site, place the stethoscope over the lower right rib cage.

PROCEDURE 22–15 *continued*

Palpating the Abdomen

Palpation is used to detect tenderness, the presence of masses or distention, and the outline and position of abdominal organs (eg, the liver, spleen, and kidneys). Two types of palpation are used: light and deep. *In some practice settings, palpation is limited to light abdominal palpation to assess tenderness and bladder palpation to assess for distention.* Before palpation, (a) ensure that the client's position is appropriate for relaxation of the abdominal muscles, and (b) warm the hands. *Cold hands can elicit muscle tension and thus impedes palpatory evaluation.*

Light Palpation

- Hold the palm of your hand slightly above the client's abdomen, with your fingers parallel to the abdomen.
- Depress the abdominal wall lightly, about 1 cm or to the depth of the subcutaneous tissue, with the pads of your fingers (Figure 22–66).
- Move the finger pads in a slight circular motion.
- If the client is extremely ticklish, place the client's hand under or over your hand. *This may decrease the degree of ticklishness and resulting muscle tenseness.*
- Note areas of slight tenderness or superficial pain, large masses, and muscle guarding. To determine areas of tenderness, ask the client to tell you about them, watch for changes in the client's facial expressions, and note areas of muscle guarding. When the client complains of overall abdominal tenderness, use a cotton wisp for palpation to help the client identify specific pain areas.

Deep Palpation

- Palpate sensitive areas last.
- Press the distal half of the palmar surface of the fingers of one hand into the abdominal wall.
  or
  Use the bimanual method of palpation discussed earlier in this chapter, page 469.
- Depress the abdominal wall about 4 to 5 cm (1.5 to 2.0 in) or an appropriate distance beyond subcutaneous tissue (Figure 22–67).
- Note masses and the structure of underlying contents. If a mass is present, determine its size, location, mobility, contour, consistency, and tenderness. Normal abdominal structures that may be mistaken for masses include the lateral borders of the rectus abdominis muscles; the feces-filled ascending, descending, or sigmoid colon; the aorta; the uterus; the common iliac artery; and the sacral promontory.

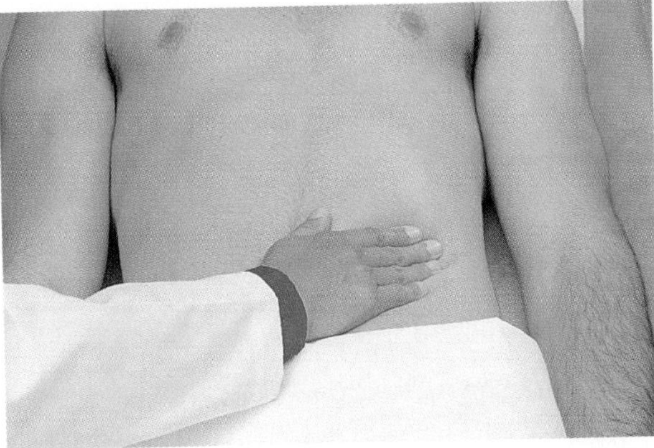

Figure 22–66 Light palpation of the abdomen.

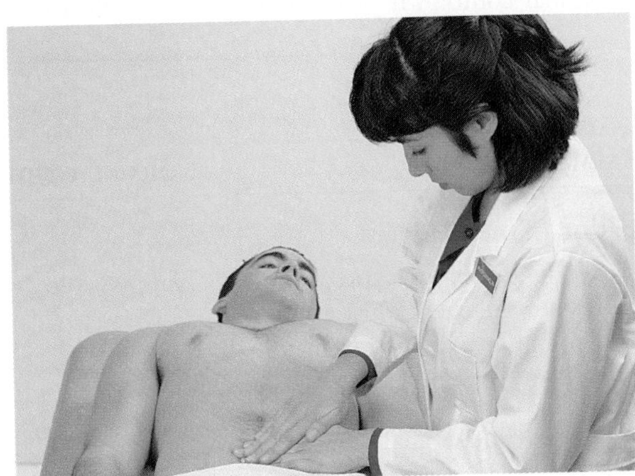

Figure 22–67 Deep palpation of the abdomen.

Palpation of the Liver **Palpate the liver to detect enlargement and tenderness.** See palpation methods in the box on page 538.	May not be palpable Border feels smooth	Enlarged (abnormal finding, even if liver is smooth and not tender) Smooth but tender; nodular or hard

PROCEDURE 22–15 ASSESSING THE ABDOMEN *continued*

Palpating the Liver

Two bimanual approaches are used in palpation of the liver. In using the *first* method, place one hand along the anterior rib cage and the other hand on the posterior rib cage.

- Stand on the client's right side.
- Place your left hand on the posterior thorax at about the eleventh or twelfth rib. This hand is used to push upward and provide support of underlying structures for the subsequent anterior palpation.
- Place your right hand along the rib cage at about a 45-degree angle to the right of the rectus abdominis muscle or parallel to the rectus muscle with the fingers pointing toward the rib cage (Figure 22–68).
- While the client exhales, exert a gradual and gentle downward and forward pressure beneath the costal margin until you reach a depth of 4 to 5 cm (1½ to 2 in). *During expiration, the abdominal wall relaxes, facilitating deep palpation.*
- Maintain your hand position, and ask the client to inhale deeply. *This makes the liver border descend and moves the liver into a palpable position.*
- While the client inhales, feel the liver border move against your hand. It should feel firm and have a regular contour. If you do not palpate the liver initially, ask the client to take two or three more deep breaths while you maintain or apply slightly more palpation pressure. Livers are harder to palpate in obese, tense, or very physically fit people.
- If the liver is enlarged (ie, palpable below the costal margin), measure the number of centimeters it extends below the costal region.

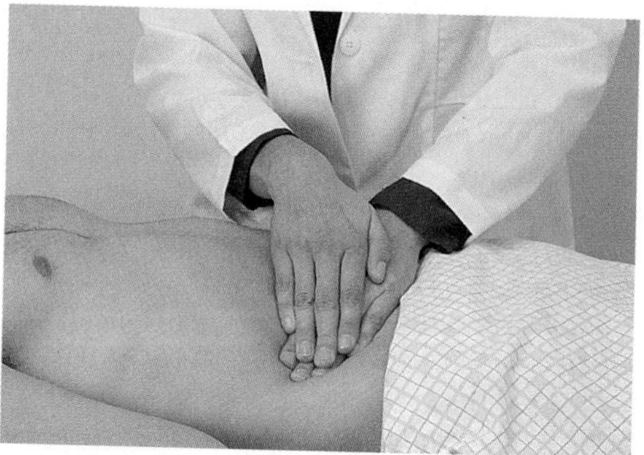

Figure 22–68 Palpating the liver.

A *second* method is the bimanual palpation method discussed on page 469, in which one hand is superimposed on the other (Figure 22–1, earlier). The techniques and principles used above apply to that method as well.

ASSESSMENT	NORMAL FINDINGS	DEVIATIONS FROM NORMAL
Palpation of the Bladder		
Palpate the area above the pubic symphysis if the client's history indicates possible urinary retention (Figure 22–69).	Not palpable	Distended and palpable as smooth, round, tense mass (indicates urinary retention)

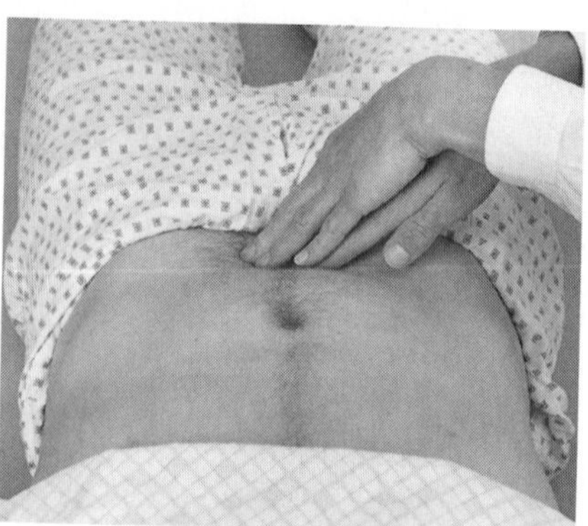

Figure 22–69 Palpating the bladder.

PROCEDURE 22–15 *continued*

THE ELDERLY: PHYSICAL CHANGES IN THE GASTROINTESTINAL TRACT

- The rounded abdomens of many older persons are due to an increase in adipose tissue and a decrease in muscle tone.
- The abdominal wall is slacker and thinner, making palpation easier and more accurate than in younger clients. Muscle wasting and loss of fibroconnective tissue occur.
- The side-effects of drugs are often manifested in the gastrointestinal tract, (eg, nausea, vomiting, and diarrhea).
- The pain threshold in the elderly is often greater; major abdominal problems such as appendicitis or other acute emergencies may therefore go undetected.
- Gastrointestinal pain needs to be differentiated from cardiac pain. Gastroinestinal pain may be located in the chest or abdomen, whereas cardiac pain is usually located in the chest. Factors aggravating gastrointestinal pain are usually related to either ingestion or lack of food intake; gastrointestinal pain is usually relieved by antacids, food, or assuming an upright position. Common factors that can aggravate cardiac pain are activity or anxiety; cardiac pain is relieved by rest or nitroglycerin.

Esophagus

- Esophageal motility may decrease and, if it is severe, it can cause discomfort as food passes through the esophagus.
- Difficulty swallowing (dysphagia), a common complaint of older adults, must be differentiated from heartburn or regurgitation. Questions about food getting "stuck in the throat" or the ability to swallow liquid foods versus solid foods can clarify these symptoms.
- Many older individuals have increased esophageal spasms and less efficient action of the lower esophageal sphincter.

Stomach

- Gastric acid secretion decreases, and emptying time of the stomach is delayed, resulting in indigestion and intolerance to certain foods. Decreases in the production of pancreatic enzymes also contribute to complaints of indigestion and anorexia.

Intestines

- Stool passes through the intestines at a slower rate in elderly clients, and the perception of stimuli that produce the urge to defecate often diminishes.
- Fecal incontinence may occur in confused or neurologically impaired older adults.
- Many older persons erroneously believe that the absence of a daily bowel movement signifies constipation. When assessing for constipation, the nurse must consider the client's diet, activity, medications, characteristics and ease of passage of feces, as well as the frequency of bowel movements.
- The incidence of colon cancer is higher among older adults than younger adults. Symptoms include a change in bowel function, rectal bleeding, and weight loss. Changes in bowel function, however, are associated with many factors, such as diet, exercise, and medications.
- Decreased absorption of oral medications often occurs with aging.

Liver

- The liver changes minimally with age, as does the gallbladder. Liver function tests are unaltered.
- Impaired metabolism of some drugs may occur with aging.

THE MUSCULOSKELETAL SYSTEM

The musculoskeletal system encompasses the muscles, bones, and joints. The completeness of an assessment of this system depends largely on the needs and problems of the individual client. The nurse usually assesses the musculoskeletal system for muscle strength, tone, size and symmetry of muscle development, and fasciculations and tremors. A **fasciculation** is an abnormal contraction (shortening) of a bundle of muscle fibers. A **tremor** is an involuntary trembling of a limb or body part. Tremors may involve large groups of muscle fibers or small bundles of muscle fibers. An **intention tremor** becomes more apparent when an individual attempts a voluntary movement, such as holding a cup of coffee. A **resting tremor** is more apparent when the client is at rest and diminishes with activity.

Bones are assessed for normal form. Joints are assessed for tenderness, swelling, thickening, crepitation (a crackling, grating sound), presence of nodules, and range of motion. The amount of joint movement can be measured by a **goniometer,** a device that measures the angle of the joint in degrees (Figure 22–70). Body posture is assessed for normal standing and sitting positions. For information about body posture, see Chapter 34.

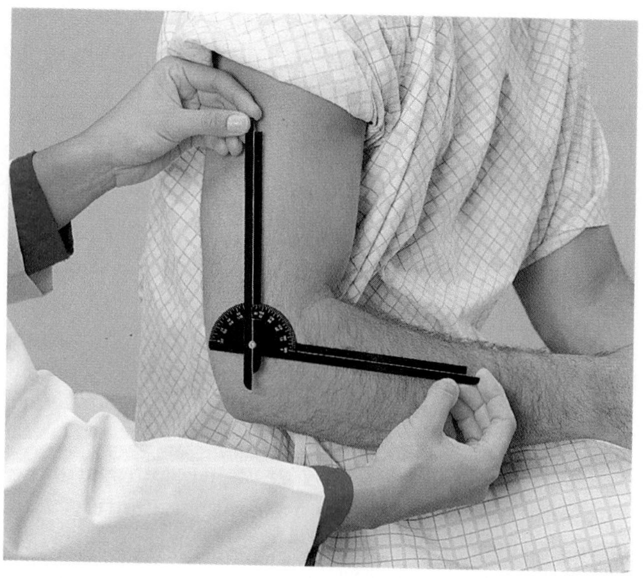

Figure 22–70 A goniometer is used to measure joint range of motion.

Procedure 22–16 describes how to assess the musculoskeletal system.

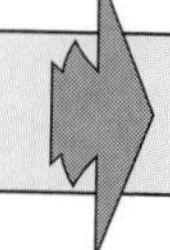

PROCEDURE 22–16 ASSESSING THE MUSCULOSKELETAL SYSTEM

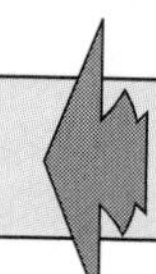

NURSING HISTORY FOCUS

History or presence of muscle pain: onset, location, character, associated phenomena (eg, redness and swelling of joints), and aggravating and alleviating factors; any limitations to movement or inability to perform activities of daily living; previous sports injuries; any loss of function without pain.

ASSESSMENT	NORMAL FINDINGS	DEVIATIONS FROM NORMAL
Muscles		
Inspect the muscles for size. Compare the muscles on one side of the body (eg, of the arm, thigh, and calf) to the same muscle on the other side. For any discrepancies, measure the muscles with a tape.	Equal size on both sides of body	**Atrophy** (a decrease in size) or **hypertrophy** (an increase in size)
Inspect the muscles and tendons for contractures (shortening).	No contractures	Malposition of body part (eg, a foot fixed in dorsiflexion)
Inspect the muscles for fasciculations and tremors. Inspect any tremors of the hands and arms by having the client hold the arms out in front of the body.	No fasciculations or tremors	Presence of fasciculation or tremor

PROCEDURE 22–16 *continued*

ASSESSMENT	NORMAL FINDINGS	DEVIATIONS FROM NORMAL
Palpate muscles at rest to determine muscle tonicity (the normal condition of tension, or tone, of a muscle at rest).	Normally firm	Atonic (lacking tone)
Palpate muscles while the client is active and passive for flaccidity, spasticity, and smoothness of movement.	Smooth coordinated movements	**Flaccidity** (weakness or laxness) or **spasticity** (sudden involuntary muscle contraction)
Test muscle strength. See tests in the box below. Compare the right side with left side.	Equal strength on each body side	25% or less of normal strength

Testing and Grading Muscle Strength

Muscle/Activity

Deltoid: Client holds arm up and resists while nurse tries to push it down.
Biceps: Client fully extends each arm and tries to flex it while nurse attempts to hold arm in extension.
Triceps: Client flexes each arm and then tries to extend it against the nurse's attempt to keep arm in flexion.
Wrist and finger muscles: Client spreads the fingers and resists as the nurse attempts to push the fingers together.
Grip strength: Client grasps the nurse's index and middle fingers while the nurse tries to pull the fingers out.
Hip muscles: Client is supine, both legs extended; client raises one leg at a time while the nurse attempts to hold it down.
Hip abduction: Client is supine, both legs extended. Nurse's hands are on the lateral surface of each knee; client is asked to spread the legs apart against the nurse's resistance.
Hip adduction: Client is in same position as for hip abduction; the nurse's hands are now placed between the knees; client is asked to bring the legs together against the nurse's resistance.
Hamstrings: Client is supine, both knees bent. Client resists while the nurse attempts to straighten them.
Quadriceps: Client is supine, knee partially extended; client resists while the nurse attempts to flex the knee.
Muscles of the ankles and feet: Client resists while the nurse attempts to dorsiflex the foot and again resists while the nurse attempts to flex the foot.

Grading Muscle Strength

0: 0% of normal strength; complete paralysis
1: 10% of normal strength; no movement, contraction of muscle is palpable or visible
2: 25% of normal strength; full muscle movement against gravity, with support
3: 50% of normal strength; normal movement against gravity.
4: 75% of normal strength; normal full movement against gravity and against minimal resistance
5: 100% of normal strength; normal full movement against gravity and against full resistance

Bones

Inspect the skeleton for normal structure and deformities.	No deformities	Bones misaligned
Palpate the bones to locate any areas of edema or tenderness.	No tenderness or swelling	Presence of tenderness or swelling (may indicate fractures, neoplasms, or osteoporosis)

PROCEDURE 22–16 ASSESSING THE MUSCULOSKELETAL SYSTEM *continued*

ASSESSMENT	NORMAL FINDINGS	DEVIATIONS FROM NORMAL
Joints		
Inspect the joints for swelling.	No swelling	One or more swollen joints
Palpate each joint for tenderness, smoothness of movement, swelling, crepitation, presence of nodules.	No tenderness, swelling, crepitation, or nodules Joints move smoothly	Presence of tenderness, swelling, crepitation, or nodules
Assess joint range of motion. Table 34–2, page 882, lists the types of joint movements. ▪ Ask the client to move selected body parts as shown in Table 34–2, page 882. Measure the amount of movement by a goniometer, as indicated.	Varies to some degree in accordance with person's genetic makeup and degree of physical activity	Limited range of motion in one or more joints

THE ELDERLY: PHYSICAL CHANGES IN THE MUSCULOSKELETAL SYSTEM

- Muscle mass decreases progressively with age, but there are wide variations among different individuals.
- The decrease in speed, strength, resistance to fatigue, reaction time, and coordination in the older person is due to a decrease in nerve conduction and muscle tone.
- The bones become more fragile, and osteoporosis leads to a loss of total bone mass. As a result, elderly people are predisposed to fractures and compressed vertebrae.
- In most elderly people, osteoarthritic changes in the joints can be observed.

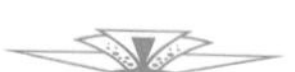

THE NEUROLOGIC SYSTEM

The nervous system integrates all other body systems, but it also depends on the appropriate functioning of peripheral organs from which it receives internal and external environmental stimuli. A thorough neurologic examination may take 1 to 3 hours; however, routine screening tests are usually done first. If the results of these tests are questionable, more extensive evaluations are made. Three major considerations determine the extent of a neurologic exam: (a) the client's chief complaints, (b) the client's physical condition (ie, level of consciousness and ability to ambulate), because many parts of the examination require movement and coordination of the extremities, and (c) the client's willingness to participate and cooperate.

Examination of the neurologic system includes assessment of (a) mental status, (b) level of consciousness, (c) the cranial nerves, (d) reflexes, (e) motor function, and (f) sensory function.

Parts of the neurologic assessment are performed throughout the health examination. For example, the nurse performs a large part of the mental status assessment during the taking of the history and when observing the client's general appearance. In addition, the nurse assesses the function of many cranial nerves. Cranial nerves II, III, IV, V (ophthalmic branch), and XI are assessed with the eyes and vision tests and cranial nerve VIII (cochlear branch) is assessed with the ears and hearing.

NURSING HISTORY FOCUS

The client is assessed for presence of pain in the head, back, or extremities: onset and aggravating and alleviating factors; disorientation to time, place, or person: speech disorder; any history of loss of consciousness, fainting, convulsions, trauma, tingling or numbness, tremors or tics, limping, paralysis, uncontrolled muscle movements, loss of memory, mood swings, or problems with smell, vision, taste, touch, or hearing.

MENTAL STATUS

Assessment of mental status reveals the client's general cerebral function. These functions include intellectual (cognitive) as well as emotional (affective) functions.

If problems with use of language, memory, concentration, thought processes, or attention span and memory are noted during the nursing history, a more extensive examination is required during neurologic assessment. Major areas of mental status assessment include language, orientation, memory, and attention span and calculation.

Language Any defects in or loss of the power to express oneself by speech, writing, or signs or to comprehend spoken or written language due to disease or injury of the cerebral cortex is called **aphasia.** Aphasias can be categorized as sensory or receptive aphasia and motor or expressive aphasia.

Sensory/receptive aphasia is the loss of the ability to comprehend written or spoken words. Two types of sensory aphasia are auditory (or acoustic) aphasia and visual aphasia. Clients with *auditory aphasia* have lost the ability to understand the symbolic content associated with sounds. Clients with *visual aphasia* have lost the ability to understand printed or written figures.

Motor/expressive aphasia involves loss of the power to express oneself by writing, making signs, or speaking. Clients may find that even though they can recall words, they have lost the ability to combine speech sounds into words.

To assess language deficits related to aphasia, the nurse does the following:

1. Point to common objects, and ask the client to name them.
2. Ask the client to read some words and to match the printed and written words with pictures.
3. Ask the client to respond to simple verbal and written commands, such as "point to your toes" or "raise your left arm."

It is also important to identify speech patterns. A pattern of repeating the same response as different questions are asked is called **perseveration. Paraphasia** is speech that is appropriately expressive but contains many incorrect words.

Orientation The nurse determines the client's orientation to *time*, *place*, and *person* by tactful questioning. Orientation is easily assessed by asking the client the city and state or residence, time of day, date, day of the week, duration of illness, and names of family members. More direct questioning may be necessary for some people, for example, "Where are you now?" "What day is it today?" Most people readily accept these questions if initially the nurse asks, "Do you get confused at times?"

Memory The nurse listens for lapses in memory, first asking the client about difficulty with memory. If problems are apparent, three categories of memory are tested: immediate recall, recent memory, and remote memory.

To assess *immediate recall*, the nurse does the following:

- Ask the client to repeat a series of three digits (eg, 7-4-3) spoken slowly.
- Gradually increase the number of digits (eg, 7-4-3-5, 7-4-3-5-6, and 7-4-3-5-6-7-2) until the client fails to repeat the series correctly.
- Start again with a series of three digits, but this time ask the client to repeat them backward. The average person can repeat a series of five to eight digits in sequence and four to six digits in reverse order.

To assess *recent memory*, the nurse carries out these steps:

- Ask the client to recall the recent events of the day, such as how the client got to the clinic. This information must be validated, however.
- Ask the client to recall information given early in the interview, such as the name of a doctor.
- Provide the client with three facts to recall (eg, a color, an object, an address) or a three-digit number, and ask the client to repeat all three. Later in the interview, ask the client to recall all three items.

To assess *remote memory*, the nurse asks the client to describe a previous illness or surgery (eg, one experienced 5 years ago) or a birthday or anniversary.

Attention Span and Calculation The nurse tests the client's ability to concentrate, or attention span, by asking the client to recite the alphabet or to count backward from 100. To test the client's ability to calculate, the nurse asks the client to subtract 7 or 3 progressively from 100; that is, 100, 93, 86, 79, or 100, 97, 94, 91. This standard test is often referred to as the *serial sevens* or *serial threes test.* Normally, an adult can complete the serial sevens test in about 90 seconds with three or fewer errors. Because educational level and language or cultural differences affect calculating ability, this test may be inappropriate for some people.

Changes in mental function in elderly people are shown in the box at the top of page 544.

THE ELDERLY: CHANGES IN MENTAL FUNCTION

- A decline in mental status is not a normal result of aging. Changes are more the result of physical or psychologic disorders (eg, fever, fluid and electrolyte imbalances).
- Intelligence and learning ability are unaltered with age. Many factors, however, inhibit learning (eg, anxiety, illness, pain, cultural barrier).
- Short-term memory is often less efficient. Long-term memory is usually unaltered.
- Because old age is often associated with loss of support persons, depression is a common disorder. It may be manifested by mood changes, weight loss, anorexia, constipation, and early morning awakening.
- The stress of being in unfamiliar situations can cause confusion in the elderly person.

LEVEL OF CONSCIOUSNESS

Level of consciousness (LOC) can lie anywhere along a continuum from a state of alertness to coma. A fully alert client responds to questions spontaneously; a comatose client may not respond to verbal stimuli. The Glasgow Coma Scale was originally developed to predict recovery from a head injury; however, it is used today to assess LOC. It tests in three major areas: eye response, motor response, and verbal response. An assessment totaling 15 points indicates the client is alert and completely oriented. A comatose client scores 7 or less. See Table 22–12.

Table 22–12 Levels of Consciousness: Glasgow Coma Scale

Faculty Measured	Response	Score*
Eye opening	Spontaneous	4
	To verbal command	3
	To pain	2
	No response	1
Motor response	To verbal command	6
	To painful stimuli:	
	▪ Localizes pain	5
	▪ Flexes and withdraws	4
	▪ Assumes decorticate posture	3
	▪ Assumes decerebrate posture	2
	▪ No response	1
Verbal response (arouse client with painful stimuli, if necessary)	Oriented, converses	5
	Disoriented, converses	4
	Uses inappropriate words	3
	Makes incomprehensible sounds	2
	No response	1

*Coma is defined as a score of 7 or less. A score of 3 or 4 indicates an 85% chance of dying or remaining vegetative. A score of 11 or more suggests an 86% chance of moderate disability or good recovery.

Source: Adapted from G Teasdale and B Bennett, Assessment of coma and impaired consciousness: A practical scale, *Lancet*, 1974, 2(7872):81.

CRANIAL NERVES

For the specific functions and assessment methods of each cranial nerve, see Table 22–13. The nurse needs to be aware of these functions to detect abnormalities. (The names and order of the cranial nerves can be recalled by remembering this sentence: "On old Olympus's treeless top, a Finn and German viewed a hop." The first letter of each word in the sentence is the same as the first letter of the names of the cranial nerves.)

REFLEXES

A **reflex** is an automatic response of the body to a stimulus. It is not voluntarily learned or conscious. The deep tendon reflex (DTR) is activated when a tendon is stimulated (tapped) and its associated muscle contracts. The quality of a reflex response varies among individuals and by age. As a person ages, reflex responses may become less intense.

Reflexes are tested using a percussion hammer. The response is described on a scale of 0 to +4. See the box below for a scale describing reflex responses. Experience is necessary to determine appropriate scoring for an individual. When assessing reflexes, it is important for the nurse to compare one side of the body with the other to evaluate the symmetry of response.

SCALE FOR GRADING REFLEX RESPONSES

0	No reflex response
+1	Minimal activity (hypoactive)
+2	Normal response
+3	More active than normal
+4	Maximum activity (hyperactive)

Table 22-13 Cranial Nerve Functions and Assessment Methods

Cranial Nerve	Name	Type	Function	Assessment Method
I	Olfactory	Sensory	Smell	Ask client to close eyes and identify different mild aromas, such as coffee, tobacco, vanilla, oil of cloves, peanut butter, orange, lemon, lime, chocolate.
II	Optic	Sensory	Vision and visual fields	Ask client to read Snellen chart; check visual fields by confrontation; and conduct an ophthalmoscopic examination.
III	Oculomotor	Motor	Extraocular eye movement (EOM); movement of sphincter of pupil; movement of ciliary muscles of lens	Assess six ocular movements and pupil reaction.
IV	Trochlear	Motor	EOM, specifically moves eyeball downward and laterally	Assess six ocular movements.
V	Trigeminal			
	Ophthalmic branch	Sensory	Sensation of cornea, skin of face, and nasal mucosa	While client looks upward, lightly touch lateral sclera of eye to elicit blink reflex; to test light sensation, have client close eyes, wipe a wisp of cotton over client's forehead and paranasal sinuses; to test deep sensation, use alternating blunt and sharp ends of a safety pin over same areas.
	Maxillary branch	Sensory	Sensation of skin of face and anterior oral cavity (tongue and teeth)	Assess skin sensation as for ophthalmic branch above.
	Mandibular branch	Motor and sensory	Muscles of mastication; sensation of skin of face	Ask client to clench teeth.
VI	Abducens	Motor	EOM; moves eyeball laterally	Assess directions of gaze.
VII	Facial	Motor and sensory	Facial expression; taste (anterior two-thirds of tongue)	Ask client to smile, raise the eyebrows, frown, puff out cheeks, close eyes tightly; ask client to identify various tastes placed on tip and sides of tongue: sugar (sweet), salt, lemon juice (sour), and quinine (bitter); identify areas of taste.
VIII	Auditory			
	Vestibular branch	Sensory	Equilibrium	Assessment methods are discussed with cerebeller functions (in next section).
	Cochlear branch	Sensory	Hearing	Assess client's ability to hear spoken word and vibrations of tuning fork.
IX	Glossopharyngeal	Motor and sensory	Swallowing ability and gag reflex, tongue movement, taste (posterior tongue)	Use tongue blade on posterior tongue while client says "ah" to elicit gag reflex; apply tastes on posterior tongue for identification; ask client to move tongue from side to side and up and down.
X	Vagus	Motor and sensory	Sensation of pharynx and larynx; swallowing; vocal cord movement	Assessed with cranial nerve IX; assess client's speech for hoarseness.
XI	Accessory	Motor	Head movement; shrugging of shoulders	Ask client to shrug shoulders against resistance from your hands and turn head to side against resistance from your hand (repeat for other side).
XII	Hypoglossal	Motor	Protrusion of tongue	Ask client to protrude tongue at midline, then move it side to side.

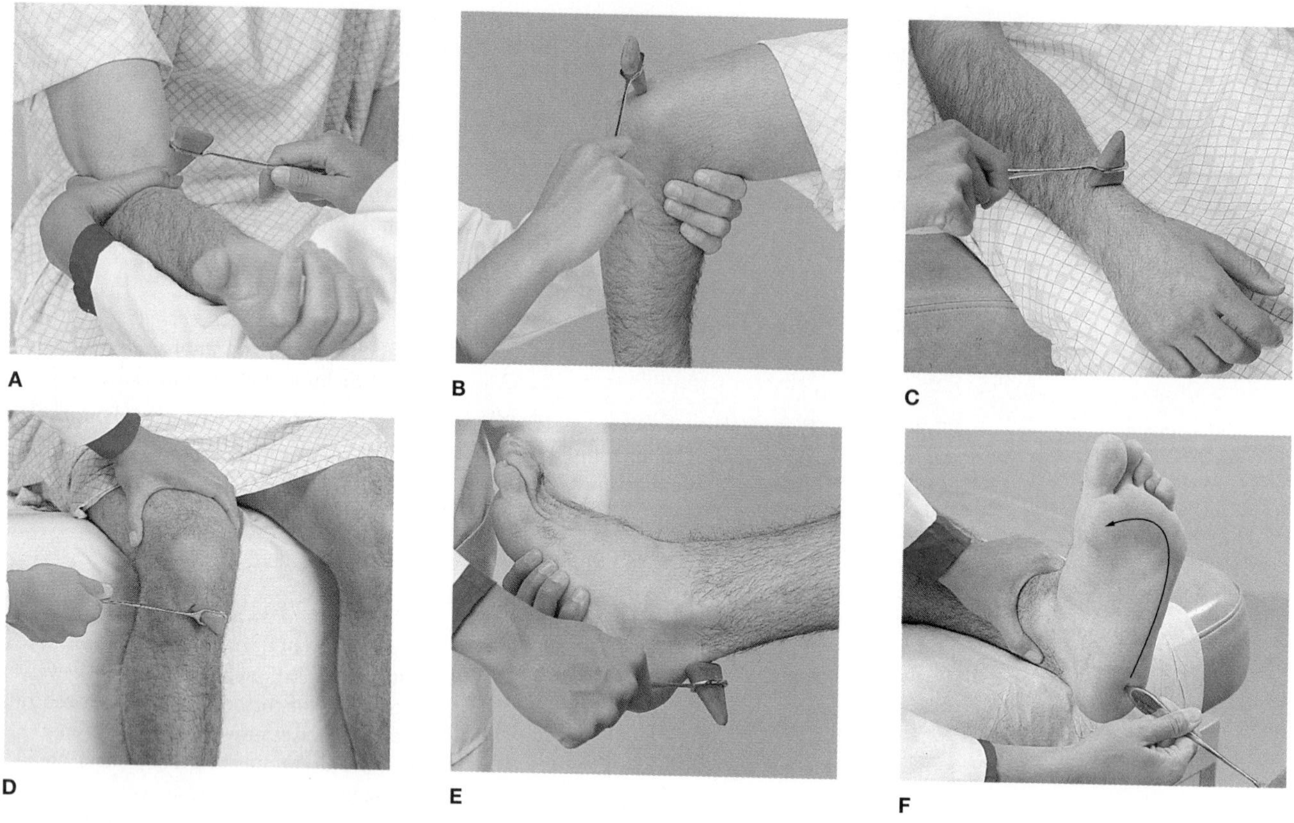

Figure 22–71 Testing reflexes: *A,* the biceps reflex; *B,* the triceps reflex; *C,* the brachioradialis reflex; *D,* the patellar reflex; *E,* the Achilles reflex; *F,* the plantar (Babinski) reflex.

Several reflexes are normally tested during a physical examination: (a) the biceps reflex, (b) the triceps reflex, (c) the brachioradialis reflex, (d) the patellar reflex, (e) the Achilles reflex, and (f) the plantar (Babinski) reflex.

Biceps Reflex This reflex tests the spinal cord level C-5, C-6.

1. Partially flex the client's arm at the elbow, and rest the forearm over the thighs, placing the palm of the hand down.
2. Place the thumb of your nondominant hand horizontally over the biceps tendon.
3. With your other hand, hold the percussion hammer between thumb and index finger.
4. Deliver a blow (slight downward thrust) with the percussion hammer to your thumb.
5. Observe the normal slight flexion of the elbow, and feel the bicep's contraction through your thumb (Figure 22–71, *A*).

Triceps Reflex This reflex tests the spinal cord level C-7, C-8.

1. Flex the client's arm at the elbow, and support it in the palm of your nondominant hand.
2. Palpate the triceps tendon about 2 to 5 cm (1 to 2 in) above the elbow.
3. Deliver a blow with the percussion hammer directly to the tendon (Figure 22–71, *B*).
4. Observe the normal slight extension of the elbow.

Brachioradialis Reflex This reflex tests the spinal cord level C-3, C-6.

1. Rest the client's arm in a relaxed position on your forearm or on the client's own leg.
2. Deliver a blow with the percussion hammer directly on the radius 2 to 5 cm (1 to 2 in) above the wrist or the styloid process, the bony prominence on the thumb side of the wrist (Figure 22–71, *C*).
3. Observe the normal flexion and supination of the forearm. The fingers of the hand may also extend slightly.

Patellar Reflex This reflex tests the spinal cord level L-2, L-3, L-4.

1. Ask the client to sit on the edge of the examining table so that the legs hang freely.
2. Locate the patellar tendon directly below the patella (kneecap).
3. Deliver a blow with the percussion hammer directly to the tendon (Figure 22–71, *D*).
4. Observe the normal extension or kicking out of the leg as the quadriceps muscle contracts.
5. If no response occurs and you suspect the client is not relaxed, ask the client to interlock the fingers and pull. This action often enhances relaxation so that a more accurate response is obtained.

Achilles Reflex This reflex tests the spinal cord level S-1, S-2.

1. With the client in the same position as for the patellar reflex, slightly dorsiflex the client's ankle by supporting the foot lightly in the hand.
2. Deliver a blow with the percussion hammer directly to the Achilles tendon just above the heel (Figure 22–71, *E*).
3. Observe and feel the normal plantar flexion (downward jerk) of the foot.

Plantar (Babinski) Reflex This plantar, or Babinski, reflex is superficial. It may be absent in adults without pathology or overridden by voluntary control.

1. Use a moderately sharp object, such as the handle of the percussion hammer, a key, or the dull end of a pin or applicator stick.
2. Stroke the lateral border of the sole of the client's foot, starting at the heel, continuing to the ball of the foot, and then proceeding across the ball of the foot toward the big toe (Figure 22–71, *F*).
3. Observe the response. Normally, all five toes bend downward; this reaction is negative Babinski. In an abnormal Babinski response the toes spread outward and the big toe moves upward. Positive Babinski is abnormal after the child ambulates.

MOTOR FUNCTION

Neurologic assessment of the motor system evaluates proprioception and cerebellar function. Structures involved in proprioception are the proprioceptors, the posterior columns of the spinal cord, the cerebellum, and the vestibular apparatus (which is innervated by cranial nerve VIII) in the labyrinth of the internal ear.

Proprioceptors are sensory nerve terminals, occurring chiefly in the muscles, tendons, joints, and the internal ear, that give information about movements and position of the body. Stimuli from the proprioceptors travel through the posterior columns of the spinal cord. Deficits of function of the posterior columns of the spinal cord result in impairment of muscle and position sense. Clients with such an impairment often must watch their own arm and leg movements to ascertain the position of the limbs.

The cerebellum (a) helps to control posture; (b) acts with the cerebral cortex to make body movements smooth and coordinated; and (c) controls skeletal muscles to maintain equilibrium.

Cerebellar disorders cause certain characteristics and common symptoms of **ataxia:** impairment of position sense, lack of muscle coordination, tremors, disturbance of equilibrium, disturbance in the timing of movements, and disturbance of gait. Tremors are especially pronounced toward the end of movements. Clients with cerebellar disease also have difficulty performing rapid skilled movements, alternating movements such as supinating and pronating the hands, and starting and stopping motions.

Procedure 22–17 describes how to assess motor function.

Text continued on page 550.

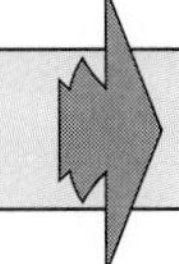

PROCEDURE 22–17 ASSESSING MOTOR FUNCTION

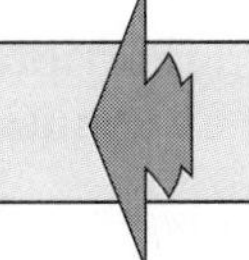

ASSESSMENT	NORMAL FINDINGS	DEVIATIONS FROM NORMAL
Gross Motor and Balance Tests There are several gross motor function and balance tests. Generally, the Romberg test and one other are used.		

PROCEDURE 22–17 ASSESSING MOTOR FUNCTION *continued*

ASSESSMENT	NORMAL FINDINGS	DEVIATIONS FROM NORMAL
Walking Gait		
Ask the client to walk across the room and back, and assess the client's gait.	Has upright posture and steady gait with opposing arm swing; walks unaided, maintaining balance	Has poor posture and unsteady, irregular, staggering gait with wide stance; bends legs only from hips; has rigid or no arm movements
Romberg Test		
Ask the client to stand with feet together and arms resting at the sides, first with eyes open, then closed. Stand close during this test to prevent the client from falling.	Negative Romberg's: May sway slightly but is able to maintain upright posture and foot stance	**Romberg's sign:** Cannot maintain foot stance; moves the feet apart to maintain stance If client cannot maintain balance with the eyes shut, client may have sensory ataxia If balance cannot be maintained whether the eyes are open or shut, client may have cerebellar ataxia
Standing on One Foot with Eyes Closed		
Ask the client to close the eyes and stand on one foot and then the other. Stand close to the client during this test.	Maintains stance for at least 5 seconds	Cannot maintain stance for 5 seconds
Heel-Toe Walking		
Ask the client to walk a straight line, placing the heel of one foot directly in front of the toes of the other foot.	Maintains heel-toe walking along a straight line	Assumes a wider foot gait to stay upright
Toe or Heel Walking		
Ask the client to walk several steps on the toes and then on the heels.	Able to walk several steps on toes or heels	Cannot maintain balance on toes or heels
Fine Motor Tests for the Upper Extremities		
Finger-to-Nose Test		
Ask the client to abduct and extend the arms at shoulder height and rapidly touch the nose alternately with one index finger and then the other. The client repeats the test with the eyes closed if the test is performed easily.	Repeatedly and rhythmically touches the nose	Misses the nose or gives lazy response

PROCEDURE 22–17 *continued*

ASSESSMENT	NORMAL FINDINGS	DEVIATIONS FROM NORMAL
Alternating Supination and Pronation of Hands on Knees		
Ask the client to pat both knees with the palms of both hands and then with the backs of the hands alternately at an ever-increasing rate.	Can alternately supinate and pronate hands at rapid pace	Performs with slow, clumsy movements and irregular timing; has difficulty alternating from supination to pronation
Finger to Nose and to the Nurse's Finger		
Ask the client to touch the nose and then your index finger, held at a distance at about 45 cm (18 in), **at a rapid and increasing rate.**	Performs with coordination and rapidity	Misses the finger and moves slowly
Fingers to Fingers		
Ask the client to spread the arms broadly at shoulder height and then bring the fingers together at the midline, first with the eyes open and then closed, first slowly and then rapidly.	As above	Moves slowly and is unable to touch fingers consistently
Fingers to Thumb (Same Hand)		
Ask the client to touch each finger of one hand to the thumb of the same hand as rapidly as possible.	Rapidly touches each finger to thumb with each hand	Cannot coordinate this fine discrete movement with either one or both hands
Fine Motor Tests for the Lower Extremities		
Ask the client to lie supine and to perform these tests.		
Heel Down Opposite Shin		
Ask the client to place the heel of one foot just below the opposite knee and run the heel down the shin to the foot. Repeat with the other foot. The client may also use a sitting position for this test.	Demonstrates bilateral equal coordination	Has tremors or is awkward; heel moves off shin
Toe or Ball of Foot to the Nurse's Finger		
Ask the client to touch your finger with the large toe of each foot.	Moves smoothly, with coordination	Misses your finger; cannot coordinate movement

SENSORY FUNCTION

Sensory functions include touch, pain, temperature, position, and tactile discrimination. The first three are routinely tested in a few locations. Generally, the face, arms, legs, hands, and feet are tested for touch and pain, although all parts of the body can be tested. If the client complains of numbness, peculiar sensations, or paralysis, the practitioner should check sensation more carefully over flexor and extensor surfaces of limbs, mapping out clearly any abnormality of touch or pain by examining responses in the area about every 2 cm (1 in). This is a lengthy procedure. Abnormal responses to touch stimuli include loss of sensation **(anesthesia);** more than normal sensation **(hyperesthesia);** less than normal sensation **(hypoesthesia);** or an abnormal sensation such as burning, pain, or an electric shock **(paresthesia).**

A more detailed neurologic examination includes position sense, temperature sense, and tactile discrimination. Three types of tactile discrimination are generally tested: **one- and two-point discrimination,** the ability to sense whether one or two areas of the skin are being stimulated by pressure; **stereognosis,** the act of recognizing objects by touching and manipulating them; and **extinction,** the failure to perceive touch on one side of the body when two symmetrical areas of the body are touched simultaneously.

To assess sensory function, the nurse needs the following equipment:

- Wisps of cotton to assess light touch sensation
- Sterile safety pin or sterile hypodermic needle to assess pain sensation
- Test tubes of hot and cold water for skin temperature assessment (optional)

Procedure 22–18 describes how to assess sensory function.

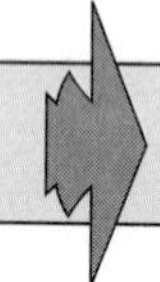

PROCEDURE 22–18 ASSESSING SENSORY FUNCTION

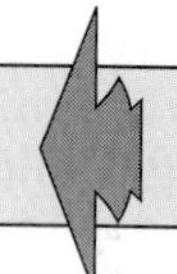

ASSESSMENT	NORMAL FINDINGS	DEVIATIONS FROM NORMAL
Light-Touch Sensation		
Compare the light-touch sensation of symmetric areas of the body. *Sensitivity to touch varies among different skin areas.*	Light tickling or touch sensation	Anesthesia, hyperesthesia, hypoesthesia, and paresthesia

- Ask the client to close the eyes and to respond by saying "yes" or "now" whenever the client feels the cotton wisp touching the skin.
- With a wisp of cotton, lightly touch one specific spot and then the same spot on the other side of the body (Figure 22–72).
- Test areas on the forehead, cheek, hand, lower arm, abdomen, foot, and lower leg. Check a specific area of the limb first (ie, the hand before the arm, and the foot before the leg), because the sensory nerve may be assumed to be intact if sensation is felt at its most peripheral part.

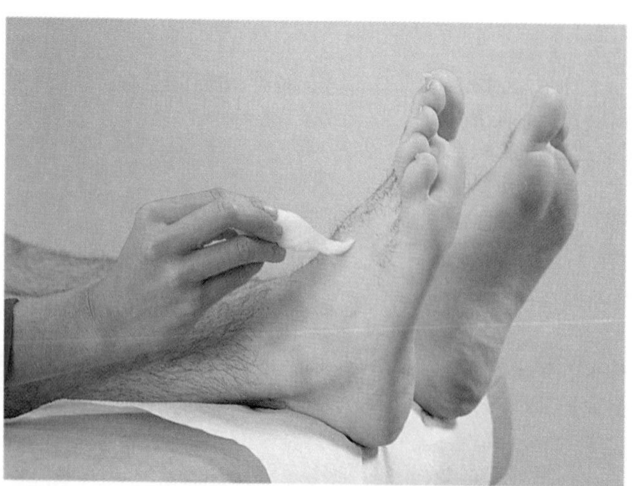

Figure 22–72 Assessing light-touch sensation.

Procedure 22–18 *continued*

ASSESSMENT	NORMAL FINDINGS	DEVIATIONS FROM NORMAL
▪ Ask the client to point to the spot where the touch was felt. *This demonstrates whether the client is able to determine tactile location (point localization)*, that is, can accurately perceive where the client was touched. ▪ If areas of sensory dysfunction are found, determine the boundaries of sensation by testing responses about every 2.5 cm (1 in) in the area. Make a sketch of the sensory loss area for recording purposes.		
Pain Sensation **Assess pain sensation.** ▪ Ask the client to close the eyes and to say “sharp,” “dull,” or “don’t know” when the sharp or dull end of the safety pin or needle is felt. ▪ Alternately use the sharp and dull end of the sterile pin or needle to lightly prick designated anatomic areas at random, such as the hand, forearm, foot, lower leg, abdomen. The face is not tested in this manner (Figure 22–73). *Alternating the sharp and dull ends of the instrument more accurately evaluates the client’s response. A sterile safety pin or needle is used to avoid the risk of infection.* 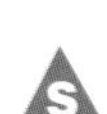 ▪ Allow at least 2 seconds between each test to prevent summation effects of stimuli (ie, several successive stimuli perceived as one stimulus).	Able to discriminate “sharp” and “dull” sensations	Areas of reduced, heightened, or absent sensation (map them out for recording purposes)
Temperature Sensation Temperature sensation is not routinely tested if pain sensation is found to be within normal limits. If pain sensation is not normal or is absent, testing sensitivity to temperature may prove more reliable.	Able to discriminate between “hot” and “cold” sensations	Areas of dulled or lost sensation (when sensations of pain are dulled, temperature sense is usually also impaired because distribution of these nerves over the body is similar)

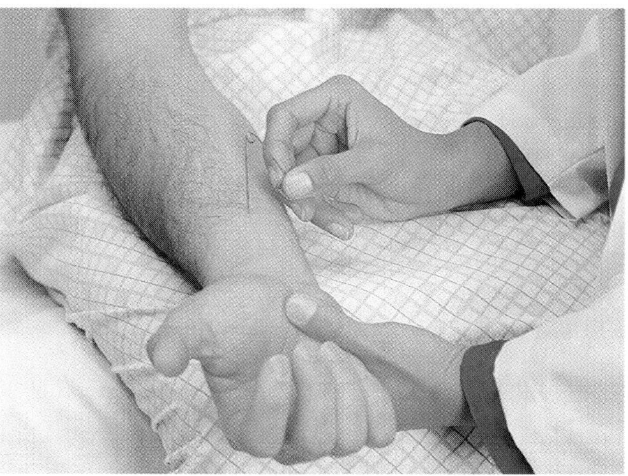

Figure 22–73 Assessing pain sensation with a pin.

PROCEDURE 22–18 ASSESSING SENSORY FUNCTION *continued*

ASSESSMENT	NORMAL FINDINGS	DEVIATIONS FROM NORMAL
▪ Touch skin areas with test tubes filled with hot or cold water. ▪ Have the client respond by saying "hot," "cold," or "don't know."		
Position or Kinesthetic Sensation		
Commonly, the middle fingers and the large toes are tested for the *kinesthetic sensation* (sense of position).	Can readily determine the position of fingers and toes	Unable to determine the position of one or more fingers or toes
▪ To test the fingers, support the client's arm with one hand, and hold the client's palm in the other; to test the toes, place the client's heels on the examining table. ▪ Ask the client to close the eyes. ▪ Grasp a middle finger or a big toe firmly between your thumb and index finger, and exert the same pressure on both sides of the finger or toe while moving it. ▪ Move the finger or toe until it is up, down, or straight out, and ask the client to identify the position. ▪ Use a series of brisk up-and-down movements before bringing the finger or toe suddenly to rest in one of the three positions.		
Tactile Discrimination		
For all tests, the client's eyes need to be closed.		
One- and Two-Point Discrimination		
Alternately stimulate the skin with two pins simultaneously and then with one pin. Ask whether the client feels one or two pinpricks.	Perception varies widely in adults over different parts of the body. Normally, a person can distinguish a one-point stimulus from a two-point stimulus within the following minimum distances: Fingertips, 2.8 mm Palms of hands, 8 to 12 mm Chest, forearm, 40 mm Back, 50 to 70 mm Upper arm, thigh, 75 mm Toes, 3 to 8 mm	Unable to sense whether one or two areas of the skin are being stimulated by pressure

PROCEDURE 22–18 *continued*

ASSESSMENT	NORMAL FINDINGS	DEVIATIONS FROM NORMAL
Stereognosis		
Place familiar objects, such as a key, paper clip, or coin, in the client's hand, and ask the client to identify them.	Able to recognize specific objects	Unable to recognize specific objects
If the client has a motor impairment of the hand and is unable to manipulate an object, write a number or letter on the client's palm, using a blunt instrument, and ask the client to identify it.	Able to identify numbers or letters written on palm	Unable to identify numbers or letters written on palm
Extinction Phenomenon		
Simultaneously stimulate two symmetric areas of the body, such as the thighs, the cheeks, or the hands.	Both points of stimulus are felt	Failure to perceive touch on one side of the body when two symmetric areas of the body are touched simultaneously (frequently noted in clients with lesions of the sensory cortex)

THE ELDERLY: CHANGES IN THE NEUROLOGIC SYSTEM

- Because older clients tire more easily than younger clients, a total neurologic assessment is often done at a time different from that of the other parts of the physical assessment.
- Although there is a progressive decrease in the number of functioning neurons in the central nervous system and in the sense organs, the older client usually functions well because of the abundant reserves in the number of brain cells.
- Impulse transmission and reaction to stimuli are slower in elderly clients.
- Many elderly clients generally have some impairment of hearing, vision, smell, temperature and pain sensation, memory, and mental endurance.
- Coordination changes in older clients, including a reduced speed of fine finger movements. Standing balance remains intact, and Romberg's test remains negative.
- Reflex responses may slightly increase or decrease in the older client. Many show loss of the Achilles reflex, and the plantar reflex may be difficult to elicit.
- When testing sensory function, the nurse needs to give the older client time to respond. Normally, older clients have unaltered perception of light touch and superficial pain, decreased perception of deep pain, and decreased perception of temperature stimuli. Many also reveal a decrease or absence of position sense in the large toes.

THE FEMALE GENITALS AND INGUINAL LYMPH NODES

The examination of the genitals and reproductive tract of adult females includes assessment of the inguinal lymph nodes and inspection and palpation of the external genitals.

Completeness of the assessment of the genitals and reproductive tract depends on the needs and problems of the individual client. *In many practice settings, nurses perform only inspection of the external genitals.*

Assessment of adolescent girls is limited to an inspection of the external genitals, unless the girl is sexually active. If so, an annual Papanicolaou test (Pap test) is advised for detecting cancer of the cervix and uterus. If the adolescent is sexually active and has an increased or abnormal vaginal discharge, specimens should be taken to check for sexually transmitted disease. The accompanying box shows the five stages of pubic hair development during puberty.

Examination of the genitals usually creates uncertainty and apprehension in females, and the lithotomy position required can cause embarrassment. The nurse must explain each part of the examination in advance and perform the examination in an objective and efficient manner. Appropriate draping is essential to prevent undue exposure of the client, and good lighting is essential for the nurse to ensure accuracy of inspection. The nurse wears disposable gloves for this genital examination to prevent the transfer of microorganisms from the client to the nurse and from the nurse to other clients. Procedure 22–19 describes how to assess the female genitals and inguinal lymph nodes.

Text continued on page 558

FIVE STAGES OF PUBIC HAIR DEVELOPMENT IN FEMALES

Stage 1 Preadolescence. No pubic hair except for fine body hair.

Stage 2 Usually occurs at ages 11 and 12. Sparse, long, slightly pigmented curly hair develops along the labia.

Stage 3 Usually occurs at ages 12 and 13. Hair becomes darker in color and curlier and develops over the pubic symphysis.

Stage 4 Usually occurs between ages 13 and 14. Hair assumes the texture and curl of the adult but is not as thick and does not appear on the thighs.

Stage 5 Sexual maturity. Hair assumes adult appearance and appears on the inner aspect of the upper thighs.

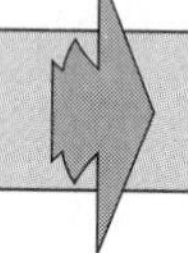

PROCEDURE 22–19 ASSESSING THE FEMALE GENITALS AND INGUINAL LYMPH NODES

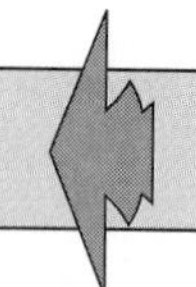

NURSING HISTORY FOCUS

Age of onset of menstruation, last menstrual period (LMP), regularity of cycle, duration, amount of daily flow, and whether menstruation is painful; incidence of pain during intercourse; vaginal discharge; number of pregnancies, number of live births, labor or delivery complications; urgency and frequency of urination at night, blood in urine, painful urination, incontinence; history of sexually transmitted disease, past and present.

ASSESSMENT	NORMAL FINDINGS	DEVIATIONS FROM NORMAL
Inspect the distribution, amount, and characteristics of pubic hair.	There are wide variations; generally kinky in the menstruating adult, thinner and straighter after menopause Distributed in the shape of an inverse triangle Hair growth should not extend over the abdomen	Scant pubic hair (may indicate hormonal problem)
Inspect the skin of the pubic area for parasites (eg, lice), **inflammation, swelling, and lesions** (eg, fissures, excoriations, scars from episiotomies, varicosities, leukoplakia). To assess pubic skin adequately, separate the labia majora and labia minora.	Pubic skin intact, no lesions Skin of vulva area slightly darker than the rest of the body Labia round, full, and relatively symmetric in adult females; labia atrophied and flatter in older females	Lice, lesions, scars, fissures, swelling, erythema, or leukoplakia

PROCEDURE 22–19 *continued*

ASSESSMENT	NORMAL FINDINGS	DEVIATIONS FROM NORMAL
Inspect the clitoris, urethral orifice, and vaginal orifice when separating the labia minora.	Clitoris does not exceed 1 cm in width and 2 cm in length Urethral orifice appears as a small slit and is the same color as surrounding tissues No inflammation, swelling, or discharge	Presence of lesions (the clitoris is a common site for syphilitic chancres in younger females and cancerous lesions in older females) Presence of inflammation, swelling, or discharge
If there is inflammation or discharge at the urethral orifice, palpate the Skene's (paraurethral) glands on either side of the urethral orifice. ▪ Insert a gloved index finger, palm uppermost, into the entrance of the vagina about 2.5 cm (1 in). ▪ While pressing gently upward, palpate for Skene's glands, then draw the finger outward (Figure 22–74). This maneuver will milk the urethra of any discharge. ▪ Observe for any discharge. ▪ If discharge is present, take a specimen, and then change gloves before proceeding with further examination.	Not palpable No discharge 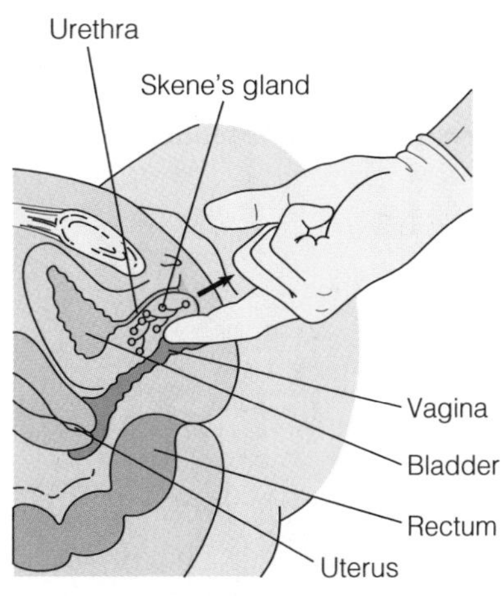 **Figure 22–74** Palpating Skene's glands.	Pain; tenderness; urethral discharge
Palpate Bartholin's glands (located on the posterior aspect of the vaginal orifice). ▪ Insert a gloved finger into the entrance of the vagina. ▪ Move the finger to the lateral and posterior aspect of the vagina. ▪ Palpate against the thumb at the posterior aspect of the labia majora (Figure 22–75). ▪ Repeat for the other side.	Not tender or palpable 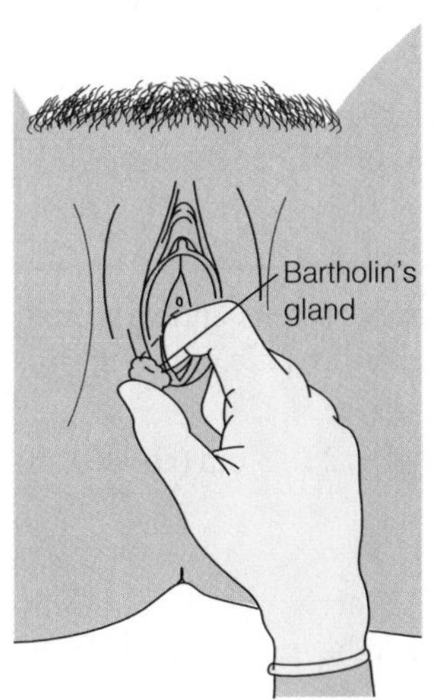 **Figure 22–75** Palpating Bartholin's gland.	Tender and palpable

PROCEDURE 22–19 ASSESSING THE FEMALE GENITALS AND INGUINAL LYMPH NODES *continued*

ASSESSMENT	NORMAL FINDINGS	DEVIATIONS FROM NORMAL
Assess the pelvic musculature while your gloved finger is in the vaginal orifice. ▪ Place two gloved fingers (index and middle finger) into the vagina. ▪ Ask the client to constrict her vaginal orifice. ▪ Ask the client to bear down while your fingers spread the vaginal wall laterally. Observe the vaginal wall for bulges.	Good tone; a **nulliparous** female (one who has never had a child) will probably have a high degree of muscle tone, whereas a **multiparous** female will have less tone Walls intact No bulges	**Cystocele** (bulging of the anterior vaginal wall as a result of a prolapse of the anterior wall and the bladder) **Rectocele** (bulging of the posterior vaginal wall as a result of a prolapse of the posterior wall and the rectum) **Enterocele** (bulging from the posterior fornix as a result of prolapse of the pouch of Douglas into the vagina)
Palpate the inguinal lymph nodes (Figure 22–76). Use the pads of the fingers in a rotary motion, noting any enlargement or tenderness.	No enlargement or tenderness	Enlargement and tenderness

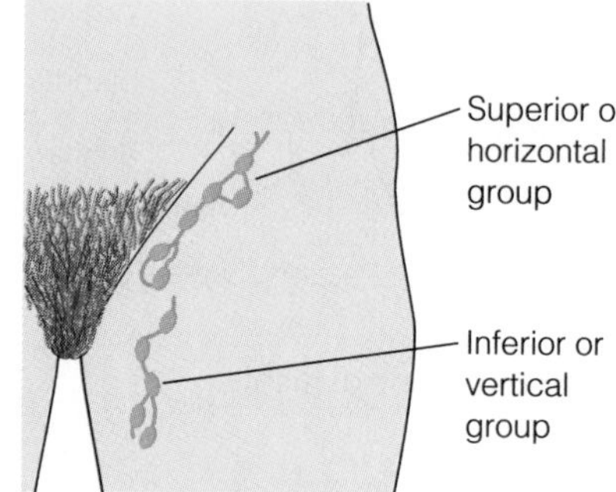

Figure 22–76 Lymph nodes of the groin area. The superior group drains the skin of the abdominal wall, the external genitals, anal canal, and lower vagina. The inferior group receives lymph from the medial aspect of the leg and foot.

ASSESSMENT	NORMAL FINDINGS	DEVIATIONS FROM NORMAL
Inspect the cervix, os, and vagina using a vaginal speculum. (Agency protocol varies as to who performs vaginal speculum examination. Determine agency policies.) See the accompanying box for steps of the technique. Observe the os for shape; the cervix for color, size, position, surface characteristics, and discharge; and the vagina for color, texture, and secretions.	**Os:** Normal nulliparous cervical os is round or oval; normal parous os is slitlike **Cervix:** *Color.* Cervix glistens and is pink in color; becomes pale after menopause *Size.* Cervix is 2 to 3 cm (about 1 in) *Position.* Cervix projects only slightly into the vaginal vault *Surface characteristics.* Cervix is smooth and intact	Hyperemia may indicate an inflammation A cervix longer than 4 cm (almost 2 in) may indicate an inflammatory condition or a tumor Cervix that projects further is indicative of uterine prolapse, and cervix that is malpositioned on a lateral wall can indicate a tumor or an adhesion. Lacerations, erosions, nodules, masses, and discharge

PROCEDURE 22–18 *continued*

Performing a Vaginal Speculum Examination

In many agencies only nurse practitioners perform this procedure. Determine agency's protocol.

- Assist the client to a lithotomy position, and drape her appropriately.
- Don gloves.
- Warm the speculum (Figure 22–77) by running warm water over it.

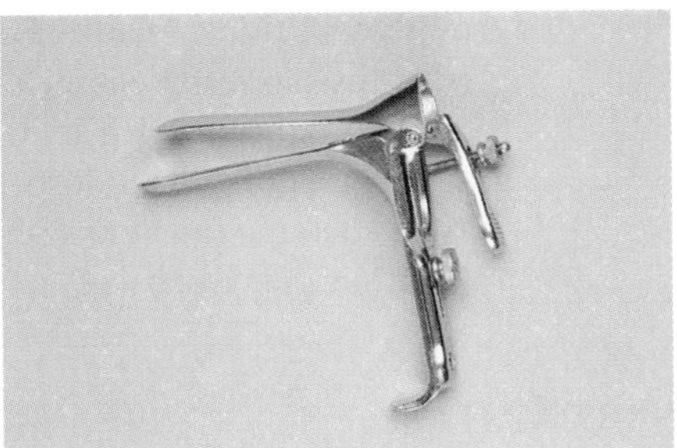

Figure 22–77 A vaginal speculum.

- Lubricate the vaginal speculum. If cytologic specimens are needed, the water serves as the lubricant; if no specimens are needed, use a water-soluble lubricant. *Lubricants can interfere with cytologic studies.*
- Place the index and middle fingers of the nondominant hand into the vaginal entrace, and exert gentle pressure down on the posterior wall.
- Insert the speculum at a 45-degree angle and downward toward the posterior wall. *This angle corresponds to the downward direction of the vagina and prevents trauma to the vaginal wall.*

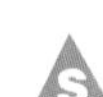

- Take care to avoid pulling pubic hair at the vaginal entrance during insertion of the speculum.
- Once the speculum is inserted beyond the wide portions of the blade, turn it so that the handle is down and the blades are in a horizontal position. The fingers are removed simultaneously.
- After full insertion, open the blades slowly, and lock the blades in the open position by closing the screw that holds the blades open.
- Observe the cervix.
- Obtain a specimen for a Papanicolaou smear, if required.
  - **a.** Collect smear samples from the three sites shown in Figure 22–78.

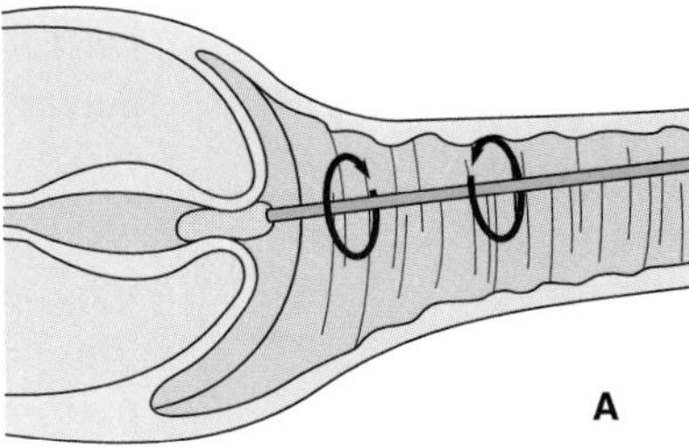

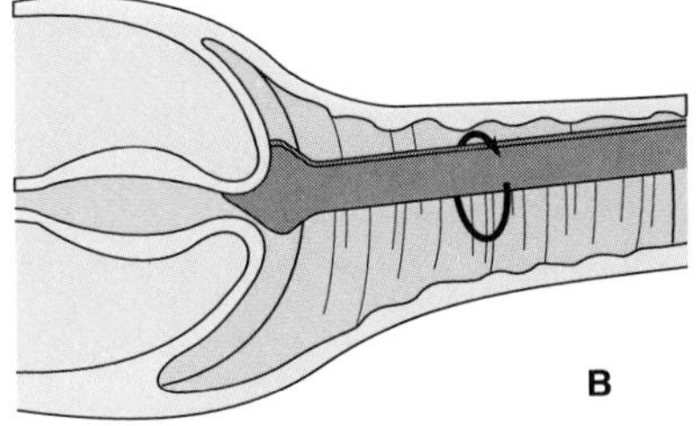

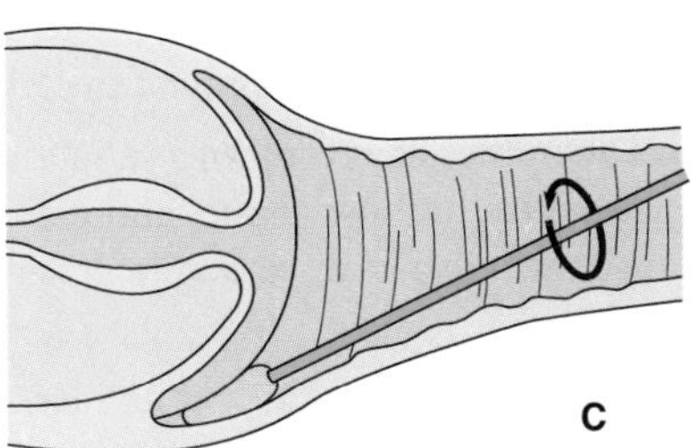

Figure 22–78 Methods of obtaining Pap smears: *A,* Endocervical. A cotton swab is inserted into the cervical os and rotated clockwise and counterclockwise in the os. *B,* Cervical scrape. An Ayre spatula with the longer end inserted into the cervical os is rotated to scrape cells from the outer surface. *C,* Vaginal smear or pool. A cotton-tipped applicator or elongated spatula is inserted along the vaginal floor.

  - **b.** Place each smear on separate glass slides labeled 1, 2, and 3, and indicate its source.
  - **c.** Fix the specimen with a fixative spray or solution.
- Withdraw the blades slowly. When the speculum is clear of the cervix, release the screws, and keep the blade open with the thumb.
- During withdrawal, carefully rotate the speculum, and inspect the vaginal walls.
- Close the blades gradually while removing the speculum, being careful not to pinch vaginal tissues or hairs in the blades. It should be closed completely when it is withdrawn from the vaginal opening.

PROCEDURE 22–19 ASSESSING THE FEMALE GENITALS AND INGUINAL LYMPH NODES *continued*

ASSESSMENT	NORMAL FINDINGS	DEVIATIONS FROM NORMAL
	Discharge. Characteristics of cervical mucus vary throughout the menstrual cycle from clear to white and from thin to thick, even stringy	Lacerations, erosions, nodules, masses, and discharge Any colored or purulent discharge
	Vagina: Color is pink, texture is consistent, and vaginal secretions are thin or mucoid and odorless.	Three common types of vaginal infections produce characteristic discharge: Monilial or yeast infections produce a thick, white, curdy, patchy discharge; trichomonal infections produce a profuse, watery, gray or green, frothy, odorous discharge; bacterial infections produce an odorous gray discharge

THE ELDERLY: CHANGES IN THE FEMALE GENITOURINARY SYSTEM

- Loss of pubic hair and a flattening of the labia occur.
- The vulva atrophies as a result of a reduction in vascularity, elasticity, adipose tissue, and estrogen levels. Because the vulva is more fragile, it is more easily irritated.
- The vaginal wall becomes thinner and less vascular, and the vagina appears pink, dry, and smooth, with fewer rugae. Atrophic vaginal tissue may readily bleed from trauma of speculum insertion.
- The vaginal environment becomes drier and more alkaline, resulting in an alteration of the type of flora present and a predisposition to vaginitis. Dyspareunia (difficult or painful coitus) is also a common occurrence.
- The cervix and uterus decrease in size. The cervix may be narrow, and the examiner may be unable to palpate the uterus during the pelvic examination.
- The fallopian tubes and ovaries atrophy.
- Ovulation and estrogen production cease.
- Vaginal bleeding unrelated to estrogen therapy is abnormal in older women.
- Prolapse of the uterus frequently occurs in older females, especially those who have had multiple pregnancies.
- Older females may be arthritic and find the lithotomy position uncomfortable. A semilithotomy position may be necessary.

THE MALE GENITALS AND INGUINAL AREA

In adult males, complete examination should include assessment of the external genitals, the presence of any hernias, and the prostate gland. As with females, *nurses in some practice settings performing routine assessment of clients may assess only the external genitals.* The male reproductive and urinary systems (Figure 22–79) share the urethra, which is the passageway for both urine and semen. Therefore, in physical assessment of the male, these two systems are frequently assessed together.

Examination of the male genital organs by a female practitioner (physician or nurse) is becoming increasingly common. Formerly, most examinations of men were done by men. Most male clients accept examination by a female, especially if she is emotionally comfortable herself about performing it and does so in a matter-of-fact and competent manner. If the female nurse does not feel comfortable about this part of the examination or if the client

Table 22–14 Five Stages of Development of Pubic Hair, Penis, and Testes/Scrotum (12 to 16 Years)

Stage	Pubic Hair	Penis	Testes/Scrotum
1 (preadolescent)	None, except for body hair like that on the abdomen	Size is relative to body size, as in childhood	Size is relative to body size, as in childhood
2	Scant, long, slightly pigmented at base of penis	Slight enlargement occurs	Becomes reddened in color and enlarged
3	Darker, begins to curl and becomes more coarse; extends over pubic symphysis	Elongation occurs	Continuing enlargement
4	Continues to darken and thicken; extends on the sides, above and below	Increase in both breadth and length; glans develops	Continuing enlargement; color darkens
5	Adult distribution that extends to inner thighs, umbilicus, and anus	Adult appearance	Adult appearance

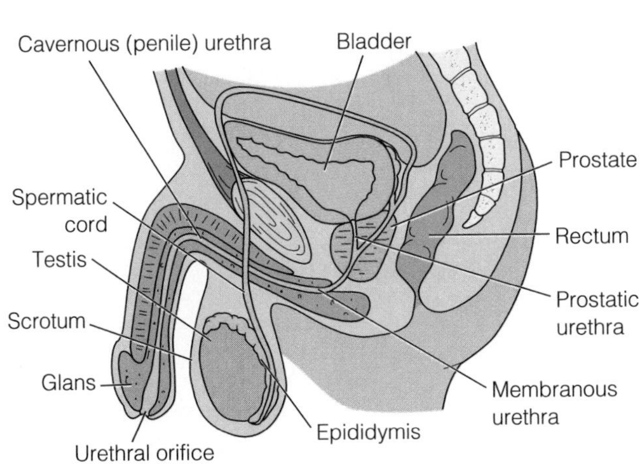

Figure 22–79 The male urogenital tract.

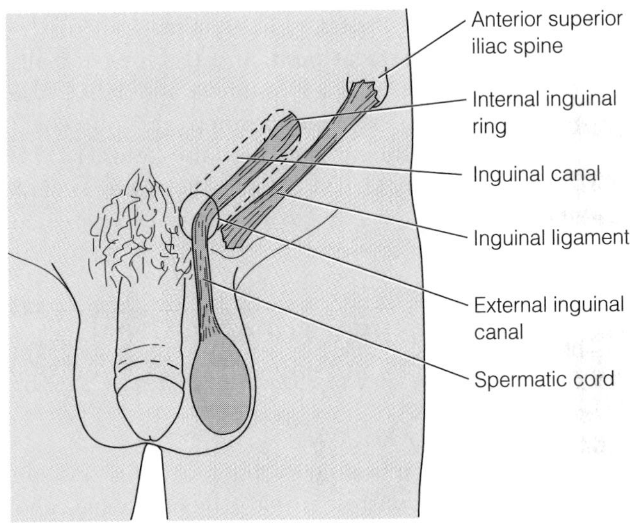

Figure 22–80 Structures of the inguinal area.

is reluctant to be examined by a female, the nurse should refer this part of the examination to a male practitioner.

The techniques of inspection and palpation are used to examine the male genitals. Equipment needed includes gloves and a penlight to transilluminate any mass. The client may be in a lying or sitting position.

Development of secondary sex characteristics is also assessed in relationship to the client's age. See Table 22–14 for the five stages of the development of pubic hair, the penis, and the testes/scrotum during puberty.

All clients should be screened for the presence of inguinal or femoral hernias. A **hernia** is a protrusion of the intestine through the inguinal wall or canal. The loop of bowel may even extend down to the scrotum. Structures of the inguinal area are shown in Figure 22–80. An *indirect inguinal hernia* is a loop of bowel that enters the internal inguinal ring. It may stay in the canal, exit through the external ring, or pass into the scrotum. A *direct inguinal hernia* enters the inguinal canal directly through a weakness in the abdominal wall just behind the external inguinal ring. It does not pass through the inguinal canal. A *femoral hernia* is more common in women. It is lower and more lateral than an inguinal hernia and may look like an enlarged lymph node.

Testicular cancer is most commonly found on the anterior and lateral surfaces of the testes. **Testicular self-examination** should be conducted monthly. The client can examine the testicles while he sits, stands, or lies down. Optimally, this exploration should take place after a hot bath or shower, because the heat causes the scrotal skin to relax and the testes to descend. Instructions for testicular self-examination are shown in the Client Teaching box at the right.

Procedure 22–20 describes how the nurse can conduct an assessment of the male genitals and inguinal area.

THE RECTUM AND ANUS

Rectal examination, an essential part of every comprehensive physical examination, involves inspection and palpation (digital examination). The extent of the assessment of the rectum and anus depends on the rectal problems stated by the client in the nursing history. *In many practice settings, the nurse performs only inspection of the anus.* An interior view of the rectum and anal canal are shown in Figure 40–4 on page 1181.

A left lateral or Sims' position with the upper leg acutely flexed is required for the examination. For females, a dorsal recumbent position with hips externally rotated and knees flexed or a lithotomy position may also be used. For males, a standing position while the client bends over the examining table may also be used. This position is commonly used to examine the prostate gland.

Text continued on page 563

CLIENT TEACHING

Testicular Self-Examination

Instruct the man to

- Examine the testicles monthly, one at a time.
- Use the fingertips to probe the surface gently, as if examining an egg for imperfections. The surface should be smooth and fairly firm.
- Use the thumb and the index and middle fingers for examination, with the thumb on top and the fingers on the underside of the scrotum.
- Roll the testicles between the thumb and fingers. The normal testicle is about 1½ to 2 inches long and feels rubbery, smooth, and firm, but not hard. It should be free of lumps.
- Palpate the epididymis, the storage tube found at the top of the testicle and extending behind it. It should feel soft, spongy, and slightly tender.
- Locate the spermatic cord, which extends from the bottom of the epididymis and up into the pelvis. It normally feels firm and smooth.

Source: Adapted from L Malasanos, V Barkauskas, and K Stoltenberg-Allen, *Health Assessment*, 4th ed. (St Louis: Mosby, 1990), p. 543.

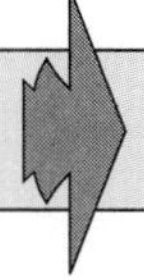

PROCEDURE 22–20 ASSESSING THE MALE GENITALS AND INGUINAL AREA

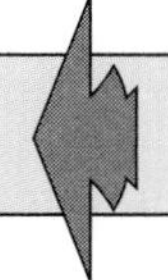

NURSING HISTORY FOCUS

Usual fluid intake and output, voiding patterns and any changes, bladder control, urinary incontinence, frequency, urgency, abdominal pain; any symptoms of sexually transmitted disease; any swellings that could indicate presence of hernia; family history of nephritis, malignancy of the prostate, or malignancy of the kidney.

ASSESSMENT	NORMAL FINDINGS	DEVIATIONS FROM NORMAL
Pubic Hair		
Inspect the distribution, amount, and characteristics of pubic hair.	Triangular distribution, often spreading up the abdomen	Scant amount or absence of hair
Penis		
Inspect the penile shaft and glans penis for lesions, nodules, swellings, and inflammation.	Penile skin intact Appears slightly wrinkled and varies in color as widely as other body skin Foreskin easily retractable from the glans penis Small amount of thick white **segma** between the glans and foreskin	Presence of lesions, nodules, swellings, or inflammation

PROCEDURE 22–20 *continued*

ASSESSMENT	NORMAL FINDINGS	DEVIATIONS FROM NORMAL
Inspect the urethral meatus for swelling, inflammation, and discharge. ▪ Compress or ask the client to compress the glans slightly to open the urethral meatus to inspect it for discharge. ▪ If the client has reported a discharge, instruct the client to strip the penis from the base to the urethra (ie, grasp the base of the penis, with the thumb at the front and finger behind, and while applying moderate pressure, move the thumb and fingers slowly down the shaft of the penis).	Pink and slitlike appearance Positioned at the tip of the penis	Inflammation; discharge Variation in meatal locations (eg, **hypospadias,** on the underside of the penile shaft, and **epispadias,** on the upper side of the penile shaft)
Palpate the penis for tenderness, thickening, and nodules. Use your thumb and first two fingers.	Smooth and semifirm Is slightly movable over the underlying structures	Presence of tenderness, thickening, or nodules Immobility
Scrotum		
Inspect the scrotum for appearance, general size, and symmetry. ▪ To facilitate inspection of the scrotum during a physical examination, ask the client to hold the penis out of the way. ▪ Inspect all skin surfaces by spreading the rugated surface skin and lifting the scrotum as needed to observe posterior surfaces.	Scrotal skin is darker in color than that of the rest of the body and is loose Size varies with temperature changes (the dartos muscles contract when the area is cold and relax when the area is warm) Scrotum appears asymmetric (left testis is usually lower than right testis)	Discolorations; any tightening of skin (may indicate edema or mass) Marked asymmetry in size
Palpate the scrotum to assess status of underlying testes, epididymis, and spermatic cord. Palpate both testes simultaneously for comparative purposes. The palpation procedure is outlined in the box on page 562.	Testicles are rubbery, smooth, and free of nodules and masses Testis is about 2 × 4 cm (0.7 × 1.5 in) Epididymis is resilient, normally tender, and softer than the spermatic cord Spermatic cord is firm	Testicles are enlarged, with uneven surface (possible tumor) Testis has swelling that transilluminates (possible hydrocele) Epididymis is nonresilient and painful

➤

PROCEDURE 22–20 ASSESSING THE MALE GENITALS AND INGUINAL AREA *continued*

Palpating the Scrotum

- Using your first two fingers and thumb, palpate each testis for size, consistency, shape, smoothness, and presence of masses. During assessment of male adolescents, establish the descent of the testicles into the scrotum; note undescended testes.
- Palpate the epididymis between your thumb and index finger. It is located at the top of the testis and extends behind it.
- Palpate the spermatic cord between thumb and index finger. It is usually found at the top lateral portion of the scrotum and feels firm.
- If swelling, iregularities, or nodules are detected during the scrotal examination, attempt to transilluminate the lesion. This is done by darkening the room and shining a flashlight behind the scrotum through the mass. Serous fluid causes the light to show with a red glow; tissue or blood does not transilluminate.
- Describe all scrotal masses in terms of their size, shape, placement, consistency, tenderness, and presence of transillumination.

ASSESSMENT	NORMAL FINDINGS	DEVIATIONS FROM NORMAL
Inguinal Area		
Inspect both inguinal areas for bulges while the client is standing, if possible. ▪ First, have the client remain at rest. ▪ Next, have the client hold the breath and strain or bear down as though having a bowel movement. *Bearing down may make the hernia more visible.*	No swelling or bulges	Swelling or bulge (possible inguinal or femoral hernia)
Palpate hernias as described in the box below.	No palpable bulge	Palpable bulge in the area

Palpating a Hernia

Direct Hernia

- Using your right hand for the client's right side or left hand for the client's left side, advance your index finger into the loose scrotal skin and over the external inguinal ring.
- Instruct the client to bear down.
- If a hernia is present, a palpable bulge will appear in the area.

Indirect Hernia

- Attempt to move the index or little finger into the path of the inguinal canal (Figure 22–80, earlier) while the client flexes the knee on the same side.
- When your finger has moved as far as possible, ask the client to bear down.
- If a hernia is present, it will be felt as a mass of tissue touching the finger and withdrawing from it.

Fermoral Hernia

- Palpate the inguinal area directly again, first while the client is at rest and then while the client bears down.
- If a hernia is present, a bulge will be felt most prominently when the client bears down.

PROCEDURE 22–20 *continued*

THE ELDERLY: CHANGES IN THE MALE GENITOURINARY SYSTEM

Genitals

- The penis decreases in size with age; the size and firmness of the testes decrease.
- Testosterone is produced in smaller amounts.
- More time and direct physical stimulation are required for the older male to achieve an erection, but the elderly man can maintain the erection for longer periods before ejaculation than he could at a younger age.
- Seminal fluid is reduced in amount and viscosity.

Urinary Bladder

- In the elderly male client, urinary frequency, nocturia, dribbling, and problems with beginning and ending the stream are usually the result of prostatic enlargement.

For all rectal examinations, the nurse should wear gloves (Malasanos et al 1990, p. 389).

Because digital examination can cause apprehension and embarrassment in the client, it is important that the nurse (a) help the client relax by encouraging the client to take slow, deep breaths (tension can cause spasms of the anal sphincters, making the examination uncomfortable), (b) inform the client about potential sensations such as feelings of defecation or passing gas, (c) assure the client that an accident is very unlikely, (d) proceed with the examination in a competent and gentle way, and (e) drape the client appropriately to prevent undue exposure of body parts. Procedure 22–21 describes how to assess the rectum and anus.

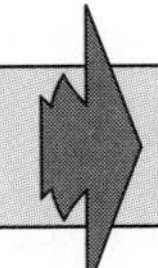

PROCEDURE 22–21 ASSESSING THE RECTUM AND ANUS

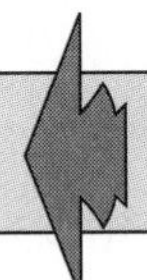

NURSING HISTORY FOCUS

History of bright blood in stools, tarry black stools, diarrhea, constipation, abdominal pain, excessive gas, hemorrhoids, or rectal pain; family history of colorectal cancer; when last stool specimen for occult blood was performed and the results; and, if not obtained during the genitourinary examination, any signs or symptoms of prostate enlargement (eg, slow urinary stream, hesitance, frequency, dribbling, and nocturia).

ASSESSMENT	NORMAL FINDINGS	DEVIATIONS FROM NORMAL
Inspect the anus and surrounding tissue for color, integrity, and skin lesions. Then, ask the client to bear down as though defecating. *Bearing down creates slight pressure on the skin that may accentuate rectal fissures, rectal prolapse, polyps, or internal hemorrhoids.* Describe the location of all abnormal findings in terms of a clock, with the 12 o'clock position toward the pubic symphysis.	Intact perianal skin; usually slightly more pigmented than the skin of the buttocks Anal skin is normally more pigmented, coarser, and moister than perianal skin and is usually hairless	Presence of fissures (cracks), ulcers, excoriations, inflammations, abscesses, protruding **hemorrhoids** (dilated veins seen as reddened protrusions of the skin), lumps or tumors, fistula openings, or **rectal prolapse** (varying degrees of protrusion of the rectal mucous membrane through the anus)

PROCEDURE 22–21 ASSESSING THE RECTUM AND ANUS *continued*

ASSESSMENT	NORMAL FINDINGS	DEVIATIONS FROM NORMAL
Palpate the rectum for anal sphincter tonicity, nodules, masses, and tenderness. See the box below for palpation technique.	Anal sphincter has good tone	Hypertonicity of the anal sphincter (may occur in the presence of an anal fissure or other lesion that causes contraction) Hypotonicity of anal sphincter (may occur after rectal surgery or result from a neurologic deficiency)
	Rectal wall is smooth and not tender	Rectal wall is tender and nodular

Palpating the Rectum

- Lubricate your index finger, and instruct the client to bear downward as though having a bowel movement. *This relaxes the anal sphincter.*
- Slowly insert your finger into the anus and into the rectum in the direction of the umbilicus. The anal canal (distance from the anal opening to the anorectal junction) is short (less than 3 cm [about 1 in]). The posterior wall of the rectum follows the curve of the coccyx and sacrum. The nurse's finger is usually able to palpate a distance of 6 to 10 cm (over 2 to 4 in).
- Never force digital insertion. If lesions are painful or bleeding occurs, discontinue the examination.
- Ask the client to tighten the anal sphincter around your finger, and note the tone of the anal sphincter.
- Rotate the pad of the index finger along the anal and the rectal walls, feeling for nodules, masses, and tenderness.
- Note the location of any abnormalities of the rectum (eg, "anterior wall, 2 cm proximal to the internal anal sphincter").

ASSESSMENT	NORMAL FINDINGS	DEVIATIONS FROM NORMAL
On withdrawing the finger from the rectum and anus, observe it for feces.	Brown color	Presence of mucus, blood, or black tarry stool
Palpate the prostate gland (if the client is male) through the anterior wall of the rectum (Figure 22–81). You should be able to feel the median sulcus, which divides the gland into two lobes.	No tenderness Edges are discrete Gland is about 4 cm (1½ in) in diameter, firm, rubbery, smooth, and mobile	Enlarged; not movable Nodular surface; tenderness

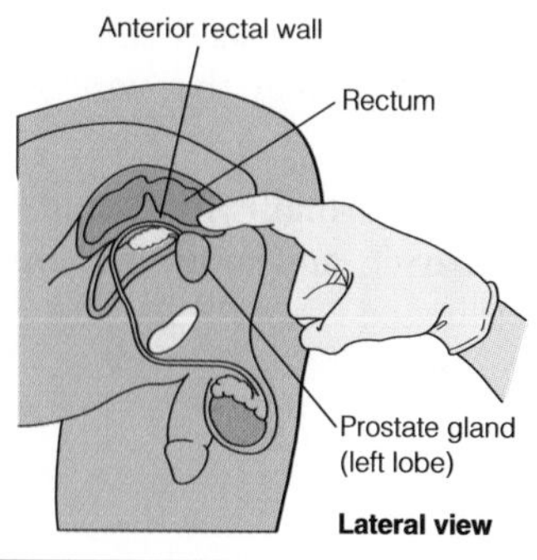

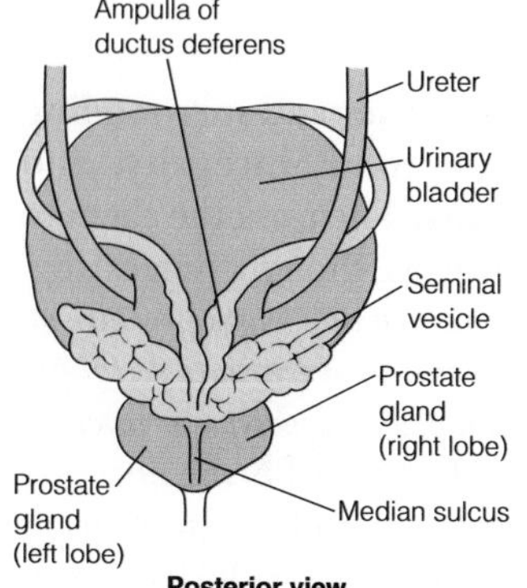

Figure 22–81 Palpating the prostate gland through the anterior wall of the rectum.

PROCEDURE 22–21 *continued*

ASSESSMENT	NORMAL FINDINGS	DEVIATIONS FROM NORMAL
Palpate the cervix (if the client is female) through the anterior rectal wall (Figure 22–82).	Smooth, round, firm, and movable; no tenderness Size is 2 to 3 cm (about 1 in)	Enlargement or tenderness of cervix; nodular surface

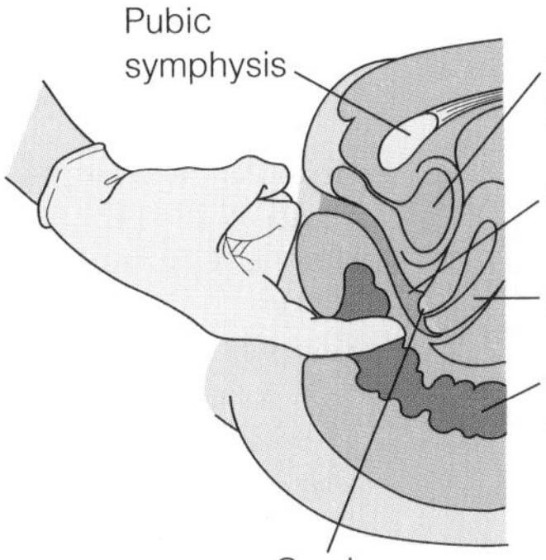

Figure 22–82 Palpating the cervix through the anterior rectal wall.

CHAPTER HIGHLIGHTS

- The health examination is conducted to assess the function and integrity of the client's body parts.
- The health examination may entail a complete head-to-toe assessment or individual assessment of a body system or body part.
- The health assessment is conducted in a systematic manner that requires the fewest position changes for the client.
- Aspects of physical assessment procedures should be incorporated in the assessment, intervention, and evaluation phases of the nursing process.
- Data obtained in the physical health examination supplement, confirm, or refute data obtained during the nursing history.
- Nursing history data help the nurse focus on specific aspects of the physical health examination.
- Data obtained in the physical health examination help the nurse establish nursing diagnoses, plan the client's care, and evaluate the outcomes of nursing care.
- Initial assessment findings provide baseline data about the client's functional abilities against which subsequent assessment findings are compared.
- Skills in inspection, palpation, percussion, and auscultation are required for the physical health examination; these skills are used in that order throughout the examination except during abdominal assessment, when auscultation follows inspection and precedes percussion and palpation.
- Knowledge of the normal structure and function of body parts and systems is an essential requisite to conducting physical assessment.

READINGS AND REFERENCES

SUGGESTED READINGS

Holmgren, C. March 1992. Perfecting the art: Abdominal assessment. *RN* 55:28–34.

The author demonstrates taking a gastrointestinal-specific history and physical examination. Observing the abdominal contours and skin are included as well as auscultation, percussion, and palpation techniques. At the end of the article are 20 multiple-choice questions.

Kuhn, JK and McGovern, M. December 1992. Peripheral vascular assessment of the elderly client. *Journal of Gerontological Nursing* 18:35–38.

The atherosclerotic process often takes its toll on the blood vessels of elderly clients, causing disabling and painful problems. These authors state that a thorough assessment of an elderly person's peripheral vascular system, combined with appropriate health teaching, can prevent or delay such problems as ischemic pain, skin ulcerations, gangrene, or amputation. The assessment includes the client interview, inspection, palpation, auscultation, and special techniques to employ if arterial or venous insufficiency is suspected.

SELECTED REFERENCES

America Cancer Society. January 1, 1994. *Summary of American Cancer Society Recommendations for Early Detection of Cancer in Asymptomatic People.* Atlanta: American Cancer Society, Inc.

Anardi, DM. October 1991. Assessment of right heart function. *Journal of Cardiovascular Nursing* 6:12–33.

Andrews, LW. November/December 1990. Neurovascular assessment. *Advancing Clinical Care* 5:5–7.

Barker, E and Moore, K. April 1992a. Neurological assessment. *RN* 55:28–35.

———. May 1992b. Cranial nerve assessment. *RN* 55:62–69.

Bates, B. 1991. *Guide to Physical Examination and History Taking.* 5th ed. Philadelphia: Lippincott.

Becker, KL. and Stevens, SA. June 1988. Performing in-depth abdominal assessment. *Nursing88* 18:59–63.

Boss, BJ. June 1991. Attention and memory systems: Nursing assessment. *AXON* 12:89–94.

Bowers, AC and Thompson, JM. 1992. *Clinical Manual of Health Assessment.* 4th ed. St Louis: Mosby-Year Book.

Burggraf, V and Donlon, B. September 1985. Assessing the elderly: System by system. *American Journal of Nursing* 85:974–84.

Eden-Kilgour, S and Miller, B. August 1993. Understanding neurovascular assessment. *Nursing93* 23:56–58.

Finesilver, C. February 1992. Perfecting the art: Respiratory assessment. *RN* 55:22–30.

Holmgren, C. March 1992. Perfecting the art: Abdominal assessment. *RN* 55:28–34.

Hunt, L. October 1992. Ophthalmic nursing assessment. *Insight* 17:9–11.

Kain, CD, Reilly, N, and Schultz, ED. December 1990. The older adult: A comparative assessment. *Nursing Clinics of North America* 25:833–48.

Malasanos, L, Barkauskas, V, and Stoltenberg-Allen, K. 1990. *Health Assessment.* 4th ed. St Louis: Mosby.

Smith, CE. February 1988. Assessing bowel sounds: More than just listening. *Nursing88* 18:42–43.

Stevens, SA and Becker, KL. January 1988a. How to perform picture-perfect respiratory assessment. *Nursing88* 18:57–63.

———. September 1988b. A simple step-by-step approach to neurological assessment. Part 1. *Nursing88* 18:53–61; Part 2. October 1988c. *Nursing88* 18:51–58.

Sullivan, J. December 1990. Neurologic assessment. *Nursing Clinics of North America* 25:795–809.

UNIT 7

Promoting Wellness Through the Life Span

STUDENT PROFILE

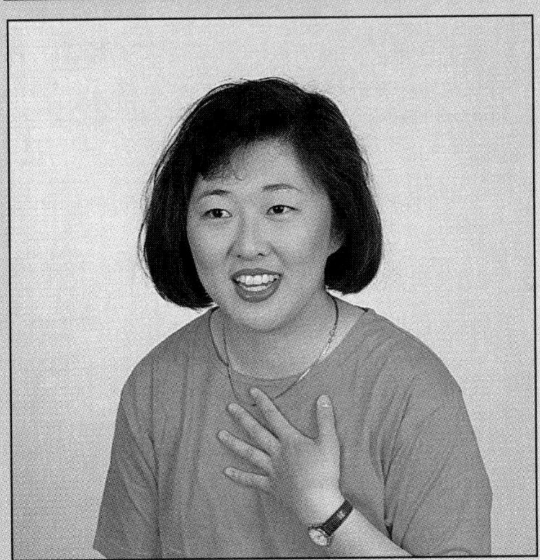

NAME	Julie Kim
SCHOOL OF NURSING	Rush University, Chicago, Illinois
HOMETOWN	Schaumburg, Illinois

WHY DID YOU ENTER THE FIELD OF NURSING?
After graduating from college with a degree in biology, I realized that I wanted a career that gave me more satisfaction and enjoyment.

WHO OR WHAT INFLUENCED THAT DECISION?
My supervisor at work was an RN. She told me great stories of her years on the floor, and her enthusiasm for nursing was contagious.

WHY DO YOU THINK THIS IS A GOOD TIME TO BE IN NURSING?
Nursing is on the verge of a major change, and the opportunities are limitless. Nurses are achieving new levels of practice and autonomy.

WHAT QUALITIES DO YOU THINK ARE NECESSARY TO BE A GOOD NURSE?
Patience, charity, organization, and diligence.

WHAT HAS BEEN YOUR MOST GRATIFYING MOMENT AS A STUDENT NURSE?
The moment I was able to hold the hand of a patient with terminal cancer and cry with her. The thank you she gave me was worth everything.

WHAT ADVICE WOULD YOU GIVE A NEW STUDENT?
Nursing is about assessment, learning about the patient, and supporting the family.

Concepts of Growth and Development

Objectives

- Describe essential facts related to growth and development.
- Differentiate growth from development.
- Describe the stages of growth and development.
- List factors that influence growth and development.
- Explain the principles of growth and development.
- Identify developmental tasks associated with Havighurst's six age periods.
- Describe characteristics and implications of Freud's five stages of development.
- Identify Erikson's eight stages of development.
- Compare Peck's and Gould's stages of adult development
- Explain Piaget's theory of cognitive development.
- Compare Kohlberg's and Gilligan's theories of moral development.
- Compare Fowler's and Westerhoff's stages of spiritual development.

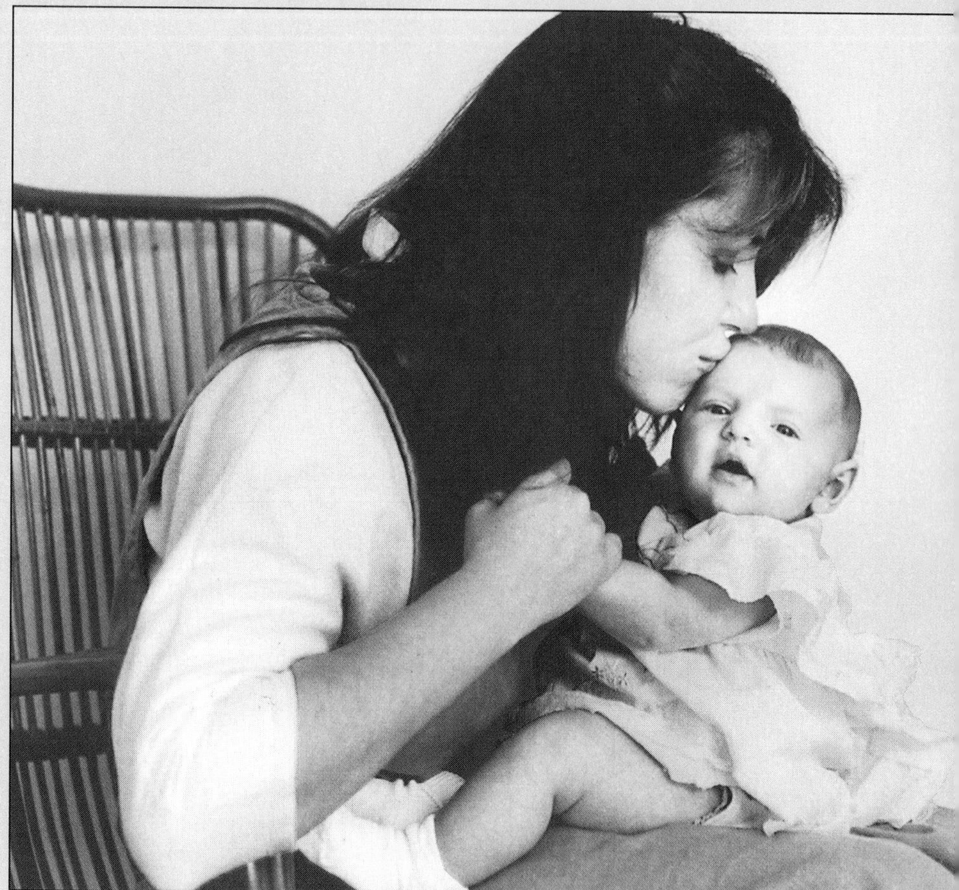

The terms *growth* and *development* both refer to dynamic processes. Often used interchangeably, these terms have different meanings. **Growth** is physical change and increase in size. Growth can be measured quantitatively. Indicators of growth include height, weight, bone size, and dentition. The pattern of physiologic growth is similar for all people. However, growth rates vary during different stages of growth and development. For example, the growth rate is very rapid during the prenatal, neonatal, infancy, and adolescent stages. The growth rate slows during childhood, and physical growth is minimal during adulthood. Specific growth trends throughout life are discussed in detail in Chapters 24, 25, and 26.

Development is an increase in the complexity of function and skill progression (Mott el al 1990, p. 117). It is the capacity and skill of a person to function. Development is the behavioral aspect of growth; for example, a person develops the ability to walk, to talk, and to run. Growth and development are independent, interrelated processes. For example, an infant's muscles, bones, and nervous system must grow to a certain point before the infant can sit up or walk. Growth generally takes place during the first 20 years of life; development continues after that. Principles of growth and development are shown in the box below.

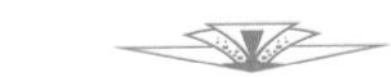

FACTORS INFLUENCING GROWTH AND DEVELOPMENT

The factors that influence growth and development are both genetic and environmental. The genetic inheritance of an individual is established at conception. This genetic inheritance remains unchanged throughout life and determines such characteristics as sex, physical stature, and race.

Many environmental factors affect an individual's growth and development. Some of these are family,

PRINCIPLES OF GROWTH AND DEVELOPMENT

- Growth and development are continuous, orderly, sequential processes influenced by maturational, environmental, and genetic factors.
- All humans follow the same pattern of growth and development.
- The sequence of each stage is predictable, although the time of onset, the length of the stage, and the effects of each stage vary with the person.
- Learning can either help or hinder the maturational process, depending on what is learned.
- Each developmental stage has its own characteristics. For example, Piaget suggests that in the sensorimotor stage (birth to 2 years) children learn to coordinate simple motor tasks.
- Growth and development occur in a **cephalocaudal** direction, that is, starting at the head and moving to the trunk, the legs, and the feet. This pattern is particularly obvious at birth, when the head of the infant is disproportionately large.
- Growth and development occur in a proximal to distal direction, that is, from the center of the body outward. For example, infants can roll over before they can grasp an object with the thumb and second finger.
- Development proceeds from simple to complex, or from single acts to integrated acts. To accomplish the integrated act of drinking and swallowing from a cup, for example, the child must first learn a series of single acts: eye-hand coordination, grasping, hand-mouth coordination, controlled tipping of the cup, and then mouth, lip, and tongue movements to drink and swallow.
- Development becomes increasingly differentiated. **Differentiated development** begins with a generalized response and progresses to a skilled specific response (eg, an infant's initial response to a stimulus involves the total body; a 5-year-old child can respond more specifically with laughter or fear).
- Certain stages of growth and development are more critical than others. It is known, for example, that the first 10 to 12 weeks after conception are critical. The incidence of congenital anomalies as a result of exposure to certain viruses, chemicals, or drugs is greater during this stage than others.
- The pace of growth and development is uneven. It is known that growth is greater during infancy than during childhood. Asynchronous development is demonstrated by rapid growth of the head during infancy and the extremities at puberty.

religion, climate, culture, school, community, and nutrition. For example, poorly nourished children are more likely to have infections than are well-fed children and may not attain their full height potential.

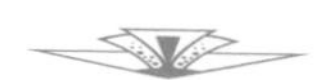

STAGES OF GROWTH AND DEVELOPMENT

The rate of a person's growth and development is highly individual; however, the sequence of growth and development is predictable. Stages of growth usually correspond to certain developmental changes. See Table 23–1.

Growth and development are commonly thought of as having five major components: physiologic, cognitive, psychosocial, moral, and spiritual. A discussion of some of the major theories relating to these components follows.

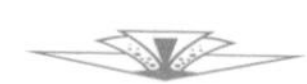

GROWTH AND DEVELOPMENT THEORIES

DEVELOPMENTAL TASK THEORY (HAVIGHURST)

Robert Havighurst believes that learning is basic to life and that people continue to learn throughout life. He describes growth and development as occurring during six stages, each associated with from six to ten tasks to be learned. See Table 23–2 on page 572. Havighurst believes that once a person learns to talk, it is mastered for life.

Havighurst promoted the concept of developmental tasks in the 1950s. A **developmental task** is "a task which arises at or about a certain period in the life of an individual, successful achievement of which leads to his happiness and to success with later tasks, while failure leads to unhappiness in the individual, disapproval by society, and difficulty with later tasks" (Havighurst 1972, p. 2).

Havighurst's developmental tasks provide a framework that the nurse can use to evaluate a person's general accomplishments. However, some nurses find that the broad categories limit its usefulness as a tool in assessing specific accomplishments, particularly those of infancy and childhood.

PSYCHOSOCIAL THEORIES

Psychosocial development refers to the development of personality. **Personality** is a complex concept that is difficult to define. It can be considered as the outward (interpersonal) expression of the inner (intrapersonal) self. It encompasses a person's temperament, feelings, character traits, independence, self-esteem, self-concept, behavior, ability to interact with others, and ability to adapt to life changes.

Many theorists attempt to account for psychosocial development in humans. Many of these theories explain the development of a person's personality and the causes of behavior. The theorists discussed in this book are Freud, Erikson, Peck, and Gould.

Freud Sigmund Freud introduced a number of concepts about development that are still used today. The concepts of the unconscious mind, defense mechanisms, and the id, ego, and superego are Freud's. The **unconscious mind** is the mental life of a person of which the person is unaware. This concept of the unconscious is one of Freud's major contributions to the field of psychiatry. **Defense mechanisms,** or **adaptive mechanisms** as they are more commonly called today, are the result of conflicts between inner impulses and the anxiety that attends these conflicts. The **id** is the source of instinctive and unconscious urges, which Freud considers chiefly sexual in nature. The id is also the source of all pleasure and gratification. The **ego** is formed by the person to make effective contact with social and physical needs. Through the ego, the id impulses are satisfied. The third aspect of the personality, according to Freud, is the **superego.** This is the conscience of the personality, a control on the id. The superego is the source of feelings of guilt, shame, and inhibition. See Chapter 32 for additional information on adaptive processes and ego defense mechanisms. Freud proposes that the underlying motivation to human development is an energy form or life instinct, which he calls **libido.**

According to Freud's theory of psychosexual development, the personality develops in five overlapping stages from birth to adulthood. The libido changes its location of emphasis within the body from one stage to another. Therefore, a particular body area has special significance to a client at a particular stage. The first three stages (oral, anal, and phallic) are called *pregenital stages.* The culminating stage is the *genital stage.* Table 23–3 on page 573 indicates characteristics and implications for each stage.

If the individual does not achieve a satisfactory resolution at each stage, the personality becomes fixated at that stage. **Fixation** is immobilization or the inability of the personality to proceed to the next stage because of anxiety. For example, nurses can assist an infant's development by making feeding a pleasurable experience and by making toilet training a positive experience, thereby enhancing the child's feeling of self-control. Freud also emphasizes the importance of infant-parent interaction. Therefore, the nurse, as a caregiver, should provide a warm, caring atmosphere for an infant and assist parents to do so also when the infant returns to their care.

Table 23–1 Stages of Growth and Development

Stage	Age	Significant Characteristics	Nursing Implications
Neonatal	Birth to 28 days	Behavior is largely reflexive and develops to more purposeful behavior.	Assist parents to identify and meet unmet needs.
Infancy	1 month to 1 year	Physical growth is rapid.	Control the infant's environment so that physical and psychological needs are met.
Toddlerhood	1 to 3 years	Motor development permits increased physical autonomy. Psychosocial skills increase.	Safety and risk-taking strategies must be balanced to permit growth.
Preschool	3 to 6 years	The preschooler's world is expanding. New experiences and the preschooler's social role are tried during play. Physical growth is slower.	Provide opportunities for play and social activity.
School age	6 to 12 years	Stage includes the preadolescent period (10 to 12 years). Peer group increasingly influences behavior. Physical, cognitive, and social development increases, and the child has increased competence in communication.	Allow time and energy for the school-age child to pursue hobbies and school activities. Recognize and support child's achievement.
Adolescence	12 to 20 years	Self-concept changes with biologic development. Values are tested. Physical growth accelerates. Stress increases, especially in face of conflicts.	Assist adolescents to develop coping behaviors. Help adolescents develop strategies for resolving conflicts.
Young adulthood	20 to 40 years	A personal life-style develops. Person establishes a relationship with a significant other, a commitment to something, and competence.	Accept adult's chosen life-style and assist with necessary adjustments relating to health. Recognize the person's commitment and the function of competence in life. Support change as necessary for health.
Middle adulthood	40 to 65 years	Life-style changes due to other changes; for example, children leave home, occupational goals change.	Assist clients to plan for anticipated changes in life, to recognize the risk factors related to health, and to focus on strengths rather than weaknesses.
Older adulthood			
Young-Old	65 to 74 years	Adaptation to retirement and changing physical abilities is often necessary. Chronic illness may develop.	Assist clients to keep physically and socially active and to maintain peer group interactions.
Middle-Old	75 to 84 years	Adaptation to decline in speed of movement, reaction time, and sensory abilities and increasing dependence on others may be necessary.	Assist clients to cope with loss (eg, hearing, eyesight, death of loved one). Provide necessary safety measures.
Old-Old	85 and over	Increasing physical problems may develop.	Assist clients with self-care as required, and with maintaining as much independence as possible.

Table 23–2 Havighurst's Age Periods and Developmental Tasks

Infancy and Early Childhood

1. Learning to walk
2. Learning to take solid foods
3. Learning to talk
4. Learning to control the elimination of body wastes
5. Learning sex differences and sexual modesty
6. Achieving psychologic stability
7. Forming simple concepts of social and physical reality
8. Learning to relate emotionally to parents, siblings, and other people
9. Learning to distinguish right from wrong and developing a conscience

Middle Childhood

1. Learning physical skills necessary for ordinary games
2. Building wholesome attitudes toward oneself as a growing organism
3. Learning to get along with age-mates
4. Learning an appropriate masculine or feminine social role
5. Developing fundamental skills in reading, writing, and calculating
6. Developing concepts necessary for everyday living
7. Developing conscience, morality, and a scale of values
8. Achieving personal independence
9. Developing attitudes toward social groups and institutions

Adolescence

1. Achieving new and more mature relations with age-mates of both sexes
2. Achieving a masculine or feminine social role
3. Accepting one's physique and using the body effectively
4. Achieving emotional independence from parents and other adults
5. Achieving assurance of economic independence
6. Selecting and preparing for an occupation
7. Preparing for marriage and family life
8. Developing intellectual skills and concepts necessary for civic competence
9. Desiring and achieving socially responsible behavior
10. Acquiring a set of values and an ethical system as a guide to behavior

Early Adulthood

1. Selecting a mate
2. Learning to live with a partner
3. Starting a family
4. Rearing children
5. Managing a home
6. Getting started in an occupation
7. Taking on civic responsibility
8. Finding a congenial social group

Middle Age

1. Achieving adult civic and social responsibility
2. Establishing and maintaining an economic standard of living
3. Assisting teenage children to become responsible and happy adults
4. Developing adult leisure-time activities
5. Relating oneself to one's spouse as a person
6. Accepting and adjusting to the physiologic changes of middle age
7. Adjusting to aging parents

Later Maturity

1. Adjusting to decreasing physical strength and health
2. Adjusting to retirement and reduced income
3. Adjusting to death of a spouse
4. Establishing an explicit affiliation with one's age group
5. Meeting social and civil obligations
6. Establishing satisfactory physical living arrangements

Source: From *Developmental Tasks and Education*, 3d ed. by Robert J Havighurst. Copyright © 1972 by Longman Publishers USA. Reprinted with permission.

Erikson Erik H Erikson adapts and expands Freud's theory of development to include the entire life span, believing that people continue to develop throughout life. He describes eight stages of development. In contrast to Freud, Erikson believes the ego to be the conscious core of the personality. See Table 23–4 on page 574.

Erikson envisions life as a sequence of levels of achievement. Each stage signals a task that must be achieved. The resolution of the task can be complete, partial, or unsuccessful. Erikson believes that the greater the task achievement, the healthier the personality of the person; failure to achieve a task influences the person's ability to achieve the next task. These developmental tasks can be viewed as a series of crises, and successful resolution of

Table 23-3 Freud's Five Stages of Development

Stage	Age	Characteristics	Implications
Oral	Birth to 1 year	Mouth is the center of pleasure. Feelings of dependence arise and can persist through life. An individual who is fixated at this stage may have difficulty in trusting others and may demonstrate nail biting, drug abuse, smoking, overeating, alcoholism, argumentativeness, and overdependence.	Feeding produces pleasure and sense of comfort and safety. Feeding should be pleasurable and provided when required.
Anal	2 and 3 years	Anus and rectum are the centers of pleasure. This stage occurs during toilet training. Fixation at the anal stage can result in obsessive-compulsive personality traits, such as obstinacy, stinginess, cruelty, and temper tantrums.	Controlling and expelling feces provide pleasure and sense of control. Toilet training should be a pleasurable experience, and appropriate praise can result in a personality that is creative and productive.
Phallic	4 and 5 years	The child's genitals are the center of pleasure. Sexual and aggressive feelings associated with genitals come into focus. Masturbation offers pleasure, and the child experiences the Oedipus or Electra complex. The Oedipus complex refers to the male child's attraction for his mother and hostile attitudes toward his father. The Electra complex refers to the female's attraction for her father and hostile attitudes toward her mother. Fixation at this stage can result in difficulties with sexual identity and problems with authority.	The child identifies with the parent of the opposite sex and later takes on a love relationship outside the family. Encourage identity.
Latency	6 to 12 years	Energy is directed to physical and intellectual activities. Sexual impulses tend to be repressed. Unresolved conflicts at this stage can result in obsessiveness and lack of self-motivation.	Encourage child with physical and intellectual pursuits.
Genital	13 years and after	Energy is directed toward attaining a mature sexual relationship. This stage involves a reactivation of the pregenital impulses. These impulses are usually displaced, and the individual passes to the genital stage of maturity. An inability to resolve conflicts can result in sexual problems, such as frigidity, impotence, and the inability to have a satisfactory sexual relationship.	Encourage separation from parents, achievement of independence, and decision making.

Source: Adapted from PH Miller, *Theories of Developmental Psychology*. Copyright © 1983 WH Freeman and Company. Used by permission.

these crises is supportive to the person's ego. Failure to resolve the crises is damaging to the ego. After attaining one stage, the person may fall back and need to approach it again.

Erikson's eight stages reflect both positive and negative aspects of the critical life periods. The resolution of the conflicts at each stage enables the person to function effectively in society. Each phase has its developmental task, and the individual must find a balance between, for example, trust versus mistrust (stage 1) or generativity versus stagnation (stage 7).

When using Erikson's developmental framework, nurses should be aware of indicators of positive and negative resolution of each stage. It is also important to be

Table 23–4 Erikson's Eight Stages of Development

Stage	Age	Central Task	Indicators of Positive Resolution	Indicators of Negative Resolution
Infancy	Birth to 18 months	Trust versus mistrust	Learning to trust others	Mistrust, withdrawal, estrangement
Early childhood	18 months to 3 years	Autonomy versus shame and doubt	Self-control without loss of self-esteem Ability to cooperate and to express oneself	Compulsive self-restraint or compliance Willfulness and defiance
Late childhood	3 to 5 years	Initiative versus guilt	Learning the degree to which assertiveness and purpose influence the environment Beginning ability to evaluate one's own behavior	Lack of self-confidence Pessimism, fear of wrongdoing Overcontrol and overrestriction of own activity
School age	6 to 12 years	Industry versus inferiority	Beginning to create, develop, and manipulate Developing sense of competence and perseverence	Loss of hope, sense of being mediocre Withdrawal from school and peers
Adolescence	12 to 20 years	Identity versus role confusion	Coherent sense of self Plans to actualize one's abilities	Confusion, indecisveness, and inability to find occupational identity
Young adulthood	18 to 25 years	Intimacy versus isolation	Intimate relationship with another person Commitment to work and relationships	Impersonal relationships Avoidance of relationship, career, or life-style commitments
Adulthood	25 to 65 years	Generativity versus stagnation	Creativity, productivity, concern for others	Self-indulgence, self-concern, lack of interests and commitments
Maturity	65 years to death	Integrity versus despair	Acceptance of worth and uniqueness of one's own life Acceptance of death	Sense of loss, contempt for others

Sources: Adapted from EH Erikson, *Childhood and Society*, 2d ed. (New York: Norton, 1963); and HS Wilson and CR Kneisl, *Psychiatric Nursing*, 4th ed. (Redwood City, CA: Addison-Wesley Nursing, 1992). Used by permission.

aware that, according to Erikson, the environment is highly influential in development. Nurses can enhance a client's development by being aware of the person's developmental stage, by providing opportunities for the individual to resolve a developmental task, and by helping the person develop coping skills relative to stressors experienced at that level. Nurses can enhance a client's positive resolution of a developmental task by providing the individual with appropriate opportunities and encouragement. For example, a 10-year-old child can be encouraged to be creative, to finish schoolwork, and to learn how to accomplish these tasks within the limitations imposed by health.

Erikson emphasizes that people must change and adapt their behavior to maintain control over their lives. In his view, no stage in personality development can be bypassed, but people can become fixated at one stage or regress to a previous stage. For example, a middle-aged woman who has never satisfactorily accomplished the task of resolving identity versus role confusion might regress to an earlier stage when stressed by an illness with which she cannot cope.

Peck Theories and models about *adult* development are relatively recent compared with theories of infant and child development. Research into adult development has been stimulated by a number of factors, including increased longevity and healthier old age. In the past, development was viewed as complete by the time of physical maturity, and aging was considered a decline following maturity. The emphasis was on the decremental aspects rather than the incremental aspects of aging. However, Peck believes that although physical capabilities and functions decrease with old age, mental and social capacities tend to increase in the latter part of life (Peck 1968).

Peck proposes three developmental tasks during old age, in contrast to Erikson's one (integrity versus despair). Peck believes that the older person must accomplish three tasks:

1. *Ego differentiation versus work-role preoccupation.* An adult's identity and feelings of worth are highly dependent on that person's work role. On retirement, some people experience feelings of worthlessness, unless they derive their sense of identity from a number of roles so that one such role can replace the work role or occupation as a source of self-esteem. For example, a man who likes to garden or golf can obtain ego rewards from those activities, replacing rewards formerly obtained from his occupation.
2. *Body transcendence versus body preoccupation.* This task calls for the individual to adjust to decreasing physical capacities and at the same time maintain feelings of well-being. Preoccupation with declining body function reduces happiness and satisfaction with life.
3. *Ego transcendence versus ego preoccupation.* Ego transcendence is the acceptance without fear of one's death as inevitable. This acceptance includes being actively involved in one's own future beyond death. Ego preoccupation, by contrast, results in holding on to life and a preoccupation with self-gratification.

Gould Gould is another theorist who has studied adult development. He believes that transformation is a central theme during adulthood: "Adults continue to change over the period of time considered to be adulthood and . . . developmental phases may be found during the adult span of life" (Gould 1972, p. 33). According to Gould, the 20s is the time when a person assumes new roles; in the 30s, role confusion often occurs; and in the 40s the person becomes aware of time limitations in relation to accomplishing life's goals. In the 50s, according to Gould, the acceptance of each stage as a natural progression of life marks the path to adult maturity. Gould's study of 524 men and women led him to describe seven stages of adult development:

- *Stage 1 (age 16–18).* Individuals consider themselves part of the family rather than individuals, and want to separate from their parents.
- *Stage 2 (ages 18–22).* Although the individuals have established autonomy, they feel it is in jeopardy; they feel they could be pulled back into their families.
- *Stage 3 (ages 22–28).* Individuals feel established as adults and autonomous from their families. They see themselves as well-defined but still feel the need to prove themselves to their parents. They see this as the time for growing and building for the future.
- *Stage 4 (ages 29–34).* Marriage and careers are well established. Individuals question what life is all about and wish to be accepted as they are, no longer finding it necessary to prove themselves.
- *Stage 5 (ages 35–43).* This is a period of self-reflection. Individuals question values and life itself. They see time as finite, with little time left to shape the lives of adolescent children.
- *Stage 6 (ages 43–50).* Personalities are seen as set. Time is accepted as finite. Individuals are interested in social activities with friends and spouse and desire both sympathy and affection from spouse.
- *Stage 7 (ages 50–60).* This is a period of transformation, with a realization of mortality and a concern for health. There is an increase in warmth and a decrease in negativism. The spouse is seen as a valuable companion (Gould 1972, pp. 525–27).

COGNITIVE THEORY (PIAGET)

Cognitive development refers to the manner in which people learn to think, reason, and use language. It involves a person's intelligence, perceptual ability, and ability to process information. Cognitive development represents a progression of mental abilities from illogical to logical thinking, from simple to complex problem solving, and from understanding concrete ideas to understanding abstract concepts.

The most widely known cognitive theorist is Jean Piaget (1896–1980). His theory of cognitive development has contributed to other theories, such as Kohlberg's theory of moral development and Fowler's theory of the development of faith, both discussed in this chapter.

According to Piaget, cognitive development is an orderly, sequential process in which a variety of new experiences (stimuli) must exist before intellectual abilities can develop. Piaget's cognitive developmental process is divided into five major phases: the sensorimotor phase, the preconceptual phase, the intuitive phase, the concrete operations phase, and the formal operations phase. A person develops through each of these phases; each phase has its own unique characteristics. See Table 23–5 on page 576.

In each phase, the person uses three primary abilities: assimilation, accommodation, and adaptation. **Assimilation** is the process through which humans encounter and react to new situations by using the mechanisms they

Table 23–5 Piaget's Phases of Cognitive Development

Phases and Stages	Age	Significant Behavior
Sensorimotor phase	Birth to 2 years	
Stage 1 Use of reflexes	Birth to 1 month	Most action is reflexive.
Stage 2 Primary circular reaction	1 to 4 months	Perception of events is centered on the body.
		Objects are extension of self
Stage 3 Secondary circular reaction	4 to 8 months	Acknowledges the external environment.
		Actively makes changes in the environment.
Stage 4 Coordination of secondary schemata	8 to 12 months	Can distinguish a goal from a means of attaining it.
Stage 5 Tertiary circular reaction	12 to 18 months	Tries and discovers new goals and ways to attain goals.
		Rituals are important.
Stage 6 Inventions of new means	18 to 24 months	Interprets the environment by mental image.
		Uses make-believe and pretend play.
Preconceptual phase	2 to 4 years	Uses an egocentric approach to accommodate the demands of an environment.
		Everything is significant and relates to "me."
		Explores the environment.
		Language development is rapid.
		Associates words with objects.
Intuitive thought phase	4 to 7 years	Egocentric thinking diminishes.
		Thinks of one idea at a time.
		Includes others in the environment.
		Words express thoughts.
Concrete operations phase	7 to 11 years	Solves concrete problems.
		Begins to understand relationships such as size.
		Understands right and left.
		Cognizant of viewpoints.
Formal operations phase	11 to 15 years	Uses rational thinking.
		Reasoning is deductive and futuristic.

Source: Adapted from J Piaget, *The Origin of Intelligence in Children.* International Universities Press, Inc. Copyright © 1966. Used by permission.

already possess. In this way, people acquire knowledge and skills as well as insights into the world around them. **Accommodation** is a process of change whereby cognitive processes mature sufficiently to allow the person to solve problems that were unsolvable before. This adjustment is possible chiefly because new knowledge has been assimilated. **Adaptation,** or coping behavior, is the ability to handle the demands made by the environment.

Nurses can employ Piaget's theory of cognitive development when developing teaching strategies. For example, a nurse can expect a toddler to be egocentric and literal; therefore, explanations to the toddler should focus on the needs of the toddler rather than on the needs of others. Further, a 13-year-old can be expected to use rational thinking and to reason; therefore, when explaining the need for a medication, a nurse can outline the consequences of taking and not taking the medication, enabling the adolescent to make a rational decision. Nurses must remember, however, that the range of normal cognitive development is very broad, despite the ages arbitrarily associated with each level. When teaching adults, nurses may become aware that some adults are more comfortable with concrete thought and slower to acquire and apply new information than are other adults.

MORAL THEORIES

Moral development, a complex process not fully understood, involves learning what ought to be and what ought not to be done. It is more than imprinting parents' rules and virtues or values upon children. The term **moral** means relating to right and wrong. The terms *morality*, *moral behavior*, and *moral development* need to be distinguished. **Morality** refers to the requirements necessary for people to live together in society; **moral behavior** is the way a person perceives those requirements and responds to them; **moral development** is the pattern of change in moral behavior with age.

Kohlberg Kohlberg's theory specifically addresses moral development in children and adults (Berkowitz & Oser 1985). The morality of an individual's decision is not Kohlberg's concern; rather, he focuses on the reasons an individual makes a decision. According to Kohlberg, moral development progresses through three levels and six stages. Levels and stages are not always linked to a certain developmental stage, because some persons progress to a higher level of moral development than others.

At Kohlberg's first level, called the *premoral* or *preconventional level*, children are responsive to cultural rules and labels of good and bad, right and wrong. However, children interpret these in terms of the physical consequences of their actions, that is, punishment or reward. At the second level, the *conventional level*, the individual is concerned about maintaining the expectations of the family, group, or nation and sees this as right. The emphasis at this level is conformity and loyalty to one's own expectations as well as society's. Level three is called the *postconventional*, *autonomous*, or *principled level*. At this level, people make an effort to define valid values and principles without regard to outside authority or to the expectations of others. For additional information about Kohlberg's levels, see Table 23–6 on page 578.

With reference to Kohlberg's six stages, Munhall writes that stage four, the "law and order" orientation, is the dominant stage of most adults (Munhall 1982, p. 14). It is recognized that there is a difference in action between nurses who act at the conventional level (level II) and those who act at the postconventional or principled level (level III). Nurses who are conventional thinkers base perceptions of moral obligations and rights on the maintenance of the social system and loyalty to established institutions and social groups. However, the postconventional nurse understands that societies and social relationships can be arranged in many ways, and that these different ways can maximize or minimize values (Munhall 1982, p. 13). Therefore, the nurse at level III questions authority and follows social norms as long as they support human values.

Gilligan Carol Gilligan (1982), after more than 10 years of research with women subjects, found that women often considered the dilemmas that Kohlberg used in his research to be irrelevant. Women scored consistently lower on his scale of moral development, in spite of the fact that they approached moral dilemmas with considerable sophistication. Gilligan believed that most frameworks do not include the concepts of caring and responsibility. Yet it is from these frameworks that most research in moral development is done. The result is that male emphasis upon individualism and autonomy is central to most moral development theories.

Gilligan describes three stages in the process of developing an "ethic of care" (Gilligan 1982, p. 74). Each stage ends with a transitional period. A *transitional period* is a time when the individual recognizes a conflict or discomfort with some present behavior and considers new approaches.

- *Stage 1. Caring for oneself.* In this first stage of development, the person is concerned only with caring for the self. The individual feels isolated, alone, and unconnected to others. There is no concern or conflict with the needs of others because the self is the most important. The focus of this stage is survival. The end of this stage occurs when the individual begins to view this approach as selfish. At this time, the person also begins to see a need for relationships and connections with other people.

- *Stage 2. Caring for others.* During this stage, the individual recognizes the selfishness of earlier behavior and begins to understand the need for caring relationships with others. Caring relationships bring with them responsibility. The definition of *responsibility* includes self-sacrifice, where "good" is considered to be "caring for others." The individual now approaches relationships with a focus of not hurting others. This approach causes the individual to be more responsive and submissive to others' needs, excluding any thoughts of meeting one's own. A transition occurs when the individual recognizes that this approach can cause difficulties with relationships because of the lack of balance between caring for oneself and caring for others.

- *Stage 3. Caring for self and others.* During this last stage, a person sees that there is a need for a balance between caring for others and caring for the self. One's concept of responsibility is now defined as including both responsibility for the self and for other people. In this final stage, care still remains the focus on which decisions are made. However, the person now recognizes the interconnections between the self and others and thus realizes that it is important to take care of one's

Table 23–6 Kohlberg's Stages of Moral Development

Level and Stage	Definition	Example
Level I *Preconventional*		
Stage 1: Punishment and obedience orientation	The activity is wrong if one is punished, and the activity is right if one is not punished.	A nurse follows a physician's order so as not to be fired.
Stage 2: Instrumental-relativist orientation	Action is taken to satisfy one's needs.	A client in hospital agrees to stay in bed if the nurse will buy the client a newspaper.
Level II *Conventional*		
Stage 3: Interpersonal concordance (good boy, nice girl)	Action is taken to please another and gain approval.	A nurse gives elderly clients in hospital sedatives at bedtime because the night nurse wants all clients to sleep at night.
Stage 4: Law and order orientation	Right behavior is obeying the law and following the rules.	A nurse does not permit a worried client to phone home because hospital rules stipulate no phone calls after 9:00 PM.
Level III *Postconventional*		
Stage 5: Social contract, legalistic orientation	Standard of behavior is based on adhering to laws that protect the welfare and rights of others. Personal values and opinions are recognized, and violating the rights of others is avoided.	A nurse arranges for an East Indian client to have privacy for prayer each evening.
Stage 6: Universal-ethical principles	Universal moral principles are internalized. Person respects other humans and believes that relationships are based on mutual trust.	A nurse becomes an advocate for a hospitalized client by reporting to the nursing supervisor a conversation in which a physician threatened to withhold assistance unless the client agreed to surgery.

Source: Adapted from R Duska and M Whelan, *Moral Development: A Guide to Piaget and Kohlberg.* Copyright © 1975 by The Missionary Society of St Paul the Apostle in the State of New York. Used by permission of Paulist Press.

own needs, because if those needs are not met, other people may also suffer.

Gilligan believes women see morality in the integrity of relationships and caring, so that the moral problems they encounter are different from those of men. Men consider what is right to be what is just, whereas for women what is right is taking responsibility for others as a self-chosen decision (Gilligan 1982, p. 140).

Gilligan feels that a blend of perspectives is necessary for a person to reach maturity. The ethic of justice, or fairness, is based on the idea of equality: that everyone should receive the same treatment. This is the development path usually followed by men. It is widely accepted by the theorists in the field. By contrast, the ethic of care is based on a premise of nonviolence: that no one should be harmed. This is the path typically followed by women. It is an approach that has been given very little attention in the literature.

In the development of maturity, according to Gilligan, both viewpoints blend "in the realization that just as inequality adversely affects both perspectives in an unequal relationship, so too violence is destructive for everyone involved" (Gilligan 1982, p. 174). The blending of these two perspectives could give rise to a new view of human development and a better understanding of human relations.

SPIRITUAL THEORIES

Fowler The spiritual component of growth and development refers to individuals' understanding of their relationship with the universe and their perceptions about the direction and meaning of life. James Fowler describes the development of faith. Fowler believes that faith, or the spiritual dimension, is a force that gives meaning to a person's life. Fowler uses the term *faith* as a form of knowing, a way of being in relation to "an ultimate environment." To Fowler, **faith** is a relational phenomenon; it is "an active 'mode-of-being-in-relation' to another or others in which we invest commitment, belief, love, risk and hope" (Fowler & Keen 1985). Fowler's stages in the development of faith are given in Table 16–2, page 314.

Fowler's theory and developmental stages were influenced by the work of Piaget, Kohlberg, and Erikson. Fowler believes that the development of faith is an interactive process between the person and the environment. In each of Fowler's stages, new patterns of thought, values, and beliefs are added to those already held by the individual; therefore the stages must follow in sequence. Faith stages, according to Fowler, are separate from cognitive stages of Piaget. Faith stages evolve from a combination of knowledge and values.

Westerhoff John Westerhoff has developed a four-stage theory of faith development based largely on his own life experiences and the interpretation of those experiences (see Table 16–3, p. 314). Westerhoff proposes that faith is a way of behaving.

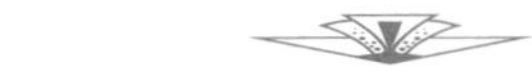

APPLYING GROWTH AND DEVELOPMENT CONCEPTS TO NURSING PRACTICE

Different theories explain one or more aspects of an individual's growth and development. Typically, theorists examine only one aspect of an individual's development, such as the cognitive, moral, or physical aspects. The area chosen for examination usually reflects the researcher's academic discipline and personal interest. The theorists may also limit the population that is studied to a particular part of the life span, such as infancy, childhood, or adulthood.

Although such theories can be useful, they also have limitations. First, the theory chosen may explain only one aspect of the growth and development process. Yet, a person does not develop in fragmented sections, but rather as a whole human being. Thus, the nurse may find it necessary to apply several theories for an adequate understanding of the growth and development of a client.

Another limitation of some theories is the suggestion that certain tasks are performed at a specific age. In most cases, the child or adult does accomplish the task at the time specified by the guidelines. In other cases, however, the nurse may find that an individual does not accomplish the task or meet the milestone at the exact time suggested by the theory. Such individual differences are not easily defined or categorized by a single theory. Human development is a complex synthesis of physiologic, cognitive, psychologic, moral, and spiritual development. Nurses should expect individual variations and take these into consideration when applying these theories about growth and development. In so doing, they will be better able to understand a client's development and plan effective nursing interventions.

In nursing, developmental theories can be useful in guiding assessment, explaining behavior, and providing a direction for nursing interventions. An understanding of a child's intellectual ability helps a nurse to anticipate and explain certain reactions, responses, and needs. Nurses can then encourage client behavior that is appropriate for that particular developmental stage.

Theories are also useful in planning a nursing intervention. For instance, choosing the appropriate toy for a 3-year-old boy requires some knowledge of the physical and cognitive development of the child, as well as a sensitivity for individual preferences.

In adult care, knowledge about the physical, cognitive, and psychologic aspects of the aging process is a fundamental aspect of administering sensitive nursing care. For example, nurses can use their familiarity with the theories of development to help clients understand and anticipate the psychosocial changes that take place after retirement or the physical limitations that come with old age.

CHAPTER HIGHLIGHTS

- Growth and development are independent, interrelated processes.
- Growth is physical change and increase in size. The pattern of physiologic growth is similar for all people.
- Development is an increase in the complexity of function and skill progression.
- The rate of a person's growth and development is highly individual, but the sequence of growth and development is predictable.
- Heredity and environment are the primary factors influencing growth and development.
- Components of growth and development are generally categorized as physiologic, psychosocial, cognitive, moral, and spiritual.

- There are several theories about the various stages and aspects of growth and development, particularly in regard to infant and child development. Theories and models about adult development are more recent.
- Each developmental stage has its own characteristics and unique problems.
- A progression of sequential steps or tasks is proposed in most theories, so that successful achievement of tasks is required in early stages before success can be achieved with later tasks.
- The nurse's major role in relation to growth and development is to assess the client's growth and development using the standards proposed in these theories, to identify and report any problem areas, and to plan and implement nursing strategies that will maintain or promote the client's development.

READINGS AND REFERENCES

SUGGESTED READINGS

Kelleher, K. April/June 1992. The afternoon of life: Jung's view of the tasks of the second half of life. *Perspectives in Psychiatric Care* 28:25–28.

Kelleher writes that Carl Jung believed middle and old age have specific developmental tasks. For the mature individual the goal is to consolidate a personality by integrating the conscious and unconscious parts of self. The article reviews relevant literature and describes Jung's quest for self.

Trocchio, J. March/April 1989. Life as a bell-shaped curve. *Geriatric Nursing* 10:71.

This brief article outlines some parallels between aging and child development. The author suggests that applying some of the principles of child care to care of the elderly may create positive results.

RELATED RESEARCH

Cantanzaro, M. May 1990. Transitions in midlife adults with long-term illness. *Holistic Nursing Practice* 4:65–73.

Gillis, AJ. April 1990. Nurses' knowledge of growth and development principles in meeting psychosocial needs of hospitalized children. *Journal of Pediatric Nursing* 5:78–87.

SELECTED REFERENCES

Berkowitz, MW and Oser, F, editors. 1985. *Moral Education: Theory and Application.* Hillsdale, NJ: Lawrence Erlbaum.

Erikson, EH. 1963. *Childhood and Society.* 2d ed. New York: Norton.

———. 1964. *Insight and Responsibility: Lectures on the Ethical Implications of Psychoanalytic Insight.* New York: Norton.

———. 1985. *The Life Cycle Completed: A Review.* New York: Norton.

Fowler, JW. 1981. *Stages of Faith: The Psychology of Human Development and the Quest for Meaning.* New York: Harper and Row.

Fowler, J and Keen, S. 1978 and 1985. *Life Maps: Conversations in the Journey of Faith.* Waco, TX: Word Books.

Freud, S. 1961. *The Ego and the Id and Other Works* Vol. 19. Strachey, J, translator. London: Hogarth Press and the Institute of Psychoanalysis.

Gilligan, C. 1982. *In a Different Voice: Psychological Theory and Women's Development.* Cambridge, MA: Harvard University Press.

Gould, RL. November 1972. The phases of adult life: A study in developmental psychology. *American Journal of Psychiatry* 129:33–43.

Havighurst, RJ. 1972. *Developmental Tasks and Education.* 3d ed. New York: David McKay.

Kegan, R. 1982. *The Evolving Self: Problem and Process in Human Development.* Cambridge, MA: Harvard University Press.

Mott, S, James, S, and Sperhac, A. 1990. *Nursing Care of Children and Families.* 2d ed. Redwood City, CA: Addison-Wesley Nursing.

Munhall, PL. June 1982. Moral development: A prerequisite. *Journal of Nursing Education* 21:11–15.

Peck, R. 1968. Psychological developments in the second half of life. In Neugarten, BL, editor. *Middle Age and Aging.* Chicago: University of Chicago Press.

Piaget, J. 1966. *Origins of Intelligence in Children.* New York: Norton.

Westerhoff, J. 1976. *Will Our Children Have Faith?* New York: Seabury Press.

24 Infancy Through Late Childhood

Objectives

- Identify tasks characteristic of different stages of development during infancy and childhood.
- Describe usual physical development throughout infancy and childhood.
- Trace psychosocial development according to Erikson through infancy and childhood.
- Explain changes in cognitive development according to Piaget throughout infancy and childhood.
- Describe moral development according to Kohlberg throughout childhood.
- Describe spiritual development according to Fowler throughout childhood.
- Identify assessment activities and expected characteristics from birth through late childhood.
- Identify nursing diagnoses for health promotion from birth through late childhood.
- List examples of health promotion goals from birth through late childhood.
- Identify essential health promotion and protection activities to meet the needs of infants, toddlers, preschoolers, and school-age children.

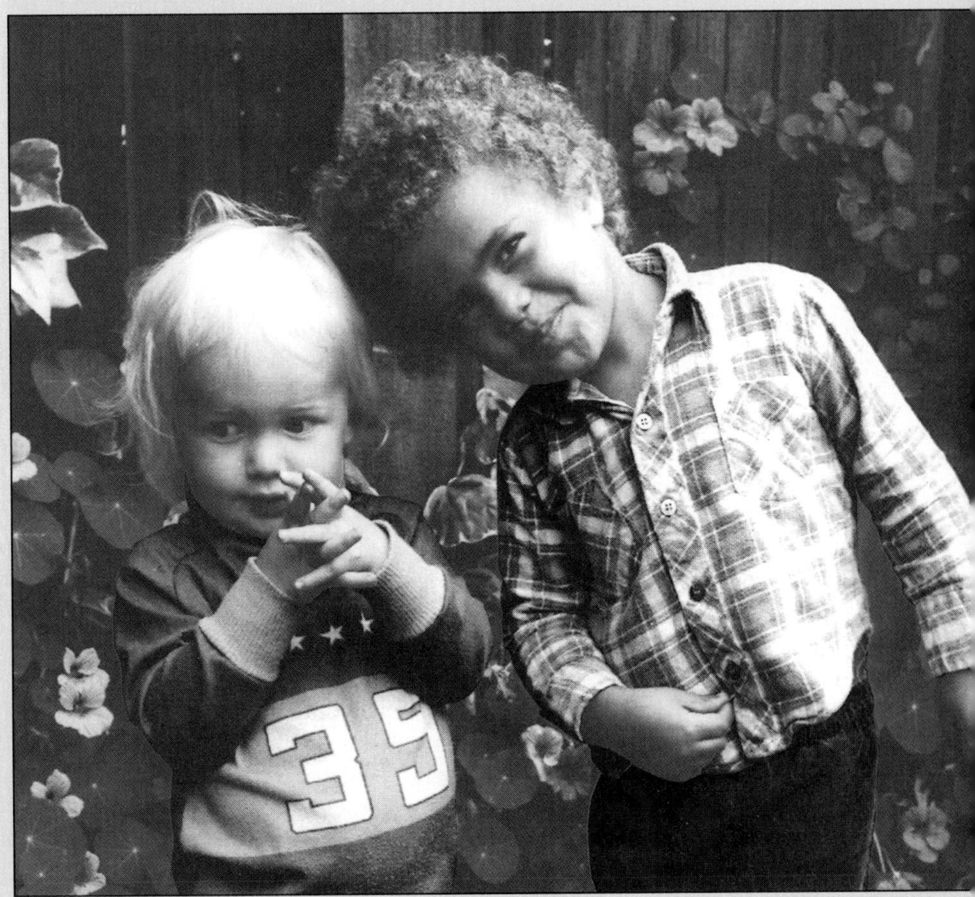

A knowledge of growth and development is essential for nurses if they are to identify developmental and health needs. This chapter applies the concepts of growth and development introduced in Chapter 23 to the infant, toddler, preschooler, and school-age child. Each developmental stage includes physical, psychosocial, cognitive, moral, and spiritual aspects. Health assessment and promotion of health and wellness are emphasized.

Infants (Birth to 1 Year)

Physiologic Growth and Development

An infant's basic task is survival, which requires breathing, sleeping, sucking, eating, swallowing, digesting, and eliminating. Because many of the infant's activities and pleasures are mouth-centered, this stage in development is often referred to as Freud's *oral* stage (see Chapter 23, page 570). Infants undergo significant physiologic change in these areas: weight, length, head growth, vision, and motor development.

Weight At birth, most babies weigh from 2.7 to 3.8 kg (6.0 to 8.5 lb); European-American infants tend to weigh more than infants of other races. Just after birth, most infants lose 5% to 10% of their birth weight because of fluid loss. This weight loss is normal, and infants usually regain that weight in about 1 week. After several days, babies usually gain weight at the rate of 5 to 7 ounces weekly for 6 months. By 5 months of age, infants usually reach twice their birth weight, and by age 12 months, three times their birth weight (Pinyerd 1992, p. 302).

Length The average length of a European-American newborn in the United States is about 50 cm (20 in). At birth, African-American infants tend to be shorter, ranging from 47.5 to 52.5 cm (19 to 21 in). Female babies are on the average smaller than male babies.

Two recumbent lengths are the crown-to-rump length (the sitting length) and the head-to-heel length (from the top of the head to the base of the heels). See Figure 24–1. Normally the crown-to-rump length is approximately the same as the head circumference. By 6 months, infants gain another 13.75 cm (5.5 in) of height. By 12 months, they add another 7.5 cm (3 in). Rate of increase in height is largely influenced by the baby's size at birth and by nutrition.

Head and Chest Circumference Assessment of head circumference is of particular importance in infants and children to determine the growth rate of the skull and the brain. An infant's head should be measured at every visit to the physician or nurse until the child is 2 years (Figure 24–2). Normal head circumference (**normocephaly**) is often related to chest circumference. At birth, the average infant's head circumference is 35 cm (14 in) and generally varies only 1 or 2 cm (0.5 in). The chest circumference of the newborn is usually less than the head circumference by about 2.5 cm (1 in). As the infant grows the chest circumference becomes larger than the head circumference. At about 9 or 10 months, the head and chest circumferences are about the same, and after 1 year of age the chest circumference is larger.

Head Molding The heads of most newborn babies are misshappen because of the molding of the head that occurs during vaginal deliveries. Molding of the head is made possible by **fontanelles** (unossified membranous gaps) in the bone structure of the skull and by overriding of the **sutures** (junction lines of the skull bones). Within a week, a newborn's head usually regains its symmetry, a fact that reassures parents. The larger anterior fontanelle (4 to 6 cm in diameter and diamond-shaped) can increase in size for several months after birth. After 6 months, the size gradually decreases until closure occurs between 9 and 18 months. The posterior fontanelle between the parietal bones and the occipital bone closes from 4 to 8 weeks after birth (Figure 24–3).

Vision The newborn can follow large moving objects and blinks in response to bright light and to sound. The pupils of the newborn respond slowly, and the eyes cannot focus on close objects. At 4 months, the infant can recognize familiar objects and follow moving ones. By 6 months, the infant can perceive colors. After 9 months, most can recognize facial characteristics and often smile in response to a familiar face. By 12 months, depth perception has developed, and the infant will be able to recognize where a change in level occurs, such as at the edge of the bed.

Hearing Newborns with intact hearing will react with a startle to a loud noise, referred to as the Moro reflex (see the discussion of reflexes, below). Within a few days, they are able to distinguish different sounds. For example, they can tell the difference between their mother's voice and

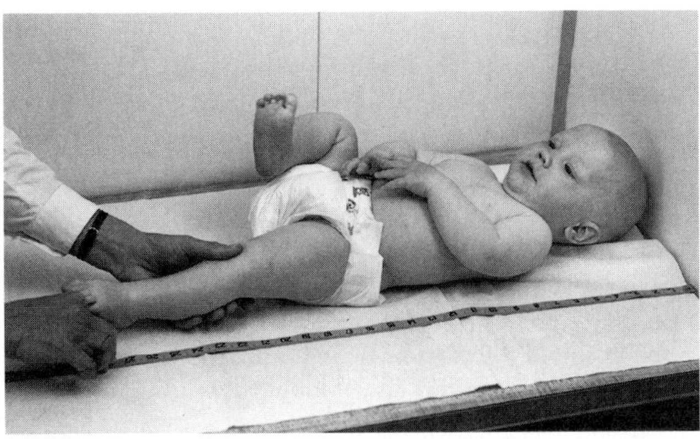

Figure 24–1 Measuring an infant, head to heel.

that of another woman (Mott et al 1990, p. 177). At about 5 months of age, the infant will pause while sucking in order to listen to the mother's voice. A 9-month-old infant is able to locate the source of sounds and recognizes familiar ones. By 1 year, the infant listens to sounds, begins to distinguish words, and responds to simple commands.

Smell and Taste The senses of smell and taste are functional shortly after birth. Newborns prefer sweet tastes and tend to decrease their sucking in response to liquids with a salty content. They are able to recognize the smell of their mother's milk and respond to this smell by turning toward the mother.

Touch The sense of touch is well developed at birth. Skin-to-skin touching is important for an infant's development. The infant responds positively to the warmth, love, and security it perceives when touched, held, and cuddled. The newborn is also sensitive to temperature extremes and pain; however, babies react diffusely and cannot isolate the discomfort. The pain of an open safety pin in the buttock, for example, is not isolated in the buttock.

Reflexes The reflexes of the newborn are unconscious, involuntary responses. They are neither learned nor consciously carried out; rather, they are nervous system responses to a number of stimuli. Reflexes normally present at birth are the rooting, sucking, Moro, palmar grasp, plantar, tonic neck, stepping, and Babinski reflexes. See the box on page 584. Infant reflexes disappear during the first year of life. In addition, the abilities to yawn, stretch, sneeze, burp, and hiccup are all present at birth.

Motor Development Motor development is the development of the baby's ability to move and to control the body. Initially, body movement is uncoordinated. At 1 month of age, the infant lifts the head momentarily when prone, turns the head when prone, and has a head lag

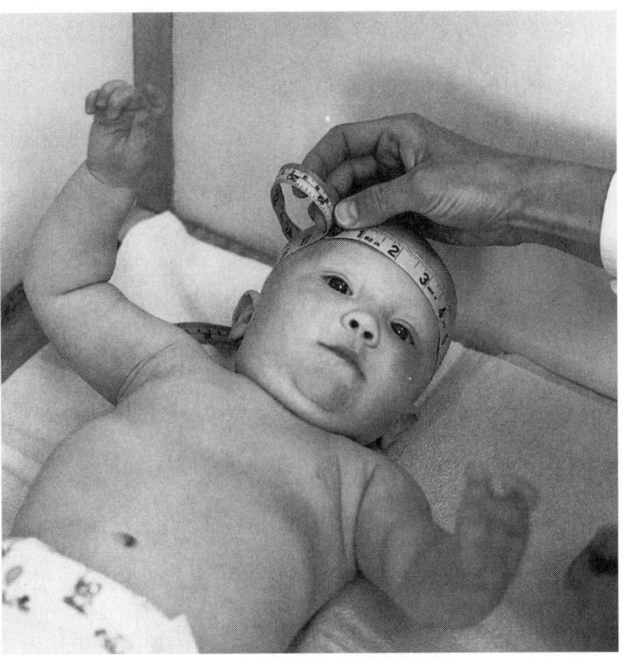

Figure 24–2 An infant's head circumference is measured around the skull, above the eyebrows.

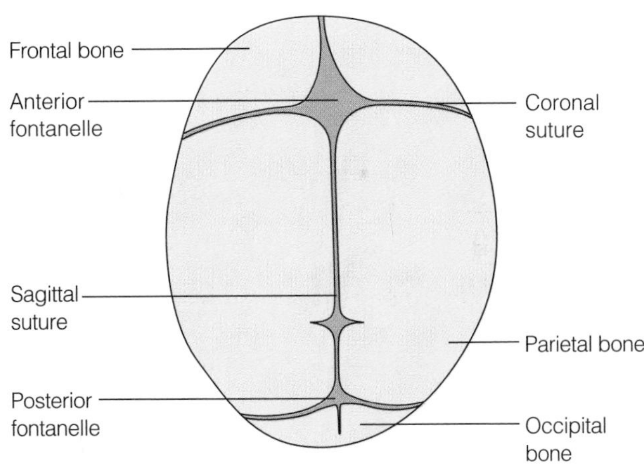

Figure 24–3 The bones of the skull, showing the fontanelles and the suture lines.

when pulled to a sitting position. By 2 months, infants can raise their heads from a prone position. After 6 months, they can sit without support (Figure 24–4, p. 584). At 9 months, they can reach, grasp a rattle, and transfer it from hand to hand. At 12 months, they can turn the pages of a book, put objects into a container, walk with some assistance, and help to dress themselves. See Table 24–1 on page 585 for details about motor development.

INFANT REFLEXES

- *Sucking reflex.* A feeding reflex that occurs when the infant's lips are touched. The reflex persists throughout infancy.
- *Rooting reflex.* A feeding reflex elicited by touching the baby's cheek, causing the baby's head to turn to the side that was touched. This reflex usually disappears after 4 months.
- *Moro reflex.* Often assessed to estimate the maturity of the central nervous system. A loud noise, a sudden change in position, or an abrupt jarring of the crib elicits this reflex. The infant reacts by extending both arms and legs outward with the fingers spread, then suddenly retracting the limbs. Often the infant cries at the same time. This reflex disappears after 4 months.
- *Palmar grasp reflex.* Occurs when a small object is placed against the palm of the hand, causing the fingers to curl around it. This reflex disappears after 3 months.
- *Plantar reflex.* Similar to the palmar grasp reflex; an object placed just beneath the toes causes them to curl around it. This reflex disappears after 8 months.
- *Tonic neck reflex (TNR) or fencing reflex.* A postural reflex. When a baby who is lying on its back turns the head to the right side, for example, the left side of the body shows a flexing of the left arm and the left leg. This reflex disappears after 4 months.
- *Stepping reflex (walking or dancing reflex).* Can be elicited by holding the baby upright so that the feet touch a flat surface. The legs then move up and down as if the baby were walking. This reflex usually disappears at about 2 months.
- *Babinski reflex.* When the sole of the foot is stroked, the big toe rises and the other toes fan out. A newborn baby has a positive Babinski. After age 1, the infant exhibits a negative Babinski; that is, the toes curl downward. A positive Babinski after age 1 indicates brain damage.

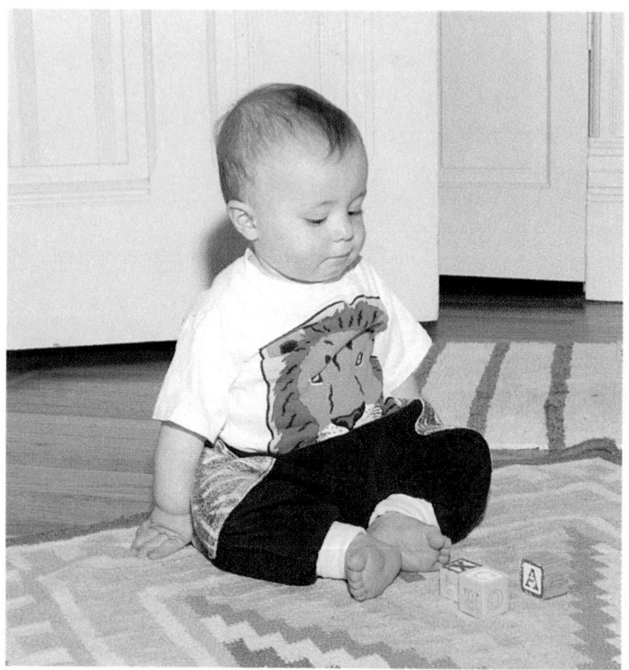

Figure 24–4 An infant sits without support at 6 months of age.

PSYCHOSOCIAL DEVELOPMENT

According to Erikson, the central crisis at this stage is *trust versus mistrust.* See Table 23–4 on page 574. Resolution of this stage determines how the person approaches subsequent developmental stages. During the first year of life, infants depend on the parents for all their physiologic and psychologic needs. Fulfillment of these needs is required for the infant to develop a basic sense of trust. Parents can enhance this sense of trust by (a) responding consistently to an infant's needs, (b) providing a predictable environment in which routines are established, and (c) being sensitive to the infant's needs and meeting these needs skillfully and promptly. Mothering behavior, such as consistent care, handling, stroking, and cuddling, is essential for healthy psychosocial development. By 8 months, most infants seem to be attached to their parents and may show displeasure when left with strangers.

The newborn reacts socially to caregivers by paying attention to the face or voice and by cuddling when held. It is able to interact with the environment by responding to various stimuli such as touch and sound. See Table 24–1 for details about social development.

Infants have no understanding of waiting and no time frame by which to measure waiting. The initial reaction of an infant to stress is crying, and crying is the infant's way of communicating stress. Infants learn gradually to tolerate stress. According to Freud, infants have an oral

Table 24–1 Motor and Social Development in Infancy

Age	Motor Development	Social Development
Newborn	Turns head from side to side when in a prone position Grasps by reflex when object is placed in palm of hand	Displays displeasure by crying and satisfaction by soft vocalizations Attends to adult face and voice by eye contact and quieting
2 months	Lifts head 45 degrees when prone Follows moving and bright objects to midline with eyes	Displays a social smile Smiles and vocalizes to a familiar voice
3 months	Actively holds object in hand Raises head and shoulders 45 to 90 degrees when in prone position	Coos and babbles Laughs aloud
4 months	Holds head steady while in sitting position Rolls over Grasps objects with both hands	Squeals Enjoys social interactions; vocalizes displeasure when left alone
5 months	Sits for longer periods when back is supported Actively grasps an object, taking it to mouth	Discriminates between strangers and family Vocalizes displeasure when desired object is removed
6 months	Lifts chest and shoulders off table when prone, bearing weight on hands Manipulates small objects	Starts to imitate sounds Vocalizes one syllable sounds: "ma ma," "da da"
7 months	Sits alone without support Bears weight on legs when held in a standing position Transfers objects from hand	Shows fear of strangers Imitates simple acts and sounds Plays "peekaboo"
8 months	Reaches for toys out of reach Feeds self with fingers Stands holding on	Reaches with open arms to be picked up Responds to the word "no"; cries when scolded Bashful and nervous with strangers
9 months	Creeps and crawls Beginner pincer grasp with thumb and forefinger Pulls self to standing position	Complies with simple verbal commands Displays fear of being left alone (eg, going to bed) Waves "bye-bye"
10 months	Stands holding on to support; sits by falling Pulls self to sitting position	Looks under an object for toy Aware of own name
11 months	Stands alone momentarily Walks while holding onto furniture Neat pincer grasp with thumb and index finger	Reacts with frustration when restricted Plays interactive games using body gestures Shakes head for "no"
12 months	Walks alone with help Uses spoon to feed self	Clings to mother in unfamiliar situations Demonstrates emotions such as anger and affection

focus, and they reduce tension by sucking and mouthing objects. Nurses and parents can also reduce the stress of an infant by maintaining the infant's routine as much as possible and limiting the number of strangers interacting with the infant.

Infants deprived of mothering, especially from months 3 to 15, will not learn to form significant relationships or to trust others. Infants who fail to establish a loving, responsive relationship with a caregiver often fail to develop normally. The disturbed parent-child relationship can result in the **failure-to-thrive syndrome.** Infants with this condition show delayed development without any physical cause. They are often malnourished and fail to gain weight and grow normally.

COGNITIVE DEVELOPMENT

According to Piaget, cognitive development is a result of interaction between an individual and the environment. Piaget refers to the initial period of cognitive development as the *sensorimotor* phase. See Table 23–5 on page 576. This phase has six stages, three of which take place during the first year. From 4 to 8 months, infants begin to have perceptual recognition. By 6 months, they respond to new stimuli, and they remember certain objects and look for them for a short time. By 12 months, infants have a concept of both space and time. They experiment to reach a goal, such as a toy on a chair.

An infant's cognitive development also proceeds from reflexive ability of the newborn to using one or two actions to attain a goal by the age of 1 year.

MORAL DEVELOPMENT

Infants associate right and wrong with pleasure and pain. What gives them pleasure is right, since they are too young to reason otherwise. When infants receive abundant positive responses from the parent such as smiles, caresses, and voice tones of approval in these early months, they learn that certain behaviors are wrong or good and that pain or pleasure is the consequence. In later months and years, children can tell easily and quickly by changes in parental facial expressions and voice tones that their behavior is either approved or disapproved.

HEALTH ASSESSMENT

Apgar Scoring Newborn babies can be assessed immediately by the **Apgar scoring system.** This provides a numeric indicator of the baby's physiologic capacities to adapt to extrauterine life. Each of five signs is assigned a maximum score of 2, so that the total score achievable is 10. A score under 7 suggests that the baby is having difficulty, and a score under 4 indicates that the baby's condition is critical. Apgar scoring is usually carried out 60 seconds after birth and is repeated in 5 minutes. Those with very low scores require special resuscitative measures and care. See Table 24–2.

Developmental Screening Tests Development can be assessed by observing the infant's behavior and by using standardized tests such as the **Denver Developmental Screening Test (DDST).** The DDST is used to screen children from birth to 6 years of age. The test is intended to estimate the abilities of a child compared to those of an average group of children of the same age and ethnic group (Wade 1992, p. 141). The DDST does not provide diagnostic information about a child's problem, does not predict how a child will develop, and should not be used to assign a child to a developmental age group. Four main areas of development are screened: *personal-social*, *fine motor adaptive*, *language*, and *gross motor.*

There are many other screening tests, for example, the Brazelton Neonatal Behavioral Assessment Scale, which focuses on neonatal behavior, and the Washington Guide to Promoting Development in Young Children. Detailed information about these tests is provided in maternal-child and pediatric textbooks.

Ongoing Nursing Assessments During ongoing assessments, the nurse examines and observes the infant, taking into account variations that occur with develop-

ASSESSMENT GUIDELINES

The Infant

In the following developmental areas, does the infant

Physical Development

- Demonstrate physical growth (weight, length, head and chest circumference) within normal range?
- Manifest appropriately sized fontanelles for age?
- Exhibit vital signs within normal range for age?

Motor Development

- Perform gross and fine motor milestones within the normal range for age?
- Exhibit reflexes appropriate for age?

Sensory Development

- Follow a moving object within normal range for age?
- Respond to sounds, such as talking or clapping hands?

Psychosocial Development

- Interact appropriately with parent through body movements and vocalizations?

Development in Activities of Daily Living

- Eat and drink appropriate amounts of breast milk, formula, and/or solid foods?
- Exhibit an elimination pattern within normal range for age?
- Exhibit a rest and sleep pattern appropriate for age?

Table 24–2 Apgar Scoring System to Assess the Newborn

	Score		
Sign	**0**	**1**	**2**
1. Heart rate	Absent	Slow (below 100 per minute)	Above 100 per minute
2. Respirations	Absent	Slow, irregular	Regular rate, crying
3. Muscle tone	Flaccid	Some flexion of extremities	Active movements
4. Reflex irritability	None	Grimace	Cries
5. Color	Body pale or cyanotic	Body pink (for African-American babies, pink mucous membranes), extremities blue	Body completely pink, pink mucous membranes in African-American babies

mental age and activity. For example, the pulse of the baby at birth is affected by the child's activity, rising up to 170 when the infant is crying and falling to as low as 70 during sleep. (See Chapter 21 for normal pulse values.)

In addition, the nurse actively listens to the parent for possible problems or areas of concern, and reviews with the parent the expected behavior or characteristics for the particular age group. This is an opportunity to allow the parent to discuss observations of the infant with the nurse. It is important for the parent to know that certain behaviors, responses, and activities of the infant are normal and expected. It is also important to discuss the many individual differences that can, quite normally, occur. The new parent needs to be given valid and accurate information to avoid undue concern with advice and comparisons from well-meaning friends.

The assessment interview is also a time to be supportive of the parent's role, to assess the attachment of the mother to the infant, and to observe the interactions between the infant and parent. Assessment guidelines for growth and development of the infant are shown in the box on page 586. Examples of NANDA nursing diagnoses, goals/outcome criteria, and nursing interventions for the infant are shown in Table 24–3.

To give adequate care to the infant, the parent or caregiver needs teaching, support, and guidance from the

Table 24–3 Examples of Nursing Diagnoses and Goals for the Infant

NANDA Diagnosis	Goal/Outcome Criteria	Interventions
Health-seeking behaviors (parental) related to the physical care of an infant	Parents will demonstrate within 1 month the ability to provide a healthy environment for infant, as evidenced by ▪ Verbalizing appropriate safety measures, skin care, toys, and nutrition. ▪ Stating the signs and symptoms of illness. ▪ Seeking protective measures, such as immunizations.	Provide parents with written and verbal guidance on basic infant care and immunizations. Schedule parents for an infant care class. Assess parental knowledge through written, verbal and/or observational feedback techniques.
Altered parenting related to parent's inability to meet infant's psychosocial needs (failure-to-thrive infant)	Parents will demonstrate within 2 weeks effective parenting skills, as evidenced by ▪ Appropriately meeting infant's oral needs (sucking, pacifier). ▪ Providing appropriate and consistent caregiving activities. ▪ Demonstration of appropriate stimulation activities.	Provide educational materials on infant growth and development. Demonstrate appropriate parenting behaviors (eg, role modeling). Refer parents to a support system (eg, parenting support group, community nursing).

nurse. The nurse may wish to discuss the following topics with the parents and also provide appropriate reading materials and references.

PROMOTING HEALTH AND WELLNESS

Protective Measures Newborns have very little resistance to infection. For this reason, parents and caregivers should be instructed to wash their hands before handling the newborn and to avoid contact with the infant if they have a cold or skin infection. In some cases, it is possible for gonorrhea organisms to be transmitted to an infant during its passage through an infected vaginal canal. Two protective measures usually carried out immediately after birth are the use of antibiotics or the placement of 2 drops of 1% silver nitrate solution into each eye to protect against the gonorrhea organisms, and the administration of Vitamin K to protect the infant against trauma. Vitamin K, which is necessary for clotting, is not produced by intestinal bacteria for several days. In the female infant, the vaginal area is protected by a thin, bluish-white mucous coating known as **smegma.** This mucous substance protects the vaginal area from fungal and bacterial infections.

Immunization against communicable diseases is a preventive health measure advocated by government agencies in the United States and Canada.

Newborn infants have limited ability to produce antibodies until they are about 3 months of age. However, during the last months of pregnancy, certain maternal antibodies pass through the placenta, thus providing the baby with some passive immunity. This immunity is temporary; it is therefore vital to practice good hygiene around infants, sterilize their formulas, and not expose them to infected people.

At 2 to 3 months of age, children should receive their first immunizations. Antigens in the form of **vaccines** (living or dead microorganisms) or **toxoids** (detoxified toxins) are administered to induce active immunity. Immunizations are needed to protect infants from the microorganisms causing diphtheria, pertussis, tetanus, poliomyelitis, measles, mumps, rubella, hepatitis B, and various infections resulting from the *Haemophilus influenzae* type B microorganism.

At age 1 year, a tuberculin test is done to determine whether the child has been exposed to the tuberculosis bacillus.

Diphtheria-pertussis-tetanus toxoid (DPT) vaccine is usually given at approximately 2, 4, and 6 months in the United States and Canada. Infants receive oral poliomyelitis vaccine at 2 and 4 months.

Measles-mumps-rubella (MMR) vaccine is usually given at 15 months of age in the United States to increase the effectiveness of antibody response; however, those infants at risk for exposure to these diseases may receive the vaccine at 1 year of age or earlier.

Haemophilus influenzae type B (Hib) is a bacterial infection that most commonly occurs in children under the age of 5 years. It is the major cause of bacterial meningitis (an infection of the covering of the brain) in this age group. Several preparations of Hib vaccine are available to prevent meningitis and other life-threatening infections in infants. These vaccines utilize different immunization schedules of 3 or 4 injections beginning at 2 months of age.

Hepatitis B is the most recently developed vaccine recommended for infants. Hepatitis B is a virus communicated by blood and blood products of infected individuals. Infection can lead to serious or fatal liver disease. The infant immunization schedule consists of a series of 3 injections beginning within the first 2 months of life (Peter 1992, p. 1797).

The risks of immunization include potential side effects and complications, contamination of the serum with microorganisms other than the desired antigens, worsening of a natural disease, failure to protect against the disease and, rarely, death. Nurses who administer immunizations must be knowledgeable about the indications, storage, dosage, preparation, and contraindications for each of the vaccines to be administered.

Health Maintenance Visits Infants should have preventive health care visits 2 weeks after birth and at 2, 4, 6, 9, and 12 months of age. These health maintenance visits are necessary for health promotion activities (eg, maintaining proper diet), health protection activities (eg, obtaining immunizations), and for early detection of problems (eg, screening for tuberculosis).

Safety Accident prevention planning is essential. Although infants are completely dependent on others for care, they soon learn to roll from side to side, put objects in their mouths, and crawl. They are oblivious to such dangers as falling or ingesting harmful substances. Accidents are the sixth leading cause of death during infancy and one of the major causes of death after the first year of life. Parents should be advised that infants need to be watched constantly.

Parents may need help in identifying potential hazards in and around the home and should be encouraged to remove any of the dangers in anticipation of the infant's development. The nurse should encourage parents to enroll in a first-aid course that includes cardiopulmonary resuscitation, interventions for airway obstruction, and the identification of common household hazards. Such education can make the parents more knowledgeable and better prepared to protect their children from accidents and injuries. Common accidents during infancy include burns, suffocation, automobile accidents, falls, poisoning, and choking. Safety measures for infants are highlighted in the box at the right.

Skin Care Sponge baths are suggested for the newborn, because daily tub baths are not considered necessary. After the bath, the infant should be immediately dried and wrapped. Parents need to be advised that the infant's ability to regulate body temperature has not yet fully developed. Infants perspire minimally, and shivering starts at a lower temperature than it does in adults; therefore, infants lose more heat before shivering begins. In addition, because the infant's body surface area is very large in relation to body mass, the body loses heat readily. Therefore, the infant should be dressed appropriately and covered with a blanket. A draft-free room with temperatures between 20.0 C and 24.4 C (60–76 F) is recommended.

Parents and caregivers must also be aware that infants can be dressed too warmly. **Miliaria rubra** (prickly heat) is a common skin problem that occurs on hot, humid days and is caused by blocked sweat glands. Prickly heat can be prevented by keeping the infant cool and dry. To reverse the rash, the caregiver can remove excess clothing, give a tepid sponge bath, or move the infant to a cooler environment.

SAFETY HIGHLIGHTS FOR NEWBORNS AND INFANTS

- Use federally approved car seat at all times (including coming home from hospital).
- Never leave infant unattended on a raised surface.
- Check temperature of infant's bath water and formula prior to using.
- Hold infant upright during feeding. Do not prop bottle. Cut food in small pieces, and do not feed peanuts or popcorn.
- Investigate infant's crib for compliance to federal safety regulations: slats no more than 2⅜ inches apart, lead-free paint, height of crib sides, tight fit of mattress to crib.
- Use a playpen with sides made of small sized netting. Never leave playpen sides in down position.
- Provide large soft toys with no small detachable or sharp-edged parts.
- Use guard rails on stairs and screens on windows. Supervise infant in walker, swing, and highchair.
- Cover electrical outlets. Coil cords out of reach.
- Place plants, household cleaners, and wastebaskets out of reach. Lock away potential poisons, such as medicines, paint, and gasoline.

Nutrition The neonate's fluid and nutritional needs are met by breast milk or formula. Fluid needs of infants are proportionately greater than those of adults because of a higher metabolic rate, immature kidneys, and greater water losses through the skin and the lungs. The last is largely due to rapid respirations. Therefore, fluid balance is a critical factor. Under normal environmental conditions, infants do not need additional water; however, neonates in very warm environments may require additional fluids. In these cases, water may be prescribed.

The total daily nutritional requirement of the newborn is about 80 to 100 mL of breast milk or formula per kilogram of body weight. The newborn infant's stomach capacity is about 90 mL, and feedings are required every 2½ to 4 hours (Snow & Fry 1990, p. 443).

The newborn infant is usually fed "on demand." **Demand feeding** usually means that the child is fed when hungry. This method tends to decrease the problem of overfeeding or underfeeding the infant. The newborn who is hungry usually cries and exhibits tension in the entire body. During feeding, the infant sucks readily and needs burping after each ounce of formula or after 5 minutes of breast feeding. Burping is done by holding the infant in an upright position while gently patting the back.  *Parents should be warned that infant bottles should never be propped up for feeding.* There is a real danger that aspiration or choking could result.

Infants demonstrate satisfaction by slowing their sucking activity or by falling asleep. Once satisfaction has been demonstrated, infants should not be coaxed into finishing the feeding. This could lead to discomfort or overfeeding. When feeding is completed, healthy infants can be placed in a lateral or supine position for sleep during the first 6 months of life to reduce the risk of sudden infant death syndrome, or SIDS (Kattwinkel et al 1992, p. 1120).

Regurgitation, or spitting up, of predigested milk during or after a feeding is a common occurrence during the first year. Although this may be of concern to parents, it does not usually result in nutritional deficiency. Demonstration of adequate weight gain should reassure parents that the infant is receiving adequate nutrition.

The addition of solid food to the diet usually takes place between 4 and 6 months of age. Six-month-old infants can consume solid food more readily because they can sit up, can hold a spoon, and have a decreased sucking reflex. Solid foods (strained or pureed) are generally introduced in the following order: cereals (rice), fruits, vegetables (yellow before green), and strained meats. Foods are introduced one at a time, usually with only one new food introduced every 5 days. With the eruption of teeth at about 7 to 9 months, the infant is ready to chew and can begin to experience different textures of food. At this time, the infant enjoys finger foods, such as pieces of skinless fruit, dry cereal, or toast.

At about 6 months of age, infants require iron supplementation to prevent iron deficiency anemia. **Iron deficiency anemia** is a form of anemia caused by inadequate supply of iron for synthesis of hemoglobin. Iron-fortified cereals are usually recommended by 6 months of age and are continued until the child reaches 18 months.

Weaning from the breast or bottle to the cup takes place gradually and is usually achieved by age 1. Some infants have difficulty in giving up the bottle, particularly at nap time or bedtime. Parents should be warned that having the bottle in bed can lead to **bottle mouth syndrome.** The term describes the decay of the teeth caused by constant contact with the sweet liquid from the bottle. Some dentists advocate brushing or cleaning the infant's teeth to prevent bottle mouth syndrome, especially for the infant who requires a bottle only at nap or bedtime. Weaning from the bottle can be facilitated by diluting the formula with water increasingly until the infant is drinking plain water. Most infants do not like to drink plain water. By the age of 1, most infants can be completely fed on table food, and milk intake is about 20 ounces per day. See Chapter 37 for additional information on nutrition.

Elimination **Meconium** is the first fecal material passed by the newborn, normally up to 24 hours after birth. It is black, tarry, odorless, and sticky. Transitional stools, which follow for about a week, are generally greenish yellow; they contain mucus and are loose.

Infants pass stool frequently, often after each feeding. Because the intestine is immature, water is not well absorbed, and the stool is soft, liquid, and frequent. When the intestine matures, bacterial flora increase. After solid foods are introduced, the stool becomes less frequent and firmer. Control is not established until the infant's neuromuscular systems are sufficiently developed. Parents need to be informed that diarrhea (very watery stools occuring more than 5 times a day) may lead to dehydration. For infants, particularly those under 6 months old, medical treatment must be sought.

Urine output varies according to fluid intake but usually is about 15 to 60 mL per day after birth, increasing to 250 to 500 mL per day during the first year. An infant may urinate as often as 20 times a day. The urine of the neonate is colorless and odorless and has a specific gravity of 1.008. Because newborns and infants have immature kidneys, they are unable to concentrate urine effectively.

Rest/Sleep Some infants sleep as long as 22 hours a day, others as little as 10 to 12 hours a day. At first, they usually awaken every 3 or 4 hours, eat, and then go back to sleep. Periods of wakefulness gradually increase by the end of the first months. By 4 months, most infants sleep through the night and establish a pattern of daytime naps that varies among individuals. They generally awaken early in the morning, however. At the end of the first year, an infant usually takes one or two naps per day and sleeps about 14 of every 24 hours.

About half of the infant's sleep time is spent in light sleep. During light sleep, the infant exhibits a great deal of activity, such as movement, gurgles, and coughing. Parents need to ascertain that infants are truly awake before picking them up for feeding and changing. Many infants begin waking up again in the middle of the night between 5 and 9 months of age. For parents who find this behavior a problem, the nurse needs to assess the infant's total sleep pattern and compare it with the parents' sleep schedule. Parents need reassurance that there is no correct way to handle this situation. The best solution is one that provides a continuous healthy environment for both the infant and the parents.

Crying Crying is of great concern to parents. When an infant's crying cannot be alleviated, parents often feel a sense of failure and frustration. A crying and fussy period lasting from 1 to 2 hours a day is usually considered normal for most infants. Parents need to be assured that this crying period is considered a source of energy release for the infant and will stop as the infant replaces this activity with more interesting interactions.

An infant who has extended periods of crying, sometimes lasting up to 8 or 10 hours a day, is described as colicky. Often the legs are extended, the body rigid, and the fists clenched. Colic is often associated with abdominal distention or passage of flatus. The cause of true colic is not known. Parents with a colicky infant are often tired and stressed. The nurse should assure them that colic is temporary and that the behavior of the infant is not a result of any inadequacy on their part.

To help relieve the colic, the nurse can assess the infant during feeding and suggest possible changes. Suggestions may include decreasing environmental stimuli during and after feeding, changing the formula or nipple, and increasing the burping frequency. Other suggestions include increasing the water intake, cuddling the infant, and finding the position that provides the infant with the most comfort.

Stimulation Through Play Caregivers can stimulate the newborn by holding, touching, and looking at the infant, providing large, colorful hanging objects over the crib, and talking to the infant in a soothing voice. Infants also like to be rocked and stroked. All of these activities are enjoyable to the infant and promote healthy language, sensory, and cognitive development. Colorful hanging toys, toys that move, and musical toys enhance eye coordination and hearing and motivate the infant to reach and grasp. Play also provides the infant with activity and ex-

HEALTH PROMOTION HIGHLIGHTS FOR INFANTS

Instruct parents about the following:

Health Maintenance Visits

- At 2 weeks and at 2, 4, 6, 9, and 12 months

Protective Measures

- Immunizations: DPT, OPV, measles-mumps-rubella (MMR), *Haemophilus influenzae* type B, and hepatitis B vaccines as recommended
- Screening for tuberculosis
- Prompt attention for illnesses
- Appropriate skin hygiene and clothing

Infant Safety

- Importance of supervision
- Car seat, crib, playpen, bath, and home environment safety measures
- Feeding measures (eg, avoid propping bottle)
- Providing toys with no small parts or sharp edges

Nutrition

- Breast and bottle feeding techniques
- Formula preparation
- Feeding schedule
- Introduction of solid foods
- Need for iron supplements at 4 to 6 months

Elimination

- Characteristics and frequency of stool and urine elimination
- Diarrhea and its effects

Rest/Sleep

- Usual sleep and rest patterns

Sensory Stimulation

- Touch: holding, cuddling, rocking
- Vision: colorful, moving toys
- Hearing: soothing voice tones, music, singing
- Play: toys appropriate for development

ercise. Playing, for the newborn, is moving the arms and legs, kicking, turning the head, and exploring the environment. Activity and exercise are enhanced by interaction from parents and others, including talking, rocking, and singing. Such toys and activities are important stimulation opportunities until about 3 months of age. Later, infants explore objects by handling them and putting them in the mouth. They should have toys that they can grasp *but not swallow,* such as plastic blocks and rings, stuffed animals, rubber or plastic cars, or boats. By age 1, they like toys that pull apart, such as large plastic beads; those with wheels that they can push back and forth, such as a cart or wagon; and those that provide them with a variety of noises, such as musical instruments, bells, and whistles. Parent education should focus on the infant's developmental landmarks and the activities that can promote this development. For example, infants at 4 months need the opportunity to sit on the parent's lap so that they can learn to support their heads when upright. At 5 months, infants begin to roll from back to stomach. Parents can place toys out of reach to encourage this activity. As the infant begins to stand, parents can place an object of appropriate height within the infant's reach.

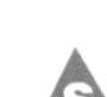

Infants need constant supervision during play and respond well to interaction and encouragement. For the young infant, a playpen provides a safe environment in which to crawl and move around. As the infant grows, a larger area is needed to promote and enhance development. Parental instruction in stimulation and other health-promotion activities during infancy are summarized in the box above.

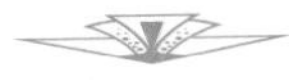

TODDLERS (1 TO 3 YEARS)

Toddlers develop from having no voluntary control to being able both to walk and speak. They also learn to control their bladder and bowels, and they acquire all kinds of information about their environment.

PHYSICAL DEVELOPMENT

Two-year-old children lose the baby look. Toddlers are usually chubby, with relatively short legs and a large head (Figure 24–5, p. 592). The face appears small when compared to the skull; but as the toddler grows, the face seems to grow from under the skull and appears better

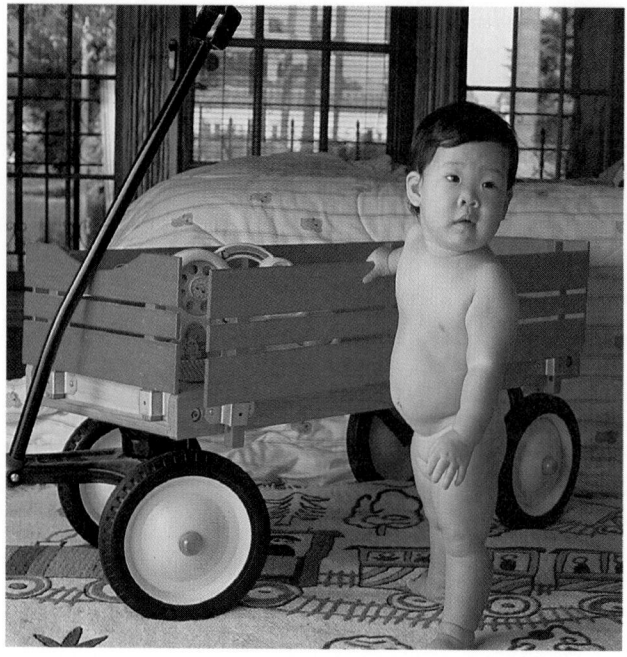

Figure 24–5 The toddler appears chubby with relatively short legs and a large head.

proportioned. Toddlers have a pronounced lumbar lordosis and a protruding abdomen. The abdominal muscles develop gradually with growth, and the abdomen flattens.

Weight Two-year-olds can be expected to weigh approximately four times their birth weight. The weight gain is about 2 kg (5 lb) between 1 year and 2 years and about 1 to 2 kg (2 to 5 lb) between 2 and 3 years. The 3-year-old weighs about 13.6 kg (30 lb).

Height A toddler's height can be measured as height or length. Height is measured while the toddler stands, and length is measured while the toddler is in a recumbent position. Although the measurements differ slightly, nurses must specify which measurement is used to avoid confusion. Between ages 1 and 2 years, the average growth in height is 10 to 12 cm (4 to 5 in), and between ages 2 and 3 years it slows to 6 to 8 cm (2½ to 3½ in).

Head Circumference The head circumference of the toddler increases on an average about 2.5 cm (1 in), and by 24 months the head is four-fifths of the average adult size. The brain is 70% of its adult size by the time the infant is 2 years old.

Sensory Abilities Visual acuity is fairly well established at 1 year; average estimates of acuity for the toddler are 20/70 at 18 months and 20/40 at 2 years of age. Accommodation to near and far objects is fairly well developed by 18 months and continues to mature with age. At 3 years of age, the toddler can look away from a toy prior to reaching out and picking it up. This ability requires the integration of visual and neuromuscular mechanisms.

The senses of hearing, taste, smell, and touch become increasingly developed and associated with each other. Hearing in the 3-year-old is at adult levels. The taste buds of the toddler are sensitive to the natural flavors of food, and the 3-year-old prefers familiar odors and tastes. Touch is a very important sense, and a distressed toddler is often soothed by tactile sensations.

Motor Abilities *Fine muscle coordination* and *gross motor skills* improve during toddlerhood. At the age of 18 months, babies can pick up small beads and place them in a receptacle. They can also hold a spoon and a cup and walk upstairs with assistance. They will probably crawl down the stairs.

At 2 years, toddlers can hold a spoon and put it into the mouth correctly. They are able to run; their gait is steady; and they can balance on one foot and ride a tricycle. By 3 years, most children are toilet trained, although they still may have the occasional accident when playing or during the night.

PSYCHOSOCIAL DEVELOPMENT

According to Freud, the ages of 2 and 3 years represent the *anal phase* of development, when the rectum and anus are the specially significant areas of the body (see Table 23–3 on page 573). Erikson sees the period from 18 months to 3 years as the time when the central developmental task is autonomy versus shame and doubt (see Table 23–4 on page 574).

Toddlers begin to develop their *sense of autonomy* by asserting themselves with the frequent use of the word "no." They are often frustrated by restraints to their behavior and between ages 1 and 3 may have temper tantrums. However, they slowly gain control over their emotions, usually with the guidance of their parents. Parents need to have a great deal of patience coupled with an understanding of the importance of this developmental milestone. To be effective, parents need to give the child some measure of control and at the same time be consistent in setting limits so that the child learns the results of misbehavior. The nurse can also assist the parents and caregivers in promoting the toddler's development by suggesting the activities summarized in the box on the next page.

Children learn to develop a sense of self through their immediate social environment, in which their parents play a significant role. If the children's social interactions with

FOSTERING THE TODDLER'S PSYCHOSOCIAL DEVELOPMENT

- Provide toys suitable for the toddler, including some toys challenging enough to motivate but not so difficult that the toddler will fail. (Failure will intensify feelings of self-doubt and shame.)
- Make positive suggestions rather than commands. Avoid an emotional climate of negativism, blame, and punishment.
- Give the toddler choices, all of which are safe; however, limit number to two or three.
- When toddler has a temper tantrum, make sure the child is safe, and then leave.
- Help the toddler to develop inner control by setting and enforcing consistent, reasonable limits.
- Praise the toddler's accomplishments.

their parents are negative (eg, constant disapproval regarding eating, toilet training, or other behavior), the children may begin to see themselves as bad. This perception is the basis of a negative self-concept. Parents need to give toddlers positive input so that they can develop a positive and healthy self-concept (Sieving & Zirbel-Donisch 1990, p. 291). With a healthy sense of self-esteem and security, the toddler is able to deal with periodic failures later in life without damage to self-esteem.

Although toddlers like to explore the environment, they always need to have a significant person nearby. Parents need to know that young children experience acute **separation anxiety,** the fear and frustration that comes with parental absences. Abandonment is their greatest fear. At this age, the child may have difficulty accepting a baby sitter or strongly resist being left by the parents at a day-care center. For example, toddlers may become highly anxious when separated from their parents and admitted to hospital. **Regression** or reverting to an earlier development stage may be indicated by bed-wetting or using baby talk. Nurses can assist parents by helping them understand that this behavior is normal and indicates that these toddlers are trying to establish their positions in the family.

Experience with separation helps the child cope with parental absences. Children need room for exploration and interaction with other children and adults. At the same time, they need to know that the parental bond of a loving and close relationship remains secure.

Toddlers assert their independence by saying no or by dawdling. During the toddler stage, receptive and expressive language skills are developing quickly. **Receptive language skill** is the ability to understand words. **Expressive language skill** refers to the ability to use or speak the words. At all ages, the ability to understand words is more advanced than the ability to express words and ideas. Children can understand words and follow directions long before they can actually form them into sentences (Castiligia 1987, p. 165). By 1 year of age, toddlers can recognize their own names.

COGNITIVE DEVELOPMENT

According to Piaget, the toddler completes the 5th and 6th stages of the *sensorimotor phase* and starts the *preconceptual phase* at about 2 years of age. See Table 23–5 on page 576. In the fifth stage, the toddler solves problems by a trial-and-error process. By stage 6, toddlers can solve problems mentally. For example, when given a new toy, the toddler will not immediately handle the toy to see how it works but will look at it carefully to think about how it works.

During Piaget's preconceptual phase, toddlers develop considerable cognitive and intellectual skills. They learn about the sequence of time. They have some symbolic thought; for example, a chair may represent a place of safety, while a blanket may symbolize comfort. Concepts start to form in late toddlerhood. A concept develops when the child learns words to represent classes of objects or thoughts. An example of a concrete concept is *table*, representing a number of articles of furniture, which are all different but all tables.

MORAL DEVELOPMENT

According to Kohlberg, the first level of moral development is the preconventional when children respond to labels of "good" or "bad" (see Table 23–6, page 578). During the second year of life, children begin to know that some activities elicit affection and approval. They also recognize that certain rituals, such as repeating phrases from prayers, also elicit approval. This provides children with feelings of security. By 2 years of age, toddlers are learning what attitudes their parents hold about moral matters.

SPIRITUAL DEVELOPMENT

According to Fowler, the toddler's stage of spiritual development is undifferentiated (see Table 16–2, page 314). Toddlers may be aware of some religious practices, but they are primarily involved in learning knowledge and emotional reactions rather than establishing spiritual beliefs. A toddler may repeat short prayers at bedtime, conforming to a ritual, because praise and affection result. This parental response enhances the toddler's sense of security.

HEALTH ASSESSMENT

Assessment activities for the toddler are similar to those for the infant in terms of measuring weight, length (height) and vital signs (see Chapter 21). Assessment guidelines for growth and development of the toddler are shown in the accompanying box. Examples of NANDA nursing diagnoses, goals/outcome criteria, and interventions for the toddler are shown in Table 24–4.

To facilitate the growth and development of the toddler and appropriate health maintenance, the nurse may choose to discuss the following topics with the parents.

ASSESSMENT GUIDELINES

The Toddler

In the following developmental areas, does the toddler

Physical Development

- Demonstrate physical growth (weight, height and head circumference) within normal range?
- Manifest vital signs within normal range for age?
- Exhibit vision and hearing abilities within normal range?

Motor Development

- Perform gross and fine motor milestones within the normal range for age? For example, by 3 years of age is the toddler able to
  - Walk up steps without assistance?
  - Balance on one foot, jump, and walk on toes?
  - Copy a circle?
  - Build a bridge from blocks?
  - Ride a tricycle?

Psychosocial Development

- Perform psychosocial developmental milestones for age? For example, by 3 years of age is the toddler able to
  - Express likes and dislikes?
  - Display curiosity and ask questions?
  - Accept separation from mother for short periods of time?
  - Begin to play and communicate with children and others outside the immediate family?
  - Understand words such as "up," "down," "cold," and "hungry"?
  - Speak in sentences of three to four words?
  - Imitate religious rituals of the family?

Development of Activities of Daily Living

- Feed self?
- Eat and drink a variety of foods?
- Begin to develop bowel and bladder control?
- Exhibit a rest and sleep pattern appropriate for age?
- Dress self?

PROMOTING HEALTH AND WELLNESS

Health Maintenance Visits and Immunizations

During the toddler period, health maintenance visits should be scheduled at 15 months and 18 months and at 2 and 3 years of age. Immunizations continue to be an important aspect of health maintenance. Routine immunizations, such as the measles-mumps-rubella vaccine (MMR), are usually given at 15 months in the United States. Diphtheria-pertussis-tetanus (DPT), oral attenuated poliomyelitis vaccine (OPV), *Haemophilus influenzae* type B and hepatitis B are other vaccines given during the toddler years as per recommended schedules.

Safety Accidents are the leading cause of mortality of toddlers. They are curious and like to feel and taste everything. Because they are also fascinated by such potential dangers as garden pools and busy streets, they need constant supervision and protection. The most common causes of fatal injuries are automobile accidents, drowning, burns, poisoning, and falls. Parents need to provide the appropriate preventive measures to guard against these health threats. For example, in the United States, many states now require the use of federally approved car restraints for young children. For children under 40 pounds or 40 inches, a safety-tested car seat is recommended; children over 40 pounds can safely use a regular seat belt with a cushion to hold the belt in position and protect the abdomen from pressure. Children should be told that the car does not move until they are properly buckled up. Parents may also wish to reassess their own behavior with respect to automobile safety and the use of seat belts.

Poisoning with lead, known as **plumbism,** remains a risk for the child under 6 years of age. Common sources of lead include paint chips from lead paint, fumes from leaded gasoline, and paper products and earthenware that have been decorated with lead paint. Parents should be aware that the ingestion of lead paint chips from windowsills and window frames painted with lead-based paint is the most common cause of lead poisoning in children.

Parents can prevent many accidents by "toddler proofing" the home or other setting where the child will be. This includes removing or securing all items that can pose a safety hazard to the child. All valuable or "precious" items should also be removed from the child's reach. Parents must keep in mind that the child's cognitive and motor skills increase quite quickly, and safety measures

Table 24–4 Examples of Nursing Diagnoses and Goals for the Toddler

NANDA Diagnosis	Goal/Outcome Criteria	Interventions
High risk for poisoning related to toddler's normal developmental behaviors (mouthing, motor activities)	Parents will demonstrate within 1 week the ability to provide a safe environment from accidental poisoning, as evidenced by ▪ Stating the common types of poisons and their location in environment (eg, kitchen and medicine cabinets). ▪ Actively taking measures to decrease risks for accidental poisoning (removing substances and locking cabinets).	Provide parents with information on accidental poisoning prevention and assistance (eg, Poison Control Center Hotline). Schedule parents for a child care class that discusses accidental poisoning. Assess parental knowledge through written, verbal and/or observational feedback techniques.
Knowledge deficit (parental) related to toilet training	Parents will demonstrate within 1 month knowledge of toilet training as evidenced by ▪ Stating the appropriate age, readiness, and procedures for training. ▪ Providing appropriate clothing (loose fitting) and equipment (step-stool, sink) for training.	Provide parents with educational guidance on toilet training and obtain written or verbal feedback to assess knowledge. Refer parents to a toddler development class.

should keep up with these new skills. Training in safety should begin at this age. For example, toddlers should be taught not to run out on the street and taught the meaning of the Mr Yuk sticker (available from the Poison Control Center) on cleaning solutions, insecticides, and other poisonous substances. See safety highlights for toddlers in the box at the right.

Vision Parents should be made aware that behaviors such as rubbing the eyes, squinting, blinking, or an inability to see things clearly may be indicative of a vision problem. During this period, the toddler should be screened for amblyopia and strabismus. **Amblyopia** (reduced visual acuity in one eye) is usually the result of strabismus. The child with amblyopia has straight eyes, whereas the child with **strabismus** (cross-eye) has a deviant eye.

To detect amblyopia, visual testing is done with one eye occluded. The optimal time for correcting amblyopia and strabismus is during early childhood. Methods of treatment include corrective surgery or the use of an eye patch over the nonaffected eye to require the deviated eye to fixate. Correction of these problems is important for future learning as well as for the optimum development of the toddler's concept of self.

Dental Health Dental caries occur frequently during the toddler period, often as a result of the excessive intake of sweets or a prolonged use of the bottle during naps and at bedtime. The nurse should give parents the following instructions for promoting and maintaining dental health:

SAFETY HIGHLIGHTS FOR TODDLERS

- Continue to use federally approved car seat or seat belts at all times. Place children in back seat when traveling in car.
- Teach child the meaning of words "no" and "don't." Make certain the child understands that these words mean danger and must be obeyed.
- Teach child not to put objects in the mouth, including pills (unless given by parent).
- Keep objects with sharp edges (such as furniture and knives) out of child's reach.
- Place hot pots on back burners with handles turned inward.
- Keep cleaning solutions, insecticides, and medicines in locked cupboards.
- Keep windows and balconies screened.
- Teach child to swim. Fence in pools, and supervise at all times. Do not overfill bathtub. Do not let toddlers play near ditches or wells.
- Teach child not to run or ride tricycle into the street.
- Obtain low bed when child begins to climb.
- Cover outlets with safety covers or plugs.

- Cleanse the child's teeth gently with a cotton ball moistened with hydrogen peroxide. This should begin when the first tooth erupts.
- Beginning at about 18 months of age, brush the child's teeth with a soft toothbrush.
- Schedule an initial dental visit for the child at about 2 years of age, and prepare the child for this experience.
- Seek professional dental attention for any problems such as discoloring of the teeth, chipping, or signs of infection such as redness and swelling.

Nutrition Because of a maturing gastrointestinal tract, toddlers can eat most foods and adjust to three meals each day. In addition, by age 3, when most of the deciduous teeth have emerged, the toddler is able to bite and chew adult table food. Toddlers' manipulative skills are sufficiently well developed for them to learn how to feed themselves. Before the age of 20 months, most toddlers require help with glasses and cups because their wrist control is limited.

Developing independence may be exhibited through the toddler's refusal of certain foods. Meals should be short because of the toddler's brief attention span and environmental distractions. Often toddlers display their liking of rituals by eating foods in a certain order, cutting foods a specific way, or accompanying certain foods with a particular drink.

The toddler is less likely to have fluid imbalances than the infant. The toddler's gastrointestinal function is more mature, and the percentage of fluid body weight is lower. A healthy toddler weighing 15 kg (33 lb) needs about 1250 mL of fluid per 24 hours (Mott et al 1990, p. 925).

During the toddler stage, the caloric requirement decreases to 900–1800 kcal per day because of a decrease in the rate of growth. From 1 to 2 years of age, the toddler may be eating a combination of prepared toddler foods and some table foods. Parents should be instructed to read labels carefully and be aware that the table foods offer more variety and are less expensive and more nutritious than prepared toddler foods. The Food Guide Pyramid should be used as a guide in discussing the toddler's diet with parents. See Chapter 37, page 1020. The need for adequate iron, calcium, vitamins C and A, which are common toddler deficiencies, should also be discussed.

Three-year-olds often use mealtime to control the family conversation and gain attention by their constant chatter and disruption. Parents may need to anticipate the child's needs, make adjustments in their food preparation, and determine the acceptable level of table manners for the child's developmental level. The following suggestions may help parents to meet the child's nutritional needs and promote effective parent-child interactions: (a) make mealtime a pleasant time by avoiding tensions at the table and discussions of bad behavior; (b) offer a variety of simple, attractive foods in small portions, and avoid meals that combine foods into one dish, such as a stew; (c) do not use food as a reward or punish a child who does not eat; (d) schedule meals, sleep, and snack times that will allow for optimum appetite and behavior; and (e) avoid the routine use of sweet desserts.

Elimination Control of the bladder and bowel is an important milestone of childhood. The average age for the completion of daytime toilet training is about 29 months; the average age for completion of day and night training is about 33 months. Parents need instruction early in the toddler period to avoid the pitfalls that can occur when toilet training is attempted too early. One-year-olds whose mothers put them on the potty every day at the right time are not trained; their mothers are trained. Toilet trained children independently go to the bathroom, undress, eliminate, and put their clothes back on. Children must be both interested and cooperative to complete this complex series of tasks. Parents need both instruction and support if they are to avoid the many frustrations that can occur in managing the first step toward the child's self-care. Children who are ready for toilet training are able to walk and balance well, climb onto the potty, and undress and dress themselves. The child also shows awareness of the need to defecate or urinate by either words or behavior. The readiness of the parent is also important. Toilet training requires time, patience, and a consistent approach. If a new sibling has entered the family or if the mother is returning to full-time work, the readiness of the child may be affected. After readiness has been determined, parents can promote and enhance development by using the following steps:

1. Introduce children to the potty chair, explain its use with words they can understand, and have them sit in it if they wish.
2. After a week or so, have the child sit in the potty chair with clothes off for 3 to 5 minutes, and explain what should be done, using the same words consistently.
3. If the child is interested, encourage potty use several times a day, praise the child's behavior, even for attempts, and do not scold or punish the child for undesired behavior.
4. When toddlers demonstrate their ability to achieve success, dress them in training pants that they can easily remove, and provide easy access to the potty chair.

Rest/Sleep The sleep requirements of toddlers decrease to 10 to 14 hours per day. Most still need an afternoon nap, but the need for midmorning naps gradually decreases. The toddler may exhibit a great deal of resistance to going to bed. Parents need assurance that if the child has had adequate attention from them during the day, maintaining a consistent approach with respect to bedtime will promote good sleep habits for the entire family.

The child who awakens at night may be afraid of the dark or have experienced night terrors or nightmares. These fears should be respected and the child can be given a night light. When children awaken, the parents should talk with them and reassure them that they are all right and that the parents are close by. Bringing the children to the bed of the parents or lying down with them to help them get to sleep can cause difficulties, because children will expect those routines to continue. There are other points the nurse should emphasize to parents:

- Allow the child to bring a soft toy or blanket to bed.
- Activities prior to bedtime should be physically quieting and emotionally soothing.
- Sleep disturbances are a normal result of the developmental level as the child begins to deal with the idea of separation (Balsmeyer 1990, p. 448).

Stimulation Through Play The child between 1 and 3 years of age seems to be engaged in endless activity. This activity is important for muscle development and the improvement of both motor skills and social skills. It is important for parents to help children pace their activity by providing outdoor games or swings and trips to the park, along with more quiet times, such as reading a book or having a nap. The main ingredient that the child needs to facilitate and enhance successful activity and play is freedom. Freedom implies that the child has adequate space to play and be active, without excess restraints on activity.

The types of play toddlers engage in can be described as **onlooker play** (eg, watching TV), **solitary play** (involvement in independent activities), **parallel play** (the child sits with other children but does not cooperate or interact with them), and **associative play** (eg, building a tower of blocks with another child).

Most of the toddler's playing time is spent in solitary play. Young children like to move constantly and to move things constantly. They may empty bookcases and drawers, rearrange kitchen cupboards, change their clothes, imitate parental behavior such as sweeping or doing dishes, or run back and forth through the house. Parents should show enthusiasm for the toddler's activities, giving them praise for the "help," and smiling and clapping at the child's accomplishments. The amount of time a child spends watching TV should be monitored by parents. Parents may want to anticipate this problem and set limits early concerning the amount of time and the quality of programs they want their children to view.

Cognitive Stimulation Parents need to be aware that the cognitive development of their child is a result of inherited ability, social interactions, and life experiences. Thus, cognitive development is enhanced by providing a variety of stimulating activities, interactions, and opportunities and by understanding the toddler's developmental skills. Parents can assist in the development of logic and reasoninig by (a) playing simple games and solving puzzles, (b) hiding objects and having the child find them, and (c) putting small objects in a container for the child to retrieve. Parents also need to be aware, and accepting, of any imaginary friends the child has created. The child often uses this make-believe behavior to do and say things that may sometimes be forbidden in the real world. Parents may experience some frustration when toddlers do not understand that they cannot have their own way or when it is difficult to understand what the child wants. Toddlers are very egocentric and do not realize that others may have thoughts that are different from their own.

Parental instruction in stimulation and other health-promotion activities for the toddler are summarized in the box at the top of the next page.

PRESCHOOLERS (4 AND 5 YEARS)

During the preschool period, physical growth slows, but control of the body and coordination increase greatly. The preschoolers' world gets larger as they meet relatives, friends, and neighbors.

PHYSICAL DEVELOPMENT

By the time children are 4 or 5 years old, they appear taller and thinner than toddlers, because children tend to grow more in height than in weight. The preschooler's brain reaches almost its adult size by 5 years. The extremities of the body grow more quickly than the body trunk, making the child's body appear somewhat out of proportion. The posture of preschoolers gradually changes as the pelvis is straightened and the abdominal muscles become stronger. Thus the preschooler appears slender with erect posture.

Weight Weight gain in preschool children is generally slow. By 5 years, they have added only another 3 to 5 kg (7 to 12 lb) to their 3-year-old weight, increasing it to somewhere between 18 and 20 kg (40 and 45 lb).

Height Preschool children grow about 5 to 6.25 cm (2.0 to 2.5 in) each year. Thus by 5 years of age, they double the birth length and measure 100 cm (40 in).

Vision Preschool children are generally **hyperopic** (farsighted), that is, unable to focus on near objects. As the eye grows in length, it becomes **emmetropic** (it refracts light normally). If the eyes become too long, the child

HEALTH PROMOTION HIGHLIGHTS FOR TODDLERS

Instruct parents about the following:

Health Maintenance Visits

- At 15 and 18 months and at 2 and 3 years

Protective Measures

- Immunizations: continuing DPT, OPV series, measles-mumps-rubella (MMR), *Haemophilus influenzae* type B, and hepatitis B vaccines as recommended
- Screenings for tuberculosis and lead poisoning

Toddler Safety

- Importance of supervision and teaching child to obey commands
- Home environment safety measures (eg, lock medicine cabinet)
- Outdoor safety measures (eg, close supervision near water)
- Appropriate toys

Nutrition

- Importance of nutritious meals and snacks
- Teaching simple mealtime manners
- Dental care

Elimination

- Toilet training techniques

Rest/Sleep

- Dealing with sleep disturbances

Play

- Providing adequate space and a variety of activities
- Toys that allow "acting on" behaviors and provide motor and sensory stimulation

becomes **myopic** (nearsighted), that is, unable to focus on objects that are far away. In severe cases of hyperopia or myopia, glasses may be prescribed. By the end of the preschool years, visual ability has improved; normal vision for the 5-year-old is approximately 20/30. The Snellen E chart (See Chapter 22, page 482) can be used to assess the preschooler's vision.

Hearing and Taste The hearing of the preschool child has reached optimal levels, and the ability to listen (attending to and comprehending what is said) has matured since the toddler age. In relation to the sense of taste, preschoolers show their preferences by asking for something "yummy," and may refuse something they consider "yucky."

Motor Abilities By 5 years of age, children are able to wash their hands and face and brush their teeth. They are self-conscious about exposing their bodies and go to the bathroom without telling others. Typically, preschool children run with increasing skill each year. By 5 years of age, they run skillfully and can jump three steps. Preschoolers can balance on their toes and dress themselves without assistance.

PSYCHOSOCIAL DEVELOPMENT

Erikson writes that the major developmental crisis of the preschooler is *initiative versus guilt.* See Table 23–4 on page 574. Preschoolers must solve problems in accordance with their consciences. Their personalities develop. Erickson views the crises at this time as important for the development of the individual's *self-concept.* According to Erikson, preschoolers must learn what they can do. As a result, preschoolers imitate behavior, and their imaginations and creativity become lively.

Parents can enhance the self-concept of the preschooler by providing opportunities for new achievements where the child can learn, repeat, and master (Sieving & Zirbel-Donisch 1990, p. 295). For example, a child obtains a two-wheel bike with safety wheels and quickly learns coordination, balance, use of the brakes, and bicycle safety. Mastery of these tasks provides the child with a sense of accomplishment. The child is soon ready for the new challenge of mastering the two-wheeler.

The self-concept of the preschooler is also based on gender identification. The preschooler is aware of the two sexes and identifies with the correct one. They often imitate sexual stereotypes and usually begin by identifying with the parent of the same sex. They may mimic the parent's behavior, attitudes, and appearance (Figure 24–6). Parents need to be aware that preschoolers are very curious about their own bodies and sexual functions, as well as those of others, and will often ask questions. Parents should not imply that a question is inappropriate or that a particular subject is bad.

Freud theorizes that the preschooler is in the *phallic stage* of development. The biologic focus of the child during this stage is the genital area. See Table 23–3 on page 573.

The phase of close emotional relationship with both parents changes to the phase Freud referred to as the Electra or Oedipus complex (Engel 1962, pp. 90–104). At this time, the child focuses feelings of love chiefly on the parent of the opposite sex, and the parent of the same sex may receive some hostile feelings. At this time, the child begins to develop sexual interests. The child becomes interested in clothes and hair styles.

During the preschool years, four *adaptive mechanisms* are learned: identification, introjection, imagination, and repression. **Identification** occurs when the child perceives the self as similar to another person and behaves like that person. For example, a boy may internalize the attitudes and gender behavior of his father. **Introjection** is similar to identification. It is the assimilation of the attributes of others. When preschoolers observe their parents, they assimilate many of their values and attitudes. **Imagination** is an important part of preschoolers' life. The preschooler has an active imagination and fantasizes in play; for example, a chair becomes a beautiful throne to a girl, and she is the ruler. **Repression** is removing experiences, throughts, and impulses from awareness. The preschooler generally represses thoughts related to the Oedipus or Electra complex.

Preschool children gradually emerge as social beings. At the age of 3 or 4, they learn to play with a small number of their peers. They gradually learn to play with more people as they grow older. Preschoolers participate more in the family than they did previously. In associations with neighbors, family guests, and baby sitters, too, they learn about social relationships.

By 4 years of age, children tend to believe that what they know is right. They tend to be dogmatic in their *speech*. Four-year-olds love nonsense words such as "jump-jump" and can string them together much to an adult's exasperation. At 4, children are aggressive in their speech and capable of long conversations, often mixing fact and fiction. By 5 years of age, speaking skills are well developed. Children use words purposefully and ask questions to acquire information. They do not merely practice speaking as 3- and 4-year-olds do, but speak as a means of social interaction. Exaggeration is common among 4- and 5-year-olds.

Preschoolers also become increasingly aware of themselves. They play with their bodies largely out of curiosity. They know where the body begins and ends as well as the correct names for the different parts. By 5 years of age, they are able to draw a person including all the features. Preschoolers also learn about their feelings; they know the words "cry," "sad," "laugh," and the feelings related to them. They also begin to learn how to control their feelings and behavior. The preschooler uses the same types of *coping mechanisms* in response to stress as the toddler does, although protest behavior (kicking, screaming) is less likely to occur in the older preschooler. Preschoolers usually have greater ability to verbalize stress.

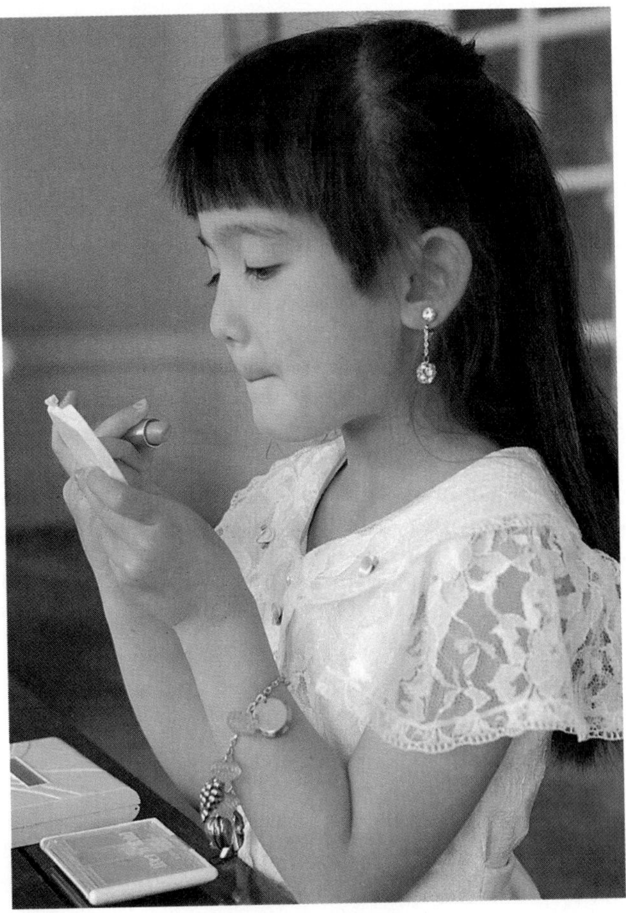

Figure 24–6 Preschoolers often identify with the parent of the same sex and like to mimic their behavior.

Preschoolers need to feel that they are loved and that they are an important part of the family. The child who has to compete with siblings for parental attention will often display jealousy. Parents should be aware that preschoolers need time to adjust to a new baby and may need additional attention or special activities to help them through this adjustment period. Preschoolers with older siblings may also experience sibling rivalry. Siblings may fight and argue and become very aggressive because of their daily close proximity or competition for parental attention. Parents who can plan some special time or activity for each child will help that child to feel loved and may decrease the sibling rivalry.

Guidance and discipline are important parts of the parental role during the preschool years. As children seek independence from adults, they often test limits by refusing to cooperate and by repeatedly ignoring parental requests. Parents find themselves both frustrated and irritated. These power struggles can sometimes be avoided by encouraging children to be responsible for their own behavior as much as possible and by setting reasonable expectations and consistent limits. When conflict does occur, parents can employ the "no-lose" method of conflict resolution, which involves mutual discussion and compromise (Mott et al 1990, p. 334).

COGNITIVE DEVELOPMENT

The preschooler's cognitive development, according to Piaget, is the phase of *intuitive thought*. See Table 23–5 on page 576. Children are still egocentric, but egocentrism gradually subsides as they encounter wider experiences. Preschoolers learn through trial and error, and they think of only one idea at a time. They do not understand relationships such as those between mother and father or sister and brother. Children start to form concepts in late toddlerhood or the early preschool years. Preschoolers become concerned about death as something inevitable, but they do not explain it. They also associate death with others rather than themselves.

Most children at the age of 5 years can count pennies; however, the opportunity to spend money usually does not occur until they attend school. Reading skills also start to develop at this age. Young children like fairy tales and books about animals and other children.

MORAL DEVELOPMENT

Preschoolers are capable of prosocial behavior, that is, any action that a person takes to benefit someone else. The term *prosocial* is synonymous with *kind* and connotes sharing, helping, protecting, giving aid, befriending, showing affection, and giving encouragement (Schulman & Mekler 1985, p. 232).

At this stage of development, preschoolers do not have fully formed consciences; however, they do develop some internal controls. Moral behavior is largely learned by *modeling*, initially after parents and later significant others. The preschooler usually behaves well in social settings.

Children who perceive their parents as strict may become resentful or overly obedient. Preschoolers usually control their behavior because they want love and approval from their parents. Moral behavior to a preschooler may mean taking turns at play or sharing. Nurses can assist parents by discussing moral development and encouraging parents to give preschoolers recognition for actions such as sharing. It is also important for parents to answer preschooler's "why" questions and discuss values with them.

ASSESSMENT GUIDELINES

The Preschooler

In the following developmental areas, does the preschooler

Physical Development

- Demonstrate physical growth (weight, height) within normal range?
- Manifest vital signs within normal range for age?
- Exhibit vision and hearing abilities within normal range?

Motor Development

- Perform gross and fine motor milestones within the normal range for age? For example, by 5 years of age is the preschooler able to
  - Jump rope and skip?
  - Climb playground equipment?
  - Ride a bicycle with training wheels?
  - Print letters and numbers?

Psychosocial Development

- Perform psychosocial developmental milestones for age? For example, by 5 years of age is the preschooler able to
  - Separate easily from parents?
  - Display imagination and creativity?
  - Enjoy playing with peers in cooperative activities?
  - Understand right from wrong and respond to others' expectations of behavior?
  - Identify four colors?
  - Exhibit increasing vocabulary using complete sentences and all parts of speech?
  - Cooperate in doing simple chores (eg, putting away toys)?
  - Identify with individuals of own sex?

Development in Activities of Daily Living

- Demonstrate development of toilet training?
- Perform simple hygiene measures?
- Dress and undress self?

Spiritual Development

Many preschoolers enroll in Sunday school or faith-oriented classes. The preschooler usually enjoys the social interaction of these classes. According to Fowler, children from the ages of 4 to 6 years are at the intuitive-projective stage of spiritual development. See Table 16–2 on page 314.

Faith at this stage is primarily a result of the teaching of significant others, such as parents and teachers. Children learn to imitate religious behavior, for example, bowing the head in prayer, although they don't understand the meaning of the behavior. Preschoolers require simple explanations, such as those in picture books, of spiritual matters. Children at this age use their imaginations to envision such ideas as angels or the devil.

Health Assessment

During assessment, the preschooler can participate in answering questions with assistance from parents when appropriate. For instance, children who attend preschool can describe the typical lunch and how much of it they usually eat. Preschoolers can also describe the types of activities that they enjoy. Assessment guidelines for growth and development of the preschooler are shown in the box at the left.

Examples of NANDA nursing diagnoses, goals/outcome criteria, and interventions for the preschooler are shown in Table 24–5.

The nurse may wish to discuss the following topics with the parents to help them facilitate optimal development of their preschool child.

Promoting Health and Wellness

Health Maintenance Visits and Immunizations Parents should schedule annual preventive health care visits and regular dental examinations during the preschool years. Immunizations that are recommended between 4 and 6 years of age include diphtheria-pertussis-tetanus toxoid (DPT), oral attenuated poliomyelitis (OPV) and measles-mumps-rubella (MMR) vaccine.

Safety Accidents continue to be the major cause of mortality among preschool children. These children are active and often clumsy and are therefore susceptible to injury. Accidents can be prevented in two ways: control of the environment and education of the child. Parents may need to learn to control the environment, for instance, by keeping matches, household medicines, and other potential poisons out of the child's reach, by teaching the child to put toys away when they are not being used and by safeguarding swimming pools and other potentially dangerous areas. The education of the preschooler may involve learning how to cross streets, what traffic signals mean, and how to ride a bicycle safely. Preschoolers like to imitate their parents, so adults can teach safety through

Table 24–5 Examples of Nursing Diagnoses and Goals for the Preschooler

NANDA Diagnosis	Goal/Outcome Criteria	Interventions
Sleep pattern disturbance related to nightmares, night fears, and awakenings	The child will be able to establish within 1 month a sleep pattern free from major disturbances, as evidenced by ▪ Ability to go to sleep willingly and readily. ▪ Ability to sleep through night.	Assess the child for sleep disturbances at each well-child visit. Provide parents with information on dealing with common sleep disturbances (eg, instituting a bedtime routine, using night lights).
Altered health maintenance related to missed well-child appointments and unimmunized child	Parents will within 1 month provide appropriate health maintenance for the preschooler, as evidenced by ▪ Keeping scheduled well-child visit appointments. ▪ Immunizations that are up-to-date or in progress. ▪ Completion of appropriate screening tests.	Provide parents with rationale and schedule for routine well-child visits and immunizations. Refer parents to social services for evaluation of financial and transportation status, as necessary.

example. For safety measures for preschoolers, see the box at the right.

Dental Health It is estimated that 80% of children in this age group have some tooth decay. Deciduous teeth guide the entrance of permanent teeth. Therefore, abnormally placed or lost deciduous teeth can cause the misalignment of permanent teeth. Fluoridation of water in the community and in school water systems can significantly reduce the number of cavities in children. If the local water supply is not fluoridated, parents can provide rinses, toothpastes, or supplements to protect their children against cavities and gum disease. Children also need instruction in the care of their teeth, such as proper brushing and the avoidance of sugary snacks. Parental supervision is needed to assure the completion of these self-care activities. See Chapter 29 for additional information.

Nutrition The preschooler eats adult foods and should have the required amounts from the four food groups. See Chapter 37 for specific information about these amounts. Parents should become informed about the diet of their child in day-care or preschool settings so that they can be sure of meeting the child's total nutritional needs. Children at this age are very active and may rush through the meal to return to playing. The 4-year-old still requires parent's help in cutting meat and may spill milk when pouring from a large container. Parents also need to teach the preschooler how to use utensils and should provide them with the opportunity to practice (eg, buttering bread). However, 4- and 5-year-olds often use their fingers to pick food up. Table manners are marginal at best. Active children often require snacks between meals. Cheese, fruits, yogurt, raw vegetables, and milk are good choices. Children at this age may enjoy helping in the kitchen, and both girls and boys should be encouraged to do so.

The preschooler is even less susceptible than the toddler to fluid imbalances. The average 5-year-old weighing 20 kg (44 lb) requires at least 75 mL of liquid per kilogram of body weight per day, or 1500 mL every 24 hours (Mott et al 1990, p. 925).

Elimination The preschooler is able to take responsibility for independent toileting. Parents need to realize that accidents do occur and the child should never be punished or chastised for this. Children often forget to wash their hands or flush the toilet and need instruction in wiping themselves. The female child should be taught to wipe from front to back to prevent contamination of the urinary tract by feces.

Rest/Sleep The preschool child requires 12 hours of sleep per night, particularly during the school year. Many children of this age dislike bedtime and resist by requesting another story, game, or television program. The 4- to 5-year-old may become restless and irritable if sleep requirements are not met. A nap or quiet time during the day may be needed to restore energy levels.

Children in this age group still require bedtime rituals. Parents can help children who resist bedtime by warning them that bedtime is approaching and by continuing to use the same firm and consistent approach as suggested for the toddler. Preschool children wake up frequently at night. Knowing how commonly this behavior occurs and that it usually decreases by age 6 may be reassuring for many parents. The cause of this nighttime wakening may be night terrors or nightmares. During a *night terror* the child screams, is in obvious distress, and is difficult to console. The child never fully wakes up but goes back to sleep in about 10 minutes with no recollection of the frightening episode. During *nightmares,* which are far more common, children wake up and can describe the details of their dreams vividly. Children who wake up at night should be consoled by their parents, reminded that the dream was not real, and encouraged to return to sleep.

Stimulation through Play The preschooler's main activity continues to be play. Children of 4 to 5 years can

SAFETY HIGHLIGHTS FOR PRESCHOOLERS

- Do not allow children to run with candy or other objects in the mouth.
- Teach children not to put small objects in the mouth, nose, and ears.
- Remove doors from unused equipment, such as refrigerators.
- Teach preschoolers to cross streets safely and obey traffic signals.
- Check Halloween treats before allowing children to eat them. Discard loose or open candy.
- Teach children to play in "safe" areas, not on streets and railroad tracks.
- Teach preschooler the dangers of playing with matches and playing near charcoal, fire, and heating appliances.
- Teach children to avoid strangers and keep parents informed of their whereabouts.
- Teach preschoolers not to walk in front of swings and not to push others off playground equipment.
- Teach children to walk quietly near animals and avoid approaching a strange animal.

separate easily from their parents and enjoy more interactive activities. Parents can facilitate their development by introducing new games to children, such as hide-and-seek, that have simple rules and require cooperation. Children also enjoy planning group activities, such as a picnic or visit to the zoo, and benefit from toys that encourage role-playing, such as construction trucks, dress-up dolls, and make-believe games. Preschoolers are able to regulate their activity and usually do well in a group setting for several sessions per week.

Social Interaction Preschoolers enjoy playing with their peers and can even take part in some activities with older children. Social interaction is important for this age group. It provides them with opportunities to learn the rules of play and cooperation, such as taking turns and following directions. Parents should be encouraged to provide these situations for the preschooler in order to enhance social development and foster school readiness.

Language The preschooler uses language to express ideas. Parents can facilitate improved language skills by

- Encouraging the child to tell stories.
- Never criticizing the child's speech and remaining patient if the child stumbles over words.
- Playing word games to teach the child new objects or names.
- Reading and discussing stories with the child.

Cognitive Stimulation According to Piaget, preschool children remain egocentric and cannot understand that other people have thoughts that are different from theirs. Parents who are aware of this will be prepared for the difficulty and the frustration that children experience when they cannot have their own way and are unable to understand that another way exists. More recent research suggests that preschoolers are able to take varying perspectives (Hauck 1991, p. 234).

Preschoolers understand the concept of time, and memory and creativity are developing. When parents discuss the activities of last week or last winter, children can usually remember the sequence of events that took place. Cognitive development can be promoted by providing opportunities for memory games and by encouraging a variety of creative play activities.

The development of moral values is closely related to the cognitive development of the child. At the preschool age, children do not have a true conscience and basically do things in their own best interest. Parents can assist in their moral development by encouraging and praising actions such as sharing and by discussing values with them.

Parental instruction in stimulation and other health-promotion activities for the preschoolers are summarized in the box at the right.

SCHOOL-AGE CHILDREN (6 TO 12 YEARS)

The school-age period starts when children are about 6 years of age, when the deciduous teeth are shed. This period includes the preadolescent (prepuberty) period. It ends at about 12 years, with the onset of puberty. Puberty is the age when the reproductive organs become functional and secondary sex characteristics develop. Because

HEALTH PROMOTION HIGHLIGHTS FOR PRESCHOOLERS

Instruct parents about the following:

Health Maintenance Visits

- At 4 and 5 years

Protective Measures

- Immunizations: DPT, OPV, measles-mumps-rubella (MMR) vaccine; other immunizations as recommended
- Screening for tuberculosis
- Vision and hearing screening
- Regular dental screenings and fluoride treatment

Preschooler Safety

- Educating child about simple safety rules (eg, crossing the street)
- Teaching child to play safely (eg, bicycle and playground safety)

Nutrition

- Importance of nutritious meals and snacks

Elimination

- Teaching proper hygiene (eg, washing hands after using bathroom)

Rest/Sleep

- Dealing with sleep disturbances (eg, nightmares)

Play

- Providing times for group play activities
- Teaching child simple games that require cooperation and interaction
- Providing toys and dress-ups for role-playing

the average age of onset of puberty is 10 for girls and 12 for boys, some people define the school-age years as 6 to 10 for girls and 6 to 12 for boys. Skills learned during this stage are particularly important in relation to work later in life and willingness to try new tasks.

Starting school is significant for a number of reasons; for one, children are able to compare their skills to those of their peers. They also receive impressions of how their skills are perceived by others: the teacher, the school nurse, and their peers. These perceptions can bolster a child's self-image or can weaken feelings of self-worth. In general, the period from 6 to 12 years is one of rapid and dramatic change.

PHYSICAL DEVELOPMENT

The school-age child gains weight rapidly and thus appears less thin than previously. Individual differences due to both genetic and environmental factors are obvious at this time.

Weight At 6 years, boys tend to weigh about 21 kg (46 lb), about 1 kg (2 lb) more than girls. The weight gain of school children from 6 to 12 years of age averages about 3.2 kg (7 lb) per year, but the major weight gains occur from age 10 to 12 for boys and from 9 to 12 for girls. By 12 years of age, boys and girls weigh on the average 40 to 42 kg (88 to 95 lb); girls are usually heavier.

Height At 6 years, both boys and girls are about the same height, 115 cm (46 in). They are about 150 cm (60 in) by 12 years. Before puberty, children of both sexes have a growth spurt, girls between 10 and 12 years and boys between 12 and 14 years. Thus, girls may well be taller than boys at 12 years, but boys are usually stronger.

The extremities tend to grow more quickly than the trunk, thus school-age children's bodies appear somewhat ill-proportioned. By 6 years of age, the thoracic curvature starts to develop, and the lordosis disappears. Full adult posture is not assumed, however, until after the complete development of the skeletal musculature during the adolescent period.

Vision The depth and distance perception of children 6 to 8 years of age is accurate. By age 6, children have full binocular vision: The eye muscles are well developed and coordinated, and both eyes can focus on one object at the same time. Because the shape of the eye changes during growth, the farsightedness of the preschool years gradually changes to 20/20 vision during the school-age years; 20/20 vision is usually well established between 9 and 11 years of age. In later childhood, myopia is not uncommon; that is, the child is able to see clearly only objects that are close. This problem is generally corrected by eyeglasses.

Hearing Auditory perception is fully developed in school-age children, who are able to identify very fine differences in voices, both in sound and in pitch. At this stage, children also have a well-developed sense of touch and are able to locate points of heat and cold on all body surfaces. They are also able to identify an unseen object, such as a pencil or a book, simply by touch. This ability is called **stereognosis.**

Prepubertal Changes Very little change takes place in the reproductive and endocrine systems until the prepuberty period. During prepuberty, at about ages 9 to 13, endocrine functions slowly increase. This change in endocrine function can result in increased perspiration and more active sebaceous glands. As a result, acne may develop, particularly on the face, neck, and back.

Certain physical changes occur in both boys and girls during prepuberty. Some of the changes in approximate sequence are as follows:

For the boy:

- The testes and scrotum increase in size.
- The skin over the scrotum changes color; it becomes reddened and stippled.
- The breasts may enlarge slightly, but this growth disappears in a few months.
- Sparse, downy pubic hair grows at the base of the penis
- The penis gradually becomes wider and longer. Development of the genitals to adult size take about 5 to 6 years.
- The boy grows taller and his shoulders widen.
- Axillary sweating begins.

For the girl:

- The pelvis and hips broaden.
- The breast tissues develop and may be tender. At first the nipple is slightly elevated, at 7½ to 8 years of age. The areolae become somewhat protuberant and enlarged between the ages of 9 and 11 years.
- Axillary sweating begins.
- The initial growth of pubic hair occurs at 8 to 14 years.
- Vaginal secretions become milky and change from an alkaline to an acid pH, and vaginal flora change from mixed to Döderlein's lactic acid–producing bacilli (Murray & Zentner 1993, pp. 332–33).

Motor Abilities During the middle years (6 to 10), children perfect their muscular skills and coordination. By 9 years, most children are becoming skilled in games of interest, such as football or baseball. These skills are often associated with school, and many of them are learned there. By 9 years most children have sufficient fine motor control for such activities as building models or sewing.

PSYCHOSOCIAL DEVELOPMENT

According to Erikson, the central task of school-age children is *industry versus inferiority*. At this time children begin to create and develop a sense of competence and perseverance. School-age children are motivated by activities that provide a sense of worth. They concentrate on mastering skills that will help them function in the adult world. Although children of this age work hard to succeed, they are always faced with the possibility of failure, which can lead to a sense of inferiority. If children have been successful in previous stages, they are motivated to be industrious and to cooperate with others toward a common goal. See Table 23–4 on page 574.

Freud describes the period from 6 through 12 years of age as the latency stage. During this time, the focus is directed toward physical and intellectual activities, while sexual tendencies seem to be repressed. See Table 23–3 on page 573.

In school, children have the restraints of the school system imposed on their behavior, and they learn to develop controls. Children compare their skills with those of their peers in a number of areas, including motor development, social development, and language. This comparison assists in the development of self-concept. Schoolchildren can sometimes be cruel in their honesty, and teachers often need to intercede to assist children who have limitations. The schoolchild develops a number of adaptive mechanisms. Four of these are regression (discussed earlier), malingering, rationalization, and ritualistic behavior. **Malingering** is a familiar mechanism to schoolchildren. It is pretending to be ill rather than facing something unpleasant; the child who feels sick the morning before a test may be malingering. **Rationalization** is an attempt to justify behavior by logical reason and explanation. A girl who does not make the swimming team may rationalize to her parents by saying she really did not try because she doesn't want swimming to interfere with her piano lessons. **Ritualistic behavior** is demonstrated by schoolchildren in many settings. For example, a child may walk down the sidewalk without stepping on a crack. Clubs and gangs often have rituals of membership. These rituals become very important to schoolchildren even though they usually do not persist for a long time. For example, the boy who must have a shower every morning may forget this ritual after a few weeks.

As they grow older, schoolchildren learn to play with more children at one time. Usually the 6- and 7-year-old is a member of a peer group. This group can be a greater influence than the family in teaching attitudes. During late childhood, children join a gang, a small group of peers, which is formed by the children themselves. It is usually informal and transitory, and the leadership changes from time to time. During this period of socialization with others, children gradually become less self-centered and selfish and more cooperative and conscious of the group.

The schoolchild's self-concept continues to mature. Children recognize similarities and differences between themselves and others. School-age children compare themselves with others and obtain feedback from teachers and peers. Children who are successful and receive recognition for their efforts feel competent and in control of themselves and of the environment. Children who feel unaccepted by their peers or who receive negative feedback and little recognition can feel inferior and worthless.

Although the focus of interest for this age group has moved to school, peers, and other activities, the home remains the crucial place for the child's development of high self-esteem.

Parents and caregivers can assist school-age children to develop psychosocially by

- Recognizing success and providing praise for achievements.
- Guiding children to perform tasks in which they are likely to succeed.
- Guiding the child to complete the task.
- Teaching the child how to get along with peers by collaborating, compromising, cooperating, and competing.
- Teaching the child how to get along with adults.

COGNITIVE DEVELOPMENT

According to Piaget, the ages 7 to 11 years mark the phase of *concrete operations*. See Table 23–5 on page 576. During this stage, the child changes from egocentric interactions to cooperative interactions (Figure 24–7, p. 606). School-age children also develop an increased understanding of concepts that are associated with specific objects, for example, environmental conservation or wildlife preservation. Children at this time develop logical reasoning from intuitive reasoning. For example, they learn to add and subtract to obtain an answer to a problem. Children also learn about cause-and-effect relationships at this age; for example, they know that a stone will not float because it is heavier than water.

Money is a concept that gains meaning for children when they start school. By the time they are 7 or 8 years old, children usually know the value of most coins. The concept of time is also learned at this age. By 6 years of age, children enter school; the schedule in school helps

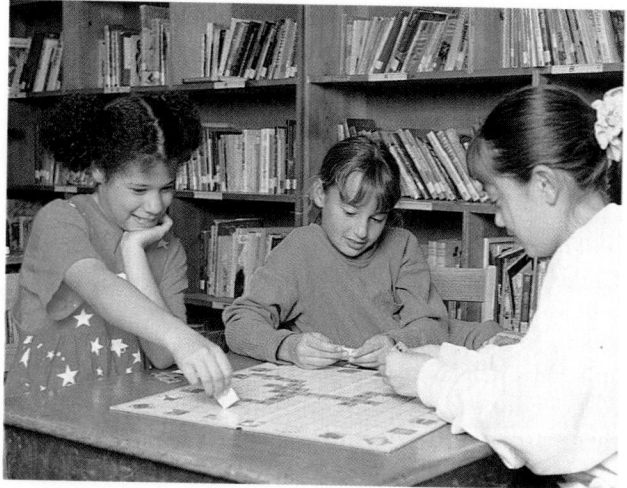

Figure 24–7 Expanding cognitive skills enable school-age children to interact cooperatively in activities of an increasingly complex nature, as shown by the children playing this board game.

them learn time periods. However, it is not until 9 or 10 years of age that children are able to understand the long periods of time in the past. Knowing the time of day and the day of the week are relatively easy for children because they relate time to routine activities. For example, a girl may go to school Monday through Friday, play on Saturday, go to Sunday school on Sunday morning, and go out with her father Sunday afternoon. Children are beginning to read a clock by the time they are 6 years old.

Later in childhood reading skills are usually well developed, and what a child reads is largely influenced by the family. By 9 years of age, most children are self-motivated. They compete with themselves, and they like to plan in advance. By 12 years, they are motivated by inner drive rather than by competition with peers. They like to talk, to discuss different subjects, and to debate.

MORAL DEVELOPMENT

Some school-age children are at Kohlberg's stage 1 of the *preconventional level* (punishment and obedience); that is, they act to avoid being punished. Some school-age children, however, are at stage 2 (*instrumental-relativist orientation*). These children do things to benefit themselves. Fairness, that is, everyone getting a fair share or chance, becomes important. Later in childhood, most children progress to the *conventional* level. This level has two stages: Stage 3 is the "good boy–nice girl" stage, and stage 4 is the *law and order orientation.* Children usually reach the conventional level between the ages of 10 and 13. The child shifts from the concrete interests of individuals to the interests of groups. The motivation for moral action at this stage is to live up to what significant others think of the child. See Table 23–6 on page 578.

SPIRITUAL DEVELOPMENT

According to Fowler, the school-age child is at stage 2 in spiritual development, the *mythical-literal stage.* Children learn to distinguish fantasy from fact. Spiritual facts are those beliefs that are accepted by a religious group,

Table 24–6 Examples of Nursing Diagnoses and Goals for the School-Age Child

NANDA Diagnosis	Goal/Outcome Criteria	Interventions
High risk for injury related to active participation in sports activities	The child will be able to remain free from injury, as evidenced by ▪ Verbalization and/or utilization by parents and child of safety measures and equipment during sports activities. ▪ No record of accidental injuries during playing of sports.	Assess school and playground rules and regulations for safety measures. Provide parents and child with information on safety equipment and measures for participating in sports activities.
Altered nutrition: more than body requirements related to dietary intake pattern, activity, and weight increase	The child will demonstrate within 2 months appropriate nutrition, as evidenced by ▪ Selection of appropriate foods for meals and snacks by child and parent. ▪ Participation in activities that encourage physical exercise. ▪ Weight within normal range for child's height.	Provide information for parents and child on appropriate nutrition for a school-age child. Refer child to peer group which engages in planned physical activities on a regular basis. Assess child's weight and dietary history each month.

whereas fantasy is thoughts and images formed in the child's mind. Parents and the minister, rabbi, or priest help the child distinguish fact from fantasy. These people still influence the child more than peers in spiritual matters. See Table 16–2 on page 314.

When children do not understand such events as the creation of the world, they use fantasy to explain them. The school-age child needs to have concepts such as prayer presented in concrete terms. For example, the child thinks of God as having human qualities, such as a kind old man or a person who punishes when behavior does not meet his standards.

School-age children may ask many questions about God and religion in these years and will generally believe that God is good and always present to help. Just before puberty, children become aware that their prayers are not always answered and become disappointed. At this age, some children reject religion, whereas others continue to accept it. This decision is largely influenced by the parents. If a child continues religious training, the child is ready to apply reason rather than blind belief in most situations.

HEALTH ASSESSMENT

During the assessment interview, the nurse responds to questions from the parent, gives appropriate feedback, and lends encouragement and support to the parent. The nurse also demonstrates interest in the child and enthusiasm for the child's strengths. Assessment guidelines for growth and development of the school-age child are shown in the accompanying box. Examples of NANDA nursing diagnoses, goals/outcome criteria, and interventions for the school-age child are shown in Table 24–6.

The school-age child can begin to take responsibility for self-care and be encouraged to utilize appropriate preventive measures, such as good nutrition and dental care. Most children in this age group still require adult supervision of their health maintenance activities. The following topics can be discussed with the parents and/or the child.

PROMOTING HEALTH AND WELLNESS

Health Maintenance Visits and Immunization The school-age child should have annual health maintenance visits as well as routine dental care. Usually, children have received all of their immunizations prior to their entry into school. Health promotion education should focus on teaching children healthy life-style habits (Igoe 1992, p. 291).

Regular dental checkups are required during these years. Permanent teeth begin to appear at about 7 years and are usually all in place except for the third molars

ASSESSMENT GUIDELINES

The School-Age Child

In the following developmental areas, does the school-age child

Physical Development

- Demonstrate physical growth (weight, height) within normal range?
- Manifest vital signs within normal range for age?
- Exhibit vision and hearing abilities within normal range?
- Demonstrate male or female prepubertal changes within normal range?

Motor Development

- Possess coordinated motor skills for age? For example, by 12 years of age, is the child able to
  - Do tricks on a bike, climb a tree, shinny up a rope?
  - Throw and catch a small ball?
  - Play a musical instrument?

Psychosocial Development

- Perform psychosocial developmental milestones for age? For example, by 12 years of age, is the child able to
  - Make friends of the same sex and establish a peer group?
  - Become less dependent on family and venture away from them?
  - Interact well with parents?
  - Control strong and impulsive feelings?
  - Participate in organized competitions?
  - Read, print, and manipulate numbers and letters easily?
  - Exhibit a concept of money and make change for small amounts of money?
  - Express self in a logical manner and talk through problems?
  - Enjoy riddles and read and understand comics?
  - Invest in a hobby or collection?
  - Like to help others?
  - Think of self as likeable and healthy?

Development in Activities of Daily Living

- Demonstrate concern for personal cleanliness and appearance?
- Express need for privacy?

SAFETY HIGHLIGHTS FOR SCHOOL-AGE CHILDREN

- Teach child safety rules for recreational and sports activities: never to swim alone; always wear a life jacket when in a boat; and wear protective helmets, knee, and elbow pads when needed.
- Supervise contact sports and activities in which child aims at a target.
- Teach child to obey all traffic and safety rules for bicycling, skateboarding, and roller skating.
- Teach child to use light or reflective clothing when walking or cycling at night.
- Teach child safe ways to use the stove, garden tools, and other equipment.
- Supervise child when the child uses saws, electrical appliances, tools, and other potentially dangerous equipment.
- Teach child not to play with fireworks, gunpowder, or firearms. Keep firearms unloaded, locked up, and out of reach.
- Teach child to avoid excavations, quarries, vacant buildings, and playing around heavy machinery.
- Teach child the effects of drugs and alcohol on judgment and coordination.

(wisdom teeth) by 12 years of age. Nurses may need to teach children and their parents about regular dental checkups and dental hygiene. See Chapter 29 for additional information.

Safety By the time children attend school, they are learning to think before they act. They often prefer adult equipment to toys. They want to be active with other children in such activities as bicycling, hiking, swimming, and boating. Although sensitive to peer pressure, the school-age child responds to rules. Children of this age engage in fantasy and magical thinking. They often imitate actions of parents and superheroes with whom they identify.

Accidents are the leading cause of death in school-age children. The most frequent causes of fatalities, in descending order, are motor vehicle accidents, drownings, fires, and firearms. School-age children are also involved in many minor accidents, frequently resulting from outdoor activities and recreational equipment such as swings, bicycles, skateboards, and swimming pools. Safety highlights for the school-age child are presented in the box at the top of the page.

Nutrition Nutrition continues to be a high priority for growing children. School-age children require a balanced diet including 2400 kcal per day. School-age children eat three meals a day and one or two nutritious snacks. Children need a protein-rich food at breakfast to sustain the prolonged physical and mental effort required at school. Studies have shown that children who skip breakfast become inattentive and restless by late morning and have decreased problem-solving ability (Baker & Henry 1987, p. 116). Undernourished children become fatigued easily and face a greater risk of infection, resulting in frequent absences from school.

The average healthy 8-year-old weighing 30 kg (66 lb) requires about 1750 mL of fluid per day (Mott et al 1990, p. 925). Many school-age children have only one meal a day with their family, at dinner. Mealtime should be a social time enjoyed by all, and parents should refrain from discussing a child's poor eating habits at this time. Parents should be aware that children learn many of their food habits by observing their parents. Eating a balanced diet should be the norm for both parent and child.

The school-age child generally eats lunch at school. The child may bring lunch from home or buy lunch at the school cafeteria. Many dietary problems stem from this independence in food choices. The children may trade their food, not eat lunch at all, or buy sweets or junk food with their lunch money. Parents should discuss with the child the foods that they should eat and continue to provide a balanced diet in the home setting. For additional information see Chapter 37.

Poor eating habits may result in obesity. Obesity in school-age children tends to result in decreased activity as well as psychosocial problems. Obese children may be ridiculed by their peers and discriminated against by peers and adults. Such behavior reinforces an already low self-esteem. Counseling should include the following:

- Reviewing the child's eating habits, including snacks
- Altering meal content
- Using rewards other than food
- Regular exercise

Elimination The school-age child's elimination system reaches maturity during this period. The kidneys double in size between ages 5 and 10. During this period, the child urinates six to eight times a day and averages one to two bowel movements per day. **Enuresis,** which is defined as the involuntary passing of urine when control should be established, can be a problem for some school-age children. About 10% of all 6-year-olds experience difficulty controlling the bladder. **Nocturnal enuresis,** or bed-wetting, is the involuntary passing of urine during sleep. Bed-wetting should not be considered a problem until after the age of 6. The incidence of nocturnal enuresis declines as the child matures. About 75% of the children with bed-wetting problems experience this problem because of a small bladder capacity.

Bed-wetting can be a very stressful situation for both parents and children. Parents need information and emotional support from the nurse to help them deal effectively with this problem. The nurse can offer the following general guidelines concerning enuresis:

- Children should not be punished for bed-wetting; they are not doing it on purpose.
- Parents should not feel that bed-wetting is their fault.
- The child should maintain proper daily hygiene and have a supply of clothes and bed linen available.
- The parents and child should come to an agreement on how to handle the laundry problem; children should have a role in this process.
- Any discussion of the problem should be limited to the parents and the child involved; the privacy and self-esteem of the child should always be an important consideration.
- The child may be helped by limiting fluids after supper and urinating prior to bedtime.

Rest/Sleep The school-age child sleeps between 8 and 12 hours a night without daytime naps. The 8-year-old requires at least 10 hours of sleep each night. As the child approaches 11 or 12 years of age, less sleep is required and bedtime may be as late as 10 PM. Although some children still experience night awakenings due to nightmares, this problem continues to decrease with age. Most school-age children have less resistance to bedtime and enjoy a quiet, private period of reading or listening to the radio before falling asleep.

Activity/Exercise Most school-age children are very active physically. During this period, motor skills increase. Children enjoy a variety of group activities, such as baseball and hockey, and individual activities, such as bicycle riding, ice-skating, and dancing. These activities help the child to develop coordination, balance, and strength and enhance social, cognitive, and personal development. Parents can support and promote growth and development by being aware of the activities in the community and by encouraging their children's participation. Children also enjoy having parents and siblings attend their games or activities. Parental supervision may sometimes be required to ascertain that children's pursuits

RESEARCH NOTE

How Do School-Age Boys and Girls Perceive Health and Manage Their Own Health Behaviors?

Social and economic influences over the last two decades have greatly decreased parental supervision and increased children's responsibility for their own health-related activities. In addition, accidents are the leading cause of death in this age group. The purpose of this study was to describe and compare health perceptions and behaviors of school-age boys and girls. Eighty-three school-age children (43 girls and 40 boys) between the ages of 6 and 12 attending an afterschool program were interviewed. The afterschool program, located in a small Southern city, was designed for children of all ethnic and socioeconomic groups. An age-appropriate interview was designed consisting of 34 open-ended questions in the areas of demographic characteristics, health status, life-style practices, nutrition, dental health, and care of minor injuries.

The results of the study indicate that the children perceived their overall health status as favorable. This finding is not unexpected, because the school-age period is one of generally good health. However, the study results indicated several areas of concern. Regarding nutrition intake, 58% of the children reported eating snacks laden with empty calories. Regarding home safety, 54% of the children reported that they had been locked out of the house on one or more occasions. Regarding seat belt use, 39% of the children reported they did not consistently wear seat belts in spite of their state having a mandatory seat belt use law. Regarding dental care, 34% of the children reported fewer dentist visits than is recommended for this age group.

Implications: This research indicates that although school-age children generally view themselves as healthy and manage their care fairly well, the areas of nutrition, home and car safety, and dental care need improvement. Health teaching should focus on areas of concern and include both parents and children. Education is especially important during this period in childhood because health habits that will persist throughout life are being established.

Source: MV Graham and CR Uphold, Health perceptions and behaviors on school-age boys and girls, *Journal of Community Health Nursing*, March/April 1992, 9:77–86.

coincide with their abilities and developmental level. In this regard, parents need to have realistic expectations about their children's abilities.

The skills, attitudes, and habits girls and boys develop during childhood, particularly during school-age, often set the groundwork for activities pursued as adults. Participation in a variety of activities during the early school-age period may help children to find one or more activities of special interest or in which they have a particular skill.

Children who learn, enjoy, and develop confidence in individual and group activities often pursue these interests throughout their college years and into adulthood. Parents should also be aware that they serve as role models for their child. Children may benefit from observing their parents' involvement in outdoor exercise and other healthy activities.

Sexuality By the age of 6, the child usually has a strong identification with the parent of the same sex. During the period from 6 to 12 years of age, children must learn the role and concepts of their gender as part of the total self-concept. In recent years, the stereotypical roles and behaviors for both sexes have changed. Many more women in North America now enter the fields of business, law, and medicine. In general, men have not entered the traditional women's professions, such as nursing and teaching, to the same extent. More men, however, are involved with child care and household tasks.

Beginning at about 8 or 9 years, children become very concerned about specific sex roles and often approach their parents with very explicit concerns about sexuality and reproduction. If parents cannot answer these questions, children will attempt to obtain the information from peers. To promote healthy development, the nurse should provide parents and children with opportunities to express their concerns and ask questions regarding sex. The nurse should answer all questions with factual data and perhaps follow up with appropriate books and other material. Parents should be advised to discuss basic information regarding sexual intercourse, menstruation, and reproduction with their children at about 10 years of age. Many parents may find it helpful to give children reading material and then discuss this material with them. Some parents may find it difficult to discuss sexual issues with their children and avoid doing so. Parents should be aware that if they do not provide such information, their children will seek answers from their peers and that the answers they obtain will frequently be incorrect or incomplete.

Social Interactions Socially, children want to be accepted by their peers and enjoy having a best friend. School-age children often ridicule those whom they perceive as different from themselves, such as children with glasses or physical defects or those who have different clothes, skills, skin color, or religion. Parents can assist school-age children in their development by teaching and reinforcing the fact they should not be cruel to children or adults that are different from themselves. Parents can also act as role models in this regard.

The school-age child has an understanding of right and wrong. Eight-year-olds know that breaking rules can

Health Promotion Highlights for School-Age Children

Instruct parents about the following:

Health Maintenance Visits

- Annual physical examination

Protective Measures

- Immunizations as recommended
- Screening for tuberculosis
- Periodic vision, speech, and hearing screenings
- Regular dental screenings and fluoride treatment
- Providing accurate information about sexual issues (eg, reproduction, AIDS)

School-Age Child Safety

- Using proper equipment when participating in sports and other physical activities (eg, helmets, pads)
- Encouraging child to take responsibility for own safety (eg, participating in bicycle and water safety courses)

Nutrition

- Importance of child not skipping meals and eating a balanced diet
- Experiences with food that may lead to obesity

Elimination

- Utilizing positive approaches for elimination problems (eg, enuresis)

Play and Social Interactions

- Providing opportunities for a variety of organized group activities
- Accepting realistic expectations of child's abilities
- Acting as role models in acceptance of other persons who may be different
- Providing a home environment that limits TV viewing and video games and encourages completion of homework

result in punishment from their parents or teachers. To avoid facing that danger, they often tell the story from their perspective. A parent who understands the normal moral behavior of the age level can deal with the child by calmly reviewing the rules and their importance and also explaining the importance of telling the truth. As children mature throughout the school-age period, they develop a better understanding of the need to tell the truth.

An issue of recent importance in some communities is whether children with acquired immune deficiency syndrome (AIDS) should be allowed to attend public schools. Schools may handle this problem in a variety of ways. In some situations, the student with AIDS has been taught at home; in other situations, only a few people are informed of the child's diagnosis. Although no casual spread of AIDS has been reported, children and their parents often face severe discrimination and harassment from frightened families.

The nurse is in a key position to assist families and to protect the child, as well as to teach the community the facts about AIDS, which can benefit the entire community. Knowledge and discussion help to decrease fears, abolish myths, and deal with necessary issues using a rational approach. The nurse should also serve as an advocate for the child and the family and facilitate decisions that will enable the child to attain optimum physical, emotional, and cognitive development.

Cognitive Stimulation The school-age child learns a variety of concepts and ideas through academic subjects such as mathematics, science, and reading and through play activities such as collections, hobbies, games, and field trips. Language skills continue to expand, and memory capabilities increase. To promote proper development of cognitive abilities, the nurse should screen the child for any vision or hearing problems. Parents can promote cognitive development by encouraging reading, showing interest in the child's work, and providing a home environment in which the child can complete home assignments. School-age children enjoy watching TV and playing video games, and parents may have to set time limits on these activities. Parents should also be aware of the child's progress in school, have realistic expectations of their child's abilities, and be encouraged to report any concerns to the teacher or to the school nurse.

School nurses play an important role in working with families to assess for learning difficulties. A nurse usually interviews the parents in the home to gather information about the family history, including learning difficulties, speech problems, or environmental problems. Nurses also interpret test results and provide ongoing counseling and support to the parent.

Parental instruction in stimulation and other health-promotion activities for the school-age child are summarized in the box on the previous page.

CHAPTER HIGHLIGHTS

- A sense of trust and security in the newborn is essential for subsequent development; the infant derives this sense from parental love, warmth, and prompt attention to physical needs.
- An essential nursing function is assessment of the newborn's physical status by the Apgar scoring system.
- Measurements of length, weight, head and chest circumferences, fontanelle size and status, reflex abilities, and motor development are important indicators of the newborn's growth and health.
- Infants from 1 month to 1 year reveal marked growth in size and stature with appropriate nutrition and care: Birth weight doubles by 5 months and triples by 12 months.
- During infancy, motor development is notable: At 3 months, infants can raise their heads from the prone position; at 6 months, they can sit unsupported; and at 12 months, they can stand momentarily and walk with help.
- To develop cognitively, the infant needs a variety of sensory and motor stimuli.
- The nurse can assess the psychosocial and motor development of infants by using the Denver Developmental Screening Test and similar tests.
- Attachment between the mother and the newborn is crucial for the optimum physical and emotional development of the infant.
- Good nutritional habits begin in infancy. The nurse should provide parents with appropriate information on the nutritional needs of the child at each developmental stage.
- Early childhood spans the period from 1 to 6 years and is subdivided into two groups: the toddler group, ages 1 to 3, and the preschool group, ages 4 and 5.

- During childhood, dramatic changes occur in physical, psychologic, and cognitive development; the child moves from being a dependent person to becoming an independent person entering school.
- As the nervous system develops, body systems mature to the point where the child can control the body, achieve finer muscle control, and perform all the activities of daily living, such as washing and dressing.
- The child also develops a unique personality and way of behaving.
- Critical to psychosocial development during childhood is the development of a sense of autonomy and initiative.
- Toddlers engage in endless activity. The types of toddler play include onlooker play, such as watching TV; solitary play, such as independent activities; parallel play, such as sitting beside other children while playing; and associative play, which is engaging in activity with others.
- During the toddler stage, parents should read labels and be aware that table foods provide more variety and are less expensive and more nutritious than prepared toddler foods.
- Estimates are that 80% of preschool children have some tooth decay. Parents should provide instruction in dental care and limit the intake of sugary snacks.
- By the end of early childhood, the child has reached the phase of intuitive thought in cognitive development, has developed some internal moral controls, and is at the undifferentiated level of spiritual development.
- The school-age period of development begins at age 6 and ends with the onset of puberty.
- School-age children perfect their muscular skills and coordination and develop a sense of competence, perseverance, and self-worth.
- During emotional development, school-age children face Erickson's conflict of industry versus inferiority.
- Peers are very important to school-age children; same-sex friendships develop.
- School-age children begin to understand relationships and change from being egocentric to having cooperative interactions; according to Piaget, they are in the concrete operations phase of cognitive development.
- Most school-age children progress to the conventional level of moral development and to the mythical-literal stage of spiritual development.
- As children reach school age, they can begin to take more responsibility for self-care and utilize appropriate preventive measures such as good nutrition and dental care.
- During the school-age period, children engage in a variety of group and individual activities that help to develop coordination, balance, and strength, as well as enhance social, cognitive, and personal development.
- During the school-age period, parents need to be aware of the child's progress in school and have realistic expectations of their child's abilities.
- Assessment activities for health promotion are related to the specific developmental stage of the child.
- During the assessment, the nurse observes the interactions of the child and the parent and listens for areas of concern or questions that the parent may have.
- Intervention for health promotion includes parent teaching in regard to the importance of regular health maintenance visits, immunizations according to suggested schedule, and screening for early detection of disorders such as tuberculosis.
- The health promotion of a child is affected by sex, racial, social, and economic factors as well as the type of family environment provided.
- The nurse assists parents in health promotion by providing information and support related to the developmental level of the child.
- Accidents are the leading cause of death in toddlers, preschool, and school-age children. Parents need specific teaching at each developmental level in relation to the potential safety hazards of the age group.
- The nurse should teach parents specific play activities for each developmental stage that promote healthy language, sensory, and cognitive development.

READINGS AND REFERENCES

SUGGESTED READINGS

Weigley, ES. September/October 1990. Changing patterns in offering solids to infants. *Pediatric Nursing* 16:439–41.
This author summarizes the historical aspects and factors that have influenced opinions about what stage to introduce solid food to infants. Currently, it is thought that developmental readiness favors beginning solids at 4 to 6 months. However, the author notes that caregivers may receive conflicting advice because of earlier practices of feeding infants solids as early as the first week of life.

Winkelstein, ML. May/June 1989. Fostering positive self-concept in the school-age child. *Pediatric Nursing* 15:229–33.
A healthy self-concept is an important component of the normal development of the school-age child. Pediatric nurses in schools and hospitals have frequent contacts with children and can be influential in fostering their positive self-concept during these years. This author describes a self-concept program consisting of three major sections and several learning objectives. A chart provides details about learning experiences and instructional materials for each objective. The nurse can use these interventions to assess the child's self-concept, provide opportunities for positive growth, and create opportunities for parental discussion.

RELATED RESEARCH

Castiglia, PT, Glenister, AM, Haughey, BP, and Kanski, GW. May/June 1989. Influences on children's attitudes toward alcohol consumption. *Pediatric Nursing* 3:263–68.

Graham, MV and Uphold, CR. March/April 1992. Health perceptions and behaviors of school-age boys and girls. *Journal of Community Health Nursing* 9:77–86.

Hauck, MR. April 1991. Mothers' descriptions of the toilet-training process: A phenomenologic study. *Journal of Pediatric Nursing* 6:80–86.

SELECTED REFERENCES

Baker, S and Henry, R. 1987. *Parents' Guide to Nutrition.* Menlo Park, CA: Addison-Wesley.

Balsmeyer, B. September/October 1990. Sleep disturbances of the infant and toddler. *Pediatric Nursing* 16:447–52.

Castiglia, PT. May/June 1987. Speech-language development. *Journal of Pediatric Health Care* 1:165–67.

Engel, GL. 1962. *Psychological Development in Health and Disease.* Philadelphia: WB Saunders.

Hauck, MR. August 1991. Cognitive abilities of preschool children: Implications for nurses working with young children. *Journal of Pediatric Nursing* 6:230–35.

Igoe, J. May/June 1992. Health promotion, health protection, and disease prevention in childhood. *Pediatric Nursing* 18:291–92.

Kattwinkel, J, Brooks, J, and Myerberg, D. June 1992. Positioning and AIDS. *Pediatrics* 89:1120–26.

Mott, SR, James, SR, and Sperhac, AM. 1990. *Nursing Care of Infants and Families.* 2d ed. Redwood City, CA: Addison-Wesley Nursing.

Murray, R and Zenter, J. 1993. *Nursing Assessment and Health Promotion Through the Life Span.* 5th ed. Englewood Cliffs, NJ: Prentice Hall.

Pinyerd, BJ. September/October 1992. Assessment of infant growth. *Journal of Pediatric Health Care* 6:302–8.

Peter, G. December 1992. Childhood immunizations. *New England Journal of Medicine* 327:1774–1800.

Schulman, M and Mekler, E. 1985. *Bringing Up a Moral Child: A New Approach for Teaching Your Child to be Kind, Just and Responsible.* Reading, MA: Addison-Wesley.

Sieving, RE, and Zirbel-Donisch, ST. November/December 1990. Development and enhancement of self-esteem in children. *Journal of Pediatric Nursing* 4:290–96.

Snow, LS, and Fry, ME. September/October 1990. Formula feeding in the first year of life. *Pediatric Nursing* 15:442–45.

Wade, G. March/April 1992. Update on the Denver II. *Pediatric Nursing* 18:140–41.

25 Adolescence Through Middle Adulthood

Objectives

Explain the essential changes in physical development from adolescence through middle adulthood.

Explain psychosocial development of adolescents, young adults, and middle-aged adults according to Erikson.

Explain the essential changes in cognitive development from adolescence through middle adulthood as postulated by Piaget.

Describe moral development of adolescents, young adults, and middle-aged adults according to Kohlberg.

Discuss spiritual development of adolescents, young adults, and middle-aged adults according to Fowler.

Identify common health hazards and concerns of adolescents, young adults, and middle-aged adults.

Discuss nursing implications related to common health concerns.

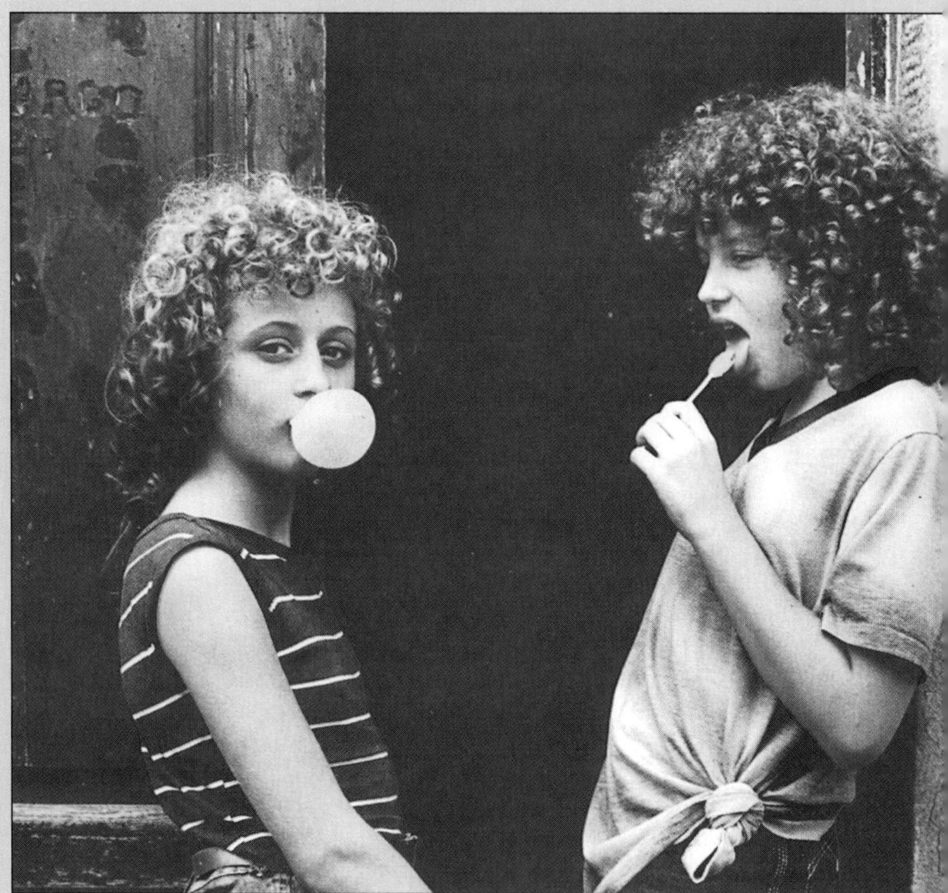

This chapter continues the health assessment and promotion of health and wellness for adolescents, young adults, and middle-aged adults. As with the previous chapter, each developmental stage includes physical, psychosocial, cognitive, moral, and spiritual aspects.

ADOLESCENCE

Adolescence is the period during which the person becomes physically and psychologically mature and acquires a personal identity. At the end of this critical period in development, the person is ready to enter adulthood and assume its responsibilities. The length of adolescence is culturally determined to some extent. In North America, adolescence is longer than in some cultures, extending to 18 to 20 years of age.

Puberty is the first stage of adolescence in which sexual organs begin to grow and mature. **Menarche** (onset of menstruation) begins in girls. **Ejaculation** (expulsion of semen) occurs in boys. For girls, puberty normally starts between 10 and 14 years; for boys, between 12 and 16 years. The adolescent period is often subdivided into three stages: early adolescence lasts from ages 12 to 13; middle adolescence extends from 14 to 16 years; and late adolescence extends from 17 to 18 or 20 years. Late adolescence is a more stable stage than the other two. In the late period, adolescents are involved mostly with planning their future and economic independence.

PHYSICAL DEVELOPMENT

During puberty, growth is markedly accelerated compared to the slow, steady growth of the child. This period, marked by sudden and dramatic physical changes, is referred to as the *adolescent growth spurt.* In boys, the growth spurt usually begins between ages 12 and 16; in girls, it begins earlier, usually between ages 10 and 14. Because the growth spurt begins earlier in girls, many girls surpass boys in height at this time.

Physical Growth Physical growth continues throughout adolescence. Growth is fastest for boys at about 14 years, and the maximum height is often reached at about 18 or 19 years. Some men add another 1 or 2 cm to their height during their 20s, as the vertebral column gradually continues to grow. During the period of 10 to 18 years of age, the average American male doubles his weight, gaining about 32 kg (72 lb), and grows about 41 cm (16 in) (James et al 1990, pp. 1917–18). The fastest rate of growth in girls occurs at about age 12; they reach their maximum height at about 15 to 16 years. During ages 10 to 18, the average American female gains about 25 kg (55 lb) and grows about 24 cm (9 in) (James et al 1990, pp. 1914–15).

Physical growth during adolescence is greatly influenced by a number of factors, such as heredity, nutrition, medical care, illness, physical and emotional environment, family size, and culture. Generally, people in the United States have grown taller in recent years. This increase in average height is thought to be due to many of the above factors.

Growth is noted first in the musculoskeletal system. This growth follows a sequential pattern: The head, hands, and feet are the first to grow to adult status. Next, the extremities reach their adult size. Because the extremities grow before the trunk, the adolescent looks leggy, awkward, and uncoordinated. After the trunk grows to full size, the shoulders, chest, and hips grow. Skull and facial bones also change proportions: The forehead becomes more prominent, and the jawbones develop.

Poor posture is a common problem during adolescence. The risk for postural problems increases among this age group because weight gains may precede a corresponding strengthening of postural muscles.

Glandular Changes The eccrine and apocrine glands increase their secretions and become fully functional during puberty. The **eccrine glands,** found over most of the body, produce sweat. The **apocrine glands** develop in the axillae, anal and genital areas, external auditory canals and around the umbilicus and the areola of the breasts. Apocrine sweat is released onto the skin in response to emotional stimuli only.

Sebaceous glands also become active under the influence of androgens in both males and females. The sebaceous glands, which secrete **sebum,** become most active on the face, neck, shoulder, upper back, chest, and genitals. When these glands become plugged and inflamed, the result is **acne,** a condition common in adolescence. Noninflammatory acne appears as open and closed **comedones** (whiteheads and blackheads). Inflammatory acne appears as inflamed skin together with pustules and papules. A **pustule** is a visible collection of pus within the epidermis. A **papule** is a superficial, circumscribed elevation of the skin. Inflammatory acne may cause scarring.

Sexual Characteristics During puberty, both primary and secondary sex characteristics develop. **Primary sexual characteristics** relate to the organs necessary for reproduction, such as the testes, penis, vagina, and uterus. **Secondary sexual characteristics** differentiate the male from the female but do not relate directly to reproduction. Examples are pubic hair growth, breast development, and voice changes.

The first noticeable sign that puberty has begun in males is the appearance of pubic hair. The milestone of male puberty is considered to be the first ejaculation, which commonly occurs at about 14 years of age. Fertility follows several months later. Sexual maturity is achieved by age 18.

Often the first noticeable sign of puberty in females is the appearance of the **breast bud,** although the appearance of hair along the labia may precede this. The milestone of female puberty is the menarche, which occurs about 2 years after the breast bud appears. At first, mentrual periods are scanty and irregular and may occur without ovulation. Ovulation is usually established 1 to 2 years after menarche. Female internal reproductive organs reach adult size about age 18 to 20.

PSYCHOSOCIAL DEVELOPMENT

According to Erikson (1963, p. 261), the adolescent seeks answers to the questions "Who am I?" and "What am I to be?" The psychosocial task of the adolescent is the *establishment of identity.* The danger of this stage is role confusion. See Table 23–4 on page 574. The inability to settle on an occupational identity commonly disturbs the adolescent. Less commonly, doubts about sexual identity arise. Because of the adolescent's dramatic body changes, the development of a stable identity is difficult. Erikson says that adolescents help one another through this identity crisis by forming cliques and a separate youth culture. These cliques often exclude all those who are "different" in skin color, cultural background, aspects of dress, gestures, and tastes.

Adolescents are usually concerned about their bodies, their appearances, and their physical abilities. Hair styling, skin care, and clothes become very important. Ingroupers of an adolescent clique can be excessively clannish and cruel in excluding out-groupers; this intolerance is a temporary defense against identity confusion (Erikson 1963, p. 236).

In their search for a new identity, adolescents have to refight the battles of many of the previous stages of development. The task of developing trust in self and others is again encountered when adolescents look for ideal persons whom they can trust and with whom they can prove trustworthy. Development of autonomy is restaged in their search for ways to express their right to choose freely. The search for an occupational role that allows expression of an autonomous, freely chosen direction is one example. Free choice and autonomy present conflicts to the adolescent. Conflict arises between behaving well in the eyes of the parents and behaving in a manner that may expose them to the ridicule of their peers. The sense of initiative is also restaged. The adolescent has unlimited imagination and ambition and aspires to great accomplishments. The sense of industry is reenacted when the adolescent chooses a career. The extent to which these tasks were achieved earlier influences the adolescent's ability to achieve a healthy self-concept and self-identity.

The adolescent needs to establish a **self-concept** that accepts both personal strengths and weaknesses. Faced with dramatic changes in body structure and function and greater expectations to assume responsibilities, many adolescents experience temporary difficulty in developing a positive self-image. Adolescents who are accepted, loved, and valued by family and peers generally tend to gain confidence and feel good about themselves. Adolescents who have difficulty forming relationships or who are perceived by peers as too different and not included in adolescent cliques may develop less favorable self-images and have low self-esteem. Adolescents need to learn to build on their strengths and not be preoccupied by such problems as acne.

Teenagers with physical handicaps or illnesses are particularly vulnerable to peer rejection. Nurses and educators can promote peer understanding and acceptance by discussing the individual's specific problems with the peer group. Adolescents gain self-concepts largely from the impressions that others have of them. If others accept defects—for example, a lost finger—teenagers accept those defects more readily. Establishing groups of peers who have similar problems can provide an opportunity for the individual to develop close relationships with others and feel valued and accepted.

Although sexual **identification** begins at about 3 or 4 years of age, it is a significant part of adolescence. The adolescent male strives to achieve a masculine sexual identity; the adolescent female, a feminine sexual identity. Because sex roles are becoming less defined in North American society, adopting masculine and feminine roles is increasingly confusing to today's adolescent. Job and family roles are less traditional and sex-specific. In forming a sexual identity, adolescents first fantasize the male or female role and then enact various aspects of that imagined role. In response to their own feelings and that of others, aspects of the role are either adopted or rejected. Later, adolescents begin to establish intimacy with a partner or partners. This intimacy lays the groundwork for the commitments of adulthood. Sexual experimentation is not part of true intimacy, but once intimacy is achieved, sexual activity is included.

Adolescents are sexually active and may engage in masturbation as well as heterosexual and homosexual activity. Homosexual activity during adolescence is not necessarily an indicator of sexual preference because both gay and nongay adolescents may experiment sexually with persons of the same and opposite sex.

About the age of 15 years, many adolescents gradually draw away from the family and gain independence. This *need for independence* combined with the need for family support sometimes creates conflict within the adolescent and between the adolescent and the family. The young person may appear hostile or depressed at times during this painful process. At this age, adolescents prefer to be with their peers rather than their parents and may seek advice from adults other than their parents. Parents sometimes are bewildered by this stage of development; instead of reducing controls, they increase them, causing the adolescent to rebel.

Adolescents also have to resolve their ambivalent feelings toward the parent of the opposite sex. As part of the resolution, adolescents may develop brief crushes on adults outside the family—teachers or neighbors, for example. Adolescents sometimes adopt some of the attributes of the adults with whom they are infatuated. This modeling can be helpful in the maturing process.

Some of the discord in the family at this time is due to the generation gap. The values of the adolescent may differ from those of the parents. This difference may be difficult for the parents to understand and to accept. Adolescents still need guidance from their parents, although they appear neither to want it nor to need it. However, adolescents need to know that their parents care about them and that their parents still want to help them. Restrictions and guidance need to be presented in a manner that makes adolescents feel loved. They need consistency in guidance and fewer restrictions than previously. They should have the independence they can handle yet know that their parents will assist them when they need help.

During adolescence, **peer groups** assume great importance (Figure 25–1). The peer group has a number of functions. It provides a sense of belonging, pride, social learning, and sexual roles. Most peer groups have well-defined, sex-specific modes of acceptable behavior. In adolescence, the peer groups change with age. They start as single-sex groups, evolve to mixed groups, and finally narrow to couples who share activities.

Dating helps prepare adolescents for marriage by teaching them how to act with members of the opposite sex. In the United States, dating starts early, often by 11 years for girls and later, perhaps 15, for boys, although dating ages vary with culture, social class, and pressures from society. Some adolescents initially date in groups of couples and eventually progress to going on dates alone.

Not all adolescents, however, are heterosexual. For homosexuals, adolescence is a difficult time. Because peer acceptance is crucial to self-acceptance, lesbian and gay adolescents usually conform to the heterosexual codes and behaviors of their peer groups even though these do not feel natural or correct. Conforming may exact a great personal cost. Adolescents who choose to be openly gay or lesbian face not only the ostracism of their peers but also the misunderstanding and hostility of parents, teachers, and other important adults.

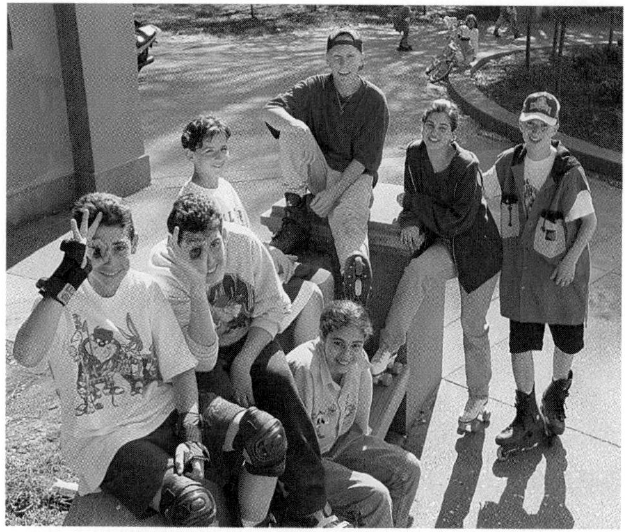

Figure 25–1 Adolescent peer group relationships enhance a sense of belonging, self-esteem, and self-identity.

Cognitive Development

Cognitive abilities mature during adolescence. Between the ages of 11 and 15, the adolescent begins Piaget's *formal operations stage* of cognitive development. See Table 23–5 on page 576. The main feature of this stage is that people can think beyond the present and beyond the world of reality. Adolescents are highly imaginative and idealistic. They consider things that do not exist but that might be and consider ways things could be or ought to be. This type of thinking requires logic, organization, and consistency.

The adolescent becomes more informed about the world and environment. Adolescents use new information to solve everyday problems and can communicate with adults on most subjects. The adolescent's capacity to absorb and use knowledge is great. Adolescents usually select their own areas for learning; they explore interests from which they may evolve a career plan. Study habits and learning skills developed in adolescence are used throughout life.

Moral Development

According to Kohlberg, the young adolescent is usually at the *conventional level* of moral development. Most still accept the Golden Rule and want to abide by social order and existing laws. Adolescents examine their values, standards, and morals. They may discard the values they have adopted from parents in favor of values they consider more suitable.

When adolescents move into the *postconventional* or *principled level,* they start to question the rules and laws of society. Right thinking and right action become a matter of personal values and opinions, which may conflict with societal laws. Adolescents consider the possibility of rationally changing the law and emphasize individual rights. Not all adolescents or even adults proceed to this postconventional level. See Kohlberg's stages of moral development in Table 23–6 on page 578.

SPIRITUAL DEVELOPMENT

According to Fowler, the adolescent or young adult reaches the synthetic-conventional stage of spiritual development. See Table 16–2 on page 314. As adolescents encounter different groups in society, they are exposed to a wide variety of opinions, beliefs, and behaviors regarding religious matters. The adolescent may reconcile the differences in one of the following ways:

- Deciding any differences are wrong
- Compartmentalizing the differences (For example, a friend may not be able to go to dances on Friday evenings because of religious observances, but the friend can share activities on other days.)
- Obtaining advice from a significant other, such as a parent or a minister

Often the adolescent believes that various religious beliefs and practices have more similarities than differences. At this stage, the adolescent's focus is on interpersonal rather than conceptual matters.

Nursing activities relative to this stage of spiritual development include

- Presenting an open, accepting attitude to adolescent's questions and statements regarding spiritual matters and their implications for health.
- Arranging for adolescents to see a member of their religious faith if this is desired. Adolescents may want to talk with members of their church peer group for support.
- Providing a comfortable environment in which adolescents can practice the rituals of their faith.

HEALTH ASSESSMENT

Assessment guidelines for growth and development of the adolescent are shown in the accompanying box. Examples of NANDA nursing diagnoses, goals/outcome criteria, and interventions for the adolescent are shown in Table 25–1.

ASSESSMENT GUIDELINES

The Adolescent

In the following developmental areas, does the adolescent

Physical Development

- Exhibit physical growth (weight, height) within normal range for age and sex?
- Demonstrate male or female sexual development consistent with standards?
- Manifest vital signs within normal range for age and sex?
- Manifest vision and hearing abilities within normal range?

Psychosocial Development

- Interact well with parents, teachers, peers, siblings, and persons in authority?
- Like self?
- Think and plan for the future, such as college or a career?
- Choose a life-style and interests that fit own identity?
- Determine own beliefs and values?
- Begin to establish a sense of identity in the family?
- Seek help from appropriate persons about problems?

Development in Activities of Daily Living

- Demonstrate knowledge of physical development, menstruation, reproduction, and birth control?
- Exhibit healthy life-style practices in nutrition, exercise, recreation, sleep patterns, and personal habits?
- Demonstrate concern for personal cleanliness and appearance?

Adolescents are usually self-directed in meeting their health needs. Because of maturation changes, however, they need teaching and guidance in the several health care areas that follow.

PROMOTING HEALTH AND WELLNESS

Health Maintenance Visits and Immunization The adolescent should receive routine health assessments, appropriate laboratory screening, and periodic dental care.

Table 25–1 Examples of Nursing Diagnoses, Goals and Interventions for the Adolescent

NANDA Diagnosis	Goal/Outcome Criteria	Interventions
Self-esteem disturbance related to diagnosis of chronic disease (diabetes)	The adolescent will demonstrate (within 1 month) increased self-esteem, as evidenced by ▪ Ability to describe self positively. ▪ Exhibiting interests that fit life-style. ▪ Interest in maintaining appearance and personal hygiene. ▪ Ability to interact appropriately with peers and parents.	Listen to the adolescent's feelings, concerns and fears, and refer to counseling as appropriate. Provide accurate information about diabetes to adolescent and peer group. Encourage adolescent to participate in self-care. Refer adolescent to peer groups who have a similar condition.
Altered nutrition: less than body requirements related to dieting pattern	The adolescent will demonstrate (within 2 months) appropriate nutrition, as evidenced by ▪ Selection of appropriate foods for meals and snacks. ▪ Weight appropriate for sex, age, and body build.	Listen to the adolescent's feelings and concerns related to body image and dieting. Provide information on foods and food intake that meet nutritional guidelines. Refer to dietitian for counseling as appropriate. Assess calorie intake and weight each month.

If immunizations required for other age periods have not been received, they should be given at this time. For adolescents who have received the appropriate immunizations, the combined tetanus and diphtheria toxoids (adult-type Td) should be given at about 14 to 16 years of age. Influenza virus vaccine, pneumococcal polysaccharide vaccine, and hepatitis B vaccine should be given to adolescents in selected high-risk groups (Murray & Zentner 1993, p. 397). Rubella (German measles) vaccine is recommended for female adolescents and women of childbearing age who are not protected against the disease. Rubella contracted during the first trimester of pregnancy may cause birth defects of the eyes, heart, and brain.

Safety Accidents are the leading cause of death and injury among adolescents. Motor vehicle accidents (automobiles, motorcycles, minibikes, and snowmobiles) and sports injuries are the most common accidents. Head injuries and fractures frequently result from these accidents. Obtaining a driver's license is an important event in the life of an adolescent in the United States and Canada, but the privilege is not always wisely handled. Teenagers may use driving as an outlet for stress, as a way to assert independence, or as a way to impress peers. When setting limits on automobile use, parents need to assess the teenager's level of responsibility, common sense, and ability to resist peer pressure. The age of the teenager alone does not determine readiness to handle this responsibility.

Adolescents are at risk for sports injuries because their coordination skills are not fully developed. However, sports activities are important to the adolescent's self-esteem and overall development. In addition to providing beneficial exercise, sports activities enhance social and personal development. They help the adolescent experience competition, teamwork, and conflict resolution.

Suicide and homicide are two other leading causes of death among teenagers. Adolescent males are more likely to commit suicide than adolescent females, and African-Americans are more likely to commit homicide than European-Americans. Suicides by firearms, drugs, and automobile exhaust gases are the most common.

Most suicidal persons give verbal or behavioral warnings prior to suicide, and certain tendencies or behavior are suspect. For example, most people who commit suicide have made previous attempts, are severely depressed, have low self-esteem, and are at odds with themselves and those close to them. Such individuals need to be referred to professional help.

Homicide is more common among the poor than other economic classes, and both killers and their victims are more likely to be men than women. Homicide is often associated with alcohol abuse and occurs most frequently at night and on weekends. Factors influencing the high homicide rate include economic deprivation, family breakup, and the availability of firearms, which are the most frequently used weapons. Cutting or stabbing tools are the next most frequently used weapons.

Health-promotion programs for adolescents need to include information about suicide, alternatives to suicide, and ways to deal with a peer who might be suicidal. Safety highlights for the adolescent are found in the box at the top of the next page.

SAFETY HIGHLIGHTS FOR ADOLESCENTS

- Have adolescents complete a driver's education course, and take practice drives with them in various kinds of weather.
- Set firm limits on automobile use, namely, never to drive after drinking or using drugs, and never to ride with a driver who has done so. Encourage adolescents to call home for a ride if they have been drinking, assuring them they can do so without a reprimand.
- Teach adolescents to wear safety helmets when riding motorcycles, scooters, and other sports vehicles. Teach safety rules for water sports.
- Encourage adolescents to use proper equipment when participating in sports. Schedule a physical examination before participation, and be certain there is medical supervision for all athletic activities.
- Encourage adolescents to swim, jog, and go boating in groups so they can obtain help in case of an accident.
- Teach rules for hunting and the proper care and use of firearms.
- Inform the adolescent of the dangers of drugs, alcohol, and unprotected sex. Be alert to changes in the adolescent's mood and behavior. Listen to and maintain open communication with the adolescent. Open communication is a powerful preventive measure.
- Set a good example of behavior that the adolescent can follow.

Skin Care Adolescents need teaching and guidance to help them deal with the changing needs of their bodies. Secretions from newly active sweat glands react with bacteria on the skin, causing a pungent odor. Teenagers need to practice good hygiene to be sure that clothes smell fresh and clean.

A frequent skin problem of the adolescent is acne. The severity of acne varies widely from a few comedones to an intense inflammatory reaction. By the end of the teenage years, it is estimated that about 70% of adolescents will have had acne (Novotny 1989, p. 247).

The nurse should respond with support, guidance, and information to prevent the physical and emotional scarring that can occur with this problem. Problems such as acne may cause teenagers to feel depressed and frustrated at a time when they are already insecure. To treat this problem, the teenagers should wash the affected area thoroughly but gently three times a day. Greasy ointments and make-up should be avoided, and the lesions should not be picked or squeezed. The role of diet and life-style in causing acne has not been determined, but the adolescent should be encouraged to eat a balanced diet and get adequate rest. A variety of oral and topical preparations, such as tetracycline and isotretinoin (Accutane), may be prescribed to treat acne. Accutane, introduced in 1982, is a very potent oral medication that is considered the wonder drug for the treatment of acne (Novotny 1989, p. 247). However, Accutane is a potent *teratogen*, an agent that causes the production of physical defects in developing embryos. The nurse who works with adolescents needs to be familiar with current therapies and their possible side-effects. Teenagers should be assured that scarring can usually be prevented if acne is treated promptly and follow-up care provided.

Nutrition The adolescent's need for nutrients and calories increases, particularly during the growth spurt. In particular, the need for protein, calcium, vitamin D, iron, and B vitamins increases during adolescence. An adequate diet for an adolescent is 1 quart of milk per day as well as appropriate amounts of meat, vegetables, fruits, breads, and cereals.

Many parents may observe that teenagers, particularly boys, seem to be eating all the time. Teenagers have active life-styles and irregular eating patterns. They tend to diet or snack frequently, often eating high-calorie foods such as doughnuts, soft drinks, ice cream, and fast foods. Parents and nurses can promote better lifelong eating habits by encouraging teenagers to eat healthy snacks. Parents can provide healthy snacks such as fruits and cheese and at the same time limit the amount of "junk food" available in the home. The teenager's food choices relate to physical, social, and emotional factors and impulses and may not be influenced by teaching. Nurses need to advise parents that adolescents must take responsibility for their decisions in many areas of life, and parents should avoid conflicts that relate to food.

Common problems related to nutrition and self-esteem among adolescents include obesity, anorexia nervosa, and bulimia. **Obesity** is a common problem of the preadolescent period and continues to be a problem in the adolescent period. It is estimated that 10% to 16% of people between the ages of 10 and 19 years are obese. Obese adolescents are frequently rejected by their peers, badgered by their parents, and ridiculed on television and in the movies. Many feel ugly and socially unacceptable. Depression is not unusual among obese adolescents. Treatment of obesity in this age group includes education on nutrition as well as assessment of psychosocial problems that may produce overeating.

Under social pressure to be slim, some adolescents severely limit their food intake to a level significantly below that required to meet the demands of normal growth. In some instances, the adolescent may develop an eating disorder, such as anorexia or bulimia. Anorexia nervosa and bulimia are severe psychophysiologic conditions usually seen in adolescent girls and young women. **Anorexia nervosa** is characterized by a prolonged inability or refusal to eat, rapid weight loss, and emaciation in persons who continue to believe they are fat. Anorexics may also induce vomiting and use laxatives and diuretics to remain thin. **Bulimia** is an uncontrollable compulsion to consume enormous amounts of food and then expel it by self-induced vomiting or by taking laxatives. These illnesses are most effectively treated in the early stages by psychotherapy. Hospitalization may be necessary when the effects of starvation become life-threatening.

Rest/Sleep Most adolescents require 8 to 10 hours of sleep each night to prevent undue fatigue and susceptibility to infections. A change in sleep pattern is common in adolescence. Children who once were early risers begin to sleep late in the mornings and occasionally take afternoon naps. The reason for daytime sleeping is not fully understood, but it is possibly a result of physical maturity and reduced nocturnal sleep.

During adolescence boys begin to experience **nocturnal emissions** (orgasm and emission of semen during sleep), known as "wet dreams," several times each month. Boys need to be informed about this normal development to prevent embarrassment and fear.

Activity/Exercise Many teenagers engage in a variety of physical activities. In the past, boys were active in team sports, whereas girls took up dancing, ice-skating, and the like. Currently, more girls and young women participate in team sports and, in some cases, try out for the boys' teams and succeed. The experience of working with a team provides physical activity, prevents obesity related to inactivity, and promotes peer group involvement. The experiences of winning and losing and accepting and working with a variety of people prepare teenagers for the team approach of the work force. Nurses and parents should encourage both sexes to develop interests that balance sedentary activity with team involvement. Girls need encouragement at an early age to gain exposure and confidence in team sports that they can pursue during their high school years. Teenagers should have regular health maintenance check-ups to ascertain that they can physically cope with the demands of the program. They should also be taught strengthening and conditioning exercises to prevent sports injuries.

Menstruation Girls need to be taught about the menstrual cycle and necessary self-care responsibilities. Initially, teenagers have irregular menstruation, which may lead to embarrassment because of stained clothing. Teenagers can be taught to be aware of more subtle signs of impending menstruation, such as a tender breast, water retention or bloating, or the appearance of skin eruptions or pimples. Girls also should be counseled regarding the variety of feminine hygiene products available (eg, sanitary pads and tampons) so that they can make intelligent choices. Parents and nurses should advise teenagers to wash their hands thoroughly before inserting a tampon, to change tampons frequently, to alternate them with sanitary pads, and to use pads at night. These measures will help to decrease infection. Thorough cleaning of the genital area and wiping from front to back will also decrease infection and prevent odors.

Dysmenorrhea (painful menstruation) is prevalent among adolescent females and causes much short-term absenteeism. Cramping, lower abdominal pain radiating to the back and upper thighs, nausea, vomiting, diarrhea, and headaches may occur for a few hours up to 3 days. Dysmenorrhea results from powerful uterine contractions, which cause ischemia and, in turn, cramping pain. The symptoms of dysmenorrhea are treated with bed rest, administration of simple analgesics such as aspirin, application of heat to the abdomen, certain exercises, biofeedback (see Chapter 32), and antiprostaglandin medications, such as ibuprofen (Motrin or Advil) and naproxen (Naprosyn).

Sexuality Adolescents want to know about sex but are often uneasy about discussing these concerns with their parents. Nurses, the schools, and the family need to provide accurate information. Parents who have established open communication regarding sexual changes and reproduction during the school-age period are more likely to be asked questions and have discussions with their teenagers regarding sexual issues. Parents and nurses need to recognize all aspects of adolescent development in planning and discussing sex education. During the nursing assessment, teenagers should be asked directly what they know about sex, contraception, and reproduction. Sometimes a lot of the teenager's information is based on popular myths and little, if any, fact. Although sex education programs for high school students are discussed in the literature, only a small percentage of teens has the opportunity to attend these sessions. The nurse should discuss factual information about sex, sexual actions and their consequences, the individual's right to make a decision regarding ways to express oneself sexually, and the responsibilities of each person with respect to sexual activity.

Sexually transmitted diseases (STDs) are the most common bacterial infections among adolescents. One universally fatal STD, acquired immune deficiency syndrome (AIDS), has increased significantly in the adolescent population. Increases in STDs are due to three factors: (a) changing sexual morals of the young, which permit increased sexual activity; (b) a sense of invulnerability; and (c) an increase in the number of sexual partners.

Because the term *sexually transmitted disease* elicits feelings of guilt, shame, and fear, adolescents frequently do not seek medical help as early as they should. Adolescents need education about these diseases, preventive measures, and early treatment. Table 17–4 on page 343 lists the common types and symptoms of STDs for which teenagers should seek medical care.

An important role of the nurse working with teenagers is to provide information regarding birth control. The nurse should inform the teenager about the various methods of birth control: pills, diaphragms, intrauterine devices (IUDs), the rhythm method, and condoms to prevent an unplanned pregnancy.

Adolescent pregnancy is reported by 1 out of 10 US women each year. The pregnant teenager is under a tremendous amount of stress and requires expert support and counseling. The teenager should be encouraged to tell her parents and her partner about the pregnancy as soon as possible. The nurse should provide information about the available options for continuing or terminating the pregnancy and refer her to appropriate and competent practitioners. Some American adolescents choose to obtain legal abortions.

Young women who choose to continue the pregnancy have a variety of special needs. Adolescents are high-risk mothers and require sensitive and expert care, both physical and emotional. Adolescent parents require continued support and teaching from the nurse. Teens who decide to give up their babies for adoption should be referred to the appropriate agencies and be provided with follow-up care and emotional support.

RESEARCH NOTE

Does Adolescents' Knowledge about AIDS Affect Their Participation in Associated Risk Behaviors?

Teenagers, because of their developmental stage, are considered to be at high risk for contracting the human immunodeficiency virus (HIV) infection. Adolescence is frequently characterized by multiple sexual partners and drug experimentation, activities that are recognized as major modes of transmission for HIV. The purpose of this study was to describe the knowledge and associated risk behaviors related to AIDS and HIV infection in suburban teenagers. A sample of 152 teenagers (73 boys and 79 girls; average age 16.3 years) attending a New Jersey high school consented to complete a 53-item questionnaire. The questionnaire addressed knowledge and attitudes about AIDS/HIV.

The results of the study indicate that this group of adolescents had the necessary knowledge for preventing the transmission of HIV infection. However, a large proportion of the teenagers indicated that they do not apply this knowledge to practical use and continue to participate in risky behaviors that could lead to HIV transmission. For example, 45% of the teenagers had had sexual intercourse at least once; 66% of the sexually experienced males reported having more than one partner, and only 60% of the males used a condom for intercourse.

Implications: Feelings of invulnerability and indestructibility in the adolescent can now, with the threat of AIDS, lead to death. Nurses can make a difference in the spread of this epidemic among adolescents. In the adolescent population, sex is a primary mode of HIV transmission, so the nurse must feel comfortable discussing sexual issues. Adolescents need accurate and up-to-date information on AIDS/HIV, specific information about condom use, and effective strategies for saying no.

Source: SH Walker, Teenagers' knowledge of the acquired immunodeficiency syndrome and associated risk behaviors, *Journal of Pediatric Nursing*, August 1992, 7:246–50.

Personal Habits Personal habits established during adolescence can greatly influence the teenager's immediate and future health. Drug and substance use and abuse are on the rise among teenagers, especially among those with problems related to self-esteem and self-concept. Many adolescents take drugs to have a new experience, to feel they belong to the group and thus relieve loneliness, or to prove they are courageous. This experimental use of drugs is usually a one-time or infrequent occurrence. Some teenagers, however, use drugs regularly. Compulsive users become dependent on drugs. Some drugs abused by teenagers are alcohol, glue and similar substances, barbiturates and amphetamines, hallucinogens, marijuana, cocaine, and crack.

Teenagers who habitually use drugs create problems for themselves and for the people with whom they associate. These teenagers may need help from nurses, physicians, and other professionals, such as psychiatrists specializing in adolescent problems.

Adolescent health-promotion programs provided by nurses should include the following information:

- The underlying reasons for drug use and more positive coping mechanisms to deal with stress
- The hazards of drug misuse and abuse
- Responsible ways to make decisions about drug use before experimentation and ways to handle peer pressure

The nurse should also be alert for signs that a teenager is misusing drugs. Some of these are a drop in school achievement, mood swings, sleepiness or fatigue, and personality changes, such as withdrawal or boisterous behavior.

Adolescents also need to be informed that *nicotine* causes many harmful physiologic effects and is a precursor to lung cancer and coronary artery disease. It is also habit forming. Some teenagers who erroneously think that *smokeless* tobacco or *chewing* tobacco is less harmful than smoking tobacco need to be informed about the potential effects of smokeless tobacco (eg, cancer of the mouth and tongue).

Health-promotion activities for the adolescent are summarized in the box below.

ADULTHOOD AND MATURITY

The age at which a person is considered an adult depends on how adulthood is described. Legally, a person in the United States can vote at 18 years. The legal age for alcohol consumption outside the home varies among states from 18 to 21 years. Another criterion of adulthood is financial independence, which is also highly variable. Some adolescents support themselves as early as 16 years of age, usually because of family circumstances. By contrast, some adults are financially dependent on their families for many years, as for example, during prolonged education.

Adulthood may also be indicated by moving away from home and establishing one's own living arrangements. Yet this independence also varies greatly. Some adolescents leave home perhaps because of family problems. In recent years, however, more young adults have been choosing to remain at home. In addition, many adults under 30 have returned to their parents' home to live. The factors contributing to this trend include high housing costs, high divorce rates, high unemployment rates, and the many problems resulting from drug abuse. Some young people who are employed full time receive only minimum wage and are unable to earn enough money to be totally self-supporting.

Maturity is the state of maximal function and integration, or the state of being fully developed. Many other characteristics are generally recognized as representative of maturity. Mature individuals are guided by an underlying philosophy of life. They take many perspectives into account and are tolerant of the views of others. A comprehensive philosophy allows a person to make sense out of life and thus helps that person maintain a sense of purpose and hope in the face of human tragedies. Mature persons are open to new experiences and continued growth; they can tolerate ambiguity, are flexible, and can adapt to change. In addition, mature people have the quality of

HEALTH PROMOTION HIGHLIGHTS FOR ADOLESCENTS

Instruct adolescent and parents about the following:

Health Maintenance Visits

- Annual physical examination

Protective Measures

- Immunizations as recommended, such as adult tetanus-diphtheria (Td) vaccine
- Screening for tuberculosis
- Periodic vision and hearing screenings
- Regular dental assessments
- Obtaining and providing accurate information about sexual issues

Adolescent Safety

- Adolescent's taking responsibility for using motor vehicles safely (eg, completing a driver's education course, wearing seat belts and helmets)
- Making certain proper physical precautions are taken during all athletic activities (eg, medical supervision, proper equipment)
- Parents' keeping lines of communication open and being alert to signs of substance abuse and emotional disturbances in the adolescent

Nutrition and Exercise

- Importance of healthy snacks and appropriate patterns of food intake and exercise
- Factors that may lead to nutritional problems (eg, obesity, anorexia nervosa, bulimia)
- Balancing sedentary activities with regular exercise

Social Interactions

- Encouraging adolescent to establish relationships that promote discussion of feelings, concerns, and fears
- Parents' encouraging adolescent peer group activities that promote appropriate moral and spiritual values
- Parents' acting as role models for appropriate social interactions
- Parents' providing a comfortable home environment for appropriate adolescent peer group activities

self-acceptance; they are able to be reflective and insightful about life and to see themselves as others see them. Mature persons also assume responsibility for themselves and expect others to do the same. They confront the tasks of life in a realistic and mature manner, make decisions, and accept responsibility for those decisions (Schuster & Ashburn 1992, p. 615).

Young Adults

The adult phase of development encompasses the years from the end of adolescence to death. Because the developmental tasks of young adults differ from those of older adults, adulthood is often divided into three phases: young adulthood, middle adulthood, and late adulthood. In this book, young adults are defined as people 20 to 40 years old; middle-aged adults, as 40 to 65; and elderly adults, over 65.

During young adulthood, people become independent of their families, establish careers, often establish a close relationship with a significant other, and decide whether to have children. The young adult is typically a busy person who faces many challenges.

Physical Development

Persons in their early 20s are in their prime years physically. The musculoskeletal system is well developed and coordinated. This is the period when athletic endeavors reach their peak. Indeed, after 40 years, most athletes are considered old. All other systems of the body (eg, circulatory and reproductive) are also functioning at peak efficiency. Although physical change during young adulthood is minimal, psychosocial development, by contrast, is great.

Psychosocial Development

According to Erikson, the central task of the young adult is *intimacy versus isolation.* Young adults are viewed as developing an intimate, lasting relationship with another person or a cause, institution, or creative effort (Erikson 1963, p. 263). The basic strength that evolves from this relationship is love; the outcome of negative resolution is exclusivity (Erikson 1982, p. 33). See Table 23–4 on page 574.

Young adults face a number of new experiences and changes in life-style as they progress toward maturity. They must make decisions for themselves, and many of the decisions made now influence the person's life-style in years to come. The expectations of the young adult are often taken for granted, because they are well defined in most cultures. Choices must be made about education and employment, about whether to marry or remain single, about starting a home, and about rearing children. Social responsibilities include forming new friendships and assuming some community activities.

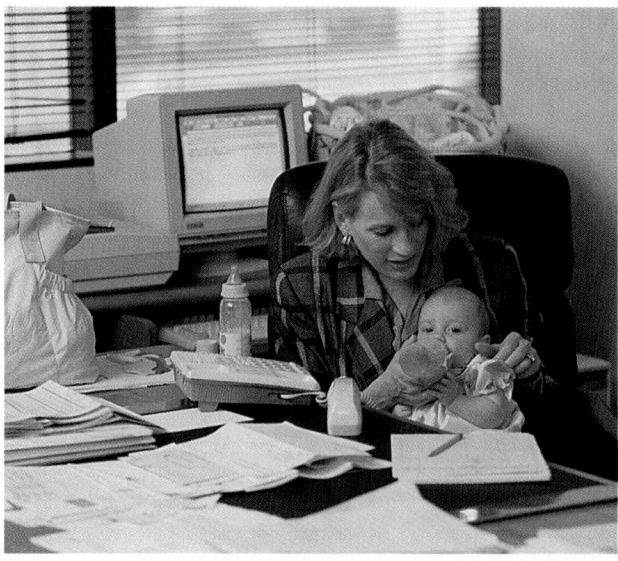

Figure 25–2 Many young women combine active careers with motherhood.

Occupational choice and education are largely inseparable. Education influences occupational opportunities; conversely, an occupation, once chosen, can determine the education needed and sought. Education enhances employment opportunities, enriches leisure time, and ensures economic survival. In the past, more young men than young women were encouraged to pursue advanced education, particularly college education. Education was deemed unnecessary for women who traditionally assumed the roles of wife and mother. This notion has changed as the role of women has changed. Many women now choose to assume active careers and civic roles in society in addition to their roles as mothers and/or wives (Figure 25–2).

Many women reenter the work force in their late 30s. This shift in family role may be met by the husband with support and flexibility or with open hostility. The husband may feel threatened by his wife's new role or by having to perform domestic chores he considers "feminine." The woman may also experience conflicts due to the change in roles. She may feel guilty because she is no longer home to nurture the family and, at the same time, anxious about the skills she may need as she enters the work force. Women reentering the job market experience considerable wage discrimination, despite current legislation and social trends that support equality.

Remaining single is becoming the life-style of more and more young adults. Many people choose to remain single, perhaps to pursue an education and then to have the freedom to pursue their chosen vocations. Some unmarried individuals choose to live with another person of the opposite or same sex and share living arrangements and certain expenses. Some unmarried people are gay or lesbian and live with or are involved with a partner to whom they are committed.

Nurses should not assume that an unmarried person has no partner. Discreet, sensitive, and unprejudiced questioning of a client can often elicit information about a friend or support person who is especially significant to the client. Because single adults may live alone or with other adults who are employed, problems can arise when single persons are ill. Finding someone to drive them to a hospital or to help with shopping and meals during recuperation can be major challenges. A support system for a single adult may take more organization than the support system of a married person.

Cognitive Development

Piaget believes that cognitive structures are complete during the *formal operations period,* from roughly 11 to 15 years. See Table 23–5 on page 576. From that time, formal operations (for example, generating hypotheses) characterize thinking throughout adulthood and are applied to more areas. Egocentrism continues to decline; however, according to Piaget, these changes do not involve a change in the structure of thought, only a change in its content and stability.

Recently, researchers in the field of psychology have suggested that a fifth and qualitatively higher stage of cognitive development may follow formal operations (Rybash et al 1986, p. 38). In addition to the adolescent ability to think in abstract terms, **post-formal operations thinkers** possess an understanding of the temporary or relative nature of knowledge. They are able to comprehend the contradictions that exist in both personal and physical reality. For instance, in a personal realm, an individual may understand that feelings toward another are not simply love or hate, but that these contrasting feelings may exist together in a relationship. Future research is needed to determine the existence of a fifth stage of cognitive development.

In recent years, cognitive psychologists have proposed an information-processing view of intelligence that seeks to explain the mental processes involved in solving a problem. **Information processing** has been described as the step-by-step mental operation that we use to solve problems. The steps of this approach include the following:

1. Encoding the items involved with a problem. This includes identifying all of the parts of a problem and determining what is already known about these parts.
2. Inferring relationships among the parts. This includes generating all of the possible links that may exist among the parts that might be helpful in solving the problem.
3. Applying relationships and justifying solutions to the problem. This involves both checking relationships and validating the information used.
4. Responding with the answer.

Individuals differ in their ability to carry out the various stages or components of this process. The best problem solvers are not necessarily the quickest. Experts often spend more time encoding a problem than do beginners, and they are often rewarded with the correct solution. Young adulthood is a time when people are most capable of forming new concepts and shifting their thinking in order to solve problems. However, other factors, such as motivation, education, memory, and maturity, also operate in the problem-solving process.

Moral Development

Young adults who have mastered the previous stages of Kohlberg's theory of moral development now enter the *postconventional level.* See Table 23–6 on page 578. At this time, the person is able to separate self from the expectations and rules of others and to define morality in terms of personal principles. When individuals perceive a conflict with society's rules or laws, they judge according to their own principles. For example, a person may intentionally break the law and join a protest group to stop hunters from killing wild animals, believing that the principle of conservation of wildlife justifies the protest action. This type of reasoning is called **principled reasoning.** See also Gilligan's *ethic of care,* page 577. Gilligan argues that as individuals approach young adulthood, men and women tend to define moral problems somewhat differently. Men use an "ethic of justice" and define moral problems in terms of rules and rights. Women, by contrast, define moral problems in terms of obligation to care and to avoid hurt.

Spiritual Development

According to Fowler, the individual enters the *individuating-reflective period* sometime after 18 years of age. See Table 16–2 on page 314. During this period, the individual focuses on reality. A 27-year-old adult may ask philosophic questions regarding spirituality and may be self-conscious about spiritual matters. The religious teaching that the young adult had as a child may now be accepted or redefined.

Health Assessment

Assessment guidelines for the growth and development of the young adult are shown in the box on the following page. Examples of NANDA nursing diagnoses, goals/

outcome criteria, and interventions for the young adult are shown in Table 25–2.

Young adults are usually interested in meeting their health needs. However, because of the many stresses and changes that occur throughout this 20-year period, the nurse needs to offer teaching and guidance in several health care areas. The nurse may wish to discuss some, or all, of the following topics with the young adult client.

PROMOTING HEALTH AND WELLNESS

Health Maintenance Visits and Immunization Although many physicians may not recommend complete annual physical examinations, the nurse should encourage young adults to request a specific health maintenance schedule from their physicians. Some physicians recommend a health risk appraisal at age 20, regular audiometry tests if the person is at risk, visual examinations every 2 to 4 years, yearly dental assessments, yearly Papanicolaou (Pap) tests for high-risk females, and a prostate examination every 5 years for males. If appropriate immunizations have not been received as recommended, they should be given at this time. Most colleges require that students show documentation of immunizations as a prerequisite to registration. Adults should receive a diphtheria and tetanus booster every 10 years and be vaccinated against influenza and hepatitis B if they are at risk of exposure. Young adults with no history of mumps should be vaccinated. Recently, public health authorities have reported an increase in the incidence of rubella among young adults due to the fact that they did not have the disease as children, were not vaccinated, or were vaccinated improperly. The nurse should assess whether the young adult is at risk for rubella. A rubella titer can be done to determine if immunity is low. A low immunity means that the client is susceptible to the disease, in which case immunization should be considered. Young women of childbearing age should be advised that rubella can cause severe complications during pregnancy. Therefore, the rubella vaccination should be given prior to pregnancy (preferably during childhood), and the client should be warned that serious side-effects could result if pregnancy occurs during the first 2 or 3 months after the rubella vaccine is administered.

ASSESSMENT GUIDELINES

The Young Adult

In the following developmental areas, does the young adult

Physical Development

- Exhibit weight within normal range for age and sex?
- Manifest vital signs (eg, blood pressure) within normal range for age and sex?
- Demonstrate visual and hearing abilities within normal range?
- Exhibit appropriate knowledge (eg, sexually transmitted diseases) and attitudes about sexuality?

Psychosocial Development

- Feel independent from parents?
- Have a realistic self-concept?
- Like self and direction life is going?
- Interact well with family?
- Cope with the stresses of change and growth?
- Have well-established bonds with significant others, such as marriage partners or close friends?
- Have a meaningful social life?
- Demonstrate emotional, social, and economic responsibility for own life?
- Have a set of values that guide behavior?

Development in Activities of Daily Living

- Have a healthy life-style?

Cancer Detection Young adult women and men need to be informed about self-examination techniques that allow for possible early detection of cancers. For women, the focus is on breast self-examination, for men, on testicular examination.

Of all cancers among women, cancer of the breast is the most frequent cause of death. Young women need to form the habit of examining their breasts monthly. **Breast self-examination** should be done once a momth. For detailed information, see Chapter 22, page 528. The earlier a breast lump is discovered, the greater the effectiveness of treatment.

Young adult females should also be screened for cervical cancer by having a routine Papanicolaou (Pap) test. A **Pap test** is done by obtaining and examining cells from the uterine cervical os. The cells are obtained during a pelvic examination. For more information on the pelvic exam, see Chapter 22, page 557. The nurse should also screen for high-risk factors for cervical cancer: sexual activity at an early age, multiple sexual partners, or a history of syphilis, herpes genitalis, or *Trichomonas* vaginitis. Many young adults are reluctant to have these examinations and screenings. Therefore, it is important for nurses to explain the purpose of the test and to encourage all young women to begin this preventive measure by age 20. See cancer screening guidelines in Chapter 22, page 467.

Table 25–2 Examples of Nursing Diagnoses, Goals, and Interventions for the Young Adult

NANDA Diagnosis	Goal/Outcome Criteria	Interventions
Health-seeking behaviors related to personal cardiovascular health	The young adult will demonstrate (within 1 month) activities that promote cardiovascular health, as evidenced by ▪ Regular participation in vigorous exercise regime. ▪ Selection of low-calorie, low-cholesterol foods. ▪ Adherence to program of weight control. ▪ Participation in stress reduction program.	Provide accurate information on the physiologic and psychologic benefits of cardiovascular health. Refer young adult to programs that promote cardiovascular health (nutrition, exercise, weight control, stress reduction). Encourage the young adult to have a periodic physical assessment that includes blood pressure and a serum cholesterol test.
Altered family processes related to loss of employment	The young adult and family will demonstrate (within 2 months) appropriate family processes, as evidenced by ▪ Attendance at weekly job counseling sessions for exploration and retraining opportunities. ▪ Ability to discuss concerns with family and plan for coping with financial difficulties. ▪ Ability of family members to provide support and encouragement to one another.	Listen to the concerns and fears of the young adult and family. Provide information on job counseling and financial assistance programs. Refer young adult and family members to mental health counseling as needed.

Testicular cancer is the most common neoplasm in men aged 20 to 34 (Malasanos et al 1990, p. 543). **Testicular self-examination,** a means of early identification of scrotal cancer, should be conducted monthly. For additional information about self-examination of the testicles, see Chapter 22, page 560.

Safety Accident prevention is an important health promotion consideration during young adulthood. Among persons 15 to 24 years old, accidents are responsible for more deaths than all other causes combined (Hales 1989, p. 474). Motor vehicle accidents are, by far, the leading cause of mortality; other causes of accidental death for young adults include drowning, fires, burns, and firearms.

One safety hazard for many young adults is exposure to natural radiation from sunbathing or outdoor activities. Exposure to the sun is directly related to skin cancer. Many young adults regard a tan not only as attractive but also as "healthy." It is the nurse's role to reinforce the negative aspects and long-term risks of sun exposure and to explain the value of sun-blocking agents, such as para-aminobenzoic acid (PABA).

Suicide is another leading cause of death in young adults. Many suicides may actually be mistaken for accidental death (automobile accidents, alcohol intoxication, and drug overdose). Suicide may result from problems with close relationships, such as those with marriage partners or parents, or from depression related to perceived occupational, academic, or financial failure. In general, suicide results from the young adult's inability to cope with the pressures, responsibilities, and expectations of adulthood.

The nurse's role in the prevention of suicide includes identifying behaviors that may indicate potential problems: depression; a variety of physical complaints, including weight loss, sleep disturbances, and digestive disorders; and decreased interest in social and work roles along with an increase in isolation. A young adult identified as at risk for suicide should be referred to a mental health professional or a crisis center. Nurses can also reduce the incidence of suicide by participating in educational programs that provide information about the early signs of suicide.

Safety highlights for the young adult are presented in the box on the next page.

Nutrition The nutritional habits established during young adulthood often lay the foundation for the patterns maintained throughout a person's life. Many young adults are aware of the four food groups but may not be knowledgeable about how many servings of each group they need or how much constitutes a serving. The nurse

Safety Highlights for Young Adults

- Reinforce motor vehicle safety: Drive defensively, use "designated drivers" if alcohol is consumed, routinely check brakes and tires, use seat and shoulder belts or car seats for all passengers.
- Remind young adult to repair potential fire hazards, such as electrical wiring.
- Reinforce water safety: Know the depth of a pool before diving; supervise backyard pools and other water activities.
- Discuss evaluating the potential for workplace injuries or death when making decisions about a career or occupation. Encourage the young adult to participate actively in programs that reduce occupational hazards.
- Discuss avoiding excessive sun radiation by limiting exposure, using sun-blocking agents, and wearing protective clothing. Learn the skin changes that may indicate a cancerous condition.
- Encourage young adults who are unable to cope with the pressures, responsibilities, and expectations of adulthood to seek counseling.

should provide the young adult client with resources such as a chart or list that contains the foods and the amounts needed in each category. (See Chapter 37 for more detailed information on dietary requirements).

Young adult females need to increase their intake of vitamin C and also maintain an adequate iron intake. A substantial number of women do not ingest sufficient dietary iron each day (Murray & Zentner 1993, p. 440). **Anemia** is defined as a condition characterized by a decrease in circulating red blood cells. To prevent anemia, females from ages 10 to 55 should ingest 18 mg of iron daily. The nurse should instruct the female client to include iron-rich foods, such as organ meats (liver and kidneys), eggs, fish, poultry, leafy vegetables, and dried fruits, in her daily diet.

The problems of obesity and hypertension may begin during young adulthood. Obesity may occur during the young adult years as the active teen becomes the sedentary adult but does not decrease caloric intake. The overweight or obese young adult is at risk for hypertension, a major health problem for this age group.

In the United States, 13% to 17% of European-Americans and 26% to 28% of African-Americans age 20 and over have both high blood pressure (hypertension) and weight problems (Edelman & Mandle 1990, p. 476). Hypertension and obesity are 2 of more than 40 risk factors that have been identified in the development of cardiovascular (CV) disease. **Risk factors** are characteristics associated with an increased chance of developing a given health problem. Preventing these risk factors and lowering the risk of CV disease are critical. Low-fat and/or low-cholesterol diets play a significant role in both the prevention and treatment of CV disease.

Exercise All young adults need sufficient physical exercise to maintain their physical fitness. The actual amount of exercise that each person needs is highly individual, because each person develops a personal idea of "fitness." Some people think that fitness is the ability to finish a marathon; others see fitness as a lean or muscular body. In general, an individual who is physically fit has the ability to meet routine physical demands with sufficient reserve to meet a sudden challenge and is able to live an active life with minimum risk of injury or disability.

Most individuals in this age group feel healthy, have busy lives with families, careers, and social activities, and in general tend to take their health for granted. It is important for the nurse to provide the young adult with information regarding fitness, explain the criteria for fitness, and discuss the need and benefits of regular exercise. In addition, the nurse should provide ongoing support and encouragement for clients about their fitness activities. See Chapter 34 for detailed information about the benefits of exercise on the body, physical fitness, preparations for exercise, and target and maximum heart rates to be achieved during exercise.

Sexuality Young adult men and women are often concerned about normal sexual response, both for themselves and their partners. Many problems arise in relationships because of basic differences in the male and female sexual response patterns. Couples need to communicate their needs to one another early in their courtship so that a successful intimate relationship can develop and grow. Young adults should also be aware that because sexual needs and responses may change, each partner should listen and respond to the needs of the other. To promote a healthy sexual relationship, both partners should focus on being patient with one another instead of "performing." The nurse should encourage the young adult couple, or individual, to discuss sexual concerns and should provide information and resources that will promote ongoing growth and understanding in this developmental area.

Sexually tansmitted diseases (STDs) such as genital herpes, AIDS, syphilis, and gonorrhea are common infections in young adults. Nursing functions are largely educational. The use of condoms greatly reduces the transfer of infectious microorganisms from one partner to another. Knowledge about the symptoms of these diseases can help the client obtain early treatment. In dealing with clients with STD, the nurse must be nonjudgmental and accepting of the client's life-style and treat any information obtained as confidential. See Table 17–4, page 343, for additional information.

Work and Career Choices During the young adult years, both men and women make career choices that they hope will give them a sense of accomplishment and help them to attain their personal goals. The job or workplace is also where young adults socialize and make new friends. However, some young adults have difficulty finding a job that is challenging and rewarding or in their area of preparation. Young women have the added burden of balancing career goals with childbearing responsibilities.

Nurses need to be aware of work-related difficulties and the resulting stress and anxiety for the young adult. Suggestions to promote health in the area of career and work life include the following:

- Encourage the young adult to discuss the problems and stresses related to the work role.
- Discuss long-term work goals, and identify specific strategies to meet those goals.
- Assist young parents in obtaining professional child care, and discuss the concept of quality time for parents and children.
- Assess the young adult for problems of work stress or potential burnout.

Personal Relationships *Divorce* separates more than a million children from their families each year. The divorce rates of young adult women are rising with the result that many young women are now heads of households. Divorce is an emotional stressor that may leave the young adult feeling angry, alone, betrayed, anxious, or depressed. These feelings may arise in the person initiating the divorce as well as the other partner. The nurse interviewing the young adult must be aware of the physical and emotional loss experienced as a result of divorce and separation. These individuals may need support and understanding from the nurse to deal with the crisis and grief. The nurse may suggest reading materials, support groups, counseling, or other resources.

The problem of *battering* or abuse of women affects families at all socioeconomic levels. Stresses that predispose to abuse may include financial problems, separation from family and community support, and physical as well as social isolation. In working with women, the nurse should (a) have open communication that will encourage them to share their problems; (b) help them to develop self-esteem that will enable them to have the courage to leave the violent situation; (c) provide information and resources, such as welfare and shelters, that will allow them to begin an alternative life-style; and (d) continue to support and educate the young women so that they can understand the causes and results of abusive and violent behavior.

Personal Habits Drug abuse is a major threat to the health of young adults. Alcohol, marijuana, amphetamines, and cocaine, for example, can bring about feelings of well-being that may be highly valued by people with adjustment problems. Prolonged use can lead to physical and psychologic dependency and subsequent health problems. For example, drug abuse during pregnancy can lead to fetal damage. Prolonged use of alcohol can lead to such diseases as cirrhosis of the liver and cancer of the esophagus.

Nursing strategies related to drug abuse include teaching about the complications of their use, changing individual attitudes toward drug abuse, and counseling regarding problems that lead to drug abuse.

Smoking is another type of drug abuse that can lead to diseases such as lung cancer and cardiovascular disease. The nurse's role regarding smoking is to (a) serve as a role model by not smoking; (b) provide educational information regarding the dangers of smoking; (c) help make smoking socially unacceptable, for example, by posting No Smoking signs in client lounges and offices; and (d) suggest resources, such as hypnosis, life-style training, and behavior modification, to clients who desire to stop smoking.

Health-promotion activities for the young adult are summarized in the box on the next page.

MIDDLE-AGED ADULTS

The middle years, from 40 to 65, have been called the years of stability and consolidation. For most people, it is a time when children have grown and moved away or are moving away from home. Thus, partners generally have more time for and with each other and time to pursue interests they may have deferred for years (Figure 25–3).

PHYSICAL DEVELOPMENT

A number of changes take place during the middle years. At 40, most adults can function as effectively as they did in their twenties. However, during ages 40 to 65, many physical changes take place. See Table 25–3 on page 631 for a summary of these changes.

Both men and women experience decreasing hormonal production during the middle years. The **menopause** refers to the so-called change of life in women, when menstruation ceases. It is said to have occurred when a woman has not had a menstrual period within a year. The menopause usually occurs anywhere between ages 40 and 55.

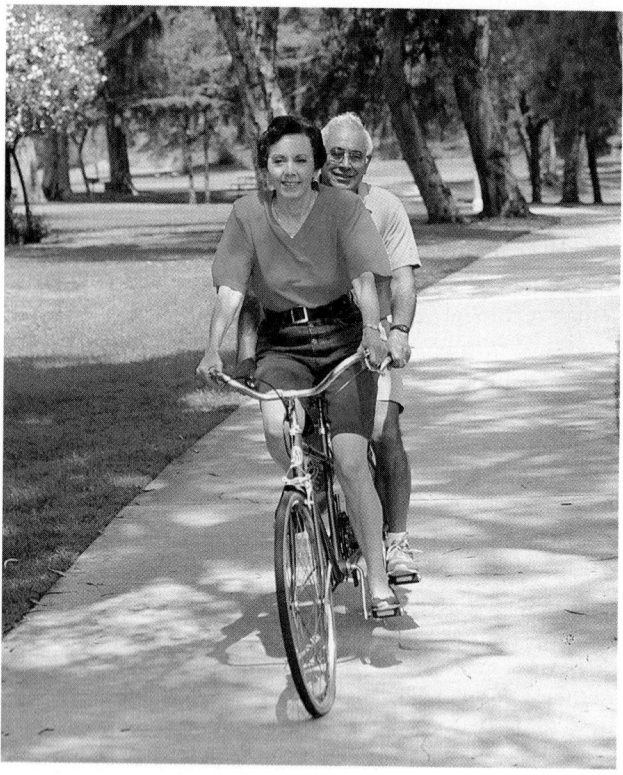

Figure 25–3 Middle-aged adults have time to pursue interests that were previously put aside for child care.

The average is about 47 years. At this time, the ovaries decrease in activity until ovulation ceases. Common symptoms are hot flashes, chilliness, a tendency of the breasts to become smaller and flabby, and a tendency to gain weight. Insomnia and headaches also occur with relative frequency. Psychologically, the menopause can be an anxiety-producing time, especially if the ability to bear children is an integral part of the woman's self-concept.

The **climacteric** (andropause) refers to the change of life in men, when sexual activity decreases. In men, there is no change comparable to the menopause in women. Androgen levels decrease very slowly; however, men can father children even in late life. The psychologic problems that men experience are generally related to the fear of getting old and to retirement, boredom, and finances.

PSYCHOSOCIAL DEVELOPMENT

Until recently, the developmental tasks of middle-aged adults have received little attention. Erikson (1963, p. 266) viewed the developmental choice of the middle-aged adult as *generativity versus stagnation*. See Table 23–4 on page 574. **Generativity** is defined as the concern for establishing and guiding the next generation. In other words, there is concern about providing for the welfare of humankind that is equal to the concern of providing for self. People in their 20s and 30s tend to be self- and family-centered. In middle age, the self seems more altruistic,

HEALTH PROMOTION HIGHLIGHTS FOR YOUNG ADULTS

Instruct the young adult about the following:

Health Maintenance Visits

- Annual physical examination

Protective Measures

- Immunizations as recommended, such as tetanus-diphtheria (Td) boosters
- Screening for tuberculosis
- Periodic vision and hearing screenings
- Regular dental assessments
- Regular cancer screenings (eg, breast or testicular self-examinations, Papanicolaou smears)
- Risk factors that lead to cardiovascular disease

Young Adult Safety

- Motor vehicle safety reinforcement (eg, using designated drivers when drinking, maintaining brakes, and tires)
- Sun protection measures
- Workplace safety measures
- Water safety reinforcement (eg, no diving in shallow water)

Nutrition and Exercise

- Importance of adequate iron intake in diet
- Nutritional and exercise factors that may lead to cardiovascular disease (eg, obesity, cholesterol and fat intake, lack of vigorous exercise)

Social Interactions

- Encouraging personal relationships that promote discussion of feelings, concerns, and fears
- Setting short- and long-term goals for work and career choices

and concepts of service to others and love and compassion gain prominence. These concepts motivate charitable and altruistic actions, such as church work, social work, political work, community fund-raising drives, and cultural endeavors. Marriage partners have more time for companionship and recreation; thus, marriage can be more satisfying in the middle years of life. There is time to work together in volunteer activities. There is time for one partner to go out for lunch and for the other to go fishing. Generative middle-aged persons are able to feel a sense of comfort in their life-style and receive gratification from charitable endeavors.

Table 25–3 Physical Changes of the Middle-Aged Adult

Category	Description
Appearance	Hair begins to thin, and gray hair appears. Skin turgor and moisture decrease, subcutaneous fat decreases, and wrinkling occurs. Fatty tissue is redistributed, resulting in fat deposits in the abdominal area.
Musculoskeletal system	Skeletal muscle bulk decreases at about age 60. Thinning of the intervertebral disks causes a decrease in height of about 1 inch. Calcium loss from bone tissue is more common among postmenopausal women. Muscle growth continues in proportion to use.
Cardiovascular system	Blood vessels lose elasticity and become thicker.
Sensory perception	Visual acuity declines, often by the late forties, especially for near vision (presbyopia). Auditory acuity for high-frequency sounds (presbycusis) also decreases, particularly in men. Taste sensations also diminish.
Metabolism	Metabolism slows, resulting in weight gain.
Gastrointestinal system	Gradual decrease in tone of large intestine may predispose the individual to constipation.
Urinary system	Nephron units are lost during this time, and glomerular filtration rate decreases.
Sexuality	Hormonal changes take place in both men and women.

Erikson believes that persons who are unable to expand their interests at this time and who do not assume the responsibility of middle age suffer a sense of boredom and impoverishment, that is, stagnation. These persons have difficulty accepting their aging bodies and become withdrawn and isolated. They are preoccupied with self and unable to give to others. Some may regress to younger patterns of behavior, for example, adolescent behavior.

Robert Peck (1968) believes that although physical capabilities and functions decrease with age, mental and social capacities tend to increase in the latter part of life. Peck recognizes four sets of developmental tasks that can be dealt with simultaneously during middle age. See the box on the following page.

The middle-aged person looks older and feels older. People usually accept the fact that they are aging; however, a few try to defy the years by their dress and even their actions. Some men and women have extramarital affairs and marry younger partners. A new freedom to be independent and follow one's individual interests arises. Prior to this period, the marriage partner or lover and other persons were crucial to a definition of self. Now the middle-aged person does not make comparisons with others, no longer fears aging or death, relaxes the sense of competitiveness, and enjoys the independence and freedom of middle age. Other people's opinions become less important, and the earlier habit of trying to please everyone is overcome. The person establishes ethical and moral standards that are independent of the standards of others. The focus shifts from inner self and being to others and doing. Religious and philosophical concerns become important.

Gail Sheehy (1976) suggests that the transition into middle life is as critical as adolescence. She outlines characteristics of the **midlife crisis** and calls the decade between the ages of 35 to 45 the "deadline decade." According to Sheehy, most women pass through the midlife crisis between 35 and 40; most men, between 40 and 45. This crisis occurs when individuals recognize that they have reached the halfway mark of life. Although people of these ages are reaching their prime, there is a beginning recognition that time is at a premium and that life is finite. Youthfulness and physical strength can no longer be taken for granted.

Hultsch and Deutsch (1981) suggest that it is not the events themselves that make midlife a crisis, but an individual's response to these life events. How will an individual respond? According to Hultsch and Deutsch, the resources of the person, the ability to use effective coping strategies, and the life stage at which an event occurs will influence any changes in behavior. Internal and external resources include physical health, family income, the social support system, intelligence, and personality (p. 293). Thus, the crisis or transitions of midlife are not just within the individual but, rather, between the individual and the individual's world (pp. 216–18).

To promote psychosocial health during midlife, the nurse should help the individual to work through the developmental changes of the period. The following can be used as guidelines.

1. Encourage both men and women to do some of the things they never had time to do previously. These may include taking up a sport such as golf, taking a cross-country trip, starting a business, joining a community or professional group, or taking a course and starting a new career.
2. Support middle-aged adults in accepting the changes of the period and adjusting to them. Discuss some of the things they can do to highlight their personal assets and make them feel attractive. For instance, they may be able to purchase some new clothes or make a change in hairstyle.
3. Assist middle-aged adults in discussing their changing role as parents. Some middle-aged parents experience emotional changes when their children leave home. They may attempt to compensate for lost opportunities or perceived failures by becoming more involved in their children's daily lives and activities. Teenagers and adult children need to have independence and be given the freedom to make their own choices. The parents' role at this time is to offer love, encouragement, and emotional support while adult children determine their own path of life.
4. Emphasize the positive outcomes of maintaining old friendships and seeking new ones. Enlarging the circle of friends and activities helps the middle-aged adult to share life experiences with others and provide positive feedback that will enhance their self-esteem.
5. Discuss the middle-aged adult's role in the care of aging parents. Allow the individual to discuss the frustrations and concerns inherent in this role reversal. Present options related to the extended care of aging parents, and allow the client to weigh the benefits and problems of each choice.
6. Review the individual's plan for retirement. Individuals and couples should be encouraged to prepare financially as well as socially for the years ahead. Proper financial arrangements require careful planning that should begin during middle adulthood. Hobbies, leisure, and travel also require planning and discussion.

PECK'S TASKS OF MIDDLE AGE

- Valuing wisdom versus physical power and attractiveness. As individuals approach middle age, physical strength and attractiveness decline. It then becomes necessary to gain satisfaction and ego strength through mental and intellectual abilities. Middle-aged persons must learn to rely more on their wisdom and accumulated experiences than on their physical powers.
- Socializing versus sexualizing. In middle age, people should begin to redefine their interpersonal relationships. It is no longer appropriate to relate to the opposite sex in terms of physical attractiveness; other criteria such as friendship, warmth, and understanding should be adopted.
- Emotional flexibility versus emotional rigidity. This task concerns the ability to become flexible, such as being able to shift emotional investment from one person to another and from one task to another. During this phase of life, the children often leave home, and parents may die. Middle-aged adults must be able to develop new roles, socially and emotionally, or they may find themselves isolated.
- Mental flexibility versus mental rigidity. Individuals often become set in their ways as they approach middle age. They may not seek new ideas or accept the novel solutions of others. To cope most effectively, however, middle-aged adults should strive to remain flexible in their thinking. The solutions of the past may not solve today's problems. New ideas and perspectives should be considered.

Source: R Peck, Psychological development in the second half of life, in BL Neugarten, editor, *Middle Age and Aging* (Chicago: University of Chicago Press, 1968), p. 89.

COGNITIVE DEVELOPMENT

The middle-aged adult's cognitive and intellectual abilities change very little. Cognitive processes include reaction time, memory, perception, learning, problem solving, and creativity. Reaction time during the middle years stays much the same or diminishes during the later part of the middle years. Memory and problem solving are maintained through middle adulthood. Learning continues and can be enhanced by increased motivation at this time in life.

Middle-aged adults are able to carry out all the strategies described in Piaget's phase of *formal operations*. See Table 23–5, page 576. Some may use post-formal operations strategies to assist them in understanding the contradictions that exist in both personal and physical aspects of reality (see the discussion on cognitive development of the young adult, page 625). The experiences of the professional, social, and personal life of middle-aged persons will be reflected in their cognitive performance. Thus, approaches to problem solving and task completion will vary considerably in a middle-aged group. The middle-aged adult can "reflect on the past and current experience and can imagine, anticipate, plan and hope" (Murray & Zentner 1993, p. 523).

MORAL DEVELOPMENT

According to Kohlberg, the adult can move beyond the *conventional level* to the *postconventional level.* See Table 23–6 on page 578. Kohlberg believes that extensive experience of personal moral choice and responsibility is required before people can reach the postconventional level. Kohlberg found that few of his subjects achieved the highest level of moral reasoning. To move from stage 4, *a law and order orientation,* to stage 5, *a social contract orientation,* requires that the individual move to a stage in which rights of others take precedence. People in stage 5 take steps to support another's rights.

SPIRITUAL DEVELOPMENT

Not all adults progress through Fowler's stages to the fifth, called the *paradoxical-consolidative stage.* At this stage, the individual can view "truth" from a number of viewpoints. See Table 16–2 on page 314. Fowler's fifth stage corresponds to Kohlberg's fifth stage of moral development. Fowler believes that only some individuals after the age of 30 years reach this stage.

In middle age, people tend to be less dogmatic about religious beliefs, and religion often offers more comfort to the middle-aged person than it did previously. People in this age group often rely on spiritual beliefs to help them deal with illness, death, and tragedy.

HEALTH ASSESSMENT

Assessment guidelines for the growth and development of the middle-aged adult are shown in the accompanying box. Examples of NANDA nursing diagnoses, goals/outcome criteria, and interventions for the middle-aged adult are shown in Table 25–4 on page 634.

Middle-aged adults usually take care of their health needs and are interested in maintaining health and preventing the acceleration of the aging process. The nurse may wish to discuss some of the following topics with the middle-aged client and offer teaching, guidance, and support in accordance with the client's needs.

ASSESSMENT GUIDELINES

The Middle-Aged Adult

In the following developmental areas, does the middle-aged adult

Physical Development

- Exhibit weight within normal range for age and sex?
- Manifest vital signs (eg, blood pressure) within normal range for age and sex?
- Manifest visual and hearing abilities within normal range?
- Exhibit appropriate knowledge and attitudes about sexuality (eg, about menopause)?
- Verbalize any changes in eating, elimination, or exercise?

Psychosocial Development

- Accept aging body?
- Feel comfortable and respect self?
- Enjoy new freedom to be independent?
- Accept changes in family roles (ie, having teenaged children and aging parents)?
- Interact well and share companionable activities with life partner?
- Expand and renew previous interests?
- Pursue charitable and altruistic activities?
- Have a meaningful philosophy of life?

Development in Activities of Daily Living

- Follow preventive health practices?

PROMOTING HEALTH AND WELLNESS

Health Maintenance Visits and Protection Middle-aged adults should be encouraged to request a specific health maintenance schedule from their physicians. Some physicians may recommend a yearly physical examination; audiometry, if the individual is in a high-risk group; yearly visual examinations; yearly dental assessments; yearly mammogram; yearly Pap test if in a high-risk group, or every 3 years if not; and yearly prostate and testicular examination.

Middle-aged clients require a tetanus booster every 10 years, as well as influenza and pneumococcal vaccinations if they are in major high-risk groups, such as those with chronic lung disease or coronary artery disease.

To maintain health, middle-aged adults should learn to recognize the signs and symptoms of cancer. Cancer accounts for considerable mortality and morbidity in both men and women. It is the second leading cause of death among people between the ages of 25 and 64 in the United States. The patterns of cancer types and incidences for men and women have changed over the past

Table 25–4 Examples of Nursing Diagnoses, Goals, and Interventions for the Middle-Aged Adult

NANDA Diagnosis	Goal/Outcome Criteria	Interventions
Knowledge deficit related to menopause	The middle-aged adult female will demonstrate (within 1 month) increased knowledge related to menopause, as evidenced by ▪ Utilization of interventions to control hot flashes and painful intercourse. ▪ Ability to differentiate the myths and facts about menopause. ▪ Seeking out gynecologic health care on a regular basis.	Provide accurate information on the physiologic and psychologic effects of menopause and appropriate remedies. Encourage the middle-aged adult female to have a periodic gynecologic examination. Encourage the middle-aged adult female and her sexual partner to seek counseling for sexual difficulties, as appropriate.
Diversional activity deficit related to a life change	The middle-aged adult will demonstrate (within 2 months) increased diversional activities, as evidenced by ▪ Seeking information from appropriate sources for at least three areas of interest and/or hobbies. ▪ Choosing at least two areas of interest and/or hobbies. ▪ Participating in at least one to two areas of interest or hobbies for a period of 4 weeks.	Assess client's interests for diversional activities. Refer client to appropriate sources of information on diversional activities: library, social interest groups, craft shops. Periodically assess client's emotional status and refer to counseling, as appropriate.

several decades. Over one-third of the deaths due to cancer occur between the ages of 35 to 64. Men have a high incidence of cancer of the lung and bladder. In women, breast cancer is highest in incidence, followed by cancer of the colon and rectum, uterus, and lung. The incidence of lung cancer is increasing in women.

Female clients may need to be reminded to perform monthly breast self-examinations and male clients to perform monthly testicular self-examination in order to detect growths. See the discussions of breast and testicular examination, earlier in this chapter and in Chapter 17. Postmenopausal women should report any vaginal bleeding. For information on sexually transmitted diseases, see Table 17–4 on page 343.

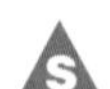

Safety Changing physiologic factors, as well as concern over personal and work-related responsibilities, may contribute to the accident rate of middle-aged persons. Motor vehicle accidents are the most common cause of accidental death in this age group. Decreased reaction times and visual acuity may make the middle-aged adult prone to accidents. Other accidental causes of death for middle-aged adults include falls, fires, burns, poisonings, and drownings (Hales 1989, p. 474). Occupational accidents continue to be a significant safety hazard during the middle years.

Safety highlights for the middle-aged adult are presented in the box on the page to the right.

Nutrition The middle-aged adult should continue to eat a healthy diet, following the recommended portions of the four food groups, with special attention to protein, calcium, and limiting cholesterol and caloric intake. See Chapter 37 for further information. There is no evidence that vitamins or other supplements are needed, unless they are specifically prescribed by a physician because of signs of nutritional deficiency or because of an insufficient diet (Murray & Zentner 1993, p. 516). Two or three liters of fluid should be included in the daily diet. Postmenopausal women need to ingest sufficient calcium and vitamin D to prevent **osteoporosis** (a decrease in bone density). See Chapter 37, page 1026.

Middle-aged adults who gain weight may not be aware of some common facts about this age period. Decreased metabolic activity and decreased physical activity mean a decrease in caloric need. The nurse's role in nutritional health promotion is to counsel clients to prevent obesity by reducing caloric intake and participating in regular exercise. Clients should also be warned that being overweight is a risk factor for many chronic diseases, such as diabetes and hypertension, and for problems of mobility, such as arthritis.

For the client who requires additional management resources, a variety of programs are frequently available. Programs may be found at hospitals, clinics, universities, industries, and in the community. Most programs use behavior modification techniques and group support to assist clients in reaching their goals. Clients should seek medical advice before considering any major changes in their diets.

During late middle age, gastric juice secretions and free acid gradually decline. As a result, some individuals may complain of "heartburn" (acid indigestion) or an increase in belching. They may determine that certain foods disagree with them. Clients should be advised to develop sensible eating habits and avoid fried or fatty foods.

Menopause **Hot flashes,** reported by 50% of women, refer to a cluster of symptoms: heat rising on the chest, spreading to the neck and face (caused by vasodilation), sweating (mild to drenching), sleep disturbances, and occasional chills. Flashes may occur 20 to 30 times a day, lasting 3 to 5 minutes (Olds et al 1992, p. 186). Because a rise in body temperature may trigger a flash, women should be advised to consider the following measures:

- Maintain a comfortable environment. Use fans, light blankets, and air conditioning if possible.
- Use measures to cool body temperature. Increase the intake of cold fluids, and take cool showers or sponge baths. Dress lightly and loosely in cotton or other natural fibers.
- Avoid food that may trigger a flash. Chocolate, red wine, and cheeses contain tyramine, an amino acid that causes the release of norepinephrine in the hypothalamus, which resets the body's thermostat and triggers a flash (McKeon 1989, p. 56).

Exercise Exercise is a key factor in delaying the aging process. Nevertheless, many middle-aged adults may not include exercise in their life-style. Many of the activities or routine chores that provided exercise in the past have been streamlined by modern devices that save time and require little if any energy, such as gas and electric lawn mowers. To promote health in relation to exercise, the nurse must assess the client's current level of activity (see Assessment Interview, p. 898) and the client's physical fitness (see components of physical fitness, p. 929). Any exercise program for the middle-aged adult should (a) begin gradually, (b) increase to a moderately strenuous level, (c) be consistent, and (d) avoid overexertion. **Overexertion** is characterized by trembling, nausea, chest pain, extreme shortness of breath, or sudden headache. Clients should stop exercising immediately if any of the symptoms of overexertion are experienced.

The exercise program for the person over 40 should focus on sports that require skill and coordination rather than speed or endurance. Persons over 50 should exercise additional caution by avoiding activities that require sudden stops and starts, and any situations or activities where they may fall. The overall objective of exercise for the middle-aged client is to increase the efficiency of the cardiovascular and respiratory system. To accomplish this objective, individuals should engage in continuous, rhythmic exercises maintained for about 30 minutes, three times per week. Walking briskly, jogging, and swimming are all highly recommended forms of exercise. For the middle-aged adult to obtain maximum benefit from an exercise program, the nurse should explain the importance of proper preparation for exercise, the concept of target heart rate (see p. 929), and the need for a warm-up and cool-down period. For additional information, see the discussion of developing a successful exercise program in Chapter 34 on page 931.

Male Climacteric The male climacteric is difficult to evaluate, because few men discuss these changes with their doctors. Although the amount of sperm produced decreases, the male maintains the capacity for fathering children throughout life. Middle-aged men are more prone to sexual dysfunction than females. They may experience a decrease in virility and a decrease in the ability to perform sexually. As a result of aging, the male may take longer to attain an erection. However, he should retain his facility for erection. To promote sexual health for the male client, the nurse should encourage him to discuss any concerns regarding changes in sexual ability or activity. The nurse should also assess the client for health risks associated with impotence: diabetes, alterations in nerves or blood supply, and medications, such as antihypertensives and muscle relaxants. See Chapter 17 for further details about sexuality.

Safety Highlights for Middle-Aged Adults

- Reinforce motor vehicle safety: Use seat belts and drive within the speed limit, especially at night. Test visual acuity periodically.
- Make certain stairways are well lighted and uncluttered.
- Equip bathrooms with hand grasps and nonskid bath mats.
- Test smoke detectors and fire alarms regularly.
- Keep all machines and tools in good working condition at work and at home. Follow safety precautions when using machinery.

HEALTH PROMOTION HIGHLIGHTS FOR MIDDLE-AGED ADULTS

Instruct the middle-aged adult about the following:

Health Maintenance Visits

- Annual physical examination

Protective Measures

- Immunizations as recommended, such as influenza and pneumococcal vaccinations
- Screening for tuberculosis
- Periodic vision and hearing screenings
- Regular dental assessments
- Regular cancer screenings (eg, breast or testicular self-examinations, Papanicolaou smears)
- Risk factors that can lead to cardiovascular disease
- Physiologic changes in middle age (eg, menopause, male climacteric)

Middle-Aged Adult Safety

- Motor vehicle safety reinforcement, especially when driving at night
- Workplace safety measures
- Home safety measures: keeping hallways and stairways lighted and uncluttered, using smoke detectors, using nonskid mats and guard rails in the bathrooms

Nutrition and Exercise

- Importance of adequate protein, calcium, and vitamin D in diet
- Nutritional and exercise factors that may lead to cardiovascular disease (eg, obesity, cholesterol and fat intake, lack of vigorous exercise)
- An exercise program that emphasizes skill and coordination

Social Interactions

- The possibility of a midlife crisis: Encourage discussion of feelings, concerns and fears
- Providing time to expand and review previous interests
- Retirement planning (financial and possible diversional activities) with partner, if appropriate

Personal Relationships Divorce is a major stressor and a potential cause of mental health alterations during middle adulthood. The first year of divorce is often considered the most stressful, and money is often the major source of disruption.

A divorce affects each member of a family differently. Women often suffer more than men with respect to emotional stress, economic status, and role loss. Men, by contrast, have more difficulties with the daily tasks involved in self-care and maintaining a comfortable living environment. The children in this situation, usually teenagers or young adults, also suffer emotionally and need support and counseling. For some couples, divorce, although difficult, provides a sense of relief from the stress and pain of living in an unhappy marital situation. The nurse can provide support by assisting each member of the family in assessing life-style and determining changes that will need to be made under the new financial structures. All family members may benefit from support groups or individual therapy to help them cope with the feelings of loss and adjust to long-term changes.

Personal Habits The excessive use of alcohol is a multifaceted problem for the individual and society. Use of the drug is part of the life-style of many Americans and Canadians. Excessive use can result in unemployment, disrupted homes, accidents, and diseases. It is estimated that four million people in the United States are dependent on alcohol and can be considered alcoholics. Nurses can help clients by providing information about the dangers of excessive alcohol use, by helping the individual clarify values about health, and by referring the client to special groups such as Alcoholics Anonymous.

Heavy smoking increases the risk of pulmonary cancer, cardiovascular disease, and chronic obstructive lung disease. See the discussion of drug abuse on page 629 for additional information. Health-promotion activities for the middle-aged adult are summarized in the box above.

CHAPTER HIGHLIGHTS

- Adolescence is a critical period of development extending from the onset of puberty to age 18 or 20.
- Rapid growth in height, development of secondary sexual characteristics, sexual maturity, and increasing independence from the family are major landmarks of adolescence.
- The dramatic physical changes of early adolescence require major adjustments in body image.
- Peer groups assume great importance during adolescence; they provide a sense of belonging and self-esteem and facilitate the development of a positive self-concept.
- Adolescents are at Fowler's synthetic-conventional stage of spiritual development.
- During the adolescent period, health promotion activities are focused on preventive interventions for the potential problems of obesity, sexually transmitted and other communicable diseases, bulimia, anorexia nervosa, unplanned pregnancy, motor vehicle accidents, sports injuries, drug abuse, and suicide.
- Late adolescence is a more stable stage, during which the adolescent is mostly involved with planning a future and economic independence.
- Adolescents between the ages of 11 to 15 begin the formal operations stage of cognitive development; they are able to think logically, rationally, and futuristically and can conceptualize things as they could be rather than as they are.
- The adolescent is at Kohlberg's conventional level of moral development, and some proceed to the postconventional or principled level.
- Maturity is the state of maximal function or the state of being fully developed. Mature persons take responsibility for their own behavior and do not expect others to make their decisions.
- The young adult is essentially in a stable period physically, but psychosocial change is great.
- Cognitive development continues throughout adulthood.
- Some young adults enter Kohlberg's postconventional level of moral development and develop principled reasoning.
- Spiritual development of young adults continues into Fowler's paradoxical-consolidative stage; young adults often feel self-conscious about spiritual matters.
- Hazards to the health of young adults include accidents, sexually transmitted diseases, suicide and homicide, substance abuse, obesity, and hypertension. Nurses can assist clients to decrease the impact of these hazards.
- The middle-aged adult needs to adjust to an aging body, the increasing dependence of parents, and the increasing independence of children; however, new independent interests can be pursued.
- Both middle-aged men and women enter a midlife crisis in which they need to reexamine their purpose and reevaluate ways to use their energies and abilities.
- Common health hazards of middle-aged adults include obesity, cardiovascular diseases, substance abuse, and cancer.
- Positive health practices can protect and promote health.

READINGS AND REFERENCES

SUGGESTED READINGS

Goolsby, MJ. January 1992. Smokeless tobacco: The consequences of snuff and chewing tobacco. *Nurse Practitioner* 17:24, 28, 31, 35–36, 38.

The use of smokeless forms of tobacco (snuff, chewing) is growing significantly in the adolescent and young adult male population. The article provides background information about the problem, reviews the health consequences, and offers interventions.

Ireland, DF. March/April 1990. New attitude/new look: An African-American adolescent health education program. *Pediatric Nursing* 16:175–78.

In developing health education programs, nurses need to consider cultural influences on the target audience. This article describes a program developed for the African-American adolescent. Health risk factors and cultural influences are incorporated into the interventions for enhancing personal attributes, self-esteem, and career development.

RELATED RESEARCH

Walker, SH. August 1992. Teenagers' knowledge of the acquired immunodeficiency syndrome and associated risk behaviors. *Journal of Pediatric Nursing* 7:246–50.

Wikbur, J, Dan, A, Hedricks, C, and Holm, K. November 1990. The relationship among menopausal status, menopausal symptoms, and physical activity in midlife women. *Family and Community Health* 13:67–78.

SELECTED REFERENCES

American Heart Association. 1989. *Exercise Diary*. Dallas, TX: AHA.

Caliandro, G and Judkins, B, editors. 1988. *Primary Nursing Practice*. Glenview, IL: Scott, Foresman.

Carpenito, LJ. 1993. *Nursing Diagnosis: Application to Clinical Practice*. 5th ed. Philadelphia: Lippincott.

Christian, JL and Greger, JL. 1994. *Nutrition for Living*. 4th ed. Redwood City, CA: Benjamin/Cummings.

Church, JL and Baer, KJ. March/April 1987. Examination of the Adolescent: A Practical Guide. *Journal of Pediatric Health Care* 1:65–72.

Edelman, C and Mandle, CL, editors. 1990. *Health Promotion Throughout the Life Span*. St Louis: Mosby.

Erikson, EH. 1963. *Childhood and Society*. 2d ed. New York: Norton.

———. 1982. *The Life Cycle Completed: A Review*. New York: Norton.

Fowler, JW. 1981. *Stages of Faith: The Psychology of Human Development and the Quest for Meaning*. New York: Harper and Row.

Fowler, J and Keen, S. 1978, 1985. *Life Maps: Conversations in the Journey of Faith*. Waco, TX: Word Books.

Gilchrist, L and Schinke, S. 1987. Adolescent pregnancy and marriage. In Van Hasselt, VB and Hersen, M, editors. *Handbook of Adolescent Psychology*. New York: Pergamon Press.

Gilligan, C. 1982. *In a Different Voice: Psychological Theory and Women's Development*. Cambridge, MA: Harvard University Press.

Gillis, A. January/February 1988. Promoting health among teenagers. *International Nursing Review* 35:42–43.

Hales, D. 1989. *An Invitation to Health*. 4th ed. Redwood City, CA: Benjamin/Cummings.

Heywood, VH. 1984. *Designs for Fitness: A Guide to Physical Fitness Appraisal and Exercise*. Minneapolis: Burgess Publishing.

Hultsch, DF and Deutsch, F. 1981. *Adult Development and Aging*. New York: McGraw-Hill.

James, S, Mott, S, and Sperhac, A. 1990. *Nursing Care of Children and Families*. Redwood City, CA: Addison-Wesley Nursing.

Kohlberg, I. 1971. *Recent Research in Moral Development*. New York: Holt, Rinehart, and Winston.

———. 1981. *The Psychology of Moral Development: Moral Stages and the Idea of Justice*. San Francisco: Harper and Row.

McKeon, VA. June 1989. Cruel myths and clinical facts about menopause. *RN* 52:52–56, 58–59.

Malasanos, L, Barkauskas, V, and Stoltenberg-Allen, K. 1990. *Health Assessment*. 4th ed. St Louis: Mosby.

Miller, PH. 1993. *Theories of Developmental Psychology*. 3d ed. New York: Freeman.

Montoye, H, Christian, J, Nagle, F, and Levin, S. 1988. *Living Fit*. Redwood City, CA: Benjamin/Cummings.

Murray, R and Zenter, J. 1993. *Nursing Assessment and Health Promotion Through the Life Span*. 5th ed. Norwalk, CT: Appleton & Lange.

Novotny, J. May/June 1989. Adolescents, acne, and the side effects of Accutane. *Pediatric Nursing* 15:247–48.

Olds, S, London, M, and Ladewig, P. 1992. *Maternal Newborn Nursing: A Family Centered Approach*. Redwood City, CA: Addison-Wesley Nursing.

Peck, R. 1968. Psychological development in the second half of life. In Neugarten, BL, editor. *Middle Age and Aging*. Chicago: University of Chicago Press.

Pender, NJ. 1987. *Health Promotion and Nursing Practice*. 2d ed. Norwalk, CT: Appleton & Lange.

Rybash, J, Hoyer, W, and Roodin, P. 1986. *Adult Cognition and Aging: Developmental Changes in Processing, Knowing, and Thinking*. New York: Pergamon Press.

Schuster, CS and Ashburn, SS. 1992. *The Process of Human Development: A Holistic Lifespan Approach*. 3d ed. Philadelphia: Lippincott.

Sheehy, G. 1976. *Passages: Predictable Crises of Adult Life*. New York: Dutton.

US Department of Health and Human Services. September 1990. *Healthy People 2000: National Health Promotion and Disease Prevention Objectives*. DHHS Pub no. (PHS) 91-50212. Washington, DC: Public Health Service.

Williams, SR. 1993. *Nutrition and Diet Therapy*. 7th ed. St. Louis: Mosby.

26 Late Adulthood

Objectives

Describe the physical changes that take place during late adulthood.

Explain essential aspects of psychosocial changes.

Describe essential aspects of cognitive changes.

Explain essential aspects of moral development.

Explain essential aspects of spiritual development

Identify common health concerns and hazards of older adults.

Discuss nursing implications of the common health concerns and hazards identified.

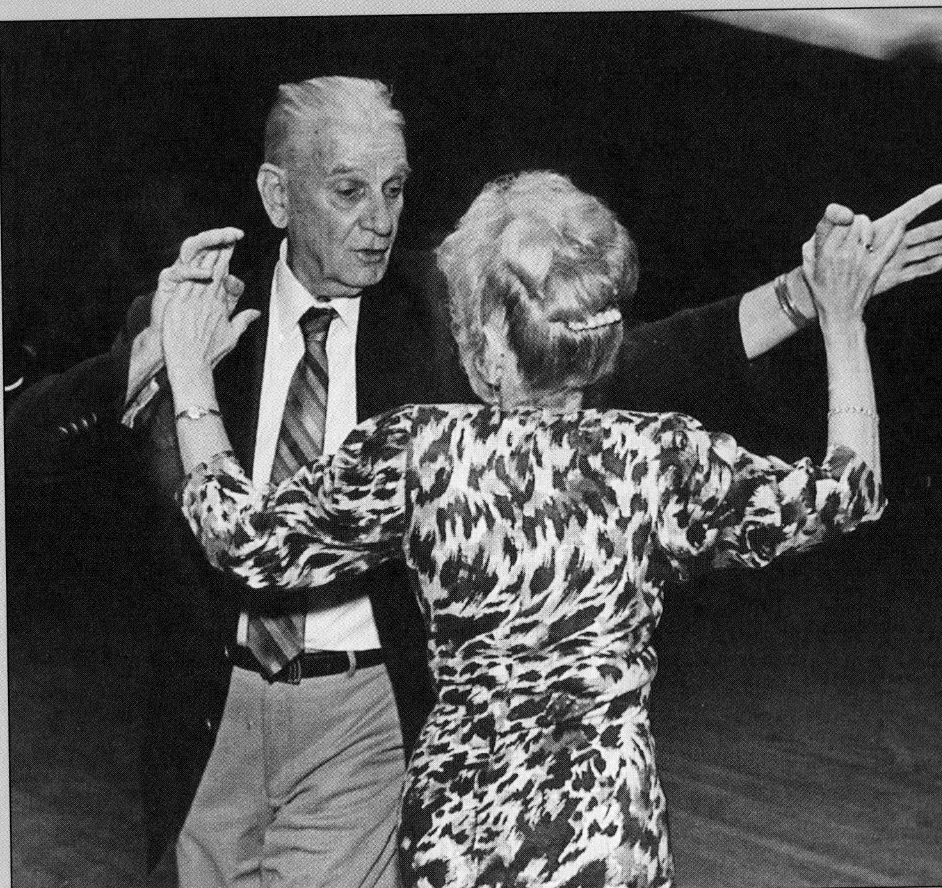

In 1990, 12.5% of the population of the United States were older than 65 years of age, and 5.3% were older than 75 years of age (US Bureau of the Census 1992). It is projected that by 2030, 21% of the population will be older than 65 years of age. As the general population grows older, nurses will have an increasing responsibility for providing health promotion care for the well elderly as well as health maintenance care for elderly clients with both chronic and acute illnesses resulting from the aging process.

Gerontology is the study of all aspects of the aging process, including biologic, psychologic, and sociologic factors. **Geriatrics** is the term for the medical specialty that addresses the diagnosis and treatment of the physical problems of the elderly person. Nursing care of the elderly may be called **geriatric, gerontologic,** or **gerontic nursing.** Nursing practice that focuses on the care of the elderly requires basic nursing knowledge and skills, combined with specialized knowledge of the diverse needs of the aging population.

The aging process begins at conception. As the individual reaches advanced years, the risk for physiologic and functional impairment increases. **Chronologic age** refers to the number of years a person has lived; it is the term used most often to describe the elderly because it is the easiest to identify and measure (Wold 1993, p. 5). Chronologic age is the basis for determining eligibility for pensions, retirement benefits, or medical support; for example, in the United States, a person of 65 years of age (chronologically) is eligible for Medicare health benefits. However, many people who are over 65 years of age are still working and are vibrant and healthy (Figure 26–1). In 1960, life expectancy at birth was about 70 years; that is, the average person born in 1960 could expect to live about 70 years. By 1991, life expectancy had increased to 72 years for males and 78.8 years for females in the United States; 73 for males and 80 for females in Canada; and in Australia, 73.9 years for males and 80 years for females. (*The World Almanac and Book of Facts* 1993, pp. 739, 940).

Various systems are used to categorize the aging population (see the box below). Another term used to describe the "old-old" or "extreme aged" is *frail elderly.* **Frail elderly,** however, is more likely to be used to describe the elderly individual who has significant physiologic and functional impairment, whatever the age.

In the past century, scientists have postulated theories of why people age. More recently, as the absolute number of elderly increases and the population percentage of elderly increases, there is renewed scientific interest in why people age, how people age, and what factors affect the physical, psychologic, and functional status of older persons. Biologic theories of aging are either intrinsic or extrinsic. **Extrinsic** theory encompasses factors in the environment; **intrinsic** theory addresses factors within the body. Table 26–1 on page 642 describes the various biologic theories of aging.

Categorizing the Aging Population

55 to 64—the older population
65 to 74—the elderly
75 to 84—the aged
85 and older—the extreme aged
or
Age 60 to 74—the young-old
Age 75 to 84—the middle-old
Age 85 and older—the old-old

Source: G Wold, *Basic Geriatric Nursing* (St Louis: Mosby-Year Book, 1993), p. 5.

Physical Changes

As the person ages, a number of physical changes occur; some are visible, some are not. See Table 26–2 on page 643 for a summary of the normal physiologic changes associated with aging.

Integument

Obvious changes occur in the integumentary system (skin, hair, nails) with age. A decrease in sebaceous gland activity, combined with the inability of the aged skin to retain fluid, results in dryness of the skin. Itching may increase because of skin dryness. The deterioration of nerve fibers and sensory endings can result in decreased sensation, especially in the lower extremities. **Lentigo senilus** (brown "age spots") commonly appear on the hands and arms and, in some instances, on the face. These are the result of the clustering of **melanocytes** (pigment-producing cells). The skin also becomes paler and loses its elasticity because of decreased vascularity. Decreased subcutaneous fat may give the face and hands a hollow or gaunt appearance. Baldness and hair loss is related to decreased vascularity of the tissue layer that produces hair follicles. The loss of hair color is due to a decrease in the number of functioning melanocytes. Fingernails and toenails be-

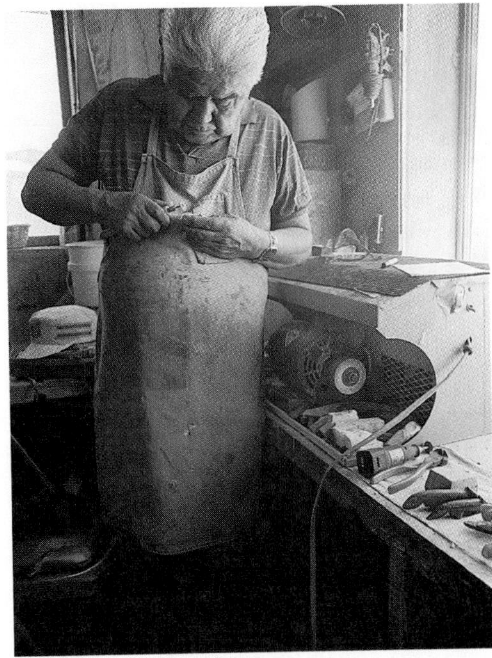

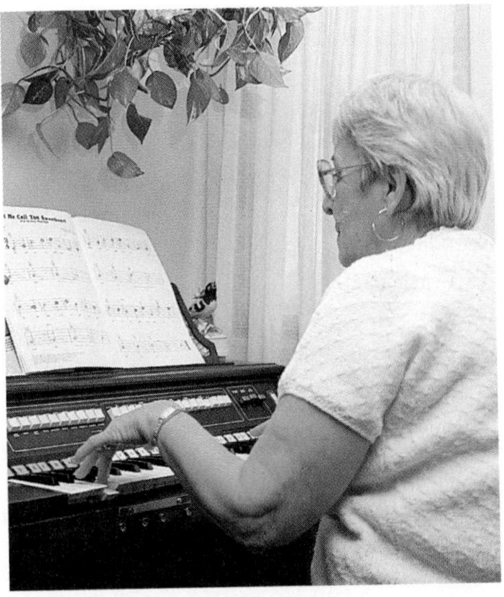

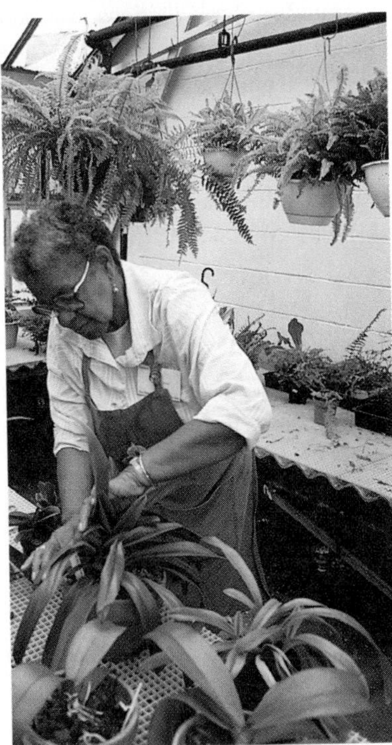

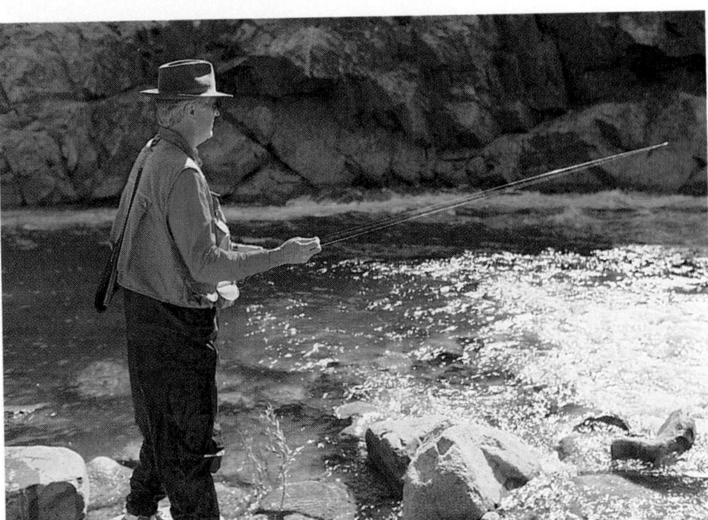

Figure 26–1 Many elderly people find creative outlets during retirement.

come thickened and brittle, and in women over 60, facial hair increases.

Responses to these changes vary among individuals and cultures. For example, one person may feel distinguished with gray hair, whereas another may feel embarrassed or depressed, interpreting gray hair as a sign of losing one's youth.

These integumentary changes accompany progressive losses of subcutaneous fat and muscle tissue, muscle atrophy, and loss of elastic fiber, resulting in a "double" chin, sagging of eyelids and earlobes, and wrinkling of skin, especially in areas exposed to sun. Bony prominences become visible. In elderly women, the breasts become smaller and may sag; if large and pendulous, they may

Table 26–1 Common Biologic Theories of Aging

Theory Type	Theory Name/Author (Date)	Description
Wear-and-tear theories	Wear-and-tear theory Pearl (1924)	Proposes that humans, like automobiles, have vital parts that run down with time, leading to aging and death.
	Rate of living theory Pearl (1928)	Proposes that the faster an organism lives, the quicker it dies.
	Stress theory Lamb (1977)	Proposes that cells wear out through exposure to internal and external stressors, including trauma, chemicals, and buildup of natural wastes.
Endocrine theory	Korenchevsky (1947)	Proposes that events occurring in the hypothalamus and pituitary are responsible for changes in hormone production and response that results in the organism's decline.
Free-radical theory	Harman (1955)	Proposes that unstable free radicals (groups of atoms) result from the oxidation of organic materials, such as carbohydrates and proteins. These radicals cause biochemical changes in the cells, and the cells cannot regenerate themselves.
Genetic theories	Programmed senescence theory Hayflick (1961)	Proposes that the organism is genetically programmed for a predetermined number of cell divisions, after which the cells/organism dies.
	Error catastrophe theory Orgel (1963)	Proposes that when damage to the protein synthesis occurs, faulty proteins will be synthesized and will gradually accumulate, causing a progressive decline in the organism.
Cross-linking theories	Collagen theory Vertzer (1957)	Proposes that the irreversible aging of proteins such as collagen are responsible for the ultimate failure of tissues and organs.
	Cross-linking theory Bjorkstein (1968)	Proposes that as cells age, chemical reactions create strong bonds, or cross-linkages, between proteins. These bonds cause loss of elasticity, stiffness, and eventual loss of function.
Immune theories	Immunologic theory Walford (1969)	Proposes that the immune system becomes less effective with age, and viruses that have incubated in the body become able to damage body organs.
	Autoimmune theory Hallgren & Yunis (1977)	Proposes that a decrease in immune function may result in an increase in autoimmune responses causing the body to produce antibodies that attack itself.

cause chafing where the skin surfaces touch. Loss of subcutaneous fat also decreases the elderly person's tolerance of cold.

BODY TEMPERATURE

Body temperture is lower in the elderly adult because of a decrease in the metabolic rate. It is not uncommon for an elderly adult to have a temperature of 35 C (95 F), particularly in the early morning, when the body's metabolism is low. Therefore, a temperature of 37.5 C (99.5 F) can represent a marked fever in some elderly people, although it represents only a mild fever in most young adults. It is important that the normal temperature of each individual person be known as a baseline for assessing changes.

One of the body's normal compensating reactions to a fall in heat production is the contraction of the surface blood vessels and shivering. Because elderly adults have a diminished shivering reflex and do not produce as much body heat from metabolic processes, they tolerate prolonged exposure to cold poorly. At the other extreme, the body compensates for higher temperatures by slowing down muscular activity to produce less heat and by

Table 26–2 Normal Physiologic Changes Associated with Aging

Integumentary System

Decreased vascularity of the dermis
Decreased melanin production
Decreased sebaceous and sweat gland function
Decreased collagen and subcutaneous fat
Decreased thickness of epidermis
Increased capillary fragility
Thinning of hair
Decreased rate of nail growth
Thickening of connective tissue

Respiratory System

Decreased number of cilia
Decreased gas exchange
Decreased lung capacity
Thickening of alveoli

Cardiovascular System

Decreased heart size
Decreased cardiac output
Increased arteriosclerosis
Thickening and fibrosis of mitral and aortic valves
Decreased elasticity of heart muscle and blood vessels

Hematopoietic and Lymph System

Increased plasma viscosity
Decreased red blood cell production
Decreased immune response

Gastrointestinal System

Decreased gag reflex
Decreased salivary production
Decreased gastric secretions
Decreased esophageal and gastrointestinal peristalsis
Decreased sphincter tone

Reproductive System

Female

Decreased estrogen levels
Decreased vaginal secretions
Decreased size of uterus and ovaries
Decreased vaginal length and width
Increased vaginal alkalinity

Male

Decreased testosterone levels
Decreased rate and force of ejaculation
Decreased speed gaining erection

Musculoskeletal System

Decreased bone calcium
Decreased blood supply to muscles
Decreased muscle mass
Decreased tissue elasticity

Nervous System

Decreased number of brain cells
Decreased reflexes
Decreased balance and coordination
Decreased motor responses
Decreased sensory perception

Sensory Changes

Visual

Decreased peripheral vision
Decreased color perception
Decreased night vision
Thickening of the lens, presbyopia
Decreased tear production
Increased sensitivity to glare

Hearing

Decreased ability to distinguish high-frequency sounds
Decreased number of hair cells in inner ear
Thickening of eardrum—decreased ability to hear

Taste and Smell

Decreased number of taste buds
Decreased number of nasal sensory receptors

Endocrine System

Decreased pituitary secretions
Decreased production of thyroid stimulating hormone—decreased basal metabolic rate
Decreased production of parathyroid hormone

Urinary System

Decreased urinary filtration rate
Increased concentration of urine
Decreased bladder capacity
Increased volume of residual urine

Changes Affecting All Body Systems

Decreased body fluid
Decreased tissue elasticity
Decreased blood supply
Decreased circulation
Decreased muscle tone

dilating surface blood vessels and sweating to increase losses of body heat. Older people, however, often have sluggish sweating and circulatory mechanisms and therefore cannot cope with heat as well as younger people. For example, they do not tolerate working in moderately high temperatures for prolonged periods. It is therefore important for the elderly adult to have a constant, comfortable environmental temperature. Many elderly persons who feel cold in rooms with a "normal" temperature wear extra clothes.

Neuromusculoskeletal Changes

With aging comes *gradual reduction in the speed and power of skeletal or voluntary muscle contractions.* The capacity for sustained muscular effort is also decreased. Great individual differences in muscular efficiency are apparent throughout life. Exercise can strengthen weakened muscles, and up to about age 50 the skeletal muscles can increase in bulk and density. After that time, there is a steady decrease in muscle fibers, ultimately leading to the typical wasted appearance of the very old person. Thus, elderly adults often complain about their lack of strength and how quickly they tire. Activities can still be carried out, but at a slower pace. Often balance is impaired with age. Prolonged muscular efforts may be sustained by older people provided they take judicious rest pauses and avoid capacity or peak performance.

The person's **reaction time** slows with age because of the diminished conduction speed of nerve fibers. Reaction time can be delayed further by decreased muscle tone as a result of diminished physical activity. Elderly people compensate for this reaction difference by being exceptionally cautious, for instance, in their driving habits, which exasperates some impatient younger drivers.

Slight loss in overall stature occurs with age due to atrophy of the discs between the spinal vertebrae. This can be exaggerated by muscular weakness resulting in a stooping posture and **kyphosis** (humpback of the upper spine). **Osteoporosis,** a decrease in bone density, along with increased brittleness of bone, make the elderly adult prone to serious fractures, some of which may be spontaneous and are called **pathologic fractures**. Osteoporosis occurs more frequently in people with insufficient intake of dietary calcium, in women after menopause, and in individuals who are immobilized or physically inactive.

Some degenerative joint changes occur, which make movement stiffer and more restricted. Stiffness is aggravated by inactivity; for example, if a person sits too long, the joints become stiff, and the person has difficulty standing and walking. A continuous program of physical activity and proper nutrition will slow bone density loss and decrease muscle atrophy and stiffness.

Cardiopulmonary Changes

Respiratory efficiency is reduced with age. The person inhales a smaller volume of air because of the musculoskeletal changes in the chest wall that reduce the size of the chest. There is a greater volume of residual air left in the lungs after expiration and a decreased capacity to cough efficiently because of weaker expiratory muscles. Mucous secretions tend to collect more readily in the respiratory tree because of decreased ciliary activity. Thus, susceptibility to respiratory infections increases in elderly adults.

Dyspnea (difficult breathing) occurs frequently with increased activity, such as running for a bus or carrying heavy parcels up stairs. This dyspnea occurs in response to an oxygen debt in the muscles. Intense exercise is followed by short, heavy, rapid breathing, which is an attempt to repay this oxygen debt in the muscles. Although this response is normal, it occurs more quickly in the aged because delivery and diffusion of oxygen to tissues is often diminished by changes in both respiratory and vascular tissues.

Blood pressure measurements often indicate a significant increase in systolic pressures and a slight increase in diastolic pressures. This is a result of the inelasticity of the systemic arteries and an increase in peripheral resistance. Because of decreased elasticity of heart muscle and blood vessels, there is a delay in the ability to adjust to rapid movement from a lying position to a standing position. This results in an abrupt drop in systolic blood pressure, known as **orthostatic hypotension.** The heart rate at normal rest does not change with age. However, the heart rate of the aged person is slow to respond to stress and slow to return to normal after periods of physical activity.

The *working capacity of the heart* diminishes with age. This is particularly evident when increased demands are made on the heart muscles, such as during periods of exercise or emotional stress. The valves of the heart tend to become harder and less pliable, resulting in reduced filling and emptying abilities. In addition, the pumping action of the heart is reduced due to changes in the coronary (cardiac) arteries, which supply progressively smaller amounts of blood to the heart muscle. These changes are evidenced by shortness of breath on exertion and pooling of blood in the systemic veins.

Changes in the *arteries* occur concurrently. The elasticity of smaller arteries is reduced by the thickening of their walls and increased calcium deposits in the muscular layer. Reduced arterial elasticity often results in diminished blood supply to, for instance, the legs and the brain, resulting in pain on exertion in the calf muscles and dizziness, respectively.

SENSORY/PERCEPTUAL CHANGES

Changes in *vision* associated with aging include the obvious changes around the eye, such as the shrunken appearance of the eyes due to loss of orbital fat, the slowed blink reflex, and the looseness of the eyelids, particularly the lower lid, due to poorer muscle tone. Other changes result in loss of visual acuity, less power of adaptation to darkness and dim light, decrease in accommodation to near and far objects, loss of peripheral vision, and difficulty in discriminating similar colors, especially blues, greens, and purples. The degenerative changes in the eyes beginning in middle age lead to the relative inflexibility of the lens, called **presbyopia.**

As the lens of the eye ages, it becomes more opaque and less elastic. By the age of 80 all elderly people have some lens opacity (**cataracts**) that reduces visual acuity and causes glare to be a problem. Surgical removal of cataracts is common at this age. Accompanying this are changes in the ciliary muscles, which control the shape of the lens. These changes reduce the power of the lens to adjust to near and far vision. The diameter of the pupil is reduced, and the amount of light entering the eye is thereby restricted. This slows the reaction time to decreases in light or illumination, a problem compounded at night with driving. Reduced blood supply due to arteriosclerosis can diminish retinal function. Reduced peripheral vision also is thought to be a result of arteriosclerosis.

The loss of *hearing* ability related to aging, called **presbycusis,** affects 13% of people over age 65 (Wold 1993, p. 85). Presbycusis comes about through changes in the structure of the inner ear: changes in nerve tissues in the inner ear and a thickening of the eardrum. Gradual loss of hearing is more common among men than women, perhaps because men are more frequently in noisy work environments. Hearing loss is greater in the higher frequencies than the lower. Thus, older adults with hearing loss usually hear speakers with low, distinct voices best. Older adults may have more difficulty compensating for hearing loss than the young, who pay closer attention to the lip movements of the speaker.

Older persons have a poorer sense of *taste and smell* and are less stimulated by food than the young. The number of taste buds in the tongue decreases, and the olfactory bulb (responsible for smell perception) at the base of the brain atrophies. This change significantly affects appetite in the older adult, contributing to poor nutrition.

Loss of skin receptors takes place gradually, producing an increased threshold for *sensations of pain and touch*. The elderly person may not be able to distinguish hot from cold or the intensity of heat. Stimuli causing severe pain in a younger person may cause only minor sensation or pressure in the elderly. This places the older adult at higher risk for burns and other injuries.

CHANGES IN DIGESTION

The digestive system is significantly less impaired by aging than are other body systems. Gradual decreases in digestive enzymes occur; examples are ptyalin in salivary secretions, which converts starch; pepsin and trypsin, which digest protein; and lipase, a fat-splitting enzyme.

There is also a decrease in the number of absorbing cells in the intestinal tract and a rise in gastric pH. These factors lower the absorption rate, slowing the absorption of nutrients and drugs. The muscle tone of the intestines also decreases, causing a decrease in peristalsis and elimination. These changes in muscle tone, digestive juices, and intestinal activity may lead to **indigestion** and **constipation** in the older adult.

CHANGES IN URINARY ELIMINATION

The excretory function of the kidney diminishes with age, but usually not significantly below normal levels unless a disease process intervenes. Blood flow can be reduced by arteriosclerotic changes, impairing renal function. With age, the number of functioning nephrons (the basic functional units of the kidney) decreases to some degree, thus impairing the kidney's filtering abilities.

More noticeable changes are those related to the bladder. Complaints of **urinary urgency** and **urinary frequency** are common. In men, these changes are often due to an enlarged prostate gland and in women to weakened muscles supporting the bladder or weakness of the urethral sphincter. The capacity of the bladder and its ability to completely empty diminish with age. This explains the need for elderly adults to arise during the night to void (**nocturnal frequency**) and the **retention** of residual urine, predisposing the elderly adult to bladder infections.

CHANGES IN SEXUAL ACTIVITY AND REPRODUCTIVE ORGANS

Sex drives persist into the 70s, 80s, and 90s, provided that health is good and an interested partner is available. Interest in sexual activity in old age depends, in large measure, on interest earlier in life (Wold 1993, p. 320). That is, people who are sexually active in young and middle adulthood will remain active during their later years. However, sexual activity does become less frequent. Many factors may play a role in the ability of an elderly person to engage in sexual activity. Physical problems such as diabetes, arthritis, and heart and respiratory conditions affect energy or the physical ability to participate in sexual activity. Also, some medications impair sexual ability in men.

Degenerative changes in the gonads are very gradual in men. Production of testosterone continues, and the testes can produce sperm well into old age, although there is a gradual decrease in the number of sperm produced. In women, the degenerative changes in the ovaries are noticed by the abrupt cessation of menses in middle age, during the menopause.

Changes in the gonads of elderly women result from diminished secretion of the ovarian hormones. Some changes, such as the shrinking of the uterus and ovaries, go unnoticed. Other changes are obvious. The breasts atrophy, and lubricating vaginal secretions are reduced. Reduced natural lubrication is the cause of painful intercourse, which often necessitates the use of lubricating jellies.

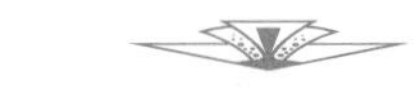

PSYCHOSOCIAL DEVELOPMENT

A number of theories explain psychosocial aging. According to **disengagement theory,** aging involves mutual withdrawal (disengagement) between the older person and others in the elderly person's environment. This withdrawal relieves the elderly person of some of society's pressures and gradually reduces the number of people with whom the elderly person interacts. According to **activity theory,** the best way to age is to stay active physically and mentally, and according to **continuity theory,** people maintain their values, habits, and behavior in old age. A person who is accustomed to having people around will continue to do so, and the person who prefers not to be involved with others will more likely disengage. This theory accounts for the great variety of behavior seen in elderly people.

According to Erikson, the developmental task at this time is *ego integrity versus despair.* See Table 23–4 on page 574. People who attain ego integrity view life with a sense of wholeness and derive satisfaction from past accomplishments. They view death as an acceptable completion of life. According to Erikson, people who develop integrity accept "one's one and only life cycle" (Erikson 1963, p. 263). By contrast, people who despair often believe they have made poor choices during life and wish they could live life over. Robert Butler sees integrity as bringing serenity and wisdom, and despair as resulting in the inability to accept one's fate. Despair gives rise to feelings of frustration, discouragement, and a sense that one's life has been worthless (Butler 1963, p. 65).

Acknowledging that the "young-old" and "old-old" differ not only in physical characteristics but also in psychosocial responses, many people have difficulty with Erikson's singular developmental task. Peck (1968) proposes three developmental tasks of the older adult in contrast to Erikson's task of ego integrity versus despair. See Chapter 23, page 574. Havighurst (1953) and Duvall (1977) have further defined the developmental tasks of the older adult. See the box at the right.

RETIREMENT

Today, a majority of the people over 65 are unemployed. However, many who are healthy continue to work on a full- or part-time basis. Work offers these people a better income, a sense of self-worth, and the chance to continue long-established routines. Some need to work for economic reasons.

Retirement can be a time when projects or recreational activities deferred for a long time can be pursued. Retired people are no longer governed by an alarm clock and can get up when they please. The enjoyment of staying up later is another luxury. Few elderly people, however, spend much time resting or sleeping. Being accustomed to activity most of their lives, most elderly find many outlets, jobs, community projects, volunteer services, intellectual or recreational pursuits, or hobbies such as stamp collecting or fishing. Travel opportunities are expanding.

The life-style of later years is to a large degree formulated in youth. This fact was recognized by Robert Browning: "Grow old along with me! / The best is yet to be, / The last of life, for which the first was made." People who attempt suddenly to refocus and enrich their lives at retirement usually have difficulty. Those who learned early in life to live well-balanced and fulfilling lives are generally more successful in retirement. The woman who has been concerned only with the accomplishments of her children or the man who has been concerned only with the paycheck and his job status can be left with a feeling of emptiness when children leave and the job no longer exists. The later years can foster a sense of integrity and continuity, or they can be years of despair.

ECONOMIC CHANGE

The financial needs of elderly people vary considerably. Though most need less money for clothing, entertainment, and work, and although some own their homes outright, costs continue to rise, making it difficult for some to manage. Food and medical costs alone are often a financial burden. Adequate financial resources enable the older person to remain independent.

Problems with income are often related to low retirement benefits, lack of pension plans for many workers, and the increased length of the retirement years. Elderly members of minority groups have greater financial problems than elderly whites. Elderly women of all ages have lower incomes than men, and the oldest women are the poorest (Ebersole & Hess 1990, p. 377). Women, as a group, receive less from pensions, less from income, and

DEVELOPMENTAL TASKS OF THE OLDER ADULT

- Adjusting to decreasing physical strength and health
- Adjusting to retirement and reduced income
- Adjusting to the death of one's spouse
- Establishing an explicit affiliation with one's age group
- Meeting social and civic obligations
- Establishing satisfactory living arrangements
- Establishing satisfactory relationships with adult children
- Finding meaning in life

less from government sources than men receive (Yurick et al 1989, p. 304–5).

Nurses should be aware of the costs of health care. For example, while assisting a client to plan a diet, the nurse must consider which foods the client can afford to buy. The nurse or the client can request the physician to order lower-priced medications. In addition, the supplies used in a client's care should be as economical as possible.

RELOCATION

During late adulthood, many people experience relocation. A variety of factors may lead to this decision. The house or apartment may be too large or too expensive. The work involved in maintaining the house may become burdensome or impossible for the aged person or couple. Some elderly persons with decreased mobility want living arrangements that are all on one floor or need more accessible bathroom facilities.

Making the decision to move is often a very stressful one. The elderly person may be moving to an apartment, which may mean leaving the comfort of the family home and the neighbors and friends of several decades. Some need to move nearer to their children for general support and supervision. For many, this decision is difficult and stressful. For others, relocation is voluntary. The person may be seeking a more moderate climate with better recreational facilities geared to a more leisurely life-style. Adjustment will be much easier for the elderly person making a voluntary move.

A small percentage of the elderly, between 5% and 7%, must relocate to long-term care facilities or nursing homes. The decision to enter a nursing home is frequently made when elderly persons can no longer care for themselves, often because of problems of mobility and memory impairment. An increasing number of nursing home residents are in the very old age group (85 years and over), and most are women (Fulmer 1988, p. 544).

The facilities in nursing homes differ in many ways and offer varying degrees of independence to the residents. All provide meals but vary in giving other services, such as assistance with hygiene and dressing, physical therapy or exercise, recreational activities, transportation services, and medical and nursing supervision.

Nurses in hospitals should find out whether a client is being discharged to a nursing home or to a private home. Many nursing homes provide nursing services to clients and require appropriate information to provide for continuity of care. Clients returning home, however, may require the assistance of a home care nurse.

FACING DEATH AND GRIEVING

Well-adjusted aging couples usually thrive on companionship. Many couples rely increasingly on their mates for this company and may have few outside friends. Great bonds of affection and closeness can develop during this period of aging together and nurturing each other. When a mate dies, the remaining partner inevitably experiences feelings of loss, emptiness, and loneliness. Many are capable and manage to live alone; however, reliance on younger family members increases as age advances and ill health occurs. Some widows and widowers remarry, particularly the latter, because widowers are less inclined than widows to maintain a household.

Women face bereavement and solitude more often than men, since women usually live longer. The brevity of life is constantly reinforced by the death of friends. It is a time when one's life is reviewed with happiness or regret. Feelings of serenity or guilt and inadequacy can arise. Independence established prior to loss of a mate makes this adjustment period easier. A person who has some meaningful friendships, economic security, ongoing interests in the community, or private hobbies and a peaceful philosophy of life copes more easily with bereavement. Successful relationships with children and grandchildren are also of inestimable value. See Chapter 33 for a discussion about facing death.

Nurses can sometimes help clients who are alone a great deal to adjust their living arrangements or life-style so that they have more companionship. Moving to a retirement home that has other people in similar circumstances and organized social activities is one example. Many communities provide social centers for the elderly, for example, drop-in centers or community centers that offer day trips for seniors. Nurses can refer clients to services and encourage them to obtain companionship.

COGNITIVE DEVELOPMENT

Piaget's phases of cognitive development end with the formal operations phase. However, considerable research on cognitive abilities and aging is currently being conducted.

Intellectual capacity includes perception, cognitive agility, memory, and learning. **Perception,** or the ability to interpret the environment, depends on the acuteness of the senses. If the aging person's senses are impaired, the ability to perceive the environment and react appropriately is diminished. Perceptual capacity may be affected by changes in the nervous system as well. **Cognitive ability**, or the ability to know, is related to perceptual ability. An older man, for example, may know that he will be retiring next year but be unable to plan for retirement. He cannot accept the knowledge psychologically because his work provides his sense of worth, self-esteem, and identity.

Changes in cognitive structures occur as a person ages. It is believed that there is progressive loss of neurons. In addition, blood flow to the brain decreases, the meninges appear to thicken, and brain metabolism slows. As yet, little is known about the effect of these physical changes on the cognitive functioning of the older adult. Neurofibrillary tangles have also been found in the hippocampal cortex, the area of the brain concerned with memory. A **neurofibrillary tangle** is an abnormal mass of fibrillar material found in the cytoplasm. Neuritic plaques are also found in the aging brain. A **neuritic plaque** is a structure composed of amyloid material surrounded by abnormal neural structures. Neurofibrillary tangles and neuritic plaques could account for some of the functional changes found in normal aging people. Another change noted in the brain of the elderly is the deposition of lipofuscin. **Lipofuscin** is a brown-colored waste material having a lipid base that accumulates within the nerves as well as cardiac and skeletal muscle tissues. The effect of lipofuscin is unknown but is postulated to affect neuronal functioning.

Memory, or the ability to retain information, is also a component of intellectual capacity and is closely related to learning. Thomas (1992) describes four stages of memory in the information processing model; sensory memory, primary memory or working memory, secondary memory, and tertiary memory. **Sensory memory,** the first stage, is the momentary perception of stimuli by the senses. New information from the visual and auditory senses is temporarily stored in sensory memory during this stage (eg, visual information is stored in visual, or *iconic*, memory; auditory information is stored in auditory, or *echoic*, memory). **Primary memory,** also called **short-term memory,** is what one has in mind at a given moment. An example of primary memory is when you call information for a telephone number and remember the number only for the brief time needed to dial the number. There is limited storage capacity and duration in primary memory. **Working memory** is the term applied to the processes of manipulating or reorganizing information in primary memory. There is generally little age difference in primary memory; however, there do appear to be age-related differences in working memory. For information to be retained, it must enter secondary memory. **Secondary memory,** also referred to as **recent memory,** includes the memory capacities that one uses on a daily basis. This includes memory about current events, a book recently read, or a movie recently viewed. Most age-related differences occur in secondary memory. The final stage of memory is **tertiary memory.** Other terms for tertiary memory are **long-term memory** and **remote memory.** Tertiary memory is the repository for information stored for very long periods (Thomas 1992, p. 168). Memories of childhood friends, teachers, and events are stored in tertiary memory. Elderly clients who remember the flowers in their wedding bouquet or the names of the boys on their dance card are drawing from tertiary memory.

Older people need additional time for learning, largely because of the problem of retrieving information. Motivation is also important. Older adults have more difficulty than younger ones in learning information they do not consider meaningful. It is suggested that the older person remain mentally active to maintain cognitive ability at the highest possible level. Lifelong mental activity, particularly verbal activity, helps the older person retain a high level of cognitive function and may help maintain long-term memory. Cognitive impairment that interferes with normal life is not considered part of normal aging. A decline in intellectual abilities that interferes with social or occupational functions should always be regarded as abnormal. Family members should be advised to seek prompt medical evaluation.

DEMENTIA

Dementia is a general term for a permanent or progressive organic mental disorder that is characterized by personality changes, confusion, disorientation, deterioration of intellectual functioning, and impaired control of memory, judgment, and impulses (Wold 1993, p. 75). There are three types of dementia: primary dementia, secondary dementia or pseudodementia, and multi-infarct dementia (MID). **Primary dementias** are diseases that directly attack brain tissue and cause the behaviors associated with dementia. Primary dementias are irreversible; that is, they can only be treated symptomatically and cannot be cured. The most common type of primary dementia, and of all types of dementias, is Alzheimer's disease (AD). Other diseases classified as primary dementias include Parkinson's disease and Huntington's disease. **Secondary dementia** refers to diseases that do not directly attack brain tissue but result in symptoms described as characteristics of dementia. Secondary dementia may result from diabetic ketoacidosis, drug intoxication, severe nutritional imbalance, severe dehydration, head trauma, severe infections, and depression. **Multi-infarct dementia** refers to dementia symptoms resulting from multiple small strokes (Thomas 1993, p. 235). Secondary dementias and multi-infarct dementias are reversible if the underlying disease process is treated promptly.

Dementia is recognized as a major public health problem in the United States, affecting approximately 5% of the population from 65 to 74 years of age, and more than 30% of those over age 80. Of the elderly residing in the community, 10% experience intellectual impairment; in the nursing home population, between 50% and 75% of the clients are affected with cognitive impairment that is thought to be dementia of the Alzheimer type (Rowe & Besdine 1988, pp. 377–81).

Alzheimer's disease affects about 3 million people in the United States. By the year 2030, that number is expected to rise to nearly 5 million. The monetary cost of care for AD clients is estimated at $30 billion annually in the United States. The symptoms of AD have been grouped into three or four stages and may vary somewhat from client to client. The most prominent symptoms are cognitive dysfunctions, including decline in memory, learning, attention, judgment, orientation, and language skills. The symptoms are progressive, and all victims experience a steady decline in cognitive and physical abilities, lasting between 7 and 15 years and ending in death. In the last stage, the client requires total assistance, is unable to communicate, is incontinent, and may be unable to walk.

Although several theories are being investigated, the cause of AD is not known. Some of the causative theories include accumulation of aluminum deposits in the neurons, changes in the immune system, active and latent viruses, and defects in the neurotransmitter system. Currently, definite diagnosis can be made only on autopsy, where the physical changes specific to AD can be validated. Scanning techniques, such as PET (positron emission tomography) and MRI (magnetic resonance imaging) are currently aiding physicians in following the clinical progression of AD. Recently, a protein designated A68 has been detected in the brain of AD victims and from the spinal fluid of AD clients. In addition, A68 is also associated with neurofibrillary tangles. If the results of further studies on A68 support these initial findings, a routine laboratory test could be developed that makes early and accurate diagnosis of AD possible.

There is no cure or specific treatment for AD. Several drugs have been developed, but none has been shown consistently to retard or reverse the progression of the disease. It is hoped that one experimental drug, tetrahydroaminocridine (THA), will allow the brain cells to function more efficiently, thereby improving cognitive function. Research is currently under way.

It is estimated that about one million people with AD are cared for in the home. The burden of care is frequently on women—wives and daughters—who are themselves aging. Hamdy et al (1990, p. xiii) state that AD is "devastating for the families and caregivers of its victims. The caregivers drive themselves to physical and emotional exhaustion while they render continuous care and experience the anguish of seeing a loved one turned into a person who no longer remembers who he or she is." The nurse's responsibility is to provide supportive nursing care, accurate information, and referral assistance, if placement in a nursing care facility becomes necessary.

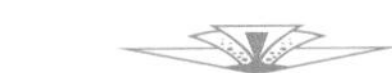

MORAL DEVELOPMENT

According to Kohlberg, moral development is completed in the early adult years. Most old people stay at Kohlberg's conventional level of moral development (see Table 23–6 on page 570), and some are at the preconventional level. An elderly person at the preconventional level obeys rules to avoid pain and the displeasure of others. At stage 1, a person defines good and bad in relation to self, whereas older persons at stage 2 may act to meet another's needs as well as their own. Elderly people at the conventional level follow society's rules of conduct in response to the expectations of others.

Wold (1992, p. 313) cautions that the value and belief patterns that are important to the elderly may have little or no significance to younger persons because they developed during a time that was very different from today. Edelman and Mandle (1990, p. 533) further point out that a large number of today's elderly are either foreign born or first-generation immigrants. Cultural background, life experiences, gender, religion, and socioeconomic status all influence one's values. The nurse must identify and consider the specific values of the older client when nursing care is planned.

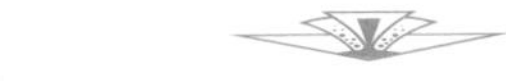

SPIRITUAL DEVELOPMENT

Murray and Zentner (1993, p. 581) write that the elderly person with a mature religious outlook strives to incorporate views of theology and religious action into thinking. Elderly people can contemplate new religious and philosophical views and try to understand ideas missed previously or interpreted differently. The elderly person

Table 26–3 Examples of Nursing Diagnoses, Goals, and Interventions for the Older Adult

NANDA Diagnoses	Goal/Outcome Criteria	Interventions
Social isolation related to inadequate individual resources	The older adult will demonstrate (within 1 month) a decrease in social isolation, as evidenced by ▪ Listing five interests or activities. ▪ Choosing two activities that can be pursued in the community. ▪ Pursuing at least one activity per week. ▪ Establishing weekly community interests.	Encourage and explore expressions of feelings about perceived social isolation. Actively listen to the client. Help the client explore causes of social isolation. Assist the client to develop a plan of action; for example, suggest possible resources and activities. Give positive reinforcement for successful involvement.
Health-seeking behaviors related to home safety measures that prevent falls	The older adult will demonstrate (within 2 weeks) a home environment that minimizes the risk of falls, as manifested by ▪ Appropriate lighting in all areas (eg, night light in hallways and bathrooms). ▪ Installation of grab bars near toilets and tub. ▪ Firmly attached rugs and carpets. ▪ Installation of handrails along stairs.	Assess the client's home for safety hazards. Provide accurate information on ways to minimize or alleviate falls in the home. Inform client of health care resources available to make necessary home adjustments (eg, bath seat). Inform client of possible financial aid available to make home safety adjustments.
Impaired home maintenance management related to inadequate social support system	The older adult will demonstrate (within 1 week) effective home maintenance management, as evidenced by ▪ Verbalizing knowledge of available resources. ▪ Following specific plans for home maintenance. ▪ Verbalizing satisfaction with maintenance of home in comfortable fashion.	Explore the health status of all family members who may assist with home maintenance management. Help client identify support system that will assist in home maintenance management. Discuss community resources for daily home maintenance. Explore role function each family member now fulfills and possible role changes. Initiate referrals for supplementing daily home maintenance. Arrange for additional support for caregiver respite.

also derives a sense of worth by sharing experiences or views. In contrast, the elderly person who has not matured spiritually may feel impoverishment or despair as the drive for economic and professional success wanes.

Carson (1989, pp. 44–45) states that religion "takes on new meaning for the elderly, who may find comfort, solace, and affirmation in religious activities." The older person's knowledge becomes wisdom, an inner resource for dealing with both positive and negative life experiences. Many elderly persons have strong religious convictions and continue to attend church services. Involvement in religion often helps the elderly person to resolve issues related to the meaning of life, to adversity, or to good fortune (Yurick et al 1989, p. 207). The "old-old" person who cannot attend formal services often continues religious participation in a more private manner. Many elderly persons watch television evangelists and some, being vulnerable to fund-raising ventures, send these organizations money that they can ill afford to spare.

According to Fowler and Keen (1985), some people enter the sixth stage of spiritual development, *universalizing*. See Table 16–2 on page 314. People whose spiritual development reaches this level think and act in a way that exemplifies love and justice.

HEALTH ASSESSMENT

Assessment guidelines for the development of the older adult are shown in box on the next page. Assessment activities may include measurement of weight, height, and vital signs (see Chapter 21); observation of the skin for hydration status or presence of lesions; examination of visual acuity using the Snellen chart; examination of hearing acuity using the whisper, Weber, and Rinne tests (see Chapter 22) and questions about the following:

- Usual dietary pattern
- Any problems with bowel or urinary elimination
- Activity/exercise and sleep/rest patterns
- Family and social activities and interests
- Any problems with reading, writing, or problem solving
- Adjustment to retirement or loss of partner

Examples of NANDA nursing diagnoses, goals/outcome criteria, and nursing interventions for the older adult are shown in Table 26–3.

According to recent research, much of the decline in health that was previously considered to be related to "old age" is caused by chronic illnesses resulting from unhealthy life-styles and poor health habits rather than aging itself (Smith 1988, p. 48). To retard the aging process, the older person must learn self-care techniques related to health promotion and disease prevention. Studies indicate that older persons are concerned about their health and are interested in information and behavioral strategies directed toward improving it. To assist the older adult in promoting health, the nurse may wish to discuss some other or all of the following topics.

ASSESSMENT GUIDELINES

The Older Adult

In the following developmental areas, does the older adult

Physical Development

- Adjust to physiologic changes (eg, appearance, sensory/perceptual, musculoskeletal, neurologic, cardiovascular)?
- Adapt life-style to diminishing energy and ability?
- Maintain vital signs (especially blood presure) within normal range for age and sex?

Psychosocial Development

- Manage retirement years in a satisfying manner?
- Participate in social and leisure activities?
- Have a social network of friends and support persons?
- View life as worthwhile?
- Have high self-esteem?
- Gain support from value system and/or spiritual philosophy?
- Accept and adjust to the death of significant others?

Development in Activities of Daily Living

- Exhibit healthy practices in nutrition, exercise, recreation, sleep patterns, and personal habits?
- Have the ability to care for self or to secure appropriate help with activities of daily living?
- Have satisfactory living arrangements and income to meet changing needs?

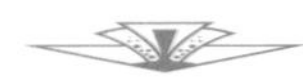

PROMOTING HEALTH AND WELLNESS

HEALTH MAINTENANCE VISITS AND IMMUNIZATION

The older adult should have routine health assessments that may involve a yearly physical examination, including a urinalysis and stool test for occult blood; yearly visual examination; yearly audiometry, if hearing ability is at risk; yearly dental assessment; yearly mammogram; Papanicolaou test every year if in a high-risk group, or every 3 years if not; and yearly testicular and prostate examination. Some physicians may also recommend a sigmoidoscopy every 5 years and certain blood tests (eg, blood lipids) on a regular basis.

The older adult should receive a diphtheria and tetanus booster every 10 years; for those at risk for hepatitis, hepatitis B vaccine is also recommended. Clients with a history of chronic respiratory or cardiac disease are usually encouraged to receive immunizations against pneumococcal pneumonia and influenza.

SAFETY

Accident prevention is a major concern for elderly people. Because vision is limited, reflexes are slowed, and bones are brittle, climbing stairs, driving a car, and even walking require caution. Driving, particularly night driving, requires caution because accommodation of the eye to light is impaired and peripheral vision is diminished. Older persons need to learn to turn the head before changing lanes and should not rely on side vision, for example, when crossing a street. Driving in a fog or other hazardous conditions should be avoided.

Fires are a hazard for the elderly person with a failing memory. The older person may forget that the iron or stove is left on or may not extinguish a cigarette completely. Because of reduced sensitivity to pain and heat, care must be taken to prevent burns when the person bathes or uses heating devices.

Many elderly persons suffer and die each year from hypothermia. **Hypothermia** is a body temperature below normal. A lowered metabolism and loss of normal insulation from thinning subcutaneous tissue decrease the elderly client's ability to retain heat. Health promotion to maintain body temperature should focus on teaching the elderly client to

- Dress warmly with layered clothing and protect head and hands when going outdoors in cold weather
- Use extra blankets at night and keep feet warm with woolen socks, which are safer than hot-water bottles.
- Eat a balanced diet, including high-energy foods such as fats and carbohydrates
- Learn to monitor the household thermostat and be sure that adequate home heating fuel is available

Because older clients who take analgesics or sedatives may become lethargic or confused, they should be monitored regularly and closely. Other measures to induce sleep should be used whenever possible. Nurses can help elderly clients make the home environment safe. Specific hazards can be identified and corrected; for example, hand rails can be installed on staircases. The nurse teaches the importance of taking only prescribed medications and contacting a health professional at the first indication of intolerance to them.

Guidelines for accident prevention for the older adult are detailed in the box on the page to the right.

NUTRITION

The older adult requires the same basic nutrition as the younger adult. However, fewer calories are needed by the older adult because of the lower metabolic rate and the decrease in physical activity. The older adult should consume approximately 1200 kcal per day. This figure may vary for each person according to the level of individual activity.

A major problem of the elderly is periodontal disease resulting in loss of teeth due to poor dental care. Poorly fitting dentures may also be a concern. These factors coupled with a decrease in salivation may cause difficulty in chewing and limit the type of food the older person can eat. As a result, the older person may avoid foods that require extensive chewing, such as meats or fresh fruits, and nutritional deficiencies may result.

A decrease in the thirst sensation, combined with a self-imposed limitation of fluids to compensate for incontinence, may result in an inadequate intake of fluids in elderly clients and **dehydration.** The nurse should instruct the older adult that about 8 glasses of water a day is needed to maintain kidney function, soften stools, prevent dehydration, and moisturize skin.

Nursing diagnoses related to diet and nutrition include **Altered nutrition: less than body requirements,** and **Altered nutrition: more than body requirements. Altered nutrition: less than body requirements** may result from a variety of physical and psychosocial factors. The elderly client may be eating empty calories rather than nutritious food, eating alone, or suffering from chronic diseases that affect food intake and metabolism, such as malignant disorders, alcoholism, or depression. Elderly clients frequently have dietary deficiencies of vitamins A, B, C, and D and the minerals of iron and calcium (Schuster & Ashburn 1992, p. 814). The nurse should assess the dietary habits of the elderly client and ascertain that intake of foods rich in these vitamins and minerals is adequate (see Chapter 37 for appropriate food sources).

Decreased exposure to sunlight and changes in the intestines and liver that interfere with metabolism are thought to contribute to vitamin D deficiency and bone disorders. **Osteomalacia** is marked by "softening of the bones," which become bent and deformed. **Osteoporosis** causes bones to become porous and less dense, resulting in an increased susceptibility to fracture and collapse. To prevent these problems, the nurse must take special care to ensure that older adults ingest sufficient amounts of vitamin D and calcium. Outdoor activities should also be encouraged to increase exposure to sunlight, a natural source of vitamin D, as well as to enhance overall well-being.

Altered nutrition: more than body requirements may result from lifelong eating patterns coupled with a lack of exercise. Retirement from work or problems with mobility due to chronic disease may also compound the problem. Other reasons cited for overeating include past habits, occupation, anxiety or nervousness, difficult life situations, mental illness, glandular imbalance, and grief or loss. Overeating may lead to chronic illness such as heart disease, high blood pressure, arteriosclerosis, and diabetes.

Guidelines for promoting nutritional health of older adults are provided in Chapter 37, page 1025.

ELIMINATION

Constipation is a common problem in the elderly population. Many elderly believe that "regularity" means a bowel movement every day. Those who do not meet this criterion often seek over-the-counter preparations to relieve what they believe to be constipation. Elderly clients should be advised that normal patterns of bowel elimination vary considerably. For some, a normal pattern may be every other day; for others, twice a day. Adequate roughage in the diet, adequate exercise, and 6 to 8 glasses of fluid daily are essential preventive measures for constipation. A cup of hot water or tea at a regular time in the morning is helpful for some. Responding to the gastrocolic reflex is also an important consideration.

The older adult should be warned that consistent use of over-the-counter preparations is thought to cause rather than cure constipation. In a few cases, moreover, they can cause serious intestinal problems. Laxatives may also interfere with the body's electrolyte balance and decrease the absorption of certain vitamins. The reasons for constipation can range from life-style habits to serious malignant disorders. The nurse should evaluate any complaints of constipation carefully for each individual. A change in bowel habits over several weeks with or without weight loss, pain, or fever should be referred to a physician for a complete medical evaluation.

A decline in bladder capacity, plus weaker muscle tone, results in an increase in frequency as well as urgency in

SAFETY HIGHLIGHTS FOR THE OLDER ADULT

Preventing Falls

- Make sure all rooms, hallways, and stairwells are adequately lighted.
- Have an easily accessible light switch next to the bed.
- Leave a night light on in the hallway or bathroom.
- Get out of bed slowly (ie, sit before standing and stand briefly before walking) to prevent dizziness from orthostatic hypotension.
- Install grab bars in the bathroom near the toilet and tub.
- Make sure rugs and carpets are firmly attached to floors and stairs.
- Make sure that electrical cords are secured against baseboards to prevent tripping.
- Keep indoor and outdoor walkways and stairs in good repair.
- Install sturdy, slip-resistant hand railings along stairs.

Preventing Burns

- Check the temperature of bath water and heating pads. Run cold water before hot water.
- Lower thermostats of water heaters to provide warm rather than very hot water.
- Avoid smoking in bed or when sleepy.
- Install smoke alarms.
- Place a hand fire extinguisher in a convenient area of the home (eg, the kitchen).
- Smother kitchen grease fires with a large lid or baking soda.
- Avoid wearing loose-fitting clothing when cooking.
- Do not overload electric circuits and keep electrical appliances in good repair.
- Keep passageways to outside doors unobstructed.

Preventing Pedestrian Accidents

- Wear reflective or light-colored clothing at night.
- Cross streets at intersections with crosswalks and traffic lights when possible; do not cross major streets in the middle of the block.
- Be sure to look both ways before stepping from the curb.

Preventing Automobile Accidents

- Have regular eye examinations to assess vision, acquire appropriate refractive corrections, and detect other problems early.
- Wear good-quality gray or green sunglasses during daytime driving to reduce glare.
- Keep car windows clean and windshield wipers in good condition.
- Place mirrors on both sides of the car and always check rearview and side mirrors before changing lanes.
- Always look behind your vehicle for people or obstacles before backing up.
- Avoid smoking when driving, especially at night. Smoke can reduce visibility.
- Follow your physician's restrictions, if any, about when and where to drive.
- Learn the effects of prescribed medications on driving ability.
- Do not drink and drive.
- Stop periodically to stretch your muscles and rest your eyes.
- Leave car windows partially open and set the radio and fans low so that you can hear sirens and horns.
- Have your ability to drive periodically reevaluated.
- Keep your automobile in good repair and keep headlights, tail lights, and turn signals clean so they are visible to others.

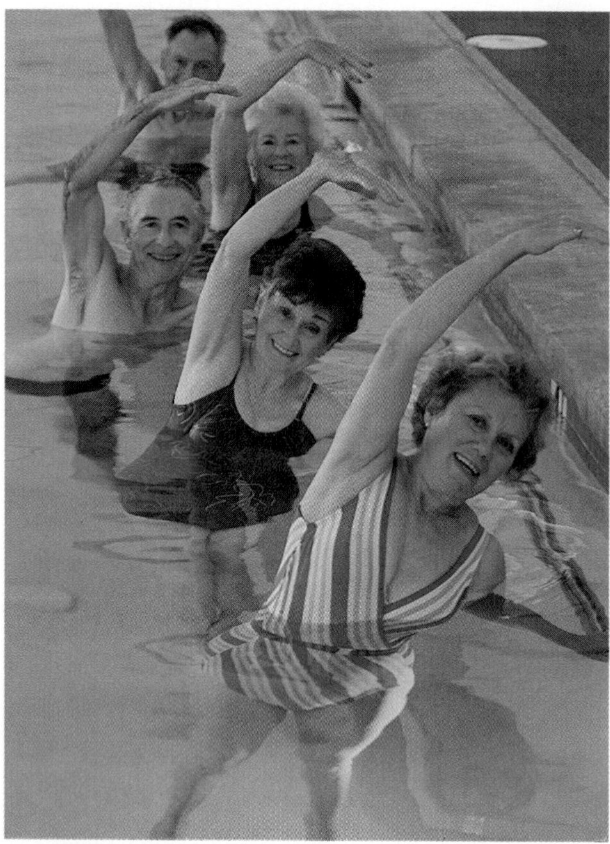

Figure 26–2 A regular program of exercise is important for maintenance of joint mobility and muscle tone and can promote socialization.

many older persons. The nurse should be aware of these changes and teach the elderly person appropriate strategies to prevent embarrassment caused by incontinence. Toilet facilities should be accessible, and elderly persons should be instructed to give themselves enough time to get to the bathroom and remove their clothing. Bladder training exercises (see Chapter 41) as well as a regular toilet schedule may also be helpful adjuncts.

Many older people learn to deal with nocturnal frequency by restricting their fluid intake in the latter part of the evening, particularly those fluids that stimulate voiding, such as coffee or alcohol. Eventually most men require prostatic surgery to relieve increasing urinary frequency throughout the day, and some women require vaginal surgery for cystoceles or rectoceles. A **cystocele** is a protrusion of the urinary bladder through the vaginal wall. A **rectocele** is the protrusion of part of the rectum through the vaginal wall. Both of these conditions produce pressure and reduce bladder capacity, thereby creating urinary urgency and frequency.

Weakness in muscle tone in the ureters and bladder also increases the elderly person's risk for urinary tract infections (UTI). Preventive measures, such as increasing fluid intake, including juices that produce an acid ash such as cranberry juice, and preventing contamination of the urinary tract should be included in the teaching plan. Elderly clients should seek medical evaluation for any of the symptoms of UTI (eg, burning on urination, frequency, and sometimes fever).

ACTIVITY AND EXERCISE

A regular program of moderate exercise is recommended for elderly adults. Walking, golfing, swimming, bowling, and bicycling are common activities (Figure 26–2). These can be performed at a leisurely pace. It is important that exercise not be too strenuous and that rest periods be taken as needed. Rapid breathing and accelerated heartbeat should disappear within a few minutes after exercise; exercise should refresh rather than fatigue. People who are too disabled to engage in active exercise can implement a program of isometric exercises to maintain joint mobility and muscle tone.

Perhaps the most significant physical benefit of regular exercise for the older adult is a decrease in the risk for cardiovascular disease. In addition, exercise maintains bone calcification, helps to maintain muscle tone throughout the body, and reduces muscle tension and muscle pain.

The nurse should suggest some safety precautions for the elderly client beginning an exercise program. These include (1) wearing proper shoes with nonstick soles; (2) avoiding slick surfaces; (3) exercising or walking in safe, well-lighted areas; (4) being aware of adverse symptoms of exercise, such as dizziness, shortness of breath, or irregular heartbeat; and (5) beginning any exercise program slowly to allow the body time to adjust. See the discussion on developing a successful exercise program on page 931 and target and maximum heart rates by age on page 929. Some physicians may recommend an exercise **stress test** to determine the type and intensity of exercise program that is best for the individual client. During a stress test, blood pressure and heart rhythm are continuously monitored while the client exercises, either on a treadmill or on a bicycle.

REST AND SLEEP

The aging process affects the amount of time spent sleeping, with the average 70-year-old getting 6 hours in a 24-hour period, 1½ hours less than the average younger adult gets. Sleep stage patterns are altered in the older adult, with the elderly experiencing less stage IV and REM sleep (see Table 35–2, p. 957). Decreases in these stages causes the elderly client to have less deep restorative sleep (Wold 1992, pp. 245–46). This results in feelings of fatigue experienced throughout the day. Elderly adults also tend to take somewhat longer to get to sleep,

CRITICAL THINKING CHALLENGE

WHAT WOULD YOU DO?

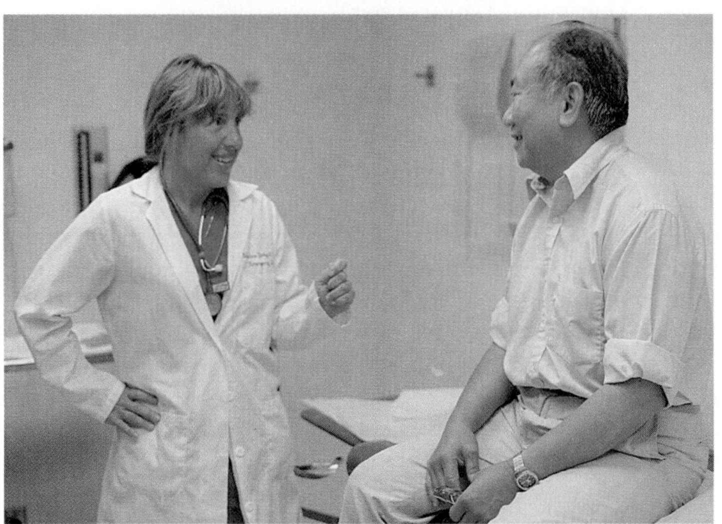

Min Leong, a 70-year-old male, visits your clinic for his annual physical. He reports that he's never felt better, stays very active, eats well, and exercises daily. Upon completing his assessment, you confirm that his physical and psychologic health appear to be very good. Mr Leong tells you that he's been training to run long distances and wants to enter a 10K race this weekend. He asks, "What do you think?"

What would you do?

wake up frequently during the night, and stay in bed longer or nap frequently throughout the day to make up for missed sleep.

The amount of sleep needed by the elderly adult varies. In general, most healthy older adults require about the same amount of sleep as they did during their middle adult years. Measures to promote rest are discussed in Chapter 35. It is valuable for the older adult who complains of sleep disturbance to keep a log of sleep, rest, and activity periods throughout the day. Often the client finds that frequent naps during the day are interfering with the ability to sustain sleep at night. Increasing daytime activity and limiting the number of naps and the amount of time napping can improve the nighttime sleep of the older adult.

Maintaining Independence and Self-Esteem

Most elderly people thrive on independence. It is important to them to be able to look after themselves even if they have to struggle to do so. Although it may be difficult for younger family members to watch the elder completing tasks in a slow, determined way, aging persons need this sense of accomplishment. Children might notice that the aging father or mother with failing vision cannot keep the kitchen as clean as before. The aging father and mother may be slower and less meticulous in carpentry tasks or gardening. To maintain the elderly adult's sense of self-respect, nurses and family members need to encourage them to do as much as possible for themselves, provided that safety is maintained (Figure 26–3). Many

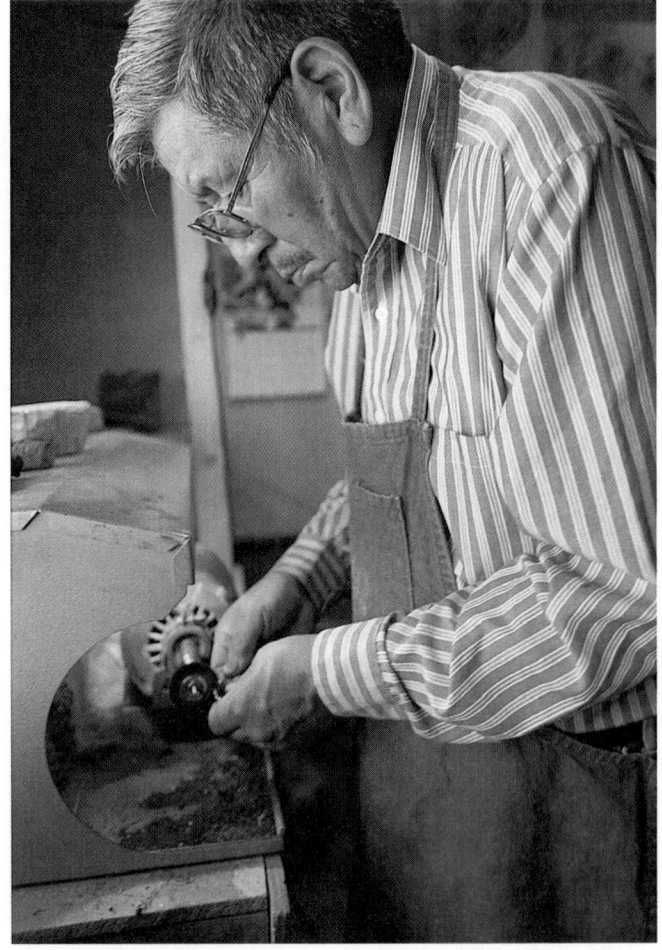

Figure 26–3 Independence fosters self-respect.

young people err in thinking that they are helpful to older people when they take over for them and do the job much faster and more efficiently.

Aging people need to be recognized for their unique individual characteristics. It can be difficult to recognize these differences, because elderly people have less energy than the young to show how they are different. Perhaps this is one reason elderly people tend to talk about past accomplishments, jobs, deeds, and experiences.

Nurses need to acknowledge the elderly client's ability to think, reason, and make decisions. Most elderly people are willing to listen to suggestions and advice, but they do not want to be ordered around. The nurse can support a decision by an elderly client even if eventually the decision is reversed because of failing health.

Older people appreciate thoughtfulness, consideration, and acceptance of their waning abilities. For example, having dinner out in a well-lighted restaurant or not expecting grandmother to baby-sit for too many hours, if at all, are actions that recognize the diminished vision and energy of older people. The values and standards held by older people need to be accepted, whether they are related to ethical, religious, or household matters. For example, it is wise to respect an older person's decision to hang the laundry outside rather than to use a dryer, or to cook on a conventional stove rather than in a microwave oven.

ELDER ABUSE

It is estimated that between one and two million elderly Americans are victims of elder abuse each year (Simon 1992, p. 1). The victims of abuse are likely to be white, female, and over 70 years of age. In addition, most victims of abuse are afflicted with substantial mental or physical impairments. Older adults who are unable to care for themselves are often cared for by family members, usually a daughter or spouse. Caring for a spouse or a parent often causes a great deal of strain and frustration in a relationship and may lead to violence and abuse.

There are many types of abuse used against the elderly. They include, (1) psychologic abuse, such as instilling fear, threatening, or making the elder perform demeaning tasks; (2) physical abuse, such as hitting, slapping, or burning; (3) financial abuse, such as taking their money or

RESEARCH NOTE

What Factors Contribute to Physical Health Impairment and Depression Among Older Adults?

This study examined factors that contribute to depression among older adults, aged 60 to 75 years. The sample included 80 white, older adults living independently in the community. Participants completed the physical health subscale and the social resources and economic resources subscales of the Older Americans Resources and Services (OARS) Multidimensional Functional Assessment Questionnaire, Pearlin's Sense of Mastery Scale, and the Center for Epidemiological Studies-Depression Scale (CESD). Participants were divided into two groups, based on their physical health impairment scores. One group consisted of participants with mild physical health impairment; the other group included participants with moderate to severe physical health impairment.

Findings revealed no significant differences in demographic characteristics (ie, age, education, employment, income, or marital status) between the two groups. However, there were significant differences in perceptions of overall health and the degree to which specific illnesses such as arthritis, hypertension, and stomach conditions impeded functioning. Group 2 participants reported (a) greater interference in their ability to do the things they wished to do, (b) increased problem drinking, (c) decreased sense of mastery (ability to control outcomes in their lives), (d) decreased social resources (fewer interactions with others, greater loneliness and less dependable help in time of need), and (e) greater scores on the depression scale. No differences in economic resources were found between the two groups. The majority (80%) in both groups reported their income to be inadequate for future needs. The findings support the empirical and theoretical links between stressful life events, specifically, physical health impairment, and depression.

Implications: In caring for physically impaired older adults, nurses need to consider the clients' social resources, economic resources, and sense of mastery, all of which according to this study are significant predictor variables of depression.

Source: TA Badger, Physical health impairment and depression among older adults, *Image: Journal of Nursing Scholarship*, Winter 1993, 25:325–30.

forcing them to sign over their assets; (4) neglect, such as withholding food, medication, or basic care; (5) infringement of personal rights, such as restraining for long periods of time against their will or isolating them from normal social interactions; and (6) sexual abuse.

The perpetrator of abuse is usually the spouse or the child of the victim. Caregivers who abuse their elderly family members are often middle-aged or older or have emotional problems such as alcoholism or substance abuse; in some cases, three or four generations may be sharing living quarters. Caregivers are often placed in the stressful situation of administering care to parents who treat them like children. Many elderly people use guilt to control their children's lives and do not give them the privacy and respect that they need. The cost of medical care may also be a burden for the caregiver, as well as the stress involved in 24-hour responsibility for another person.

To prevent abuse, the nurse should spend time counseling families prior to their making the decision to care for their elderly parent. The nurse should also be aware that ongoing support is needed for the caregiver as well as for the elderly client. Frequent visits should be made to the home of an elderly client to assess the home situation for factors that may lead to an abusive situation. The elderly in general are unwilling and/or often unable to report abuse. They may feel guilty that they have raised a child who has mistreated them, or they may feel that they have no other place to go. In some cases, the abused persons may be cognitively impaired and unable to advocate in their own behalf.

The nurse who suspects an abusive situation has an obligation to report it. Nurses should be familiar with the laws of their particular state regarding reporting of suspected or known abuse. The legally competent adult cannot be forced, however, to leave the abusive situation and in many cases may decide to stay. If the elderly client is not legally competent, court proceedings to attain guardianship can be initiated.

Drug Use and Misuse

In the past several decades, the pharmaceutical industry has developed hundreds of prescription and nonprescription drugs that are now available to the public. Elderly adults frequently suffer from one or more chronic diseases that often require medication. Episodes of acute illness may require additional medications. Clients may purchase over-the-counter (OTC) drugs to remedy common discomforts related to aging, such as constipation, sleep disturbance, and joint pain. The complexities involved in the self-administration of medication may lead to a variety of misuse situations, including taking too much or too little medication, combining alcohol and medication, combining prescribed medications with over-the-counter drugs, taking medications at the wrong time, or taking someone else's medication. "Problems related to medications are common in the elderly, and they are costly in terms of both time and money" (Wold 1992, p. 328). Other potential misuse situations occur when more than one physician prescribes medications and the client fails to tell each doctor what has been previously prescribed.

Additionally, in the past medications have not been tested for their specific effect in elderly populations. Currently, senior citizens groups are advocating for such testing with the Food and Drug Administration (FDA).The pharmacodynamics of drugs are altered in the elderly. The variations in absorption, distribution, metabolism, and excretion of drugs are related to physiologic changes associated with aging. Decreased secretion of gastric acid and enzymes and decreased esophageal and gastrointestinal motility delay absorption of drugs. Decreased cardiac output and decreased serum albumin for binding of drugs for transport delays the distribution. Diminished liver metabolism interfere with the breakdown and metabolism of drugs already in the body, and decreased renal filtration delays excretion of drugs.

To prevent drug misuse, the nurse should assess the drug history of the elderly person carefully and determine a realistic teaching plan. Elderly clients should be given written instructions, in large print and in language that they can understand. In addition, the side effects of each drug should be listed and reviewed with the client. In simple terms, elderly clients should be taught the importance of maintaining a schedule for important medications (eg, digitoxin, insulin) and the risks involved in skipping a dose or "running out" of pills. Forgetful persons may need to use a pill organizer to ensure accurate medication ingestion. The nurse should also discuss any over-the-counter drugs the elderly client may use and explain potential risk and side effects of self-medication and multiple medications. In some cases, the nurse can offer conservative measures, such as relaxation techniques or soothing baths, to replace tranquilizers or pain medications. Health promotion activities, such as diet and exercise, may also be helpful adjuncts to reduce the need for medications for chronic disease.

Alcoholism

Edelman and Mandle (1990, p. 539) suggest that the alcohol problems among older adults are hidden and have been underestimated. Miller (1991) found that 14% of older males and 1.5% of older females had alcohol problems. In general, people tend to consume less alcohol as they get older. Elderly alcoholics include those who began drinking alcohol in their youth and those who began excessive alcohol use later in life. Alcoholics who begin drinking later in life do so to help them cope with the changes and problems of their older years. Many late-onset alcoholics are widowers.

Chronic drinking has major effects on all body systems, causes progressive liver and kidney damage, damages the stomach and related organs, and slows mental response, frequently leading to accidents and death. Alcohol interacts with various drugs, altering the normal effect of the medication on the body. Some medications have an increased effect when taken with alcohol (eg, anticoagulants and narcotics), whereas the action of other medications (eg, antibiotics) is inhibited. For the elderly person who has a chronic illness and takes many medications, the combination of drugs and alcohol can lead to serious drug overdose.

Elderly alcoholic clients should not be stereotyped or prejudged by the nurse. Rather, they should be accepted, listened to, and offered help. The nurse should assess the number and type of alcoholic beverages consumed as well as the pattern and frequency of consumption. It is important that the nurse discuss any medications the client is taking and review the side effects and interaction effects of alcohol and medication. The role of the nurse is to act as a client advocate and facilitate the treatment of the drinking problem in addition to the prevention of possible complications.

CHAPTER HIGHLIGHTS

- The life expectancy of North Americans is increasing to the point that it has become useful to divide late adulthood into three periods: the elderly, or "young-old" (60 or 65 to 74 years); the aged, or "middle-old" (75 to 84 years); and the extreme aged, or "old-old" (85 years and over).
- Several theories have been proposed to account for the biologic aging process: wear-and-tear, rate of living, stress, endocrine, free-radical, genetic, programmed senescence, error catastrophe, collagen, cross-linking, immunologic, and autoimmune theories.
- Psychosocial theories about aging include the disengagement, activity, and continuity theories.
- Many physical changes occur with aging and involve all body systems: the integument; body temperature; and the neuromusculoskeletal, cardiopulmonary, hematopoietic, immune, sensory/perceptual, digestive, urinary, endocrine, and reproductive systems.
- The older adult has to adjust to possible psychosocial changes, including retirement (which ne cessitates financial and social adjustments), relocation, increasing dependence on others, and coping with losses and death.
- Intellectual abilities of the healthy elderly person undergo minimal change. Of the four types of memory (sensory, primary, secondary, and tertiary), secondary memory is most affected by the aging process.
- A decline in memory and cognitive abilities (dementia) caused by such factors as depression, infection, and thyroid disorder are reversible if prompt diagnosis and treatment are obtained. Dementia caused by Alzheimer's disease, repeated strokes, and Parkinson's disease are irreversible at this time.
- The moral concerns of elderly people tend to be interpersonal rather than social or legalistic.
- Spiritual maturity can provide the elderly person with inner resources for dealing with life experiences.
- Much of the decline in health during late adulthood is due to chronic illnesses resulting from unhealthy life-styles and poor health habits, rather than the aging process itself.
- Health promotion and protection activities of the older adult focus on regular health maintenance visits and immunization; accident prevention; ensuring adequate nutrition; prevention of elimination problems; encouraging appropriate exercise, rest, and sleep; and maintaining the person's self-esteem and independence to the maximum potential.
- Elder abuse, drug use and misuse, and alcoholism are situations that require sensitive assessment and counseling by the nurse.

READINGS AND REFERENCES

SUGGESTED READINGS

Maas, M, Buckwalter, KC, and Hardy, M. 1991. *Nursing Diagnoses and Interventions for the Elderly.* Redwood City, CA: Addison-Wesley Nursing.

The authors discuss the application of selected NANDA-approved nursing diagnoses and appropriate interventions to the care of dependent elderly clients. Additional nursing diagnoses that have not been approved by NANDA such as "Impaired swallowing" and "Translocation syndrome," are also included because of their significance in the care of the dependent elderly. Normal changes of aging related to each functional health pattern are described, and case studies throughout the text highlight the material.

National Institute on Aging. 1987. *Bound for Good Health.* Washington, DC: US Government Printing Office.

This publication is a compilation of NIA's Age Pages, which provide information for laypersons as well as health professionals on topics of health and safety. Published in large print, with written permission for unlimited reproduction included, these documents are excellent for client education. The topics covered include nutrition, sexuality, accidents, cancer, crime, diabetes, and exercise.

RELATED RESEARCH

Badger, TA. Winter 1993. Physical health impairment and depression among older adults. *Image: Journal of Nursing Scholarship* 25:325–30.

Conn, VS, Taylor, SG, and Kelley, S. Winter 1991. Medication regimen complexity and adherence among older adults. *Image: Journal of Nursing Scholarship.* 23:231-35.

SELECTED REFERENCES

Bjorksten, J. 1974. Crosslinkage and the aging process. In Rockstein, MM, Sussman, M, and Chesky, J, editors. *Theoretical Aspects of Aging.* New York: Academic Press.

Burggraf, V and Donlon, B. September/October 1985. Assessing the elderly system by system. *American Journal of Nursing* 85:974–84, 1103–12.

Burggraf, V and Stanley, M. 1989. *Nursing the Elderly: A Care Plan Approach.* Philadelphia: Lippincott.

Burnside, IM. 1988. *Nursing and the Aged: A Self-Care Approach.* 3d ed. New York: McGraw-Hill.

Butler, R. 1963. The life review: An interpretation of reminiscence in the aged. *Psychiatry* 26:65.

Carson, VB. 1989. *Spiritual Dimensions in Nursing Practice.* Philadelphia: WB Saunders.

Ciocon, J and Potter, J. October 1988. Age related changes in human memory: Normal and abnormal. *Geriatrics* 43:43–48.

Conn, VS, Taylor, SG, and Kelley, S. Winter 1991. Medication regimen complexity and adherence among older adults. *Image: Journal of Nursing Scholarship* 23:231–35.

Duvall, EM. 1977. *Family Development.* 5th ed. Philadelphia: Lippincott.

Ebersole, P and Hess, P. 1990. *Toward Healthy Aging: Human Needs and Nursing Response.* St Louis: Mosby.

Edelman, C and Mandle, CL. 1990. *Health Promotion Throughout the Life Span.* 2d ed. St Louis: Mosby.

Erickson EH, 1963. *Childhood and Society:* 2d ed. New York: Norton.

______. 1982. *The Life Cycle Completed: A Review.* New York: Norton.

Fowler, J and Keen, S. 1985. *Life Maps: Conversations in the Journey of Faith.* Waco, TX: Word Books.

Fulmer, T. 1988. The older adult. In Caliandro, G, and Judkins, B, editors. pp. 543–57. *Primary Nursing Practice.* Glenview, IL: Scott, Foresman.

Hallgren, HM and Unis, EJ. June 1977. Suppressor lymphocytes in young and aged humans. *Journal of Immunology* 118(6):2004.

Hamdy, RC, Turnbull, JM, Norman, LD, and Lancaster, MM. 1990. *Alzheimer's Disease: A Handbook for Caregivers.* St Louis: Mosby-Year Book.

Havighurst, RJ. 1953. Older People. New York: Longmans, Green.

Hayflick, L. Cell aging. 1977. In Cherkin, A et al, editors. *Physiology and Cell Biology of Aging.* New York: Raven Press.

______. October 1988. Why do we live so long? *Geriatrics* 43:77–87.

Jarvis, C. 1992. *Physical Examination and Health Assessment.* Philadelphia: WB Saunders.

Job, S and Anema, M. December 1988. Elder care: Ethical dimensions. *Journal of Gerontological Nursing* 14:16–19.

Kart, CS, Metress, EK, and Metress, SP. 1992. *Human Aging and Chronic Disease.* Boston, MA: Jones and Bartlett.

Kohlberg, L. 1971. *Recent Research in Moral Development.* New York: Holt, Rinehart and Winston.

Kozier, B, Erb, G, and Blais K. 1992. *Concepts and Issues in Nursing Practice.* 2d ed. Redwood City, CA: Addison-Wesley Nursing.

Lamb, M. 1977. *Biology of Aging.* New York: Wiley.

Lenihan, AA. July/August 1988. Identification of self care behaviors in the elderly: A nursing assessment tool. *Journal of Professional Nursing* 4:285–88.

Lyles, DC, Larisey, MM and Morrill, LS. May/June 1988. Health promotion for the elderly: A student experience. *Nurse Educator* 13:23–26.

Maas, M. Buckwalter, KC, and Hardy, M. 1991. *Nursing Diagnoses and Interventions for the Elderly.* Redwood City, CA; Addison-Wesley Nursing.

McCracken, AL. October 1988. Sexual practice by elders: The forgotten aspect of functional health. *Journal of Gerontological Nursing* 14:13–18.

Matteson, MA and McConnell, ES. 1988. *Gerontological Nursing: Concepts and Practice.* Philadelphia: WB Saunders.

Miller, NS. 1991. Alcohol and drug dependence. In Sadovoy, J, Lazarus, LW, and Jarvik, LF, editors. *Comprehensive Review of Geriatric Psychiatry.* Washington, DC: American Psychiatric Association.

Murray, RB, and Zentner, JP 1993. *Nursing Assessment and Health Promotion Strategies Through the Life Span.* 5th ed. Norwalk, CT: Appleton & Lange.

National Center for Health Statistics. 1993. *Health United States 1992 and Healthy People 2000 Review.* Hyattsville MD: Public Health Service.

National Institute on Aging. No date. *Answers about Aging: New Pieces to an Old Puzzle.* Silver Springs, MD: National Institute on Aging.

Nesbitt, B. July 1988. Nursing diagnosis: Age related changes. *Journal of Gerontological Nursing* 14:6–12.

Peck, R. 1955. Psychological developments in the second half of life. In Anderson, J, editor. *Psychological Aspects of Aging.* Washington, DC: American Psychological Association.

______. 1968. Psychological development in the second half of life. In Neugarten, BL, editor. *Middle Age and Aging.* Chicago: University of Chicago Press.

Pender, NJ. 1987. Health promotion and nursing practice. 2d ed. Norwalk, CT: Appleton & Lange.

Person, JE. 1993. *Statistical Forecasts of the United States.* Detroit: Gale Research.

Reed, AT and Birge, SJ. July 1988. Screening for osteoporosis. *Journal of Gerontological Nursing* 14:18–20.

Rowe, J and Besdine, R. 1988. *Geriatric Medicine.* 2d ed. Boston: Little, Brown.

Rybash, J, Hoyer, W, and Roodin, P. 1986. *Adult Cognition and Aging.* New York: Pergamon Press.

Rybash, JM, Roodin, PA, and Hoyer, WJ. 1983. Expressions of moral thought in later adulthood. *Gerontologist* 23:254–59.

Saxon, SV and Etten MJ. 1987. *Physical Change and Aging: A Guide for the Helping Professions.* 2d ed. New York: Tiresias Press.

Schuster, CS and Ashburn, SS. 1992. *The Process of Human Development: A Holistic Life-Span Approach.* 3d ed. Boston: Little, Brown.

Scura, KW. October 1988. Audiological assessment program. *Journal of Gerontological Nursing* 14:19–25.

Simon, ML. 1992. *An Exploratory Study of Adult Protective Services Programs' Repeat Elder Abuse Clients.* Washington, DC: American Association of Retired Persons.

Smith, DL. September/October 1988. Health promotion for older adults. *Health Values* 12:46–51.

Thomas, JL. 1992. *Adulthood and Aging.* Needham Heights, MA: Allyn & Bacon.

Trice, LB. Winter 1990. Meaningful life experience to the elderly. *Image: Journal of Nursing Scholarship* 22:248–51.

Tzirides, E. April 1988. Health outreach program: Marketing the "Health Way." *Nursing Management* 19:557.

US Bureau of the Census. 1992. *Statistical Abstract of the United States.* 112th ed. Washington, DC: US Government Printing Office.

Utley, QE, Hawkins, JE, Igou, JF, and Johnson, FF. June 1988. Giving and getting support at the wellness center. *Journal of Gerontological Nursing* 14:23–25.

Vander-Zanden, J. 1985. *Human Development.* 3d ed. New York: Knopf.

Walford, RL. 1980. Immunology and aging. *American Journal of Clinical Pathology* 74:247.

Webster, JA. December 1988. Key to healthy aging: Exercise. *Journal of Gerontological Nursing* 14:8–15.

Wold, G. 1993. *Basic Geriatric Nursing.* St Louis: Mosby-Year Book.

The World Almanac and Book of Facts. 1993. New York: Press Publishing Co.

Yurick, A, Spier, B, Robb, S, and Ebert, N. 1989. *The Aged Person and the Nursing Process.* Norwalk, CT: Appleton & Lange.

UNIT

8

PROTECTING HEALTH

STUDENT PROFILE

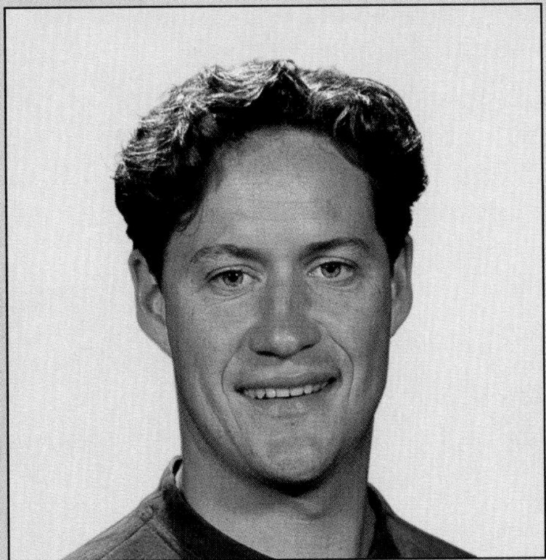

NAME Darren McLean

SCHOOL OF NURSING James Cook University, Townsville, Australia

HOME TOWN Melbourne, Australia

WHY DID YOU ENTER THE FIELD OF NURSING?
I wanted a career that offered diversity, the opportunity for advancement, and work which I felt was important and worthwhile.

WHY DO YOU THINK THIS IS A GOOD TIME TO BE IN NURSING?
There are important advances being made today toward establishing nursing as a true and recognized profession. Through research, education, policy formation, and advanced clinical competence, nurses are becoming more professional and autonomous, both individually and collectively.

WHAT HAS BEEN YOUR MOST GRATIFYING MOMENT AS A STUDENT NURSE?
Helping a middle-aged man with severe depression during one of my mental health practicums. Through deliberate and consistent interaction, I believe I was able to establish rapport and trust. When he broke down in tears during one of our conversations, it was gratifying to think that he felt comfortable enough to openly express his emotions.

WHAT ADVICE WOULD YOU GIVE TO A NEW STUDENT?
Make a commitment to your study, learn to be self-directed, persevere through the difficult times, and keep a positive attitude. Remember to take care of yourself, make time for your other interests and especially for other people. Above all else, enjoy what you are doing.

27

Preventing the Transfer of Microorganisms

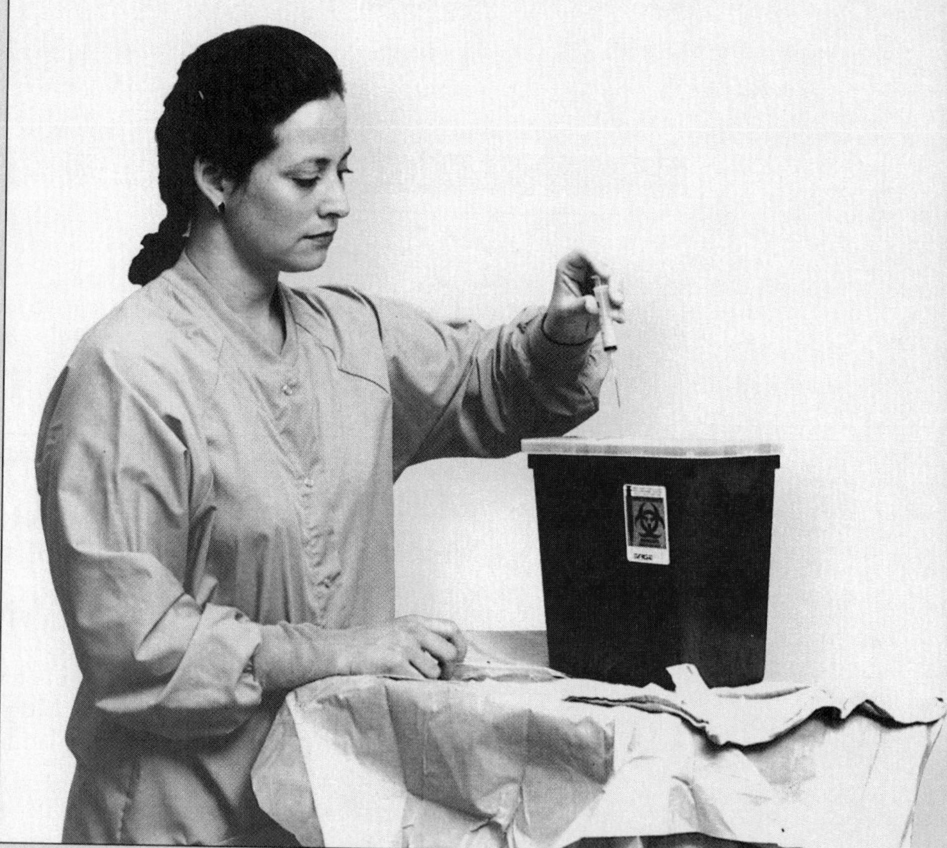

Objectives

- Describe the importance of biologic safety.
- Identify anatomic and physiologic barriers that defend the body against microorganisms.
- Describe the difference between nonspecific and specific defenses of the body.
- Differentiate active from passive immunity.
- Identify six links in the chain of infection.
- Identify measures that break each link in the chain of infection.
- Identify factors influencing a microorganism's capability to produce an infectious process.
- Identify people at risk for acquiring an infection.
- Describe four stages of an infectious process.
- Identify risks for nosocomial infections.
- Identify signs of localized and systemic infections.
- Identify relevant nursing diagnoses and contributing factors for clients at risk for infection and who have an infection.
- Develop outcome criteria to evaluate a client's response to nursing interventions and achievement of goals.
- Explain the concepts of medical and surgical asepsis.
- Identify interventions to reduce risks for infections.
- Compare and contrast category-specific, disease-specific, universal, and body substance isolation precaution systems.
- Discuss methods for evaluating the effectiveness of protective measures.
- Correctly implement aseptic practices, including hand washing, donning and removing a face mask, gowning, donning and removing disposable gloves, bagging articles, managing equipment used for isolation clients, and assessing vital signs.

Nurses are directly involved in providing a biologically safe environment and promoting health. Microorganisms exist everywhere in the environment: in water, soil, and on body surfaces such as the skin, intestinal tract, and other areas open to the outside (eg, mouth, upper respiratory tract, vagina, and lower urinary tract). Most microorganisms are harmless, and some are even beneficial in that they perform essential functions in the body. Some microorganisms found in the intestines (eg, enterobacteria) produce substances called **bacteriocins,** which are lethal to related strains of bacteria. Others produce antibiotic-like substances and toxic metabolites that repress the growth of other microorganisms. Some microorgainsms are normal **flora** (the collective vegetation in a given area) in one part of the body and produce infection in another. For example, *Escherichia coli* is a normal inhabitant of the large intestine but a common cause of infection of the urinary tract. Two pathogens that may be found in an infected person's blood are hepatitis B virus (HBV) and human immunodeficiency virus (HIV).

An **infection** is an invasion of body tissue by microorganisms and their proliferation there. Such a microorganism is called an infectious agent. If the microorganism produces no clinical evidence of disease, the infection is called *asymptomatic* or *subclinical.* Some subclinical infections can cause significant damage to the host, for example, cytomegalovirus (CMV) infection in a pregnant woman. A detectable alteration in normal tissue function, however, is called **disease.** Microorganisms vary in their **virulence** (ie, their ability to produce disease). In general, five groups of microorganisms normally can cause disease: bacteria, viruses, fungi, protozoa, and *Rickettsia.*

Microorganisms also vary in the severity of the diseases they produce and their degree of communicability. For example, the common cold virus is more readily transmitted than the bacillus that causes leprosy (*Mycobacterium leprae*). If the infectious agent can be transmitted to an individual by direct or indirect contact, through a vector or vehicle, or as an airborne infection, the resulting condition is called a **communicable disease.**

Trauma is injury to the body. Trauma can be physical, such as a cut by a piece of glass; trauma also describes injury caused by invading microorganisms. Thus, an infectious process can be described as trauma. Often, the trauma of infection follows physical trauma, as when a cut becomes infected.

Pathogenicity is the ability to produce disease; thus, a pathogen is a microorganism that causes disease. No microorganism produces disease 100% of the time. However, many microorganisms that are normally harmless can cause disease under certain circumstances. A "true" pathogen causes disease or infection in a healthy individual. An **opportunistic pathogen** causes disease only in a susceptible individual.

Etiology is the study of causes; the etiology of an infectious process is the identification of the invading microorganisms. Infectious diseases are the major cause of death worldwide, and a leading cause of illness and death in the United States (US Department of Health and Human Services, Public Health Division 1993). The control of the spread of microorganisms and the protection of people from communicable diseases and infections are carried out on the international, national, state, community, and individual level. The World Health Organization is the major regulatory agency at the international level. In the United States, the Centers for Disease Control and Prevention (CDC) is the principal public health agency at the national level concerned with disease prevention and control.

One way infectious disease is controlled at the international level is to require immunization against certain diseases, such as cholera, before travel to certain countries. Similarly, health regulations govern the immunizations required of US and Canadian citizens returning home. National regulations govern, for example, the interstate and interprovincial transportation of food. These regulations protect people from receiving contaminated food. Also, national regulations attempt to control pollution of water, the air, and the environment, subjects currently receiving much publicity. At the state and provincial level, health departments track epidemics and illnesses as reports are made throughout that area. At the community level, the disposal of sewage and the purity of drinking water, for example, are regulated to protect residents from infectious disease. Protection from infection is also an individual responsibility. Individuals protect themselves not only by practicing good hygiene (see Chapter 29) but also by eating a balanced diet and exercising.

Normal Body Defenses

The human normally has microbial flora that reside in and outside the body, for example, on the skin, on mucous membranes, inside the respiratory passages, and inside the gastrointestinal tract. These microorganisms are called **resident flora** because they are always present, usually in numbers compatible with the individual's health. See Table 27–1 on page 664. In contrast to resident flora, **transient flora** are microorganisms that are present episodically.

Table 27–1 Normal Organisms of the Body

Body Area	Bacteria	Comment
Skin	*Staphylococcus epidermidis*	Normally nonpathogenic
	Propionibacterium acnes	Use skin fat and oil for growth; involved in acne
	Staphylococcus aureus	Potential pathogen of surgical wounds
	Corynebacterium xerosis	Most numerous in axillae
	Pityrosporum oxale (yeast)	Found on scalp and oily skin
Nasal passages	*Staphylococcus aureus*	Potential pathogen
	Staphylococcus epidermidis	
Oropharynx	*Streptococcus pneumoniae*	Potential pathogen
Bronchi, lungs	None	
Mouth	*Streptococcus mutans*	Adhere to tooth enamel, cause caries
		Component of plaque
	Lactobacillus	Involved in tooth decay
	Bacteroides	Increased with gum disease
	Actinomyces	May cause deposition of calcium salts in plaque
Stomach	None	
Esophagus	None	
Small intestine	(See large intestine)	Fewer microorganisms than in large intestine
Large intestine	*Bacteroides*	Ferment food residues
	Fusobacterium	
	Eubacterium	
	Lactobacillus	Produce lactic acid
	Streptococcus	Low pathogenicity
	Enterobacteriaceae	Produce bacteriocins
	Shigella	
	Escherichia coli	
Urethral orifice	*Staphylococcus epidermidis*	
Urethra (lower)	*Proteus*	
Bladder	None	
Ureters	None	
Kidneys	None	
Vagina	*Lactobacillus*	Balance can be upset by antibiotics
	Bacteroides	
	Clostridium	
	Candida albicans	Yeast
Nervous system	None	
Blood, lymph system	None	

Individuals normally have defenses that protect the body from infection. These defenses can be categorized as nonspecific and specific. **Nonspecific defenses** protect the person against all microorganisms, regardless of prior exposure. **Specific (immune) defenses,** by contrast, are directed against identifiable bacteria, viruses, fungi, or other infectious agents.

NONSPECIFIC DEFENSES

Nonspecific body defenses include anatomic and physiologic barriers. *Intact skin and mucous membranes* are the body's first line of defense against microorganisms. Unless the skin and mucosa become cracked and broken, they are an effective barrier against bacteria. Fungi can live on the skin, but they cannot penetrate it. The dryness of the skin also is a deterrent to bacteria. They are most plentiful in moist areas of the body, such as the perineum and axillae. Another deterrent is sebum, which contains an unsaturated fatty acid that kills some bacteria. Resident bacteria of the skin also prevent other bacteria from multiplying. They use up the available nourishment, and the end products of their metabolism inhibit other bacteria. Normal secretions make the skin slightly acidic; acidity also inhibits bacterial growth.

The *nasal passages* have a defensive function. As entering air follows the tortuous route of the passage, it comes in contact with moist mucous membranes and small hairlike projections called *cilia.* These trap microorganisms, dust, and foreign materials. The *lungs* have alveolar **macrophages** (large phagocytes). **Phagocytes** are cells, eg, white blood cells, that ingest microorganisms, other cells, and foreign particles. Healthy lungs are free of microorganisms. The central nervous system is protected by the skull and spinal column, which prevent microbial entry.

Each body orifice also has protective mechanisms. The *oral cavity* regularly sheds mucosal epithelium to rid the mouth of colonizers. The flow of saliva and its partially buffering action help prevent infections. Saliva contains microbial inhibitors, such as lactoferrin, lysozyme, and secretory IgA. **Lactoferrin** is an iron-binding protein that inhibits the growth of invading microorganisms by making iron unavailable to them. The enzyme **lysozyme,** present in saliva and tears, functions as an antibacterial agent. Secretory IgA (SIGA) is an immunoglobulin that coats bacteria and thus prevents them from attaching to the oral epithelium and to the teeth.

The *eye* is protected from infection by tears, which continually wash microorganisms away and contain inhibiting lysozyme. The *gastrointestinal tract* also has defenses against infection. The high acidity of the stomach normally prevents microbial growth. The role that the normal microorganisms of the small intestine play in the body's defense is unknown. However, the resident flora of the large intestine help prevent the establishment of disease-producing microorganisms. Many enterobacteria produce bacteriocins that are lethal to closely related bacterial strains. Some enterobacteria release an antibiotic-like substance that kills or inhibits the growth of some bacteria.

The *vagina* also has natural defenses against infection. When a girl reaches puberty, lactobacilli ferment sugars in the vaginal secretions, creating a vaginal pH of 3.5 to 4.5. This low pH inhibits the growth of many disease-producing microorganisms. A reasonably healthy female normally has a relatively constant number of these lactobacilli in the vagina. However, antibiotic therapy can upset the bacterial balance because the lactobacilli are highly susceptible to antibiotics. **Colonization** (the process by which strains of bacteria become resident flora) by *Candida albicans* (yeast) often results. The *entrance to the urethra* normally harbors many microorganisms, such as "coagulase negative staph" (*Staphylococcus epidermidis* coagulase from the skin) and *Escherichia coli* (from feces). It is believed that the urine has a flushing and bacteriostatic action that keeps the bacteria from ascending the urethra.

Inflammation is a local and nonspecific defensive response of the tissues to injury or infection. It is an adaptive mechanism that destroys or dilutes the injurious agent, prevents further spread of the injury, and promotes the repair of damaged tissue. It is characterized by five signs: (a) pain, (b) swelling, (c) redness, (d) heat, and (e) impaired function of the part, if the injury is severe. Commonly, words with the suffix *-itis* describe an inflammatory process. For example, *appendicitis* means inflammation of the appendix; *gastritis* means inflammation of the stomach.

Injurious stressors (inflammatory agents) to body tissues can be categorized as physical agents, chemical agents, and microorganisms. *Physical agents* include mechanical objects causing trauma to tissues, excessive heat or cold (causing burns or frostibite), and radiation. *Chemical agents* include external irritants (eg, strong acids, alkalis, poisons, and irritating gases) and internal irritants (substances manufactured within the body such as excessive hydrochloric acid in the stomach due to altered function). *Microorganisms* include the broad groups of bacteria, viruses, fungi, protozoa, and *Rickettsia.*

The inflammatory response involves a series of dynamic events commonly referred to as the three stages of the inflammatory response:

First stage: Vascular and cellular responses

Second stage: Exudate

Third stage: Reparative

At the start of the *first stage,* constriction of the blood vessels occurs at the site of injury, lasting only a few moments. This initial constriction is rapidly followed by dilation of small blood vessels (occurring as a result of histamine released by the injured tissues). Thus, more blood flows to the injured area. This marked increase in blood supply is referred to as **hyperemia** and is responsible for the characteristic signs of redness and heat.

Vascular permeability is increased at the injured site with the dilation of the vessels in response to tissue necrosis, the release of chemical mediators (eg, bradykinin, serotonin, and prostaglandin), and the release of histamine. The result of this altered permeability is an outpouring of fluid, proteins, and leukocytes into the interstitial spaces, clinically manifested by the characteristic inflammatory signs of swelling (edema) and pain. The pain is caused by the pressure of accumulating fluid on local nerve endings and the chemical mediators, which are thought to irritate the nerve endings. Too much fluid pouring into areas such as the pleural or pericardial cavity can seriously affect organ function. In other areas, such as joints, mobility is impaired.

During the first stage of the inflammatory response, blood flow slows in the dilated vessels. This altered rate of flow facilitates the mobilization of the increased number of **leukocytes** (white blood cells) to the injured tissues. Mobilization of leukocytes includes the two processes of margination and emigration. Normally, blood cells (erythrocytes, leukocytes, and platelets) flow along the center of a blood vessel, while a cell-less stream of plasma flows around them against the walls of the blood vessel. When the blood flow slows, leukocytes aggregate or line up along this inner surface of the blood vessels. This process is known as **margination.** Leukocytes then move through the blood vessel wall into the affected tissue spaces, a process called **emigration.**

The actual passage of blood corpuscles through the blood vessel wall is referred to as **diapedesis.** Leukocytes are attracted to injured cells by **chemotaxis.** The action of chemotaxis is not fully understood, but basically leukocytes are drawn toward the source of chemicals released in the injured cells (positive chemotaxis), or they are propelled away from released chemicals (negative chemotaxis).

In a compensatory response to the exit of leukocytes from the blood vessels, the bone marrow produces large numbers of leukocytes and releases them into the bloodstream (**leukocytosis**). The exact mechanism stimulating this increase is unknown, but it is another sign associated with inflammation. A normal leukocyte count of 4500 to 11,000 per cubic millimeter of blood can rise to 20,000 or more when inflammation occurs.

In the *second stage* of inflammation, fluid that escaped from the blood vessels, dead phagocytic cells, as well as dead tissue cells and products that they release, produce the inflammatory **exudate.** A plasma protein called **fibrinogen** (which is converted to fibrin when it is released into the tissues), thromboplastin (a product released by injured tissue cells), and platelets together form an interlacing network to form a barrier, wall off the area, and prevent its spread. During the second stage, the injurious agent is overcome, and the exudate is cleared away by lymphatic drainage.

The nature and amount of exudate vary in accordance with the tissue involved and the intensity and duration of the inflammation. The major types of exudate are serous, purulent, and hemorrhagic (sanguineous). A **serous exudate** is composed chiefly of serum (the clear portion of the blood) derived from the blood and serous membranes of the body, such as the peritoneum, pleura, pericardium, and meninges. It is watery in appearance and has few cells. An example is the fluid in a blister from a burn.

A **purulent exudate** is thicker than serous exudate due to the presence of pus. It consists of leukocytes, liquefied dead tissue debris, and dead and living bacteria. The process of pus formation is referred to as **suppuration,** and the bacteria that produce pus are called **pyogenic bacteria.** Not all microorganisms are pyogenic. Purulent exudates vary in color, some acquiring tinges of blue, green, or yellow. The color may depend on the causative organism.

A **sanguineous (hemorrhagic) exudate** consists of large amounts of red blood cells, indicating damage to capillaries that is severe enough to allow the escape of red blood cells from plasma. This type of exudate is frequently seen in open wounds. Nurses often need to distinguish whether the sanguineous exudate is dark or bright. A bright sanguineous exudate indicates fresh bleeding, whereas dark sanguineous exudate denotes older bleeding. Mixed types of exudates are often observed. A **serosanguineous exudate** (consisting of clear and blood-tinged drainage) is commonly seen in surgical incisions.

The *third stage* of the inflammatory response, also referred to as the *reparative phase,* involves the repair of injured tissues by regeneration or replacement with fibrous tissue (scar) formation. **Regeneration** is the replacement of destroyed tissue cells by cells that are identical or similar in structure and function. It involves not only replacement of damaged cells one by one but also organization of these cells so that the architectural pattern of the tissue and function are restored.

The **stroma** is the tissue that forms the framework (connective tissue) or ground substance of an organ. The **parenchyma** comprises the essential functional elements of an organ. Functional cells must have proper relationships between stroma and parenchyma, and among their blood vessels, lymph vessels, nerves, and ducts. All must regenerate concurrently. If one component lags behind the others, a normal product will not be formed.

The ability to reproduce cells varies considerably from one type of tissue to another. For example, epithelial tissues of the skin and of the digestive and respiratory tracts have a good regenerative capacity, provided that their underlying support structures are intact. The same holds true for osseous, lymphoid, and bone marrow tissues. Tissues that have little regenerative capacity include nervous, muscular, and elastic tissues.

When regeneration is not possible, repair occurs by *fibrous tissue formation.* **Fibrous (scar) tissue** has the capacity to proliferate under the unusual conditions of ischemia and altered pH. The inflammatory exudate with its interlacing network of fibrin provides the framework for this tissue to develop. Damaged tissues are replaced with the connective tissue elements of collagen, blood capillaries, lymphatics, and other tissue-bound substances. In the early stages of this process, the tissue is called **granulation tissue.** It is a fragile, gelatinous tissue, appearing pink or red because of the many newly formed capillaries. Later in the process, the tissue shrinks (the capillaries are constricted, even obliterated) and the collagen fibers contract, so that a firmer fibrous tissue remains. This is called a **cicatrix,** or scar.

Although scar tissue has the positive attribute of repairing the injured area, it also can present problems. It can reduce the functional capacity of the tissue or organ. For example, scar tissue in cardiac muscle renders that area of the heart weaker. Mechanical obstructions can also arise, for example, in the healing of a duodenal ulcer. Sometimes the pyloric sphincter becomes stenosed as granulation tissue contracts into scar tissue.

SPECIFIC DEFENSES

Specific defenses of the body involve the immune system, which responds to foreign protein in the body (eg, bacteria or transplanted tissues) or, in some cases, even the body's own proteins. Foreign proteins in the body are called **antigens** and are considered invaders. If the proteins originate in a person's own body, the antigen is called an **autoantigen. Immunity** is the specific resistance of the body to infection (pathogens or their toxins). There are two major types of immunity: active and passive. See Table 27–2. Through **active immunity,** the host produces its own antibodies in response to natural antigens (eg, infection) or artificial antigens (eg, vaccines). With **passive immunity,** the host receives natural (eg, from a nursing mother) or artificial (eg, from an injection of immune serum) antibodies produced by another source.

Table 27–2 Types of Acquired Immunity

Type	Antigen or Antibody Source	Duration
1. Active	Antibodies are produced by the body in response to infection	Long
a. Natural	Antibodies are formed in the presence of active infection in the body	Lifelong
b. Artificial	Antigens (vaccines or toxoids) are administered to the person to stimulate antibody production	Many years: the immunity must be reinforced by booster inoculations
2. Passive	Antibodies are produced by another source, animal or human	Short
a. Natural	Antibodies are transferred naturally from an immune mother to her baby through the placenta or in colostrum	6 months to 1 year
b. Artificial	Immune serum (antibody) from an animal or another human is injected	2 to 3 weeks

The immune response has two components: antibody-mediated defenses and cell-mediated defenses. These two systems provide distinct but overlapping protection. The *antibody-mediated defense* is also referred to as **humoral (circulating) immunity,** since it resides ultimately in the B lymphocytes and is mediated by antibodies produced by B cells. **Antibodies,** also called **immunoglobulins,** are part of the body's plasma proteins. B cells are one type of lymphocyte; they comprise 30% of blood lymphocytes and are short-lived, having a life span of 15 days. The antibody-mediated response defends primarily against the extracellular phases of bacterial and viral infections.

B cells are activated when they recognize a foreign invader, an antigen. They then differentiate into plasma cells, which secrete antibodies, and serum proteins, which bind specifically to the foreign substance and initiate a variety of elimination responses. The B cell response to an antigen may produce antibody molecules of five classes of immunoglobulins designated by the letters M, G, A, D, and E, usually written as follows: IgM, IgG, IgA, IgD, and IgE. The presence of IgM on laboratory analysis shows current infection. Before an antibody response, the phagocytic cells of the blood bind and ingest foreign substances. The rate of binding and phagocytosis increases if IgG antibodies (which indicate past infection and subsequent immunity) are present.

The first interaction between an antigen and antibody is known as the **primary immune response.** The principal characteristics of this response are a latent period before the appearance of an antibody, the production of only a small amount of antibody (chiefly IgM), and, most importantly, the creation of a large number of memory cells capable of responding to the same antigen in the future. The **secondary immune (booster) response** takes place on sebsequent encounters with the same antigen. The principal characteristics of this response are: rapid proliferation of B cells, rapid differentiation of B cells into plasma cells that promptly produce large quantities of antibody (chiefly class IgG), and release of antibody into the blood and other body tissues, where it can react with the antigen.

The **cell-mediated defenses** or **cellular immunity,** occurs through the T cell system.

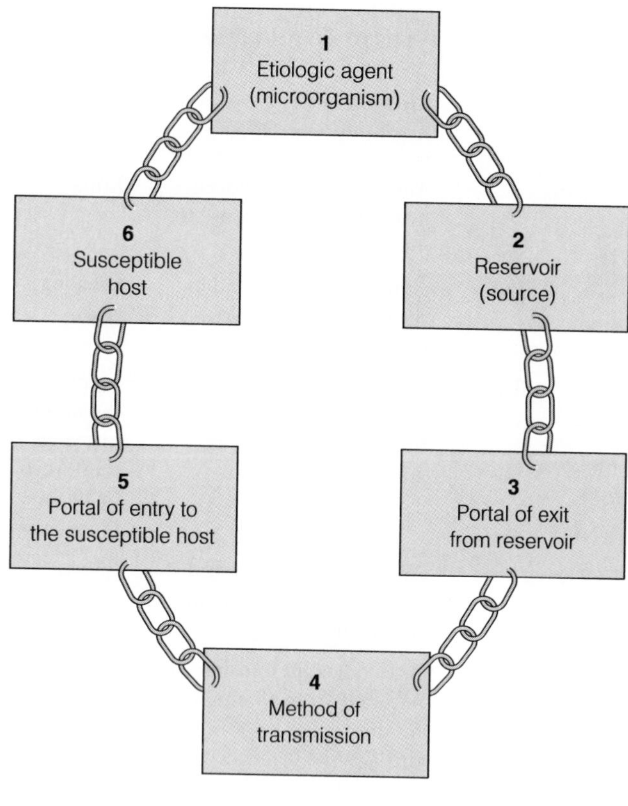

Figure 27–1 The chain of infection.

On exposure to an antigen, the T lymphocytes of the lymphoid tissue release large numbers of activated T cells into the lymph system. These T cells pass into the general circulation. There are three main groups of T cells: (a) helper T cells, which help in the functions of the immune system; (b) cytotoxic T cells, which attack and kill micoorganisms and sometimes the body's own cells; and (c) suppressor T cells, which can suppress the functions of the helper T cells and the cytotoxic T cells. It is believed that they help regulate immune reactions. When cell-mediated immunity is lost, as occurs with human immunodeficiency virus (HIV) infection, the individual is "defenseless" against most viral, bacterial, and fungal infections.

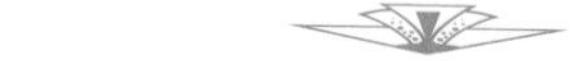

CHAIN OF INFECTION

There are six links in the chain of infection (Figure 27–1): the etiologic agent, or microorganism; the place where the organism naturally resides (reservoir); a portal of exit from the reservoir; a method (mode) of transmission; a portal of entry into a host; and the susceptibility of the host.

ETIOLOGIC AGENT

A **parasite** is a microorganism that lives in or on another and obtains its nourishment from it. All viruses are parasites. The extent to which any microorganism or parasite is capable of producing an infectious process depends on the number of organisms present, the virulence and potency of the organisms (pathogenicity), the ability of the organisms to enter the body, the susceptibility of the host, and the ability of the organisms to live in the host's body.

Some microorganisms, such as the smallpox virus, have the ability to infect almost all susceptible people after exposure. By contrast, microorganisms such as the tuberculosis bacillus infect a relatively small number of the population who are susceptible and exposed, usually people who are poorly nourished and living in crowded conditions. The presence of organisms in body secretions or excretions that does not cause illness is called **colonization.** A **carrier** is a person or animal that harbors a specific infectious agent and serves as a potential source of infection yet does not manifest any clinical signs of disease.

The carrier state may also exist in the incubation period, convalescence, and postconvalescence of an individual with a clinically recognizable disease. This type of carrier is referred to as an *incubatory* or *convalescent carrier.* Under either circumstance, the carrier state may be of short duration (*temporary* or *transient carrier*) or long duration (*chronic carrier*) (Beneson 1990, p. 497).

RESERVOIR

There are many **reservoirs,** or sources of microorganisms. Common sources are other humans, the client's own microorganisms, plants, animals, or the general environment. See Table 27–3. People are the most common source of infection for others and for themselves. The person with, for example, an influenza virus frequently spreads it to others. When resistance is lowered by fatigue and other factors, an infection emerges.

Insects, birds, and other animals are common reservoirs of infection. The *Anopheles* mosquito carries the malaria parasite. Food, water, milk, and feces also can be reservoirs. An example is contaminated chicken at a club luncheon. The reservoir must have certain characteristics for the organisms to live and grow. Among these characteristics are: food, water, oxygen (or, for some organisms, absence of oxygen), optimal temperature and pH, and minimal light.

PORTAL OF EXIT FROM RESERVOIR

Before an infection can establish itself in a host, the microorganisms must leave the reservoir. If the reservoir is

Table 27–3 Human Reservoirs and Methods of Transmission of Common Microorganisms

Body Area (Source)	Transport Vehicle	Common Infectious Organisms
Respiratory tract	Droplets expelled while sneezing and coughing	Parainfluenza virus *Klebsiella* species *Staphylococcus aureus*
Gastrointestinal tract	Vomitus, feces, drainage (such as from the gallbladder), saliva	Hepatitis A virus *Shigella* species *Salmonella* species
Urinary tract	Urine	*Escherichia coli* enterococci *Pseudomonas aeruginosa*
Reproductive tract (including genitals)	Urine and semen	*Neisseria gonorrhoeae* *Treponema pallidum* Herpes simplex virus type 2 Hepatitis B virus
Blood	Blood sample, needle used for venipuncture	Hepatitis B virus (HBV) Human immunodeficiency virus (HIV) *Staphylococcus aureus* *Staphylococcus epidermidis*
Tissue	Drainage from a cut or wound	*Staphylococcus aureus* *Escherichia coli* *Proteus* species

within a human, the microorganisms have a number of exits, depending on the site of the reservoir. Common human reservoirs and their associated portals of exit are summarized in Table 27–4.

METHOD OF TRANSMISSION

After a microorganism leaves its source or reservoir, it requires a means of transmission to reach another person or host through a *receptive portal of entry.* There are three mechanisms:

1. *Direct transmission.* Direct transmission involves immediate and direct transfer of microorganisms from person to person through touching, biting, kissing, or sexual intercourse. Droplet spread is also a form of direct contact but can occur only if the source and the host are within 3 feet of each other. Sneezing, coughing, spitting, singing, or talking can project droplet spray into the conjunctiva or onto the mucous membranes of the eye, nose, or mouth of another person.
2. *Indirect transmission.* Indirect transmission may be either vehicle-borne or vector-borne.
   a. **Vehicle-borne transmission.** A *vehicle* is any substance that serves as an intermediate means to transport and introduce an infectious agent into a susceptible host through a suitable portal of entry. *Fomites* (inanimate materials or objects), such as handkerchiefs, toys, soiled clothes, cooking or eating utensils, and surgical instruments or dressings, can act as vehicles. For example, an intravenous needle can be a vehicle for transmission of microorganisms from the reservoir to the host. Water, food, milk, blood, serum, and plasma are other vehicles. For example, food or water may become contaminated by a food

Table 27–4 Human Reservoirs and Portals of Exit

Reservoir	Portals of Exit
Respiratory tract	Nose/mouth through sneezing, coughing, breathing, or talking; endotracheal tubes or tracheostomies
Gastrointestinal tract	Mouth: through saliva, vomitus, anus/ostomies: feces, drainage tubes (eg, nasogastric or T-tubes)
Urinary tract	Urethral meatus and urinary diversion ostomies
Reproductive tract	Vagina: vaginal discharge; may be further transported by urine; urinary meatus: semen, urine
Blood	Open wound, needle puncture site, any disruption of intact skin or mucous membrane surfaces

Table 27–5 Nursing Interventions that Break the Chain of Infection

Link	Interventions	Rationale
Etiologic agent (microorganism)	Ensure that articles are correctly cleaned and disinfected or sterilized before use.	Correct cleaning, disinfecting, and sterilizing reduce or eliminate microorganisms.
	Educate clients and support persons about appropriate methods to clean, disinfect, and sterilize articles.	Knowledge of ways to reduce or eliminate microorganisms reduces the numbers of microorganisms present and the likelihood of transmission.
Reservoir (source)	Change dressings and bandages when they are soiled or wet.	Moist dressings are ideal environments for microorganisms to grow and multiply.
	Assist clients to carry out appropriate skin and oral hygiene.	Hygienic measures reduce the numbers of resident and transient microorganisms and the likelihood of infection.
	Dispose of damp, soiled linens appropriately.	Damp, soiled linens harbor more microorganisms than dry linens.
	Dispose of feces and urine in appropriate receptacles.	Urine and feces in particular contain many microorganisms. Feces may also be the source of certain microorganisms, such as the hepatitis A virus in asymptomatic carriers.
	Ensure that all fluid containers, such as bedside water jugs and suction and drainage bottles, are covered or capped.	Prolonged exposure increases the risk of contamination and promotes microbial growth.
	Empty suction and drainage bottles at the end of each shift or before they become full, or according to agency policy.	Drainage harbors microorganisms that, if left for prolonged periods, proliferate and can be transmitted to others.
Portal of exit from the reservoir	Avoid talking, coughing, or sneezing over open wounds or sterile fields, and cover the mouth and nose when coughing and sneezing.	These measures limit the number of microorganisms that escape from the respiratory tract.
Method of transmission	Wash hands between client contacts, after touching body substances, and before performing invasive procedures or touching open wounds. Instruct clients and support persons to wash hands before handling food or eating, after eliminating, and after touching infectious material.	Hand washing is an important means of controlling and preventing the transmission of microorganisms.

handler who transports the hepatitis A virus. The food is then ingested by a susceptible host.

b. **Vector-borne transmission.** A *vector* is an animal or flying or crawling insect that serves as an intermediate means of transporting the infectious agent. Transmission may occur by injecting salivary fluid during biting or by depositing feces or other materials on the skin through the bite wound or a traumatized skin area.

3. *Airborne transmission.* **Airborne transmission** occurs when **droplet nuclei** (residue of evaporated droplets that may remain in the air for long periods of time) emitted by an infected host (eg, one with tuberculosis) or dust particles containing the infectious agent (eg, *Clostridium difficile* spores from the soil) are transmitted by air currents to a suitable portal of entry, usually the respiratory tract, of another person.

PORTAL OF ENTRY TO THE SUSCEPTIBLE HOST

Before a person can become infected, microorganisms must enter the body. The skin is a barrier to infectious agents; however, any break in the skin can readily serve as

Table 27–5 *continued*

Link	Interventions	Rationale
	Place discarded soiled materials in moistureproof refuse bags.	Moistureproof bags prevent the spread of microorganisms to others.
	Hold used bedpans steadily to prevent spillage, and dispose of urine and feces in appropriate receptacles.	Urine and feces in particular contain many microorganisms.
	Initiate and implement aseptic precautions for all clients.	All clients may harbor potentially infectious microorganisms that can be transmitted to others.
	Wear masks and eye protection when in close contact with clients who have infections transmitted by droplets from the respiratory tract.	Masks and eyewear reduce the spread of droplet-transmitted microorganisms.
	Wear gloves when handling infectious secretions and excretions. Wear gowns if there is danger of soiling clothing with body substances.	Gloves and gowns prevent soiling of the hands and clothing.
	Wear masks and eye protection when sprays of body fluid are possible (eg, during irrigation procedures).	Masks and eye protection provide protection from microorganisms in clients' body substances.
Portal of entry to the susceptible host	Use sterile technique for invasive procedures, such as injections and catheterizations.	Invasive procedures penetrate the body's natural protective barriers to microorganisms.
	Use sterile technique when exposing open wounds or handling dressings.	Open wounds are vulnerable to microbial infection.
	Place used disposable needles and syringes in puncture-resistant containers for disposal.	Injuries from needles contaminated by blood or body fluids from an infected client or carrier are a primary cause of hepatitis B virus (HBV) and human immunodeficiency virus (HIV) transmission to health care workers.
	Provide all clients with their own personal care items.	People have less resistance to another person's microorganisms than to their own.
Susceptible host	Maintain the integrity of the client's skin and mucous membranes.	Intact skin and mucous membranes protect against invasion by microorganisms.
	Ensure that the client receives a balanced diet.	A balanced diet supplies essential proteins and vitamins necessary to build or maintain body tissues.
	Educate the public about the importance of immunizations.	Immunizations protect people against virulent infectious diseases.

a portal of entry. Microorganisms can enter the body through the same routes they use to leave the body. Often, microorganisms enter the body of the host by the same route they used to leave the source.

SUSCEPTIBLE HOST

A **susceptible host** is any person who is at risk for infection. **Compromised hosts** are persons "at increased risk," individuals who for one or more reasons are more likely than others to acquire an infection. Impairment of the body's natural defenses and a number of other factors can affect susceptibility to infection.

BREAKING THE CHAIN OF INFECTION

Various practices break the chain of infection or interrupt the infectious disease process. For example, the first link in the chain, the etiologic agent, is interrupted by the use of **antiseptics** (agents that inhibit the growth of some microorganisms) and **disinfectants** (agents that destroy pathogens other than spores), and by sterilization. Nurses carry out practices that break other links in the chain. See Table 27–5. The aim of most isolation precautions and

Table 27–6 Commonly Used Antiseptics and Disinfectants

Agent	Uses
Antiseptics	
Povidone iodine	Kills bacteria; applied to skin, in wounds, and for irrigations
Chlorhexidine gluconate (Hibiclens)	Kills gram-positive bacteria; skin cleansing and irrigations
Hydrogen peroxide (3%)	Decomposes necrotic tissues; wound irrigations
Disinfectants	
Isopropyl alcohol	Kills bacteria but not spores, virus, or fungi
Chlorine	Kills most microorganisms; used to clean countertops

many hospital practices for infection prevention and control is breaking the chain during the transmission phase of the cycle.

CLEANING AND DISINFECTING

Cleanliness inhibits the growth of microorganisms. An object that is not free of infectious or potentially infectious agents is considered contaminated or dirty. When cleaning visibly soiled objects, nurses must always wear gloves to avoid direct contact with infectious microorganisms. Most objects used in the care of clients, whether artery forceps or drawsheets, can be cleaned by rinsing them in cold water to remove any organic material, washing them with hot soapy water, then rinsing them again to remove the soap. The following steps should be followed when cleaning objects in a hospital or in a home where infectious agents exist.

1. Rinse the article with cold water to remove organic material. Hot water coagulates the protein of organic material and tends to make it adhere. Examples of organic material are blood and pus.
2. Wash the article in hot water and soap. The emulsifying action of soap reduces surface tension and facilitates the removal of dirt. Washing dislodges the emulsified dirt.
3. Use an abrasive, such as a stiff-bristled brush, to clean equipment with grooves and corners. Friction helps dislodge foreign material.
4. Rinse the article well with warm-hot water.
5. Dry the article; it is now considered clean.
6. Clean the brush, gloves, and sink. These are considered soiled until they are cleaned appropriately, usually with a disinfectant.

Noninfectious organisms may or may not be completely eliminated by disinfection. A disinfectant is a chemial preparation, such as phenol or iodine compounds, used to treat inanimate objects. Disinfectants are frequently caustic and toxic to tissues. An antiseptic is a chemical preparation used on skin or tissue. Disinfectants and antiseptics are often have similar chemical components, but the disinfectant is a more concentrated solution.

Both antiseptics and disinfectants are said to have bactericidal or bacteriostatic properties. A *bactericidal* preparation destroys bacteria, whereas a *bacteriostatic* preparation prevents the growth and reproduction of some bacteria. See Table 27–6 for commonly used antiseptics and disinfectants.

STERILIZING

Sterilization is a process that destroys *all* microorganisms, including spores and viruses. Before one chooses a method for disinfecting or sterilizing it is important to consider the following:

1. The type and number of infectious organisms. Some microorganisms are readily destroyed, whereas others require longer contact with the disinfectant. Also, a large number of organisms requires a proportionately longer disinfecting time.
2. The recommended concentration of the disinfectant and the duration of contact. A lesser concentration or shorter exposure could be ineffective.
3. The temperature of the environment. Most disinfectants are intended for use at room temperature. In lower temperatures, the exposure must usually be increased.
4. The presence of soap. Some disinfectants are ineffective in the presence of soap or detergent. Such disinfectants are cationic and react with the anions in the soap rather than the bacterial membrane.
5. The presence of organic materials. The presence of saliva, blood, pus, or excretions can readily inactivate many disinfectants. The disinfectant acts on the nonmicrobial organic matter, reducing its antimicrobial action. It is therefore important to wash off the organic material before disinfecting.
6. The limitations of the available methods.
7. The surface areas to be treated. The sterilizing or disinfecting agent must come into contact with all surfaces and areas.

Four commonly used methods of sterilization are moist heat, gas, boiling water, and radiation.

Moist Heat For sterilizing, moist heat (steam) can be employed in two ways: as steam under pressure or as free steam. Steam under pressure attains temperatures higher than the boiling point. Autoclaves supply steam under pressures of 15 to 17 pounds and temperatures of 121 to 123 C (250 to 254 F).

Free steam, 100 C (212 F), is used to sterilize objects that would be destroyed at the higher temperature and pressure of the autoclave. Usually, it is necessary to steam the article for 30 minutes on 3 consecutive days. The intervals are required so that unkilled spores will return to their vegetative state and again become vulnerable to the heat.

One example of free steam used in a hospital is the bedpan flusher. Because the temperature of the flusher never exceeds 100 C, it does not really sterilize bedpans but washes away some microorganisms. Some viruses, such as the virus that causes hepatitis A, can survive this free steam application.

Gas Ethylene oxide gas destroys microorganisms by interfering with their metabolic processes. It is also effective against spores. Its advantages are good penetration and effectiveness for heat-sensitive items. Its major disadvantage is its toxicity to humans.

Boiling Water This is the most practical and inexpensive method for sterilizing in the home. The main disadvantage is that spores and some viruses are not killed by this method. The water temperature rises no higher than 100 C (212 F). Boiling a minimum of 15 minutes is advised for disinfection of articles in the home.

Radiation Both ionizing and nonionizing radiation can be used for disinfection and sterilization. Ultraviolet light, a type of nonionizing radiation, can be used for disinfection. Its main drawback is that the ultraviolet rays do not penetrate deeply. Ionizing radiation is used effectively in industry to sterilize foods, drugs, and other items that are sensitive to heat. Its main advantage is that it is effective for items difficult to sterilize; its chief disadvantage is that the equipment is very expensive.

Nurses should be familiar with the cleaning, disinfecting, and sterilizing protocols of the agency in which they practice.

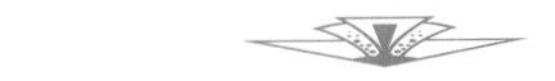

Risk Factors for Infection

Whether a microorganism causes an infection depends on a number of factors already mentioned. One of the most important factors is host susceptibility, which is affected by age, heredity, level of stress, nutritional status, immunization status, current medical therapy, preexisting disease processes, and some past or recent surgical interventions.

Age is a factor influencing the risk of infection. Newborns and elderly people have reduced defenses against infection. Infections are a major cause of death of newborns, who have immature immune systems and are protected only for the first 2 or 3 months by immunoglobulins passively received from the mother. Between 1 to 3 months of age, infants begin to synthesize their own immunoglobulins; about 40% of adult levels are reached by 1 year of age (Wong 1991, p. 539). Immunizations against diphtheria, tetanus, and pertussis are usually started at 2 months, when the infant's immune system can respond.

With advancing age, the immune responses again become weak. The immune response (cell-mediated immunity) is reduced. Lymphocytes become more diverse with age, and there is a progressive loss of cellular regulation in the body. Although there is still much to learn about aging, it is known that immunity to infection decreases with advancing age. For example, recent reports confirm that urinary tract infections increase with age in both men and women (Nicolle 1992, p. S261). Because of the prevalence of influenza and its potential for causing death, the CDC recommends immunization against influenza for the elderly and for persons with chronic cardiac, respiratory, metabolic, and renal disease. Pneumococcal vaccine is also recommended. Immunization is usually provided in early October or November; annual boosters are required to maintain immunity.

Heredity is a factor influencing the development of infection in that some people have a genetic susceptibility to certain infections. For example, some people may be deficient in serum immunoglobulins, which play a significant role in the internal defense mechanism of the body. The nature, number, and duration of physical and emotional *stressors* can influence susceptibility to infection. Stressors elevate blood cortisone. Prolonged elevation of blood cortisone decreases anti-inflammatory responses, depletes energy stores, leads to a state of exhaustion, and decreases resistance to infection. For example, a person recovering from a major operation or injury is more likely to develop an infection than a healthy person.

Resistance to infection depends on adequate *nutritional status*. Because antibodies are proteins, the ability of the body to synthesize antibodies may be impaired by inadequate nutrition, especially when protein reserves are depleted (eg, as a result of injury, surgery, or debilitating diseases such as cancer). Some *medical therapies* predispose a person to infection. For example, radiation treatments for cancer destroy not only cancerous cells but also some normal cells, thereby rendering them more vulnerable to infection.

Certain *medications* also increase susceptibility to infection. Antineoplastic (anticancer) medications may depress bone marrow function, resulting in inadequate production of white blood cells and lymphocytes necessary to combat infections. Anti-inflammatory medications, such as adrenal corticosteroids, inhibit the inflammatory response, an essential defense against infection. Even some antibiotics used to treat infections can have adverse effects. Antibiotics may kill resident flora, allowing the proliferation of strains that would not grow and multiply in the body under normal conditions. Certain antibiotics can also induce resistance in some strains of organisms. Some *diagnostic procedures* may also predispose the client to an infection, especially when the skin is broken or sterile body cavities are penetrated during the procedure.

Any *disease* that lessens the body's defenses against infection places the client at risk. Examples are chronic pulmonary disease, which impairs ciliary action and weakens the mucous barrier; peripheral vascular disease, which inhibits blood flow; burns, which impair skin integrity; chronic or debilitating diseases, which deplete protein reserves; and such immune system diseases as leukemia and aplastic anemia, which alter the production rate of white blood cells. Diabetes mellitus is a major underlying disease predisposing clients to infection, since compromised peripheral vascular status and increased serum glucose levels increase susceptibility. All surgical interventions place the client at risk for infection. Some procedures, however, may place the client at long-term risk of infection; one example is mastectomy (breast removal) in which lymph nodes are removed.

STAGES OF AN INFECTIOUS PROCESS

The course of an infection has four stages: the incubation period, the prodromal period, the illness period, and the convalescent period.

Incubation Period The incubation period is the time between the entry of the microorganisms into the body and the onset of the symptoms. During this time, the organism adapts to the person and multiplies sufficiently to produce an infection. The length of incubation varies greatly, depending on the microorganism. For example, rubella (measles) develops in 10 to 14 days, whereas tetanus (lockjaw) takes from 4 to 21 days to develop. In many viral diseases (eg, chickenpox and measles), persons can transmit infection during the incubation period. A person with hepatitis A is most infectious *before* the onset of any symptoms.

Prodromal Period The prodromal period is the time from the onset of nonspecific symptoms, such as fatigue, malaise, elevated temperature, and irritability, until the specific symptoms of the infection appear. Infected persons are most infectious and most likely to spread the infecting organisms during this stage. Because the symptoms are general, precautions to prevent spread are often not taken at this time. A prodromal stage usually lasts a short time, hours or days at the most.

Illness Period During the illness period, specific symptoms develop and become evident. The symptoms of most infectious processes are manifested both in the affected body organ or area (the local inflammatory response or **localized symptoms**) and in the entire body **(systemic symptoms).** During this period, the person often has fever and headache and feels fatigued. Sometimes a skin rash **(exanthema)** or a rash of the mucous membrane **(enanthema)** appears at this stage. The severity of the symptoms and the length of the illness vary with the susceptibility of the person to the etiologic agent.

Convalescent Period The convalescent period extends from the time the symptoms start to abate until the person returns to a normal state of health. Depending on the severity of the illness and the person's general health, convalescence can last from a few days to months. Often it is longer than the person expects.

NOSOCOMIAL INFECTIONS

Nosocomial infections are classified as infections that are associated with the delivery of health care services in a health care facility. Nosocomial infections can either develop during a client's stay in a facility or manifest after discharge. Nosocomial organisms may also be acquired by health personnel working in the facility (eg, hepatitis B infection and HIV infection) and can cause significant illness and time lost from work.

All nosocomial infections have received increasing attention in recent years and are believed to involve about 2 million clients per year. The most common settings where nosocomial infections develop are surgical or medical intensive care units (Mylotte et al 1993, p. 116). A report of data from the National Nosocomial Infection Surveillance (NNIS) System revealed that the surgical site was the most common nosocomial infection site (Horan et al 1993, p. 73).

The microorganisms that cause nosocomial infections can originate from the clients themselves (an **endogenous** source) or from the hospital environment and hospital personnel (**exogenous** sources). Most nosocomial infections appear to have endogenous sources. The National Nosocomial Infection Surveillance (NNIS) System reports that between 1979 and 1983, *Escherichia coli* was the most common infecting organism, followed by *Staphylococcus aureus* and enterococci (Pickering & DuPont 1986, p. 28).

A number of factors contribute to nosocomial infections. **Iatrogenic** infections (those that are due to any aspect of medical therapy) are the direct result of a diagnostic or therapeutic procedures. One example of an iatrogenic infection is bacteremia that results from an intravascular line. Not all nosocomial infections (eg, the development of a respiratory infection in an immobilized elderly female) are iatrogenic, nor are all nosocomial infections preventable.

Another factor contributing to the development of nosocomial infections is the *presence of compromised hosts*, that is, clients whose normal defenses have been lowered by surgery or illness. The hands of personnel are a common vehicle for the spread of microorganisms. *Insufficient hand washing* is thus an important factor contributing to the spread of nosocomial organisms, especially those from gastrointestinal infections. Personnel can acquire microorganisms from infected clients and pass them on to other clients.

The cost of nosocomial infections to the client, the facility, and funding sources (eg, insurance companies and federal, state, or local governments) is very great. Nosocomial infections extend hospitalization time, increase clients' time away from work, cause disability and discomfort, and even result in loss of life. On average, four extra hospital days are required to control a nosocomial infection, with an additional charge of more than $2000 (Mylotte et al 1993, p. 116).

Assessing

Nursing History

During the nursing history, the nurse assesses (a) the degree to which a client is at risk of developing an infection and (b) any client complaints suggesting the presence of an infection. To identify clients at risk, the nurse reviews the client's chart and structures the nursing interview to collect data regarding the factors influencing the development of infection, especially existing disease process, history of recurrent infections, current medications and therapeutic measures, current emotional stressors, nutritional status, and history of immunizations. See the accompanying box for a sample assessment interview.

To obtain subjective data that may indicate the presence of an infection, the nurse asks whether the client has experienced loss of energy, loss of appetite, nausea, headache, or other signs associated with specific body systems (eg, difficulty urinating, urinary frequency, or a sore throat).

ASSESSMENT INTERVIEW

Clients at Risk for Infections

- When were you last immunized for diphtheria, tetanus, poliomyeletis, rubella, measles, influenza, and pneumococcal pneumonia?
- When did you last have a tuberculin skin test?
- What infections have you had in the past, and how were these treated?
- Have any of these infections recurred?
- Are you taking any antineoplastic, anti-inflammatory, or antibiotic medications?
- Have you had any recent diagnostic procedure or therapy that penetrated through your skin or a body cavity?
- What past surgeries have you had?
- How would you describe your nutritional status in terms of a well-balanced diet?
- On a scale of 1 to 10, how would you rate the stress you have experienced in the last 6 months?

Physical Health Data

Signs and symptoms of an infection may be either localized or systemic. The signs of *localized infection* vary according to the body area involved (see Table 27–7, p. 676) and are caused by the inflammatory response. Commonly the skin and mucous membranes are involved, resulting in

- Localized swelling
- Localized redness
- Pain or tenderness with palpation or movement
- Palpable heat at the infected area
- Loss of function of the body part affected, depending on the site and extent of involvement

In addition, open wounds may exude drainage of various colors. For additional information regarding localized responses and description of exudate, see the discussion about inflammatory responses, earlier in this chapter.

Signs of *systemic infection* include

- Fever
- Increased pulse and respiratory rate, if the fever is high

Table 27–7 Guide to Detect Infection of Various Body Parts

Body Part	Common Signs and Symptoms
Respiratory Tract	
Nose and sinuses	Sneezing; watery or mucoid discharge from nose; swollen and inflamed nasal turbinates; nasal stuffiness; sensation of pressure over infected sinus; palpable tenderness over involved sinus (eg, in the cheek for maxillary sinus, in the nasal bridge or around the eyes for ethmoid sinus)
Throat and pharynx	Inflamed throat and pharynx; dry, scratchy, or sore throat; reddened and enlarged tonsils with accumulation of leukocytes, dead cells, and bacteria in the crypts; possible swollen cervical lymph nodes; fever; chills
Larynx	Hoarseness or loss of voice; feeling of roughness or tickling in throat; dry cough; possible fever
Bronchi	Productive cough; burning substernal sensation that may be aggravated by a deep breath; auscultatory crackles, rhonchi, and wheeze; malaise
Lungs	Hacking cough initially, followed by productive cough with sputum; possible hemoptysis; chills; severe pleural pain; rapid, shallow respirations; fever; malaise; weakness
Gastrointestinal Tract	
Stomach	Epigastric discomfort; bloating; anorexia; nausea; vomiting; eructation; abdominal cramps; possible diarrhea
Intestines	Diarrhea; watery or purulent stools; abdominal cramps; nausea and vomiting
Urinary Tract	
Urethra and bladder	Reddened and inflamed urethra; discomfort with urination; urinary frequency; possible stress incontinence; suprapubic tenderness; cloudy or discolored urine; fever; fatigue
Kidneys	Severe pain or constant dull aching over the flank area; fever and chills; nausea and vomiting

- Lassitude, malaise, and loss of energy
- Anorexia and, in some situations, nausea and vomiting
- Enlargement and tenderness of lymph nodes that drain the area of infection

LABORATORY DATA

Laboratory data that indicate the presence of an infection include the following:

1. Elevated leukocyte (white blood cell or WBC) count (4500 to 11,000/cu mm is normal).
2. Increases in specific types of leukocytes as revealed in the differential white blood cell count. Specific types of white blood cells are increased or decreased in certain infections. Normal values are cited for the adult.
   a. **Neutrophils** are increased in acute suppurative infections but may be decreased in acute bacterial infection, especially in older people. Normal range is 55% to 75%.
   b. **Lymphocytes** are increased in chronic bacterial and viral infections. Normal is 20% to 40%.
   c. **Monocytes** are increased in some protozoal and rickettsial infections and in tuberculosis. Normal is 2% to 8%.
   d. **Eosinophils** are generally unaltered in an infectious process. Normal is 1% to 4%.
   e. **Basophils** are generally unaltered in an infectious process. Normal is 0.5% to 1% (Pagana & Pagana 1992, p. 787).
3. Elevated **erythrocyte sedimentation rate (ESR),** commonly referred to as sedimentation rate. The ESR is a measure of the speed with which red blood cells in anticoagulated whole blood settle to the bottom of a calibrated tube. Sedimentation normally takes place slowly, but the rate increases in the presence of an inflammatory process.
4. Urine, blood, sputum, or other drainage **cultures** (cultivations of microorganisms in a special growth medium) that indicate the presence of pathogenic microorganisms.

DIAGNOSING

The NANDA nursing diagnosis label that relates to problems associated with the transmission of microorganisms is **High risk for infection.**

When using this diagnosis, the nurse should identify the specific focus of the inadequate primary or secondary defense or immunity alteration. This diagnosis, with definitions and related risk factors, is shown in the the box at the top of the next page. A high-risk diagnosis is not evidenced by signs and symptoms, because the problem has not actually occurred. Clinical applications of this and some associated diagnoses are shown in Table 27–8 on the facing page.

Clients who have or are at risk for an existing infection are prime candidates for other physical and psychologic problems. Examples of other nursing diagnoses that may apply to some associated physical and psychologic problems follow. These diagnoses are discussed in detail in other chapters of this book.

NURSING DIAGNOSES

CLIENTS AT RISK FOR INFECTION

NURSING DIAGNOSIS: High risk for infection: The state in which an individual is at an increased risk for invasion by pathogens

Risk Factors

- Inadequate primary defenses, including broken skin, traumatized tissue, decreased ciliary action, stasis of body fluids, change in pH of secretions, altered peristalisis
- Inadequate secondary defenses, including decreased hemoglobin, leukopenia, immunosuppression, or suppressed inflammatory response
- Inadequate acquired immunity
- Tissue destruction and increased environmental exposure
- Chronic disease
- Invasive procedures
- Malnutrition
- Pharmaceutical agents that alter the immune system
- Rupture of amniotic membranes
- Insufficient knowledge to avoid exposure to pathogens

Sources: LJ Carpenito, *Nursing Diagnosis: Application to Clinical Practice*, 4th ed. (Philadelphia: Lippincott, 1992), pp. 503–4; M Gordon, *Manual of Nursing Diagnosis 1993–1994* (St Louis: Mosby-Year Book, 1993) p. 71; MJ Kim, GK McFarland, and AM McLane, *Pocket Guide to Nursing Diagnoses*, 5th ed. (St Louis: Mosby-Year Book, 1993), pp. 33–34; GK McFarland, and EA McFarlane, *Nursing Diagnosis and Intervention: Planning for Patient Care*, 2d ed. (St Louis: Mosby, 1993), p. 48; North American Nursing Diagnosis Association, *NANDA Nursing Diagnoses: Definitions and Classification 1992–1993* (NANDA, 1992), pp. 12–13; and JR Lederer, GL Marculescu, B Mocnik, and N Seaby, *Care Planning Pocket Guide—A Nursing Diagnosis Approach*, 5th ed. (Redwood City, CA: Addison-Wesley Nursing, 1993), p. 106.

- **Altered oral mucous membranes** (Chapter 29, page 754)
- **High risk for altered body temperature** (hyperthermia) (Chapter 21, page 427)
- **Impaired skin integrity** (Chapter 30, page 792) or **Impaired tissue integrity**
- **Impaired physical mobility** (Chapter 34, page 904)
- **Altered nutrition: less than body requirements** (Chapter 37, page 1035)
- **Pain** (Chapter 36, page 990)
- **Social isolation**
- **Diversional activity deficit**
- **Self-esteem disturbance** (Chapter 31, page 813)
- **Anxiety** (Chapter 32, page 842)
- **Fear**
- **Hopelessness** (Chapter 33, page 866)

PLANNING

The major outcomes for clients susceptible to infection are to maintain or restore defenses, avoid the spread of infectious organisms, and reduce or alleviate problems associated with the infection. Specific outcome criteria are shown in the Care Planning Guide on page 678.

Table 27–8 Clinical Application: Examples of Assessment Data Clusters and Related Nursing Diagnoses

Data Cluster	Nursing Diagnosis
Kim Bradley, a 40-year-old shipyard worker, was admitted to emergency with a puncture wound on his foot. He reports stepping on a rusty nail that penetrated his shoe. Wound is 6 mm in diameter, unclean, and inflamed with slight serosanguineous discharge. Reports no immunization since childhood.	**High risk for infection** related to lack of immunization (tetanus) and impaired skin integrity
Kuniko Tanaka, 12 years old, has had diagnosis of chickenpox confirmed and must stay home from school until her lesions are dry. She anticipates "feelings of boredom," missing her friends and school, and, in particular, missing her art classes.	**Diversional activity deficit** related to confinement for communicable disease
Grant Madigan, a 28-year-old teacher who has AIDS, reports an increasing sense of aloneness. His health status does not allow him to work, and most of his former colleagues and friends no longer visit him.	**Social isolation** related to misinformation by others about the transmission of the AIDS virus

CARE PLANNING GUIDE

CLIENTS AT RISK FOR INFECTION

NURSING DIAGNOSIS: High risk for infection

Outcome Criteria	Nursing Interventions	Rationale
The client		
▪ Verbalizes understanding of individual risk factors associated with potential for infection.	Discuss risk factors which place the client at risk for developing an infection See the box on page 677.	Personal knowledge of risk behaviors may result in behavior changes that reduce risk.
▪ Verbalizes understanding of precautionary measures being implemented to prevent or reduce the risk of infection.	Instruct the client about ▪ Purpose of medications (eg, prophylactic antibiotic therapy). ▪ Monitoring of health status (eg, vital signs, lung auscultation). ▪ Dressing changes and other intervention protocols (eg, frequent repositioning and turning; deep-breathing exercises). ▪ Isolation precautions and/or body substance precautions.	Understanding facilitates compliance and overall participation of the client in the therapeutic regimen.
▪ Remains free of nosocomial infection during hospitalization, as manifested by	Implement appropriate aseptic precautions as warranted (eg, body substance precautions, surgical asepsis).	Appropriate precautions reduce the risk of transmission of microorganisms to and from the client.
a. Absence of signs of *systemic* infection (has normal vital signs, normal leukocyte and erythrocyte sedimentation rate, and no chills, malaise, or lethargy).	Monitor vital signs and skin color at least every shift, or more frequently, for changes that might indicate the presence of an infection.	Increased body temperature, skin flushing, and increased pulse and respiratory rates may indicate systemic infection.
	Assess laboratory blood values for indications of infection. Note: Agency protocol may require blood cultures for a temperature elevation to 38 C (100.5 F) or above.	An elevated leukocyte count, elevated erythrocyte sedimentation rate, and a positive blood culture are indicative of infection.

IMPLEMENTING

Nursing strategies to prevent the spread of an infection include use of meticulous medical and surgical asepsis. **Asepsis** is the freedom from infection or infectious material. Hands washed with soap and water or an antiseptic can be considered aseptic, that is, free from infectious organisms. However, some microorganisms in all probability are still present on washed hands. There are two basic types of asepsis: medical and surgical. **Medical asepsis** includes all practices intended to confine a specific microorganism to a specific area, limiting the number, growth, and transmission of microorganisms.

In medical asepsis, objects are often referred to as clean or dirty. **Clean** denotes the absence of almost all microorganisms. **Dirty** (soiled, contaminated) denotes the likely presence of microorganisms, some of which may be capable of causing infection. Aseptic measures are protective as they are designed to reduce the number of potentially infectious agents.

Surgical asepsis, or sterile technique, refers to those practices that keep an area or objects free of all microorganisms; it includes practices that destroy all microorganisms and spores. (A **spore** is a round or oval structure enclosed in a tough capsule. Some microorganisms assume this structure in response to adverse conditions; in this form, they are highly resistant to destruction.) Surgical

Outcome Criteria	Nursing Interventions	Rationale
	Ask the client about the presence of subjective clinical signs of infection (eg, chills, malaise, lethargy).	These signs are commonly associated with systemic infections.
b. Absence of *local* signs of infection (has clear breath sounds; clear, pale yellow urine; intact skin without inflammation or drainage; negative cultures of sputum, urine, wound or other drainage).	Assess and document clinical signs of infection every 4 hours or in accordance with agency protocol:	Regular assessment allows early detection of infectious process and early therapy.
	▪ Auscultate lungs and inspect urine, sputum, and any other drainage for alterations in color and consistency.	Auscultated "crackles" or "gurgles" indicate fluid or mucus in the air passages. Cloudy malodorous urine and discolored foul-smelling sputum or other drainage may indicate the presence of bacteria.
	▪ Inspect the skin for signs of inflammation and impaired tissue integrity.	Inflammation signals a localized infection. Impaired skin integrity places the client at high risk for infection.
	▪ Collect wound, sputum, urine, and other specimens as ordered for culture and sensitivity, and report abnormalities.	
▪ Implements appropriate practices to promote wellness, support body defenses, and prevent an infection (eg, adequate diet, fluid intake, and rest; proper hygiene; appropriate immunization).	Assess the client's immunization status and life-style practices.	Immunizations provide appropriate antibodies to combat communicable diseases. A balanced diet and fluid intake of 2500 mL/day enhances the health of all body tissues and enables tissues to maintain and rebuild themselves. Adequate rest and sleep are essential to health maintenance. Appropriate body and oral hygiene practices remove transient microorganisms, thereby reducing the likelihood of infection.
	As required, develop and implement a plan to teach client about proper nutrition (high-protein, high-vitamin diet), adequate fluid intake, proper hygiene, and the importance of rest.	

asepsis is required for invasive procedures, such as injections, intravenous therapy, or urinary catheterization.

ISOLATION PRECAUTIONS

Isolation refers to measures designed to prevent the spread of infections or potentially infectious microorganisms to health personnel, clients, and visitors. A variety of infection control measures are used to decrease the risk of transmission of microorganisms in hospitals.

CDC ISOLATION PRECAUTIONS (1983 AND 1987)

In 1983 the Centers for Disease Control and Prevention (CDC) established isolation guidelines that allowed health facilities to choose between two systems: category-specific or disease-specific isolation.

Category-specific isolation precautions are based on seven categories: strict isolation, contact isolation, respiratory isolation, tuberculosis isolation, enteric precautions, drainage/secretions precautions, and blood/body fluid precautions.

Disease-specific isolation precautions provide for precautions for specific diseases. For example, pulmonary

CLINICAL GUIDELINES

Universal Precautions (CDC 1987)*

- Wear masks and protective eyewear or face shields in situations (eg, wound irrigation) where droplets of blood or other body fluids (containing blood) may spray onto the mucous membranes of the eyes, nose, or mouth.
- Wear gloves when in contact with blood or other body fluids containing blood and when handling supplies and equipment or surfaces soiled with blood or other body fluids. Change gloves after client contact.
- Wear gowns in situations where it is likely that droplets of blood or body fluids will be sprayed.
- Immediately and thoroughly wash hands or other skin surfaces that come into contact with blood or other body fluids.
- To prevent needlestick injuries, deposit used needles in a puncture-resistant container that has a secure lid and has been placed near the area where the needles were used. Do not recap, break, or bend needles after use.
- Use mouthpieces, resuscitation bags, or other ventilation equipment when providing resuscitation. This reduces the need for mouth-to-mouth contact.
- Do not provide direct client care when you have open or exudative skin lesions.

* These precautions apply to blood and to other fluids associated with the transmission of bloodborne pathogens. These precautions do not apply to saliva, sputum, nasal secretions, sweat, tears, feces, urine, or vomitus, unless they are visibly contaminated with blood.

tuberculosis precautions specify putting the client in a private room with special ventilation or having the client share a room with other clients who are infected with the same organism, and the use of masks for nurses entering the room and gowning only to prevent gross soilage of clothes. Gloves are not indicated. Special masks (disposable dust/mist particulate respirators) are also recommended by the CDC (Gardner 1993, p. 66).

In 1987, the CDC presented recommendations (revised in 1988 for **universal precautions (UP)** on *all clients* to decrease the risk of transmitting unidentified pathogens (US Department of Health and Human Services 1987, pp. 35–85).

Universal precautions apply to those body fluids associated with **bloodborne pathogens,** namely hepatitis B virus, hepatitis C virus, and HIV. This includes blood and other body fluids containing visible blood. While blood is the single most important source of HIV and other bloodborne pathogens, these precautions also apply to other body fluids such as semen and vaginal secretions, cerebrospinal fluid, synovial fluid, pleural fluid, pericardial fluid, peritoneal fluid, amniotic fluid, saliva, body fluids containing blood, and body fluids where it is difficult to differentiate among body fluids. Universal precautions do not apply to feces, nasal secretions, sputum, sweat, tears, urine, and vomitus unless they contain visible blood (USDHHS 1988, p. 378) because these fluids are not normally associated with the transmission of bloodborne pathogens. A summary of universal precautions is provided in the box at the left.

The CDC did *not* recommend that universal precautions replace disease-specific or category-specific precautions, but that they be used in conjunction with them. Special precautions have been recommended for high-risk areas such as the laboratory and for invasive procedures.

BODY SUBSTANCE ISOLATION (BSI) SYSTEM (1991)

Body substance isolation (BSI) employs generic infection control precautions for *all* clients except those with the few diseases transmitted through the air (Lynch et al 1990, p. 2). The body substance isolation system, conceptualized in 1984 (Jackson & Lynch 1984, pp. 208–10), is a system based on three premises (Jackson & Lynch 1991, p. 448):

1. All people have an increased risk for infection from microorganisms placed on their mucous membranes and nonintact skin.
2. All people are likely to have potentially infectious microorganisms in all of their moist body sites and substances.
3. An unknown portion of clients and health care workers will always be colonized or infected with potentially infectious microorganisms in their blood and other moist body sites and substances.

The purposes of the BSI are similar to those of all precaution systems: (a) to prevent cross-transmission of microorganisms and (b) to protect the health care worker from microorganisms harbored by clients.

The exact protective barriers used for BSI depend on the type of intervention employed, but they are applied to all clients. The term *body substance* includes not only blood and some body fluids, but also urine, feces, wound drainage, oral secretions, and any other body substance.

When BSI precautions are used, category-specific and disease-specific precautions are not required. BSI is sufficient for all clients except those who have certain airborne diseases, such as pulmonary tuberculosis and varicella (chicken pox). It is necessary to place these clients in a private room and to keep the door closed. (Some clients can share a room with another client who is infected by the same microorganism, however.) In addition, a "stop alert" sign is placed on the door advising visitors to consult with the nurse before entering. Depending on the microorganism involved, visitors and health personnel may be advised to wear protective coverings (eg, masks). The following are main elements of BSI:

1. Wash hands thoroughly before and after client care and when gloves are removed. Wearing gloves does not eliminate the need to wash the hands.
2. Wear clean gloves before contact with any body fluids, mucous membranes, nonintact skin, and any moist areas (eg, site of an indwelling venous catheter).
3. Wear gowns, plastic aprons, masks, protective eyewear (eg, goggles), hair covers, and shoe covers as required to keep moist body substances (eg, blood, serous drainage) off clothing, skin, hair, and mucous membranes.
4. Discard all needles and sharp instruments in a puncture-proof container at the place of use.
5. Bag soiled linen securely before it is transported to the laundry area.
6. Place disposable trash in plastic bags and dispose of it according to agency protocol.
7. Handling and reprocessing practices are the same for all equipment used on all clients.
8. Place all specimens in plastic bags, seal the bags, and arrange for transport to the laboratory.

OSHA Standards for Bloodborne Pathogen Exposure (1991)

In late 1991, the Occupational Safety and Health Administration (OSHA) established regulations to protect health care workers from occupational exposure to bloodborne pathogens (Department of Labor, OSHA, 1991). See the discussion of infection control for health care workers later in this chapter. OSHA's guidelines adapt the CDC's Universal Precautions as revised in 1988.

In addition to other actions and precautions discussed in this chapter, significant emphasis is placed on avoiding injury due to sharp instruments (see Chapter 43), measures to be taken in case of exposure to bloodborne pathogens, and communication of biohazards to employees. Federal regulations require that in most cases warning labels be affixed to containers of regulated waste and to refrigerators and freezers containing blood or other potentially infectious materials. The labels required are

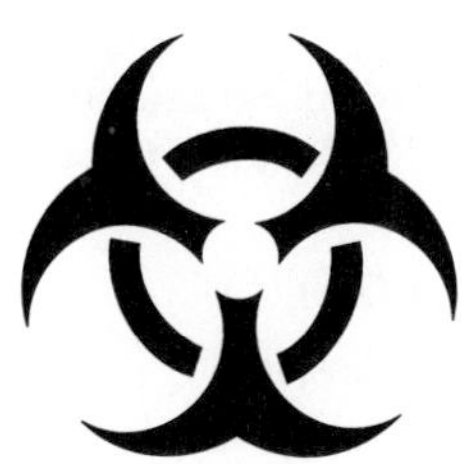

Figure 27–2 Biohazard alert. **Source:** US Department of Labor, Occupational Safety and Health Administration, Occupational exposure to bloodborne pathogens: Final Rule (29 CFR Part 1910.1030), *Federal Register,* December 6, 1991, 56(235):64175–82.

fluorescent orange or orange-red and feature the biohazard legend shown in Figure 27–2.

CDC (HICPAC) Isolation Precautions (1996: Updated 18 February 1997)

The Hospital Infection Control Practices Advisory Committee (HICPAC) of the CDC presented new guidelines for isolation precautions in hospitals in 1996. These latest guidelines designate two tiers of precautions:

Tier 1: Standard Precautions

Tier 2: Transmission-Based Precautions

Standard Precautions

These precautions are used in the care of all hospitalized persons regardless of their diagnosis or possible infection status. They apply to blood, all body fluids, secretions, and excretions *except sweat* (whether or not blood is present or visible), nonintact skin, and mucous membranes.

Thus they combine the major features of UP (Universal Precautions) and BSI (Body Substance Isolation). Recommended practices for Standard Precautions are shown in Table 27–9.

Transmission-Based Precautions

These precautions are used in addition to Standard Precautions for clients with known or suspected infection that are spread in one of three ways: by airborne or droplet transmission, or by contact. The three types of transmission-based precautions may be used alone or in combination but always **in addition** to Standard Precautions. They encompass all the conditions or diseases previously listed in the category-specific or disease specific classifications developed by the CDC in 1983.

Airborne Precautions are used for clients known or suspected to have serious illnesses transmitted by airborne droplet nuclei smaller than 5 microns. Examples of such illnesses include

Table 27–9 Recommended Isolation Precautions in Hospitals (HICPAC) (1996, revised February 17, 1997)

Standard Precautions (Tier One)

- Designed for *all* clients in hospital.
- These precautions apply to 1) blood; 2) all body fluids, excretions, and secretions except sweat; 3) nonintact (broken) skin; and 4) mucous membranes.
- Designed to reduce risk of transmission of microorganisms from recognized and unrecognized sources.

1. Wash hands after contact with blood, body fluids, secretions, excretions, and contaminated objects whether or not gloves are worn.
   - Wash hands immediately after removing gloves.
   - Use a nonantimicrobial soap for routine handwashing.
   - Use an antimicrobial agent or an antiseptic agent for the control of specific outbreaks of infection.
2. Wear clean gloves when touching blood, body fluids, secretions, excretions, and contaminated items (ie, soiled gowns).
   - Clean gloves can be unsterile unless it is intended to prevent the entrance of microorganisms into the body. See the discussion of sterile gloves in this chapter.
   - Remove gloves before touching noncontaminated items and surfaces.
   - Wash hands immediately after removing gloves.
3. Wear a mask, eye protection, or a face shield if splashes or sprays of blood, body fluids, secretions, or excretions can be expected.
4. Wear a clean, nonsterile gown if client case is likely to result in splashes or sprays of blood, body fluids, secretions, or excretions. The gown is intended to protect clothing.
   - Remove a soiled gown carefully to avoid the transfer of microorganism to others (ie, clients or other health care workers).
   - Wash hands after removing gown.
5. Handle client care equipment that is soiled with blood, body fluids, secretions, or excretions carefully to prevent the transfer of microorganisms to others and to the environment.
   - Make sure reusable equipment is cleaned and reprocessed corrrectly.
   - Dispose of single-use equipment correctly.
6. Handle transport and process linen that is soiled with blood, body fluids, secretions, or excretions in a manner to prevent contamination of clothing and the transfer of microorganisms to others and to the environment.
7. Prevent injuries from used equipment, ie scalpels or needles, and place in puncture-resistant containers.

Transmission-Based Precautions (Tier Two)

Airborne Precautions

Use the Tier One precautions as well as the following:

1. Place client in a private room that has negative air pressure; 6 to 12 air changes per hour and discharge of air to the outside or a filtration system for the room air.
2. If a private room is not available, place client with another client who is infected with the same microorganism.
3. Wear a respiratory device (N95 respirator) when entering the room of a client who is known or suspected of having primary tuberculosis.
4. Susceptible people should not enter the room of a client who has rubella (measles) or varicella (chicken pox). If they must enter they should wear a respirator.
5. Limit movement of client outside the room to essential purposes. Place a surgical mask on the client if possible.

Droplet Precautions

Use the Tier One precautions as well as the following:

1. Place client in private room.
2. If a private room is not available, place client with another client who is infected with the same microorganism.
3. Wear a mask if working within 3 feet of the client.
4. Transport client outside of the room only when necessary and place a surgical mask on the client if possible.

Contact Precautions

Use the Tier One precautions as well as the following:

1. Place client in private room.
2. If a private room is not available, place client with another client who is infected with the same microorganism.
3. Wear gloves as described in standard precautions.
   - Change gloves after contact with infectious material.
   - Remove gloves before leaving client's room.
   - Wash hands immediately after removing gloves. Use an antimicrobial agent.
   - After handwashing do not touch possibly contaminated surfaces or items in the room.
4. Wear a gown (see Standard Precautions) when entering a room if there is a possibility of contact with infected surfaces or items, or if the client is incontinent, has diarrhea, a colostomy, or wound drainage not contained by a dressing.
   - Remove gown in the client's room.
   - Make sure clothing does not contact possible contaminated surfaces.
5. Limit movement of client outside the room.
6. Dedicate the use of noncritical client care equipment to a single client or to clients with the same infecting microorganisms.

Source: Adapted from JS Garner and the Hospital Infection Control Practices Advisory Committee (HICPAC), Guidelines for isolation precautions in hospitals, *Infection Control Hospital Epidemiology*, 1996, 17:53–80 and NCID Home Page, February 18, 1997, and *American Journal of Infection Control*, 1996, 24:24–52.

- Measles
- Varicella (including disseminated zoster)
- Tuberculosis (note the CDC has prepared special guidelines for preventing the transmission of tuberculosis in health care facilities)

Droplet Precautions are used for clients known or suspected to have serious illnesses transmitted by particle droplets larger than 5 microns. Such illnesses include

- Invasive *Haemophilus influenzae* type b disease, including meningitis, pneumonia, epiglottitius, and sepsis
- Invasive *Neisseria meningitidis* disease, including meningitis, pneumonia, and sepsis
- Other serious bacterial respiratory infections spread by droplet transmission, including:
  a. Diphtheria (pharyngeal)
  b. Mycoplasma pneumonia
  c. Pertussis
  d. Pneumonic plague
  e. Streptococcal pharyngitis, pneumonia, or scarlet fever in infants and young children
- Serious viral infections spread by droplet transmission, including:
  a. Adenovirus
  b. Influenza
  c. Mumps
  d. Parvovirus B19
  e. Rubella

Contact Precautions are used for clients known or suspected to have serious illnesses easily transmitted by direct client contact or by contact with items in the client's environment. According to the Centers for Disease Control (1996), such illesses include

- Gastrointestinal, respiratory, skin, or wound infections or colonization with multidrug-resistant bacteria judged by the infection control program, based on current state, regional, or national recommendations, to be of special clinical and epidemiologic significance
- Enteric infections with a low infectious dose or prolonged environmental survival, including
  a. *Clostridium difficile*
  b. For diapered or incontinent patients: enterohemorrhagic *Escherichia coli* 0157:H7, *Shigella*, hepatitis A, or rotavirus
- Respiratory syncytial virus, parainfluenza virus, or enteroviral infections in infants and young children
- Skin infections that are highly contagious or that may occur on dry skin, including
  a. Diphtheria (cutaneous)
  b. Herpes simplex virus (neonatal or mucocutaneous)
  c. Impetigo
  d. Major (noncontained) abscesses, cellulitis, or decubiti
  e. Pediculosis
  f. Scabies
  g. Staphylococcal furunculosis in infants and young children
  h. Staphylococcal scaled skin syndrome
  j. Zoster (disseminated or in the immunocompromised host)
- Viral/hemorrhagic conjunctivitis
- Viral hemorrhagic fevers (Lassa fever or Marburg virus)

Recommended practices for Transmission-Based Precautions are shown in Table 27–9.

BARRIER TECHNIQUE (REVERSE ISOLATION)

Compromised clients (ie, highly susceptible to infection) are often infected by their own microorganisms, by microorganisms on the inadequately washed hands of health care personnel, and by nonsterile items (food, water, air, and client-care equipment). Clients who are severely compromised include those who

- Have diseases, such as leukemia, that depress the client's resistance to infectious organisms
- Have extensive skin impairments, such as severe dermatitis or major burns, that cannot be effectively covered with dressings

The 1996 and 1997 CDC guidelines for severely compromised (immunocompromised) clients include the following (Garner 1996, pp. 24–52):

- Use Standard Precautions as described earlier
- Use Transmission-Based Precautions for specified clients

PSYCHOLOGIC ASPECTS OF ISOLATION

Clients requiring isolation precautions can develop several problems as a result of the separation from others and of the special precautions taken in their care. Two of the most common are sensory deprivation and decreased self-esteem related to feelings of inferiority. *Sensory deprivation* occurs when the environment lacks normal stimuli for the client, for example, frequent communications with others. Nurses should therefore be alert to common clinical signs of sensory deprivation: boredom, inactivity, slowness of thought, daydreaming, increased sleeping, thought disorganization, anxiety, hallucinations, and panic.

Chapter 31 provides information on the development of self-esteem and self-esteem disturbances. A client's *feeling of inferiority* can be due to the perception of the infection itself or to the required precautions. In North America, many people place a high value on cleanliness, and the idea of being "soiled," "contaminated," or "dirty" can give clients the feeling that they are at fault and substandard. While this is obviously not true, the infected persons may feel "not as good" as others and blame themselves.

Nurses need to provide care that prevents these two problems and/or deals with them positively. Nursing interventions include the following:

1. Assess the individual's need for stimulation.
2. Initiate measures to help meet the need, including regular communication with the client and diversionary activities, such as toys for a child and books, television, or radio for an adult; provide a variety of foods to stimulate the client's sense of taste; stimulate the client's visual sense by providing a view or an activity to watch.
3. Explain the infection and the associated procedures to help clients and their support persons understand and accept the situation.
4. Demonstrate warm, accepting behavior. Avoid conveying to the client any sense of annoyance about the precautions or any feelings of revulsion about the infection.

IMPLEMENTING ISOLATION PRECAUTIONS

Initiation of precautions to prevent the transmission of microorganisms is generally a nursing responsibility and is based on a comprehensive assessment of the client. This assessment takes into account the status of the client's normal defense mechanisms, the client's ability to implement necessary precautions, and the source and mode of transmission of the infectious agent. The nurse then decides whether to wear gloves, gowns, masks, or protective eyewear. In all client situations, nurses must *wash their hands before and after giving care.*

In addition to the precautions cited within this chapter, the nurse implements aseptic precautions when performing many specific therapies discussed throughout this book. The following are some examples:

- Use strict aseptic technique when performing any invasive procedure (eg, inserting an intravenous needle or catheter, suctioning an airway, and inserting a urinary catheter) and when changing surgical dressings. See Chapters 38, 39, 41, and 44.
- Handle needles and syringes carefully to avoid needle prick injuries. See Chapter 43.
- Change intravenous tubing and solution containers according to hospital policy (eg, every 48 to 72 hours); check intravenous solutions for expiration date and clarity. See Chapter 38.
- Prevent urinary infections by maintaining a closed urinary drainage system with a downhill flow of urine; do not irrigate a catheter unless ordered to do so; provide regular catheter care; clean the perineal area with soap and water; and keep the drainage bag and spout off the floor. See Chapter 41.
- Implement measures to prevent impaired skin integrity, (see Chapter 30) and to prevent accumulation of secretions in the lungs (for example, encourage the client to move, cough, and breathe deeply at least every 2 hours).

Hand Washing Hand washing is important in every setting, including hospitals. It is considered one of the most effective infection control measures. Any client may harbor microorganisms that are currently harmless to the client yet potentially harmful to another person or to the same client *if they find a portal of entry.* It is important that hands be washed at the following times to prevent the spread of microorganisms: before eating, after using the bed pan or toilet, and after the hands have come in contact with any body substances, such as sputum or drainage from a wound. In addition, health care workers should wash their hands before and after giving care.

For routine client care, the CDC recommends a vigorous hand washing under a stream of water for at least 10 seconds using bar soap, granule soap, soapfilled tissues, or antimicrobial liquid soap (Garner & Favero 1985, p. 7). Liquid soaps are frequently supplied in dispensers at the sink. Antimicrobial soaps are usually provided in high-risk areas, such as the newborn nursery. In the following situations, the CDC recommends *antimicrobial* hand-washing agents with any chemical germicides listed with the Environmental Protection Agency:

- When there are known multiple resistant bacteria
- Before invasive procedures
- In special care units, such as nurseries and ICUs

The hands are held down (below the elbows) when they are soiled with body substances and during routine hand washing so that the microorganisms are washed directly into the sink. For surgical asepsis, this text further recommends that the hands be held above the elbows so that the water runs from the cleanest to the least clean area. Nurses usually dry their hands with paper towels, discarding them in an appropriate container immediately after use. Procedure 27–1 provides more detailed instructions for hand washing.

Face Masks Masks are worn to reduce the risk for transmission of organisms by the droplet contact, airborne routes, and splatters of body substances. The CDC recommends that masks be worn under the following conditions (USDHHS 1988, pp. 337–88):

1. Only by those close to the client if the infection (eg, measles, mumps, or acute respiratory diseases in children) is transmitted by large-particle aerosols

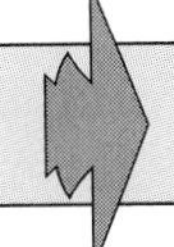

PROCEDURE 27–1 HAND WASHING

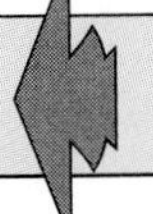

PURPOSES

- To reduce the number of microorganisms on the hands
- To reduce the risk of transmission of microorganisms to clients
- To reduce the risk of cross-contamination among clients
- To reduce the risk of transmission of infectious organisms to oneself

EQUIPMENT

☐ Soap ☐ Warm running water ☐ Towels

INTERVENTION

1. Prepare and assess the hands.

- File the nails short. *Short nails are less likely to harbor microorganisms, scratch a client, or puncture gloves. Long nails are hard to clean.*
- Remove all jewelry. Some nurses prefer to slide their watches up above their elbows. Others pin the watch to the uniform. *Microorganisms can lodge in the settings of jewelry and under rings (Larson 1989a, p. 936). Removal facilitates proper cleaning of the hands and arms.*

- Check hands for breaks in the skin, such as hangnails or cuts. Report cuts to the instructor or nurse in charge before beginning work, or check agency policy about cuts. Use lotions to prevent hangnails and cracked, dry skin. A nurse who has open sores may have to change work assignments or wear gloves for protection.

2. Turn on the water, and adjust the flow.

- There are four common types of faucet controls:
  a. Hand-operated handles.
  b. Knee levers. Move these with the knee to regulate flow and temperature. (Figure 27–3).
  c. Foot pedals. Press these with the foot to regulate flow and temperature. (Figure 27–4).
  d. Elbow controls. Move these with the elbows instead of the hands.
- Adjust the flow so that the water is warm. *Warm water removes less of the protective oil of the skin than hot water.*

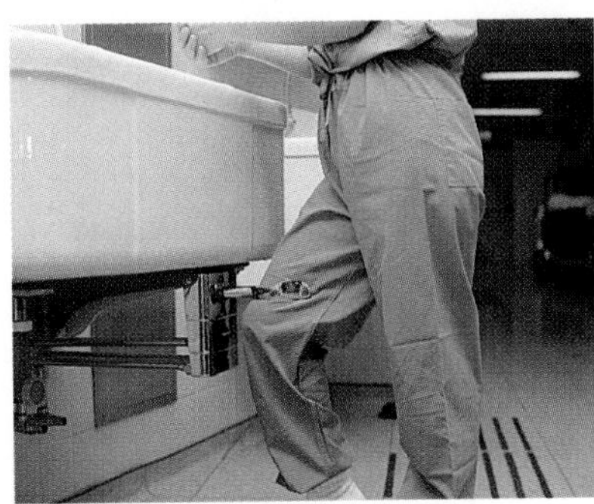

Figure 27–3 A knee-lever faucet control.

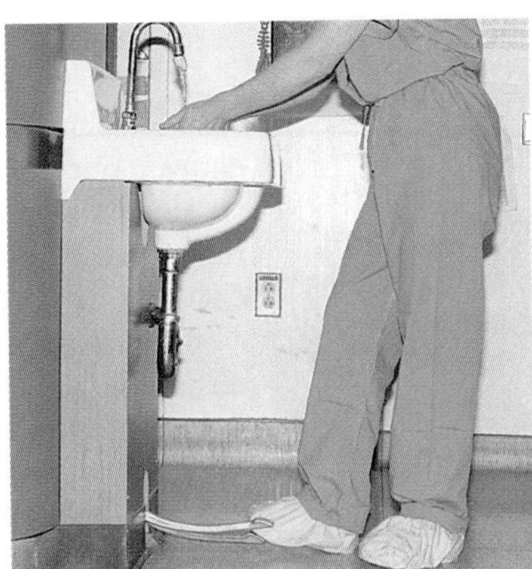

Figure 27–4 A foot pedal faucet control.

3. Wet the hands thoroughly by holding them under the running water, and apply soap to the hands.

- Hold the hands lower than the elbows so that the water flows from the arms to the fingertips. *The water should flow from the least contaminated to the most contaminated area; the hands are generally considered more contaminated than the lower arms.*
- If the soap is liquid, apply 2 to 4 mL (1 tsp). If it is bar soap, rub it firmly between the hands.

4. Thoroughly wash and rinse the hands.

- Use firm, rubbing, and circular movements to wash the palm, back, and wrist of each hand. Interlace the fingers and thumbs, and move the hands back and forth (Figure 27–5). Then continue this motion for 10 seconds. *The circular action helps remove microorganisms mechanically. In-*

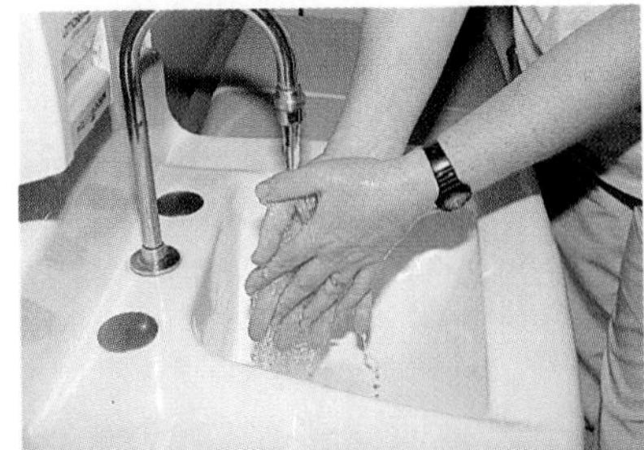

Figure 27–5 Interlacing the fingers during hand washing.

Procedure 27–1 Hand Washing *continued*

terlacing the fingers and thumbs cleans the interdigital spaces.

- Rinse the hands.
- Wash hands for a minimum of 10 seconds. For a more thorough washing, extend the time for wetting, washing, and rinsing.

5. Thoroughly dry the hands and arms.

- Dry hands and arms thoroughly with a paper towel. *Moist skin becomes chapped readily; chapping produces lesions.*
- Discard the paper towel in the appropriate container.

6. Turn off the water.

- Use paper towels to grasp a hand-operated control (Figure 27–6). *This prevents the nurse from picking up microorganisms from the faucet handles.*

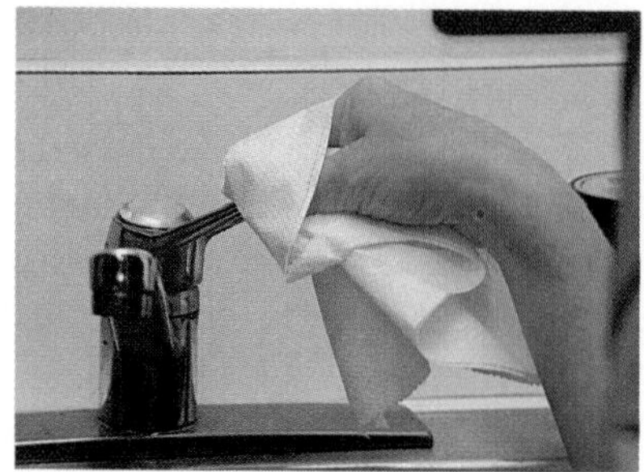

Figure 27–6 Using a paper towel to grasp the handle of a hand-operated faucet.

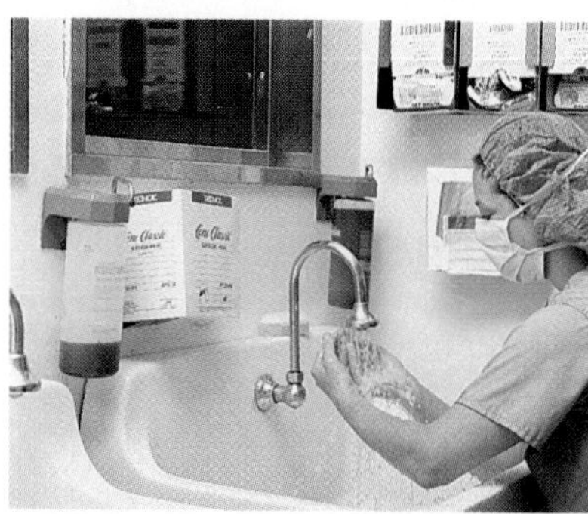

Figure 27–7 The hands are held higher than the elbows during a hand wash before sterile technique.

Variation: Hand Washing before Sterile Techniques

- Hold the hands higher than the elbows during this hand wash. Wet the hands and forearms under the running water, letting it run from the fingertips to the elbows so that the hands become cleaner than the elbows (Figure 27–7). *In this way, the water runs from the area with the fewest microorganisms to areas with a relatively greater number.*
- Apply the soap and wash as described earlier in step 4, maintaining the hands uppermost.
- After washing and rinsing, use a towel to dry one hand thoroughly in a rotating motion from the fingers to the elbow. Use a clean towel to dry the other hand and arm. *A clean towel prevents the transfer of microorganisms from one elbow (least clean area) to the other hand (cleanest area).*

(droplets). Large-particle aerosols are transmitted by close contact and generally travel short distances (about 1 m, or 3 ft).

2. By all persons entering the room if the infection (eg, pulmonary tuberculosis) is transmitted by small-particle aerosols (droplet nuclei). Small-particle aerosols remain suspended in the air and thus travel greater distances by air. Special masks that provide a tighter face seal and better filtration may be used for these infections. The CDC recommends using a disposable dust/mist particulate respirator when caring for any client who has pulmonary tuberculosis. The National Institute for Occupational Safety and Health (NIOSH) recommends that caregivers wear battery-powered respirators that cover most of the face (Gardner 1993, p. 66).

Various types of masks available today differ in their filtration effectiveness and fit. Single-use disposable masks are effective for use while the nurse provides care to most clients but should be changed if they become wet or soiled. These masks are discarded in the waste container after use. *Nondisposable surgical masks* used in the operating room are effective for droplet transmission and splatters but are *not* effective against airborne microorganisms.

During certain techniques requiring surgical asepsis, sterile technique masks are worn (a) to prevent droplet contact transmission of exhaled microorganisms to the sterile field or to a client's open wound and (b) to protect the nurse from splashes of body substances from the client.

Because the effectiveness of disposable masks and nondisposable surgical masks against airborne microorganisms is questionable, agencies usually do not assign *susceptible* caregivers to clients with the specific airborne disease in question. However, caregivers who are immune to specific diseases (eg, chicken pox, tuberculosis, measles, mumps, and rubella) can provide care to clients with these diseases. Guidelines for donning and removing face masks are shown in the box on page 687.

CLINICAL GUIDELINES

Using Disposable Masks

- Ensure that the mask covers the mouth and the nose, because air moves into and out of both.
- If the mask has a metal strip, adjust this firmly over the bridge of the nose. A secure fit prevents both the escape and the inhalation of microorganisms around the edges of the mask and the fogging of eyeglasses.
- If glasses are worn, fit the upper edge of the mask under the glasses. Keeping the edge of the mask under the glasses helps prevent them from clouding.
- Avoid unnecessary talking and, if possible, sneezing or coughing when caring for an at-risk client (eg, when exposing an open wound).
- Wear the mask only once, and do not wear any mask longer than the manufacturer recommends or once it becomes wet. A mask should be used only once because it becomes ineffective when moist.
- When removing a mask with strings, first untie the *lower* strings of the mask. This prevents the top part of the mask from falling onto the chest.
- Discard a disposable mask in the waste container.
- Wash the hands if they have become contaminated by accidentally touching the soiled part of the mask.

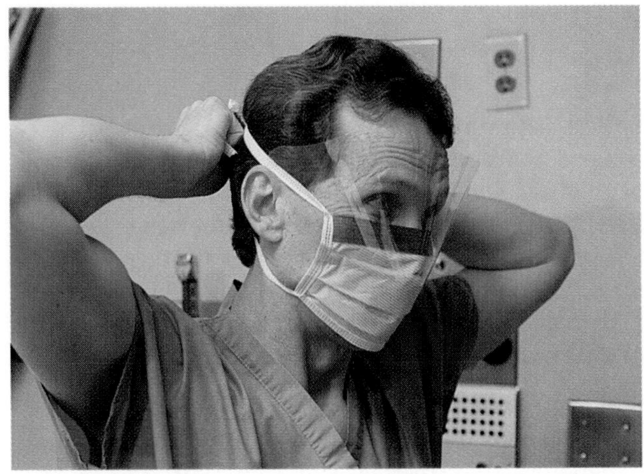

Figure 27–8 A face mask and eye protection covering the nose, mouth, and eyes.

Eyewear Protective eyewear (goggles or glasses) and masks may be indicated in situations where body substances may splatter the face. Figure 27–8 shows an eye shield and mask.

CLINICAL GUIDELINES

Gowning

Donning a Clean Gown

- Pick up a clean gown, and allow it to unfold in front of you without allowing the inside of the gown to touch any area visibly soiled with body substances.
- Fasten the ties at the neck to keep the gown in place.
- Overlap the gown at the back as much as possible, and fasten the waist ties or belt (Figure 27–9). Overlapping securely covers the uniform at the back. Waist ties keep the gown from falling away from the body and prevent inadvertent soiling of the uniform.

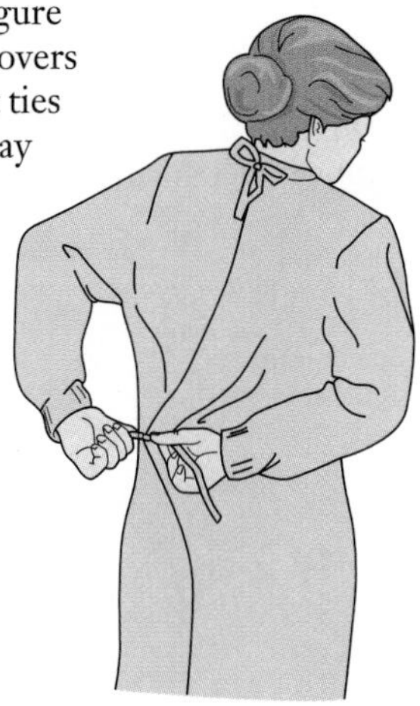

Figure 27–9 Overlapping the gown at the back to cover the nurse's uniform.

Removing a Grossly Soiled Gown

- Avoid touching soiled parts on the outside of the gown, if possible. The top part of the gown may be soiled, for example, if you have been holding an infant with a respiratory infection.
- Roll up the gown with the soiled part inside, and discard it in the appropriate container.

Gowns Clean or disposable gowns or plastic aprons are worn during procedures when the nurse's uniform is likely to become soiled. *Single-use gown technique* (using a gown only once before it is discarded or laundered) is the usual practice in hospitals. After the gown is worn, the nurse discards it (if it is paper) or places it in a laundry hamper. Before leaving the client's room, the nurse washes his or her hands.

Sterile gowns may be indicated when the nurse changes the dressings of a client with extensive wounds (eg, burns).

No special precautions are required to don a clean gown or to remove a gown that is not visibly soiled with body substances. However, many nurses take precautions when removing a grossly soiled gown so that they do not soil their uniform. Check agency protocol. Guidelines are shown in the box above.

CLINICAL GUIDELINES

Removing Disposable Gloves

- Remove the first glove by grasping it on its palmar surface just below the cuff, taking care to touch only glove to glove (Figure 27–10). This keeps the soiled parts of the used gloves from touching the skin of the wrist or hand.
- Pull the first glove completely off by inverting or rolling the glove inside out.
- Continue to hold the inverted removed glove by the fingers of the remaining gloved hand. Place the first two fingers of the bare hand inside the cuff of the second glove (Figure 27–11). Touching the outside of the second soiled glove with the bare hand is avoided.
- Pull the second glove off to the fingers by turning it inside out. This pulls the first glove inside the second glove. The soiled part of the glove is folded to the inside to reduce the chance of transferring any microorganisms by direct contact.
- Using the bare hand, continue to remove the gloves, which are now inside out, and dispose of them in the refuse container (Figure 27–12).
- Wash hands.

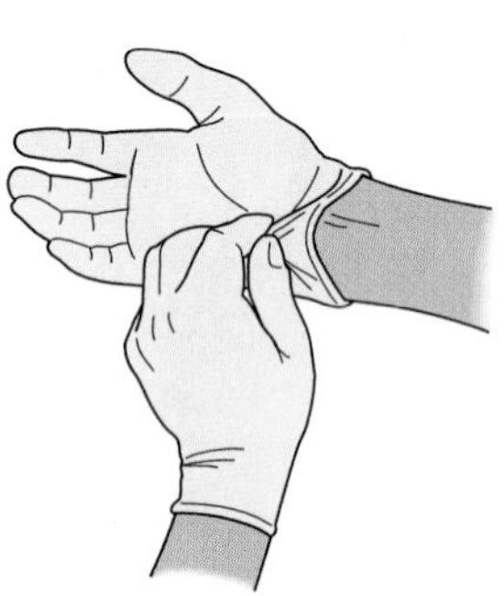

Figure 27–10 Plucking the palmar surface below the cuff of a contaminated glove.

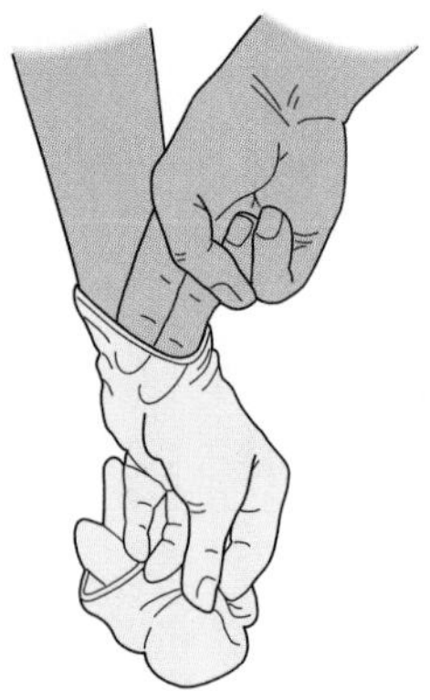

Figure 27–11 Inserting fingers to remove the second contaminated glove.

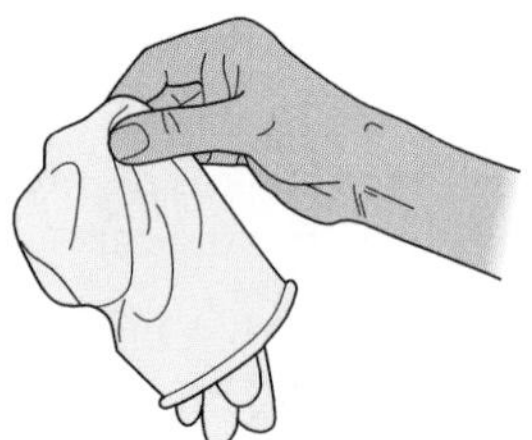

Figure 27–12 Holding contaminated gloves, which are inside out.

Gloves Gloves are worn to protect the hands when the nurse is likely to handle any body substances, for example, blood, urine, feces, sputum, mucous membranes, and nonintact skin. Gloves also reduce the likelihood of nurses' transmitting their own endogenous microorganisms to individuals receiving care. Nurses who have open sores or cuts on the hands must wear gloves for protection. For most activities, disposable *clean* gloves are used. Sterile gloves are used when the hands will come in contact with an open wound or when the hands might introduce microorganisms into a body orifice (See Procedure 27–3 on page 698). No special technique is required to don disposable gloves.

If a gown is worn, the nurse pulls the gloves up to cover the cuffs of the gown. If a gown is not worn the nurse pulls up the cuffs to cover the wrists.

No special technique is usually required to remove the gloves, and the hands are always washed afterward. If, however, there is a reason to prevent soilage of the hands (eg, if the nurse has a cut), the nurse follows the steps in the box above.

Soiled Equipment and Supplies Many pieces of equipment are supplied for single use only and disposed of after use. Some items, however, are reusable. Agencies have specific policies and procedures for handling soiled equipment (eg, disposal, cleaning, disinfecting, and sterilizing); the nurse needs to become familiar with these practices in the employing agency. Appropriate handling of soiled equipment and supplies is essential

- To prevent inadvertent exposure of health care workers to articles contaminated with body substances
- To prevent contamination of the environment

For information about cleaning, disinfecting, and sterilizing, see pages 672 to 673, earlier in this chapter.

Bagging Most articles do not need to be bagged unless they are contaminated, or likely to be contaminated, with infective material such as pus, blood, body fluids, feces, or respiratory secretions. Soiled articles need to be enclosed in a sturdy bag impervious to microorganisms before they are removed from the room or cubicle of any client. Some agencies use labels or bags of a particular color that designates them as infective wastes. Check agency policy.

The 1988 CDC guidelines recommend the following methods (USDHHS 1988, pp. 337–88):

- A single bag, if it is sturdy and impervious to microorganisms, and if the contaminated articles can be placed in the bag without soiling or contaminating its outside
- Double-bagging if the above conditions are not met

Follow agency protocol, or use the following CDC guidelines to handle and bag soiled items (USDHHS 1988, pp. 337–88)

- Place garbage and soiled *disposable* equipment, including dressings and tissues, in the plastic bag that lines the waste container. Some agencies separate dry and wet waste material and incinerate dry items, such as paper towels and disposable items. No special precautions are required for disposable equipment that is not contaminated.
- Place *nondisposable* or *reusable* equipment that is visibly soiled in a labeled bag before removing it from the client's room or cubicle, and send it to a central processing area for decontamination. Some agencies may require that glass bottles or jars and metal items be placed in separate bags from rubber and plastic items. Glass and metal can be sterilized in an autoclave, but rubber and plastic are damaged by this process and must be cleaned by other methods, such as gas sterilization.
- Disassemble *special procedure trays* into component parts. Some components can be discarded; others need to be sent to the laundry or central services for cleaning and decontaminating.
- Bag soiled *clothing* before sending it home or to the agency laundry.
- Use two bags for articles if the single bag is not sturdy or impervious to microorganisms or is soiled on the outside.

Linens Handle soiled linen as little as possible and with the least agitation possible before placing it in the client's laundry hamper. This prevents gross microbial contamination of the air and/or persons handling the linen.

Tie the bag closed before sending it to the laundry in accordance with agency practice. Some agencies use hot-water-soluble plastic bags for contaminated linen to elminate the need for touching the linen after it is placed in the bag. This type of bag dissolves in hot washing water.

Laboratory Specimens Laboratory specimens, if placed in a leak-proof container with a secure lid, need no special precautions. Use care when collecting specimens to avoid contaminating the outside of the container. Clean or disinfect specimen containers that are visibly contaminated on the outside before sending them to the laboratory. This prevents personnel from having hand contact with potentially infective material.

Dishes Dishes require no special precautions. Soiling of dishes can largely be prevented by encouraging clients to wash their hands before eating. Some agencies use paper dishes for convenience, which are disposed of in the refuse container.

Blood Pressure Equipment Blood pressure equipment needs no special precautions unless it becomes contaminated with infective material. If contaminated, follow agency practice. Cleaning procedures vary according to whether it is a wall or portable unit.

Thermometers Nondisposable used thermometers are generally disinfected after use. Check agency practice.

Disposable Needles, Syringes, and Sharps Place needles and syringes and "sharps" (eg, lancets, scalpels, and broken glass) into a puncture-resistant container. To avoid puncture wounds, do not detach needles from the syringe or recap the needle before disposal. See Chapter 43, page 1318, for how to prevent needlestick injuries.

Toys Personal toys that are visibly contaminated are bagged and sent home. Agency toys, if visibly soiled, may require terminal cleaning. Check agency practice. Depending on the type of microorganism and its transmission and the child's hygiene behaviors, special precautions may be required. For example, the nurse may prevent a child who has an enteric infection that may be spread by contact transmission or by fomites from sharing toys with others.

Client Placement Clients who have infections transmitted by the airborne route require a private room. A private room may also be needed for an individual who soils the environment with body substances.

Some facilities provide "special rooms" for clients with airborne infections, such as active pulmonary tuberculosis; these rooms are equipped with negative pressure and adequate air changes and exhaust.

In some situations, placing an infected client in a room with another client is unavoidable. It is preferable if both clients have the same infectious disease and are infected with the same microorganisms. For all people, the key to preventing transmission of microorganisms is washing hands between contacts with body substances.

Transporting Clients with Infections Transporting clients with infections (eg, chicken pox) outside their own rooms is avoided unless absolutely necessary. If a client

WELLNESS TEACHING

Preventing Infections in the Home

- Wash your hands before handling foods, before eating, after toileting, before and after any required home care treatment, and after touching any infected body substances (eg, wound drainage).
- Keep your fingernails short, clean, and well-manicured to eliminate rough edges or hangnails, which can harbor microorganisms.
- Use your own personal care items: toothbrush, washcloths, and towels.
- Wash raw fruits and vegetables before eating them.
- Refrigerate all opened and nonpackaged foods.
- Clean used equipment (eg, emesis basin) with soap and water, and disinfect it with a chlorine bleach solution.
- Place contaminated dressings and other disposable items containing infectious body fluids in moistureproof plastic bags.
- Put used needles in a puncture-resistant container with a screw-top lid. Label so as not to discard in the garbage.
- Clean obviously soiled linen separately from other laundry. Rinse in cold water, wash in hot water if possible, and add a cup of bleach or Lysol to the wash.
- Avoid coughing, sneezing, or breathing directly on others. Cover the mouth and nose to prevent the transmission of airborne microorganisms.
- Be aware of any signs or symptoms of an infection, and report these immediately to your health care contact person.
- Maintain a sufficient fluid intake to promote urine production and output. This helps flush the bladder and urethra of microorganisms.

must be moved, the nurse provides the client with a special particulate mask and takes precautions to prevent soilage of the environment. For example, the nurse ensures that any draining wound is securely covered. In addition, the nurse notifies personnel at the "receiving" area of any infection risk so that they can maintain necessary precautions. Follow agency protocol.

SUPPORTING DEFENSES OF A SUSCEPTIBLE HOST

People are constantly in contact with microorganisms in the environment. Normally, a person's natural defenses ward off the development of an infection. *Susceptibility* is the degree to which an individual can be affected, that is, the likelihood of an organism causing an infection in that person. The following measures can reduce a person's susceptibility. See also the box at the left.

Hygiene Maintaining the intactness of the skin and mucous membranes retains one barrier against microorganisms entering the body. In addition, oral care, including flossing the teeth, reduces the likelihood of an oral infection. Regular and thorough bathing and shampooing remove microorganisms and dirt that harbor microorganisms and can result in an infection.

Immunizations The immunologic system is a major defense against infections. Keeping up to date with immunizations is an important preventive measure. See discussions of specific defenses earlier in this chapter, and Chapters 24 and 25 for immunizations at various ages.

Nutrition A balanced diet enhances the health of all body tissues, helps keep the skin intact, and promotes the skin's ability to repel microorganisms. Adequate nutrition enables tissues to maintain and rebuild themselves and helps keep the immune system functioning well.

Fluid An adequate fluid intake permits a fluid output that flushes out the bladder and urethra, removing microorganisms that could cause an infection.

Rest and Sleep Adequate rest and sleep are essential to health and to renewing energy. See Chapter 35.

Stress Stress predisposes people to infections. Nurses can assist clients to learn stress-reducing techniques. See Chapter 32.

INFECTION CONTROL FOR HEALTH CARE WORKERS

The Occupational and Safety Health Administration (OSHA) provides regulations to protect health care workers from occupational exposure to bloodborne pathogens in the workplace. **Occupational exposure** is defined by OSHA as reasonably anticipated skin, eye, mucous membrane, or parenteral contact with blood or other potentially infectious materials that may result from the performance of an employee's duties (Department of Labor, OSHA 1991).

There are three major modes of transmission of infectious fluids in the clinical setting:

- *Puncture wounds* from contaminated needles or other sharps.
- *Skin contact*, which allows infectious fluids to enter through wounds, broken or damaged skin, and cuts.
- *Mucous membrane* contact, which allows infectious fluids to enter through mucous membranes of the eyes, mouth, and nose.

CRITICAL THINKING CHALLENGE

WHAT WOULD YOU DO?

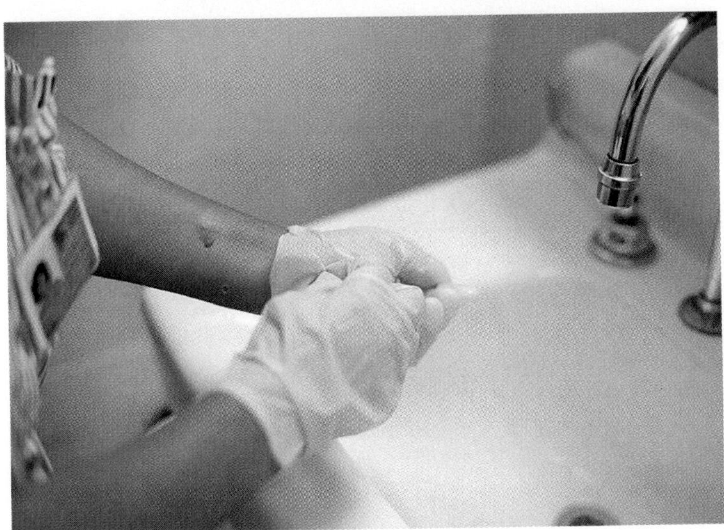

An intravenous infusion has been ordered for your client, Nivea Castro. Having started the infusion, you are removing your gloves when you notice a small amount of blood on your left forearm.

What would you do?

Using proper precautions with general medical asepsis, appropriately using personal protective equipment (gloves, masks, gowns, goggles, shoe covers, special resuscitative equipment), and avoiding carelessness in the clinical area will place the caregiver at significantly less risk for injury. To avoid injury due to sharp instruments, see Chapter 43, page 1318. Measures to be taken in case of exposure to hepatitis B and HIV are outlined in the box at the right.

OSHA also advises that health care employers make available the hepatitis B vaccine and vaccination series to all employees. Other vaccinations may also be made available (eg, nurses working in an obstetric area should be vaccinated against rubella to protect pregnant clients and their fetuses).

STEPS TO FOLLOW AFTER EXPOSURE TO BLOODBORNE PATHOGENS

- Wash the exposed area immediately!
- Report the incident immediately to appropriate personnel within the agency, and consult a doctor.
- Complete an injury report.
- Seek appropriate evaluation and follow-up. This includes the following:
  - Identification and documentation of the source individual when feasible and legal
  - Testing of the source individual's blood when feasible and consent is given
  - Making results of the test available to the person's health care provider
  - Collection and testing of blood of exposed health care provider (with consent)
  - Post exposure prophylaxis, if medically indicated (eg, hepatitis B vaccine for HBV, or zidovudine—or recommended agent—for HIV)
  - Medical counseling regarding personal risk of infection or risk of infecting others

Source: US Department of Labor, Occupational Safety and Health Administration, Occupational exposure to bloodborne pathogens: Final rule (29 CFR Part 1910.1030), *Federal Register*, December 6, 1991, 56(235):64175–82.

SURGICAL ASEPSIS

An object is sterile only when it is free of all microorganisms. It is well known that surgical asepsis is practiced in operating rooms, labor and delivery rooms, and special diagnostic areas. Less known perhaps is that surgical asepsis is also employed for many procedures in general care areas (ie, procedures such as administering injections, changing wound dressings, performing urinary catheterizations, and administering intravenous therapy). In these situations, all of the principles of surgical asepsis are applied as in the operating or delivery room; however, not all of the sterile techniques that follow are always required. For example, before an operating room procedure, the "scrub" nurse generally puts on a mask and cap,

Table 27–10 Principles and Practices of Surgical Asepsis

Principles	Practices
All objects used in a sterile field must be sterile.	All articles are sterilized appropriately by dry or moist heat, chemicals, or radiation before use.
	Sterile articles can be stored for only a prescribed time; after that, they are considered unsterile.
	Always check a package containing a sterile object for intactness, dryness, and expiration date. Any package that appears already open, torn, punctured, or wet is considered unsterile. Never assume an item is sterile.
	Storage areas should be clean, dry, off the floor, and away from sinks.
	Always check the sterilization dates and periods on the labels of wrapped items before using the items.
	Always check chemical indicators of sterilization before using a package. The indicator is often a tape used to fasten the package or contained inside the package. The indicator changes color during sterilization, indicating that the contents have undergone a sterilization procedure. If the color change is not evident, the package is considered unsterile. Commercially prepared sterile packages may not have indicators but are marked with the word *sterile.*
Sterile objects become unsterile when touched by unsterile objects.	Handle sterile objects that will touch open wounds or enter body cavities only with sterile forceps or sterile gloved hands.
	Discard or resterilize objects that come into contact with unsterile objects.
	Whenever the sterility of an object is questionable, assume the article is unsterile.
Sterile items that are out of vision or below the waist level of the nurse are considered unsterile.	Once left unattended, a sterile field is considered unsterile.
	Sterile objects are always kept in view. Nurses do not turn their backs on a sterile field.
	Only the front part of a sterile gown (from the waist to the shoulder) and 2 inches above the elbows to the cuff of the sleeves are considered sterile.
	Always keep sterile gloved hands in sight and above waist level; touch only objects that are sterile.
	Sterile draped tables in the operating room or elsewhere are considered sterile only at surface level.
	Once a sterile field becomes unsterile, it must be set up again before proceeding.
Sterile objects can become unsterile by prolonged exposure to airborne microorganisms.	Keep doors closed and traffic to a minimum in areas where a sterile procedure is being performed, because moving air can carry dust and microorganisms.
	Keep areas in which sterile procedures are carried out as clean as possible by frequent damp cleaning with detergent germicides to minimize contaminants in the area.
	Keep hair clean and short or enclose it in a net to prevent hair from falling on sterile objects. Microorganisms on the hair can make a sterile field unsterile.
	Wear surgical caps in operating rooms, delivery rooms, and burn units.
	Refrain from sneezing or coughing over a sterile field. This can make it unsterile, because droplets containing microorganisms from the respiratory tract can travel 3 feet. Some nurses recommend

performs a surgical hand scrub, and then dons a sterile gown and gloves. In a general care area, the nurse may only perform a hand wash and don sterile gloves. The nine basic principles of surgical asepsis, and practices that relate to each principle, appear in Table 27–10.

STERILE FIELD

A **sterile field** is a microorganism-free area, including free of spores. Nurses often establish a sterile field by using the innermost side of a sterile wrapper or by using a sterile drape. When the field is established, sterile supplies and sterile solutions can be placed on it. Sterile forceps are used in many instances to handle and transfer the sterile supplies.

So that its sterility can be maintained, equipment is wrapped in a variety of materials. Commercially prepared items are frequently wrapped in plastic, paper, or glass. Commercially prepared sterile liquids for both internal and external use are often supplied in plastic or glass con-

Table 27–10 ***continued***

Principles	Practices
	that masks covering the mouth and the nose should be worn by anyone working over a sterile field or an open wound.
	Nurses with mild upper respiratory tract infections refrain from carrying out sterile procedures or wear masks.
	When working over a sterile field, keep talking to a minimum. Avert the head from the field if talking is necessary.
	To prevent microorganisms from falling over a sterile field, refrain from reaching over a sterile field unless sterile gloves are worn and refrain from moving unsterile objects over a sterile field. Always reach around a sterile field or carefully turn it by reaching under the wrapper or by touching the wrapper edges.
Fluids flow in the direction of gravity.	Unless gloves are worn, always hold wet forceps with the tips below the handles. When the tips are held higher than the handles, fluid can flow onto the handle and become contaminated by the hands. When the forceps are again pointed downward, the fluid flows back down and contaminates the tips.
	During a surgical hand wash, hold the hands higher than the elbows to prevent contaminants from the forearms from reaching the hands.
Moisture that passes through a sterile object draws microorganisms from unsterile surfaces above or below to the sterile surface by capillary action.	Sterile moistureproof barriers are used beneath sterile objects. Liquids (sterile saline or antiseptics) are frequently poured into containers on a sterile field. If they are spilled onto the sterile field, the barrier keeps the liquid from seeping beneath it.
	Keep the sterile covers on sterile equipment dry. Damp surfaces can attract microorganisms in the air.
	When pouring sterile solutions into sterile containers, take care to avoid dampening the sterile field.
	Replace sterile drapes that do not have a sterile barrier underneath when they become moist.
The edges of a sterile field are considered unsterile.	A 2.5-cm (1-in) margin at each edge of an opened drape is considered unsterile, because the edges are in contact with unsterile surfaces.
	Place all sterile objects more than 2.5-cm (1-in) inside the edges of a sterile field.
	Any article that falls outside the edges of a sterile field is considered unsterile.
The skin cannot be sterilized and is unsterile.	Wear sterile gloves and/or use sterile forceps to handle sterile items.
	Prior to a surgical aseptic procedure, wash the hands to reduce the number of microorganisms on them.
Conscientiousness, alertness, and honesty are essential qualities in maintaining surgical asepsis.	When a sterile object becomes unsterile, it does not necessarily change in appearance.
	The person who sees a sterile object become contaminated must correct or report the situation.
	Do not set up a sterile field ahead of time for future use.

tainers. Plastics are often pliable, usually transparent, impervious to dust, and relatively resistant to tearing. Liquids used in hospitals may be prepared commercially or in the hospital. In the past, it was not unusual for sterile liquids (eg, sterile water for irrigations) to be supplied in large glass containers and used many times. This practice is today considered undesirable because once a container has been opened, there can be no assurance that it is sterile. Liquids are preferably packaged in amounts adequate for one use only. Any leftover liquid is discarded. Hospital-packaged liquids are often sterilized in reusable containers; commercially packaged liquids are supplied in disposable containers. These containers normally have a seal over the cap, and often the word *sterile* is clearly marked on the top. If the cap has been tampered with or if the seal is broken, the liquid is considered unsterile. All containers should also be inspected for cracks.

Procedure 27–2 on page 694 describes how to establish and maintain a sterile field.

Text continued on page 697

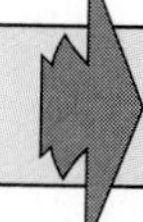

Procedure 27–2 Establishing and Maintaining a Sterile Field

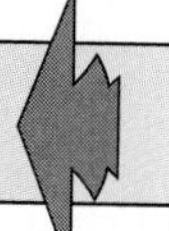

Purpose

- To maintain the sterility of supplies and equipment

Equipment

- ☐ Package containing a sterile drape
- ☐ Sterile equipment as needed (eg, wrapped sterile gauze, wrapped sterile bowl, antiseptic solution, sterile forceps)

INTERVENTION

1. Confirm the sterility of the package.

- Ensure that the package is clean and dry; if moist, it is considered contaminated and must be discarded.
- Check the sterilization expiration dates on the package, and look for any indications that it has been previously opened.
- Follow agency practice about the disposal of possibly contaminated packages.

2. Open the package.

To Open a Wrapped Package on a Surface

- Place the package in the center of the work area so that the top flap of the wrapper opens away from you. *This position prevents the nurse from subsequently reaching directly over the exposed sterile contents, which could contaminate them.*
- Reaching around the package (not over it), pinch the first flap on the outside of the wrapper between the thumb and index finger (Figure 27–13). With some folded packages, it may be necessary to grasp the uppermost flap at each corner. *Touching only the outside of the wrapper maintains the sterility of the inside of the wrapper.* Pull the flap open, laying it flat on the far surface.
- Repeat for the side flaps, opening the top one first. Use the right hand for the right flap, and the left hand for the left flap (Figure 27–14). *By using both hands, the nurse avoids reaching over the sterile contents.*
- Pull the fourth flap toward you by grasping the corner that is turned down (Figure 27–15). Make sure that the flap does not touch your uniform. *If the inner surface touches any unsterile article, it is contaminated.*

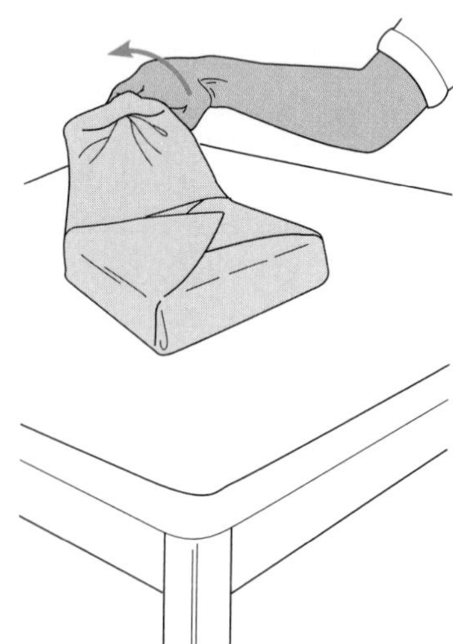

Figure 27–13 Opening the first flap of a sterile wrapped package.

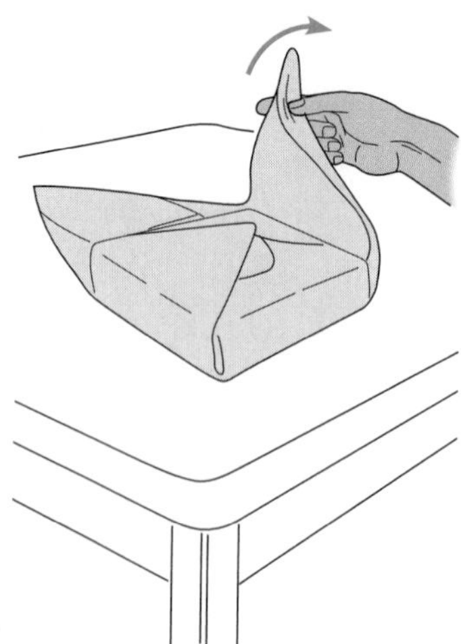

Figure 27–14 Opening the second flap to the side.

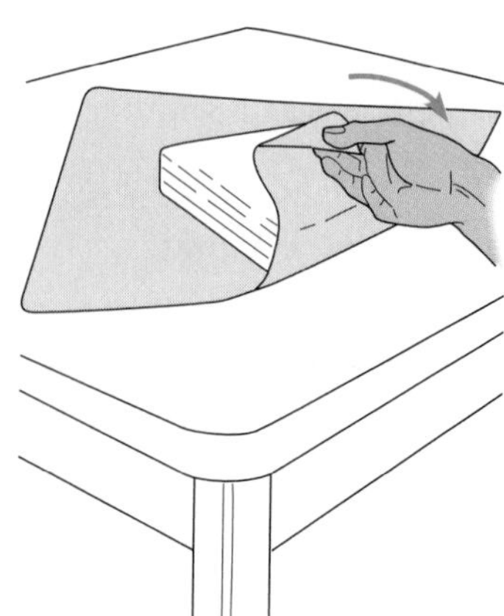

Figure 27–15 Pulling the last flap toward oneself by grasping the corner.

PROCEDURE 27–2 *continued*

To Open a Wrapped Package While Holding It

- Hold the package in one hand with the top flap opening away from you.
- Using the other hand, open the package as described above, pulling the corners of the flaps well back (Figure 27–16). *The hands are considered contaminated, and at no time should they touch the contents of the package.*

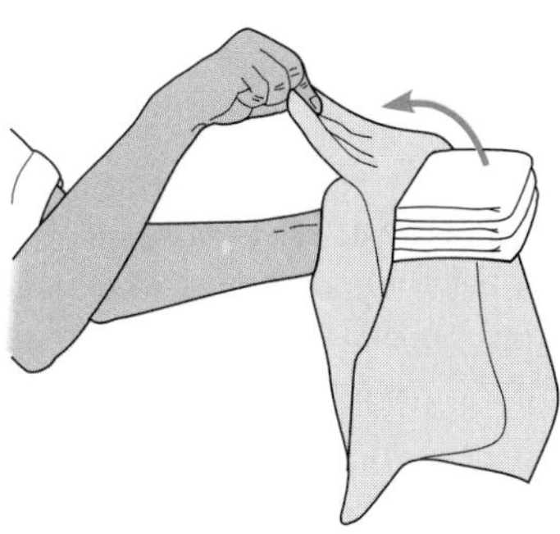

Figure 27–16 Opening a wrapped package while holding it.

To Open Commercially Prepared Packages

Commercially prepared sterile packages and containers usually have manufacturer's directions for opening.

- If the flap of the package has an unsealed corner, hold the container in one hand, and pull back on the flap with the other hand (Figure 27–17).
- If the package has a partially sealed edge, grasp both sides of the edge, one with each hand, and pull apart gently (Figure 27–18).

3. Rewrap the sterile package as required (eg, for transport to the bedside).

- Rewrap in the *reverse* order to unwrapping. Close the proximal flap first to prevent reaching across the sterile field, the side flaps next, and the distal flap last.

4. Establish a sterile field by using a drape.

- Open the package containing the drape as described above.
- With one hand, pluck the corner of the drape that is folded back on the top.
- Lift the drape out of the cover, and allow it to open freely without touching any objects (Figure 27–19). *If the drape touches the outside of the package, the uniform or any unsterile surface, it is considered contaminated.*
- Discard the cover.
- With the other hand, carefully pick up another corner of the drape, holding it well away from yourself.
- Lay the drape on a clean and dry surface, placing the bottom (ie, the freely hanging side) farthest from you (Figure 27–20). *By placing the lowermost side farthest away, the nurse avoids leaning over the sterile field and contaminating it.*

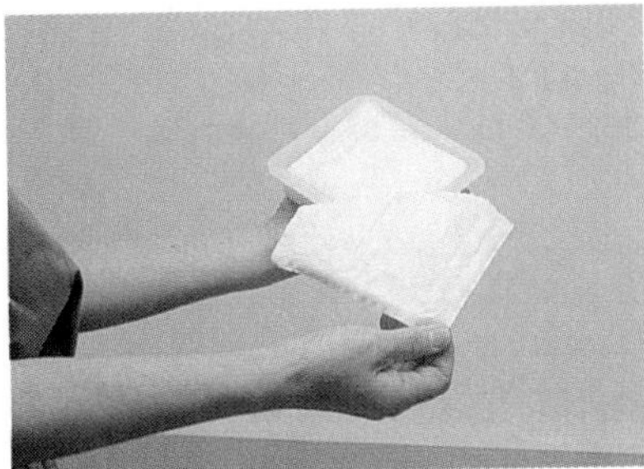

Figure 27–17 Opening a sterile package that has an unsealed corner.

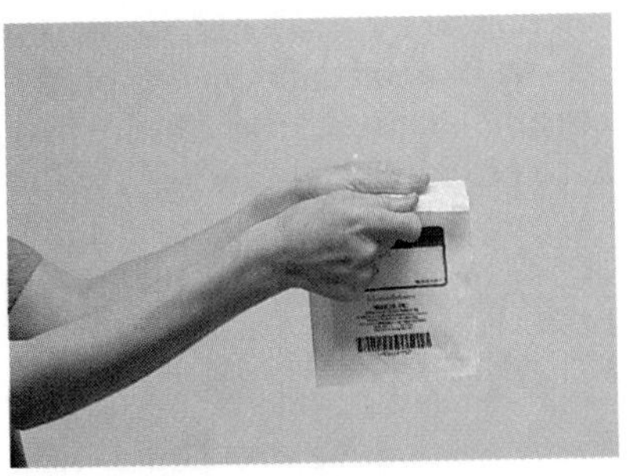

Figure 27–18 Opening a sterile package that has a partially sealed edge.

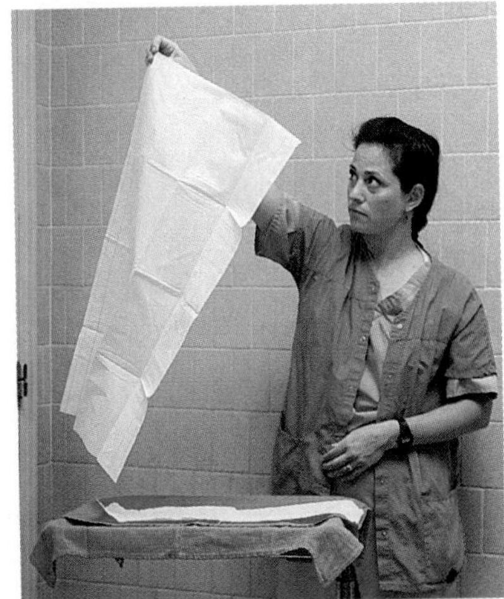

Figure 27–19 Allowing a drape to open freely without touching any objects.

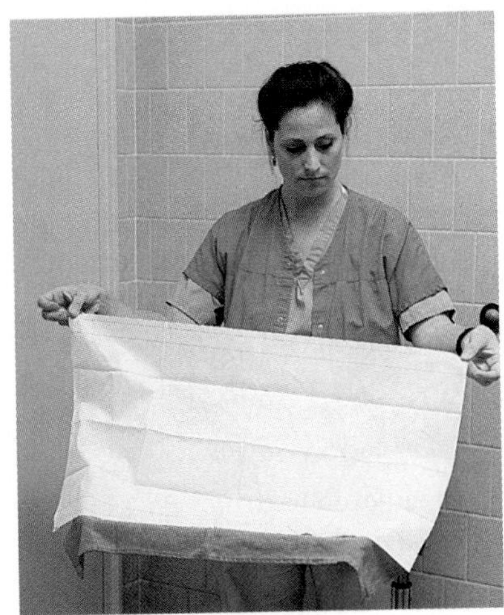

Figure 27–20 Placing a drape on a surface.

PROCEDURE 27–2 ESTABLISHING AND MAINTAINING A STERILE FIELD *continued*

5. Add necessary sterile supplies.

To Add Wrapped Supplies to a Sterile Field

- Open each wrapped package as described in the preceding steps.
- With the free hand, grasp the corners of the wrapper, and hold them against the wrist of the other hand (Figure 27–21). *The unsterile hand is now covered by the sterile wrapper.*

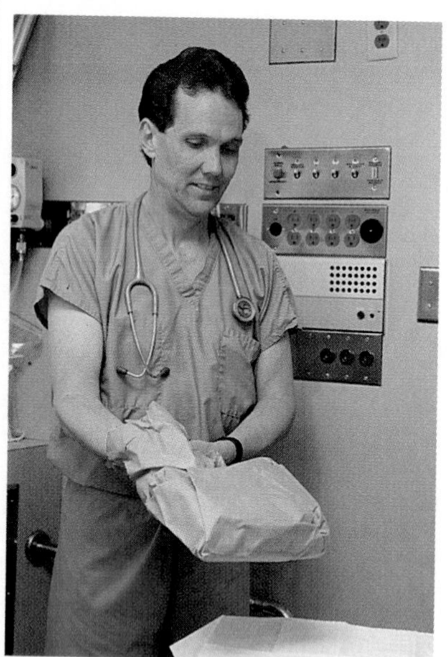

Figure 27–21 Adding wrapped sterile supplies to a sterile field.

- Place the sterile bowl, drape, or other supply on the sterile field by approaching from an angle rather than holding the arm over the field.
- Discard the wrapper.

To Add Commercially Packaged Supplies to a Sterile Field

- Open each package (eg, gauze) as described above.
- Hold the package 15 cm (6 in) above the field, and allow the contents to drop on the field (Figure 27–22). Keep in mind that 2.5 cm (1 in) around the edge of the field is considered contaminated. *At a height of 15 cm (6 in), the outside of the package is not likely to touch and contaminate the sterile field.*

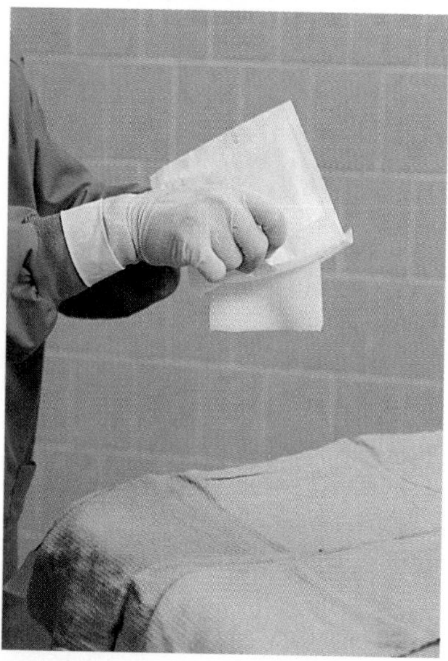

Figure 27–22 Adding commercially packaged gauze to a sterile field.

To Add Sterile Solution to a Sterile Bowl

Sterile liquids (eg, normal saline) frequently need to be poured into metal or nonabsorbent containers within a sterile field. Unwrapped bottles or flasks that contain sterile solution are considered sterile on the inside and contaminated on the outside, because the bottle may have been handled. Bottles used in an operating room may be sterilized on the outside as well as the inside, however, and these are handled with sterile gloves.

- Before pouring any liquid, read the label three times to make sure you have the correct solution.
- Obtain the exact amount of solution, if possible. *Once a sterile container has been opened, its sterility cannot be ensured for future use unless it is used again immediately.*
- Read the label to confirm both the name of solution and its strength.
- Remove the lid or cap from the bottle, and invert the lid before placing it on a surface that is not sterile. *Inverting the lid maintains the sterility of the inside surface because it is not allowed to touch an unsterile surface.*
- Hold the bottle so that the label is uppermost. *Any solution that flows down the outside of the bottle during pouring will not damage or obliterate the label.*
- Hold the bottle of fluid at a height of 10 to 15 cm (4 to 6 in) over the bowl and to the side of the sterile field so that as little of the bottle as possible is over the field. *At this height, there is less likelihood of contaminating the sterile field by touching the field or by reaching an arm over it.*
- Pour the solution gently to avoid splashing the liquid. *If the sterile drape is on an unsterile surface, any moisture will contaminate the field by facilitating the movement of microorganisms through the sterile drape.*
- Replace the lid securely on the bottle if you plan to use it again, and provide the date and time of opening. Check agency protocol. *Replacing the lid immediately maintains the sterility of the inner aspect of the lid and the solution.* In many agencies a sterile container of solution that is opened is used only once and then discarded.

PROCEDURE 27–2 *continued*

6. Use sterile forceps to handle certain sterile supplies.

Forceps are commonly used for such techniques as changing a sterile dressing and shortening a drain. Transfer forceps are usually used to move a sterile article from one place to another, for example, transferring sterile gauze from its package to a sterile dressing tray. Forceps are usually packaged and discarded or resterilized after use. Commonly used forceps include hemostats, or artery forceps (Figure 27–23), and tissue forceps (Figure 27–24).

- Keep the tips of wet forceps lower than the wrist at all times, unless you are wearing sterile gloves (Figure 27–25). *Gravity prevents liquids on the tips of the forceps from flowing to the handles and later back to the tips, thus making the forceps unsterile. The handles are unsterile once they are held by the bare hand.*
- Hold sterile forceps above waist level. *There is less danger of contamination if the forceps are held near to eye level.*
- Hold sterile forceps within sight. *While out of sight, forceps may unknowingly become unsterile. Any such forceps should be considered unsterile.*
- When using forceps to lift sterile supplies out of a commercially prepared package, be sure that the forceps do not touch the edges or outside of the wrapper. *The edges and outside of the package are exposed to the air and handled and are thus unsterile.*
- When placing forceps whose handles were in contact with the bare hand, position the handles outside the sterile area. *The handles of these forceps harbor microorganisms from the bare hand.*
- Deposit a sterile item on a sterile field without permitting moist forceps to touch the sterile field when the surface under the absorbent sterile field is unsterile and a barrier drape is not used. A *barrier drape* is resistant to moisture (eg, blood and antiseptics) and should be used whenever a procedure involves the use of liquids. *Made of chemically treated cotton or synthetic materials, barrier drapes prevent a sterile field from becoming unsterile when the drape becomes wet. It is known that a sterile cloth becomes unsterile when dampened (even with sterile water) if it is on an unsterile surface or has contact with any unsterile object. Microorganisms can move through a damp sterile cloth from an unsterile surface, contaminating the field. If the underlying surface is sterile (eg, a plastic container), the field will not become unsterile when moist.*

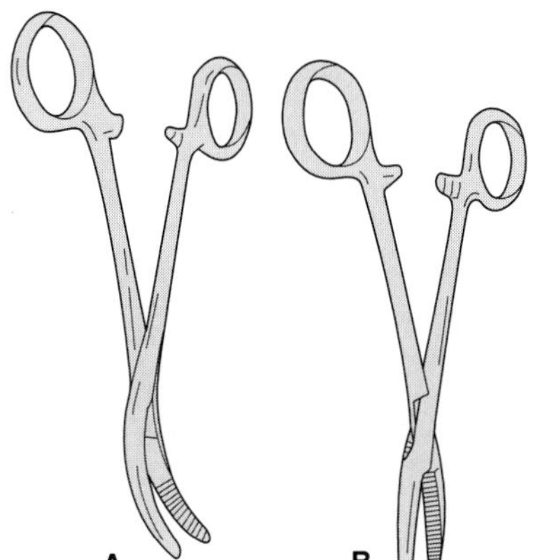

Figure 27–23 Hemostats: *A,* curved; *B,* straight.

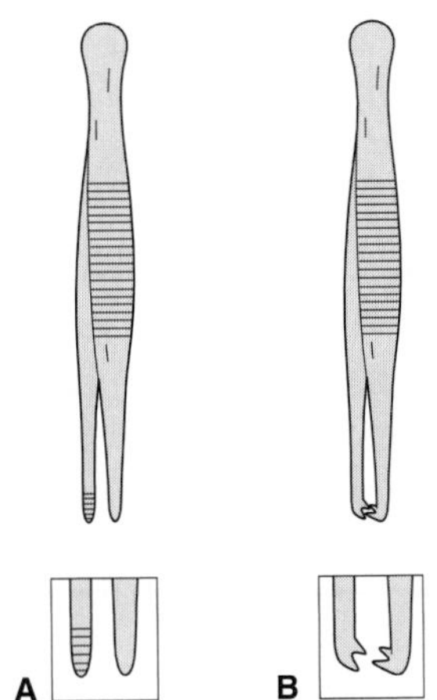

Figure 27–24 Tissue forceps: *A,* plain; *B,* toothed.

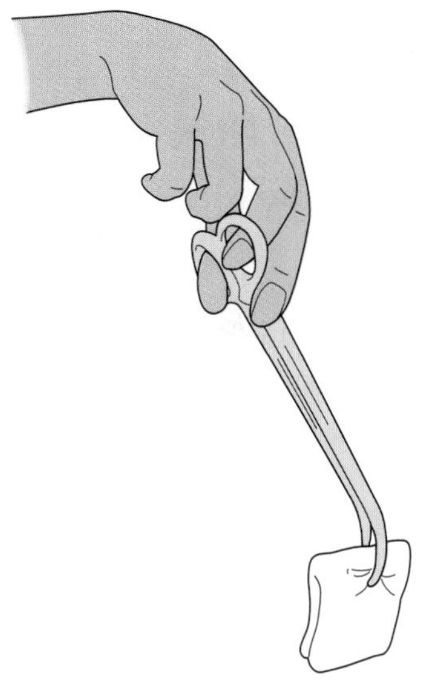

Figure 27–25 Holding forceps with an ungloved hand, keeping the tips lower than the handles.

STERILE GLOVES

Sterile gloves may be donned by the open method or the closed method. The open method is most frequently used outside the operating room, since the closed method requires that the nurse wear a sterile gown. Gloves are worn during many sterile procedures to maintain the sterility of equipment and protect a client's open wound.

Sterile gloves are packaged with a cuff often about 5 cm (2 in) and with the palms facing upward when the package is opened. The package usually indicates the size of the glove (eg, size 6 or 7½). Gloves may or may not be used with sterile forceps. For example, when inserting a catheter, the nurse generally wears gloves and uses sterile forceps; when changing a dressing, the nurse uses sterile forceps but may not wear gloves.

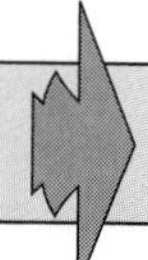

Latex and vinyl gloves are available to protect the nurse from contact with blood and body fluids. *Latex* is more flexible than vinyl, molds to the wearer's hands, allows freedom of movement, and has the added feature of resealing tiny punctures automatically. Korniewicz et al (1991, p. 39) recommend that nurses wear latex gloves when performing tasks (a) that demand flexibility; (b) that place stress on the material (eg, turning stopcocks, handling sharp instruments or tape); and (c) that involve a high risk of exposure to pathogens (eg, in intensive care units, the operating room, labor and delivery areas, infectious disease units, and emergency departments). *Vinyl* gloves should be chosen for tasks unlikely to stress the glove material, requiring minimal precision, and with minimal risk of exposure to pathogens (eg, in ambulatory care settings, postoperative eye surgery units, and outpatient psychiatric units).

Procedure 27–3 describes how to don and remove sterile gloves by the open method.

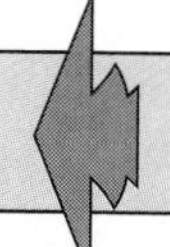

PROCEDURE 27–3 DONNING AND REMOVING STERILE GLOVES (OPEN METHOD)

PURPOSES

- To enable the nurse to handle sterile objects freely
- To prevent clients at risk (eg, those with open wounds) from becoming infected by microorganisms on the nurse's hands

EQUIPMENT

☐ Package of sterile gloves

INTERVENTION

1. Open the package of sterile gloves.

- Place the package of gloves on a clean dry surface. *Any moisture on the surface could contaminate the gloves.*
- Some gloves are packed in an inner as well as an outer package. Open the outer package without contaminating the gloves or the inner package. See Procedure 27–2.
- Remove the inner package from the outer package.
- Open the inner package as above or according to the manufacturer's directions. Some manufacturers provide a numbered sequence for opening the flaps and folded tabs to grasp for opening the flaps. If no tabs are provided, pluck the flap so that the fingers do not touch the inner surfaces. *The inner surfaces, which are next to the sterile gloves, will remain sterile.*

2. Put the first glove on the dominant hand.

- If the gloves are packaged so that they lie side by side, grasp the glove for the dominant hand by its cuff (on the palmar side) with the thumb and first finger of the nondominant hand. Touch only the inside of the cuff (Figure 27–26). *The hands are not sterile. By touching only the inside of the glove, the nurse avoids contaminating the outside.*
  or
  If the gloves are packaged one on top of the other, grasp the cuff of the top glove as above, using the opposite hand.

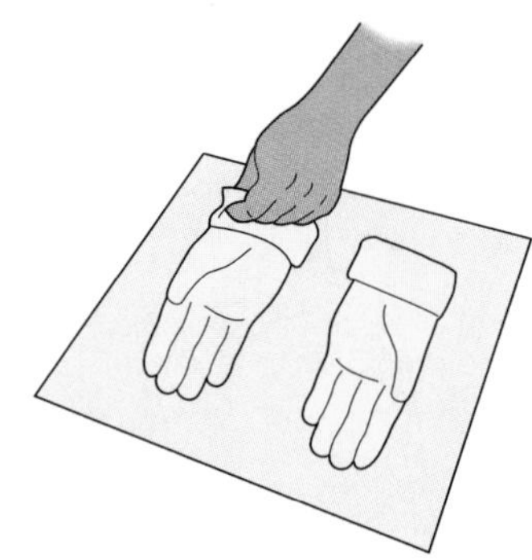

Figure 27–26 Picking up the first sterile glove.

- Insert the dominant hand into the glove and pull the glove on. Keep the thumb of the inserted hand against the palm of the hand during insertion (Figure 27–27). *If the thumb is kept against the palm, it is less likely to contaminate the outside of the glove.*
- Leave the cuff turned down.

PROCEDURE 27–3 *continued*

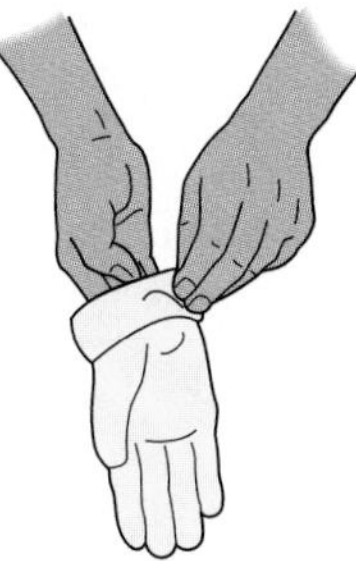

Figure 27–27 Putting on the first sterile glove.

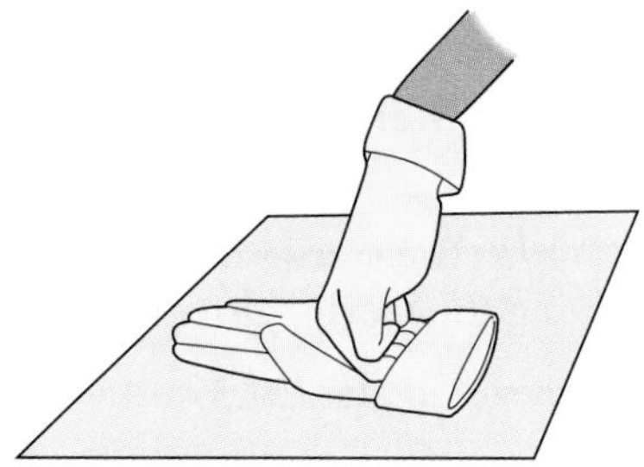

Figure 27–28 Picking up the second sterile glove.

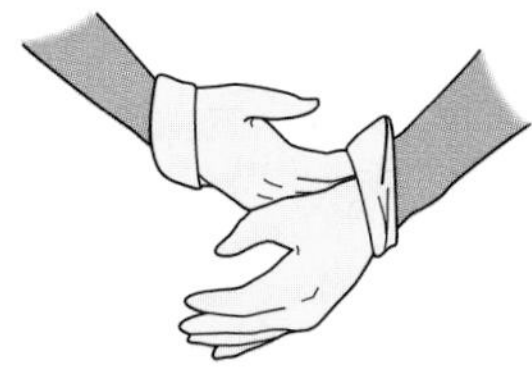

Figure 27–29 Putting on the second sterile glove.

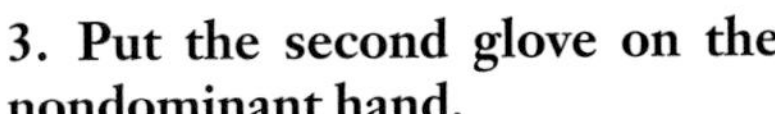

3. Put the second glove on the nondominant hand.

- Pick up the other glove with the sterile gloved hand, inserting the gloved fingers under the cuff and holding the gloved thumb close to the gloved palm (Figure 27–28). *This helps prevent accidental contaminattion of the glove by the bare hand.*
- Pull on the second glove carefully. Hold the thumb of the gloved first hand as far as possible from the palm (Figure 27–29). *In this position, the thumb is less likely to touch the arm and become contaminated.*
- Adjust each glove so that it fits smoothly, and carefully pull the cuffs up by sliding the fingers under the cuffs.

4. Remove and dispose of used gloves.

- There is no special technique for removing sterile gloves. If they are soiled with secretions, remove them by turning them inside out. See removal of disposable gloves, on page 688.

STERILE GOWNS

Sterile gowning and closed gloving are chiefly carried out in operating or delivery rooms, where surgical asepsis is necessary. The closed method of gloving can be used only when a sterile gown is worn because the gloves are handled through the sleeves of the gown. In some agencies, gown and gloves are provided in a single sterile pack; in others, the gloves are provided in a separate package. Prior to these procedures, the nurse dons a hair cover and a mask, and performs a surgical hand wash.

Procedure 27–4 describes the steps in donning a sterile gown and sterile gloves by the closed method.

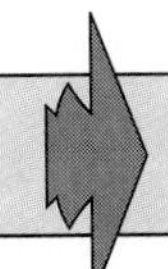

PROCEDURE 27–4 DONNING A STERILE GOWN AND STERILE GLOVES (CLOSED METHOD)

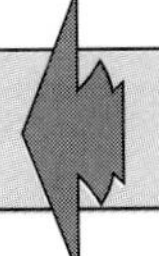

PURPOSES

- To enable the nurse to work close to a sterile field and handle sterile objects freely
- To prevent clients at risk from becoming infected

EQUIPMENT

☐ A sterile pack containing a sterile gown and sterile gloves

PROCEDURE 27-4 DONNING A STERILE GOWN AND STERILE GLOVES *continued*

INTERVENTION

Donning a Sterile Gown

1. Open the sterile pack.

- Remove the outer wrap from the sterile gloves, and drop the gloves in their inner sterile wrap on the sterile field established by the sterile outer wrapper. *If the inner wrapper is not touched, it will remain sterile.* See Procedure 27–2, step 2, page 694.

2. Wash and dry hands carefully.

- See Variation at the end of Procedure 27–1, page 686, and determine agency practice.

3. Put on the sterile gown.

- Grasp the sterile gown at the crease near the neck, hold it away from you, and permit it to unfold freely without touching anything, including the uniform. *The gown will be unsterile if its outer surface touches any unsterile objects.*
- Put the hands inside the shoulders of the gown, and work the arms partway into the sleeves without touching the outside of the gown (Figure 27–30).
- If donning sterile gloves by using the *closed* method (see below), work the hands down the sleeves only to the proximal edge of the cuffs.

  or

  If donning sterile gloves by using the *open* method, work the hands down the sleeves and through the cuffs.
- Have a co-worker wearing a hair cover and mask grasp the neck ties without touching the outside of the gown and pull the gown upward to cover the neckline of your uniform in front and back. The coworker ties the neck ties. Gowning continues at step 7.

Donning Sterile Gloves (Closed Method)

4. Open the sterile wrapper containing the sterile gloves.

- Open the sterile glove wrapper while the hands are still covered by the sleeves (Figure 27–31).

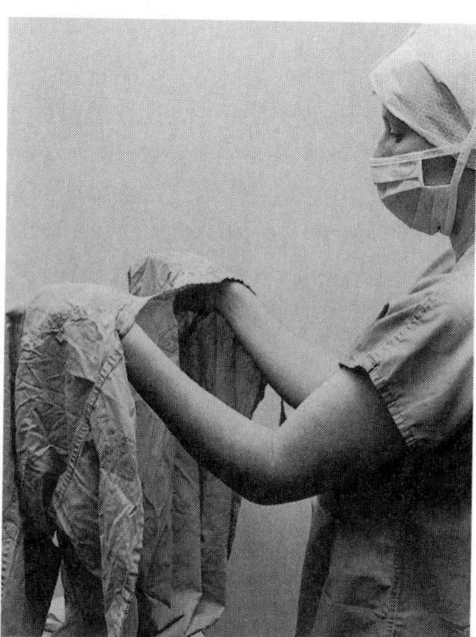

Figure 27–30 Putting on a sterile gown.

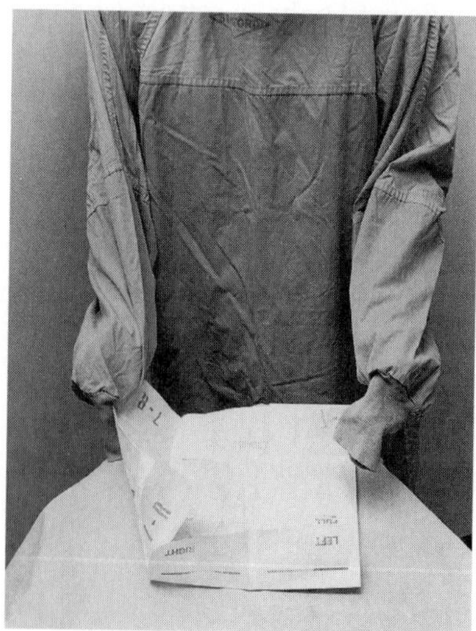

Figure 27–31 Opening the sterile glove wrapper.

5. Put the glove on the nondominant hand. ***In this case, the right hand.***

- With the *dominant* hand, pick up the *opposite* glove with the thumb and index finger, handling it through the sleeve.
- Lay the glove on the opposite gown cuff, thumb side down, with the glove opening pointed toward the fingers (Figure 27–32). Position the nondominant hand palm upward inside the sleeve.

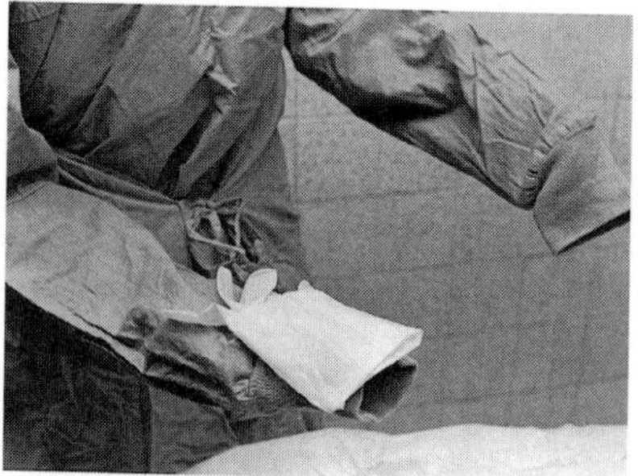

Figure 27–32 Positioning the first sterile glove for the nondominant hand.

- Use the nondominant hand to grasp the cuff of the glove through the gown cuff, and firmly anchor it.
- With the dominant hand working through its sleeve, grasp the upper side of the glove's cuff, and stretch it over the cuff of the gown.
- Pull the sleeve up to draw the cuff over the wrist as you extend the fingers of the nondominant hand into the glove's fingers (Figure 27–33).

6. Put the glove on the dominant hand. ***In this case, the left hand.***

- Place the fingers of the gloved hand under the cuff of the remaining glove.

PROCEDURE 27–4 *continued*

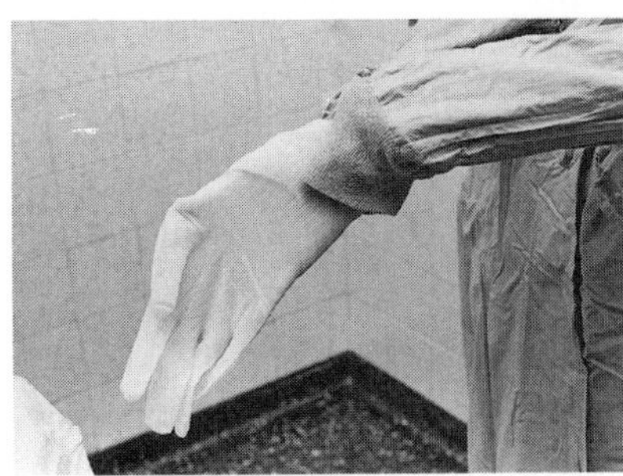

Figure 27–33 Pulling on the first sterile glove.

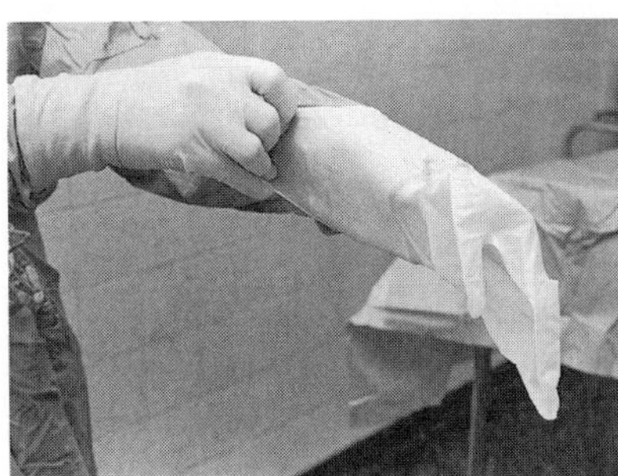

Figure 27–34 Extending the fingers into the second glove of the dominant hand.

- Place the glove over the cuff of the second sleeve.
- Extend the fingers into the glove as you pull the glove up over the cuff (Figure 27–34).

Completion of Gowning

7. Complete gowning as follows.

- Have a co-worker who is masked and whose hair is covered hold the waist tie of your gown, using sterile gloves or a sterile forcep or drape. *This approach keeps the ties sterile.*
- Make a three-quarter turn, then take the tie, and secure it in front of the gown.

or

Have a co-worker wearing sterile gloves take the two ties at each side of the gown and tie them at the back of the gown, making sure that your uniform is completely covered. *Both methods ensure that the back of the gown remains sterile.*

- When worn, sterile gowns should be considered *sterile* in front from the waist to the shoulder. The sleeves should be considered sterile from 2 inches above the elbow to the cuff, since the arms of a scrubbed person must move across a sterile field. Moisture collection and friction areas such as the neckline, shoulders, underarms, back, and sleeve cuffs should be considered unsterile (AORN 1991, p. 482).

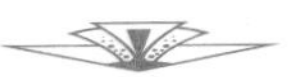

EVALUATING THE EFFECTIVENESS OF PROTECTIVE MEASURES

Using data collected during care—vital signs, breath sounds, skin status, characteristics of urine or other drainage, laboratory blood values, and so on—the nurse judges whether client outcomes have been achieved.

If outcomes are not achieved, the nurse may need to consider questions such as the following:

- Is the client's fluid intake and diet adequate?
- Were appropriate measures implemented to prevent skin breakdown and lung infection?
- Was strict aseptic technique implemented for invasive procedures?
- Are prescribed medications affecting the immune system?
- Is client placement appropriate to reduce the risk of transmission of microorganisms?
- Did the client and visitors misunderstand or fail to comply with necessary instructions?

CHAPTER HIGHLIGHTS

- Microorganisms are everywhere. Most are harmless and some are beneficial; however, many can cause infection in susceptible persons.
- Effective control of infectious disease is an international, national, community, and individual responsibility.
- Asepsis is the freedom from infection or infectious material.
- Medical aseptic practices limit the number, growth, and transmission of microorganisms.
- Surgical aseptic practices keep an area or objects free of all microorganisms.

- An infection can develop if the six links in the chain of infection—infectious agent, reservoir, portal of exit, mode of transmission, portal of entry, and susceptible host—are not interrupted.
- Aseptic practices can be used to break most of the six links in the chain of infection. They do not affect host susceptibility.
- Humans have both nonspecific and specific defenses that combat infectious agents.
- Intact skin and mucous membranes are the body's first line of defense against microorganisms.
- Some normal body flora release bacteriocins and antibiotic-like substances that inhibit microbial growth and destroy foreign bacteria.
- Some body secretions (eg, saliva and tears) contain enzymes that act as antibacterial agents.
- The inflammatory response limits physical, chemical, and microbial injury and promotes repair of injured tissue.
- Immunity is the specific resistance of the body to infectious agents.
- Acquired immunity is active or passive and in either case may be naturally or artificially induced.
- Especially at risk of acquiring an infection are the very young or old; those with poor nutritional status, a deficiency of serum immunoglobulins, multiple stressors, insufficient immunizations, or an existing disease process; and those receiving certain medical therapies.
- The incidence of nosocomial infections is significant. Major sites for these infections are the respiratory and urinary tracts, the bloodstream, and surgical or open wounds.
- Factors that contribute to nosocomial infection risks are invasive procedures, medical therapies, the existence of a large number of susceptible persons, inappropriate use of antibiotics, and insufficient hand washing after client contact and after contact with body substances.
- Preventing infections in healthy or ill persons and preventing the transmission of microorganisms from infected clients to others are major nursing functions.
- The nurse must be knowledgeable about sources and modes of transmission of microorganisms.
- Microorganisms are invisible, and nurses have an ethical obligation to ensure that appropriate aseptic measures are taken to protect clients, support persons, and health personnel, including themselves.

READINGS AND REFERENCES

SUGGESTED READINGS

Bruning, LM. February 1993. The bloodborne pathogens final rule: Understanding the regulation. *AORN Journal* 57:437, 439, 441+.
This article focuses on providing an understanding of the regulations established by the Occupational Safety and Health Administration in 1991.

Korniewicz, DM, Kirwin, M, and Larson, E. June 1991. Do your gloves fit the task? *American Journal of Nursing* 91:38–40.
The authors discuss guidelines for selecting gloves and maximizing the safety and effectiveness of gloves currently in use.

RELATED RESEARCH

Butz, AM, Laughton, BE, Gullette, DL, and Larson, EL. April 1990. Alcohol-impregnated wipes as an alternative in hand hygiene. *American Journal of Infection Control* 18:70–76.

LeClair, SM, Schicker, JM, Duthie, EH, Hoffman, RG, and Franson, TR. August 1988. Survey of nursing personnel attitudes toward infections and their control in the elderly. *American Journal of Infection Control* 16:159–66.

SELECTED REFERENCES

AORN. February 1991. Proposed recommended practices: Aseptic technique. *AORN Journal* 53:480–87.

Benenson, AS, editor. 1990. *Control of Communicable Diseases in Man.* 15th ed. Washington DC: The American Public Health Association.

Brown, BL and Brown, JW. January 1993. OSHA regulations demand strict documentation, compliance. *Provider* 19:37–38.

Bruning, LM. February 1993. The bloodborne pathogens final rule: Understanding the regulation. *AORN Journal* 57:437, 439, 441+.

Carpenito, LJ. 1992. *Nursing Diagnosis: Application to Clinical Practice.* 4th ed. Philadelphia: Lippincott.

Centers for Disease Control. 1987. Recommendations for prevention of HIV transmission in health-care settings. *Morbidity and Mortality Weekly Report* (suppl) 36:3s–18s.

———. June 24, 1988. Recommendations for prevention of HIV transmission in health care settings. *Morbidity and Mortality Weekly Report* 37:1–7.

———. 1994. Guidelines for preventing the transmission of tuberculosis in health care facilities. *Federal Register* 59 (208).

______. 1996. Guideline for isolation precautions in hospitals, Part I: Evolution of isolation practices. *American Journal of Infection Control* 24(1): 24–31.

______. 1996. Guideline for isolation precautions in hospitals, Part II: Recommendations for isolation precautions in hospitals. *American Journal of Infection Control* 24(1): 32–52.

Cox, H, Hinz, M, Lubno, M, Newfield, S. Ridenour, N, Slater, M, and Sridaromont, K. 1993. *Clinical Applications of Nursing Diagnosis: Adult, Child, Women's, Psychiatric, Gerontic, and Home Health Considerations.* 2d ed. Philadelphia: FA Davis.

Doenges, ME, and Moorhouse, MF. 1993. *Nurse's Pocket Guide: Nursing Diagnoses with Interventions.* 4th ed. Philadelphia: FA Davis.

Durham, J and Cohen, F, editors. 1991. *The Person with Aids—Nursing Perspectives.* 2d ed. New York: Springer Publishing.

Gardner, J. October 1993. Guarding your airway against TB. *Nursing93* 23:66.

Garner, JS and Favero, MS. 1985. *Guidelines for Handwashing and Hospital Environmental Control 1985.* Washington, DC: US Government Printing Office.

Garner, JS and Simmons, BP. July/August 1983. CDC guidelines for isolation precautions in hospitals. *Infection Control* (special supplements) 4:245–325.

Gerberding, JL. December 1989. Risks to health care workers from occupational exposure to hepatitis B virus, human immunodeficiency virus, and cytomegalovirus. *Infectious Disease Clinics of North America* 3:735–45.

Gill, J and Slater, J. December 11–17, 1991. Building barriers against infection . . . use of protective clothing. *Nursing Times* 87:53–54.

Groah, L. 1990. *Operating Room Nursing—Perioperative Practice.* Norwalk, CT: Appleton & Lange.

Haiduven, DJ, DeMaio, TM, and Stevens, DA. May 1992. A five-year study of needlestick injuries: Significant reduction associated with communication, education, and convenient placement of sharp containers. *Infection Control and Hospital Epidemiology* 13:265–271.

Horan, TC, Culver, DH, Gaynes, RP, Jarvis, W, Edwards, J, and Reid, C. February 1993. Nosomocomial infections in surgical patients in the United States, January 1986–June 1992. *Infection Control and Hospital Epidemiology* 14:73–80.

Jackson, MM and Lynch, P. February 1984. Infection control: Too much or too little? . . . undiagnosed cases. *American Journal of Nursing* 84: 208–10.

______. July 1991. An attempt to make an issue less murky: A comparison of four systems for infective precautions. *Infection Control and Hospital Epidemiology* 12:448–50.

Jackson, MM, Lynch, P, McPherson, DC, Cummings, MJ, and Greenawalt, NC. September 1987. Why not treat all body substances as infectious? *American Journal of Nursing* 87:1137–39.

Kim, MJ, McFarland, GK, and McLane, AM. 1993. *Pocket Guide to Nursing Diagnoses.* 5th ed. St Louis: Mosby-Year Book.

Kneedler, J and Dodge, G. 1991. *Perioperative Patient Care.* 2d ed. Boston: Jones and Bartlett.

Korniewicz, DM, Kirwin, M, and Larson, E. June 1991. Do your gloves fit the task? *American Journal of Nursing* 91:38–40.

Larson, E. July 1989a. Handwashing: It's essential—even when you use gloves. *American Journal of Nursing* 89:934–39.

______. 1989b. Infection control. In Vol 7, *Annual Review of Nursing Research*, pp. 95–113. New York: Springer.

Lederer, JR, Marculescu, GL, Mocnik, B, and Seaby, N. 1993. *Care Planning Pocket Guide—A Nursing Diagnosis Approach.* 5th ed. Redwood City, CA: Addison-Wesley Nursing.

Lynch, P, Cummings, MJ, Roberts, PL, Herriott, MJ, Yates, B, and Stamm, WE. February 1990. Implementing and evaluating a system of generic infection precautions: Body substance isolation. *American Journal of Infection Control* 18:1–12.

McDonald, L. September 1993. The influence of the Occupational Safety and Health Administration on infection control practice. *Nursing Clinics of North America* 28:613–24.

McFarland, GK and McFarlane, EA. 1993. *Nursing Diagnosis and Intervention: Planning for Patient Care.* 2d ed. St Louis: Mosby.

Mylotte, JM, Niederman, MS, and Summer, WR. February 15, 1993. Staying on top of hospital infections. *Patient Care* 27(3):116–37.

Nicolle, LE. 1992. Urinary tract infection in the elderly: How to treat and when? *Infection* 20:(suppl. 4):S261–65.

North American Nursing Diagnosis Association. 1992. *NANDA Nursing Diagnoses: Definitions and Classifications 1992–1993.* Philadelphia: NANDA.

Norton, CF. 1986. *Microbiology.* 2d ed. Reading, MA: Addison-Wesley.

Pagana, KD and Pagana, TJ. 1992. *Mosby's Diagnostic and Laboratory Test Reference.* St Louis: Mosby-Year Book.

Perceval, A. May 1993. Wash hands, disinfect hands, or don't touch: Which, when, and why? *Infection Control and Hospital Epidemiology* 14:273–75.

Pereira, LJ, Lee, GM, and Wade, KJ. December 1990. The effect of surgical handwashing routines on the microbial counts of operating room nurses. *American Journal of Infection Control* 18:354–70.

Pickering, LK and DuPont, HL. 1986. *Infectious Diseases of Children and Adults: A Step By Step Approach to Diagnosis and Treatment.* Menlo Park, CA: Addison-Wesley Nursing.

Roup, BJ. March 1993. OSHA's new standard: Exposure to bloodborne pathogens. *AAOHN Journal* 41:136–42, 158–60.

Satterfield, N. January 1993. Infection control in long-term care facilities: The hospital-based practitioner's role. *Infection Control and Hospital Epidemiology* 14:40–47.

Simmons, BP. August 1983. CDC guidelines for the prevention and control of nosocomial infections: Guidelines for prevention of surgical wound infections. *American Journal of Infection Control* 11:133–41.

Simmons, B, Bryant, J, Neiman, K, Spencer, L, and Arheart, K. November 1990. The role of handwashing in prevention of endemic intensive care unit infections. *Infection Control and Hospital Epidemiology* 11:589–94.

Turnbull, GB and Balic, A. March 1993. An innovative option to comply with 1992 OSHA guidelines. *Infection Control and Hospital Epidemiology* 14:153–54.

US Department of Health and Human Services, Public Health Service. August 21, 1987. Recommendations for prevention of HIV transmission in health-care settings. *Morbidity and Mortality Weekly Report* 36:2S–17S.

______. June 24, 1988, and June 23, 1989. Update: Universal precautions for prevention of transmission of human immunodeficiency virus, hepatitis B virus, and other blood-borne pathogens in health care settings. *Morbidity and Mortality Weekly Report* 37:377–82, 387–88; 38(S-6):9–18.

______. April 16, 1993. Emerging infectious diseases. *Morbidity and Mortality Weekly Report* 42:257–63.

US Department of Labor, Occupational Safety and Health Administration. December 6, 1991. Occupational exposure to bloodborne pathogens: Final rule. 29 CFR Part 1910.1030. *Federal Register* 56(235):64175–82.

Walker, A and Donaldson, B. January 13–19, 1993. Dressing for protection. *Nursing Times* 89:60–62.

Williams, WW. July/August 1983. CDC guidelines for infection control in hospital personnel. *Infection Control* 4:326–49.

______. February 1984. CDC guidelines for the prevention and control of nosocomial infections: Guidelines for infection control in hospital personnel. *American Journal of Infection Control* 12:34–57.

Wong, DL. 1993. *Whaley and Wong's Essentials of Pediatric Nursing.* 4th ed. St Louis: Mosby.

28 Providing for Safety

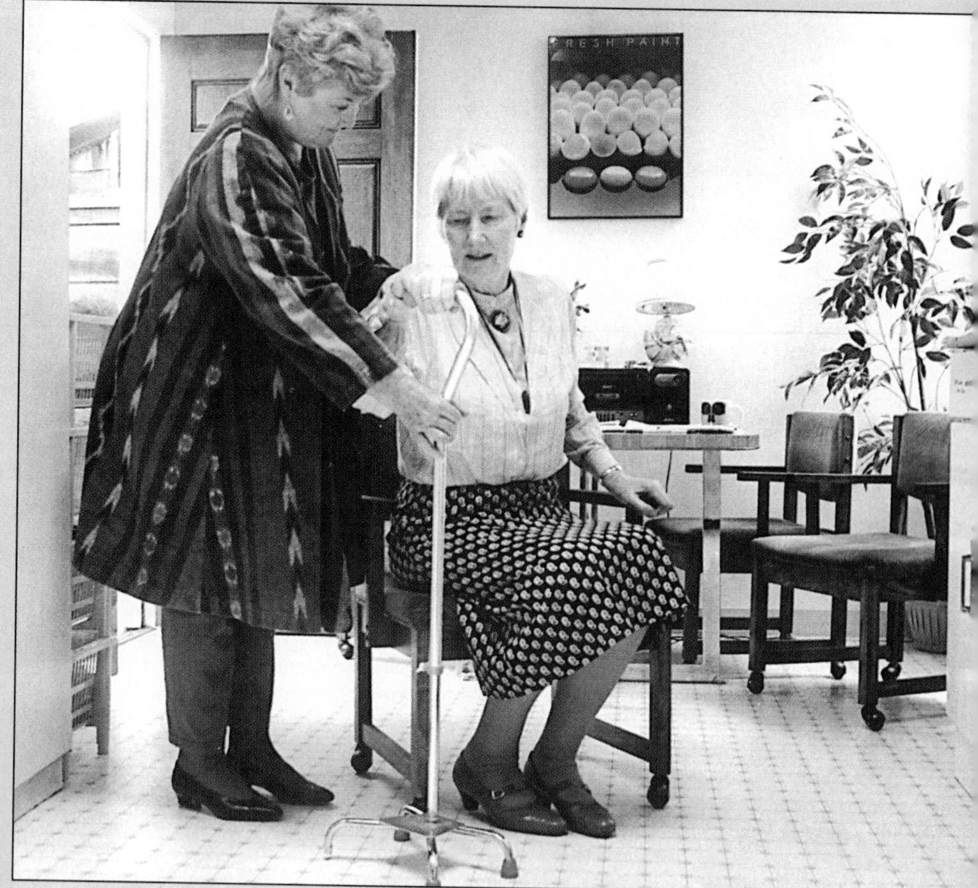

Objectives

- Identify clients at risk of physical injury.
- Identify common hazards in the home.
- Give examples of nursing diagnoses for clients at risk for accidental injury.
- List outcome criteria for evaluating selected strategies for preventing injury.
- Describe nursing responsibilities regarding fires.
- Identify common causes of scalds and burns in home and hospital settings.
- Identify precautions to prevent falls of hospitalized clients.
- Describe legal implications of restraining clients.
- Identify various alternatives to restraints.
- State guidelines for selecting and applying restraints.
- Identify essential precautions to prevent poisoning.
- Identify measures to reduce electrical hazards.
- Describe measures to minimize noise.
- List precautions to prevent exposure to radiation.

People's need for safety is lifelong. The environment contains many hazards, both seen and unseen. The automobile, which may run down a pedestrian, is an obvious hazard. Microorganisms and radiation are unseen hazards.

The need for a safe environment is a national, community, and individual concern. Nurses are voicing their thoughts individually and collectively about such issues as air and water pollution and the safety of foods, cosmetics, and medications. The need for safety on the highways is underscored by newspaper reports of morbidity and mortality from automobile accidents. Increasingly, governments are being pressed to take action and legislate in these areas to make the environment safer. In addition, people are also becoming aware of safety hazards in their communities. Regulations to control the speed of boats on lakes used for swimming, local ordinances curbing the burning of refuse, and stricter local regulation of industrial pollution are all indications of increasing awareness of the need for safety in the environment.

Traditionally, nurses have thought of safety in relation to a client's immediate environment, and this awareness is no less important today in spite of the broader focus on human protection. A primary concern of nurses is awareness of what constitutes a safe environment for a particular person and how this environment can be achieved. The blind person may need railings; the crawling baby, a protective gate at the head of the stairs; and the elderly person, secure footing and an uncluttered floor. Nurses thus focus attention on preventing accidents and injury as well as on assisting the injured.

Accidents are a leading cause of death. In the United States, the causes of accidental death, in order of occurrence, are motor vehicle accidents, falls, drowning, fire and burns, poisoning, inhalation and ingestion of foreign objects, and firearm use. (US Department of Commerce, 1990)

SPECIFIC HAZARDS TO SAFETY

Fire Fire is a constant danger in homes and hospitals. Common causes of hospital fires are smoking in bed and faulty electrical equipment. Hospital fires are particularly hazardous to clients who are incapacitated and unable to leave the building without assistance. Many health care agencies have therefore instituted no-smoking policies to decrease the chances of fire as well as to promote employee health.

A fire can burn only if three elements are present: sufficient heat to start the fire, a combustible material, and sufficient oxygen to support the fire. To prevent fires, the nurse controls the environment to ensure that the three essential elements are not simultaneously present.

Nurses need to become familiar with the fire-prevention practices of their employing agency. When a fire occurs, the nurse has two major goals:

1. To protect clients from injury
2. To contain and put out the fire

Scalds and Burns A **scald** is a burn from a hot liquid or vapor, such as steam. A **burn** results from excessive exposure to thermal, chemical, electrical, or radioactive agents.

Common home hazards causing scalds include the following:

- Pot handles that protrude over the edge of a stove
- Electrical appliances used to heat liquids or oils, especially those with dangling cords that are within reach of crawling infants and young children
- Excessively hot bath water

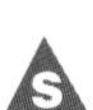

In health care agencies, the risk of scalds and burns is greater for clients whose skin sensitivity to temperature is impaired. Scalds can occur from overly hot bath water or from overly hot moist dressings. Heat lamps can cause burns. (The therapeutic application of heat is discussed in Chapter 44.) It is important for the nurse to assess how well clients can protect themselves and what special precautions, if any, need to be taken.

Falls People of any age can fall, but infants and the elderly are particularly prone to falling and incurring serious injury. See the box on page 710.

Many falls are caused by clutter and wet spots on floors, equipment crowded around beds or chairs, and furniture or equipment obstructing access to bed, chairs, bathrooms, or railings in corridors. Overbed tables, bedside stands, and call lights placed out of reach frequently lead to falls. An ordered and uncluttered environment in which objects are placed within reach are thus essential to safety.

The adequacy of lighting is another factor contributing to falls. Dimness or glare can impair sight and thus be a safety hazard. In an adequately lighted environment, both dimness and glare are absent, as are deep shadows.

Night lights, for example, help prevent falls, allowing people to walk to the bathroom safely, especially in unfamiliar surroundings. Night lights should light walkways, yet not shine in sleepers' eyes.

SELECTED POISONOUS PLANTS*

Avocado (leaves)	Morning glory
Azaleas	Mushrooms (some varieties)
Boston Ivy	Narcissus
Buttercups	Oleander
Cherries (pits)	Philodendron
Crocus, autumn	Poison hemlock
Daffodil	Poison ivy
English ivy	Poison oak
Foxglove	Poppy (California poppy excepted)
Holly berries	Potato (sprouts)
Horsetail reed	Rhododendron
Hyacinth	Rhubarb (leaves)
Hydrangea	Tobacco
Iris	Tomato (except fruit)
Ivy (Boston, English, and others)	Tulip
Larkspur	Wisteria
Lily-of-the-valley	Yew berries
Lobelia	
Mistletoe	

* These plants are considered poisonous and possibly dangerous. They contain a wide variety of poisons, and symptoms of ingestion may vary from a mild stomachache, skin rash, and swelling of the mouth and throat to involvement of the heart, kidneys, or other organs. Many plants are not toxic unless ingested in very large amounts.

Poisoning A **poison** is any substance that injures or kills through its chemical action when inhaled, injected, applied, or absorbed in relatively small amounts. For certain poisons, specific antidotes or treatments are available; for many, there is no specific therapy.

In response to the ever-increasing number of poison hazards, many countries have established poison centers. The American and Canadian Association of Poison Control Centers is a network of poison control centers and concerned individuals, who work together and with government and industry to make life safer from the hazards of poisons. Poison control centers provide accurate, up-to-date information about potential hazards and recommend treatment as needed. Selected poisonous plants are shown in the box above. Additional information is available from poison control centers.

The major reasons for poisoning in children are inadequate supervision and improper storage of many household toxic substances (over 500 in the average home). Adolescent and adult poisonings are usually caused by insect or snake bites and drugs used for recreation or in suicide attempts. Poisoning in elderly people usually results from accidental ingestion of a toxic substance (eg, due to failing eyesight) or an overdose of a prescribed medication (eg, due to impaired memory).

CLIENT TEACHING

Preventing Poisoning

- Place potentially toxic agents, including drugs and cleaning agents, out of reach of crawling infants.
- Lock cleaning agents in a cupboard, or attach special plastic hooks to the inside of cabinet doors to keep them securely closed. Unlatching these hooks requires firmer thumb pressure than small children can usually exert.
- Avoid storing toxic liquids or solids in food containers, such as soft drink bottles, peanut butter jars, or milk cartons.
- Do not remove container labels or reuse empty containers to store different substances. Laws mandate that the labels of all poisons specify antidotes.
- Keep poisonous house plants out of reach of young children. Be able to identify the poisonous plants in your neighborhood.
- Do not rely on cooking to destroy toxic chemicals in plants. Never use anything prepared from nature as a medicine or "tea."
- Teach children never to eat any part of an unknown plant or mushroom and not to put leaves, stems, bark, seeds, nuts, or berries from any plant into their mouths.
- Place poison warning stickers designed for children on containers of bleach, lye, kerosene, solvent, and other toxic substances.
- Do not take medications in front of children. They may imitate you.
- Never call medicine candy when giving medications to children.
- Read and follow label directions on all products before using them.
- Keep syrup of ipecac on hand at all times. Syrup of ipecac is a nonprescription emetic available in single-dose 15-mL vials in all drugstores. Use it only after advice from the local poison control center or the family physician.
- Display the phone number of the poison control center near or on all telephones in the home so that it is available to baby-sitters, family, and friends.

Nurses can intervene by educating the public about what to do in the event of poisoning: Identify the specific poison by searching for an opened container, empty bottle, or other evidence. Contact the poison control center, indicate the exact quantity of poison the person ingested, and state the person's age and apparent symptoms. Keep the person as quiet as possible on one side or with head placed between the legs to prevent aspiration of vomitus.

The box above provides additional guidelines in teaching clients to prevent poisoning.

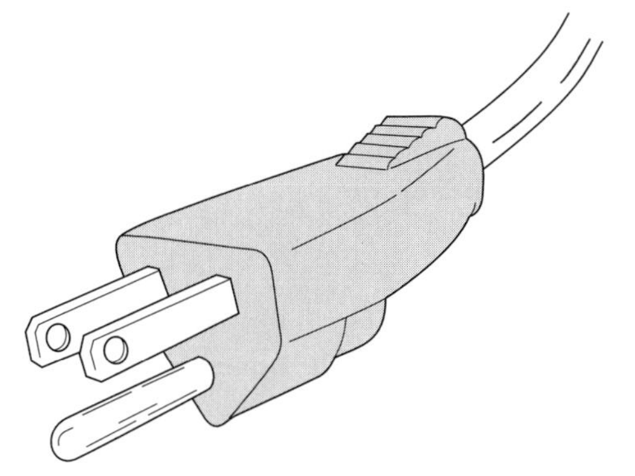

Figure 28–1 Three-pronged grounded plug.

CLIENT TEACHING

Reducing Electrical Hazards

- Check cords for fraying or other signs of damage before using an appliance. Do not use if damage is apparent.
- Avoid overloading outlets and fuse boxes with too many appliances.
- Use only grounded outlets and plugs.
- Always pull a plug from the wall outlet by firmly grasping the plug and pulling it straight out. Pulling a plug by its cord can damage the cord and plug unit.
- Never use electrical appliances near sinks, bathtubs, showers, or other wet areas since water readily conducts electricity.
- Keep electrical cords and appliances out of the reach of young children.
- Place protective covers over wall outlets to protect young children.
- Have all noninsulated wiring in the home altered to meet safety standards.
- Carefully read instructions before operating electrical equipment. Clients who do not understand how to operate the equipment should seek advice.
- Always disconnect appliances before cleaning or repairing them.
- Unplug any appliance that has given a tingling sensation or shock and have an electrician evaluate it for stray current.
- Keep electrical cords coiled or taped to the ground away from areas of traffic to prevent others from damaging the cord or tripping over it.

Electric Shock Nurses need to use electrical equipment that is properly **grounded** (that transmits an electric current from an object or surface to the ground). The electrical plug of grounded equipment has three prongs. The two short prongs transmit the power to the equipment. The third, longer prong is the grounding device, which carries short circuits or stray electric current to the ground (Figure 28–1). Grounding prongs offer a path of least resistance to stray electric currents.

Faulty equipment (eg, equipment with a frayed cord) presents a danger of electric shock or may start a fire. For example, an electric spark near certain anesthetic gases or a high concentration of oxygen can cause a serious fire.

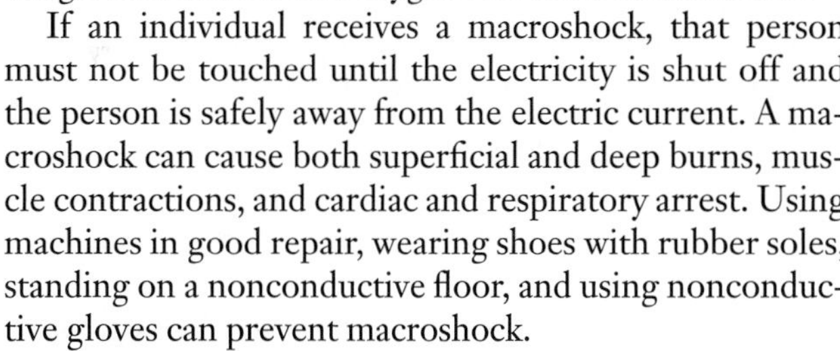

If an individual receives a macroshock, that person must not be touched until the electricity is shut off and the person is safely away from the electric current. A macroshock can cause both superficial and deep burns, muscle contractions, and cardiac and respiratory arrest. Using machines in good repair, wearing shoes with rubber soles, standing on a nonconductive floor, and using nonconductive gloves can prevent macroshock.

To prevent explosions caused by the buildup of static electricity in operating rooms, surgery personnel do not use nylon, Dacron, or other materials that tend to build up static charges. Also, the air is humidified, and antistatic sprays are used in such areas. Actions to reduce electrical hazards are described in the box at the right.

Excessive Noise Excessive noise is a health hazard that can cause hearing loss, depending on (a) the overall level of noise, (b) the frequency range of the noise, and (c) the duration of exposure and individual susceptibility. Sound levels above 120 decibels (units of loudness) are painful and may cause hearing damage even if a person is exposed for only a short period. Exposure to 85 to 95 decibels for several hours a day can lead to progressive or permanent hearing loss. Noise levels below 85 decibels usually do not affect hearing.

Tolerance of noise is largely individual. The rural dweller may find the city noisy, whereas the city dweller may be oblivious to urban sounds. Adults often find teenager's music uncomfortably loud. Noise has psychosocial effects, such as feelings of annoyance, disrupted sleep and relaxation, and interruption of thought and conversation patterns. Noise can also interfere with job performance and safety.

The ill and injured are frequently sensitive to noises that normally would not disturb them. Loud voices, the clatter of dishes, and even a nearby television can disturb clients, some of whom react angrily. Physiologic effects of noise include (a) increased heart and respiratory rates, (b) increased muscular activity, (c) nausea, and (d) hearing loss, if the noise is sufficiently loud.

Noise can be minimized in several ways. Acoustic tile on ceilings, walls, and floors as well as drapes and carpeting absorb sound. Background music can mask noise and have a calming effect on some people. It is important for nurses to minimize noise in the hospital setting and to encourage clients to protect their hearing as much as possible.

Radiation Radiation as a health hazard is a recent source of concern. Nurses are concerned specifically with those radioactive materials used in diagnostic and therapeutic procedures. Radiation injury can occur from overexposure or from exposure to radiation that treats specific tissues and at the same time injures other tissues.

Radioactive materials are used in diagnostic procedures such as radiography, fluoroscopy, and nuclear medicine. In nuclear medicine, radioactive isotopes that have an affinity for specific tissues are given orally or intravenously. The following are some of the isotopes of the elements used:

- Calcium, which has an affinity for bones
- Iodine, which is attracted to the thyroid gland
- Phosphorus, which is attracted to blood

Radioactive materials are provided in sealed sources and unsealed liquid sources. For example, cobalt implants are sealed; iodine 131 and phosphorus 32 are unsealed liquids. Principles governing the degree of exposure to radiation are as follows:

- The longer the time in the presence of radiation, the greater the exposure.
- The closer a person is to the radioactive source, the greater the exposure.
- The more extensive the use of lead and other radiation shields, the greater the protection against radiation.

Often nurses help care for clients treated or diagnosed with radioactive substances. The client diagnosed through radiography or fluoroscopy generally receives minimal exposure, and few precautions are necessary. The nurse restraining a small child during radiography needs to wear a lead apron. Clients with radioactive implants are a source of radiation to the immediate environment. The nurse who is in close contact with such clients also needs to wear a lead apron.

Nurses must deal safely with radioactive body discharges by wearing gloves and in some instances placing excreta in containers for special disposal. The nurse must wash gloved hands well before and after removing the gloves and place contaminated materials in a special container for disposal.

Hospitals in which radioactive materials are used usually have a radioisotope committee. This committee establishes policies and procedures to be used in the care of clients who receive radioactive materials. Nurses must be cognizant of these policies.

One important aspect of caring for clients receiving radiation treatment is making sure they understand the treatment and the precautions they need to take. Often such clients are restricted to bed or to a confined area to protect others. These clients need emotional support to deal with the precautions and will likely accept treatments and precautions better when they know what will happen, when, and why.

Suffocation or Choking Suffocation, or asphyxiation, is lack of oxygen due to interrupted breathing. Suffocation can occur if the air source is cut off, for example, if the victim is under water or has a plastic bag around the head. Suffocation can also be caused by a foreign body (eg, a piece of food) in the upper respiratory tract that acts as a barrier to the movement of air into and from the lungs. Acute swelling of the pharyngeal tissues can also block the flow of air.

If the victim does not obtain immediate relief, interrupted breathing leads to respiratory and cardiac arrest and subsequent death. However, most incidents of suffocation in the community and hospital are preventable. It is important to educate the public about accident prevention. The following are some aspects of such a prevention program.

1. Encourage people either to lock or to remove doors from old refrigerators, freezers, and so on, so that children cannot trap themselves inside.
2. Teach the public to keep plastic away from infants and young children and to avoid using plastic in cribs.
3. Teach children and adults to take suitable safety precautions, such as wearing life jackets when boating and fishing.
4. Encourage children to learn to swim. Educate adults not to leave young children unsupervised near pools or at beaches.
5. Encourage the use of nonskid surfaces in bathtubs, particularly those used by elderly people.
6. In hospitals, always supervise tub baths for clients at risk, for example, those who have epilepsy, hypertension, or brain tumors.
7. Maintain suction equipment at the bedsides of clients who might choke, such as those who have difficulty swallowing.

If a person begins to suffocate, any obstruction to the air passages must be removed immediately and cardiopulmonary resuscitation (CPR) established if cardiac or respiratory arrest has occurred.

Equipment-Related Accidents As the use of highly complex equipment in the health care setting increases, so does the danger of injury from equipment that does not function well or is incorrectly used. It is important that nurses recognize equipment malfunction and report this to the correct authority. In addition, nurses must learn to use the equipment correctly. Before using unfamiliar equipment on a client, the nurse must obtain information about its use from another health professional.

Procedure-Related Accidents Most procedures carried out by nurses have the potential for error. Whether giving a medication or assisting a client out of bed, nurses should follow safeguards to prevent errors or accidents. Most health care agencies establish protocols that are designed to prevent accidents. When in doubt about a course of action, the nurse should confer with another nurse or consult the appropriate written guidelines before proceeding.

When an accident or error does occur, most agencies require that the incident be reported. The nurse completes the report immediately after notifying the charge nurse and taking whatever action is required to safeguard the client. For additional information about incident reports, see Chapter 12, page 234.

FACTORS AFFECTING SAFETY

The ability of people to protect themselves from injury is affected by a number of factors, such as age, life-style, sensory perception, awareness, mobility, emotional state, ability to communicate, and safety knowledge. Nurses need to assess each of these factors when they plan care or teach clients to protect themselves.

SELECTED SAFETY HAZARDS THROUGHOUT THE LIFE SPAN*

- *Developing fetus:* Exposure to maternal smoking, alcohol consumption, addictive drugs, X rays (first trimester), certain pesticides
- *Newborns and infants:* Falling, suffocation in crib, choking from aspirated milk or ingested objects, burns from both water or spilled hot liquids, automobile accidents, crib or playpen injuries, electric shock, poisoning
- *Toddlers:* Physical trauma from falling, banging into objects, or getting cut by sharp objects; automobile accidents, burns, poisoning, drowning, and electric shock
- *Preschoolers:* Injury from traffic, playground equipment, and other objects; choking, suffocation, and obstruction of airway and ear canal by foreign objects; poisoning; drowning; fire and burns; harm from other people or animals
- *Adolescents:* Vehicle (automobile, bicycle) accidents, recreational accidents, firearms, substance abuse
- *Older adults:* Falling, burns, and pedestrian and automobile accidents

* Preventive measures are discussed in Chapters 24 through 26.

Age Through knowledge and accurate assessment of the environment, people learn to protect themselves from many injuries. Children walking to school learn to stop before crossing the street and wait for oncoming traffic. They also learn not to touch a hot stove. For the very young, learning about the environment is essential. Only through knowledge and experience do children learn what is potentially harmful.

Elderly people also can have special problems protecting themselves from injury. Often the balance of elderly people is impaired by their flexed posture, which places their center of gravity forward. Once balance is lost, it is not readily regained. An elderly person may need to learn to stand up slowly, thus avoiding the fall that can result from a quick, sudden movement. Slowness of movement and diminished sensual acuity also contribute to the likelihood of injury. Elderly persons may neither see nor hear an oncoming car. They may not see a footstool. They may also be unable to pull themselves out of a bathtub safely.

Specific age-related potential hazards and preventive measures are discussed in Chapters 24 through 26. The box at the upper right summarizes selected hazards for each age group.

Life-Style Life-style factors that place people at risk are unsafe work environments, where workers are in danger from machinery, industrial belts and pulleys, and chemicals; residence in neighborhoods with high crime rates; access to guns and ammunition; insufficient income to buy safety equipment or make necessary repairs; and access to illicit drugs, which may also be contaminated by harmful additives. Risk-taking behavior is a factor in accidents. For example, some people disregard safety recommendations by driving automobiles at high speeds and refusing to wear seat belts in automobiles, headgear on motorcycles, or flotation jackets in boats.

Mobility Status Persons who have impaired mobility due to paralysis, muscle weakness, and poor balance or coordination are obviously prone to injury. Clients with spinal cord injury and paralysis of both legs may be unable to move even when they perceive discomfort. Hemiplegic clients or clients with leg casts often have poor balance and fall easily. Clients weakened by illness or surgery are not always fully aware of their condition. It is not uncommon for clients to believe themselves able to walk and fall while trying.

Sensory/Perceptual Alterations Accurate sensory perception of environmental stimuli is vital to safety. People with impaired touch perception, hearing, taste, smell, and vision are highly susceptible to injury. A person who does not see well may trip over a toy or not see a signal cord at a hospital bed unit. Deaf persons do not hear a siren in traffic, and persons with impaired olfactory sense may not smell burning food or escaping gas. Paralysis and other neurologic impairments diminish touch perceptions. A paralyzed person may not feel a burn from a burning hot-water bottle, and a person whose sense of taste is impaired may not detect contaminated food.

Some neurologic diseases cause changes in kinesthetic sense and tactile perceptions. Disease of the inner ear, for example, can cause loss of kinesthetic sense. Spinal cord injuries and cerebrovascular accidents cause paralysis and loss of tactile perception. Certain problems create sensations that do not arise from normal external or internal stimuli. For example, a client who has a disease of the auditory nerve may hear sounds that correspond to no external stimulus. Hallucinations (perceptions of external stimuli in the absence of such stimuli) can result, for example, from a disease process or hallucinogenic drugs. Illusions are misinterpretations of external stimuli. For example, a person may interpret a shadow cast by a lamp as a person.

Level of Awareness Awareness is the ability to perceive environmental stimuli and body reactions and to respond appropriately through thought and action. The normal, alert person assimilates many kinds of information at one time, perceives reality accurately, and acts on those perceptions. Most people do this with little or no awareness of the mental processes involved.

Clients with impaired awareness include persons lacking in sleep, unconscious or semiconscious persons, disoriented persons (ie, those who may not understand where they are or what to do to help themselves), persons who perceive stimuli that do not exist, and persons whose judgment is altered by disease or medications, such as narcotics, tranquilizers, hypnotics, and sedatives.

Mildly confused hospitalized clients may momentarily forget they are not at home, wander from their rooms, misplace personal belongings, and so forth. Severely confused people do not know where they are or what time of day or day of the week it is. Some may not know family members or may think the nurse is a relative. Such persons may act atypically: Confused, usually docile people may become combative with nurses and others.

Emotional State Extreme emotional states can alter the ability to perceive environmental hazards. The acutely anxious or angry person has reduced perceptual awareness. They may become absent-minded or lose their sense of direction. Often these episodes are due to stressful situations that reduce a person's level of concentration, cause errors of judgment, and decrease awareness of external stimuli.

Depressed persons may think and react to environmental stimuli more slowly than usual. People worried about their own or loved ones' illnesses are less aware than usual of potential dangers in the environment, such as a street curb or an oncoming automobile.

Ability to Communicate People with diminished ability to receive and convey information are also at risk for injury. Aphasic clients, people with language barriers, and those unable to read are among them. For example, the person unable to interpret the sign "No smoking—oxygen in use" may cause a fire.

Knowledge of Safety Precautions Information is crucial to safety. Clients in hospitals and other unfamiliar environments frequently need specific safety information. Lack of knowledge about unfamiliar equipment, such as oxygen tanks, intravenous tubing, and hot packs, is a potential hazard. Nurses need to teach clients what safety precautions to take when oxygen is in use and how to maintain intravenous infusions. Healthy clients need knowledge about water safety, car safety, fire prevention, ways to prevent the ingestion of harmful substances, and many preventive measures related to specific age-related hazards.

RISK FACTORS FOR FALLS

- Age greater than 65 years
- Previous history of falls in the home or hospital
- Difficulty walking (altered gait or posture)
- Difficulty getting out of bed or a chair
- Episodes of dizziness or seizures
- Difficulty asking someone for help
- Use of ambulatory devices (cane, crutches, walker, braces, wheelchair)
- Impaired vision or hearing
- Weakness from disease process or therapy
- Altered mental state (confusion/disorientation, impaired memory or judgment, inability to follow directions)
- Current medication regimen that includes sedatives, hypnotics, tranquilizers, analgesics, diuretics, or laxatives

RESEARCH NOTE

A Concise Risk Tool Developed to Prevent Falls

In this study, the authors developed a 26-item risk assessment tool (RAT) for falls. They based this tool on a literature review and an analysis of causative factors of falls that had occurred over a 3-month period at an 1100-bed acute and extended care facility. Results indicated that only *four* variables were statistically related to falls. Specific categories of medications (eg, diuretics, central nervous system suppressants) were *not* statistically related to client falls. It is assessment of the client's response to medications that is most crucial in determining risk for falls.

Based on these findings, the RAT was revised and shortened to four elements, any one of which categorizes the client at risk for falls. It was also renamed the *Reassessment Is Safe "Kare" (RISK) Tool.* These are the four elements:

- Unsteady gait/dizziness/imbalance
- Impaired memory or judgment
- Weakness
- History of falls

In addition, the results revealed that the client who is identified at high risk for falls is at an even greater risk if the client uses a wheelchair.

Implications: Nurses can use this RISK tool to quickly assess clients at risk for falls and to feel assured that essential data has been obtained.

Source: LK Brians, K Alexander, P Grota, RWH Chen, and V Dumas. The development of the RISK tool for fall prevention, *Rehabilitation Nursing*, March/April 1991, 16(2):67–69.

ADULT HOME HAZARD APPRAISAL

Assess the following:

- *Walkways and stairways (inside and outside).* Note uneven sidewalks or paths, broken or loose steps, absence of hand rails or placement on only one side of stairways, insecure hand rails, congested hallways or other traffic areas, and adequacy of lighting at night.
- *Floors.* Note uneven and highly polished or slippery floors and any unanchored rugs or mats.
- *Furniture.* Note hazardous placement of furniture with sharp corners. Note chairs or stools that are too low to get into and out of or that provide inadequate support.
- *Bathroom(s).* Note presence of grab bars around tubs and toilets, nonslip surfaces in tubs and shower stalls, adequacy of night lighting, adequacy of lighting for medicine cabinet, and need for raised toilet seat or bath chair in tub or shower.
- *Kitchen.* Note pilot lights (gas stove) in need of repair, inaccessible storage areas, and hazardous furniture.
- *Bedrooms.* Note adequacy of lighting, in particular the availability of night lights and accessibility of light switches. Assess floors and furniture as above.
- *Electrical.* Note unanchored and/or frayed electrical cords and overloaded outlets or those near water.
- *Fire protection.* Note presence or absence of smoke detectors, fire extinguisher, and fire escape plan, improper storage of combustibles (eg, gasoline) or corrosives (eg, rust remover [phosphoric acid]), and accessibility of emergency telephone numbers (fire, police).
- *Toxic substances.* Note medications kept beyond date of expiration and improperly labeled cleaning solutions.

ASSESSING

Assessing clients at risk for injury involves (a) using specifically developed risk assessment tools and (b) appraising the client's environment to detect potential hazards.

Risk Assessment Tools Many risk assessment tools are available to determine clients at risk for falling. These tools summarize specific data contained in the client's nursing history and physical examination. Essential data are summarized in the box on page 710.

Home Hazard Appraisal Hazards in the home are major causes of falls, fire, poisoning, suffocation, and other accidents, such as those caused by improper use of household equipment (eg, tools and cooking utensils). The appraisal of such hazards is an essential nursing function. See the box at the top of this column for a home hazard appraisal for an adult. See Chapters 24 and 25 for potential hazards and preventive actions for children and adolescents.

NURSING DIAGNOSES

CLIENTS AT RISK FOR INJURY OR ACCIDENTS

NURSING DIAGNOSIS: High risk for injury: The state in which an individual is at risk for injury as a result of environmental conditions interacting with the individual's adaptive and defensive resources

Risk Factors

Perceptual or physiologic deficit (eg, impaired physical mobility, altered thought processes, impaired sensory function); developmental age; lack of awareness of environmental hazards (eg, household, automotive, fire, thermal, chemical hazards); insufficient knowledge of safety precautions; substance abuse (eg, alcohol, drugs); unfamiliar setting

NURSING DIAGNOSIS: High risk for poisoning: The state in which an individual is at accentuated risk of accidental exposure to or ingestion of drugs or dangerous substances in amounts sufficient to cause poisoning

Risk Factors

Individual (internal) factors

Reduced vision; verbalization of occupational setting without adequate safeguards; lack of safety or drug education or precautions; cognitive or emotional difficulties

Environmental (external) factors

Large supplies of drugs in house; medicines stored in unlocked cabinets accessible to children or confused persons; dangerous products placed or stored within reach of children or confused persons; availability of illicit drugs potentially contaminated by poisonous additives; flaking, peeling paint or plaster in presence of young children; chemical contamination of food and water; unprotected contact with heavy metals or chemicals, paint, lacquer, and other toxic substances in poorly ventilated areas or without effective protection; presence of poisonous vegetation; presence of atmospheric pollutants

Sources: LJ Carpenito, *Nursing Diagnosis: Application to Clinical Practice*, 4th ed. (Philadelphia: Lippincott, 1992), pp. 525–53; MJ Kim, GK McFarland, and AM McLane, *Pocket Guide to Nursing Diagnoses*, 5th ed. St Louis: Mosby-Year Book, 1993), pp. 34–35, 43–44, 59; GK McFarland and EA McFarlane, *Nursing Diagnosis and Interventions: Planning for Patient Care* (St Louis: Mosby, 1989), pp. 62–84; North American Nursing

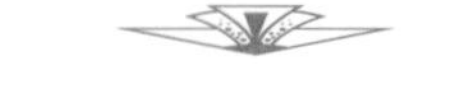

DIAGNOSING

The nursing diagnostic category applicable to clients at risk for physical injury is **High risk for injury**. Four subcategories of this diagnostic label are accepted by NANDA:

- **High risk for poisoning**
- **High risk for suffocation**
- **High risk for trauma**
- **High risk for aspiration** (see Chapter 39)

The etiologies and interventions for poisoning, suffocation, and trauma are included under the broad category **High risk for injury.** However, these subcategory diagnoses may be preferred when the nurse wants to isolate interventions for a specific category, such as poisoning.

The above diagnoses, with definitions, contributing factors, and defining characteristics, are shown in the accompanying box. Note that these diagnoses do not have defining characteristics because they are potential or high-risk diagnoses. Clinical applications of these diagnoses are shown in Table 28–1.

PLANNING

The nurse planning health protective measures must consider the age, knowledge, and sensory deficits of the client. Potential hazards and preventive measures for people of all ages are discussed in Chapters 24, 25, and 26. The nursing care plan should include two aspects: (a) educating clients about preventive actions and (b) modifying the environment to make it safe.

Education is a major factor in preventing accidents. It is directed toward helping people identify potential hazards and changing their health practices and habits accordingly.

NURSING DIAGNOSIS: High risk for suffocation: The state in which an individual is at accentuated risk of accidental suffocation (inadequate air available for inhalation)

Risk Factors

Individual (internal) factors

Reduced olfactory sensation; reduced motor abilities; lack of safety education and/or precautions; cognitive or emotional difficulties; disease or injury process

Environmental (external) factors

Pillow placed in infant's crib; vehicle warming in closed garage; children playing with plastic bags or inserting small objects into their mouths or noses; discarded or unused refrigerators or freezers without doors removed; children left unattended in bathtubs or pools; household gas leaks; smoking in bed; use of fuel-burning heaters not vented to outside; low-strung clothesline; pacifier hung around infant's neck; eating of large mouthfuls of food; propped bottle placed in infant's crib

NURSING DIAGNOSIS: High risk for trauma: The state in which an individual is at accentuated risk for accidental tissue injury (eg, wound, burn, fracture)

Risk Factors

Perceptual or physiologic deficit (eg, impaired physical mobility, altered thought processes, impaired sensory function); developmental age; lack of awareness of environmental hazards (eg, household automotive, fire, thermal, chemical hazards); insufficient knowledge of safety precautions; substance abuse (eg, alcohol, drugs); unfamiliar setting

Diagnosis Association, *NANDA Nursing Diagnoses: Definitions and Classification 1992–1993* (Philadelphia: NANDA, 1992), pp. 28–32; JR Lederer, GL Marculescu, B Mocnik, and N Seaby, *Care Planning Pocket Guide—A Nursing Diagnosis Approach*, 5th ed. (Redwood City, CA: Addison-Wesley Nursing, 1993), pp. 108–9, 146–47, 204.

To provide a safe environment, the nurse and/or client may have to modify the environment. Modification can involve not only arranging the environment but also limiting it in some ways.

Older clients with sensory deficits are particularly susceptible to injury. As a result, they may require assistance from nurses in taking precautions to prevent accidents. A client with loss of vision may require assistance walking. A nurse should stand on the client's nondominant side about one step ahead of the client. A blind person should grasp the nurse's arm with the nondominant arm. In addition, nurses can make the environment safe by

Table 28–1 Clinical Application: Assessment Data Clusters and Related Nursing Diagnoses for Clients at High Risk for Injury

Data Clusters	Nursing Diagnosis
Edith Dalton, an elderly widow, lives alone in her own home. She has a history of glaucoma, for which she takes eye drops twice daily. She reports difficulty in focusing, loss of side vision, and inability to adjust to darkness.	**High risk for injury** related to sensory deficit (impaired visual ability)
David Gagnon suffered a stroke one month ago and has been discharged to his apartment. Home assessment revealed lack of bathroom safety (no grab bars or nonskid shower floor), unanchored rugs, inadequate light at night, and several cluttered traffic areas.	**High risk for injury** related to altered mobility and lack of home safety precautions

CARE PLANNING GUIDE

CLIENTS AT RISK FOR INJURY OR ACCIDENTS

NURSING DIAGNOSIS: High risk for injury from falling

Outcome Criteria	Nursing Interventions	Rationale
The client ▪ Avoids personal injury from falling during hospitalization	Reassess the client for the presence of risk factors biweekly or as the client's condition or therapy indicate (see "Risk Factors for Falls" box on page 710).	Client condition and therapy change continually.
	Document and report risk factors and client susceptibility; put alert signs at the bedside, on the room door, and in the client's record in accordance with agency policy.	All health care professionals involved with the client need to be informed of the client's risk for falls to ensure continuity of care and the client's safety.
	Modify the client's environment to make it safe: ▪ Keep the bed in the low position with side rails up; keep the call light and frequently used articles within reach. ▪ Provide a bedside walker, wheelchair, commode, or even an Ambularm if client is unable to comply with safety precautions.	Modifications alert the client to safety precautions (eg, side rails), provide security or limits to ambulation (eg, walker, Ambularm), enable the client to maintain some independence (eg, articles within reach) and enable the client to seek assistance when needed (eg, call light).
	Monitor the client frequently during the first 3 days of hospitalization (eg, whenever passing the room) and at least every 2 hours during the night.	Frequent supervision reduces client anxiety and unsafe behavior, and prevents the likelihood of falls.
	Teach the client and support persons. ▪ To use the call light to call for assistance. ▪ That side rails are kept up to remind them to obtain assistance in getting out of bed.	Instruction about needed precautions enlists the cooperation of client and support persons in preventing injury.

(a) arranging furniture and other objects so the client will not trip over them and explaining the location of furniture and (b) leaving bedside articles as the client arranges them and within easy reach.

The client whose level of consciousness is altered also requires special protection. Side rails to prevent falls, appropriate positioning in bed, appropriate lighting, and reduced noise level are all common measures nurses employ to ensure client safety. If the client is unconscious, necessary nursing interventions include bathing, giving skin care, feeding, and meeting elimination needs. If the client is disoriented but conscious, the nurse may need to give instructions on how to perform these activities. Unless the person is totally incapacitated, nurses should foster independence and feelings of self-worth by helping the individuals care for themselves.

Planning also involves the development of outcome criteria to evaluate the effectiveness of nursing interventions.

The major outcome is to prevent injury by helping the client to identify hazards and to take related safety measures. Specific outcome criteria follow. See also the accompanying Care Planning Guide for clients at high risk for injury.

NURSING DIAGNOSIS: High risk for injury from falling *continued*

Outcome Criteria	Nursing Interventions	Rationale
	▪ To wear rubber- or crepe-soled shoes. ▪ That the hospital may seem unfamiliar at night and that they should use a night light. ▪ That medications, preparations for diagnostic tests, or surgery may cause drowsiness and/or weakness.	

NURSING DIAGNOSIS: High risk for poisoining (of children)

Outcome Criteria	Nursing Interventions	Rationale
The parent		
▪ Identifies potential hazards.	Determine parent's present level of knowledge about poison hazards and safety precautions indicated.	This enables the nurse to identify misinformation and to focus on information the client requires.
	Instruct parents about potential hazards (eg, medicines and dangerous products within reach of children, flaking paint, poisonous vegetation).	Awareness of potential hazards promotes safety-conscious behavior.
▪ Verbalizes understanding of essential safety precautions.	See Client Teaching box on page 706.	Instruction about necessary precautions alerts parents to essential practices that will prevent accidental ingestion of poisonous substances.
▪ Reports satisfaction with changes made to home environment; reports responses of child to instruction.	Explore parent's feelings about home modifications and behavior of the child.	Dissatisfaction or unresolved problems require additional nursing interventions.

The client

- Remains free of or avoids personal injury
  a. During hospitalization.
  b. In the home setting.
- Identifies environmental hazards that increase the potential for injury (trauma, poisoning, suffocation).
- Identifies preventive measures for specific hazards (eg, falls, fire, electric shock, poisoning, burns, suffocation).
- Reports use of appropriate countermeasures to protect self from injury (trauma, poisoning, suffocation).
- Alters physical environment as indicated to reduce the risk of injury.
- Seeks instruction to implement safe child-rearing practices.

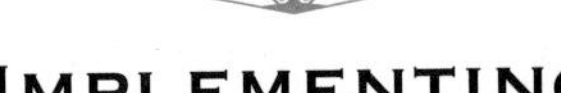

IMPLEMENTING

Providing measures to ensure safety is one important aspect of planning nursing care. Teaching about safety is

FIRE PROTECTION PRACTICES IN HEALTH CARE AGENCIES

- Telephone numbers of emergency services are displayed on all telephones.
- Personnel know the location of fire exits.
- Personnel know the location and types of fire extinguishers and how to operate them.
- Fire drill or fire evacuation procedure is in place.
- Hallways remain free of unnecessary furniture and equipment.
- Signs are posted on elevator doors regarding the use of stairs in the event of fire.
- Location of fire exits is clearly marked.

another important aspect, and nurses usually have opportunities to teach while providing client care.

Table 28–2 Types of Fire Extinguishers and Indications for Use

Type of Extinguisher	Class of Fire*	Precautions/Comments
Water pump	A	Do not use on electrical or flammable liquid fires (eg, grease); water conducts electricity and causes grease to splatter, thus spreading the fire.
Carbon dioxide (CO_2)	B and C	Because it has a limited range, the extinguisher must be used close to the flames. Used for small surface fires only.
Dry chemical	B and C	Causes grease to splatter. Used for small surface fires only.
Multipurpose	A, B, and C	Good anywhere in the home because they put out most types of fires.
Foam	B	For home use this type of extinguisher could be placed in a garage or basement.
Special dry powder	D	Dry powders absorb heat. Use only for designated metals.

* Class A: Paper, wood, upholstery, rags, ordinary rubbish
Class B: Flammable liquids and gases
Class C: Electrical
Class D: Designated metals

MAINTAINING FIRE SAFETY

Fires are always a possibility in health care agencies and hospitals. Agency fires have usually resulted from smoking in bed, malfunctioning electrical equipment, or combustion of anesthetic gas. In the home, fires most frequently result from careless disposal of burning cigarettes, from grease, or from faulty electrical wiring of appliances.

Health Care Agency Agencies usually provide orientations regarding fire prevention. These orientations alert personnel to many of the practices listed in the box above. Agency protocols to follow in case of fire usually include many of the following:

- Evacuate clients who are in immediate danger. First, direct ambulatory clients to a safe area, or enlist their help in moving clients in wheelchairs. This clears the area for the evacuation of nonambulatory clients, who can be moved in a stretcher or bed, carried, or dragged on sheets and blankets.
- Activate the fire alarm if one is nearby.
- Notify the hospital switchboard of the location of the fire.
- If the fire is small, use the fire extinguisher on the fire.
- Close windows and doors in the area of the fire to reduce ventilation.
- Turn off oxygen and any electrical appliances in the vicinity of the fire.
- Clear fire exits, if necessary.
- Contain smoke as necessary by placing damp cloths or blankets around the outside edges of doors.
- Protect clients from smoke inhalation by giving them wet washcloths through which to breathe.

Containing the Fire Fires are categorized into four classes according to the type of material burning. Several types of fire extinguishers are in use today. The right type of extinguisher must be used to fight a fire. See Table 28–2 for various types of extinguishers and indications for their use. Fire extinguishers are now commonly labeled with picture symbols showing which fires they should and should not be used on. Directions for use are also attached to the extinguisher.

Home Health teaching regarding fires in the home stresses prevention as well as what to do when a fire occurs. Preventive measures include the following:

- Keep emergency numbers near the telephone.
- Be aware of the nearest exits from different locations in the home.
- Use a fire extinguisher if one is available, and keep extinguishers in good working order.
- Close windows and doors.
- Use stairs instead of an elevator.

PREVENTING FALLS

The chief causes of falls in a home include poor lighting, slippery floors, and poorly fitted slippers or clothing. Falls commonly occur in bathrooms, in kitchens, and on stairs.

Installing hand rails on bath tubs helps reduce the incidence of slipping and may be particularly advisable for the elderly. In health care agencies, side rails on beds and stretchers help prevent clients, particularly those who are disoriented, unconscious, or confused, from rolling off.

Other methods for preventing falls in hospitals are provided in the accompanying box. Some agencies have their own protocols for preventing falls. Procedure 28–1 describes how to use the Ambularm safety monitoring device.

RESTRAINING CLIENTS

Restraints are protective devices used to limit the physical activity of the client or a part of the body.

Restraints can be classified as physical or chemical. *Physical restraints* are any manual method or physical or mechanical device, material, or equipment attached to the client's body; they cannot be removed easily and they restrict the client's movement. *Chemical restraints* are medications such as neuroleptics, anxiolytics, sedatives, and

CLINICAL GUIDELINES

Preventing Falls in Hospitals

- Orient clients on admission to their surroundings, and explain the call system.
- Carefully assess the client's ability to ambulate and transfer; provide walking aids and assistance as required.
- Closely supervise clients at risk for falls during the first few days, especially at night.
- Encourage the client to use call bell to request assistance; ensure that the bell is within easy reach.
- Place bedside tables and overbed tables near the bed or chair so that clients do not overreach and consequently lose their balance.
- Always keep hospital beds in the low position when not providing care so that clients can move in or out of bed easily.
- Encourage clients to use grab bars mounted in toilet and bathing areas and railings along corridors.
- Make sure nonskid bath mats are available in tubs and showers.
- Encourage the client to wear nonskid footwear.
- Keep the environment tidy; especially keep light cords from underfoot and furniture out of the way.
- Reduce poor lighting and glare, which causes clients to squint.
- Attach side rails to the beds of confused, sedated, restless, and unconscious clients, and keep the rails in place when the client is unattended. See also stretcher precautions in Chapter 34.

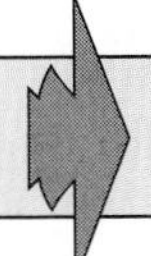

PROCEDURE 28–1 USING AN AMBULARM SAFETY MONITORING DEVICE

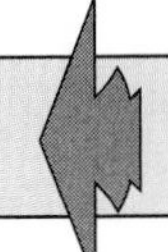

The Ambularm is an electronic device with a position-sensitive switch that triggers an audio alarm when the client attempts to get out of bed unassisted. When activated, the alarm alerts the nurse and provides an opportunity for the nurse to intervene.

PURPOSES

- To alert the nurse that the client is attempting to get out of bed
- To help decrease the risk of client falls

ASSESSMENT FOCUS

Mobility status; judgment about ability to get out of bed safely; skin integrity of leg to which band is applied; vascular status of leg; proximity of client's room to nurses' station; position of side rails and functioning status of call light.

EQUIPMENT

- ☐ Alarm device
- ☐ Leg band of appropriate size
- ☐ Ambularm sticker

PROCEDURE 28–1 USING AN AMBULARM SAFETY MONITORING DEVICE *continued*

INTERVENTION

1. Explain to client and support persons the purpose and procedure for using safety monitoring.

- Explain that the device does not limit mobility in any manner; rather, it alerts the staff when the client is about to get out of bed.
- Explain that the nurse must be called when the client needs to get out of bed.

2. Measure for proper size of leg band. Measure thigh circumference just above the knee with the tape measure:

- For a thigh circumference of up to 18 inches, use a regular sized band.
- For a thigh circumference of 18 inches or larger, use a large sized band.

3. Test the battery device and alarm sound. Touch alarm snaps on the Ambularm device to the corresponding snaps on the leg band (Figure 28–2). *This ensures that the device is functioning properly prior to use.*

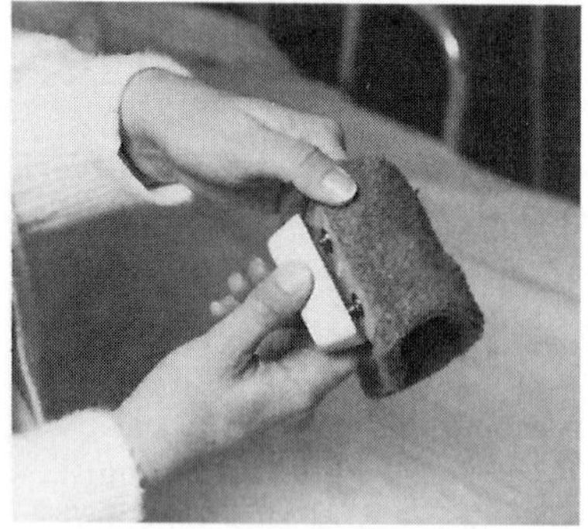

Figure 28–2 Testing an Ambularm by contacting corresponding snaps on the leg band.

4. Apply the Ambularm.

- Place the leg band just above the knee (Figure 28–3).

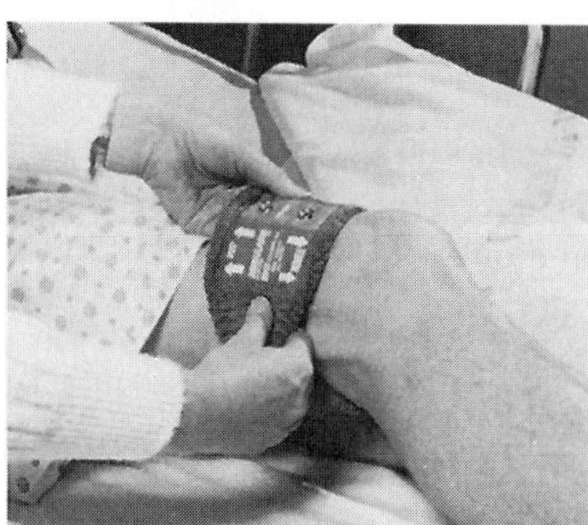

Figure 28–3 Placing the leg band around the leg just above the knee.

- Securely snap the Ambularm onto the leg band at the corresponding snap junctions (Figure 28–4). *This activates the position-sensitive alarm device.*

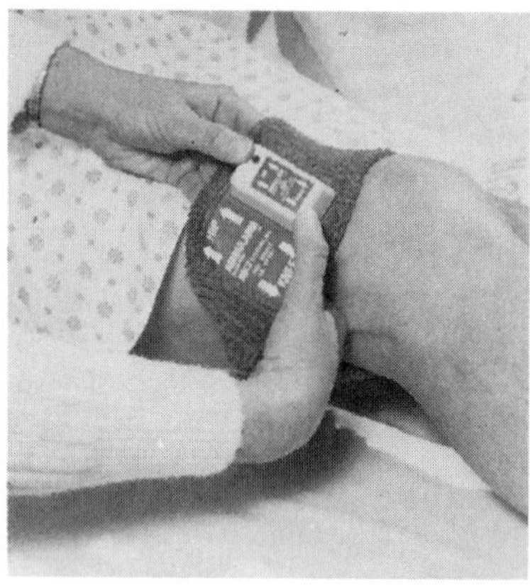

Figure 28–4 Attaching the Ambularm to the leg band.

- Place the client's leg in a straight horizontal position. *The alarm device is position-sensitive; that is, when it approaches a near-vertical position (such as in walking, crawling, or kneeling as the client attempts to get out of bed), the audio alarm is triggered, causing a sharp, shrill sound* (Figure 28–5).

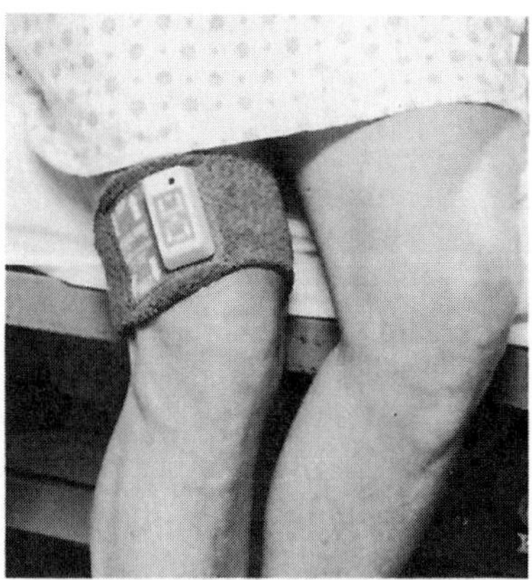

Figure 28–5 Triggering of the alarm when the leg is in a near-vertical position.

5. Instruct the client to call the nurse when the client wants or needs to get up, and assist as required.

- When assisting the client to rise, deactivate the alarm by unsnapping the alarm device from the elastic band (Figure 28–6).

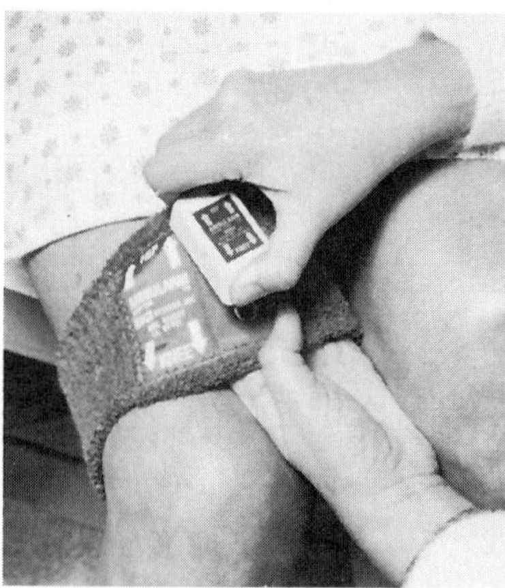

Figure 28–6 Detaching the Ambularm from the leg band.

- Assist the client back to bed, and reattach the alarm device to the leg band.

PROCEDURE 28–1 *continued*

6. Ensure client safety with additional safety precautions.

- Place call light within client reach, lift all side rails, and lower the bed to its lowest position. *The alarm device is not a substitute for other precautionary measures.*
- Periodically assess the skin and vascular status of leg being used.
- Place ambulation monitoring stickers on the client's door, chart, and Kardex.

7. Document relevant data.

- Record that ambulation device is intact when applied.
- Record all assessments.
- Record all safety precautions and interventions discussed and employed.

EVALUATION FOCUS
Status of the Ambularm device; effectiveness of safety precautions.

ALTERNATIVES TO RESTRAINTS

- Assign nurses in pairs to act as "buddies" so one can observe the client when the other leaves the unit.
- Place unstable clients in an area that is constantly or closely supervised.
- Prepare clients before a move to limit relocation shock and resultant confusion.
- Frequently assist confused clients to the toilet to prevent falls during attempts to climb out of bed to use the bathroom.
- Discuss with the physician the administration time of laxatives and diuretics; if possible, peak action should occur when the client may easily be assisted to the bathroom.
- Stay with clients using a bedside commode or bathroom if the client is confused or sedated or has a gait disturbance or a high risk score for falling.
- Monitor all of the client's medications and, if possible, attempt to lower or eliminate dosages of sedatives or psychotropics.
- Position beds at their lowest level to the floor to facilitate getting in and out of bed.
- Replace full-length side rails with half- or three-quarter-length rails to prevent confused clients from climbing over rails or falling from the end of the bed.
- Use rocker chairs or frequent walks to help confused clients expend some of their energy so that they will be less inclined to wander.
- Wedge pillows or pads against the sides of wheelchairs to keep clients properly positioned.
- Place a removable lap tray on a wheelchair to provide support and keep the client in place.
- To quiet agitated clients, try a warm beverage, soft lights, a back rub, or a walk.
- Use "environmental restraints," such as pieces of furniture or large plants as barriers, to keep clients from wandering beyond appropriate areas.
- Place a picture or other personal item on the client's door to help the client identify their room.
- Try to determine possible causes of the client's *sundowner's syndrome* (nocturnal wandering and disorientation as darkness falls, associated with dementia), such as poor hearing, poor eyesight, or pain.
- Establish ongoing assessment to monitor changes in physical and cognitive functional abilities and risk factors.

psychotropic agents used to control socially disruptive behavior.

In the past decade, restraint practices have been seriously questioned. Reducing the use of restraints and using safe alternatives are being emphasized. See the box immediately above.

Numerous complications have occurred from the use or misuse of restraints. Physical complications associated with immobility include pressure ulcers, skin tears, urinary retention or incontinence, and fecal impaction. Deaths have also been reported, especially with application of the jacket-type restraint. Most jacket-restraint deaths were due to asphyxiation and strangulation that occurred when the clients slid down and attempted to free themselves from the device. Psychologically, clients who are restrained suffer loss of self-esteem, confusion, forgetfulness, a sense of abandonment, depression, humiliation, fear, and anger (Weick 1992, p. 74).

Nurses have stated that they use restraints to prevent clients from

- Falling out of a bed or chair.
- Pulling out an intravenous line, feeding tube, catheter, or other such device.
- Breaking open sutures.
- Unsafe ambulation.
- Wandering and entering an unsafe place.
- Infringing on the rights of others and/or causing harm to others (Varone et al 1992, p. 271).

Experience, however, has shown that restraints do not prevent falls or injury (Evans & Strumpf 1990, p. 124).

To safeguard clients in long-term care facilities, the US government, as part of the 1987 Omnibus Budget Reconciliation Act (OBRA), regulated the use of mechanical restraints. OBRA clearly states that *restraints should be applied only as a last resort.* Regulations also require (a) that restraints be *applied only under a physician's written order,* one that specifies why the restraint is used and for how long it will be used; (b) that the client agree to be restrained; and (c) that clients be free of physical restraints *not* required to treat the client's medical symptoms.

In November 1991, the FDA made similar recommendations, which apply to acute care as well as to long-term care.

Legal Implications of Restraints Because restraints restrict a person's ability to move freely, their use has legal implications. Inappropriate decisions about the application of restraints may subject the nurse to allegations of false imprisonment, battery, and lack of informed consent. Before applying any restraint, the nurse must weigh its benefits against the risks to the client. It is necessary on the one hand to foster the client's independence and autonomy as much as possible and, on the other hand, to protect the client from personal injury or injury to others.

To protect clients and to avoid legal problems, the nurse should follow these guidelines:

- Know the agency's restraint policies. Policies should cover all types of physical and chemical restraints and specify how and when to apply them and what procedures to follow. For example, general criteria may specify that restraints be applied to clients who are comatose, confused, disoriented, sedated, paralyzed, or recovering from anesthesia. Age is *not* an objective criterion (Feutz-Harter 1990, p. 8); for example, the fact that a client is over 70 years of age is not in itself enough to require that side rails be raised at all times.
- When determining the need for a restraint, always assess the underlying reason for a client's restlessness, agitation, or confusion.
- Apply restraints only when necessary for the client's health and safety, not for convenience or to cope with understaffing.
- Avoid being influenced by a family member's advice not to restrain the client, even when the person offers to sit with the client. Nurses cannot legally delegate responsibility to a family member.
- Try to obtain a physician's order before applying a restraint. If the client needs to be restrained immediately, apply the restraint and then notify the physician as soon as possible. In many agencies, standing orders allow the use of restraints under certain circumstances, provided that a written order is obtained from the physician within 24 hours.
- Recognize the competent adult's right to make decisions regarding personal care and treatment, and obtain appropriate consent. Check agency policies if necessary restraint is refused. An agency may require the client to sign a release of liability should injury result; otherwise, the agency has the option of refusing to continue care. For clients who are declared legally incompetent, obtain consent from an appointed guardian or surrogate as permitted under law.
- Keep in mind the *principle of least restriction;* that is, restrain the client only to the extent necessary to accomplish the restraint's purpose.
- Make sure that a physical restraint fits properly.
- When a restraint is applied, document
  a. The specific behavior that made it necessary.
  b. The type of restraint used.
  c. The substance of explanations given to the client and support persons.
  d. The client's consent.
  e. The exact times the restraint was applied and removed.
  f. The client's behavior while the restraint was applied.
  g. The care given while the restraint was applied and removed (eg, assessment of circulation and range-of-motion exercises).
  h. Notification of the physician.
- Periodically reevaluate the need for the restraint.

Selecting a Restraint Before selecting a restraint, nurses need to understand its purpose clearly and measure it against the following five criteria:

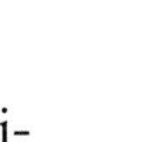

1. *It restricts the client's movement as little as possible.* If a client needs to have one arm restrained, do not restrain the entire body.
2. *It is the least obvious to others.* Both clients and visitors are often embarrassed by a restraint, even though they

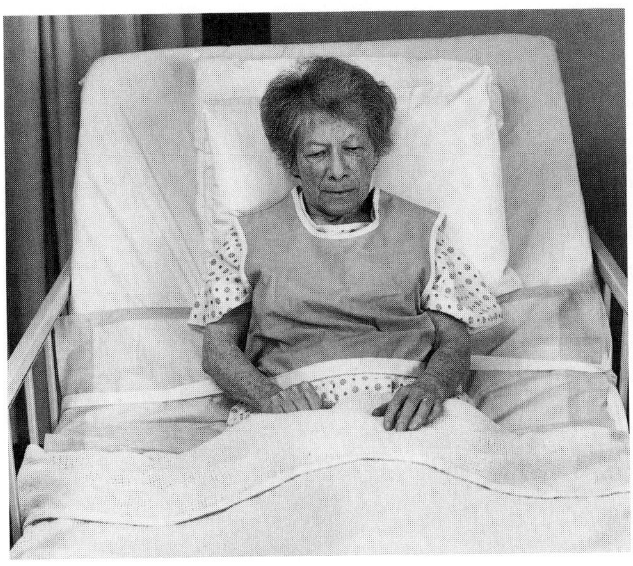

Figure 28–7 A poncho-type jacket restraint.

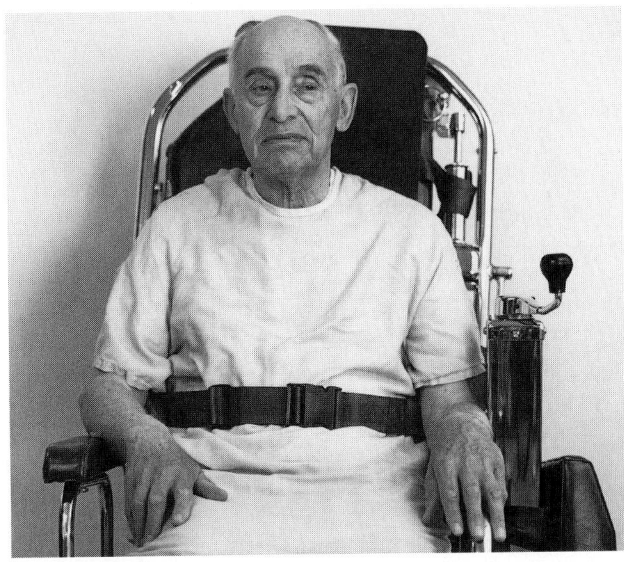

Figure 28–8 A belt restraint.

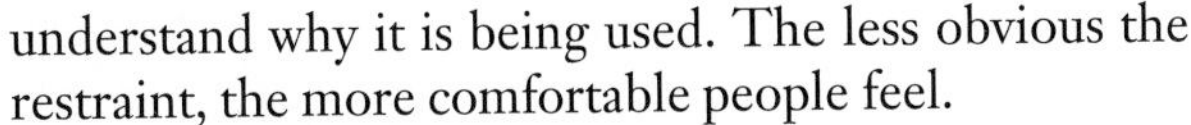

understand why it is being used. The less obvious the restraint, the more comfortable people feel.

3. *It does not interfere with the client's treatment or health problem.* If a client has poor blood circulation to the hands, apply a restraint that will not aggravate that circulatory problem.
4. *It is readily changeable.* Restraints need to be changed frequently, especially if they become soiled. Keeping other guidelines in mind, choose a restraint that can be changed with minimal disturbance to the client.
5. *It is safe for the particular client.* Choose a restraint with which the client cannot self-inflict injury. For example, a physically active child could incur injury trying to climb out of a crib if one wrist is tied to the side of the crib. A jacket restraint would restrain the child more safely.

Kinds of Restraints There are several kinds of restraints. Among the most common are the jacket restraint, the belt restraint, the mitt or hand restraint, limb restraints, elbow restraints, mummy restraints, and crib nets. Geri chairs and wheelchairs used to confine client activity can also be considered restraints. There are several types of *jacket restraints,* but all are essentially sleeveless jackets (vests) with straps (tails) that can be tied to the bed frame under the mattress or to the legs of a chair (Figure 28–7). The jacket may be put on with the ties at the front or at the back, depending on the type. Jackets intended to open at the front must be applied in this manner. These body restraints are used to ensure the safety of confused or sedated clients in beds or wheelchairs.

Belt or safety strap body restraints (Figure 28–8) are used to ensure the safety of all clients who are being moved on stretchers or in wheelchairs. Some wheelchairs have a soft padded safety bar that attaches to side brackets that are installed under the arm rests. To prevent the person from slumping forward, the nurse then attaches a shoulder "Y" strap to the bar and over the client's shoulders to the rear handles. Other safety belt models have a three-loop design. One loop surrounds the person's waist and attaches to the rear handles. If such restraints are unattainable, the nurse can place a folded towel or small sheet around the client's waist and fasten it at the back of the wheelchair. Belt restraints may also be used for certain clients confined to bed or to chairs.

A *mitt or hand restraint* (Figure 28–9) is used to prevent confused clients from using their hands or fingers to scratch and injure themselves. For example, a confused client may need to be prevented from pulling at intravenous tubing or a head bandage following brain surgery.

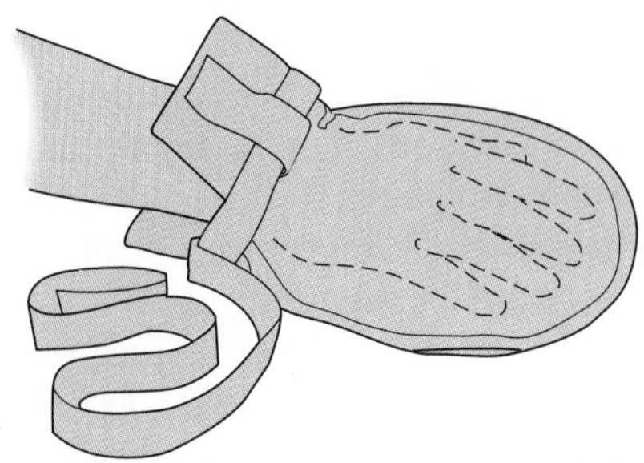

Figure 28–9 A commercially made mitt restraint.

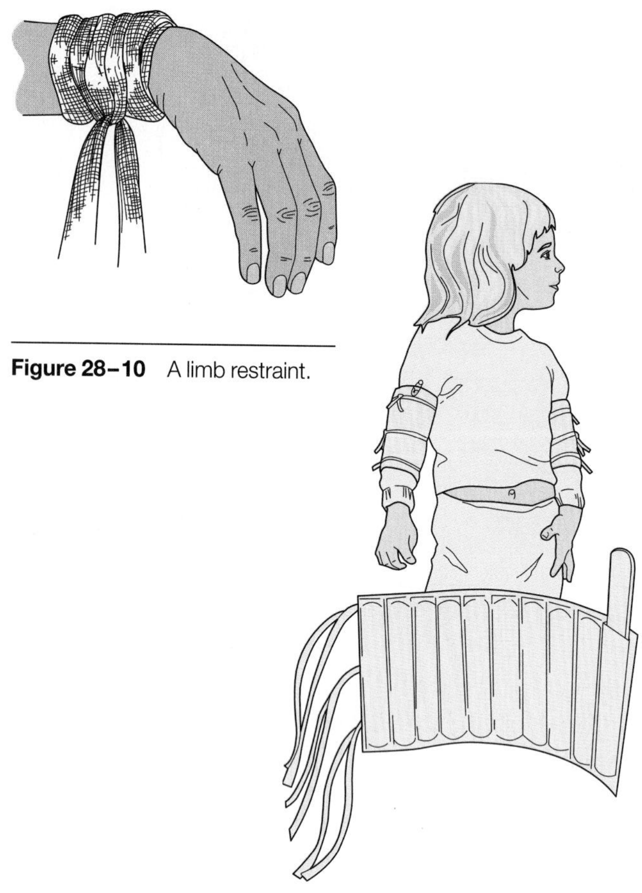

Figure 28–10 A limb restraint.

Figure 28–11 An elbow restraint for a young child.

Hand or mitt restraints allow the client to be ambulatory and/or to move the arm freely rather than be confined to a bed or a chair. Mitt restraints are commercially available. Also, nurses can make hand restraints using large dressings and stockinette. See Procedure 28–2. Mittens need to be removed at least every two hours to permit the client to wash and exercise the hands. The nurse also needs to take off the mitten regularly to check the circulation to the hand.

Limb restraints (Figure 28–10), which are generally made of cloth, may be used to immobilize a limb, primarily for therapeutic reasons (eg, to maintain an intravenous infusion). Some commercially prepared restraints are available. Nurses can also improvise a clove hitch limb restraint using padded dressing and gauze.

Elbow restraints (Figure 28–11) are used to prevent infants or small children from flexing their elbows to touch or scratch a skin lesion or to reach the head when a scalp vein infusion is in place. This restraint consists of a piece of material with pockets into which plastic or wooden tongue depressors are inserted to provide rigidity.

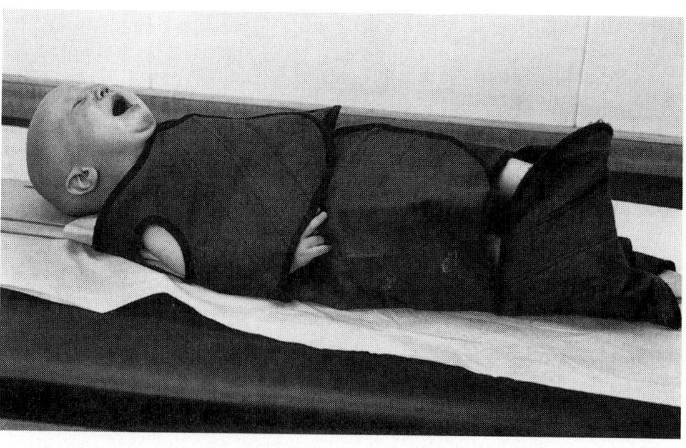

Figure 28–12 A commercially made mummy restraint.

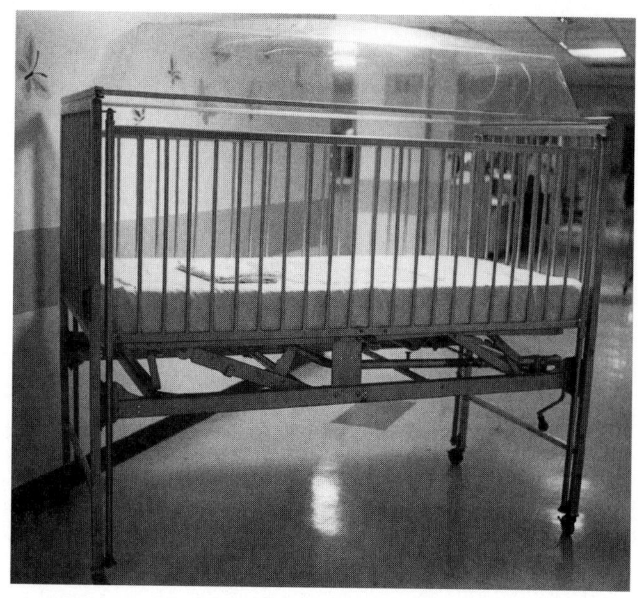

Figure 28–13 A crib dome.

The *mummy restraint* (Figure 28–12) is a special folding of a blanket or sheet around the child to prevent movement during a procedure such as gastric washing, eye irrigation, or collection of a blood specimen. A *crib net* or *dome* (Figure 28–13) is simply a device placed over the top of a crib to prevent active young children from climbing out of the crib. At the same time, it allows them freedom to move about in the crib. The crib net or dome is not attached to the movable parts of the crib so that the caregiver can have access to the child without removing the dome or net.

When using restraints, the nurse may find the guidelines in the accompanying box helpful. See Procedure 28–2 for applying restraints.

Text continued on page 726

CLINICAL GUIDELINES

Applying Restraints

- Obtain consent from the client or guardian.
- Ensure that a physician's order has been provided, or, in an emergency, obtain one within 24 hours after applying the restraint.
- Assure the client and the client's support persons that the restraint is temporary and protective. A restraint must never be applied as punishment for any behavior or merely for the nurse's convenience.
- Apply the restraint in such a way that the client can move as freely as possible without defeating the purpose of the restraint.
- Ensure that limb restraints are applied securely but not so tightly that they impede blood circulation to any body area or extremity.
- Pad bony prominences (eg, wrists and ankles) before applying a restraint over them. The movement of a restraint without padding over such prominences can quickly abrade the skin.
- Always tie a limb restraint with a knot (eg, a clove hitch) that will not tighten when pulled.
- Tie the ends of a body restraint to the part of the bed that moves when the head is elevated. Never tie the ends to a side rail or to the fixed frame of the bed if the bed position is to be changed.
- Assess the restraint every 30 minutes. Some facilities have specific forms to be used to record ongoing assessment.
- Release all restraints at least every 2 to 4 hours, and provide range-of-motion (ROM) exercises (see Chapter 34) and skin care (see Chapter 30).
- Reassess the continued need for the restraint every 8 hours. Include an assessment of the underlying cause of the behavior necessitating use of the restraints.
- When a restraint is temporarily removed, do not leave the client unattended.
- Immediately report to the nurse in charge and record on the client's chart any persistent reddened or broken skin areas under the restraint.
- At the first indication of cyanosis or pallor, coldness of a skin area, or a client's complaint of a tingling sensation, pain, or numbness, loosen the restraint and exercise the limb.
- Apply a restraint so that it can be released quickly in case of an emergency and with the body part in a normal anatomic position.
- Provide emotional support verbally and through touch.

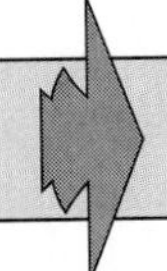

PROCEDURE 28–2 APPLYING RESTRAINTS

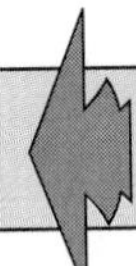

PURPOSE

- To enable the client to receive treatment and to allow the treatment to proceed without client interference (eg, to prevent movements that would disrupt therapy to a limb connected to tubes or appliance.)

ASSESSMENT FOCUS

Behavior indicating the possible need for a restraint; underlying cause for assessed behavior (to ascertain what other protective measures may be implemented before applying a restraint); status of skin to which restraint is to be applied; circulatory status of extremities; effectiveness of other available safety precautions.

EQUIPMENT

Select the kind and size of restraint required by the client. See "Selecting a Restraint," earlier in this chapter. If a commercial hand, wrist, or ankle restraint is not available, the supplies that follow are needed.

Mitt Restraint

- ☐ Four large padded dressings (eg, ABD pads)
- ☐ Pieces of thick gauze
- ☐ Stockinette dressing or elastic bandage
- ☐ Adhesive tape

Wrist or Ankle Restraint

- ☐ Padded or thick gauze dressing, (eg, an ABD pad)
- ☐ Strip of gauze bandage or cloth tie 5 to 8 cm (2 to 3 in) wide and 90 to 120 cm (3 to 4 ft) long

PROCEDURE 28–2 APPLYING RESTRAINTS *continued*

INTERVENTION

1. Explain to client and support persons the purpose and procedure for using restraint.

2. Apply the selected restraint.

Belt Restraint (Safety Belt)

- Determine that the safety belt is in good order. If a Velcro safety belt is to be used, make sure that both pieces of Velcro are intact.
- If the belt has a long portion and a shorter portion, place the long portion of the belt behind (under) the bedridden client and secure it to the movable part of the bed frame. *The long attached portion will then move up when the head of the bed is elevated and will not tighten around the client.* Place the shorter portion of the belt around the client's waist, over the gown. There should be a finger's width between the belt and the client.

  or

  Attach the belt around the client's waist, and fasten it at the back of the chair.

  or

  If the belt is attached to a stretcher, secure the belt firmly over the client's hips or abdomen. Belt restraints need to be applied to all clients on stretchers even when the side rails are up.

Jacket Restraint

- Place vest on client, with opening at the front or the back, depending on the type.
- Pull the tie on the end of the vest flap across the chest, and place it through the slit on the opposite side of the chest.
- Repeat for the other tie.
- Use a half-bow knot to secure each tie around the movable bed frame or behind the chair to a chair leg (Figure 28–14). *A half-bow knot does not tighten or slip when the attached end is pulled but unties easily when the loose end is pulled.*

  or

  Fasten the ties together behind the chair using a square (reef) knot (Figure 28–15). *This knot does not tighten with pulling and does not slip when pressure is released.*
- Ensure that the client is positioned appropriately to enable maximum chest expansion for breathing.

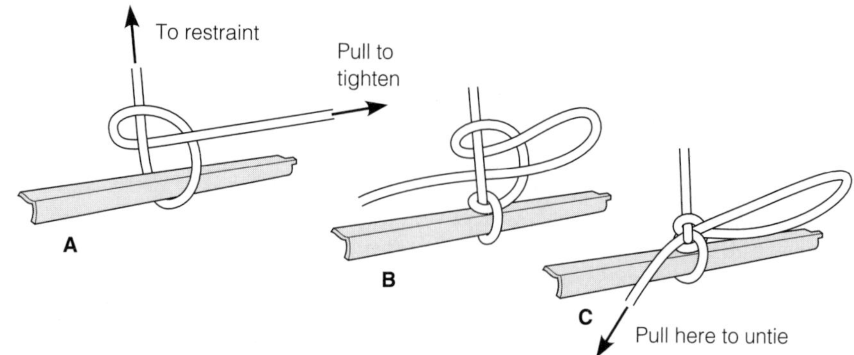

Figure 28–14 To make a half-bow knot, first place the restraint tie under the side frame of the bed (or around a chair leg). *A,* Bring the free end up, around, under, and over the attached end of the tie, and pull it tight. *B,* Again take the free end over and under the attached end of the tie, but this time make a half-bow loop. *C,* Tighten the free end of the tie and the bow until the knot is secure. To untie the knot, pull the end of the tie, and then loosen the first cross over the tie.

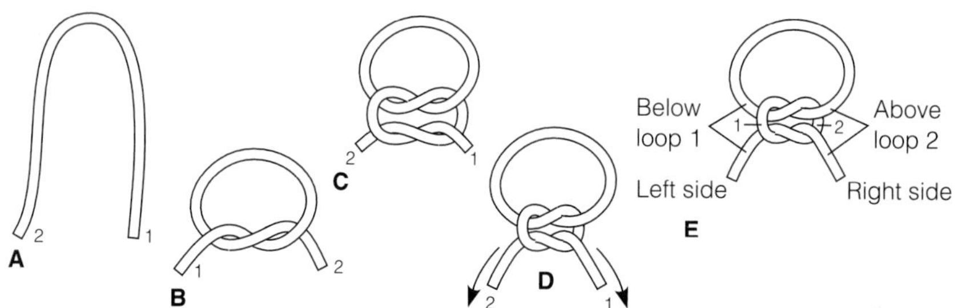

Figure 28–15 To make a square (reef) knot: *A,* Form a "U" loop. *B,* Pass one end (1) over and under the other. *C,* Take the same end (1), and pass it over, under, and over the other. *D,* Pull knot tight. *E,* When the knot is tied correctly, the ties on each side are both either above or below the loop.

Mitt Restraint

- Apply the commercial thumbless mitt (Figure 28–9, earlier) to the hand to be restrained. Make sure the fingers can be slightly flexed and are not caught under the hand.
- Follow the manufacturer's directions for securing the mitt.
- If there is no commercial mitt, make a mitt as follows:
  a. Place a large folded dressing, such as an abdominal (ABD) pad, in the client's palm. Ensure that the hand is in a natural position with the fingers slightly flexed.

PROCEDURE 28–2 *continued*

b. Separate the fingers with pieces of large dressing or thick gauze. *This prevents skin abrasion.*
c. Put a padded dressing around the client's wrist. *This prevents pressure and skin abrasion.*
d. Place two large dressings (ABD pads) over the hand. Place the first one from the back of the hand over the fingers to the palm; then wrap the other from side to side around the hand.
e. Cover these dressings by placing a stockinette dressing over the hand or wrapping them with an elastic bandage, using a recurrent pattern. See Chapter 44, pages 1389 and 1390. See also page 1388 for basic turns used in bandaging.
f. Secure the stockinette or elastic bandage with adhesive tape.

- If a mitt is to be worn for several days, remove it at least every 2 to 4 hours. Wash and exercise the client's hand, then reapply the mitt. Check agency practices about recommended intervals for removal.
- Assess the client's circulation to the hands shortly after the mitt is applied and at regular intervals. *Feelings of numbness or discomfort or inability to move the fingers could indicate impaired circulation to the hand.*

Wrist or Ankle Restraint

- Apply the padded portion of a commercially prepared restraint around the ankle or wrist.

  or

  Improvise a restraint as follows:

  a. Cushion the wrist or ankle with a padded or thick gauze dressing (eg, an ABD pad).

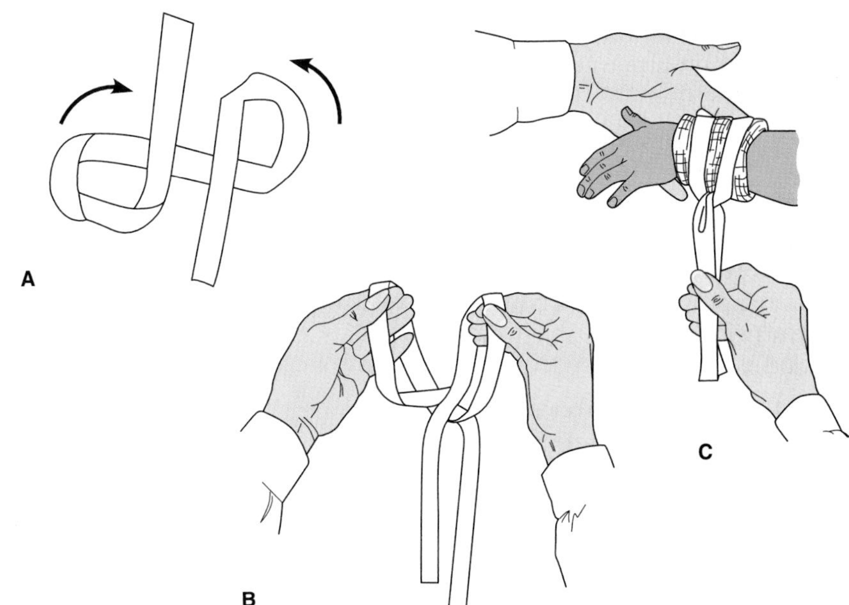

Figure 28–16 To make a clove hitch: *A*, make a figure-eight; *B*, pick up the loops; *C*, put the limb through the loops, and secure it.

  b. Wrap a long, narrow strip of gauze bandage or a cloth tie around the padding.

- Pull the tie of the commercially made restraint through the slit in the wrist portion or through the buckle.

  or

  Use a clove hitch to secure the gauze strip or cloth tie of the improvised restraint (Figure 28–16). *The clove hitch knot does not tighten with pulling and is readily released.*
- Using a half-bow knot or a square knot as appropriate, attach the other end of the commercial restraint (or the two ends of the improvised restraint) to the movable portion of the bed frame. *If the ties are attached to the movable portion, the wrist or ankle will not be pulled when the bed position is changed.*

Elbow Restraint

- Examine the restraint to make sure that the tongue depressors are intact, that is, all in place and not broken.
- Place the infant's elbow in the center of the restraint. Make sure that the ends of the tongue depressors are covered by the padded material. *This prevents them from irritating the skin.*
- Wrap the restraint smoothly around the arm.
- Secure the restraint, using safety pins, ties, or tape. Ensure that it is not so tight that it obstructs blood circulation.
- (Optional) After the restraint is applied, pin it to the child's shirt. *This prevents it from sliding down the arm.*

Mummy Restraint

- Obtain a blanket or sheet large enough so that the distance between opposite corners is about

PROCEDURE 28–2 *continued*

twice the length of the infant's body. Lay the blanket or sheet on a flat dry surface.

- Fold down one corner, and place the baby on it in the supine position.
- Fold the right side of the blanket over the infant's body, leaving the left arm free (Figure 28–17, *A*). The right arm is in a natural position at the side.
- Fold the excess blanket at the bottom up under the infant (Figure 28–17, *B*[2]).
- With the left arm in a natural position at the baby's side, fold the left side of the blanket over the infant, including the arm, and tuck the blanket under the body (Figure 28–17, *B*[3]).
- Remain with the infant who is in a mummy restraint until the specific procedure is completed.

Crib Net

- Place the net over the sides and ends of the crib.

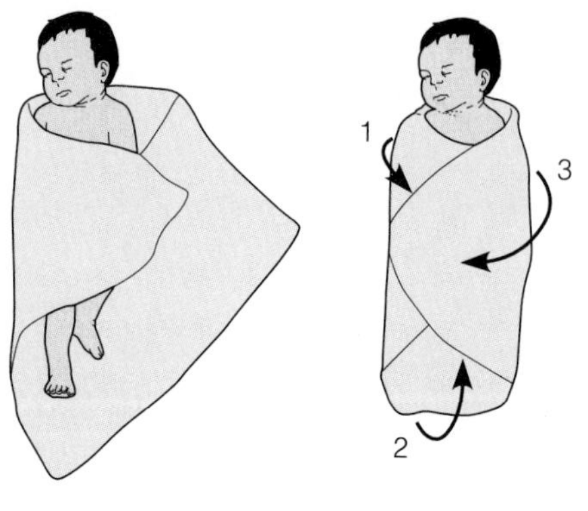

Figure 28–17 Making a mummy restraint.

- Secure the ties to the springs or frame of the crib. *The crib sides can then be freely lowered without removing the net.*
- Test with your hand to ascertain that the net will stretch if the child stands in the crib against it.

3. Document relevant information for all types of restraints.

- Record on the client's chart the time the physician was notified, the type of restraint applied, the time it was applied, the reason for its application, the client's response to the restraint, and the times that the restraints are removed and skin care given.
- Record any other interventions, assessments, and explanations to client and significant others.
- Adjust the nursing care plan as required, for example, to include releasing the restraint q2h, providing skin care, and providing range-of-motion exercises.

EVALUATION FOCUS
Client response to restraint; circulatory status of restrained limbs; skin status beneath restraints.

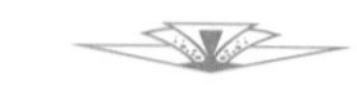

EVALUATING

Using data collected during care, the nurse judges whether the client outcomes have been achieved. If the outcomes have *not* been achieved, the nurse should explore the reasons. Examples of questions the nurse might consider are

- Have precautions been taken to prevent trauma?
- What precautions does the client desire and know about?
- Did the client agree to follow any precautions?
- Did the nurse write and implement a teaching plan for the client?
- Do the support persons understand and agree to follow the precautions?
- Are any medications affecting the client's abilities?

CHAPTER HIGHLIGHTS

- Education is a major health protection strategy in preventing accidents.
- When planning to meet safety needs of clients, nurses need to consider physical factors in the en-

vironment and the psychologic and physiologic state of the individual.

- Accidents are a major cause of death among individuals of all ages in the United States and Canada. The seven major causes of accidental deaths in the United States are motor vehicle accidents, falls, drowning, fire and burns, poisoning, inhalation and ingestion of foreign objects, and firearms. Most accidents are due to negligence and are preventable.
- Nurses must be familiar with the fire procedures in the health care agency where they practice. In the event of a fire, the nurse must protect clients from injury and contain and put out the fire.
- Falls are a common cause of injury among the very young, the elderly, and the ill or injured.
- To prevent falls, the nurse must provide constant surveillance for infants and young children and carefully assess older clients' safety needs.
- Poisoning from numerous plants, household chemicals, and medications is a major threat to young, curious children.
- Major reasons for poisoning in children are inadequate supervision and improper storage of household toxic substances.
- Faulty electrical equipment and improper grounding pose health hazards in the hospital and the home.
- Electrical accidents can be prevented by using grounded outlets and plugs, putting protective covers over outlets, keeping appliances in good repair, and making sure that electrical wiring and circuits meet safety standards.
- Prolonged exposure to excessive noise can produce hearing loss.
- In hospitals, radioactive substances are used for both diagnostic and treatment purposes; agency policy should be followed to safeguard clients and staff from inadvertent exposure.
- Suffocation can occur when foreign objects are swallowed or inhaled, cutting off the person's oxygen supply.
- Nursing assessment of the mobility status of clients at risk includes assessment of age, life-style, sensory alterations, level of awareness, and emotional state.
- Nursing diagnoses for clients at risk for accidental injury can be categorized as **High risk for injury,** with four subcategories: **High risk for trauma, High risk for poisoning, High risk for suffocation,** and **High risk for aspiration.**
- Nursing intervention must include education in accident prevention and modification of the environment to make it safe.
- Side rails and hand rails protect hospitalized clients from falls; restraints keep clients from falling and from inflicting injuries on themselves and others.
- Because restraints restrict a client's basic freedom to move, careful assessment and accurate, complete documentation are important when restraints are used.
- Various alternatives to restraints must be used before a restraint is applied.

READINGS AND REFERENCES

SUGGESTED READINGS

Cutchins, CH. July 1991. Blueprint for restraint-free care. *American Journal of Nursing* 91:36–42.

This article explains how to identify and carry out changes in the environment and in clinical practice to give clients maximum protection from falls and other accidents. The author also identifies people at risk of falling and describes how the nursing staff at one agency monitored falls and adjusted its environment.

Kallmann, SL, Denine-Flynn, M, and Blackburn, DM. May/June 1992. Comfort, safety, and independence: Restraint release and its challenges. *Geriatric Nursing* 13:142–48.

This article describes the challenge that nurses face in implementing a restraint release program as mandated by the Omnibus Budget Reconciliation Act (OBRA). Further, the authors describe a program of client assessment and interventions that one long-term care unit established to provide safety while reducing the use of restraints.

RELATED RESEARCH

Morse, JM and McHutchion, E. June 1991. Releasing restraints: Providing safe care for the elderly. *Research in Nursing and Health* 14:187–96.

Varone, L, Tappen, RM, Dixon-Antonio, E, Gonzales, I, and Glussman, B. September/October 1992. To restraint or not to restrain? The decision-making dilemma for nursing staff. *Geriatric Nursing* 13:269–72.

SELECTED REFERENCES

Barbieri, EB. March 1983. Patient falls are not patient accidents. *Journal of Gerontological Nursing* 9:164–73.

Berger, ME and Hubner, KF. August 1983. Hospital hazards: Diagnostic radiation. *American Journal of Nursing* 83:1155–59.

Blakeslee, JA, Goldman, BD, Papougenis, D, and Torell, CA. February 1991. Making the transition to restraint-free care. *Journal of Gerontological Nursing* 17:4–8.

Brower, HT. February 1991. The alternatives to restraints. *Journal of Gerontological Nursing* 17:18–22.

Calfree, BE. December 1991. Protecting yourself from allegations of nursing negligence. *Nursing* 21:34–40.

Carpenito, LJ. 1992. *Nursing Diagnosis: Application to Clinical Practice.* 4th ed. Philadelphia: Lippincott.

Coberg, A, Lynch, D, and Mavretish, MS. May/June 1991. Harnessing ideas to release restraints. *Geriatric Nursing* 12(3):133–34.

Craighead, J, Fletcher, R, and Maxwell, J. May 1991. Seven steps for fall prevention. *Dimensions in Health Service* 68(4):25–26.

Croft, W and Foraker, S. November 1992. Taking charge: Working together to prevent falls. *RN* 55:17–18, 20.

Crutchins, CH. July 1991. Blueprint for restraint-free care. *American Journal of Nursing* 91:36–44.

Dowd, SB. Fall 1991. The basics of radiation protection for hospital workers: Considerations and procedures. *Hospital Topics* 69(4):31–35.

Easterling, ML. January 1990. Which of your patients is headed for a fall? *RN* 53:56–59.

Eigsti, DG and Vrooman, V. January 1992. Releasing restraints in the nursing home: It can be done. *Journal of Gerontological Nursing* 18:21–23.

Evans, LK and Strumpf, NE. Summer 1990. Myths about elder restraint. *Image: Journal of Nursing Scholarship* 22:124–27.

———. January 1991. Myths and facts . . . about restraints for the elderly. *Nursing* 21:24.

Feutz-Harter, SA. October 1990. Legal implications of restraints. *Journal of Nursing Administration* 20:8–9.

FDA Medical Alert. November 16, 1991. *Potential Hazards with Restraint Devices.* Medical Bulletin. Washington, DC: Public Health Service.

George, JE and Quattrone, MS. February 1993. Restraining patients: Can you be sued? Part 2. *Journal of Emergency Nursing* 19:57.

Gibbs, J. July 3–9, 1991. Radiation hazards. *Nursing Times* 87(27):46–47.

Ginter, SF and Mion, LC. November 1992. Falls in the nursing home: Preventable or inevitable? *Journal of Gerontological Nursing* 18:43–48, 57–58.

Harry, A and Kopetsky, D. September/October 1991. Unrestrained pride: Development of a protocol for a restraint-free environment. *Canadian Journal of Nursing Administration* 4(3):12–16.

Jech, AO. January/February 1992. Preventing falls in the elderly. *Geriatric Nursing* 13(1):43–44.

Johnson, BP. March 1992. Legal answer. *Nursing Management* 23:20.

Johnson, D. January/February 1991. Make your own chairbound alternatives! *Geriatric Nursing* 12(1):18–19.

Jones, WJ, Simpson, JA, and Pieroni, RE. Summer 1991. Preventing falls in hospitals: The roles of patient age and diagnostic status in predicting falls. *Hospital Topics* 69(3):30–33.

Kallmann, SL, Denine-Flynn, M, and Blackburn, DM. May/June 1992. Comfort, safety, and independence: Restraint release and its challenges. *Geriatric Nursing* 13(3):143–48.

Kim, MJ, McFarland, GK, and McLane, AM. 1993. *Pocket Guide to Nursing Diagnoses.* 5th ed. St Louis: Mosby-Year Book.

Lederer, JR, Marculescu, GL, Mocnik, B, and Seaby, N. 1993. *Care Planning Pocket Guide—A Nursing Diagnosis Approach.* 5th ed. Redwood City, CA: Addison-Wesley Nursing.

McFarland, GK and McFarlane, EA. 1989. *Nursing Diagnosis and Interventions: Planning for Patient Care.* St Louis: Mosby.

McHutchion, E and Morse, JM. February 1989. Releasing restraints: A nursing dilemma. *Journal of Gerontological Nursing* 15:16–21.

Manoquerra, AS. October 1992. Pediatric poisoning. *Emergency* 24:19–24.

Mayhew, MS. December 1991. Strategies for promoting safety and preventing injury. *Nursing Clinics of North America* 26:885–93.

Mion, LC and Mercurio, AT. November 1992. Methods to reduce restraints: Process, outcomes, and future directions. *Journal of Gerontological Nursing* 18:5–11.

North American Nursing Diagnosis Association. 1992. *NANDA Nursing Diagnoses: Definitions and Classification 1992–1993.* Philadelphia: North American Nursing Diagnosis Assocation.

Omnibus Budget Reconciliation Act. 1987. 4201(C)(1)(A)(II)(Medicare) codified at 42 USC 1395i-3(C)(I)(A)(II)(supp 1991), and Public Law 100 203 4211 (C)(1)(A)(II)(Medicaid) codified at 42 USC 1396r-3 (C)(1)(A)(II)(supp 1991). Washington, DC: Health Care Financing Administration.

Press, MM. December 1991. Restraints: Protection or abuse? *Canadian Nurse* 87:29–30.

Rader, J. February 1991. Modifying the environment to decrease use of restraints. *Journal of Gerontological Nursing* 17:9–13.

Rader, J and Donius, M. March/April 1991. Restraints in the 90s: Leveling off restraints. *Geriatric Nursing* 12(2):71–73.

Rogers, B and Travers, P. March 1992. Legally speaking: Nursing can be hazardous to your health. *RN* 55:67–68, 71, 73–74.

Ross, JER. September 1991. Iatrogenesis in the elderly: Contributors to falls. *Journal of Gerontological Nursing* 17:19–23.

Scherer, YK. February 1991. The nursing dilemma of restraints. *Journal of Gerontological Nursing* 17:14–17.

Stilwell, EM. February 1991. Nurses' education related to the use of restraints. *Journal of Gerontological Nursing* 17:23–26.

Strumpf, NE and Evans, LK. November 1992. Alternatives to physical restraints. *Journal of Gerontological Nursing* 18:4.

———. February 1991. The ethical problems of prolonged physical restraint. *Journal of Gerontological Nursing* 17:27–30.

Tammelleo, AD. April 1992. Legally speaking. Restraints: A legal catch-22? *RN* 55:71–72, 75–76.

Varone, L, Tappen, RM, Dixon-Antonio, E, Gonzales, I, and Glussman, B. September/October 1992. To restrain or not to restrain? The decision-making dilemma for nursing staff. *Geriatric Nursing* 13(5):269–72.

Weick, MD. November 1992. Physical restraints: an FDA update. *American Journal of Nursing* 92:74, 76–80, 80.

Wood, L and Cunningham, G. July/August 1992. Fall risk protocol and nursing care plan. *Geriatric* Nursing 13(4):205–6.

29 Assisting with Hygiene

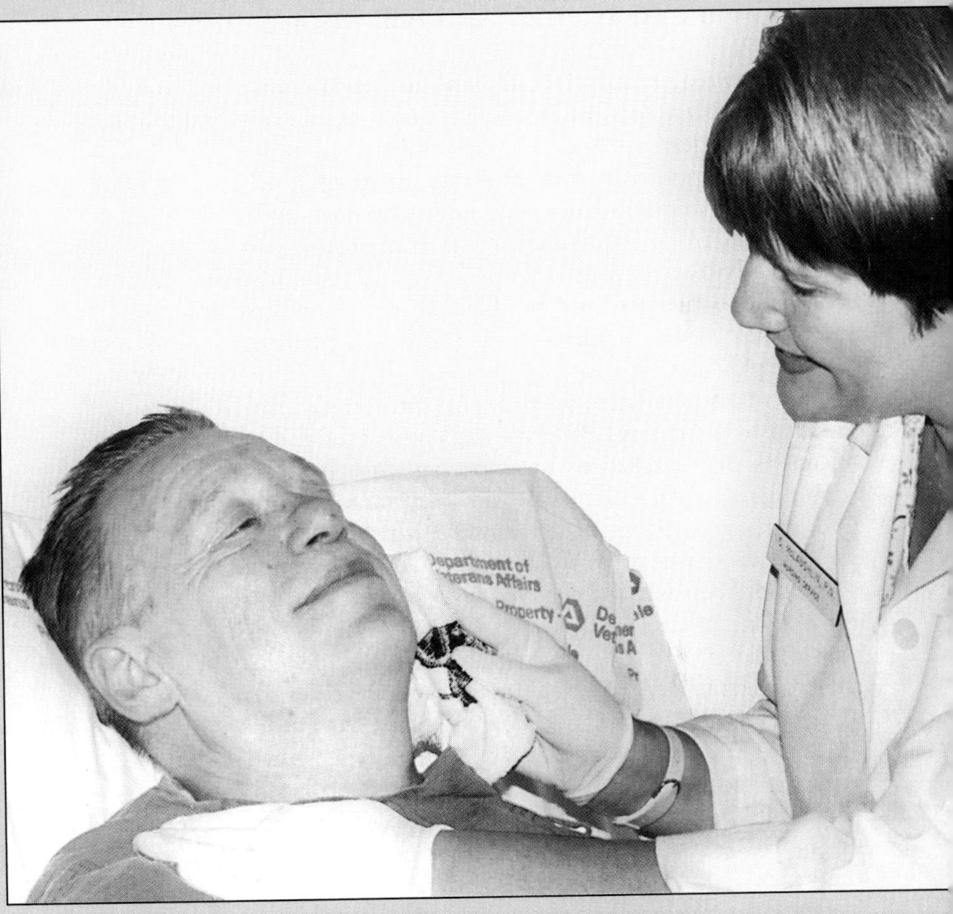

Objectives

- Describe kinds of hygienic care nurses provide to clients.
- Identify factors influencing personal hygiene.
- Identify normal and abnormal findings obtained during inspection and palpation of the skin, feet, nails, mouth, hair, eyes, ears, and nose.
- Describe variations in the appearance of the skin, nails, and mucous membranes of light-skinned and dark-skinned clients.
- Identify common problems of the skin, feet, nails, mouth, hair, eyes, ears, and nose and formulate related nursing diagnoses.
- Describe guidelines for planning and implementing nursing interventions for the skin, feet, nails, mouth, hair, eyes, ears, and nose.
- List outcome criteria to evaluate goal achievement.
- Identify the purposes of bathing.
- Describe various types of baths.
- Describe steps in perineal and genital care.
- Explain specific ways in which nurses help hospitalized clients with oral hygiene.
- Identify steps in removing contact lenses and inserting and removing artificial eyes.
- Describe steps in inserting and removing hearing aids.
- Identify safety and comfort measures underlying bedmaking procedures.

Hygiene is the science of health and its maintenance. Personal hygiene is the self-care by which people attend to such functions as bathing, toileting, general body hygiene, and grooming. Hygiene is a highly personal matter determined by individual values and practices. Hygiene involves care of the skin, hair, nails, teeth, oral and nasal cavities, eyes, ears, and perineal and genital areas. It serves a number of purposes (See Procedure 29–1 on page 739).

HYGIENIC CARE

Clients may require assistance to carry out many hygienic activities. It is important for nurses to know exactly how much a client can safely do and how much assistance is required. Clients may require care after urinating or defecating, after vomiting, and whenever they become soiled, for example, from wound drainage or from profuse perspiration. Nurses must keep the hygiene needs and personal practices of clients in mind and assist them whenever indicated. See Table 29–1 for factors influencing hygiene practices.

Nurses commonly use the following terms to describe kinds of hygienic care. *Early morning care* is provided to clients as they awaken in the morning. In a hospital, nurses on the night shift may provide early morning care. This care helps clients ready themselves for breakfast or for early diagnostic tests. Usually, it consists of providing a urinal or bedpan to the client confined to bed, washing the face and hands, and giving oral care. *Morning care* is provided after clients have breakfast. It usually includes the provision of a urinal or bedpan (to clients who are not ambulatory), a bath or shower, perineal care, back massages, and oral, nail, and hair care. Making the client's bed is part of morning care. *Afternoon care* may be provided, for example, when clients return from physiotherapy or diagnostic tests. Providing a bedpan or urinal, washing the hands and face, and assisting with oral care refresh clients. *Hour of sleep (HS) care* is provided to clients before they retire for the night. It usually involves providing for elimination needs, washing face and hands, giving oral care, and giving a back massage. *As-needed (prn) care* is provided as required by the client. For example, a client who is *diaphoretic* (sweating profusely) may need bathing and changes of clothes and linen frequently.

SKIN

The skin is the largest organ of the body. It serves five major functions:

Table 29–1 Factors Influencing Individual Hygienic Practices

Factor	Variables
Culture	North American culture places a high value on cleanliness. Many North Americans bathe or shower once or twice a day, whereas people from some other cultures bathe once per week. Some cultures consider privacy essential for bathing, whereas others practice communal bathing. Body odor may be offensive in some cultures and accepted as normal in others.
Religion	Ceremonial washings are practiced by some religions.
Environment	Finances may affect the availability of facilities for bathing. For example, homeless people may not have warm water available; soap, shampoo, shaving lotion, and deodorants may be too expensive for people who have limited resources.
Developmental level	Children learn hygiene in the home. Practices vary according to the individual's age; for example, preschoolers can carry out most tasks independently with encouragement.
Health and energy	Ill people may not have the motivation or energy to attend to hygiene. Some clients who have neuromuscular impairments may be unable to perform hygienic care.
Personal preferences	Some people prefer a shower to a tub bath.

1. It protects underlying tissues from injury by preventing the passage of microorganisms. The skin and mucous membranes are considered the body's first line of defense.
2. It regulates the body temperature. Cooling the body occurs through the heat loss processes of evaporation of perspiration, and by radiation and conduction of heat from the body when the blood vessels of the skin are vasodilated. Body heat is conserved through lack of perspiration and vasoconstriction of the blood vessels. See Chapter 21, page 429, for a detailed discussion of body heat losses and gains.
3. It secretes **sebum,** an oily substance that (a) softens and lubricates the hair and skin, (b) prevents the hair from becoming brittle, and (c) decreases water loss

from the skin when the external humidity is low. Because fat is a poor conductor of heat, sebum (d) lessens the amount of heat lost from the skin. Sebum also (e) has a **bactericidal** (bacteria-killing) action.

4. It transmits sensations through nerve receptors, which are sensitive to pain, temperature, touch, and pressure.
5. It produces and absorbs vitamin D in conjunction with ultraviolet rays from the sun, which activate a vitamin D precursor present in the skin.

The normal skin of a healthy person has transient microorganisms that are not usually harmful. Adults usually have some resident micrococci, bacteria of the genera *Corynebacterium* and *Propionibacterium*, and a genus of fungi, *Pityrosporon*. Children also have gram-positive, spore-forming rods and *Neisseria* bacteria. Transient microorganisms vary considerably from one person to another. They do not maintain themselves on the skin because of (a) the chemical effects of the fatty acids in the sebum and (b) the normal skin pH of 5 to 6, which is too acidic for many microorganisms.

Sudoriferous (sweat) glands are on all body surfaces except the lips and parts of the genitals. The body has from two to five million, which are all present at birth. They are most numerous on the palms of the hands and the soles of the feet. Sweat glands are classified as apocrine and eccrine. The **apocrine glands,** located largely in the axillae and anogenital areas, begin to function at puberty under the influence of androgens. Although their secretion is produced almost constantly, apocrine glands are of little use in thermoregulation. The secretion of these glands is odorless, but when decomposed or acted upon by bacteria on the skin, it takes on a musky, unpleasant odor. The **eccrine glands** are important physiologically. They are more numerous than the apocrine glands and are found chiefly on the palms of the hands, the soles of the feet, and forehead. The sweat they produce cools the body through evaporation. Sweat is made up of water, sodium, potassium, chloride, glucose, urea, and lactate.

DEVELOPMENTAL CHANGES

In early embryonic life, the skin is a single layer of cells. Other layers develop quickly. The fetus's skin is covered by a substance called **vernix caseosa,** whitish, cheesy material seen on newborns. It usually disappears in the first day. The skin of an infant is thinner than an adult's, is usually mottled, and in light-skinned babies varies from pink to red and becomes ruddy when the baby cries. Babies who are genetically dark-skinned are lightly pigmented at birth. Sweat glands of babies begin to function at about 1 month of age. The skin of children gradually becomes more resistant to injury and infection with age.

In adolescence, the **sebaceous glands** (oil-supplying glands) increase in activity as a result of increased levels of hormones (androgens). This is thought to be one factor responsible for the development of acne, a common skin problem of adolescents. Secretions from the sebaceous glands are maintained during adolescence to about 50 years.

The older adult also experiences skin changes. The skin tends to be thinner, drier, somewhat inelastic, and thus subject to fine wrinkling. This process usually begins any time after age 40. The elderly person's skin typically shows wrinkles, sagging, pigmentations, and keratotic spots, usually on areas exposed to the sun. The skin is less resilient; that is, when pinched, it returns to place more slowly than the skin of a younger person does.

ASSESSING

Assessment of the client's skin and hygienic practices includes (a) a nursing history to determine the client's skin care practices, self-care abilities, and past or current skin problems; (b) physical assessment of the skin; and (c) identification of clients at high risk for developing skin impairments.

Nursing History Data about the client's *skin care practices* enable the nurse to incorporate the client's needs and preferences as much as possible in the plan of care and to determine necessary learning needs. Assessment of the client's *self-care abilities* determines the amount of nursing assistance and the kind of bath (bed, tub, or shower) the client requires. Important considerations include the client's balance (for tub and shower), ability to sit unsupported (in the tub or bed), activity tolerance, coordination, adequate muscle strength, appropriate joint range of motion, and vision. Cognition and motivation are also essential. Clients whose cognitive function is impaired or whose illness alters energy levels and motivation will also need assistance. It is important for the nurse to determine the client's functional level to maintain and promote as much client independence as possible. This also enables the nurse to identify the client's potential for growth and rehabilitation. There are several models of functional levels of self-care. One example is shown in Table 29–2.

The *presence of past or current skin problems* alerts the nurse to specific nursing interventions or referrals the client may require. The client may provide descriptions of these problems during the nursing history, or the nurse may observe some during the physical examination that follows. Common skin problems and implications for nursing interventions are shown in Table 29–3. Frequently encountered skin problems are also shown in the color section on skin lesions, following page 474. Questions to elicit data about the client's skin care practices, self-care abilities, and skin problems are shown in the box on page 733.

Table 29–2 Definitions and Descriptors for Functional Level

	Totally Dependent	Moderately Dependent	Semidependent
Bathing	Client needs complete bath; cannot assist at all.	Nurse supplies all equipment; positions client; washes back, legs, perineum, and all other parts, as needed. Client can assist.	Nurse provides all equipment; positions client in bed/bathroom. Client completes bath, except for back and feet.
Dressing/ grooming	Client needs to be dressed and cannot assist the nurse; nurse combs client's hair.	Nurse combs client's hair; assists with dressing; buttons and zips clothing, ties shoes.	Nurse gathers items for client; may button, zip, or tie clothing. Client dresses self.
Toileting	Client is incontinent; nurse places client on bedpan or commode.	Nurse provides bedpan; positions client on or off bedpan; places client on bedside commode.	Client can walk to bathroom/commode with assistance.

Source: JR Lederer, GL Marculescu, B Mocnik, and N Seaby. *Care Planning Pocket Guide: A Nursing Diagnosis Approach*, 5th ed. (Redwood City, CA: Addison-Wesley Nursing, 1993), p. 164.

Table 29–3 Common Skin Problems

Problem and Appearance	Nursing Implications
Abrasion Superficial layers of the skin are scraped or rubbed away. Area is reddened and may have localized bleeding or serous weeping.	1. Prone to infection; therefore, wound should be kept clean and dry. 2. Do not wear rings or jewelry when providing care to avoid causing abrasions to clients. 3. Lift, do not pull, a client across a bed. See Chapter 34.
Excessive Dryness Skin can appear flaky and rough.	1. Prone to infection if the skin cracks; therefore, provide alcohol-free lotions to moisturize the skin and prevent cracking. 2. Bathe client less frequently; use no soap, or limit use of nonirritating soap. Rinse skin thoroughly, because soap can be irritating and drying. 3. Encourage increased fluid intake if health permits to prevent dehydration.
Ammonia Dermatitis (Diaper Rash) Caused by skin bacteria reacting with urea in the urine. The skin becomes reddened and is sore.	1. Keep skin dry and clean by applying protective ointments containing zinc oxide to areas at risk (eg, buttocks and perineum). 2. Boil an infant's diapers or wash them with an antibacterial detergent to prevent infection. Rinse diapers well, because detergent is irritating to an infant's skin.
Acne Inflammatory condition with papules and pustules.	1. Keep the skin clean to prevent secondary infection. 2. Treatment varies widely.
Erythema Redness associated with a variety of conditions, such as rashes, exposure to sun, elevated body temperature.	1. Wash area carefully to remove excess microorganisms. 2. Apply antiseptic spray or lotion to prevent itching, promote healing, and prevent skin breakdown.
Hirsutism Excessive hair on a person's body and face, particularly in women.	1. Remove unwanted hair by using depilatories, shaving, electrolysis, or tweezing. 2. Enhance client's self-concept. See Chapter 31.

ASSESSMENT INTERVIEW

Skin Hygiene

Skin Care Practices

- What are your usual showering or bathing times?
- What hygienic products do you routinely use (eg, bath oils, powder, facial cleansing creams, body lotions or creams, deodorants, antiperspirants)?
- What facial cosmetic products do you use?
- How and when do you clean make-up applicators and puffs? (Applicators should be kept clean, and products used around the eyes, in particular, should be discarded after 4 months to prevent bacterial and fungal infections.)
- What hygienic or cosmetic products do you not use because of the skin problems they create (eg, skin dryness or allergic reactions)?

Self-Care Abilities

- Do you have any problems managing your hygienic practices (eg, baths and facial care)? If so, what are these?
- How can the nurses best help you?

Skin Problems

- Do you have any tendency toward skin dryness, itchiness, rashes, bruising, excessive perspiration, or lack of perspiration? Have you had skin or scalp lesions in the past?
- Do you have any allergic tendencies? If so, what?

Positive responses to any of these require further exploration in terms of duration (when did it start?) frequency (how often have you had this?); description of lesion or rash; any associated signs, such as fever or nausea; aggravating factors (eg, season of the year, stress, occupation, medication, recent travel, housing, personal contact); alleviating factors (eg, medications, lotions, home remedies); and any family history of the problem.

Table 29–4 Clinical Application: Assessment Data Clusters and Related Nursing Diagnoses for Clients with Skin Problems

Data Cluster	Nursing Diagnosis
Stan Bailey, 75 years old, suffered a "stroke" 2 weeks ago resulting in paralysis of his left side. States, "I don't want a bath. I can wash myself. I just want to be left alone." Is withdrawn and uncommunicative.	**Self care deficit: bathing/hygiene** related to paralyzed left upper and lower limbs and lack of motivation
Mark Drake, a 15-year-old, has facial pustules and papules. Facial skin is inflamed. States, "I hate going to school or anywhere looking like this. I don't think any girl wants to go out with me. Can you do something to get rid of this?"	**Self-esteem disturbance** related to acne

Physical Assessment Physical assessment of the skin, which involves inspection and palpation, is described in Chapter 22, pages 474 to 477. A systematic head-to-toe assessment facilitates collection of data about skin color, uniformity of color, texture, turgor, temperature, intactness, and lesions.

DIAGNOSING

Self-care deficit diagnoses are used for clients who have problems performing hygiene care. Three of NANDA's four self-care deficit diagnoses, specified as **Self-care deficit: bathing/hygiene, Self-care deficit: dressing/grooming,** and **Self-care deficit: toileting** are discussed in this chapter. The fourth diagnosis, **Self-care deficit: feeding** is discussed in Chapter 37. The box on page 734 provides definitions, related factors, and defining characteristics of the first three diagnoses. Clinical examples of assessment data clusters and related nursing diagnoses are shown in Table 29–4.

Other associated diagnoses include the following:

- **Knowledge deficit** related to
  a. Lack of experience with skin condition (acne) and need to prevent secondary infection
  b. New therapeutic regimen to manage skin problem
  c. Lack of experience in providing hygiene care to dependent person
  d. Unfamiliarity with devices available to facilitate sitting on or rising from toilet
- **Self-esteem disturbance** related to
  a. Visible skin problem (eg, acne or alopecia)
  b. Body odor

The diagnoses **High risk for impaired skin integrity** and **Impaired skin integrity** are discussed in Chapter 30.

PLANNING

In planning care, the nurse identifies nursing interventions that will assist the client to achieve the major outcomes of maintaining or improving skin cleanliness,

NURSING DIAGNOSES

CLIENTS WITH HYGIENE PROBLEMS

NURSING DIAGNOSIS: Self-care deficit: bathing/hygiene: A state in which one experiences an impaired ability to perform or complete bathing/hygiene activities for oneself

Defining Characteristics

Inability to

- Wash body or body parts
- Obtain or get to water source
- Regulate water temperature or flow

Related Factors

Activity intolerance; weakness, pain, or discomfort; mental impairment; sensory impairment (eg, visual); neuromuscular or skeletal impairment; psychologic or motivation impairment (eg, depression, severe anxiety); medically prescribed restriction.

NURSING DIAGNOSIS: Self-care deficit: dressing/grooming: A state in which one experiences an impaired ability to perform or complete dressing and grooming activities for oneself

Defining Characteristics

Impaired ability to

- Put on or take off necessary items of clothing
- Obtain or replace articles of clothing
- Fasten clothing
- Maintain appearance at satisfactory level

Related Factors

As above

NURSING DIAGNOSIS: Self-care deficit: toileting: A state in which the individual experiences an impaired ability to perform or complete toileting activities for oneself

Defining Characteristics

Inability to

- Get to toilet or commode
- Sit on or rise from toilet or commode
- Manipulate clothing for toileting
- Carry out proper toilet hygiene
- Flush toilet or empty commode

Related Factors

As above

Sources: LJ Carpenito, *Nursing Diagnosis: Application to Clinical Practice*, 4th ed. (Philadelphia: Lippincott, 1992) pp. 684-86; MJ Kim, GK McFarland, and AM McLane, *Pocket Guide to Nursing Diagnoses*, 5th ed. (St Louis: Mosby-Year Book, 1993), p. 49; GK McFarland and EA McFarlane, *Nursing Diagnosis and Interventions: Planning for Patient Care* (St Louis: Mosby, 1989), p. 382; North American Nursing Diagnosis Association, *NANDA Nursing Diagnoses: Definition and Classification 1992-1993* (Philadelphia: NANDA, 1993), pp. 62-63; JR Lederer, GL Marculescu, B Mocnik, and N Seaby, *Care Planning Pocket Guide—A Nursing Diagnosis Approach*, 5th ed. (Redwood City, CA: Addison-Wesley Nursing, 1993), pp. 164-65.

---

maintaining circulation to the skin, and improving or maintaining a sense of well-being. Nursing interventions may include assisting dependent clients with bathing, skin care, and perineal care, providing back massages to promote circulation, and instructing clients about appropriate hygienic practices and therapies to prevent skin lesions. Although the nursing interventions discussed in this chapter focus on hygienic measures, the etiology of the nursing diagnoses established may point to other interventions that promote circulation, promote self-esteem, restore nutritional status, correct fluid deficits or excesses, or prevent problems associated with immobility. Nursing strategies to deal with these etiologies are provided in other chapters.

Planning to assist a client with personal hygiene includes consideration of the client's personal preferences, health, and limitations; the best time to give the care; and the equipment, facilities, and personnel available. Clients' personal preferences—about when and how to bathe, for example—should be followed as long as they are compatible with the clients' health and the equipment available. Nurses need to provide whatever assistance the client requires, either directly or by delegating this task to other nursing personnel. Examples of outcome criteria, nursing interventions, and rationales are shown in the Care Planning Guide on page 736.

IMPLEMENTING

General Guidelines for Skin Care

1. *An intact, healthy skin is the body's first line of defense.* Nurses need to ensure that all skin care measures prevent injury and irritation. Scratching the skin with jewelry or long, sharp fingernails is avoided. Harsh rubbing or use of rough towels and washcloths can cause tissue damage, particularly when the skin is irritated or when circulation or sensation is diminished. Bottom bedsheets are kept taut and free from wrinkles to reduce friction and abrasion to the skin. Top bed linens are arranged to prevent undue pressure on the toes. When necessary, bed cradles or footboards are used to keep bedclothes off the feet.
2. *The degree to which the skin protects the underlying tissues from injury depends on the general health of the cells, the amount of subcutaneous tissue, and the dryness of the skin.* Skin that is poorly nourished and dry is less able to protect and more vulnerable to injury. When the skin is dry, lotions or creams with lanolin are applied, and bathing is limited to once or twice a week. For back rubs, lotion is used rather than alcohol. The greater the amount of subcutaneous tissue, the more padding there is, particularly over bony prominences. Nurses also assess the client's nutritional and fluid intake. When either one is deficient, measures are taken to improve it.
3. *Moisture in contact with the skin for a period of time can result in increased bacterial growth and irritation.* After a bath, the client's skin is dried carefully. Particular attention is paid to areas such as the axillae, the groin, beneath the breasts, and between the toes, where the potential for irritation is greatest. A nonirritating dusting powder, such as cornstarch, tends to reduce moisture and can be applied to these areas after they are dried. Clients who are incontinent of urine or feces or who perspire excessively are provided with immediate skin care to prevent skin irritation.
4. *Body odors are caused by resident skin bacteria acting on body secretions.* Cleanliness is the best deodorant. Commercial deodorants and antiperspirants can be applied only after the skin is cleaned. Deodorants diminish odors, whereas antiperspirants reduce the amount of perspiration. Neither is applied immediately after shaving, because of the possibility of skin irritation, nor are they used on skin that is already irritated.
5. *Skin sensitivity to irritation and injury varies among individuals and in accordance with their health.* Generally speaking, skin sensitivity is greater in infants, very young children, and the elderly. A person's nutritional status also affects sensitivity. Emaciated or obese persons tend to experience more skin irritation and injury. The same tendency is seen in individuals with poor dietary habits and insufficient fluid intake. Even in healthy persons, skin sensitivity is highly variable. Some people's skin is sensitive to chemicals in skin care agents and cosmetics. Hypoallergenic cosmetics and soaps or soap substitutes are now available for these people. The nurse needs to ascertain whether the client has any sensitivities and what agents are appropriate to use.
6. *Agents used for skin care have selective actions and purposes.* Commonly used agents are described in Table 29–5.

Table 29–5 Agents Commonly Used on the Skin

Type	Description
Soap	Lowers surface tension and thus helps in cleaning. Some soaps contain antibacterial agents, which can change the natural flora of the skin.
Detergent	Used instead of soap for cleaning. Some people who are allergic to soaps may not be allergic to detergents, and vice versa.
Bath oil	Used in bath water; provides an oily film on the skin that softens and prevents chapping. Oils can make the tub surface slippery, and clients should be instructed about safety measures (eg, using nonskid tub surface or mat). 
Skin cream, lotion	Provides a film on the skin that prevents evaporation and therefore chapping.
Powder	Can be used to absorb water and prevent friction. For example, powder under the breasts can prevent skin irritation. Some powders are antibacterial.
Deodorant	Masks or diminishes body odors.
Antiperspirant	Reduces the amount of perspiration.

CARE PLANNING GUIDE

CLIENTS WITH HYGIENE PROBLEMS

NURSING DIAGNOSIS: Self-care deficit: bathing/hygiene, dressing/grooming, toileting

Outcome Criteria	Nursing Interventions	Rationale
The client		
▪ Makes decisions and states preferences regarding hygienic care appropriate for health limitations.	Discuss the agency's bathing routines with the client, and consider the client's personal preferences (eg, tub or shower if bed bath not indicated), desired grooming products, and best time for care. Consider other care the client is receiving (eg, physiotherapy).	A sense of control enhances self-respect and self-esteem.
▪ Participates in self-care to optimal level of capacity.	Clearly identify the client's functional level for bathing/hygiene, dressing/grooming, and toileting (see Table 29–2, page 732).	This prevents overtaxing the client's energy level and capacities and promotes as much independence as possible.
	Explore use of appropriate assistive devices, particularly for tub and toileting (eg, tub transfer seat, commode grab bars, raised toilet seat).	Appropriate devices can increase the client's independence and self-sufficiency.
	Provide pain medications as indicated before care.	Discomfort and pain decrease capacity to perform self-care.
	Assist the client as needed to bathe, use the bedpan or commode, and dress and comb hair, in accordance with functional level.	Appropriate assistance prevents client fatigue and injury.
	Encourage the client to do as much as possible for self (eg, dress self, with the nurse only obtaining clothing from closet and laying out clothing in the proper order).	This maintains functional capacity and self-esteem.
	Monitor all self-care activities to determine energy expenditure and activity tolerance; assess vital signs and observe the client for signs of fatigue or discouragement.	Adverse signs indicate the need for more assistance.
	Observe for signs of readiness to increase the amount of self-care.	Revision of functional level status is necessary to ensure optimal self-care activity.
▪ Demonstrates optimal hygiene, as evidenced by clean, soft, odor-free, intact skin and pleasant grooming.	Assess outcomes of the client's self-care (eg, skin cleanliness and integrity, and grooming).	Early detection of problems promotes prompt nursing intervention.
	Teach the client about specific skin problems and care (eg, dryness, rash, acne) as indicated. See the Client Teaching box on page 744.	Knowledge may enhance use of preventive measures to avoid a recurrence of problems or complications.
	Dry the skin thoroughly after each cleaning, and apply lotion after the bath.	Retained moisture can cause skin maceration. Lotion softens the skin and prevents excessive dryness.
	Give perineal care after voiding and defecation as required.	Accumulated secretions cause odor and act as a reservoir for infection.

Bathing and Skin Care Bathing removes accumulated oil, perspiration, dead skin cells, and some bacteria. The nurse can appreciate the quantity of oil and dead skin cells produced when observing a person after the removal of a cast that has been on for 6 weeks. The skin is crusty, flaky, and dry underneath the cast. Applications of oil over several days are usually necessary to remove the debris.

Excessive bathing, however, can interfere with the intended lubricating effect of the sebum, causing dryness of the skin. This is an important consideration, especially for the elderly, who produce less sebum.

In addition to cleaning the skin, bathing also stimulates circulation. A warm or hot bath dilates superficial arterioles, bringing more blood and nourishment to the skin. Vigorous rubbing has the same effect. Rubbing with long smooth strokes from the distal to proximal parts of extremities (from the point farthest from the body to the point closest) is particularly effective in facilitating venous blood flow.

Bathing also produces a sense of well-being. It is refreshing and relaxing and frequently improves morale, appearance, and self-respect. Some people take a morning shower for its refreshing, stimulating effect. Others prefer an evening bath because it is relaxing. These effects are more evident when a person is ill. For example, it is not uncommon for clients who have had a restless or sleepless night to feel relaxed, comfortable, and sleepy after a morning bath.

Bathing offers an excellent opportunity for the nurse to assess ill clients. The nurse can observe the condition of the client's skin and physical conditions such as sacral edema or rashes. While assisting a client with a bath, the nurse can also assess the client's psychosocial needs, such as orientation to time and ability to cope with the illness. Learning needs, such as a diabetic client's need to learn foot care, can also be assessed.

Because of the increasing acuity of hospitalized clients, many clients receive intravenous therapy. Easy-to-remove gowns are now available that have velcro or snap fasteners along the sleeves. If a special gown is not available, the nurse needs to pay special attention when changing the client's gown after the bath (or whenever the gown becomes soiled). General Guidelines are provided in the accompanying box. These guidelines do not apply if the client has an IV pump or controller. In this situation, use a special gown or do not put the sleeve of a gown over the client's involved arm.

CHANGING A HOSPITAL GOWN FOR A CLIENT WITH AN INTRAVENOUS INFUSION

- Slip the gown completely off the arm without the infusion and onto the tubing connected to the arm with the infusion.
- Holding the container above the client's arm, slide the sleeve up over the container to remove the used gown.
- Place the clean gown sleeve for the arm with the infusion over the container as if it were an extension of the client's arm, from the inside of the gown to the sleeve cuff.
- Rehang the container. Slide the gown carefully over the tubing toward the client's hand.
- Guide the client's arm and tubing into the sleeve, taking care not to pull on the tubing.
- Assist the client to put the other arm into the second sleeve of the gown, and fasten as usual.
- Count the rate of flow of the infusion to make sure it is correct before leaving the bedside.

There are generally two categories of baths given to clients: cleaning and therapeutic. *Cleaning baths* are given chiefly for hygiene purposes and include these types:

- *Complete bed bath.* The nurse washes the entire body of a dependent client in bed.
- *Self-help bed bath.* Clients confined to bed are able to bathe themselves with help from the nurse for washing the back and perhaps the feet.
- *Partial bath (abbreviated bath).* Only the parts of the client's body that might cause discomfort or odor, if neglected, are washed: the face, hands, axillae, perineal area, and back. Omitted are the arms, chest abdomen, legs, and feet. The nurse provides this care for dependent clients and assists self-sufficient clients confined to bed by washing their backs. Some ambulatory clients prefer to take a partial bath at the sink. The nurse can assist them by washing their backs.
- *Tub bath.* Tub baths are preferred to bed baths, because it is easier to wash and rinse in a tub. Tubs are also used for therapeutic baths. The amount of assistance the nurse offers depends on the abilities of the client. Many agencies have specially designed tubs for dependent clients. These tubs greatly reduce the work of the nurse in lifting clients in and out of the tub and offer greater benefits than a sponge bath in bed.
- *Shower.* Many ambulatory clients are able to use shower facilities and require only minimal assistance from the nurse.

The water should feel comfortably warm to the client. People vary in their sensitivity to heat; generally, the temperature should be 43 to 46 C (110 to 115 F). Most clients will verify a suitable temperature. The water for a bed bath should be changed at least once.

Therapeutic baths, which are usually ordered by a physician, are given for physical effects, such as to soothe

CRITICAL THINKING CHALLENGE

WHAT WOULD YOU DO?

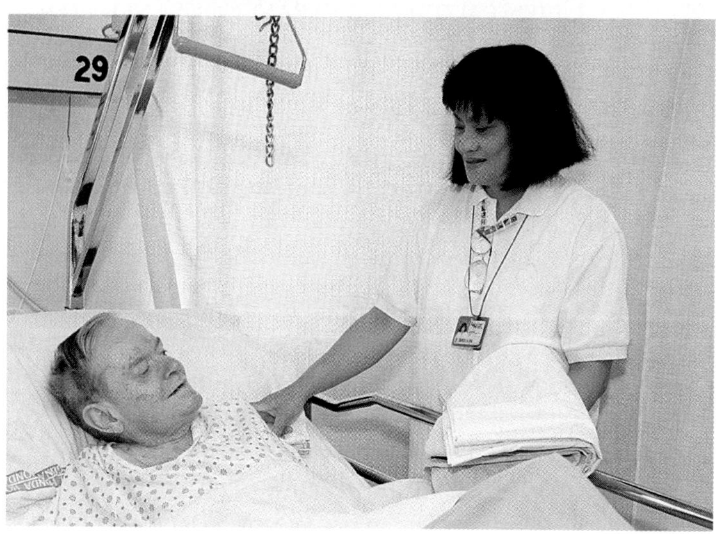

Ian Witkowski, a 62-year-old male, is assigned to your care. He is ambulatory and able to perform self-care for bathing and toileting. He has completed his morning care and is resting comfortably in bed. When you ask to change his bed linens, he responds, "They are just fine, and I'd rather rest."

What would you do?

Table 29–6 Types of Therapeutic Baths

Bath Solution	Directions	Uses
Saline	4 mL (1 tsp) sodium chloride (NaCl) to 500 mL (1 pt) water.	Has a cooling effect. Cleans. Decreases skin irritation.
Oatmeal or Aveeno	720 mL (3 cups) cooked oatmeal in a cheesecloth bag. Tie the bag securely and twirl it in the tub until the water is opalescent.	Soothes skin irritations. Softens and lubricates dry, scaly skin.
Cornstarch	0.45 kg (1 lb) cornstarch in sufficient cold water to dissolve it; then add boiling water until the mixture is thick. Add to the tub water.	Soothes skin irritation.
Sodium bicarbonate	4 mL (1 tsp) sodium bicarbonate to 500 mL (1 pt) water, or 120–360 mL (4–12 oz) to 120 liters (30 gal).	Has cooling effect. Relieves skin irritation.
Potassium permanganate ($KMnO_4$)	Available in tablets, which are crushed, dissolved in a little water, and added to the bath.	Cleans and disinfects. Treats infected skin areas.

irritated skin or to treat an area (eg, the perineum). Medications may be placed in the water. A therapeutic bath is generally taken in a tub one-third or one-half full, about 114 liters (30 gal). The client remains in the bath for a designated time, often 20 to 30 minutes. If the client's back, chest, and arms are to be treated, these areas need to be immersed in the solution. The bath temperature is generally included in the order; 37.7 to 46 C (100 to 115 F) may be ordered for adults and 40.5 C (105 F) is usually ordered for infants. See Table 29–6 for types of therapeutic baths. Procedure 29–1 provides guidelines for bathing clients.

Text continued on page 742

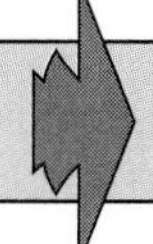

PROCEDURE 29–1 BATHING AN ADULT OR PEDIATRIC CLIENT

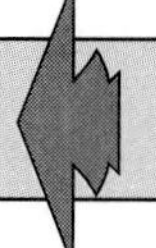

Before bathing a client, determine: (a) the type of bath the client needs and what assistance the client requires; (b) other care the client is receiving, such as roentgenography or physiotherapy, so that the bath can be coordinated with those activities to prevent undue fatigue; and (c) the bed linen required.

When bathing a client who is HIV positive, the caregiver should wear gloves when in the presence of body fluids or open lesions.

PURPOSES

- To remove transient microorganisms, body secretions and excretions, and dead skin cells
- To stimulate circulation to the skin
- To produce a sense of well-being
- To promote relaxation and comfort
- To prevent or eliminate unpleasant body odors

ASSESSMENT FOCUS

Condition of the skin (color, texture and turgor, presence of pigmented spots, temperature, lesions, excoriations, and abrasions); fatigue; presence of pain and need for adjunctive measures (eg, an analgesic) before the bath; range of motion of the joints and any other aspects of health that affect the bathing process.

EQUIPMENT

- ☐ Bedpan or urinal
- ☐ Changing table
- ☐ Bath blanket
- ☐ Gloves (if giving perineal care)
- ☐ Washcloth
- ☐ Soap
- ☐ Basin
- ☐ Water between 43 and 46 C (110 and 115 F) for adults, 38 and 40 C (100 and 105 F) for children
- ☐ Two bath towels
- ☐ Additional bed linen and towels, if required
- ☐ Hygiene supplies such as lotion, powder, and deodorant
- ☐ Clean gown or pajamas as needed

INTERVENTION

1. Prepare the client and the environment.

- Invite a parent or family member to participate if desired.
- Close the windows and doors to make sure that the room is free from drafts. *Air currents increase loss of heat from the body by convection.*
- Provide privacy by drawing the curtains or closing the door. *Hygiene is a personal matter.* Some agencies provide signs indicating the need for privacy.
- Offer the client a bedpan or urinal or ask whether the client wishes to use the toilet or commode. *The client will be more comfortable after voiding, and voiding before cleaning the perineum is advisable.*
- During the bath, assess each area of the skin carefully.

For a Bed Bath

2. Prepare the bed, and position the client appropriately.

- Place the bed in the high position. Place an infant or small child on a changing table or elevated crib. *This avoids undue strain on the nurse's back.*
- Remove the top bed linen, and replace it with the bath blanket. If the bed linen is to be reused, place it over the bedside chair. If it is to be changed, place it in the linen hamper.
- Assist the client to move near you. *This facilitates access without undue reaching and straining.*
- Remove the gown.

3. Make a bath mitt with the washcloth (Figure 29–1, p. 740). *A bath mitt retains water and heat better than a cloth loosely held.*

- Triangular method: (1) Lay your hand on the washcloth; (2) fold the top corner over your hand; (3,4) fold the side corners over your hand; (5) tuck the second corner under the cloth on the palmar side to secure the mitt.
- Rectangular method: (1) Lay your hand on the washcloth, and fold one side over your hand; (2) fold the second side over your hand; (3) fold the top of the cloth down; and (4) tuck it under the folded side against your palm to secure the mitt.

4. Wash the face.

- Place one towel across the client's chest.

PROCEDURE 29–1 BATHING AN ADULT OR PEDIATRIC CLIENT *continued*

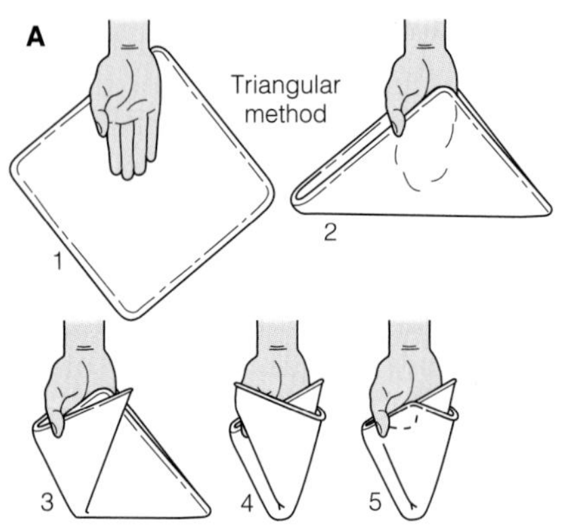

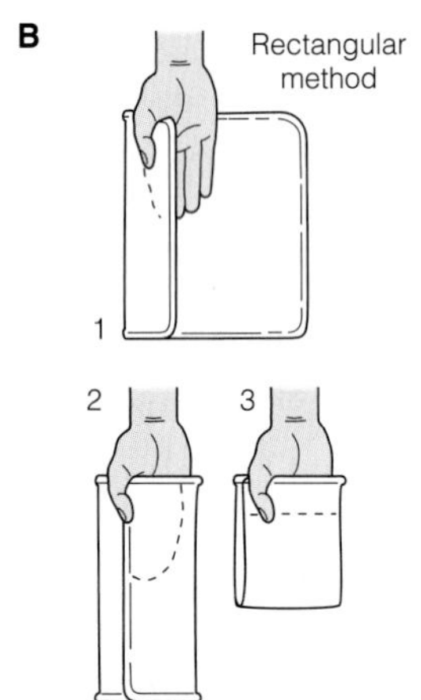

Figure 29–1 Making a bath mitt: *A*, triangular method; *B*, rectangular method.

- Wash the client's eyes with water only, and dry them well. Use a separate corner of the washcloth for each eye. *Using separate corners prevents transmitting microorganisms from one eye to the other.* Wipe from the inner to the outer canthus. *Cleaning from the inner to the outer canthus prevents secretions from entering the nasolacrimal ducts.*
- Ask whether the client wants soap used on the face. *Soap has a drying effect, and the face, which is exposed to the air more than other body parts, tends to be drier.*
- Wash, rinse, and dry the client's face, neck, and ears.

5. Wash the arms and hands.

- Place the bath towel lengthwise under the arm. *It protects the bed from becoming wet.*
- Wash, rinse, and dry the arm, using long, firm strokes from distal to proximal areas (from the point farthest from the body to the point closest. *Firm strokes from distal to proximal areas increase venous blood return.*
- Wash the axilla well. Repeat for the other arm. (Omit the arms for a partial bath.) Exercise caution if an intravenous infusion is present, and check its flow after moving the arm.
- Place a towel directly on the bed, and put the basin on it. Place the client's hands in the basin. *Many clients enjoy immersing their hands in the basin and washing themselves.* Assist the client as needed to wash, rinse, and dry the hands, paying particular attention to the spaces between the fingers.

6. Wash the chest and abdomen.

- Fold the bath blanket down to the client's pubic area, and place the towel alongside the chest and abdomen.
- Wash, rinse, and dry the chest and abdomen, giving special attention to the skinfold under the breasts. Keep the chest and abdomen covered with the towel between the wash and the rinse.
- Replace the bath blanket when the areas have been dried. (Omit the chest and abdomen for a partial bath. However, the creases under a woman's breasts may require bathing if they are irritated.) Avoid undue exposure when washing the chest and abdomen. For some clients, it may be preferable to wash the chest and the abdomen separately. In that case, place the bath towel horizontally across the abdomen first and then across the chest.

7. Wash the legs and feet.

- Wrap one of the client's legs and feet with the bath blanket, ensuring that the pubic area is well covered (Figure 29–2).

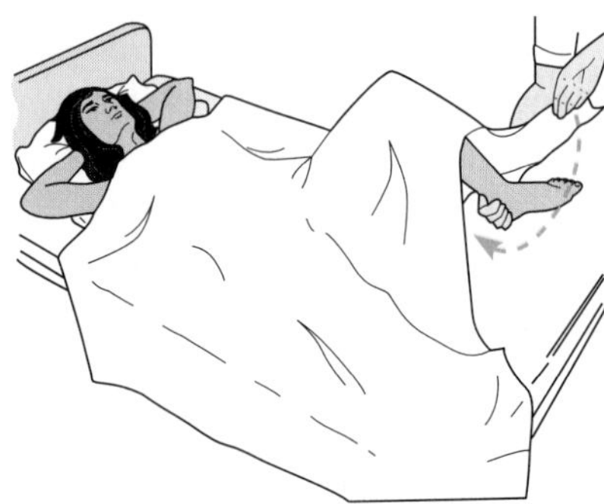

Figure 29–2 Draping one leg of the client.

- Place the bath towel lengthwise under the other leg, and wash that leg. Use long, smooth, firm strokes, washing from the ankle to the knee to the thigh. *Washing from distal to proximal areas stimulates venous blood flow.*
- Rinse and dry that leg, reverse the coverings, and repeat for the other leg. (Omit legs and feet for a partial bath.)
- Wash the feet by placing them in the basin of water.
- Dry each foot. Pay particular attention to the spaces between the toes. If you prefer, wash one foot after that leg, before washing the other leg.
- Obtain fresh, warm bath water now or when necessary. *Water may become dirty or cold.* Because surface skin cells are removed with washing, the bath water from dark-skinned clients may be dark; however this does not mean the client is dirty.

PROCEDURE 29–1 *continued*

8. Wash the back and then the perineum.

- Assist the client to turn to a prone position or side-lying position facing away from you, and place the bath towel lengthwise alongside the back and buttocks.
- Wash and dry the back, buttocks, and upper thighs, paying particular attention to the gluteal folds. Avoid undue exposure of the client, as for the abdomen and chest. See above.
- Assist the client to the supine position, and determine whether the client can wash the perineal–genital area independently. If the client cannot do so, drape the client as shown in Figure 29–3 on page 743, and wash the area. See Procedure 29–2.

9. Assist the client with grooming aids such as powder, lotion, or deodorant.

- Use powder sparingly. Release as little as possible into the atmosphere. *This will avoid irritation of the respiratory tract by powder inhalation.*
- Help the clients to put on a clean gown or pajamas.
- Assist the client to care for hair, mouth, and nails. Some people prefer or need mouth care prior to the bath.

10. Document pertinent data.

- Record assessments, such as excoriation in the folds beneath the breasts or reddened areas over bony prominences as well as progress in relief of the client's previous problems.
- Record the type of bath given (ie, complete, partial, or self-help). This is usually recorded on a flow sheet.

For a Tub Bath or Shower

11. Prepare the client and the tub.

- Fill the tub about one-third to one-half full of water at 43 to 46 C (110 to 115 F). *Sufficient water is needed to cover the perineal area.*
- Cover all intravenous catheters or wound dressings with plastic coverings, and instruct client to prevent wetting area if possible.
- Secure assistance with holding a pediatric client as indicated. *Holding minimizes contamination of open skin areas.*

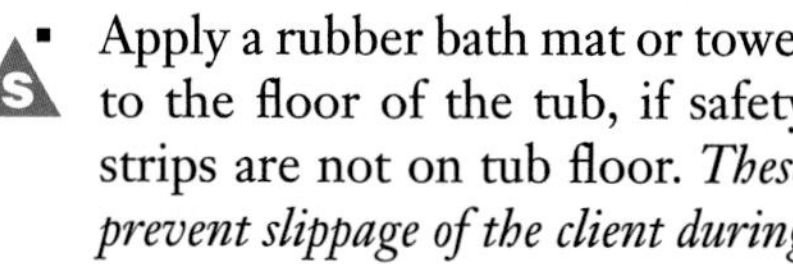

- Apply a rubber bath mat or towel to the floor of the tub, if safety strips are not on tub floor. *These prevent slippage of the client during the bath or shower.*
- Use a small basin or large sink for a small child. *Smaller containers decrease the danger of slippage of an active child and possible drowning.*

12. Assist the client into the shower or tub.

- Assist the client taking a standing shower with the initial adjustment of the water temperature and water flow pressure, as needed. Some clients need a chair to sit in the shower because of weakness. Elderly people often feel faint under hot water.
- If the client requires considerable assistance with a tub bath, a second nurse may be needed. To provide support as the client sits down in the tub, fold a towel lengthwise, and place it around the chest under both axillae; then hold the ends securely at the back as the client sits. It may be helpful to seat the client on the edge of the tub or on a chair beside the tub before transferring the client into the tub.

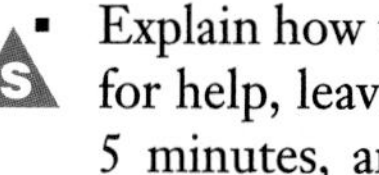

- Explain how the client can signal for help, leave the client for 2 to 5 minutes, and place an "occupied" sign on the door.

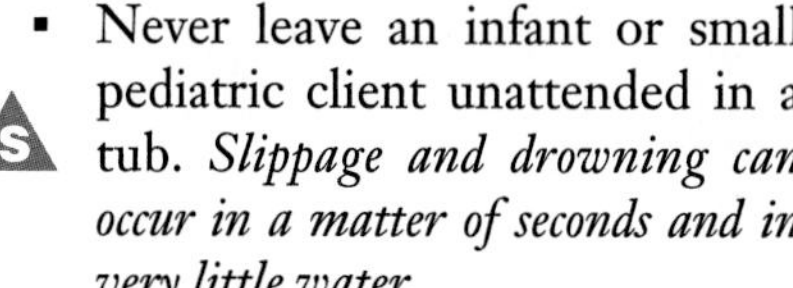

- Never leave an infant or small pediatric client unattended in a tub. *Slippage and drowning can occur in a matter of seconds and in very little water.*

13. Assist the client with washing and getting out of the tub.

- Wash the client's back, lower legs, and feet, if necessary.
- Assist the client out of the tub. If the client is unsteady, drain the tub of water before the client attempts to get out of it, and place a bath towel over the client's shoulders. *Draining the water first lessens the likelihood of a fall. The towel prevents chilling.*

14. Dry the client, and assist with follow-up care.

- Follow step 9.
- Assist the client back to the room.
- Clean the tub or shower in accordance with agency practice, discard used linen in the laundry hamper, and place the "unoccupied" sign on the door.

15. Document pertinent data.

- Follow step 10.

EVALUATION FOCUS

Client tolerance of procedure (note respiratory rate and effort, and pulse rate); status of skin (dryness, turgor, lesions, and so on); client strength and percentage of bath done without assistance.

Perineal–Genital Care Perineal–genital care is also referred to as *perineal care* or *peri-care*. Perineal care is a part of the bed bath that may be an embarrassing procedure for many clients. Nurses also may find it embarrassing initially, particularly with clients of the opposite sex. Most clients who require a bed bath from the nurse are able to clean their own genital areas with minimal assistance. The nurse may need to hand a moistened washcloth and soap to the client, rinse the washcloth, and provide a towel.

Because some clients are unfamilir with terminology for the genitals and perineum, it may be difficult for nurses to explain what is expected. Most clients, however, understand what is meant if the nurse simply says, "I'll give you a washcloth to finish your bath." Older clients may be familiar with the term *private parts*. Whatever expression the nurse uses, it needs to be one that the client understands and one that is comfortable for the nurse to use.

The nurse needs to provide perineal care efficiently and matter-of-factly. Some nurses wear gloves while providing this care for the comfort of the client and to protect themselves from infection. Procedure 29–2 explains how to provide perineal–genital care.

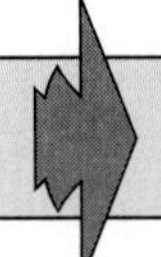

PROCEDURE 29–2 PROVIDING PERINEAL–GENITAL CARE

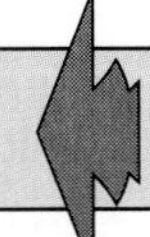

PURPOSES

- To remove normal perineal secretions and odors
- To prevent infection (eg, when an indwelling catheter is present)
- To promote client comfort

ASSESSMENT FOCUS

Presence of irritation, excoriation, inflammation, swelling; excessive discharge; odor; pain or discomfort; presence of urinary or fecal incontinence; recent rectal or perineal surgery; presence of indwelling catheter; perineal–genital hygiene practices; self-care abilities.

EQUIPMENT

Perineal–genital care provided in conjunction with the bed bath

- ☐ Bath towel
- ☐ Bath blanket
- ☐ Disposable gloves
- ☐ Bath basin two-thirds filled with water at 43 to 46 C (110 to 115 F)
- ☐ Soap
- ☐ Washcloth
- ☐ Protective ointment as required

Special perineal–genital care

- ☐ Bath towel
- ☐ Bath blanket
- ☐ Disposable gloves
- ☐ Cotton balls or swabs
- ☐ Solution bottle, pitcher, or container filled with warm water or a prescribed solution
- ☐ Bedpan to receive rinse water
- ☐ Moisture-resistant bag or receptacle for used cotton swabs
- ☐ Perineal pad

INTERVENTION

1. Prepare the client.

- Offer the client an appropriate explanation, being particularly sensitive to any embarrassment felt by the client.
- Determine whether the client is experiencing any discomfort in the perineal–genital area.
- Fold the top bed linen to the foot of the bed, and fold the gown up to expose the genital area.
- Place a bath towel under the client's hips so that the lower end can be used to dry the anterior perineum, while the upper end can dry the rectal area. *The bath towel also prevents the bed from becoming soiled.*

2. Position and drape the client, and clean the upper inner thighs.

For Females

- Position the female in a back-lying position, with the knees flexed and spread well apart (abducted).
- Cover her body and legs with the bath blanket. Drape the legs by tucking the bottom corners of the bath blanket under the inner sides of the legs (Figure 29–3). *Minimum exposure lessens embarrassment and helps to provide warmth.* Bring the middle portion of the base of the blanket up over the pubic area.

- Don gloves, and wash and dry the upper inner thighs.

PROCEDURE 29–2 *continued*

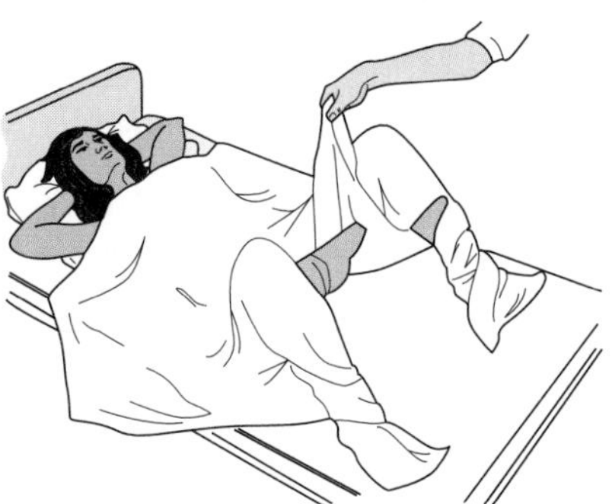

Figure 29–3 Draping the client for perineal–genital care.

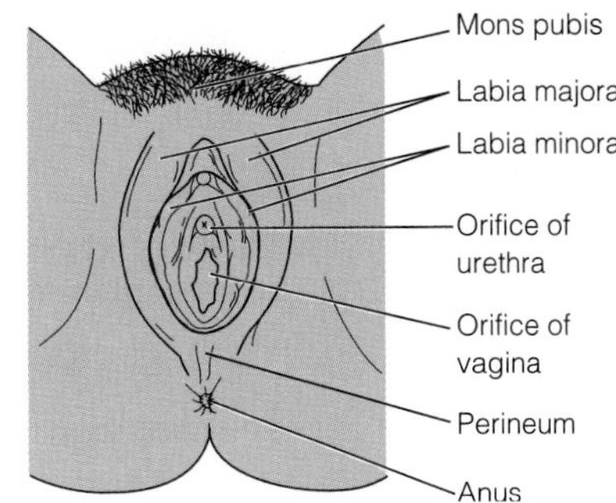

Figure 29–4 Female genitals.

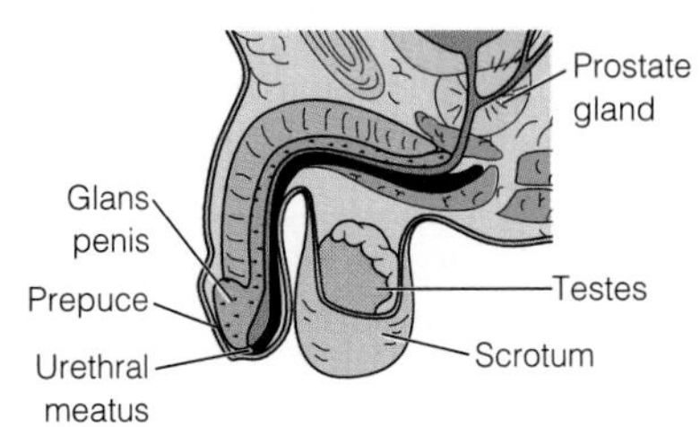

Figure 29–5 Male genitals.

For Males

- Position the male client in a supine position with knees slightly flexed and hips slightly externally rotated.
- Don gloves, and wash and dry the upper inner thighs.

3. Inspect the perineal area.

- Note particular areas of inflammation, excoriation, or swelling, especially between the labia in females and the scrotal folds in males.
- Also note excessive discharge or secretions from the orifices and the presence of odors.

4. Wash and dry the perineal–genital area.

For Females

- Clean the labia majora. Then spread the labia to wash the folds between the labia majora and the labia minora (Figure 29–4). *Secretions that tend to collect around the labia minora facilitate bacterial growth.*
- Use separate quarters of the washcloth for each stroke, and wipe from the pubis to the rectum. For menstruating women and clients with indwelling catheters, use cotton balls or gauze. Take a clean ball for each stroke. *Using separate quarters of the washcloth or new cotton balls or gauzes prevents the transmission of microorganisms from one area to the other. Wipe from the area of least contamination (the pubis) to that of greatest (the rectum).*
- Rinse the area well. You may place the client on a bedpan and pour a pitcher of warm water over the area. Dry the perineum thoroughly, paying particular attention to the folds between the labia. *Moisture supports the growth of many microorganisms.*

For Males

- Wash and dry the penis, using firm strokes. *Handling the penis firmly may prevent an erection.*
- If the client is uncircumcised, retract the prepuce (foreskin) to expose the glans penis (the tip of the penis) for cleaning. Replace the foreskin after cleaning the glans penis (Figure 29–5). *Retracting the foreskin is necessary to remove the smegma that collects under the foreskin and facilitates bacterial growth.*
- Wash and dry the scrotum. The posterior folds of the scrotum may need to be cleaned with the buttocks. *The scrotum tends to be more soiled than the penis because of its proximity to the rectum; thus it is usually cleaned after the penis.*

5. Inspect perineal orifices for intactness.

- Inspect particularly around the urethra in clients with indwelling catheters. *A catheter may cause excoriation around the urethra.*
- Apply protective ointment, if necessary.

6. Clean between the buttocks.

- Assist the client to turn on the side facing away from you.
- Pay particular attention to the anal area and posterior folds of the scrotum in males. Clean the anus with toilet tissue before washing it, if necessary.
- Dry the area well.
- Apply protective ointments, such as petroleum jelly, if necessary.
- For postdelivery or menstruating females, apply a perineal pad as needed from front to back. *This prevents contamination of vagina and urethra from anal area.*

7. Document any assessments (redness, swelling, discharge).

EVALUATION FOCUS
Perineal–genital skin integrity; presence of inflammation, excoriation, swelling, discharge; localized areas of tenderness.

CLIENT TEACHING

Skin Problems and Care

Dry Skin

- Use cleansing creams to clean the skin rather than soap or detergent, which cause drying and, in some cases, allergic reactions.
- Use bath oils, but take precautions to prevent falls caused by slippery tub surfaces.
- Thoroughly rinse soap or detergent, if used, from the skin.
- Bathe less frequently when environmental temperature and humidity are low.
- Increase fluid intake.
- Humidify the air with a humidifier or by keeping a tub or sink full of water.
- Use moisturizing or emollient creams that contain lanolin, petroleum jelly, or cocoa butter to retain skin moisture.

Skin Rashes

- Keep the area clean by washing it with a mild soap. Rinse the skin well, and pat it dry.
- To relieve itching, try a tepid bath or soak. Some over-the-counter preparations, such as Caladryl lotion, may help but should be used with full knowledge of the product.
- Avoid scratching the rash to prevent inflammation, infection, and further skin lesions.
- Choose clothing carefully. Too much can cause perspiration and aggravate a rash.
- Consult a physician if symptoms persist.

Acne

- Wash the face frequently with soap or detergent and hot water to remove oil and dirt.
- Avoid using oily creams, which aggravate the condition.
- Avoid using cosmetics that block the ducts of the sebaceous glands and the hair follicles.
- Never squeeze or pick at the lesions. This increases the potential for infection and scarring.
- Avoid foods such as chocolate, nuts, and colas, *if* they exaggerate the problem after they are ingested.
- Obtain adequate rest and moderate exercise.
- Consult a physician if the problem is severe.

Table 29–7 Examples of Evaluating Outcome Achievement for Clients with Bathing/Hygiene Self-Care Deficits

Outcome Criteria	Evaluation Activities	Evaluation Statements
Makes decisions and states preferences regarding hygiene care appropriate for health limitation.	Check client's records for documentation of this data.	Chose tub bath over shower. Verbalized need for help in and out of tub. Stated brought own grooming aids (soap, lotion). Dec. 1/94
Participates in self-care to optimal level of capacity.	Observe what hygiene care client is able and not able to carry out.	Completed all bathing/hygiene self-care except back and feet. Dec. 2/94
Demonstrates optimal hygiene with assistance, as manifested by clean, soft, odor-free, intact skin and pleasant grooming.	Inspect all skin surfaces and grooming.	Skin intact, warm, smooth and soft. Daughter did client's hair and applied make-up. Dec. 2/94

Client Teaching Clients often need information about dry skin, skin rashes, diaper rash, and acne (described in Chapter 25, page 620). The box at the left provides some guidelines for these problems.

EVALUATING

Using data collected during care, the nurse judges whether client outcomes have been achieved. Table 29–7 includes examples of evaluation activities associated with the outcome criteria established in the planning phase.

If the outcomes are not achieved, the nurse explores reasons why, for example:

- Did the nurse overestimate the client's functional abilities (physical, mental, emotional) for self-care?
- Were provided instructions not clear?
- Were appropriate assistive devices or supplies not available to the client?
- Did the client's condition change?
- Were required analgesics provided before hygienic care?

- What currently prescribed medications and therapies could affect the client's abilities or tissue integrity?
- Is the client's fluid and food intake adequate or appropriate to maintain skin and mucous membrane moisture and integrity?

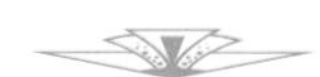

THE FEET

The feet are essential for ambulation and merit attention even when people are confined to bed. Each foot contains 26 bones, 107 ligaments, and 19 muscles. These structures function together for both standing and walking.

DEVELOPMENTAL VARIATIONS

At birth, a baby's foot is relatively unformed. The arches are supported by fatty pads and do not take their full shape until 5 to 6 years of age. During childhood, the bones and small muscles of the feet are easily damaged by tight, binding stockings and ill-fitting shoes. For normal development, it is important that the arches be supported and that the bony structure and the feet grow with no external restrictions. Feet are not fully grown until about age 20. Healthy feet remain relatively unchanged during life. However, the elderly often require special attention for their feet. For example, reduced blood supply and accompanying arteriosclerosis can make a foot prone to infection following trauma.

ASSESSING

Nursing History The nurse determines the client's history of (a) normal nail and foot care practices; (b) type of footwear worn; (c) self-care abilities; (d) presence of factors that place the client at risk for foot problems; (e) any foot discomfort; and (f) any perceived problems with foot mobility. To elicit such data, the nurse asks the client the questions in the box at the right.

ASSESSMENT INTERVIEW

Foot Hygiene

Foot Care Practices

- How often do you wash your feet and cut your toenails?
- What hygiene products do you usually use on your feet (eg, soap, foot powder or deodorant, lotion, or cream)?
- What type of shoes and socks (stockings) do you wear?
- How often do you change your socks or put on clean socks?
- Do you ever go barefoot? If so, when, where, and how often?

Self-Care Abilities

- Do you have any problems managing your foot care? If so, what are these?
- How can the nurses best help you?

Foot Problems and Risk Factors

- Do you have any problems with foot odor?
- Do you have any foot discomfort? If so, where? When does this occur? What do you do to relieve the discomfort? Does this discomfort affect how you walk?
- Have you noticed any problems with foot mobility (eg, joint stiffness)?
- Do you have diabetes, any circulatory problems with feet (eg, swelling, changes in skin color, arthritis), or any instances of prolonged exposure to chemicals or water?

Physical Assessment Each foot and toe is inspected for shape, size, and presence of lesions and is palpated to assess areas of tenderness, edema, and circulatory status. Normally, the toes are straight and flat. See Table 29–8 on page 746 for physical assessment methods for the feet. Common foot problems include calluses, corns, unpleasant odors, plantar warts, fissures between the toes, and fungal infections, such as athlete's foot.

A **callus** is a thickened portion of epidermis, a mass of keratotic material. Calluses are usually painless and flat and found on the bottom or side of the foot over a bony prominence. Calluses are usually caused by pressure from shoes. They can be softened by soaking the foot in warm water with Epsom salts, and they can be abraded by pumice stones or similar abrasives. Creams with lanolin help to keep the skin soft and prevent the formation of calluses.

A **corn** is a keratosis caused by friction and pressure from a shoe. It commonly occurs on a toe, usually the fourth or fifth toe, and usually on a bony prominence such as a joint. Corns are usually conical (circular and raised). The base is the surface of the corn and the apex is in deeper tissues, sometimes even attached to bone. Corns are generally removed surgically. They are prevented from reforming by relieving the pressure on the area (ie, wearing comfortable shoes), and massaging the tissue to promote circulation. The use of oval corn pads should be avoided, since they increase pressure and decrease circulation.

Table 29–8 Assessment of the Feet

Method	Normal Findings	Deviations from Normal
Inspect all skin surfaces, particularly between the toes, for cleanliness, odor, dryness, inflammation, swelling, abrasions, or other lesions.	Intact skin Absence of swelling or inflammation	Excessive dryness Areas of inflammation or swelling (eg, corns, calluses) Fissures Scaling and cracking of skin (eg, athlete's foot) Plantar warts
Palpate anterior and posterior surfaces of ankle and feet for edema.	No swelling	Swelling or pitting edema. See Chapter 22, page 476.
Palpate dorsalis pedis pulse on dorsal surface of foot just above longitudinal arch.	Strong, regular pulses in both feet	Weak or absent pulses
Compare skin temperatures of two feet.	Warm skin temperature	Cool skin temperature in one or both feet

Unpleasant odors occur as a result of perspiration and its interaction with microorganisms. Regular and frequent washing of the feet and wearing clean hosiery help to minimize odor. Foot powders and deodorants also help to prevent this problem.

Plantar warts appear on the sole of the foot. These warts are caused by the virus papovavirus hominis. They are moderately contagious. The warts are frequently painful and often make walking difficult. The physician may curettage the warts, freeze them with solid carbon dioxide several times, or apply salicylic acid.

Fissures, or deep grooves, frequently occur between the toes as a result of dryness and cracking of the skin. The treatment of choice is good foot hygiene and application of an antiseptic to prevent infection. Often a small piece of gauze is inserted between the toes in applying the antiseptic and left in place to assist healing by allowing air to reach the area.

Athlete's foot, or **tinea pedis** (ringworm of the foot), is caused by a fungus. The symptoms are scaling and cracking of the skin, particularly between the toes. Sometimes small blisters form, containing a thin fluid. In severe cases, the lesions may also appear on other parts of the body, particularly the hands. Treatments vary from potassium permanganate soaks, using a 1:8000 solution, to application of commercial antifungal ointments or powders. Prevention is important. Common preventive measures are keeping the feet well ventilated, drying the feet well after bathing, wearing clean socks or stockings, and not going barefoot in public showers.

An **ingrown toenail,** the growing inward of the nail into the soft tissues around the nails, most often results from improper nail trimming. Pressure applied to the area causes localized pain. Treatment involves frequent, hot antiseptic soaks and surgical removal of the portion of nail embedded in the skin. Prevent of recurrence involves appropriate instruction and adherence to proper nail-trimming techniques.

DIAGNOSING

A number of nursing diagnoses may apply to clients with foot or foot care problems. The most common diagnoses, along with possible contributing factors, are as follows:

- **Self-care deficit** related to
  a. Visual impairment
  b. Impaired hand coordination
  c. Other contributing factors (see the Nursing Diagnoses box on page 754)
- **High risk for impaired skin integrity** related to
  a. Altered tissue perfusion: peripheral (associated with edema, inadequate arterial circulation)
  b. Poorly fitting shoes
- **Impaired skin integrity** related to
  a. Ineffective hygiene practices
  b. Altered tissue perfusion: peripheral
- **High risk for infection** related to
  a. Impaired skin integrity (ingrown toenail, corn, trauma)
  b. Deficient nail or foot care
- **Pain** related to Impaired skin integrity (corn, ingrown toenail)
- **Knowledge deficit** (diabetic foot care) related to
  a. Lack of exposure to information
  b. Newly established medical diagnosis (diabetes) and necessary foot hygiene practices
- **Impaired physical mobility** related to
  a. Painful foot lesion (corn, ingrown toenail, plantar wart)
  b. Altered foot alignment (contracture)

Examples of assessment data clusters and related nursing diagnoses are shown in Table 29–9.

PLANNING

Planning involves (a) identifying nursing interventions that will help the client maintain or restore healthy foot care practices and (b) establishing specific outcome criteria for each client. Interventions may include teaching the client about correct nail and foot care, proper foot wear, and ways to prevent potential foot problems (eg, infection, injury, and decreased circulation). For clients with self-care difficulties, the nurse plans a schedule for soaking the client's feet and assisting with regular cleaning and trimming of nails (if not contraindicated). Foot and nail care is often provided during the client's bath but may be provided at any time in the day to accommodate the client's preference. The frequency of foot care is determined by the nurse and client and is based on objective assessment data and the client's specific problems. For some clients, the feet need to be bathed daily; for those whose feet perspire excessively, bathing more than once a day may be necessary. Examples of outcome criteria to evaluate the achievement of goals and effectiveness of nursing interventions are shown below.

The client

- Participates in self-care (foot hygiene) to optimal level of capacity (specify).
- Describes hygienic and other interventions to maintain skin integrity, prevent infection, and maintain peripheral tissue perfusion.
- Demonstrates optimal hygiene, as evidenced by
  a. Intact, pink, smooth, soft, hydrated, and warm skin.
  b. Intact cuticles and skin surrounding nails.
  c. Correct foot care and nail care practices.
- Verbalizes less pain or discomfort when walking.

IMPLEMENTING

Procedure 29–3 describes how to provide foot care. See also the discussion of nails. During these procedures, the nurse has the opportunity to teach the client appropriate methods for foot care, that is, those designed to prevent tissue injury and infection. Because of reduced peripheral circulation to the feet, clients with diabetes or peripheral vascular disease are particularly prone to infection if skin breakage occurs. Many foot problems can be prevented by teaching the client simple foot care guidelines. See the box on page 749.

Table 29–9 Clinical Application: Assessment Data Clusters and Related Nursing Diagnoses for Clients with Foot Problems

Data Cluster	Nursing Diagnosis
Sally Brown, an 83-year-old widow, lives alone. Has homemaker services twice per week and Meals-On-Wheels service daily. Manages a shower once per week with daughter's help. Has pronounced hand tremors and obvious cataracts. States, "I can't see well enough to cut my nails, and even if I could see, my hands shake so badly."	**Self-care deficit:** (foot) **hygiene** related to impaired hand coordination and visual impairment
Kyle Stevens, 14-year-old, lives with his mother and eight sisters and brothers in a three-room walk-up. Bathroom down the hall is shared with other tenants in the building. Shoes are ragged and fit poorly. States, "I can't get new ones."	**High risk for impaired skin integrity** related to poorly fitting shoes and limited access to bathing facilities
Jim Wakefield, 64 years old, was recently diagnosed with diabetes mellitus. States has heard of "diabetes" and is worried, since a friend of his father's had diabetes and, after cutting his foot, had his leg amputated.	**Knowledge deficit** (diabetic foot care) related to misinterpretation of information

EVALUATING

See Evaluating on page 744.

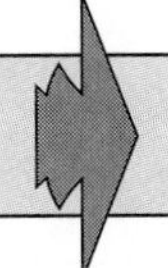

PROCEDURE 29–3 PROVIDING FOOT CARE

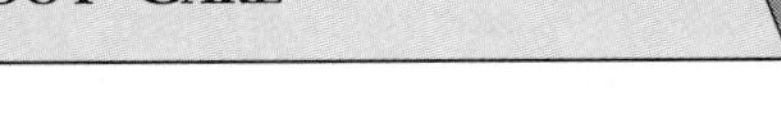

PURPOSES

- To maintain the skin integrity of the feet
- To prevent foot infections
- To prevent foot odors
- To maintain foot function

ASSESSMENT FOCUS
Skin surfaces; presence of edema or tenderness; circulatory status; usual foot care practices; self-care abilities.

PROCEDURE 29–3 PROVIDING FOOT CARE *continued*

EQUIPMENT

- ☐ Washbasin containing warm water
- ☐ Pillow
- ☐ Moisture-resistant disposable pad
- ☐ Towels
- ☐ Soap
- ☐ Washcloth
- ☐ Toenail cleaning and trimming equipment
- ☐ Lotion or foot powder

INTERVENTION

1. Prepare the equipment and the client.

- Fill the washbasin with warm water at about 40 to 43 C (105 to 110 F). *Warm water promotes circulation, comforts, and refreshes.*
- Assist the ambulatory client to a sitting position in a chair, or the bed client to a supine or semi-Fowler's position.
- Place a pillow under the bed client's knees. *This provides support and prevents muscle fatigue.*
- Place the washbasin on the moisture-resistant pad at the foot of the bed for a bed client or on the floor in front of the chair for an ambulatory client.
- For a bed client, pad the rim of the washbasin with a towel. *This towel prevents undue pressure on the skin.*

2. Wash the foot, and soak it as required.

- Place one of the client's feet in the basin, and wash it with soap, paying particular attention to the interdigital areas.
- Rinse the foot well to remove soap. *Soap irritates the skin if not properly removed.*
- Rub callused areas of the foot with the washcloth. *This helps remove dead skin layers.*
- If the nails are brittle or thick and require trimming, replace the water and allow the foot to soak for 10 to 20 minutes. *Soaking softens the nails and loosens debris under them.*
- Clean the nails as required with an orange stick or the blunt end of a toothpick. *This removes excess debris that harbors microorganisms.*
- Remove the foot from the basin, and place it on the towel.

3. Dry the foot thoroughly, and apply lotion or foot powder.

- Blot the foot gently with the towel to dry it thoroughly, particularly between the toes. *Harsh rubbing can damage the skin. Thorough drying reduces the risk of infection.*
- Apply lotion or lanolin cream. *This lubricates dry skin.*

  or
- Apply a foot powder containing a nonirritating deodorant if the feet tend to perspire excessively. *Foot powders have greater absorbent properties than regular bath powders; some also contain menthol, which makes the feet feel cool.*

4. If agency policy permits, trim the nails of the first foot while the second foot is soaking.

- See the discussion on nails for the appropriate method to trim nails. Note that in many agencies toenail trimming is contraindicated for clients with diabetes mellitus, toe infections, and peripheral vascular disease, unless performed by a podiatrist or general practice physician.

5. Document any foot problems observed.

- Foot care is not generally recorded unless problems are noted.
- Record any signs of inflammation, infection, breaks in the skin, corns, troublesome calluses, bunions, and pressure areas. This is of particular importance for clients with peripheral vascular disease and diabetes.

EVALUATION FOCUS

Skin color and temperature; presence of foot odor; foot comfort; tenderness.

CLIENT TEACHING

Foot Care

- Wash the feet daily, and dry them well, especially between the toes.
- When washing, check the skin of the feet for breaks or red or swollen areas.
- To prevent burns, check the water temperature before immersing the feet.
- Use creams or lotions to moisten the skin, or soak the feet in warm water with Epsom salts to avoid excessive drying of the skin of the feet. Lotion will also soften calluses. A lotion that reduces dryness effectively is a mixture of lanolin and mineral oil.
- To prevent or control an unpleasant odor due to excessive foot perspiration, wash the feet frequently, and change socks and shoes at least daily. Special deodorant sprays or absorbent foot powders are also helpful.
- File the toenails rather than cutting them to avoid skin injury. File the nails straight across the ends of the toes. If the nails are too thick or misshapen to file, consult a podiatrist.
- Wear clean stockings or socks daily. Avoid socks with holes or darns that can cause pressure areas.
- Wear correctly fitting shoes that neither restrict the foot nor rub on any area; rubbing can cause corns and calluses. Check worn shoes for rough spots in the lining. Break in new shoes gradually by increasing the wearing time 30 to 60 minutes each day.
- Avoid walking barefoot, since injury and infection may result. Wear slippers in public showers and change areas to avoid contracting athlete's foot or other infections.
- Several times each day, exercise the feet to promote circulation. Point the feet upward, point them downward, and move them in circles.
- Avoid wearing constricting garments such as kneehigh elastic stockings or sitting with the legs crossed at the knees, which may decrease circulation.
- When the feet are cold, use extra blankets and wear warm socks rather than using heating pads or hot water bottles, which may cause burns. Test bathwater before stepping into it.
- Wash any cut on the foot thoroughly, apply a mild antiseptic, and notify the physician.
- Avoid self-treatment for corns or calluses. Pumice stones and some callus and corn applications are injurious to the skin. Consult a podiatrist.

ASSESSMENT INTERVIEW

Nail Hygiene

- What are your usual nail care practices?
- Do you have any problems managing your nail care? If so, what are these?
- Have you had any problems associated with your nails (eg, inflammation of the tissue surrounding the nail, injury, prolonged exposure to water or chemicals, circulatory problems)?

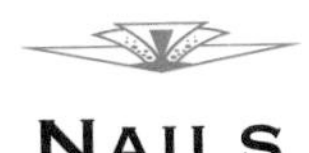

NAILS

Nails are normally present at birth. They continue to grow throughout life and change very little until people are old. At that time, the nails tend to be tougher, more brittle, and in some cases thicker. The nails of an elderly person normally grow less quickly than those of a younger person and may be ridged and grooved.

ASSESSING

During the nursing history, the nurse explores the client's usual nail care practices, self-care abilities, and any problems associated with them. See the assessment box above. Physical assessment involves inspection of the nails (see also Chapter 22, page 479).

DIAGNOSING

Nursing diagnoses related to nail care and nail problems include **Self-care deficit, High risk for infection,** and **Pain.** Examples of these nursing diagnoses and contributing factors are shown below.

- **Self-care deficit: grooming** related to
  a. Impaired vision
  b. Impaired hand coordination
- **High risk for infection** around the nail bed related to
  a. Impaired skin integrity of cuticles
  b. Altered peripheral circulation
- **Pain** related to inflamed cuticle and/or skin surrounding the nails

PLANNING

The nurse identifies measures that will assist the client to develop or maintain healthy nail care practices. A schedule of nail care needs to be established. Examples of

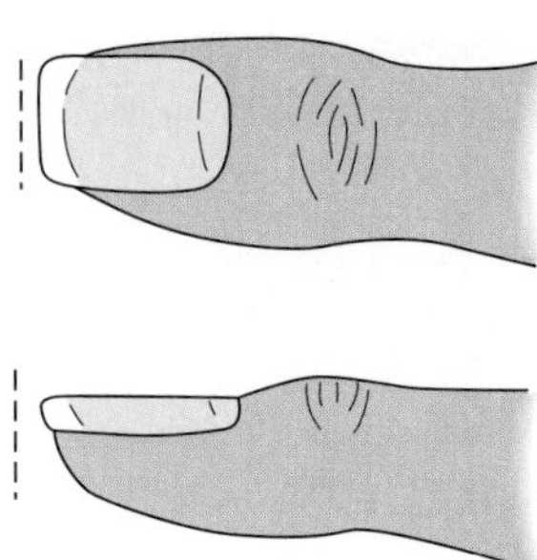

Figure 29–6 Fingernails are trimmed straight across.

outcome criteria to evaluate the effectiveness of nursing interventions are shown below.

The client

- Demonstrates healthy nail care practices, as evidenced by
  a. Clean, short nails with smooth edges.
  b. Intact cuticles and hydrated surrounding skin.
- Describes factors contributing to the nail problem.
- Describes preventive interventions for the specific nail problem.
- Demonstrates nail care as instructed.
- Has pink nail beds and quick return of nail bed color after blanch test.

IMPLEMENTING

To provide nail care, the nurse needs a nail cutter or sharp scissors, a nail file, an orange stick to push back the cuticle, hand lotion or mineral oil to lubricate any dry tissue around the nails, and a basin of water to soak the nails if they are particularly thick or hard.

One hand or foot is soaked, if needed, and dried; then the nail is cut or filed straight across beyond the end of the finger or toe. See Figure 29–6. Avoid trimming or digging into nails at the lateral corners. This predisposes the client to ingrown toenails. Clients who have diabetes or circulatory problems should have their nails filed, rather than cut; inadvertent injury to tissues can occur if scissors are used. After the initial cut or filing, the nail is filed to round the corners, and the nurse cleans under the nail. The nurse then gently pushes back the cuticle, taking care not to injure it. The next finger or toe is cared for in the same manner. Any abnormalities, such as an infected cuticle or inflammation of the tissue around the nail, are recorded and reported.

EVALUATING

See Evaluating on page 744.

MOUTH

DEVELOPMENTAL VARIATIONS

Teeth usually appear 5 to 8 months after birth. Each tooth has a number of parts: the crown, the root, and the pulp cavity (Figure 29–7). The **crown** is the exposed part of the tooth, which is outside the gum. It is covered with a hard substance called **enamel.** The ivory-colored internal part of the crown below the enamel is the **dentin.** The root of a tooth is embedded in the jaw and covered by a bony tissue called **cementum.** The **pulp cavity** in the center of the tooth contains the blood vessels and nerves.

By the time children are 2 years old, they usually have all 20 of their temporary teeth (Figure 29–8). At about age 6 or 7, children start losing their deciduous teeth, and these are gradually replaced by the 32 permanent teeth (Figure 29–9). By age 25, most people have all their permanent teeth.

The incidence of periodontal disease increases during pregnancy, because an increase in female hormones affects gingival tissue and increases its reaction to bacterial plaque. Many pregnant women manifest increased bleeding from the gingival sulcus during brushing and increased redness and swelling of the **gingiva** (the gum).

Some elderly people may have few permanent teeth left, and some have **dentures.** Most people have lost all their own teeth by age 70, mainly because of **periodontal disease** (gum disease) rather than **dental caries** (cavities); however, caries are also common in middle-aged adults.

Some receding of the gums and a brownish pigmentation of the gums occur with age. Because saliva production decreases with age, dryness of the oral mucosa is a common finding in older people.

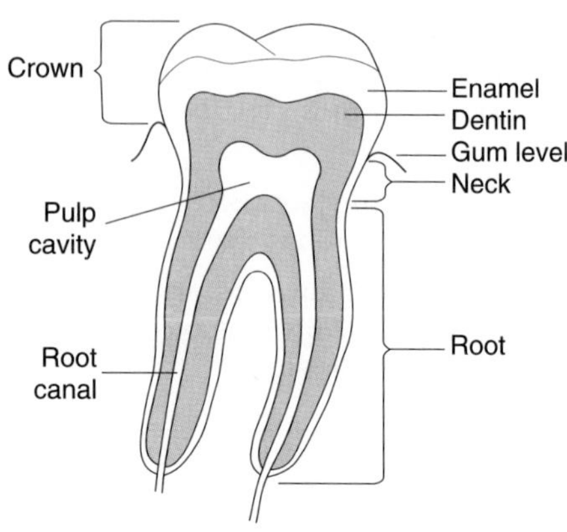

Figure 29–7 The anatomic parts of a tooth.

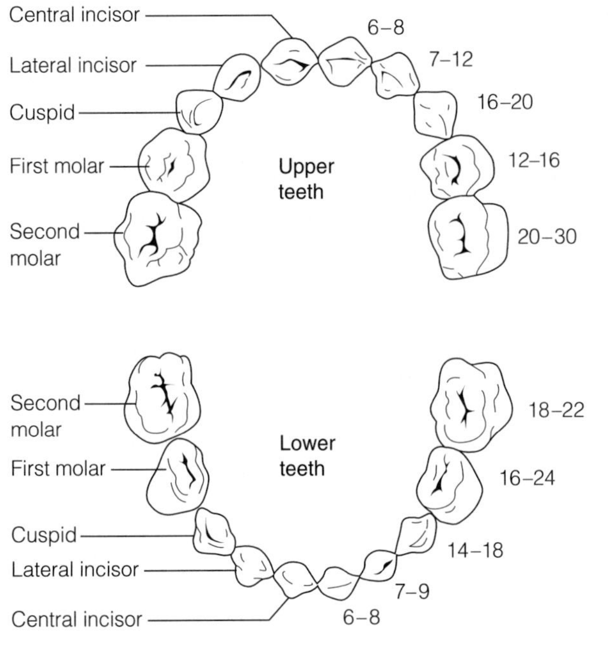

Figure 29–8 Temporary teeth and their times of eruption (stated in months).

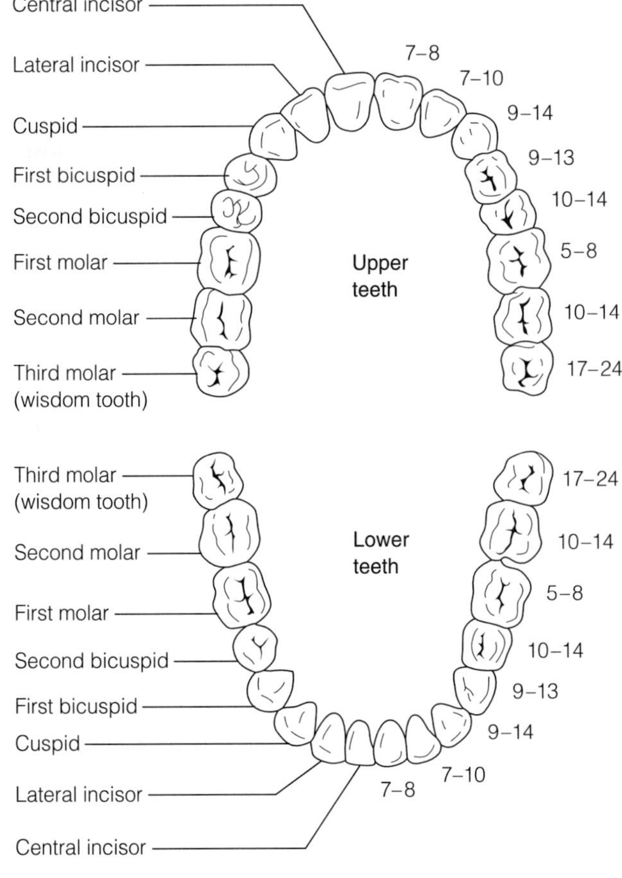

Figure 29–9 Permanent teeth and their times of eruption (stated in years).

> ### DEFINITIONS AND DESCRIPTIONS FOR FUNCTIONAL LEVEL (ORAL HYGIENE)
>
> - *Totally dependent:* Nurse completes the entire procedure.
> - *Moderately dependent:* Nurse prepares brush; rinses client's mouth; positions client.
> - *Semidependent:* Nurse provides equipment; client performs the task.
>
> **Source:** JR Lederer, GL Marculescu, B Mocnik, and N Seaby, *Care Planning Pocket Guide: A Nursing Diagnosis Approach*, 5th ed. (Redwood City, CA: Addison-Wesley Nursing, 1993), p. 164.

ASSESSING

Assessment of the client's mouth and hygiene practices includes (a) a nursing history, (b) physical assessment of the mouth, and (c) identification of clients at risk for developing oral problems.

Nursing History During the nursing history, the nurse obtains data about the client's oral hygiene practices, including dental visits, self-care abilities, and past or current mouth problems. Data about the client's oral hygiene helps the nurse determine learning needs and to incorporate the client's needs and preferences in the plan of care. Assessment of the client's *self-care abilities* determines the amount and type of nursing assistance to provide. See the box above for definitions and descriptions of functional level. Clients whose hand coordination is impaired, whose cognitive function is impaired, whose illness alters energy levels and motivation, or whose therapy imposes restrictions on activities will need assistance from the nurse. Data about *past or current problems* alert the nurse to specific interventions required or referrals that may be necesary. Questions to elicit the above data are shown in the box on page 752.

Physical Assessment For information about mouth assessment, see Chapter 22, pages 498 to 502. Dental caries (cavities) and peridontal disease (pyorrhea) are two problems that most frequently affect the teeth. Both problems are commonly associated with plaque and tartar deposits. **Plaque** is an *invisible* soft film that adheres to the enamel surface of teeth; it consists of bacteria, molecules of saliva, and remnants of epithelial cells and leukocytes. When plaque is unchecked, tartar (dental calculus) is formed. **Tartar** is a visible, hard deposit of plaque and dead bacteria that forms at the gum lines. Tartar buildup

ASSESSMENT INTERVIEW

Oral Hygiene

Oral Hygiene Practices

- What are your usual mouth care and/or denture care practices?
- What oral hygiene products do you routinely use (eg, mouthwash, type of toothpaste, dental floss, denture cleaner)?
- When was your last dental examination, and how often do you see your dentist?

Self-Care Abilities

- Do you have any problems managing your mouth care?

Past or Current Mouth Problems

- Have you had or do you have any problems such as bleeding, swollen or reddened gums, ulcerations, lumps, or tooth pain?

can alter the fibers that attach the teeth to the gum and eventually disrupt bone tissue. Periodontal disease is characterized by **gingivitis** (red, swollen gingiva), bleeding, receding gum lines, and the formation of pockets between the teeth and gums. In advanced periodontal disease, the teeth are loose, and pus is evident when the gums are pressed.

Other problems nurses may see are **glossitis** (inflammation of the tongue), **stomatitis** (inflammation of the oral mucosa), and **parotitis** (inflammation of the parotid salivary gland). The accumulation of foul matter (food, microorganisms, and epithelial elements) on the teeth and gums is referred to as **sordes.** See also Table 29–10 for common problems of the mouth.

RESEARCH NOTE

Do You Know How to Assess Oral Health?

Oral care and basic hygiene are fundamental client care tasks. On a daily basis, they are practiced by nurses in a multitude of clinical settings with clients of all ages. Given these facts, it is important to consider the level of oral health knowledge possessed by practicing nurses.

In this study, Adams sought to evaluate the oral health knowledge of Registered Nurses practicing in medical and geriatric inpatient settings. The author hypothesized that nurses lack adequate knowledge of oral health and that this knowledge results in inadequate oral care.

Using a questionnaire comprised of a mixture of open-ended and closed style questions, Adams evaluated the level of knowledge and the oral care practices of 34 registered nurses. Nurses included in the sample were either employed on a geriatric unit or on one of three medical wards in a general hospital in the United Kingdom. Data were collected over a one-month time span. The 34 nurses sampled had a wide range of clinical experience.

Adams' hypotheses were supported by her data. In particular, she found numerous gaps in knowledge of oral care procedures and inadequate oral health assessment. In addition, many nurses failed to document their assessment findings or the care rendered.

Implications: This study demonstrates the need for ongoing learning in the area of oral health. Although oral hygiene is a basic skill, it should not be neglected as students and practicing nurses take on additional skills and more complex assessments.

Source: R Adams, Qualified nurses lack adequate knowledge related to oral health, resulting in inadequate oral care of patients on medical wards, *Journal of Advanced Nursing*, September 1996, 24(3):552–60.

Identifying Clients at Risk Certain clients are prone to oral problems often because of lack of knowledge or the inability to maintain oral hygiene. Among these are seriously ill, confused, comatose, depressed, and dehydrated clients. In addition, persons with nasogastric tubes or receiving oxygen are likely to develop dry oral mucous membranes, especially if they breathe through their mouths. Clients who have had oral or jaw surgery must have meticulous oral hygiene care to prevent the development of infections. Related factors are presented in the box on page 754.

Healthy-appearing individuals, too, may be at risk. High-risk variables such as inadequate nutrition, excessive intake of refined sugars, and family history of periodontal disease also need to be identified. Some elderly people may also be at risk, for example, those who choose salty and enamel-eroding sugary foods because of a decline in their number of taste buds. The decreased saliva production in the aged, which produces a dry mouth and

Table 29–10 Common Problems of the Mouth

Problem	Description	Nursing Implications
Halitosis	Bad breath	Teach or provide regular oral hygiene.
Glossitis	Inflammation of the tongue	As above
Gingivitis	Inflammation of the gums	As above
Periodontal disease	Gums appear spongy and bleeding	As above
Reddened or excoriated mucosa		Check for ill-fitting dentures.
Excessive dryness of the buccal mucosa		Increase fluid intake as health permits.
Cheilosis	Cracking of lips	Lubricate lips, use antimicrobial ointment to prevent infection.
Dental caries	Teeth have darkened areas, may be painful	Advise client to see a physician and/or dentist.

thinning of the oral mucosa, is another factor (Pettigrew 1989, p. 22).

A dry mouth can be aggravated by poor fluid intake, heavy smoking, alcohol use, high salt intake, anxiety, and many medications. Medications that can cause dryness of the mouth include diuretics; laxatives, if used excessively; and tranquilizers, such as chlorpromazine (Thorazine) and diazepam (Valium). Some chemotherapeutic agents used to treat cancer also cause oral dryness and oral lesions.

DIAGNOSING

Three nursing diagnoses related to problems with oral hygiene and the oral cavity are **Self-care deficit, Altered oral mucous membrane,** and **Knowledge deficit.** Note that NANDA includes oral hygiene with the diagnostic label **Self-care deficit: bathing/hygiene.** In this book the diagnosis **Self-care deficit: oral hygiene** will be used for clients unable to perform oral care independently. The Nursing Diagnoses box on page 754 provides definitions, contributing factors, and defining characteristics of the first two diagnoses. **Knowledge deficit** is discussed in detail in Chapter 19.

The following diagnoses may also apply:

- **Impaired tissue integrity** related to
  a. Radiation therapy involving the oral cavity
  b. Medication
  c. Ill-fitting dentures
- **High risk for infection** related to
  a. Ineffective oral hygiene practices
  b. Impaired oral mucosa
- **Knowledge deficit (correct oral hygiene practices)** related to lack of exposure to information on correct oral hygiene

Table 29–11 Clinical Application: Assessment Data Clusters and Related Nursing Diagnoses for Clients with Oral Cavity Problems

Data Cluster	Nursing Diagnosis
Mary Brown, 77 years old, suffered a cerebrovascular accident. Is unconscious and breathing through the mouth via O_2 face mask. 2500 mL intravenous fluid ordered daily.	**Self care deficit:** (oral) **hygiene** related to cognitive inability (unconsciousness)
Joe Kwan, 46 years old, was admitted with a fractured femur. Teeth stained from heavy smoking. One large cavity evident in 2nd lower left molar, tartar buildup along gum margins, and pronounced halitosis. Gums are reddened in some areas and bleed when flossed. States, "I can't remember when I last saw a dentist."	**Altered oral mucous membrane** related to ineffective oral hygiene

Clinical examples of assessment data clusters and related nursing diagnoses are shown in Table 29–11.

PLANNING

The nurse identifies interventions that will assist the client to maintain or improve oral hygiene practices and

NURSING DIAGNOSES

CLIENTS WITH ORAL PROBLEMS

NURSING DIAGNOSIS: Self-care deficit: (oral) hygiene: The state in which one experiences an impaired ability to perform oral self-care

Defining Characteristics	Related Factors
Inability to brush or floss teeth or clean dentures	Altered level of consciousness; impaired mobility of upper extremities; impaired cognitive ability. See also related factors for other self-care deficits in the box on page 734.

NURSING DIAGNOSIS: Altered oral mucous membrane: The state in which an individual experiences disruptions in the tissue layers of the oral cavity

Defining Characteristics	Related Factors
Coated tongue; dry mouth; dental caries; halitosis; gingivitis; oral plaque, pain, discomfort, erythema, lesions or ulcers; lack of or decreased salivation.	Inadequate oral hygiene; physical injury or drying effect (eg, mouth breathing, oxygen therapy, decreased salivation, temperature extreme, NPO); mechanical trauma (eg, surgery, injury from oral tube, broken teeth or ill-fitting dentures); chemical trauma (eg, side-effects of medications); radiation injury.

maintain or restore the integrity of the oral mucous membrane. Nursing interventions may include assisting dependent clients to clean their teeth and oral cavity, and teaching clients about good oral hygiene practices and other measures to prevent tooth decay (eg, use of fluoride, adequate nutrition, and regular visits to a dentist). Examples of outcome criteria are outlined below.

The client

- Performs oral hygiene according to instructions with assistance (specify).
- Demonstrates optimal oral hygiene, as evidenced by
  a. Pink, moist, and intact mucosa, tongue, and lips.
  b. Absence of debris and plaque on dental surfaces.
  c. Verbalizing feeling of oral cleanliness.
- Identifies reasons for alteration in oral mucosa.
- Manifests oral tissue integrity, as evidenced by
  a. Intact, smooth, well-hydrated oral mucosa of uniform color.
  b. Absence of inflammation of the oral mucosa.
  c. Firm, well-hydrated, nonbleeding gums of uniform color.
  d. Well-hydrated tongue without inflammation.
  e. Smooth and well-hydrated lips.
  f. No oral discomfort.

Nursing interventions with rationales associated with these outcomes are provided in the Care Planning Guide for Clients with Oral Hygiene and Mouth Problems, at the right.

IMPLEMENTING

Good oral hygiene includes daily stimulation of the gums, mechanical brushing and flossing of the teeth, flushing of the mouth, and regular checkups by a dentist. The nurse is often in a position to help people to maintain oral hygiene by helping or teaching them to clean the teeth and oral cavity, by inspecting whether clients (especially children) have done so, or by actually providing mouth care to clients who are ill or incapacitated. The nurse can also be instrumental in identifying and referring problems that require the intervention of a dentist or oral surgeon. Specific measures to prevent tooth decay and periodontal disease are shown in the box on page 757.

Brushing and Flossing the Teeth Thorough brushing of the teeth is important in preventing tooth decay. The mechanical action of brushing removes food particles that can harbor and incubate bacteria. It also stimulates circulation in the gums, thus maintaining their healthy firmness. Children need to be shown how to brush their

CARE PLANNING GUIDE

CLIENTS WITH ORAL PROBLEMS

NURSING DIAGNOSIS: Oral hygiene self-care deficit

Outcome Criteria	Nursing Interventions	Rationale
The client		
▪ Performs oral hygiene according to instructions.	Assess the client's functional ability to perform oral care, and document the functional level. See the box on page 751.	Appropriate assessment guides the amount of assistance required to maintain client independence and ensure optimal care.
	Assess current oral hygiene practices, and provide teaching as required, such as brushing or flossing technique or measures to prevent tooth decay (see page 757).	Knowledge of current practices enables the nurse to determine required health-promoting behavior.
	Establish an oral hygiene schedule after meals and at bedtime, for example: ▪ Use sulcular technique and soft toothbrush. ▪ Rinse with preferred mouthwash or solution of warm water and salt or baking soda (1/2 tsp to 1 pint water). ▪ Floss once a day.	Oral care after meals removes food debris that can harbor microorganisms. Brushing mechanically removes debris and stimulates gum circulation. Flossing prevents plaque formation. Rinsing removes dislodged particles and dentifrice and may have antiseptic properties.
▪ Demonstrates optimal oral hygiene, as evidenced by a. Pink, moist, and intact mucosa, tongue, and lips. b. Absence of debris and plaque on dental surfaces. c. Verbalizing feeling of oral cleanliness.	Inspect all surfaces of oral cavity each shift, including color and moistness of mucosa, presence of debris and odor, status of gum tissue, and presence of lesions.	Regular inspection allows early detection of problems and prompt correction.

NURSING DIAGNOSIS: Altered oral mucous membrane

Outcome Criteria	Nursing Interventions	Rationale
The client		
▪ Identifies reasons for alteration in oral mucosa.	Explain the etiology of the problem (eg, lack of oral hygiene or use of chemotherapeutic drugs). See other etiologies in the box on page 754.	Understanding of the underlying cause increases the client's awareness and may enhance motivation to improve oral hygiene or follow a therapeutic regimen.
▪ Manifests oral tissue integrity as evidenced by: a. Intact, smooth, well-hydrated oral mucosa of uniform color. b. Absence of inflammation of the oral mucosa. c. Firm, well-hydrated, nonbleeding gums of uniform color.	Assess all surfaces of oral mucosa for irritation, ulceration, and inflammation, daily or each shift or q4h (specify), and report alterations.	This allows the nurse to detect changes.

➤

CLIENTS WITH ORAL PROBLEMS CONTINUED

NURSING DIAGNOSIS: Altered oral mucous membrane *continued*

Outcome Criteria	Nursing Interventions	Rationale
d. Well-hydrated tongue without inflammation. e. Smooth and well-hydrated lips. f. No oral discomfort.		
	Establish a mouth care regimen: before meals if exudate is excessive, and after meals and at bedtime or more often as condition warrants (eg, q2h).	Oral care before meals removes exudate and stimulates appetite; after meals and at bedtime it removes food debris and prevents infection.
	Provide or use appropriate supplies (specify):	
	▪ Child's soft toothbrush or, if a toothbrush is contraindicated, use a gloved finger wrapped in gauze or a bulb syringe and suction catheter to irrigate.	This avoids further injury to mucosa.
	▪ Nonabrasive toothpaste.	
	▪ Normal saline or sodium bicarbonate solution for rinsing.	Normal saline is nonirritating, and sodium bicarbonate helps remove thick mucus.
	▪ Toothettes or disposable foam swabs.	This stimulates the gums.
	▪ Floss except when there is excessive bleeding.	
	▪ Lubricant, such as lanolin or petroleum jelly.	This maintains the texture of the lips.
▪ Verbalizes absence of or a reduction of oral pain.	Instruct client to	
	▪ Avoid tobacco, alcohol, extremes of temperature in food, excessive seasoning, commercial mouthwashes with alcohol, citrus fruit juices, foods high in roughage.	These substances are irritating to the oral mucosa and may cause discomfort and further damage.
	▪ Remove dentures as needed.	Ill-fitting dentures can irritate oral tissues.
	▪ Eat bland, soft foods if able.	Nonirritating, soft foods maintain the current status of oral mucous membrane.
	▪ Drink 2 to 3 liters of fluid per day.	Adequate hydration maintains the moisture of oral tissues and prevents cracking of lips and other injury.
	Consult with dietitian as needed to modify the diet.	
	Administer prescribed analgesics, or consult with physician to obtain one.	

WELLNESS TEACHING

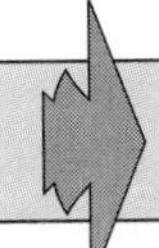

Measures to Prevent Tooth Decay

- Brush the teeth thoroughly after meals and at bedtime. Assist children or inspect their mouths to be sure the teeth are clean. If the teeth cannot be brushed after meals, vigorous rinsing of the mouth with water is recommended.
- Floss the teeth daily.
- Ensure an adequate intake of nutrients, particularly calcium, phosphorus, vitamins A, C, and D, and fluoride.
- Avoid sweet foods and drinks between meals. Take them in moderation at meals.
- Eat coarse, fibrous foods (cleansing foods), such as fresh fruits and raw vegetables.
- Take a fluoride supplement daily until age 14 or 16, unless the drinking water is fluoridated.
- Have topical fluoride applications as prescribed by the dentist.
- Have a checkup by a dentist every 6 months.
- A child's first visit to the dentist should occur at about age 2½ or 3, so that the child learns not to fear such visits.

teeth by age 2, when their teeth appear. Until the child can manipulate the toothbrush effectively, however, parents need to help the child. The technique most recently recommended for brushing teeth is called the **sulcular technique,** which removes plaque and cleans under the gingival margins. Many toothpastes are marketed, any of which can be used. An effective dentifrice can also be made by combining two parts of table salt to one part of baking soda.

When providing mouth care for the client, the nurse should wear gloves to guard against infections such as acquired immune deficiency syndrome (AIDS). Other required equipment includes a curved basin that fits snugly under the client's chin (eg, a kidney basin) to receive the rinse water and a towel to protect the client and the bedclothes. See Procedure 29–4.

Caring for Artificial Dentures Some people have artificial teeth in the form of a plate—a complete set of teeth for one jaw. A person may have a lower plate and/or an upper plate. When only a few artificial teeth are needed, the individual may have a bridge rather than a plate. A bridge may be fixed or removable. Artificial teeth are fitted to the individual and usually will not fit another person. People who wear dentures or other types of oral

Text continued on page 759

PROCEDURE 29–4 BRUSHING AND FLOSSING THE TEETH

PURPOSES

- To remove food particles from around and between the teeth
- To remove dental plaque
- To enhance the client's feelings of well-being
- To prevent sordes and infection of the oral tissues

ASSESSMENT FOCUS

Self-care abilities; presence of tooth caries; gum inflammation; halitosis; status of oral mucosa and lips; usual mouth care practices.

EQUIPMENT

- ☐ Towel
- ☐ Gloves
- ☐ Curved basin (emesis basin)
- ☐ Toothbrush
- ☐ Cup of tepid water
- ☐ Dentifrice
- ☐ Mouthwash
- ☐ Dental floss, at least two pieces 20 cm (8 in) in length
- ☐ Floss holder (optional)

INTERVENTION

1. Prepare the client.

- Explain the procedure.
- Assist the client to a sitting position in bed, if health permits. If not, assist the client to a side-lying position with the head on a pillow so that the client can spit out the rinse water.

PROCEDURE 29-4 BRUSHING AND FLOSSING THE TEETH *continued*

2. Prepare the equipment.

- Place the towel under the client's chin.
- Don gloves. *Wearing gloves while providing mouth care prevents the nurse from acquiring infections, such as AIDS, particularly if oral bleeding is present. Gloves also prevent transmission of microorganisms to the client.*
- Moisten the bristles of the toothbrush with tepid water, and apply the dentifrice to the toothbrush.
- Use a soft toothbrush (a small one for a child) and the client's choice of dentifrice. For the person who does not have dentifrice, use a mixture of salt and baking soda.
- For the client who must remain in bed, place or hold the curved basin under the client's chin, fitting the small curve around the chin or neck.
- Inspect the mouth and teeth.

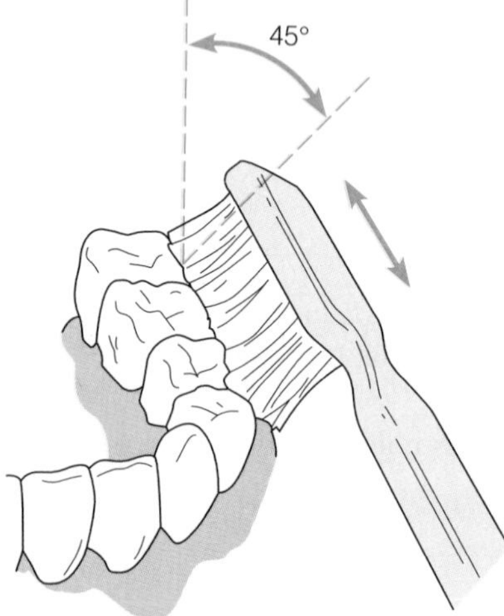

Figure 29–10 The sulcular technique: placing the bristles at a 45-degree angle against the teeth.

3. Brush the teeth.

- Hand the toothbrush to the client, or brush the client's teeth as follows.
  a. Hold the brush against the teeth with the bristles at a 45-degree angle (Figure 29–10). The tips of the outer bristles should rest against and penetrate under the gingival sulcus (Figure 29–11). The brush will clean under the sulcus of two or three teeth at one time. *This sulcular technique removes plaque and cleans under the gingival margins.*
  b. Move the bristles back and forth using a vibrating or jiggling motion, from the sulcus to the crowns of the teeth.
  c. Repeat until all outer and inner surfaces of the teeth and sulci of the gums are cleaned.
  d. Clean the biting surfaces by moving the brush back and forth over them in short strokes (Figure 29–12).
  e. If the tongue is coated, brush it gently with the toothbrush. *Brushing removes accumulated materials and coatings. A coated tongue may be caused by poor oral hygiene and low fluid intake. Brushing gently and carefully helps prevent gagging or vomiting.*
- Hand the client the water cup or mouthwash to rinse the mouth vigorously. Then ask the client to spit the water and excess dentifrice into the basin. Some agencies supply a standard mouthwash. Alternatively, a mouth rinse of normal saline or diluted hydrogen peroxide can be an effective cleaner and moisturizer. *Vigorous rinsing loosens food particles and washes out already loosened particles.*
- Repeat the steps above until the mouth is free of dentifrice and food particles.
- Remove the curved basin, and help the client wipe the mouth.

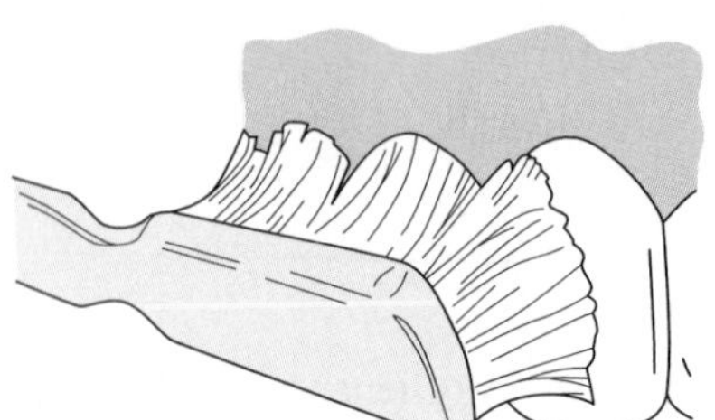

Figure 29–11 Directing the tips of the outer bristles under the gingival margins.

4. Floss the teeth.

- Assist the client to floss independently, or floss the teeth as follows. Waxed floss is less likely to fray than unwaxed floss; particles between the teeth attach more readily to unwaxed floss than to waxed floss. Some believe that waxed floss leaves a residue on the teeth and that plaque then adheres to the wax.
  a. Wrap one end of the floss around the third finger of each hand (Figure 29–13).
  b. To floss the upper teeth, use your thumb and index finger to stretch the floss (Figure 29–14). Move the floss up and down between the teeth from the tops of the crowns to the gum and along the gum lines

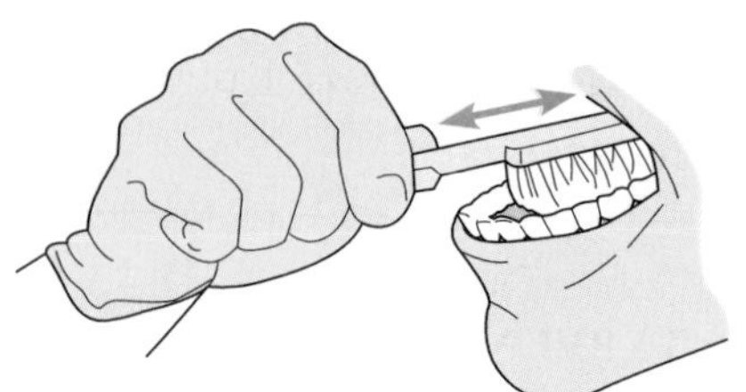

Figure 29–12 Brushing the biting surfaces.

PROCEDURE 29–4 *continued*

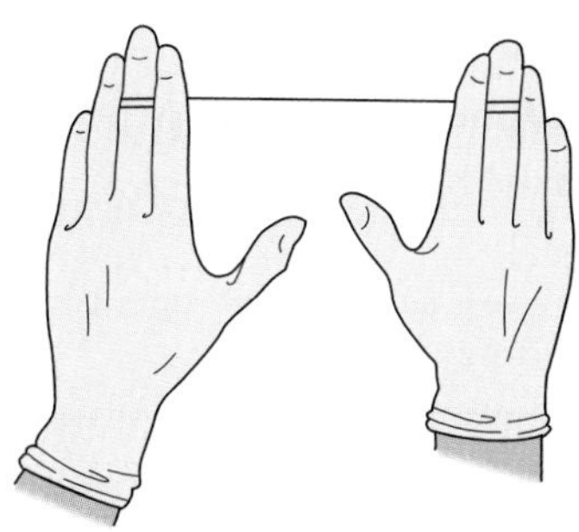

Figure 29–13 Stretching the floss between the third finger of each hand.

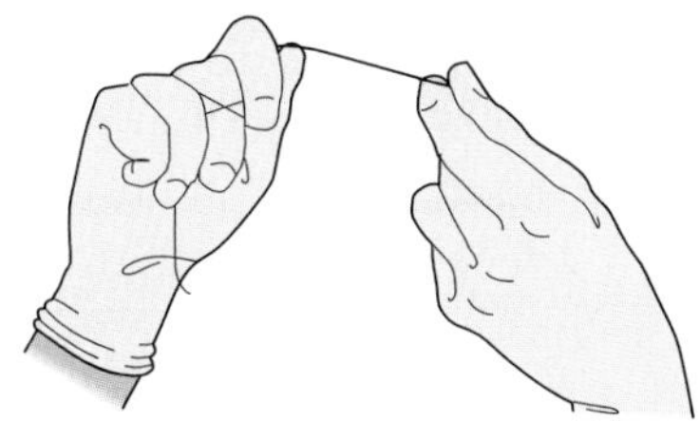

Figure 29–14 Flossing the upper teeth by using the thumbs and index fingers to stretch the floss.

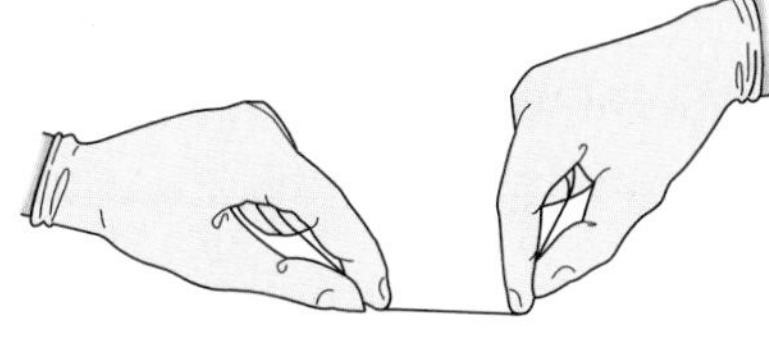

Figure 29–15 Flossing the lower teeth by using the index fingers to stretch the floss.

as far as possible. Make a "C" with the floss around the tooth edge being flossed. Start at the back on the right side and work around to the back of the left side, or work from the center teeth to the back of the jaw on either side.

c. To floss the lower teeth, use your index fingers to stretch the floss (Figure 29–15).

- Give the client tepid water or mouthwash to rinse the mouth and a curved basin in which to spit the water.
- Assist the client in wiping the mouth.

5. Remove and dispose of equipment appropriately.

- Remove and clean the curved basin.
- Remove and discard the gloves.

6. Document assessment of the teeth, tongue, gums, and oral mucosa. Include any problems such as sordes or inflammation and swelling of the gums. Brushing and flossing teeth are not usually recorded.

EVALUATION FOCUS
Health status of teeth, gums, tongue, oral mucosa, and lips.

prostheses should be encouraged to use them. Those who do not wear their prostheses are prone to shrinkage of the gums, which results in further tooth loss.

Most people prefer privacy when they take their artificial teeth out to clean them. Many do not like to be seen without their teeth; one of the first requests of many postoperative clients is "May I have my teeth in, please?"

Like natural teeth, artificial dentures collect microorganisms and food. They need to be cleaned regularly, at least once a day. They can be removed from the mouth, scrubbed with a toothbrush, rinsed, and reinserted. Some people use a dentifrice, while others use commercial cleaning compounds for plates. Procedure 29–5 describes how to clean artificial dentures.

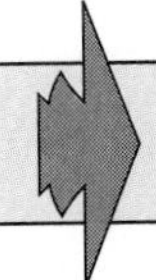

PROCEDURE 29–5 CLEANING ARTIFICIAL DENTURES

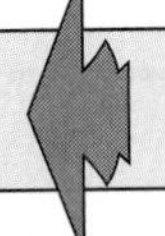

Before commencing to clean artificial dentures, determine (a) areas in the mouth that require ongoing assessment, and (b) whether the client has upper and lower dentures.

PURPOSES

- To remove food particles and microorganisms from artificial teeth
- To prevent infection of the oral tissues
- To enhance the client's feelings of well-being

ASSESSMENT FOCUS
Health status of gums, oral mucosa, and tongue; condition of dentures.

PROCEDURE 29–5 CLEANING ARTIFICIAL DENTURES *continued*

EQUIPMENT

- ☐ Gloves
- ☐ Tissue or piece of gauze
- ☐ Denture container
- ☐ Clean washcloth
- ☐ Toothbrush or stiff-bristled brush
- ☐ Dentifrice or denture cleaner
- ☐ Tepid water
- ☐ Container of mouthwash
- ☐ Curved basin (emesis basin)
- ☐ Towel

INTERVENTION

1. Prepare the client.

- Assist the client to a sitting or side-lying position.

2. Remove the dentures.

- Don gloves. *Wearing gloves protects the nurse from infection.*
- If the client cannot remove the dentures, take the tissue or gauze, grasp the upper plate at the front teeth with your thumb and second finger, and move the denture up and down slightly (Figure 29–16). *The slight movement breaks the suction that holds the plate on the roof of the mouth.*

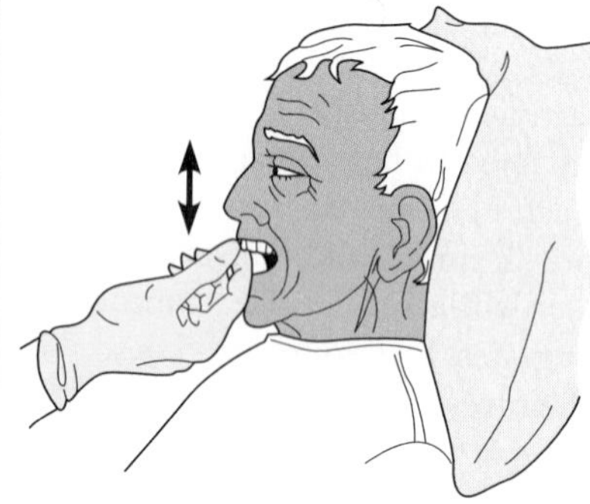

Figure 29–16 Removing the top dentures by first breaking the suction.

- Lower the upper plate, move it out of the mouth, and place it in the denture container.
- Lift the lower plate, turning it so that the left side, for example, is slightly lower than the right, to remove the plate from the mouth without stretching the lips. Place the lower plate in the denture container.
- Remove a partial denture by exerting equal pressure on the border of each side of the denture, not on the clasps, which can bend or break.

3. Clean the dentures.

- Take the denture container to a sink. Take care not to drop the dentures. *They may break.* Place a washcloth in the bowl of the sink. *A washcloth prevents damage if the dentures are dropped.*
- Using a toothbrush or special stiff-bristled brush, scrub the dentures with the cleaning agent and tepid water. *Hot water is not used, because heat will change the shape of some dentures.*
- Rinse the dentures with tepid running water. *Rinsing removes the cleaning agent and food particles.*
- If the dentures are stained, soak them in a commercial cleaner. Be sure to follow the manufacturer's directions. To prevent corrosion, dentures with metal parts should not be soaked overnight. The following mixtures are substitutes for commercial cleaner:
  a. 5 to 10 mL (1 to 2 tsp) white vinegar and 240 mL (1 cup) warm water.
  or
  b. 5 mL (1 tsp) chlorine bleach, 10 mL (2 tsp) water softener, and 240 mL (1 cup) warm water. It is essential to mix water softener with the bleach to prevent denture corrosion and to rinse well before replacing in the mouth.

4. Inspect the dentures and the mouth.

- Observe the dentures for any rough, sharp, or worn areas that could irritate the tongue or mucous membranes of the mouth, lips, and gums.
- Inspect the mouth for any redness, irritated areas, or indications of infection.
- Assess the fit of the dentures. People who have them should see a dentist at least once a year to check the fit, occlusion, and the presence of any irritation to the soft tissues of the mouth. Clients who need repairs to their dentures or new dentures may need a referral for financial assistance to correct problems.

5. Return the dentures to the mouth.

- Offer some mouthwash and a curved basin to rinse the mouth. If the client cannot insert the dentures independently, insert the plates one at a time. Hold each plate at a slight angle while inserting it, to avoid injuring the lips (Figure 29–17).

PROCEDURE 29–5 *continued*

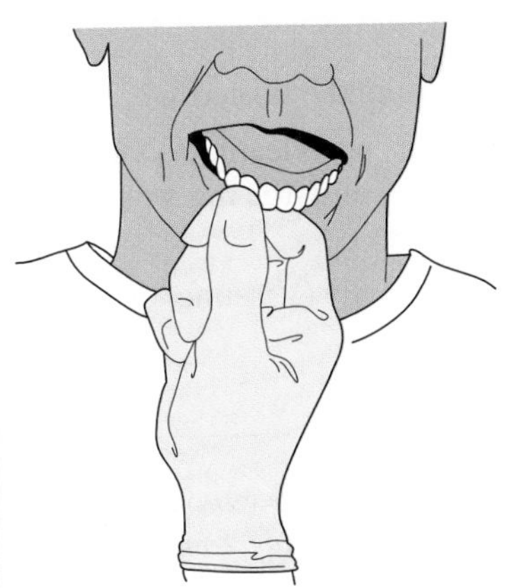

Figure 29–17 Inserting the dentures at a slight angle.

6. Assist the client as needed.
   - Wipe the client's hands and mouth with the towel.
   - If the client does not want to or cannot wear the dentures, store them in a denture container with water. Label the cup with the client's name and identification number.

7. Remove and discard gloves.

8. Document all relevant information.
   - Document all assessments, and include any problems, such as an irritated area on the mucous membrane.

EVALUATION FOCUS
Condition of the oral mucosa, gums, tongue, and lips; condition of the dentures.

Special Oral Care For the client who is unconscious or has excessive dryness, sores, or irritations of the mouth, it may be necessary to clean the oral mucosa and tongue, in addition to cleaning the teeth. Agency practices differ in regard to special mouth care and the frequency with which it is provided. Depending on the health of the client's mouth, special care may be needed every 2 to 8 hours.

Mouth care for unconscious people is very important, because their mouths tend to become dry and consequently predisposed to infections. Dryness occurs because the client cannot take fluids by mouth, is often breathing through the mouth, or may be receiving oxygen, which tends to dry the mucous membranes.

The nurse can use commercially prepared applicators of lemon juice and oil to clean the mucous membranes. If these are unavailable, a gauze square wrapped around a tongue blade and dipped into lemon juice and oil or into mouthwash solution usually suffices. Long-term use can lead to further dryness of the mucosa and changes in tooth enamel, however. Applicator swabs may also be used. Mineral oil is generally contraindicated, because aspiration of it can initiate an infection (lipid pneumonia). 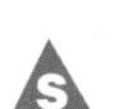 Hydrogen peroxide can be used prior to the lemon juice and oil, if necessary. This agent, which should be diluted 1:1 with water, is effective in removing encrustations that coat the tongue.

Procedure 29–6 focuses on oral care for the unconscious person but may be adapted for conscious persons who are seriously ill or have mouth problems.

EVALUATING

See Evaluating on page 744.

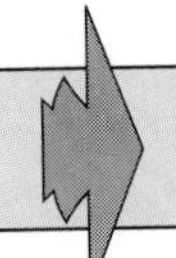

PROCEDURE 29–6 PROVIDING SPECIAL ORAL CARE

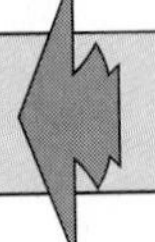

PURPOSES
- To maintain the continuity of the lips, tongue, and mucous membranes of the mouth
- To prevent oral infections
- To clean and moisten the membranes of the mouth and lips

ASSESSMENT FOCUS
Status of the oral mucosa, lips, tongue, and teeth; presence of halitosis.

PROCEDURE 29–6 PROVIDING SPECIAL ORAL CARE *continued*

EQUIPMENT

- ☐ Towel
- ☐ Curved basin (emesis basin)
- ☐ Gloves
- ☐ Bite-block to hold the mouth open and teeth apart (optional)
- ☐ Toothbrush
- ☐ Cup of tepid water
- ☐ Dentifrice or denture cleaner
- ☐ Tissue or piece of gauze to remove dentures (optional)
- ☐ Denture container as needed
- ☐ Mouthwash
- ☐ Rubber-tipped bulb syringe
- ☐ Applicators and cleaning solution for cleaning the mucous membranes
- ☐ Petroleum jelly (Vaseline) or cold cream

INTERVENTION

1. Prepare the client.

- Position the unconscious client in a side-lying position, with the head of the bed lowered. *In this position, the saliva automatically runs out by gravity rather than being aspirated into the lungs.* This position is the one of choice for the unconscious client receiving mouth care. If the client's head cannot be lowered, turn it to one side. *The fluid will readily run out of the mouth or pool in the side of the mouth, where it can be suctioned.*
- Place the towel under the client's chin.
- Place the curved basin against the client's chin and lower cheek to receive the fluid from the mouth (Figure 29–18).

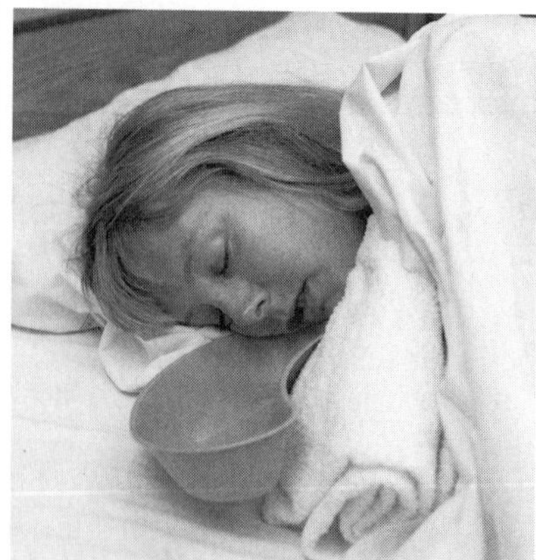

Figure 29–18 Position of client and placement of curved basin when providing special mouth care.

- Don gloves.

2. Clean the teeth, and rinse the mouth.

- If the person has natural teeth, brush the teeth as described earlier. Brush gently and carefully to avoid injuring the gums. If the client has artificial teeth, clean them as described earlier.
- Rinse the client's mouth by drawing about 10 mL of water or mouthwash into the syringe and injecting it gently into each side of the mouth. *If the solution is injected with force, some of it may flow down the client's throat and be aspirated into the lungs.*
- Watch carefully to make sure that all the rinsing solution has run out of the mouth into the basin. If not, suction the fluid from the mouth. See the section on oropharyngeal suctioning in Chapter 39, page 1149. *Fluid remaining in the mouth may be aspirated into the lungs.*
- Repeat rinsing until the mouth is free of dentifrice, if used.

3. Inspect and clean the oral tissues.

- If the tissues appear dry or unclean, clean them with the applicators or gauze and cleaning solution. If hydrogen peroxide is used, rinse the mouth thoroughly before applying oil and lemon juice. *The gums and mucosa can become spongy from prolonged action of hydrogen peroxide.* Oil and lemon juice are recommended for short-term use only.
- Picking up one oil applicator, wipe the mucous membrane of one cheek. If no commercially prepared applicators are available, wrap a small gauze square around a tongue blade and moisten it with oil and lemon solution. Discard the applicator or tongue blade in a waste container, and with a fresh one clean the next area. *Using separate applicators for each area of the mouth prevents the transfer of microorganisms from one area to another.*
- Clean all the mouth tissues in an orderly progression, using separate applicators: the cheeks, roof of the mouth, base of the mouth, and tongue.
- Observe the tissues closely for inflammation and dryness.
- Rinse the client's mouth as described above.
- Remove and discard gloves.

4. Ensure client comfort.

- Remove the basin, and dry around the client's mouth with the towel. Replace artificial dentures, if indicated.
- Lubricate the client's lips with petroleum jelly or cold cream.

PROCEDURE 29-6 *continued*

Lubrication prevents cracking and subsequent infection.

5. **Document pertinent data.**

- Record special oral hygiene and pertinent observations.
- Report problems to the nurse in charge.

EVALUATION FOCUS
Status of oral tissues, lips, and tongue; any irritation, dryness, or lesions.

HAIR

The appearance of the hair often reflects a person's feelings of well-being. A person who feels ill may not groom hair as before. The hair may also reflect state of health (eg, endocrine changes can affect the pattern of hair growth, and color changes may reflect aging). In addition, hair texture can also reflect health status (eg, excessive coarseness and dryness may be associated with endocrine disorders such as hypothyroidism).

Each person has particular ways of caring for hair, influenced by a number of factors. Some shampoo it daily; others shampoo once a week or even less often. Black-skinned people often need to oil their hair daily because it tends to be dry. Oil prevents the hair from breaking and the scalp from drying. A wide-toothed comb is usually used, because finer combs pull and break the hair. Some people brush their hair vigorously before retiring, others comb their hair frequently.

ASSESSMENT INTERVIEW

Hair Care

Hair Care Practices

- What are your usual hair care practices?
- What hair care products do you routinely use (eg, hair spray, lubricant, shampoo, conditioners, hair dye, curling or straightening preparations)?

Self-Care Abilities

- Do you have any problems managing your hair?

Past or Current Hair Problems

- Have you had any of the following conditions or therapies: recent chemotherapy, hypothyroidism, radiation of the head, unexplained loss of hair, growth of excessive body hair?

DEVELOPMENTAL VARIATIONS

Newborns may have **lanugo** (the fine hair on the body of the fetus, also referred to as *down* or *woolly hair*) over their shoulders, back, and sacrum. This generally disappears, and the hair distribution on the eyebrows, head, and, eyelashes of young children subsequently becomes noticeable. Some newborns have hair on their scalps; others are free of hair at birth but grow hair over the scalp during the first year of life.

Pubic hair usually appears in early puberty followed in about 6 months by the growth of axillary hair. Boys develop facial hair in later puberty.

In adolescence, the sebaceous glands increase in activity as a result of increased hormone levels. As a result, hair follicle openings enlarge to accommodate the increased amount of sebum, which can make the adolescent's hair more oily.

In elderly people, the hair is generally thinner, grows more slowly, and loses its color as a result of aging tissues and diminishing circulation. Men often lose their scalp hair and may become completely bald. This phenomenon may occur even when a man is relatively young. The older person's hair also tends to be drier than normal. With age, axillary and pubic hair becomes finer and scanter, in contrast to the eyebrows, which become bristly and coarse. Many women develop hair on their faces, which may be a concern to them.

ASSESSING

Nursing History During the nursing history, the nurse elicits data about usual hair care, self-care abilities, history of hair or scalp problems, and conditions known to affect the hair. Chemotherapeutic agents and radiation of the head may cause **alopecia** (hair loss). Hypothyroidism may cause the hair to be thin, dry, and/or brittle. Use of some hair dyes and curling or straightening preparations can cause the hair to become dry and brittle. Questions to elicit these data are shown in the Interview box above.

Physical Assessment Physical assessment of the hair is discussed in Chapter 22, page 478. Problems include dandruff, hair loss, ticks, pediculosis, scabies, and hirsutism.

Dandruff Dandruff appears as a diffuse scaling of the scalp often accompanied by itching. In severe cases it involves the auditory canals and the eyebrows. Mild cases of dandruff can usually be treated effectively with a commercial shampoo specifically recommended for dandruff. In severe or persistent cases, the client may need the advice of a physician.

Hair Loss Hair loss and growth are continual processes. Some permanent thinning of hair normally occurs with aging. Baldness, common in men, is thought to be a hereditary problem for which there is no known remedy other than the wearing of a hairpiece or a costly surgical hair transplant, in which hair is taken from the back or the sides of the scalp and surgically moved to the hairless area. Although some external medications are being developed, their long-term outcomes are unknown.

Ticks Ticks are small parasites that bite into tissue and suck blood. They take many forms and can adapt themselves to various conditions. The genera *Ornithodoros* and *Dermacentor* are found in North America. They can attach to human beings and are found frequently in the hair. They can be as large as 1.3 cm (0.5 in) and appear gray-brown. They attach to a person with the apparatus by which they suck blood. The tick should be pulled out quickly as soon as it bites. If the sucking apparatus remains in the tissue, pour oil on the tick. This causes it to lose its hold because it is deprived of oxygen, and it withdraws its sucker.

Ticks transmit several diseases to people, in particular Rocky Mountain spotted fever and Lyme disease.

Pediculosis (Lice) Lice are parasitic insects that infest mammals. Infestion with lice is called **pediculosis.** Hundreds of varieties of lice infest humans. Three common kinds are *Pediculus capitis* (the head louse), *Pediculus corporis* (the body louse), and *Pediculus pubis* (the crab louse).

Pediculus capitis is found on the scalp and tends to stay hidden in the hairs; similarly, *Pediculus pubis* stays in pubic hair. *Pediculus corporis* tends to cling to clothing, so that when a client undresses, the lice may not be in evidence on the body; these lice suck blood from the person and lay their eggs on the clothing. The nurse can suspect their presence in the clothing if (a) the person habitually scratches, (b) there are scratches on the skin, and (c) there are hemorrhagic spots on the skin where the lice have sucked blood.

Head and pubic lice lay their eggs on the hairs; the eggs look like oval particles, similar to dandruff, clinging to the hair. Bites and pustular eruptions may also be noticed at the hair lines and behind the ears.

Lice are very small, grayish white, and difficult to see. The crab louse in the pubic area has red legs. Lice may be contracted from infested clothes and direct contact with an infested person.

The treatment now used in most areas is gamma benzene hexachloride (Kwell), available as a cream, a lotion, and a shampoo. If the client has head lice, the hair is washed with the shampoo and the bed linens are changed. This treatment is repeated 12 to 24 hours later if needed. A client with pubic or body lice takes a bath or shower, dries, and applies the lotion or cream—to the entire body surface for body lice, and to the pubic area and adjacent areas for pubic lice. After 12 to 24 hours, the lotion is washed off, and clean clothing and linens are supplied.

Scabies is a contagious skin infestation by the itch mite. The characteristic lesion is the burrow produced by the female mite as it penetrates into the upper layers of the skin. Burrows are short, wavy, brown or black thread-like lesions most commonly observed between the webs of the fingers and the folds of the wrists and elbows. The mites cause intense itching that is more pronounced at night because the increased warmth of the skin has a stimulating effect on the parasites. Secondary lesions caused by scratching include vesicles, papules, pustules, excoriations, and crusts. Treatment involves thorough cleansing of the body with soap and water to remove scales and debris from crusts, and then an application of a scabicide lotion. All bed linens and clothing should be washed in very hot or boiling water.

Hirsutism is the growth of excessive body hair. The acceptance of body hair in the axillae and on the legs is largely dictated by culture. In North America, the well-groomed woman, as depicted in magazines, has no hair on her legs or under her axillae (although this idea is changing). In many European cultures, it is not customary for well-groomed women to remove this hair.

Excessive facial hair on a woman is thought unattractive in most Western and Asian cultures. For example, some Japanese brides follow the custom of shaving their faces the day before the wedding.

The cause of excessive body hair is not always known. Elderly women may have some on their faces, and women during menopause may also experience the growth of facial hair. These conditions may be due to the action of the endocrine system. It is also throught heredity influences both the pattern of hair distribution and the production of androgens by the adrenal glands.

DIAGNOSING

Nursing diagnoses related to hair hygiene and hair and scalp problems include **Self-care deficit: grooming, Impaired skin integrity, High risk for infection,** and **Body image disturbance.** Examples of these nursing diagnoses with contributing factors are shown below.

- **Self-care deficit: grooming** related to
  a. Activity intolerance
  b. Imposed immobility (bed rest)
  c. Pain in upper extremities
  d. Altered level of consciousness
  e. Lack of motivation associated with depression
- **Impaired skin integrity** related to
  a. Scalp laceration
  b. Insect bite
- **Potential for infection** related to
  a. Scalp laceration
  b. Insect bite
- **Body image disturbance** related to alopecia

PLANNING

In planning care, the nurse identifies nursing interventions that will assist the client to improve hair texture, growth, and cleanliness; maintain or improve a sense of well-being; and prevent specific hair and scalp problems. Plans for assisting the client should take into account the client's personal preferences, health, and energy resources as well as the time, equipment, and personnel available. Often, clients like to receive hair care after a bath, before receiving visitors, and/or before retiring. At some agencies, shampoos can be given to clients only after a physician's order. Examples of outcome criteria to evaluate the the effectiveness of nursing interventions are shown below.

The client

- Performs hair grooming with assistance (specify).
- Has clean, well-groomed, resilient hair with a healthy sheen.
- Has reduced or absent scalp lesions or infestations.
- Describes contributing factors, interventions, and preventive measures for specific hair problem (eg, dandruff).

IMPLEMENTING

Brushing and Combing Hair To be healthy, hair needs to be brushed daily. Brushing has three major functions: It stimulates the circulation of blood in the scalp, it distributes the oil along the hair shaft, and it helps to arrange the hair, although many people use a comb for that purpose.

Long hair may present a problem for hospitalized clients. A brush with stiff bristles provides the best stimulation to blood circulation in the scalp. The bristles should not be so sharp that they injure the client's scalp, however. To prevent hair from matting, the client or nurse needs to comb it at least daily. A comb with dull, even teeth is advisable. A comb with sharp teeth might injure the scalp; combs that are too fine can pull and break the hair. Some clients are pleased to have their hair tied neatly in the back or braided until other assistance is available or until they feel better and can look after it. Others may consider such styles unattractive or juvenile. The nurse should work with the client to find an acceptable style.

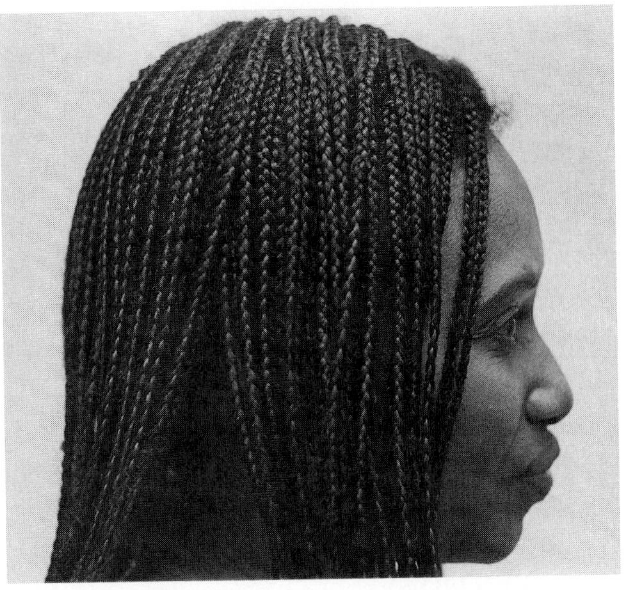

Figure 29–19 An African-American's hair styled with braids.

Dark-skinned people often have thicker, drier, curlier hair than light-skinned people. Spiraled or very curly hair may stand out from the scalp. Although the shafts of spiraled hair look strong and wiry, they have less strength than straight hair shafts and can break easily.

Some African-Americans have their spiraled hair straightened. Even if straightened, the hair tends to tangle and mat easily, especially at the back and the sides if the client is confined to bed. Other African-Americans style their hair in small braids (Figure 29–19). These braids do not have to be unbraided for shampooing and washing. The nurse should obtain the client's permission before any such unbraiding. Some African-American clients need to oil their hair daily because it tends to be dry. Oil also prevents the hair strands from breaking and the scalp from becoming too dry.

Neat, well-groomed hair usually gives clients a sense of well-being and improves their appearance. Appearance is often particularly important to clients when they have visitors. Procedure 29–7 describes how to provide hair care.

Shampooing the Hair When a client is hospitalized for extended periods or the hair becomes soiled, the nurse needs to help shampoo the client's hair. There are several ways to shampoo clients' hair, depending on their health,

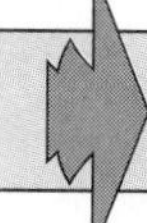

PROCEDURE 29–7 PROVIDING HAIR CARE

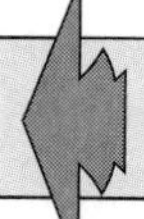

PURPOSES

- To stimulate the blood circulation to the scalp
- To distribute hair oils and provide a healthy sheen
- To increase the client's sense of well-being
- To discover or monitor hair or scalp problems (eg, matted hair or dandruff)

ASSESSMENT FOCUS
Usual hair care practices; routinely used hair care products; self-care abilities; any scalp problems.

EQUIPMENT

- ☐ Even-toothed comb
- ☐ Personal hair care products (optional)

INTERVENTION

1. Position and prepare the client appropriately.

- Assist the client who can sit to move to a chair. *Hair is more easily brushed and combed when the client is in a sitting position.* If health permits, assist a client confined to bed to a sitting position by raising the head of the bed. Otherwise, assist the client to alternate side-lying positions, and do one side of the head at a time.
- If the client remains in bed, place a clean towel over the pillow and the client's shoulders. Place it over the sitting client's shoulders. *The towel collects any removed hair, dirt, and scaly material.*
- Remove any pins or ribbons in the hair.

2. Comb the hair.

- Depending on the client's hair style, texture, and length, either start at the neckline and lift and fluff hair outward, moving upward toward the forehead (Figure 29–20) *or* begin at the hairline and comb downward and outward, toward the neck and shoulders.
- Continue fluffing the hair outward and upward until all of the hair is combed on one half of the head. Repeat the procedure for the other half.

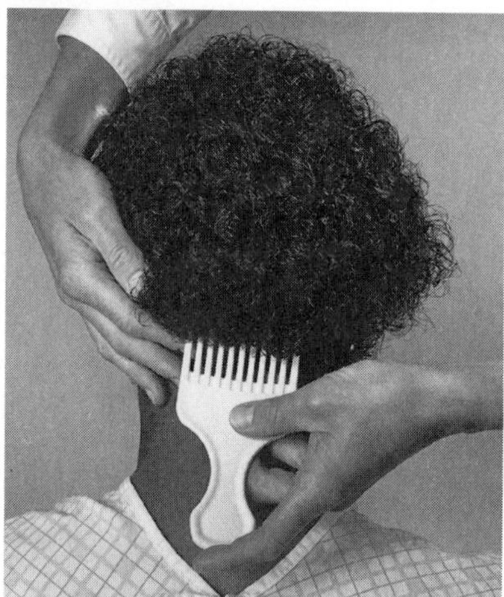

Figure 29–20 Using a large open-toothed comb to comb an African-American's client's hair from the neckline upward toward the forehead.

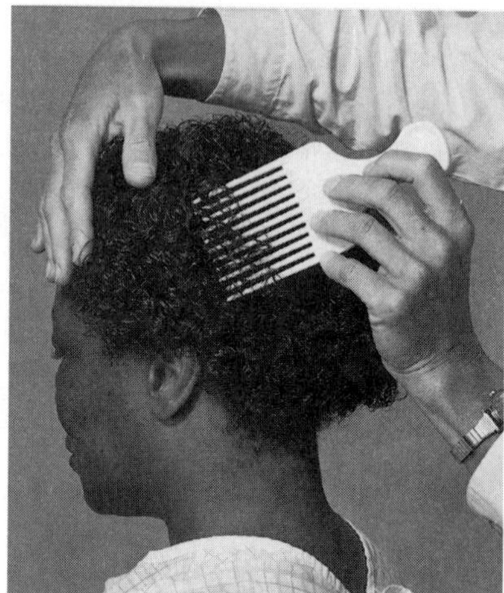

Figure 29–21 Removing tangles with a long-toothed comb.

3. Remove tangles gradually.

- Support the hair securely at the base of the scalp, if possible, to prevent pulling and discomfort. Insert a long-toothed comb into the ends of the hair and carefully comb out the ends of the tangles (Figure 29–21).
- Repeat this step, each time working the comb farther up the hair shaft toward the scalp, until the hair is untangled.

4. Document assessments and special nursing interventions.

- Daily combing and brushing of hair are not normally recorded.
- Record problems such as excessive dandruff, very dry or very oily hair, or the presence of lice.

EVALUATION FOCUS
Problems such as dandruff, alopecia, pediculosis, scalp lesions, or excessive dryness or mats.

strength, and age. The client who is well enough to take a shower can shampoo while in the shower. The client who is unable to shower may be given a shampoo while sitting on a chair in front of a sink. The back-lying client who can move to a stretcher can be given a shampoo on a stretcher wheeled to a sink. The client who must remain in bed can be give a shampoo with water brought to the bedside. This method is the least convenient. Some hospitals have volunteer beauticians with portable shampoo chairs who assist with hair care.

Shampoo basins to catch the water and direct it to the washbasin or other receptacle are usually made of plastic or metal. If one is not available, a plastic drawsheet can be rolled up on three sides to make edges about 7 cm (3 in) high. These edges will guide the water to the receptacle, in which the unrolled fourth edge of the sheet is placed. A pail or large washbasin can be used as a receptacle for the shampoo water. If possible, the receptacle should be large enough to hold all the shampoo water so that it does not have to be emptied during the shampoo.

Water used for the shampoo should be 40.5 C (105 F) for an adult or child to be comfortable and not injure the scalp. Usually, the person will supply a liquid or cream shampoo. If the shampoo is being given to destroy lice, the physician or agency protocol will indicate the shampoo to be used.

How often a person needs a shampoo is highly individual, depending to a large degree on the person's activities and the amount of sebum secreted by the scalp. Oily hair tends to look stringy and dirty, and it feels unclean to the person. Procedure 29–8 explains how to provide a shampoo for a client confined to bed.

Beard and Mustache Care Beards and mustaches also require daily care. The most important aspect of the care is to keep them clean. Food particles tend to collect in beards and mustaches, and they need washing and combing periodically. Clients may also wish a beard or mustache trim to maintain a well-groomed appearance. A beard or mustache should not be shaved off without the client's consent.

Male clients often shave or are shaved after a bath. Frequently clients supply their own electric or safety razors. See the box above for the steps involved in shaving a beard with a safety razor.

USING A SAFETY RAZOR TO SHAVE FACIAL HAIR

- Apply shaving cream or shaving soap and water first to soften the bristles and make the skin more pliable.
- Hold the razor so that the blade is at a 45-degree angle to the skin, and shave in short, firm strokes in the direction of hair growth.
- Hold the skin taut, particularly around creases, to prevent cutting the skin.
- After shaving the entire area, wipe the client's face with a wet washcloth to remove any remaining shaving cream and hair.
- Dry the face well, then apply aftershave lotion or powder as the client prefers.
- To prevent irritating the skin, pat on the lotion with the fingers and avoid rubbing the face.

EVALUATING

See Evaluating on page 744.

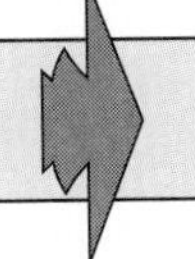

PROCEDURE 29–8 SHAMPOOING THE HAIR OF A CLIENT CONFINED TO BED

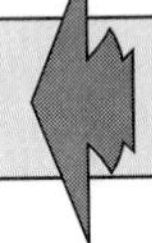

PURPOSES

- To stimulate the blood circulation to the scalp through massage
- To clean the hair and increase the client's sense of well-being

ASSESSMENT FOCUS

Routinely used shampoo products; any scalp problems; activity tolerance of the client.

EQUIPMENT

- ☐ Comb and brush
- ☐ Plastic sheet or pad
- ☐ Two bath towels
- ☐ Shampoo basin
- ☐ Washcloth or pad
- ☐ Bath blanket
- ☐ Receptacle for the shampoo water
- ☐ Cotton balls (optional)
- ☐ Pitcher of water
- ☐ Bath thermometer
- ☐ Liquid or cream shampoo
- ☐ Hair dryer

PROCEDURE 29–8 SHAMPOOING THE HAIR OF A CLIENT CONFINED TO BED *continued*

INTERVENTION

1. Verify agency policy and the physician's order.

- Determine whether a physician's order is needed before a shampoo can be given. *Some agencies require an order.*
- Determine the type of shampoo to be used (eg, medicated shampoo).

2. Prepare the client.

- Determine the best time of day for the shampoo. Discuss this with the client. A person who must remain in bed may find the shampoo tiring. Choose a time when the client is rested and can rest after the procedure.
- Assist the client to the side of the bed from which you will work.
- Remove pins and ribbons from the hair, and brush and comb it to remove any tangles.

3. Arrange the equipment.

- Put the plastic sheet or pad on the bed under the head. *The plastic keeps the bedding dry.*
- Remove the pillow from under the client's head, and place it under the shoulders. *This hyperextends the neck.*
- Tuck a bath towel around the client's shoulders. *This keeps the shoulders dry.*
- Place the shampoo basin under the head, putting a folded washcloth or pad where the client's neck rests on the edge of the basin. If the client is on a stretcher, the neck can rest on the edge of the sink with the washcloth as padding. *Padding supports the muscles of the neck and prevents undue strain and discomfort.*
- Fanfold the top bedding down to the waist, and cover the upper part of the client with the bath blanket. *The folded bedding will stay dry, and the bath blanket, which can be discarded after the shampoo, will keep the client warm.*
- Place the receiving receptacle on a table or chair at the bedside. Put the spout of the shampoo basin over the receptacle.

4. Protect the client's eyes and ears.

- Place a damp washcloth over the client's eyes (Figure 29–22). *The washcloth protects the eyes from soapy water. A damp washcloth will not slip.*

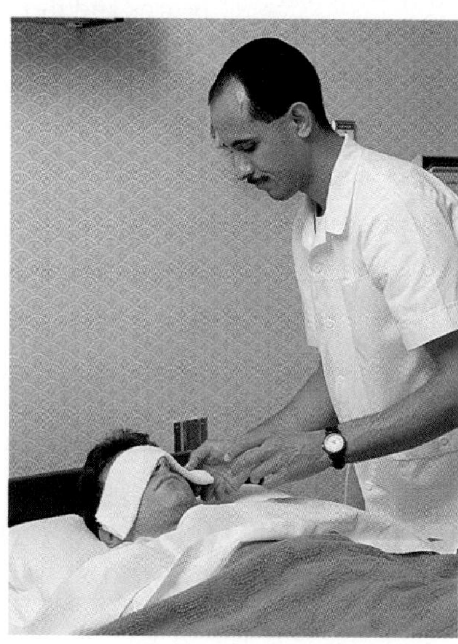

Figure 29–22 Using a damp washcloth to protect the eyes from soapy water.

- Place cotton balls in the client's ears if indicated. *These keep water from collecting in the ear canals.*

5. Shampoo the hair.

- Wet the hair thoroughly with the water.
- Apply shampoo to the scalp. Make a good lather with the shampoo while massaging the scalp with the pads of your fingertips. Massage all areas of the scalp systematically, for example, starting at the front and working toward the back of the head. *Massaging stimulates the blood circulation in the scalp. The pads of the fingers are used so that the fingernails will not scratch the scalp.*
- Rinse the hair briefly, and apply shampoo again.
- Make a good lather and massage the scalp as before.
- Rinse the hair thoroughly this time to remove all the shampoo. *Shampoo remaining in the hair may dry and irritate the hair and scalp.*
- Squeeze as much water as possible out of the hair with your hands.

6. Dry the hair thoroughly.

- Rub the client's hair with a heavy towel.
- Dry the hair with the dryer. Set the temperature at "warm."
- Continually move the dryer to prevent burning the client's scalp.

7. Ensure client comfort.

- Assist the person confined to bed to a comfortable position.
- Arrange the hair using a clean brush and comb.

8. Document the shampoo and any assessments.

- Report problems noted to the nurse in charge.

EVALUATION FOCUS
Any scalp problems or intolerance to procedure.

EYES

Normally, eyes require no special hygiene, since lacrimal fluid continually washes the eyes, and the eyelids and lashes prevent the entrance of foreign particles. Special interventions are needed, however, for unconscious clients and for clients recovering from eye surgery or having eye injuries, irritations, or infections. In unconscious clients, the blink reflex may be absent, and excessive drainage may accumulate along eyelid margins. In clients with eye trauma or eye infections, excessive discharge or drainage is common. Excessive secretions on the lashes need to be removed before they dry on the lashes as crusts. Clients who wear eyeglasses, contact lenses, or an artificial eye also may require instruction from and care by the nurse.

ASSESSING

Nursing History During the nursing history, the nurse obtains data about the client's eyeglasses or contact lenses, recent examination by an ophthalmologist, and any history of eye problems and related treatments. Questions to elicit these data are shown in the box at the right.

Physical Assessment In physical assessment, all external eye structures are inspected for signs of inflammation, excessive drainage, encrustations, or other obvious abnormalities. Inspection of the external eye structures is discussed in Chapter 22, page 483.

DIAGNOSING

Nursing diagnoses related to eye problems may include **Self-care deficit, High risk for infection,** and **High risk for injury.** Examples of these diagnoses and possible contributing factors are shown below.

- **Self-care deficit** (contact lens insertion, removal, and cleaning) related to
  a. Knowledge deficit
  b. Impaired vision associated with cataracts
- **High risk for infection** related to
  a. Improper contact lens hygiene
  b. Accumulation of secretions on eyelids
- **High risk for injury** related to
  a. Prolonged wearing of contact lenses
  b. Absence of blink reflex associated with unconsciousness

PLANNING

In planning care, the nurse identifies nursing interventions that will assist the client to maintain the integrity of the cornea, conjunctiva, and/or a prosthesis and to prevent eye injury and infection from contact lenses. Nursing interventions may include teaching clients about proper insertion, cleaning, and removal of contact lenses or a prosthesis and ways to protect the eyes from injury and strain. Examples of outcome criteria to evaluate the effectiveness of nursing interventions are shown below.

The client

- Has clear conjunctiva and white sclera without inflammation.

ASSESSMENT INTERVIEW

Eyes

For Clients Who Wear Eyeglasses

- When were the glasses/lenses prescribed?
- What is your vision like with and without the corrective device?

For Clients Who Wear Contact Lenses

- How often do you wear lenses? Daily? On special occasions?
- How long do you wear your lenses in a given day, including sleep time?
- Do you have any problems with the lenses (eg, cleaning, insertion, removal, damage)?
- Do you carry an emergency identification label to alert others to remove the lenses and ensure appropriate care in an emergency? (If not, advise the client to acquire one.)
- What are your insertion and removal procedures?
- What are your cleaning and storage procedures?
- Have you had any problems with either or both eyes or eyelids, such as excessive tearing, burning, redness, sensitivity to light, swelling, or feelings of dryness? Describe them.
- Are you using any eyedrops or ointments? (These medications can combine chemically with *soft* lenses and cause lens damage and eye irritation.)

For All Clients

- When did you last visit an ophthalmologist?
- Are you currently taking any eye medication? If so, provide name, dosage, and frequency.
- Do you have any of the following eye problems: difficulty reading or seeing objects, blurring of vision, tearing, spots or floaters, photophobia (sensitivity to light), burning, itching, pain, double vision, flashing lights, or halos around lights?

EYE CARE FOR THE COMATOSE CLIENT

When a comatose client's corneal reflex is impaired, eye care is essential to keep moist the areas of the cornea that are exposed to air.

- Administer moist compresses to cover the eyes as ordered (eg, every 2 to 4 hours).
- Clean eyes with saline solution and cotton balls. Wipe from the inner to outer canthus. This prevents debris from being washed into the nasolacrimal duct.
- Use a new cotton ball for each wipe. This prevents extending infection in one eye or to the other eye.
- Instill ophthalmic ointment into the lower lids. This keeps the eyes moist.
- Close the client's eyelids, and then put a small amount of mineral oil on the outer eyelids to lubricate and protect the skin.
- If the client's corneal reflex is absent, keep the eyes closed by placing an eye pad soaked in the saline solution over each eye and securing these with nonallergenic tape. These pads should *not* be so tight as to provide pressure on the eyes.

- Has reduced secretions on eyelids.
- Experiences no tearing.
- Verbalizes no eye discomfort.
- Demonstrates appropriate methods of caring for contact lenses.
- Describes interventions to prevent eye injury and infection.

IMPLEMENTING

Eye Care Dried secretions that have accumulated on the lashes need to be softened and wiped away. Soften dried secretions by placing a sterile cotton ball moistened with sterile water or normal saline over the lid margins. Wipe the loosened secretions from the inner canthus of the eye to the outer canthus to prevent the particles and fluid from draining into the lacrimal sac and nasolacrimal duct.

If the client is unconscious and lacks a blink reflex or cannot close the eyelids completely, drying and irritation of the cornea must be prevented. Lubricating eye drops may be administered if ordered by the physician. An eye patch may also be placed over the affected eye or eyes. See the box above for providing eye care for the comatose client.

Eyeglass Care It is essential that the nurse exercise caution when cleaning eyeglasses to prevent breaking or scratching the lenses. Glass lenses can be cleaned with warm water and dried with a soft tissue that will not scratch the lenses. Plastic lenses are easily scratched and require special cleaning solutions and drying tissues. When not being worn, all glasses should be placed in a case labeled appropriately, and stored in the client's bedside table drawer.

Contact Lens Care Contact lenses, thin curved discs of hard or soft plastic, fit on the cornea of the eye directly over the pupil. They float on the tear layer of the eye. For some people, contact lenses offer several advantages over eyeglasses: (a) they cannot be seen and thus have cosmetic value; (b) they are highly effective in correcting some astigmatisms; (c) they are safer than glasses for some physical activities; (d) they do not fog, as eyeglasses do; and (e) they provide better vision in many cases.

Contact lenses may be either hard or soft or a compromise between the two types—gas-permeable lenses. *Hard contact lenses* are made of a rigid, unwettable, airtight plastic that does not absorb water or saline solutions. They usually cannot be worn for more than 12 to 14 hours and are rarely recommended for first-time wearers.

Soft contact lenses cover the entire cornea. Being more pliable and soft, they mold to the eye for a firmer fit. The duration of extended-wear varies by brand from 1 to 30 days or more. Eye specialists recommend that long-wear brands be removed and cleaned at least once a week. These lenses require scrupulous care and handling.

Gas-permeable lenses are rigid enough to provide clear vision but are more flexible than the traditional hard lens. They permit oxygen to reach the cornea, thus providing greater comfort, and will not cause serious damage to the eye if left in place for several days.

Most clients normally care for their own contact lenses. In general, each lens manufacturer provides detailed cleaning instructions. Depending on the type of lens and cleaning method used, warm tap water, normal saline, or special rinsing or soaking solutions may be used.

All users should have a special container for their lenses. Some contain a solution so that the lenses are stored wet; in others, the lenses are dry. Each lens container has a slot with a label indicating whether it is for the right or left lens. It is essential that the correct lens be stored in the appropriate slot so that it can be worn in the correct eye.

Removing Contact Lenses *Hard* contact lenses must be positioned directly over the cornea for proper removal. If the lens is displaced, the nurse asks the client to look straight ahead, and gently exerts pressure on the upper and lower lids to move the lens back onto the cornea. Figure 29–23 shows the steps needed to remove a hard lens.

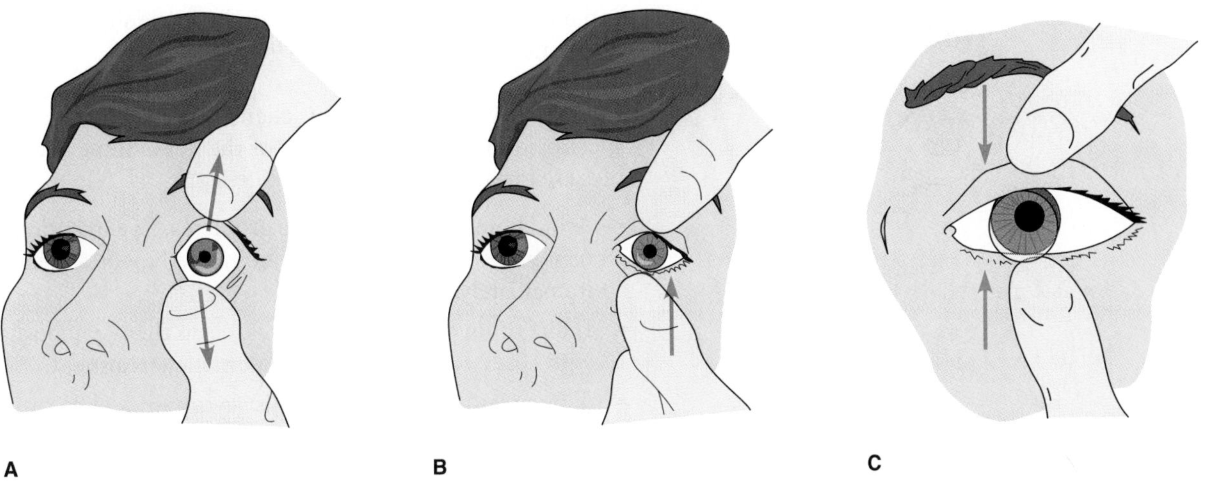

Figure 29–23 Removing hard contact lenses: *A,* Separate the eyelids until they are beyond the edges of the lens. *B,* Hold the top eyelid stationary at the edge of the lens, and lift the bottom edge of contact lens by pressing the lower lid at its margin. *C,* After the lens is slightly tipped, slide the lens out of the eye by moving both eyelids toward each other.

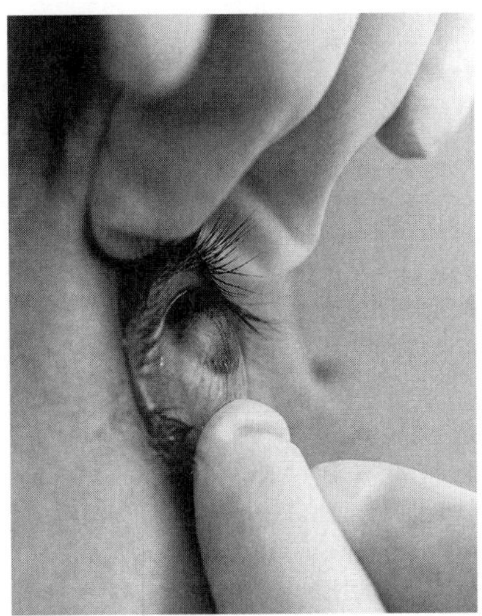

Figure 29–24 Moving a soft lens down to the inferior part of the sclera.

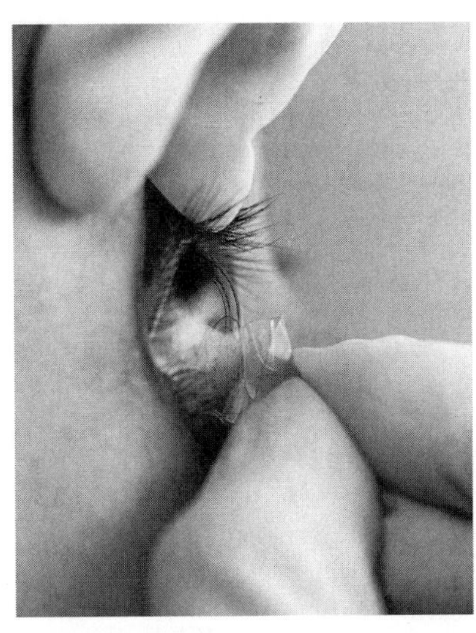

Figure 29–25 Removing a soft lens by pinching it between the pads of the thumb and index finger.

To avoid lens mix-ups, the nurse places the first lens in its designated cup in the storage case before removing the second lens.

Removal of *soft* lenses varies in two ways First, after separating the eyelids with the nondominant hand, move the lens down to the inferior part of the sclera using the pad of the dominant index finger (Figure 29–24). This reduces the risk of damage to the cornea. Second, remove the lens by gently pinching the lens between the pads of the thumb and index finger of your dominant hand (Figure 29–25). Pinching causes the lens to double up, so that air enters underneath the lens, overcoming the suction and allowing removal. Use the pads of the fingers to prevent scratching the eye or the lens with the fingernails.

Inserting Contact Lenses Seriously ill clients whose contact lenses have been removed will not need them reinserted until they become more active in their care and require the lenses to see properly. Contact lenses need to be lubricated in a sterile, nonirritating wetting solution (usually a saline solution) before they are inserted. The wetting solution helps the lens to glide over the cornea, thus reducing the risk of injury. Most clients, when well, will reinsert the lenses independently.

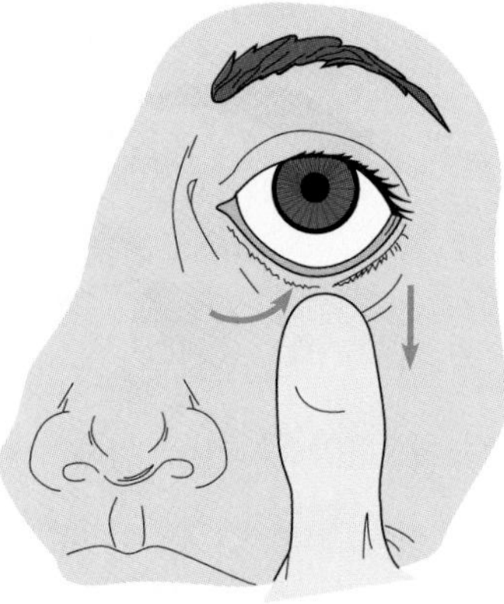

Figure 29–26 Removing an artificial eye by retracting the lower eyelid and exerting slight pressure below the eyelid.

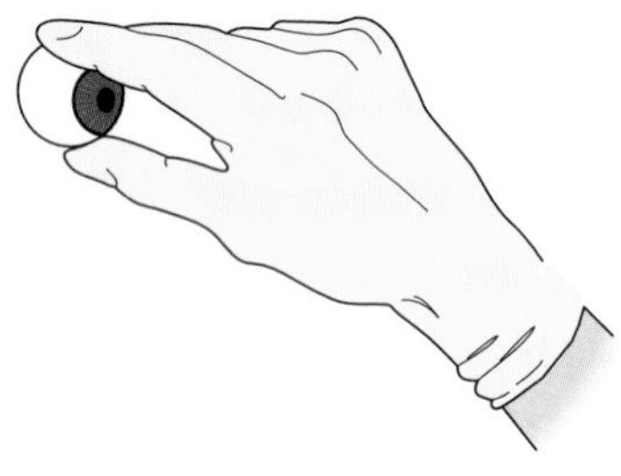

Figure 29–27 Holding an artificial eye between the thumb and index finger for insertion.

Artificial Eyes Artificial eyes are usually made of glass or plastic. Some are permanently implanted; others are removed regularly for cleaning. Most clients who wear a removable artificial eye follow their own care regimen. Even for an unconscious client, daily removal and cleaning are not necessary.

To remove an artificial eye, the nurse dons clean gloves and uses the dominant thumb to pull the client's lower eyelid down over the infraorbital bone, exerting slight pressure below the eyelid to overcome the suction (Figure 29–26). An alternative method is to compress a small rubber bulb and apply the tip directly to the eye. As the nurse gradually releases the finger pressure on the bulb, the suction of the bulb counteracts the suction holding the eye in the socket and draws the eye out of the socket.

The eye is cleaned with warm normal saline and placed in a container filled with water or saline solution. The socket and tissues around the eye are usually cleaned with cotton wipes and normal saline. To reinsert the eye, the nurse uses the thumb and index finger of one hand to retract the eyelids, exerting pressure on the supraorbital and infraorbital bones. Holding the eye between the thumb and index finger of the other hand, the nurse slips the eye gently into the socket (Figure 29–27).

General Eye Care Many clients may need to learn specific information about care of the eyes. Some examples are given below.

- Avoid home remedies for eye problems. Eye irritations or injuries at any age should be treated medically and immediately.
- If dirt or dust gets into the eyes, clean them copiously with clean, tepid water as an emergency treatment.
- Take measures to guard against eyestrain and to protect vision, such as maintaining adequate lighting for reading and obtaining shatterproof lenses for glasses.
- Schedule regular eye examinations, particularly after age 40, to detect problems such as cataracts and glaucoma.

EVALUATING

See Evaluating on page 744.

EARS

Normal ears require minimal hygiene. Clients who have excessive **cerumen** (earwax) and dependent clients who have hearing aids may require assistance from the nurse. Hearing aids are usually removed before surgery.

Cleaning the Ears The auricles of the ear are cleaned during the bed bath. The nurse or client must remove excessive cerumen that is visible or that causes discomfort or hearing difficulty. Visible cerumen may be loosened and removed by retracting the auricle downward. If this measure is ineffective, irrigation is necessary (see the section on otic irrigation in Chapter 43). Clients need to be advised never to use bobby pins, toothpicks, or cotton-tipped applicators to remove cerumen. Bobby pins and toothpicks can injure the ear canal and rupture the tympanic membrane; cotton-tipped applictors can cause wax to become impacted within the canal.

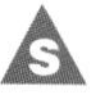

Care of Hearing Aids A hearing aid is a battery-powered, sound-amplifying device used by hearing-impaired persons. It consists of a microphone that picks up sound and converts it to electric energy, an amplifier that magnifies the electric energy electronically, a receiver that converts the amplified energy back to sound energy, and an earmold that directs the sound into the ear. There are several types of hearing aids:

- *Behind-the-ear (BTE, or postaural) aid.* This is the most widely used type, because it fits snugly behind the ear.

The hearing aid case, which holds the microphone, amplifier, and receiver, is attached to the earmold by a plastic tube (Figure 29–28).

- *In-the-ear aid.* This one-piece aid has all its components housed in the earmold (Figure 29–29).
- *In-the-canal (ITC) aid.* This is the most compact and least visible aid, fitting completely inside the ear canal. In addition to having cosmetic appeal, the ITC does not interfere with telephone use or the wearing of eyeglasses. However, it is not suitable for clients with progressive hearing loss; it requires adequate ear canal diameter and length for a good fit; and it tends to plug with cerumen more than other aids.
- *Eyeglasses aid.* This is similar to the behind-the-ear aid, but the components are housed in the temple of the eyeglasses. A hearing aid can be in one or both temples of the glasses.
- *Body hearing aid.* This pocket-sized aid, used for more severe hearing losses, clips onto an undergarment, shirt pocket, or harness carrier supplied by the manufacturer. The case, containing the microphone and amplifier, is connected by a cord to the receiver, which snaps into the earpiece.

For correct functioning, hearing aids require appropriate handling during insertion and removal, regular cleaning of the earmold, and replacement of dead batteries. With proper care, hearing aids generally last 5 to 10 years. Earmolds generally need readjustment every 2 to 3 years.

Procedure 29–9 describes how to remove, clean, and insert a hearing aid.

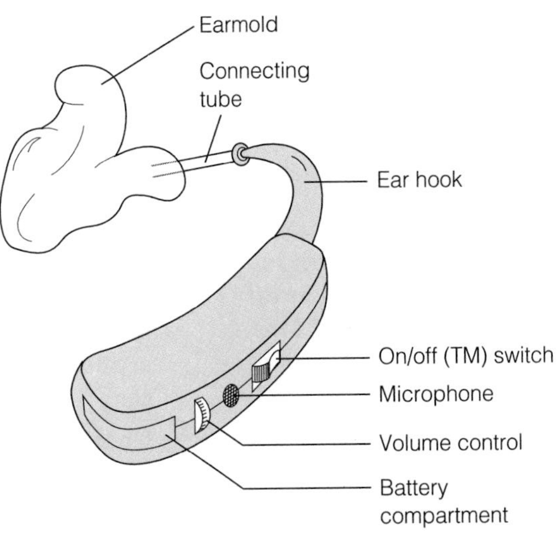

Figure 29–28 A behind-the-ear hearing aid.

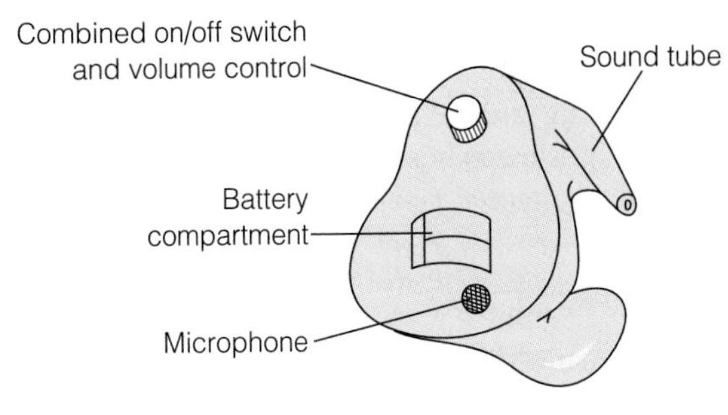

Figure 29–29 An in-the-ear hearing aid.

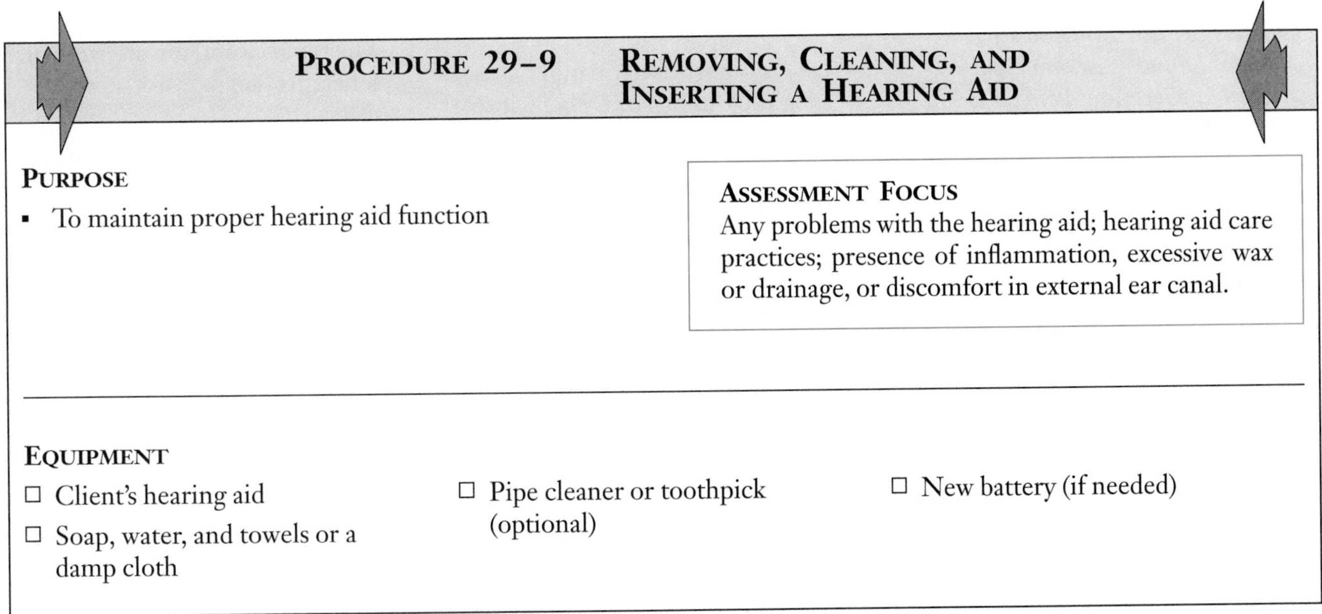

PROCEDURE 29–9 REMOVING, CLEANING, AND INSERTING A HEARING AID

PURPOSE

- To maintain proper hearing aid function

ASSESSMENT FOCUS

Any problems with the hearing aid; hearing aid care practices; presence of inflammation, excessive wax or drainage, or discomfort in external ear canal.

EQUIPMENT

- ☐ Client's hearing aid
- ☐ Soap, water, and towels or a damp cloth
- ☐ Pipe cleaner or toothpick (optional)
- ☐ New battery (if needed)

PROCEDURE 29–9 REMOVING, CLEANING, AND INSERTING A HEARING AID *continued*

INTERVENTION

1. Remove the hearing aid.

- Turn the hearing aid off, and lower the volume. The on/off switch may be labeled "O" (off), "M" (microphone), "T" (telephone), or "TM" (telephone/microphone). *The batteries continue to run if the aid is not turned off.*
- Remove the earmold by rotating it slightly forward and pulling it outward.
- If the aid is not to be used for several days, remove the battery. *Removal prevents corrosion of the aid from battery leakage.*
- Store the hearing aid in a safe place. Avoid exposure to heat and moisture. *Proper storage prevents loss or damage.*

2. Clean the earmold.

- Detach the earmold *if possible.* Disconnect the earmold from the receiver of a body hearing aid or from the hearing aid case of behind-the-ear and eyeglasses aids where the tubing meets the hook of the case. Do not remove the earmold if it is glued or secured by a small metal ring. *Removal facilitates cleaning and prevents inadvertent damage to the other parts.*
- If the earmold is *detachable*, soak it in a mild soapy solution. Rinse and dry it well. Do not use isopropyl alcohol. *Alcohol can damage the hearing aid.*
- If the earmold is *not detachable* or is for an in-the-ear aid, wipe the earmold with a damp cloth.
- Check that the earmold opening is patent. Blow any excess moisture through the opening or remove debris (eg, earwax) with a pipe cleaner or toothpick.
- Reattach the earmold if it was detached from the rest of the hearing aid.

3. Insert the hearing aid.

- Determine from the client if the earmold is for the left or the right ear.
- Check that the battery is inserted in the hearing aid. Turn off the hearing aid, and make sure the volume is turned all the way down. *A volume that is too loud is distressing.*
- Inspect the earmold to identify the ear canal portion. Some earmolds are fitted for only the ear canal and concha; others are fitted for all the contours of the ear. The canal portion, common to all, can be used as a guide for correct insertion.
- Line up the parts of the earmold with the corresponding parts of the client's ear.
- Rotate the earmold slightly forward, and insert the ear canal portion.
- Gently press the earmold into the ear while rotating it backward.
- Check that the earmold fits snugly by asking the client if it feels secure and comfortable.
- Adjust the other components of a behind-the-ear or body hearing aid.
- Turn the hearing aid on, and adjust the volume according to the client's needs.

4. Correct problems associated with improper functioning.

- If the sound is weak or there is no sound:
  a. Ensure that the volume is turned high enough.
  b. Ensure that the earmold opening is not clogged.
  c. Check the battery by turning the aid on, turning up the volume, cupping your hand over the earmold, and listening. A constant whistling sound indicates the battery is functioning. If necessary, replace the battery. Be sure that the negative (−) and positive (+) signs on the battery match those on the aid.
  d. Ensure that the ear canal is not blocked with wax, which can obstruct sound waves.
- If the client reports a whistling sound or squeal after insertion:
  a. Turn the volume down.
  b. Ensure that the earmold is properly attached to the receiver.
  c. Reinsert the earmold.

5. Document pertinent data.

- The removal and the insertion of a hearing aid are not normally recorded.
- Report and record any problems the client has with the hearing aid.

EVALUATION FOCUS
Absence of inflammation; wax buildup or discomfort in external ear canal; adequacy of hearing acuity with aid inserted; comfort of aid when inserted.

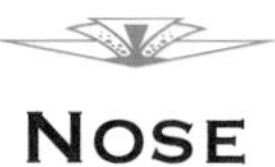

NOSE

Nurses usually need not provide special care for the nose, because clients can ordinarily clear nasal secretions by blowing gently into a soft tissue. When the external pores are encrusted with dried secretions, they should be cleaned with a cotton-tipped applicator or moistened with saline or water. The applicator should not be inserted beyond the length of the cotton tip; inserting it further may cause injury to the mucosa.

SUPPORTING A HYGIENIC ENVIRONMENT

Because ill persons are confined to bed, sometimes for week or months, the bed unit becomes an important element in the client's life. A unit that is clean, safe, and comfortable contributes to the client's ability to rest and sleep and to a sense of well-being. Basic furniture in a hospital bed unit includes the bed, bedside table, overbed table, one or more chairs, and a storage space for clothing. Hospitals vary in the equipment provided as part of the bed unit. Basic to all are a call light, light fixtures, electrical outlets, and hygienic equipment in the bedside table. Long-term care facilities may have very little additional equipment, whereas an acute care facility may have several commonly used devices built into each unit. Three types of equipment are often installed on the wall at the head of the bed: a *suction outlet* for several kinds of suction, an *oxygen outlet* for most oxygen equipment, and a *sphygmomanometer* to measure the client's blood pressure. Some long-term care agencies also permit clients to have *personal furniture*, such as a television, a chair, and lamps, at the bedside.

HOSPITAL BEDS

Hospital beds can be adjusted to a variety of positions. When the gatches, or joints of the bed, are flexed, the client is raised to a sitting position with the knees elevated. The cranks that operate the gatches are usually at the bottom or side of the bed. Manual cranks are left in the retracted position under the bed when they are not being used. Otherwise, people walking by the bed might easily hit their legs against the cranks. Many hospital beds have electric motors to operate the gatches. The motor is activated by pressing a button or moving a small lever, located either at the side of the bed or on a small panel separate from the bed but attached to it by a cable, which the client can readily use. Common bed positions are shown in Table 29–12 on page 776.

Hospital beds are usually 66 cm (26 in) high and 0.9 m (3 ft) wide, narrower than the usual bed, so that the nurse can reach the client from either side of the bed without undue stretching. The length is usually 1.9 m (6.5 ft). Some beds can be extended in length to accommodate very tall clients. Long-term care facilities for ambulatory clients usually have low beds to facilitate movement in and out of bed. Most hospital beds have "high" and "low" positions that can be adjusted either mechanically or electrically by a button or lever. The high position permits the nurse to reach the client without undue stretching or stooping. The low position allows the client to step easily to the floor.

Mattresses Most mattresses used in hospitals have innersprings, which give even support to the body. When changing a bed, nurses need to note any unevenness of the mattress surface, which might indicate a broken spring. Mattresses are usually covered with a water-repellent material that resists soiling and can be cleaned easily. Most mattresses have handles on the sides called lugs by which the mattress can be removed.

Many special mattresses are also used in hospitals to relieve pressure on the body's bony prominences, such as the heels. They are particularly helpful for clients confined to bed for a long time. For additional information about mattresses, see Table 30–4, page 795.

Side Rails Side rails, or safety sides, are used on both hospital beds and stretchers. They are of various shapes and sizes and are usually made of metal. Devices to raise and lower them differ. Often one or two knobs are pulled to release the side and permit it to be moved. When side rails are being used, it is important that the nurse *never* leave the bedside while the rail is lowered. Some side rails have two positions: up and down. Others have three: high, intermediate, and low. The down and low positions are employed when a side rail is not needed. With some models, the bed foundation (the mattress and frame supporting it) must be raised before the side rail can be put in the low position; otherwise, the side rail might hit the floor and be damaged. The intermediate position is used when the bed is in the low position and the nurse is present. The up or high side rail position is used when a client is in bed and requires protection from falling. Some hospitals have a release form that the client can sign if the use of side rails is refused.

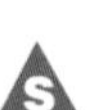

Footboards A footboard is a flat panel, often made of wood or plastic, placed at the foot of a bed. It serves three purposes:

1. To provide support for the client's feet and maintain a natural foot position while the client is in bed (Figure 29–30, p. 776).

Table 29–12 Commonly Used Bed Positions

Position	Description	Indications for Use
Flat Head of bed Foot of bed	Mattress is completely horizontal.	Client sleeping and a variety of bed positions, such as back-lying, side-lying, and prone (face down) To maintain spinal alignment for clients with spinal injuries To assist clients to move and turn in bed Bed-making by nurse
Fowler's position	Semisitting position in which head of bed is raised to angle of at least 45 degrees. Knees may be flexed or horizontal.	Convenient for eating, reading, visiting, watching TV Relief from lying positions To promote lung expansion for client with respiratory problem To assist a client to a sitting position on the edge of the bed
Semi-Fowler's position	Head of bed raised only to 30-degree angle.	Relief from lying position To promote lung expansion
Trendelenburg's position	Head of bed lowered and the foot raised in a straight incline.	To promote venous circulation in certain clients To provide postural drainage of basal lung lobes
Reverse Trendelenburg's position	Head of bed raised and the foot lowered. Straight tilt in direction opposite to Trendelenburg's position.	To promote stomach emptying and prevent esophageal reflex in clients with hiatal hernia

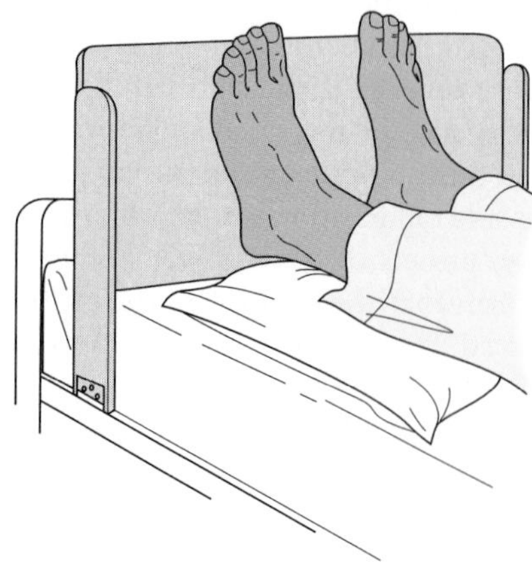

Figure 29–30 A footboard that can be adjusted to the client's height.

2. To keep the top bed covers off the client's feet, relieving the pressure of the weight of the covers.
3. To make the foot comfortable (for example, when a client has a painful foot).

Without the support of a footboard, a client's feet drop from their normal right angle to the legs and assume a plantar flexion position with the toes pointing toward the foot of the bed (Figure 29–31). Prolonged assumption of this position results in permanent shortening of the muscles and tendons at the back of the legs. When that happens, the clients is unable to stand flat-footed on the floor, and walking is seriously impaired.

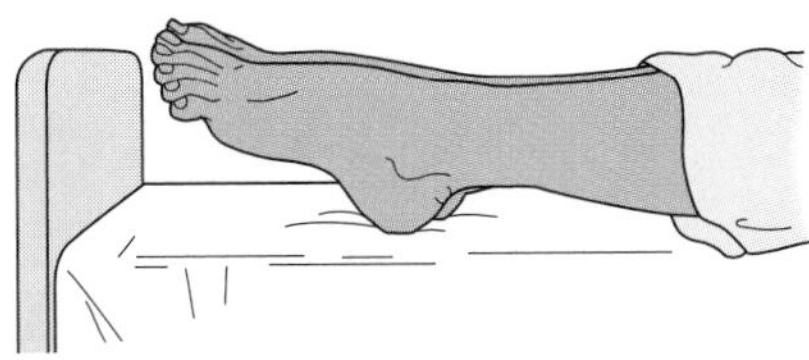

Figure 29–31 Feet in plantar flexion.

Footboards are often made in an L shape so that the base of the L fits under the foot of the mattress. Some footboards can be moved along the mattress to adjust to the client's height. If a board cannot be adjusted, sandbags and rolled pillows or blankets can be used to fill the space between the client's feet and the board.

Bed Cradles A bed cradle, sometimes called an *Anderson frame,* is a device designed to keep the top bedclothes off the feet, legs, and even abdomen of a client. The bedclothes are arranged over the device and may be pinned in place. There are several types of bed cradles. One of the most common is a curved metal rod that fits over the bed. Part of the cradle fits under the mattress, and small metal brackets press down on each side of the mattress to keep the cradle in place. The frame of some cradles extends over half of the width of the bed, above one leg.

Intravenous Rods Intravenous rods (poles, stands, standards), usually made of metal, support intravenous (IV) infusion containers while fluid is being administered to a client. These rods were traditionally freestanding on the floor beside the bed. Now, intravenous rods are often attached to the hospital beds. Some hospital units have overhead hanging rods on a track for IVs.

Specialized Beds Whenever a client's body alignment must be strictly maintained, a specially designed bed that rotates on an axis is used to turn the client from the supine to the prone position and vice versa. Two such beds are the Stryker wedge frame and the CircOlectric bed. The Stryker wedge frame, which is manually operated by the nurse, turns the client laterally through the side-lying position. The CircOlectric bed, which is operated electrically by the nurse using a push button, rotates the client vertically through the standing position. These turning frames are used for clients with certain types of spinal injuries, such as extensive burns, arthritis, and pressure sores, who require position changes that cannot be effectively managed in the standard bed.

MAKING BEDS

Nurses need to be able to prepare hospital beds in different ways for specific purposes. In most instances, beds are made after the client receives certain care and when beds are unoccupied. At times, however, nurses need to make an occupied bed or prepare a bed for a client who is having surgery (an anesthetic, postoperative, or surgical bed). Regardless of what type of bed equipment is available, whether the bed is occupied or unoccupied, or the purpose for which the bed is being prepared, certain guidelines pertain to all bed making. These are summarized in the box above.

An *unoccupied bed* can be either closed or open. Generally the top covers of an open bed are folded back *(open bed)* to make it easier for a client to get in. Open and closed beds are made the same way, except that the top sheet, blanket, and bedspread of a *closed* bed are drawn up to the top of the bed and under the pillows.

Hospital beds are often changed after bed baths. The linen can be collected before the bath. Nurses in some hospitals do not change all the linen unless it is soiled. Check the policy at each clinical agency. Unfitted sheets, blankets, and bedspread are mitered at the corners of the bed. The purpose of mitering is to secure the bedclothes while the bed is occupied. Figure 29–32 on page 778 shows how to miter the corner of a bed.

Procedure 29–10 explains how to change an unoccupied bed.

Text continued on page 781

CLINICAL GUIDELINES

Bed-Making

- Wash hands thoroughly after handling a client's bed linen. Linens and equipment that have been soiled with secretions and excretions harbor microorganisms that can be transmitted to others directly or by the nurse's hands or uniform.
- Hold soiled linen away from uniform.
- Linen for one client is *never* (even momentarily) placed on another client's bed.
- Soiled linen is placed directly in a portable linen hamper or tucked into a pillow case at the end of the bed before it is gathered up for disposal in the linen hamper or linen chute.
- Soiled linen is never shaken in the air because shaking can disseminate secretions and excretions and the microorganisms they contain.
- When stripping and making a bed, conserve time and energy by stripping and making up one side as completely as possible before working on the other side.
- To avoid unnecessary trips to the linen supply area, gather all needed linen before starting to strip a bed.

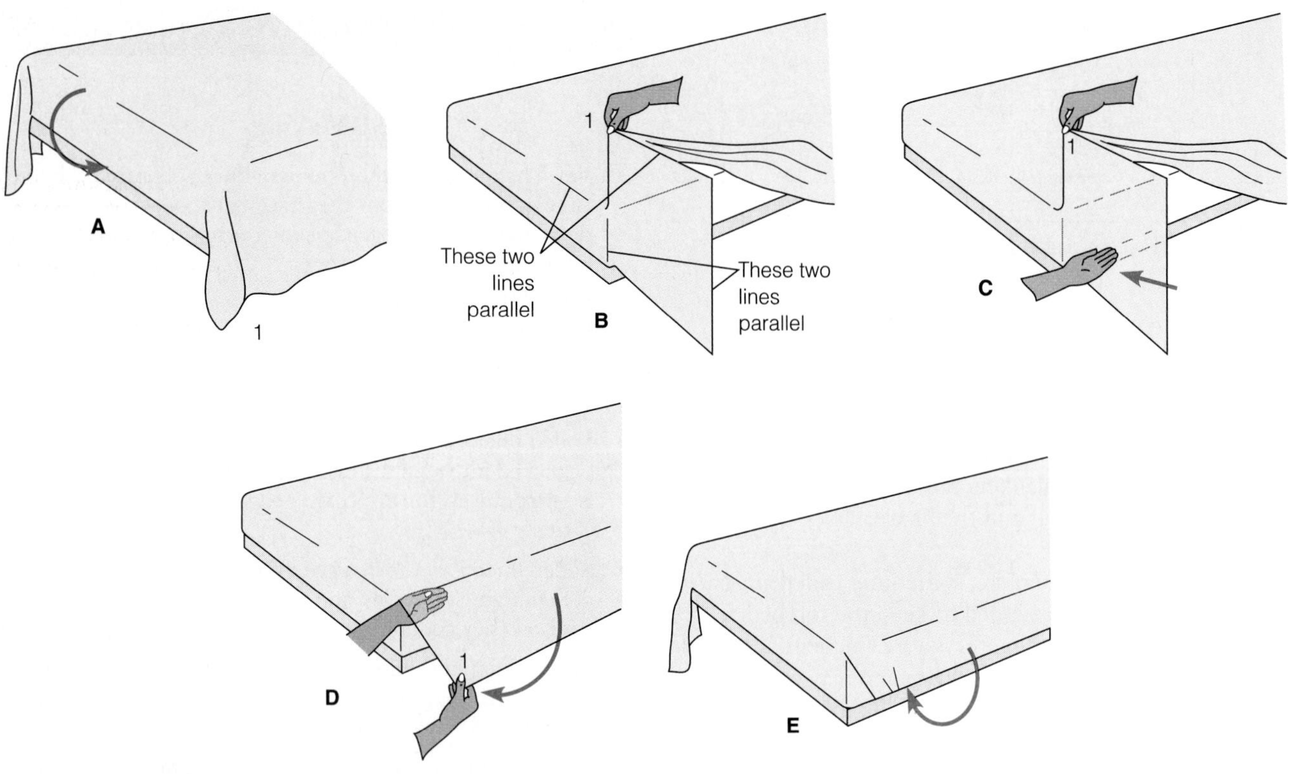

Figure 29–32 Mitering the corner of a bed: *A,* Tuck in the bedcover (sheet, blanket, and/or spread) firmly under the mattress at the bottom or top of the bed. *B,* Lift the bedcover at point 1 so that it forms a triangle with the side edge of the bed, and the edge of the bedcover is parallel to the end of the bed. *C,* Tuck the part of the cover that hangs below the mattress under the mattress while holding the cover at point 1 against the mattress. *D,* Bring point 1 down toward the floor while the other hand holds the fold of the cover against the side of the mattress. *E,* Remove the hand, and tuck the remainder of the cover under the mattress, if appropriate. The sides of the top sheet, blanket, and bedspread may be left hanging freely rather than tucked in. The bedspread is mitered separately and left hanging freely if the top sheet and blanket are tucked in.

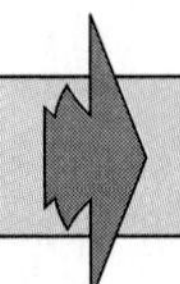

PROCEDURE 29–10 CHANGING AN UNOCCUPIED BED

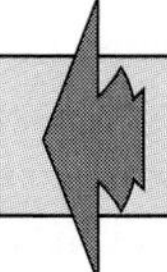

PURPOSES

- To promote the client's comfort
- To provide a clean, neat environment for the client
- To provide a smooth, wrinkle-free bed foundation, thus minimizing sources of skin irritation

EQUIPMENT

- ☐ Two large sheets
- ☐ Cloth drawsheet (optional)
- ☐ One blanket
- ☐ One bedspread
- ☐ Waterproof drawsheet or waterproof pads (optional)
- ☐ Pillowcase(s) for the head pillow(s)
- ☐ Portable linen hamper, if available

PROCEDURE 29–10 *continued*

INTERVENTION

1. Place the fresh linen on the client's chair or overbed table; do not use another client's bed. *This prevents cross-contamination (the movement of microorganisms from one client to another) via soiled linen.*

2. Assess and assist the client out of bed.

- Make sure that this is an appropriate and convenient time for the client to be out of bed.
- Assess the client's health status to determine that the person can safely get out of bed. In some hospitals it is necessary to have a written order if the client has been in bed continuously.
- Assess the client's pulse and respirations if indicated.
- Assist the client to a comfortable chair.

3. Strip the bed.

- Check bed linens for any items belonging to the client, and detach the call bell or any drainage tubes from the bed linen.
- Loosen all bedding, starting at the head of the bed, moving down the bed, working around the foot, and moving up to the other side of the head. *Moving around the bed systematically prevents stretching and reaching and possible muscle strain.*
- Remove the pillowcases, if soiled, and place the pillows on the bedside chair near the foot of the bed.
- Fold reusable linens, such as the bedspread and top sheet on the bed, into fourths. First, fold the linen in half by bringing the top edge even with the bottom edge, and then grasp it at the center of the middle fold and bottom edges (Figure 29–33). *Folding linens on the bed prevents strain on the nurse's arms and saves time and energy when reapplying the linens on the bed.*

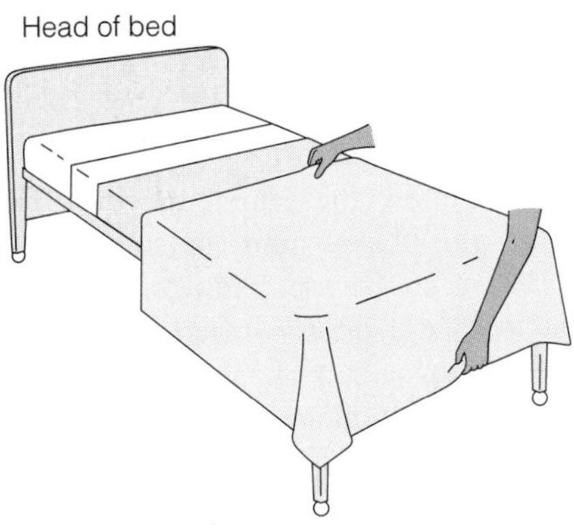

Figure 29–33 Folding reusable linens into fourths when removing them from the bed.

- Remove the waterproof pad, and discard it if soiled.
- Roll all soiled linen inside the bottom sheet, hold it away from your uniform, and place it directly in the linen hamper. *These actions are essential to prevent the transmission of microorganisms to the nurse and others.*
- Grasp the mattress securely, using the lugs if present, and move the mattress up to the head of the bed.

4. Apply the bottom sheet and drawsheet.

- Place the folded bottom sheet with its center fold on the center of the bed. Make sure the sheet is hemside down for a smooth foundation. Spread the sheet out over the mattress, and allow a sufficient amount of sheet at the top to tuck under the mattress. *The top of the sheet needs to be well tucked under to remain securely in place, especially when the head of the bed is elevated.* Place the sheet along the edge of the mattress at the foot of the bed, and do not tuck it in (unless it is a contour sheet).
- Miter the sheet at the top corner on the near side (Figure 29–32, earlier), and tuck the sheet under the mattress, working from the head of the bed to the foot.
- If a waterproof drawsheet is used, place it over the bottom sheet so that the center fold is at the center line of the bed and the top and bottom edges will extend from the middle of the client's back to the area of the mid thigh or knee. Fanfold the uppermost half of the folded drawsheet at the center or far edge of the bed, and tuck in the near edge.
- Lay the cloth drawsheet over the waterproof sheet in the same manner described above.
- *Optional:* Before moving to the other side of the bed, place the top linens on the bed, hemside up, unfold them, tuck them in, and miter the bottom corners. *Completing the entire side of the bed saves time and energy.*

5. Move to the other side, and secure the bottom linens.

- Tuck in the bottom sheet under the head of the mattress, pull the sheet firmly, and miter the corner of the sheet.
- Pull the remainder of the sheet firmly so that there are no wrinkles. *Wrinkles can cause discomfort for the client.* Tuck the sheet in at the side.
- Complete this same process for the drawsheet(s).

PROCEDURE 29–10 CHANGING AN UNOCCUPIED BED *continued*

6. Apply or complete the top sheet, blanket, and spread.

- Place the top sheet, hemside up, on the bed so that its center fold is at the center of the bed and the top edge is even with the top edge of the mattress.
- Unfold the sheet over the bed.
- *Optional:* Make a vertical or a horizontal toe pleat in the sheet to provide additional room for the client's feet.
  a. *Vertical toe pleat:* Make a fold in the sheet 5 to 10 cm (2 to 4 in) perpendicular to the foot of the bed (Figure 29–34).

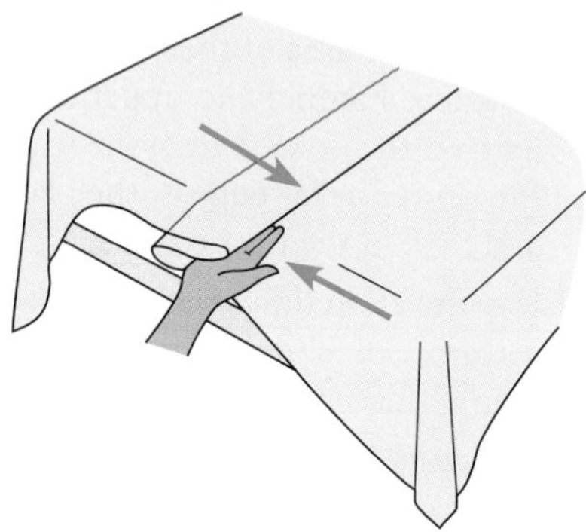

Figure 29–34 A vertical toe pleat.

  b. *Horizontal toe pleat:* Make a fold in the sheet 5 to 10 cm (2 to 4 in) across the bed near the foot (Figure 29–35).

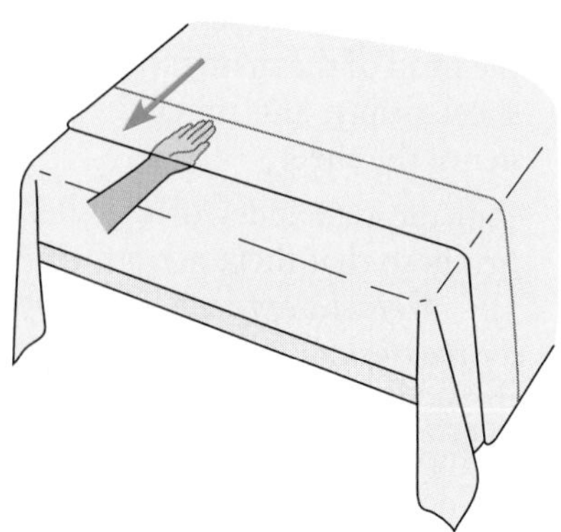

Figure 29–35 A horizontal toe pleat.

Loosening the top covers around the feet after the client is in bed is another way to provide additional space.

- Follow the same procedure for the blanket and the spread, but place the top edges about 15 cm (6 in) from the head of the bed to allow a cuff of sheet to be folded over them.
- Tuck in the sheet, blanket, and spread at the foot of the bed, and miter the corner, using all three layers of linen. Leave the sides of the top sheet, blanket, and spread hanging freely unless toe pleats were provided.
- Fold the top of the top sheet down over the spread, providing a cuff of about 15 cm (6 in). *The cuff of sheet makes it easier for the client to pull the covers up.*
- Move to the other side of the bed, and secure the top bedding in the same manner.

7. Put clean pillowcases on the pillows as required.

- Grasp the closed end of the pillowcase at the center with one hand.
- Gather up the sides of the pillowcase, and place them over the hand grasping the case. Then grasp the center of one short side of the pillow through the pillowcase (Figure 29–36).
- With the free hand, pull the pillowcase over the pillow.
- Adjust the pillowcase so that the pillow fits into the corners of the case and the seams are straight. *A smoothly fitting pillowcase is more comfortable than a wrinkled one.*
- Align and place the pillows at the head of the bed in the center.

8. Provide for client comfort and safety.

- Attach the signal cord so that the client can conveniently use it. Some cords have clamps that attach to the sheet or pillowcase. Others are attached by a safety pin.
- If the bed is currently being used by a client, either fold back the top covers at one side or fanfold them down to the center of the bed. *This makes it easier for the client to get into the bed.*
- Place the bedside table and the overbed table so that they are available to the client.
- Leave the bed in the high position if the client is returning by stretcher, or place in the low position if the client is returning to bed after being up.
- After changing a crib, leave both side rails in the highest position.

9. Document and report pertinent data.

- Bed-making is not normally recorded.
- Record any nursing assessments, such as the client's physical status and pulse and respiratory rates before and after being out of bed, as indicated.

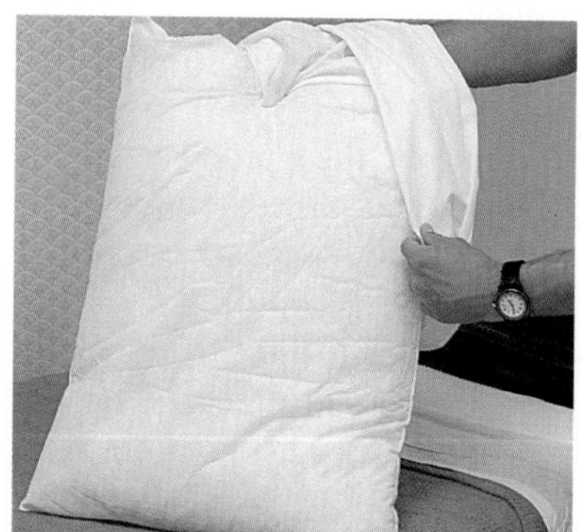

Figure 29–36 Method for putting a clean pillowcase on a pillow.

CHANGING AN OCCUPIED BED

Some clients may be too weak to get out of bed. Either the nature of their illness may contraindicate their sitting out of bed, or they may be restricted in bed by the presence of traction or other therapies. When changing an *occupied* bed, the nurse works quickly and disturbs the client as little as possible to conserve the client's energy, using the following guidelines:

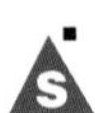

- Maintain the client in good body alignment. Never move or position a client in a manner that is contraindicated by the client's health. Obtain help if necessary to ensure safety.
- Move the client gently and smoothly. Rough handling can cause the client discomfort and abrade the skin.
- Throughout the procedure, explain what you plan to do before you do it. Use terms that the client can understand.
- Use the bed-making time, like the bed bath time, to assess and meet the client's needs.

Procedure 29–11 describes how to change an occupied bed.

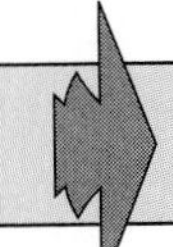

PROCEDURE 29–11 CHANGING AN OCCUPIED BED

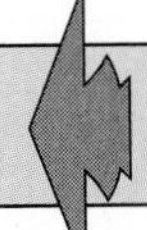

PURPOSES

- To conserve the client's energy and maintain current health status
- To promote client comfort
- To provide a clean, neat environment for the client
- To provide a smooth, wrinkle-free bed foundation, thus minimizing sources of skin irritation

ASSESSMENT FOCUS

Specific orders or precautions for moving and positioning the client; presence of incontinence or excessive drainage from other sources indicating the need for protective waterproof pads; skin condition and need for special mattress (eg, egg crate), footboard, or heel protectors.

EQUIPMENT

- ☐ Two large sheets
- ☐ Cloth drawsheet (optional)
- ☐ One blanket
- ☐ One bedspread
- ☐ Waterproof drawsheet or waterproof pads (optional)
- ☐ Pillowcase(s) for the head pillow(s)
- ☐ Portable linen hamper, if available

INTERVENTION

1. Remove the top bedding.

- Remove any equipment attached to the bed linen, such as a signal light.
- Loosen all the top linen at the foot of the bed, and remove the spread and the blanket.
- Leave the top sheet over the client (the top sheet can remain over the client if it is being changed and if it will provide sufficient warmth), *or* replace it with a bath blanket as follows:
  a. Spread the bath blanket over the top sheet.
  b. Ask the client to hold the top edge of the blanket.
  c. Reaching under the blanket from the side, grasp the top edge of the sheet and draw it down to the foot of the bed, leaving the blanket in place.
  d. Remove the sheet from the bed and place it in the soiled linen hamper.

2. Move the mattress up on the bed.

- Place the bed in the flat position, if the client's health permits.
- Grasp the mattress lugs, and, using good body mechanics, move the mattress up to the head of the bed. Ask the client to assist, if permitted, by grasping the head of the bed and pulling as you push. If the client is heavy, you may need help from another nurse.

3. Change the bottom sheet and drawsheet.

- Assist the client to turn on the side facing away from the side where the clean linen is.

- Raise the side rail nearest the client. *This protects the client from falling.* If there is no side rail,

PROCEDURE 29–11 CHANGING AN OCCUPIED BED *continued*

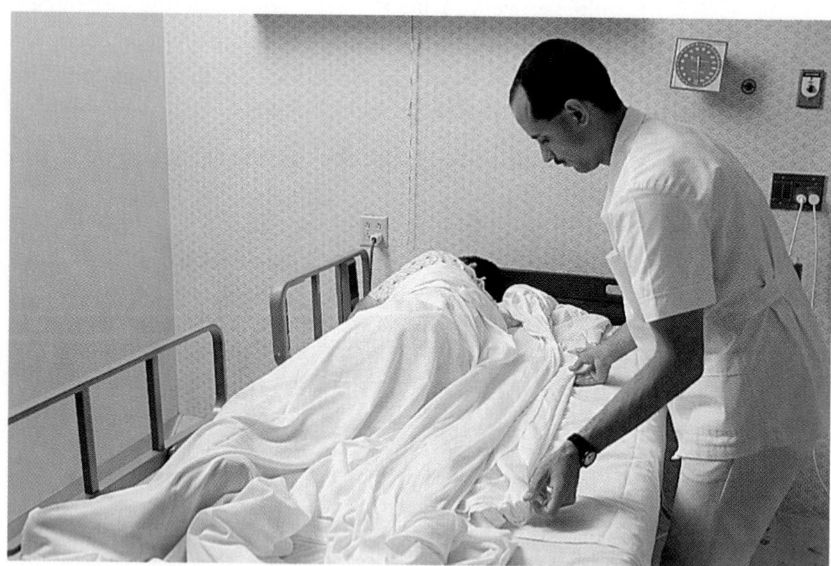

Figure 29–37 Fanfolding soiled linen as close to the client as possible.

have another nurse support the client at the edge of the bed.

- Loosen the foundation linen on the side of the bed near the linen supply.
- Fanfold the drawsheet and the bottom sheet at the center of the bed (Figure 29–37), as close to the client as possible. Doing this leaves the near half of the bed free to be changed.
- Place the new bottom sheet on the bed, and vertically fanfold the half to be used on the far side of the bed as close to the client as possible. Tuck the sheet under the near half of the bed, and miter the corner if a contour sheet is not being used.
- Place the clean drawsheet on the bed with the center fold at the center of the bed. Fanfold the uppermost half vertically at the center of the bed, and tuck the near side edge under the side of the mattress.
- Assist the client to roll over toward you onto the clean side of the bed. The client rolls over the fanfolded linen at the center of the bed.
- Move the pillows to the clean side for the client's use. Raise the side rail before leaving the side of the bed.
- Move to the other side of the bed, and lower the side rail.
- Remove the used linen, and place it in the portable hamper.
- Smooth out the mattress cover to remove any wrinkles. Unfold the fanfolded bottom sheet from the center of the bed.
- Facing the side of the bed, use both hands to pull the bottom sheet so that it is smooth, and tuck the excess under the side of the mattress.
- Unfold the drawsheet fanfolded at the center of the bed, and pull it tightly with both hands. Pull the sheet in three sections: (a) face the side of the bed to pull the middle section; (b) face the far top corner to pull the bottom section; and (c) face the far bottom corner to pull the top section.
- Tuck the excess drawsheet under the side of the mattress.

4. Reposition the client in the center of the bed.

- Reposition the pillows at the center of the bed.
- Assist the client to the center of the bed. Determine what position the client requires or prefers, and assist the client to that position.

5. Apply or complete the top bedding.

- Spread the top sheet over the client, and ask the client to hold the top edge of the sheet or tuck it under the shoulders. The sheet should remain over the client when the bath blanket or used sheet is removed.
- Complete the top of the bed.

S **6. Ensure continued safety of the client.**

- Raise the side rails. Place the bed in the low position before leaving the bedside.
- Attach the signal cord to the bed linen within the client's reach.
- Put items used by the client within easy reach.

EVALUATION FOCUS

Client comfort and safety; patency of all drainage tubes; client's ability to summon help when needed.

CHAPTER HIGHLIGHTS

- Clients' hygiene is influenced to a large degree by their sociocultural background.
- When clients cannot meet their hygiene needs, the nurse usually assumes them.
- The major functions of the skin are to help regulate body temperature, to protect underlying tissues, to secrete sebum, and to contain nerve receptors that act in sensory perception.
- While assisting a client with hygiene measures, the nurse has an opportunity to assess the client's health.
- While planning hygiene care, the nurse must take the client's preferences into consideration.
- The back rub is an essential part of hygiene care for clients confined to bed.
- Nurses provide perineal-genital care for clients who are unable to do so for themselves.
- Nurses can often teach clients how to prevent foot problems.
- Oral hygiene should include daily dental flossing and mechanical brushing of the teeth.
- Regular dental checkups and fluoride supplements are recommended to maintain healthy teeth.
- Nurses provide special oral care to clients who are helpless (eg, unconscious) and who have oral problems.
- Hair care includes daily combing and brushing and regular shampooing.
- African-American clients' hair may require special care.
- Nurses may need to assist helpless clients with their artificial eyes, eyeglasses, and contact lenses.
- The deaf client may require nursing assistance with his or her hearing aid.
- Changing beds is a part of maintaining hygiene.
- It is important to keep beds clean and comfortable for clients.

READINGS AND REFERENCES

Suggested Readings

Osterman, HM and Stuk, RM. November/December 1990. The aging foot. *Orthopaedic Nursing* 9:43–47, 76.

The aging person may experience changes in the feet that affect mobility. Common foot pathologies are heel pain, metatarsalgia, hammertoes and clawtoes, bunions, hallux rigidus, corns and calluses, nail pathologies, arthritis, and neuropathies. This article familiarizes the nurse with these conditions and discusses their prevention, conservative treatment, surgical procedures, nursing interventions, and client education.

Tolson, D. May 1, 1991. Making sense of . . . hearing aids. *Nursing Times* 87:36–38.

This question-and-answer article discusses types of hearing aids; how they operate; how to apply hearing aid molds, behind-the-ear aids, and body-worn aids; cleaning methods; and other helpful hints.

Related Research

McMahon, R and Buckeldee, J. October 1992. Skin problems beneath the breasts of in-patients: The knowledge, opinions, and practices of nurses. *Journal of Advanced Nursing* 17:1243–50.

Pierson, MA. February 1991. Nurses' knowledge and perceptions related to foot care for older persons. *Journal of Nursing Education* 30:57–62.

Selected References

Barnett, J. September 1991. A reassessment of oral healthcare. *Professional Nurse* 6:703–4, 706–8.

Brodie, BS. September/October 1989. Community health and foot health. *Canadian Journal of Public Health* 80:331–33.

Carden, RG. February 1985. The ins and outs of contact lenses. *RN* 48:48–50.

Carpenito, LJ. 1992. *Nursing Diagnosis: Application to Clinical Practice.* 4th ed. Philadelphia: Lippincott.

Chovaz, C. March 1989. Nursing the hearing impaired patient. *Canadian Nurse* 85:34–36.

Davis, M. April 1977. Getting to the root of the problem . . . Hair-grooming techniques for black patients. *Nursing 77* 7:60–65.

Echavarria, KH, Bezon, J, and Black, JR. November/December 1988. A team approach to foot care. *Geriatric Nursing* 9:338–40.

Edelstein, JE. December 1988. Foot care for the aging. *Physical Therapy* 68:1882–86.

Eliopoulos, C, editor. 1990. *Health Assessment of the Older Adult.* 2d ed. Redwood City, CA: Addison-Wesley Nursing.

Freinkel, RK. July 1988. Caring for your skin. *Diabetes Forecast* 41:76–78, 81.

Giles, SF. 1972. Hair, the nursing process and the black patient. *Nursing Forum* 11(1):78–88.

Gooch, J. October 1989. Skin hygiene. *Professional Nurse* 5(1):13,16,18.

Hauk, L. September/October 1986. Enabling clients to manage dentures. *Geriatric Nursing* 7:254–55.

Holder, I. April 1982. Hearing aids: Handle with care. *Nursing 82* 12:64–67.

Kamenir, S and Fothergill, R. December 1982. Hands-on skills for dealing with hearing aids. *Canadian Nurse* 78:44–45.

Kelechi, T and Lukacs, K. September 1991. Nursing foot care for the aged. *Journal of Gerontological Nursing* 17:40–43.

Kim, MJ, McFarland, GK, and McLane, AM. 1993. *Pocket Guide to Nursing Diagnoses.* 5th ed. St Louis: Mosby-Year Book.

Lederer, JR, Marculescu, GL, Mocnik, B, and Seaby, N. 1993. *Care Planning Pocket Guide—A Nursing Diagnosis Approach.* 5th ed. Redwood City, CA: Addison-Wesley Nursing.

Longman, AL and Dewalt, EM. September/October 1986. A guide for oral assessment: Nursing assistants working in long-term care facilities. *Geriatric Nursing* 7:252–53.

Maas, M, Buckwalter, KC, and Hardy, M. 1991. *Nursing Diagnoses and Interventions for the Elderly.* Redwood City, CA: Addison-Wesley Nursing.

McCord, F and Stalker, A. March 30, 1988. Brushing up on oral care. *Nursing Times* 84:40–41.

McFarland, GK and McFarlane, EA. 1989. *Nursing Diagnosis and Intervention: Planning for Patient Care.* St Louis: Mosby.

Marieb, EN. 1992. *Human Anatomy and Physiology.* 2d ed. Redwood City, CA: Benjamin/Cummings.

North American Nursing Diagnosis Association. 1992. *NANDA Nursing Diagnoses: Definitions and Classification 1992–1993.* Philadelphia: NANDA.

Ophthalmic issues. April 1988. Facts and myths: Misconceptions about eye care. *American Association of Occupational Health Nurses Journal* 36:174–77.

Osguthorpe, NC. October 1984. If your patient has contact lenses. *American Journal of Nursing* 84:1255–56.

Parrott, TE. September/October 1987. Care of long hair. *Associate Degree Nurse* 2:8–10.

Pettigrew, D. January/February 1989. Investigating in mouth care. *Geriatric Nursing* 10:22–24.

Sawaya, ME and Stough, DB IV. May 15, 1992. Untangling misconceptions about hair. *Patient Care* 26:193–202, 204–5.

Thompson, J. February 1990. Foot and leg care. *Community Outlook* 14, 16–17.

Travis, SS. March/April 1990. Personalizing self-care. *Geriatric Nursing* 11:72–73.

Wagnild, G and Manning, RW. December 1985. Convey respect during bathing procedures. *Journal of Gerontological Nursing* 11:6–10.

Yetzer, EA and Sullivan, RL. September 1992. The foot at risk: Identification and prevention of skin breakdown. *Rehabilitation Nursing* 17:243–52.

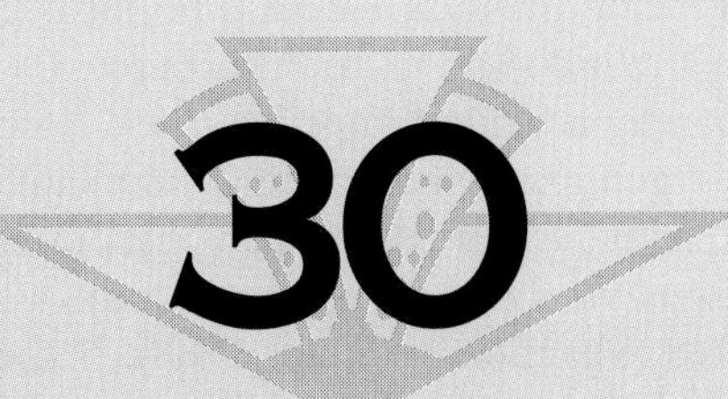

30 Maintaining Skin Integrity

Objectives

Describe three major factors predisposing clients to pressure ulcers.

Identify risk factors contributing to the formation of pressure ulcers.

Describe the four stages of pressure ulcer development.

Identify clients at risk for pressure ulcer formation.

Compare selected risk assessment tools.

Describe how to assess common pressure sites and an existing pressure ulcer.

Identify etiologies and defining characteristics of NANDA diagnoses associated with impaired skin integrity.

Identify appropriate outcome criteria for clients at risk for or with impaired skin integrity.

Discuss measures to prevent pressure ulcer formation.

List guidelines for treating pressure ulcers.

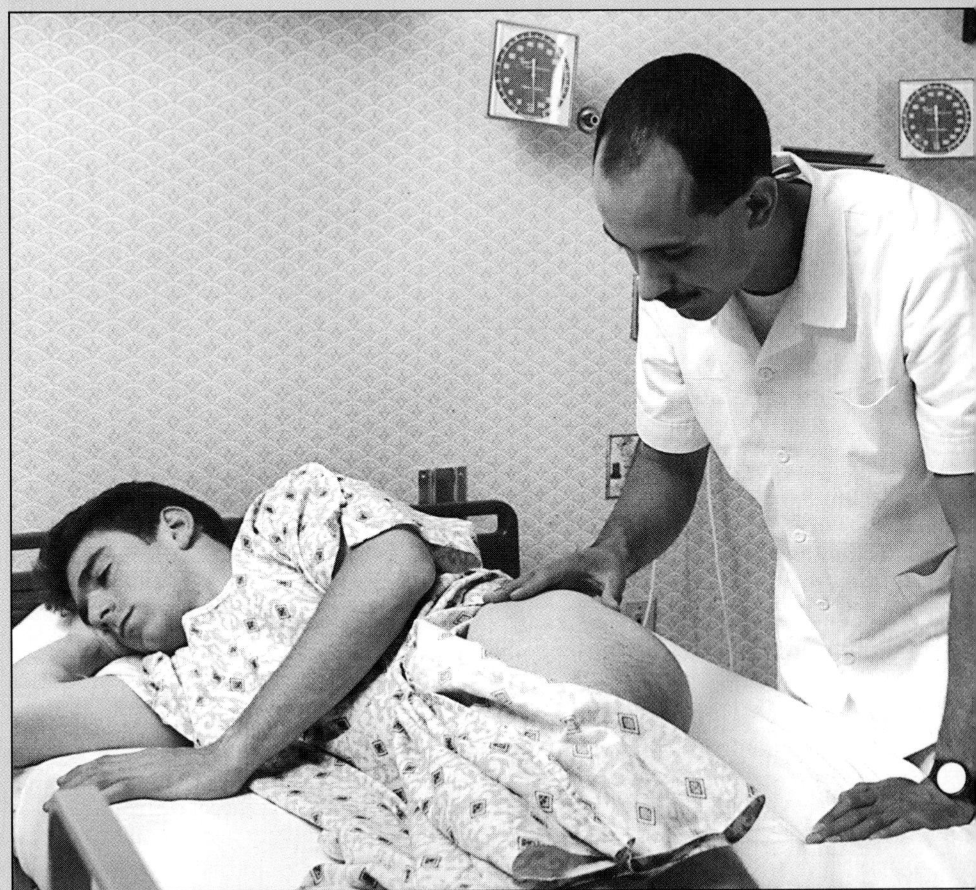

Maintaining skin integrity is an important independent function of nursing. Nurses must use consistent planned observations and skin care measures to prevent abrasions and subsequent tissue breakdown. Impaired skin integrity is not normally a problem in healthy people but it is a threat to the elderly and to clients who have restricted mobility or chronic illness. The development of a pressure ulcer adds to a client's recovery time and costs. It is estimated that a pressure ulcer can increase the costs of a client's nursing care by 50% (Maklebust 1987, p. 359).

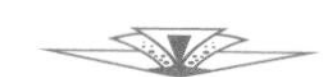

PRESSURE ULCERS

Pressure ulcers are also called **decubitus ulcers,** *pressure sores, bedsores,* or *distortion sores.* A pressure ulcer is defined as any lesion caused by unrelieved **pressure** (a compressing downward force on a body area) that results in damage to underlying tissue (US Department of Health and Human Services 1992, p. 1).

Pressure ulcers are a problem in both acute-care settings and long-term care settings, including homes. The incidence of pressure ulcers in hospital settings has been reported by some as 3.5% (Shannon & Skorga 1989, p. 38) and by others as 9.2% (Meehan 1990, p. 14). A few client populations are thought to be at greater risk of developing pressure sores because of immobility: orthopedic clients with fractures (Versluysen 1985, p. 10), the elderly with femoral fractures (Versluysen 1986, p. 1131), and clients in nursing home settings. Studies in the latter settings have shown that the incidence of pressure ulcers increases with length of stay (Brandeis et al 1991, p. 1688).

ETIOLOGY OF PRESSURE ULCERS

Pressure ulcers are due to localized **ischemia,** a deficiency in the blood supply to the tissue. The tissue is caught between two hard surfaces, usually the surface of the bed and the bony skeleton. When blood cannot reach the tissue, the cells are deprived of oxygen and nutrients, the waste products of metabolism accumulate in the cells, and the tissue consequently dies. Prolonged, unrelieved pressure also damages the small blood vessels.

Pressure ulcers usually occur over bony prominences. After the skin has been compressed, it appears white, as if the blood had been squeezed out of it. A white person's skin loses its pink color in the affected area, and a dark-skinned person's skin is also less pink, although the change is more difficult to see.

When pressure is relieved, the skin takes on a bright red flush, called **reactive hyperemia,** which is the body's mechanism for preventing pressure ulcers. The flush is due to vasodilation; extra blood floods to the area to compensate for the preceding period of impeded blood flow. The blood carries oxygen and removes the accumulated metabolic wastes. Reactive hyperemia usually lasts one-half to three-quarters as long as the duration of impeded blood flow to the area (Shannon & Miller 1988). If the redness disappears in that time, no tissue damage can be anticipated. If, however, the redness does not disappear, then tissue damage has occurred.

Two other factors frequently act in conjunction with pressure to produce pressure ulcers: friction and shearing force. **Friction** is a force acting parallel to the skin. For example, when a client pulls up in bed, the skin rubbing against the sheet creates friction. Friction can abrade the skin, that is, remove the superficial layers, making it more prone to breakdown.

Shearing force is a combination of friction and pressure. It occurs commonly when a client assumes a Fowler's position in bed. In this position, the body tends to slide downward toward the foot of the bed. This downward movement is transmitted to the sacral bone and the deep tissues. At the same time, the skin over the sacrum tends not to move because of the friction between the skin and the bedsheets. The skin and superficial tissues are thus relatively unmoving in relation to the bed surface, whereas the deeper tissues are firmly attached to the skeleton and move downward. This causes a shearing force in the area where the deeper tissues and the superficial tissues meet. The force damages the blood vessels and tissues in this area.

RISK FACTORS

Several factors contribute to the formation of pressure ulcers: immobility and inactivity, inadequate nutrition, fecal and urinary incontinence, decreased mental status, diminished sensation, excessive body heat, and advanced age.

Immobility and Inactivity Although pressure is the major cause of pressure ulcers, immobility and inactivity are also important risk factors. **Immobility** refers to an alteration in the amount and control of movement a person has (Kelley & Mobily 1991, p. 26). Normally, people move when they experience discomfort due to pressure on an area of the body. Healthy people rarely exceed their tolerance to pressure. However, paralysis, extreme weakness, or immobility brought about by the presence of a cast or traction can hinder a person's ability to change positions independently and relieve the pressure, even if the person can perceive the pressure.

Inactivity refers to an alteration in a person's ability to ambulate independently (Kelley & Mobily 1991, p. 26). Some elderly clients and others who have chronic health problems, such as neuromuscular, cardiac, or respiratory disease, have decreased agility and energy and cannot ambulate without assistance.

Inadequate Nutrition Nutritional factors are crucial in the development of pressure ulcers. Generally, prolonged inadequate nutrition causes weight loss, muscle atrophy, and the loss of subcutaneous tissue. These three reduce the amount of padding between the skin and the bones, thus increasing the risk of pressure sore development. More specifically, inadequate intakes of protein, carbohydrates, fluids, and vitamin C contribute to pressure ulcer formation.

Hypoproteinemia (abnormally low protein content in the blood), due either to inadequate intake or abnormal loss, results in negative nitrogen balance, which predisposes the client to dependent edema. The presence of edema makes skin more prone to injury by decreasing its elasticity, resilience, and vitality. Edema increases the distance between the capillaries and the cells, thereby slowing the diffusion of oxygen to the tissue cells and of metabolites away from the cells. Inadequate intake of carbohydrates creates low levels of blood glucose and breakdown of tissue proteins. Inadequate fluid intake results in skin that is dry, has decreased tissue tolerance and is less resistant to trauma. Vitamin C aids in the absorption and use of iron and is essential for protein collagen formation; a lack of vitamin C can thus impede healing of tissue damaged by pressure.

Fecal and Urinary Incontinence Moisture from incontinence promotes skin **maceration** (tissue softened by prolonged wetting or soaking) and makes the epidermis more easily eroded and susceptible to injury. Digestive enzymes in feces also contribute to skin excoriation. Any accumulation of secretions or excretions is irritating to the skin, harbors microorganisms, and makes an individual prone to skin breakdown and infection.

Decreased Mental Status Individuals with a reduced level of awareness, for example, those who are unconscious or heavily sedated by analgesics, barbiturates, or tranquilizers, are at risk for pressure ulcers because they are less able to recognize and respond to pain associated with prolonged pressure.

Diminished Sensation Paralysis or other neurologic disease may cause loss of sensation in a body area. Loss of sensation reduces a person's ability to discern injurious heat and cold and to feel the tingling ("pins and needles") that signals loss of circulation. This loss makes the person prone to skin damage.

Excessive Body Heat Body heat is another factor in the development of pressure sores. An elevated body temperature increases the body's metabolic rate, thus increasing the need of the cells for oxygen. This increased need is particularly severe in the cells of the area under pressure, which are already oxygen deficient. Therefore, severe infections with accompanying elevated body temperatures may affect the body's ability to deal with the effects of tissue compression.

Advanced Age The aging process brings about several changes in the skin and its supporting structures, making the older person more prone to impaired skin integrity. These changes include the following (Kelley & Mobily 1991, p. 25; Bryant et al 1992, p. 116):

- Loss of lean body mass.
- Generalized thinning of the epidermis.
- Decreased strength and elasticity of the skin due to changes in the collagen fibers of the dermis.
- Decreased vascularity of the dermis due to a reduction in the number of epithelial cells and blood vessels. For example, when a person sits on an unpadded surface, the blood flow to the area of the ischial tuberosity decreases. Studies have shown that this decrease in blood flow is greater in the geriatric population than in other populations. Without essential nutrients carried by the blood, tissues of the skin are vulnerable to breakdown.
- Reduced skin turgor due to loss of elastic fiber.
- Increased dryness and scaliness due to a decrease in the amount of oil produced by the sebaceous glands.
- Diminished pain perception due to a reduction in the number of cutaneous end organs responsible for the sensation of pressure and light touch.

Other Factors Other factors contributing to the formation of pressure sores are poor lifting techniques, incorrect positioning, repeated injections in the same area, hard support surfaces, and incorrect application of pressure-relieving devices. See Figure 30–1 on page 788 for pressure areas in selected positions.

Stages of Pressure Ulcer Formation

There are four recognized stages in pressure ulcer formation related to observable tissue damage (USDHHS 1992, p. 8).

Stage I: Nonblanchable erythema of intact skin; this is the heralding lesion of skin ulceration (Figure 30–2,*A*).

Stage II: Partial-thickness skin loss involving epidermis and/or dermis. The ulcer is superficial and presents

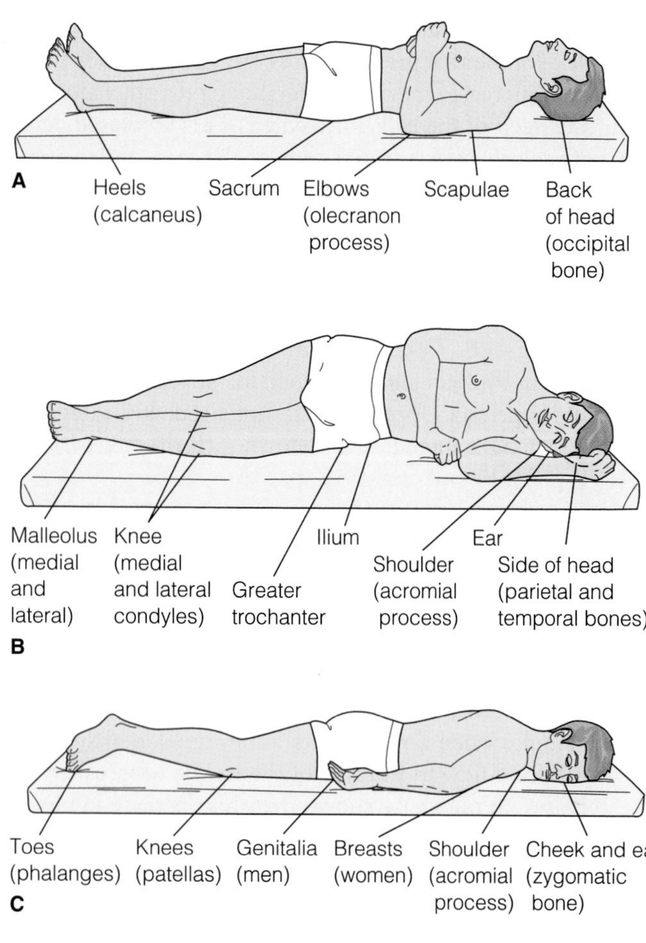

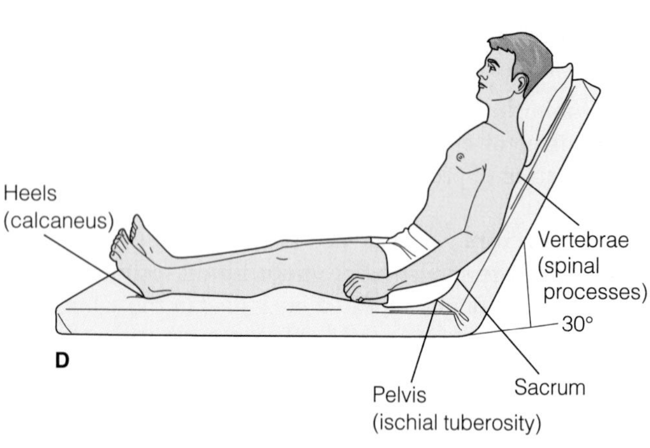

Figure 30–1 Body pressure areas in *A,* supine position; *B,* lateral position; *C,* prone position; *D,* Fowler's position.

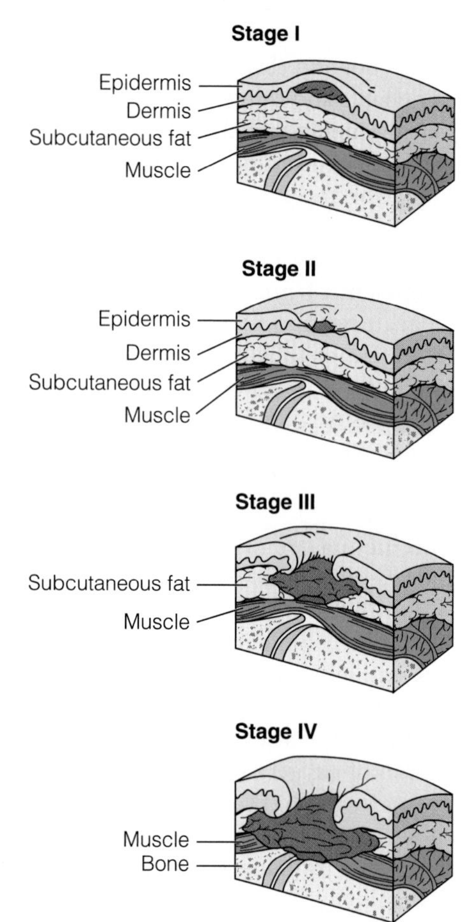

Figure 30–2 Four stages of pressure ulcers. **Source:** US Department of Health and Human Services, Clinical practice guideline, *Pressure Ulcers in Adults: Prediction and Prevention,* Pub no. 9-0047 (Rockville, MD: Public Health Service, 1992), p. 8.

clinically as an abrasion, blister, or shallow crater (Figure 30–2,*B*).

Stage III: Full-thickness skin loss involving damage or necrosis of subcutaneous tissue that may extend down to, but not through, underlying fascia. The ulcer presents clinically as a deep crater with or without undermining of adjacent tissue (Figure 30–2,*C*).

Stage IV: Full-thickness skin loss with extensive destruction, tissue necrosis or damage to muscle, bone, or supporting structures, such as a tendon or joint capsule (Figure 30–2,*D*). Undermining and sinus tracts may also be associated with stage IV pressure ulcers.

Also see color photographs on pages 474a and 474b.

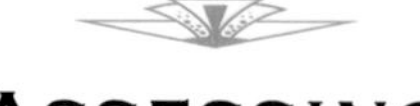

ASSESSING

In assessing clients for pressure ulcer development, the nurse identifies clients at risk by using a risk assessment tool; meticulously examines common pressure area sites; and conducts a detailed inspection of any pressure ulcer present.

Table 30–1 Norton's Pressure Area Risk Assessment Form (Scoring System)

A General Physical Condition		B Mental State		C Activity		D Mobility		E Incontinence	
Good	4	Alert	4	Ambulatory	4	Full	4	Absent	4
Fair	3	Apathetic	3	Walks with help	3	Slightly limited	3	Occasional	3
Poor	2	Confused	2	Chairbound	2	Very limited	2	Usually urinary	2
Very bad	1	Stuporous	1	Bedfast	1	Immobile	1	Double	1

Source: D Norton, R McLaren, and AN Exton-Smith, *An Investigation of Geriatric Nursing Problems in Hospital* (Edinburgh: Churchill Livingstone, 1962). Reissued, 1975. Used by permission.

Table 30–2 Shannon's Scoring System to Identify Clients at Risk for Developing Pressure Sores*

	Mental Status	Continence	Mobility	Activity	Nutrition	Circulation	Temperature	Medications
4	Alert	Continent	Fully mobile	Ambulatory	Good	Immediate capillary refill	36.6 to 37.2 C (98 to 99 F)	No analgesics, tranquilizers, or steroids
3	Apathetic	Incontinent of urine (without catheter)	Slightly limited	Walks with assistance	Fair	Delayed capillary refill	37.2 to 37.7 C (99 to 100 F)	One of the above
2	Confused	Incontinent of feces	Very limited	Confined to wheelchair	Poor	Mild edema	37.7 to 38.3 C (100 to 101 F)	Two of the above
1	Stuporous or comatose	Incontinent of urine and feces	Immo-bile	Bedridden	Cachectic	Moderate to severe edema	**>38.3 C (>101 F)	All of the above

* Evaluate clients for each of the above categories, then assign appropriate score. Clients with a score of 16 or less on this assessment scale are at significant risk of developing pressure sores.

** > greater than

Source: Reprinted, with permission, from ML Shannon EdD, RN, Five famous fallacies about pressure sores, *Nursing84*, October 1984, 14:37,

Risk Assessment Tools

Several risk assessment tools are available that provide the nurse with a systematic means of identifying clients at high risk for pressure ulcer development. For example, Norton et al (1962) have developed a guide that includes five categories: physical condition, mental condition, activity, mobility, and incontinence. See Table 30–1. Their study showed that only 5% of clients in good general condition developed pressure sores. Among clients with a score of 12 and below, almost 50% developed pressure sores (Norton 1975, p. 65). In 1987, Norton revised her guide to include medications and concluded that scores of 15 or 16 should be viewed as indicators, not predictors, of risk (Anthony 1987, p. 6).

Shannon (1984) has also created a scoring system for identifying clients at risk. This system includes eight categories. See Table 30–2. Clients with a score of 16 or less are at significant risk of developing pressure sores.

Waterlow (1985) developed a risk assessment card that includes six categories: build (weight for height), visual skin type, continence, mobility, sex and age, and appetite. Further research indicates that nutritional status is an important factor in pressure sore development (Osborne 1987, p. 75).

BRADEN SCALE FOR PREDICTING PRESSURE SORE RISK

Patient's Name ____________________ Evaluator's Name ____________________

					Date of Assessment			
SENSORY PERCEPTION Ability to respond meaningfully to pressure-related discomfort	**1. Completely Limited:** Unresponsive (does not moan, flinch, or grasp) to painful stimuli, due to diminished level of consciousness or sedation, OR limited ability to feel pain over most of body surface.	**2. Very Limited:** Responds only to painful stimuli. Cannot communicate discomfort except by moaning or restlessness, OR has a sensory impairment which limits the ability to feel pain or discomfort over 1/2 of body.	**3. Slightly Limited:** Responds to verbal commands but cannot always communicate discomfort or need to be turned, OR has some sensory impairment which limits ability to feel pain or discomfort in 1 or 2 extremities.	**4. No Impairment:** Responds to verbal commands. Has no sensory deficit which would limit ability to feel or voice pain or discomfort.				
MOISTURE Degree to which skin is exposed to moisture	**1. Constantly Moist:** Skin is kept moist almost constantly by perspiration, urine, etc. Dampness is detected every time patient is moved or turned.	**2. Moist:** Skin is often but not always moist. Linen must be changed at least once a shift.	**3. Occasionally Moist:** Skin is occasionally moist, requiring an extra linen change approximately once a day.	**4. Rarely Moist:** Skin is usually dry; linen requires changing only at routine intervals.				
ACTIVITY Degree of physical activity	**1. Bedfast:** Confined to bed.	**2. Chairfast:** Ability to walk severely limited or nonexistent. Cannot bear own weight and/or must be assisted into chair or wheelchair.	**3. Walks Occasionally:** Walks occasionally during day but for very short distances, with or without assistance. Spends majority of each shift in bed or chair.	**4. Walks Frequently:** Walks outside the room at least twice a day and inside room at least once every 2 hours during waking hours.				
MOBILITY Ability to change and control body position	**1. Completely Immobile:** Does not make even slight changes in body or extremity position without assistance.	**2. Very Limited:** Makes occasional slight changes in body or extremity position but unable to make frequent or significant changes independently.	**3. Slightly Limited:** Makes frequent though slight changes in body or extremity position independently.	**4. No Limitations:** Makes major and frequent changes in position without assistance.				
NUTRITION Usual food intake pattern	**1. Very Poor:** Never eats a complete meal. Rarely eats more than 1/3 of any food offered. Eats 2 servings or less of protein (meat or dairy products) per day. Takes fluids poorly. Does not take a liquid dietary supplement, OR is NPO and/or maintained on clear liquids or IV's for more than 5 days.	**2. Probably Inadequate:** Rarely eats a complete meal and generally eats only about 1/2 of any food offered. Protein intake includes only 3 servings of meat or dairy products per day. Occasionally will take a dietary supplement, OR receives less than optimum amount of liquid diet or tube feeding.	**3. Adequate:** Eats over half of most meals. Eats a total of 4 servings of protein (meat, dairy products) each day. Occasionally will refuse a meal, but will usually take a supplement if offered, OR is on a tube feeding or TPN regimen, which probably meets most of nutritional needs.	**4. Excellent:** Eats most of every meal. Never refuses a meal. Usually eats a total of 4 or more servings of meat and dairy products. Occasionally eats between meals. Does not require supplementation.				
FRICTION AND SHEAR	**1. Problem:** Requires moderate to maximum assistance in moving. Complete lifting without sliding against sheets is impossible. Frequently slides down in bed or chair, requiring frequent repositioning with maximum assistance. Spasticity, contractures, or agitation leads to almost constant friction.	**2. Potential Problem:** Moves feebly or requires minimum assistance. During a move skin probably slides to some extent against sheets, chair, restraints, or other devices. Maintains relatively good position in chair or bed most of the time but occasionally slides down.	**3. No Apparent Problem:** Moves in bed and in chair independently and has sufficient muscle strength to lift up completely during move. Maintains good position in bed or chair at all times.					
					Total Score			

Figure 30–3 Braden Scale for Predicting Pressure Sore Risk. **Source:** US Department of Health and Human Services, Clinical practice guideline, *Pressure Ulcers in Adults: Prediction and Prevention,* Pub no. 9-0047 (Rockville, MD: Public Health Service, 1992), pp. 16–17. Copyright © Barbara Braden and Nancy Bergstrom, 1988. Reprinted with permission.

In 1987, Bergstrom et al published the Branden Scale for Predicting Pressure Sore Risk. Their scale consists of six subscales (Figure 30–3). Five of the six subscales are rated from 1 (least favorable) to 4 (most favorable). The friction subscale is rated from 1 to 3. A total of 23 points is possible. An adult client who scores 16 or below is considered at risk; an older person may be at risk with a score of 17 or 18 (Bergstrom et al 1987, p. 124).

Risk assessment tools need to be completed when the client is admitted to hospital, repeated 24 to 48 hours after admission, and repeated thereafter whenever the client's condition changes.

PHYSICAL ASSESSMENT

The nurse conducts a physical examination to assess (a) common pressure sites and (b) the characteristics of an existing pressure ulcer. The box at the right outlines guidelines for assessing common pressure sites. When a pressure ulcer is present, the nurse notes the following:

- Location of the lesion.
- Size of lesion in centimeters. Measure length, width and depth, beginning with length (head to toe) and then width (side to side). To measure depth, insert a cotton swab at the deepest part of the wound, and then measure the swab against a measuring guide.
- Stage of the ulcer (see page 787).
- Color of the wound bed and location of necrosis.
- Condition of the wound margins.
- Integrity of surrounding skin.
- Clinical signs of infection, such as redness, warmth, swelling, pain, odor, and exudate (note color of exudate).
- The amount of time the lesion has been known to exist.
- Any previously used treatments.

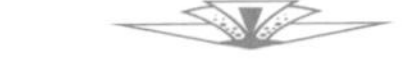

DIAGNOSING

The NANDA nursing diagnoses that relate to clients who have skin wounds or who are at risk for skin breakdown are **High risk for impaired skin integrity, Impaired skin integrity,** and **Impaired tissue integrity. Impaired skin integrity** commonly applies to stage I and II pressure ulcers and to superficial wounds extending through the epidermis but not through the dermis. **Impaired tissue integrity** applies to stage III and IV pressure ulcers and to wounds extending into subcutaneous tissue, muscle, or bone (Krasner 1992, p. 36). The diagnoses **High risk for impaired skin integrity** and **Impaired skin integrity,** with definitions, contributing factors, and defining characteristics, are shown in the box on page 792.

CLINICAL GUIDELINES

Assessing Common Pressure Sites

- Be sure there is good lighting, preferably natural or fluorescent, because incandescent lights can create a transilluminating effect.
- Regulate the environment prior to beginning assessment so that the room is neither too hot nor too cold. Heat can cause the skin to flush; cold can cause the skin to blanch or become cyanotic.
- Inspect pressure areas (see Figure 30–1) for any whitish or reddened spots; discoloration can be caused by impaired blood circulation to the area. It should disappear in a few minutes when rubbing restores circulation.
- Inspect pressure areas for abrasions and excoriations. An **abrasion** (wearing away of the skin) can occur when skin rubs against a sheet (eg, when the client is pulled). **Excoriations** (loss of superficial layers of the skin) can occur when the skin has prolonged contact with body secretions or excretions or with dampness in skin folds.
- Palpate the surface temperature of the skin over the pressure areas (warm the hands first). Normally, the temperature is the same as that of the surrounding skin. Increased temperature is abnormal and may be due to inflammation or blood trapped in the area.
- Palpate over bony prominences and dependent body areas for the presence of edema, which feels spongy.

Clinical applications of these diagnoses are shown in Table 30–3 on page 792.

PLANNING

The major outcomes for clients at risk for pressure sore development are to maintain skin integrity and to avoid potential associated risks. Clients with **Impaired skin integrity** need to demonstrate progressive wound healing and regain intact skin. Specific outcome criteria, nursing interventions, and rationales are shown in the Care Planning Guide on page 793.

IMPLEMENTING

PREVENTING PRESSURE ULCERS

To reduce the likelihood of pressure ulcer development, the nurse employs a variety of preventive measures to

NURSING DIAGNOSES

CLIENTS WITH POTENTIAL OR ACTUAL SKIN PROBLEMS

Nursing Diagnosis: High risk for impaired skin integrity: The state in which an individual's skin is at risk of being adversely altered (NANDA)

Risk or Related Factors

External

Immobilization; excessive heat or cold; chemical substance; mechanical factors (shearing forces, pressure, restraint); radiation; presence of excretions or secretions.

Internal

Alterations in nutritional state (emaciation, obesity); circulation; metabolic state; sensation; pigmentation; skin turgor.

Nursing Diagnosis: Impaired skin integrity: A state in which the individual's skin is adversely altered (NANDA)

Defining Characteristics

- Disrupted skin surface
- Destroyed skin layers
- Invasion of body structures

Risk or Related Factors

Medications; immunologic deficit; skeletel prominence; edema. See also risk factors for **Impaired skin integrity,** above.

Sources: LJ Carpenito, *Nursing Diagnosis: Application to Clinical Practice,* 4th ed. (Philadelphia: Lippincott, 1992), pp. 857–58; MJ Kim, GK McFarland, AM McLane, *Pocket Guide to Nursing Diagnoses,* 5th ed. (St Louis: Mosby-Year Book, 1993), pp. 54–55; GK McFarland, and EA McFarlane, *Nursing Diagnosis and Intervention: Planning for Patient Care.* (St Louis: Mosby, 1989), pp. 202–4, 210, 211; NANDA, *Nursing Diagnoses: Definitions and Classification 1992–1993.* (Philadelphia: NANDA), pp. 34–35; JR Lederer, GL Marculescu, B Mocnik, and N Seaby, *Care Planning Pocket Guide—A Nursing Diagnosis Approach,* 5th ed. (Redwood City, CA: Addison-Wesley Nursing, 1993), pp. 182–84.

---

maintain the skin integrity (ie, skin hygiene) and instructs the client, support persons, and caregivers in how to prevent pressure ulcers.

Ongoing assessment of risk factors (see page 788) is essential to preventing pressure ulcers. In addition, all clients who are at risk should have a systematic skin inspection at least daily, with special attention to bony prominences. Findings from the skin inspection should be documented.

Providing Nutrition Because an inadequate intake of calories, protein, and iron is believed to be a risk factor for pressure ulcer development, nutritional supplements should be considered for nutritionally compromised clients. It is recommended that the diet be supplemented with calories (specifically, from protein and carbohydrates), vitamin C, and zinc to maintain skin integrity (USDHHS 1992, p. 21).

Maintaining Skin Hygiene Skin must be cleansed at routine intervals and at times of soiling. The client's skin should be kept clean and dry and free of irritation and

Table 30–3 Clinical Application: Assessment Data Clusters and Related Nursing Diagnoses for Clients at Risk for or with Impaired Skin Integrity

Data Cluster	Nursing Diagnosis
Juanita Perez, an 85-year-old, is newly admitted to the hospital. Is pale, emaciated, and listless. Weight 90 lb. Is incontinent of urine, has no bowel control, and is bedridden.	**High risk for impaired skin integrity** related to incontinence and immobility
Matthew Brown, an obese 70-year-old hemiplegic, complains of discomfort in his left heel after attempting to move in bed. Superficial skin abrasion 1.2 cm in diameter present at base of left heel.	**Impaired skin integrity** (stage II pressure ulcer) related to friction

CARE PLANNING GUIDE
CLIENTS WITH POTENTIAL OR ACTUAL SKIN PROBLEMS

NURSING DIAGNOSIS: High risk for impaired skin integrity

Outcome Criteria	Nursing Interventions	Rationale
The client		
▪ Maintains intact skin tissue	Monitor the client for risk factors (see page 789).	The presence of risk factors increases the possibility of pressure ulcer development.
	Inspect the client's skin for baseline data and thereafter at least once a day. Pay particular attention to any prominences.	Baseline data provide criteria to measure against subsequent skin assessments.
	Keep the skin clean and dry; lubricate excessively dry skin. Apply protective barrier (ointment/cream) to perineal region as needed. See also the discussion of incontinence care, Chapter 41, page 1242.	The presence of urine, feces, sweat, water (eg, from incomplete drying after a bath), soap, alcohol, and excessive dryness cause skin irritation and maceration, thus decreasing tissue tolerance and making the skin more vulnerable to breakdown.
	Provide appropriate protective and pressure-relieving devices and measures (see page 794 and Table 30–4, page 795). Avoid using donuts for suspect areas.	Pressure is the major causative factor in pressure ulcer formation. Donuts increase pressure and damage tissue.
	Establish a repositioning schedule. Reposition bed-bound and chair-bound clients every 1 to 2 hours as indicated (see sample positioning schedule in Chapter 34, page 911). Encourage the client to change position frequently even if only slightly.	Changes in position relieve and alternate body pressure areas.
	Implement appropriate measures to lift and move clients to avoid friction and shearing forces (see page 794).	Friction and shearing forces in concert with gravity are significant factors contributing to ulcer formation.
▪ Demonstrates optimal nutritional intake, as evidenced by ideal body weight and good skin color and turgor.	Ensure adequate nutritional and fluid intake (2500 mL/day).	If the diet is deficient in calories, protein, and fluid, tissue tolerance decreases, and tissue becomes more vulnerable to lower amounts of pressure.
	Compare actual weight to ideal weight, observe for signs of dehydration (dry skin, sunken eyeballs, poor skin turgor), and assess weight daily. Consult the dietitian as needed for a nutritional assessment.	Dietary supplements may be needed by some clients.
▪ Maintains optimal circulation to all body areas.	Provide assistive devices to increase movement (eg, overbed trapeze, walkers, canes). Ambulate the client whenever possible.	Activity stimulates the circulation.

➤

POTENTIAL OR ACTUAL SKIN PROBLEMS CONTINUED

NURSING DIAGNOSIS: High risk for impaired skin integrity *continued*

Outcome Criteria	Nursing Interventions	Rationale
	Avoid using massage over bony prominences and reddened areas. Avoid using heat lamps.	Massage can cause additional skin trauma. Heat lamps dry the skin and decrease tissue tolerance.
	Encourage the client to do active range-of-motion (ROM) exercises every 2 to 3 hours.	Muscle contractions stimulate circulation to the skin.
▪ Verbalizes understanding of a. Risk factors that increase the chance of skin breakdown. b. Measures to prevent skin breakdown.	Teach the client and support persons self-care measures to prevent pressure ulcers (see page 795).	Knowledge of risk factors, turning schedules, skin care routines, and nuotrition facilitates cooperation in preventing pressure ulcers.
▪ Demonstrates optimal self-care measures to prevent pressure ulcers.	Have client/support persons demonstrate necessary preventive measures.	This enables the nurse to determine the abilities of the client/support persons to provide care.

maceration by urine, feces, sweat, incomplete drying after a bath, soap, or alcohol. When bathing the client, the nurse should minimize the force and friction applied to the skin, using mild cleansing agents that minimize irritation and dryness and that do not disrupt the skin's "natural barriers." Also, the nurse should avoid hot water, which increases skin dryness and irritation. Nurses can also minimize dryness by avoiding exposure to cold and to low humidity. Dry skin is best treated with moisturizing lotions.

In addition, massage over bony prominences should be avoided. Traditionally, nurses have used massage to stimulate blood circulation, with the intention of preventing pressure sores. However, scientific evidence does not support this belief; in fact, massage may lead to deep tissue trauma (USDHHS 1992, p. 19).

Avoiding Skin Trauma Providing the client with a smooth, firm, and wrinkle-free foundation on which to sit or lie helps prevent skin trauma. To prevent injury due to friction and shearing forces, clients must be positioned, transferred, and turned correctly (see Chapter 34). Friction injuries can be reduced by applying a thin layer of cornstarch to the bedsheet or wheelchair seat cover or by using protective films, such as transparent dressings and skin sealants. For bedridden clients, shearing force can be reduced by elevating the head of the bed to no more than 30 degrees, if this position is not contraindicated by the client's condition (for example, clients with respiratory disorders may find it easier to breathe in Fowler's position). When the head of the bed is raised, the skin and superficial fascia stick to the bed linen while the deep fascia and skeleton slide downward toward the bottom of the bed. As a result, blood vessels in the sacral area become twisted, and the tissues in the area can become ischemic and necrotic (Reichel 1958, p. 763). Frequent shifts in position, even if only slight, effectively change pressure points. The client should shift weight every 15 to 30 minutes and, whenever possible, exercise or ambulate to stimulate blood circulation.

When lifting a client to change position, nurses should use a lifting device such as a trapeze rather than dragging the client across or up in bed. The friction that results from dragging the skin against a sheet can cause blisters and abrasions, which may contribute to more extensive tissue damage. Therefore, using devices that lift the client's weight off the bed surface is the method of choice.

Any at-risk client confined to bed—even when a special support mattress is used—should be repositioned at least every 2 hours, depending on the client's need, to allow another body surface to bear the weight. Six body positions (discussed in Chapter 34, page 910), can usually be used: prone, supine, right and left lateral (side-lying), and right and left Sims' positions. When the lateral position is used, the nurse should avoid positioning the client directly on the trochanter and instead position the client off the trochanter, on an angle. A written schedule should be established for turning and repositioning. For a sample turning schedule, see Chapter 34, page 911.

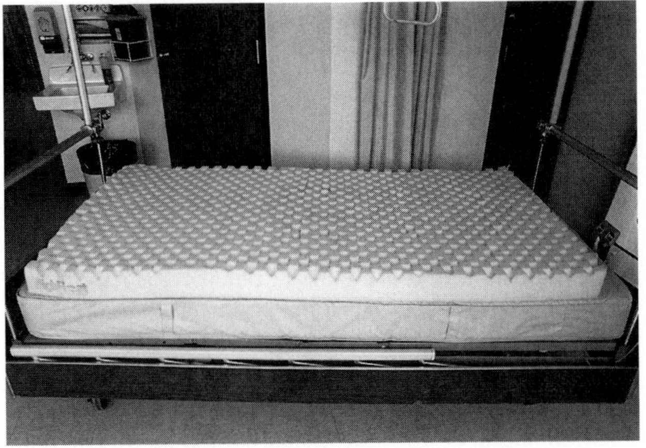

Figure 30–4 An egg crate mattress provides comfort and helps to distribute the body weight evenly, thus helping to reduce pressure on bony prominences.

Providing Supportive Devices For clients confined to bed, special support surfaces and positioning devices can be used to protect bony prominences. There are three types of support surfaces that can be used to relieve pressure. The *overlay mattress* is applied on top of the standard bed mattress. An example is the egg crate mattress (Figure 30–4). A *replacement mattress* is a mattress that replaces the standard mattress; most are made of foam and gel combinations. *Specialty beds* replace hospital beds. They provide pressure relief, eliminate shearing and friction, and decrease moisture. Examples are high air loss (HAL) beds, low air loss (LAL) beds, and beds that provide kinetic therapy. Kinetic beds (eg, RotoRest) provide continuous passive motion or oscillation therapy, which is intended to counteract the effects of a client's immobility. See Table 30–4 for selected mechanical devices for reducing pressure on body parts.

When a client is confined to bed or to a chair, pressure-reducing devices, such as pillows made of foam, gel, air, or a combination of these, can be used. When the client is sitting, weight should be distributed over the entire seating surface so that pressure does not center on just one area. To protect a clients' heels in bed, supports such as wedges or pillows can be used to raise the heels completely off the bed. Donut-type devices should not be used (USDHHS 1992, p. 23).

Client Teaching Clients and support persons need an understanding about the following in order to effectively participate in or to independently carry out measures to prevent pressure ulcers:

- Causes of pressure ulcers
- Individual risk factors
- Skin inspection for redness, temperature, blistering, and pulses

Table 30–4 Mechanical Devices for Reducing Pressure on Body Parts

Device	Description/Comments
Gel flotation pads	Polyvinyl, silicone, or Silastic pads filled with a gelatinous substance similar to fat.
Sheepskins (natural and artificial)	Some manufacturers produce mixed natural and synthetic pads; artificial pads are less likely to be damaged by washing but are more likely to make the client hot than natural skins.
Pillows and wedges (foam, gel and air, foam and fluid)	Can raise a body part (eg, heels) off the bed surface.
Heel protectors (sheepskin boots, padded splints, foam wedges)	Limit pressure on heels when client is in bed.
Egg crate mattress	Polyurethane foam mattress resembling an egg crate; some types are flammable
Foam mattress	Foam molds to the body.
Alternating pressure mattress	Composed of a number of cells in which the pressure alternately increases and decreases; utilizes a pump.
Water bed	Special mattress filled with water; controls temperature of water.
Air-fluidized (AF) bed (static high air loss [HAL] bed)	Forced temperature-controlled air is circulated around millions of tiny silicone-coated beads, producing a fluidlike movement. Provides uniform support to body contours. Decreases skin maceration by its drying effect. Moisture from the client penetrates the bed sheet and soaks the beads. Air flow forces the beads away from the client and rapidly dries the sheet. A major disadvantage is that the head of the bed cannot be elevated.
Static low air loss (LAL) bed	Consists of many air-filled cushions divided into four or five sections. Separate controls permit each section to be inflated to a different level of firmness; thus pressure can be reduced on bony prominences but increased under other body areas for support.
Active or second-generation low air loss (LAL) bed.	Like the static LAL, but in addition gently pulsates or rotates from side to side, thus stimulating capillary blood flow and facilitating movement of pulmonary secretions.

RESEARCH NOTE

Does Increased Availability of Pressure-Relieving Mattresses Meet the Need for Pressure Sore Prevention?

In response to the expanded use of pressure-redistributing (PR) mattresses, this study investigated how it has affected the incidence of pressure sores. Data were gathered within one health district over a 4-year period to compare the incidence of pressure sores with the availability of PR mattresses. The investigation included these objectives:

- To define the current incidence of pressure sores within the surveyed hospitals and to compare how this incidence (and the characteristics of the encountered sores) changed between 1986 and 1989
- To identify changes in the availability of PR mattresses in the same period
- To consider whether sufficient resources are available to match current demand

A total of 102 pressure sores were examined and classified. The sites most commonly affected were the sacrum, the heels, and the greater trochanters. Other sites were the ischial tuberosities, lower leg, shoulder, elbow, ankle, external ear, toes, and spine.

Findings revealed (a) that the incidence of pressure sores increased from between 6% and 8% in 1986 to 14.2% in 1989; (b) that the total availability of PR mattresses, bed-sized sheepskin overlays, and silicone-coated bed overlays increased in this 4-year period, and (c) that the increased availability of PR mattresses did *not* result in a reduction in the incidence of pressure sores.

Implications: The use of PR mattresses does not replace other forms of nursing care, such as manual repositioning and monitoring of pressure areas. More information is required to determine the relative effectiveness of PR mattresses and their suitability for particular clients. In addition, PR mattresses need to be checked for functioning and correct use.

Source: M Clark, and N Cullum, Matching patient need for pressure sore prevention with the supply of pressure redistributing mattresses, *Journal of Advanced Nursing*. March 1992. 17:310–16.

- Skin care plan to keep the skin clean, lubricated, and protected from secretions and excretions
- Need to keep pressure off the skin and bony prominences as much as possible
- Selection of pressure-relieving devices that may be used

CLINICAL GUIDELINES

Treating Pressure Sores

- Minimize direct pressure on the sore. Reposition the client at least every 2 hours. Make a schedule, and record position changes on the client's chart.
- Clean the pressure sore daily. The method of cleaning depends on the stage of the ulcer and agency protocol. For example, a whirlpool bath may be indicated for a stage I ulcer and a wound irrigation for a stage IV ulcer. See Chapter 44, page 1378.
- Clean and dress the sore using surgical asepsis. Refrain from using antiseptics, such as alcohol, that are vasoconstrictors and reduce blood flow to the area.
- If the pressure sore is *infected*, obtain a sample of the drainage for culture and sensitivity to antiseptic agents.
- Reduce friction by applying a small amount of cornstarch on the bedsheet.
- Reduce shearing force by keeping the head of the bed flat or elevated to a maximum of 30 degrees, unless contraindicated by the client's condition.
- If the client cannot keep weight off the pressure sore, use pressure-relieving devices, such as an egg crate mattress.
- Teach the client to move, if only slightly, to relieve pressure.
- Encourage ambulation or sitting in a wheelchair as the client's condition permits.
- Provide range-of-motion (ROM) exercises as the client's condition permits.

- Schedule for repositioning the client and demonstration of desired positions and positioning devices to keep bony prominences from direct contact with others
- Importance of maintaining or increasing correct activity level
- Avoidance of massage, donuts, and heat lamps
- Need to contact the physician when there is skin reddening, blister formation, or breakdown

TREATING PRESSURE ULCERS

Pressure sores are a challenge for nurses because of the number of variables involved (eg, risk factors, types of ulcers, and degrees of impairment) and the numerous treatment measures advocated. Existing and potential infections are the most serious complications of pressure sores. In treating pressure sores, nurses should follow the agency protocols and/or the physician's orders. Prompt

Table 30–5 Dressings for Pressure Ulcers

Dressing	Mechanism of Action	Stage I	Stage II	Stage III	Stage IV
Dry gauze	Wicks drainage away from wound surface	No	No	Yes	Yes
Moist gauze	Maintains a moist wound environment while wicking drainage away from surface	No	No	?	?
Moist-to-dry gauze	Debrides necrotic and healthy tissue nonselectively	No	No	?	?
Polyurethane film (eg, Tegaderm, Opsite)	Traps serous exudate and provides a moist wound environment	Yes	Yes	No	No
Hydrocolloid (eg, DuoDerm intact)	Reacts with wound fluid to create a soft gel that promotes granulation and epithelialization	Yes	Yes	?	No
Polyurethane foam (eg, Lyofoam, Allevyn)	Absorbs exudate and maintains a moist wound environment	No	Yes	?	No
Absorptive dressing (eg, Bard Absorption Dressing, Sorbsan, Kaltostat)	Absorbs exudate and debris while maintaining a moist environment	No	No	Yes	?
Hydrogel (eg, Vigilon, Geliperm)	Maintains a moist environment	No	Yes	Yes	No

Source: J Maklebust and M Sieggreen, *Pressure Ulcers: Guidelines for Prevention and Nursing Management* (West Dundee, IL: S-N Publications, 1991), as cited in J Maklebust, Pressure ulcer update, *RN*, December 1991, 54:61. Used with permission.

pressure ulcer treatment can prevent further tissue damage and pain and facilitate wound healing. Dressing wounds is discussed in Chapter 44. See the box at the left for clinical guidelines regarding treating pressure ulcers, and Table 30–5 for dressings for pressure ulcers.

EVALUATING

To judge whether client outcomes have been achieved, the nurse uses data collected during care, such as skin status over bony prominences and perineal area, nutritional and fluid intake, mental status, signs of healing if an ulcer is present, and so on. If outcomes are *not* achieved, the nurse should explore the reasons why:

- Has the client's physical condition changed?
- Were risk factors correctly identified?
- Were appropriate lifting devices and techniques used?
- Did the client fail to comply with instructions about moving and turning? Why?
- Were appropriate pressure-relieving devices used, and were they applied correctly?
- Was the repositioning schedule adhered to?
- Is the client's diet and fluid intake adequate?
- Were appropriate measures used to control incontinence and protect the client's skin?
- If an ulcer is present, was the wound treated appropriately?
- If the client is at home, were support services adequate? Did the support person have the ability to perform required care?

CHAPTER HIGHLIGHTS

- Maintaining skin integrity is an important independent function of nursing.
- A pressure ulcer is any lesion caused by unrelieved pressure that results in damage to underlying tissues. Pressure ulcers usually occur over bony prominences.
- Two other factors that act in conjunction with pressure to produce a pressure ulcer are friction and shearing forces.

- Several factors increase the risk for the development of pressure ulcers: immobility and inactivity, inadequate nutrition, fecal and urinary incontinence, decreased mental status, diminished sensation, excessive body heat, and advanced age.
- There are four stages of pressure ulcer development, which vary according to the degree of tissue damage.
- Several risk assessment tools are available to identify clients at risk for pressure ulcer development. They include scoring systems to evaluate a person's degree of risk.
- Meticulous skin examination of common pressure ulcer sites by the nurse is an important ongoing assessment activity for clients at risk.
- When a pressure ulcer is present, the nurse describes the ulcer in terms of location, size, depth, stage, color, status of wound margins and surrounding skin, and specific signs of infection, if present.
- The NANDA nursing diagnoses **High risk for impaired skin integrity, Impaired skin integrity,** and **Impaired tissue integrity** apply to clients at risk for developing pressure ulcers and to those with stage I to stage IV pressure ulcers.
- Major goals/outcomes for clients at risk for developing pressure ulcers are to maintain skin integrity and to avoid potential associated risks. Clients with impaired skin/tissue integrity need to demonstrate wound healing.
- Nursing interventions to prevent the formation of pressure ulcers include conducting ongoing assessment of risk factors and skin status; providing skin care to maintain skin integrity; ensuring adequate nutrition; implementing measures to avoid skin trauma; providing supportive devices; and client teaching.
- Treatment for pressure ulcers varies according to the stage of the ulcer and agency protocol.

READINGS AND REFERENCES

SUGGESTED READINGS

Alterescue, V and Alterescu, KB. March/April 1992. Pressure ulcers: Assessment and treatment. *Orthopaedic Nursing* 11:37–39.
This article discusses both the assessment and treatment of pressure ulcers. Topics addressed include the etiology of pressure ulcers, skin physiology, wound healing, pathophysiology of unhealthy wounds, major categories of dressings, and other treatment modalities.

Maklebust, J. December 1991. Pressure ulcer update. *RN* 54:56–63.
This article includes guidelines for assessing clients at risk for developing pressure ulcers, a quick guide to prevention, a pictorial display of the National Pressure Ulcer Advisory Panel's staging system, and various treatments used in managing pressure ulcers. A multiple-choice test follows the article.

RELATED RESEARCH

Burd, C, Langemo, DK, Olson, B, Hanson, D, Hunter, S, and Sauvage, T. September 1992. Skin problems: Epidemiology of pressure ulcers in a skilled-care facility. *Journal of Gerontological Nursing* 18:29–41.

Clark, M and Cullum, N. March 1992. Matching patient need for pressure sore prevention with the supply of pressure redistributing mattresses. *Journal of Advanced Nursing* 17:310–16.

SELECTED REFERENCES

Alterescu, V and Alterescu, KB. March/April 1992. Pressure ulcers: Assessment and treatment. *Orthopaedic Nursing* 11:37–49.

Anthony, D. August 26, 1987. Norton revises risk scores. *Nursing Times* 83:6.

Barnes, HR. March 1993. Alternating transparent and hydrocolloid dressings: A difficult case. *Nursing93* 23:59–61.

Beckel, J. March/April 1992. Implementation of a standardized protocol for treating pressure ulcers in a nursing home. *Geriatric Nursing* 13:84–89.

Bergstrom, N, Braden, JB, Laguzza, A, and Holman, V. July/August 1987. The Braden Scale for predicting pressure sore risk. *Nursing Research* 36:205–10.

Brandeis, GH, Morris, JM, Nash, DJ, and Lipsitz, LA. December 1, 1990. The epidemiology and natural history of pressure ulcers in elderly nursing home residents. *Journal of the American Medical Association.* 264:2905–909.

Bryant, RA, Shannon, ML, Pieper, B, Braden, BJ, and Morris, DJ. 1992. Pressure ulcers. In Bryant, RA, editor. pp. 105–63. *Acute and Chronic Wounds: Nursing Management.* St Louis: Mosby-Year Book.

Burd, C, Langemo, DK, Olson, B, Hanson, D, Hunter S, and Sauvage, T. September 1992. Skin problems: Epidemiology of pressure ulcers in a skilled-care facility. *Journal of Gerontological Nursing* 18:29–41.

Carpenito, LJ. 1992. *Nursing Diagnosis: Application to Clinical Practice.* 4th ed. Philadelphia: Lippincott.

Clark, M and Cullum, N. March 1992. Matching patient need for pressure sore prevention with the supply of pressure redistributing mattresses. *Journal of Advanced Nursing* 17:310–16.

Clinical guidelines: How to predict and prevent pressure ulcers. July 1992. *American Journal of Nursing* 92:52, 54–56, 58–60.

Collier, M. October 1990. A sore point: Prevention of pressure sores. *Community Outlook* pp. 29–30, 32.

Cullum, N and Clark, M. April 1992. Intrinsic factors associated with pressure sores in elderly people. *Journal of Advanced Nursing* 17:427–31.

Dugan, MC. November 1992. Pressure areas: Standard protocols improve care. *Nursing Management* 23:78,80.

Goodridge, DM. January 1993. Pressure ulcer risk assessment tools: What's new for gerontological nurses. *Journal of Gerontological Nursing* 19:23–27.

Green, E and Katz, J. February 1991. Practice guidelines for management of pressure ulcers. *Decubitus* 4:36,38,40,42.

Griffiths, G. September 4–10, 1991. Choosing a dressing. *Nursing Times* 87:84,86,88,90.

Guthrie, J. March 31–April 6, 1993. Using air fluidized therapy. *Nursing Times* 89:82–88.

Kelley, LS and Mobily, PR. September 1991. Iatrogenesis in the elderly: Impaired skin integrity. *Journal of Gerontological Nursing* 17:24–29.

Kim, MJ, McFarland, GK, and McLane, AM. 1993. *Pocket Guide to Nursing Diagnoses.* 5th ed. St Louis: Mosby-Year Book.

Krasner, D. December 1992. The 12 commandments of wound care. *Nursing92* 12:34–42.

Lederer, JR, Marculescu, GL, Mocnik, B, and Seaby, N. 1993. *Care Planning Pocket Guide—A Nursing Diagnosis Approach.* 5th ed. Redwood City, CA: Addison-Wesley Nursing.

Lovell, HW, and Anderson, CL. May 1990. Put your patient on the right bed. *RN* 53:66–72.

McFarland, GK and McFarland, EA. 1989. *Nursing Diagnosis and Interventions: Planning for Patient Care.* St Louis: Mosby.

Maklebust, J. June 1987. Pressure ulcers: Etiology and prevention. *Nursing Clinics of North America* 22:359–77.

______. December 1991. Pressure ulcer update. *RN* 54:56–63.

Malone, C. September 2–8, 1992. Intensive pressures . . . reduce the incidence of pressure sores. *Nursing Times* 88:57–60.

Meehan, M. November 1990. Multisite pressure ulcer prevalance survey. *Decubitus* 3:14–17.

North American Nursing Diagnosis Association. 1992. *NANDA Nursing Diagnoses: Definitions and Classification 1992–1993.* Philadelphia: NANDA.

Norton, D. February 13, 1975. Research and the problem of pressure sores. *Nursing Mirror* 140:65–67.

Norton, D, McLaren, R, and Exton-Smith, AN. 1962, 1975. An investigation of geriatric nursing problems in hospital. Edinburgh: Churchill Livingstone.

Osborne, S. February 18–24, 1987. A quality circle . . . reducing the incidence of pressure sores: Investigations. *Nursing Times* 83:73,75–76.

Reichel, SM. February 15, 1958. Shearing force as a factor in decubitus ulcers in paraplegics. *Journal of the American Medical Association* 166:762–63.

Shannon, ML. October 1984. Five famous fallacies about pressure sores. *Nursing84* 14:34–41.

Shannon, ML and Miller, BM. May/June 1988. Pressure sore treatments: A case in point. *Geriatric Nursing* 9:154–57.

Shannon, ML and Skorga, P. November 1989. Pressure ulcer prevalence in two general hospitals. *Decubitus* 2:38–43.

Spurgin, S and Clinch, K. September 4–10, 1991. A new dressing for pressure sores. *Nursing Times* 87:82,84.

Tudor, R and Gupta, R. September 2–8, 1992. Factors to focus on . . . wound healing. *Nursing Times* 88:62,64.

US Department of Health and Human Services. 1992. Clinical practice guideline. *Pressure Ulcers in Adults: Prediction and Prevention.* Pub no. 9-0047. Rockville, MD: Public Health Service.

Versluysen, M. January 1985. Pressure sores in elderly patients: The epidemiology related to hip operations. *Journal of Bone and Joint Surgery* (Br Ed) 67:10–13.

______. May 1986. How elderly patients with femoral fractures develop pressure sores in hospital. *British Medical Journal* (Clin Res Ed) 17:1311–13.

Wardman, C. March 27–April 2, 1991. Norton V. Waterlow. *Nursing Times* 87:74,76,78.

Waterlow, J. November 27–December 3, 1985. A risk assessment card. *Nursing Times* 81:49,51,55.

Williams, C. September 4–10, 1991. Comparing Norton and Medley . . . pressure sore risk assessment systems. *Nursing Times* 87:66–68.

UNIT 9

Promoting Psychosocial Health

STUDENT PROFILE

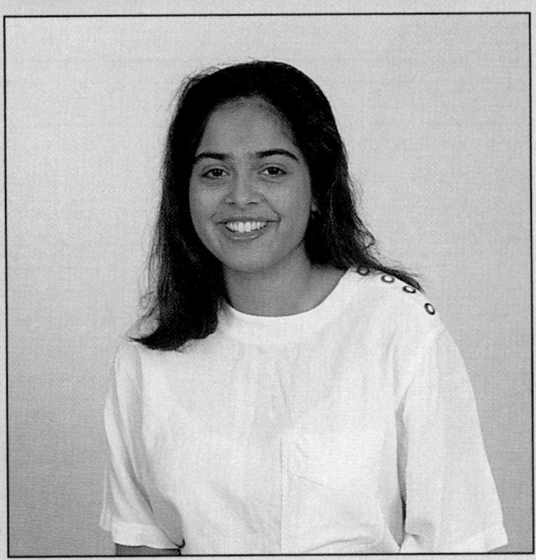

NAME Amna Khan

SCHOOL OF NURSING Baptist Memorial Hospital School of Nursing, Memphis, Tennessee

HOMETOWN Memphis

WHY DID YOU ENTER THE FIELD OF NURSING?
I have always wanted to work in the medical sciences. Nursing provided an avenue for me to explore different fields of medicine, a broad scope of practice, and it confirmed that I want a "hands-on" patient-care career.

WHY DO YOU THINK THIS IS A GOOD TIME TO BE IN NURSING?
Nurses play a key role in guiding the future of the health care delivery system as the scope of practice broadens and new opportunities arise. Being a part of this historic change is both challenging and exciting.

WHAT QUALITIES DO YOU THINK ARE NECESSARY TO BE A GOOD NURSE?
Patience, open-mindedness, excellent communication skills, enthusiasm, intelligence, and professionalism are all components of a "good nurse."

WHAT HAS BEEN YOUR MOST GRATIFYING MOMENT AS A STUDENT NURSE?
When a patient recuperates as a direct result of nursing care and intervention, and when families of patients express sincere hugs and tears of thanks, the rewards of the profession are invaluable.

WHAT ADVICE WOULD YOU GIVE A NEW STUDENT?
Hang in there.

31

Self-Concept and Role Relationships

Objectives

- Differentiate *self-concept* from *self-esteem.*
- Describe the components of self-concept.
- Give Erikson's explanation of the effects of psychosocial crises on self-concept and self-esteem.
- Describe the effects of communication/coping styles on self-esteem.
- Identify four areas involved in the nursing assessment of self-concept.
- Describe key data to be included when assessing self-perception.
- Describe the essential aspects of assessing role relationships.
- List important assessment data to be included when identifying clients' stressors and coping strategies.
- Identify common stressors affecting self-concept and coping strategies.
- List behaviors that could indicate altered self-concept.
- Identify nursing diagnoses related to altered self-concept.
- Select appropriate goals for clients with altered self-concept.
- Describe nursing actions designed to achieve identified goals for clients with altered self-concept.
- Describe ways to enhance the self-esteem of older adults.
- Identify outcome criteria that permit evaluation of clients with altered self-concept.
- Identify strategies for promoting professional self-concept.

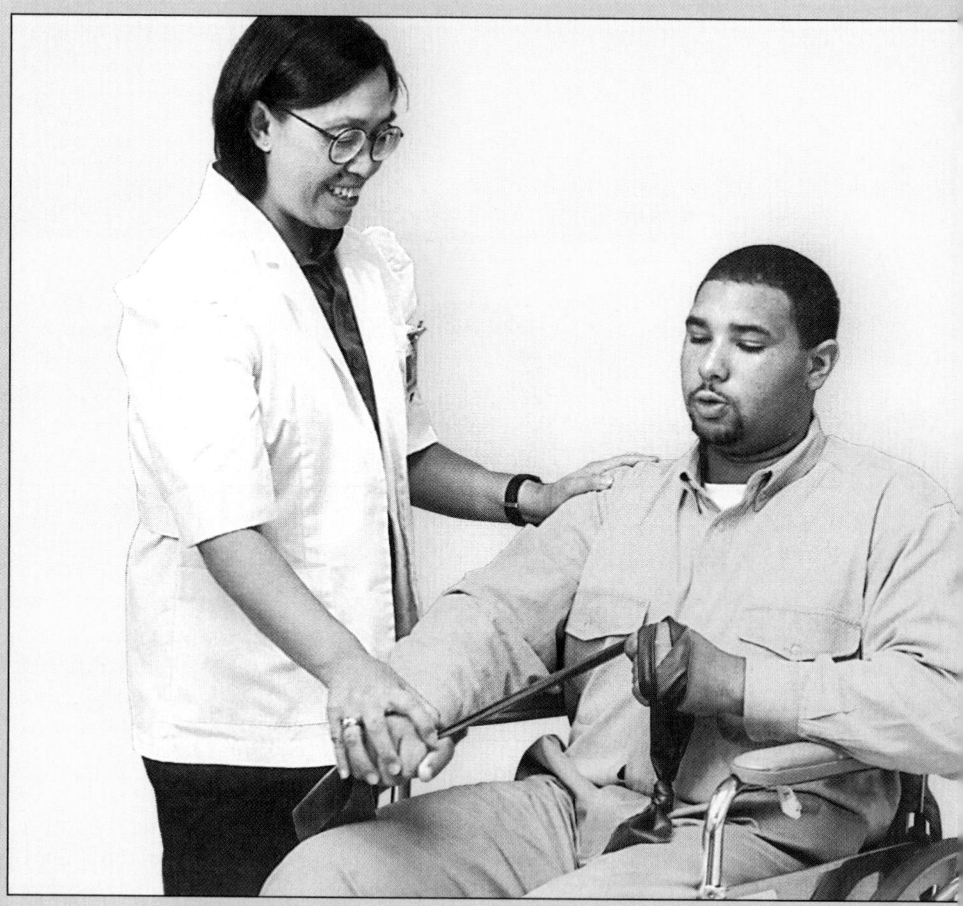

Self-concept, self-esteem, and self-image are essential to a person's mental and physical health. Individuals with a positive self-concept or high self-esteem are better able to develop and maintain warm interpersonal relationships and resist psychologic and physical illness. A healthy self-concept enables a person to find happiness in life and to cope with life's disappointments and changes. Failure to achieve a positive self-image presents major obstacles in the treatment of common disorders such as depression, eating disorders, postvictimization syndrome (abuse or rape), and crisis reactions. One of the nurse's major responsibilities is to identify persons with a negative self-concept or low self-esteem and to assist them in developing a more positive view of themselves. People who do not have a healthy self-concept are less able to live as fully or be as happy as they might be. People with an unhealthy self-concept generally express feelings of worthlessness, self-dislike or self-hatred, and, on some occasions, hatred for others. They often feel sad or hopeless and are drained of energy.

Self-concept or self-esteem influences a person in these ways (Sanford & Donovan 1984, p. 3):

- It affects everything one thinks, says, or does.
- It affects how others in the world see and treat one.
- It affects the choices one makes, such as the choice of mate and the choice of career.
- It affects one's ability to give and receive love.
- It affects one's ability to take action to change things that need to be changed.

The nurse's own self-concept is also important. Nurses who have difficulty meeting their own needs have difficulty meeting the needs of clients. Nurses who understand the different dimensions of themselves, by contrast, are better able to understand the needs, desires, feelings, and conflicts of their clients. Nurses who feel positive about themselves are better equipped to assist others in meeting their needs. Such nurses feel well, look good, are effective and productive, and respond to people (including themselves) in healthy and positive ways.

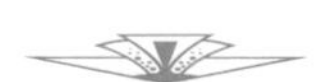

Concept of Self and Self-Esteem

The terms *self-concept, self-image, self-esteem, self-worth, sense of self-worth, self-respect,* and *self-love* are often used interchangeably. *Self-concept* has been referred to as the *cognitive* component of the self system, and *self-esteem* as the *affective* component (Hamachek 1987). Lindberg et al (1990, p. 87) describe **self-concept** as the "collection of notions, feelings, and beliefs about ourselves with which we identify and through which we relate and communicate with others and interact with the environment." Klose and Tinius (1992, p. 5) define **self-esteem** as "confidence in one's abilities and judgment." In other words, self-concept is "how I *see* myself," and self-esteem is "how I *feel about* myself." Stanwyck (1983, p. 11), however, maintains that these two constructs are inseparable, because self-esteem is based on self-concept. To Stanwyck, self-esteem is "how I feel about how I see myself," even though most researchers use the terms interchangeably.

Three positions of self-concept have been delineated:

1. *Cognized self,* or self as known to the individual: "How I am," or, "How I perceive me."
2. *Other self,* or social self: "How I perceive others perceiving me."
3. *Ideal self:* "How I would like to be."

People who value most "how I perceive me" can be termed "me-centered." They try hard to live up to their own expectations and compete only with themselves, not others. In contrast, "other-centered" people have a high need for approval from others and try hard to live up to the expectations of others, constantly comparing, competing, and evaluating themselves in relation to others. They tend to avoid personal shortcomings, are unable to assert themselves, and continually fear disapproval. The healthy self-concept, therefore, is me-centered and is formed without reference to other persons.

Global and Specific Self-Concept

The term **global self** refers to the collective beliefs and images one holds about oneself. It is the most complete description that individuals can give of themselves at any one time. It is also a person's frame of reference for experiencing and viewing the world. Some of these beliefs and images represent statements of fact, for example, "I am a woman"; "I am a mother"; "I am Irish"; "I am short"; "I am a student"; "I am poor." Others refer to less tangible aspects of self, for instance, "I am stupid"; "I am competent"; "I am clumsy"; "I am lovable"; "I am no good"; "I am shy"; "I am strong"; "I am outgoing."

Each separate image and belief one holds about oneself has a bearing on self-concept. However, self-concept is not simply a sum of its parts, for the various images and beliefs persons hold about themselves are not given equal weight and prominence (Sanford & Donovan 1984, p. 9). Each person's self-concept is like a collage. At the center of the collage are the beliefs and images that are most vital to the person's identity and self-esteem. They constitute

core self-concept. For example: "I am competent/incompetent"; "I am pretty/ugly"; "I am rich/poor"; "I am male/female." Images and beliefs that are less important to the person are on the periphery. For example: "I am left-/right-handed"; "I am athletic/unathletic"; "I am a good/poor cook"; "I have brown/blue eyes."

According to Goldin (1985, p. 33), people base their self-concept on how they perceive and evaluate themselves in these areas:

- Vocational performance
- Intellectual functioning
- Personal appearance and physical attractiveness
- Sexual attractiveness and performance
- Being liked by others
- Ability to cope with and resolve problems
- Independence
- Particular talents

In children, self-concept includes the child's self-esteem, sense of control, body concept, and sex role (Edelman & Mandle 1990, p. 418). Self-esteem involves the following:

- Family relationships
- Peer relationships
- School performance
- Body image
- Physical ability
- Emotional well-being

A person's self-perception in any of these areas becomes a self-fulfilling prophecy: Individuals actually behave as they perceive themselves (Goldin 1985, p. 34).

COMPONENTS OF SELF-CONCEPT

There are four components of self-concept: body image, role performance, personal identity, and self-esteem.

Body Image The image of physical self, or body image is how a person perceives the size, appearance, and functioning of the body and its parts. According to Arnold and Boggs (1989, p. 73), body image has both cognitive and affective self-understandings. The cognitive is the knowledge of the material body and its attachments; the affective includes the sensations of the body. The Roy adaptation model describes the physical self as composed of body image and body sensation. Body image is "how one views oneself physically and one's view of one's appearance" (Andrews 1991, p. 270). Body image encompasses the functioning of the body and its parts. It includes clothing, make-up, hairstyle, jewelry, and other things intimately connected to the person. It also includes body prostheses, such as artificial limbs, dentures, and hairpieces, as well as devices required for functioning, such as wheelchairs, canes, and eyeglasses. Body sensation describes "how one feels and experiences oneself as a physical being" (Andrews 1991, p. 270) and includes sensory perceptions such as pain, pleasure, fatigue, and physical movement.

A person's body image develops partly from others' attitudes and responses to that person's body and partly from the individual's own exploration of the body. For example, body image develops in infancy as the parent or caregivers respond to the child with smiles, holding, and touching and also as the child explores its own body sensations during breast-feeding, thumb sucking, and the bath. Cultural and societal values also influence a person's body image. For example, in the United States, being tall and being thin are considered by many as parameters of physical beauty. A person who is unusually short or obese may experience negative responses or even discrimination from others. Because a person's body image has developed over a lifetime, actual or potential alterations in body image can create considerable anxiety.

Role Performance Throughout life people undergo numerous role changes. A **role** is a set of expectations about how the person occupying one position behaves toward a person occupying another position (Roy & Andrews 1991, p. 348). Expectations, or standards of behavior, are set by society or the smaller group to which the person belongs. Each person usually has several roles, such as husband, parent, brother, son, employee, friend, golf club member. Some roles are assumed for only limited periods, such as client/nurse, student/instructor, and ill person.

To act appropriately, people need to know who they are in relation to others and what society expects for the positions they hold. When there is **role ambiguity**, expectations are unclear, and people do not know what to do or how to do it and are unable to predict the reactions of others to their behavior. This creates confusion and stress. To relate or interact appropriately with others, people also need to know the role positions that others occupy.

Role performance relates what a person does in a particular role in relation to the behaviors expected of that role. **Role mastery** means that the person's behaviors meet social expectations. Failure to master a role creates frustration and feelings of inadequacy, often with consequent lowered self-esteem.

Self-concept is also affected by role strain and role conflicts. Persons undergoing **role strain** are frustrated because they feel or are made to feel inadequate or unsuited to a role. Role strain often is associated with sex role stereotypes. For example, women in occupations traditionally held by men may be thought less knowledgeable and less competent than men in the same roles. As a result, these women feel the need to surpass the level expected for role mastery by male counterparts.

Role conflicts arise from opposing or incompatible expectations. In an *interpersonal conflict*, different people have different expectations about a particular role. For example, a mother's parents may have different expectations about how the mother should care for her children. In an *interrole conflict*, one person's or group's role expectations differ from the expectations of another person or group. For example, a woman who works in an office 8 hours a day may have a role conflict if her husband expects her to be home with the children. In a **person-role conflict,** role expectations violate the beliefs or values of the role occupant. For example, a woman who values her right to choose abortion will have a conflict if this right is denied.

Personal Identity A person's personal identity, or **self-identity,** is the conscious sense of individuality and uniqueness that is continually evolving throughout life. People often view their identity in terms of name, sex, age, race, ethnic origin or culture, occupation or roles, talents, and other situational characteristics (eg, marital status and education). People usually first identify themselves by name and occupation or roles. When interactions progress beyond the superficial, other characteristics may be revealed, such as special talents or interests. Self-identity also includes a person's beliefs and values, personality, and character. For instance, is the person outgoing, friendly, reserved, generous, kind, honest, ruthless, selfish? Self-identity thus encompasses both the tangible and factual, such as name and sex, and the intangible, such as values and beliefs. In brief: Identity is what distinguishes self from others.

RESEARCH NOTE

Does Treatment for Breast Cancer Affect Women's Body Image?

Body image was compared in four groups of women who received the most common types of treatment for a first incidence of breast cancer: mastectomy without breast reconstruction, mastectomy with delayed breast reconstruction, mastectomy with immediate breast reconstruction, and conservative surgery. The total sample size was 257 women. The questionnaires used to solicit data from the study participants were the Body Image Scale (Berscheid et al 1972) and the Tennessee Self-Concept Scale (TSCS) (Roid & Fitts 1988).

Comparison of the groups indicated that women treated with conservative surgery reported greater satisfaction with their bodies than women treated either with mastectomy or immediate reconstruction. No differences in self-concept were evident among the four groups, although TSCS scores for physical self were lower in all four treatment groups than norms for the general population.

Implications: Nurses need to be aware that women who have been diagnosed with breast cancer are likely to have diminished self-image regardless of the type of surgical treatment. Nursing strategies should be implemented to assist clients to express feelings and to improve self-image.

Source: V Mock, Body image in women treated for breast cancer, *Nursing Research*, May/June 1993, 42:153–57.

Self-Esteem The way one perceives and structures one's self-concept can result in either positive or negative self-esteem. There are two types of self-esteem: global and specific (Sanford & Donovan 1984, p. 9). **Global self-esteem** is how much one likes one's perceived self as a whole. **Specific self-esteem** is how much one approves of a certain part of oneself (Sanford & Donovan 1984, p. 9). Global self-esteem is influenced by specific self-esteem. For example, if a man values his looks, then how he looks will strongly affect his global self-esteem. By contrast, if a man places little value on his cooking skills, then how well or badly he cooks will have little influence on his global self-esteem.

Maintenance and Evaluation of Self-Esteem

By the time people reach adulthood, their *basic* self-concept and *basic* level of self-esteem are relatively well established, and they already have some idea about their **perceived self,** that is, how they see themselves and how they are seen by others. In addition, they have an idea about their **ideal self,** that is, how they should be or would prefer to be. Sometimes this ideal self is realistic; sometimes it is not. Klose and Tinius (1992, p. 5) state that "an adequate self-esteem is seen as an acceptance of oneself despite mistakes, defeats, and failures made in life." When perceived self is close to ideal self, people do not wish to be much different from what they believe they already are. A discrepancy between ideal self and perceived self can be an incentive to self-improvement. However, when the discrepancy is large, low self-esteem can result.

Basic self-esteem refers to the foundation for self-esteem that is established during early life experiences, usually within the family. However, an adult's functional level of overall self-esteem may change markedly from day to day and moment to moment. *Functional self-esteem* is a result of the person's ongoing evaluation of interactions with people and objects. Functional self-esteem can exceed basic self-esteem, or it can regress to a level below that of basic self-esteem. Severe stress—for example, stress related to prolonged illness or unemployment—can substantially lower a person's basic self-esteem.

Perceptions of self (both as is and as desired) generally arise from self-evaluation in accordance with certain criteria. The following are four basic criteria by which people judge themselves:

1. *Power*—the ability to influence significant others and control events that are personally important
2. *Significance*—the acceptance, attention, and affection of others who communicate to the person a clear sense of being valued and cared about as a worthwhile human being
3. *Competence*—successfully meeting demands for achievement, particularly personally important goals
4. *Virtue*—adherence to moral and ethical standards

Self-evaluation is usually a covert mental process. Frequently, people label themselves negatively or project failures into the future. Positive self-credit is usually less frequent.

DEVELOPMENT OF SELF-ESTEEM

Four elements of experience that are pertinent to the development of self-esteem are (a) significant others, (b) social role expectations, (c) crises of psychosocial development, and (d) communication/coping style (Stanwyck 1983, p. 13).

Significant Others Most social psychologists acknowledge that social interaction plays a crucial role in the development of self-esteem. Because some people exert more influence than others on the development of an individual's self-esteem, Sullivan's term *significant other* has been generally accepted (Sullivan 1950). A **significant other** is an individual or group that takes on special importance for the development of self-esteem during a particular life stage. Significant others may include parents, siblings, peers, teachers, and the like. During various stages of development, one or several significant others may be identified. Through social interaction with significant others and the resultant interpreted feedback on the perceptions of others, one develops attitudes toward oneself. Put more simply, "as a person is judged by others, so he comes to judge himself" (Burns 1979, p. 184). Many components of a person's self-evaluation are established early in life under the influence of significant others. These values often get so strongly reinforced that they are difficult to change later, even though it may benefit the person to do so.

Social Role Expectations At the various stages of life, people are strongly influenced by general societal expectations regarding role-specific behavior. The larger society and smaller societal groups have expectations that differ in clarity and are communicated with varying degrees of force. Expectations differ by age, sex, socioeconomic status, ethnicity, religious background, and career identification. Smaller societal groups, such as the family, school, armed forces, work groups, and recreational groups, also expect certain behaviors and performance levels of people. Success in meeting such expectations has profound implications for self-esteem.

Because North American society is highly oriented toward achievement, everything a person does is evaluated, for example, earning capacity, social skills, performance at school, athletic performance, and sexual performance. A high level of performance is rewarded; poor performance is belittled. As a result, people tend to focus on their failures and shortcomings rather than on their strengths. In many instances a person's actual performance is superior to the person's *perception* of that performance. Compliance with the social expectations for role-specific behavior therefore leads to judgments of personal worth; noncompliance often leads to judgments of personal worthlessness.

Crises of Psychosocial Development Throughout life people face certain developmental tasks that, if not successfully achieved, may lead to problems with self, self-concept, and self-esteem. Several developmental theories are discussed in Chapter 23. The eight psychosocial stages described by Erikson (1963) provide a convenient and familiar theoretical framework with obvious implications for self-esteem. The success with which a person copes with these developmental crises largely determines the development of self-concept. Inability to cope results in self-concept problems, at the time and, often, later in life. See Table 31–1 for behaviors indicating successful and unsuccessful resolution of these developmental crises.

Communication/Coping Styles A person's choice of strategies to cope with a stress-producing situation is important in determining how successfully a person adapts to that situation and whether self-esteem is maintained, enhanced, or decreased. Some coping mechanisms for dealing with stress are presented in Chapter 32. Other reactions to stressful situations that threaten self-esteem include problem-solving reactions, assertive reactions, and defensive reactions.

Problem-Solving Reactions Problem solving is a conscious, action-oriented response in which the person uses

Table 31–1 Examples of Behaviors Associated with Erikson's Stages of Psychosocial Development

Stage: Developmental Crisis	Behaviors Indicating Positive Resolution	Behaviors Indicating Negative Resolution
Infancy: Trust vs mistrust	Requesting assistance and expecting to receive it Expressing belief of another person Sharing time, opinions, and experiences	Restricting conversation to superficialities Refusing to provide a person with information Being unable to accept assitance
Toddlerhood: Autonomy vs shame and doubt	Accepting the rules of a group but also expressing disagreement when it is felt Expressing one's own opinion Easily accepting deferment of a wish fulfillment	Failing to express needs Not expressing one's own opinion when opposed Overconcern about being clean
Early childhood: Initiative vs guilt	Starting projects eagerly Expressing curiosity about many things Demonstrating original thought	Imitating others rather than developing independent ideas Apologizing and being very embarrassed over small mistakes Verbalizing fear about starting a new project
Early school years: Industry vs inferiority	Completing a task once it has been started Working well with others Using time effectively	Not completing tasks started Not assisting with the work of others Not organizing work
Adolescence: Identity vs role confusion	Asserting independence Planning realistically for future roles Establishing close interpersonal relationships	Failing to assume responsibility for directing one's own behavior Accepting the values of others without question Failing to set goals in life
Early adulthood: Intimacy vs isolation	Establishing a close, intense relationship with another person Accepting sexual behavior as desirable Making a commitment to that relationship, even in times of stress and sacrifice	Remaining alone Avoiding close interpersonal relationships
Middle-aged adults: Generativity vs stagnation	Being willing to share with another person Guiding others Establishing a priority of needs, recognizing both self and others	Talking about oneself instead of listening to others Showing concern for oneself in spite of the needs of others Being unable to accept interdependence
Elderly adults: Integrity vs despair	Using past experience to assist others Maintaining productivity in some areas Accepting limitations	Crying and being apathetic Not accepting changes Demanding unnecessary assistance and attention from others

cognitive skills to deal with a stressor. First the person cognitively appraises the threatening situation by asking questions such as these:

- What is the exact nature of the threatening situation?
- What unfavorable consequences can I expect from the situation should it occur?
- What courses of action can I use to cope with the threat?
- What courses of action are most likely to succeed, that is, cause the least personal loss or concern?

After a realistic appraisal, the person chooses the most effective course of action, for example, talking to a friend, calling a crisis center, doing nothing, or seeking out professional help.

Assertive Reactions Everyday interpersonal interactions can produce stress. In such situations, assertive

CLINICAL GUIDELINES

Assertive Techniques

- Include positive and negative information in a statement: "I like your plan, but. . . ."
- Start the statement with "I," and avoid generalizations such as "we all believe" or "it seems like a good idea."
- Express your own beliefs and rights: "I believe that. . . ."
- Express your thoughts and feelings directly to reinforce your identity "I feel you are . . ." or "I want you to. . . ."
- When replying negatively, state, "I won't . . ." not "I can't. . . ." The latter implies lack of power, whereas the former communicates assumption of responsibility.
- Make assertive statements:
  a. Simple assertive: "I think. . . ."
  b. Empathic assertive: "I realize you are very tired, but. . . ."
  c. Confrontive assertive: "You said you could bathe Mr Greene, but you didn't. . . ."
  d. Soft assertive: "I am very grateful you did that for me, and I think. . . ."
  e. Persuasive assertive: "I agree with most of what you said, but I also think. . . ."

When an individual says something that the nurse perceives as negative or a "put-down," the following assertive responses can be given to provide time:

- "I need to think about this for a few minutes."
- "It seems to me that . . ." followed by a clear statement of personal feelings.
- Silence as an answer (giving no verbal response).

---

behavior is useful. **Assertiveness** involves expressing oneself confidently and comfortably while respecting the rights of others (Smith 1992, p. 8). It provides feelings of control and self-confidence for the communicator and is based on the belief that each person is important. Assertive people are able to present their feelings and values, stand up for themselves, and claim their rights. Assertiveness is prerequisite to building self-esteem. Because it enables the person to cope with a stressful event actively, it enhances self-esteem.

Assertiveness with individuals and groups facilitates

- Prompt coping with problems.
- Achievement of group goals.
- Communication of power within oneself.
- Communication of competence and self-confidence.
- Reduction of anxiety or tenseness in key situations.

Assertive behavior can be described as falling between nonassertiveness and aggressive behavior on a continuum. Nonassertive or passive persons appear hesitant and unsure of themselves. Their feelings are hidden, for fear of hurting others or being hurt. Because nonassertive persons do not ask or know how to ask, they often do not obtain what they want and thus become frustrated. After a time, this frustration often results in explosively aggressive behavior, which helps the person feel better, but only briefly. Through **aggressiveness,** at the other extreme, people can make their feelings known, but often at others' expense. Although this behavior can result in change, it can be harmful to the individual eventually, as others respond negatively to the aggressive behavior.

According to Smith (1992, p. 8), communicating assertively means:

- Being skilled in a variety of communication strategies for expressing thoughts and feelings in a way that protects the rights of all involved.
- Having a positive attitude about communicating in a forthright and fair way.
- Feeling comfortable and in control of negative feelings, such as anxiety, tenseness, shyness, or fear.
- Feeling confident that one can conduct oneself in a self-respecting and other-respecting way.
- Keeping the rights of all equally paramount.

Nurses, too, can benefit from using assertive responses. The example that follows illustrates the different types of responses in a typical nursing situation. Additional communication techniques are discussed in Chapter 18.

Situation
Charge Nurse: Ms Eammons, why can't you ever take your blood pressures on time? This is the fourth day this week that they have not been taken.

Aggressive response
Nurse: It's not my fault they are late. You're always interrupting my work with extra duties.

Nonassertive response
Nurse: Yes, I'm sorry. We've been short staffed, and I have a very heavy load.

Assertive response
Nurse: I didn't know that all the blood pressures were late. I'd like to check that further. Could we discuss a way to resolve this problem so that it doesn't recur? Perhaps, in your office before you leave today?

The techniques shown in the box at the upper left can help the nurse develop skills in communicating assertively.

Three assertive methods of coping with criticism are fogging, negative assertion, and negative inquiry. *Fogging* is agreeing in principle to a statement made by another. In this technique, the nurse listens carefully to the criticism and accepts it without becoming defensive or anxious.

Client: You can't do anything right.

Nurse: You're not satisfied with my work, Mr Milos.

Negative assertion is the assertive expression of those attributes that are negative about oneself:

Client: You didn't give that injection well.

Nurse: I didn't give it very smoothly.

Negative inquiry asks for additional information about the critical statements:

Charge Nurse: You look messy today.

Nurse: What do you mean?

Charge Nurse: You look untidy.

Nurse: Do you mean my uniform is wrinkled?

To learn assertiveness, nurses can take workshops or study articles on the subject.

Defensive Reactions Defensive responses are generally used when other responses have been unsuccessful in adapting to the stressful event and anxiety or other feelings remain high. Specific defensive coping behaviors are called ego-defense mechanisms (see Chapter 32, page 836).

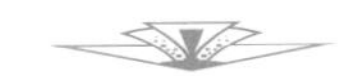

ASSESSING

Assessing problems related to self-concept is normally indicated if (a) the client or support persons present cues that could reflect problems or (b) the client's illness is one often associated with self-concept problems. Problems with self-concept and self-esteem are frequently manifested by expressions of anxiety, fear, anger, hostility, guilt, and/or powerlessness. Behaviors reflecting excessive role conflict may also indicate the need for meaningful intervention by nurses.

A trusting client-nurse relationship is essential for an effective assessment of self-concept. Clients tend not to share personal feelings unless the nurse has established an empathetic, nonjudgmental relationship. Potential disclosure of personal data can be threatening. Some people, particularly those with low self-esteem, may fear that the nurse will not accept or like them if they reveal their true performance capabilities, thoughts, and feelings.

The nursing assessment involves four areas: (a) self-perception or self-awareness, (b) role performance and relationships, (c) major stressors and coping strategies, (d) behaviors suggestive of low self-esteem.

SELF-PERCEPTION

Assessment of self-perception involves (a) determining the client's perceptions of physical and personal self and (b) observing for nonverbal cues that reflect the client's self-perception.

To determine the client's perception of *physical self*, or body image, the nurse either listens to comments the client makes about the physical self or asks the client questions such as those shown in the box on page 810. Responses such as "I feel ugly," "I'm awkward and clumsy," "I can't do anything now," "No one will like me now," and "I'm afraid my husband won't love me any more" indicate that the client's self-esteem is threatened or low. The client is focusing on particular disabilities or shortcomings and blocking out accurate perception of the total self.

In regard to *personal self*, some people may volunteer clearly self-deprecating or overly-critical comments indicating low self-esteem—for example, "People don't like me," or "I'm no good." For other clients, consider some of the questions shown in the first box on page 810.

Nonverbal behaviors—such as body posture, movements, gestures, tone of voice, speech pattern, and general appearance—tend to be more spontaneous than verbal messages and can provide important clues to the person's self-concept. Nonverbal cues that can indicate low self-esteem include stooped shoulders, lack of attention to hygiene or grooming, avoiding eye contact, hesitant speech, and withdrawing from social interaction. Nonverbal cues can help the nurse confirm the reliability of the client's verbal messages.

ROLE RELATIONSHIPS

The nurse assesses the client's satisfactions and dissatisfactions associated with role responsibilities and relationships: family roles, work roles, student roles, social roles. Family roles are especially important to clients, since family relationships are particularly close. Relationships can be supportive and growth-producing or, at the opposite extreme, highly stressful if violence and abuse permeate relationships. Assessment of family role relationships may begin with structural aspects such as number in the family group, ages, and residence location. For more information on the family, see Chapter 14. To obtain data related to the client's family relationships and satisfaction or dissatisfaction with work roles and social roles, the nurse might ask some of the questions shown in the second box on page 810, keeping in mind, however, that questions need to be tailored to the individuals and their age and situation.

MAJOR STRESSORS AND COPING STRATEGIES

The nurse needs to identify stressors that challenge the client's self-worth. Most people face numerous stress-

ASSESSMENT INTERVIEW

Self-Perception

Physical Self

- How do you feel about your personal appearance (or physical features)?
- What do others say about your personal appearance (or physical features)?
- How would you describe your physical movements?
- What changes in your body do you expect as a result of this illness (or surgery, or treatment)?
- What changes have you noticed in how your body looks (or functions)?
- How have important persons in your life (eg, spouse, parent, partner) reacted to changes in your body?
- How do you think the important people in your life will react to the anticipated change in your body?

Personal Self

- How would you describe your personal characteristics? or, How do you see yourself as a person?
- What do you like about yourself?
- How do others describe you as a person?
- What do you do well?
- What are your personal strengths, talents, and abilities?
- What would you change about yourself if you could?
- Does it bother you a great deal if you think someone doesn't like you?
- Is it difficult for you to say no when you want to say no?
- How do you feel about your educational accomplishments?
- Do you ever feel inadequate with certain people? Who?
- How easily can you express your opinion when it differs from that of others?
- Do you make friends easily?
- Generally, do you feel liked by your peers and coworkers?
- How do you feel about your occupation?
- Do you feel appreciated by your employer?

ASSESSMENT INTERVIEW

Role Relationships

Family Relationships

- Tell me about your family.
- What is home like?
- Who are you closest to in the family?
- Who are you most distant from in the family?
- What are your relationships like with your other relatives?
- What are your responsibilities in the family?
- How well do you feel you accomplish what is expected of you?
- What about your role or responsibilities would you like changed?
- Do you see yourself as frequently getting the short end of things and coming out second best?
- Are you proud of your family members?
- Do you feel your family members are proud of you?
- Tell me how you spend your time each day.

Work Roles and Social Roles

- Do you like your work?
- How do you get along at work?
- What about your work would you like to change if you could?
- How do you spend your free time?
- Are you involved in any community groups?
- Are you most comfortable alone, with one other person, or in a group?
- Who is most important to you?
- Whom do you seek out for help?

producing events simultaneously. Illness and hospitalization can compound the effects. Common stressors that influence a client's self-concept and self-esteem are shown in the first box on page 811. Additional information about stress and coping can be found in Chapter 32.

When stressors are identified, the nurse needs to determine how the client perceives the stressor. A positive, growth-oriented perception of stressful events reinforces self-worth; a negative, hopeless, defeatist perception leads to decreased self-esteem. The nurse also should identify the client's coping style and determine whether or not this style is effective by asking the client such questions as the following:

STRESSORS AFFECTING SELF-CONCEPT AND SELF-ESTEEM

Body-Image Stressors

- Loss of body parts (eg, amputation, mastectomy, hysterectomy)
- Loss of body functions (eg, from heart disease, renal disease, spinal cord injury, cerebrovascular accident, neuromuscular disease, arthritis, declining mental or sensory abilities)
- Disfigurement (eg, through pregnancy, severe burns, facial blemishes, colostomy, ileostomy, tracheostomy, laryngectomy)

Role Stressors

- Loss of parent, spouse, child, or close friend
- Change or loss of job
- Retirement
- Divorce or separation
- Illness
- Hospitalization
- Ambiguous role expectations
- Conflicting role expectations
- Inability to meet role expectations

Identity Stressors

- Change in physical appearance
- Declining physical, mental, or sensory abilities
- Inability to achieve goals
- Relationship concerns
- Sexuality concerns
- Unrealistic ideal self
- Membership in a minority group

- When you have a problem or face a stressful situation, how do you usually deal with it?
- Do these methods work?

BEHAVIORS SUGGESTING LOW SELF-ESTEEM

Some of the verbal and nonverbal behaviors that can indicate altered self-concept or low self-esteem were discussed earlier in this section. Other behaviors associated with low self-esteem are listed in the box at the right.

BEHAVIORS ASSOCIATED WITH LOW SELF-ESTEEM

The client

- Avoids eye contact.
- Stoops in posture and moves slowly.
- Is poorly groomed and has an unkempt appearance.
- Is hesitant or halting in speech.
- Is overly critical of self (eg, "I'm no good," "I'm ugly," or "People don't like me").
- May be overly critical of others.
- Is unable to accept positive remarks about self.
- Encourages reprimands from others, to punish self.
- Apologizes frequently.
- Verbalizes feelings of hopelessness, helplessness, and powerlessness, such as "I really don't care what happens," "I'll do whatever anyone wants," "Whatever is destined will happen."
- Verbalizes feelings of worthlessness, such as "Nobody cares about me," "I'm just a burden to everyone," "I'm not worth all that trouble."
- Withdraws from or changes social involvements or relationships.
- Fails to complete or follow through with activities.
- Avoids initiating conversation or interaction with others.
- Exhibits self-destructive behavior, such as excessive use of alcohol, drugs.
- Has negative feelings about own body, for example, avoids looking at or touching body part, or hides body part; emphasizes previous appearance or function; talks excessively about loss or change.
- Is indecisive (eg, "I can't make up my mind what to do," "I don't understand what's happening").
- Cannot solve problems effectively and does not ask for help.
- Displays overdependence, for example, asks for assistance unnecessarily, seeks attention by speaking loudly, asks irrelevant questions, seeks approval and praise.
- Displays lack of energy (eg, "I feel tired all the time").
- Verbalizes inability to cope.
- Expresses or manifests anxiety, fear, anger.
- Does not meet role expectations.

People with low self-esteem generally exhibit illogical and **distorted thinking.** Some cognitive therapists (Ellis & Harper 1975, p. 100; Beck 1979, p. 54) assert that illogical and distorted thinking causes or perpetuates low self-esteem. Common types of irrational, illogical, or muddled thinking include the following (Crouch & Straub, 1983, p. 72):

- **Catastrophizing,** the tendency to think the worst. For example, the persons says, "If something bad can happen it will," or, "Things are bad now, but they will get worse."
- **Minimizing** and **maximizing,** the tendency to minimize the positive, to overlook partial successes, to magnify the significance or meaning of the negative, and to emphasize mistakes.
- **Black-and-white thinking,** the tendency to attribute things to one of two extremes. Things are either perfect or no good. Activities must be performed without mistake or the performance is a failure.
- **Overgeneralization,** the tendency to believe that something that applied in one situation or that happened once will apply in all situations.
- **Self-reference,** the tendency to believe that what others are thinking, saying, or doing relates to self. The person believes that others are highly concerned with that person's thoughts and actions and are particularly aware of the person's shortcomings and mistakes.
- **Filtering,** the tendency to support beliefs or conclusions by selectively pulling certain details out of context and neglecting other facts. Usually, it is the negative details that are selected while positive facts are neglected.

Table 31–2 Clinical Application: Assessment Data Clusters and Related Nursing Diagnoses: Self-Concept and Role Problems

Data Cluster	Nursing Diagnosis
Frank Sawyers had a permanent colostomy 7 days ago for cancer of the sigmoid colon. When the nurse was changing the colostomy appliance, Frank said, "My wife will be repulsed by this." He avoided looking at the stoma and put his arm over his eyes.	**Body image disturbance** related to disfigurement
Sofie Ferraro, a 73-year-old with right-sided (dominant) hemiplegia, says, "Although the Rehabilitation Center taught me so much about how to manage in my home, my poor husband has to do a lot to help me with cooking meals and cleaning the house."	**Altered role performance** related to change in physical capacity
George Kawazi, a first-year college student, is studying liberal arts and the sciences. George states that even though he attends all his classes and studies every day and on weekends, his grades do not please his father, who expects straight A's. "I've always had trouble measuring up to Father's expectations. He never thought I was as good as my older brother."	**Chronic low self-esteem** related to unrealistic parental expectations

DIAGNOSING

The nursing diagnoses identified by NANDA (1992) relating specifically to self-concept include the following:

- **Body image disturbance**
- **Altered role performance**
- **Self-esteem disturbance**

These diagnoses, with definitions, contributing factors, and defining characteristics, are shown in the box on page 813. Clinical applications of these diagnoses are shown in Table 31–2.

Additional nursing diagnoses that may apply to clients with problems of self-concept include the following:

- **Personal identity disturbance**
- **Anxiety** related to changed physical appearance (eg, amputation, mastectomy)
- **Impaired adjustment** to changed physical functioning or appearance
- **Ineffective individual coping** with role change related to death of spouse
- **Anticipatory grieving** or **dysfunctional grieving** related to change in physical appearance
- **Hopelessness**
- **Powerlessness**
- **Parental role conflict**
- **Rape-trauma syndrome**
- **Sleep pattern disturbance**
- **Social isolation**
- **Spiritual distress**
- **Altered thought processes**

Some of these nursing diagnoses are discussed in other chapters of this book.

NURSING DIAGNOSES

CLIENTS WITH SELF-CONCEPT ALTERATIONS

NURSING DIAGNOSIS: Body image disturbance: The state in which one experiences or is at risk of experiencing a disruption in the perceptions, beliefs, and knowledge possessed about one's own body structure, function, appearance, and limits

Defining Characteristics

- Negative verbal or behavioral response to actual or perceived change in body structure and/or function
- Inability to look at or touch altered body site
- Avoidance or refusal of social contact
- Verbalization of feelings of helplessness, hopelessness, powerlessness
- Lack of self-care
- Depersonalization or excessive personalization of altered body part

Related Factors

- Obvious changes in body structure or functioning related to disease, surgery, accident or treatment; deviations from norms of appearance as defined by society or culture; negative perceptions of self; societal prejudices regarding handicapping conditions; transitional life stages (eg, adolescence, menopause, aging); eating disorders; pain.

NURSING DIAGNOSIS: Altered role performance: A state in which one experiences a change, conflict, or denial of role responsibilities or inability to perform role responsibilities

Defining Characteristics

- Inability or refusal to perform new or usual roles
- Lack of knowledge about or difficulty in learning about role
- Different perception of role
- Inadequate problem-solving skills
- Confusion or frustration about role performance
- Changes in usual patterns of responsibility
- Change in physical ability to perform role

Related Factors

- Situational or maturational crises; physical or mental illness; substance abuse; decline in physical strength or ability; lack of adequate role model; inadequate resources or social supports; cultural transition.

NURSING DIAGNOSIS: Self-esteem disturbance: A state in which one experiences a disruption in self-perception or the unrealistic self-evaluation or feelings about self or one's capabilities

Defining Characteristics

- Self-deprecating verbalizations
- Expressions of shame or guilt
- Rejection of positive feedback and/or exaggeration of negative feedback
- Social withdrawal
- Verbalizations of or behaviors indicating lack of self-confidence
- Avoidance of new situations
- Inability to perform self-care

Related Factors

- Physical illness; changes in physical appearance or functioning; maturational or situational crises; loss of control; psychiatric illness; substance abuse; cognitive or perceptual problems; inadequate coping or problem-solving skills; isolation from one's cultural or spiritual group; spiritual crisis.

Sources: LJ Carpenito, *Nursing Diagnosis: Application to Clinical Practice*, 4th ed. (Philadelphia: Lippincott, 1992); M Gordon, *Manual of Nursing Diagnosis 1993–1994* (St Louis: Mosby, 1993), and GK McFarland and EA McFarlane, *Nursing Diagnosis and Intervention: Planning for Patient Care*, 2d ed. (St Louis: Mosby, 1993).

PLANNING

The nurse develops plans in collaboration with the client and significant support persons when possible, according to the client's state of health, level of anxiety, support resource, coping mechanisms, and sociocultural and religious affiliation. The nurse who has little experience in intervening with clients with altered self-concept may wish to consult with a clinical specialist or a more experienced nurse to develop effective plans. The nurse and client set goals to enhance the client's self-concept.

The overall client goal for clients with disturbances in self-concept is to restore or improve self-concept. Goals should emphasize strengths rather than weaknesses or impairments. See the Care Planning Guide below for clients experiencing self-concept alterations. The following are some suggested outcome criteria.

The client

- Verbalizes concerns about altered self-concept regarding
  a. Body image
  b. Personal identity

CARE PLANNING GUIDE

CLIENTS WITH SELF-CONCEPT ALTERATIONS

NURSING DIAGNOSIS: Body image disturbance

Outcome Criteria	Nursing Interventions	Rationale
The client		
▪ Expresses feelings about body image.	Provide privacy and assist the client to express feelings. Support the client in expressing feelings of grief or anger related to changed body image. Spend time with the client.	Clients will feel more free to express feelings in a supportive environment. Expressing feelings enables the client to deal with feelings and resolve problems. Spending time with the client and allowing the client to express feelings show support and acceptance.
▪ Verbalizes realistic understanding of body image and/or functioning.	Provide reliable information about altered appearance and its effect on physical functioning. Provide information about appropriate supportive devices or prostheses. Clarify any misunderstandings the client may have regarding appearance.	Providing accurate information reduces misconceptions, minimizes the client's fears, and helps client adapt to changes in appearance or functioning.
▪ Acknowledges changes in physical appearance and/or functioning.	Support the client in efforts to view and touch changes in body appearance. Support the client in efforts to adapt to changes in physical functioning.	Supporting the client in acknowledging changes in appearance and/or function conveys acceptance and provides a foundation on which to develop skills for adjusting to changes.
	Teach significant others necessary skills for assisting the client.	Significant others must accept changes in the client's appearance and/or functioning. Involving significant others in care shows acceptance of the client.
	Offer praise and encouragement to the client and significant others.	Praise and encouragement promote learning and acceptance of changes.
▪ Integrates changes in physical appearance and/or functioning into adapted life-style.	Teach client new self-care necessary for adaptation. Reinforce instruction in occupational and vocational skills necessary for adaptation.	Teaching new self-care skills and reinforcing the instruction of other health professionals promote the client's independence and encourages a positive perception of the client's body image.

NURSING DIAGNOSIS: Body image disturbance *continued*

Outcome Criteria	Nursing Interventions	Rationale
	Provide information on resources available for assistance. Encourage the client to participate in social activities. Praise and encourage the client and significant others.	In this way, the nurse provides support for the client in resolving needs; decreases feelings of social isolation and increases independence; and helps the client accept changes and view self more positively.

NURSING DIAGNOSIS: Altered role performance

Outcome Criteria	Nursing Interventions	Rationale
The client		
▪ Verbalizes feelings about role changes.	Assist the client to express feelings about role changes. Support the client in grieving over role loss.	In this way the nurse provides an outlet for the expression of anger, anxiety, grief or other feelings so that the client can move on to more constructive adaptation to role changes.
▪ Verbalizes accurate knowledge of role expectations and requirements.	Help the client accurately assess role loss or change. Help the client differentiate perceived from actual role requirements. Provide resources for role modeling or instruction regarding role change. Demonstrate role behaviors that the client needs to learn.	These actions promote accurate understanding of role expectations and requirements on which to develop more realistic goals for role achievement.
▪ Demonstrates role competence.	Provide opportunities for practicing new role behaviors. Praise and encourage the client when success in new role performance is demonstrated.	Practice increases the client's confidence in ability to perform new roles.
▪ Verbalizes satisfaction with role performance.	Provide opportunities for discussing new role.	Discussion increases client's confidence in ability to perform new roles.

NURSING DIAGNOSIS: Self-esteem disturbance

Outcome Criteria	Nursing Interventions	Rationale
The client		
▪ Verbalizes realistic perceptions of self.	Encourage client to identify personal strengths. Recognize client's past accomplishments and knowledge. Discourage client from focusing on past weaknesses and/or failures.	In this way, the nurse enables the client to maximize personal strengths.
	Maintain a caring and nonjudgmental attitude.	In conveying such an attitude, the nurse provides support for the client's self-reflection.

➤

SELF-CONCEPT ALTERATIONS CONTINUED

NURSING DIAGNOSIS: Self-esteem disturbance *continued*

Outcome Criteria	Nursing Interventions	Rationale
▪ Participates in activities to improve self-esteem.	Provide information about activities and support groups that promote self-esteem. Assist the client to choose satisfying and rewarding activities. Encourage participation in activities to promote self-esteem (eg, exercise; support groups; social, creative, and recreational, activities; self-help; community service; and self-care activities).	These actions provide positive reinforcement of the client's worth.
	When prescribed, encourage client's participation in individual or group psychotherapy.	Therapy enables the client to explore self-perceptions, beliefs, values, and relationship to others in a supportive environment.
▪ Describes positive relationships with significant others.	Help the client determine factors that interfere with positive interpersonal relationships.	Recognizing negative behaviors enables the client to correct those that interfere with interpersonal relationships.
	Teach the client appropriate interaction techniques. Teach significant others appropriate interaction techniques.	Knowledge of appropriate interaction techniques helps the client maintain positive self-esteem and promotes positive interaction between the client and significant others.
▪ Verbalizes improved self-esteem.	Listen attentively. Provide a supportive environment. Acknowledge the client's growth and accomplishments.	These actions reinforce the client's self-esteem.

Sources: LJ Carpenito, *Nursing Diagnosis: Application to Clinical Practice*, 4th ed. (Philadelphia: Lippincott, 1992); GK McFarland and EA McFarlane, *Nursing Diagnosis and Intervention: Planning for Patient Care*, 2d ed. (St Louis: Mosby, 1993).

   c. Role performance
   d. Self-esteem
- Verbalizes understanding of
   a. Factors related to altered self-concept
   b. Effect of changes in body image on function
   c. Maturational changes in body image and functioning
   d. Self as separate from but related to others
   e. Role expectations and obligations
   f. Personal strengths and weaknesses
   g. Effective personal coping strategies
- Expresses satisfaction with
   a. Appearance and functioning
   b. Interpersonal relationships
   c. Role performance
   d. Self-worth
- Expresses realistic perceptions of
   a. Body image
   b. Physical functioning

A critical pathway (p. 823) may also be used to individualize client care.

IMPLEMENTING

Assisting people with self-concept disturbances requires skills in communicating and in developing helping relationships (see Chapter 18). Helping clients with self-concept disturbances is akin to promoting health, as discussed in Chapter 13. Because stressful situations can result in situational self-concept disturbances, the nurse should know stress management techniques (see Chapter 32).

The client assumes responsibility for implementing the plans. The nurse provides information, education, and ongoing support; suggests strategies to encourage behavioral change; and implements techniques that help the client gain a realistic and acceptable view of self. Selected interventions to help clients with self-concept disturbances follow. Numerous community self-improvement programs are also available, many of which emphasize the need for individuals to take charge of their lives, to take responsibility for their actions, to think positively rather than negatively, and to become more assertive.

It is important for both the nurse and the client to realize that changes in self-concept require an extended period of time. Although varying from person to person, this may take several months or years. It is essential for the client to learn that self-concept or self-image is not fixed; it can change and improve in progressive small steps, particularly if the client desires such change.

IDENTIFYING AREAS OF STRENGTH

Healthy people often perceive their problems and weaknesses more clearly than their assets and strengths. Average well-functioning persons with some college education, when asked to write down their strengths, are able to list only five or six; however, the same persons can list three to four times as many problems or areas of weakness (Otto 1965, p. 34).

Because people with low self-esteem tend to focus on their limitations, they may list even fewer strengths and many more problems. When a client has difficulty identifying personality strengths and assets, the nurse must provide the client with a framework to follow. Interests, abilities, and past accomplishments and experiences need to be included. An abbreviated framework for identifying personality strengths has been developed at the University of Utah. See the box on page 818. Such an inventory has the following advantages:

- It can result in a more well-rounded self-concept and more positive self-esteem.
- It can help mobilize health and regenerative processes.
- It can help the person to become more aware of the strengths of others and thus facilitate relationships. The person begins to see others' previously unrecognized strengths or "good side."

DEVELOPING BEHAVIOR SPECIFICITY

Many people overgeneralize and think in unspecific ways. The nurse can assist clients to think more clearly and to become more behavior specific in language and thought. Crouch and Straub (1983, p. 71) offer the following strategies for developing behavior specificity.

1. *Define goals clearly.* For example, in response to the question "In what ways would you like to feel differently about yourself?" the client may give an unspecific, subjective, and unmeasurable answer such as "better," "happier," or "not so uptight." To help the client, the nurse needs to bring unspecific answers into focus. This can be done by inquiring, for example, "How will you know you are better?" or "What do you mean by 'uptight'?" or "If I were to observe you now in your usual activities and then after you had made these changes, how could I tell you had achieved them?" Open-ended questions that probe into the who, what, how much, when, where, and how of thought and behavior help the client and the nurse develop a clearer understanding of the individual, the problem, and the goals.

   When formulating goals and strategies for achieving them, the nurse needs to assess the client's ideal self and perceived self, along with the amount of discrepancy between them. Teaching clients about perceived self and ideal self can assist them in exploring areas in which they may be unduly biased. It is also of value for subsequent exploration and assessment. For example, if a client expresses discouragement about the client's behavior in a situation, the nurse could say, "Ideally, how do you think you should have acted or reacted?" and then "How do you perceive you actually acted?" Some situations involve complications that are beyond the person's control; such questioning will help clarify that for the client.

2. *Help the client think clearly.* Clients with low self-esteem tend to think negatively and irrationally. For example, a client with low self-esteem who has followed through on homework for 3 out of 7 days might say, "There was no excuse; I failed," or "I didn't follow through; I can't do anything right." When responding, the nurse should avoid contradicting the client but need not accept the client's evaluation as accurate. The nurse might ask, "What exactly did you not follow through with?" or "How does not doing the homework perfectly mean you can't do anything right?"

CHANGING LANGUAGE PATTERNS

Helping clients to change language patterns from passive phrases to more active phrases can help them assume greater responsibility for their power. Examples of passive phrases and alternate active phrases follow:

It makes me . . . (passive)
I choose to . . . *or* I do (active)

I have to . . . (passive)
I want to . . . (active)

I can't . . . (passive)
I won't . . . *or* I choose not to . . . (active)

FRAMEWORK FOR IDENTIFYING PERSONALITY STRENGTHS

- *Spectator sports and similar activities.* The rationale here is that the client's current interest or participation in spectator sports, as well as past interests which are recalled with pleasure, constitutes a vital spark, is evidence of a creative engagement with life, and, in most instances, presages a movement in the direction of health.
- *Sports and activities.* Taking part in a program of bodybuilding, conditioning, or rehabilitative exercises or similar physical regimens, including an interest (and anticipated future participation) in sports and outdoor activities.
- *Hobbies and crafts.* Participating, or having participated in, some hobby or craft activity, and having the desire to start or resume a hobby, craft, or similar pursuit.
- *Expressive arts.* Past or current interest in writing, painting, sketching, or music appreciation with a desire to participate in one of the expressive arts.
- *Health status.* Desire to maintain or regain health, as well as having an interest or ability to carry through with regimens and treatments designed to foster and facilitate health.
- *Education, training, and related areas.* Any education is seen as a personality asset—vocational trade or technical training, scholastic honors, self-education or a desire to obtain further education or training.
- *Work, vocation, job, or position.* Successful on-the-job performance or enjoyment in work, a sense of pride in work or duties, earned seniority or recognition for work performed.
- *Special aptitudes or resources.* Included are such diverse factors as sales ability, aptitude for mathematics or some other subject, ability to fix mechanical things, a "green thumb," ability to construct or teach, knowing how to make a good impression on people.
- *Strengths through family and others.* Such sources of strengths as a spouse or children, relationships with parents, in-laws, or relatives who give love and understanding.
- *Intellectual strengths.* Ability to apply reason to problem solving, do original, creative, and critical thinking, accept new ideas, work on broadening one's mind through reading, conversation, and sharing ideas; the capacity to learn and enjoy learning.
- *Aesthetic strengths.* Recognizing and enjoying beauty, and being able to use the sense of beauty to enhance the physical environment.
- *Organizational strengths.* Capacity for systematic planning, developing sound short- and long-range goals, and organizing resources, energy, and time to achieve such goals; the ability to assign and carry out priorities and to coordinate or lead the efforts and labor of others in relation to specific tasks.
- *Imaginative and creative strengths.* Such characteristics as creativity, imagination, and inventiveness for the development of new and different ideas regarding home, family, work, or social relationships.
- *Relationship strengths.* Ability to make people feel comfortable and the capacity to enjoy being with people, being aware of people's needs and feelings, being able to listen, and being patient with children as well as with adults.
- *Spiritual strengths.* Religious faith or love of God, membership and participation in church and related activities, and the capacity to express moral and religious values in living, that is, "living what one believes."
- *Emotional strengths.* Capacity to give and receive warmth, affection, and love; ability to "take" anger and to feel and express a wide range of emotions; capacity for empathy.
- *Other strengths.* Included here are the ability to use humor, to "laugh" at oneself and take "kidding"; having a liking for adventure or pioneering; having stick-to-itiveness, perseverance, and the drive or will needed to get things done.

Source: HA Otto, The human potentialities of nurses and patients, *Nursing Outlook*, August 1965, 13:32–35. Reprinted with permission.

Changing language patterns does not alter a person's beliefs, but the process of recognizing and modifying language helps the person consider habitual as well as alternative ways of thinking and believing. To encourage the use of more active language, the nurse may have the client initially listen for passive language without modifying it and then deliberately notice passive language and modify it. It is also important for clients to gain awareness of their overall feeling states when using passive or active language.

ENCOURAGING POSITIVE SELF-EVALUATION

Persons with high self-esteem express positive self-evaluation more frequently than negative self-evaluation. Persons with low self-esteem, by contrast, frequently make negative self-evaluations and rarely give themselves positive feedback. Therefore, clients with low self-esteem need help in developing more positive thoughts and images about themselves. Strategies include modeling, praise or recognition, positive self-feedback, and visualization.

Modeling The nurse can model positive self-statements for the client by saying such things as "I did a good job painting my recreation room last weekend," or "I am improving my cooking," or "I am proud of the produce I'm getting from my vegetable garden."

Praise To help the client make the transition to self-recognition, the nurse provides honest, positive feedback. For example, the nurse might say, "I think you did a really fine job," or "It sounds like you worked very hard and have done well."

Positive Self-Feedback To help clients begin making positive self-statements, the nurse may implement some of the following strategies.

1. Ask the client: "Tell me some things you have done recently that you feel good about," or "Tell me some things you like about yourself."
2. Ask clients to develop a list of accomplishments they feel good about and a list of characteristics they like about themselves. Accomplishments, behaviors, and characteristics that hold high significance for the person are preferred, since they incorporate a sense of competence, virtue, and power. Frequent reference to this list or to one attribute on the list is encouraged.
3. Reduce negative self-feedback through thought-stopping techniques. For example, every time the client begins to think negatively about self, ask the client to say mentally, "Stop," or "No," or "Think about now," and then attend to the details of the present experience.

Visualization Because strong positive images or expectations often become self-fulfilling, visualization, or imagery procedures, can be used to enhance self-esteem. Positive images of desired changes are consciously imagined. This can be a powerful tool for achieving goals and gaining a positive self-concept. To strengthen goals with visualization, the client:

1. Sets a positive goal or image, such as "I am talking with someone at a party" or "I am saying to my family that I need some help from them to be able to manage work and home responsibilities."
2. Relaxes and slowly repeats the goal-phrase several times.
3. Closes the eyes and visualizes the goal-phrase on a written page.
4. Envisions self as having accomplished the goal.

Because a person's receptivity to positive suggestions is greater when that person is deeply relaxed, deep-breathing exercises, progressive relaxation techniques, meditation, and self-hypnosis are often introduced before imagery techniques are used in self-involvement programs. Some of these techniques are discussed in Chapter 32. The nurse may refer clients to specific community programs.

ENHANCING SELF-ESTEEM IN CHILDREN AND ADOLESCENTS

Hamachek (1987, p. 248) describes the key ingredients for helping children develop high self-esteem: love, acceptance, firmness, consistency, and the establishment of expectations. Love and acceptance indicate to the child that parents, teachers, and caregivers care and want the best for the child. Firmness and consistency provide the rules and the consequences for breaking them. Such limits provide a safe and predictable world in which to live. Establishing high but reasonable expectations for the child indicates confidence in the child's abilities. As the child succeeds in meeting those expectations, self-confidence increases.

The roles of parents and teachers are of great significance in determining children's self-concept. Children are able to grow in self-confidence, personal competence, and independence if they can develop five basic attitudes, involving (a) security and trust, (b) identity, (c) belonging, (d) purpose, and (e) personal competence (Reasoner 1983, p. 55). Parents and teachers have specific roles and responsibilities in helping children develop these five basic attitudes. The nurse can be instrumental in helping parents learn their supportive role.

Security and Trust This first step in helping the child develop self-esteem is to set well-defined limits, that is, what is expected in terms of behavior and what has to be done to get approval. Limits need to be enforced consistently by all involved adults. Inconsistency tends to create anxiety and weakens feelings of security. Rules or standards need to be reasonable and broad enough to serve as general guidelines in new situations, such as in a neighbor's house, a friend's yard, or school classroom. Standards needs to be established for the treatment of others, respect for the property of others, the value of honesty, and routines such as getting ready for school in the morning, doing homework, completing chores, and going to bed at night.

Systems such as checklists, charts, and calendars can serve as reminders of what is expected and also enable children to monitor their own performance. Conforming to expectations builds positive self-esteem. Self-monitoring builds a sense of pride and provides opportunities for positive recognition as opposed to only negative feedback for uncompleted chores.

Preparing the child for what to expect if standards are *not* met is also effective in encouraging desired behavior and discouraging misbehavior. Restricting privileges tends to be more effective than scolding or lecturing and helps children learn the consequences of their behavior.

To feel secure, children also need to believe that the adults responsible for them are dependable and can be counted on. Adults, therefore, must serve as role models for appropriate behavior.

Identity The second step in developing self-esteem is a strong sense of identity. Children need to feel they are unique. A child's identity is strengthened when the child is given positive feedback, recognition of strengths, love and acceptance, and help in assessing strengths and shortcomings.

Children need positive feedback from the people of greatest significance to them: parents, grandparents, older siblings, teachers, and close friends. The kind of feedback given can be more significant than the child's actual level of performance. Positive feedback enhances a child's sense of identity and self-concept. The absence of feedback is likely to make a child hesitant and unsure in new situations. Predominantly negative feedback can give a child a negative self-image.

Adults foster a strong self-concept by recognizing a child's strengths. Parents and teachers who focus on the child's shortcomings and devote extra time to only those areas considered weak contribute to the child's negative feelings. Adults need to point out the child's special talents and qualities, such as an attractive smile, skill at playing games, desire to help others, and a strong sense of right and wrong.

Before they can accept themselves, children need to feel loved and accepted. Adults can demonstrate this by taking time to be with the child, to listen, to read, to play, or to just be there. Physical contact—such as a hand on the shoulder or a hug—usually conveys warmth and caring more effectively than words.

Children need to learn to assess their own level of performance and to build confidence in their own judgment. Even though positive feedback from others is always important, children also need to learn to rely on their own judgment. They can be encouraged to evaluate their performance through test results, grades, or other objective measures.

Belonging Feeling socially accepted is important to children. Just as children need to feel unique, so do they need to feel just like everyone else. They need to dress the same, talk the same, and be in the same club. A sense of belonging can be developed through a family that is united. The family unit enables children to learn how to function as group members, to learn that they cannot always be first or have their way, and to learn that they need to handle their own share of responsibilities. In the family unit and in groups, children learn sensitivity and concern for others. Parents and group leaders can foster this concern by encouraging children to express empathy for others and to find ways to help others. Learning how to be of service to others and how to be a friend builds a sense of belonging and reduces feelings of alienation.

Purpose Children need a sense of purpose to provide direction to their lives and a basis for success, fulfillment, and, therefore, a positive self-concept. Adults can help a child develop a sense of purpose by setting reasonable expectations, by helping the child set realistic goals, by conveying faith and confidence in the child's ability to achieve the goals, and by helping the child expand interests, talents, and abilities.

Children tend to work toward expectations that are set for them by parents or teachers, especially if the goals are within their capabilities and the adults are confident the children can achieve them. If expectations are too high or too low, motivation is reduced. Expectations that are long term and relatively general put less pressure on the child and tend to enhance motivation. For example, expecting a child to improve general math skills is more motivating and less stressful than expecting an A on the next math test. To encourage children to try new challenges and reach new levels of performance, adults can expose children to new experiences. For instance, watching a demonstration on how to cook nutritious and tasty food, observing a highly skilled gymnast's performance, or talking with a firefighter can help children identify their own goals. The more opportunities children have, the more likely they will be motivated to learn and to acquire new skills.

Children need to help to be specific in defining what they want to learn or how to solve a problem. Parents can help by assisting children to identify the sequence of steps needed to achieve a goal or solve a problem. When a child sets a goal, involved adults should convey faith in the child's ability to achieve the goal. Children who sense a parent's or teacher's confidence in them tend to increase their efforts toward, and their chances for, success.

Personal Competence A sense of personal competence grows out of a sequence of successes. This gives the child a feeling of being able to cope with problems or meet goals. Children with a sense of personal competence have a positive approach to solving problems, tend to achieve success, and feel responsible for their own actions. Children who lack a sense of personal competence are overwhelmed by problems and may attribute lack of success to fate or being victimized. Parents can foster a feeling of competence by helping the child achieve the goals. To do this, the parent needs to do the following:

1. Develop a plan of action by having the child list the steps to be taken or review alternatives for achieving the goals. Parents should avoid prescribing what to do. Directing tends to foster dependence rather than independence. The child needs the freedom to make final decisions on how a plan should proceed.
2. Provide encouragement and support while monitoring the child's progress. From time to time, the parent needs to check on the child's progress, helping assess what might still need to be done, fostering consideration of other resources, or—most important—praising the child's efforts and achievement.
3. Provide feedback that will help the child determine whether the goal has been achieved. This should include more sharing of the joy of accomplishment and factual comparative information than judgment or praise, although some children value an extrinsic reward more highly. However, children need to learn to become less dependent on extrinsic or tangible rewards. Excessive praise also can make some children more dependent rather than less dependent (Reasoner 1983, p. 62).

ENHANCING SELF-ESTEEM IN OLDER ADULTS

There is a wide variation in the way older adults perceive themselves; most, however, benefit from having their independence fostered. Low self-esteem is often associated with the dependence that accompanies the declining physical and mental capacities related to aging. The nurse can foster the older adult's independence and a more positive self-concept by doing the following:

1. Encourage clients to participate in planning their care, and involve them in decision making. For example, encourage clients to choose what to wear or what activities to participate in, and consult them about food preferences.
2. Encourage clients to keep photographs and other significant objects around them. These establish one's territory or physical space as one's own and help to maintain memory.
3. Ask permission before moving or putting the client's clothing (eg, dressing gown, nightclothes) or other objects into the client's locker or closet. To do so without permission would limit the client's sense of control over personal space and can be perceived as disrespectful.
4. Listen to what the client is saying. Elderly people need to know their comments are valued.
5. Allow the client sufficient time to complete an interaction or activity. Older adults are often slow to respond. Attempts to hurry their responses can create anxiety and embarrassment and can lower self-esteem.
6. Receive contributions of thanks or appreciation (eg, candy or fruit) graciously and sincerely. Having something to contribute helps older adults maintain or enhance their self-esteem.
7. Permit able elderly clients to perform tasks or participate in planning social or recreational activities. Having something to do or participating in decision making provides a sense of control and increases self-esteem.

EVALUATING

To determine whether client outcomes have been achieved, the nurse uses data collected during interactions with the client and significant others. To elicit such data, the nurse requires communication and interviewing skills, such as listening attentively and asking open-ended questions. Observation skills are also essential for evaluating changes in behavior and appearance. If outcomes are not achieved, the nurse should explore the reasons, considering questions such as the following:

- Have old situations recurred, triggering feelings or behaviors associated with low self-esteem?
- Have new stressful situations occurred with which the client feels unable to cope, resulting in continuing or recurrent low self-esteem?
- Are new or additional roles causing increased stress in adapting?
- Are significant others supporting the client adequately in attempts to improve self-esteem?
- Have physical complications occurred that resulted in delayed or impaired healing of body sites associated with altered body image or functioning?
- Did the client follow through on referrals to appropriate support agencies? Did the agencies provide the expected services?
- Did the client maintain intervention strategies to promote self-esteem when not directly supervised by health professionals?
- Were the client's expectations too high in relation to the time needed for successful resolution of self-esteem problems?
- Should the nursing diagnosis be reevaluated?
- Should the selected intervention strategies be reevaluated?

Nurse, client, and significant others need to understand that to change beliefs, feelings, and behaviors affecting self-esteem requires time and ongoing effort. Unlike physical problems (eg, wounds), where healing can be quickly observed, improving one's self-concept can be a continuing concern and is not so easily evaluated. New crises can cause the client to doubt self and revert to former feelings of inadequacy. People can learn from each new situation and gain new strategies for feeling satisfied with self.

PROFESSIONAL SELF-CONCEPT

Strasen (1992, p. 2) defines **professional self-concept** as the set of beliefs and images held to be true as a result of specific professional socialization. The development of professional self-concept is based on one's personal self-concept. An individual's personal self-concept and professional self-concept affect one another. As nurses develop a sense of commitment to nursing, their many life roles overlap. For example, for nurses who are parents, it is impossible not to view their sick child from their role as nurse. The nurse's life roles as individual, as spouse, as child, and as professional often become inseparable.

Leddy and Pepper (1993, pp. 66–67) state that "the kind of professional a person becomes depends on the person's self-system." How one thinks and what one believes affect one's self-concept. Understanding self and working to view self positively leads to more professional success and productivity (Jenny 1990). During socialization to the profession, exposure to traditional views of nurses as subservient to the physician and hospital administration may contribute to a low professional self-concept. As nurses become more autonomous and come to view the profession more positively, however, recognition for professional accomplishments can help enhance not only the self-esteem of the individual nurse, but also the image of the nursing profession.

Strasen (1992) states that nursing students can develop a professional self-image by

- Assuming responsibility for and accepting accountability for personal and professional beliefs and actions.
- Identifying personal and professional life goals.
- Refusing to blame other individuals or events for what has happened in the past or present or what will happen in the future.
- Developing a professional appearance through proper grooming, nutrition, and exercise.
- Acknowledging personal and professional accomplishments.
- Seeking out a role model or mentor who is positive, experienced, and competent and who will provide constructive feedback as the nurse grows and develops professionally. The characteristics of experienced professional nurses are identified in the box at the top of this page.

Nurses who seek to maintain or improve both their personal and professional selves are more effective in caring for their clients. They are also more effective in communicating with other health professionals and in promoting a positive image of nursing in the community.

CHARACTERISTICS OF EXPERIENCED PROFESSIONAL NURSES

Experienced professional nurses

- Are confident, self-controlled role models.
- Make independent decisions on behalf of their clients, department, and organization in new or difficult situations.
- Take full responsibility and accountability for the outcomes of their nursing practice and never blame, rationalize, or justify.
- Are internally driven and require little direction and supervision.
- Take responsibility for their ongoing, lifelong learning.
- Look for opportunities to make a contribution to the profession, their departments, and their organizations.
- Function as mentors for inexperienced nurses.

Source: LL Strasen, *The Image of Professional Nursing: Strategies for Action* (Philadelphia: Lippincott, 1992), pp. 86–87.

CRITICAL PATHWAY FOR HELEN MORTON

ASSESSMENT DATA

Nursing Assessment

Mrs Helen Morton, 36 years old, was admitted for a right radical mastectomy. She had a positive biopsy for breast cancer two weeks prior to admission. On admission to the surgical unit, Mrs Morton asked the nurse, "Will I ever look normal again?" She also told the nurse, "I don't want any visitors after surgery, I don't want anyone to see how I look." The day following surgery, Mrs Morton states, "I don't want to look at it," when the physician starts the dressing change.

Physical Examination

Height: 167.6 cm (5′6″)
Weight: 65 kg (143 lb)
Temperature: 37 C (98.6 F)
Pulse rate: 76 bpm
Respirations: 20 per minute
Blood pressure: 120/80 mm Hg
Skin warm, dry, pink, and pale
Mastectomy incision clean, dry, and well-approximated

Diagnostic Data

RBC: 4.2 million/μL
Hgb: 12.2 g/dL
Hct: 39%
Urine: negative

CRITICAL PATHWAY FOR CLIENT FOLLOWING RADICAL MASTECTOMY

Expected length of stay 3 to 4 days

	Date ________ First 24 hours postoperative	Date ________ 48 hours postoperative	Date ________ 3–4 days postoperative
Daily outcomes	Client will ▪ be afebrile. ▪ have clean, dry dressing. ▪ recover from anesthesia as evidenced by: VS return to baseline, awake, alert, and oriented. ▪ verbalize understanding and demonstrate cooperation with turning, coughing, deep breathing, and splinting. ▪ tolerate ordered diet without nausea and vomiting. ▪ verbalize control of incisional pain. ▪ verbalize ability to cope.	Client will ▪ be afebrile. ▪ have clean, dry wound with edges well-approximated, healing by first intention. ▪ demonstrate cooperation with turning, coughing, deep breathing, and splinting. ▪ tolerate ordered diet without nausea and vomiting. ▪ ambulate 4 times per day in hallway. ▪ verbalize control of incisional pain. ▪ verbalize beginning ability to cope with changes in body image. ▪ verbalize ability to cope. ▪ verbalize beginning understanding of home care instructions.	Client ▪ is afebrile. ▪ has clean, dry wound with edges well-approximated, healing by first intention. ▪ manages pain with oral medications and/or nonpharmacologic measures. ▪ is independent in self-care. ▪ is fully ambulatory. ▪ has resumed preadmission urine and bowel elimination pattern. ▪ verbalizes home care instructions. ▪ tolerates usual diet. ▪ verbalizes ability to cope with changes in body image and ongoing stressors. ▪ demonstrates progressive upper extremity exercises that include external rotation and abduction of the affected shoulder when the stitches are removed 7 to 10 days after surgery.

	First 24 hours postoperative *continued*	48 hours postoperative *continued*	3–4 days postoperative *continued*
Tests and treatments	Vital signs and O_2 saturation, neurovascular assessment, dressing and wound drainage assessment q15min × 4; q30min × 4; q1h × 4 and then q4h if stable. NO BLOOD PRESSURES OR VENIPUNCTURE ON AFFECTED ARM. Assess respiratory status q4h and prn. Incentive spirometer q2h. Intake and output q shift. Assess voiding—if unable to void, try suggestive voiding techniques or catheterize q8h or prn.	Vital signs and dressing and would drainage assessment q4h. NO BLOOD PRESSURES OR VENIPUNCTURE ON AFFECTED ARM. Assess respiratory status q4h. Incentive spirometer q2h until fully ambulatory. Intake and output q shift. Assess voiding pattern q shift. Dressing change by surgeon.	Vital signs and dressing and wound drainage assessment q4–8h. NO BLOOD PRESSURES OR VENIPUNCTURE ON AFFECTED ARM. Assess respiratory status q4–8h. Assess wound and apply dry sterile dressing q day and prn.
Knowledge deficit	Orient to room and surroundings. Provide simple, brief instructions. Review preoperative preparation including hospital and specific postoperative care: turning, coughing, deep breathing, incentive spirometer, mobilization, intravenous, pain management (PCA or prn medications).	Review plan of care and importance of early mobilization. Begin discharge teaching regarding wound care/dressing change, diet, and activity. Review written discharge instructions with client and significant other.	Complete discharge teaching to include wound care, diet, follow-up care, signs and symptoms to report, activity, and medication: frequency, dose, route, and side effects. Provide client with written discharge instructions including upper arm and shoulder exercises for affected arm.
Diet	Clear to full liquids as tolerated.	Full liquids to usual diet to tolerance.	Usual diet to tolerance.
Activity	Provide safety precautions. Ambulate 4 times in room. Encourage finger, wrist, and elbow movement and use of affected arm for ADLs and personal hygiene.	Fully ambulatory in room. Walk in hall 4 to 6 times per day. Encourage finger, wrist, and elbow movement and use of affected arm for ADLs and personal hygiene. Instruct client in progressive upper arm exercises.	Fully ambulatory. Encourage finger, wrist, and elbow movement and use of affected arm for ADLs and personal hygiene. Reinforce instructions regarding progressive exercises.
Medications	IM or IV/PCA analgesics IV antibiotics IV fluids	PO, IM or IV/PCA analgesics IV antibiotics Intermittent IV device	PO analgesics D/C IV device
Body image	Establish a trusting relationship with client. Encourage client and significant others to verbalize their feelings about the mastectomy.	Maintain trusting relationship with client. Encourage client and significant others to verbalize their feelings about the mastectomy.	Provide opportunities to verbalize ongoing concerns regarding changes in body image and self-concept.

	First 24 hours postoperative *continued*	**48 hours postoperative** *continued*	**3–4 days postoperative** *continued*
Body image *continued*	Listen to client and significant others and show interest and concern rather than giving advice. Allow the client to respond to loss of body part and changed body image with denial, shock, anger, depression, and other grieving behaviors. Support the client's strengths and assist her to look at herself in totality.	Listen to client and significant others and show interest and concern rather than giving advice. Allow the client to respond to loss of body part and changed body image with denial, shock, anger, depression, and other grieving behaviors. Support the client's strengths and assist her to look at herself in totality.	Encourage and provide opportunities for self-care of wound and dressing. Provide opportunity for client to meet with volunteer from Reach to Recovery. Assist client to obtain temporary breast prosthesis. Answer questions and provide information re: breast reconstruction.
Psycho-social	Assess coping status. Use active listening. Provide a nonthreatening environment. Determine support persons and resources available to the client. Assess responses of support persons. Allow for client's input regarding sequence of care. Be supportive of client's effective coping behaviors.	Assess coping status. Use active listening. Provide a nonthreatening environment. Assist client to identify and develop support system and resources. Assess responses of support persons. Allow for client's input regarding sequence of care. Be supportive of client's effective coping behaviors.	Assess coping status. Use active listening. Provide a nonthreatening environment. Determine support persons and resources available to the client. Assess responses of support persons. Allow for client's input regarding sequence of care. Be supportive of client's effective coping behaviors.
Transfer/ discharge plans	Determine discharge needs with client and significant others. Begin home care instructions.	Review progress toward discharge goals. Finalize discharge plans. Refer to Reach to Recovery.	Complete discharge instructions.

CHAPTER HIGHLIGHTS

- A healthy self-concept, or positive self-esteem, is essential to a person's physical and psychologic well-being.
- Self-concept is sometimes referred to as the cognitive component of the self system, and self-esteem as the affective component.
- Components of self-concept include body image, role performance, personal identity, and self-esteem.
- A person's self-perception can differ from the person's perception of how others see the person and from how the person would like to be.
- From the hour of birth, interactions with significant others create the conditions that influence self-esteem throughout life.
- When individuals are able to conceptualize the self, they begin a lifelong process of deciding whether and to what extent they are valuable and worthy.
- Individuals who grow up in families whose members value each other are likely to feel good about themselves.
- Most individuals feel good about themselves in some ways and bad in other ways.

- The development of self-esteem can be seen as a process of establishing a sense of security, a sense of identity, and a sense of belonging.
- When children feel secure and accepted, they can be encouraged to set goals for themselves.
- If adults help children to accomplish goals that are important to them, children are more likely to develop a sense of personal competence and independence.
- Four elements of experience that affect the development of self-esteem are significant others, social role expectations, psychosocial development crises, and communications/coping styles.
- Adults base their self-concept on how they perceive and evaluate their performance in the areas of work, intellect, appearance, sexual attractiveness, particular talents, ability to cope and to resolve problems, independence, and interpersonal interactions.
- An individual's functional level of overall self-esteem may change markedly from day to day and moment to moment.
- Because a healthy self-concept is basic to health, one of the nurse's major responsibilities is to assist clients whose self-concept is disturbed to develop a more positive and realistic image of themselves.
- A trusting client-nurse relationship is essential for the effective assessment of a client's self-concept, for providing help and support, and for motivating client behavior change.
- The nurse's personal self-concept and professional self-concept are interrelated.
- Nurses who seek to maintain or improve their professional self-concept are more effective in providing care and in promoting a positive image of nursing in the community.

READINGS AND REFERENCES

SUGGESTED READINGS

Roy, C and Andrews, HA. 1991. *The Roy Adaptation Model: The Definitive Statement.* Norwalk, CT: Appleton & Lange.

This text describes Roy's adaptation model of nursing. Two of the four modes of the Roy model, the self-concept mode and the role function mode, are discussed in detail.

Strasen, LL. 1992. *The Image of Professional Nursing: Strategies for Action.* Philadelphia: Lippincott.

This book provides strategies for assisting nursing students and experienced nurses to improve their professional self-concept by viewing themselves and their profession more positively.

RELATED RESEARCH

Heidrich, SM and Ward, SE. October 1992. The role of the self in adjustment to cancer in elderly women. *Oncology Nursing Forum* 19:1491–96.

Pletsch, PK, Johnson, MD, Tosi, CB, Thurston, CA, and Riesch, SK. April 1991. Self-image among early adolescents: Revisited. *Journal of Community Health Nursing* 8:215–31.

SELECTED REFERENCES

Andrews, HA. 1991. Overview of the self-concept mode. In Roy, C and Andrews, HA. *The Roy Adaptation Model: The Definitive Statement.* Norwalk, CT: Appleton & Lange.

Arnold, E and Boggs, K. 1989. *Interpersonal Relationships: Professional Communication Skills for Nurses.* Philadelphia: WB Saunders.

Barry, PD. 1989. *Psychosocial Nursing Assessment and Intervention: Care of the Physically Ill Person.* 2d ed. Philadelphia: Lippincott.

Beck, AT. 1979. *Cognitive Theory of Depression.* New York: Guilford Press.

Berscheid, E, Walster, E, and Bohrnstedt, G. February, 1972. Body image: A *Psychology Today* questionnaire. *Psychology Today* 6(2): 57–64.

Burns, RB. 1979. *The Self Concept in Theory, Measurement, Development, and Behavior.* London: Longman Group Ltd.

Carpenito, LJ. 1992. *Nursing Diagnosis: Application to Clinical Practice.* 4th ed. Philadelphia: Lippincott.

Crosby, R. September 1982. Self-concept development. *Journal of School Health* 52:432–36.

Crouch, MA, and Straub, V. August 1983. Enhancement of self-esteem in adults. *Family and Community Health* 6:65–78.

Edelman, CL and Mandle, CL. 1990. *Health Promotion Throughout the Life Span.* 2d ed. St Louis: Mosby.

Ellis, A and Harper, RA. 1975. *A New Guide to Rational Living.* North Hollywood, CA: Wilshire Book Co.

Erikson, EH. 1963. *Childhood and Society.* 2d ed. New York: Norton.

Goldin, J. November/December 1985. The influence of self-image upon the performance of nursing home staff. *Nursing Homes* 34:33–38.

Gordon, M. 1993. *Manual of Nursing Diagnosis 1993–1994.* St Louis: Mosby-Year Book.

Hamachek, DE. 1987. *Encounters with the Self.* 3d ed. Chicago: Holt, Rinehart and Winston.

Husted, GL, Miller, MC, and Wilczynski, EM. May 1990. Five ways to build your self-esteem. *Nursing90* 20:152, 154.

Jenny, J. October 1990. Self-esteem: A problem for nurses. *Canadian Nurse* 86 (10):19–21.

Klose, P and Tinius, T. 1992. Confidence builders: A self-esteem group at an inpatient psychiatric hospital. *Journal of Psychosocial Nursing* 30 (7):5–9.

Leddy, S. and Pepper, JM. 1993. *Conceptual Bases of Professional Nursing.* 3d ed. Philadelphia: Lippincott.

Lindberg, JB, Hunter, ML, and Kruszewski, AZ. 1990. *Introduction to Nursing: Concepts, Issues, and Opportunities.* Philadelphia: Lippincott.

McFarland, GK and McFarlane, EA. 1993. *Nursing Diagnosis and Intervention: Planning for Patient Care.* 2d ed. St Louis: Mosby-Year Book.

McKay, SA. April 1993. Powering up our professional image. *Canadian Nurse* 89 (4):35–37.

Mixson, K. November/December 1989. How to enhance our self-esteem. *Advanced Clinical Nursing* 4:12–14.

Mock, V. May/June 1993. Body image in women treated for breast cancer. Nursing Research 42:153–57.

Nelson, PB. February 1990. Intrinsic/extrinsic religious orientation of the elderly: Relationship to depression and self-esteem. *Journal of Gerontological Nursing* 16:29–37.

North American Nursing Diagnosis Association. 1992. NANDA Nursing Diagnoses: Definitions and Classification 1992–1993. Philadelphia: NANDA.

Otto, HA. August 1965. The human potentialities of nurses and patients. *Nursing Outlook* 13:32–35.

Reasoner, RW. August 1983. Enhancing self-esteem in children and adolescents. *Family and Community Health* 6:51–64.

Roid, GH and Fitts, WH. 1988. *Tennessee Self-Concept Scale: Revised Manual.* Los Angeles: Western Psychological Services.

Roy, C and Andrews, HA. 1991. *The Roy Adaptation Model: The Definitive Statement.* Norwalk, CT: Appleton & Lange.

Sanford, LT, and Donovan, ME. 1984. *Women and Self-Esteem.* New York: Penguin Books.

Smith, MJ. 1975. *When I Say No, I Feel Guilty.* New York: Bantam Books.

Smith, S. 1992. *Communications in Nursing: Communicating Assertively and Responsibly in Nursing.* St Louis: Mosby-Year Book.

Stanwyck, DJ. August 1983. Self-esteem through the life span. *Family and Community Health* 6:11–28.

Strasen, LL. 1992. *The Image of Professional Nursing: Strategies for Action.* Philadelphia: Lippincott.

Sullivan, HS. 1950. *The Interpersonal Theory of Psychiatry.* New York: Norton.

Sundeen, SJ, Stuart, GW, Rankin, EAD, and Cohen, SA. 1989. *Nurse-Client Interaction.* 4th ed. St Louis: Mosby.

32 Stress and Coping

Objectives

- Differentiate the concepts of stress as a stimulus, as a response, and as a transaction.
- Identify Selye's definition of stress.
- Describe the three stages of Selye's general adaptation syndrome.
- Describe essential aspects of the Lazarus stress model.
- Identify physiologic and psychologic (cognitive, verbal, and motor) manifestations of stress.
- Identify behaviors related to specific ego defense mechanisms.
- Differentiate four levels of anxiety.
- Describe the relationship of anger to anxiety.
- Give examples of constructive and destructive anger.
- Give examples of three modes of adaptation.
- Identify characteristics of adaptive responses.
- Identify examples of nursing diagnoses related to stress.
- Identify general guidelines to minimize a client's anxiety and stress.
- Describe interventions to help clients cope with stress.
- Describe outcome criteria that can be used to evaluate whether a client is effectively coping with a stressful problem.
- Describe ways in which nurses can cope with professional and personal stressors.

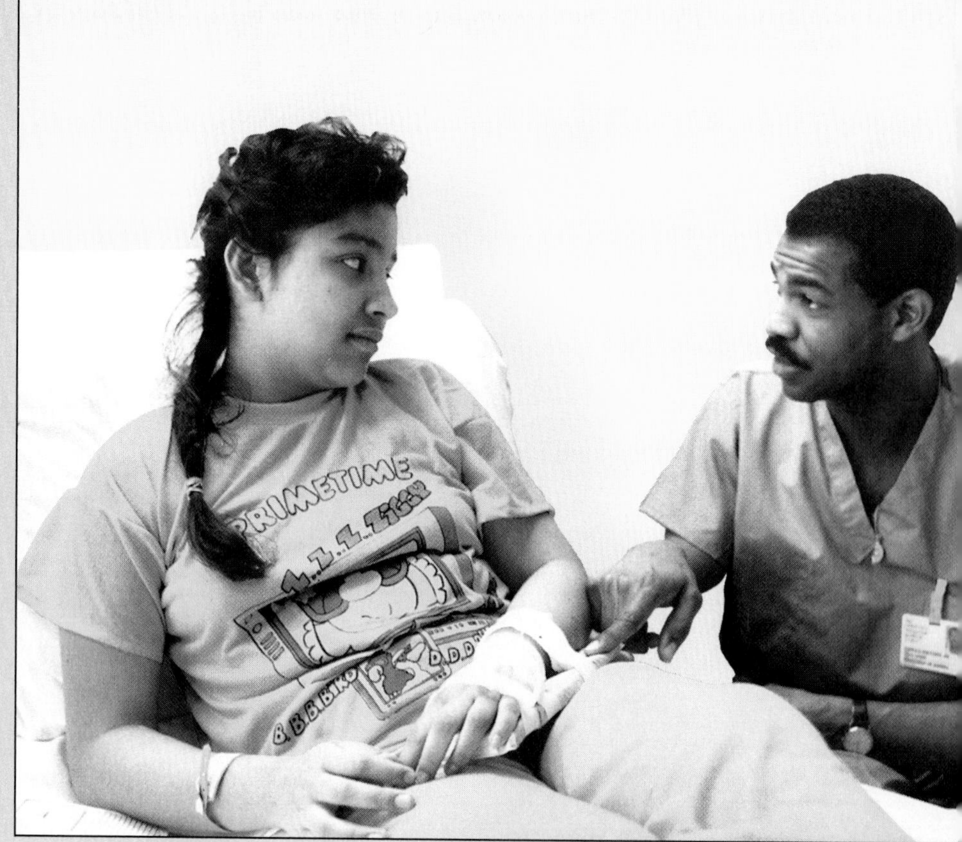

Stress is a universal phenomenon. All people experience it. Parents refer to the stress of raising children; working people talk of the stress of their jobs; and students at all levels talk of the stress of school. The concept of stress is important because it provides a way of understanding the person as a unified being who responds in totality (mind, body, and spirit) to a variety of changes that take place in daily life.

Concept of Stress

Stress can have physical, emotional, intellectual, social, and spiritual consequences. Usually, the effects are mixed, because stress affects the whole person. Physically, stress can threaten a person's physiologic homeostasis (see Chapter 14). Emotionally, stress can produce negative or nonconstructive feelings about self. Intellectually, stress can influence a person's perceptual and problem-solving abilities. Socially, stress can alter a person's relationships with others. Spiritually, stress can challenge one's beliefs and values. Many illnesses have been linked to stress (Figure 32–1). Stress is defined in a number of ways: as a stimulus, as a response, and as a transaction.

Stress as a Stimulus

Stress may be defined as a **stimulus,** a life event (sometimes called a "life change") or set of circumstances causing a disrupted response (Lyon & Werner 1987) that

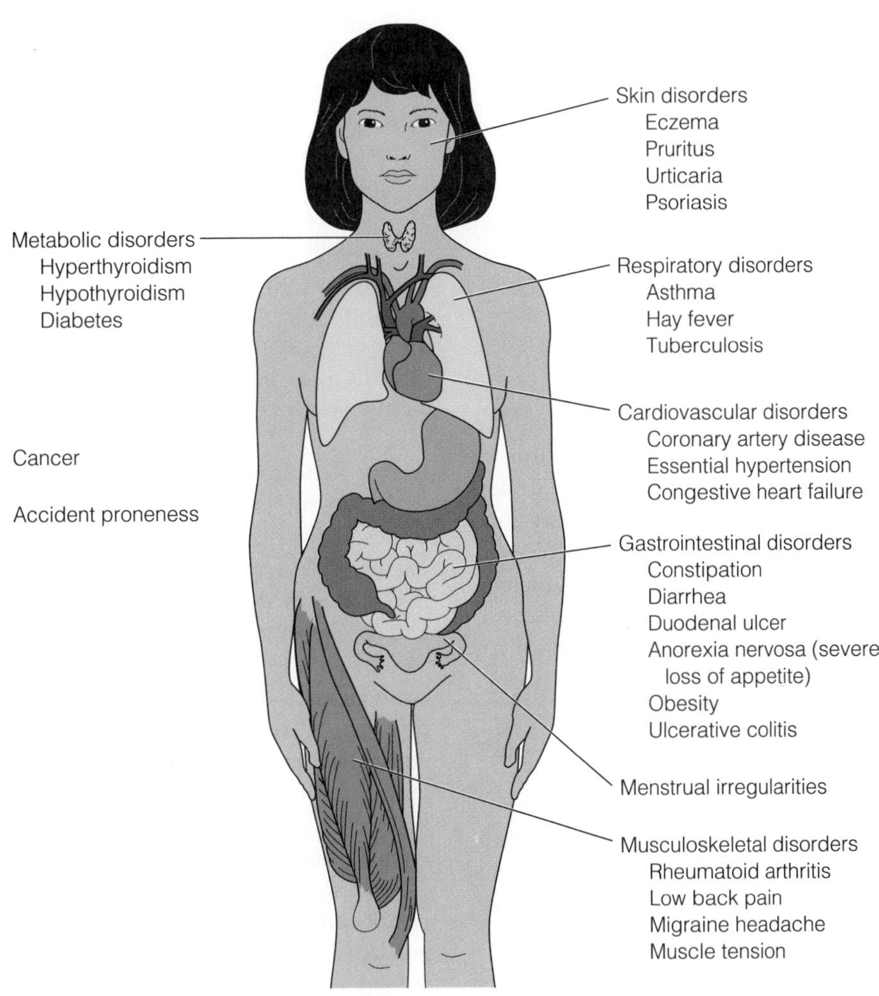

Figure 32–1 Some disorders that can be caused or aggravated by stress. **Source:** Adapted from G Edlin and E Golanty, *Health and Wellness: A Holistic Approach,* 4th ed. (Boston: Jones and Bartlett, 1992), p. 210.

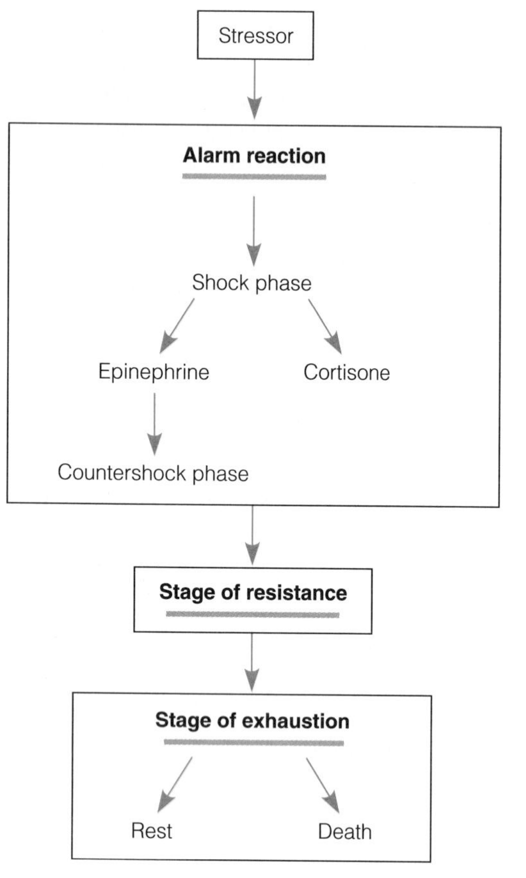

Figure 32–2 The three stages of adaptation to stress: the alarm reaction, the stage of resistance, and the stage of exhaustion.

increases the individual's vulnerability to illness. Holmes and Rahe (1967) assigned a numerical value to 43 life changes or events. The scale of stressful life events is used to document a person's relatively recent experiences, such as divorce, pregnancy, and retirement. In this view, both positive and negative events are considered stressful.

Since 1967, similar scales have been developed, including scales for measuring stress in nurses (Kinzel 1982, pp. 54–55) and in hospitalized clients (Volicer & Burns 1975, p. 358). Burgess and Lazare (1976, p. 58) caution people in the use of such scales. They emphasize that the degree of stress the event presents can be highly individual. For example, a divorce may be highly traumatic to one person and cause relatively little anxiety to another. What is important is that research has shown that people who have a high level of stress are often more prone to illness and have lowered ability to cope with illness and subsequent stress.

STRESS AS A RESPONSE

Stress may also be defined as a **response,** the disruption caused by a noxious stimulus or stressor (Lyon & Werner 1987). In this definition of stress, reactions rather than events are the focus. Schafer (1992, p. 9) defines stress as the "arousal of mind and body in response to demands made upon them." The response view was developed by Hans Selye (1956, 1976). He defined stress as "the nonspecific response of the body to any kind of demand made upon it" (1976, p. 1). Regardless of the cause, situation, or psychologic interpretation of a demanding situation, Selye's stress response is characterized by the same chain or pattern of physiologic events. This nonspecific response was called the **general adaptation syndrome (GAS)** or **stress syndrome.**

To differentiate the cause of stress from the response to stress, Selye created the term **stressor** (1976, p. 51) to denote any factor that produces stress and disturbs the body's equilibrium. Because stress is a state of the body, it can be observed only by the changes it produces in the body. This response of the body, the stress syndrome or general adaptation syndrome, occurs with the release of certain adaptive hormones and subsequent changes in the structure and chemical composition of the body. Body organs affected by stress are the gastrointestinal tract, the adrenal glands, and the lymphatic structures. With prolonged stress, the adrenal glands enlarge considerably; the lymphatic structures, such as the thymus, spleen, and lymph nodes, atrophy (shrink); and deep ulcers appear in the lining of the stomach. In addition to adapting globally, the body can also react locally; that is, one organ or a part of the body reacts alone. This is referred to as the **local adaptation syndrome (LAS).** One example of the LAS is inflammation. See the section on the inflammatory response, in Chapter 27. Selye proposed that both the GAS and the LAS had three stages (1976, p. 38): alarm reaction, resistance, and exhaustion (Figure 32–2).

Alarm Reaction (AR) The initial reaction of the body is the alarm reaction (AR), which alerts the body's defenses against the stressor, whether the stressor is heat, bacteria, or a verbal or physical attack from someone. Selye divided this stage into two parts: the shock phase and the countershock phase.

During the **shock phase,** the stressor may be perceived consciously or unconsciously by the person. In any case, the autonomic nervous system reacts, and large amounts of epinephrine (adrenaline) and cortisone are released into the body. The person is then ready for "fight or flight." This primary response is short lived, lasting from 1 minute to 24 hours.

The second part of the alarm reaction is called the **countershock phase.** During this time, the body changes produced during the shock phase are reversed. It is, therefore, during the shock phase of the alarm reaction that a person is best mobilized to react.

Stage of Resistance (SR) It's during the second stage in the GAS and LAS syndromes that the stage of resistance (SR), the body's adaptation, takes place. In other words, the body attempts to cope with the stressor and to limit the stressor to the smallest area of the body that can deal with it.

Stage of Exhaustion (SE) During the third stage, the stage of exhaustion (SE), the adaptation that the body made during the second stage cannot be maintained. This means that the ways used to cope with the stressor have been exhausted. If adaptation has not overcome the stressor, the stress effects may spread to the entire body. At the end of this stage, the body may either rest and return to normal, or death may be the ultimate consequence. The end of this stage depends largely on the adaptive energy resources of the individual, the severity of the stressor, and the external adaptive resources that are provided, such as oxygen.

Selye's general adaptation syndrome encompasses a range of *physiologic* responses to stressors in the body as a whole (Figure 32–3). Stressors stimulate the sympathetic nervous system, which in turn stimulates the hypothalamus. The hypothalamus releases corticotropin-releasing hormone (CRH), which stimulates the anterior pituitary gland to release adrenocorticotropin (ACTH). During stress, the adrenal medulla, which is functionally related to the sympathetic nervous system, secretes epinephrine and norepinephrine in response to sympathetic stimulation. Significant body responses to epinephrine include the following:

1. Increased myocardial contractility, which increases cardiac output and blood flow to active muscles
2. Bronchial dilation, which allows increased oxygen intake
3. Increased blood clotting
4. Increased cellular metabolism
5. Increased fat mobilization to make energy available and to synthesize other compounds needed by the body

The principal effect of norepinephrine is decreased blood to the kidneys and increased secretion of renin. *Renin* is an enzyme that hydrolyzes one of the blood proteins to produce *angiotensin*. Angiotensin tends to increase the blood pressure by constricting arterioles. The sum of all these adrenal hormonal effects permits the person to perform far more strenuous physical activity than would otherwise be possible.

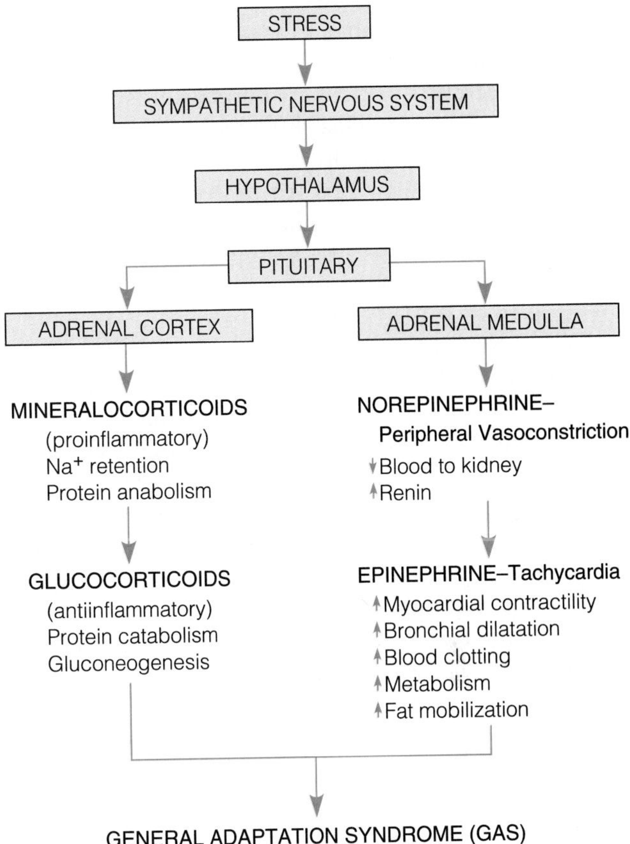

A stress syndrome, termed the General Adaptation Syndrome (GAS) by Hans Selye, evolves in three stages. Stages 1 and 2 are continuously repeated throughout a lifetime cycle. If resistance cannot be sustained, exhaustion (Stage 3), with its altered psychophysiologic functioning, occurs.

Figure 32–3 Physiologic response to stress: general adaptation syndrome. **Source:** MJ Smith and H Selye, Stress: Reducing the negative effects of stress, *American Journal of Nursing*, November 1979, 79:1954. Used by permission.

STRESS AS A TRANSACTION

Transactional theories of stress are based on the work of Lazarus (1966), who states that the stimulus theory and the response theory do not consider individual differences. Neither explains which factors lead some persons and not others to respond effectively nor interprets why some persons are able to adapt over longer periods than others. According to Lazarus, "Stimulus definitions focus on events in the environment such as natural disasters, illness, or termination of employment. This approach assumes that certain situations are normatively stressful but does not allow for individual differences in the evaluation of events. Response definitions refer to a state of stress; the person is spoken of as reacting with stress, being under stress, and so on. Stimulus and response definitions have limited utility, because a stimulus gets defined as stressful only in terms of a stress response" (Lazarus & Folkman 1984, p. 21).

Although Lazarus recognizes that certain environmental demands and pressures produce stress in substantial numbers of people, he emphasizes that people and groups differ in their sensitivity and vulnerability to certain types of events, as well as in their interpretations and reactions. For example, in terms of illness, one person may respond with denial, another with anxiety, and still another with depression. To explain variations among individuals under comparable conditions, the Lazarus model takes into account cognitive processes that intervene between the encounter and the reaction, and the factors that affect the nature of this process. In contrast to Selye, who focuses on physiologic responses, Lazarus includes mental and psychologic components or responses as part of his concept of stress.

The Lazarus **transactional stress theory** encompasses a set of cognitive, affective, and adaptive (coping) responses that arise out of person-environment transactions. The person and the environment are inseparable; each affects and is affected by the other. Stress "refers to any event in which environmental demands, internal demands, or both tax or exceed the adaptive resources of an individual, social system, or tissue system" (Monat & Lazarus 1991, p. 3). The individual responds to perceived environmental changes by adaptive or coping responses. **Cognitive appraisal** is an evaluative process that determines why and to what extent a particular transaction or series of transactions between the person and the environment is stressful.

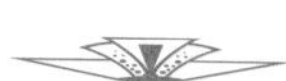

MANIFESTATIONS OF STRESS

Manifestations of the stress experience, both physiologic and psychologic, may be considered coping strategies or mechanisms. According to Folkman and Lazarus (1991, p. 210) **coping** is "the cognitive and behavioral effort to manage specific external and/or internal demands that are appraised as taxing or exceeding the resources of the person." Coping can be adaptive or maladaptive. Adaptive coping helps the person to deal effectively with stressful events and minimizes distress associated with them. Maladaptive coping can result in unnecessary distress for the person and others associated with the person or stressful event (Schafer 1992, p. 198).

Coping may be described as dealing with problems and situations, or contending with them successfully. A **coping strategy (coping mechanism)** is an innate or acquired way of responding to a changing environment or specific problem or situation. In nursing literature, effective and ineffective coping are often differentiated. *Effective coping* results in adaptation; *ineffective coping* results in maladaptation. Although coping behavior may not always seem appropriate, the nurse needs to remember that coping is always purposeful.

Coping strategies vary among individuals and are often related to the individual's perception of the stressful event. Schafer (1992, pp. 200–201) describes three approaches to coping with stress: alter the stressor, adapt to the stressor, or avoid the stressor. A person's coping strategies often change with a reappraisal of a situation. There is never only one way to cope. Some people choose avoidance; others confront a situation as a means of coping. Still others seek information or rely on religious beliefs as a means of coping. Bell (1977, p. 137) places coping strategies into two groups: long term and short term. Long-term coping strategies can be constructive and realistic. For example, in certain situations talking with others about the problem and trying to find out more about the situation are long-term strategies.

Short-term coping strategies can reduce stress to a tolerable limit temporarily but are in the long run ineffective ways to deal with reality. They may even have a destructive or detrimental effect on the person (Bell 1977, p. 137). Examples of short-term strategies are using alcoholic beverages or drugs, daydreaming and fantasizing, and relying on the belief that everything will work out.

PHYSIOLOGIC MANIFESTATIONS

Physiologic manifestations may or may not occur in clients experiencing stress, depending on the way the client perceives the stressful event and on the effectiveness of the client's coping strategies. There is considerable evidence that a person's cognitive coping strategies mediate blood pressure and heart rates. For example, when a person cognitively attends to the stressor or threat, the heart rate decreases. Specific physiologic manifestations are presented in the box on page 833.

PSYCHOLOGIC MANIFESTATIONS

Psychologic manifestations of stress include anxiety, fear, anger, depression, cognitive behaviors, verbal and motor responses, and unconscious ego defense mechanisms. Some of these coping patterns are helpful; others are a hindrance, depending on the situation and the length of time they are used or experienced. Indeed, anxiety is often considered to be a response to a stressful event rather than a coping mechanism, since it may impede action to remove the stressor.

Anxiety This common reaction to stress is a state of mental uneasiness, apprehension, dread, or foreboding or a feeling of helplessness related to an impending or anticipated unidentified threat to self or significant relationships. Anxiety can be experienced at the conscious, subconscious, or unconscious levels. It differs from fear in four ways:

1. The source of anxiety is not identifiable; the source of fear is identifiable.
2. Anxiety is related to the future, that is, to an anticipated event. Fear is related to the present.
3. Anxiety is vague, whereas fear is definite.
4. Anxiety is the result of psychologic or emotional conflict; fear is the result of a discrete physical or psychologic entity.

All people experience anxiety to some degree most of the time. Mild or moderate anxiety is needed to accomplish developmental tasks and motivate goal-directed behavior. In this sense, anxiety is an effective coping strategy. For example, mild anxiety motivates students to study. Excessive anxiety, however, often has destructive effects.

Anxiety may be manifested on four different levels:

1. *Mild anxiety*, which produces a slight arousal state that enhances perception, learning, and productive abilities. Most healthy persons experience mild anxiety, perhaps as a feeling of mild restlessness that prompts a person to seek information and ask questions.
2. *Moderate anxiety*, which increases the client's arousal state to a point where the person expresses feelings of tension, nervousness, or concern. Perceptual abilities are narrowed. Attention is focused more on a particular aspect of a situation than on peripheral activities.
3. *Severe anxiety*, which consumes most of the person's energies and requires intervention. Perception is further decreased. The person, unable to focus on what is really happening, focuses on only one specific detail of the situation generating the anxiety.
4. *Panic*, which is an overpowering, frightening level of anxiety causing the person to lose control. It is less frequently experienced than other levels of anxiety. The perception of a panicked person can be altered to the point where the person distorts events. See Table 32–1 on page 834 for signs of these levels.

Fear Fear is "a mild to severe feeling of apprehension about some perceived threat" (Schafer 1992, p. 107). The fear may be in response to something that has already occurred, in response to an immediate or current threat, or in anticipation of something the person believes will happen. The object of fear may or may not be based in reality. For example, the beginning nursing student may be fearful in anticipation of the first experience in a client care setting. The student may fear that the client will not want

PHYSIOLOGIC MANIFESTATIONS OF STRESS*

- Pupils dilate to increase visual perception when serious threats to the body arise.
- Sweat production (diaphoresis) increases to control elevated body heat due to increased metabolism.
- The heart rate increases, which leads to an increased pulse rate to transport nutrients and byproducts of metabolism more efficiently.
- Skin is pallid because of constriction of peripheral blood vessels, an effect of norepinephrine.
- Blood pressure increases because of
  a. Constriction of vessels in blood reservoirs, such as the skin, kidneys, and most large interior organs.
  b. Increased secretion of renin, an effect of norepinephrine.
  c. Increased sodium and water retention due to release of mineralocorticoids, which results in increased blood volume.
  d. Increased cardiac output.
- The rate and depth of respirations increase because of dilation of the bronchioles, promoting hyperventilation.
- Urinary output decreases.
- The mouth may be dry.
- Peristalsis of the intestines decreases, resulting in possible constipation and flatus.
- For serious threats, mental alertness improves.
- Muscle tension increases to prepare for rapid motor activity or defense.
- Blood sugar increases because of release of glucocorticoids and gluconeogenesis.
- Lethargy, mental lassitude, inactivity (parasympathetic dominance) may ensue.
- There may be decreased physiologic functioning and loss of skeletal muscle tone (parasympathetic dominance).

*All signs are the result of increased activity of the sympathetic nervous system unless indicated otherwise.

Table 32–1 Signs of Mild, Moderate, and Severe Anxiety

Sign	Mild	Moderate	Severe (Panic)
Verbalization changes	Expresses feelings of increased arousal and concern Increased questioning or information seeking	Expresses feelings of unfocused tension, apprehension, nervousness, or concern Verbalized expectation of danger Voice tremors and pitch changes Increased rate and quantity of verbalization	Expresses feelings of severe dread, apprehension, nervousness, concern, helplessness, and isolation Absence of verbalization Inappropriate verbalization, such as false cheerfulness or laughing while discussing a serious subject
Motor activity changes	Mild restlessness	Pacing Hand tremor or shakiness Increased muscle tension	Immobilization Purposeless activity Increased muscle tension Rigid posture Fixed or scattered perceptual focus
Perception and attention changes	Increased awareness Increased attending Ability to focus on most of what is really happening	Narrowed focus of attention Ability to focus on most of what is really happening	Intellectualizing about a subject, for example, explaining the pathophysiology of leukemia rather than describing own feelings Intent and fearful watching of everything going on Inability to focus on what is really happening Inability to focus on reality, for example, denial, saying, "I don't want to talk about it"
Respiratory and circulatory changes	Nil	Rapid pulse Increased respiratory rate	Tachycardia Palpitations Hyperventilation
Other changes	Nil	Diaphoresis Sleep or eating disturbances (eg, insomnia, somnolence, overeating, or anorexia) Irritability	Diaphoresis Dilated pupils Pallor Clammy hands and skin Dry mouth Sullenness, withdrawal

Sources: Compiled from M Gordon, *Manual of Nursing Diagnosis* (St Louis: Mosby, 1993), pp. 253–61; and Anxiety: Recognition and intervention (programmed instruction) *American Journal of Nursing*, September 1965, 65:129–52. Copyright © 1965 The American Journal of Nursing Company; LJ Carpenito, *Nursing Diagnosis: Application to Clinical Practice*, 4th ed. (Philadelphia: Lippincott, 1992), pp. 140–54; and GK McFarland and EA McFarlane, *Nursing Diagnosis and Intervention: Planning for Patient Care*, 2d ed. (St Louis: Mosby-Year Book, 1993), pp. 492–98.

to be cared for by the student or that the student might inadvertently harm the client. Although the feeling of fear is real and may elicit a stress response, the instructor's structure of the student's first client assignment is such that the student's anticipated fears are unlikely to occur.

Anger Anger is an emotional state consisting of a subjective feeling of animosity or strong displeasure. Many people feel guilty when they feel anger, because they have learned that to feel angry is wrong. In fact, anger, hostility, violence, and aggression differ. Anger can be expressed in a nonalienating verbal manner; it is then considered a positive emotion and a sign of emotional maturity, since growth and beneficial interactions result from it.

Anger is commonly manifested in altered voice tone as a communication to desist from some action or other.

Verbal expression of anger can therefore be considered a signal to others of one's internal psychologic discomfort and a call for assistance to deal with perceived stress. In contrast, *hostility* is usually marked by overt antagonism and harmful or destructive behavior; *aggression* is an unprovoked attack or a hostile, injurious, or destructive action or outlook; and *violence* is the exertion of physical force to injure or abuse. Verbally expressed anger differs from hostility, aggression, and violence, but it can lead to destructiveness and violence if the anger persists unabated.

Clearly expressed verbal communication of anger, when the angry person tells the other person about the anger and carefully identifies the source, is constructive. This clarity of communication gets the anger out into the open so that the other person can deal with it and help to alleviate it. The angry person "gets it off his chest" and prevents an emotional buildup. Constructive expressions of anger have three elements (Duldt 1981, p. 516):

1. *Alerting*, the act of engaging another's attention
2. *Describing*, the process of delineating the source of the angry person's feelings, that is, what has happened here and now
3. *Identifying*, the act of seeking a response and support from others

The following are examples of constructive anger:

- "Darn! (Alerting) This electric drill won't work. (Describing) What am I doing wrong?" (Identifying)
- "Robert! (Alerting) Your going to the football game this afternoon infuriates me. You said yesterday you'd clean the car for me before I have to drive my friends to the church social tonight. (Describing) Now what am I going to do?" (Identifying)

Unclear communication of anger is destructive. It is similar to constructive expressions only in the alerting behavior. Then the person fails to describe the source of the feelings adequately and denies any responsibility for the anger by blaming others or by generalizing to other people or past situations. Thus, those in the presence of the angry person are unable to respond helpfully. The following are examples of unclearly expressed anger:

- "Darn it! (Alerting) A woman can never win." (Generalizing)
- "You weasel! (Alerting) You're always leaving me in the lurch." (Generalizing, blaming)

Depression Depression is a common reaction to events that seem overwhelming or negative. Buckwalter and Babich (1990, p. 947) state that "10% to 15% of adults will suffer symptoms of a major depressive episode and another 20% to 30% will experience significant depressive symptoms" at some time during life. The signs and symptoms of depression and the severity of the problem vary with the client and the significance of the precipitating event. Emotional symptoms can include feelings of tiredness, sadness, emptiness, or numbness. Behavioral signs of depression include irritability, inability to concentrate, difficulty making decisions, loss of sexual desire, crying, sleep disturbance, and social withdrawal. Physical signs of depression may include loss of appetite, weight loss, constipation, headache, and dizziness. Many people may experience short periods of depression in response to overwhelming stressful events, such as the death of a loved one or loss of a job; prolonged depression, however, is a cause for concern and may require treatment.

COGNITIVE MANIFESTATIONS

Cognitive manifestations of stress are thinking responses that include problem solving, structuring, self-control or self-discipline, suppression, fantasy, and prayer. *Problem solving* involves thinking through the threatening situation, using specific steps, similar to those of the nursing process, to arrive at a solution. The person assesses the situation or problem, analyzes or defines it, chooses alternatives, carries out the selected alternative, and evaluates whether the solution was successful.

Structuring is the arrangement or manipulation of a situation so that threatening events do not occur. For example, a nurse can structure or control an interview with a client by asking only direct, closed questions. This strategy avoids information or questions that may be threatening to the nurse's knowledge or values. Structuring, however, can be productive in certain situations. A person who schedules a dental examination semiannually to prevent severe dental disease is using productive structuring.

Self-control (discipline) is assuming a manner and facial expression that convey a sense of being in control or in charge, no matter what the situation is. When self-control prevents panic and harmful or nonproductive actions in a threatening situation, it is a helpful response that conveys strength. Self-control carried to an extreme, however, can delay problem solving and prevent a person from receiving the support of others, who may perceive the person as handling the situation well, as cold, or as unconcerned.

Suppression is consciously and willfully putting a thought or feeling out of mind: "I won't deal with that today. I'll do it tomorrow." This response relieves stress temporarily but does not solve the problem. A man who keeps ignoring a toothache, pushing it out of his mind because he fears the pain of having a filling, will not relieve his symptoms or find the solution.

Fantasy or *daydreaming* is likened to make-believe. Unfulfilled wishes and desires are imagined as fulfilled, or a threatening experience is reworked or replayed so that it ends differently from reality. Experiences can be relived, everyday problems solved, and plans for the future made. The outcome of current problems may also be fantasized.

For example, a client who is awaiting the results of a breast biopsy may fantasize the surgeon as saying, "You do not have cancer." Fantasy responses can be helpful if they lead to problem solving. For example, the client awaiting breast biopsy results might say to herself, "Even if the doctor doesn't say, 'You do not have cancer,' as long as he says I won't need mutilating surgery, I can accept that." Fantasies can be destructive and nonproductive if a person uses them to excess and retreats from reality.

Prayer often involves identifying and describing the problem, suggesting solutions, and reaching out for support and help. For example, a young woman may pray: "Please help me. The doctor says I have headaches and hypertension because I'm overweight (describing problem). What I need is to discipline myself to exercise more and go on a diet" (suggesting solutions). If these first two problem-solving steps lead to action, prayer can be a constructive response, aside from the support and meaning the person derives from it.

VERBAL AND MOTOR MANIFESTATIONS

Verbal or motor manifestations of stress may be the first responses evident. Among these responses are crying, verbal abuse, laughing, screaming, hitting and kicking, and holding and touching. *Crying* releases tension in situations perceived as painful, joyful, or sad and when the situation cannot yet be managed cognitively. As a response, crying tends to be more socially acceptable in women and in certain cultures, for instance, among Hispanics/Latinos or Mediterranean people. People often cry when they perceive that others care. Crying is beneficial as a release of tension and if it is followed by problem solving. It is not helpful without problem solving.

Verbal abuse is another release mechanism most often expressed toward stress-producing objects and events, such as nonfunctional equipment, misplaced or lost items, and rainy weather. *Laughing* is also an anxiety-reducing response that can lead to constructive problem solving. People may laugh at small incidents and at the way they handled a situation. For example, a preoccupied, stressed man whose wife has been injured in an accident may laugh at having put on one black shoe and one brown shoe before rushing to the emergency room.

Screaming is a response to fear or intense frustration and anger. One may scream in response to a person appearing suddenly out of the dark or in response to a family member who keeps planning other activities to avoid cleaning the garage. Screaming, like other verbal responses, reduces tension but can be harmful if the person is unable to control it and becomes hysterical. The hysterical, frightened person needs to be moved to a quiet place and assured that the threat is over. The hysterical, frustrated person needs a more effective coping strategy (eg, problem solving).

Hitting and *kicking* can be spontaneous responses to physical threats or to feelings of frustration. Adults who are socialized to control such responses toward people may direct them toward objects by pounding a table with a fist or kicking a wastebasket. Preschoolers, however, have not matured enough to develop control and may, for example, hit or kick a nurse who is administering an injection. Of grave concern are stress responses that result in child, spouse, or elder abuse. Hitting or kicking can be helpful in reducing tension provided the person or object is not damaged and provided they lead to more effective coping techniques.

Holding and *touching* are often responses to joyful, painful, or sad events. Holding or touching another is a gesture of support and comfort. Holding and touching responses vary considerably, however, among cultures and among individuals in a culture. Verbal communication can also convey caring. "Crisis lines" or close friends often provide meaningful and supportive verbal communication that conveys caring by phone or in person.

UNCONSCIOUS EGO DEFENSE MECHANISMS

Unconscious ego defense mechanisms are psychologic defensive (adaptive) mechanisms or, in the words of Sigmund Freud (1946), mental mechanisms, which develop as the personality attempts to defend itself, establish compromises among conflicting impulses, and allay inner tensions. Defense mechanisms are the unconscious mind working to protect the person from anxiety. They can be considered precursors to conscious cognitive coping mechanisms that will ultimately solve the problem. Like some verbal and motor responses, defense mechanisms release tension. Table 32–2 describes these mechanisms and lists examples of their adaptive and maladaptive use.

FACTORS INFLUENCING THE MANIFESTATIONS OF STRESS

The degree to which a stressor affects an individual depends on the nature of the stressor, perception of the stressor, number of simultaneous stressors, duration of exposure to the stressor, experiences with a comparable stressor (Byrne & Thompson 1978, p. 3), age, and support people available. The *nature of the stressor* refers to its magnitude. Obviously, a fall from the roof of a building is more stressful than a fall from a chair. Similarly, angry remarks from a loved one are more stressful than those from a stranger.

Perception of the stressor (what the stressor means to the person) can be as important as the actual magnitude of the

Table 32–2 Unconscious Ego Defense Mechanisms

Mechanism	Description	Adaptive Use	Maladaptive Use
Denial	Blocking painful or anxiety-producing aspects of reality out of consciousness. Reality is either completely disregarded or transformed so that it is no longer threatening.	A man does not acknowledge that he has cancer even though the physician has told him the results of the biopsy. A child insists his mother is not dead, just "out of town for a few days."	A woman who has had a heart attack refuses to acknowledge illness and does not follow prescribed therapy.
Rationalization	Often referred to as the "sour-grapes" or "half-truth" mechanism. Good reasons, acceptable to the conscious mind, are given for behavior or circumstances instead of the real reason. The person often disparages some goal that in reality the person would like to attain.	A student who fails an examination because she doesn't understand the material says that the teacher did not clarify the material sufficiently or she did not prepare adequately. A client whose work is interrupted by illness prematurely gives up the work and says he wouldn't have been successful in that field anyway.	A man always gives reasons for not attaining his goals and refuses to accept self-responsibility for not achieving them.
Compensation	Substituting an activity for one that the person really would like to do or cannot do.	A short man shows aggressive, dominating traits to suggest strength and authority that his stature does not convey. A boy who cannot participate in athletics studies hard and attains high grades.	A woman abuses alcohol and drugs to make up for feelings of inadequacy.
Repression	Excluding from consciousness desires, impulses, thoughts, memories, and strivings that conflict with self-image or that involve guilt, shame, or lowering of self-esteem. The painful events cannot be recalled or recognized. Repression is the underlying basis of all defense mechanisms.	A woman forgets a repugnant work assignment. A young woman who was raped and was brought to the outpatient clinic by her roommate says she feels very anxious but cannot remember the events of the past few hours.	A woman excludes a number of events from memory (amnesia).
Regression	Adopting behavior that was comforting earlier in life to overcome the discomfort and insecurity of the present situation.	A toilet-trained preschooler begins bed-wetting after his mother returns home with a new baby. A hospitalized elderly woman becomes more dependent on the nurse than is physically warranted.	A teenager assumes the fetal position for prolonged periods or plays with the genitals.

stressor. Because perception is a subjective phenomenon, there are wide differences in how people regard a stressor. Being late can create a greater stress response in a punctual person than a nonpunctual person. Some clients associate hospitals solely with dying friends and relatives. To such clients, being admitted to the hospital is particularly stressful, because they worry about dying.

The *number of stressors* a person is experiencing at one time can greatly affect the responses. This often explains why a stressor that the nurse considers small can elicit a disproportionate response. For example, a hospitalized client who is coping with separation from her family, the unknown outcome of her illness, and financial problems can react angrily when the nurse brings her the wrong fruit juice. Normally, this woman would not be upset whichever juice was served; however, she is using up her

Table 32–2 Unconscious Ego Defense Mechanisms *continued*

Mechanism	Description	Adaptive Use	Maladaptive Use
Sublimation	Redirecting libidinal drives (sexual and aggressive) into socially acceptable channels.	A person channels, to a limited degree, a sex drive into athletic activity, work, poetry, or music. A man who is fired goes to the gym and punches a punching bag to express rage at his boss.	A person has extreme difficulty in communicating with others.
Identification	Assuming the attitudes, ideas, and behavior patterns of another person or persons; it is an important growth mechanism for children. It is unconscious and differs from imitation, which is conscious.	A teenager changes her hairstyle to that of an idolized movie star. After having surgery, a young boy decides to become a doctor.	A man imitates socially unacceptable or harmful behavior.
Projection	Attributing to others characteristics and feelings that one does not want to admit are one's own.	A woman criticizes a neighbor for being a terrible gossip when in fact the woman herself gossips. A wife with illicit sexual wishes claims that all husbands are unfaithful and not to be trusted.	A person fails to take any responsibility for own behavior.
Conversion	Transforming a mental conflict into a physical symptom.	Before taking a math exam, a student develops a headache. A woman develops a "lump in her throat" at a sad event.	A man experiences paralysis of his punching arm to avoid letting his anger get out of control and punching his boss. A girl develops an inability to speak in the context of protecting a sexually abusive father. A pregnant woman develops pathologic vomiting to express the forbidden desire not to have the baby.
Displacement	Transferring an emotion or feeling from the actual object to a less dangerous or threatening substitute.	A child directs hostility toward a parent to a teacher. A woman who has had an unpleasant experience with a man with red hair reacts strongly against all men with red hair.	A man is verbally or physically aggressive toward all authority or oppressive figures.
Reaction formation	Acting oppositely to what the person truly feels.	A woman shows great interest and concern for her mother-in-law, whom she dislikes. A man strongly criticizes pornographic literature when he has a desire to read it.	A young woman is always unnaturally sweet and loving and is unable to consider the possibility of being angry. A person with strong sadistic tendencies becomes an ardent opponent of research on animals.

Source: Adapted with permission from P Solomon and VI Patch, *Handbook of Psychiatry*, 3d ed. (Los Altos, CA: Lange Medical Publications, 1974), pp. 500–505.

coping energies on the other problems and has little left to adapt to this incident.

The *duration of exposure to the stressor* can also influence the manifestations of stress. If the duration of the stressor extends a person's stage of resistance beyond the person's coping powers, the person becomes exhausted, developing an increased susceptibility to complications and can eventually die. An example is a man admitted to a hospital with a fractured femur. The client survives the surgery and is healing well but develops an acute pain in the gallbladder, necessitating another operation. By this time, the client's energy reserves have been used up, and, although the operation is successful, the client develops an infection that delays his return home.

Previous *experience with a comparable stressor* can be useful both in predicting how the person will react and in reducing stress in the current situation. A person who has successfully adjusted to a situation once before is more likely to do so again in a similar situation than a person who is adjusting to the situation for the first time. Such people are strengthened by knowledge that they handled the situation successfully before. A client who has had an unsuccessful interaction with a physician and other health care personnel once before is more likely to experience stress during a second interaction. Determining what a particular event means to a person can help the nurse plan care.

The *age* of the individual affects response and adaptation to stressors. Infants, for example, have poorly developed immune mechanisms and cannot tolerate large fluid losses. Elderly people may have declining physical and mental resources to cope with increased stressors. *Support people* can assist a person coping with stress to maintain psychologic and physical integrity. They provide emotional support, often help in decision making, and, by sharing the experience, can relieve the intensity of the stress response.

Friedman and Rosenman (1974) identify two personality types: type A and type B. People with type A personality share such characteristics as impatience, competitiveness, aggressiveness, insecurity, a sense of urgency, and an inability to relax. In contrast, people with type B personality have a more relaxed and unhurried approach to life, which enables them to enjoy both work and play. See the box at the right for more characteristics associated with type A and type B personalities.

The research of Friedman and Rosenman found that clients with type A personalities were more prone to cardiovascular illness than clients with type B personalities. Subsequent researchers have disagreed about whether there is a correlation between type A personality and cardiovascular disease: Some studies have reported a correlation between type A behavior and cardiovascular disease (Blumenthal et al 1978; Frank et al 1978; Abbott & Sutherland, 1990) whereas other studies have reported little relationship (Shekelle et al 1985; Case et al 1985). This controversy has led to the identification of a third personality type, called type C, the coping personality (Nuernberger 1981, p. 12).

The person with type C personality experiences considerable stress but has learned to cope with it. Nuernberger believes many people are type C, because most people share some of the characteristics of types A and B. The type C person, however, uses personality characteristics as coping strategies. Kobasa (1984) describes these coping characteristics as challenge, commitment, and control.

CHARACTERISTIC BEHAVIOR PATTERNS OF TYPE A AND TYPE B PERSONALITIES

Type A Behaviors

- Hurried speech
- Constant, rapid movement/eating
- Aggression, ambition, and competitive spirit
- Inability to delegate authority
- Preoccupation with deadlines
- Chronic sense of time urgency
- Impatience with the rate at which things occur and the way others operate
- Career orientation, lack of hobbies
- Little satisfaction with accomplishments
- Restlessness and feelings of guilt during periods of relaxation
- Tendency to think and perform several things at once
- Obsession with money and numbers
- Tendency to dominate conversation, determine topics
- Preoccupation with own thoughts when others are talking
- Overconcern with getting things worth having, less concern with becoming things worth being
- Facade of self-assurance and confidence to hide insecurity about status
- Tendency to measure self-worth by number of achievements
- Nervous gestures: tics, clenched fist or jaw, tooth grinding

Type B Behaviors

- Freedom from all type A traits
- No sense of time urgency
- Ability to relax without guilt
- Ability to work without agitation
- Belief that the purpose of play is fun and relaxation, not to demonstrate superiority
- Tendency to discuss achievements and accomplishments only when situation demands it

Sources: Adapted from M Friedman and R Rosenman, *Type A Behavior and Your Heart* (Greenwich, CT: Fawcett, 1974) and P Nuernberger, *Freedom from Stress: A Holistic Approach* (Honesdale, PA: The Himalayan International Institute of Yoga Science and Philosophy, 1981).

Challenge is the ability to view change as an opportunity for personal growth. *Commitment* is described as a strong sense of inner purpose and confidence. It is the ability to become involved and still maintain the emotional distance to recognize when dedication or desire is becoming harmful. *Control* is the recognition that people have power over their own lives and attitudes. Type C people are proactive rather than reactive; that is, they make their own decisions rather than let circumstances or others make decisions for them.

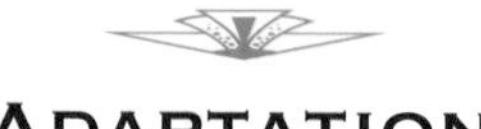

ADAPTATION

Adaptation is the basis of homeostasis and resistance to stress. According to Monsen et al (1992, p. 28), **adaptation** "results when the individual is able to effect a series of behaviors and mental processes to neutralize the stress experience and reestablish integrity of function. Adaptation involves achieving a balance between perceived demands (stress) and marshaled resources (coping), a state of reduced anxiety and enhanced well-being." To adapt is to modify to meet new, changing, or different conditions. Because it is a phenomenon of all living things, adaptation is studied in many disciplines, such as plant biology, physics, psychology, education (personality adaptation), biochemistry, psychiatry, and ecology. In all disciplines, adaptation denotes interaction and change. The change is viewed as positive, for the better, or healthy.

MODES OF ADAPTATION

Human adaptation occurs in three interrelated modes: physiologic, psychologic, and sociocultural.

Physiologic Mode Physiologic or **biologic adaptation** occurs in response to increased or altered demands placed on the body and results in compensatory physical changes (eg, increased muscle size and strength plus increased capacity of the heart and lungs following prolonged exercise, and immunity to a specific disease following the invasion of a specific microorganism).

Psychologic and Sociocultural Modes **Psychologic adaptation** involves a change in attitude and behavior (eg, coping strategies) toward emotionally stressful situations. Examples include changing a life-style pattern (such as eating a balanced diet, exercising regularly, or balancing leisure time with work), using problem solving in decision making instead of anger or other nonconstructive responses, and stopping smoking.

Adaptation in the psychologic mode may also be maladaptive. For example, abusing alcohol or drugs and constantly giving in to others to avoid their anger are maladaptive.

Sociocultural adaptation involves changes in the person's behavior in accordance with the norms, conventions, and beliefs of various groups, such as family, society, ethnic group, religious group, professional group, and economic group. Examples include becoming socialized into a profession or military group, or living in a new country and learning to speak the language.

CHARACTERISTICS OF ADAPTIVE RESPONSES

All adaptive responses, whether physiologic, psychologic, or sociocultural, have common characteristics:

1. All adaptive responses are attempts to maintain homeostasis (see Chapter 14).
2. Adaptation is a whole body or total organism response.
3. Adaptive responses have limits. Physiologic adaptive responses are more limited than psychologic or social responses.
4. Adaptation requires time. A person adapts to an inadequate cardiac output that occurs gradually because the heart increases its pumping rate and the size of the ventricles. In the psychologic realm, people are able to think more rationally in controlled or expected situations than in emergencies.
5. Adaptability varies from person to person. The person who is physically healthy has greater resources to adapt. The person who is flexible, responds readily to change, and uses a wide range of coping strategies is more likely to adapt than the person who does not tolerate change and responds in a limited way.
6. Adaptive responses may be inadequate or excessive. For example, the inflammatory response to bacterial invasion may not be sufficient to overcome an infection without antibiotic therapy. The inflammatory response to an allergic reaction can be excessive and create other problems.
7. Adaptive responses are egocentric and tiring because they require body energy and tax physical and psychologic resources. Adapting can consume a person's energy to the point that the person overlooks or is unable to meet the needs of others and fails to give the support they require.

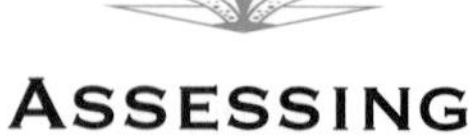

ASSESSING

How a person perceives and responds to stressors is highly individual. Vulnerability to stressors is largely related to previous learning, stage of development, life events, health, and coping methods. The nurse can help the client recognize stress and support effective coping

ASSESSMENT INTERVIEW

Stress and Coping Patterns

- On a scale of one to ten, how would you rate the stress you are experiencing in the following areas?
  a. Home
  b. Work or school
  c. Finance
  d. Recent illness or loss of loved one
  e. Your health
  f. Family responsibilities
  g. Ethnic or cultural group
  h. Religion
  i. Relationships with friends
  j. Relationship with parents or children
  k. Relationship with partner
  l. Recent hospitalization
  m. Other (specify)
- How long have you been dealing with the above stressor(s)?
- How do you usually handle stressful situations?
  a. Cry?
  b. Get angry?
  c. Become verbally abusive?
  d. Talk to someone (who)?
  e. Withdraw from the situation?
  f. Structure and control others or situation?
  g. Go for a walk or physical exercise?
  h. Try to arrive at a solution?
  i. Pray for wisdom and courage?
  j. Laugh, joke, or use some other expression of humor?
  k. Meditate or use some other relaxation technique such as yoga, guided imagery, etc.?
  l. Other (specify)?
- How does your usual coping strategy work?

Table 32–3 Selected Stressors Associated with Developmental Stages

Developmental Stage	Stressors
Child	Resolving conflict between independence and dependence Beginning school Establishing peer relationships and adjustments Coping with peer competition
Adolescent	Accepting changing body physique Developing heterosexual or other relationships Achieving independence Choosing a career
Young adult	Getting married Leaving home Managing a home Getting started in an occupation Continuing one's education Rearing children
Middle adult	Accepting physical changes of aging Maintaining social status and standard of living Helping teenage children to become independent Adjusting to aging parents
Older adult	Accepting decreasing physical abilities and health Accepting changes in residence Adjusting to retirement and reduced income Adjusting to death of spouse and friends

strategies or teach the client new and more effective ways of handling stress.

Assessment relative to a client's stress and coping patterns includes (a) a stress and coping pattern history and (b) clinical examination of the client for indicators of stress. Questions to elicit data about the client's stress and coping patterns are shown in the box above. In addition, the nurse should be aware of expected developmental transitions (predictable tasks that must be accomplished if the person is to grow psychologically as well as physically; see Chapter 23). This knowledge helps the nurse identify additional stressors that are present and the client's response to them. Table 32–3 provides an overview of these developmental stressors.

Indicators of stress were discussed earlier in this chapter. See the box titled "Physiologic Manifestations of Stress" on page 833 and Table 32–1 for descriptions of levels of anxiety. Observe the client also for verbal, motor, and cognitive manifestations. Remember, however, that clinical signs and symptoms may not occur when cognitive coping is effective.

DIAGNOSING

The nursing diagnoses identified by NANDA (1992) relating specifically to clients experiencing stress include the following:

NURSING DIAGNOSES

CLIENTS EXPERIENCING STRESS

NURSING DIAGNOSIS: Anxiety: A vague, uneasy feeling manifested by physiologic arousal and varying patterns of behavior, the source of which is often nonspecific or unknown to the individual

Defining Characteristics

- Increased heart rate, respiratory rate, and blood pressure
- Increased palmar sweating
- Verbalization of fear, apprehension, worry, or nervousness
- Palmar sweating and increased perspiration
- Hand tremors
- Increased muscle tension
- Urinary frequency and urgency
- Restlessness, agitated body movements
- Focused on self

Related Factors

Perceived threat to self-concept, health status, socioeconomic status, role functioning, interaction patterns, or environment; perceived threat of death; threatened loss of relationships through relocation, divorce, separation, or death; threatened role changes, such as loss of job, marriage, new baby, or children leaving household; unmet needs, such as security; lack of control over events; ethical or emotional conflict.

NURSING DIAGNOSIS: Ineffective individual coping: Impairment of adaptive behaviors and problem-solving abilities for meeting life's demands and roles. (Usual strategies for handling stressful life situations are insufficient to control anxiety, fear, or anger.)

Defining Characteristics

- Verbalization of inability to cope
- Inability to solve problem effectively; inappropriate or ineffective use of defense mechanisms
- Feelings of anxiety, fear, anger, irritability, tension
- Physiologic disturbances associated with stress (eg, increased heart rate, respiratory rate, blood pressure, perspiration, chronic fatigue, sleep pattern disturbance)
- Presence of life stress
- Inability to meet role expectations
- Inability to meet basic needs
- Excessive smoking, alcohol consumption, drug use, or food intake
- Excessive risk-taking behavior, such as speeding when driving, participating in dangerous activities, or not using appropriate safety precautions when participating in high-risk activities
- Change in social participation

Related Factors

Situational crises, such as natural disasters or loss of loved ones through separation, divorce, or death; maturational crises, such as marriage, career pressures, changes in financial status, or retirement; problem-solving skills deficit; physiologic or psychologic alteration or impairment; inaccurate appraisal of stressful event; inappropriate use of coping resources.

Sources: LJ Carpenito, *Nursing Diagnosis: Application to Clinical Practice*, 4th ed. (Philadelphia: Lippincott, 1992), pp. 140–55, 268–91; M Gordon, *Manual of Nursing Diagnosis 1993–1994* (St Louis: Mosby, 1993), pp. 253, 355; GK McFarland and EA McFarlane, *Nursing Diagnosis and Intervention: Planning for Patient Care*, 2d ed. (St Louis: Mosby, 1993), pp. 492–98, 686–94.

- **Anxiety**
- **Ineffective individual coping**

These diagnoses, with definitions, contributing factors, and defining characteristics, are shown in the box above. Clinical applications of these diagnoses are shown in Table 32–4.

Alternative diagnoses in which responses to stressful situations or events may be an etiology include the following:

- **Fear** related to anticipated treatment (eg, surgery, chemotherapy) or language barrier
- **Defensive coping**

- **Family coping: potential for growth**
- **Ineffective family coping: compromised**
- **Ineffective family coping: disabling**
- **Decisional conflict** related to conflict with personal values/beliefs or an ethical dilemma

PLANNING

The nurse develops plans in collaboration with the client and significant support persons when possible, according to the client's state of health (eg, ability to return to work), level of anxiety, support resources, coping mechanisms, and sociocultural and religious affiliation. The nurse with little experience intervening with clients undergoing stress may wish to consult with a clinical specialist or a more experienced nurse to develop effective plans. The nurse and client set goals to change the existing client responses to the stressor or stressors.

The overall client goals for persons experiencing stress-related responses are to decrease anxiety and fear and to increase the ability to manage or cope with stressful events or circumstances. See the Care Planning Guide on page 844 for clients experiencing stress. Some suggested outcome criteria follow.

The client

- Verbalizes a reduced level of anxiety.
- Develops realistic goals.
- Expresses feelings in a positive way.
- Verbalizes feelings to another.
- Develops effective coping mechanisms in managing stress:
  a. Identifies alternative strategies for coping with stress.
  b. Selects appropriate strategies.
  c. Receives adequate support for coping.
  d. Expresses ability to cope with multiple life changes.

IMPLEMENTING

Although stress accompanies every disease and illness, it is also highly individual; a situation that to one person is a major stressor may not affect another. Some methods to help reduce stress will be effective for one person; other methods will be appropriate for a different person. A nurse who is sensitive to clients' needs and reactions can choose those methods of intervention that will be most effective for each individual.

Table 32–4 Clinical Application: Assessment Data Clusters and Related Nursing Diagnoses: Stress and Coping Abilities

Data Cluster	Nursing Diagnosis
Darryl Johnson, a 47-year-old accountant, was admitted to the emergency department with a heart attack. He says, "I'm scared about this. My dad died of a heart attack when he was 48 years old." He appears restless, questions everything that is going on, and is hyperventilating.	**Anxiety** related to change in health status and threat of dying
Sonia Park, a 33-year-old mother of three, returned to nursing after taking a refresher course. She says, "I'm so tired since I started work. I'm not keeping up with housekeeping the way I should, and I'm not spending as much time with the kids. I'm too tired to shop and go to my son's baseball game. Tom and all the kids are helping out and not complaining, but I just keep thinking they wish I still baked cookies and played more with them. I'm sure not sleeping well, and I'm having awful headaches."	**Ineffective individual coping** related to work overload and unrealistic expectations

MINIMIZING ANXIETY

One way to reduce or perhaps eliminate anxiety is for the nurse and client to establish goals that are attainable. Clients must first recognize that they are anxious. This recognition is best brought about in an atmosphere of warmth and trust. Sometimes anxious clients react negatively to nurses because of personal frustration. It is important for nurses to understand this response and react to the behavior in a calm, accepting, and confident manner.

After clients realize that they are anxious, it is important to discuss all the possible reasons for their anxiety. Perley (1984, p. 362) categorizes three underlying states of mind associated with anxiety: *helplessness*, such as that in the person who has recently had a stroke and is unable to perform previous functions; *isolation*, such as that in an adolescent who fears rejection because of a sexually transmitted disease; and *insecurity*, such as that in a person

CARE PLANNING GUIDE

CLIENTS EXPERIENCING STRESS

NURSING DIAGNOSIS: Anxiety related to stress (specify)

Outcome Criteria	Nursing Interventions	Rationale
The client		
▪ Describes cause and level of anxiety.	Help the client determine sources of anxiety. Help the client determine level of anxiety (mild, moderate, severe, panic).	These actions help the client establish realistic understanding of the nature and cause of the anxiety. Once the stress is accurately understood, the anxiety may decrease, and the client can more readily identify strategies for coping.
▪ Verbalizes feelings related to anxiety.	Encourage the client to verbalize feelings and express emotions (cry, shout).	Sharing concerns and expressing emotions can decrease the client's feelings of being alone or overwhelmed by stressful situations.
▪ Describes usual coping patterns.	Help the client recognize usual coping patterns and their effectiveness.	Identifying usual coping strategies enables the client to determine the effectiveness of existing coping mechanisms and consider developing new coping strategies more appropriate to the present situation.
▪ Verbalizes an increase in emotional and physical comfort.	Provide reassurance and comfort. Stay with the client. Support present coping strategies. Speak slowly and calmly. Convey a sense of caring and empathy.	Providing a reassuring presence decreases the client's sense of aloneness and supports the client in coping.
	Decrease sensory stimulation.	Excessive sensory stimulation may increase the client's anxiety.

NURSING DIAGNOSIS: Ineffective individual coping

Outcome Criteria	Nursing Interventions	Rationale
The client		
▪ Appraises accurately the stressful event or circumstance.	Help the client determine the nature of the stressful event or circumstance.	This provides the client with a more realistic understanding of the nature of the stress.
▪ Identifies personal strengths and usual coping patterns.	Help the client determine personal strengths and differentiate positive from negative coping mechanisms.	Identifying personal sources of strength and differentiating ineffective or harmful coping patterns from effective coping patterns improve the client's self-concept and sense of ability to manage stress.
▪ Verbalizes feelings related to emotional state.	Support positive expressions of emotions.	Expressing emotions can decrease the perceived intensity of the stressor.
▪ Develops new coping strategies for managing stress.	Help the client identify new strategies for managing stress (eg, relaxation, exercise, imagery, massage).	New coping strategies can enable the client to manage present and future stressful situations in a more effective manner.

who is worried about being unable to earn a living or pay medical bills. When clients can identify the cause of their anxiety, they may find it helpful to explore the cause with the objective of learning better coping strategies. General nursing guidelines to minimize the client's anxiety and stress follow:

- *Support the client and family at a time of illness.* By conveying caring and understanding, the nurse can help clients reduce their stress. Feeling that someone else cares is a source of support to stressed people. Often families require time to talk about their worries and anxieties before they can feel assured and less stressed.
- *Orient the client to the hospital or agency.* The nurse helps the client adjust to the role change from, for example, independent wage earner to relatively dependent client. The nurse can help family members by giving information, for instance, about visiting hours and specific unit policies.
- *Give the client in a hospital some way of maintaining identity.* A person's name and clothes are important parts of the person's uniqueness as an individual. Nurses can help clients maintain identity by addressing them by the name they prefer and by assisting them to wear their own clothes in a hospital setting, when this is possible.
- *Provide information when the client has insufficient information.* Fear of the unknown and incorrect information can frequently cause stress. Stressed clients often misunderstand facts related by health personnel. Additional information or clarification can allay stress.
- *Repeat information when the client has difficulty remembering.* Nurses can assist clients by repeating information when it is requested and assisting people to apply it when they so desire. This problem is particularly prevalent among elderly people who are stressed by a change of setting as well as by their illness.
- *Encourage the client to participate in the plan of care.* Loss of the right to determine their own destiny can be very stressful to some people, particularly adults who function independently or who assume responsibility for others in their daily lives.
- *Give the client time to express feelings and thoughts.* Allow time for clients to describe their feelings and worries if they wish. Nurses should be sensitive to clients' needs and neither probe with prying questions nor be too busy to listen.
- *Ensure that expectations are within the client's capabilities.* Whatever the activity, whether an exercise or recreation, the nurse should make sure that it is possible for the client to accomplish it. If an activity is beyond the client's ability, the client is likely to be more stressed by not achieving the goal.
- *Be sensitive to specific situations and experiences that increase anxiety and stress for clients.* For example, a man might appear highly stressed each time he receives an intramuscular injection. A careful remark by the nurse about the stress may elicit information that the nurse can use to assist the client.
- *Assist a client to make a correct appraisal of a situation.* Sometimes, through a lack of knowledge or misinterpretation of a sequence of events, people draw incorrect conclusions. Having valid information might relieve the client's stress.
- *Provide an environment in which a person can function independently to some degree without assistance.* It may be difficult and stressful for an adult to assume the dependent client role even for a short time. By restoring some degree of independent functioning, such as by adapting eating utensils so that the clients can feed themselves, nurses can lower clients' stress levels.
- *Reinforce positive environmental factors and recognize negative ones to help reduce stress.* Dwelling on problems and difficulties increases stress, but focusing on what can be accomplished positively usually decreases stress.
- *Arrange for other clients with similar experiences to visit.* Clients with colostomies or similar conditions may be highly stressed and feel that they will never be able to live a normal life again. Meeting another person who has successfully adjusted to a colostomy can lower the stress greatly.
- *Bring clients and their support persons into contact with people in community agencies who can help them make valid plans.* Social workers are familiar with discharge planning and arrangements that a client may need to make. Often people are stressed needlessly because they do not know what help is available to them in the community.
- *Communicate competence, understanding, and empathy rather than stress and anxiety.* When a nurse conveys stress or anxiety, the client and support persons may be concerned about the nurse's ability to function where the client's health and life are involved. To reduce a client's stress, nurses need to know themselves well and be able to function in a nondefensive manner that conveys competence and empathy.
- *Encourage humor as a means of coping with stressors.* According to Simon (1988), humor has both psychologic and physical benefits. Psychologically, humor relieves tension and anxiety, reduces aggression, and distracts from sadness or guilt. This promotes a feeling of relaxation and well-being. The physiologic benefits include alternating states of stimulation and relaxation. During laughter, stimulation causes increases in respiratory rate, heart rate, muscular tension, and oxygen exchange. A state of relaxation follows laughter, during

which heart rate, blood pressure, respiration, and muscle tension decrease. Humor stimulates production of catecholamines and hormones and increases pain tolerance by releasing endorphins (Fry 1979).

MEDIATING ANGER

Often nurses find clients' anger difficult to handle. Caring for the client who is angry is difficult for two reasons (Gluck 1981, p. 9):

- Clients rarely state, "I feel angry or frustrated," and rarely indicate the reason for their anger. Instead, they may refuse treatment, become verbally abusive or demanding, may threaten violence, or become overly critical. Their complaints rarely reflect the cause of their anger.
- Anger from clients can elicit fear and anger in the nurse, who may respond in a manner that intensifies the client's anger, even to the point of violence. The majority of nurses respond in a way that reduces their own stress rather than the client's stress (Gluck 1981, p. 11).

Responses whose main purpose is reducing a nurse's stress include defending, providing reassurance, offering advice or persuading, and retaliating aggressively. For example, this response to a client's demands is defensive: "I can't take care of everyone at once! We've been very busy this evening." This response does not recognize the client's problem and increases the client's tension and anger. A reassuring response, such as "You'll feel better as soon as you are up and about," is a way to recognize the problem and calm the client; however, it does not encourage the person to talk about the problem. Responses meant to offer advice or persuade often begin with the words "Yes, but, . . ." By offering advice or persuading, nurses focus on their own values and ideas, thus increasing the client's sense of powerlessness. Aggressive responses indicate disapproval of the client's behavior. For example, a nurse might say, "You're spoiled. You could do that yourself." Or a nurse might say, "What do *you* want *now?* Some people here are a lot sicker than you and need my help."

Responses that reduce the client's anger and stress include offering help, apologizing, asking relevant questions, and conveying understanding. For example, the nurse might respond by saying, "I guess it's pretty frustrating being alone and having to wait for others to do things for you." Gluck (1981, p. 10) suggests that nurses wishing to provide understanding responses to clients follow these guidelines:

- Focus on the feeling words of the client.
- Note the general content of the message.
- Restate the feeling and content of what the client has communicated.
- Observe the client's body language.
- Ask, "If I were in the client's shoes, what would I be feeling?"

In addition to these general guidelines for minimizing stress, several health promotion strategies are often appropriate as interventions for clients with stress related nursing diagnoses. Among these are physical exercise and recreation, optimal nutrition, adequate rest and sleep, time management, and relaxation techniques.

MASSAGE

A variety of massage strokes or movements may be used singly or in combination, depending on the outcome desired. These include **effleurage** (stroking), friction, pressure, **petrissage** (kneading or large, quick pinches of the skin, subcutaneous tissue, and muscle), vibration, and percussion.

Historically, the back massage has been used by nurses to enhance or induce relaxation before sleep or to stimulate skin circulation in association with hygienic measures. Support persons, too, can provide the technique to loved ones. See Procedure 35–1, page 965, for a back massage technique that includes a combination of massage strokes.

The duration of a massage ranges from 5 to 20 minutes, in accordance with the client's tolerance. Before offering a massage, the nurse must ensure that the environment is free of distractions and interruptions and that the room temperature is comfortable for the client with the back uncovered. The nurse must also feel relaxed and convey an attitude that the massage will alleviate pain, stress, and physical and mental tension. Because cultural and religious beliefs regarding personal touch may cause the client emotional discomfort during massage therapy, the nurse must, in addition, ensure that the client is receptive to the therapy.

PROGRESSIVE RELAXATION

Relaxation techniques have been used extensively to reduce high levels of stress and chronic pain. Using relaxation techniques enables the client to exert control over the body's responses to tension and anxiety. For many years, nurses on maternity units have encouraged women in labor to relax and breathe rhythmically.

Progressive relaxation requires that the client (a) tense and then relax successive muscle groups, and (b) focus attention on discriminating the feelings experienced when the muscle group is relaxed in contrast to when it was tense. Jacobsen (1938), the originator of the progressive relaxation technique, found that tension of a muscle

A TOTAL BODY RELAXATION TECHNIQUE

- Inhale. Send breath down to your toes and relax them. Send breath to the soles of your feet and ankles, and relax them. Exhale. Your feet are now fully relaxed.
- Inhale. Send breath to the muscles of your lower legs from the ankles to the knees and relax them. First the left leg; then the right leg. Exhale. Feel the relaxation from your toes to the tops of your legs.
- Inhale. Send breath to your buttocks and groin and relax them. Exhale.
- Inhale. Send breath to your stomach and lower back muscles. Relax them. Exhale.
- Inhale. Send breath to your chest and upper back muscles. Relax them. Exhale.
- Inhale. Send breath to your shoulders, arms, and to the tips of your fingers. Relax them. Exhale.
- Inhale. Send breath to your forehead, cheeks, eyelids, and jaw muscles. Let jaw drop. Feel a comfortable letting go as these muscles are relaxed. Let this feeling of deep relaxation spread to your neck, throat, and tongue muscles. Exhale.
- Breathe very slowly and easily throughout this exercise, allowing breathing to match rhythms of the relaxed body.

Source: RB Murray and MM Huelskoetter, *Psychiatric/Mental Health Nursing: Giving Emotional Care* (Englewood Cliffs, NJ: Prentice Hall, 1983), p. 413. Used with permission.

group before its relaxation actually achieved a greater degree of relaxation than simply commanding oneself to relax. This technique can result in decreased body oxygen consumption, metabolism, respiratory rate, cardiac rate, muscle tension, and systolic and diastolic blood pressures.

Procedures for teaching progressive relaxation vary. The method for relaxing muscle groups, the specific muscle groups to be relaxed, the number of sessions involved, and the role of the instructor (taped versus live instructions) may differ. The box above provides an example of a total body relaxation technique.

GUIDED IMAGERY

Guided imagery involves the use of self-chosen or instructor-suggested positive images to achieve specific health-related goals. Imagery is "the formation of a mental representation of an object that is usually only perceived through the senses" (Sodergren 1985, p. 104). Images can have visual, auditory, olfactory, gustatory, or

Table 32–5 Types of Images

Type	Example
Visual	A valley scene with its many shades of greenery
Auditory	Ocean waves breaking rhythmically upon a beach
Olfactory	Freshly baked bread
Gustatory	A juicy hamburger
Tactile-proprioceptive	Stroking a soft, furry cat

tactile-proprioceptive qualities. For examples of the different types of images used to assist in acute and chronic pain control and to augment relaxation techniques, see Table 32–5. Images often evoke more than one sense. For example, the image of waves breaking upon a shore may combine the visual picture with the sound of the waves and the smell of the salt air. Such images focus the mind *away from* the body.

Imagery can be used to enhance other forms of medical and nursing therapies to improve the body's response to therapy (eg, chemotherapy and radiation therapy). In these instances, an image of power, such as a crocodile, a knight on a white horse, or an intergalactic battleship may be selected to control or eradicate the problem (eg, a tumor). Such images focus the mind internally, or *toward* the body.

The nurse and client may explore together what images will be effective in achieving the desired goal. The client's religious and/or spiritual beliefs should be considered when determining helpful images. Images of religious or spiritual bliss can produce physical relaxation and mental peace. Images that are meaningful to the client need to be used.

BIOFEEDBACK

Biofeedback is a technique that brings under conscious control bodily processes normally thought to be beyond voluntary command. In the past, most physiologic processes were considered involuntary. However, it has been discovered that many of these processes are partially subject to voluntary control. Studies show that muscle tension, heartbeat, blood flow, peristalsis, and skin temperature, for example, can be controlled voluntarily. The feedback is usually provided through temperature meters that indicate skin temperature changes or an electromyogram (EMG) that shows the electric potential created by the contraction of muscles. Reduced EMG activity reflects muscle relaxation. Biofeedback teaches clients to

RESEARCH NOTE

Does Thermal Biofeedback Combined with Progressive Muscle Relaxation Training Reduce Blood Pressure in Clients with Essential Hypertension?

This study measured the effect of thermal biofeedback training combined with progressive relaxation training in the treatment of female clients who were diagnosed with essential hypertension. The sample consisted of 19 adult women 30 to 59 years of age who were not taking antihypertensive medication. Blood pressure decline was measured on the treatment group of 11 clients, who underwent thermal biofeedback combined with progressive muscle relaxation training, and on the control group of 8 clients, who underwent only progressive muscle relaxation training.

For both groups, baseline blood pressure was measured four times for 2 weeks. For the treatment group, blood pressure was measured twice, once before and once after each of the eight sessions of thermal biofeedback training for 4 weeks. For the control group, blood pressure was measured at every other visit to a clinic for progressive muscle relaxation self-training, twice before and after the self-training. On average, the treatment group experienced a decline in systolic blood pressure of 20.6 mm Hg and a decline in diastolic blood pressure of 14.4 mm Hg. In the control group, both systolic and diastolic blood pressures tended to increase.

Implications: Nurses should be knowledgeable about thermal biofeedback and progressive muscle relaxation techniques so that they can teach clients effective ways to manage essential hypertension in conjunction with other physician-prescribed treatments.

Source: YB Hahn, YJ Ro, HH Song, NC Kim, HS Kim, and YS Yoo. The effect of thermal biofeedback and progressive relaxation training in reducing blood pressure of patients with essential hypertension, *Image: Journal of Nursing Scholarship*, Fall 1993, 25:204–7.

achieve a generalized state of relaxation characterized by parasympathetic dominance and antagonistic to the pattern of physicologic arousal manifested in stress-related disorders.

THERAPEUTIC TOUCH

Therapeutic touch (TT) is a process by which energy is transmitted or transferred from one person to another with the intent of potentiating the healing process of one who is ill or injured. It is derived from, but not the same as, the "laying on of hands" associated with Eastern, European, and religious philosophies. Delores Krieger (1979), who coined the term *therapeutic touch*, refers to TT as a healing meditation, because the primary act of the nurse (healer) is to "center" the self and to maintain that center (mental concentration and focusing) throughout the process.

Basic to therapeutic touch are the concepts that the human being has an energy field—or, more properly, *is* an energy field (human field)—and that energy can be intentionally channeled from one person to another. The human field extends beyond the level of the skin and is perceptible to the trained sense (primarily touch) of a healer. This energy field can be most clearly "felt" within several feet of the body. An everyday experience that may demonstrate this field phenomenon is the feeling of having one's space invaded when someone stands too close in a crowded elevator, even though there is no physical contact.

The body and the environment are considered open systems and constantly exchange energy and matter. The pattern and organization of the human field are constantly affected by the flow of energy from the environment. In situations of disease, illness, or pain, the pattern and organization of the field are disrupted; there may be a loss of energy, a disruption in the flow, an accumulation, or a blockage (Wright 1987, p. 708).

The therapeutic touch process consists of the following four steps (Snyder 1985, p. 203):

1. *Centering* is a meditative step in which the person directs attention inward to achieve a sense of detachment, sensitivity, and balance.
2. *Assessing* is a head-to-toe scanning process in which the nurse holds the palms of both hands 2 to 3 inches over the client's skin surface. This process can be performed by one nurse or two. One nurse scans the client's front while the second nurse simultaneously scans the client's back. The purpose of the assessment is to detect asymmetric differences in the client's energy flow, such as heat, cold, tingling, congestion, pressure, emptiness, or other sensations.
3. *Unruffling* is a process in which an identified congestive energy field is "unruffled," or mobilized, to make the client's energy field more receptive and to enhance the transfer of energy from the nurse to the client. The nurse accomplishes this step by moving the hands (palms facing the client) in a sweeping motion from the area where pressure was perceived down along the long bones of the body.
4. *Transferring energy* is the process in which the actual transference of energy from the nurse to the client occurs. The nurse must know which form of energy to use, how to modulate energy, and where to apply energy. The form of energy has different effects and is

related to colors: Blue energy is sedating; yellow energy is stimulating and energizing; and green energy is harmonizing. The nurse modulates these energy forms by mentally visualizing the color, for example, visualizing light through a blue stained-glass window. The nurse may apply energy directly over an identified area of congestion or to one of the *chakras* (special channels that serve as entry areas for energy from the environment). These are located in the thoracic or solar plexus. Energy transference helps restore the balance of the energy field and provides additional energy to promote self-healing.

EVALUATING

To evaluate the achievement of client goals, the nurse collects data in accordance with the outcome criteria established earlier. Evaluation activities may include the following:

- Observing the client for absence or reduction of manifestations of fear and/or anxiety
- Measuring blood pressure and pulse rate
- Listening to the client's reports of increased physiologic or psychologic comfort, decreased emotional responsiveness, or verbalizations of fears and concerns
- Asking the client about personal strengths or coping resources identified
- Questioning the client about effective and ineffective coping responses and consequences
- Discussing situations in which the client has used specific adaptive coping methods and the client's perception of their effectiveness
- Asking the clients about specific resources used, including support persons

Examples of evaluative statements indicating goal achievement are "The client identified four personal strengths for coping with stressful events," "The client verbalized the ability to channel feelings of anger into assertive behaviors and exercise," and "The client attended a time-management seminar on July 20 and stated it was valuable."

STRESS MANAGEMENT FOR NURSES

Nurses, like clients, are susceptible to experiencing anxiety and crises. In recent years, more attention has been given to the occupational stress nurses experience. Nursing practice involves many stressors related to both clients and the work environment. Kinzel (1982, p. 55) devised a 20-item, 24-hour scale to help nurses measure their stress levels. All 20 items fall into five main categories: inadequate knowledge, inadequate support from peers and supervisors, dealing with death, poor communication, and salary and staffing problems. The purpose of such a scale is to make nurses aware of the source of negative feelings and frustration on the job, to help them make adjustments, and to support colleagues.

Nurses can manage stress by using all of the techniques discussed for clients. In addition, Hamilton (1984), Scully (1980), and Wilson (1989) suggest the following:

1. First recognize that you are stressed. Become attuned to feelings of being overwhelmed, fatigue, angry outbursts, and physical illness. Also be aware of increases in smoking, drinking coffee, or other substance abuse, and determine whether you are distancing yourself from client interaction.
2. When attuned to your reactions to stress, determine when the reactions occur.
3. When attuned to your stress and when it occurs, determine alternative actions to deal with it constructively. Some suggestions follow:
   a. Plan a daily relaxation program with meaningful quiet times to reduce tension.
   b. Establish an activity program to direct energy outward.
   c. Become more assertive to overcome feelings of powerlessness in relationships with others. Learn to say no.
   d. Manage time better by delegating to others and combining tasks.
   e. Take a course in biofeedback, yoga, meditation, or some other advanced relaxation technique.
   f. Learn to accept failures and learn from them.
   g. Learn to ask for help, and share your feelings with colleagues.
   h. Learn to support your colleagues in times of need. Give them a chance to "ventilate" feelings and listen to their concerns.
   i. Learn to handle problems constructively instead of defensively.
   j. Accept what cannot be changed. There are certain limitations in every situation.
   k. If working in an intensive care or similar unit (ICU), establish a structured emotional support group. These groups are identified by various names: ventilation groups, discussion forums, or regular staff meetings for the purpose of dealing with feelings and anxieties generated in the work setting.

Finally, nurses must learn to laugh and have fun. **Humor** is defined as the ability to discover, express, or appreciate the ludicrous or absurdly incongruous, to be amused by one's own imperfections or the whimsical aspects of life, and to see the fun side of an otherwise serious situation (Murray & Huelskoetter 1983, p. 192). Fay's research (1983) indicated that individuals most effective in coping with stress had the greatest ability to appreciate humor.

CHAPTER HIGHLIGHTS

- Stress is a state of physiologic or psychologic tension that affects the whole person—physically, emotionally, intellectually, socially, and spiritually.
- A person's response to stressors varies according to the way the stressor is perceived, its intensity and duration, the number of stressors, previous experience, coping mechanisms used, support people available, and age.
- A common psychologic response to stress is anciety, which is manifested in a variety of cognitive, verbal, and motor responses that reduce tension.
- Unconscious psychologic defense mechanisms, such as denial, rationalization, compensation, and sublimation, also protect the individual from tension.
- Both physiologic and psychologic responses to stressors can be adaptive or maladptive.
- Adaptation is a process of change in response to stress. It occurs in three interrelated modes: physiologic, psychologic, and sociocultural.
- Coping is a more immediate response to stress than adaptation.
- Coping strategies can be either effective or ineffective and result in adaptation or maladaptation, respectively.
- The nurse can help clients recognize stress and support clients' effective coping mechanisms.
- Nursing interventions for stress are aimed at reducing anxiety, at promoting clients' physical and mental well-being so that they handle stress more effectively, and at helping clients learn more effective coping mechanisms.
- Stress management strategies include massage, progressive relaxation exercises, guided imagery, biofeedback, and therapeutic touch.
- The nurse, too, is prone to occupational stress and needs to learn effective stress-management techniques.

READING AND REFERENCES

SUGGESTED READINGS

Cheneveret, M. 1993. *The Pro-Nurse Handbook.* 2d ed. St Louis: Mosby-Year Book.

Throughout this handbook, the author provides strategies for nurses to manage the stresses of professional life and prevent burnout.

Peddicord, K. December 1991. Strategies for promoting stress reduction and relaxation. *Nursing Clinics of North America* 26:867-74.

This article explores the Roy adaptation model and its application to various stress-reduction interventions to facilitate an understanding of the nurse's role in the management and prevention of stress-related problems.

RELATED RESEARCH

Kelley, SJ. Winter 1993. Caregiver stress in grandparents raising grandchildren. *Image: Journal of Nursing Scholarship* 25:331–37.

Younger, JB. March/April 1993. Development and testing of the Mastery of Stress Instrument. *Nursing Research* 42:68–73.

SELECTED REFERENCES

Abbott, J and Sutherland, C. 1990. Cognitive, cardiovascular and haematological responses of type A and type B individuals prior to and following examinations. *Journal of Social Behavior and Personality* 5(special issue) (1):343–68.

Anspaugh, DJ, Hamrick, MH, and Rosato, FD. 1991. *Concept and Applications: Wellness.* St Louis: Mosby-Year Book.

Bell, JM. March/April 1977. Stressful life events and coping methods in mental-illness and wellness behaviors. *Nursing Research* 26:136–40.

Blumenthal, JA, Williams, RS, King, Y, Schanberg, SM, and Thompson, L. 1978. Type A behavior pattern and coronary atherosclerosis. *Circulation* 58:634–39.

Breakwell, GM. August 1990. Are you stressed out? *American Journal of Nursing* 90:31–33.

Buckwalter, KC and Babich, KS. December 1990. Psychologic and physiologic aspects of depression. *Nursing Clinics of North America* 25:945–54.

Burgess, AW and Lazare, A. 1976. *Community Mental Health: Target Populations.* Englewood Cliffs, NJ: Prentice Hall.

Byrne, ML and Thompson, LF. 1978. *Key Concepts for the Study and Practice of Nursing.* St Louis: Mosby.

Caplan, G. February 1990. Loss, stress, and mental health. *Community Mental Health Journal* 26:27–48.

Caroselli-Dervan, C. September 1989. Modifying stress in cardiovascular patients: Nursing intervention. *Journal of Advanced Medical-Surgical Nursing* 1:11–20.

Carpenito, LJ. 1992. *Nursing Diagnosis: Application to Clinical Practice.* 4th ed. Philadelphia: Lippincott.

Case, RB, Heller, SS, Case, NB, and Moss, AJ. March 21, 1985. Type A behavior and survival after acute myocardial infarction. *New England Journal of Medicine* 312:634–39.

Detherage, KS and Johnson, SS. 1990. Stress reduction and crisis intervention. In Edelman, C and Mandle, CL, editors. *Health Promotion Throughout the Life Span.* 2d ed. St Louis: Mosby.

Duldt, BW. September 1981. Anger: An occupational hazard for nurses. *Nursing Outlook* 29:510–18.

Fay, R. October 1983. The defensive role of humor in the management of stress. *Dissertation Abstracts International* 44:1219B.

Folkman, S and Lazarus, RS. 1991. Coping and emotion. In Monat, A and Lazarus, RS. *Stress and Coping.* New York: Columbia University Press.

Frank, KA, Heller, SS, Kornfield, DS, Sporn, AA, and Weiss, MB. 1978. Type A behavior pattern and coronary angiographic findings. *Journal of the American Medical Association* 240:761–63.

Freud, S. 1946. *The Ego and the Mechanisms of Defense.* New York: International Universities Press.

Friedman, M and Rosenman, R. 1974. *Type A Behavior and Your Heart.* Greenwich, CT: Fawcett.

Fry, W. 1979. Humor and the human cardiovascular system. In Mindness, H and Turek, J, editors. *The Study of Humor.* Los Angeles: Antioch University.

Gluck, M. March 1981. Learning a therapeutic verbal response to anger. *Journal of Psychiatric Nursing and Mental Health Services* 19:9–12.

Gordon, M. 1993. *Manual of Nursing Diagnosis 1993–1994.* St Louis: Mosby-Year Book.

Hahn, YB, Ro, YJ, Song, HH, Kim, NC, Kim, HS, and Yoo, YS. Fall 1993. The effect of thermal biofeedback and progressive relaxation training in reducing blood pressure of patients with essential hypertension. *Image: Journal of Nursing Scholarship* 25:204–07.

Hales, D. 1992. *An Invitation to Health: Taking Charge of Your Life.* 5th ed. Redwood City, CA: Benjamin/Cummings.

Hamilton, JM. July/August 1984. Effective ways to relieve stress. *Nursing Life* 4:24–27.

Holmes, TH and Rahe, RH. August 1967. The social readjustment rating scale. *Journal of Psychomatic Research* 11:213–18.

Jacobsen, E. 1938. *Progressive Relaxation.* Chicago: University of Chicago Press.

Johnson, JE and Lauver, DR. January 1989. Alternative explanations of coping with stressful experiences associated with physical illness. *Advances in Nursing Science* 11:39–52.

Kinzel, SL. March/April 1982. What's your stress level? *Nursing Life* 2:54–55.

Kobasa, S. July 1984. How much stress can you survive? *American Health* 5:64–77.

Krieger, D. 1979. *The Therapeutic Touch: How to Use Your Hands to Help or Heal.* Englewood Cliffs, NJ: Prentice Hall.

Lazarus, RS. 1966. *Psychological Stress and the Coping Process.* New York: McGraw-Hill.

Lazarus, RS and Folkman, S. 1984. *Stress, Appraisal, and Coping.* New York: Springer.

Lyon, BL and Werner, J. 1987. Stress. In Fitzpatrick, JJ and Taunton, RI, editors. *Annual Review of Nursing Research.* Vol 5, pp. 3–22. New York: Springer.

McFarland, GK and McFarlane, EA. 1993. *Nursing Diagnosis and Intervention: Planning for Patient Care.* 2d ed. St Louis: Mosby-Year Book.

Monat, A and Lazarus, RS, editors. 1991. *Stress and Coping.* 3d ed. New York: Columbia University Press.

Monsen, RB, Floyd, RL, and Brookman, JC. October/December 1992. Stress-coping-adaptation: Concepts for nursing. *Nursing Forum* 27:27–32.

Murray, RB and Huelskoetter, MM. 1983. *Psychiatric/Mental Health Nursing: Giving Emotional Care.* Englewood Cliffs, NJ: Prentice Hall.

North American Nursing Diagnosis Association. 1992. *NANDA Nursing Diagnoses: Definitions and Classification 1992–1993.* Philadelphia: NANDA.

Nuernberger, P. 1981. *Freedom from Stress: A Holistic Approach.* Honesdale, PA: The Himalayan International Institute of Yoga Science and Philosophy.

Peddicord, K. December 1991. Strategies for promoting stress reduction and relaxation. *Nursing Clinics of North America* 26:867–74.

Perley, NZ. 1984. Problems in self-consistency: Anxiety. In Roy, C, editor. *Introduction to Nursing: An Adaptation Model.* Englewood Cliffs, NJ: Prentice Hall.

Perrez, M and Reicherts, M. 1992. *Stress, Coping, and Health.* Seattle: Hogrefe & Huber.

Schafer, W. 1992. *Stress Management for Wellness.* 2d ed. Philadelphia: Harcourt Brace Jovanovich.

Scully, R. May 1980. Stress in the nurse. *American Journal of Nursing* 80:912–14.

Selye, H. 1956. *The Stress of Life.* New York: McGraw-Hill.

______. 1976. *The Stress of Life,* revised ed. New York: McGraw-Hill.

Shekelle, RB, Hulley, S, Neaton, J, Billings, J, Borhani, N, Gerace, T, Jacobs, D, Lasser, N, Mittlemark, M, and Stamler, J. 1985. The MRFIT behavioral pattern study: II. Type A behavior pattern and incidence of coronary heart disease. *American Journal of Epidemiology* 122:559–70.

Simon, JM. August 1988. The therapeutic value of humor in aging adults. *Journal of Gerontological Nursing* 14:8–13.

Snyder, M. 1985. *Independent Nursing Interventions.* New York: Wiley.

Sodergren, KM. 1985. Guided imagery. In Snyder, M. pp. 103–24. *Independent Nursing Interventions.* New York: Wiley.

Volicer, BJ and Burns, MW. September/October 1975. A hospital stress rating scale. *Nursing Research* 24:358.

Whitley, GG. October/December 1992. Concept analysis of fear. *Nursing Diagnosis* 3(4):107–16.

Wilson, LK. December 1989. Professional growth section: High-gear nursing: How it can run you down and what you can do about it. *Nursing89* 19:81–82, 84, 86, 88.

Wright, SM. September 1987. The use of therapeutic touch in the management of pain. *Nursing Clinics of North America* 22:705–13.

______. July/September 1992. Concept analysis of anxiety. *Nursing Diagnosis* 3:107–16.

Younger, JB. March/April 1993. Development and testing of the Mastery of Stress Instrument. *Nursing Research* 42:68–73.

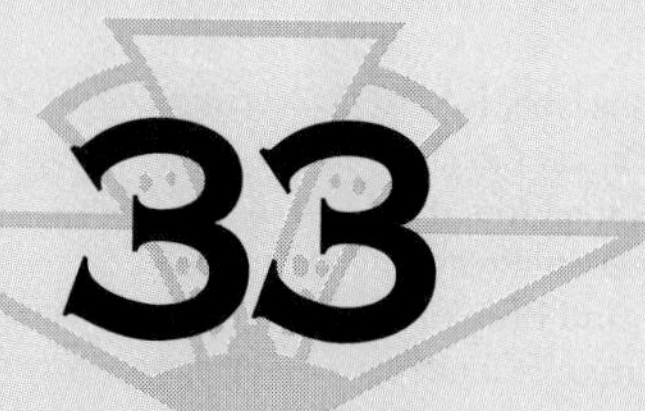

33 Loss, Grieving, and Death

Objectives

- Discuss selected frameworks for identifying stages of grieving.
- Identify clinical symptoms of grief.
- Discuss factors affecting a loss reaction.
- Recognize common fears associated with dying.
- Identify factors contributing to unresolved grief.
- Describe guidelines for helping clients to die with dignity.
- Identify measures that facilitate the grieving process.
- List clinical signs of impending and imminent death and of death itself.
- List changes that occur in the body after death.
- Describe nursing measures for care of the body after death.

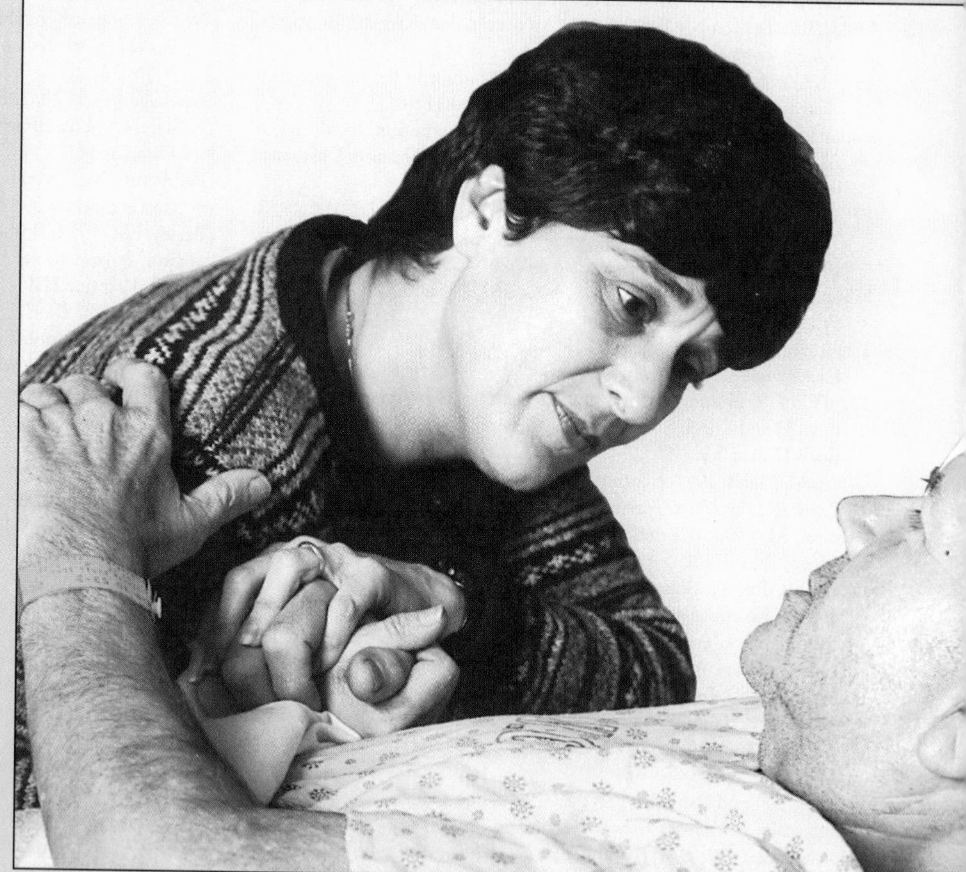

Loss, grieving, and death are experienced by everyone at some time during their life. People may suffer the loss of valued relationships through life changes, such as moving from one city to another, separation, divorce, or the death of parent, spouse or friend. People may grieve changing life roles as they watch grown children leave home, or they retire from their lifelong work. The loss of valued material objects through theft or natural disaster can evoke feelings of grief and loss. When people's lives are influenced by civil or national strife, they may grieve the loss of valued ideals such as safety, freedom, or democracy.

In the clinical setting the nurse encounters clients who may be experiencing grief related to decreasing health, loss of a body part, terminal illness, or the impending death of self or a significant other. The nurse may also work with clients in community settings who are grieving losses related to personal crisis (eg, divorce, separation) or natural disaster (earthquakes, floods, or hurricanes). Therefore, it is important that the nurse understand the significance of loss and develop the ability to assist clients as they work through the grieving process.

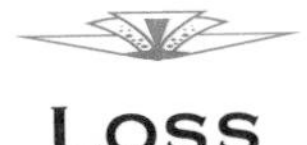

Loss

Loss is an actual or potential situation in which something that is valued is changed, no longer available, or gone. People can experience the loss of body image, a significant other, a sense of well-being, a job, personal possessions, beliefs, a sense of self, and so on. Illness and hospitalization often produce losses.

Death is a fundamental loss, both for the dying person and for those who survive. Although death is inevitable for everyone, it is a lonely experience that each person ultimately faces alone. Yet even death, like loss, can stimulate people to grow in perception of both themselves and others. Death can be viewed not simply as loss of life, but as the dying person's final opportunity to experience life in ways that bring meaning and fulfillment.

Types and Sources of Loss

There are two general types of loss, actual and perceived. Both actual losses and perceived losses can be anticipatory. An **actual loss** can be identified by others and can arise either in response to or in anticipation of a situation. For example, a woman whose husband is dying may experience actual loss in anticipation of his death. A **perceived loss** is experienced by one person but cannot be verified by others. Psychologic losses are often perceived losses, in that they are not directly verifiable. For example, a woman who leaves her employment to care for her children at home may perceive a loss of independence and freedom. An **anticipatory loss** is experienced before the loss really occurs.

There are many sources of loss: (a) loss of an aspect of oneself—a body part, a physiologic function, or a psychologic attribute, (b) loss of an object external to oneself, (c) separation from an accustomed environment, and (d) loss of a loved or valued person.

Aspect of Self The loss of an aspect of self changes a person's body image, even though the loss may not be obvious to others. A face scarred from a burn is generally obvious to people; loss of part of the stomach or loss of ability to feel emotion may not be as obvious. The degree to which these losses affect a person largely depends on the integrity of the person's body image (part of self-concept). Sometimes, changes in self-image affect a person's social roles, such as the roles of employee, father, and husband. Any change that the person perceives as negative in the way the person relates to the environment can be considered a loss of self.

Losses such as divorce can have considerable impact. A divorce may mean loss of financial security, a home, daily routines, and one's role as spouse. Therefore, even when the divorce was desired, the sense of loss can last for some time afterward.

During old age, dramatic changes occur in physical and mental capabilities. Again the self-image is vulnerable, and support and reassurance are important. Old age is when people usually experience many losses: of employment, of usual activities, of independence, of health, of friends, and of family.

External Objects Loss of external objects includes (a) loss of inanimate objects that have importance to the person, such as the loss of money for a person without financial means, or the burning down of a family's house, and (b) loss of animate objects such as pets that provide love and companionship.

Accustomed Environment Separation from an environment and people who provide security can result in a sense of loss. The 6-year-old sheltered by home and family is likely to feel loss when first attending school and relating to more people. The university student who moves away from home for the first time also experiences a sense of loss.

Loved Ones The loss of a loved one or valued person through illness, separation, or death can be very disturbing. In illness such as brain damage from viral infection or stroke, a person may undergo personality changes that make friends and family feel they have lost that person.

The death of a loved one is a permanent and complete loss. In primitive societies, death was considered a normal, natural event, and life was seldom long. In contemporary North American society, death is denied. People are uncomfortable with talking about death and being around people who are dying. Death usually occurs in private. Death often happens in a hospital or in a home in the presence of immediate family. There is a tendency to prolong and preserve life. The culture reveres youthfulness; although people expect to live to old age, this is not considered as attractive as youth.

LOSS AS CRISIS

Loss can be viewed as either a situational or a developmental crisis. The loss of one's job, the death of a child, or the loss of functional ability as a result of acute illness or injury, for example, are unexpected situational crises. Losses that occur in the process of normal development—such as the departure of grown children from the home, retirement from a career, and the death of aged parents—are developmental crises that can be anticipated and, to some extent, prepared for.

How individuals deal with loss is closely related to their stage of development, personal resources, and social support systems. When caring for clients who are experiencing loss of functional ability resulting from acute or chronic illness, who have experienced loss of a body part (eg, amputation of a limb, mastectomy), or who are in the process of dying, the nurse needs to consider the influence of these factors not only on the client, but also on the client's family and loved ones. All persons concerned experience the loss and may exhibit different expressions of grieving.

GRIEF AND BEREAVEMENT

Grief is the total response to the emotional experience related to loss. Grief is manifested in thoughts, feelings, and behaviors associated with overwhelming distress or sorrow. **Bereavement** is the subjective response experienced by the surviving loved ones after the death of a person with whom they have shared a significant relationship. **Mourning** is the behavioral process through which grief is eventually resolved or altered; it is often influenced by culture, religious experience, and custom. Grief and mourning are experienced not only by the person who faces the death of a loved one, but also by the person who suffers other kinds of losses.

Normal bereavement can last as long as a year or more. Dealing with loss caused by death is complex and intensely emotional and should not be oversimplified.

AGE AND THE IMPACT OF LOSS

Age affects a person's understanding of and reaction to loss. With experience, people usually increase their understanding and acceptance of life, loss, and death. As in other aspects of human development, children show more rapid and dramatic variation and changes in their understanding of death. Table 33–1 outlines the development of the concept of death through the life span.

People do not usually experience the loss of life or loved ones at regular intervals. As a result, preparation for these experiences is difficult. Coping with other of life's losses, such as the loss of a pet, the loss of a friend, and the loss of youth or a job, can help people anticipate the more severe loss of death by teaching them successful coping strategies.

Childhood Children differ from adults not only in their understanding of loss and death, but also in how they are affected by the loss of others. The child's patterns progress rapidly; adult patterns of growth and development are generally stable. The loss of a parent or other significant person can threaten the child's ability to develop, and regression sometimes results. Assisting the child with the grief experience includes helping the child regain the normal continuity and pace of emotional development.

Some adults may assume that children do not have the same need as an adult to grieve the loss of others. In situations of crisis and loss, children are sometimes pushed aside or protected from the pain. They can feel afraid, abandoned, and lonely. Careful work with bereaved children is especially necessary, because experiencing a loss in childhood can have serious effects later in life.

Early and Middle Adulthood As people grow, they come to experience loss as part of normal development. By middle age, for example, the loss of a parent through death seems a normal occurrence compared to the death of a younger person. Coping with the death of an aged parent has even been viewed as a necessary developmental task of the middle-aged adult.

For the middle-aged adult, the loss of a parent can signal the disintegration of the family of origin. It is also a forceful reminder that the adult child is part of the older generation and therefore closer to death. The challenge of this developmental crisis for adult children is to assess the psychologic legacy of the parent, integrating what is valuable into their own identity. If the relationship with the parent was full of conflict, the parent's death can help release the child's energy for more productive use.

The middle-aged adult can experience losses other than death of a loved one. For example, losses resulting from impaired health or body function and losses of various role functions can be difficult for the middle-aged adult. For the middle-aged adult, the ability to carry out the tasks associated with raising a family and developing a successful work role can be especially important. Murphy and Osband (1991, p. 603) state that "physical changes that result from illness or accidents have the capacity to frustrate a sense of accomplishment." How the middle-aged adult responds to such losses is influenced by previous experiences with loss, the person's sense of self-esteem, and the strength and availability of support.

Late Adulthood For older adults, the loss through death of a long-time mate is profound. Although individuals differ in their ability to deal with such a loss, research suggests that health problems for widows and widowers increase during the first year following the death of the spouse. (Richter 1984). Because the majority of deaths occur among the elderly, and because the number of elderly is increasing in North America, nurses will need to be especially alert to the potential problems of older grieving adults.

Additional losses experienced by the elderly include loss of health, loss of mobility, loss of independence, and loss of work role. Limited income and the need to change one's living accommodations can also lead to feelings of loss and grieving.

Educating the Nurse About Death

People in North America are socialized to think of death as the worst occurrence in life. They therefore do their best to avoid thinking or talking about death—especially their own. Death is thought about rarely, and almost exclusively in negative terms. Nurses are not immune to such attitudes. They need to take time to analyze their own feelings about death before they can effectively help others with a terminal illness. Nurses who are unconsciously uncomfortable with dying clients tend to impede the clients' attempts to discuss dying and death in these ways:

- Changing the subject (eg, "Let's think of something more cheerful," or "You shouldn't say things like that")
- Offering reassurance (eg, "You are doing very well")
- Denying what is happening (eg, "You don't really mean that," or "You're going to live until you're a hundred")
- Being fatalistic (eg, "Everyone dies sooner or later," or "God will take you when He wants you")
- Blocking discussion (eg, "I don't think things are really that bad"), conveying an attitude that stops further discussion of the subject
- Being aloof and distant or avoiding the client
- "Managing" the client's care and making the client feel increasingly dependent and powerless

Caring for the dying and the bereaved is one of the nurse's most complex and challenging responsibilities,

Table 33–1 Development of the Concept of Death

Age	Beliefs/Attitudes
Infancy to 5 years	Does not understand concept of death Infant's sense of separation forms basis for later understanding of loss and death Believes death is reversible, a temporary departure, or sleep Emphasizes immobility and inactivity as attributes of death
5 to 9 years	Understands that death is final Believes own death can be avoided Associates death with aggression or violence Believes wishes or unrelated actions can be responsible for death
9 to 12 years	Understands death as the inevitable end of life Begins to understand own mortality, expressed as interest in afterlife or as fear of death Expresses ideas about death gathered from parents and other adults
12 to 18 years	Fears a lingering death May fantasize that death can be defied, acting out defiance through reckless behaviors, (eg, dangerous driving, substance abuse) Seldom thinks about death, but views it in religious and philosophic terms May seem to reach "adult" perception of death but be emotionally unable to accept it May still hold concepts from previous developmental stages
18 to 45 years	Has attitude toward death influenced by religious and cultural beliefs
45 to 65 years	Accepts own mortality Encounters death of parents and some peers Experiences peaks of death anxiety Death anxiety diminishes with emotional well-being
65 years +	Fears prolonged illness Encounters death of family members and peers Sees death as having multiple meanings, (eg, freedom from pain, reunion with already deceased family members)

Table 33–2 Client Responses and Nursing Implications in Kübler-Ross's Stages of Grieving

Stage	Behavioral Responses	Nursing Implications
Denial	Refuses to believe that loss is happening Is unready to deal with practical problems, such as prosthesis after loss of leg May assume artificial cheerfulness to prolong denial	Verbally support client's denial for its protective function. Examine your own behavior to ensure that you do not share in client's denial.
Anger	Client or family may direct anger at nurse or hospital staff, about matters that normally would not bother them	Help client understand that anger is a normal response to feelings of loss and powerlessness. Avoid withdrawal or retaliation with anger; do not take anger personally. Deal with needs underlying any angry reaction. Provide structure and continuity to promote feelings of security. Allow clients as much control as possible over their lives.
Bargaining	Seeks to bargain to avoid loss May express feelings of guilt or fear of punishment for past sins, real or imagined	Listen attentively, and encourage client to talk to relieve guilt and irrational fear. If appropriate, offer spiritual support.
Depression	Grieves over what has happened and what cannot be May talk freely (eg, reviewing past losses such as money or job), or may withdraw	Allow client to express sadness. Communicate nonverbally by sitting quietly without expecting conversation. Convey caring by touch. Help support persons understand importance of being with the client in silence.
Acceptance	Comes to terms with loss May have decreased interest in surroundings and support persons May wish to begin making plans (eg, will, prosthesis, altered living arrangements)	Help family and friends understand client's decreased need to socialize and need for short, quiet visits. Encourage client to participate as much as possible in the treatment program.

bringing into play all the skills needed for holistic physiologic and psychosocial care. To be effective, nurses must come to grips with their own attitudes toward loss, death, and dying, because these attitudes will directly affect their ability to provide care.

The curricula of many nursing schools include education about death. Agencies and associations sponsor continuing education programs aimed at reducing death anxiety among nursing staff. Other programs help nurses explore the specific problems of direct contact with terminally ill clients and around-the-clock responsibility for their care. In all such programs, nurses learn not only their own attitudes and concerns but also ways to support and comfort each other when they experience anger and frustration in the grief that follows the death of clients whom they not only cared for but also cared about.

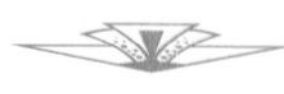

GRIEF

Grieving, the normal response to loss, is essential for good mental and physical health. It permits the individual to cope with the loss gradually and to accept it as part of reality. Grief is a social process; it is best shared and carried out with the assistance of others.

Working through one's grief is important, because bereavement has been shown to have potentially devastating effects on health. Among the symptoms that can accompany grief are anxiety, depression, weight loss, difficulties in swallowing, vomiting, fatigue, headaches, dizziness, fainting, blurred vision, skin rashes, excessive sweating, menstrual disturbances, palpitations, chest pain, dyspnea, and infection. The bereaved may also experience alterations in libido, concentration, and patterns of eating, sleeping, activity, and communication.

Although bereavement can threaten health, a positive resolution of the grieving process can enrich the individual with new insights, values, challenges, openness, and sensitivity. This applies to both the dying person and surviving loved ones, for the dying person is also living. If the quality of life permits, the dying person also should have the opportunity to grow emotionally and spiritually in the time that remains.

STAGES OF GRIEVING

Many authors have described stages or phases of grieving, perhaps the most famous of them being Kübler-Ross, who has described five stages: denial, anger, bargaining, depression, and acceptance (Kübler-Ross 1969, pp. 38–137). See Table 33–2. Engel (1964, pp. 94–96) has identified six stages of grieving: shock and disbelief, developing awareness, restitution, resolving the loss, idealization, and outcome. See Table 33–3. More recently, Sanders (1989) has described five phases of bereavement: shock, awareness, conservation/withdrawal, healing, and renewal. See Table 33–4 on page 858.

Nurses also have written about the components of grief. Clark (1984) describes a three-phase course through which the bereaved progresses, lasting 6 months to 2 years. Martocchio (1985) discusses five clusters of grief and maintains that there is no single correct way, nor a correct timetable, by which a person progresses through the grief process. Whether a person can succeed in integrating the loss and how this is accomplished are related to that person's individual development and personal makeup. And individuals responding to the very same loss cannot be expected to follow the same pattern or schedule in resolving their grief, even while they support each other. Martocchio's five clusters of grief include the following:

1. *Shock and disbelief.* A feeling of numbness is a common response immediately following the death of a loved one. The bereaved may feel depressed, angry, guilty, and sad. Disbelief or denial may persist even though the loss has been accepted intellectually.
2. *Yearning and protest.* The anger that the bereaved feel may be directed at the deceased for having died, at God, at others whose loved ones are still alive, or at the caregivers. The bereaved may begin to fear their own mental deterioration and withdraw from sharing their thoughts and feelings with others.
3. *Anguish, disorganization, and despair.* When the reality of the loss is genuinely admitted, depression can set in. Weeping is common at this time. The bereaved lose interest and motivation in pursuing the future, are unable to make decisions, and lack confidence and purpose. Activities that were once enjoyed with the deceased are now without attraction. Coping strategies such as excessive drinking may compromise health.
4. *Identification in bereavement.* The bereaved may take on the behavior, personal traits, habits, and ambitions of the deceased. Sometimes they may also experience the same symptoms of physical illness.

Table 33–3 Engel's Stages of Grieving

Stage	Behavioral Responses
Shock and disbelief	Refusal to accept loss
	Stunned feelings
	Intellectual acceptance but emotional denial
Developing awareness	Reality of loss begins to penetrate consciousness
	Anger may be directed at hospital, nurses, etc.
	Crying and self-blame
Restitution	Rituals of mourning (eg, funeral)
Resolving the loss	Attempts to deal with painful void
	Still unable to accept new love object to replace lost person
	May accept more dependent relationship with support person
	Thinks over and talks about memories of the dead person
Idealization	Produces image of dead person that is almost devoid of undesirable features
	Represses all negative and hostile feelings toward deceased
	May feel guilty and remorseful about past inconsiderate or unkind acts to deceased
	Unconsciously internalizes admired qualities of deceased
	Reminders of deceased evoke fewer feelings of sadness
	Reinvests feelings in others
Outcome	Behavior influenced by several factors: importance of lost object as source of support, degree of dependence on relationship, degree of ambivalence toward deceased, number and nature of other relationships, and number and nature of previous grief experiences (which tend to be cumulative)

Source: GL Engel, Grief and grieving, *American Journal of Nursing*, September 1964, 64:93–98. Used by permission.

Table 33–4 Sanders's Phases of Bereavement

Phase	Description	Characteristics
Shock	Survivors are left with feelings of confusion, unreality, and disbelief that the loss has occurred. They are often unable to process the normal thought sequences. Phase may last from a few minutes to many days.	Disbelief Confusion Restlessness Feelings of unreality Regression and helplessness State of alarm Physical symptoms: dryness of mouth and throat, sighing, weeping, loss of muscular control, uncontrolled trembling, sleep disturbance, and loss of appetite. Psychologic symptoms: preoccupation with thoughts of the deceased and psychologic distancing
Awareness of loss	After the funeral, friends and family resume normal activities. The bereaved experience the full significance of their loss.	Separation anxiety Conflicts Acting out emotional expectations Prolonged stress Physical symptoms: crying and sleep disturbance Psychologic symptoms: anger, guilt, frustration, shame, oversensitivity, disbelief and denial, dreaming, sense of presence of the deceased, and fear of death
Conservation/withdrawal	During this phase, survivors feel a need to be alone to conserve and replenish both physical and emotional energy. The social support available to the bereaved has decreased, and they may experience despair and helplessness.	Physical symptoms: weakness, fatigue, need for more sleep, and a weakened immune system Psychologic symptoms: withdrawal, obsessional review, grief work, and ultimately a renewal of hope
Healing: the turning point	During this phase, the bereaved move from distress about living without their loved one to learning to live more independently.	Assuming control Identity restructuring Relinquishing roles, such as spouse, child, or parent Physical symptoms: increased energy, sleep restoration, immune system restoration, and physical healing Psychologic symptoms: forgiving, forgetting, searching for meaning, and hope
Renewal	In this phase, survivors move on to a new self-awareness, an acceptance of responsibility for self, and learning to live without the deceased.	Functional stability Revitalization Assumption of responsibility for self-care needs Psychologic symptoms: loneliness, anniversary reactions, and a reaching out to others

Source: Adapted from CM Sanders, *Grief: The Mourning After: Dealing with Adult Bereavement*, (New York: Wiley, 1989).

5. *Reorganization and restitution.* Achieving stability and a sense of reintegration can take a period of time that ranges widely, from less than a year to several years. Although the bereaved are able to experience a sense of well-being and can resume most normal patterns of functioning, the feelings of grief do not simply cease. For many the pain of loss, though diminished, recurs for the rest of their lives.

A normal grief reaction may be abbreviated or anticipatory. *Abbreviated grief* is brief but genuinely felt. The lost object may not have been sufficiently important to the grieving person or may have been replaced immediately by another, equally esteemed object. *Anticipatory grief* is experienced in advance of the event. The wife who grieves before her ailing husband dies is anticipating the loss. A beauty queen may grieve in advance of an operation that will leave a scar on her body. Because many of the normal symptoms of grief will have already been expressed in anticipation, the reaction when the loss actually occurs may be quite abbreviated.

Unhealthy grief—that is, *pathologic* or *dysfunctional grief*—may be unresolved or inhibited. Both normal and unhealthy grief may be delayed. Many factors can contribute to dysfunctional grief, including a prior traumatic loss in childhood and the circumstances of the present loss. For instance, the sudden, untimely death of an adolescent or young adult can complicate the expression and resolution of grief. Other influences include family or cultural barriers to the emotional expression of grief.

Unresolved grief is extended in length and severity. The same signs are expressed as with normal grief, but the bereaved may also have difficulty expressing the grief, may deny the loss, or may grieve beyond the expected time. With *inhibited grief*, many of the normal symptoms of grief are suppressed, and other effects, including somatic, are experienced instead.

Burgess and Lazare (1976, p. 100) state that dysfunctional grief may be inferred from the following data or observations:

- The client fails to grieve following the death of a loved one; for example, a husband does not cry at, or absents himself from, his wife's funeral.
- The client becomes recurrently symptomatic on the anniversary of a loss or during holidays (especially Thanksgiving and Christmas).
- The client avoids visiting the grave and refuses to participate in religious memorial services of a loved one, even though these practices are a part of the client's culture.
- The client develops persistent guilt and lowered self-esteem.
- Even after a prolonged period, the client continues to search for the lost person. Some make the search while in fugue states. Others may wander from town to town or act as if they were expecting the deceased to return. Some may consider suicide to effect reunion.
- A relatively minor event triggers symptoms of grief.
- Even after a period of time, the client is unable to discuss the deceased with equanimity; for example, the client's voice cracks and quivers, eyes become moist.
- An interview of the client is characterized by themes of loss.
- After the normal period of grief, the client experiences physical symptoms similar to those of the person who died.
- The client's relationships with friends and relatives worsen following the death.

Many factors contribute to *unresolved grief*:

- Ambivalence (intense feelings of both love and hate) toward the lost person. The bereaved is often afraid to grieve for fear of discovering unacceptable negative feelings.
- A perceived need to be brave and in control; fear of losing control in front of others.
- Endurance of multiple losses, such as the loss of an entire family, which the bereaved finds too overwhelming to contemplate.
- Extremely high emotional value (overcathexis) invested in the dead person. Failure to grieve in this instance helps the bereaved avoid the reality of the loss.
- Uncertainty about the loss—for example, when a loved one is "missing in action."
- Lack of support persons.
- Subjection to socially unacceptable loss that cannot be spoken about, such as suicide, abortion, or giving a child up for adoption.

ASSESSING LOSS AND GRIEVING

To gather a complete database that allows accurate analysis and identification of appropriate nursing diagnoses for clients experiencing losses and grieving, the nurse first needs to recognize the state of awareness the client and family manifest, the symptoms of grief, and the factors influencing a loss reaction.

States of Awareness In cases of terminal illness, the state of awareness shared by the dying person and the family affects the nurse's ability to communicate freely with clients and other health care team members and to assist in the grieving process. Three types of awareness that have been described are closed awareness, mutual pretense, and open awareness.

In **closed awareness,** the client and family are unaware of impending death. They may not completely understand why the client is ill, and they believe the client will recover. The physician may believe it is best not to communicate a diagnosis or prognosis to the client or family. Nursing personnel are confronted with an ethical problem in this situation, and they have several choices. One course is to answer questions evasively or falsely. But ultimately the client and family will know the truth, and when they do they may recognize that information given them earlier was false. See Chapter 11 for further information on ethical dilemmas.

With **mutual pretense,** the client, family, and health personnel know that the prognosis is terminal but do not talk about it and make an effort not to raise the subject. Sometimes the client refrains from discussing death to protect the family from distress. The client may also sense discomfort on the part of health personnel and therefore not bring up the subject. Mutual pretense permits the client a degree of privacy and dignity, but it places a heavy burden on the dying person, who then has no one in whom to confide fears.

With **open awareness,** the client and people around know about the impending death and feel comfortable about discussing it, even though it is difficult. This awareness provides the client an opportunity to finalize affairs and even participate in planning funeral arrangements.

Not all people can handle open awareness. For example, a 45-year-old man who knows he is dying may be unable to discuss his forthcoming death without becoming angry at people around him. Whether to inform dying clients that their condition is terminal is a difficult issue for physicians. Some authorities believe that terminal clients acquire knowledge of their condition even if they are not directly informed. Others believe that many clients remain unaware of their condition until the end. It is difficult, however, to distinguish what clients know from what they are willing to accept. Cappon (1970) asked groups of healthy persons, physically ill clients, psychiatric clients, and dying clients whether they would like to know if a serious illness was terminal. The majority responded yes; however, of the four groups, the dying least desired this information (33% did not want to be told). Cappon concluded that physicians should be cautious and not give more information than the client wants.

Symptoms of Grief The nurse assesses the grieving client and/or family members following a loss to determine the phase or stage of grieving. Clinical symptoms of grief include the following:

- Repeated somatic distress
- Tightness in the chest
- Choking or shortness of breath
- Dryness of the mouth and throat
- Sighing
- Empty feeling in the abdomen
- Loss of muscular control
- Uncontrolled trembling
- Loss of appetite
- Sleep disturbance
- Intense subjective distress

Physiologically, the body responds to a current or anticipated loss with a stress reaction. The nurse can assess the clinical signs of this response. See Chapter 32. See also coping mechanisms and responses in Chapter 32.

Factors Influencing a Loss Reaction The influence of age and developmental level on a person's reaction to loss has already been discussed. Other factors include the personal significance of the loss, culture, spiritual beliefs, sex role, and socioeconomic status.

Significance of the Loss The significance of a loss depends on the perceptions of the individual experiencing the loss. One person may experience a great sense of loss over a divorce; another may find it only mildly disrupting. A number of factors affect the significance of the loss:

- Age of the person
- Value placed on the lost person, body part, and so on
- Degree of change required because of the loss
- The person's beliefs and values

Expectations can also greatly affect significance. For elderly people who have already encountered many losses (eg, the loss of family, health, independence), an anticipated loss such as their own death may not be important; they may be apathetic about it instead of reactive. More than fearing death, some may fear loss of control or becoming a burden.

Culture Culture influences an individual's reaction to loss. How grief is expressed is often determined by the customs of the culture. In the United States and Canada, unless an extended family structure exists, grief is handled by the nuclear family, which, because of its small size, emphasizes self-reliance and independence. The death of a family member in a typical nuclear European American family leaves a great void, because the same few individuals fill most of the roles (Ross 1984). In cultures where several generations and extended family members either reside in the same household or are physically close, the impact of a family member's death may be softened, because the roles of the deceased are quickly filled by other relatives (Ross 1984).

Many Americans appear to have internalized the belief that grief is a private matter to be endured internally. Therefore, feelings tend to be repressed and may remain unidentified. People who have been socialized to "be strong" and "make the best of the situation" may not express deep feelings or personal concerns when they experience a serious loss.

Some cultural groups value social support and the expression of loss. In some groups, the expression of grief through wailing, crying, physical prostration, and other outward demonstrations are acceptable and encouraged as part of the resolution of grief. Other groups may frown on this demonstration as a loss of control, favoring a more quiet and stoic expression of grief. In cultural groups where strong kinship ties are maintained, physical and emotional support and assistance are provided by family members.

Spiritual Beliefs Spiritual beliefs and practices greatly influence both a person's reaction to loss and subsequent behavior. Most religious groups have practices related to dying, which are often important to the client and support persons. For additional information, see Chapter 16. To provide support at a time of death, nurses need to understand the client's particular beliefs and practices.

Sex Role The sex roles into which many people are socialized in the United States and Canada affect their reactions at times of loss. Men are frequently expected to "be strong" and show very little emotion during grief, whereas it is acceptable for women to show grief by crying. Often when a wife dies, the husband, who is the chief mourner, is expected to repress his own emotions and to comfort sons and daughters in their grieving.

Sex roles also affect the significance of body image changes to clients. A man might consider a facial scar to be "macho," but a woman might consider it ugly. Thus, the woman, but not the man, would see it as a loss.

Socioeconomic Status The socioeconomic status of an individual often affects the support system available at the time of a loss. A pension plan or insurance, for example, can offer a widowed or disabled person choices of ways to deal with a loss: A person who loses a hand and can no longer carry out work-related tasks may be able to pursue vocational reeducation; a wealthy person whose spouse has died may decide to take a cruise or visit relatives in Europe. Conversely, a person who is confronted with both severe loss and economic hardship may not be able to cope with either.

Table 33–5 Clinical Application: Assessment Data Clusters and Related Nursing Diagnoses: Clients Who Are Grieving

Data Cluster	Nursing Diagnosis
Teresa Jimenez's son Ramon, age 15, has cystic fibrosis of the lungs. Mother and son are waiting for an appropriate donor for a heart-lung transplant. She says, "We've been called to the transplant unit twice, but things didn't work out. Ramon gets his hopes all geared up, and then he's deflated. I'm worried that they won't get the right donor in time. I can't eat or sleep worrying. I don't know what I'll do if he doesn't get that transplant. He's all I've got since my husband left us 6 years ago."	**Anticipatory grieving** related to perceived potential loss of loved one
Tom Bauer's wife died 14 months ago of a ruptured aortic aneurysm at age 59. He lives alone, has no children, and refuses to see friends. He reports frequent headaches, inability to concentrate at work, little interest in food, and early morning insomnia. These symptoms increase at the time of his wife's birthday and their anniversary. He says, "I still can't find it in myself to visit her grave. There are times when I'd just like to die and be with her."	**Dysfunctional grieving** related to lack of adequate social support

DIAGNOSING

The nursing diagnoses identified by NANDA (1992, p. 72) relating specifically to grieving include the following:

- **Grieving** related to an actual or perceived loss
- **Anticipatory grieving**
- **Dysfunctional grieving**

These diagnoses, with definitions, contributing factors, and defining characteristics, are shown in the box on page 862. Clinical applications of these diagnoses are shown in Table 33–5.

Alternative diagnoses in which loss, grieving, one's impending death, or the actual or impending death of a loved one is the etiology include the following:

- **Impaired adjustment** related to incomplete grieving over loss of physical function (paraplegia)
- **Social isolation** related to death of spouse
- **Altered family processes** related to death of child

Impaired adjustment may be the diagnosis for clients with loss of a body part or physiologic function. It is the "state in which the individual is unable to modify his/her behavior or lifestyle in a manner consistent with a change in health status" (Carpenito 1992, p. 131). Such clients may verbalize nonacceptance of the change in health status, lack movement toward independence, or be unable to limit expectations of self. This diagnosis can be applied either to the person suffering the loss or to a significant other. For instance, the husband of a woman hospitalized with a life-threatening illness may feel unable to assume unaccustomed domestic duties, such as child care, and he may feel resentment because the disease has removed the person who maintained the stability of family life. The athlete who suffers a sudden heart attack might also be diagnosed with **Impaired adjustment.** The reduced capacity for physical exertion that the condition imposes may threaten self-image and self-esteem.

Social isolation occurs when the painful nature of grief causes those experiencing it to withdraw from their

NURSING DIAGNOSES

CLIENTS EXPERIENCING GRIEF AND LOSS

NURSING DIAGNOSES: Grieving related to an actual or perceived loss: A state in which an individual or family experiences an actual or a perceived loss (person, object, function, status, relationship); **Anticipatory grieving:** The state in which an individual/group experiences feelings in response to an expected significant loss; **Dysfunctional grieving:** The state in which an individual or group experiences prolonged unresolved grief and as a result engages in detrimental activities

Defining Characteristics

Major

- Verbalization of an actual or perceived loss
- Expressed distress at potential loss **(Anticipatory grieving)**
- Unsuccessful adaptation to loss **(Dysfunctional grieving)**
- Prolonged denial, depression **(Dysfunctional grieving)**

Minor

- Crying
- Denial
- Anger
- Despair
- Guilt
- Sleep disturbance
- Loss of appetite
- Inability to concentrate
- Sense of loss of personal identity
- Social withdrawal
- Decreased energy
- Feelings of loss and loneliness
- Irritability
- Dyspnea, choking, hyperventilation, or other respiratory difficulty
- Signs and symptoms of depression
- Suicidal thoughts

Related Factors

Loss of function (actual or potential) related to a disease of a body system; loss of function or body part related to trauma; surgery or treatment that alters body appearance (eg, mastectomy, amputation, chemotherapy); situational crises (eg, divorce, death of a loved one, loss of job, terminal illness); maturational losses associated with aging (eg, retirement, loss of income).

Sources: LJ Carpenito, *Nursing Diagnosis: Application to Clinical Practice*, 4th ed. (Philadelphia: Lippincott, 1992), pp. 399–419; M Gordon, *Manual of Nursing Diagnosis 1993–1994*, (St Louis: Mosby-Year Book, 1992), pp. 287–91; GK McFarland and EA McFarlane, *Nursing Diagnosis and Intervention: Planning for Patient Care*, 2d ed. (St Louis: Mosby-Year Book, 1993), pp. 585–98; and North American Nursing Diagnosis Association, *NANDA Nursing Diagnoses: Definitions and Classification 1992–1993*, (Philadelphia: NANDA, 1992), p. 72.

normal social support systems. These clients may have a sad, dull affect, be uncommunicative and withdrawn, express feelings of loneliness, and lack supportive others. Some people feel the need to display mastery of the situation or wish not to burden friends. They may be afraid to test the strength of friendships. A new widow, for example, might feel awkward maintaining a social relationship in the circle of married couples she had participated in with her husband.

Social support is a major positive influence on the successful resolution of grief. **Social isolation,** as a nursing diagnosis, can therefore be useful in directing nursing interventions that help the client to build the necessary support network. **Altered family processes** occur when a family that normally functions effectively experiences a dysfunction. See the discussion about this diagnosis in Chapter 14.

PLANNING

The overall goals for clients who are grieving the loss of body function or a body part are to adjust to the changed ability and to redirect both physical and emotional energy into rehabilitation. The goals for clients who are grieving the loss of a loved one are to remember that person without feeling intense pain and to redirect emotional energy into one's own life and regain the capacity to love. Examples of outcome criteria for clients experiencing loss and grief are shown on page 863 in the accompanying Care Planning Guide.

CARE PLANNING GUIDE

CLIENTS EXPERIENCING GRIEF AND LOSS

NURSING DIAGNOSIS: Grieving related to actual or perceived loss

Outcome Criteria	Nursing Intervention	Rationale
The client		
▪ Discusses thoughts and feelings related to loss.	Plan time to be available for the client.	Making oneself available to the client lets the client know the nurse cares.
▪ Describes the personal meaning of loss or death.	Use therapeutic communication strategies of attentive listening, silence, providing general leads, using open-ended questions, and so on. See the discussion of communication techniques, in Chapter 18.	Therapeutic communication skills enhance the exploration of personal thoughts and feelings and the emotional expression of grief.
▪ Expresses grief.	Respect racial, cultural, religious, and personal values of the client/family in their expressions of grief.	Expressions of grief vary among races, cultures, religious groups, and individuals.
	Assure the client that intense feelings and reactions are normal initially.	Clients are more comfortable expressing grief in an accepting, caring environment.
▪ Identifies phases of the grief process.	Provide information about the grief process and what to expect: that is, labile emotions that will stabilize as time passes, and feelings of sadness, guilt, anger, fear, aloneness.	Knowledge of the grief process helps the client understand that personal thoughts and feelings are normal/acceptable.
▪ Shares thoughts and feelings with significant others.	Encourage the client to express grief with family, friends, and support persons.	Clients sometimes are reluctant to share grief with loved ones because they don't want to burden them. Communication of mutual concerns/fears, plans, and hopes with significant others acknowledges the grief of loved ones, reinforces a sense of sharing, and assists them through the grief process.
▪ Maintains constructive interpersonal relationships.	Acknowledge the client's family and support persons in their own grief and their desire to help their loved one.	Acknowledging the grief of loved ones promotes a cohesive family support structure.
▪ Establishes new relationships.	Encourage the development of new relationships.	Clients may be fearful or guilty about developing new relationships.
▪ Selects and uses appropriate resources.	Provide information about available resources.	Clients are often unaware of available resources and/or may feel uncomfortable using them.
	Encourage client to explore available resources (eg, clergy, work-related employee assistance programs)	Clients may have unique support systems of which they are unaware. Many personal support systems are available at no cost (eg, clergy).
		Utilizing community or personal resources can decrease the intensity of grief, help the client make necessary readjustments in life-style, and form new relationships and promote a more rapid recovery.

➤

GRIEF AND LOSS CONTINUED

Nursing Diagnosis: Grieving related to actual or perceived loss *continued*

Outcome Criteria	Nursing Intervention	Rationale
	Encourage the client to explore support groups for individuals who have experienced a similar loss (eg, Reach for Recovery, support groups for parents who have lost a child)	Clients may feel less alone when they can talk about their feelings with those who have already experienced similar feelings.
▪ Verbalizes decrease in grief-related physical and psychologic symptoms.	Assess client well-being: vital signs, appetite, sleep patterns, concentration, desire to return to normal activities.	Physical and psychologic status are indicators of resolution of grief.
▪ Resumes normal routine.	Suggest that client resume normal activities on a schedule that promotes physical and psychologic health.	Clients may try to return to normal activities too quickly before they have resolved their grief. They may experience a recurrence of grief symptoms.

Implementing

The skills most relevant to situations of loss and grief are attentive listening, silence, open and closed questioning, paraphrasing, clarifying and reflecting feelings, and summarizing. Less helpful to clients are responses that give advice and evaluation, those that interpret and analyze, and those that give unwarranted reassurance. To ensure effective communication, the nurse must make an accurate assessment of what is appropriate for the client.

Communication with grieving clients needs to be relevant to their stage of grief. Whether the client is angry or depressed affects how the client hears messages and how the nurse interprets the client's statements. Implications for nurse-client communication are related to Kübler-Ross's five stages in Table 33–2, earlier.

The guidelines in the first box on page 865 can assist nurses in helping the bereaved.

Evaluating

Evaluating the effectiveness of nursing care of the grieving client is difficult because of the long-term nature of the life transition. Criteria for evaluation must be based on goals set by the client and family. A follow-up visit to the surviving family members may be an appropriate nursing measure not only to obtain information for evaluation but also to assist nurses in working through their own grief by expressing their continuing concern for the family.

Examples of evaluative statements indicating goal achievement are "the client expressed anger over diagnosis of AIDS and is concerned about his relationship with his family," and "The client requested visitation from the hospital chaplain."

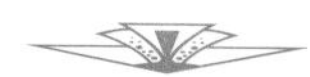

Care of the Dying Client

Assessing

Nursing care and support for the dying client and family include making an accurate assessment of the physiologic signs of approaching death. In addition to signs related to the client's specific disease, certain other physical signs are indicative of impending death. The four main characteristic changes are loss of muscle tone, slowing of the circulation, changes in vital signs, and sensory impairment. See the second box on page 865 for indications of impending clinical death.

Various consciousness levels occur just before death. Some clients are alert, whereas others are drowsy, stuporous, or comatose. Hearing is thought to be the last sense lost.

The traditional *clinical signs of death* were cessation of the apical pulse, respirations, and blood pressure. However, since the advent of artificial means to maintain respirations and blood circulation, identifying death is more difficult. In 1968, the World Medical Assembly adopted the following guidelines for physicians as indications of death (Benton 1978, p. 18):

- Total lack of response to external stimuli
- No muscular movement, especially breathing

ASSISTING CLIENTS WITH GRIEF

- Provide opportunity for the persons involved to express their feelings.
- Listen attentively.
- Avoid euphemisms. Learn to be comfortable with hearing and saying such words as *death, die, cancer,* and so on.
- Recognize and accept the varied expressions of emotion that people exhibit in response to loss and grief. Do not be judgmental.
- Provide support for the expression of difficult feelings, such as anger and guilt.
- Include children in the grieving process.
- Encourage the bereaved to maintain established relationships.
- Connect clients and other involved persons with appropriate support groups.
- Encourage self-care by family members, especially the primary caregiver.
- Provide time for family members and other loved ones to be with their loved one both before and after death.
- Assist family members and loved ones to make decisions, providing time for contemplation.
- Provide follow-up for family members and/or significant others. Sending a note or card or making a telephone call can decrease feelings of abandonment.

- No reflexes
- Flat encephalogram

In instances of artificial support, absence of electric currents from the brain (measured by an electroencephalogram) for at least 24 hours is an indication of death. Only a physician can pronounce death, and only after this pronouncement can life-support systems be shut off.

Another definition of death is **cerebral death,** which occurs when the higher brain center, the cerebral cortex, is irreversibly destroyed. The client may still be able to breathe but is irreversibly unconscious. People who support this definition of death believe the cerebral cortex, which holds the capacity for thought, voluntary action, and movement, *is* the individual.

SIGNS OF IMPENDING CLINICAL DEATH

Loss of muscle tone

- Relaxation of the facial muscles (eg, the jaw may sag)
- Difficulty speaking
- Difficulty swallowing and gradual loss of the gag reflex
- Decreased activity of the gastrointestinal tract, with subsequent nausea, accumulation of flatus, abdominal distention, and retention of feces, especially if narcotics or tranquilizers are being administered
- Possible urinary and rectal incontinence due to decreased sphincter control
- Diminished body movement

Slowing of the circulation

- Diminished sensation
- Mottling and cyanosis of the extremities
- Cold skin, first in the feet and later in the hands, ears, and nose (the client, however, may feel warm because of elevated temperature)

Changes in vital signs

- Decelerated and weaker pulse
- Decreased blood pressure
- Rapid, shallow, irregular, or abnormally slow respirations; Cheyne-Stokes respirations; noisy breathing, referred to as the *death rattle,* due to collecting of mucus in the throat; mouth breathing, which leads to dry oral mucous membranes.

Sensory impairment

- Blurred vision
- Impaired senses of taste and smell

DIAGNOSING

The full range of nursing diagnoses, addressing both physiologic and psychosocial needs, can be applied to the dying client, depending on the assessment data. Three diagnoses that may be particularly appropriate are **Fear, Hopelessness,** and **Powerlessness.**

Many fears are associated with death, and the nurse needs to determine a client's specific fears. Gonda and Ruark (1984, pp. 31–32) discuss three objects of the dying person's fear: the process of dying, nonexistence, and what comes after death. The nurse is usually better able to assist a client with the complex process of dying than with the spiritual fears of nonexistence and the hereafter.

Schulz (1978, p. 27) outlines the following fears related to a person's own death: pain, body misfunction, humiliation, rejection or abandonment, nonbeing, punishment, interruption of goals, and negative impact on survivors (eg, psychologic suffering, economic hardship).

NURSING DIAGNOSES

CLIENTS WHO ARE DYING

NURSING DIAGNOSIS: Hopelessness: The subjective state in which an individual sees limited or no alternatives or personal choices available and cannot mobilize energy on own behalf

Defining Characteristics

Major

- Passivity, decreased verbalization
- Decreased affect
- Verbal cues indicating despondency ("I can't," sighing)

Minor

- Lack of initiative
- Decreased response to stimuli
- Turning away from speaker
- Closing eyes
- Shrugging in response to speaker
- Decreased appetite
- Altered sleep pattern
- Lack of involvement in or passively allowing care

Related Factors

Abandonment; prolonged activity restriction creating isolation; long-term stress; loss of spiritual belief.

NURSING DIAGNOSIS: Powerlessness: Perception that one's own action will not significantly affect an outcome; a perceived lack of control over a current situation or immediate happening

Defining Characteristics

Severe

- Verbal expressions of having no control or influence over the situation or outcome of self-care
- Depression over physical deterioration that occurs despite patient compliance with regimens
- Apathy

Moderate

- Nonparticipation in care or decision making when opportunities are provided
- Expressions of dissatisfaction and frustration over inability to perform previous tasks and/or activities
- Does not monitor progress
- Expression of doubt regarding role performance
- Reluctance to express true feelings, fearing alienation from caregivers
- Inability to seek information regarding care
- Dependence on others that may result in irritability, resentment, anger, and guilt
- Does not defend self-care practices when challenged

Low

- Passivity
- Expressions of uncertainty about fluctuating energy levels

Related Factors

Health care environment; chronic or terminal illness; interpersonal interaction; treatment regimen; life-style characterized by helplessness.

Sources: LJ Carpenito, *Nursing Diagnosis: Application to Clinical Practice*, 4th ed. (Philadelphia: Lippincott, 1992), pp. 379–98, 680–81; M Gordon, *Manual of Nursing Diagnosis 1993–1994*, (St Louis: Mosby-Year Book, 1993), pp. 265, 267–69; MJ Kim, GK McFarland, and AM McLane, *Pocket Guide to Nursing Diagnoses*, 5th ed. (St Louis: Mosby-Year Book, 1993), pp. 23–26; GK McFarland and EA McFarlane, *Nursing Diagnosis and Intervention: Planning for Patient Care*, 2d ed. (St Louis: Mosby, 1993), pp. 499 and 505; North American Nursing Diagnosis Association, *NANDA Nursing Diagnoses: Definitions and Classification 1992–1993*, (Philadelphia: NANDA, 1992), pp. 32, 53–56; and JR Lederer, GL Marculescu, B Mocnik, and N Seaby, *Care Planning Pocket Guide—A Nursing Diagnosis Approach*, 5th ed. (Redwood City, CA: Addison-Wesley Nursing, 1993), pp. 76–83.

Sheehy (1981, pp. 27–62), in his discussion about common fears of dying, includes fear of pain, loneliness, dependence, the moment of death, and annihilation. Although there is no pain at the moment of death and the transition from life to death seems easy, many people fear this moment. Sheehy believes that fear of the moment of death is the result of the emotional sting and pain experienced during the death of a parent. People remember this

Table 33–6 Clinical Application: Assessment Data Clusters and Related Nursing Diagnoses: Clients Who Are Dying

Data Cluster	Nursing Diagnosis
Keisha Washington, who has multiple sclerosis and is paralyzed from the neck down, has appealed for someone to help her commit suicide. Her mind and speaking ability are unimpaired. She states, "I dread the same fate as my sister, who also had multiple sclerosis and before death had pain and became blind and mute."	**Hopelessness** related to deteriorating physiologic condition
John Yee, age 63, has metastatic carcinoma of the bowel. He has noticed a rapid deterioration in energy in the past week and feels bloated and nauseated. He has become increasingly jaundiced and says, "I know I haven't long to live. Why can't they just give me a big dose of morphine and get it over with?"	**Powerlessness** related to terminal illness and inability to terminate life.

previous pain and, therefore, believe that dying is painful. Fear of annihilation, or being reduced to nothingness after death, and questions about immortality need to be faced. Does immortality rest in what the individual achieved in this life, or does the soul survive after death? Whatever a person believes about life after death, both body and mind may be viewed as reentering the universe and becoming part of it as some form of energy.

The diagnoses of **Hopelessness** and **Powerlessness,** with definitions, contributing factors and defining characteristics, are shown in the box on page 866. Examples of assessment data clusters and related nursing diagnoses are shown in Table 33–6.

PLANNING

Major goals of dying clients are (a) maintaining physiologic and psychologic comfort and (b) achieving a dignified and peaceful death. When planning care with these clients, the Dying Person's Bill of Rights can be a useful guide (see the box at the right). Some outcome criteria for clients with diagnoses of **Fear, Hopelessness,** and **Powerlessness** are shown below.

The client

- Is free of pain.
- Participates in self-care activities in accordance with health status.
- Makes choices related to care and treatment.
- Verbalizes feelings of anger, sorrow, or loss.
- Maintains open relationship with support persons and staff.
- Identifies areas of personal control.
- Expresses sense of control over the present situation.
- Expresses feelings of optimism about the present and future.
- Expresses positive feelings about relationships with significant others.

THE DYING PERSON'S BILL OF RIGHTS

I have the right to be treated as a living human being until I die.

I have the right to maintain a sense of hopefulness, however changing its focus may be.

I have the right to be cared for by those who can maintain a sense of hopefulness, however changing this might be.

I have the right to express my feelings and emotions about my approaching death in my own way.

I have the right to participate in decisions concerning my care.

I have the right to expect continuing medical and nursing attention even though "cure" goals must be changed to "comfort" goals.

I have the right not to die alone.

I have the right to be free from pain.

I have the right to have my questions answered honestly.

I have the right not to be deceived.

I have the right to have help from and for my family in accepting my death.

I have the right to die in peace and dignity.

I have the right to retain my individuality and not be judged for my decisions which may be contrary to beliefs of others.

I have the right to discuss and enlarge my religious and/or spiritual experiences, whatever these may mean to others.

I have the right to expect that the sanctity of the human body will be respected after death.

I have the right to be cared for by caring, sensitive, knowledgeable people who will attempt to understand my needs and will be able to gain some satisfaction in helping me face my death.

Source: AJ Barbus, The dying person's bill of rights, © 1975, American Journal of Nursing Company. Reprinted with permission from the *American Journal of Nursing,* 75:99, January 1975.

- Shares values and personal meaning of life.
- Reminisces and reviews personal life positively.
- Accepts limitations and seeks help as needed.

IMPLEMENTING

The major nursing responsibility for clients who are dying is to assist the client to a peaceful death. More specific responsibilities are the following:

1. To provide relief from loneliness, fear, and depression
2. To maintain the client's sense of security, self-confidence, dignity, and self-worth
3. To maintain hope
4. To help the client accept losses
5. To provide physical comfort

People facing death need help facing the fact that they will have to depend on others. Some dying clients require only minimal care and can be cared for at home; others need continuous attention and the services of a hospital and its staff. People need help, well in advance of death, in planning for the period of dependence. They need to consider what will happen and how and where they would like to die.

Helping Clients Die with Dignity Dignity may be defined as the ability to function as a significant and integrated person. True dignity comes from within. Generally, dependence on others and loss of control over oneself and interactions with the environment are associated with loss of dignity. Nurses need to ensure that the client is treated with dignity, that is, with honor and respect. Dying clients often feel they have lost control over their lives and over life itself. By introducing options available to the client and significant others, nurses can restore and support feelings of control. Some choices that clients can make are the location of care (eg, hospital, home, or hospice); times of appointments with health professionals; activity schedule; use of health resources; and times of visits from relatives and friends.

Most clients interviewed about dying indicate that they want to be able to manage the events preceding death so they can die peacefully. Nurses can help clients to find meaning and completeness and to determine their own physical, psychologic, and social priorities. Dying people often strive for self-fulfillment more than self-preservation, and they need to find meaning in continuing to live while suffering. Part of the nurse's challenge, then, is to help maintain, day to day, the client's will and hope.

Salter (1982, p. 21) believes it is important for nurses and clients to focus not on the end, but on three stages of living fully until death:

1. *Developing and growing.* In this stage, the client can be assisted to paint, sculpt, go to a library, visit an art gallery, etc. An occupational therapist can help clients do what they still can do and what is pleasurable.
2. *Lying fallow.* In this stage, physiotherapy measures, such as breathing exercises and passive exercises, help the client to relax and enhance self-esteem.
3. *Letting go and becoming dependent.* In this stage, nursing intervention is usually required to meet both physical and psychologic needs.

Often nurses have difficulty discussing death with clients who are dying. Although it is natural for people to be uncomfortable discussing death, there are steps that can be taken to make such discussions easier for both the nurse and the client. Callanan (1994, pp. 22–23) lists the following strategies:

- Identify personal feelings about death and how they may influence interactions with clients. Acknowledge personal fears about death, and discuss them with a friend or colleague.
- Focus on the client's needs. The client's fears and beliefs may be different from the nurse's. It is important that the nurse avoid imposing personal fears and beliefs on the client or family.
- Understand the client and how the client copes. Talk to the client or the family about how the client usually copes with stress. Clients will use their usual coping strategies for dealing with impending death. For example, if they are usually quiet and reflective, they will become more quiet and withdrawn when facing terminal illness.
- Establish a communication relationship that shows concern for and commitment to the client. Communication strategies which let the client know the nurse is available to talk about death include the following:
  a. Describing what the nurse sees, for example, "You seem sad. Would you like to talk about what's happening to you?"
  b. Clarifying the nurse's concern, for example, "I'd like to know better how you feel and how I may help you."
  c. Acknowledging the client's struggle, for example, "It must be difficult to feel so uncomfortable. I care about you and would like to help you be more comfortable."
  d. Providing a caring touch. Holding the client's hand or offering a comforting massage can encourage the client to verbalize feelings.
- Determine what the client knows about the illness and prognosis.
- Respond with honesty and directness to the client's questions about death.
- Make time to be available to the client to provide support, listen, and respond.

Hospice and Home Care Hospice care, palliative care, and home care focus on support and care of the dying person and family, with the goal of facilitating a peaceful and dignified death. **Hospice care** is based on holistic concepts that emphasize care to improve the quality of life rather than cure. The hospice movement was founded by Dr Cecily Saunders in London, England, in 1967 and was later extended to the United States by Dr Sylvia Lack. Its goals are

- To control and relieve pain and symptoms of the illness.
- To provide physical comfort for the terminally ill.
- To provide social, emotional, and spiritual comfort for the client, family, and friends throughout the final stage of illness, at the time of death, and during the bereavement period of the survivors.

The principles of hospice care can be carried out in a variety of settings, the most common being the autonomous hospice and the hospital-based **palliative care** unit. Palliative care is special care that is challenging and requires skillful interpersonal relationships and compassion. Services range from fully comprehensive to a focus on selected areas, such as symptom control and pain management, in some palliative care units. Home care services for the dying client maintain the client in the natural home environment until that is no longer possible or until death. Hospice care is always provided by a team of both health professionals and nonprofessionals to ensure a full range of care services. In the United States, these services have been delivered primarily through autonomous, community-based hospices. In Canada, most hospice programs are hospital-based.

Meeting Physiologic Needs of the Dying Client

The physiologic needs of the dying are related to a slowing of body processes and to homeostatic imbalances. Interventions include providing personal hygiene measures; controlling pain; relieving respiratory difficulties; assisting with movement, nutrition, hydration, and elimination; and providing measures related to sensory changes. See also Table 33–7 on page 870.

Pain control is essential to enable clients to maintain quality life activities, including eating, moving, and sleeping. Many drugs have been used to control the pain associated with terminal illness: morphine, heroin, methadone, alcohol, marijuana, and LSD. Usually the physician determines the dosage, but the client's opinion should be considered; the client is the one ultimately aware of personal pain tolerance and fluctuations of internal states. Because physicians usually prescribe dosage ranges for pain medication, nurses use their own judgment as to the amount and frequency of pain medication in providing client relief. See also the discussion of patient-controlled analgesia in Chapter 36. Because of decreased blood circulation, analgesics may be administered by intravenous infusion rather than subcutaneously or intramuscularly.

RESEARCH NOTE

What Attributes and Skills Are Associated with Expert Care of the Dying?

Nursing is intimately timed to pivotal transitions (eg, birth, illness, loss, and death) in the human experience. Much has been written about the nurse's role in care of sick and healthy clients, and, more recently, renewed emphasis has been placed on the nurse's role in care of the dying.

This qualitative study explored expert nursing behaviors in care of the dying adult in the intensive care unit. The sample included 10 intensive care unit nurses identified by their peers as experts in the care of dying clients. Expert nurses were either employed in a surgical intensive care unit at a tertiary care hospital or at a medical–surgical intensive care unit in a community hospital. Both facilities were located in a western Canadian city.

Lengthy interviews with the expert nurses were transcribed and analyzed. Themes were identified via constant comparative analysis.

The authors identified a variety of behaviors associated with expert nursing care of the dying. These behaviors included: responding after death has occurred; responding to the family; responding to anger; responding to colleagues; providing comfort care; and enhancing personal growth.

Implications: This study provides a foundation to examine nursing care of the dying. Delineation of specific nursing interventions in terminal care helps nurses improve their role in care of the dying.

Source: SE McClement and LF Degner, Expert nursing behaviors in care of the dying adult in the intensive care unit, *Heart & Lung: Journal of Critical Care,* September/October 1995, 24(5):408–19.

Spiritual Support Spiritual support is of great importance in dealing with death. Although not all clients identify with a specific religious faith or belief, the majority have a need for meaning in their lives, particularly as they experience a terminal illness. Jacik (1989, pp. 271–73) describes the spiritual needs of the dying as follows:

- Forgiveness from and reconciliation with God and past human relationships
- Prayer and religious services, such as sacraments or blessings

Table 33–7 Physiologic Needs of Dying Persons

Problem	Nursing Interventions
Ineffective airway clearance	Fowler's position: conscious clients
	Throat suctioning: conscious clients
	Lateral position: unconscious clients
	Oxygen therapy as needed
Self-care deficit: Bathing/hygiene	Frequent baths and linen changes if diaphoretic
	Encourage wearing of daytime clothes
	Clean eyelids with absorbent cotton and saline if secretions gather in eyelids
	Mouth care as needed for dry mouth
Impaired physical mobility	Assist client out of bed periodically, if client able
	Regularly change bedridden client's position
	Support client's position with pillows, blanket rolls, or towels as needed
	Lateral position in bed, to decrease aspiration of saliva
	Elevate client's legs when sitting up, to prevent pooling of blood
Altered nutrition: less than body requirements	Antiemetics or small amount of alcoholic beverage to stimulate appetite
	High-calorie, high-vitamin diet
Fluid volume deficit, actual or high risk for	Encourage fluids
	Semisolid, soft, or liquid foods because of decreased gag reflex
	Continuing assessment of gag reflex
Constipation	Dietary fiber as tolerated
	Laxatives as needed to prevent constipation
Altered urinary elimination	Skin care in response to incontinence of urine or feces
	Bedpan, urinal, or commode chair within easy reach
	Call light within reach for assistance onto bedpan or commode
	Absorbent pads placed under incontinent client; linen changed as often as needed
	Catheterization, if necessary
	Keep room as clean and odor-free as possible
Sensory/perceptual alteration: visual, tactile	Clients prefer a light room
	Hearing is *not* diminished; speak clearly and do not whisper
	Touch is diminished, but client will feel pressure of touch

- Spiritual assistance at the time of death from clergy, family, or health care providers
- Peace and tranquility of spirit

The nurse has a responsibility to ensure that the client's spiritual needs are attended to, either through direct intervention or by arranging access to individuals who can provide spiritual care. Nurses need to be aware of their own comfort with spiritual issues and be clear about their own ability to interact supportively with the client. Nurses have a responsibility to not impose their own religious/spiritual beliefs on a client, but to respond to the client in relation to the client's own background and needs. Communication skills are most important in helping the client articulate needs and in developing a sense of caring and trust.

Specific interventions may include facilitating expressions of feeling, prayer, meditation, reading, and discussion with appropriate clergy/spiritual advisor. It is important for nurses to establish an effective interdisciplinary relationship with spiritual support specialists. For a further discussion of spiritual issues, see Chapter 16. Death-related beliefs and practices of selected religious groups are shown in Table 33–8 on pages 872 and 873.

Evaluating

To evaluate the achievement of client goals, the nurse collects data in accordance with the outcome criteria established earlier. Evaluation activities may include the following:

- Listening to the client's reports of feeling in control of the environment surrounding death, such as control over pain relief, visitation of family and support persons, or treatment plans
- Observing the client's relationship with significant others
- Listening to the client's thoughts and feelings related to hopelessness or powerlessness

Examples of evaluative statements indicating goal achievement are "The client expressed his desire to have family members with him at the time of death," and "The client discussed wishes for his funeral with family members." Examples of outcome criteria are listed on page 867.

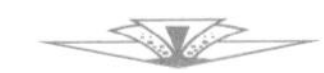

Care of the Body After Death

Body Changes

Rigor mortis is the stiffening of the body that occurs about 2 to 4 hours after death. It results from a lack of adenosine triphosphate (ATP), which is not synthesized because of a lack of glycogen in the body. ATP is necessary for muscle fiber relaxation. Its lack causes the muscles to contract, which in turn immobilizes the joints. Rigor mortis starts in the involuntary muscles (heart, bladder, and so on) then progresses to the head, neck, and trunk, and finally reaches the extremities.

Because the deceased's family often wants to view the body, and because it is important that the deceased appear natural and comfortable, nurses need to position the body, place dentures in the mouth, and close the eyes and mouth *before* rigor mortis sets in. Rigor mortis usually leaves the body about 96 hours after death.

Algor mortis is the gradual decrease of the body's temperature after death. When blood circulation terminates and the hypothalamus ceases to function, body temperature falls about 1 C (1.8 F) per hour until it reaches room temperature. Simultaneously, the skin loses its elasticity and can easily be broken when removing dressings and adhesive tape.

After blood circulation has ceased, the skin becomes discolored. The red blood cells break down, releasing hemoglobin, which discolors the surrounding tissues. This discoloration, referred to as **livor mortis,** appears in the lowermost or dependent areas of the body.

Tissues after death become soft and eventually liquefied by bacterial fermentation. The hotter the temperature, the more rapid the change. Therefore, bodies are often stored in cool places to delay this process. Embalming reverses the process through injection of chemicals into the body to destroy the bacteria.

Legal Aspects of Death

Of the many legal ramifications of human death, the most basic for the nurse is that death must be certified by a physician. In circumstances of unusual death, an **autopsy (postmortem examination)** may be required. Nurses have a responsibility to be aware of the legal ramifications of death in the jurisdiction in which they practice. Chapter 12 provides legal information about death certificates, labeling the deceased, autopsy, organ donation, and inquest. Wills, euthanasia, and the right to die (living wills) are also discussed in Chapter 12.

Nursing Intervention

Nursing personnel may be responsible for care of a body after death. If the deceased's family or friends wish to view the body, it is important to make the environment as clean and pleasant as possible and to make the body appear natural and comfortable. All equipment and supplies should be removed from the bedside. Some agencies require that all tubes in the body be clamped and remain in place; in other agencies, tubes may be cut to within 2.5 cm (1 in) of the skin and taped in place. Soiled linen is removed so that the room is free from odors. Postmortem care should be carried out according to the policy of the hospital or extended care facility. Because care of the body may be influenced by religious law, the nurse should check the client's religion and make every attempt to comply. See Table 33–8 on pages 872 and 873.

Normally, the body is placed in a supine position with the arms either at the sides, palms down, or across the abdomen. The wristband is left on unless it is too tight. One pillow is placed under the head and shoulders to prevent blood from discoloring the face by settling in it. The eyelids are closed and held in place for a few seconds so they remain closed. If they will not stay closed, a moistened cotton fluff will hold them in place. Dentures are usually inserted to help give the face a natural appearance. The mouth is then closed; a rolled towel under the chin will hold it closed.

Soiled areas of the body are washed; however, a complete bath is not necessary, since the body will be washed by the **mortician** (also referred to as an **undertaker**), a person trained in care of the dead. Absorbent pads are placed under the buttocks to take up any feces and urine released because of relaxation of the sphincter muscles. A clean gown is placed on the client, and the hair is brushed and combed. All jewelry is removed, except a wedding

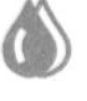

Text continued on page 874

Table 33–8 Death-Related Beliefs and Practices of Selected Religious Groups

Group	Afterlife	Rituals/Funerals
Native American	Beliefs vary	Practices vary; most want family present
Black Muslim		Special procedures for washing and shrouding the dead; special funeral rites
Buddhist in America	Reincarnation; after reaching state of enlightenment, may attain nirvana	Last rite; chanting at bedside
Church of Christ Scientist	Yes	No last rites
Church of Jesus Christ of Latter Day Saints (Mormon)	Yes	Baptism of those who have died outside the faith essential; may preach gospel to the spirit of the dead
Eastern Orthodox (Greek and Russian Orthodox)	Yes	Last rites and administration of Holy Communion (obligatory for some)
Episcopal (Anglican)	Yes	Last rites not mandatory
Hindu	Reincarnation; after leading a perfect life, may join Brahma	Priest pours water into mouth of corpse and ties string around wrist or neck as sign of blessing; string must not be removed; family washes body
Islam (Moslem, Muslim)	May join Allah by being a good Moslem and observing rituals daily	Dying person must confess sins and ask forgiveness in presence of family; family washes and prepares body (female body cannot be washed by male) and turns body toward Mecca
Jehovah's Witness	Immortality is reward for faithfulness	
Judaism	Dead will be resurrected with coming of Messiah; man lives on through survival of memory	Body ritually washed by members of Ritual Burial Society; burial as soon as possible after death; dead not left unattended; five stages of mourning extending over a year; no embalming; no flowers at funeral (because flowers are a symbol of life)
Lutheran, Methodist, Presbyterian	Yes	Last rites or Scripture reading optional
Roman Catholicism	Yes; resurrection with second coming of Christ	Rites for anointing the sick not mandatory; receiving Holy Communion mandatory
Seventh-day Adventist	Dead are asleep until return of Christ, when final rewards and punishments will be given	
Unitarian	Beliefs vary	

Sources: HM Ross, Societal/cultural views regarding death and dying, *Topics in Clinical Nursing*, 1981, 3(3):1–16; HM Ross and JB Pumphrey (consultant), Recognizing your patient's spiritual needs, *Nursing77*, December 1977, 7:64–70; LJ Carpenito, *Nursing Diagnosis: Application to Clinical*

Autopsy	Organ Donation	Cremation	Prolonging Life
Prohibited	Practices vary		
			Encouraged
No restriction	Considered an act of mercy and encouraged	No restriction	Permit euthanasia in hopeless illness
Only in sudden death	No	Individual decision	Unlikely to use medical means to prolong life
No restriction	No restriction	Discouraged	No restriction
Discouraged		Discouraged	Encouraged
No restriction	No restriction	No restriction	
No restriction	No restriction	Preferred; ashes cast in holy river	No restriction
May oppose	Prohibited	Prohibited	Encouraged
Prohibited unless required by law. No body parts may be removed	Prohibited	No restriction	
Orthodox prohibit; some liberals permit; no body parts removed	Beliefs vary	Largely prohibited; beliefs vary	Generally opposed after irreversible brain damage
No restriction	No restriction	No restriction	
Permitted, but all body parts must be given appropriate burial	No restriction	No restriction	Discouraged
No restriction	No restriction	No restriction	
No restriction	No restriction	Encouraged	Support for death with dignity and self-determination in dying

Practice, 4th ed. (Philadelphia: Lippincott, 1992), pp. 806–10; and MM Andrews and PA Hanson, Religious beliefs: Implications for nursing practice. In JS Boyle and MM Andrews, *Transcultural Concepts in Nursing Care*, (Boston: Scott, Foresman, 1989), pp. 357–418.

band in some instances, which is taped to the finger. The top bed linens are adjusted neatly to cover the client to the shoulders. Soft lighting and chairs are provided for the family. All the client's valuables, including clothing, are listed and placed in a safe storage area for the family to take away.

After the body has been viewed by the family, additional identification tags are applied, one to the ankle and one to the wrist if the client's wrist identification band was not left in place. The body is wrapped in a **shroud,** a large rectangular or square piece of plastic or cotton material used to enclose a body after death. Another identification band is then applied to the outside of the shroud. The body is taken to the morgue for cooling, if arrangements have not been made to have a mortician pick it up from the client's room. Agencies vary in their policies about transporting bodies. Some close all room doors before transporting a deceased client through corridors, and service elevators are often used.

CHAPTER HIGHLIGHTS

- Nurses help clients deal with all kinds of losses, including loss of body image, loss of a loved one, loss of a sense of well-being, and loss of a job.
- Loss, especially loss of a loved one or a valued body part, can be viewed as a crisis event, either situational or developmental, and either actual or perceived (both of which can be anticipatory).
- How an individual deals with loss is closely related to the individual's stage of development, personal resources, and social support systems.
- Caring for the dying and the bereaved is one of the nurse's most complex and challenging responsibilities.
- Nurses' attitudes about death and dying directly affect their ability to provide care.
- Nurses must consider the entire family as the client of care in situations involving loss, especially during the crisis of death.
- Grieving is a normal, subjective emotional response to loss; it is essential for mental and physical health. Grieving allows the bereaved person to cope with loss gradually and to accept it as part of reality.
- Knowledge of different stages or phases of grieving and factors that influence the loss reaction can help the nurse understand the responses and needs of clients.
- Nurses caring for clients who are suffering loss or dying need effective communication skills.
- Dying clients require physical help and emotional support to ensure a peaceful and dignified death.

READINGS AND REFERENCES

SUGGESTED READINGS

Miles, A. December 1993. Caring for the family left behind. *American Journal of Nursing* 93:34–36.

The author, a hospital chaplain, provides strategies for assisting the families and loved ones of dying or deceased clients with their grief.

Sanders, CM. 1989. *Grief: The Mourning After: Dealing with Adult Bereavement.* New York: Wiley.

The author discusses five phases of bereavement, describing characteristics and physical and psychologic symptoms of each phase and identifying tasks for successful resolution.

RELATED RESEARCH

Sowell, RL, Bramlett, MH, Gueldner, SH, Gritzmacher, D and Martin, G. Summer 1991. The lived experience of survival and bereavement following the death of a lover from AIDS. *Image: Journal of Nursing Scholarship* 23:89–94.

SELECTED REFERENCES

Alexander, J and Kiely, J. March/April 1986. Working with the bereaved. *Geriatric Nursing* 7:85–86.

Andrews, MM and Hanson, PA. 1989. Religious beliefs: Implications for nursing practice. In Boyle, JS and Andrews, MM. pp. 357–418. *Transcultural Concepts in Nursing Care.* Boston: Scott, Foresman.

Ardery, G. 1992. Terminal care. In Bulechek, GM and McCloskey, JC. pp. 366–78. *Nursing Interventions: Essential Nursing Treatments.* 2d ed. Philadelphia: WB Saunders.

Benoliel, JQ. June 1985. Loss and terminal illness. *Nursing Clinics of North America* 20:439–48.

Benton, RE. 1978. *Death and Dying: Principles and Practices in Patient Care.* New York: Van Nostrand.

Betz, CL and Poster, EC. June 1984. Children's concepts of death: Implications for pediatric practice. *Nursing Clinics of North America* 19:341–49.

Burgess, AW and Lazare, A. 1976. *Community Mental Health: Target Populations.* Englewood Cliffs, NJ: Prentice Hall.

Callanan, M. January 1994. Dealing with death: Breaking the silence. *American Journal of Nursing* 94:22–23.

Cappon, D. February 1970. Attitudes towards death. *Coast Graduate Medicine* 47:257.

Carpenito, LJ. 1992. *Nursing Diagnosis: Application to Clinical Practice.* 4th ed. Philadelphia: Lippincott.

Clark, C, Curley, A, and Hughes, A. December 1988. Hospice care: A model for caring for the person with AIDS. *Nursing Clinics of North America* 23:851–62.

Clark, MD. December 1984. Healthy and unhealthy grief behaviors. *Occupational Health Nursing* 32:633–35.

Demi, AS and Miles, MS. 1986. Bereavement. *Annual Review of Nursing Research* 4:105–23.

Dobratz, MC. April 1990. Hospice nursing: Present perspectives and future directives. *Cancer Nursing* 13:116–22.

Engel, GL. September 1964. Grief and grieving. *American Journal of Nursing* 64:93–98.

Fetsch, SH. November/December 1984. The 7- to 10-year-old child's conceptualization of death. *Oncology Nurses' Forum* 11:52–56.

Gabriel, RM and Kirschling, JM. 1989. Assessing grief among the bereaved elderly: A review of existing measures. *Hospice Journal* 5:29–54.

Gifford, BJ and Cleary, BB. February 1990. Supporting the bereaved. *American Journal of Nursing* 90:48–55.

Giger, JN and Davidhizar, RE. 1991. *Transcultural Nursing: Assessment and Intervention.* St Louis: Mosby-Year Book.

Gonda, TA. and Ruark, JE. 1984. *Dying Dignified: The Health Professional's Guide to Care.* Menlo Park, CA: Addison-Wesley Nursing.

Gordon, M. 1993. *Manual of Nursing Diagnosis 1993–1994.* St Louis: Mosby-Year Book.

Health and Welfare Canada. 1981. *Palliative Care Services in Hospitals: Guidelines.* Ottawa: Ministry of National Health and Welfare.

Hoff, LA. 1989. *People in Crisis: Understanding and Helping.* 3d ed. Redwood City, CA: Addison-Wesley.

Jacik, M. 1989. Spiritual care of the dying adult. In Carson, VB. pp. 254–88. *Spiritual Dimensions of Nursing Practice.* Philadelphia: Saunders.

Kim, MJ, McFarland, GK, and McLane, AM. 1993. *Pocket Guide to Nursing Diagnoses.* 5th ed. St Louis: Mosby-Year Book.

Kübler-Ross, E. 1969. *On Death and Dying.* New York: Macmillan.

______. 1974. *Questions and Answers on Death and Dying.* New York: Macmillan.

______. 1975. *Death: The Final Stage of Growth.* Englewood Cliffs, NJ: Prentice Hall.

______. 1978. *To Live Until We Say Good-bye.* Englewood Cliffs, NJ: Prentice Hall.

McFarland, GK and McFarlane, EA. 1993. *Nursing Diagnosis and Intervention: Planning for Patient Care.* 2d ed. St Louis: Mosby-Year Book.

Martocchio, BC. June 1985. Grief and bereavement: Healing through hurt. *Nursing Clinics of North America* 20:327–41.

Masson, V. September/October 1989. On hearing the news of a patient's death. *Nursing Outlook* 37:245.

Miles, A. December 1993. Caring for the family left behind. *American Journal of Nursing* 93:34–36.

Murphy, SA and Osband, BA. 1991. Loss. In Creasia, JL and Parker, B. pp. 593–607. *Conceptual Foundations of Professional Nursing Practice.* St Louis: Mosby-Year Book.

North American Nursing Diagnosis Association. 1992. *NANDA Nursing Diagnoses: Definitions and Classification 1992–1993.* Philadelphia: NANDA.

Richter, JM. July 1984. Crisis of mate loss in the elderly. *American Nursing Society* 6(4):45–54.

Ross, HM. 1981. Societal/cultural views regarding death and dying. *Topics in Clinical Nursing* 3(3):1–16.

Salter, R. March 1982. The art of dying. *Canadian Nurse* 78:20–21.

Sanders, CM. 1989. *Grief: The Mourning After: Dealing with Adult Bereavement.* New York: Wiley.

Schulz, R. 1978. *The Psychology of Death, Dying and Bereavement.* Reading, MA: Addison-Wesley.

Seventh-day Adventists Believe . . . 1988. Silver Spring, MD: General Conference of Seventh-day Adventists.

Sheehy, PF. 1981. *On Dying with Dignity.* New York: Pinnacle Books.

Sowell, RL, Bramlett, MH, Gueldner, SH, Gritzmacher, D and Martin, G. Summer 1991. The lived experience of survival and bereavement following the death of a lover from AIDS. *Image: Journal of Nursing Scholarship* 23:89–94.

Spector, RE. 1991. *Cultural Diversity in Health and Illness.* 3d ed. Norwalk, CT: Appleton & Lange.

Strauss, AL, and Glasser, BG. 1970. Awareness of dying. In Schoenberg, B, Carr, AC, Peretz, D, and Kutcher, AH, editors. *Loss and Grief.* New York: Columbia University Press.

Sumner, L and Hurula, J. August 1993. Pediatric hospice nursing: Making the most of each moment. *Nursing93* 23:50–55.

Taylor, PB and Ferszt, GG. January 1994. Letting go of a loved one. *Nursing94* 24:54–56.

UNIT 10

Promoting Physiologic Health

STUDENT PROFILE

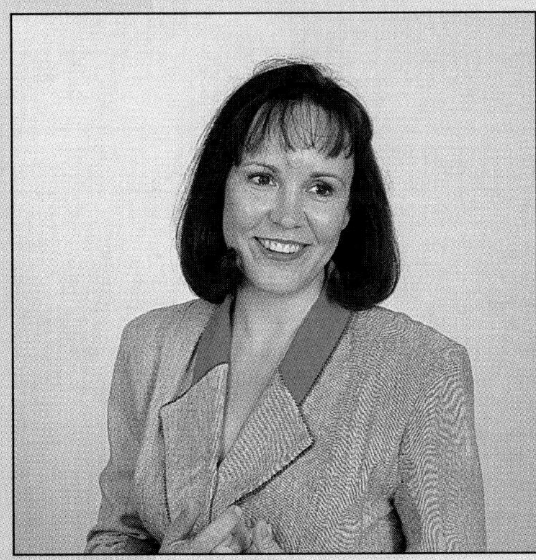

NAME Pam Smith

SCHOOL OF NURSING Rogers State College, Claremore, Oklahoma

HOMETOWN Claremore, Oklahoma

WHY DID YOU ENTER THE FIELD OF NURSING?
I had reached a point in my life where it was time for a change; in my job, in my goals, and in my future. The varied and exciting career that nursing offered appealed to me. The field of nursing will allow me to enter the world as a professional.

WHO OR WHAT INFLUENCED THAT DECISION?
A friend inspired me, "Yes, you can take that first step." I took that step and many more and have not regretted a day.

WHAT IS THE MOST CHALLENGING ASPECT OF NURSING FOR YOU?
The vast amount of information and high degree of skills needed by a nurse today.

WHAT QUALITIES DO YOU THINK ARE NECESSARY TO BE A GOOD NURSE?
Caring, sharing, compassion, love.

WHAT HAS BEEN YOUR MOST GRATIFYING MOMENT AS A STUDENT NURSE?
When a terminal patient shared the story of her life, which included a secret desire to be a nurse, and then thanked me for my care and concern.

WHAT ADVICE WOULD YOU GIVE A NEW STUDENT?
Be like a sponge and absorb all you can. Don't be afraid to ask questions.

34 Activity and Exercise

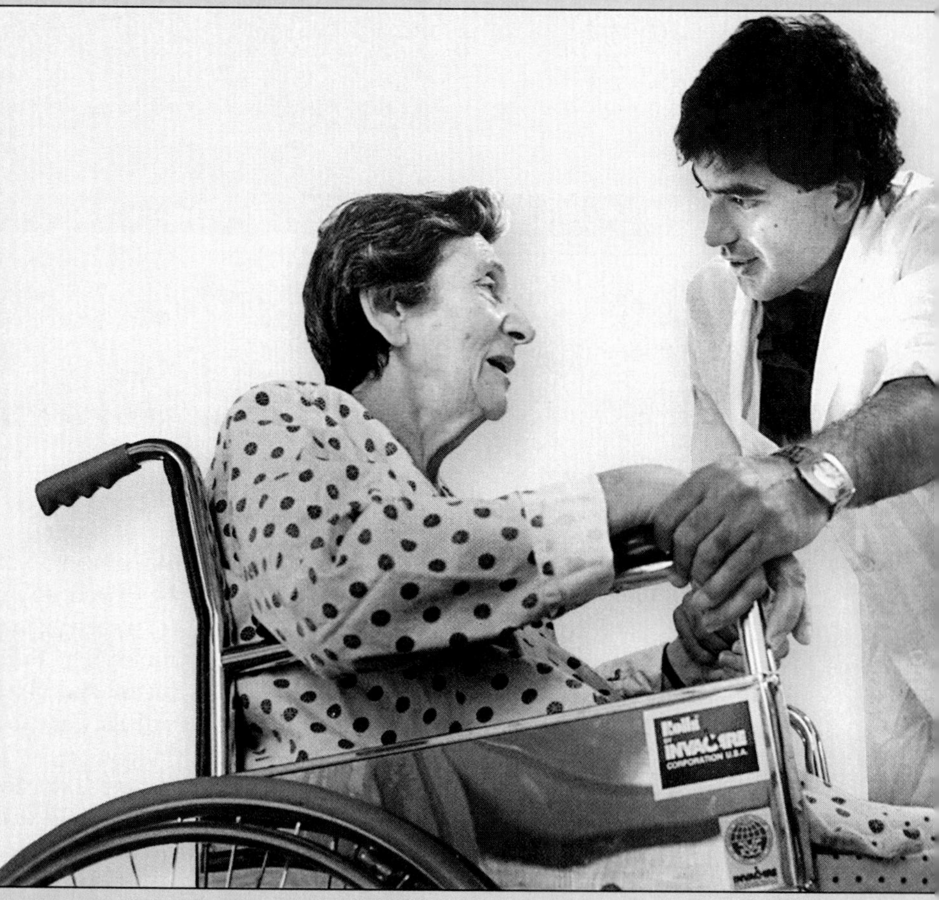

Objectives

Identify the importance, for both clients and nurses, of maintaining good body alignment and using good body mechanics.

Describe the three basic elements of body mechanics.

Identify principles or concepts for safe and effective body movement.

Identify factors influencing a person's body alignment and mobility.

Compare the effects of immobility and exercise on body systems.

Identify information to obtain in a health history to assess a client's activity/exercise pattern.

Describe essential aspects of assessing a client's posture, gait, joint appearance and movement, capabilities and limitations for movement, muscle mass and strength, activity tolerance, and problems related to immobility.

Describe examples of nursing diagnoses related to activity/exercise problems.

List outcome criteria to evaluate the client's responses to strategies implemented to promote activity/exercise.

Identify appropriate interventions to prevent musculoskeletal problems and pressure areas in various bed positions described in this chapter.

Describe essential steps and rationales of techniques to move and turn clients in bed and to transfer clients from bed to chair or to stretcher.

Describe five major kinds of exercise that may be implemented to maintain or improve physical fitness.

Describe purposes of three kinds of joint range-of-motion exercises.

Assist clients to ambulate safely with or without assistive devices.

Assist clients to design an effective exercise program.

The ability to move freely, easily, rhythmically, and purposefully in the environment is an essential part of living. **Activity** can be described as energetic action or as being in a state of movement. People must move to obtain food and water, to protect themselves from trauma, and to meet other basic needs. Mobility is vital to independence; a fully immobilized person is as vulnerable and dependent as an infant.

People often define their health and physical fitness by their activity, because mental well-being and the effectiveness of body functioning depend largely on their mobility status. For example, when a person is upright, the lungs expand more easily, intestinal activity (peristalsis) is more effective, and the kidneys are able to empty completely. In addition, motion is essential for proper functioning of bones and muscles.

The ability to move also influences self-esteem and body image, both components of self-concept. For most people, self-esteem depends on a sense of independence and a feeling of usefulness or being needed. People with mobility impairments may feel helpless and burdensome to others. Body image can be altered by paralysis, amputations, or any motor impairment. The reaction of others to impaired mobility can also alter self-esteem and body image significantly.

Body Mechanics

Good body mechanics is the efficient, coordinated, and safe use of the body to produce motion and maintain balance during activity. Proper movement promotes body musculoskeletal functioning, reduces the energy required to move and maintain balance, therefore reducing fatigue, and decreasing the risk of injury.

The major purpose of proper body mechanics is to facilitate safe and efficient use of appropriate groups of muscles. Good body mechanics is essential to both clients and nurses to prevent strain, injury, and fatigue.

Body mechanics involves three basic elements: Body alignment (posture), balance (stability), and coordinated body movement.

Body Alignment

Body alignment is the geometric arrangement of body parts in relation to each other. Good alignment promotes optimal balance and maximal body function in whatever position the client assumes: standing, sitting, or lying down. Good body alignment and good **posture** are synonymous terms. When the body is well aligned, balance is achieved without undue strain on the joints, muscles, tendons, or ligaments. Skeletal muscles are usually in a state of slight tension or contraction **(tonus)** when the body is healthy and well aligned. This state requires minimal muscular force and yet supports the internal framework and organs.

Proper body alignment enhances lung expansion and promotes efficient circulatory, renal, and gastrointestinal functions. Conversely, poor body alignment detracts from a pleasing appearance and affects an individual's health adversely. A person's posture is one criterion for assessing general health, physical fitness, and attractiveness. Posture reflects the mood, self-esteem, and personality of an individual.

Balance

Balance is a state of equipoise (equilibrium) in which opposing forces counteract each other. Good body alignment is essential to body balance. It is difficult to differentiate balance from body alignment, although balance is the result of proper alignment. A person maintains balance as long as the **line of gravity** (an imaginary vertical line drawn through an object's center of gravity) passes through the **center of gravity** (the point at which all of the mass of an object is centered) and the **base of support** (the foundation on which an object rests).

The center of gravity of a well-aligned standing adult is located slightly anterior to the upper part of the sacrum (Figure 34–1, p. 880). Standing posture can be unstable because of a narrow base of support, a high center of gravity, and a constantly shifting line of gravity. For greatest balance and stability, a standing adult must center body weight symmetrically along the line of gravity.

In a well-aligned standing person, the center of gravity remains fairly stable. When the person moves, however, the center of gravity shifts continuously in the direction of the moving body parts. Balance depends on the interrelationship of the center of gravity, the line of gravity, and the base of support. When a person moves, the closer the line of gravity is to the center of the base of support, the greater the person's stability (Figure 34–2, *A*, p. 880). Conversely, the closer the line of gravity is to the edge of the base of support, the more precarious the balance (Figure 34–2, *B*). If the line of gravity falls outside the base of support, the person falls (Figure 34–2, *C*).

The broader the base of support and the lower the center of gravity, the greater the stability and balance. Body balance, therefore, can be greatly enhanced by (a) widening the base of support and (b) lowering the center of gravity, bringing it closer to the base of support. The base of support is easily widened by spreading the feet farther apart. The center of gravity is readily lowered by flexing the hips and knees until a squatting position is achieved.

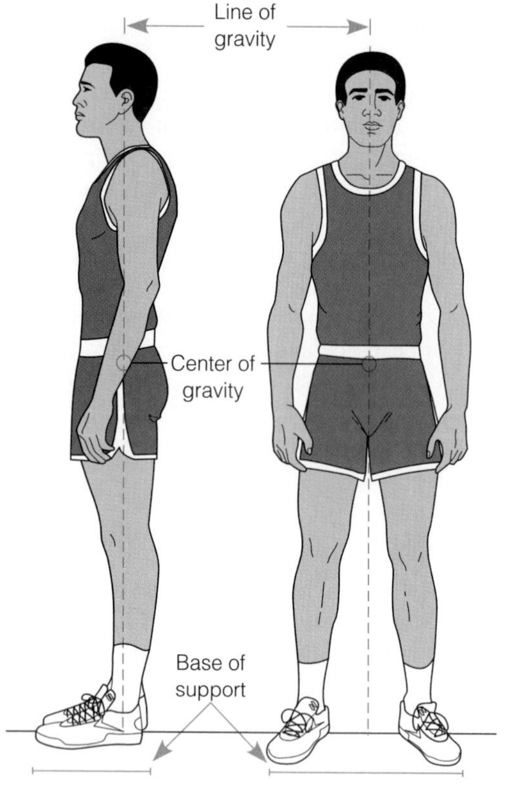

Figure 34–1 The center of gravity and the line of gravity influence standing alignment.

The importance of these alterations cannot be overemphasized for nurses.

When a person rests in a chair or bed, the feet of the chair or bed form a considerably wider base of support. The center of gravity is lower, and the line of gravity is less mobile. Thus, a person has greater stability and balance in a sitting or lying position than in a standing position.

COORDINATED BODY MOVEMENT

Body mechanics involves the integrated functioning of the musculoskeletal and nervous systems as well as joint mobility. Muscle tone, the neuromuscular reflexes (including the visual and proprioceptive reflexes), and the coordinated movements of opposing voluntary muscle groups (the antagonistic, synergistic, and antigravity muscles) play important roles in producing balanced, smooth, purposeful movement.

Muscles contract and relax. When a muscle contracts, it becomes shorter, bringing the bones to which it is attached closer. At the same time, muscles on the other side of the joint relax or lengthen, to permit the movement. Each muscle normally has an *antagonist muscle*, which acts in the opposite manner. For example, the hamstring muscles flex the leg (bend the knee) and the quadriceps femoris muscles extend the leg (straighten the knee).

Synergistic muscles prevent undesirable movements. They aid the action of a prime mover by effecting the

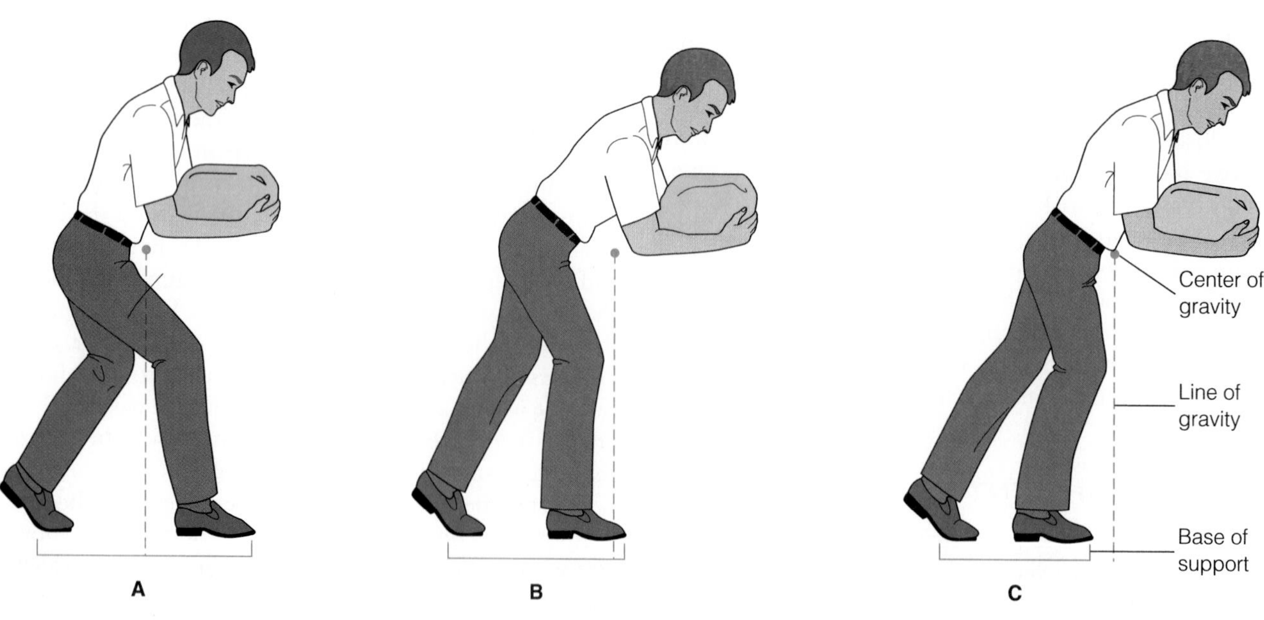

Figure 34–2 *A,* Balance is maintained when the line of gravity falls close to the base of support. *B,* Balance is precarious when the line of gravity falls at the edge of the base of support. *C,* Balance cannot be maintained when the line of gravity falls outside the base of support.

Table 34–1 Types of Synovial Joint Movements

Movement	Action
Flexion	Decreasing the angle of the joint (eg, bending the elbow)
Extension	Increasing the angle of the joint (eg, straightening the arm at the elbow)
Hyperextension	Further extension or straightening of a joint (eg, bending the head backward)
Abduction	Movement of the bone away from the midline of the body
Adduction	Movement of the bone toward the midline of the body
Rotation	Movement of the bone around its central axis
Circumduction	Movement of the distal part of the bone in a circle while the proximal end remains fixed
Eversion	Turning the sole of the foot outward by moving the ankle joint
Inversion	Turning the sole of the foot inward by moving the ankle joint
Pronation	Moving the bones of the forearm so that the palm of the hand faces downward when held in front of the body
Supination	Moving the bones of the forearm so that the palm of the hand faces upward when held in front of the body
Protraction	Moving a part of the body forward in the same plane parallel to the ground
Retraction	Moving a part of the body backward in the same plane parallel to the ground

same movement or by stabilizing joints across which the prime mover acts. For example, the flexor muscles of the fingers cross both the wrist and the phalangeal joints, but the fingers can be flexed without bending the wrist because synergistic muscles stabilize the wrist joint.

Continuous action of postural muscles sustains humans in an upright position against the force of gravity. The extensor muscles, often referred to as the *antigravity* muscles, carry the major load. Sustained contraction of the muscles supporting this upright position is called **postural tonus.** Numerous postural or **righting reflexes** stimulate and maintain postural tonus.

1. *Labyrinthine sense.* Sensory organs of the inner ear stimulate postural tonus through impulses that arise when the head is moved. These impulses are transmitted to the cerebellum.
2. *Tonic neck-righting reflexes.* Movement of the head from side to side affects tonic neck reflexes. Tonus of the neck muscles seems most affected when the head is thrown backward.
3. *Visual or optic reflexes.* Visual impressions are important in maintaining erect posture. Visual sensations help the person establish spatial relationships to objects in the environment.
4. *Proprioceptor or kinesthetic sense.* The kinesthetic sense, sometimes referred to as the sixth sense, is activated when nerve endings in muscles, tendons, and fascia are stimulated by movements of joints. Individuals become aware of their position when the brain is informed of the location of a limb or body part at any given moment.
5. *Extensor or antigravity (stretch) reflexes.* This reflex is best developed in the extensor muscles, which counteract the tendency of the body to flex at the hip and the knees because of its own weight. If, for example, the knees begin to buckle under the influence of gravity, the extensor muscles of the knee joint are stretched, straightening the knee joint and maintains upright posture.
6. *Plantar reflexes.* Pressure against the sole of the foot by the ground elicits a reflexive contraction of the extensor muscles of the lower legs.

JOINT MOBILITY

A joint is the functional unit of the musculoskeletal system. The bones of the skeleton articulate at the joints. Most of the skeletal muscles attach to the two bones at the joint. These muscles are categorized according to the type of joint movement they produce on contraction. Muscles are therefore called flexors, extensors, internal rotators, and the like. The flexor muscles are stronger than the extensor muscles. Thus, when a person is inactive, the joints are pulled into a flexed (bent) position. If this tendency is not counteracted with exercise and position changes, the muscles permanently shorten, and the joint becomes fixed in a flexed position. The types of synovial joint movement are shown in Table 34–1.

Table 34–2 Joint Movements

Movement	Normal Range	Major Muscle(s)	Illustration
Temporomandibular Joint (TMJ)			
TMJ opening. Open mouth.	3 to 6 cm (1 to 2.3 in)		
TMJ closure. Close mouth.	Complete closure	Masseter and temporalis	
Protrusion. Jut chin out (Figure 1).		Pterygoideus lateralis	Figure 1
Retrusion. Tuck chin in (Figure 1).			
Lateral motion. Move jaw from side to side (Figure 2).	1 to 2 cm (0.3 to 0.7 in) from midline	Pterygoideus lateralis and pterygoideus medialis	Figure 2
Neck—Pivot Joint			
Flexion. Move the head from the upright midline position forward, so that the chin rests on the chest (Figure 3).	45° from midline	Sternocleidomastoideus	
Extension. Move the head from the flexed position to the upright position (Figure 3).	45° from midline	Trapezius	Figure 3
Hyperextension. Move the head from the upright position back as far as possible.	10°	Trapezius	
Lateral flexion. Move the head laterally to the right and left shoulders, while facing front (Figure 4).	40° from midline	Sternocleidomastoideus	Figure 4
Rotation. Turn the face as far as possible to the right and left (Figure 5).	70° from midline	Sternocleidomastoideus and trapezius	Figure 5

A **synovial joint** is freely movable, has space between the articulating bone surfaces, and characteristically has a cavity enclosed by a capsule. Within this capsule is a lining of synovial membrane, which secretes synovial fluid to lubricate the joint. Cartilage provides a smooth surface on which the bone glides during movement.

Range of Motion The *range of motion* of a joint is the maximum movement that is possible for that joint. Joint range of motion varies from individual to individual and is determined by genetic makeup, developmental patterns, the presence or absence of disease, and the amount of physical activity in which the person normally engages. Table 34–2 shows the various joint movements and the normal ranges of motion.

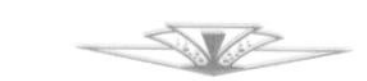

PREVENTING BACK INJURY

Many factors increase the potential for lower back injuries. A major contributor is habitually poor standing and sitting posture, which produces an exaggerated curvature

Text continued on page 887

Table 34–2 ***continued***

Movement	Normal Range	Major Muscle(s)	Illustration
Shoulder—Ball-and-Socket Joint			
Flexion. Raise each arm from a position by the side forward and upward to a position beside the head (Figure 6).	180° from the side	Pectoralis major, coracobrachialis, and deltoideus	
Extension. Move each arm from a vertical position beside the head forward and down to a resting position at the side of the body (Figure 6).	180° from vertical position beside the head	Latissimus dorsi, deltoideus, and teres major	Figure 6
Hyperextension. Move each arm from a resting side position to behind the body (Figure 6).	50° from side position	Latissimus dorsi, deltoideus, and teres major	
Abduction. Move each arm laterally from a resting position at the sides to a side position above the head, palm of the hand away from the head. (Figure 7).	180°	Deltoideus and supraspinatus	
Adduction (anterior). Move each arm from a position beside the head downward laterally and across the front of the body as far as possible (Figure 8).	230°	Pectoralis major and teres major	Figure 7
Adduction (posterior). Move each arm from a position beside the head downward laterally and across behind the body as far as possible.	230°	Latissimus dorsi and teres major	
Horizontal flexion. Extend each arm laterally at shoulder height and move it through a horizontal plane across the front of the body as far as possible (Figure 9).	130° to 135°	Pectoralis major and coracobrachialis	Figure 8
Horizontal extension. Extend each arm laterally at shoulder height and move it through a horizontal plane as far behind the body as possible (Figure 9).	45°	Latissimus dorsi, teres major, and deltoideus	
Circumduction. Move each arm forward, up, back, and down in a full circle (Figure 10).	360°	Deltoideus, coracobrachialis, latissimus dorsi, and teres major	Figure 9
External rotation. With each arm held out to the side at the shoulder level and the elbow bent to a right angle, fingers pointing down, move the arm upward so that the fingers point up (Figure 11, p. 884).	90°	Infraspinatus and teres minor	Figure 10

Table 34–2 Joint Movements *continued*

Movement	Normal Range	Major Muscle(s)	Illustration
***Shoulder—Ball-and-Socket Joint** continued*			
Internal rotation. With each arm held out to the side at shoulder level and the elbow bent to a right angle, fingers pointing up, bring the arm forward and down so that the fingers point down (Figure 11).	90°	Subscapularis, pectoralis major, latissimus dorsi, and teres major	Figure 11
Elbow—Hinge Joint			
Flexion. Bring each lower arm forward and upward so that the hand is at the shoulder (Figure 12).	150°	Biceps brachii, brachialis, and brachioradialis	
Extension. Bring each lower arm forward and downward, straightening the arm (Figure 12).	150°	Triceps brachii	Figure 12
Rotation for supination. Turn each hand and forearm so that the palm is facing upward (Figure 13).	70° to 90°	Biceps brachii and supinator	
Rotation for pronation. Turn each hand and forearm so that the palm is facing downward (Figure 13).	70° to 90°	Pronator teres and pronator quadratus	Figure 13
Wrist—Condyloid Joint			
Flexion. Bring the fingers of each hand toward the inner aspect of the forearm (Figure 14).	80° to 90°	Flexor carpi radialis and flexor carpi ulnaris	
Extension. Straighten each hand to the same plane as the arm (Figure 14).	80° to 90°	Entensor carpi radialis longus	Figure 14
Hyperextension. Bend the fingers of each hand back as far as possible (Figure 15).	70° to 90°	Extensor carpi radialis longus extensor, carpi radialis brevis, and extensor carpi ulnaris	Figure 15
Radial flexion (abduction). Bend each wrist laterally toward the thumb side with hand supinated (Figure 16).	0 to 20°	Extensor carpi radialis longus	
Ulnar flexion (adduction). Bend each wrist laterally toward the fifth finger with the hand supinated.	30° to 50°	Extensor carpi ulnaris	Figure 16
Hand and Fingers: Metacarpophalangeal Joints—Condyloid; Interphalangeal Joints—Hinge			
Flexion. Make a fist with each hand (Figure 17).	90°	Interossei dorsales manus and flexor digitorum superficialis	
Extension. Straighten the fingers of each hand (Figure 17).	90°	Extensor indicis and extensor digiti minimi	Figure 17
Hyperextension. Bend the fingers of each hand back as far as possible.	30°	Extensor indicis and extensor digiti minimi	

Table 34–2 *continued*

Movement	Normal Range	Major Muscle(s)	Illustration
***Hand and Fingers: Metacarpophalangeal Joints—Condyloid; Interphalangeal Joints—Hinge** continued*			
Abduction. Spread the fingers of each hand apart (Figure 18).	20°	Interossei dorsales manus, abductor digiti minimi manus, and op ponens digiti minimi	Figure 18
Adduction. Bring the fingers of each hand together (Figure 18).	20°	Interrossei palmares	
Thumb—Saddle Joint			
Flexion. Move each thumb across the palmar surface of the hand toward the fifth finger (Figure 19).	90°	Flexor pollicis brevis and opponens pollicis	Figure 19
Extension. Move each thumb away from the hand.	90°	Extensor pollicis brevis and extensor pollicis longus	
Abduction. Extend each thumb laterally (Figure 20).	30°	Abductor pollicis brevis and abductor pollicis longus	Figure 20
Adduction. Move each thumb back to the hand (Figure 20).	30°	Adductor pollicis	
Opposition. Touch each thumb to the tip of each finger of the same hand. The thumb joint movements involved are abduction, rotation, and flexion (Figure 21).		Opponens pollicis and flexor pollicis brevis	Figure 21
Hip—Ball-and-Socket Joint			
Flexion. Move each leg forward and upward. The knee may be extended or flexed (Figure 22).	Knee extended, 90°; knee flexed, 120°	Psoas major and iliacus	Figure 22
Extension. Move each leg back beside the other leg (Figure 23).	90° to 120°	Gluteus maximus, adductor magnus, semitendinosus, and semimembranosus	
Hyperextension. Move each leg back behind the body (Figure 23).	30° to 50°	Gluteus maximus semitendinosus, and semimembranosus	

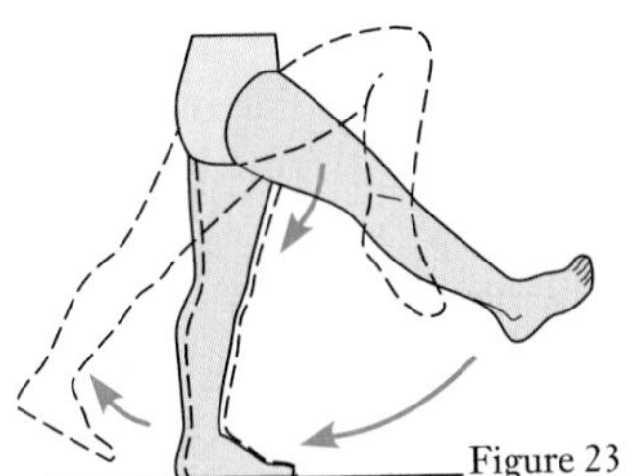
Figure 23

Table 34–2 Joint Movements *continued*

Movement	Normal Range	Major Muscle(s)	Illustration
***Hip—Ball-and-Socket Joint** continued*			
Abduction. Move each leg out to the side (Figure 24).	45° to 50°	Gluteus medius and gluteus minimus	
Adduction. Move each leg back to the other leg and beyond in front of it (Figure 24).	20° to 30° beyond other leg	Adductor magnus, adductor brevis, and adductor longus	Figure 24
Circumduction. Move each leg backward, up, to the side, and down in a circle (Figure 25).	360°	Psoas major, gluteus maximus, gluteus medius, and adductor magnus	
Internal rotation. Turn each foot and leg inward so that the toes point as far as possible toward the other leg (Figure 26).	90°	Gluteus minimus and tensor fasciae latae	
External rotation. Turn each foot and leg outward so that the toes point as far as possible away from the other leg (Figure 26).	90°	Obturator externus, obturator internus, and quadratus femoris	Figure 25
			Figure 26
Knee—Hinge Joint			
Flexion. Bend each leg bringing the heel toward the back of the thigh (Figure 27).	120° to 130°	Biceps femoris, semitendinosus, and semimembranosus	
Extension. Straighten each leg, returning the foot to its position beside the other foot (Figure 27).	120° to 130°	Rectus femoris, vastus lateralis, vastus medialis, and vastus intermedius	Figure 27
Ankle—Hinge Joint			
Extension (plantar flexion). Point the toes of each foot downward (Figure 28).	45° to 50°	Gastrocnemius and soleus	
Flexion (dorsiflexion). Point the toes of each foot upward (Figure 28).	20°	Peroneus tertius and tibialis anterior	Figure 28
Eversion. Turn the sole of each foot laterally (Figure 29).	5°	Peroneus longus and peroneus brevis	
Inversion. Turn the sole of each foot medially.	5°	Tibialis posterior and tibialis anterior	Figure 29

Table 34–2 *continued*

Movement	Normal Range	Major Muscle(s)	Illustration
Foot and Toes: Interphalangeal Joints—Hinge; Metatarsophalangeal Joints—Hinge; Intertarsal Joints—Gliding			
Flexion. Curve the toe joints of each foot downward (Figure 30).	35° to 60°	Flexor hallucis brevis, lumbricales pedis, and flexor digitorum brevis	
Extension. Straighten the toes of each foot (Figure 30).	35° to 60°	Extensor digitorum longus, extensor digitorum brevis and extensor hallucis longus	Figure 30
Abduction. Spread the toes of each foot apart.	0 to 15°	Interossei dorsales pedis and abductor hallucis	
Adduction. Bring the toes of each foot together.	0 to 15°	Adductor hallucis and interossei plantares	
Trunk—Gliding Joint			
Flexion. Bend the trunk toward the toes (Figure 31).	70° to 90°	Rectus abdominis, psoas major, and psoas minor	
Extension. Straighten the trunk from a flexed position (Figure 31).	70° to 90°	Longissimus thoracis, iliocostalis thoracis, iliocostalis lumborum, erector spinae, and longissimus cervicis	Figure 31
Hyperextension. Bend the trunk backward.	20° to 30°	Longissimus thoracis, iliocostalis thoracis, iliocostalis lumborum, erector spinae, and longissimus cervicis	
Lateral flexion. Bend the trunk to the right and to the left (Figure 32).	35° on each side	Quadratus lumborum	Figure 32
Rotation. Turn the upper part of the body from side to side (Figure 33).	30° to 45°	Erector spinae	Figure 33

of the lumbar spine, called **lordosis.** Overweight individuals who carry their extra weight over their abdomen, pregnant women, and women who consistently wear high-heeled shoes are at risk because of the exaggerated lumbar curvature these situations produce. Sedentary persons are at greater risk because of weak back and abdominal muscles.

Lower back injuries are preventable. Some guidelines for preventing back injuries are presented in the box on page 888.

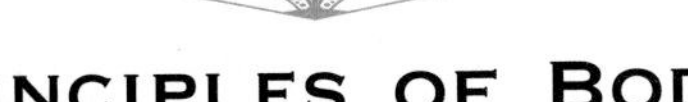

PRINCIPLES OF BODY MECHANICS

The concepts of center of gravity, line of gravity, and base of support were discussed earlier in relation to body alignment and balance. In addition to these concepts, the nurse needs to consider the concepts of **leverage, force, friction,** and **inertia** when moving clients or objects. These

WELLNESS TEACHING

Preventing Back Injuries

- Become consciously aware of your posture and body mechanics.
- Make a conscious effort to improve your posture and body mechanics. Seek assistance if you need it.
- Minimize lumbar lordosis as much as possible:
  a. When standing for a period of time, periodically flex one hip and knee and rest your foot on an object if possible.
  b. When sitting, keep your knees slightly higher than your hips.
  c. Unless you have a pillow or other support beneath your abdomen, avoid sleeping in the prone position.
- Use a firm mattress that provides good body support at natural body curvatures.
- Exercise regularly to maintain overall physical condition; include exercises that strengthen the pelvic, abdominal, and lumbar muscles.
- Avoid exercises that cause pain or require spinal flexion with straight legs (eg, toe-touching and sit ups) or spinal rotation (twisting).
- Avoid activities that require an excessive arching of the spine (eg, hockey) and spinal rotation (eg, golf or tennis) *unless* you are physically fit.
- Apply principles of body mechanics when moving objects. For example:
  a. Spread your feet apart to provide a wide base of support.
  b. Place your feet appropriately in the direction in which the movement occurs.
  c. Keep objects to be moved close to the body.
  d. Push, pull, roll, or slide objects rather than lifting them, whenever possible.
  e. When pushing or pulling an object, use the body's weight to counteract the weight of the object.
  f. Avoid twisting the spine by pushing or pulling objects directly away from or toward the body and squarely facing the direction of movement.
  g. When lifting objects, distribute the weight between large muscles of the legs and arms.
- Plan ahead how you will move a load and where you will move it. Make sure the area is free of obstructions.
- Wear clothing that allows you to use good body mechanics and comfortable low-heeled shoes that provide good foot support and will not cause you to slip, stumble, or turn your ankle.

Table 34–3 Concepts Applicable to Moving Clients

Concept	Definition
Friction	Force that opposes the motion of an object as it is slid across the surface of another object.
Force	The energy or power required to accomplish movement.
Inertia	The tendency of an object at rest to remain at rest and an object in motion to remain in motion.
Fulcrum	A fixed point (eg, elbow) about which a lever moves.
Lever (first class)	A rigid piece that transmits or modifies motion or force. When force (energy) is applied to the rigid arm with a fixed point (fulcrum), an object at the other end of the rigid arm can be lifted more easily.

concepts are defined and discussed in Tables 34–3 and 34–4.

Two movements to avoid because of their potential for causing back injury are twisting (rotation) of the thoracolumbar spine and acute flexion of the back with hips and knees straight (stooping). Undesirable twisting of the back can be prevented by squarely facing the direction of movement, whether pushing, pulling, or sliding, and moving the object directly toward or away from one's center of gravity.

LIFTING

When a person lifts or carries an object, the weight of the object becomes part of the person's body weight. This weight affects the location of the person's center of gravity, which is displaced in the direction of the added weight. To counteract this potential imbalance, body parts move in a direction away from the weight. In this way, the center of gravity is maintained over the same point in the base of support. By holding the center of gravity of the lifted object as close as possible to the body's center of gravity, the lifter avoids undue displacement of the center of gravity and achieves greater stability.

Although there are three types of **levers,** the type nurses use most frequently in lifting is the third class lever (Figure 34–3, *A*, on page 890). In the body, the joints are the **fulcrums,** and the bones of the skeleton act as levers. The force, or effort, provided by muscle contraction is applied where a muscle attaches to bone. When the nurse lifts objects, the resisting force or weight is held in the hands or on the forearms, the fulcrum is the elbow, and the force is applied by contraction of the flexor muscles of the forearm (Figure 34–3, *B*). The lifting power is

Table 34–4 Summary of Principles and Guidelines Related to Body Mechanics

Principles	Guidelines
Balance is maintained and muscle strain is avoided as long as the line of gravity passes through the base of support.	Start any body movement with proper alignment. Stand as close as possible to the object to be moved. Avoid stretching, reaching, and twisting, which may place the line of gravity outside the base of support.
The wider the base of support and the lower the center of gravity, the greater the stability. Objects that are close to the center of gravity are moved with the least effort.	Before moving objects, increase your stability by widening your stance and flexing your knees, hips, and ankles. Adjust the working area to waist level, and keep the body close to the area. Elevate adjustable beds and overbed tables or lower the side rails of beds to prevent stretching and reaching.
Balance is maintained with minimal effort when the base of support is enlarged in the direction in which the movement will occur.	When *pushing* an object, enlarge the base of support by moving the front foot forward. When *pulling* an object, enlarge the base of support by either moving the rear leg back if facing the object or moving the front foot forward if facing away from the object.
The greater the preparatory isometric tensing, or contraction of muscles, before moving an object, the less the energy required to move it, and the less the likelihood of musculoskeletal strain and injury.	Before moving objects, contract your gluteal, abdominal, leg, and arm muscles to prepare them for action.
The synchronized use of as many large muscle groups as possible during an activity increases overall strength and prevents muscle fatigue and injury.	To move objects below your center of gravity, begin with the back and knees flexed. Use your gluteal and leg muscles rather than the sacrospinal muscles of your back to exert an upward thrust when lifting the weight. Distribute the work load between both arms and legs to prevent back strain. Always face the direction of the movement to prevent twisting of the spine and ineffective use of major muscle groups.
The closer the line of gravity to the *center* of the base of support, the greater the stability.	When moving or carrying objects, hold them as close as possible to your center of gravity. Pull an object toward you rather than pushing it away to control its movement and keep it close to your center of gravity.
The greater the friction against the surface beneath an object, the greater the force required to move the object. Pulling creates less friction than pushing. The heavier an object, the greater the force needed to move the object.	Provide a firm, smooth, dry bed foundation before moving a client in bed. Pull clients rather than push them whenever possible. Encourage clients to assist as much as possible by pushing or pulling themselves to reduce the muscular effort of the nurse. Use arms as levers whenever possible to increase lifting power. Use own body weight to counteract the weight of the object. For example, lean forward when pushing an object, and rock your body weight backward when pulling an object or client toward you. Obtain the assistance of other persons or use mechanical devices to move objects that are too heavy.
Moving an object along a level surface requires less energy than moving an object up an inclined surface or lifting it against the force of gravity.	Avoid working against gravity. Pull, push, roll, or turn objects instead of lifting them. Lower the head of the client's bed before moving client up in bed.
Continuous muscle exertion can result in muscle strain and injury.	Alternate rest periods with periods of muscle use to help prevent fatigue.

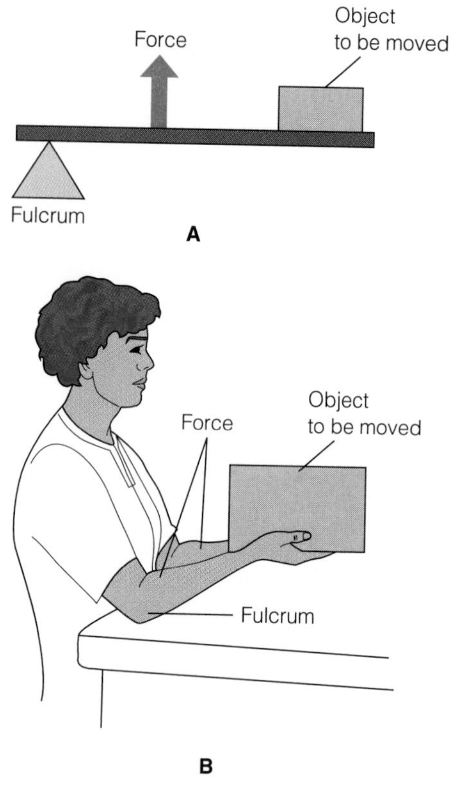

Figure 34–3 *A*, A third-class lever. *B*, Using the arm as a lever.

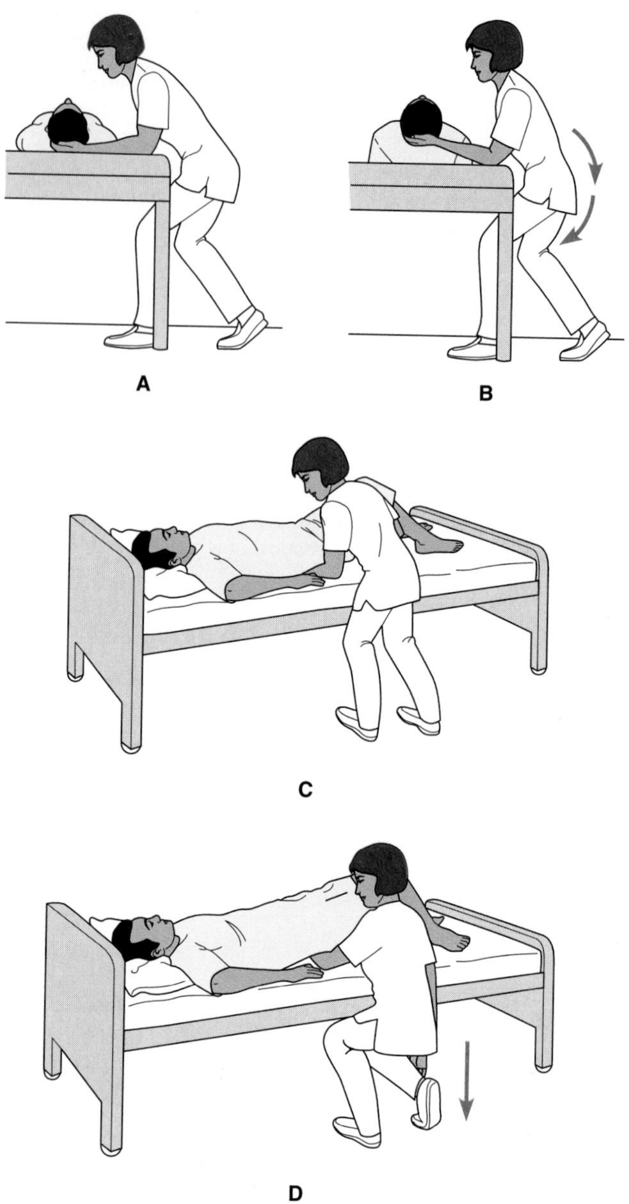

Figure 34–4 This nurse uses her arms as levers and employs her body weight to lift a client: *A*, position before lifting; *B*, position after lifting; *C* and *D*, the nurse uses positions *A* and *B* to lift a client's buttocks.

increased when the elbow (fulcrum) is supported on a bed surface or a countertop. People can lift more weight when they use this lever than when they do not. Use of the arms as levers is often applied in clinical practice when the nurse needs to raise the head or buttocks of a client in bed, for example, to assist the client onto a bedpan or to give back care to a client in traction. Figure 34–4 illustrates this lifting technique.

Because lifting involves movement against gravity, the nurse must use major muscle groups of the thighs, knees, upper and lower arms, abdomen, and pelvis to prevent back strain. The nurse can increase overall muscle strength by synchronized use of as many muscle groups as possible during an activity. For instance, when the arms are used in an activity, dividing the work between the arms and legs helps prevent back strain. The nurse further enhances lifting power by using body weight to counteract the client's weight. The nurse increases hip and knee flexion to lower the center of gravity. As the nurse does so, the forearms and hands supporting the client automatically rise (Figure 34–4, *C* and *D*).

Another technique based on the principle of leverage is also recommended. In this technique, the back and knees are flexed until the load is at thigh level, at which point the knees are flexed more to provide thrust as the back begins to straighten (Figure 34–5). This technique provides for better balance, leverage, and synchronized use of muscles, which help avoid back pain and injury. When one lifts an object to knee level, the shoulder and arm muscles pull, the abdominal and lumbar muscles contract for leverage and pull, and the thigh and leg muscles exert the upward thrust to bring the object off the floor. When one lifts an object from mid-thigh to waist level, force is provided essentially by the leg and thigh muscle groups, but the back and lumbar muscles remain contracted.

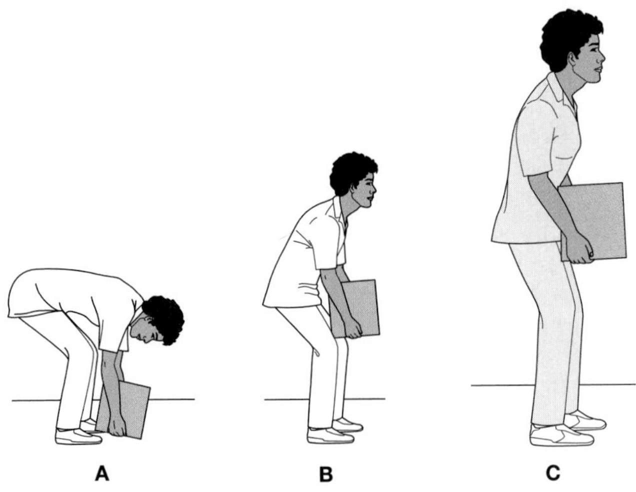

Figure 34–5 Stages in lifting an object to the waist: *A,* Move close to the object, and begin with the back and knees flexed to grasp the object. *B,* Start the lift by keeping the back flexed while the knees begin to straighten so that the leg muscles can exert an upward thrust. *C,* Keep the back and knees in a less flexed, but not straight, position (Owen 1980, p. 895).

In all positions, it is important to maintain a distance of at least 30 cm (12 in) between the feet and to keep the load close to the body, especially when it is at knee level (Owen 1985, p. 457). Before attempting the lift, the nurse must ensure that there are no hazards on the floor, that there is a clear path for moving the object, and that the nurse's base of support is secure.

PULLING AND PUSHING

When pulling or pushing an object, a person maintains balance with least effort when the base of support is enlarged in the direction in which the movement is to be produced or opposed. For example, when pushing an object, a person can enlarge the base of support by moving the front foot forward. When pulling an object, a person can enlarge the base of support by (a) moving the rear leg back if the person is facing the object; or (b) moving the front foot forward if the person is facing away from the object. It is easier and safer to pull an object toward one's own center of gravity than to push it away, as the person can exert more control of the object's movement when pulling it.

PIVOTING

Pivoting is a technique in which the body is turned in a way that avoids twisting of the spine. To pivot, place one foot ahead of the other, raise the heels very slightly, and put the body weight on the balls of the feet. When the weight is off the heels, the frictional surface is decreased and the knees are not twisted when turning. Keeping the body aligned, turn (pivot) about 90 degrees in the desired direction. The foot that was forward will now be behind. The box on page 888 presents guidelines for teaching how to maintain good body mechanics when moving objects.

FACTORS AFFECTING BODY ALIGNMENT AND MOBILITY

A number of factors affect an individual's body alignment and mobility. These include growth and development, physical health, mental health, nutrition, life-style, personal values, fatigue and stress, and certain external factors.

Growth and Development A person's age and musculoskeletal and nervous system development affect posture, body proportions, body mass, and body movements. Developmental variations are presented in Chapters 24, 25, and 26 and in Table 34–5, page 899.

Physical Health Problems of the musculoskeletal and/or nervous system often affect mobility and body alignment. One example is **osteoporosis,** a condition in which the bones become brittle and fragile due to calcium depletion. Osteoporosis is common in older women and primarily affects the weight-bearing joints of the lower extremities and the back.

Degenerative arthritis, or **osteoarthritis,** is another common cause of damage to the skeletal system. This disorder, common among the elderly, also affects the weight-bearing joints of the lower extremities and the back. Frequently, the knee and hip joints degenerate or develop bony spurs that cause pain on movement. In the back, degeneration of the vertebrae may produce painful narrowing of disc spaces or bony spurs on the edges of a vertebra.

Disorders of the nervous system that impair movement occur less frequently but are often more serious. Inner ear infections and dizziness can impair balance with movement. Parkinson's disease, multiple sclerosis, central nervous system tumors, cerebral vascular accidents (strokes), and spinal cord injuries can leave muscle groups weakened, paralyzed, **spastic** (with too much muscle tone), or **flaccid** (without muscle tone).

Problems of other body systems can also affect movement and body posture. For example, the unconscious client is often completely immobile, and the client who has abdominal pain often lies with knees drawn up to the abdomen.

Mental Health Mental health, too, can affect a person's appearance and movement. For example, the depressed person often appears slumped, with head bowed; may lack enthusiasm for taking part in any activity; and may even lack energy for usual hygienic practices. Furthermore, facial expression may be absent (lack of affect). By contrast, confident, happy people usually stand erect and have an animated facial expression.

Nutrition Both undernutrition and overnutrition can influence body alignment and mechanics. Poorly nourished people may have muscle weakness and fatigue. Inadequate calcium intake increases the risk of osteoporosis. Obesity can distort movement, and an obese person usually expends extra energy to move. Furthermore, obesity can adversely affect posture and balance.

Life-Style A person's life-style can affect posture and mobility. Postures repeatedly assumed during work can result in permanent postural defects; for example, a mail carrier may walk for years leaning to one side from carrying a heavy bag, or an assembly line worker may sit for hours hunched over a bench. Repeated physical activity, such as weight lifting, can produce muscle hypertrophy and concomitant alignment changes to accommodate the hypertrophy. Continual inactivity and resulting poor physical fitness can produce muscle atrophy and concomitant alignment changes to accommodate the atrophy, possibly resulting in back injuries. Repeatedly performed movements, especially twisting or bending of the back, can result in permanent disability. Repeatedly walking on slippery or uneven surfaces can result in disabling falls. The person who leads an overly busy, stressful, and active life can become careless and is at risk of injury.

Personal Values Personal values about body alignment and the use of good body mechanics are important influences. Tall adolescents may slouch because they do not value being taller than peers. Some people value good posture and intentionally try to maintain body alignment for reasons of health or appearance. Persons who value their appearance and health are more likely to practice good body mechanics and gait to protect their backs and prevent falls.

Fatigue and Stress Stress can deplete a person's energy to such a degree that it becomes difficult for the person to deal with day-to-day life. In addition, the person may feel too tired to exercise, which in itself could increase energy. Conversely, excessive exercise can fatigue a person and cause injury to the body.

External Factors Many external factors affect a person's mobility. Excessively high temperature and high humidity discourage activity, whereas comfortable temperature and humidity are conducive to activity, such as a brisk walk or a game of tennis. The availability of recreational facilities also influences activity; for example, lack of money may prohibit a client from joining an exercise group or swimming in an indoor pool. Neighborhood safety promotes outdoor activity, whereas an unsafe environment discourages people from going out of doors.

BENEFITS OF BED REST

- Reduces the needs of the body cells for oxygen because of reduced metabolism secondary to reduced activity
- Directs energy resources toward the healing process rather than toward activity
- Reduces pain in some instances, thereby decreasing the need for analgesics

EFFECTS OF IMMOBILITY AND EXERCISE ON BODY SYSTEMS

There are varying degrees of immobility. The unconscious client is often completely immobile, whereas the client with a fractured leg is only partially immobile. In addition, some clients restrict activity for health reasons. For example, a client who is short of breath may be advised not to walk up stairs.

Nurses use the term **bed rest** to describe a client's degree of immobility. The term has different meanings in different nursing settings. For example, in some settings, "complete bed rest" means that the client never moves from the bed and does not go to the bathroom or sit in a chair. "Bed rest," in contrast, may mean that the client stays in bed except when using a bedside commode or going to the bathroom. Nurses should be familiar with the meaning of such terms in their practice setting. See the box above for some of the common benefits of bed rest.

Whether bed rest causes any problems often depends on the duration of the bed rest, the client's health, and the client's sensory awareness. Exercise and joint movement also have many positive effects on body systems. Promoting exercise to maintain a client's muscle tone, joint mobility, and cardiovascular function is an important nursing function. For additional information regarding the effects of exercise, see Table 34–15 on page 932.

MUSCULOSKELETAL SYSTEM

Problems Related to Immobility The most obvious signs of prolonged immobility are often manifested in the musculoskeletal system. Clients experience a significant decrease in muscular strength whenever they do not maintain a moderate amount of physical activity. Common musculoskeletal problems resulting from prolonged immobility include the following:

- *Disuse osteoporosis.* Without the stress of weight-bearing activity, the bones demineralize. They are depleted chiefly of calcium, which gives the bones strength and density. Regardless of the amount of calcium in a person's diet, the demineralization process, known as **osteoporosis,** continues with immobility. The bones become spongy and may gradually deform and fracture easily.
- *Disuse atrophy.* Unused muscles **atrophy** (decrease in size), losing most of their strength and normal function.
- *Contractures.* When the muscle fibers are no longer able to shorten and lengthen, **contractures** form, limiting joint mobility. This process eventually involves the tendons, ligaments, and joint capsules; it is irreversible except by surgical intervention. Joint deformities such as foot drop and external hip rotation occur when a stronger muscle dominates the opposite muscle.
- *Stiffness and pain in the joints.* Without movement, the collagen (connective) tissues at the joint become **ankylosed** (permanently immobile). In addition, as the bones demineralize, excess calcium may deposit in the joints, contributing to stiffness and pain.

Effects of Exercise The size, shape, tone, and strength of muscles (including the heart muscle) are maintained with mild exercise and increased with strenuous exercise. With strenuous exercise, muscles **hypertrophy** (enlarge), and the efficiency of muscular contraction increases. Hypertrophy is commonly seen in the arm muscles of a tennis player, the leg muscles of a skater, the arm and hand muscles of a carpenter, and the body muscles of weight lifters.

Exercise also helps maintain joint mobility. Moreover, bone density is maintained through weight-bearing. The stress of weight-bearing maintains a balance between *osteoblasts* (bone-building cells) and *osteoclasts* (bone-resorption and breakdown cells).

CARDIOVASCULAR SYSTEM

Problems Related to Immobility

- *Diminished cardiac reserve.* Prolonged immobility weakens the cardiovascular system, which cannot fully meet the demands placed on it. Decreased mobility creates an imbalance in the autonomic nervous system, resulting in a preponderance of sympathetic activity over cholinergic activity that increases heart rate. Resting heart rate increases approximately 0.5 beats/minute per each day of immobilization (Kottke et al 1990, p. 1124).

  In a mobile, active person with a slow heart rate, the diastolic phase of the cardiac cycle is longer than the systolic phase. Because blood flow through coronary vessels occurs primarily during the diastolic phase, there is sufficient time for adequate blood flow through the coronary arteries. During immobility, however, the rapid heart rate reduces diastolic pressure, coronary blood flow, and the capacity of the heart to respond to any metabolic demands above the basal levels. Because of this diminished cardiac reserve, the immobilized person may experience tachycardia and angina with even minimal exertion.
- *Increased use of the Valsalva maneuver.* The Valsalva maneuver refers to holding the breath and straining against a closed glottis while moving. For example, clients tend to hold their breath when attempting to move up in a bed or sit on a bedpan. This builds up sufficient pressure on the large veins in the thorax to interfere with the return blood flow to the heart and coronary arteries. When the client exhales and the glottis again opens, pressure is suddenly released, and a surge of blood flows to the heart. Tachycardia and cardiac arrhythmias can result, if the client has cardiac disease.
- *Orthostatic (postural) hypotension.* Orthostatic hypotension is a common sequel of immobilization. Under normal conditions, sympathetic nervous system activity causes automatic vasoconstriction in the blood vessels in the lower half of the body when a mobile person changes from a horizontal to a vertical posture. Vasoconstriction prevents pooling of the blood in the legs and effectively maintains central blood pressure to ensure adequate perfusion of the heart and brain. During any prolonged immobility, this reflex becomes dormant. When the immobile person attempts to sit or stand, this reconstricting mechanism fails to function properly in spite of increased adrenalin output. The blood pools in the lower extremities, and central blood pressure drops. Cerebral perfusion is seriously compromised, and the person feels dizzy or lightheaded and may even faint. This sequence is usually accompanied by a sudden and marked increase in heart rate, the body's effort to protect the brain from an inadequate blood supply.
- *Venous vasodilation and stasis.* The skeletal muscles of an active person contract with each movement, compressing the blood vessels in those muscles and helping to pump the blood back to the heart against gravity. The tiny valves in the leg veins, which remain constricted, aid in venous return to the heart by preventing backward flow of blood and pooling. In an immobile

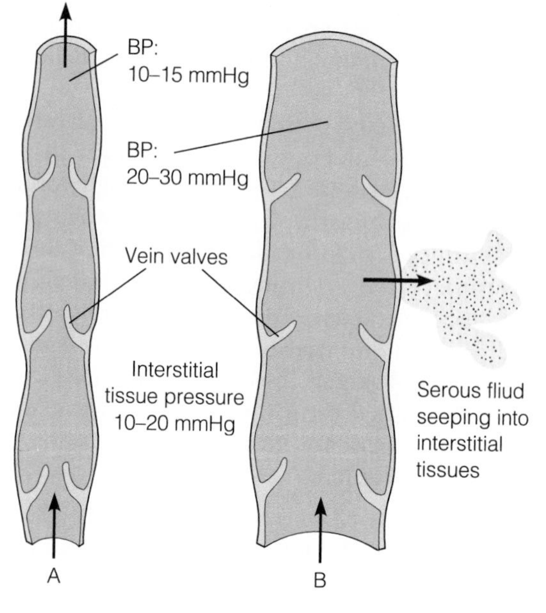

Figure 34–6 Leg veins: *A,* in a mobile person; *B,* in an immobile person.

person, the skeletal muscles do not contract sufficiently, and the muscles atrophy. The skeletal muscles can no longer assist in pumping blood back to the heart against gravity. Blood pools in the leg veins, causing vasodilation and engorgement. The valves in the veins can no longer work effectively to prevent backward flow of blood and pooling (Figure 34–6). This phenomenon is known as *incompetent valves.* As the blood continues to pool in the veins, its greater volume increases venous blood pressure, which can become much higher than that exerted by the tissues surrounding the vessel.

- *Dependent edema.* When the venous pressure is sufficiently great, some of the serous part of the blood is forced out of the blood vessel into the interstitial spaces surrounding the vessel, causing edema. Edema is most common in parts of the body positioned below heart level and maintained in that position. Dependent edema is most likely to occur around the sacrum or heels of a client who sits up in bed or in the feet and lower legs of a client who sits on the side of the bed. Edema further impedes venous return of blood to the heart, causing more pooling and more edema. Edematous tissue is uncomfortable and more susceptible to injury than normal tissue.
- *Thrombus formation.* Three factors, known as *Virchow's triad,* collectively predispose a client to the formation of a *thrombophlebitis* (a clot that is loosely attached to an inflamed vein wall). These are impaired venous return to the heart, hypercoagulability of the blood, and injury to a vessel wall.

A thrombus is particularly dangerous if it breaks loose from the vein wall to enter the general circulation as an *embolus* (a clot that has moved from its place of origin, causing obstruction to circulation elsewhere). Large emboli that enter the pulmonary circulation may occlude the vessels that nourish the lungs to cause an infarcted (dead) area of the lung. If the infarcted area is large, pulmonary function may be seriously compromised, or death may ensue. Emboli traveling to the coronary vessels or brain can produce a similarly dangerous outcome.

Effects of Exercise With adequate exercise, the heart rate increases, arterial (systolic) blood pressure increases, and blood is shunted from the nonexercising tissues to the heart and the muscles. Cardiac output (the amount of blood pumped by the heart) increases due to the redirection of the blood flow. Exercise can increase cardiac output to 22 L/min in the average person (Guyton 1991, p. 237). Normal cardiac output is 5 to 7 L/min. See also Table 34–15 on page 932.

RESPIRATORY SYSTEM

Problems Related to Immobility

- *Decreased respiratory movement.* In a recumbent, immobile client, ventilation of the lungs is passively altered. The rigid bed presses against the body and curtails chest movement. The abdominal organs push against the diaphragm, further restricting chest movement and making it difficult to expand the lungs fully. An immobile recumbent person rarely sighs, partly because overall muscle atrophy also affects the respiratory muscles and partly because there is no need to do so without the stimulus of activity. Without these periodic stretching movements, the cartilaginous intercostal joints may become fixed in an expiratory phase of respiration, further restricting the potential for maximal ventilation. These changes produce shallow respirations and reduce vital capacity significantly. **Vital capacity** is the maximum amount of air that can be exhaled after a maximum inhalation. An immobile, paralyzed client can lose as much as 25% to 50% of normal vital capacity (Kottke et al 1990, p. 1128).
- *Pooling of respiratory secretions.* Secretions of the respiratory tract are normally expelled by changing positions or posture and by coughing. Inactivity allows secretions to pool by gravity (Figure 34–7), interfering with the normal diffusion of oxygen and carbon dioxide in the alveoli. The ability to cough up secretions may also be hindered by loss of respiratory muscle tone, dehydration (which thickens secretions), or sedatives that depress the cough reflex. Poor oxygenation and retention of carbon dioxide in the blood can, if al-

lowed to continue, predispose the person to respiratory acidosis, a potentially lethal disorder.

- *Atelectasis.* When ventilation is decreased, pooled secretions may accumulate in a dependent area of a bronchiole and effectively block it. As a result of changes in regional blood flow, bed rest decreases the amount of surfactant produced. (Surfactant enables the alveoli to remain open.) The combination of decreased surfactant and blockage of a bronchiole with mucus can cause atelectasis (the collapse of a lobe or of an entire lung) distal to the mucous blockage. Immobile elderly, postoperative clients are at greatest risk of atelectasis.
- *Hypostatic pneumonia.* Pooled (hypostatic) secretions provide excellent media for bacterial growth. Under these conditions, a minor upper respiratory infection can evolve rapidly into a severe infection of the lower respiratory tract. Hypostatic pneumonia caused by static respiratory secretions can severely impair oxygen-carbon dioxide exchange in the alveoli and is a fairly common cause of death among weakened, immobile persons, especially heavy smokers.

Effects of Exercise Ventilation (the amount of air circulating into and out of the lungs) increases. In strenuous exercise, the intake of oxygen increases to as much as 20 times normal intake (Guyton 1991, p. 945). Normal ventilation is about 5 or 6 L/min. Adequate exercise also prevents pooling of secretions in the bronchi and bronchioles, decreases breathing effort, and improves diaphragmatic excursion.

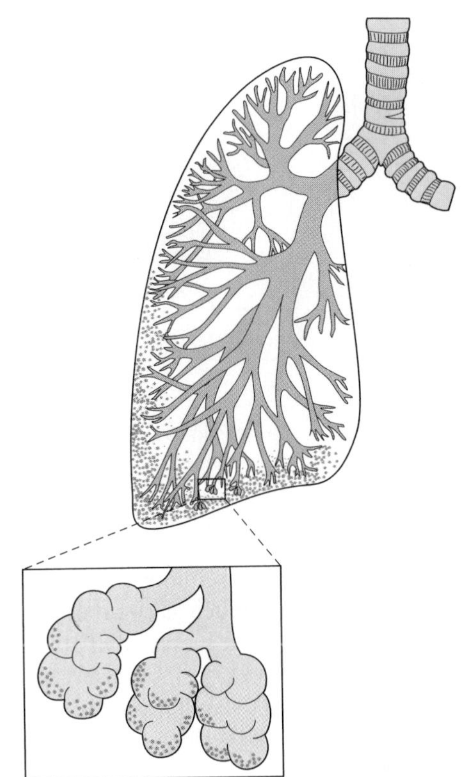

Figure 34–7 Pooling of secretions in the lungs of an immobile person.

METABOLIC SYSTEM

Problems Related to Immobility

- *Decreased metabolic rate.* **Metabolism** refers to all physical and chemical processes of the body. **Basal metabolism** is the minimal energy expended for the maintenance of these processes. The metabolic rate is the rate of basal metabolism expressed in calories per hour per square meter of body surface. In immobile clients, the basal metabolic rate decreases as the energy requirements of the body decrease. Gastrointestinal motility and secretions of various digestive glands are also reduced.
- *Negative nitrogen balance.* In an active person, there is a balance between protein synthesis *(anabolism)* and protein breakdown *(catabolism)*. Immobility creates a marked imbalance, and the catabolic processes exceed the anabolic processes. Over time, more nitrogen is excreted than is ingested, producing a negative nitrogen balance. Catabolized muscle mass is the source of this excreted nitrogen. Excessive amounts are excreted in the urine, reaching peak levels at about the sixth to tenth day of immobilization (Kottke et al 1990, p. 1125). The negative nitrogen balance represents a depletion of protein stores that are essential for building muscle tissue and for wound healing.
- *Anorexia.* Loss of appetite (anorexia) occurs as a result of the decreased metabolic rate and the increased catabolism that accompany immobility. Reduced caloric intake is usually a response to the decreased energy requirements of the inactive person. If protein intake is reduced, the nitrogen imbalance may become more pronounced, sometimes so severely that malnutrition ensues.
- *Negative calcium balance.* A negative calcium balance occurs as a direct result of immobility. Greater amounts of calcium are extracted from bone than can be replaced. The absence of weight-bearing and of stress on the musculoskeletal structures is the direct cause of the calcium loss from bones. Weight-bearing and stress, absent during immobility, are also required for calcium to be replaced in bone. A similar process occurs with the body's stores of phosphate to cause a negative phosphate balance to develop during immobility.

Effects of Exercise Exercise elevates the metabolic rate, thus increasing the production of body heat and

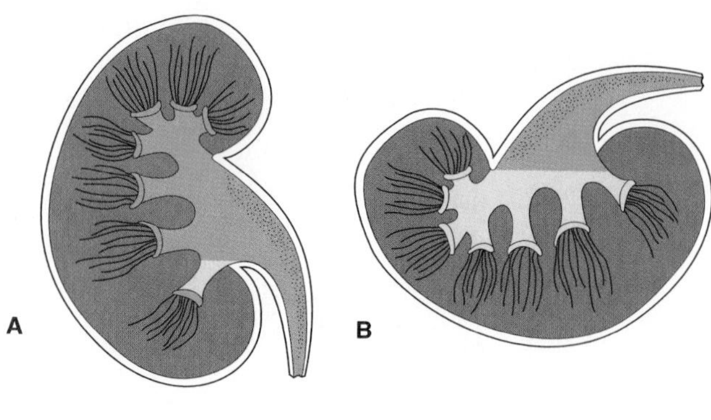

Figure 34–8 Pooling of urine in the kidney: *A,* The client is in an upright position; *B,* the client is in a back-lying position.

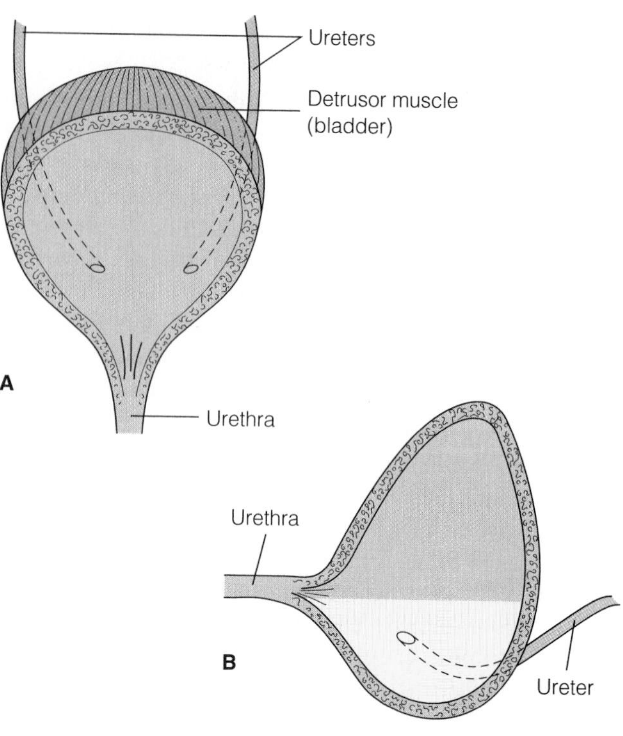

Figure 34–9 Pooling of urine in the urinary bladder: *A,* The client is in an upright position; *B,* the client is in a back-lying position.

waste products. During very strenuous exercise, the metabolic rate can increase to as much as 20 times the normal rate. Lying in bed and eating an average diet utilizes 1,850 calories per day (Guyton 1991, p. 793). Exercise also increases the use of triglycerides and fatty acids, resulting in a reduced level of serum triglycerides.

URINARY SYSTEM

Problems Related to Immobility

- *Urinary stasis.* In mobile persons, gravity plays an important role in the emptying of the kidneys and the bladder. The shape and position of the kidneys and active kidney contractions are important in completely emptying the urine from the calyces, renal pelvis, and ureters (Figure 34–8, *A*). The shape and position of the urinary bladder (the detrusor muscle) and active bladder contractions are also important in achieving complete emptying (Figure 34–9, *A*).

  When the person remains in a horizontal position, gravity impedes the emptying of urine from the kidneys and the urinary bladder. To urinate, the person who is supine (in a back-lying position) must push upward, against gravity (Figures 34–8, *B* and 34–9, *B*). The renal pelvis may fill with urine before it is pushed into the ureters. Emptying is not as complete, and **urinary stasis** occurs after a few days of bed rest. Because of the overall decrease in muscle tone during immobilization, including the tone of the detrusor muscle, bladder emptying is further compromised.
- *Renal calculi.* In a mobile person, calcium in the urine remains dissolved because calcium and citric acid are balanced in an appropriately acid urine. With immobility and the resulting excessive amounts of calcium (and phosphate) in the urine, this balance is no longer maintained. The urine becomes more alkaline, and the calcium salts precipitate out as crystals to form renal calculi (stones). In an immobile person in a horizontal position, the renal pelvis filled with stagnant, alkaline urine is an ideal location for calculi to form. The stones usually develop in the renal pelvis and pass through the ureters into the bladder. As the stones pass along the long, narrow ureters, they cause extreme pain and bleeding and can sometimes obstruct the urinary tract.
- *Urinary retention.* The immobile person may suffer from urinary retention, bladder distention, and occasionally **urinary incontinence** (involuntary urination). The decreased muscle tone of the urinary bladder inhibits its ability to empty completely, and the immobilized person is unable to relax the perineal muscles sufficiently to urinate. The discomfort of using a bedpan or urinal, the embarrassment and lack of privacy associated with this function, and the unnatural position for urination combine to make it difficult for the client to relax the perineal muscles sufficiently to urinate while lying in bed.

  When urination is not possible, the bladder gradually becomes distended with urine. The bladder may stretch excessively, eventually inhibiting the urge to void. When bladder distention is considerable, some involuntary urinary "dribbling" may occur *(retention with overflow)*. This does not relieve the urinary distention, because most of the stagnant urine remains in the bladder.
- *Urinary infection.* Static urine provides an excellent medium for bacterial growth. The flushing action of nor-

mal, frequent urination is absent, and urinary distention often causes minute tears in the bladder mucosa, allowing infectious organisms to enter. The increased alkalinity of the urine caused by the hypercalcuria supports bacterial growth. The organism most commonly causing urinary tract infections is *Escherichia coli*, which normally resides in the colon. The normally sterile urinary tract may be contaminated by improper perineal care, the use of an indwelling urinary catheter, or occasionally **urinary reflux** (backward flow). During reflux, contaminated urine from an overly distended bladder backs up into the renal pelvis to contaminate the kidney pelvis as well.

Effects of Exercise Because adequate exercise promotes efficient blood flow, the body excretes wastes more effectively. Also, stasis (stagnation) of urine in the bladder is usually prevented.

GASTROINTESTINAL SYSTEM

Problems Related to Immobility Constipation is a frequent problem for immobilized persons. Adrenalin production increases, resulting in decreased peristalsis and colon motility and more tightly constricted sphincters (Kottke et al 1990, p. 1128). The overall skeletal muscle weakness affects the abdominal and perineal muscles used in defecation. When the stool becomes very hard, more strength is required to expel it. The immobile person may lack this strength.

The bedfast person's unnatural and uncomfortable position on the bedpan does not facilitate elimination. The backward-leaning posture does not promote effective use of the muscles used in defecation. Some persons are reluctant to use the bedpan in the presence of others. The embarrassment, lack of privacy, dependence on others to assist with the bedpan, and disruption of normal bowel habits may cause the individual to postpone or ignore the urge for elimination. Repeated postponement eventually suppresses the urge and weakens the defecation reflex.

Some persons may make excessive use of the Valsalva maneuver by straining at stool in an attempt to expel the hard stool. This effort dangerously increases intra-abdominal and intrathoracic pressures and places undue stress on the heart and circulatory system.

Effects of Exercise Exercise improves the appetite and increases gastrointestinal tract tone, improving digestion and elimination.

INTEGUMENTARY SYSTEM

Problems Related to Immobility

- *Reduced skin turgor.* The skin can atrophy as a result of prolonged immobility. Shifts in body fluids between the fluid compartments can affect the consistency and health of the dermis and subcutaneous tissues in dependent parts of the body, eventually causing a gradual loss in skin **turgor** (elasticity).
- *Skin breakdown.* Normal blood circulation relies on muscle activity. Immobility impedes circulation and diminishes the supply of nutrients to specific areas. As a result, skin breakdown and formation of pressure ulcers can occur. See Chapter 30.

Effects of Exercise By improving blood circulation throughout the body, exercise promotes the delivery of nutrients and oxygen and the removal of waste products. These processes result in an improvement in the health of integumentary structures, such as the skin and hair.

PSYCHONEUROLOGIC SYSTEM

Problems Related to Immobility People who are unable to carry out the usual activities related to their roles (eg, as breadwinner, husband, mother, or athlete) become aware of an increased dependence on others. These factors lower the person's self-esteem. Frustration and the decrease in self-esteem may in turn provoke exaggerated emotional reactions. Emotional reactions vary considerably. Some individuals become apathetic and withdrawn; some regress; and some become angry and aggressive.

Because the immobilized person's participation in life becomes much narrower and the variety of stimuli decreases, the person's perception of time intervals deteriorates. Problem-solving and decision-making abilities often deteriorate as a result of lack of intellectual stimulation and the stress of the illness and immobility. In addition, the loss of control over events can cause anxiety.

Immobility can impair the social and motor development of young children.

Effects of Exercise Exercise improves a person's tolerance to stress. It produces a sense of relaxation and restores well-being. Exercise is also thought to reduce a tendency to depression and improve one's body image. In addition, exercise improves sleep and increases a person's energy and appearance.

ASSESSING

Assessment relative to a client's activity/exercise includes a nursing history and physical examination of body alignment, gait, joint appearance and movement, capabilities and limitations for movement, muscle mass and strength, activity tolerance, physical fitness, and problems related to immobility.

ASSESSMENT INTERVIEW

Activity/Exercise

Daily Activity Level

- What activities do you usually carry out during a routine day?
- Are you able to carry out the following activities of daily living (ADLs)—tasks of daily life—independently?
  - Eating
  - Dressing
  - Bathing
  - Toileting
  - Achieving urinary continence
  - Achieving bowel continence
  - Ambulating
  - Using a wheelchair
  - Transferring (a) from bed to chair, (b) in and out of bath, and (c) in and out of car
  - Communicating
- Where problems exist in your functional abilities to carry out ADLs:
  - Would you rate yourself as partially or totally dependent?
  - How is the ADL achieved (by family, friend, agency, or through the use of specialized equipment)?

Activity Tolerance

- How much and what types of activities make you tired?
- Do you ever experience dizziness, shortness of breath, marked increase in respiratory rate, or other problems following mild or moderate activity?

Exercise

- What type of exercise do you carry out to enhance your physical fitness?
- What is the frequency and length of this exercise session?
- Do you believe exercise is beneficial to health? Explain.

Factors Affecting Mobility

Environmental factors. Do stairs, lack of railings or other assistive devices, or an unsafe neighborhood impede your mobility or exercise regimen?
Health problems. Do any of the following physical or mental health problems, past or current, affect your muscle strength or endurance: heart disease, lung disease, stroke, cancer, neuromuscular problems, musculoskeletal problems, visual or mental impairments, trauma, or pain?
Financial factors. Are your finances adequate to obtain equipment or other aids that you require to enhance your mobility?

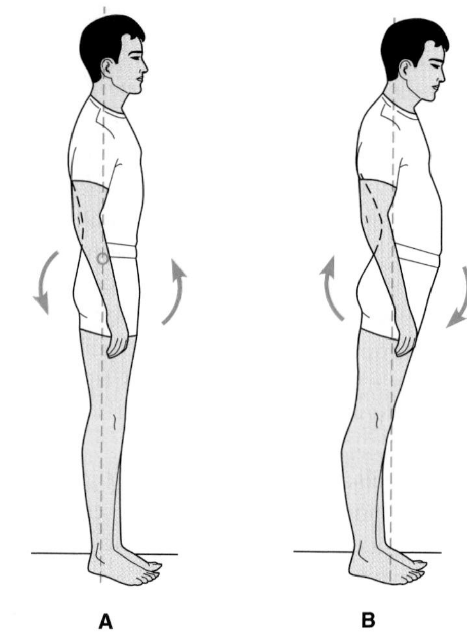

Figure 34–10 A standing person with *A,* good trunk alignment; *B,* poor trunk alignment. The arrows indicate the direction in which the pelvis is tilted.

The nurse collects information from the client, from other nurses, and from the client's records. The examination and history are important sources of information about disabilities affecting the musculoskeletal system, such as contractures, edema, pain in the extremities, or generalized fatigue, that affect the planning of nursing interventions for that client. A review of the recent nurses' notes is also useful.

NURSING HISTORY

An activity/exercise history is usually part of the comprehensive nursing history form and includes daily activity level, activity tolerance, type and frequency of exercise, and factors affecting mobility. If the client indicates a recent pattern change or difficulties with mobility, a more detailed history is required. This detailed history should include the specific nature of the problem, when it first began and its frequency, causes if known, how the problem affects daily living, what the client is doing to cope with the problem, and whether these methods have been effective. Examples of interview questions to elicit this data are shown in the accompanying box.

PHYSICAL EXAMINATION

Body Alignment Assessment of body alignment includes an inspection of the client while the client stands and sits. The purpose of body alignment assessment is to identify the following:

Table 34–5 Developmental Variations in Body Alignment

Age Group	Characteristics	Implications
Newborns	Usual posture is horizontal rather than upright; the spine is straight and lacks the anteroposterior curves of the adult but can be flexed; the abdomen is rounded and prominent; all extremities are generally flexed but can be passively moved through a full range of motion; the feet are usually *inverted* (toes point inward) but can be passively *everted* (toes point outward).	The congenital condition *metatarsus adductus* may be present if inversion of feet occurs in early infancy, especially if the lower legs are straight. Inversion is normally the result of internal *tibial torsion,* or inward rotation of the lower legs.
Infants (1 year)	Usually stands with legs slightly bowed, feet far apart, toes turned outward, and knees hyperextended; the head and upper part of the trunk are carried forward, and the arms are abducted to enhance balance; has an exaggerated lumbar curvature and a "pot belly."	Balance is precarious as the infant learns to stand and walk; may fall backward.
Toddlers	Marked lumbar lordosis and protruding abdomen; slight outward rotation of hips and eversion of feet.	Child commonly widely abducts arms for balance. Growth should produce inward rotation of hips and correct foot eversions.
Preschoolers	Protrusion of abdomen less exaggerated; extremities more proportionate to trunk.	Developing coordination and refining gross motor skills.
School-age children	Legs have straightened and toes point straight ahead; appears more steady and evenly balanced on the feet. Scoliosis screening should be performed.	Usually has excellent posture, often best during lifetime.
Adolescents	Posture is highly individual and determined to a large extent by the person's self-image and the significant changes in body proportions and contour; postural problems are common at this age.	Growth spurts may result in awkwardness, which may be manifested in posture. Postural habits formed during adolescence often persist into adulthood.
Older adults	Tend to have some contractures of flexor muscles; may show kyphosis with disappearance of earlier lumbar lordosis; osteoporosis common among older women and may cause compression fractures of the vertebrae, resulting in a forward-leaning, stooped posture, sometimes call *dowager's hump.*	Deterioration of postural reflexes may require conscious widening of base of support to maintain balance; use of bifocals may result in hyperextension of cervical spine and may cause injury to nearby ligaments and joints.

- Normal changes resulting from growth and development. (Normal developmental variations in posture are shown in Table 34–5.)
- Poor posture and learning needs to maintain good posture
- Factors contributing to poor posture, such as fatigue or low self-esteem
- Muscle weakness or other motor impairments

Stance To assess **stance** (the manner in which a person stands), the nurse views the client from lateral, anterior, and posterior perspectives.

Lateral View Normally, when viewed laterally:

- The line of gravity falls along the ears, along the center of the knees, and in front of the ankles (Figure 34–10, *A*).
- The head is erect.
- The chest is upward and forward.
- The lumbar spine is elongated; neither the thoracic nor lumbar curvature is exaggerated.
- The abdomen is held upward.
- The pelvis is "tucked under." This tensed trunk alignment, in which the pelvis is tucked under, is referred to as the **pelvic tilt,** using a *long midriff,* or putting on an *internal girdle.*
- The knees are extended.
- The feet are at right angles to the lower legs.

When one segment of the body deviates from proper alignment, compensatory deviations occur in other body segments; the result is strain and damage to the maligned ligaments and joint structures supporting body weight.

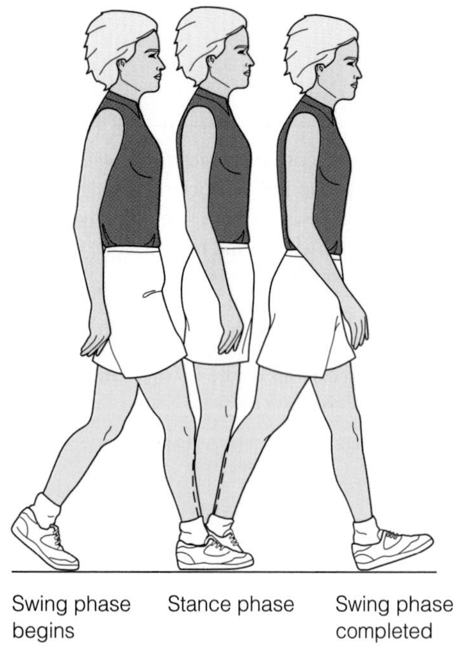

Figure 34–11 The stance and swing phases of a normal gait.

The "slumped" posture (Figure 34–10, *B*) is the most common problem that occurs when people stand. The neck is flexed far forward, the abdomen protrudes, the pelvis is thrust forward to create lordosis (an exaggerated curvature of the lumbar spine), and the knees are markedly hyperextended. Lower back pain and fatigue occur quickly in people with poor posture.

Anterior View Normally, when viewed anteriorly:

- A vertical line from the body's center of gravity (located on the midline halfway between the umbilicus and the pubic symphysis) falls between the feet (the body's base of support) and extends upward through the middle of the forehead (Figure 34–1, earlier).
- The shoulders and hips are level.
- The toes point forward.
- The line drawn through the patella and the middle of the ankle ends at the second or third toe.

Posterior View Normally, when viewed posteriorly:

- The shoulder and hips are level.
- The spine is straight, not curved to either side.
- The main body weight is borne well forward on the outer sides of the feet.

Sitting Alignment To assess sitting alignment, the nurse views the client from the lateral perspective. Normally, the head and trunk are the same as in the standing position, but the lumbar curve is less anteriorly convex because of hip flexion. The weight of the body is centered on the buttocks and thighs. Both feet are on the floor (one foot may be in front of the other), and the forearms are supported to prevent upward or downward pulling of the shoulder girdle. The popliteal spaces should be at least 2.5 cm (1 in) away from the edge of the chair to avoid pressure on the blood vessels and the nerves of the legs. Persons who have peripheral vascular problems should avoid crossing the legs for this reason.

Sitting with one leg crossed over the other creates a C shape, or postural **scoliosis,** of the lumbar-thoracic spine. Habitually sitting with the same leg crossed over the other can eventually contribute to permanent postural scoliosis. Slouching while sitting may be relaxing for short periods, but habitual slouching can contribute to permanent postural abnormalities.

Gait The characteristic pattern of a person's **gait** (walk) is assessed to determine the client's mobility and risk for injury due to falling. Two phases of normal gait are stance and swing (Figure 34–11). In the *stance phase,* (a) the heel of the right foot strikes the ground, and (b) body weight is spread over the ball of the right foot while the left heel pushes off and leaves the ground. In the *swing phase,* the leg from behind moves in front of the body. When one leg is in the swing phase, the other is in the stance phase.

The nurse assesses gait as the client walks into the room or asks the client to walk a distance of 10 feet down a hallway and observes for the following:

- Head is erect, gaze is straight ahead, and vertebral column is upright.
- Toes and kneecaps point forward.
- Heel strikes the ground before the toe.
- Feet are dorsiflexed in the swing phase.
- Arm opposite the swing-through foot moves forward at the same time.
- Instep fails along the line of gravity; that is, feet are parallel.
- Steps are appropriate.
- Gait is smooth, coordinated, and rhythmic, with even weight borne on each foot.
- Gait produces minimal body swing from side to side and directs movement straight ahead.
- Gait starts and stops with ease.

The nurse may also assess **pace** (the number of steps taken per minute). A normal walking pace is 70 to 100 steps per minute. The pace of an elderly person may slow to about 40 steps per minute. A person can increase pace by moving the center of gravity slightly forward, lengthening the stride, and increasing the pushing force of the toes at the end of each weight-bearing phase of a step.

The nurse should also note the client's need for a prosthesis or assistive device, such as a cane or walker. For a client who uses assistive aids, the nurse assesses gait without the device and compares the assisted and unassisted gaits.

Joint Appearance and Movement Physical examination of the joints involves inspection; palpation; assessment of range of active motion; and, if active motion is not possible, assessment of range of passive motion. The following joints may be given special attention: temporomandibular joint, neck, shoulder, elbow, wrist, hip, knee, and ankle.

The nurse should assess the following:

- Any joint swelling or redness, which could indicate the presence of an injury or an inflammation.
- Any deformity, such as a bony enlargement or contracture, and symmetry of involvement.
- The muscle development associated with each joint and the relative size and symmetry of the muscles on each side of the body.
- Any reported or palpable tenderness.
- Crepitation (palpable or audible crackling or grating sensation produced by joint motion).
- Increased temperature over the joint. The nurse palpates the joint using the backs of the fingers and compares the temperature with that of the symmetric joint.
- The degree of joint movement. Ask the client to move selected body parts as shown in Table 34–2, earlier. As indicated, measure the amount of movement by a goniometer, a device that measures the angle of the joint in degrees. See Figure 22–70 on page 540.

Assessment of range of motion should not be unduly fatiguing, and the joint movements need to be performed smoothly, slowly, and rhythmically. No joint should be forced. Uneven, jerky movement and forcing can injure the joint and its surrounding muscles and ligaments.

Capabilities and Limitations for Movement The nurse needs to obtain data that may indicate hindrances or restrictions to the client's movement and the need for assistance, including the following:

- How the client's illness influences the ability to move and whether the client's health contraindicates any exertion, position, or movement.
- Assistive devices required, such as overhead trapeze, pull and/or turn sheet, roller bar, transfer or sliding bar, transfer belt, canes, walker, crutches, braces. If the client is using assistive devices, determine the strength of the upper extremities (See next section).
- Encumbrances to movement, such as an intravenous line in place or a heavy cast on one leg.
- Mental alertness and ability to follow directions. The nurse checks whether the client is receiving medications that hinder the ability to walk safely (eg, narcotics, sedatives, tranquilizers, and antihistamines cause drowsiness, dizziness, weakness, and orthostatic hypotension).
- Balance and coordination, if the client is to be transferred from the bed.
- Presence of orthostatic hypotension before transfers. Specifically, the nurse assesses for any increase in pulse rate, marked fall in blood pressure, dizziness, lightheadedness, and dimming of vision when the client moves from a supine to a vertical posture.
- Degree of comfort. People who have pain may not want to move and require an analgesic before they are moved.
- Weight. Moving obese people may require the assistance of another person or a hydraulic lifter.
- Vision. Is it adequate to prevent falls?
- The nurse's own skill and physical strength.

The nurse also assesses the amount of assistance the client requires for the following:

- Moving in the bed. In particular, the nurse observes for the amount of assistance the client requires for turning
  a. From a supine position to a lateral position.
  b. From a lateral position on one side to a lateral position on the other.
  c. From a supine position to a prone position.
  d. From a supine position to a sitting position in bed.
- Rising from a lying position to a sitting position on the edge of the bed. The client can normally rise without support from the arms; however, a client with muscle weakness may roll to the side and push with the arms or pull with the arms on side rails or nearby furniture to rise.
- Rising from a chair to a standing position. Normally this can be done without pushing with the arms; however, a person with weak muscles may use the arms to push upward and may thrust the upper body forward before rising.
- Range of motion of joints needed to complete transfer movements (see previous section).
- Coordination and balance. The nurse determines the client's abilities to hold the body erect, to bear weight and keep balance in a standing position on both legs or only one, to take steps, and to push off from a chair or bed.

Muscle Mass and Strength Before the client undertakes a change in position or attempts to ambulate, it is essential that the nurse assess the client's strength and ability to move. Providing appropriate assistance lowers the risk of muscle strain and body injury to both the client and nurse. Assessment of upper extremity strength is

Table 34–6 Guidelines for Appropriate Girth Measurements

	Males	Females
Chest or bust	Same size as hips	Same size as hips
Waist	About 13 to 18 cm less than chest	About 25 cm less than bust
Upper arm	Twice the wrist size	Twice the wrist size
Thigh	20 to 25 cm less than abdomen	15 cm less than abdomen
Calf	18 to 20 cm less than thigh	15 to 18 cm less than thigh
Ankle	15 to 18 cm less than calf	13 to 15 cm less than calf

Source: N J Pender, *Health Promotion in Nursing Practice*, 2d ed. (Norwalk, CT: Appleton & Lange, 1987), p. 112. Used by permission.

especially important for clients who use ambulation aids, such as walkers and crutches. For information on how to determine muscle mass and strength in lower and upper extremities, see Chapter 22, page 541.

Activity Tolerance By determining an appropriate activity level for a client, the nurse can predict whether a client has the strength and endurance to participate in activities that require similar expenditures of energy. This assessment is useful in encouraging increasing independence in persons who (a) have a cardiovascular or respiratory disability, (b) have been completely immobilized for a prolonged period, (c) have decreased muscle mass or a musculoskeletal disorder, (d) have experienced inadequate sleep, (e) have experienced pain, or (f) are depressed, anxious, or unmotivated.

The most useful measures in predicting activity tolerance are heart rate, strength, and rhythm; respiratory rate, depth, and rhythm; and blood pressure. These data are obtained at the following times:

- Before the activity starts (baseline data), while the client is at rest
- During the activity
- Immediately after the activity stops
- Three minutes after the activity has stopped and the client has rested

The activity should be stopped immediately in the event of any physiologic change indicating the activity is too strenuous or prolonged for the client. These changes include the following:

- Sudden facial pallor
- Feelings of dizziness or weakness
- Heart rate or respiratory rate that significantly exceeds baseline or preestablished levels
- Change in heart and/or respiratory rhythm from regular to irregular
- Weakening of the pulse
- Dyspnea, shortness of breath, or chest pain
- Diastolic blood pressure change of 10 mm/Hg or more

If, however, the client tolerates the activity well, and if the client's heart rate returns to baseline levels within 5 minutes after the activity ceases, the activity is considered safe. This activity, then, can serve as a standard for predicting the client's tolerance for similar activities.

Physical Fitness Assessment of physical fitness includes girth measurements, skinfold measurements, the step test, computation of fitness index, assessment of muscle strength and endurance, and assessment of joint flexibility.

The nurse takes *girth measurements* of the chest, waist, hips, upper arm (biceps), thigh, calf, and ankle. Guidelines for body proportions are shown in Table 34–6.

Skinfold measurements indicate the amount of body fat. To take skinfold measurements, the nurse grasps the skinfold (skin layers and subcutaneous fat) between the thumb and forefinger and measures the skinfold with special calipers. Skinfold sites are the triceps, subscapula, suprailiac, and thigh. See Chapter 37 for further information about skinfold procedures and norms.

For the Harvard *step test*, the client steps up and down a 17-inch step for 3 minutes if able. The following movements constitute one step: left foot up, right foot up, left foot down, right foot down. The rate should be at least 24 steps per minute.

Before the test, the nurse takes a resting pulse to obtain baseline data. After the test, the client sits in a chair while the nurse assesses the pulse rate for 15 seconds at prescribed intervals:

- 15 to 30 seconds
- 60 to 75 seconds
- 120 to 135 seconds
- 180 to 195 seconds

To compute the person's *fitness index*, that is, cardiovascular fitness:

1. Multiply each of the 15-second heart rates by 4 to obtain the beats per minute.
2. Add the per-minute heart rates after exercise.
3. Divide 30,000 by that number.

Ratings of 65 to 80 are average (Edlin & Golanty 1992, p. 566).

There are several tests of *muscle strength and endurance.* One is performing sit-ups with knees bent (bent-knee sit-ups). Women are asked to do these for 1 minute; men, for 2 minutes. The average rate for women is about 20 to 25 sit-ups per minute; for men, 50 to 60 per 2 minutes.

Joint flexibility can be assessed quickly by asking the person to touch the toes several times. The average touch point is 1 to 3 inches in front of the toes. See page 881 for detailed discussion of joint range of motion.

Problems Related to Immobility When collecting data pertaining to the problems of immobility, the nurse uses the assessment methods of inspection, palpation, and auscultation; checks results of laboratory tests; and takes measurements, including body weight, fluid intake, and fluid output. Specific techniques for assessing immobility problems and abnormal assessment findings related to the complications of immobility are listed in Table 34–7.

It is extremely important to obtain and record baseline assessment data soon after the client first becomes immobile. These baseline data serve as the standard against which all data collected throughout the period of immobilization are compared.

Because a major nursing responsibility is to prevent the complications of immobility, the nurse needs to identify clients at risk of developing such complications before problems arise. Clients at risk include those who (a) are poorly nourished; (b) have decreased sensitivity to pain, temperature, or pressure; (c) have existing cardiovascular, pulmonary, or neuromuscular problems; and (d) are unconscious.

DIAGNOSING

NANDA nursing diagnoses that relate to activity/mobility problems include: **Activity intolerance, High risk for activity intolerance, Impaired physical mobility,** and **High risk for disuse syndrome.** These diagnoses, with definitions, contributing factors, and defining characteristics, are shown in the box on page 904.

Gordon (1993, p. 165) delineates four levels of **Activity intolerance** and **Impaired physical mobility** that describe the extent of the client's problems. The level can be specified after the diagnostic label.

- **Activity intolerance**
  - Level I: Walks at regular pace on level indefinitely; walks upstairs one flight or more, but more short of breath than normally
  - Level II: Walks one city block 500 feet on level; climbs one flight slowly without stopping

Table 34–7 Assessing Problems of Immobility

Assessment	Problem
Musculoskeletal System	
Measure arm and leg circumferences	Decreased circumference due to decreased muscle mass
Palpate and observe body joints	Stiffness or pain in joints
Take goniometric measurements of joint ROM	Decreased joint ROM, joint contractures
Cardiovascular System	
Auscultate the heart	Increased heart rate
Measure blood pressure	Orthostatic hypotension
Palpate and observe sacrum, legs, and feet	Peripheral dependent edema Increased peripheral vein engorgement
Palpate extremity pulses	Weak peripheral pulses
Measure calf muscle circumferences	Edema
Observe calf muscle for redness, tenderness, and swelling	Thrombophlebitis
Respiratory System	
Observe chest movements	Asymmetric chest movements; dyspnea
Auscultate chest	Diminished breath sounds, crackles, wheezes, and increased respiratory rate
Metabolic System	
Measure height and weight	Weight loss due to muscle atrophy and loss of subcutaneous fat
Take anthropometric measurements	Loss of body muscle and subcutaneous fat
Observe wound healing	Slow wound healing
Palpate body skin	Generalized edema due to low blood proteins
Urinary System	
Measure intake and output	Dehydration
Observe urine output	Cloudy, dark urine, high specific gravity
Palpate urinary bladder	Distended urinary bladder due to urinary retention
Gastrointestinal System	
Observe stool	Hard, dry, small stool
Auscultate bowel sounds	Decreased bowel sounds due to decreased intestinal motility
Integumentary System	
Observe skin for intactness	Break in skin integrity

NURSING DIAGNOSES

CLIENTS WITH ACTIVITY/MOBILITY PROBLEMS

Nursing Diagnosis: Activity intolerance: A state in which an individual has insufficient physiologic or psychologic energy to endure or complete required or desired daily activities

Defining Characteristics

- Verbalization of fatigue or weakness
- Abnormal responses to activity, for example, heart rate, blood pressure or electrocardiographic changes that reflect arrhythmias or ischemia
- Discomfort or dyspnea with exertion

Related Factors

Bed rest, immobility; sedentary life-style; generalized weakness; imbalance between oxygen supply and demand.

Nursing Diagnosis: High risk for activity intolerance: A state in which the individual is at risk of experiencing insufficient physiologic or psychologic energy to endure or complete required or desired daily activities

Risk Factors

History of previous intolerance; deconditioned health status or bed rest; presence of circulatory/respiratory problems or pain; inexperience with the activity.

Nursing Diagnosis: Impaired physical mobility: A state in which the individual experiences a limitation of ability for independent physical movement

Defining Characteristics

- Inability to move purposefully within the bed or the environment; inability to transfer or ambulate
- Limited active joint range of motion
- Decreased muscle strength or control
- Imposed movement restriction (medical or mechanical)
- Impaired coordination

Related Factors

Intolerance to activity; decreased strength and endurance; pain/discomfort; neuromuscular impairment; musculoskeletal impairment; cognitive impairment; depression or severe anxiety.

Nursing Diagnosis: High risk for disuse syndrome: A state in which an individual is at risk for deterioration of body systems (see the discussion of complications of immobility, on page 892) as a result of prescribed or unavoidable musculoskeletal inactivity

Risk Factors

Paralysis; prescribed or mechanical immobilization; severe pain; altered level of consciousness.

Sources: LJ Carpenito, *Nursing Diagnosis: Application to Clinical Practice*, 4th ed. (Philadelphia: Lippincott, 1992), pp. 379–398, 680–80; M Gordon, *Manual of Nursing Diagnosis 1993–1994*, 6th ed. (St Louis: Mosby-Year Book, 1993), pp. 159, 161, 165, 169; MJ Kim, GK McFarland, and AM McLane, *Pocket Guide to Nursing Diagnoses*, 5th ed. (St Louis: Mosby-Year Book, 1993), pp. 2, 20, 36–37; GK McFarland, and EA McFarlane, *Nursing Diagnosis and Intervention: Planning for Patient Care*, 2d ed. (St Louis: Mosby, 1993), pp. 322, 329–30, 335; North American Nursing Diagnosis Association, *NANDA Nursing Diagnoses: Definitions and Classification 1992–1993* (Philadelphia: NANDA, 1992), pp. 32, 53–56; and JR Lederer, GL Marculescu, B Mocnik, and N Seaby, *Care Planning Pocket Guide—A Nursing Diagnosis Approach*, 5th ed. (Redwood City, CA: Addison-Wesley Nursing, 1993), pp. 2, 60, 112.

Level III: Walks no more than 50 feet on level without stopping; unable to climb one flight of stairs without stopping
Level IV: Dyspnea and fatigue at rest

- **Impaired physical mobility**
  Level I: Requires use of equipment or device
  Level II: Requires assistance, supervision, or teaching from another person(s)
  Level III: Requires help from another person(s) and equipment device
  Level IV: Is dependent and does not participate in movement

Because mobility affects many areas of human functioning, the diagnoses **Impaired physical mobility** and **Activity intolerance** may themselves be the etiology of other diagnoses, for example, **Self-care deficit, High risk for injury, Impaired home maintenance management,** and **Altered health maintenance.** Another diagnoses that may pertain to mobility status is **Fear** (of falling). Examples of assessment data clusters and related nursing diagnoses are shown in Table 34–8.

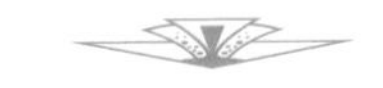

PLANNING

The major outcomes for clients with potential or actual problems related to mobility or activity are to avoid any complications associated with immobility, to restore or improve the capability to ambulate or take part in activity, and to avoid injury from falling or improper use of body mechanics. Specific outcome criteria, nursing interventions, and rationales are shown in the Care Planning Guide on page 906.

Positioning, transferring, and ambulating clients are almost always independent nursing functions. Although certain activity orders are medically prescribed, the physician rarely writes specific directions to indicate how the order is to be accomplished. The physician usually orders specific body positions only after surgery, anesthesia, or trauma involving the nervous and musculoskeletal systems. The client's current "activity order" contains data essential for planning nursing interventions for body alignment. All clients should have an activity order written by their physician when they are admitted to the agency for care. Examples of common activity orders are shown in the box on page 910.

As part of planning, the nurse is responsible for identifying those clients who need assistance with body alignment and determining the degree of assistance they need. The nurse must be sensitive to the client's need to function as independently as possible yet provide assistance when the client needs it. Clients who are not very mobile and can help themselves only minimally may also have low energy levels.

Most clients require some nursing guidance and assistance to learn about, achieve, and maintain proper body

Text continued on page 910

Table 34–8 Clinical Application: Data Clusters and Related Nursing Diagnoses

Data Cluster	Nursing Diagnoses
Mrs Ivy Snowfield, a frail-appearing 82-year-old, has an unsteady gait and increasing difficulty maintaining her balance. Pace is slow (20 steps per minute). Posture is stooped. Leg and arm muscle strength is symmetric but weak. Has difficulty rising from a sitting to a standing position. No mechanical assistive devices are used.	**Impaired physical mobility** related to decreased motor agility and muscle weakness associated with advanced age
Peter Brown, a 69-year-old accountant being treated for congestive heart failure, states he has dyspnea with mild activity ("I cannot climb a flight of stairs without stopping and resting and become breathless even when walking on level ground"). Rales present in both lungs. ECG reveals an enlarged heart. Prefers the orthopneic position.	**Activity intolerance** (Level III) related to imbalance between oxygen supply and demand secondary to **Decreased cardiac output**
Florence Grayson was admitted to hospital with a cerebrovascular accident 2 days ago. She weighs 46 kg (101 lb), is stuporous, is anorexic and malnourished, has flaccid paralysis of her left arm and leg, and is incontinent of urine. Is unable to move without help.	**High risk for disuse syndrome** related to neuromuscular impairment (hemiplegia), altered level of consciousness, and inactivity.
Mr Tim Cherry, a 93-year-old widower, has chronic obstructive lung disease. States, "I can't breathe properly when I move about. I cannot maintain the house the way my wife did. All I can do is feed myself. Luckily, I have a nice neighbor who shops for me every week."	**Impaired home maintenance management** related to chronic debilitating disease, activity intolerance, and lack of familiarity with neighborhood resources

CARE PLANNING GUIDE

CLIENTS WITH ACTIVITY/MOBILITY PROBLEMS

NURSING DIAGNOSIS: High risk for disuse syndrome

Outcome Criteria	Nursing Interventions	Rationale
The client		
▪ Maintains normal musculoskeletal function, as evidenced by usual range of motion in all body joints and maintenance of baseline muscle mass and strength.	Implement appropriate exercise program (active, isotonic, or passive exercises) at least every 4 hours to arms, legs, and neck as indicated. See pages 926 to 933.	Isotonic exercises prevent contractures and muscle atrophy. Isometric exercises maintain muscle tone. Passive exercises maintain joint mobility.
	Encourage active participation in self-care activities.	Self-care activities involve active movement of body joints and muscles.
	Compare muscle size and strength (see p. 901) to baseline data and on each side of body daily.	Early detection of muscle atrophy or decreased strength facilitates early intervention to correct the problem.
	Position clients in good alignment.	Good alignment prevents contractures and maintains structural integrity of muscles and joints.
	Ambulate client as tolerated, or assist to stand at bedside.	Weight-bearing prevents disuse osteoporosis.
▪ Experiences minimal cardiovascular alterations, as evidenced by maintenance of baseline vital signs and signs of adequate venous blood flow (absence of edema, calf pain, inflammation, venous distention, skin changes).	Monitor vital signs according to client needs and/or agency protocol (eg, bid or tid).	Regular monitoring enables the nurse to detect alterations early.
	Instruct client how and when to avoid the Valsalva maneuver.	The Valsalva maneuver increases the stress on the heart.
	Apply antiemboli stocking as indicated.	Use of antiemboli stockings prevents thrombus formation, venous engorgement, dependent edema, and orthostatic hypotension.
	Elevate legs several time each day for 20 minutes.	Elevation increases peripheral venous circulation.
	Implement measures to prevent orthostatic hypotension (see p. 937).	
	Assess skin of lower limbs, and measure calf circumferences as indicated.	Regular inspection and measurement enable the nurse to detect changes.
	See also interventions for musculoskeletal function.	These interventions also stimulate blood circulation and prevent cardiovascular complications.
▪ Maintains normal respiratory function, as evidenced by normal breath sounds during auscultation; normal chest expansion; and absence of chest pain, fever, or other respiratory signs indicative of pulmonary infarction, emboli, or atelectasis.	Assess breath sounds and chest expansion at least every 8 hours.	This allows the nurse to detect onset of abnormal breath sounds and inadequate chest expansion.
	Teach clients to take five deep breaths and to cough every waking hour.	Deep breaths and coughing increase alveolar expansion, prevent stasis of secretions, promote adequate gaseous exchange, and maintain a patent airway.
	Establish a position schedule, and alter client's position every 2 hours. Ambulate client if possible, or place client in chair.	Changes in position allow previously dependent lung areas to expand and promote movement and subsequent removal of secretions by coughing.

Outcome Criteria	Nursing Interventions	Rationale
▪ Maintains appropriate nutritional and fluid pattern, as evidenced by maintenance of baseline weight, adequate tissue turgor, balanced fluid intake and output, and normal serum protein values.	Monitor the client's weight, tissue turgor, fluid intake and output, and serum protein values.	Normal or baseline findings of these assessments indicate adequate hydration and nutritional intake.
▪ Maintains normal elimination pattern, as evidenced by clear amber urinary output of at least 1500 mL per day; urine specific gravity of 1.010 to 1.025; an acidic urine; absence of signs of urinary retention or infection; and excretion of formed semisolid stool at least every 2 or 3 days.	Monitor color, clarity, amount, acidity, and specific gravity of urine; color and characteristics of feces; and frequency of defecation. Ask whether client has pain when urinating.	Decreased urinary output, cloudy urine, and painful urination are indicative of urinary retention and infection. Alkaline urine increases the risk for calculi. Constipation is associated with immobility.
	Refer to Chapter 40 for interventions to prevent constipation. Teach clients to select high-fiber foods.	High-fiber foods promote intestinal peristalsis and defecation. See Chapter 37 for foods high in fiber.
▪ Maintains intact integument, as evidenced by clean, intact, well-hydrated skin and absence of pressure signs (pallor, redness, increased warmth or tenderness) over pressure areas.	See Care Planning Guide in Chapter 30, page 793.	
▪ Maintains social, emotional, and intellectual well-being, as evidenced by active participation and decision making in care, verbalization of concerns, maintaining positive relationships with others, and performing satisfying activities.	Encourage the client to make as many decisions as possible, such as placement of personal items, daily plan of activities, clothes to wear.	Decision making enhances self-esteem.
	Plan time to be available to the client other than task-oriented time.	Making oneself available for the client may encourage open expression of feelings.
	Explore diversional activities of interest to the client, and develop a daily activity plan.	A satisfying daily activity prevents boredom and gives the client something to look forward to.

NURSING DIAGNOSIS: Activity intolerance

Outcome Criteria	Nursing Interventions	Rationale
The client		
▪ Identifies activities and factors that contribute to activity intolerance.	Explore with client known activities causing activity intolerance (eg, self-care, exercise, and leisure activities) and signs indicating the intolerance.	This helps the nurse and client establish baseline data and enables the nurse to specify level of activity intolerance.
	Determine possible contributing factors (see examples on p. 904).	Identification of contributing factors enables the nurse and client to focus interventions appropriately.
▪ Maintains pulse, respirations, and blood pressure within predetermined ranges during planned activities.	Monitor the client's response to present activities. See the discussion of assessing activity tolerance, page 902.	Monitoring enables the nurse and client to determine current tolerance and either increase or decrease present activities.

➤

ACTIVITY/MOBILITY PROBLEMS CONTINUED

NURSING DIAGNOSIS: Activity intolerance *continued*

Outcome Criteria	Nursing Interventions	Rationale
▪ Develops an activity and rest pattern that promotes optimal independence and minimizes fatigue.	Assist the client to identify activities that can now be performed without adverse signs, and encourage the client to perform them.	Identifying activities that can be performed enables the client to participate as much as possible in required activities and maintain a degree of independence and self-esteem.
	Intersperse rest periods (napping, relaxing in a chair) with activity periods and in accordance with the client's daily schedule.	Adequate rest replenishes energy reserves.
	Assess and adjust the client's daily schedule as indicated (eg, postpone a morning tub bath if the client is scheduled for a diagnostic test).	Adapting care and treatments to the client's limitations preserves energy for its expenditure during activity.
	Implement measures to conserve the client's energy during activity; for example, administer pain medications before activity, provide walking aids as required, and administer oxygen if ordered.	Measures to conserve the client's energy enable the client to increase activity tolerance.
▪ Increases activity tolerance to level required or desired.	Suggest that the client perform activities more slowly and for shorter time periods, resting more often, and using more assistance as required.	Shorter activity periods performed more slowly and more frequent rest periods promote optimal performance and achievement levels. Appropriate assistance ensures safety and prevents falling.
	Provide positive reinforcement for increased activity.	Positive reinforcement provides an incentive to achieve goals.
	Include the family or support persons in assisting the client with ADLs.	Support helps to maintain a desired life-style.
▪ Verbalizes fears about activity intolerance, increasing level of activity, and/or effects of activity intolerance on role function and responsibilities.	Plan time to be with the client, and listen attentively to the client's concerns.	Anxiety and fear deplete energy reserves and reduce the client's capacity to perform desired activities.
▪ Accepts help and selects and uses appropriate resources.	Provide information about available resources to help with ADLs and home maintenance management.	Using community resources can decrease anxiety and feelings of frustration in completing necessary activities.

NURSING DIAGNOSIS: Impaired physical mobility

Outcome Criteria	Nursing Interventions	Rationale
The client		
▪ Describes factors that contribute to impaired physical mobility.	Assess causative factors, such as trauma, debilitating disease, pain, and so on (see examples of contributing factors on p. 904).	Identifying contributing factors enables the nurse and client to focus on appropriate interventions.

Outcome Criteria	Nursing Interventions	Rationale
▪ Maintains optimal musculoskeletal functioning.	Instruct client and monitor active ROM exercises for all joints at least two times daily.	Active ROM exercises maintain joint mobility, improve muscle tone, and maintain and improve cardiovascular function, depending on intensity and duration.
	Perform passive ROM exercises if active exercises are not possible.	Passive ROM exercises maintain joint mobility and prevent contractures.
	Encourage client to participate actively in self-care activities as much as possible.	Performing self-care activities uses joints and muscles, helping maintain their function.
	Encourage optimal ambulation within physical limitations.	Ambulation provides stress in bones and prevents many of the respiratory, circulatory, skin, and elimination, complications associated with immobility. See page 892.
	See also interventions for **High risk for disuse syndrome.**	
▪ Uses assistive devices correctly and independently (or with supervision) to move and ambulate safely.	Instruct client in correct use of assistive device (trapeze, cane, walker, crutches). See Client Teaching boxes on pages 938 and 939.	Knowing how to use these devices appropriately facilitates mobility without injury to the body.
	Supervise all mobilization attempts as required.	Appropriate supervision ensures safe performance of activities.
	Provide positive reinforcement during activities.	Positive reinforcement provides incentive to become as independent as possible.
▪ Transfers safely between bed and chair, commode, or wheelchair; between wheelchair and toilet; and to standing position.	Teach the client safe methods of transfer. *or* Assist client to make transfers safely as required.	Safe methods of transfer prevent falls and body injury.
▪ Uses safety measures to minimize potential for injury.	Inform client of safety precautions (wearing shoes or slippers with nonskid soles, ensuring that rubber tips on canes and crutches are intact, locking wheelchair before transfers, etc).	Knowledge of safety precautions alerts the client to potential hazards for injury.
▪ Discusses concerns and abilities to manage in the home.	Assess need for home care assistance and need for medical equipment (eg, raised toilet seat, bath seat). Consult with occupational therapist and/or physical therapist as indicated.	Appropriate assistance and equipment enable the client to maintain an optimal degree of independence and self-esteem.

CLINICAL ALERT

Before planning outcome criteria and nursing interventions for a specific client, the nurse must assess the contributing factors and adapt the outcome criteria and interventions to the individual and the specific etiology. For example, if the client's etiology for **Impaired physical mobility** is painful arthritis in the joints the nurse would not implement active joint ROM exercises until severe pain and joint swelling subside or as the physician indicates. Outcome criteria and interventions would need to include pain management and measures to protect the acutely affected joints.

EXAMPLES OF ACTIVITY ORDERS

- *BR (bed rest) or CBR (complete bed rest).* This order indicates that the client is not to get out of bed for any reason.
- *BRP (bathroom privileges).* This order indicates that the client is not to get out of bed except to urinate or defecate.
- *Up ad lib.* This order indicates that the client may be in and out of bed as the client wishes.
- *HOB 30 continuously.* This order indicates that the head of the bed is to be elevated 30 degrees (in semi-Fowler's position) both day and night.

mechanics. The nurse should also plan to teach clients applicable skills. For example, a client with a back injury needs to learn how to get out of bed safely and comfortably; a client with an injured leg needs to learn how to transfer from bed to wheelchair safely; and a client with a newly acquired walker needs to learn how to use it safely. Nurses often teach family members or caregivers in the home safe moving, lifting, and transfer techniques.

A critical pathway (see p. 945) can be useful in planning client care.

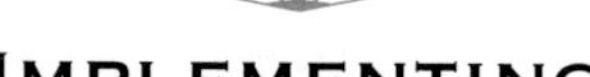

IMPLEMENTING

MAINTAINING GOOD POSTURE

As noted earlier, many problems concerning alignment, body mechanics, and ambulation are preventable and/or treatable. General exercise promotes good *standing alignment.* The nurse who practices good postural habits can be a significant role model and motivator. When prolonged standing is unavoidable, the client should elevate one foot onto a support to straighten the spine. Periodically changing the foot that is elevated prevents undue strain to one side of the spinal column at the expense of the other. Flexion of the hip and knee straightens the lumbar spine and reduces lordosis.

Nursing interventions to promote good *sitting alignment* apply whether the client is sitting in a chair, in a wheelchair, or on the side of the bed. When the client is sitting, alignment problems frequently affect not only the back but also the top extremities. For certain clients (eg, those who have musculoskeletal impairments of the arm and shoulder), support of the arm is essential. If the armrests of a chair are too high, the person's shoulder girdle may be forced upward into an uncomfortable position. In this case, placing pillows on the chair seat to elevate the body improves alignment. When the armrests of the chair are too low, the person's shoulder girdle is pulled downward, causing the shoulders and back to slump when the person attempts to rest the arms on the chair armrests. Padding to raise the level of the armrests improves alignment.

A chair seat that is too high creates undue pressure against the thighs, especially in the popliteal area behind the knees, since the lower legs and feet are unsupported. Prolonged pressure can damage the nerves and blood vessels in the popliteal space.

POSITIONING CLIENTS

Positioning a client in good body alignment and changing the position regularly and systematically are essential aspects of nursing practice. Clients who can move easily automatically reposition themselves for comfort. Such people generally require minimal positioning assistance from nurses, other than guidance about ways to maintain body alignment and to exercise their joints. However, people who are weak, frail, in pain, paralyzed, or unconscious rely on nurses to provide or assist with position changes. For all clients, it is important to assess the skin and provide skin care before and after a position change.

Any position, correct or incorrect, can be detrimental if maintained for a prolonged period. Frequent change of position helps to prevent muscle discomfort, undue pressure resulting in pressure ulcers, damage to superficial nerves and blood vessels, and **contractures** (permanent shortening of a muscle). Position changes also maintain muscle tone and stimulate postural reflexes.

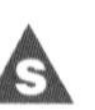

When the client is not able to move independently or assist with moving, the *preferred method is to have two or more nurses move or turn the client.* Appropriate assistance reduces the risk of muscle strain and body injury to both the client and nurse.

When positioning clients in bed, the nurse can do a number of things to ensure proper alignment and promote client comfort and safety:

- Before placing the client in bed, make sure the mattress is firm and level yet has enough give to fill in and support natural body curvatures. A sagging mattress, a mattress that is too soft, or an underfilled water bed used over a prolonged period can contribute to the development of hip flexion contractures and low back strain and pain. Bed boards made of plywood and placed beneath a sagging mattress are increasingly recommended for clients who have back problems or are prone to them. Some bed boards are hinged across the middle so that they will bend as the head of the bed is raised. It is particularly important in the home setting to inspect the mattress for support.

SUPPORT DEVICES

- *Pillows.* Different sizes are available. Used for support or elevation of a body part, (eg, an arm). Specially designed dense pillows can be used to elevate the upper body.
- *Mattresses.* There are two types of mattresses: ones that fit on the bed frame (eg, standard bed mattress) and mattresses that fit *on* the standard bed mattress (eg, egg crate mattress). Mattresses should be evenly supportive. See Chapter 29, page 775, for additional information and Table 30–4, page 795, for devices that reduce pressure on body parts.
- *Bed boards.* The boards are usually made of wood and are placed under the mattress to provide support.
- *Chair beds.* These beds can be placed into the position of a chair for clients who cannot move from the bed but require a sitting position.
- *Trapeze bar.* This bar is suspended from an overhead frame that extends from the foot to the head of the bed. The client can grasp the bar to raise the trunk off the bed surface or to move up in bed.
- For additional supportive devices, see Chapter 30, page 795.

- Ensure that the bed is kept clean and dry. Wrinkled or damp sheets increase the risks of pressure ulcer formation. See Chapter 30. Make sure extremities can move freely whenever possible. For example, the top bedclothes need to be loose enough for the client to move the feet.
- Place support devices in specified areas according to the client's position. See the box above for commonly used support devices. Use only those support devices needed to maintain alignment and to prevent stress on the client's muscles and joints. If the person is capable of movement, too many devices limit mobility and increase potential for muscle weakness and atrophy. Common alignment problems that can be corrected with support devices include the following:
  a. Flexion of the neck
  b. Internal rotation of the shoulder
  c. Adduction of the shoulder
  d. Flexion of the wrist
  e. Anterior convexity of the lumbar spine
  f. External rotation of the hips
  g. Hyperextension of the knees
  h. Plantar flexion of the ankle
- Avoid placing one body part, particularly one with bony prominences, directly on top of another body part. Excessive pressure can damage veins and predispose the client to thrombus formation. Pressure against the popliteal space may damage nerves and blood vessels in this area.

SAMPLE SCHEDULE FOR POSITION CHANGES

Time		Position
10:00 AM	(1000 hr)	Left lateral
Noon	(1200 hr)	Fowler's or chair
2:00 PM	(1400 hr)	Right lateral
4:00 PM	(1600 hr)	Right Sims'
6:00 PM	(1800 hr)	Fowler's or chair
8:00 PM	(2000 hr)	Left lateral
10:00 PM	(2200 hr)	Left Sims'
Midnight	(2400 hr)	Supine
2:00 AM	(0200 hr)	Right lateral
4:00 AM	(0400 hr)	Right Sims'
6:00 AM	(0600 hr)	Supine
8:00 AM	(0800 hr)	Fowler's

- Plan a *systematic 24-hour schedule* for position changes. See the box above. Frequent position changes are essential to prevent pressure ulcers in immobilized clients. Such clients should be repositioned every 2 hours throughout the day and night and more frequently when there is a risk for skin breakdown. See Chapter 30. This schedule is usually outlined on the client's nursing care plan. Schedule periods throughout the day during which the client assumes positions that provide full extension of the neck, hips, and knees to prevent flexion contractures of these joints.
- Always elicit information from the client to determine which position is most comfortable and appropriate. Seeking information from the client about what feels best is a useful guide when aligning persons and is an essential aspect of evaluating the effectiveness of an alignment intervention. Sometimes a person who appears well-aligned may be experiencing real discomfort. Both appearance, in relation to alignment criteria, and comfort are important in achieving effective alignment. To promote comfort, the nurse may administer prescribed analgesics approximately 30 minutes before moving or ambulating the client.

Fowler's Position Fowler's position, or semisitting position, is a bed position in which the head and trunk are raised 45 to 90 degrees. In **low-Fowler's,** or **semi-Fowler's,** position, the head and trunk are raised 15 to 45 degrees (Figure 34–12); in **high-Fowler's position,** the head and trunk are raised 90 degrees. See Table 34–9. In this position, the knees may or may not be flexed.

Table 34–9 Fowler's Position

Unsupported Position	Problem to be Prevented	Corrective Measure*
Bed-sitting position with upper part of body elevated 30 to 90 degrees commencing at hips	Posterior flexion of lumbar curvature	Pillow at lower back (lumbar region) to support lumbar region
Head rests on bed surface	Hyperextension of neck	Pillow to support head, neck and upper back
Arms fall at sides	Shoulder muscle strain, possible dislocation of shoulders, edema of hands and arms with flaccid paralysis; flexion contracture of the wrist	Pillows under forearms to eliminate pull on shoulder and assist venous blood flow from hands and lower arms
Legs lie flat and straight on lower bed surface	Hyperextension of knees	Small pillow under thighs to flex knees
Legs are externally rotated	External rotation of hips	Trochanter roll lateral to femur (Figure 34–13)
Heels rest on bed surface	Pressure on heels	Pillow under lower legs
Feet are in plantar flexion	Plantar flexion of feet (foot drop)	Footboard to provide support for dorsal flexion

* The amount of support depends on the needs of the individual client.

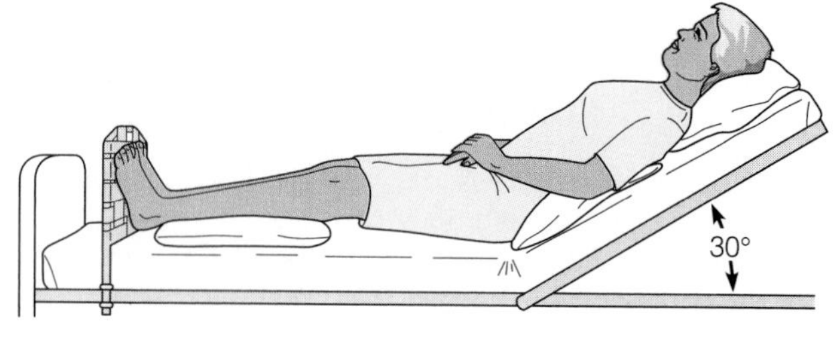

Figure 34–12 Low-Fowler's (semi-Fowler's) position (supported). Note that arm support is omitted in this instance.

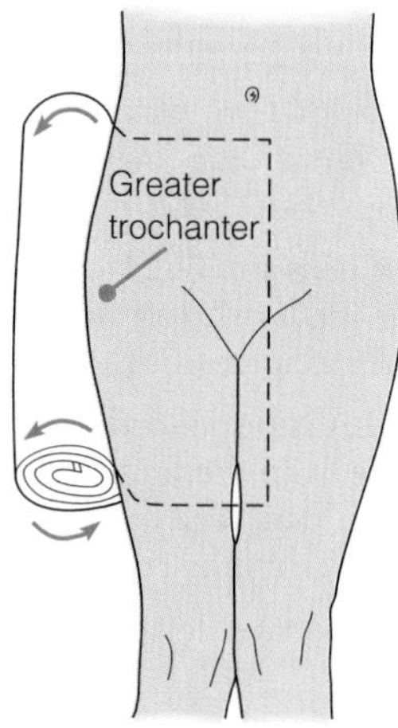

Figure 34–13 Making a trochanter roll: (1) Fold the towel in half lengthwise. (2) Roll the towel tightly, starting at one narrow edge and rolling within approximately 30 cm (1 ft) of the other edge. (3) Invert the roll. Then palpate the greater trochanter of the femur and place the roll with the center at the level of the greater trochanter; place the flat part of towel under the client; then roll the towel snugly against the hip.

Nurses need to clarify the meaning of the term *Fowler's position* in a particular agency. In some hospitals, *Fowler's position* refers to elevation of the upper part of the body without knee flexion, and the term *semi-Fowler's* is used to refer to the sitting position with knee flexion.

Fowler's position is the position of choice for people who have difficulty breathing and for some people with heart problems. When the client is in this position, gravity pulls the diaphragm downward, allowing greater chest expansion and lung ventilation. Clients confined to bed but capable of eating, reading, watching television, or visiting find this position comfortable.

A common error nurses make when aligning clients in Fowler's position is placing an overly large pillow or more than one pillow behind the client's head. These errors promote the development of neck flexion contractures. If a client desires several head pillows, the nurse should encourage the client to rest without a pillow for several hours each day to extend the neck fully and counteract the effects of poor neck alignment.

Orthopneic Position An adaptation of high-Fowler's position is the orthopneic position. The client sits either in bed or on the side of the bed with an overbed table across the lap (Figure 34–14). This position facilitates respiration by allowing maximum chest expansion. It is particularly helpful to clients who have problems exhaling, because they can press the lower part of the chest against the edge of the overbed table.

Dorsal Recumbent Position In the dorsal recumbent (back-lying) position, the client's head and shoulders are slightly elevated on a small pillow (Figure 34–15). In some agencies, the terms *dorsal recumbent* and *supine* are used interchangeably; strictly speaking, however, in the **supine** or **dorsal position** the head and shoulders

Table 34–10 Dorsal Recumbent Position

Unsupported Position	Problem to be Prevented	Corrective Measure
Head is flat on bed surface	Hyperextension of neck in thick-chested person	Pillow of suitable thickness under head and shoulders if necessary for alignment
Lumbar curvature of spine is apparent	Posterior flexion of lumbar curvature	Roll or small pillow under lumbar curvature
Legs may be externally rotated	External rotation of legs	Roll or sandbag placed laterally to trochanter of femur (optional)
Legs are extended	Hyperextension of knees	Small pillow under thigh to flex knee slightly
Feet assume plantar flexion position	Plantar flexion (foot drop)	Footboard or rolled pillow to support feet in dorsal flexion
Heels on bed surface	Pressure on heels	Pillow under lower legs

Table 34–11 Prone Position

Unsupported Position	Problem to Be Prevented	Corrective Measure
Head is turned to side and neck is slightly flexed	Flexion or hyperextension of neck	Small pillow under head unless contraindicated because of promotion of mucous drainage from mouth
Body lies flat on abdomen accentuating lumbar curvature	Hyperextension of lumbar curvature; difficulty breathing; pressure on breasts (women); pressure on genitals (men)	Small pillow or roll under abdomen just below diaphragm
Toes rest on bed surface; feet are in plantar flexion	Plantar flexion of feet (foot drop)	Allow feet to fall naturally over end of mattress, or support lower legs on a pillow so that toes do not touch the bed

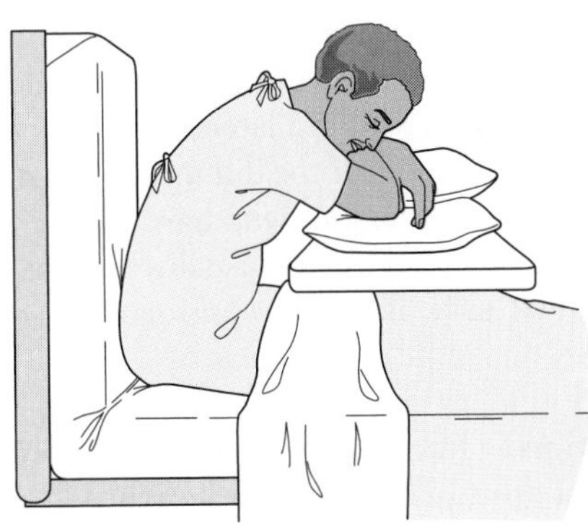

Figure 34–14 Orthopneic position.

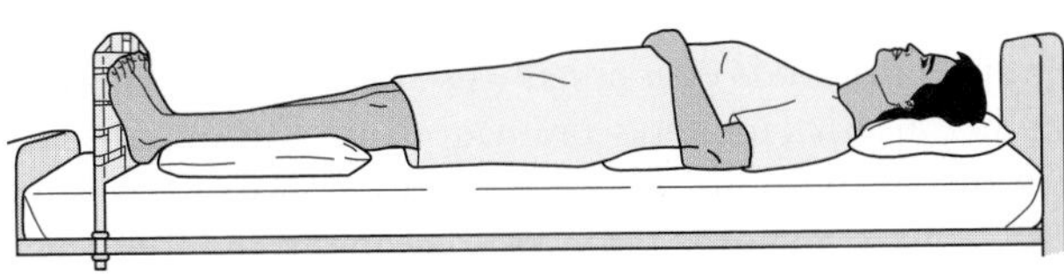

Figure 34–15 Dorsal recumbent position (supported).

are not elevated. In both positions, the client's forearms may be elevated on pillows or placed at the client's sides. Supports are similar in both positions, except for the head pillow. See Table 34–10. The dorsal recumbent position is used to provide comfort and to facilitate healing following certain surgeries and/or anesthetics (eg, spinal).

Prone Position In the prone position, the client lies on the abdomen with the head turned to one side. The hips are not flexed. Both children and adults often sleep in this position, sometimes with one or both arms flexed over their heads (Figure 34–16). This position has several advantages. It is the only bed position that allows full extension of the hip and knee joints. When used periodically, the prone position helps to prevent flexion contractures of the hips and knees, thereby counteracting a problem caused by all other bed positions. The prone position also promotes drainage from the mouth and is especially useful for unconscious clients or those clients recovering from surgery of the mouth or throat. See Table 34–11.

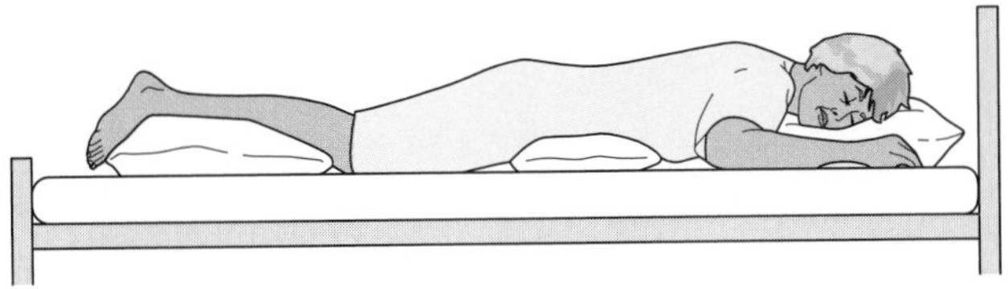

Figure 34–16 Prone position (supported).

Table 34–12 Lateral Position

Unsupported Position	Problem to Be Prevented	Corrective Measure
Body is turned to side, both arms in front of body, weight resting primarily on lateral aspects of scapula and ilium	Lateral flexion and fatigue of sternocleidomastoid muscles	Pillow under head and neck to provide good alignment
Upper arm and shoulder are rotated internally and adducted	Internal rotation and adduction of shoulder and subsequent limited function; impaired chest expansion	Pillow under upper arm to place it in good alignment; lower arm should be flexed comfortably
Upper thigh and leg are rotated internally and adducted	Internal rotation and adduction of femur; twisting of the spine	Pillow under leg and thigh to place them in good alignment; shoulders and hips should be aligned

The prone position poses some distinct disadvantages. The pull of gravity on the trunk produces a marked lordosis in most persons, and the neck is rotated laterally to a significant degree. For this reason, the prone position may not be recommended for persons with problems of the cervical or lumbar spine. This position also causes plantar flexion. Some clients with cardiac or respiratory problems find the prone position confining and suffocating, because chest expansion is inhibited during respirations. The prone position should be used only when the client's back is correctly aligned, only for short periods, and only for persons with no evidence of spinal abnormalities.

Lateral Position In the lateral (side-lying) position, the person lies on one side of the body (Figure 34–17).

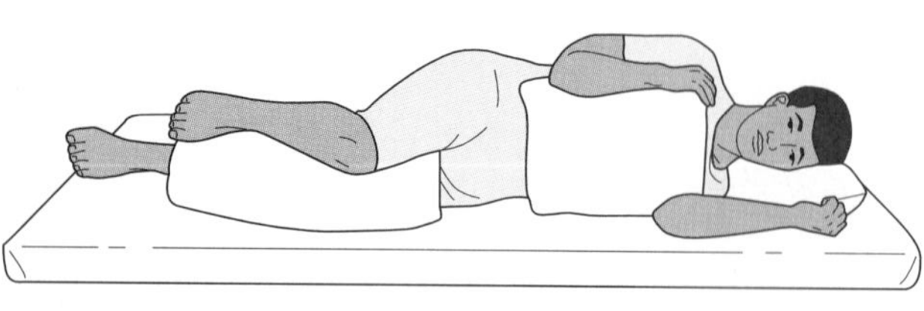

Figure 34–17 Lateral position (supported).

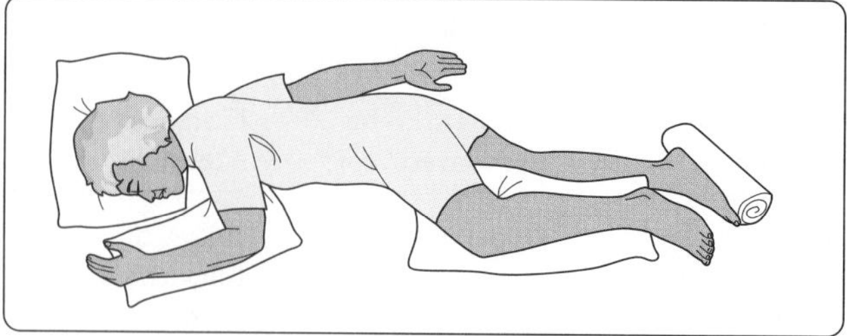

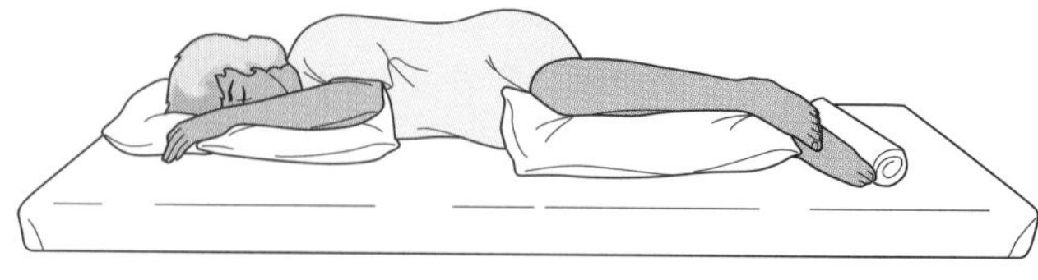

Figure 34–18 Sims' position (supported).

Flexing the top hip and knee and placing this leg in front of the body creates a wider, triangular base of support and achieves greater stability. The greater the flexion on the top hip and knee, the greater the stability and balance in this position. This flexion reduces lordosis and promotes good back alignment. For this reason, the lateral position is good for resting and sleeping clients. The lateral position helps to relieve pressure on the sacrum and heels in persons who sit for much of the day or who are confined to bed and rest in Fowler's or dorsal recumbent positions much of the time. In the lateral position, most of the body's weight is borne by the lateral aspect of the lower scapula, the lateral aspect of the ilium, and the greater trochanter of the femur. Persons who have sensory or motor deficits on one side of the body usually find that lying on the uninvolved side is more comfortable. See Table 34–12.

Sims' Position In Sims' (semiprone) position, the client assumes a posture halfway between the lateral and the prone positions (Figure 34–18). In Sims' position, the lower arm is positioned behind the client, and the upper arm is flexed at the shoulder and the elbow. Both legs are flexed in front of the client. The upper leg is more acutely flexed at both the hip and the knee than the lower one is.

Sims' position is occasionally used for unconscious clients because it facilitates drainage from the mouth and prevents aspiration of fluids. It is also used for paralyzed (paraplegic or hemiplegic) clients because it reduces pressure over the sacrum and greater trochanter of the hip. It is often used for clients receiving enemas and occasionally for clients undergoing examinations or treatments of the perineal area. Many people, especially pregnant women, find Sims' position comfortable for sleeping. Persons with sensory or motor deficits on one side of the body usually

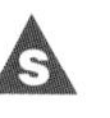

Table 34–13 Sims' Position (Semiprone Position)

Unsupported Position	Problem to Be Prevented	Corrective Measure
Head rests on bed surface; weight is borne by lateral aspects of cranial and facial bones	Lateral flexion of neck	Pillow supports head, maintaining it in good alignment unless drainage from the mouth is required
Upper shoulder and arm are internally rotated	Internal rotation of shoulder and arm; pressure on chest, restricting expansion during breathing	Pillow under upper arm to prevent internal rotation
Upper leg and thigh are adducted and internally rotated	Internal rotation and adduction of hip and leg	Pillow under upper leg to support it in alignment
Feet assume plantar flexion	Foot drop	Sandbags to support feet in dorsal flexion

find that lying on the uninvolved side is more comfortable. See Table 34–13.

MOVING AND TURNING CLIENTS IN BED

Although healthy people usually take for granted that they can change body position and go from one place to another with little effort, ill people may have difficulty moving even in bed. How much assistance clients require depends on their own ability to move and their health status. In general, nurses should be sensitive to both the need of people to function independently and their need for assistance to move.

When a nurse assists a person to move, correct body mechanics need to be employed so that the nurse is not injured. Actions and rationales common to the lifting and moving procedures that follow are outlined in the accompanying box. Correct body alignment for the client must also be maintained so that undue stress is not placed on the musculoskeletal system.

SUMMARY OF ACTIONS AND RATIONALES APPLICABLE TO MOVING AND LIFTING PROCEDURES*

- Before moving a client, assess the degree of exertion permitted, the client's physical abilities (ie, muscle strength, presence of paralysis), ability to understand instructions, degree of comfort or discomfort when moving, client's weight, presence of orthostatic hypotension (particularly important when client will be standing), and your own strength and ability to move the client.
- Raise the height of the bed to bring the client close to your center of gravity.
- Lock the wheels on the bed, and raise the rail on the side of the bed opposite you to ensure client safety.
- Face the direction of the movement to prevent spinal twisting.
- Assume a broad stance to increase stability and provide balance.
- Incline your trunk forward, and flex your hips, knees, and ankles to lower your center of gravity, increase stability, and ensure use of large muscle groups during movements.
- Tighten your gluteal, abdominal, leg, and arm muscles to prepare them for action and prevent injury.
- Rock from the front leg to the back leg when pulling or from the back leg to the front leg when pushing to overcome inertia, counteract the client's weight, and help attain a balanced, smooth motion.
- After moving the client, determine the client's comfort, body alignment, tolerance of the activity (eg, check pulse rate, blood pressure), and safety precautions required (eg, side rails).

* See also the discussion of principles of body mechanics on page 879.

Moving a Client Up in Bed Clients who have slid down in bed from the Fowler's position or been pulled down by traction need assistance to move up in bed. See Procedure 34–1 on page 916. The client should be encouraged to accomplish this movement independently whenever health permits.

Moving a Client to the Side of the Bed in Segments

This movement is used in preparation for moving the client onto a stretcher, in preparation for turning the client to the lateral (side-lying) position, or when changing the client's bed. See Procedure 34–2 on page 917. Whenever capable of assisting with this movement, the client lifts the body by holding onto the raised side rail or by using the overhead trapeze. In this movement, the nurse's weight is used to counteract the client's weight; the nurse's arms serve as connecting bars between the client and the nurse.

Text continued on page 918

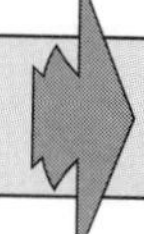

PROCEDURE 34–1 MOVING A CLIENT UP IN BED

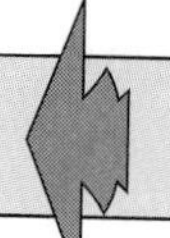

INTERVENTION

1. Adjust the bed and the client's position.

- Adjust the head of the bed to a flat position or as low as the client can tolerate. *Moving the client upward against gravity requires more force and can cause back strain.*
- Raise the bed to the height of your center of gravity.
- Lock the wheels on the bed and raise the rail on the side of the bed opposite you.
- Remove all pillows, then place one against the head of the bed. *This pillow protects the client's head from inadvertent injury against the top of the bed during the upward move.*

2. Elicit the client's help in lessening your workload.

- Ask the client to flex the hips and knees and position the feet so that they can be used effectively for pushing. *Flexing the hips and knees keeps the entire lower leg off the bed surface, preventing friction during movement, and ensures use of the large muscle groups in the client's legs when pushing, thus increasing the force of movement.*
- Ask the client to
  a. Grasp the head of the bed with both hands and pull during the move.
  or
  b. Raise the upper part of the body on the elbows and push with the hands and forearms during the move.
  or
  c. Grasp the overhead trapeze with both hands and lift and pull during the move. *Client assistance provides additional power to overcome inertia and friction during the move. These actions also keep the client's arms partially off the bed surface, reducing friction during movement, and make use of the large muscle groups of the client's arms to increase the force during movement.*

3. Position yourself appropriately, and move the client.

- Face the direction of the movement, and then assume a broad stance, with the foot nearest the bed behind the forward foot and weight on the forward foot. Incline your trunk forward from the hips. Flex hips, knees, and ankles.
- Place your near arm under the client's thighs. *This supports the heaviest part of the body (the buttocks).* Push down on the mattress with the far arm (Figure 34–19). *The far arm acts as a lever during the move.*

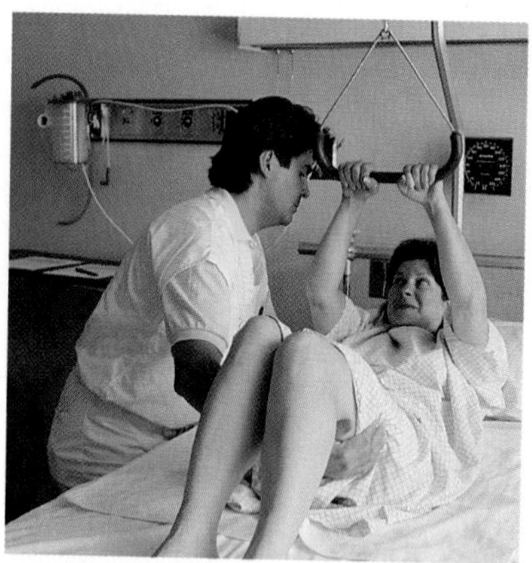

Figure 34–19 Moving a client up in bed.

- Tighten your gluteal, abdominal, leg, and arm muscles, and rock from the back leg to the front leg and back again. *Then* shift the weight to the front leg as the client pushes with the heels and pulls with the arms, moving the client toward the head of the bed.

4. Ensure client comfort.

- Elevate the head of the bed and provide appropriate support devices for the client's new position.
- See the sections on positioning clients earlier in this chapter.

Variation: A Client Who Has Limited Strength of the Upper Extremities

- Assist the client to flex the hips and knees as above. Place the client's arms across the chest. *This keeps them off the bed surface and minimizes friction during movement.* Ask the client to flex the neck during the move and keep the head off the bed surface.
- Position yourself properly (as above), and place one arm under the client's back and shoulders and the other arm under the client's thighs. *This placement of the arms distributes the client's weight and supports the heaviest part of the body (the buttocks).* Shift your weight as above.

Variation: Pulling a Client up in Bed

This method emphasizes pulling the client up toward the head of the bed rather than lifting the client. It is designed to create less back strain for the nurse than a method that utilizes lifting. The steps are as follows:

- After lowering the head of the bed and removing all pillows, move the client to the edge of the bed closest to your body. (Procedure 34–2 describes this action.)
- Ask the client to assist (see step 2 above), or, if the client has limited strength of the upper ex-

PROCEDURE 34–1 *continued*

tremities, place the client's arms across the chest and ask the client to flex the neck during the move.

- Stand toward the head of the bed, and face the foot of the bed. Position yourself appropriately, and place both hands together beneath the client's coccyx. Align your body so that it is directly in line with your hands. Your elbow closest to the client will be beneath the client's upper back. Both elbows should rest on the surface of the bed. *This placement of the arms, beneath the heaviest part of the client's body, allows you to pull the client directly toward your center of gravity, preventing spinal twisting. Pulling from the client's center of gravity directly toward your own center of gravity requires less force than lifting and allows greater control over the movement.*
- Coordinating your efforts with those of the client, rock backward and shift weight from the forward to the backward foot, pulling the client directly toward you while the client pushes with the heels and pulls with the arms. The hip closest to the bed should slide along the side of the mattress. Your elbows should slide along the bed surface.
- Raise the side rail and move to the opposite side of the bed. Move or pull the client as above, and move again to the opposite side of the bed. Move or pull the client back to the center of the bed. Raise the side rail.

Variation: Two Nurses Using a Hand-Forearm Interlock

Two people are required to move clients who are unable to assist because of their condition or weight. Using the technique described in step 3, with the second nurse on the opposite side of the bed, both of you interlock your forearms under the clients thighs and shoulders and lift the client up in bed (Figure 34–20).

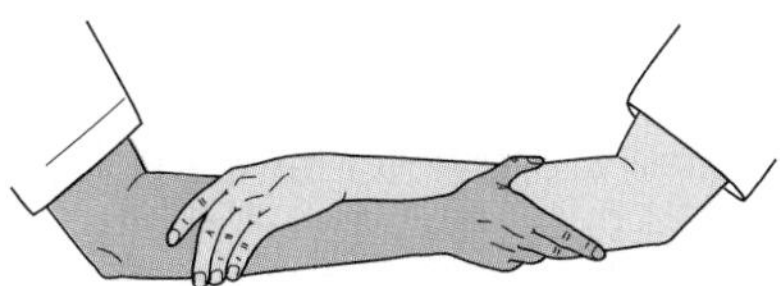

Figure 34–20 Two nurses using a hand-forearm interlock.

Variation: Two Nurses Using a Turn Sheet

Two nurses can use a turn sheet to move a client up in the bed. *A turn sheet distributes the client's weight more evenly, decreases friction, and exerts a more even force on the client during the move. In addition, it prevents injury of the client's skin, because the friction created between two sheets when one is moved is less than that created by the client's body moving over the sheet.*

- Place a drawsheet or a full sheet folded in half under the client, extending from the shoulders to the thighs. Each of you rolls up or fanfolds the turn sheet close to the client's body on either side.
- Both of you then grasp the sheet close to the shoulders and buttocks of the client. *This draws the weight closer to the nurses' center of gravity and increases the nurses' balance and stability, permitting a smoother movement.* Then follow the method of moving clients with limited upper extremity strength, described earlier.

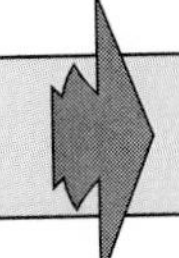

PROCEDURE 34–2 MOVING A CLIENT IN SEGMENTS TO THE SIDE OF THE BED

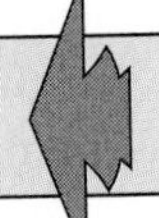

INTERVENTION

1. Position yourself and the client appropriately before performing the move.

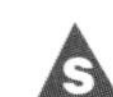

- Stand as close as possible at the side of the bed toward which the client will be moved and opposite the client's chest. *This position lessens the client's fear of falling and places your center of gravity close to the client's.*
- Place the client's near arm across the chest. *This avoids friction and resistance to movement and prevents injury to the arm.*
- Incline your trunk forward from the hips. Flex your hips, knees, and ankles. Assume a broad stance, with one foot forward and the weight placed upon this forward foot.

2. Move the client's head and trunk.

- Place your arms and hands with palms facing upward close together beneath the client's scapulae. *This focuses the force for movement under the heaviest part of*

PROCEDURE 34–2 MOVING A CLIENT IN SEGMENTS TO THE SIDE OF THE BED *continued*

the upper trunk. Placing the arms close together reduces the friction of the client's body against the bed, making the pull easier.

- Flex your fingers around the client's far shoulder, and rest your elbows on the surface of the bed. *This prevents inadvertent lifting.*
- If the client cannot support the head during the movement, position your arm nearest the head of the bed so that it cradles the client's head.
- Tighten your gluteal, abdominal, leg, and arm muscles, rock backward, and shift your weight from the forward to the backward foot, while pulling the client's shoulders directly toward you.

3. Move the client's buttocks.

- Place your arms and hands close together beneath the client's buttocks, and pull the buttocks to the side of the bed as described above.

4. Move the client's legs and feet.

- Place your hands close together beneath the client's ankles, and repeat the steps above, pulling the client's legs and feet to the side of the bed.

- Elevate the side rail next to the client. *This prevents the client from falling off the bed.*

Variation: Using a Pull Sheet

Use a pull sheet beneath the client's trunk and thighs to pull the client to the side of the bed. Roll up the sheet as close as possible to the client's body, and pull the client's shoulders, then the buttocks, to the side of the bed. Move the legs and feet as described above.

Turning a Client to a Lateral or Prone Position in Bed Movement to a lateral (side-lying) position may be necessary when placing a bedpan beneath the client, when changing the client's bed linen, or when repositioning the client. See Procedure 34–3.

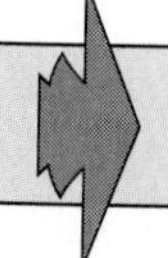

PROCEDURE 34–3 TURNING A CLIENT TO A LATERAL OR PRONE POSITION IN BED

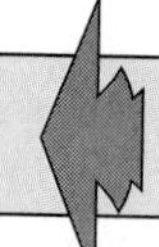

INTERVENTION

1. Position yourself and the client appropriately before performing the move.

- Move the client closer to the side of the bed opposite the side the client will face when turned. See Procedure 34–2. *This ensures that the client will be positioned safely in the center of the bed after turning.*
- While standing on the side of the bed nearest the client, place the client's near arm across the chest. Abduct the client's far shoulder slightly from the side of the body. *Pulling the one arm forward facilitates the turning motion. Pulling the other arm away from the body prevents that arm from being caught beneath the client's body during the roll.*
- Place the client's near ankle and foot across the far ankle and foot. *This facilitates the turning motion. Making these preparations on the side of the bed closest to the client helps the nurse prevent unnecessary reaching.*

- Raise the side rail next to the client before going to the other side of the bed. *This ensures that the client, who is close to the edge of the mattress, will not fall.*
- Position yourself on the side of the bed toward which the client will turn, directly in line with the client's waistline and as close to the bed as possible.
- Incline your trunk forward from the hips. Flex your hips, knees, and ankles. Assume a broad stance with one foot forward and the weight placed upon this forward foot.

2. Pull or roll the client to a lateral position.

- Place one hand on the client's far hip and the other hand on the client's far shoulder (Figure 34–21, *A*). *This position of the hands supports the client at the two heaviest parts of the body, providing greater control in movement during the roll.*
- Tighten your gluteal, abdominal, leg, and arm muscles; rock backward, shifting your weight from

PROCEDURE 34–3 *continued*

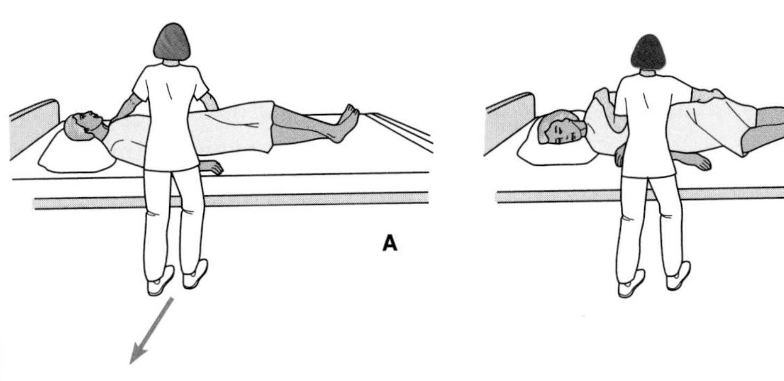

Figure 34–21 Moving a client to a lateral position.

the forward to the backward foot; and roll client onto the side of the body to face you (Figure 34–21, *B*).

Variation: Turning the Client to a Prone Position

To turn a client to the prone position, follow all of the above steps, with two exceptions:

- Instead of abducting the far arm, keep the client's arm alongside the body for the client to roll over. *Keeping the arm alongside the body prevents it from being pinned under the client when the client is rolled.*
- Roll the client completely onto the abdomen. *It is essential to move the client as close as possible to the bed edge before the turn so that the client will be lying on the center of the bed after rolling.* Never pull a client across the bed while the client is in the prone position. *Doing so can injure a woman's breasts or a man's genitals.*

Logrolling a Client Logrolling is a technique used to turn a client whose body must at all times be kept in straight alignment (like a log). See Procedure 34–4. An example is the client with a spinal injury. Considerable care must be taken to prevent additional injury. This technique requires two nurses or, if the client is large, three nurses. *For the client who has a cervical injury, one nurse must maintain the client's head and neck alignment.*

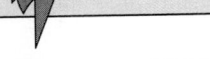

PROCEDURE 34–4 LOGROLLING A CLIENT

INTERVENTION

1. Position yourselves and the client appropriately before the move.

- Stand on the same side of the bed, and assume a broad stance with one foot ahead of the other.

- Place the client's arms across the chest. *Doing so ensures that they will not be injured or become trapped under the body when the body is turned.*
- Incline your trunk, and flex your hips, knees, and ankles.
- Place your arms under the client as shown in Figure 34–22 or Figure 34–23, depending on the client's size. *Each nurse then has a major weight area of the client centered between the arms.*

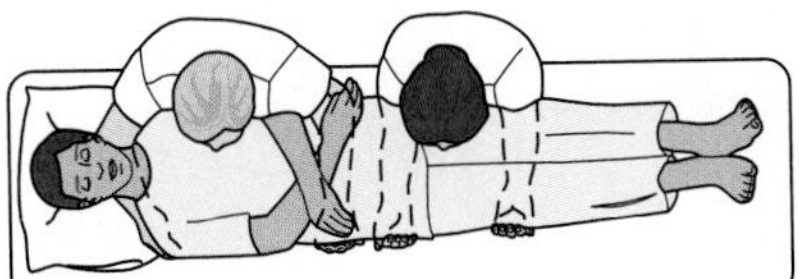

Figure 34–22 Correct arm placement for moving a client to the side of the bed: two nurses.

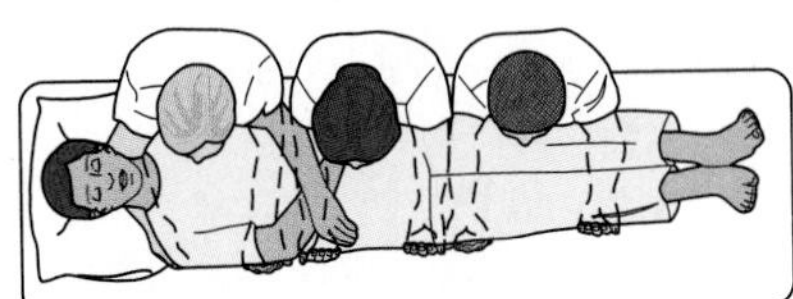

Figure 34–23 Correct arm placement for moving a client to the side of the bed: three nurses.

- Tighten your gluteal, abdominal, leg, and arm muscles.

2. Pull the client to the side of the bed.

- One nurse counts, "One, two, three, go." Then, at the same time, all nurses pull the client to the side of the bed by shifting weight to the back foot. *Moving the client in unison maintains the client's body alignment.*

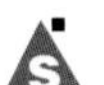

- Elevate the side rail on this side of the bed. *This prevents the client from falling while lying so close to the edge of the bed.*

Procedure 34–4 Logrolling a Client *continued*

3. Move to the other side of the bed, and place supportive devices for the client when turned.

- Place a pillow where it will support the client's head after the turn. *The pillow prevents lateral flexion of the neck and ensures alignment of the cervical spine.*
- Place one or two pillows between the client's legs to support the upper leg when the client is turned. *This pillow prevents adduction of the upper leg and keeps the legs parallel and aligned.*

4. Roll and position the client in proper alignment.

- All nurses flex the hips, knees, and ankles and assume a broad stance with one foot forward.
- All nurses reach over the client and place hands as shown in Figure 34–24. *Doing so centers a major weight area of the client between each nurse's arms.*
- One nurse counts, "One, two, three, go." Then, at the same time, all nurses roll the client to a lateral position.
- Place pillows to maintain the client's lateral position. See the discussion of the lateral position on page 914.

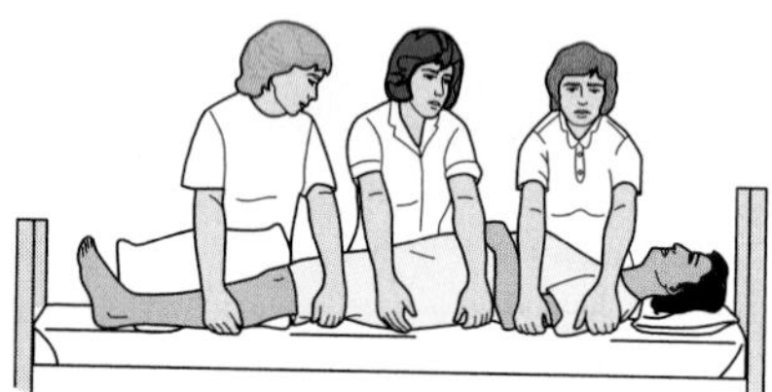

Figure 34–24 Correct hand placement for logrolling a client.

Variation: Using a Turn or Lift Sheet

- Use a turn sheet to facilitate logrolling. First, stand with another nurse on the same side of the bed. Assume a broad stance with one foot forward, and grasp half of the fanfolded or rolled edge of the turn sheet. On a signal, pull the client toward both of you (Figure 34–25).
- Before turning the client, place pillow supports for the head and legs, as described in step 3 above. This helps maintain the client's alignment when turning. Then go to the other side of the bed (farthest from the client), and assume a stable stance. Reaching over the client, grasp the far edges of the turn sheet, and roll the client toward you (Figure 34–26). The second nurse (behind the client) helps turn the client and provides pillow supports to ensure good alignment in the lateral position.

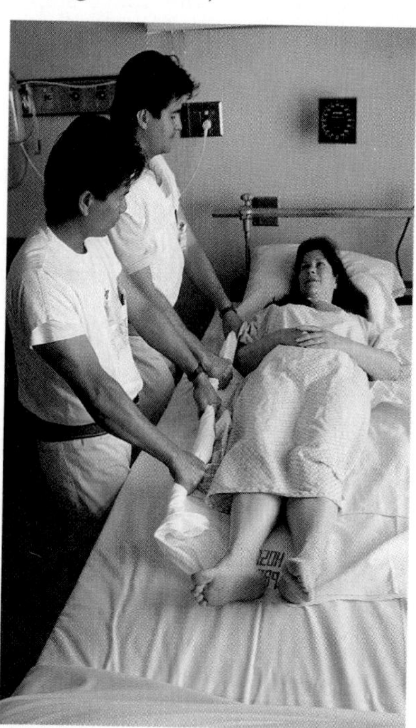

Figure 34–25 Using a turn sheet, the nurses pull the sheet with the client on it to the edge of the bed.

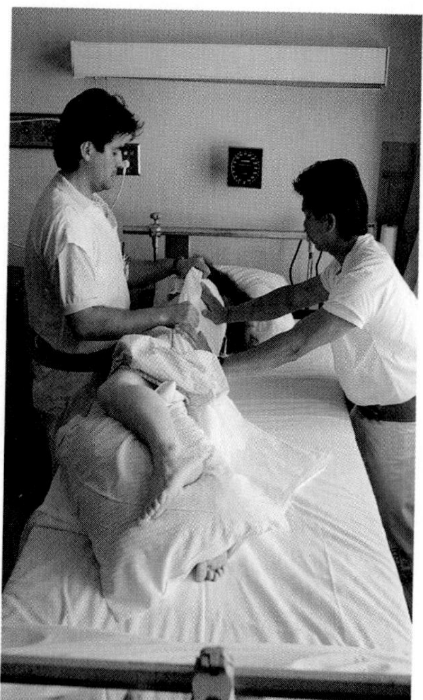

Figure 34–26 The nurse on the left uses the far edge of the sheet to roll the client toward him; the nurse on the right remains behind the client and assists with turning.

Assisting a Client to a Sitting Position in Bed A client may need assistance in raising the head and shoulders while the nurse rearranges pillows or provides back care. If the client needs to rise to a sitting position in bed, the easiest method is simply to raise the head of the bed to the desired height. If the client is not in a hospital bed that can be raised mechanically, the nurse may need to assist the client. See Procedure 34–5.

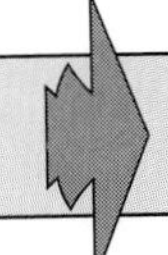
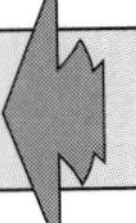

PROCEDURE 34–5 ASSISTING A CLIENT TO A SITTING POSITION IN BED

INTERVENTION

1. Position yourself and the client appropriately before performing the move.

- Ask the client to place arms at the sides with the palms of the hands against the surface of the bed. *In this way, the client can push against the bed surface to provide additional power for the lift.*
- Face the head of the bed, and stand at the side of the bed beside the client's buttocks. Assume a broad stance with the foot farthest from the bed forward and body weight on this foot.

2. Lift the client to a sitting position.

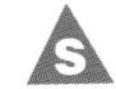

- Place the hand nearest the client over the client's far shoulder to rest between the shoulder blades. *This hand position enables you to pull the client's upper body directly toward your center of gravity and prevents spinal twisting.*
- Place the hand of your free arm on the edge of the surface of the bed near the client's shoulder, and use it to push during the lift (Figure 34–27, *A*). *This provides balance and leverage.*

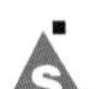

- Have the client lift with you simultaneously on your signal. Lift by pulling with the arm and hand over the client's shoulder, pushing on the bed surface with the other hand, and shifting your weight from the forward to the back foot in a rocking motion (Figure 34–27, *B*). *Pushing with the muscles of one arm while pulling with the muscles of the other arm distributes the workload and increases lifting power.* The client simultaneously pushes with the hands and arms.

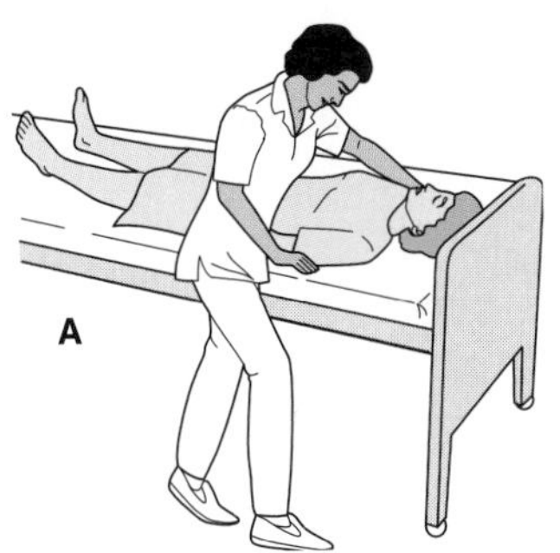

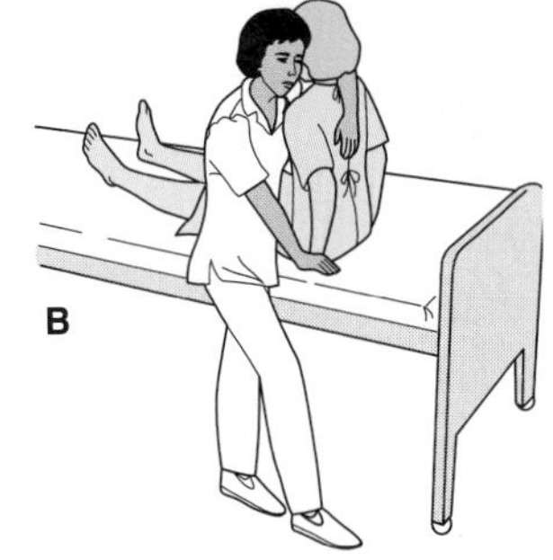

Figure 34–27 Assisting a client to a sitting position in bed.

Moving a Client to a Sitting Position on the Edge of the Bed The client assumes a sitting position on the edge of the bed before walking, moving to a chair or wheelchair, eating, or performing other activities. See Procedure 34–6.

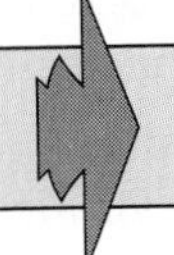
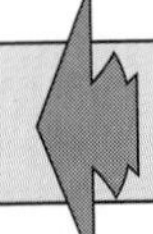

PROCEDURE 34–6 MOVING A CLIENT TO A SITTING POSITION ON THE EDGE OF THE BED

ASSESSMENT FOCUS
Client's physical ability to assist and then maintain this position, ability to comprehend instructions, degree of discomfort when moving; vital signs before ambulating; presence of postural hypotension; the nurse's own strength and ability.

INTERVENTION

1. Position yourself and the client appropriately before performing the move.

- Assist the client to a lateral position facing you. See Procedure 34–3.
- Raise the head of the bed slowly as high as it will go. *This decreases the distance that the client needs to move to sit up on the side of the bed.*
- Position the client's feet and lower legs at the edge of the bed. *This enables the client's feet to move easily off the bed during the movement, and the client is aided by gravity into a sitting position.*
- Stand beside the client's hips and face the far corner of the bottom of the bed (the angle in which movement will occur). Assume a

PROCEDURE 34–6 MOVING A CLIENT TO A SITTING POSITION ON THE EDGE OF THE BED *continued*

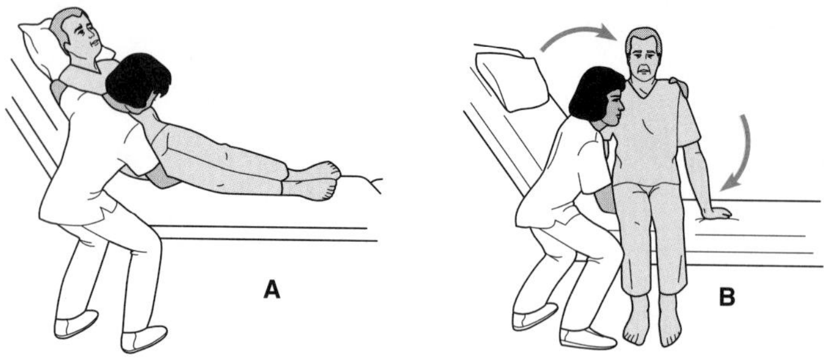

Figure 34–28 Assisting a client to a sitting position on the edge of the bed.

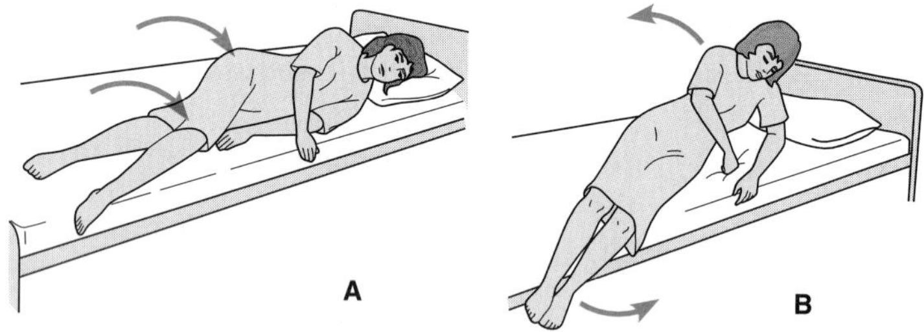

Figure 34–29 Moving to a sitting position independently.

broad stance, placing the foot nearest the client forward. Incline your trunk forward from the hips. Flex your hips, knees, and ankles (Figure 34–28, *A*).

2. Move the client to a sitting position.

- Place one arm around the client's shoulders and the other arm beneath both of the client's thighs near the knees (Figure 34–28, *A*). *Supporting the client's shoulders prevents the client from falling backward during movement. Supporting the client's thighs reduces friction of the thighs against the bed surface during the move and increases the force of the movement.*
- Tighten your gluteal, abdominal, leg, and arm muscles.
- Lift the client's thighs slightly. *This reduces the friction of the client's thighs and the nurse's arm against the bed surface.*
- Pivot on the balls of your feet in the desired direction facing the foot of the bed while pulling the client's feet and legs off the bed (Figure 34–28, *B*). *Pivoting prevents twisting of the nurse's spine. The weight of the client's legs swinging downward increases downward movement of the lower body and helps make the client's upper body vertical.*
- Keep supporting the client until the client is well balanced and comfortable. *This movement may cause some clients to faint.*

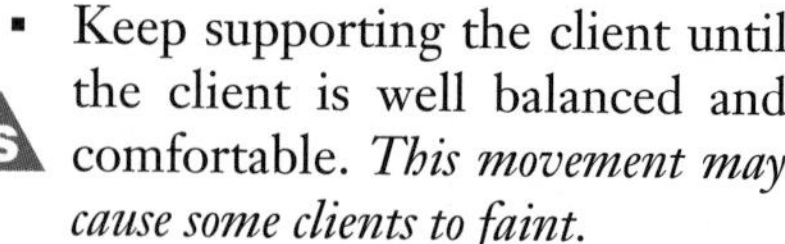

- Assess vital signs (eg, pulse, respirations and blood pressure) as indicated by client's health status.

Variation: Teaching a Client How to Sit on the Side of the Bed Independently

A client who has had recent abdominal surgery or who is weak may have too much abdominal pain or too little strength to sit straight up in bed. This person can be taught to assume a "dangle" position without assistance. Instruct the client to

- Roll to the side and lift the far leg over the near leg (Figure 34–29, *A*).
- Grasp the mattress edge with the lower arm and push the fist of the upper arm into the mattress (Figure 34–29, *B*).
- Push up with the arms as the heels and legs slide over the mattress edge (Figure 34–29, *B*).
- Maintain the sitting position by pushing both fists into the mattress behind and to the sides of the buttocks.

TRANSFERRING CLIENTS

Many clients require some assistance in transferring between bed and chair or wheelchair, between wheelchair and toilet, and between bed and stretcher. Before transferring any client, however, the nurse must determine the client's physical and mental capabilities to participate in the transfer technique. In addition, the nurse must mentally analyze and organize the activity. General guidelines for transfer techniques are included in the box on page 923.

Because wheelchairs and stretchers are unstable, they can predispose the client to falls and injury. Guidelines for the safe use of wheelchairs and stretchers are shown in the boxes on page 923.

CLINICAL GUIDELINES

Transferring Clients

- Plan what to do and how to do it. Determine the space in which the transfer is maneuvered (bathrooms, for instance, are usually cramped); the number of assistants (1 or 2) needed to accomplish the transfer safely; the skill and strength of the nurse(s); and client's capabilities.
- Obtain essential equipment before starting (eg, transfer belt, wheelchair), and check its function.
- Remove obstacles from the area used for the transfer.
- Explain the transfer to the client, including what the client should do.
- Explain the transfer to the nursing personnel who are helping; specify who will give directions (one person needs to be in charge).
- Always support or hold the client rather than the equipment.
- During the transfer, explain step-by-step what the client should do, for example, "Move your right foot forward."
- Make a written plan of the transfer, including the client's tolerance (eg, pulse and respiratory rates).

Transferring a Client between a Bed and a Wheelchair A client may need to be transferred between the bed and a wheelchair or chair, the bed and the commode, or a wheelchair and the toilet. There are numerous variations of the technique; several are described in Procedure 34–7 on page 924. Which variation the nurse selects depends on a number of factors: the client's disabilities and body size, the technique with which the client is familiar, the space in which the transfer is maneuvered (bathrooms, for instance, are usually cramped), the number of assistants (1 or 2) needed to accomplish the transfer safely, and the skill and strength of the nurse(s).

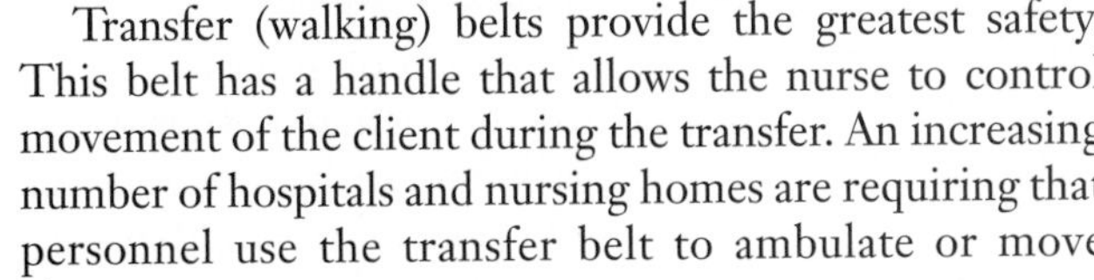

Transfer (walking) belts provide the greatest safety. This belt has a handle that allows the nurse to control movement of the client during the transfer. An increasing number of hospitals and nursing homes are requiring that personnel use the transfer belt to ambulate or move clients.

Transferring a Client between a Bed and a Stretcher The stretcher, or gurney, is used to transfer supine clients from one location to another. Whenever the client is capable of accomplishing the transfer from bed to stretcher independently, either by lifting onto it or by rolling onto it, the client should be encouraged to do so. If the

Text continued on page 926

CLINICAL GUIDELINES

Wheelchair Safety

- Always lock the brakes on both wheels of the wheelchair when the client transfers in or out of it.
- Raise the footplates before transferring the client into the wheelchair.
- Lower the footplates after the transfer, and place the client's feet on them.
- Ensure the client is positioned well back in the seat of the wheelchair.
- Use seat belts that fasten behind the wheelchair to protect confused clients from falls.
- Back the wheelchair into or out of an elevator, rear large wheels first.
- Place your body between the wheelchair and the bottom of an incline.

CLINICAL GUIDELINES

Safe Use of Stretchers

- Lock the wheels of the bed and stretcher before the client transfers in or out of them.
- Fasten safety straps across the client on a stretcher, and raise the side rails.
- Never leave a client unattended on a stretcher unless the wheels are locked and the side rails are raised on both sides and/or the safety straps are securely fastened across the client.
- Always push a stretcher from the end where the client's head is positioned. This position protects the client's head in the event of a collision.
- If the stretcher has two swivel wheels and two stationary wheels:
  - Always position the client's head at the end with the stationary wheels
    and
  - Push the stretcher from the end with the stationary wheels. The stretcher is maneuvered more easily when pushed from this end.
- Maneuver the stretcher when entering the elevator so that the client's head goes in first.

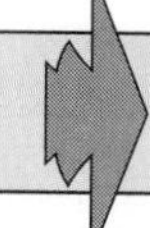

PROCEDURE 34–7 TRANSFERRING A CLIENT BETWEEN A BED AND A WHEELCHAIR

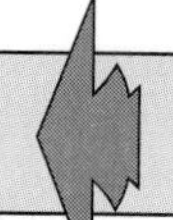

INTERVENTION

1. Position the equipment appropriately.

- Lower the bed to its lowest position so that the client's feet will rest flat on the floor. Lock the wheels of the bed.
- Place the wheelchair parallel to the bed as close to the bed as possible (Figure 34–30). Lock the wheels of the wheelchair, and raise the footplate.

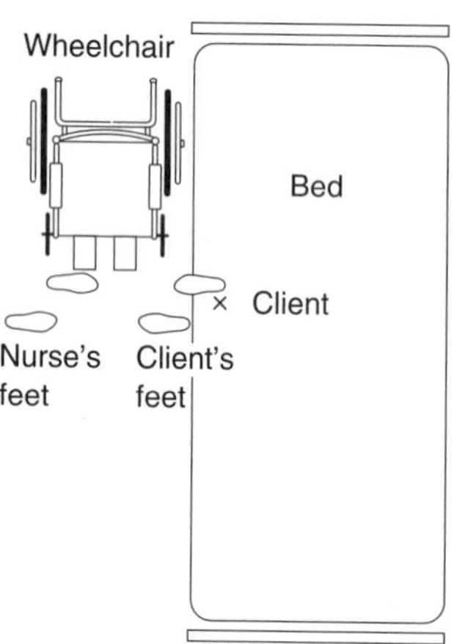

Figure 34–30 The wheelchair is placed parallel to the bed as close to the bed as possible. Note that placement of the nurse's feet mirrors that of the client's feet.

2. Prepare and assess the client.

- Assist the client to a sitting position on the side of the bed. See Procedure 34–6.
-  Assess the client for orthostatic hypotension before moving the client from the bed.
- Assist the client in putting on a bathrobe and nonskid slippers or shoes.
- 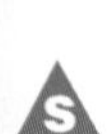 Place a transfer belt snugly around the client's waist. Check to be certain that the belt is securely fastened.

3. Give explicit instructions to the client. Ask the client to

- Move forward and sit on the edge of the bed. *This brings the client's center of gravity closer to the nurse's.*
- Lean forward slightly from the hips. *This brings the client's center of gravity more directly over the base of support and positions the head and trunk in the direction of the movement.*
- Place the foot of the stronger leg beneath the edge of the bed and put the other foot forward. *In this way, the client can use the stronger leg muscles to stand and power the movement. A broader base of support makes the client more stable during the transfer.*
- Place the hands on the bed surface or on your shoulders so that the client can push while standing. *This provides additional force for the movement and reduces the potential for strain on the nurse's back.*  The client should not grasp your neck for support. *Doing so can injure the nurse.*

4. Position yourself correctly.

- Stand directly in front of the client. Incline the trunk forward from the hips. Flex the hips, knees, and ankles. Assume a broad stance, placing one foot forward and one back. Mirror the placement of the client's feet, if possible. *This helps prevent loss of balance during the transfer.*
- 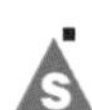 Encircle the client's waist with your arms, and grasp the transfer belt at the client's back (Figure 34–31) with thumbs pointing downward. *The belt provides a secure handle for holding onto the client and controlling the movement.*

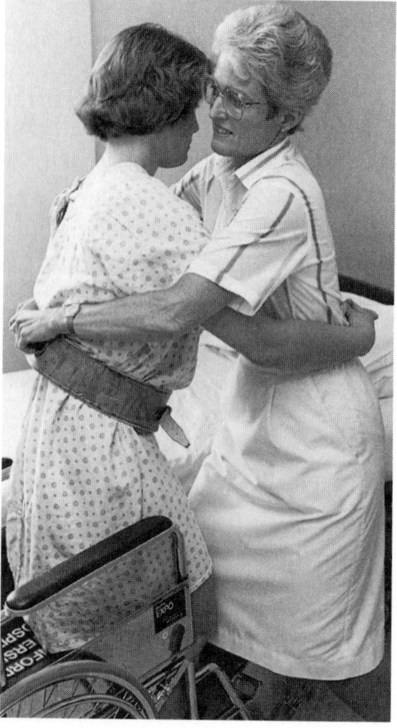

Figure 34–31 Using a transfer (walking) belt.

Downward placement of the thumbs prevents potential wrist injury as the nurse lifts (Leinweber 1978). By encircling the client in this manner, you keep the client from tilting backward during the transfer.

- Tighten your gluteal, abdominal, leg, and arm muscles.

5. Assist the client to stand, and then move together toward the wheelchair.

- On the count of three:
  a. Ask the client to push with the back foot, rock to the forward foot, extend (straighten) the joints of the lower extremities, and push or pull up with the hands, while
  b. You push with the forward foot, rock to the back foot, extend the joints of the lower extremities, and pull the client

Procedure 34–7 *continued*

(directly toward your center of gravity) into a standing position.

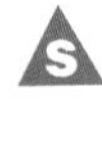

- Support the client in an upright standing position for a few moments. *This allows the nurse and the client to extend the joints and provides the nurse with an opportunity to ensure that the client is all right before moving away from the bed.*
- Together, pivot or take a few steps toward the wheelchair.

6. Assist the client to sit.

- Ask the client to
  a. Back up to the wheelchair and place the legs against the seat. *Having the client place the legs against the wheelchair seat minimizes the risk of the client's falling when sitting down.*
  b. Place the foot of the stronger leg slightly behind the other. *This supports body weight during the movement.*
  c. Keep the other foot forward. *This provides a broad base of support.*
  d. Place both hands on the wheelchair arms or on your shoulders. *This increases stability and lessens the strain on the nurse.*
- Stand directly in front of the client. Place one foot forward and one back.
- Tighten your grasp on the transfer belt, and tighten your gluteal, abdominal, leg, and arm muscles.
- On the count of three:
  a. Have the client shift the body weight by rocking to the back foot, lower the body onto the edge of the wheelchair seat by flexing the joints of the legs and arms, and place some body weight on the arms, while
  b. You shift your body weight by stepping back with the forward foot and pivoting toward the chair while lowering the client onto the wheelchair seat.

7. Ensure client safety.

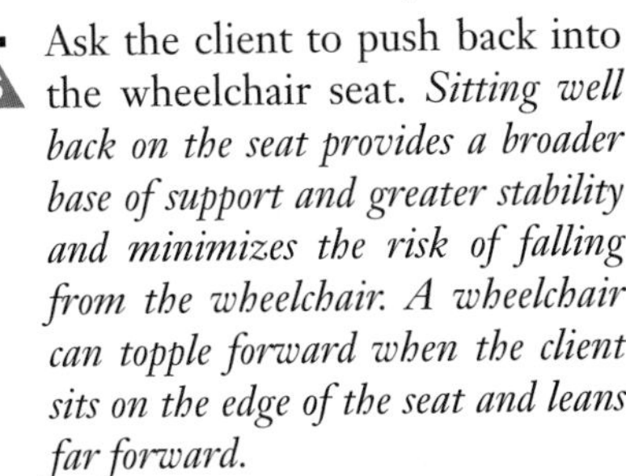

- Ask the client to push back into the wheelchair seat. *Sitting well back on the seat provides a broader base of support and greater stability and minimizes the risk of falling from the wheelchair. A wheelchair can topple forward when the client sits on the edge of the seat and leans far forward.*
- Lower the footplates, and place the client's feet on them.
- Apply a seat belt as required.

Variation: Angling the Wheelchair

For clients who have difficulty walking, place the wheelchair at a 45 degree angle to the bed. *This enables the client to pivot into the chair and lessens the amount of body rotation required.*

Variation: Transferring Without a Belt

- For clients who need minimal assistance, place the hands against the sides of the client's chest (not at the axillae) during the transfer (Figure 34–32). For clients who require more assistance, reach through the client's axillae, and place the hands on the client's scapulae during the transfer. Avoid placing hands or pressure on the axillae, especially for clients who have upper extremity paralysis or paresis.

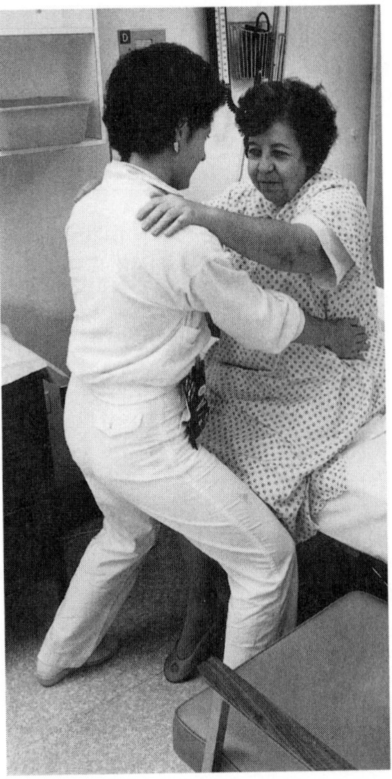

Figure 34–32 Transferring without a belt.

- Follow the steps described previously.

Variation: Transferring with a Belt and Two Nurses

- When the client is able to stand, position yourselves on both sides of the client, facing the same direction as the client. Flex your hips, knees, and ankles; grasp the client's transfer belt with the hand closest to the client; and with the other hand support the client's elbows.
- Coordinating your efforts, all three of you stand simultaneously, pivot, and move to the wheelchair. Reverse the process to lower the client onto the wheelchair seat.

Procedure 34–7 Transferring a Client between a Bed and a Wheelchair *continued*

Variation: Transferring a Client with an Injured Lower Extremity

When the client has an injured lower extremity, movement should always occur toward the client's unaffected (strong) side. For example, if the client's right leg is injured and the client is sitting on the edge of the bed preparing to transfer to a wheelchair, position the wheelchair on the client's left side. *In this way, the client can use the unaffected leg most effectively and safely.*

Variation: Using a Sliding Board

Have a client who cannot stand use a sliding board to move without nursing assistance. This method not only promotes the client's sense of independence but preserves your energy (Figure 34–33).

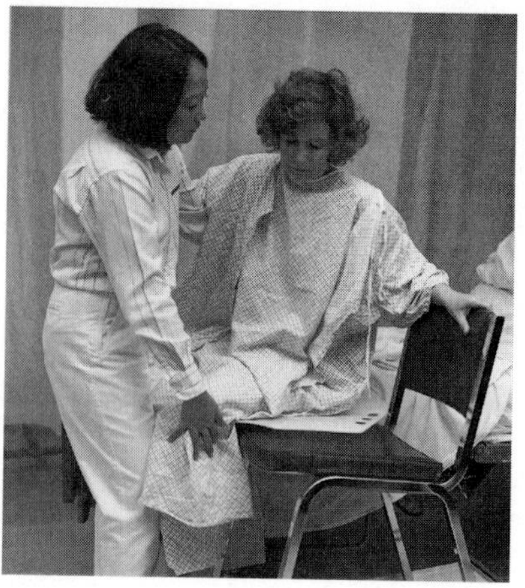

Figure 34–33 Using a sliding board.

client cannot move onto the stretcher independently, at least two nurses are needed to assist with the transfer; more are needed if the client is totally helpless or heavy. See Procedure 34–8.

Moving a Client Using a Hydraulic Lift Hydraulic lifts, such as the Hoyer lift, are used primarily for clients who cannot help themselves or who are too heavy for others to lift safely. The lift can be used in transferring the client between the bed and a wheelchair, the bed and the bathtub, and the bed and a stretcher. The Hoyer lift consists of a base on casters, a hydraulic mechanical pump, a mast boom, and a sling (Figure 34–34). The sling may consist of a one-piece or two-piece canvas seat. The one-piece seat stretches from the client's head to the knees. The two-piece seat has one canvas strap to support the client's buttocks and thighs and a second strap extending up to the axillae to support the back. It is important to be familiar with the model used and the practices that accompany use. Before using the lift, the nurse ensures that it is in working order and that the hooks, chains, straps, and canvas seat are in good repair. *Most agencies recommend that two nurses operate a lift.* Check agency policy.

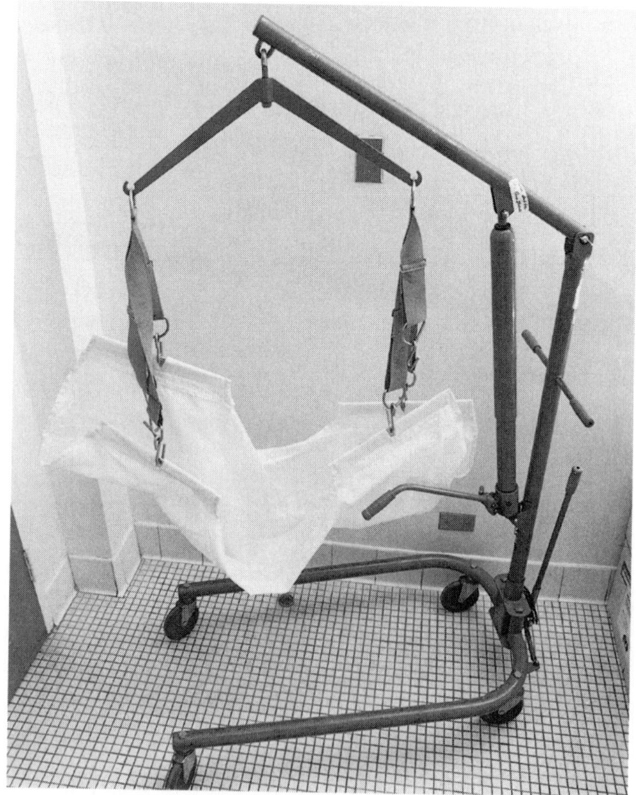

Figure 34–34 A one-piece seat hydraulic lift.

Exercise

Exercise is the active contraction and relaxation of muscles. Exercises can be classified according to the type of muscle contraction (isotonic, isometric, or isokinetic) and according to the source of energy (aerobic or anaerobic).

Isotonic (dynamic) exercises are those in which muscle tension is constant and the muscle shortens to produce muscle contraction and movement. Because the muscles contract, the size, shape, and strength of the muscles, and joint mobility are maintained. Most physical conditioning exercises—running, walking, swimming, cycling, and other such activities—are isotonic, as are activities of daily living (ADLs) and active ROM exercises. Examples of isotonic bed exercises are pushing or pulling against a

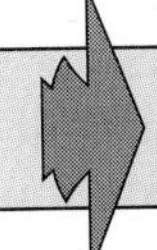

PROCEDURE 34–8 TRANSFERRING A CLIENT BETWEEN A BED AND A STRETCHER

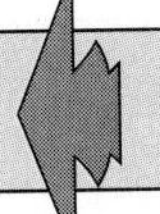

EQUIPMENT

☐ Stretcher

☐ Roller bar (optional)

INTERVENTION

1. Adjust the client's bed in preparation for the transfer.

- ower the head of the bed until it is flat or as low as the client can tolerate.
- Raise the bed so that it is slightly higher than the surface of the stretcher. *It is easier and requires less effort for the client to move down an incline.*
- Ensure that the wheels on the bed are locked.
- Pull the drawsheet out from both sides of the bed.

2. Move the client to the edge of the bed, and position the stretcher.

- Roll the drawsheet as close to the client's side as possible.
- Pull the client to the edge of the bed, and cover the client with a sheet or bath blanket to maintain comfort.
- Place the stretcher parallel to the bed, next to the client, and lock its wheels.
- Fill the gap that exists between the bed and the stretcher loosely with bath blankets (optional).

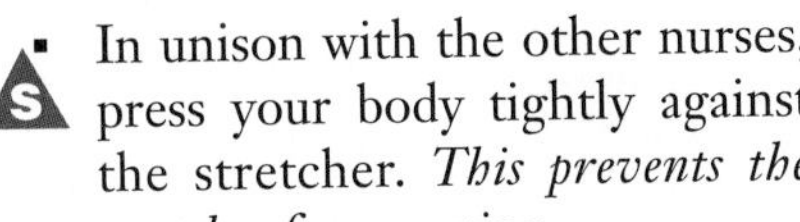

3. Transfer the client securely to the stretcher.

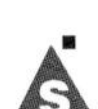

- In unison with the other nurses, press your body tightly against the stretcher. *This prevents the stretcher from moving.*
- Roll the pull sheet tightly against the client. *This achieves better control over client movement.*
- Flex your hips, and pull the client on the pull sheet in unison directly toward you and onto the stretcher. *Pulling downward requires less force than pulling along a flat surface.*

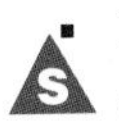

- Ask the client to flex the neck during the move, if possible, and place arms across the chest. *This prevents injury to these body parts.*

4. Ensure client comfort and safety.

- Make the client comfortable, unlock the stretcher wheels, and move the stretcher away from the bed.
- Immediately raise the stretcher side rails and/or fasten the safety straps across the client. *Because the stretcher is high and narrow, the client is in danger of falling unless these safety precautions are taken.*

Variation: Using a Roller Bar During the Transfer

A roller bar is a metal frame covered with longitudinal rollers. Place the bar over the gap between the bed and the stretcher. Using a pull sheet, pull the client onto the roller bar, and roll the client easily onto the stretcher.

Variation: Using a Long Board

The long board, which may be referred to as the Smooth Mover or Easyglide, is a lacquered or smooth polyethylene board measuring 45 to 55 cm (18 to 22 in) by 182 cm (72 in) with handholds along its edges. This device may be used by one nurse alone or up to four nurses together. Turn the client to a lateral position away from you, position the board close to the client's back, and roll the client onto the board. Pull the client and board across the bed to the stretcher. Safety belts may be placed over the chest, abdomen, and legs.

stationary object, pressing the feet against a footboard, using a trapeze to lift the body off the bed, lifting the buttocks off the bed by pushing with the hands against the mattress, and pushing the body to a sitting position.

Isotonic exercises increase muscle strength and endurance and can improve cardiorespiratory function. During isotonic exercise, both heart rate and cardiac output quicken to increase blood flow to all parts of the body. Little or no change in blood pressure occurs.

Isometric (static or setting) exercises are those in which there is a change in muscle tension but no change in muscle length. No muscle or joint movement occurs. These exercises are useful for strengthening abdominal, gluteal, and quadriceps muscles used in ambulation but are not useful in preventing joint contracture, because joint movement is absent. When an immobilized client's leg is confined in a cast or traction, isometric exercises may help maintain muscle strength in the affected limb. Isometric exercises may be useful for strengthening arm muscles in preparation for crutch-walking.

Isometric exercises produce a moderate increase in heart rate and cardiac output, but no appreciable increase in blood flow to other parts of the body. A marked increase in blood pressure occurs with isometric exercise, and use of the Valsalva maneuver is essentially unavoidable. This combination can pose real danger for any cardiac client, who should be taught to *exhale* when performing these exercises. (The *Valsalva Maneuver* is forced

RESEARCH NOTE

Which Nursing Tasks Impose Great Stress on the Back?

The purpose of this study was to reduce back stress for nursing personnel by changing the physical demands of the job. The goals were (a) to determine the most stressful client handling tasks, (b) to conduct an ergonomic evaluation of these tasks, (c) to find less stressful methods for carrying out these tasks, and (d) to apply the less stressful methods in the clinical setting. The latter goal has not yet been completed.

The ergonomic process involved identifying the jobs and specific tasks within those jobs that impose great stress on the back; studying and pilot testing ways to change the task demands; and implementing these changes in the work setting.

The study took place in two settings: a nursing home/long-term care facility in which 38 nursing assistants (two were males) ranging in age from 19 to 61 years participated, and a laboratory in a university school of nursing in which six senior nursing students participated. Participants listed the client handling tasks they perceived as most stressful in their duties. An ergonomic evaluation was then completed on the ten tasks perceived as most stressful.

The tasks ranked as most stressful were transferring the client on and off the toilet and in and out bed, and the transfers involved in bathing and weighing clients. The participants reported that they felt the greatest amount of exertion in the lower back. Problems encountered in the transfers were the presence of railings around toilets, unequal heights of toilet and wheelchair seats, and stress levels related to the use of hoists. Problems with the use hoists resulted from body postures the nurses needed to assume in order to position the slings and the effort needed to push the hoist with the client in it.

Of the manual lifting techniques used, the method of lifting the client under the axilla was perceived to be the most stressful; the walking belt was rated the least stressful. The most commonly used assistive device was the walking belt.

Implications: To minimize back pain, nurses need to explore ways to change environmental impediments, such as altering railings around the toilet and raising toilet seat levels. Furthermore, nurses need to learn to use transfer devices effectively.

Source: BD Owen and A Garg, Reducing the risk for back pain in nursing personnel. *AAOHN Journal*, January 1991, 39:24–33.

exhalation against a closed glottis, which increases intrathoracic pressure and thus interferes with the return of venous blood to the heart. It commonly occurs when a person strains to defecate and holds the breath.)

Isokinetic (resistive) exercises involve muscle contraction and joint movement. They can be either isotonic or isometric. During isokinetic exercise, the person moves (isotonic) or tenses (isometric) against resistance. Special machines or devices provide the resistance to the movement. These exercises are used in physical conditioning and are often done to build up certain muscle groups; for example, the pectorals (chest muscles) may be increased in size and strength by lifting weights. A client who pushes the feet against a footboard placed in the bed is also performing an isokinetic exercise.

Aerobic exercise is an activity in which the amount of oxygen taken into the body is greater than or equal to the amount the body requires. Walking briskly and swimming are common aerobic exercises. These exercises improve cardiovascular fitness. **Anaerobic exercise** is activity in which the amount of oxygen taken into the body is insufficient to meet the body's need. In this case, the oxygen need is made up later. An example of an anaerobic exercise is running up three flights of stairs. Anaerobic exercises are usually done to develop muscle tone and to improve cardiorespiratory function. In addition, anaerobic exercises involving joint movement can improve joint mobility.

Range of motion (ROM) is the totality of movement a joint is capable of doing. Table 34–2, page 882, describes the normal range of motion of the body joints. When people are ill, they often need to perform ROM exercises until they regain their normal activity levels.

Active ROM exercises are isotonic exercises in which the client moves each joint in the body through its complete range of movement, maximally stretching all muscle groups within each plane, over the joint. These exercises maintain or increase muscle strength and endurance and help to maintain cardiorespiratory function in an immobilized client. They also prevent deterioration of joint capsules, ankylosis, and contractures. Instructions for the client performing active ROM exercises are shown in the box on page 929.

Full ROM does not occur spontaneously in the immobilized individual who independently achieves ADLs, independently moves about in bed, independently transfers between bed and wheelchair or chair, or independently ambulates a short distance, because only a few muscle groups are maximally stretched during these activities. Although the client may successfully achieve some active ROM movements of the upper extremities while combing the hair, bathing, and dressing, the immobilized client is very unlikely to achieve any active ROM movements of the lower extremities when these are not used in their normal functions of standing and walking about. For this reason, most wheelchair and many ambulatory clients need active ROM exercises until they regain their normal activity levels.

A physician's order for ROM exercises is usually required if a client has an abnormal or injured musculoskeletal part or if the client's overall condition could be compromised by exercise. A nursing order to carry out preventive exercises is expected for the client whose musculoskeletal system is otherwise normal but who is suffering from the consequences of immobility. At first, the nurse may need to help the client perform the needed ROM exercises; eventually, the client may be able to accomplish these independently, with only periodic guidance from the nurse.

During **passive ROM exercises,** another person moves each of the client's joints through their complete range of movement, maximally stretching all muscle groups within each plane over each joint. Since the client does not contract the muscle, passive ROM exercises are of no value in maintaining muscle strength but are useful in maintaining joint flexibility. For this reason, passive ROM exercises should be performed only when the client is unable to accomplish the movements actively.

Passive ROM exercises should be accomplished for each movement of the arms, legs, and neck *that the client is unable to achieve actively.* As with active ROM exercises, passive ROM exercises should be accomplished to the point of slight resistance, but not beyond, and never to the point of discomfort. The movements should be systematic, and the same sequence should be followed during each exercise session. Each exercise should consist of three repetitions, and the series of exercises should be done twice daily (Kottke et al 1990, p. 444). Performing one series of exercises along with the bath is helpful. Passive ROM exercises are accomplished most effectively when the client lies supine in bed.

General guidelines for providing passive exercises are shown in the box on page 930. Refer to the *Procedures Supplement* that accompanies this text for details about how to perform these exercises.

During **active-assistive ROM exercises,** the client uses a stronger, opposite arm or leg to move each of the joints of a limb incapable of active motion. The client learns to support and move the weak arm or leg with the strong arm or leg as far as possible. Then the nurse continues the movement passively to its maximal degree. This activity increases active movement on the strong side of the client's body and maintains joint flexibility on the weak side. Such exercise is especially useful for stroke victims who are hemiplegic (paralyzed on one half of the body). Some clients who begin with passive ROM exercises after a disability progress to active-assistive ROM exercises and, finally, to active ROM exercises.

CLIENT TEACHING

Active ROM Exercises

- Perform each ROM exercise as taught to the point of slight resistance, but not beyond, and never to the point of discomfort.
- Perform the movements systematically, using the same sequence during each session.
- Perform each exercise three times.
- Perform each series of exercises twice daily.

For the Elderly

- For elderly clients, it is not essential to achieve full range of motion in all joints. Instead, emphasize achieving a sufficient range of motion to carry out ADLs, such as walking, dressing, combing hair, showering, and preparing a meal.

Components of Physical Fitness The four main components of physical fitness are muscle strength and endurance, cardiorespiratory fitness, flexibility, and body composition.

Muscle Strength and Endurance Muscle strength is the amount of force a person can exert with the muscles against resistance. Three kinds of exercise improve muscle strength: isotonic (eg, lifting weights), isometric (eg, contracting the thigh muscles without moving the legs), and isokinetic (eg, using an exercise machine such as a Cybex, in which the client not only lifts the weights up but also must pull it back down). These exercises may or may not offer aerobic benefit.

Endurance is the ability of the muscles to be used over a period of time without becoming fatigued. Whereas good muscle strength means a person can lift more, good muscle endurance means a person can lift longer.

Cardiorespiratory Fitness Endurance exercises that improve cardiorespiratory fitness include activities such as walking, cycling, or jogging. The person attempts to keep moving for at least 20 minutes even if it is necessary to slow down. The goal is to work up to and sustain a target heart rate during the exercise. The target heart rate is based on the person's age. For suggested rates, see Table 34–14 on page 931. One of the simplest methods of assessing achievement of the target is to take the pulse. As the fitness level improves, the person can elect either to go on to a higher heart rate or to continue for a longer time at the same rate.

Exercise to achieve cardiovascular endurance, or aerobic exercise, is strenuous exercise that does not leave the

CLINICAL GUIDELINES

Providing Passive ROM Exercise

- Ensure that the client understands the reason for doing ROM exercises.
- If there is a possibility of hand swelling, make sure rings are removed.
- Clothe the client in a loose gown, and cover the body with a bath blanket.
- Use correct body mechanics when providing ROM exercise to avoid muscle strain or injury to both yourself and the client.
- Position the bed at an appropriate height.
- Expose only the limb being exercised to avoid embarrassing the client.
- Support the client's limbs above and below the joint as needed to prevent muscle strain or injury (Figure 34–35). This may also be done by cupping joints in the palm of the hand or cradling limbs along the nurse's forearm (Figure 34–36). If a joint is painful (eg, arthritic), support the limb in the muscular areas above and below the joint.
- Use a firm, comfortable grip when handling the limb.
- Move the body parts smoothly, slowly, and rhythmically. Jerky movements cause discomfort and, possibly, injury. Fast movements can cause *spasticity* (sudden, prolonged involuntary muscle contraction) or *rigidity* (stiffness or inflexibility).
- Avoid moving or forcing a body part beyond the existing range of motion. Muscle strain, pain, and injury can result. This is particularly important for people with flaccid (limp) paralysis, whose muscles can be stretched and joints dislocated without their awareness. 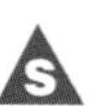
- If muscle spasticity occurs during movement, stop the movement temporarily, but continue to apply slow, gentle pressure on the part until the muscle relaxes; then proceed with the motion.
- If a contracture is present, apply slow firm pressure without causing pain, to stretch the muscle fibers.
- If rigidity occurs, apply pressure against the rigidity, and continue the exercise slowly.

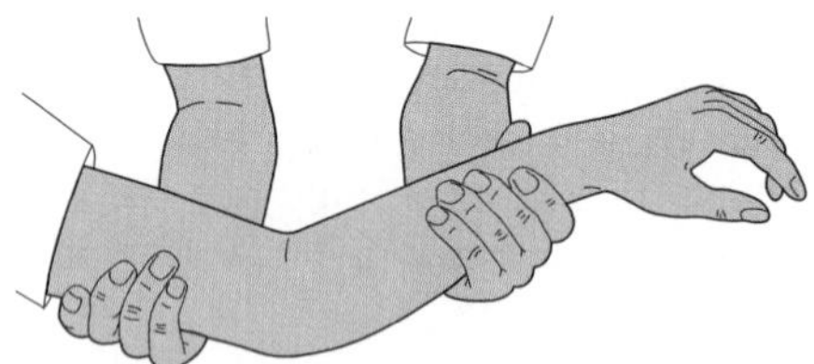

Figure 34–35 Supporting a limb above and below the joint for passive exercise.

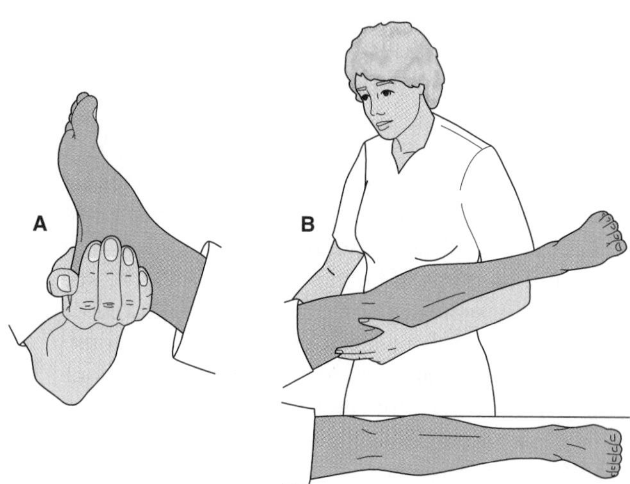

Figure 34–36 Holding limbs for support during passive exercise: *A*, cupping; *B*, cradling.

person breathless. The box on page 931 describes types of exercise, frequency, intensity, and duration recommended for healthy adults and elderly people.

Joint Flexibility Flexibility is the ability to use a muscle fully through its maximum range of motion. Loss of flexibility leads to shortened muscles and tendons and can contribute to an imbalance in muscle strength of opposing pairs of muscles and subsequent joint injury. To improve flexibility, the person must stretch the muscles further than they are usually stretched. Specific warm-up and cool-down activities, such as some forms of dance, yoga, and t'ai chi, involve stretching.

Functional joint flexibility is also maintained in the performance of activities of daily living (ADLs). The following are examples:

- Eating, shaving, grooming, and bathing exercise the elbow (flexion and extension) and shoulder (abduction).
- Activities requiring fine motor skills, such as writing and eating, exercise fingers (flexion, extension, adduction, abduction) and the thumb (opposition).
- Walking exercises the shoulders (flexion, extension), hip (flexion, extension, hyperextension), the knee (flexion, extension), and ankle (plantar flexion and dorsiflexion).

Table 34–14 Target and Maximum Heart Rates

Age (years)	Target HR Zone 50–75% (beats per min)	Average Max HR 100%
20	100-150	200
25	98-146	195
30	95-142	190
35	93-138	185
40	90-135	180
45	88-131	175
50	85-127	170
55	83-123	165
60	80-120	160
65	78-116	155
70	75-113	150

Source: Reproduced with permission. *Exercise Diary, 1993.* Copyright American Heart Association. (Dallas: American Heart Association, 1993), p. 5.

- Reaching for articles exercises the shoulders (flexion, extension, and perhaps slight abduction or adduction).
- Dressing involves many joint movements.

Body Composition Body composition refers to the recommended proportion of fat to lean body tissue. Because muscle movement is fueled by food energy, the more vigorous and sustained the exercise, the larger the caloric expenditure per hour. Thus, general principles of nutrition apply to people involved in exercise programs, who require adequate intakes of vitamins, protein, and fluids (see Chapters 37 and 38). Physical fitness in daily life encompasses both caloric balance and functional fitness, and a person can use both exercise and diet efficiently together to reduce body weight. (Approximately 3500 calories equal 1 pound of body fat). The following are examples of activities that burn up 100 calories:

- Walk briskly for 15 to 20 minutes
- Bicycle 8 km/h for 20 minutes
- Run 15 km/h for 7 minutes
- Swim crawl 20 m/min for 20 minutes
- Dance (at a moderate pace) for 25 to 30 minutes
- Play tennis for 15 minutes

Developing a Successful Exercise Program for Wellness All people require sufficient exercise to maintain physical fitness. Benefits of exercise and a comparison of the physically fit person to the physically unfit person

WELLNESS TEACHING

Exercising to Develop and Maintain Cardiovascular Fitness

Healthy Adults

Type of Exercise:

Any endurance exercise that uses large muscle groups, can be performed continuously, and is rhythmic and aerobic in nature, such as walking, jogging, running, bicycling, dancing, cross-country skiing, jumping rope, rowing, swimming, and skating

Frequency:

3 to 5 days per week

Intensity:

60% to 90% of maximum heart rate. See the American Heart Association Guidelines (Table 34 – 14). Alternatively, calculate your maximum heart rate by subtracting your current age in years from 220, and then obtain the target heart rate by taking 60% to 90% of the maximum. Another simple and quick method is the "talk test": If it is possible to *converse normally* during exercise without running out of breath, the pace of the program is probably safe and realistic.

Duration:

20 to 60 minutes of continuous activity

Elderly Adults

- Consult with your physician before beginning an exercise program.
- Start slowly, and gradually increase intensity and duration to reach the desired goals.

Type of Exercise:

Aerobic (walking, biking, swimming)

Intensity:

At least 60% of maximum heart rate

Frequency:

At least every 42 hours

Duration:

At least 20 minutes

Sources: American College of Sports Medicine, The recommended quantity and quality of exercise for developing and maintaining cardiorespiratory and muscular fitness in healthy adults, *Medicine and Science in Sports and Exercise,* 1990, 22:265; JM Schilke, Slowing the aging process with physical activity, *Journal of Gerontological Nursing,* June 1991, 17:6.

Table 34–15 Benefits of Exercise on Body: Comparison of Physically Fit and Unfit Person

System	Physically Fit Person	Physically Unfit Person
General	Percentage of body fat is less than 15% in men, 25% in women Increased sense of well-being, improved self-concept, and ability to cope with stress Improved energy level and work performance Improved quality of sleep	Percentage of body fat is more than 16% in men, 26% in women Tendency toward depression, nervous tension, and anxiety reactions Decreased energy level and work performance Decreased quality of sleep
Cardiovascular	During exertion: Increased strength of heart muscle contraction Increased heart rate Increased blood supply to heart and muscle Decreased potential for irregular heart rate Faster recovery time following exertion At rest: Decreased heart rate Decreased systolic and diastolic blood pressure	During exertion: Increased heart rate Shortness of breath Chest and skeletal muscle pain, which indicate inadequate perfusion Danger of irregular heart rate At rest: Increased heart rate Increased systolic and diastolic blood pressure
Musculoskeletal	Firm muscle tone Increased strength and endurance Increased joint flexibility and range of motion Increased balance and coordination	Flabby muscle tone Decreased strength and endurance Decreased joint flexibility and range of motion Decreased balance and coordination
Respiratory	Increased vital and functional capacity Increased oxygen diffusion and consumption	Decreased vital and functional capacity Decreased oxygen diffusion and consumption
Gastrointestinal	Increased motility of gastrointestinal tract	Decreased gastrointestinal tract motility, increasing potential for constipation
Metabolic	Decreased serum triglyceride and cholesterol levels	Increased serum triglyceride and cholesterol levels, increasing potential for heart desease

are shown in Table 34–15. Any exercise program should (a) be designed for the individual, (b) incorporate activities of daily living (ADLs), and (c) be put in writing and give specific instructions.

Nurses help the client as follows:

- Explore client goals and choose a feasible exercise by considering the client's current fitness level, the benefit of the activity, time involved, equipment and expense required, necessary precautions, and risks. For example, jogging produces cardiovascular fitness but does little for increasing flexibility. Choice of activity must also be tailored to person's interests, capabilities, and resources.
- Obtain medical consultation before initiating exercise program for any client who is older than 35 years and sedentary or who has any cardiovascular problem.
- Start the exercise program gradually. Movements should not be painful or forced but enable the body to accommodate to the new stress.
- Start the exercise session with a *warm-up period.* An 8 to 10 minute warm-up period (eg, slow jogging or brisk walking) slightly raises the heart rate, increases the body's internal temperature, and increases the circulation (oxygen flow) to the muscles, making them more flexible for stretching. Increasing the range of motion of the joints helps avoid injuries and muscle tears and pulls.
- Work within the target heart range to identify a safe pace for the program (see the box on page 931 for recommended intensity, frequency, and duration).
- End the exercise session with a *cool-down period.* To cool down after the exercise, keep moving with light activity similar to those performed in the warm-up for at least another 5 minutes. The cool-down period decreases peripheral blood pooling. Extensive blood pooling can result in insufficient blood supply to the brain, heart, or intestine and cause symptoms such as vertigo, syncope, arrhythmias, or nausea. The major purposes of cool-down are to (a) reduce pulse rate, (b) return blood to the heart in sufficient quantities to rid the muscles of lactic acid, and (c) slowly stretch muscles that have been contracting vigorously (Edmunds 1991, p. 862). Longer cool-down periods may be needed for seden-

CRITICAL THINKING CHALLENGE

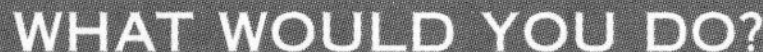

WHAT WOULD YOU DO?

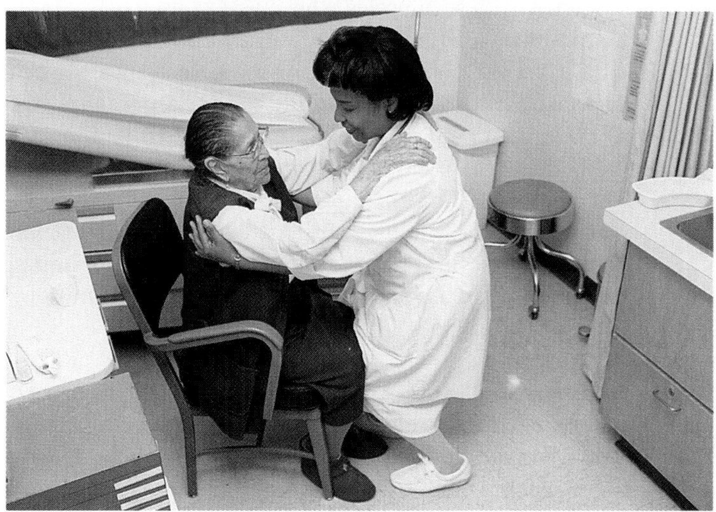

Teresa Martinez, a 79-year-old female, is recovering from a mild stoke (cerebrovascular accident). She is receiving daily physical therapy and has some residual right-sided weakness. The physician has ordered that Mrs Martinez be ambulated three times a day. Mrs Martinez states that she feels dizzy when she stands and is fearful that she will fall.

What would you do?

---

tary or older people or when exercises are performed in a hot environment.

- When possible, incorporate a variety of exercise activities to achieve goals of cardiovascular fitness, joint flexibility, and so on.
- Instruct the client to avoid possible hazards to prevent injury, for example:
  a. Wear comfortable support shoes and well-fitting socks. Proper footgear prevents blisters and injury.
  b. Avoid running or walking on hard surfaces or in hilly areas. Running on hard surfaces can jar the joints. Also avoid areas of high pollution or smog.
  c. Avoid exercising on hottest or most humid days. Body temperature may become overly elevated.
  d. Wait 1½ to 2½ hours after a meal. After that time, blood flow will be directed to the muscles rather than to the alimentary tract.
  e. Drink ample fluid before exercising. Adequate intake prevents dehydration due to fluid loss through perspiration. Schedule regular fluid breaks during heavy exercise. Glucose provides energy for exercise, so choose fluids containing glucose (or sucrose), in sufficient amounts. Fluids consumed should have less than 2.5 grams per 100 mL of water (Hill & Smith 1990, p. 252). Electrolyte replacement drinks are generally not recommended.
  f. Stop exercise immediately and consult your health care provider if you experience pain or pressure in the center of the chest, irregular heart action, dizziness, fainting, light-headedness, or blackout.
  g. Scale down your program or take more rest periods if you experience prolonged rapid heart action more than 15 minutes after stopping moderate exercise, prolonged breathlessness after moderate exercise, nausea or vomiting after exercise, insomnia, or prolonged fatigue.
  h. Check your equipment or check with a health adviser if arthritis, knee, or back problems recur, or you experience pulled muscles, muscle cramps or charley horse, or shin splints or pain of any type.
- Encourage and complement the program with everyday activities requiring exercise. For example, walk to work rather than ride. Walk upstairs rather than using the elevator.
- Find an exercise partner who will participate and support the exercise program as a regular part of life.

AMBULATING CLIENTS

Ambulation (the act of walking) is a function that most people take for granted. However, when people are ill they are often confined to bed and are thus nonambulatory. The longer clients are in bed, the more difficulty they have walking.

Even 1 or 2 days of bed rest can make a person feel weak, unsteady, and shaky when first getting out of bed. A client who has had surgery, is elderly, or has been immobilized for a longer time will feel more pronounced weakness. The potential problems of immobility are far less likely to occur when clients become ambulatory as soon

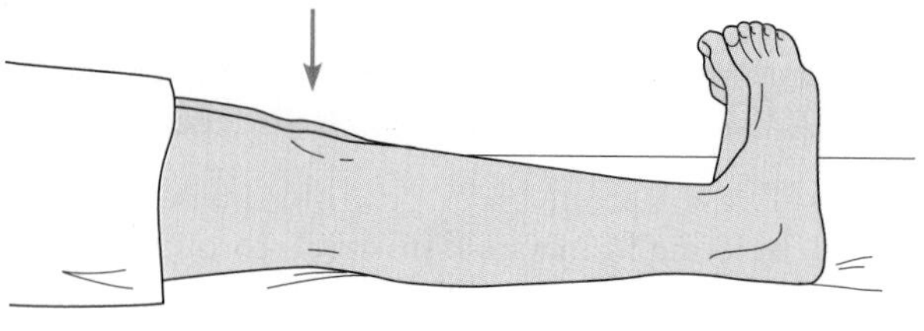

Figure 34–37 Tensing the quadriceps femoris muscles before ambulation.

as possible. The nurse can assist clients to prepare for ambulation by helping them become as independent as possible while in bed. Nurses should encourage clients to perform ADLs, maintain good body alignment, and carry out active range-of-motion exercises to the maximum degree possible yet within the limitations imposed by their illness and recovery program.

Preambulatory Exercises Clients who have been in bed for long periods often need a plan of muscle tone exercises to strengthen the muscles used for walking before attempting to walk. One of the most important muscle groups is the quadriceps femoris, which extends the knee and flexes the thigh. This group is also important for elevating the legs, for example, for walking upstairs. To strengthen these muscles, the client consciously tenses them, drawing the kneecap upward and inward. The client pushes the popliteal space of the knee against the bed surface, relaxing the heels on the bed surface (Figure 34–37). On the count of 1, the muscles are tensed; they are held during the counts of 2, 3, 4; and they are relaxed at the count of 5. The exercise should be done within the client's tolerance, that is without fatiguing the muscles. Carried out several times an hour during waking hours, this simple exercise significantly strengthens the muscles used for walking.

Assisting Clients to Ambulate Clients who have been immobilized for even a few days may require assistance with ambulation. The amount of assistance will depend on the client's condition, including age, health status, and length of inactivity. Assistance may mean walking alongside the client while providing physical support (see Procedure 34–9) or providing instruction to the client about the use of assistive devices such as a cane, walker, or crutches (see the next section).

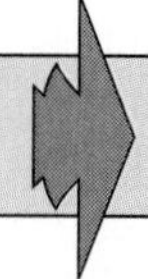

PROCEDURE 34–9 ASSISTING A CLIENT TO WALK

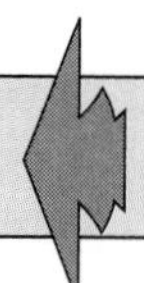

A physician's order for ambulation is usually required, especially if the client has been immobilized in bed for any length of time.

PURPOSES

- To increase muscle strength and joint mobility
- To prevent some potential problems of immobility
- To increase the client's sense of independence and self-esteem

ASSESSMENT FOCUS

Length of time in bed and time up previously; pulse rate, respiratory rate, and blood pressure for baseline data before walking, especially if this is the client's first time up; range of motion of joints needed for ambulating (eg, hips, knees, ankles); muscle strength of lower extremities; need for ambulation aids (eg, cane, walker, crutches); client's intake of medications (eg, narcotics, sedatives, tranquilizers, and antihistamines) that may cause drowsiness, dizziness, weakness, and orthostatic hypotension and seriously hinder the client's ability to walk safely; presence of joint inflammation, fractures, muscle weakness, or other conditions that impair physical mobility; ability to understand directions; need for the assistance of another nurse.

EQUIPMENT

□ Walking belt (optional)

PROCEDURE 34–9 *continued*

INTERVENTION

1. Prepare the client for ambulation.

- Apply elastic (antiemboli) stockings as required. See page 1407.
- Assist the client to sit on the edge of the bed.
-  Assess the client carefully for signs and symptoms of orthostatic hypotension (dizziness, lightheadedness, pallor, or a sudden increase in heart rate) prior to leaving the bedside.
-  Ensure that the client is appropriately dressed to walk and wears shoes or slippers with nonskid soles. *Proper attire and footwear prevent chilling and falling.*
- Assist the client to stand by the side of the bed until the client feels secure.
- Plan the length of the walk with the client, in light of the nursing or physician's orders. Be prepared to shorten the walk according to the person's activity tolerance.

One Nurse

 **2. Ensure client safety while assisting the client to ambulate.**

- Encourge the client to ambulate independently if the client is able, but walk beside the client.
- Remain physically close to the client in case assistance is needed at any point.
- Use a transfer or walking belt if the client is slightly weak and unstable. Make sure the belt is pulled snugly around the client's waist and fastened securely. Grasp the belt at the client's back, and walk behind and slightly to one side of the client (Figure 34–38).
- If it is the client's first time out of bed following surgery, injury, or an extended period of immobility, or if the client is quite weak or unstable, have an assistant follow you and the client with a wheelchair in the event that it is needed quickly.
- If the client is moderately weak and unstable, interlock your forearm with the client's closest forearm, and walk on the client's weaker side. Encourage the client to press the forearm against your hip or waist for stability if desired. In addition, have the client wear a transfer or walking belt so that you can quickly grab the belt and prevent a fall if the client feels faint.
- If the client is very weak and unstable, place your near arm around the client's waist, and with your other arm support the client's near arm at the elbow. Walk on the client's stronger side. Again, have the client wear a transfer or walking belt in case of an emergency.
- Encourage the client to assume a normal walking stance and gait as much as possible.

3. Protect the client who begins to fall while ambulating.

- If a client begins to experience the signs and symptoms of orthostatic hypotension or extreme weakness, quickly assist the client into a nearby wheelchair or other chair, and help the client to lower the head between the knees. *Lowering the head facilitates blood flow to the brain.*
- Stay with the client. *A client who faints while in this position could fall, head first, out of the chair.*
- When the weakness subsides, assist the client back to bed.
- If a chair is not close by, assist the client to a horizontal position on the floor before fainting occurs (Figure 34–39). *A vertical position may increase feelings of faintness.*

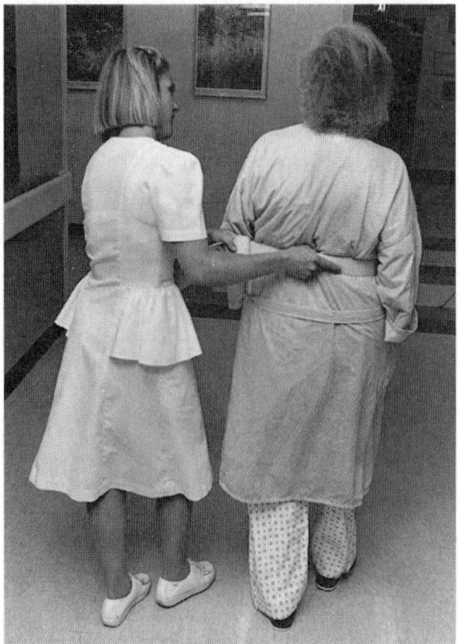

Figure 34–38 Using a transfer (walking) belt to support the client.

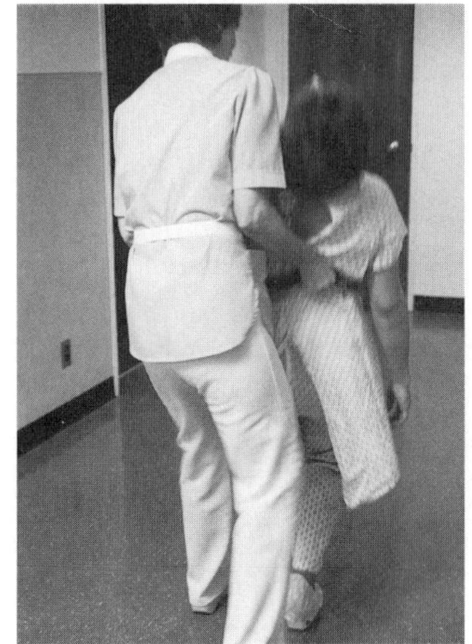

Figure 34–39 Lowering a client who feels faint to the floor.

PROCEDURE 34–9 ASSISTING A CLIENT TO WALK *continued*

a. Assume a broad stance with one foot in front of the other. *A broad stance widens the nurse's base of support for stability. Placing one foot behind the other allows the nurse to rock backward and use the femoral muscles when supporting the client's weight and lowering the center of gravity (see the next step), thus preventing back strain.*

b. Bring the client backward so that your body supports the person. *Clients who do faint or start to fall and cannot regain their strength or balance usually drop straight downward or pitch slightly forward because of the momentum of ambulating; thus, their head, hips, and knees are most vulnerable to injury. Bringing the client's weight backward against the nurse's body allows gradual movement to the floor without injury to the client.*

c. Allow the client to slide down your leg, and lower the person gently to the floor, making sure the client's head does not hit any objects.

Two Nurses

4. Prepare the client.

- See step 1 above.

5. Ensure client safety.

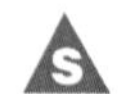

- After the client stands, assume a position with one nurse at either side. Grasp the inferior aspect of the client's upper arm with your nearest hand and the client's lower arm or hand with your other hand (Figure 34–40). *This provides a secure grip for each nurse.*

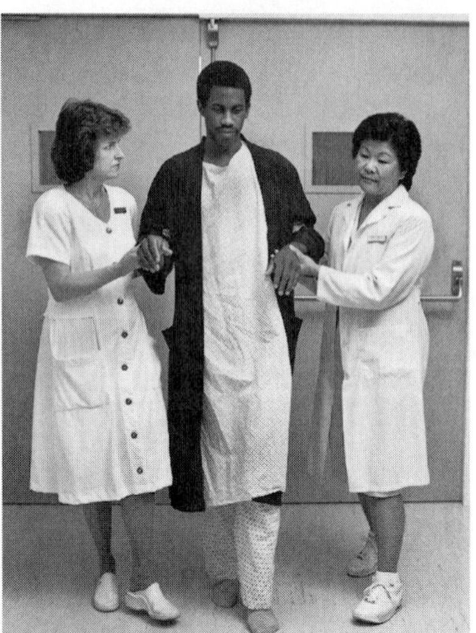

Figure 34–40 Two nurses supporting an ambulatory client.

- *Optional:* Place a walking belt around the client's waist. Each nurse grasps the side handle with the near hand and the lower aspect of the client's upper arm with the other hand.
- Walk in unison with the client, using a smooth, even gait, at the same speed and with steps the same size as the client's. *This gives the client a greater feeling of security.*
- If the client starts to fall and cannot regain strength or balance, slip your arms under the client's axillae, grasp the client's hands, and lower the person gently to the floor or to a nearby chair (Figure 34–41). *Placing the nurses' arms under the client's axillae evenly balances the client's weight between the two nurses, preventing injury to both the nurses and the client.*

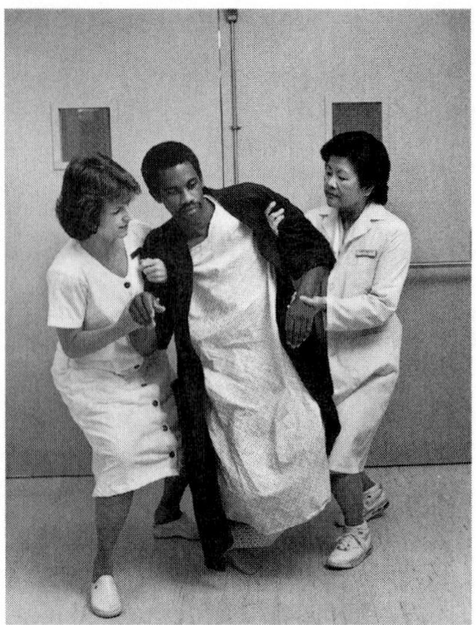

Figure 34–41 Two nurses lowering a fainting client to the floor.

6. Document all relevant information.

- Document the time of the walk, the distance walked or time taken, and all nursing assessments.

EVALUATION FOCUS

The client's gait (including body alignment) when walking; the client's pace; activity tolerance when walking (eg, pulse rate, facial color, any shortness of breath, feelings of dizziness, or weakness); distance walked and degree of support required; pulse rate, respiratory rate, and blood pressure after an initial ambulation to compare with baseline data.

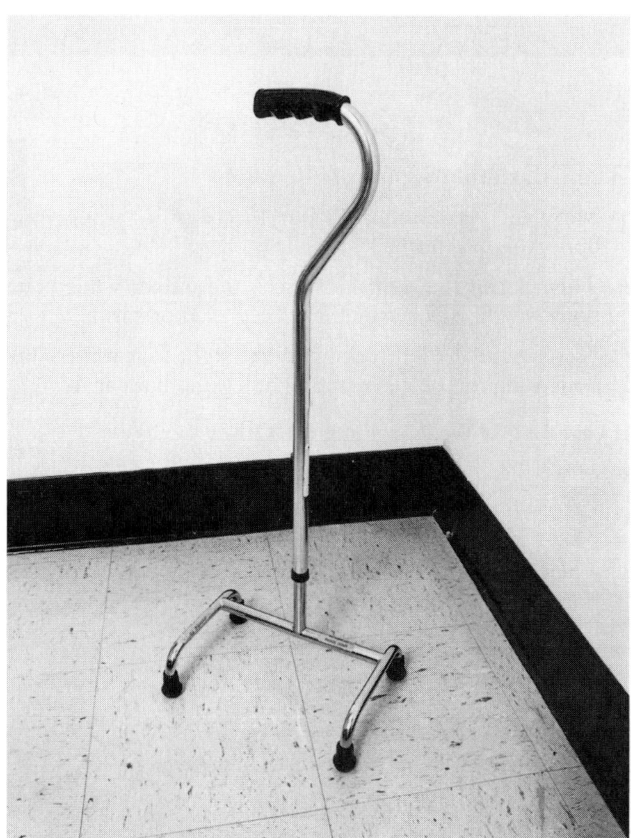

Figure 34–42 A quad cane.

Some clients experience postural, (orthostatic) hypotension on assuming a vertical position from a lying position (see p. 893) and may need to be given information about ways to control this problem (see the box at the right). The client may exhibit some or all of the following symptoms: pallor, diaphoresis, nausea, tachycardia, and dizziness. If any of these are present, the client should be assisted to a supine position in bed and closely assessed.

TEACHING CLIENTS TO USE MECHANICAL AIDS FOR WALKING

Canes Three types of canes are used today; the standard straight-legged cane; the tripod or crab cane, which has three feet; and the quad cane, which has four feet and provides the most support (Figure 34–42). Cane tips should have rubber caps to improve traction and prevent slipping. The standard cane is 91 cm (36 in) long; some aluminum canes can be adjusted from 56 to 97 cm (22 to 38 inches). The length should permit the elbow to be slightly flexed. Clients may use either one or two canes, depending on how much support they require. The box on page 938 provides instructions for clients regarding the use of a cane.

CLIENT TEACHING

Controlling Postural Hypotension

- Sleep with the head of the bed elevated 8 to 12 inches. This position makes the person's position change on rising less severe.
- Avoid sudden changes in position. Arise from bed in three stages:
  a. Sit up in bed for 1 minute.
  b. Sit on the side of the bed with legs dangling for 1 minute.
  c. Stand with care, holding onto the edge of the bed or another nonmovable object for 1 minute. Gradual changes in position stimulate renin (a kidney enzyme that has a role in regulating blood pressure), which prevents a dramatic drop in pressure.
- Never bend down all the way to the floor or stand up too quickly after stooping. Baroreceptors (sensory nerve endings in the walls of blood vessels) cannot accommodate rapid change.
- Postpone activities, such as shaving and hair grooming, for at least 1 hour after rising. Baroreceptor reflexes are slow to respond after a night of recumbency during sleep.
- Wear elastic stockings at night to inhibit venous pooling in the legs.
- Be aware that the symptoms of hypotension are most severe
  a. 30 to 60 minutes after a heavy meal.
  b. 1 to 2 hours after taking an antihypertension medication.
- Get out of a hot bath very slowly, because high temperatures can lead to venous pooling.
- Use a rocking chair to improve circulation in the lower extremities. Even mild leg conditioning can strengthen muscle tone and enhance circulation.
- Refrain from any strenuous activity that results in holding the breath and bearing down. This Valsalva maneuver slows the heart rate, leading to subsequent lowering of blood pressure.

Source: Adapted from L Aaronson, W Carlon-Wolfe, and S Schoener. Pressures that fall on rising: Ways to control postural hypotension, *Geriatric Nursing*, March/April 1991, 12:67.

Walkers Walkers are mechanical devices for ambulatory clients who need more support than a cane provides. There are many types of walkers of different shapes and sizes, with devices suited to individual needs. The standard type is made of polished aluminum. It has four legs with rubber tips and plastic hand grips (Figure 34–43, p. 938). Many walkers have adjustable legs.

CLIENT TEACHING

Using Canes

- Hold the cane with the hand on the stronger side of the body to provide maximum support and appropriate body alignment when walking.
- Position the tip of a standard cane (and the nearest tip of other canes) about 15 cm (6 in) to the side and 15 cm (6 in) in front of the near foot, so that the elbow is slightly flexed.

When Maximum Support Is Required

- Move the cane forward about 30 cm (1 ft), or a distance that is comfortable while the body weight is borne by both legs.
- Then, move the affected (weak) leg forward to the cane while the weight is borne by the cane and stronger leg.
- Next, move the unaffected (stronger) leg forward ahead of the cane and weak leg while the weight is borne by the cane and weak leg.
- Repeat the steps. This pattern of moving provides at least two points of support on the floor at all times.

As You Become Stronger and Require Less Support

- Move the cane and weak leg forward at the same time, while the weight is borne by the stronger leg.
- Move the stronger leg forward, while the weight is borne by the cane and the weak leg.

CLIENT TEACHING

Using Walkers

When Maximum Support Is Required

- Move the walker ahead about 15 cm (6 in) while your body weight is borne by both legs.
- Then, move the right foot up to the walker while your body weight is borne by the left leg and both arms.
- Next, move the left foot up to the right foot while your body weight is borne by the right leg and both arms.

If One Leg Is Weaker Than the Other

- Move the walker and the weak leg ahead together about 15 cm (6 in) while your weight is borne by the stronger leg.
- Then, move the stronger leg ahead while your weight is borne by the affected leg and both arms.

The standard walker needs to be picked up to be used. The client therefore requires partial strength in both hands and wrists; strong elbow extensors, such as the triceps brachii; and strong shoulder depressors, such as the pectoralis minor. The client also needs the ability to bear at least partial weight on both legs.

Four-wheeled and two-wheeled models of walkers (roller walkers) do not need to be picked up to be moved, but they are less stable than the standard walker. They are used by clients who are too weak or unstable to pick up and move the walker with each step. Some roller walkers have a seat at the back so the client can sit down to rest when desired. An adaptation of the standard and four-wheeled walker is one that has two tips and two wheels. This type provides more stability than the four-wheeled model yet still permits the client to keep the walker in contact with the ground all the time. The client tilts the walker toward the body, lifting the tips while the wheels remain on the ground, then pushes the walker forward.

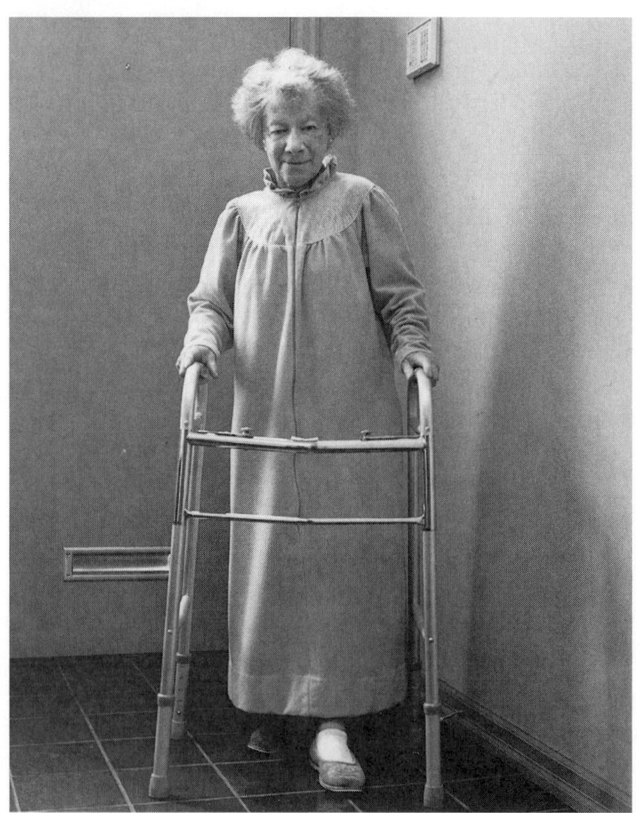

Figure 34–43 A standard walker.

The nurse may need to adjust the height of a client's walker so that the hand bar is just below the client's waist and the client's elbows are slightly flexed. This position helps the client assume a more normal stance. A walker that is too low causes the client to stoop; one that is too high makes the client stretch and reach. Instructions for using walkers are provided in the box above.

Crutches Crutches may be a temporary need for some people and a permanent one for others. Crutches should enable a person to ambulate independently; therefore, it is important to learn to use them properly. Sometimes clients are discouraged when they attempt crutch walking. Clients confined to bed are often unaware of weakness that becomes apparent when they try to stand or walk. Clients realize that they can no longer take balance for granted when they must cope with the weight of a heavy cast or a paralyzed limb. Frequently, progress may be slower than the client anticipated. Encouragement from the nurse and the setting of realistic goals are especially important.

There are several kinds of crutches. The most frequently used are the underarm crutch, or *axillary crutch* with hand bars, and the *Lofstrand crutch*, which extends only to the forearm. The underarm crutch can be extended. It has double uprights, an underarm bar, and a hand bar (Figure 34–44, *A*). The Lofstrand crutch is a single adjustable tube of aluminum to which are attached a curved piece of steel, a rubber-covered hand bar, and a metal forearm cuff (Figure 34–44, *B*). This type of crutch is most useful as a substitute for a cane. The metal cuff around the forearm and the metal bar stabilize the wrists and thus make walking safer and easier. The person can release the hand bar to use his or her hand, and the metal cuff will hold the crutch in place, while a cane would fall.

The *Canadian*, or *elbow extensor crutch*, like the Lofstrand, is made of a single tube of aluminum with lateral attachments, a hand bar, and a cuff for the forearm, but it also has a cuff for the upper arm (Figure 34–44, *C*). This crutch is usually used by clients who require support for weak extensor muscles of the arm (eg, weak triceps brachii).

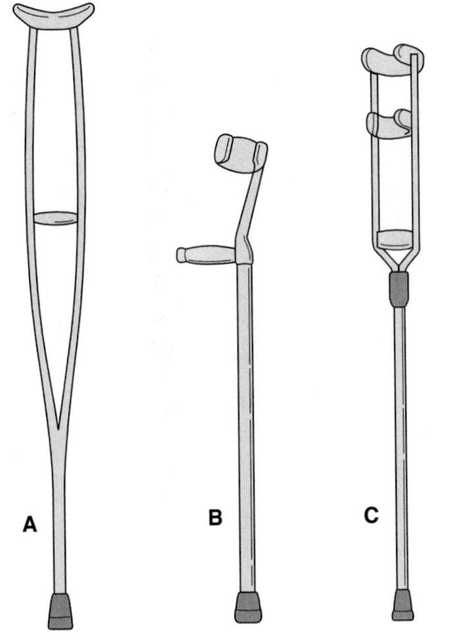

Figure 34–44 Three types of crutches: *A*, axillary crutch; *B*, Lofstrand crutch; *C*, Canadian, or elbow extensor, crutch.

CLIENT TEACHING

Using Crutches

- Follow the plan of exercises developed for you to strengthen your arm muscles before beginning crutch walking.
- Have a health care professional establish the correct length for your crutches and the correct placement of the handpieces. Crutches that are too long force your shoulders upward and make it difficult for you to push your body off the ground. Crutches that are too short will make you hunch over and develop an improper body stance.
- The weight of your body should be borne by the arms rather than the axillae (armpits). Continual pressure on the axillae can injure the radial nerve and eventually cause *crutch palsy*, a weakness of the muscles of the forearm, wrist, and hand.
- Maintain an erect posture as much as possible to prevent strain on muscles and joints and to maintain balance.
- Each step taken with crutches should be a comfortable distance for you. It is wise to start with a small rather than large step.
- Inspect the crutch tips regularly, and replace them if worn.
- Keep the crutch tips dry and clean to maintain their surface friction. If the tips become wet, dry them well before use.
- Wear a tie shoe with a low heel that grips the floor.

All crutches require suction tips, usually made of rubber, which help to prevent the crutches from slipping on a floor surface. Suggested client instructions for using crutches are provided in the box above.

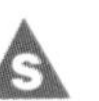

Exercises for Crutch Walking In crutch walking, the client's weight is borne by the muscles of the shoulder girdle and the upper extremities. Before beginning crutch walking, the following exercises are recommended:

- Flexing and extending the arms in several directions.
- Moving from a supine position to a sitting position by flexing the elbows and pushing the hands against the bed surface (Figure 34–45). This exercise strengthens the flexor and extensor muscles of the arms and the muscles that dorsiflex the wrists.

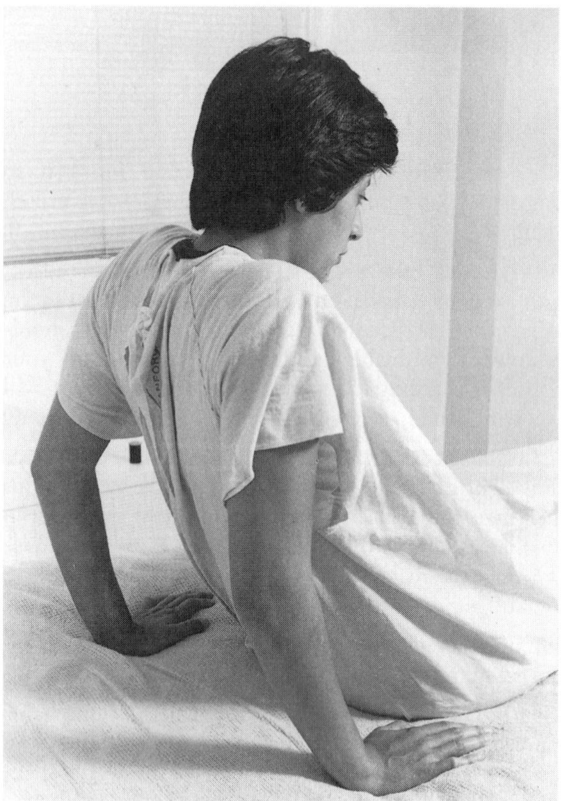

Figure 34–45 Strengthening the flexor and extensor muscles of the arms and the muscles that dorsiflex the wrist.

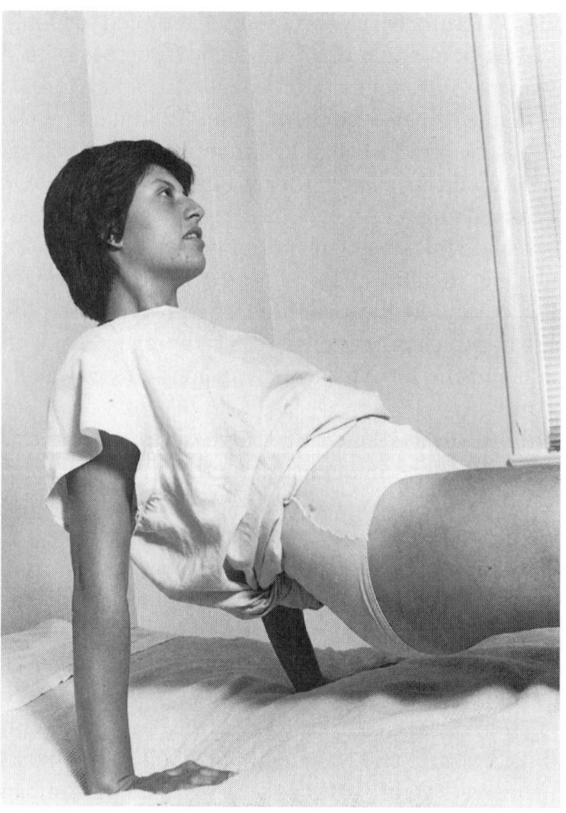

Figure 34–46 Strengthening the extensor muscles of the arms in preparation for crutch walking.

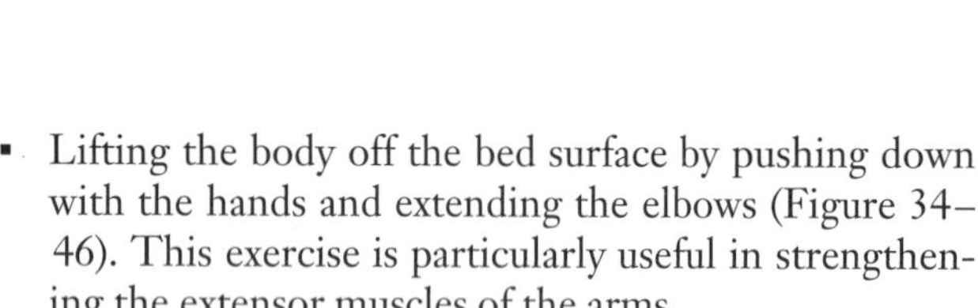

- Lifting the body off the bed surface by pushing down with the hands and extending the elbows (Figure 34–46). This exercise is particularly useful in strengthening the extensor muscles of the arms.
- Tensing the quadriceps femoris muscles (Figure 34–37, p. 934).
- Straight leg exercises. The client lies supine with one knee bent and the other leg straight. The client tightens the quadriceps muscle in the straight leg and slowly raises it until it is parallel with the flexed leg. Hold the leg in this position for the count of 5, then slowly lower the leg. Repeat with the opposite leg and do this 5 times (Lane & Le Blanc 1990, p. 33).
- Squeezing a rubber ball or a gripper with the hands. This exercise strengthens the flexor muscles of the fingers.

Measuring Clients for Crutches When nurses measure clients for axillary crutches, it is most important to obtain the correct length for the crutches and the correct placement of the hand piece. There are two methods of measuring crutch length:

1. The client lies in a supine position, and the nurse measures from the anterior fold of the axilla to the heel of the foot and adds 2.5 cm (1 in) (Figure 34–47).
2. The client stands erect and positions the crutch as shown in Figure 34–48. The nurse makes sure the shoulder rest of the crutch is at least 3 finger widths, that is, 2.5 to 5 cm (1 to 2 in), below the axilla.

To determine the correct placement of the hand bar:

1. The client stands upright and supports the body weight by the hand grips of the crutches.

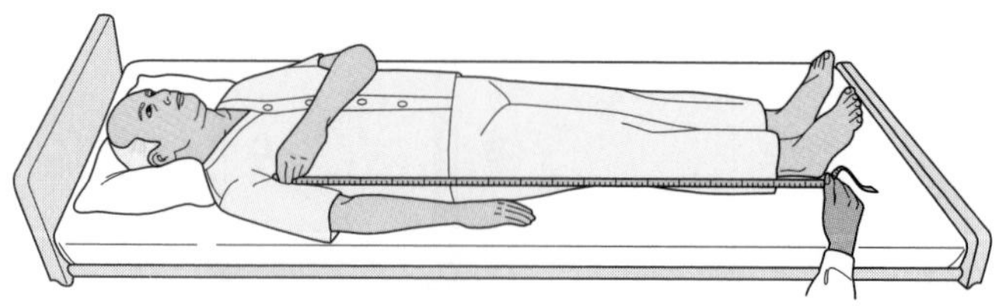

Figure 34–47 Measuring for crutch length while the client is in the supine position.

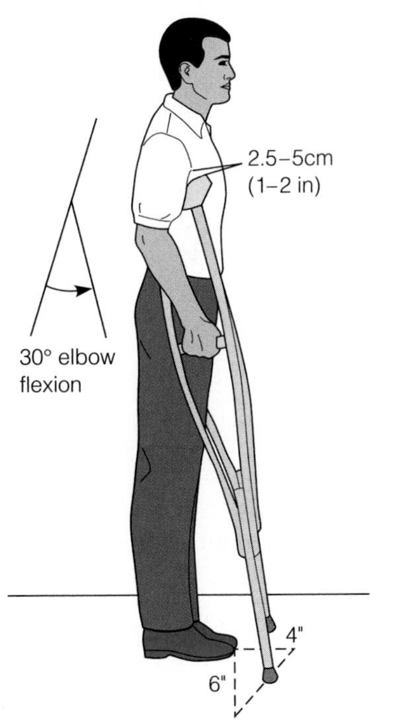

Figure 34–48 The standing position for measuring the correct length for crutches.

2. The nurse measures the angle of elbow flexion. It should be about 30 degrees. A goniometer (Figure 22–70, p. 540) may be used to verify the correct angle.

Crutch Gaits The crutch gait is the gait a person assumes on crutches by alternating body weight on one or both legs and the crutches. Five standard crutch gaits are the four-point gait, three-point gait, two-point gait, swing-to gait, and swing-through gait. The gait used depends on the following individual factors: (a) the ability to take steps, (b) the ability to bear weight and keep balance in a standing position on both legs or only one, and (c) the ability to hold the body erect.

A physiotherapist or a physician usually decides which crutch gait is best for a particular client. Nurses are increasingly involved in these decisions, however. Often, a physiotherapist teaches the crutch gait initially, but nurses give follow-through lessons. In some instances, nurses alone teach the client the technique.

Clients also need instruction about how to get into and out of chairs and go up and down stairs safely. All of these crutch skills are best taught before the client is discharged and preferably before the client has surgery.

Crutch Stance (Tripod Position) Before crutch walking is attempted, the client needs to learn facts about posture and balance. The proper standing position with crutches is called the **tripod (triangle) position** (Figure 34–49).

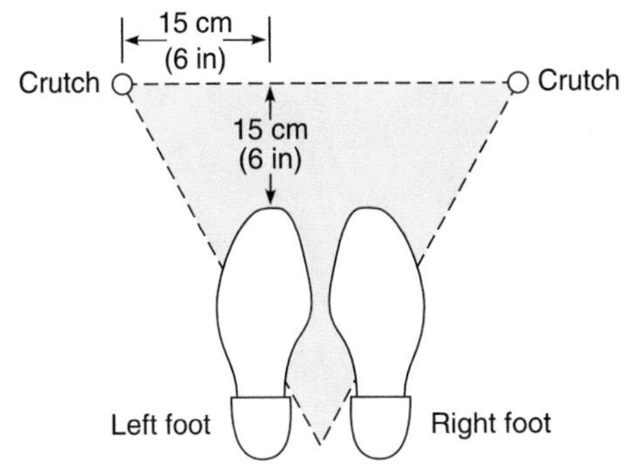

Figure 34–49 The tripod position.

The crutches are placed about 15 cm (6 in) in front of the feet and out laterally about 15 cm (6 in), creating a wide base of support. The feet are slightly apart. A tall person requires a wider base than a short person. Hips and knees are extended, the back is straight, and the head is held straight and high. There should be no hunch to the shoulders and thus no weight borne by the axillae. The elbows are extended sufficiently to allow weight bearing on the hands. If the client is unsteady, the nurse places a walking belt around the client's waist and grasps the belt from above, not from below. A fall can be prevented more effectively if the belt is held from above.

Sometimes clients are discouraged when they attempt crutch walking. Clients confined to bed are often unaware of weakness that becomes apparent when they try to stand or walk. Clients realize that they can no longer take balance for granted when they must cope with the weight of a heavy cast or a paralyzed limb. Frequently, progress may be slower than the client anticipated. Encouragement from the nurse and the setting of realistic goals are especially important.

Four-Point Alternate Gait This is the most elementary and safest gait, providing at least three points of support at each time, but it requires coordination. Clients can use it when walking in crowds because it does not require much space. To use this gait, the client needs to be able to bear weight on both legs (Figure 34–50, p. 942, reading from bottom to top). The nurse asks the client to

1. Move the right crutch ahead a suitable distance, such as 10 to 15 cm (4 to 6 in).
2. Move the left front foot forward, preferably to the level of the left crutch.
3. Move the left crutch forward.
4. Move the right foot forward.

Three-Point Gait To use this gait, the client must be able to bear entire body weight on the unaffected leg. The two crutches and the unaffected leg bear weight alternately

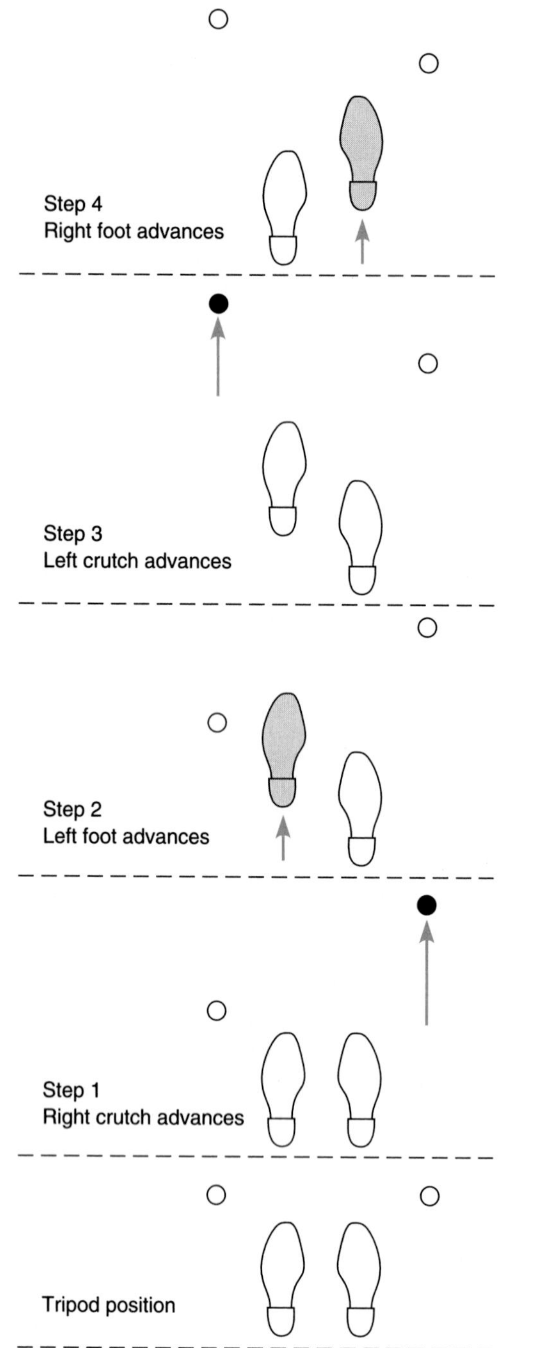

Figure 34–50 The four-point alternate crutch gait.

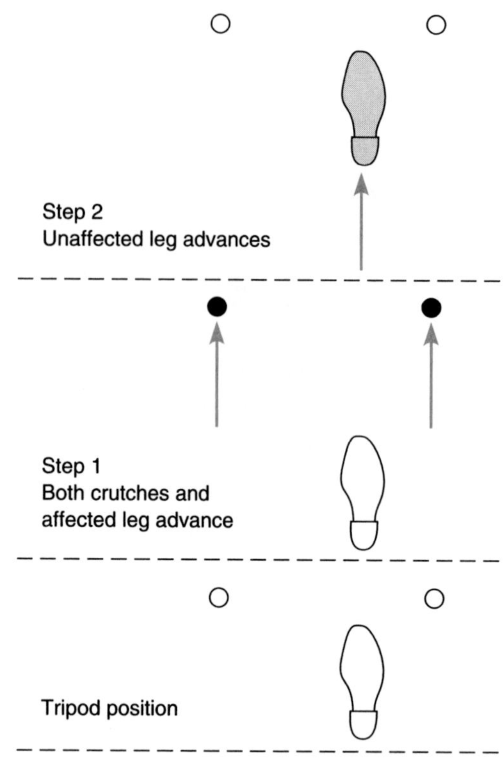

Figure 34–51 The three-point crutch gait.

(Figure 34–51, reading from bottom to top). The nurse asks the client to

1. Move both crutches and the weaker leg forward.
2. Move the stronger leg forward.

Two-Point Alternate Gait This gait is faster than the four-point gait. It requires more balance, because only two points support the body at one time; it also requires at least partial weight bearing on each foot. In this gait, arm movements with the crutches are similar to the arm movements during normal walking (Figure 34–52, reading from bottom to top). The nurse asks the client to

1. Move the left crutch and the right foot forward together.
2. Move the right crutch and the left foot ahead together.

Swing-To Gait The swing gaits are used by clients with paralysis of the legs and hips. Prolonged use of these gaits results in atrophy of the unused muscles. The swing-to gait is the easier of these two gaits (Figure 34–53). The nurse asks the client to

1. Move both crutches ahead together.
2. Lift body weight by the arms and swing *to* the crutches.

Swing-Through Gait This gait requires considerable skill, strength, and coordination (Figure 34–54). The nurse asks the client to

1. Move both crutches forward together.
2. Lift body weight by the arms and swing *through and beyond* the crutch.

Getting into a Chair Chairs that have armrests and are secure or braced against a wall are essential for clients using crutches. For this procedure the nurse instructs the client to

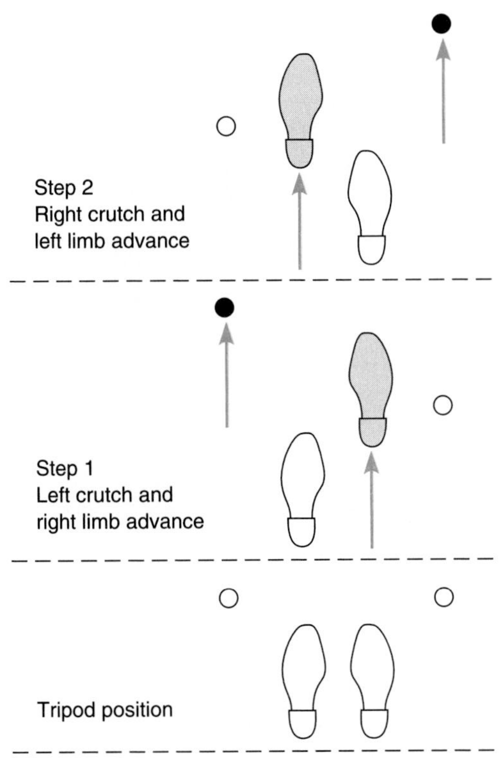

Figure 34–52 The two-point alternate crutch gait.

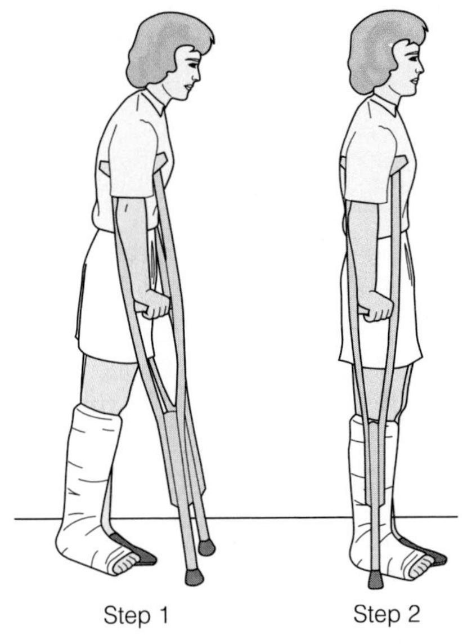

Figure 34–53 The swing-to crutch gait.

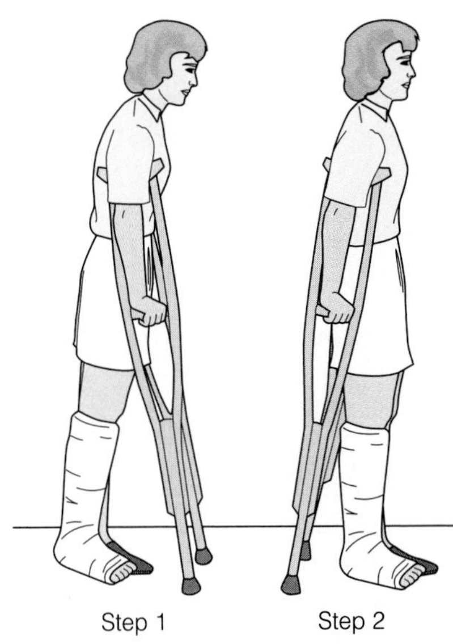

Figure 34–54 The swing-through crutch gait.

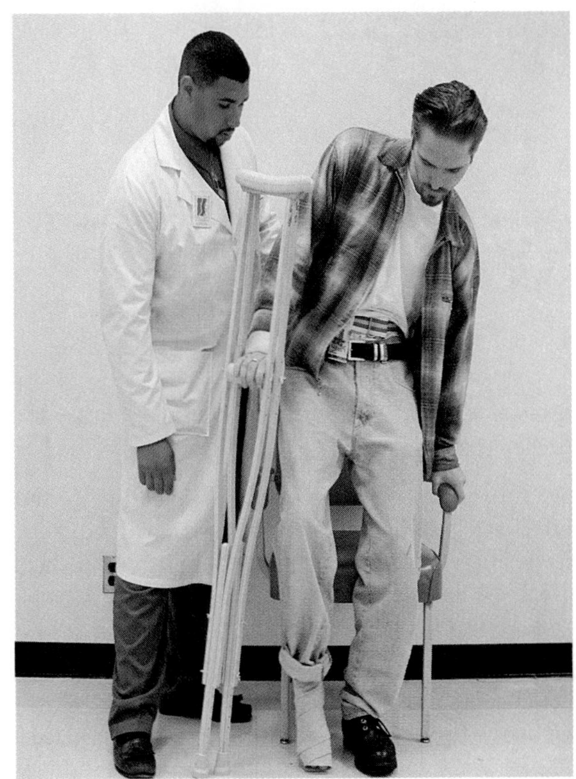

Figure 34–55 A client using crutches getting into a chair.

1. Stand with the back of the unaffected leg centered against the chair. The chair helps support the client during the next steps.
2. Transfer the crutches to the hand on the affected side and hold the crutches by the hand bars. The client grasps the arm of the chair with the hand on the unaffected side (Figure 34–55). This allows the client to support the body weight on the arms and the unaffected leg.
3. Lean forward, flex the knees and hips, and lower into the chair.

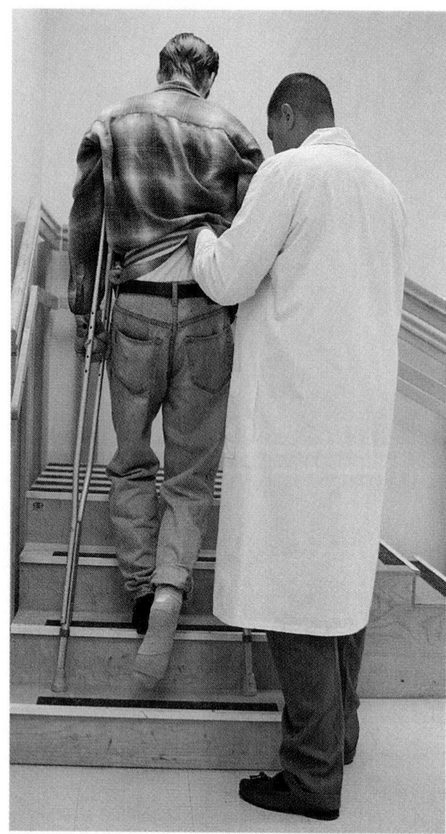

Figure 34–56 Climbing stairs: placing weight on the crutches while first moving the unaffected leg onto a step.

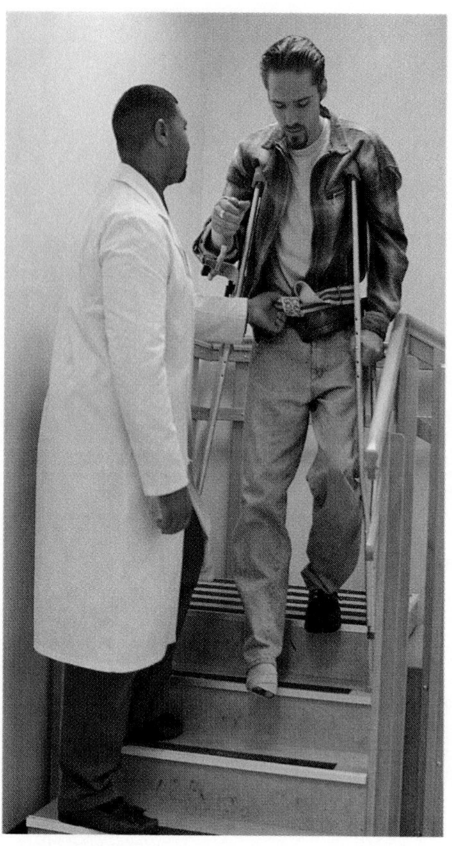

Figure 34–57 Descending stairs: moving the crutches and affected leg to the next step.

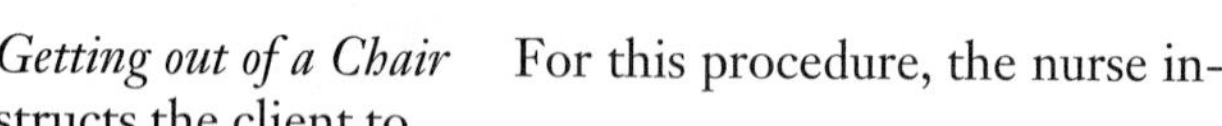

Getting out of a Chair For this procedure, the nurse instructs the client to

1. Move forward to the edge of the chair and place the unaffected leg slightly under or at the edge of the chair. This position helps the client stand up from the chair and achieve balance, since the unaffected leg is supported against the edge of the chair.
2. Grasp the crutches by the hand bars in the hand on the affected side, and grasp the arm of the chair by the hand on the unaffected side. The body weight is placed on the crutches and the hand on the armrest to support the unaffected leg when the client rises to stand.
3. Push down on the crutches and the chair armrest while elevating the body out of the chair.
4. Assume the tripod position before moving.

Going up Stairs For this procedure, the nurse stands behind the client and slightly to the affected side if needed. The nurse instructs the client to

1. Assume the tripod position at the bottom of the stairs.
2. Transfer the body weight to the crutches and move the unaffected leg onto the step (Figure 34–56).
3. Transfer the body weight to the unaffected leg on the step and move the crutches and affected leg up to the step. The affected leg is always supported by the crutches.
4. Repeat steps 2 and 3 until the client reaches the top of the stairs.

Going down Stairs For this procedure, the nurse stands one step below the client on the affected side if needed. The nurse instructs the client to

1. Assume the tripod position at the top of the stairs.
2. Shift the body weight to the unaffected leg, and move the crutches and affected leg down onto the next step (Figure 34–57).
3. Transfer the body weight to the crutches, and move the unaffected leg to that step. The affected leg is always supported by the crutches.
4. Repeat steps 2 and 3 until the client reaches the bottom of the stairs.

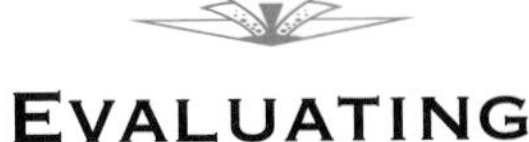

Evaluating

To evaluate whether client goals have been achieved, the nurse collects data relevant to the outcome criteria previously established. For instance, the nurse may ask the client to report adherence to a planned exercise program, demonstrate specific exercises, measure muscle size, observe the client's activity tolerance when performing self-care activities, measure vital signs before and after exercise and ambulation, auscultate the lungs for absence of adventitious breath sounds, palpate extremities for temperature and edema, ask the client about any discomfort, observe times of fecal elimination, and check fluid balance and laboratory records.

The nurse can most easily observe and evaluate body alignment by doing the following:

1. Standing directly in front of the person to evaluate the frontal plane of standing and sitting positions or by standing at the foot of the bed to evaluate the bed positions
2. Standing at the side of the person, chair, or bed to inspect the lateral view
3. Asking how comfortable the client feels in that position

The quality of the client's ambulation is evaluated according to how well the client achieves stability in gait without falling and whether preset goals have been achieved. For example, the nurse determines whether "the client walked independently with the aid of a walker from the bed to the nursing station three times a day" or whether "the client stood erect when walking" or whether "the client demonstrated correct use of a four-point crutch gait."

The quality of a client's body mechanics in daily activities can be evaluated only by observing how well the person conforms to the principles of body mechanics and prevents back injury.

If the client outcomes are not achieved, the nurse should ask the following questions to determine why:

- Has the client's physical or mental condition changed?
- Were contributing or risk factors identified correctly?
- Were appropriate range-of-motion exercises implemented?
- Was the client encouraged to participate in self-care activities as much as possible?
- Was the positioning schedule adhered to?
- Did the client fail to perform deep-breathing exercises as instructed.
- Was the client's nutritional and fluid intake adequate to maintain desired weight, tissue turgor, fluid balance, and normal serum protein values?
- Were all measures to stimulate blood circulation implemented?
- Were appropriate measures implemented to prevent constipation?
- Was the client encouraged to make as many decisions as possible, develop a daily activity plan, and verbalize concerns to maintain emotional and social well-being?
- Were appropriate assistive devices selected for the client to move and ambulate safely?
- Did the nurse provide appropriate supervision and monitoring?
- Was the client informed of necessary safety precautions for ambulation?
- Were needs for home care assistance and available community resources correctly identified or selected?
- Were family or support persons included to assist the client with ADLs?

Critical Pathway for Kevin Andrews

Assessment Data

Nursing Assessment

Kevin Andrews, a 17-year-old high school student gymnast, fell from the parallel bars and fractured his left fibula and tibia. He was admitted via the emergency room after having undergone an emergency open reduction and internal fixation of the fractures and cast application. He is ordered on bedrest for 36 hours. Because of painful muscle spasms and fear, he often refuses to turn or move voluntarily. He often refuses his hospital meals and thus has a poor appetite. He needs encouragement to cough and deep breathe.

Physical Examination

Height: 175.3 cm (5′9″)
Weight: 70 kg (155 lb) on admission
Temperature: 37 C (98.6 F)
Pulse rate: 80 bpm
Respirations: 16 per minute
Blood pressure: 114/70 mm Hg

Diagnostic Data

Chest X-ray film: negative
Urine: negative
Hgb: 12.2 g/dL
Hct: 37%

Critical Pathway for Client Following Open Reduction and Internal Fixation of Lower Leg Fracture

Expected length of stay 3–4 days following surgery

	Date ________ **Operative day**	**Date ________** **1st Postoperative day**
Daily outcomes	Client will ▪ be afebrile. ▪ recover from anesthesia as evidenced by: VS return to baseline, be awake, alert, & oriented, with clear lungs. ▪ verbalize understanding and demonstrate cooperation with turning, coughing, deep breathing, and prescribed activity level. ▪ state pain controlled with ordered medication. ▪ tolerate ordered diet without nausea and vomiting. ▪ verbalize ability to cope.	Client will ▪ be afebrile. ▪ have stable vital signs with clear lungs, and be alert & oriented. ▪ verbalize understanding and demonstrate cooperation with turning, coughing, deep breathing, and prescribed activity level. ▪ state pain controlled with ordered medication. ▪ tolerate ordered diet without nausea and vomiting. ▪ verbalize ability to cope.
Tests and treatments	Hct/Hgb. Vital signs and O_2 saturation, neurovascular assessment and cast assessment q15min × 4; q30min × 4; q1h × 4; and then q4h if stable. Head to toe assessment* q4–8h. Incentive spirometer q2h. Intake and output q shift.	Vital signs and O_2 saturation, neurovascular assessment and cast assessment q4h if stable. Head to toe assessment* q shift and prn. Incentive spirometer q2h. Intake and output q shift.
Knowledge deficit	Orient to room and surroundings. Provide simple, brief instructions. Review plan of care and importance of specific postoperative care: turning, coughing, deep breathing, incentive spirometer, mobilization, possible tubes and intravenous), pain management (IV/PCA or IM prn medications).	Review plan of care and importance of early mobilization. Begin discharge teaching regarding cast care and mobility.
Psycho-social	Assess anxiety related to diagnosis and surgery. Assess fears of the unknown and surgery. Encourage verbalization of concerns. Provide information regarding surgical experience. Minimize external stimuli (eg, noise, movement).	Assess level of anxiety. Encourage verbalization of concerns. Provide information. Provide ongoing support and encouragement.
Diet	Advance from clear liquids to full liquids to tolerance. Baseline nutritional assessment.	Advance from full liquids to regular diet as tolerated. Offer supplemental feedings high in protein and vitamins.

* Head to toe assessment: This assessment should address major body systems affected by immobility including musculoskeletal, cardiovascular, respiratory, metabolic and nutritional, urine and endocrine, fecal elimination, integumentary, and neurosensory.

	Operative day *continued*	**1st Postoperative day** *continued*
Activity	Provide safety precautions. Reposition q2h and prn. Assist client with full range of motion to all unaffected extremities 3 or 4 × daily. Teach the client isometric exercises for lower limb. Encourage client to participate in activities of daily living as much as possible. Provide overhead trapeze and encourage use q3h.	Provide safety precautions. Reposition q2h and prn. Assist client with full range of motion to all unaffected extremities 3 or 4 × daily. Encourage client to perform isometric exercises for lower limb. Encourage client to participate in activities of daily living as much as possible. Encourage use of overhead trapeze q3h.
Medications	IV/PCA or IM analgesic IV antibiotics IV fluids	IV/PCA or IM analgesic IV antibiotics IV fluids or intermittent IV device
Transfer/ discharge plans	Assess discharge plans and support system.	Determine needs at time of discharge. Begin home care teaching.

	Date ________ **2d Postoperative day**	**Date ________** **3d–4th Postoperative day**
Daily outcomes	Client will ▪ be afebrile and have clear lungs. ▪ demonstrate cooperation with turning, coughing, deep breathing, and prescribed activity level. ▪ state pain controlled with ordered medication. ▪ tolerate ordered diet without nausea and vomiting. ▪ ambulate with crutches 2–3 × daily. ▪ verbalize beginning understanding of home care instructions.	Client ▪ is afebrile, has stable vital signs and clear lungs. ▪ has intact neurovascular status to affected extremity. ▪ manages pain with oral medications. ▪ is independent in self-care. ▪ is independent in transfers and ambulatory with crutches. ▪ has resumed preadmission urine and bowel elimination pattern. ▪ verbalizes home care instructions. ▪ tolerates usual diet ▪ verbalizes ability to cope with ongoing stressors.
Tests and treatments	Vital signs q4h. Head to toe assessment* q shift and prn. Incentive spirometer q2h until fully ambulatory. Intake and output q shift.	Vital signs assessment q4h. Neurovascular assessment q4h and prn. Head to toe assessment* q shift. Incentive spirometer q2h until fully ambulatory. D/C intake and output if taking adequate fluids and balanced with output.

* Head to toe assessment: This assessment should address major body systems affected by immobility including musculoskeletal, cardiovascular, respiratory, metabolic and nutritional, urine and endocrine, fecal elimination, integumentary, and neurosensory.

	2d Postoperative day *continued*	**3d–4th Postoperative day** *continued*
Knowledge deficit	Initiate discharge teaching regarding diet, signs and symptoms to report, and activity level. Begin instructions regarding crutch walking. Review written discharge instructions.	Provide client with written discharge instructions that discuss: (1) weight bearing on affected extremity, (2) signs and symptoms of infection related to internal fixation device, (3) importance of regular follow-up care, (4) care of cast, (5) monitoring neurovascular status, and (6) use of assistive devices. Complete discharge teaching to include diet, follow-up care, signs and symptoms to report, activity, and medications: dose, frequency, route, and side effects.
Psycho-social	Encourage verbalization of concerns. Provide ongoing support and encouragement.	Encourage verbalization of concerns. Provide ongoing support and encouragement.
Diet	Regular diet to tolerance. Encourage fluid intake of 2000 mL per day when IV fluids D/C. Offer supplemental feedings high in protein and vitamins.	Regular diet as tolerated. Encourage fluids to 2000 mL/24 hours. Offer supplemental feedings high in protein and vitamins.
Activity	Provide safety precautions. Assist client with full range of motion to all unaffected extremities 3 or 4 × daily. Encourage the client to perform isometric exercises for lower limb. Encourage the client to participate in activities of daily living as much as possible. Encourage use of overhead trapeze q3h. Refer to physical therapy to begin non–weight bearing crutch walking. Assist out of bed 2–3 × daily to tolerance.	Provide safety precautions. Assist client with full range of motion to all unaffected extremities 3 or 4 × daily. Encourage the client to perform isometric exercises for lower limb. Encourage client to participate in activities of daily living as much as possible. Encourage client to use overhead trapeze q3h. Continue to work with physical therapy to promote non–weight bearing crutch walking 4 × daily and begin stair training.
Medications	IV/PCA, IM or PO analgesics IV antibiotics Intermittent IV device	PO analgesic D/C intermittent IV device
Transfer/ discharge plans	Complete discharge plans. Continue home care instructions.	Complete discharge instructions.

CHAPTER HIGHLIGHTS

- The nurse acts as a role model and teacher of good body alignment and mechanics.
- Good body mechanics is the efficient, coordinated, and safe use of the body to produce motion and maintain balance during activity.
- Maintaining good body alignment and using good body mechanics are essential for good body function and for preventing discomfort, fatigue, and injury to body structures.
- Falls and back injuries are the most common and serious consequences of improper body mechanics.
- Body mechanics involves three basic elements: body alignment, balance, and coordinated body movement.
- Numerous postural reflexes stimulate and maintain postural tonus: labyrinthine sense, tonic neck-righting reflexes, visual reflexes, proprioceptor or kinesthetic sense, extensor or antigravity (stretch) reflexes, and plantar reflexes.
- A person maintains balance as long as the line of gravity passes through the center of gravity and the base of support.
- The broader the base of support and the lower the center of gravity, the greater the stability and balance achieved.
- When lifting, pushing, or pulling clients or objects, the nurse needs to consider the concepts of leverage, force, friction, and inertia.
- To prevent spinal twisting, the nurse faces the direction of movement and moves objects directly toward or away from the nurse's center of gravity.
- Squatting, in contrast to stooping or partially flexing the hips and knees, is essential when moving objects.
- Factors influencing body alignment and mobility include growth and development, physical and mental health, life-style, and fatigue and stress.
- Immobility affects almost every body organ and system adversely; complications also include psychosocial problems. Exercise, by contrast, provides many benefits to the same body organs and systems.
- Exercise is classified as either isotonic, isometric, or isokinetic and as either aerobic or anaerobic.
- The nurse has responsibilities (a) to prevent the complications of immobility and reduce the severity of any problems resulting from immobility and (b) to design exercise programs for clients that promote wellness.
- Assessment relative to a client's activity/exercise includes a nursing history and physical examination of body alignment, (stance and sitting alignment) gait, joint appearance and movement, capabilities and limitations for movement, muscle mass and strength, activity tolerance, and problems related to immobility.
- An activity/exercise history includes daily activity level, activity tolerance, type and frequency of exercise, and factors affecting mobility.
- NANDA nursing diagnoses that relate to activity/mobility problems include: **Activity intolerance, High risk for activity intolerance, Impaired physical mobility,** and **High risk for disuse syndrome.** Other relevant diagnoses are **Self-care deficit, High risk for injury, Impaired home maintenance management, Altered health maintenance,** and **Fear** (of falling).
- The major outcomes for clients with potential or actual problems related to mobility or activity are to avoid any complications associated with immobility, to restore or improve ambulatory or activity capability, and to avoid injury from falling or improper use of body mechanics.
- The nurse who practices good postural habits can be a significant role model and motivator. Clients for whom prolonged standing is unavoidable need to learn ways to prevent undue strain on the lumbar spine and reduce lordosis. Clients who have musculoskeletal impairments of the arm and shoulder need appropriate arm supports when sitting to protect the shoulder muscles.
- Positioning a client in good body alignment and changing the position regularly and systematically are essential aspects of nursing practice.
- Before positioning dependent clients, the nurse should plan a systematic 24-hour schedule for

position changes, including positions that provide for full extension of the neck, hips, and knees. The nurse also uses appropriate supportive devices to maintain alignment and prevent strain on the client's muscles and joints.

- Before moving, turning, or transferring a client, the nurse must consider the client's health status and degree of exertion permitted, physical ability to assist, ability to comprehend instruction, degree of discomfort, client's weight, and the nurse's own strength and ability.
- Assistance from others or the use of mechanical lifting aids is essential for clients who are too heavy for the nurse to move or lift safely.
- Safety measures must always be employed when the nurse uses a wheelchair or stretcher to move and transfer clients.
- The nurse assists clients with appropriate exercise programs to maintain physical fitness.
- Ambulating techniques that facilitate normal walking gait yet provide needed support are most effective.
- The nurse can assist clients to prepare for ambulation by helping them become as independent as possible while in bed.
- Preambulatory exercises that strengthen the muscles for walking are essential for clients who have been immobilized for prolonged periods.
- Clients need specific instructions about appropriate use of canes, walkers, and crutches.
- Safety precautions and the use of appropriate body mechanics are essential whenever the nurse assists clients to move.

READINGS AND REFERENCES

SUGGESTED READINGS

Moore, SR. July 1991. Walking for health: A nurse-managed activity. *Journal of Gerontological Nursing* 15:26–28.

The author describes a multifaceted walking program for seniors that is managed by nurses and provides health-promotion measures such as blood pressure, blood cholesterol, and blood sugar screenings; educational programs; weight-reduction classes; and health consultation.

Norman, GM and Gibbs, JA. August 1991. Why walk when you can ride? Clinical ambulation incentives for the immobile elderly. *Journal of Gerontological Nursing* 17:28–33.

In long-term care settings, many residents use wheelchairs as their primary mode of mobility. This article discusses steps to follow to develop a successful ambulation incentive program.

RELATED RESEARCH

Bonheur, B and Young, SW. February 1991. Exercise as a health-promoting lifestyle choice. *Applied Nursing Research* 4:2–6.

Owen, BD. January 1991. Reducing the risk for back pain in nursing personnel. *American Association of Occupational Health Nursing Journal* 39:24–33.

SELECTED REFERENCES

Aaronson, L, Carlon-Wolfe, W, and Schiener, S. March/April 1991. Pressures that fall on rising: Ways to control postural hypotension. *Geriatric Nursing* 12:67.

American College of Sports Medicine. 1990. The recommended quantity and quality of exercise for developing and maintaining cardiorespiratory and muscular fitness in healthy adults. *Medicine and Science in Sports and Exercise* 22:265.

Braun, LT. March 1991. Exercise physiology and cardiovascular fitness. *Nursing Clinics of North America* 26:135–47.

Carpenito, LJ. 1992. *Nursing Diagnosis: Application to Clinical Practice*. 4th ed. Philadelphia: Lippincott.

Edlund, G and Golanty, E. 1992. *Health and Wellness: A holistic approach*. 4th ed. Boston: Jones and Bartlett.

Edmunds, MW. December 1991. Strategies for promoting physical fitness. *Nursing Clinics of North America* 26:855–66.

Eustace, C. June 1991. Back up and wait. *RN* 54:49–51.

Farmer, P. July 15–21, 1987. Mechanical aids: Easyslide lifting aid. *Nursing Times* 83:36–37.

Freed, MM, Hofkosh, J, Kaplan, LI, and Neuhauser, C. October 1987a. Choosing ambulatory aids. *Patient Care* 21:20–23, 26–27, 30–32.

———. October 1987b. Using ambulatory aids. *Patient Care* 21:36–40, 42, 45–47.

Gates, S. May 1988. On-the-job back exercises. *American Journal of Nursing* 88:656–59.

Gordon, M. 1993. *Manual of Nursing Diagnosis 1993–1994*. 6th ed. St Louis: Mosby-Year Book.

Guyton, AC. 1991. *Textbook of Medical Physiology*. 8th ed. Philadelphia: Saunders.

Haley, E and Colgate, W. November 1990. Standing up for your back. *Canadian Nurse* 86:26–27.

Harber, P et al. July 1985. Occupational low-back pain in hospital nurses. *Journal of Occupational Medicine* 27:518–24.

———. February 1986. Abstract. Oh, my aching back. *American Journal of Nursing* 86:118.

Heeschen, S. May/June 1989. Getting a handle on patient mobility. *Geriatric Nursing* 10:146–47.

Hill, L and Smith, N. 1990. *Self Care Nursing Promotion of Health*. 2d ed. Norwalk, CT: Appleton & Lange.

Hogstel, M and Kashka, M. January/February 1989. Staying healthy after 85. *Geriatric Nursing* 10:16–18.

Holm, K and Walker, J. May/June 1990. Osteoporosis: Treatment and prevention update. *Geriatric Nursing* 11:140–42.

Kim, MJ, McFarland, GK, and McLane, AM. 1993. *Pocket Guide to Nursing Diagnoses.* 5th ed. St Louis: Mosby-Year Book.

Kisner, C and Colby, L. 1990. *Therapeutic Exercise: Foundations and Techniques.* 2d ed. Philadelphia: FA Davis.

Kottke, F, Stillwell, G, and Lehmann, J, editors. 1990. *Krusen's Handbook of Physical Medicine and Rehabilitation.* 4th ed. Philadelphia: WB Saunders.

Lane, PL and Le Blanc, R. September/October 1990. Crutch walking. *Orthopaedic Nursing* 9:31–38.

Lederer, JR, Marculescu, GL, Mocnik, B, and Seaby, N. 1993. *Care Planning Pocket Guide—A Nursing Diagnosis Approach.* 5th ed. Redwood City, CA: Addison-Wesley Nursing.

Leinweber, E. December 1978. Belts to make moves smoother. *American Journal of Nursing* 78:2080–81.

McConnell, EA. July 1990. Placing your patient in the lateral position. *Nursing90* 20:65.

McFarland, GK and McFarlane, EA. 1993. *Nursing Diagnosis and Intervention: Planning for Patient Care.* 2d ed. St Louis: Mosby.

Madson, S. September 1989. How to reduce the risk of postmenopausal osteoporosis. *Journal of Gerontological Nursing* 15:20–23.

Mather, D and Bennett, B. March 1987. How to move patients the easy way . . . and save your back. *Nursing87* 17:55–57.

Milde, FK. March 1988. Impaired physical mobility. *Journal of Gerontological Nursing* 14:20–24.

Mobily, PR and Kelly, LS. September 1991. Iatrogenesis in the elderly: Factors of immobility. *Journal of Gerontological Nursing* 17:5–11.

Moore, S. July 1989. Walking for health: A nurse-managed activity. *Journal of Gerontological Nursing* 15:26–28.

Neville, K. January/February 1988. Promoting health for seniors. *Geriatric Nursing* 9:42–43.

Norman, GM and Gibbs, JA. August 1991. Why walk when you can ride? Clinical ambulation incentives for the immobile elderly. *Journal of Gerontological Nursing* 17:28–33.

North American Nursing Diagnosis Association. 1992. *NANDA Nursing Diagnoses: Definitions and Classification 1992–1993.* Philadelphia: NANDA.

Olson, EV, Johnson, BJ, and Thompson, LF. March 1990. The hazards of immobility. *American Journal of Nursing* 90:43–44, 46–48.

O'Neill, K and Reid, G. November/December 1991. Perceived barriers to physical activity by older adults. *Canadian Journal of Public Health* 82:392–96.

Owen, BD. May 1980. How to avoid that aching back. *American Journal of Nursing* 80:894–97.

______. November 1985. The lifting process and back injury in hospital nursing personnel. *Western Journal of Nursing Research* 7:445–59.

______. April 1989. The magnitude of low-back problems in nursing. *Western Journal of Nursing Research* 11:234–42.

Owen, BD and Garg, A. January 1991. Reducing risk for back pain in nursing personnel. *American Association of Occupational Health Nursing Journal* 39:24–33.

Perry, G. May/June 1988. Living with osteoporosis. *Geriatric Nursing* 9:174–76.

Robertson, JF. June 1991. Promoting health among the institutionalized elderly. *Journal of Gerontological Nursing* 17:15–19.

Rubin, M. January 1988a. How bedrest changes perception. *American Journal of Nursing* 88:55–56.

______. January 1988b. The physiology of bedrest. *American Journal of Nursing* 88:50–55.

Ryan, S. September/October 1988. Exercise to reduce cardiovascular risk. *Cardiovascular Nursing* 97:1077–82.

Schilke, JM. June 1991. Slowing the aging process with physical activity. *Journal of Gerontological Nursing* 17:4–8, 44–45.

Swinford, PA and Webster, JA. 1989. *Promoting Wellness: A Nurse's Handbook.* Rockville, MD: Aspen Publishers.

Thomas, DF. November 1986. An ambulation assessment system you can count on. *Nursing86* 16:58–59.

Urrows, S, Freston, M, and Pryor, D. December 1991. Profiles in osteoporosis. *American Journal of Nursing* 91:33–37.

Wightwick, S. June 1987. Canadian padded transfer board. *Physiotherapy* 73:309–10.

35 Rest and Sleep

Objectives

Explain the physiologic basis of sleep.

Identify the characteristics of NREM and REM sleep.

Identify the four stages of NREM sleep.

Identify developmental variations in sleep patterns.

Identify interventions that promote sleep at various ages.

Identify factors that affect normal sleep.

Describe common sleep disorders.

Identify the components of a sleep assessment.

Identify defining characteristics and related factors of the nursing diagnosis **Sleep pattern disturbance.**

Identify interventions that promote normal sleep.

Identify outcome criteria for evaluating a client's response to interventions employed to promote sleep.

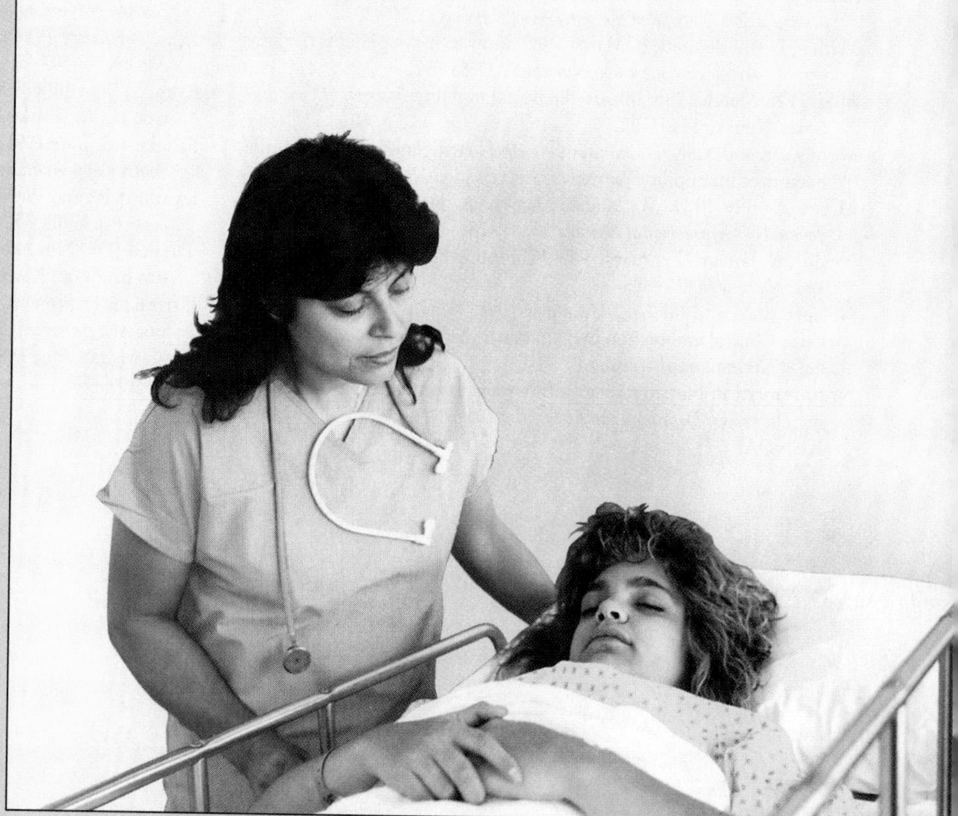

Rest and sleep are essential for health. People who are ill frequently require more rest and sleep than normal. Often, debilitated people expend unusual amounts of energy just to regain health or maintain the activities of daily living. As a result, such people experience increased and frequent fatigue and thus need more rest and sleep than usual. Providing a restful environment for clients is an important function of nurses.

The meaning of rest and the need for rest vary among individuals. **Rest** implies calmness, relaxation without emotional stress, and freedom from anxiety. Therefore, rest does not always imply inactivity; in fact, some people find some activities such as walking in fresh air restful. When rest is prescribed for a client, both nurse and client must know whether the client is to be inactive and whether that inactivity involves the whole body or a body part (eg, an arm).

Rest restores a person's energy, allowing the individual to resume optimal functioning. When people are deprived of rest, they are often irritable, depressed, and tired, and they may have poor control over their emotions.

Sleep is a basic human need (Maslow 1970, p. 92); it is a universal process common to all people. Historically, sleep was considered to be a state of unconsciousness. More recently, **sleep** has come to be considered a state of consciousness in which the individual's perception and reaction to the environment are decreased. Sleep is characterized by minimal physical activity, variable levels of consciousness, changes in the body's physiologic processes, and decreased responsiveness to external stimuli. Some environmental stimuli, such as a smoke detector alarm, will awaken a sleeper, whereas other noises will not. It appears that individuals respond to meaningful stimuli while sleeping and selectively disregard unmeaningful stimuli.

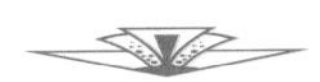

PHYSIOLOGY OF SLEEP

The cyclic nature of sleep is thought to be controlled by centers located in the lower part of the brain. These centers actively inhibit wakefulness thus causing sleep. This active inhibitory process replaces an earlier theory that the brain, including the reticular activating system (RAS), simply fatigued and sleep resulted (Guyton 1991, p. 660).

CIRCADIAN RHYTHMS

Biorhythmology, the study of the biologic rhythms of the body, is receiving increasing attention from biologists and health professionals. **Biorhythms** (rhythmic biologic clocks) exist in plants, animals, and humans. In humans, these are controlled from within the body and synchronized with environmental factors, such as light and darkness, gravity, and electromagnetic stimuli. The most familiar biorhythm is the *circadian rhythm.* The term *circadian* is from the Latin *circa dies*, meaning "about a day."

Sleep is a complex biological rhythm. When a person's biological clock coincides with sleep-wake patterns, the person is said to be in **circadian synchronization;** that is, the person is awake when the physiologic and psychologic rhythms are most active and is asleep when the physiologic and psychologic rhythms are most inactive.

Circadian regularity approaching that of adults begins by the 3d week of life and may be inherited. Babies are awake most often in the early morning and the late afternoon. After 4 months of age, infants enter a 24-hour cycle in which they sleep mostly during the night. By the end of the 5th or 6th month, infants' sleep-wake patterns are almost like those of adults.

PHYSIOLOGIC CHANGES DURING NREM SLEEP

- Arterial blood pressure falls.
- Pulse rate decreases.
- Peripheral blood vessels dilate.
- Activity of the gastrointestinal tract occasionally increases.
- Skeletal muscles relax.
- Basal metabolic rate decreases 10% to 30%.

Source: AC Guyton, *Textbook of Medical Physiology*, 8th ed. (Philadelphia: WB Saunders, 1991), p. 659.

STAGES OF SLEEP

The **electroencephalogram (EEG)** provides a good picture of what occurs during sleep. Electrodes are placed on various parts of the sleeper's scalp. The electrodes transmit electric energy from the cerebral cortex to pens that record the **brain waves** (fluctuations in energy) on graph paper.

Two types of sleep have been identified: **NREM** (non-REM) sleep and **REM** (rapid eye movement) sleep.

NREM Sleep NREM sleep is also referred to as slow-wave sleep, because the brain waves of a sleeper are slower than the alpha and beta waves of a person who is awake or alert. Most sleep during a night is NREM sleep. It is a deep, restful sleep and brings a decrease in some physiologic functions. See the box above.

NREM sleep is divided into four stages. *Stage I* is the stage of very light sleep. During this stage, the person

Table 35–1 Characteristics of NREM Sleep

Stage	Characteristics
Stage 1	Relaxed and drowsy Profound restfulness Usually lasts only a few minutes Floating sensation Eyes roll from side to side
Stage II	Lightly asleep Easily aroused Constitutes 40% to 45% of total sleep time
Stage III	Less easily aroused Medium-depth sleep Muscles totally relaxed Blood pressure lowers Body temperature lowers
Stage IV	Deepest sleep stage Rarely moves Muscles completely relaxed Difficult to arouse Occurs 30 to 40 minutes following sleep onset

CHARACTERISTICS OF REM SLEEP

- Active dreaming occurs, and dreams are remembered.
- The sleeper may be difficult to arouse or may wake spontaneously.
- Muscle tone is depressed.
- Heart rate and respiratory rate often are irregular.
- A few irregular muscle movements occur—in particular, rapid eye movements.
- Brain metabolism increases.
- The lower jaw relaxes.

feels drowsy and relaxed, the eyes roll from side to side, and the heart and respiratory rates drop slightly. The sleeper can be readily awakened and this stage lasts only a few minutes.

Stage II is the stage of light sleep during which body processes continue to slow down. The eyes are generally still, the heart and respiratory rates decrease slightly, and body temperature falls. Stage II lasts only about 10 to 15 minutes.

During *stage III*, the heart and respiratory rates, as well as other body processes, slow further because of the domination of the parasympathetic nervous system. The sleeper becomes more difficult to arouse. The person is not disturbed by sensory stimuli; the skeletal muscles are very relaxed; reflexes are diminished; and snoring may occur.

Stage IV signals deep sleep. The sleeper's heart and respiratory rates drop 20% to 30% below those exhibited during waking hours. The sleeper is very relaxed, rarely moves, and is difficult to arouse. Stage IV is thought to restore the body physically. During this stage, the eyes usually roll, and some dreaming occurs. See Table 35–1 for the characteristics of NREM sleep.

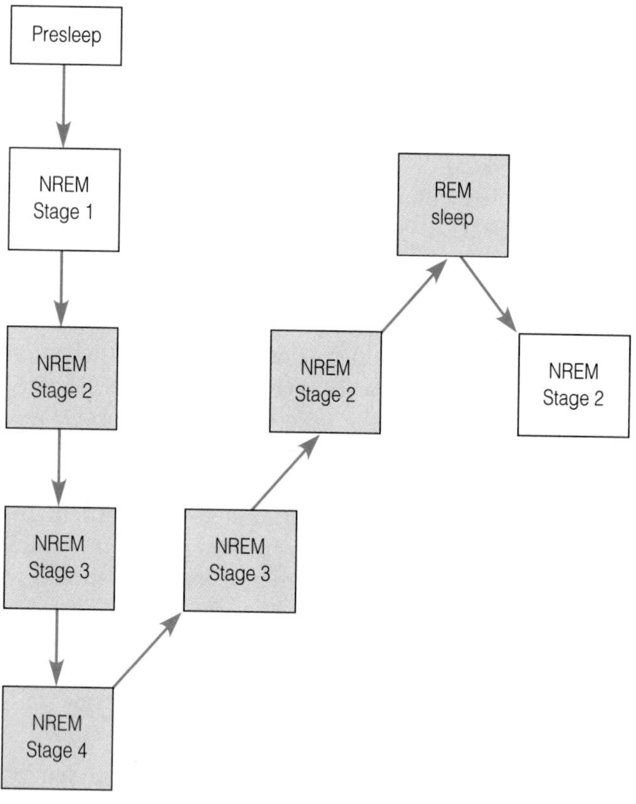

Figure 35–1 The adult sleep cycle. The shaded areas are repeated 4 or 5 times during a night's sleep.

REM Sleep REM sleep constitutes about 25% of the sleep of a young adult. It usually recurs about every 90 minutes and lasts 5 to 30 minutes. REM sleep is not as restful as NREM sleep, and most dreams take place during REM sleep. Furthermore, these dreams are usually remembered; that is, they are consolidated in the memory (Guyton 1991, p. 659).

During REM sleep, the brain is highly active, and brain metabolism may increase as much as 20%. This type of sleep is also called *paradoxical sleep* because it seems a paradox that sleep can take place simultaneously with this type of brain activity. See the box at the top of this page for the characteristics of REM sleep. When a person is very tired, the duration of each REM sleep is very short or even absent. As the person becomes more rested

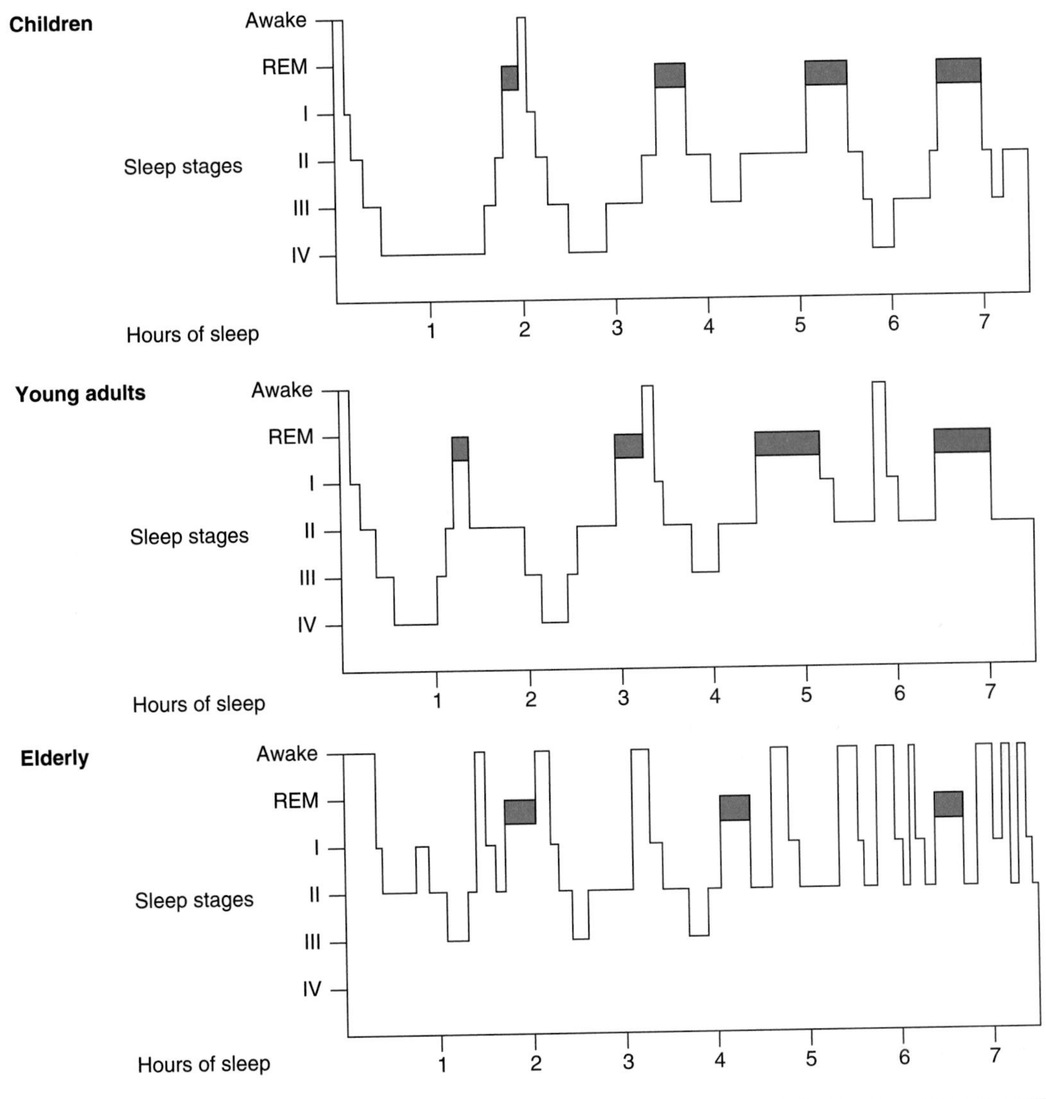

Figure 35–2 Normal sleep cycles of children, young adults, and elderly adults. Children and young adults show early preponderance of NREM stages III and IV, progressive lengthening of the first three REM periods, and infrequent awakenings. In elderly adults, there is little or no NREM stage IV sleep, REM periods are fairly uniform in length, and awakenings are frequent and often lengthy. **Source:** A Kales, Sleep and dreams: Recent research in clinical aspects, *Annals of Internal Medicine,* May 1968, 68:1078. Used with permission.

through the night, the duration of the REM sleep increases (Guyton 1991, p. 660).

SLEEP CYCLES

During a sleep cycle, people pass through the four stages of NREM sleep, usually lasting about 1 hour in adults. A sleeper passes from stage I NREM sleep through stages II and III to stage IV in about 20 to 30 minutes. Stage IV may last about 30 minutes. These stages are then followed by stage III and II, in that order. Thereafter the first REM stage occurs, lasting about 10 minutes. This sequence completes the first sleep cycle (Figure 35–1). The usual sleeper experiences four to six cycles of sleep during 7 to 8 hours. Each cycle lasts about 70 minutes. The sleeper who is awakened during any stage must begin anew at stage I NREM sleep and proceed through all the stages to REM sleep. As the person becomes rested, the cycles become longer.

The duration of NREM stages and REM sleep varies throughout the 8-hour sleep period. As the night progresses, the sleeper becomes less tired and spends less time in stages III and IV of NREM sleep. REM sleep increases, and dreams tend to lengthen. If the sleeper is very tired, REM cycles are often short—for example, 5 minutes instead of 20—during the early portion of sleep. Before sleep ends, periods of near wakefulness occur, and stages I and II NREM sleep and REM sleep predominate.

The ratio of NREM to REM sleep varies with age (Figure 35–2).

FUNCTIONS OF SLEEP

Sleep exerts physiologic effects on both the nervous system and other body structures. Sleep in some way restores normal levels of activity and normal balance among parts of the nervous system (Guyton 1991, p. 661). The effects of sleep on the body are not understood, but it is known that the activity of the sympathetic nervous system is greater while the person is awake, as are the impulses to the body's muscles, which increase muscle tone. During sleep, however, the activity of the parasympathetic nervous system increases, causing the physiologic changes described in the box on page 953. Sleep is also necessary for protein synthesis, which allows repair processes to occur (Dorociak 1990, p. 40).

It has been suggested that maintaining a regular sleep-wake rhythm is more important than the number of hours actually slept. Some people, for example, can function well on as little as 5 hours sleep each night. It then follows that reestablishing a disrupted sleep-wake cycle (eg, because of surgery) is an important aspect of nursing (Dorociak 1990, p. 39).

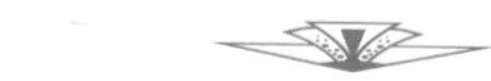

FACTORS AFFECTING SLEEP

Both the quality and the quantity of sleep are affected by a number of factors. *Quality of sleep* means the individual's ability to stay asleep and to get appropriate amounts of REM and NREM sleep. *Quantity of sleep* is the total time the individual sleeps.

Age Age is probably one of the most important factors affecting a person's sleep and rest needs. See Table 35–2 for sleep pattern variations that occur with age.

Environment Environment can promote or hinder sleep. Any change—for example, in the noise level in the environment—can inhibit sleep. The absence of usual stimuli or the presence of unfamiliar stimuli can keep people from sleeping. Most people sleep best in their home environment.

Fatigue It is thought that a person who is moderately fatigued usually has a restful sleep. Fatigue can also affect a person's sleep pattern. The more tired the person is, the shorter the first period of paradoxical (REM) sleep. As the person rests, the REM periods become longer.

Life-Style A person who does shift work and changes shifts frequently must arrange activities so that the person is ready to sleep at the right time. Moderate exercise usually is conducive to sleep, but excessive exercise can delay sleep. The person's ability to relax before retiring is an important factor affecting the ability to fall asleep.

Psychologic Stress Anxiety and depression frequently disturb sleep. A person preoccupied with personal problems may be unable to relax sufficiently to get to sleep. Anxiety increases the norepinephrine blood levels through stimulation of the sympathetic nervous system. This chemical change results in less stage IV NREM and REM sleep and more stage changes and awakenings (Closs 1988, p. 49).

Alcohol and Stimulants People who drink an excessive amount of alcohol often find their sleep disturbed. Excessive alcohol disrupts REM sleep, although it may hasten the onset of sleep. While making up for lost REM sleep after some of the effects of the alcohol have worn off, clients often experience nightmares. Tolerance to alcohol also affects sleep; the alcohol-tolerant person may be unable to sleep well and may become irritable as a result.

Caffeine-containing beverages act as stimulants of the central nervous system, thus interfering with sleep.

Diet Weight loss and weight gain have been thought to affect sleep. Weight loss has been associated with reduced total sleep time as well as broken sleep and earlier awakening. Weight gain, on the other hand, was associated with an increase in total sleep time, less broken sleep, and later waking.

The amino acid L-tryptophan is thought to affect sleep. Dietary L-tryptophan—found, for example, in cottage cheese, milk, beef, and canned tuna—may induce sleep, a fact that might explain why warm milk helps some people get to sleep.

Smoking Nicotine has a stimulating effect on the body, and smokers often have more difficulty falling asleep than nonsmokers. Smokers are usually easily aroused and often describe themselves as light sleepers. By refraining from smoking after the evening meal, the person usually sleeps better; moreover, many former smokers report that their sleeping patterns improved once they stopped smoking.

Motivation The desire to stay awake can often overcome a person's fatigue. For example, a tired person can probably stay alert while attending an interesting concert. When a person is bored and does not have the motivation to stay awake, by contrast, sleep often readily ensues.

Illness People who are ill require more sleep than normal, and the normal rhythm of sleep and wakefulness is often disturbed. People deprived of REM sleep subse-

Table 35–2 Sleep Patterns According to Age

Developmental Level	Normal Sleep Pattern
Newborn	Sleeps 14 to 18 hours a day 50% REM sleep Most remaining time spent in Stages III and IV NREM sleep Sleep cycles last 45 to 60 minutes
Infant	Sleeps 12 to 14 hours a day 20% to 30% REM sleep Sleeps longer at night (8 to 10 hours) and has a scheduled pattern of naps At 12 months, naps once or twice a day
Toddler	Sleeps about 10 to 12 hours a day 25% REM sleep Most sleep during the night Midmorning naps decrease Normal sleep-wake cycle is established by most at age 2 or 3 years.
Preschooler	Sleeps about 11 hours at night 20% REM sleep Second nap eliminated by most at age 3 At age 5, daytime naps are relinquished, except in cultures where an afternoon nap or siesta is customary
School-age child	Sleeps about 10 hours at night 18.5% REM sleep Sleep time remains relatively constant
Adolescent	Sleeps about 8.5 hours a day 20% REM sleep
Young adult	Most sleep 7 to 9 hours a day but time varies 20 to 25% REM sleep 5 to 10% Stage I sleep 50% Stage II sleep 10 to 20% Stage III and IV
Middle-aged adult	Sleeps about 7 hours a day About 20% REM sleep May have insomnia
Elderly adult	Sleeps about 6 hours a day 20 to 25% REM sleep Stage IV sleep is markedly decreased and sometimes absent First REM period is longer May awaken more often during the night Takes longer to fall asleep

Sources: L Malasanos, V Barkauskas, M Moss, and K Stoltenberg-Allen, *Health Assessment*, 4th ed. (St Louis: Mosby, 1990), pp. 95–98; DL Wong, *Essentials of Pediatric Nursing*, 4th ed. (St Louis: Mosby, 1993), pp. 181, 291, 355, 378, 459; and C Hoch and C Reynolds, Sleep disturbances and what to do about them, *Geriatric Nursing*, January/February 1986, 7:25.

quently spend more sleep time than normal in this stage. Pain also can affect sleep—either preventing sleep or awakening the sleeper.

Respiratory conditions can disturb an individual's sleep. Shortness of breath often makes sleep difficult, and people who have nasal congestion or sinus drainage may have trouble breathing and hence a difficult sleep. Research also indicates that hypoxia and hypercapnia may interfere with normal sleep (Closs 1988, p. 50).

People who have gastric or duodenal ulcers may find their sleep disturbed because of pain, often a result of the increased gastric secretions that occur during REM sleep. Certain endocrine disturbances can also affect sleep. Hyperthyroidism lengthens presleep time, often making it difficult for a client to fall asleep. Hypothyroidism, conversely, decreases stage IV sleep. Elevated body temperatures can cause some reduction in stages III and IV NREM sleep and REM sleep.

The need to urinate during the night (enuresis) also disrupts sleep, and people who awaken at night to urinate sometimes have difficulty getting back to sleep.

Medications Some medications affect the quality of sleep. Hypnotics (eg, secobarbital) can interfere with stages III and IV NREM sleep and suppress REM sleep. Beta-blockers have been known to cause insomnia and nightmares. Narcotics, such as meperidine hydrochloride (Demerol) and morphine, are known to suppress REM sleep and to cause frequent awakenings and drowsiness. Tranquilizers interfere with REM sleep. Amphetamines and antidepressants decrease REM sleep abnormally. A client withdrawing from any of these drugs gets much more REM sleep than usual and as a result may experience upsetting nightmares.

COMMON SLEEP DISORDERS

A knowledge of common sleep disorders helps nurses obtain and recognize pertinent data. Sleep disorders may be categorized as primary disorders, secondary disorders, and the parasomnias. **Primary sleep disorders** are those in which the person's sleep problem is the main disorder. These disorders include insomnia, hypersomnia, narcolepsy, sleep apnea, and parasomnias. **Secondary sleep disorders** are sleep disturbances caused by another clinical disorder, such as thyroid dysfunction, depression, or alcoholism.

Insomnia Insomnia, the most common sleep disorder, is the inability to obtain an adequate amount or quality of sleep. People suffering from insomnia do not feel refreshed on arising. There are three types of insomnia:

1. Difficulty in falling asleep (initial insomnia)
2. Difficulty in staying asleep because of frequent or prolonged waking (intermittent or maintenance insomnia)
3. Early morning or premature waking (terminal insomnia)

Some insomniacs have been observed to fall asleep and obtain more sleep than they say they do. This type of insomnia is referred to by some as *subjective* or *imaginary insomnia.* Such a condition is no less distressing than the above types of insomnia and may lead to increased wakefulness.

Insomnia can result from physical discomfort but more often is a result of mental overstimulation due to anxiety. People sometimes become anxious because they think they might not be able to sleep. People who become habituated to drugs or who drink large quantities of alcohol are likely to have insomnia.

Treatment for insomnia frequently requires the client to develop new behavior patterns that induce sleep. The usefulness of sleeping medications is questionable. Such medications do not deal with the cause of the problem, and their prolonged use can create drug dependencies.

Hypersomnia Hypersomnia, the opposite of insomnia, is excessive sleep, particularly in the daytime. The afflicted person often sleeps until noon and takes many naps during the day. Hypersomnia can be caused by medical conditions, for example, central nervous system damage and certain kidney, liver, or metabolic disorders, such as diabetic acidosis and hypothyroidism. In many instances, a person uses hypersomnia as a coping mechanism to avoid facing the responsibilities of the day.

PARASOMNIAS

- **Somnambulism.** Somnambulism (sleepwalking) occurs during stages III and IV of NREM sleep. It is episodic and usually occurs 1 to 2 hours after falling asleep. Sleepwalkers tend not to notice dangers (eg, stairs) and often need to be protected from injury.
- **Sleeptalking.** Talking during sleep occurs during NREM sleep before REM sleep. It rarely presents a problem to the person unless it becomes troublesome to others.
- **Nocturnal enuresis.** Bedwetting during sleep usually occurs in children over 3 years. More males than females are affected. It often occurs 1 to 2 hours after falling asleep, when rousing from NREM stages III to IV.
- **Nocturnal erections.** Nocturnal erections and emissions occur during REM sleep. They begin during adolescence and do not present a sleep problem.
- **Bruxism.** Usually occurring during stage II NREM sleep, this clenching and grinding of the teeth can eventually erode dental crowns and cause teeth to come loose.

Narcolepsy *Narcolepsy*—from the Greek *narco,* meaning "numbness," and *lepsis,* meaning "seizure"—is a sudden wave of overwhelming sleepiness that occurs during the day; thus it is referred to as a "sleep attack." Its cause is unknown, although it is believed to be a genetic defect of the central nervous system in which REM sleep cannot be controlled. In narcoleptic attacks, sleep starts with the REM phase. Even though people who have narcolepsy sleep well at night, they nod off several times a day even when conversing with someone or driving a car. Narcolepsy is often controlled by central nervous system stimulants, such as pemoline or deanol.

Sleep Apnea Sleep apnea is the periodic cessation of breathing during sleep. This disorder needs to be assessed by a sleep expert, but it is often suspected when the person has loud snoring, frequent nocturnal awakenings, excessive daytime sleepiness, insomnia, morning headaches, intellectual deterioration, irritability or other personality changes, and physiologic changes such as hypertension and cardiac arrhythmias (Weaver & Millman 1986, p. 148). It is most frequent in men over 50 and in postmenopausal women.

Table 35–3 Types, Causes, and Signs of Sleep Deprivation

Type	Causes	Clinical Signs
REM deprivation	Alcohol, barbiturates, shift work, jet lag, extended ICU hospitalization, morphine, meperidine hydrochloride (Demerol)	Excitability, restlessness, irritability, and increased sensitivity to pain Confusion and suspiciousness Emotional lability
NREM deprivation	All of the above plus diazepam (Valium) flurazepam hydrochloride (Dalmane), hypothyroidism, depression, respiratory distress disorders, sleep apnea, and age (common in the elderly)	Withdrawal, apathy, hyporesponsiveness Feeling physically uncomfortable Lack of facial expression Speech deterioration Excessive sleepiness
Both REM and NREM deprivation	As above	Decreased reasoning ability (judgment) and ability to concentrate Inattentiveness Marked fatigue manifested by blurred vision, itchy eyes, nausea, headache Difficulty performing activities of daily living Lack of memory, mental confusion, visual or auditory hallucinations, and illusions

The periods of apnea, which last from 10 seconds to 2 minutes, occur during REM or NREM sleep. Frequency of episodes ranges from 50 to 600 per night. These apneic episodes drain the person of energy and lead to excessive daytime sleepiness.

Three common types of sleep apnea are obstructive apnea, central apnea, and mixed apnea. *Obstructive apnea* occurs when the structures of the pharynx or oral cavity block the flow of air. The person continues to try to breathe; that is, the chest and abdominal muscles move. The movements of the diaphragm become stronger and stronger until the obstruction is removed. Enlarged tonsils, a deviated nasal septum, and nasal polyps predispose the client to obstructive apnea.

Central apnea is thought to involve a defect in the respiratory center of the brain. All actions involved in breathing, such as chest movement and air flow, cease. Clients who have brain stem injuries and muscular dystrophy, for example, often have central sleep apnea. At this time there is no available treatment. *Mixed apnea* is a combination of central apnea and obstructive apnea.

An episode of sleep apnea begins with snoring; thereafter, breathing ceases, followed by marked snorting as breathing resumes. Toward the end of each apneic episode, increased carbon dioxide levels in the blood cause the client to wake up. Treatment can be directed at the cause of the apnea; for example, enlarged tonsils may be removed. The use of a nasal continuous positive airway pressure (CPAP) device at night is often effective.

Sleep apnea profoundly affects a person's work or school performance. In addition, prolonged sleep apnea can cause a sharp rise in blood pressure and may also lead to cardiac arrest. Over time, apneic episodes can cause cardiac arrhythmias, pulmonary hypertension, and subsequent left-sided heart failure.

Parasomnias Parasomnias refers to a cluster of waking behaviors that may interfere with sleep. The box on page 958 describes five kinds of parasomnias.

Sleep Deprivation A prolonged disturbance results in decreases in amount, quality, and consistency of sleep and can lead to a syndrome referred to as sleep deprivation. This is not a sleep disorder in itself but a result of sleep disturbances. It produces a variety of physiologic and behavioral symptoms, the severity of which depends on the degree of the deprivation. Two major types of sleep deprivation are REM deprivation and NREM deprivation. A combination of the two increases the severity of symptoms. Table 35–3 shows the causes and clinical signs of sleep deprivation.

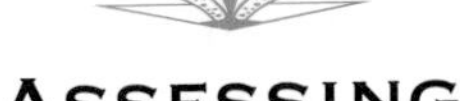

ASSESSING

Assessment relative to a client's sleep includes a sleep history, a sleep diary, and physical examination.

SLEEP HISTORY

A brief general sleep history, which is usually part of the comprehensive nursing history form, is obtained for all clients entering a health care facility. This enables the nurse to incorporate the client's needs and preferences in the plan of care. A general sleep history often includes the following:

- Usual sleeping pattern, specifically sleeping and waking times; hours of undisturbed sleep; quality of or satisfaction with sleep (eg, effect on energy level for daily functioning); and time and duration of naps.
- Bedtime rituals performed to help the person fall asleep (eg, a glass of hot fluid, reading or other method of relaxing, and special equipment or positioning aids).
- Use of sleep medications. Sleep can be disturbed by a variety of drugs, such as stimulants or steroids, if they are taken close to bedtime. Hypnotics and sedating antidepressants may cause excessive daytime sleepiness.
- Sleep environment (eg, dark room, cool or warm temperature, noise level, nightlight).
- Recent changes in sleep patterns or difficulties in sleeping.

If the client indicates a recent pattern change or difficulties in sleeping, a more detailed history is required. This detailed history should explore the exact nature of the problem and its cause, when it first began and its frequency, how it affects daily living, what the client is doing to cope with the problem, and whether these methods have been effective. Questions the nurse might ask the client with a sleeping disturbance are shown in the accompanying box.

ASSESSMENT INTERVIEW

Sleep Disturbances

- How would you describe your sleeping problem? What changes have occurred in your sleeping pattern? How often does this happen?
- Do you have difficulty falling asleep?
- Do you wake up often during the night? If so, how often?
- Do you wake up earlier in the morning than you would like and have difficulty falling back to sleep?
- How do you feel when you wake up in the morning?
- Do you sleep more than usual? If so, how often do you sleep?
- Do you have periods of overwhelming tiredness? If so, when does this happen?
- Have you ever suddenly fallen asleep in the middle of a daytime activity? If so, has any muscle weakness or paralysis occurred?
- Has anyone ever told you that you snore, walk in your sleep, talk in your sleep, or stop breathing for a while when sleeping?
- What have you been doing to deal with this sleeping problem? Does it help?
- What do you think might be causing this problem? Do you have any medical condition that might be causing you to sleep more (or less)? Are you receiving medications for an illness that might alter your sleeping pattern? Are you experiencing any stressful or upsetting events or conflicts that may be affecting your sleep?
- How is your sleeping problem affecting you?

SLEEP DIARY

Sometimes clients with a sleeping problem can provide more precise information if they keep a written record of their sleep pattern and the habits associated with it. Such a sleep diary or log can be kept by clients who are sleeping at home and should be maintained for at least 1 week. A sleep diary may include all of the following information or selected aspects of it that pertain to the client's specific problem:

- Total number of sleep hours per day
- Activities performed 2 to 3 hours before bedtime (type, duration, and time)
- Bedtime rituals (eg, ingestion of food, fluid, or medication) before going to bed
- Time of (a) going to bed, (b) trying to fall asleep, (c) falling asleep (approximate), (d) any instances of waking up and duration of these periods, and (e) waking up in the morning
- Any worries that the client believes may affect sleep
- Factors that the client believes have a positive or negative affect on sleep

Keeping such a diary may become stressful for some clients and further affect their sleep. The nurse needs to advise the client to obtain the assistance of a bed partner in keeping the diary or to discontinue the diary if it presents a problem. When a diary is completed, the nurse and client can develop flow charts or graphs that will assist in organizing the data and identifying the specific problem.

PHYSICAL EXAMINATION

Examination of the client includes observation of the client's facial appearance, behavior, and energy level.

NURSING DIAGNOSES
CLIENTS WITH SLEEP PROBLEMS

NURSING DIAGNOSIS: Sleep pattern disturbance: The state in which the individual experiences a disruption in the amount or quantity of sleep, causing discomfort or interference with desired life-style

Defining Characteristics

- Complaints of difficulty falling asleep, awakening earlier or later than desired, interrupted sleep, or not feeling well-rested
- Behavior changes: increasing irritability, restlessness, listlessness, lethargy, decreased attention span, frequent daytime napping, disorientation
- Physical signs: dark circles under eyes, frequent yawning, postural changes, slight hand tremor, mild nystagmus, and expressionless face

Related Factors

Worries about actual or anticipated loss of a loved one, loss of a job, loss of life due to serious disease process, or worry about a family member's behavior or illness; frequent changes in sleep time due to shift work or overtime; specific illness that affects the sleep cycle; pain and discomfort associated with a disease process; inability to cope with multiple stresses; changes in sleep environment or bedtime rituals (eg, noise or overstimulation of hospital environment; alcohol or other drug dependency; drug withdrawal; misuse of sedatives prescribed for insomnia; effects of medications such as steroids or stimulants (specify).

Sources: LJ Carpenito, *Nursing Diagnosis: Application to Clinical Practice*, 4th ed. (Philadelphia: Lippincott, 1992), pp. 776–77; M Gordon, *Manual of Nursing Diagnosis 1993–1994*, 6th ed. (St Louis: Mosby-Year Book, 1993), pp. 219–21; MJ Kim, GK McFarland, and AM McLane, *Pocket Guide to Nursing Diagnoses*, 5th ed. (St Louis: Mosby-Year Book, 1993), p. 56; GK McFarland, and EA McFarlane, *Nursing Diagnosis and Intervention: Planning for Patient Care*, 2d ed. (St Louis: Mosby, 1993), pp. 421–22; North American Nursing Diagnosis Association, *NANDA Nursing Diagnoses: Definitions and Classification 1992–1993*, (Philadelphia: NANDA, 1992), p. 56; and JR Lederer, GL Marculescu, B Mocnik, and N Seaby, *Care Planning Pocket Guide—A Nursing Diagnosis Approach*, 5th ed. (Redwood City, CA: Addison-Wesley Nursing, 1993), p. 192.

Darkened areas around the eyes, puffy eyelids, reddened conjunctiva, glazed or dull-appearing eyes, and limited facial expression are indicative of sleep insufficiency. Behaviors such as irritability, restlessness, inattentiveness, slowed speech, slumped posture, hand tremor, yawning, rubbing the eyes, withdrawal, confusion, and incoordination are also suggestive of sleep problems. Lack of energy may be noted by observing whether the client appears physically weak, lethargic, or fatigued.

In addition, the nurse assesses whether the client has a deviated nasal septum, enlarged neck, or is obese. These findings may be associated with obstructive sleep apnea and/or snoring.

DIAGNOSTIC STUDIES

Sleep is measured objectively in a sleep disorder laboratory by **polysomnography;** an electroencephalogram (EEG), electromyogram (EMG), and electro-oculogram (EOG) are recorded simultaneously. This simultaneous recording divides sleep into REM and NREM sleep. Electrodes are placed on the center of the scalp to record brain waves (EEG), on the outer canthus of each eye to record eye movement (EOG), and on the chin muscles to record the structural electromyogram (EMG). The following may also be monitored, depending on findings of the initial interview: respiratory effort and airflow, ECG, leg movements, and oxygen saturation. Oxygen saturation is determined by monitoring arterial blood or by an *oximeter*, a light-sensitive cell that attaches to the ear or a finger. Oxygen saturation and ECG assessments are of particular importance if sleep apnea is suspected. Through polysomnography, the client's activity (movements, struggling, noisy respirations) during sleep can be assessed. Such activity of which the client is unaware may be the cause of arousal during sleep.

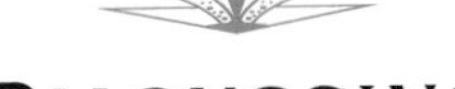

DIAGNOSING

Sleep pattern disturbance is the NANDA nursing diagnosis given to clients with sleep problems. See the box above for its definition, defining characteristics, and related factors. After assessment data are grouped, patterns emerge that will enable the nurse to specify this diagnosis and perhaps provide an etiology. Examples of assessment data clusters and related nursing diagnoses for primary sleep disturbances are shown in Table 35–4 on page 962.

Table 35–4 Clinical Application: Assessment Data Clusters and Related Nursing Diagnoses for Clients with Sleep Problems

Data Cluster	Nursing Diagnoses
Gillian Marks, a 51-year-old woman, states she has a problem falling asleep since her mastectomy 2 months ago. Says fears of prognosis become prominent when she is not active and busy. Has tried reading or watching TV but neither make her sleepy or relaxed. Appears agitated and restless.	**Sleep pattern disturbance: insomnia (difficulty falling asleep)** related to fear of prognosis and difficulty relaxing
Joseph Mintz, an 83-year-old man was admitted to a four-bed room in extended care unit 3 days ago. States he falls asleep about 10 PM but is awakened by roommate's snoring. States, "At home I used to have a hot cup of Ovaltine whenever I awakened."	**Sleep pattern disturbance: insomnia (difficulty staying asleep)** related to change in sleep environment and sleep-time rituals.
Plooney Larsh states he was fired from his job because of alcohol abuse. Has joined Alcoholics Anonymous but has been unable to get any work for the past 2 years. States, "Every day I wake up at 4 AM (full of self-reproach and self-punitive thinking) and can't get back to sleep."	**Sleep pattern disturbance: insomnia (early morning waking)** related to low self-esteem secondary to loss of job and inability to obtain employment.
Marny Closky, a high school student whose father and mother recently divorced, broke up with her boyfriend 2 weeks ago. States she doesn't have the energy to get up in the morning and just wants to sleep all the time. She has Grade 12 examinations next week.	**Sleep pattern disturbance** related to inability to cope with multiple stresses
Thomas Strep states that recent shortage of firefighters has resulted in extensive overtime, frequent "double shifts" and rotations from his usual 2 weekly 7–3 and 3–7 shifts. States, "All I want to do is go to sleep when I get home, but I can't. I guess I'm too riled up."	**Sleep pattern disturbance: altered sleep-wake pattern** related to frequent shift changes and overtime

Sleep pattern disturbances may also be stated as the *etiology* of another diagnosis, in which case the nursing interventions are directed toward the sleep disturbance itself. Examples include the following:

- **High risk for injury** related to somnambulism
- **Self-esteem disturbance** related to nocturnal enuresis
- **Ineffective individual coping** related to sleep deprivation
- **Fatigue** related to insomnia
- **High risk for impaired gas exchange** related to sleep apnea
- **Knowledge deficit** (nonprescription remedies for insomnia) related to misinformation
- **Altered thought processes** related to chronic insomnia
- **Anxiety** related to sleep apnea and fear of death
- **Activity intolerance** related to sleep deprivation
- **Impaired social interaction** related to excessive daytime sleeping secondary to sleep deprivation

PLANNING

The major goal/outcome for clients with sleep disturbances is to maintain (or develop) a sleeping pattern that provides sufficient energy for daily activities. The nurse plans specific nursing interventions based on the etiology of each nursing diagnosis. These interventions may include reducing environmental distractions; promoting bedtime rituals; providing comfort measures; scheduling nursing care to provide for uninterrupted sleep periods; teaching stress reduction, relaxation techniques, or ways to develop good sleep habits; and promoting self-esteem. If the sleep disturbance is the etiology of the nursing diagnosis, the nurse plans specific strategies to relieve insomnia and deal with sleep deprivation. Specific outcome criteria, nursing interventions, and rationales are shown in the Care Planning Guide.

A critical pathway can also be useful for planning client care (see p. 968).

IMPLEMENTING

For hospitalized clients, sleep problems are often related to the hospital environment or their illness. Assisting the client to sleep in such instances can be challenging to a nurse, often involving scheduling activities, administering analgesics, and providing a supportive environment. Explanations and a supportive relationship are essential for the fearful or anxious client.

CARE PLANNING GUIDE

CLIENTS WITH SLEEP PROBLEMS

NURSING DIAGNOSIS: Sleep pattern disturbance

Outcome Criteria	Nursing Interventions	Rationale
The client		
▪ Participates in identifying possible causes of sleeping problem.	Assess and document the client's daytime and nighttime sleeping patterns, and compare the current pattern with usual sleep habits before this sleep disturbance episode.	Accurate assessment enables the nurse and client to determine the exact nature of the change.
	Discuss possible causes that contribute to the sleep pattern disturbance (eg, fear, unresolved problems and conflicts, medications, and so on). See the discussion of related factors in the Nursing Diagnoses box on page 961.	Identifying possible causes helps the nurse and client plan appropriate interventions to promote sleep.
	Include the spouse or significant other in care planning.	Participating in care planning enhances the support persons' understanding of specific plans and encourages their cooperation.
▪ Participates in identifying measures that will promote an optimal sleep pattern.	Explore sleep-promoting techniques and life-style changes that may contribute to an optimal sleep period.	Client involvement may enhance compliance to planned interventions.
▪ Verbalizes satisfaction with quality and amount of sleep, for example: a. Falls asleep within 30 to 45 minutes of going to bed. b. Sleeps specified number of hours per night or for longer intervals between nursing care functions. c. Reports feelings of being rested or refreshed after waking.	Provide client's desired comfort measures or sleeping aids at or before bedtime, such as appropriate positioning and supports, pain medication, back rub, soft music, warm bedclothes and linens, reading material, warm milk, or prescribed sedative.	Relaxation measures help induce sleep.
	Provide a quiet, peaceful environment during sleep periods. Avoid loud noises, use of overhead lights, and other interruptions during sleep periods.	A quiet, peaceful environment promotes restful sleep.
	Inform the client of necessary care interruptions ahead of time. Organize care to allow for sleep cycles of at least 90 minutes; for example, when the client is awakened for medication, obtain necessary vital signs, and administer treatments at that time.	Preparing the client for awakenings and planning to minimize awakenings decrease unnecessary stress and anxiety that may prevent subsequent sleep. A sleep time of at least 90 minutes helps the client maintain normal sleep time and promotes REM sleep.
	Implement measures as indicated to prevent frequent voiding at night, such as decreasing fluid intake before bedtime, assisting the client as needed to void at bedtime, and avoiding the ingestion of caffeine for 4 hours before sleep.	These measures prevent the need to waken for frequent voiding.

➤

SLEEP PROBLEMS CONTINUED

NURSING DIAGNOSIS: Sleep pattern disturbance *continued*

Outcome Criteria	Nursing Interventions	Rationale
	Plan satisfying activities for the client during the daytime.	Satisfying daytime activities stimulate wakefulness and discourage daytime napping, which can disrupt circadian rhythms and nighttime sleep.
	Encourage the client to express concerns when unable to sleep.	Verbalizing concerns may help allay anxiety and promote relaxation.
	Ensure a compatible roommate, if possible.	Incompatibilities create stress and conflict that disturb rest periods.

REDUCING ENVIRONMENTAL DISTRACTIONS

- Close window curtains if street lights shine through.
- Close curtains between clients in semiprivate and larger rooms.
- Reduce or eliminate overhead lighting; provide a night-light at the bedside or in the bathroom.
- Close the door of the client's room.
- Adhere to agency policy about times to turn off communal televisions or radios.
- Lower the ring tone of nearby telephones.
- Discontinue use of the paging system after a certain hour (eg, 2100 hours), or reduce its volume.
- Keep required staff conversations at low levels; conduct nursing reports or other discussions in a separate area away from client rooms.
- Wear rubber-soled shoes.
- Ensure that all cart wheels are well oiled.
- Perform only essential nursing tasks during sleeping hours.

CREATING A RESTFUL ENVIRONMENT

To create a restful environment, the nurse needs to reduce environmental distractions, reduce sleep interruptions, ensure a safe environment, and provide a room temperature that is satisfactory to the client. Environmental distractions such as bright lighting and noise are particularly troublesome for hospitalized clients. There are three general types of noises in the hospital setting: environmental noises, procedural noises, and staff communication noises (Walgenbach 1990, p. 279). Environmental noises include the sound of paging systems, telephones, and call lights; doors slamming; and pieces of furniture squeaking. Procedural noises include those associated with emptying catheter bags, distributing fluids, crushing pills, and wheeling drug or linen carts through corridors. Staff communication is a major factor creating noise, particularly at staff change of shift. Some interventions to reduce environmental distractions, especially noise, are listed in the box in the left column.

SAFETY MEASURES FOR SLEEP

- Use night-lights.
- Place the bed in low position.
- Employ side rails if appropriate.
- Place the call bell within easy reach.
- Instruct the client on how to obtain assistance.
- Instruct the client who is attached to intravenous tubing or drainage tubing on how to move about.
- Provide tubing long enough to permit the client to move.

The environment must also be safe so that the client can relax. People who are unaccustomed to narrow hospital beds may feel more secure with side rails. See the box above for additional safety measures. See also the section on promoting comfort and relaxation, later in this chapter.

SUPPORTING BEDTIME RITUALS

Most people are accustomed to bedtime rituals or presleep routines that are conducive to comfort and relaxation. Altering or eliminating such routines can affect a client's sleep. Common prebedtime activities of adults include an evening stroll, listening to music, taking a soothing bath, and praying. Children, too, are socialized into presleep routines such as a bedtime story, or holding on to a favorite toy or blanket. Sleep is also usually preceded by hygienic routines, such as washing the face and hands (or bathing), brushing the teeth, and voiding.

In addition, the snacks of some sort that many people take before bedtime to allay hunger may interfere with sleep. Some high-protein beverages and snacks such as a hot milky drink, cheese, or nuts are thought to promote sleep when taken before bedtime. These are thought to promote sleep because they contain the amino acid L-tryptophan, a sleep inducer. Excessive fluid intake before retiring should also be avoided. This prevents the need to use the bathroom during sleeping hours.

People need to learn to avoid excessive physical exercise and excessive mental stimulation such as office work or dealing with family problems before bedtime. Such activity prolongs falling asleep. Exercise performed 2 hours before bedtime, however, can promote sleep because it contributes to physical fatigue and invites sleep. Adherence to a consistent time for sleep and getting up at the same time each morning is also important in establishing a healthy sleep pattern.

PROMOTING COMFORT AND RELAXATION

Comfort measures are essential to help the client fall asleep and stay asleep, especially if the effects of the person's illness interfere with sleep. A concerned, caring attitude, along with the following interventions, can significantly promote client comfort and sleep:

- Provide loose-fitting nightwear.
- Assist clients with hygienic routines.
- Make sure the bed linen is smooth, clean, and dry.
- Assist or encourage the client to void before bedtime.
- Offer to provide a back massage before sleep (see Procedure 35–1).
- Position dependent clients appropriately to aid muscle relaxation, and provide supportive devices to protect pressure areas.
- Schedule medications, especially diuretics, to prevent nocturnal awakenings.
- For clients who have pain, administer analgesics 30 minutes before sleep, or apply warm or cool applications or supportive dressings or splints to painful areas.

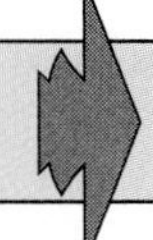

PROCEDURE 35–1 PROVIDING A BACK MASSAGE

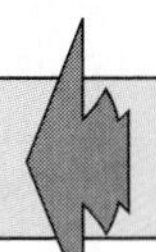

See the box at the right for types of massage strokes.

PURPOSES

- To relieve muscle tension
- To promote physical and mental relaxation
- To improve muscle and skin functioning
- To relieve insomnia
- To provide relief from pain

TYPES OF MASSAGE STROKES

- *Effleurage:* stroking the body
- *Petrissage:* kneading or making large quick pinches of the skin, subcutaneous tissue, and muscle

ASSESSMENT FOCUS

Vital signs; signs of stress (eg, muscle tension); receptability of the client to therapy.

EQUIPMENT

- ☐ Lotion or oil

PROCEDURE 35–1 PROVIDING A BACK MASSAGE *continued*

INTERVENTION

1. Select an appropriate time free of interruptions and distractions.

- Provide massage following the morning bath, before sleeping, and at other times as necessary to achieve relaxation and comfort for the client.
- Assist the client to a prone position in bed. Remove the client's gown, or open the back of the hospital gown.

2. Warm the massage lotion or oil before use.

- Warm the lotion or oil by pouring it into your hands before applying it to the client's back. *Cold lotion may startle the client and increase discomfort.*

3. Effleurage the entire back.

- Place your hands next to the lower spine. Using your palms and fingers, slowly massage upwards to the neck, gradually decreasing pressure as you get close to the neck. Circle your hands over the shoulder blades, and then slowly move them gently down the lateral surface of the back. *Effleurage has a relaxing, sedative effect if slow movement and light pressure are used.*

4. Apply friction strokes next to the spine.

- Use your thumbs to apply friction strokes (strong circular motions).
- Massage the back, moving from side to side in smooth, tiny circles, starting at the neck and ending at the waist.

5. Optional: Petrissage the back and shoulders of the client.

- Petrissage first up the vertebral column and then over the entire back. *Petrissage is stimulating, especially if done quickly and with firm pressure.*
- Observe the client carefully to ensure that petrissage does not cause pain or discomfort. If the client grimaces or withdraws from the touch, ease the kneading pressure.

6. Apply hand pressure movements up the back.

- Using moderate pressure, walk your hands up the outer edges of the back from the hips to the neck.

7. Optional: Effleurage and petrissage the upper back and shoulders, using long soothing strokes. *This area often experiences the most tension.*

8. Apply pressure strokes along the spinal column.

- Place one hand on top of the other, and move slowly from the lower spine to the top of the spine, using light to moderate pressure.
- Observe the client carefully to ensure that the pressure strokes are not causing the client pain or discomfort.

9. Using gentle pressure, apply large circular movements to the back.

- Start at the outer side of the back at the waistline. Move from the waistline to the lower hip, then across the hip and up the spine.

10. Complete the massage by using light effleurage to the entire back.

- With each massage stroke, lessen the pressure.

11. Assist the client to a position of comfort.

12. Document the massage and the client's response.

EVALUATION FOCUS

Signs of relaxation and/or decreased pain (eg, relaxed breathing, decreased muscle tension, drowsiness, and peaceful affect); verbalizations of freedom from pain and tension; areas of redness, broken skin, bruises, or other signs of skin breakdown.

- For clients who have breathing problems, administer prescribed medications such as bronchodilators before bedtime and position clients appropriately (eg, semi-Fowler's position) to facilitate breathing.
- Listen to the client's concerns and deal with problems as they arise.

People of any age, but especially older adults, are unable to sleep well if they feel cold. Changes in circulation, metabolism, and body tissue density reduce the older person's ability to generate and conserve heat. To compound this problem, hospital gowns have short sleeves and are made of thin polyester. Bedsheets also are often made of

RESEARCH NOTE

Is Music an Effective Calming Agent for Clients with Dementia?

This study was conducted to investigate the effects of selected dinner music on demented clients institutionalized in a nursing home. Three different types of music were played during dinner for three separate two-week periods. A control period (during which no music was played) followed the six weeks of music. The reactions of five demented clients were recorded on videotape.

Each client responded to the music. Soothing music was noted to have the most effect. For example, one agitated client became unusually calm and another fed herself more than usual. All spent more time at dinner and ate more calmly when soothing music was played.

Implications: Although this study was conducted with a small sample size, it appears that music may positively affect restless and agitated clients. Music is a simple and inexpensive tool that may be worth using with agitated or demented clients.

Source: H Ragneskog, M Kihlgran, I Karlsson, and A Norberg, Dinner music for demented patients: Analysis of video-recorded observations, *Clinical Nursing Research*, August 1996, 5(3):262–82.

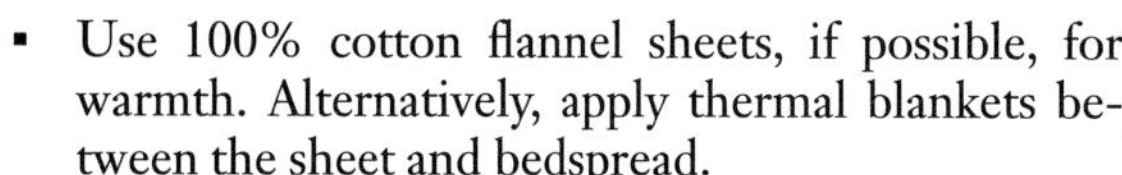

HELPING ELDERLY CLIENTS KEEP WARM IN BED

- Before the client goes to bed, warm the bed with hot water bottles or prewarmed bath blankets. Remove the hot water bottle before the client gets into bed to avoid the risk of a burn.
- Use 100% cotton flannel sheets, if possible, for warmth. Alternatively, apply thermal blankets between the sheet and bedspread.
- Encourage the client to bring clothing from home, such as flannel nightgown or pyjamas, loose-fitting jogging suit, thermal socks, leg warmers, long underwear, sleeping cap (if scalp hair is sparse), sweater, or a favorite quilt or blanket.

polyester rather than a warm fabric, such as cotton flannel. Interventions to keep elderly clients warm during sleep are shown in the box above at the right.

Emotional stress obviously interferes with a person's ability to relax, rest, and sleep, inability to sleep further aggravates feelings of tension. Sleep rarely occurs until a person is relaxed. Relaxation techniques can be encouraged as part of the nightly routine. Slow, deep breathing for a few minutes followed by slow, rhythmic contraction and relaxation of muscles can alleviate tension and induce calm. Imagery, meditation, and yoga can also be taught. See specialized stress-reduction techniques in Chapter 32, pages 843–849, and distraction techniques in Chapter 36, page 1004.

ADMINISTERING SLEEP MEDICATIONS

Sleep medications often prescribed on a prn basis for clients include sedative-hypnotics, which induce sleep, and antianxiety drugs or tranquilizers, which decrease anxiety and tension. Because a tolerance to the sleep-inducing properties develops after several weeks, clients at home may increase the dosage or complement the drug with alcohol.

Nurses need to teach clients about the action and side effects of such drugs and the risks of overreliance and to caution clients about taking drugs with alcohol. The use of nonprescription sleeping medications should be discouraged. When administering prescribed drugs to clients in hospital, the nurse must be knowledgeable about expected side-effects and administer them only when indicated. Elderly clients, in particular, are prone to side effects because of their altered rates of gastrointestinal absorption, decreased ability to metabolize and excrete drugs, and, in some cases, increased body fat. Whenever possible, nonpharmacologic interventions to induce and maintain sleep are preferred interventions.

CLIENT TEACHING

Many insomniacs or people suffering from sleep deprivation can benefit from instructions about good sleep habits and factors that interfere with sleep. Most people also need instruction about the safe use of sleep medications. Client teaching for promoting sleep is shown in the box on page 968.

EVALUATING

To evaluate whether client outcomes have been achieved, the nurse may observe the duration of the client's sleep, observe the client for signs of REM and NREM sleep deprivation, ask how the client feels on awakening, or question the client about the effectiveness of specific interventions, such as the use of relaxation techniques, adherence to a consistent sleep-wake cycle, or ingestion of milk products before bedtime.

If outcomes are *not* achieved, the nurse should explore the reasons, which may include answers to the following questions:

- Were etiologic factors correctly identified?
- Has the client's physical condition or medication therapy changed?
- Did the client comply with instructions about establishing a regular sleep-wake pattern?
- Did the client avoid ingesting caffeine?
- Did the client participate in stimulating daytime activities to avoid daytime naps?
- Were all possible measures taken to provide a restful environment for the client?
- Were bedtime rituals supported?
- Were the comfort and relaxation measures provided effective?
- Were administered sleep medications ineffective?

See also the evaluation checklist in Table 8–3 on page 158.

WELLNESS TEACHING

Promoting Rest and Sleep

- Establish a regular bedtime and wake-up time to prevent disruptions in your biologic rhythm. If a daytime nap is necessary, take it at the same time each day.
- Use the bed mainly for sleep, so that you associate it with sleep.
- Get adequate exercise during the day to reduce stress, but avoid stimulating activity before bedtime.
- Set aside time each day for restful, enjoyable activities.
- Avoid alcohol and caffeine-containing foods and beverages (coffee, tea, chocolate) during the afternoon and evening.
- Establish a regular routine before sleep, such as taking part in a relaxing pastime and/or having a snack.
- Go to bed only when you are sleepy and not when you are wakeful.
- If you use sleeping pills, take them judiciously (eg, three times a week).
- When you are unable to sleep, pursue some relaxing activity until you feel drowsy.
- If you are unable to sleep in the early morning, get up and pursue nonstrenuous activity that provides a sense of accomplishment.

CRITICAL PATHWAY FOR JACK HARRIS

ASSESSMENT DATA

Nursing Assessment

Jack Harris is a 36-year-old police officer assigned to a high-crime police precinct. He was admitted to the hospital following a bullet wound to his arm that resulted in a fracture. He was admitted for an open reduction and internal fixation of the fracture with removal of bullet fragments. While speaking to the nurse, he mentions that he has recently been promoted to the rank of detective and has assumed new responsibilities. He states that since his promotion, he has experienced an increasing amount of difficulty falling asleep and sometimes staying asleep. Mr Harris expresses considerable concern over the danger of his occupation and also his desire to do well in his new position. He complains of waking up feeling tired and of becoming quite irritable.

Physical Examination

Height: 185.4 cm (6′1″)
Weight: 85.7 kg (189 lb)
Temperature: 37 C (98.6 F)
Pulse rate: 80 bpm
Respirations: 18 per minute at rest
Blood pressure: 114/88 mm Hg
Pale, drawn with dark circles under eyes

Diagnostic Data

CBC within normal range
X-ray film of left arm: open fracture of humerus with bullet fragment lodged in bone with soft tissue injury

Critical Pathway for Client following Open Reduction and Internal Fixation of Upper Arm Fracture

Expected length of stay 3–4 days following surgery

	Date _________ Operative day	**Date _________ 1st Postoperative day**
Daily outcomes	Client will ▪ be afebrile. ▪ recover from anesthesia as evidenced by: VS return to baseline, awake, alert and oriented, with clear lungs. ▪ verbalize understanding and demonstrate cooperation with turning, coughing, deep breathing, and prescribed activity level. ▪ state pain controlled with ordered medication. ▪ tolerate ordered diet without nausea and vomiting. ▪ verbalize ability to cope. ▪ identify two factors that contribute to insomnia.	Client will ▪ be afebrile. ▪ have stable vital signs, with clear lungs, and be alert and oriented. ▪ verbalize understanding and demonstrate cooperation with turning, coughing, deep breathing, and prescribed activity level. ▪ state pain controlled with ordered medication. ▪ tolerate ordered diet without nausea and vomiting. ▪ verbalize ability to cope. ▪ identify two measures that promote sleep.
Tests and treatments	Hct/Hgb Vital signs and O_2 saturation, neurovascular assessment and cast assessment q15min × 4; q30min × 4; q1h × 4; and then q4h if stable. Head to toe assessment* q4–8h. Incentive spirometer q2h. Intake and output q shift.	Vital signs and O_2 saturation, neurovascular assessment and cast assessment q4h if stable. Head to toe assessment* q shift and prn. Incentive spirometer q2h. Intake and output q shift.
Knowledge deficit	Orient to room and surroundings. Provide simple, brief instructions. Review plan of care and importance of specific postoperative care: turning, coughing, deep breathing, incentive spirometer, mobilization, possible tubes and intravenous pain management (IV/PCA or IM prn medications).	Review plan of care and importance of early mobilization. Begin discharge teaching regarding cast care and mobility.
Psycho-social	Assess anxiety related to diagnosis and surgery. Assess fears of the unknown and surgery. Encourage verbalization of concerns. Provide information regarding surgical experience. Minimize external stimuli (eg, noise, movement).	Assess level of anxiety. Encourage verbalization of concerns. Provide information. Provide ongoing support and encouragement.
Sleep/rest	Assist client to identify factors that cause or contribute to insomnia. Encourage client to establish and maintain a bedtime routine. Offer sleep aids such as reading, back rub, or listening to soft music.	Instruct in relaxation techniques. Instruct client to avoid caffeine stimulants in the evening before bedtime. Offer sleep aids. Encourage bedtime routine.

* Head to toe assessment: This assessment should address major body systems affected by immobility including musculoskeletal, cardiovascular, respiratory, metabolic and nutritional, urine and endocrine, fecal elimination, integumentary, and neurosensory.

	Operative day *continued*	**1st Postoperative day** *continued*
Diet	Advance from clear liquids to full liquids to tolerance. Baseline nutrtional assessment	Advance from full liquids to regular diet as tolerated. Offer supplemental feedings high in protein and vitamins.
Activity	Provide safety precautions. Reposition q2h and prn. Assist client with full range of motion to all unaffected extremities 3 or 4 × daily. Teach the client isometric exercises for upper arm. Ecourage client to participate in activities of daily living as much as possible.	Provide safety precautions. Encourage client to participate in activities of daily living as much as possible. Ambulate in room 4 × daily.
Medications	IV/PCA or IM analgesic IV antibiotics IV fluids Tetanus toxoid if indicated	IV/PCA or IM analgesic IV antibiotics IV fluids or intermittent IV device
Transfer/ discharge plans	Assess discharge plans and support system.	Determine needs at time of discharge. Begin home care teaching.

	Date ________ **2d Postoperative day**	**Date ________** **3d–4th Postoperative day**
Daily outcomes	Client will ▪ be afebrile and have clear lungs. ▪ demonstrate cooperation with turning, coughing, deep breathing, and prescribed activity level. ▪ state pain controlled with ordered medication. ▪ tolerate ordered diet without nausea and vomiting. ▪ verbalize ability to cope. ▪ verbalize beginning understanding of home care instructions. ▪ practice relaxation techniques.	Client ▪ is afebrile, has stable vital signs and clear lungs. ▪ has intact neurovascular status to affected extremity. ▪ manages pain with oral medications. ▪ is independent in self-care. ▪ is fully ambulatory. ▪ has resumed preadmission urine and bowel elimination pattern. ▪ verbalizes home care instructions. ▪ tolerates usual diet. ▪ verbalizes ability to cope with ongoing stressors. ▪ demonstrates less irritability and verbalizes a greater sense of well-being. ▪ establishes a bedtime routine and awakens feeling rested.

	2d Postoperative day *continued*	**3d-4th Postoperative day** *continued*
Tests and treatments	Vital signs q4h. Head to toe assessment* q shift and prn. Incentive spirometer q2h until fully ambulatory. Intake and output q shift.	Vital signs assessment q4h. Neurovascular assessment q4h and prn. Head to toe assessment* q shift. Incentive spirometer q2h until fully ambulatory. D/C intake and output if taking adequate fluids and balanced with output.
Knowledge deficit	Initiate discharge teaching regarding diet, signs and symptoms to report, and activity level. Review written discharge instructions.	Provide client with written discharge instructions that discuss: (1) signs and symptoms of infection related to internal fixation device, (2) importance of regular follow-up care, (3) care of cast, and (4) monitoring neurovascular status. Complete discharge teaching to include diet, follow-up care, signs and symptoms to report, activity, and medications: dose, frequency, route, and side effects.
Psycho-social	Encourage verbalization of concerns. Provide ongoing support and encouragement.	Encourage verbalization of concerns. Provide ongoing support and encouragement.
Sleep/rest	Reinforce instructions in relaxation techniques. Encourage client to avoid caffeine stimulants. Offer sleep aids. Encourage bedtime routine.	Reinforce instructions in relaxation techniques. Encourage client to avoid caffeine stimulants. Offer sleep aids. Encourage bedtime routine.
Diet	Regular diet to tolerance. Encourage fluid intake of 2000 mL per day when IV fluids D/C. Offer supplemental feedings high in protein and vitamins.	Regular diet as tolerated. Encourage fluids to 2000 mL/24 h. Offer supplemental feedings high in protein and vitamins.
Activity	Provide safety precautions. Encourage client to participate in activities of daily living as much as possible. Ambulate ad lib.	Provide safety precautions. Encourage ambulation ad lib. Encourage client to participate in activities of daily living as much as possible.
Medications	IV/PCA, IM or PO analgesics IV antibiotics Intermittent IV device	PO analgesic D/C intermittent IV device
Transfer/ discharge plans	Complete discharge plans. Continue home care instructions.	Complete discharge instructions.

* Head to toe assessment: This assessment should address major body systems affected by immobility including musculoskeletal, cardiovascular, respiratory, metabolic and nutritional, urine and endocrine, fecal elimination, integumentary, and neurosensory.

CHAPTER HIGHLIGHTS

- Sleep is a conscious state in which a person's perception and reaction to the environment are decreased.
- The sleep cycle is controlled by specialized areas in the brain stem and is affected by the individual's circadian rhythm.
- During a normal night's sleep, an adult has four to six sleep cycles, each with NREM sleep and REM sleep.
- NREM (slow-wave) sleep consists of four stages, progressing from stage I, very light sleep, to stage IV, deep sleep.
- REM sleep recurs about every 90 minutes, is less restful than NREM sleep, and is often associated with dreaming.
- NREM sleep constitutes most of a sleep cycle.
- The ratio of NREM to REM sleep varies with age.
- Many factors can affect sleep, including age, environment, life-style, psychologic stress, alcohol and stimulants, diet, smoking, motivation, illness, and medications.
- Common sleep disorders include insomnia, hypersomnia, narcolepsy, sleep apnea, and parasomnias, such as somnambulism, talking during sleep, nocturnal enuresis, nocturnal erections, and bruxism.
- Assessment of a client's sleep includes obtaining a sleep history, reviewing a sleep diary, and conducting a physical examination.
- Nursing responsibilities to help clients sleep include (a) creating a restful environment, (b) supporting bedtime rituals, (c) promoting comfort and relaxation, (d) administering prescribed sleep medications, and (e) teaching clients ways to enhance sleep and rest.

READINGS AND REFERENCES

SUGGESTED READINGS

Balsmeyer, B. September/October 1990. Sleep disturbances of the infant and toddler. *Pediatric Nursing* 16:447–52.

Two common sleep disorders of infants and toddlers are sleeplessness and arousal disorders. This article discusses methods to reduce the impact of these problems on the family.

Metzler, D and Finesilver, C. March 1990. When to worry if your patient can't sleep. *RN* 53:52–57.

The authors discuss three types of sleep apnea, assessment of the client's sleep pattern, polysomnography, and treatment options.

RELATED RESEARCH

Gall, K, Petersen, T, and Riesch, SK. October 1990. Nightlife: Nocturnal behavior patterns among hospitalized elderly. *Journal of Gerontological Nursing* 168:31–35.

Skipper, JK, Jung, FD, and Coffey, LC. July 1990. Nurses and shiftwork: Effects on physical health and mental depression. *Journal of Advanced Nursing* 15:835–42.

SELECTED REFERENCES

Balsmeyer, B. September/October 1990. Sleep disturbances of the infant and toddler. *Pediatric Nursing* 16:447–52.

Boomer, H and Deakin, A. March 20–26, 1991. Getting children to sleep. *Nursing Times* 87:40–43.

Carpenito, LJ. 1992. *Nursing Diagnosis: Application to Clinical Practice.* 4th ed. Philadelphia: Lippincott.

Closs, J. January 6–12 and 13–20, 1988. Patients' sleep-wake rhythms in hospital. Parts I and II, *Nursing Times* 84:48–50; 54–55.

———. July 1988. Assessment of sleep in hospital patients: A review of methods. *Journal of Advanced Nursing* 13:501–10.

Cohen, FL. September 1988. Narcolepsy: A review of a common, life-long sleep disorder. *Journal of Advanced Nursing* 13:546–56.

Davidhizar, R and Cosgray, R. November/December 1990. Helping the wanderer. Both over- and understimulation can cause wandering in the confused patient. Here's what to watch for. *Geriatric Nursing* 16:280–81.

Dorociak, Y. December 19–26, 1990. Aspects of sleep. *Nursing Times* 86:38–40.

Emra, KL and Herrera, CO. September 1989. When your patient tells you he can't sleep. *RN* 52:79–80, 82, 84.

Gordon, M. 1993. *Manual of Nursing Diagnosis 1993–1994.* 6th ed. St Louis: Mosby-Year Book.

Guyton, AC. 1991. *Textbook of Medical Physiology.* 8th ed. Philadelphia: WB Saunders.

Hoch, C and Reynolds, C. January/February 1986. Sleep disturbances and what to do about them. *Geriatric Nursing* 7:24–27.

Holtzclaw, BJ. July/August 1993. Keeping patients warm in bed. *Geriatric Nursing* 14:180–81.

Kim, MJ, McFarland, GK, and McLane, AM. 1993. *Pocket Guide to Nursing Diagnoses.* 5th ed. St Louis: Mosby-Year Book.

Knapp, M. May 1993. Night shift: The restorative sleep specialists. *Journal of Gerontological Nursing* 19:38–42.

Lederer, JR, Marculescu, GL, Mocnik, B, and Seaby, N. 1993. *Care Planning Pocket Guide—A Nursing Diagnosis Approach.* 5th ed. Redwood City, CA: Addison-Wesley Nursing.

Locsin, RC. November/December 1988. Sleeplessness among the elderly. *Rehabilitation Nursing* 13:340–41.

McFarland, GK and McFarlane, EA. 1993. *Nursing Diagnosis and Intervention: Planning for Patient Care.* 2d ed. St Louis: Mosby.

Malasanos, L, Barkauskas, V, Moss, M, and Stoltenberg-Allen, K. 1990. *Health Assessment.* 4th ed. St Louis: Mosby.

Marieb, EN. 1992. *Human Anatomy and Physiology.* 2d ed. Redwood City, CA: Benjamin/Cummings.

Maslow, A. 1970. *Motivation and Personality.* New York: Harper and Row.

Meek, SS. Spring 1993. Effects of slow stroke back massage on relaxation in hospice clients. *Image: Journal of Nursing Scholarship* 25:17–20.

Metzler, D and Finesilver, C. March 1990. When to worry if your patient can't sleep. *RN* 53:52–57.

North American Nursing Diagnosis Association. 1992. *NANDA Nursing Diagnoses: Definitions and Classification 1992–1993.* Philadelphia: NANDA.

Quine, L, Wade, K, and Hargreaves, R. November 27–December 3, 1991. Learning to sleep. *Nursing Times* 87:41–43.

Roberts, A. March 14–20, 1990. Senior systems . . . older patients and their medication . . . sleep and sleep difficulties in later life, Part 46. *Nursing Times* 86:61–64.

Stewart, A. November 1991. The sleep apnea/hypopnea syndrome. *Canadian Nurse* 87:25–27.

Walgenbach, JC. November/December 1990. Lullabye and not a good night? *Geriatric Nursing* 11:278–79.

Weaver, T, and Millman, RP. February 1986. Broken sleep. *American Journal of Nursing* 86:146–50.

36 Comfort and Pain

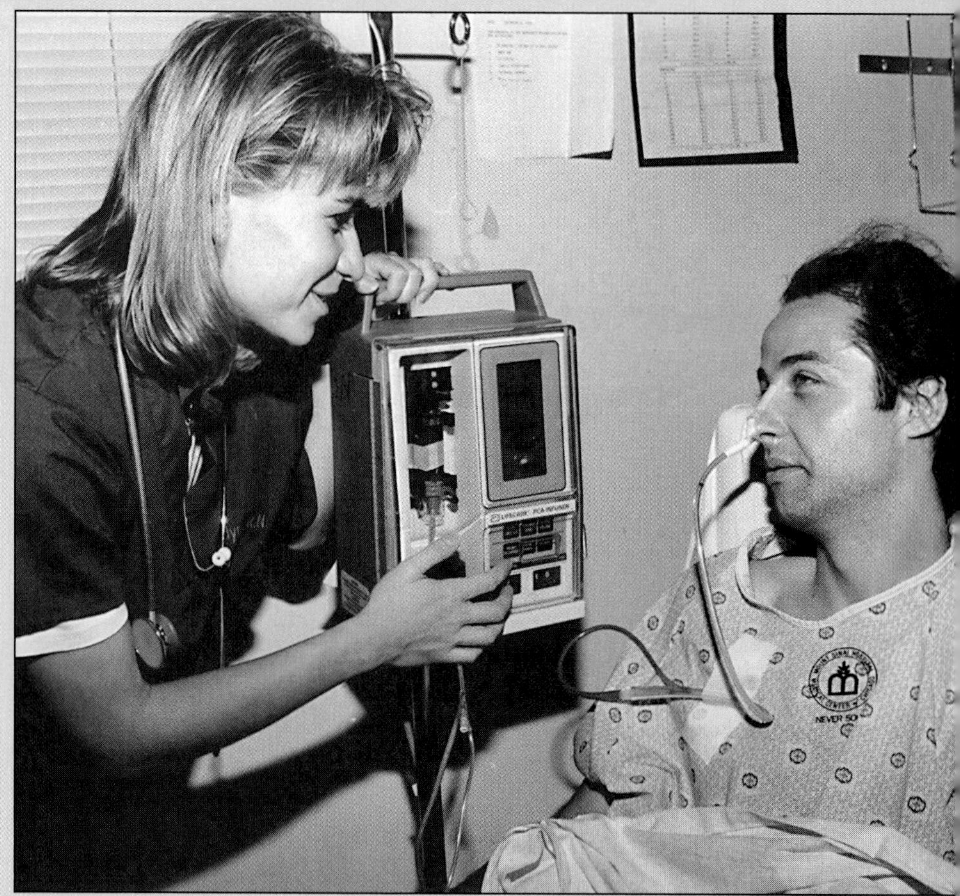

Objectives

- Differentiate various types/categories of pain according to origin, cause, and acuteness or chronicity.
- Differentiate pain threshold from pain tolerance.
- Describe pain transmission, perception, and interpretation.
- Describe the gate control theory.
- Describe the body's natural analgesic system.
- Identify subjective and objective data to be collected and analyzed when assessing pain.
- Identify examples of nursing diagnoses for clients with pain.
- State outcome criteria by which to evaluate a client's response to interventions for pain.
- Differentiate three types of analgesics: opioids, nonsteroidal anti-inflammatory drugs (NSAIDs), and adjuvant drugs.
- Describe the World Health Organization's ladder step approach to cancer pain management.
- Identify rationales for using various pain delivery routes.
- Describe nonpharmacologic pain

Pain is a highly unpleasant and very personal sensation that cannot be shared with others. It can occupy all a person's thinking, direct all activities, and change a person's life. Yet pain is a difficult concept for a client to communicate. A nurse can neither feel nor see a client's pain.

Pain is known to be the most common reason people seek help from a physician. One 1985 study found that of 1254 people contacted, most had pain within that year; headache, backache, joint pain, and stomach/abdominal pain occurred with the greatest frequency (Donovan 1990, p. 851). However, no two people experience pain in exactly the same way. In addition, the differences in individual pain perception and reaction, as well as the many causes of pain, present the nurse with a complex situation when developing a plan to relieve pain and provide comfort. Effective pain management is an important aspect of care.

The last two decades have seen a gradual shift in focus toward pain control and pain management independent of the cause of the pain. Severe pain is now being viewed as an emergency situation deserving anticipation and prompt treatment. Pain is more than a symptom of a problem; it is a high-priority problem in itself. Pain presents both physiologic and psychologic dangers to health and recovery. Pain increases morbidity and mortality. According to Bocchino (1992, p. 167), "Actual physical damage can result from unresolved pain, and ineffective pain management can inhibit recovery, prolong hospitalization, and contribute to increased health care costs." St. Marie (1991, p. 334) adds, "Driving this greater preoccupation with pain and its suppression is the recognition that pain is not just a side effect of other physiological problems: it can directly impair health and prolong recovery from surgery, disease, and trauma, all of which are accompanied by pain."

RESEARCH NOTE

How Does Ethnicity Affect Nurses' Judgments about Pain?

A study was conducted to evaluate the pain response of Mexican American and Anglo-American women who had undergone a cholecystectomy (gallbladder surgery). Responses to pain, as indicated by vital signs, rating of pain, and amount of medication used for pain, were similar for both cultural groups. However, findings did reveal a difference in the nurses' evaluation of pain in the two cultural groups. Nurses evaluated Anglo-American women as experiencing more pain than Mexican-American women. Further, nurses judged those clients to be in more pain who were (a) blue collar or professional workers, rather than unskilled workers or homemakers; (b) more educated; (c) born in the United States versus Mexico; (d) English speaking versus Spanish speaking; and (e) Protestant versus Catholic. All clients, regardless of their cultural background, evaluated their pain as more severe than did the nurses. It was also found that the ethnic background of the nurse affected the evaluation of the client's pain. Nurses of northern European background thought clients were experiencing less physical pain and distress; nurses of eastern European, southern European, or African backgrounds thought clients were experiencing more pain and psychologic distress.

Implications: Nurses' judgments about the pain their clients experience can be affected by the nurses' own beliefs and those of their cultures. Nurses need to become more aware of the influence of personal values on their assessments of a client's pain.

Source: E Calvillo and J Flaskerud, Evaluation of the pain response by Mexican American and Anglo American women and their nurses, *Journal of Advanced Nursing,* March 1993, 18:451–59.

THE NATURE OF PAIN

Although pain is a universal experience, its exact nature remains a mystery. There are a number of definitions of pain. Geach (1987, p. 12) defines **pain** as "the noxious stimulation of threatened or actual tissue damage." It is known that pain is highly subjective and individual and that it is one of the body's defense mechanisms indicating that there is a problem. McCaffery (1979, p. 11) defines pain as "whatever the experiencing person says it is, existing whenever he (or she) says it does." Basic to this definition is the caregiver's willingness to believe that the client is experiencing pain and that the client is the real authority about that pain.

MISCONCEPTIONS AND BIASES

Because pain is so difficult to understand, there are many misconceptions and biases about it. Taylor et al (1984, pp. 4–8) studied the responses of a group of registered nurses who were asked about a hypothetical client who was having pain. Some of the nurses' biases and misconceptions are described in the box on page 976.

ORIGINS AND CAUSES OF PAIN

Pain can be categorized according to its origin as cutaneous, deep somatic, or visceral. **Cutaneous pain** originates in the skin or subcutaneous tissue. A paper cut causing a sharp pain with some burning is an example of cutaneous

COMMON MISCONCEPTIONS ABOUT PAIN

Misconception	*Correction*
Clients experience severe pain only when they have had major surgery.	Even after minor surgery, clients can experience intense pain.
The nurse or other health professionals are the authorities about a client's pain.	The person who experiences the pain is the only authority about its existence and nature.
Administering analgesics regularly for pain will lead to addiction.	Clients are unlikely to become addicted to an analgesic provided to treat pain.
The amount of tissue damage is directly related to the amount of pain.	Pain is a subjective experience, and the intensity and duration of pain vary considerably among individuals.
Visible physiologic or behavioral signs accompany pain and can be used to verify its existence.	Even with severe pain, periods of physiologic and behavioral adaptation can occur.

TYPES OF PAIN

Pain is described in various ways. It can be described as either acute or chronic, based on its duration and intensity. *Acute pain* may have a sudden or slow onset; it varies from mild to severe, may last up to 6 months, and subsides as healing takes place (McCaffrey & Beebe 1989, p. 19). Acute pain is protective in that it reflects potential or present tissue damage. *Chronic pain* lasts 6 months or longer and often limits normal functioning. See Table 36–1 for a comparison of acute and chronic pain.

Pain may also be described according to where it is experienced in the body. **Radiating pain** is perceived at the source of the pain and extends to nearby tissues. For example, cardiac pain may be felt not only in the chest but also along the left shoulder and down the arm. **Referred pain** is pain felt in a part of the body that is considerably removed from the tissues causing the pain. For example, pain from one part of the abdominal viscera may be perceived in an area of the skin remote from the organ causing the pain (Figure 36–1).

Intractable pain is pain that is highly resistant to relief. One example is the pain from an advanced malignancy. Often nurses are challenged to use a number of methods, such as imagery and patient-controlled analgesia (PCA), to provide a client with pain relief. See page 1000 for additional information. **Phantom pain** is a painful sensation perceived in a missing body part (eg, an amputated leg) or in body part paralyzed from a spinal cord

pain. **Deep somatic pain** arises from ligaments, tendons, bones, blood vessels, and nerves. It is diffuse and tends to last longer than cutaneous pain. An ankle sprain is an example of deep somatic pain. **Visceral pain** results from stimulation of pain receptors in the abdominal cavity, cranium, and thorax. Visceral pain tends to appear diffuse and often feels like deep somatic pain, that is, burning, aching, or a feeling of pressure. Visceral pain is frequently caused by stretching of the tissues, ischemia, or muscle spasms.

Pain can have a physical cause (eg, a broken femur) or a psychogenic cause (that is, a physical cause cannot be identified). It has been suggested that pain rarely results from just a single cause and that most pain has both physical and psychogenic origins. Also, many believe that pain resulting from emotional trauma is just as intense as pain resulting from a physical cause.

The National Institutes of Health (NIH) Consensus Development Conference (1987, p. 35) suggested three categories of pain that are based on the pain's cause: (1) pain following acute injury, disease or some type of surgery **(acute pain);** pain associated with cancer or other progressive disorders **(chronic malignant pain);** and pain in persons whose tissue injury is nonprogressive or healed **(chronic nonmalignant pain).**

Table 36–1 Comparison of Acute and Chronic Pain

Acute Pain	Chronic Pain
Mild to severe Sympathetic nervous system responses: Increased pulse rate Increased respiratory rate Elevated blood pressure Diaphoresis Dilated pupils	Mild to severe Parasympathetic nervous system responses: Vital signs normal Dry, warm skin Pupils normal or dilated
Related to tissue injury; resolves with healing	Continues beyond healing
Client appears restless and anxious	Client appears depressed and withdrawn
Client reports pain	Client often does not mention pain unless asked
Client exhibits behavior indicative of pain: crying, rubbing area, holding area	Pain behavior often absent

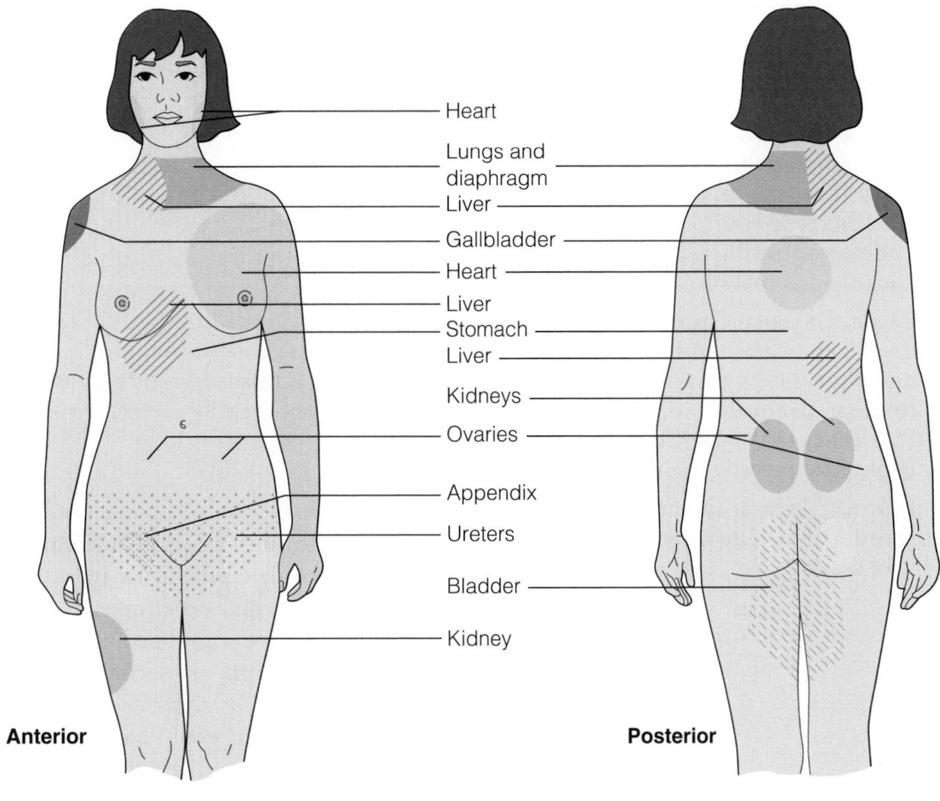

Figure 36–1 Common sites of referred pain from various body organs.

injury (Davis 1993, p. 80). It can be distinguished from a **phantom sensation,** that is, the feeling that the missing body part is still present.

Phantom pain is thought to result from stimulation of a severed dendrite rather than the stimulation of the pain receptor. It occurs most frequently in clients who experienced pain before the removal of the body part.

CONCEPTS ASSOCIATED WITH PAIN

When an individual perceives pain from injured tissue, the pain threshold is reached. An individual's **pain threshold** is the amount of pain stimulation a person requires in order to feel pain. People's pain threshold is generally fairly uniform; however, it can change. For example, the same stimuli that once produced mild pain can at another time produce intense pain. Excessive sensitivity to pain is called *hyperalgesia.*

Two additional terms used in the context of pain are pain sensation and pain reaction. **Pain sensation** can be considered the same as pain threshold; **pain reaction** includes the autonomic nervous system and behavioral responses to pain. The autonomic nervous system response is the automatic reaction of the body that often protects the individual from further harm, for example, the automatic withdrawal of the hand from a hot stove. The behavioral response is a learned response used as a method of coping with the pain.

Pain tolerance is the maximum amount and duration of pain that an individual is willing to endure. Some clients are unable to tolerate even the slightest pain, whereas others are willing to endure severe pain rather than be treated for it. Thus, pain tolerance varies greatly among people and is widely influenced by psychologic and sociocultural factors. Pain tolerance appears to increase with age.

PAIN SYNDROMES

Certain pain syndromes have been identified to describe conditions associated with prolonged severe pain. Three of these syndromes are described in the box on the left on page 978.

PHYSIOLOGY OF PAIN

How pain is transmitted and perceived is still incompletely understood. Whether pain is perceived or not and to what degree depend on the interaction between the body's analgesia system and the nervous system's transmission and interpretation of stimuli.

THREE PAIN SYNDROMES

- *Postherpetic neuralgia.* An episode of herpes has two phases: a vesicular eruption and neuralgic pain that encircles the body. The pain ranges from mild to severe. In the postherpetic syndrome, severe pain persists for months or years with lightning-like pain in the area of the original eruption.
- *Headache.* This common somatic pain can be caused by either intracranial or extracranial problems. To establish a plan to prevent or treat headache, the nurse needs to assess the quality, location, onset, duration, and frequency of the pain, as well as any signs and symptoms that precede the headache.
- *Cancer pain syndrome.* These syndromes can result from the progression of the disease or from efforts to cure or control the disease.

Source: Adapted from NT Meinhart and M McCaffery, *Pain: A Nursing Approach to Assessment and Analysis,* (Norwalk, CT: Appleton-Century-Crofts, 1983).

STIMULATION OF NOCICEPTORS

When a pain threshold has been reached and there is injured tissue, substances that stimulate the pain receptors called **nociceptors,** are released. These pain receptors can be stimulated by serotonin, histamine, potassium ions, acids, and some enzymes (Guyton 1991, p. 521). **Bradykinin,** a powerful vasodilator that also increases capillary permeability, is released at the site of an injury and in turn causes the release of inflammatory chemicals such as histamine. These two chemicals (bradykinin and histamine) cause the area to redden, swell, and become tender. Bradykinin also stimulates the release of prostaglandins. These compounds sensitize the pain receptors and enhance the effects of bradykinin and histamine. Another chemical, **substance P,** may act as a stimulant to the nociceptors as well as be involved in the inflammatory response of the tissues. In addition, substance P is known to be a neurotransmitter that enhances the movement of impulses across the nerve synapse from the primary afferent neuron to the second-order neuron (Figure 36–2).

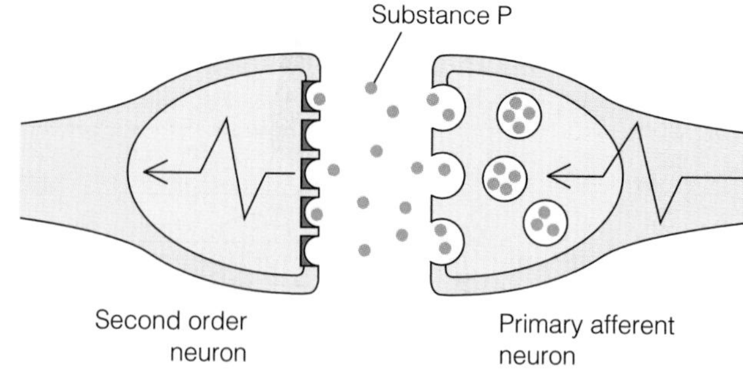

Figure 36–2 Substance P assists the transmission of impulses across the synapse from the primary afferent neuron to a second-order neuron.

Nociceptors are stimulated either directly, by damage to the receptor cell, or secondarily, by the release of chemicals such as bradykinin. Basically, there are three types of stimuli that excite corresponding types of nociceptors: mechanical, thermal, and chemical. See Table 36–2.

Some body tissues, such as the brain and the alveoli, have no nociceptors. Other tissues, such as the skin and certain internal tissues—the periosteum, the joint surfaces, and the arterial walls, for example—have many receptors. Most other deep tissues have few pain receptors. Although all nociceptors are structurally similar, they respond differently to noxious stimuli according to their body location. For example, a cut in the skin causes acute pain, but a similar injury in the viscera does not. Similarly, moderate stretching produces visceral pain but not skin pain.

TYPES OF PAIN FIBERS

Type of Fiber	*Description of Pain*
"Fast" fibers	Sharp, pricking, acute, electric
"Slow" fibers	Burning, aching, throbbing, nauseous, chronic

TRANSMISSION OF PAIN STIMULI

There are two separate pathways that transmit pain impulses to the brain. One pathway (made up of type A-delta fibers) carries **fast pain** (sharp pain) to the spinal cord. The second pathway (made up of type C fibers) carry the **slow pain** (chronic pain) impulse to the spinal cord. See the box above for information about fast and slow pain fibers. The pain fibers enter the spinal cord through the dorsal horn (Figure 36–3). Here they synapse with second-order neurons.

This first synapse is considered to be the pain gate. (See the discussion of the gate control theory of pain, p. 980.) If the pain stimuli are strong enough, they will pass the pain gate and be carried to the brain. The fast A fibers primarily conduct impulses from mechanical and thermal pain. They synapse with second-order neurons

Table 36–2 Types of Pain Stimuli

Stimulus Type	Physiologic Basis
Mechanical	
1. Trauma to body tissues (eg, surgery)	Tissue damage; direct irritation of the pain receptors; inflammation
2. Alterations in body tissues (eg, edema)	Pressure on pain receptors
3. Blockage of a body duct	Distention of the lumen of the duct
4. Tumor	Pressure on pain receptors; irritation of nerve endings
5. Muscle spasm	Stimulation of pain receptors (also see chemical stimuli)
Thermal	
Extreme heat or cold (eg, burns)	Tissue destruction; stimulation of thermosensitive pain receptors
Chemical	
1. Tissue ischemia (eg, blocked coronary artery)	Stimulation of pain receptors because of accumulated lactic acid (and other chemicals, such as bradykinin and enzymes) in tissues
2. Muscle spasm	Secondary to mechanical stimulation (see above), causing tissue ischemia

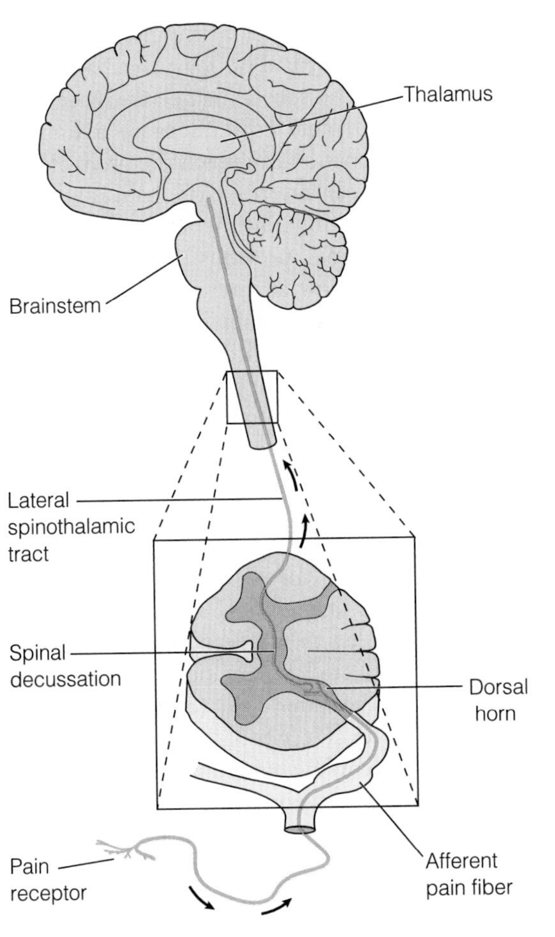

Figure 36–3 The pain impulse is transmitted along a primary afferent pain fiber to the dorsal horn of the spinal cord. The fiber synapses with a second-order neuron, which crosses over at the other side of the spinal cord and ascends to the thalamus.

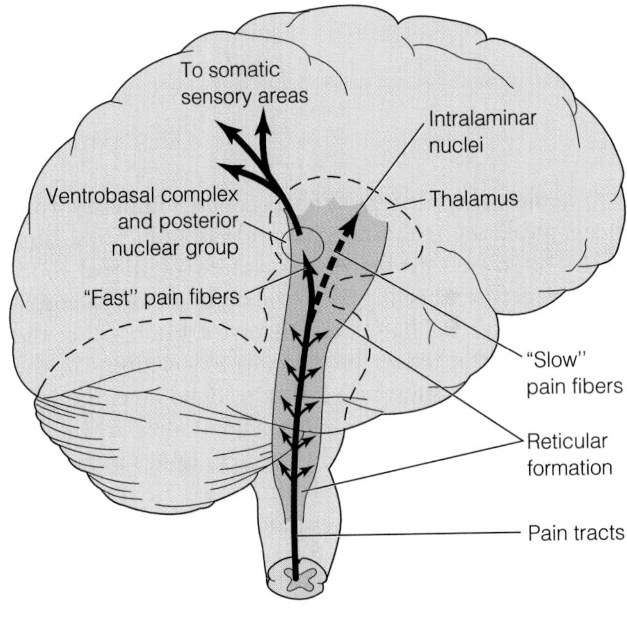

Figure 36–4 The transmission of pain signals to the higher brain centers.

(long fibers), which cross immediately to the opposite side of the spinal cord and then enter the neospinothalamic tract and ascend to the brain. A few fibers terminate in the reticular areas of the brain stem, but most terminate in the thalamus. From there signals are sent to the basal areas of the brain and to the somatic sensory cortex (Figure 36–4).

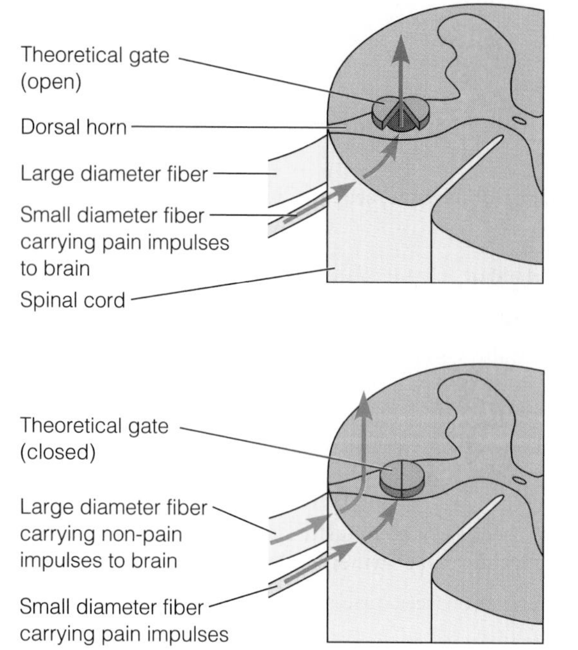

Figure 36–5 A schematic illustration of the gate control theory.

The slow chronic type C fibers conduct impulses from mechanical, thermal, and chemical stimuli. These impulses often pass through one or more additional short neurons before traveling up to the brain by the paleospinothalamic tract. The C fibers release substance P as the synaptic transmitter to the second-order neurons in the spinal cord. This substance is slow to build up at the synaptic junction of the two neurons and slow to be destroyed. This is probably why pain continues to be perceived even after the painful stimuli has been removed (Guyton 1991, p. 523). Most of the second-order neurons of the slow chronic type C fibers end in the brain stem (eg, the medulla, pons, and mesencephalon), with only one-tenth to one-fourth of them passing all the way to the thalamus (Guyton 1991, p. 523). Additional neurons communicate the pain impulses from the brain stem to the thalamus, the hypothalamus, and other areas of the brain.

PAIN PERCEPTION

Pain perception is the point at which the person becomes aware of the pain. The pain stimuli transmitted along the nerve fibers as described earlier, enter the spinal cord, and ascend the cord to the thalamus reticular formation. Conscious perception of the pain probably occurs initially at the brain stem and thalamic level. Interpretation and localization of the pain is thought to occur in the cerebral cortex (Guyton 1991, p. 523). The cerebral cortex is thought to play a role in interpreting the quality of the pain even though pain perception may be a function of lower centers such as the thalamus and reticular formation (Guyton 1991, p. 523).

GATE CONTROL THEORY

In 1965, Melzack and Wall proposed the gate control theory (1982, p. 232). According to this theory, peripheral nerve fibers carrying pain to the spinal cord can have their input modified at the spinal cord level before transmission to the brain. Synapses in the dorsal horns act as gates that close to keep impulses from reaching the brain or open to permit impulses to ascend to the brain.

According to the gate control theory, small-diameter nerve fibers carry pain stimuli through a gate, but large-diameter nerve fibers going through the same gate can inhibit the transmission of those pain impulses—that is, close the gate (Figure 36–5). The gate mechanism is thought to be situated in the substantia gelatinosa cells in the dorsal horn of the spinal cord. Because a limited amount of sensory information can reach the brain at any given time, certain cells can interrupt the pain impulses. The brain also appears to influence whether the gate is open or closed. For example, previous experiences with pain are known to affect how an individual responds to pain. The involvement of the brain helps explain why painful stimuli are interpreted differently by people. Although the gate control theory is not unanimously accepted, it does help explain why electrical and mechanical interventions as well as heat and pressure can relieve pain. For example, a back massage may stimulate impulses in large nerves, which in turn, close the gate to back pain.

The original gate control theory has been adapted to encompass new findings and clinical applications. The gate control theory has led to the recognition that pain can be reduced or modulated at four points: (a) the peripheral site of pain, (b) the spinal cord, (c) the brain stem, and (d) the cerebral cortex (Herr & Mobily 1992, p. 348). The theory remains incomplete but is used as the basis for many pain management interventions.

The pain gate in the spinal cord can be shut in several different ways:

- *Stimulation of touch fibers (mechanoreceptors).* Stimulation of the tactile fibers of the skin inhibits the transmission of pain signals from the same area of the body or even from other areas of the body (Guyton 1991, p. 525). These touch fibers are stimulated by rubbing, stroking, massage, vibration, and application of liniments and other ointments.

- *Release of endogenous opioids.* Natural mechanisms (neuromodulators) within the body are thought to modulate pain transmission and pain perception. This pain control system is called an **analgesia system** (Guyton 1991, p. 524). It releases morphinelike drugs into the body. These **endogenous opioids** are produced in various parts of the central nervous system. They are thought to decrease or block the pain impulses at the dorsal horn level of the spinal cord and at other levels of the central nervous system. Certain pain relief therapies, such as acupuncture, are thought to stimulate the release of endogenous opioids. To date, about one dozen of these substances have been found. The more important of these substances are met-enkephalin, leu-enkephalin, β-endorphin, and dynorphin.
- *Electrical stimulation.* Electrical stimulation of the skin's sensory nerve fibers inhibits pain. The electrodes can be placed around the painful area or over the spinal cord. The client controls the amount of stimulation to achieve the best level of pain control. A description of the transcutaneous electrical nerve stimulation (TENS) unit for pain management is provided later in this chapter.
- *Morphine and other opioid drugs.* The opioid drugs bind to the opioid receptors of the nerve cells in the dorsal horn of the spinal cord where the pain is transmitted. This binding alters the function of the nerve cell, and transmission of the pain signal is inhibited or blocked completely. Opioids also bind to opioid receptors in the brain responsible for perception and interpretation of pain.
- *Normal and excessive sensory stimuli.* Sensory stimulation may also relieve pain by competing with the pain stimuli for attention. The client "tunes out" the pain. The brain stem can inhibit incoming stimuli, including pain, if the person is receiving sufficient or excessive sensory input (McCaffery and Beebe 1989, p. 36). The brain stem may be able to close the pain gate with inhibitory impulses. Such things as music, application of heat and cold, imagery, and elaborate distractions such as video games can all be used to close the pain gate. A nonstimulating, monotonous environment tends to open the pain gate, increasing pain perception.
- *Cerebral cortex and thalamic inhibition of pain.* The gate control theory suggests that pain can be relieved by inhibitory signals from the cerebral cortex and the thalamus (McCaffery 1989, p. 37). Pain may be relieved by reducing anxiety and fear and teaching the client about the pain and helping the client feel capable of controlling the pain. The fear and anxiety that result from not knowing what to expect and feeling helpless tend to open the gate, increasing pain perception.

Table 36–3 Responses to Pain

Sympathetic Responses	Parasympathetic Responses
Increased pulse rate	Decreased pulse rate
Increased systolic blood pressure	Decreased systolic blood pressure; syncope
Increased respiratory rate	Variable breathing pattern
Diaphoresis	Nausea/vomiting
Increased muscle tension	Warm, dry skin
Pallor	Prostration
Pupil dilation	Pupil constriction
Rapid speech/elevated pitch	Slow, monotonous speech
Increased alertness	Withdrawal

Responses to Pain

The body's response to pain is a complex process rather than a specific action. It involves physiologic and psychosocial aspects. Initially the sympathetic nervous system responds, resulting in the fight-or-flight response. See Table 36–3. As pain continues, the body adapts as the parasympathetic nervous system takes over, reversing many of the initial physiologic responses. This adaptation to the pain occurs after several hours or days of pain. The actual pain receptors adapt very little and continue to transmit the pain message. This serves the purpose of keeping the person continually aware of the damaging stimuli causing the pain (Guyton 1991, p. 521). The person may learn to cope with the pain through cognitive and behavioral activities, such as diversions, imagery, and excessive sleeping. The individual may respond to pain by seeking out physical interventions to manage the pain, such as analgesics, massage, and exercise.

There is also a proprioceptive reflex that occurs with the stimulation of pain receptors. Impulses travel along sensory pain fibers to the spinal cord. There they synapse with motor neurons, and the impulses travel back via motor fibers to a muscle near the site of the pain (Figure 36–6, p. 982). The muscle then contracts in a protective action. For example, when a person touches a hot stove the hand reflexively draws back from the heat even before the person is aware of the pain.

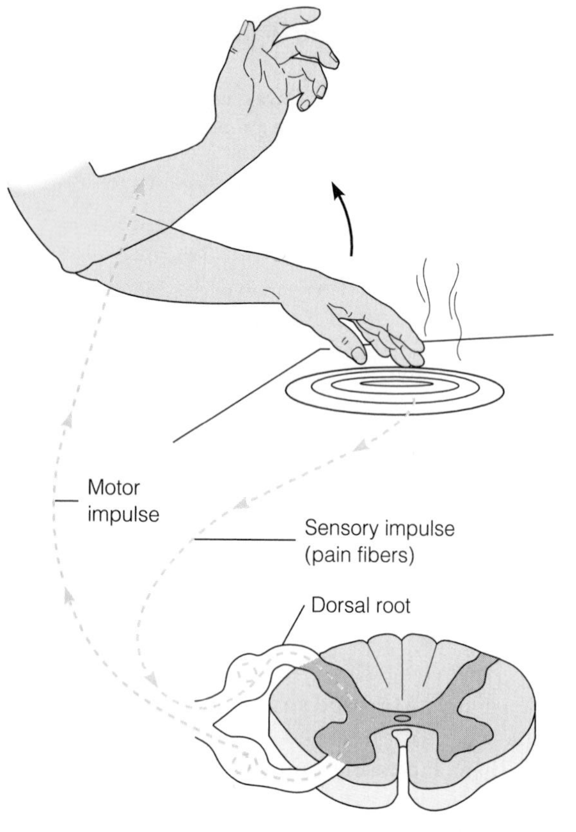

Figure 36–6 Proprioceptive reflex to a pain stimulus.

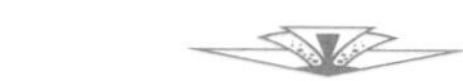

FACTORS AFFECTING THE PAIN EXPERIENCE

Numerous factors can affect a person's perception and reaction to pain. These include the ethnic/cultural values, age, environment and support persons, and anxiety and stress.

Ethnic/Cultural Values In some cultures, pain may be considered a punishment for bad deeds; the individual is, therefore, to tolerate pain without complaint in order to atone for sins. In some Middle Eastern and African cultures, self-infliction of pain is a sign of mourning or grief. In other groups, pain may be anticipated as a part of the ritualistic practices of passage ceremonies, and therefore tolerance of pain signifies strength and endurance. The meaning of pain will affect the individual's perception of pain, tolerance of painful stimuli, and the expression of or reaction to pain.

Age Age is an important variable that influences how people admit or describe pain and how they behave. See Table 36–4.

Environment and Support Persons A strange environment such as a hospital, with its noises, lights and activity, can compound pain. In addition, the lonely person who is without a support network may perceive pain as severe, whereas the person who has supportive people around may not perceive the pain as greatly. Some people prefer to withdraw when they are in pain, whereas others prefer the distraction of people and activity around them.

Some clients use pain to acquire secondary gains, that is, special attention from support persons and nurses. If the situation becomes difficult for the support persons, the nurse can intervene and discuss the problem before the support persons become angry and avoid the client.

Expectations of significant others can affect a person's perceptions of and responses to pain. In some situations, for example, girls may be permitted to express pain more openly than boys. Family role can also affect how a person perceives or responds to pain. For instance, a single mother supporting three children may ignore pain because of her need to stay on the job. The presence of support persons often changes a client's reaction to pain. For example, toddlers often tolerate pain more readily when supportive parents or nurses are nearby.

Anxiety and Stress Anxiety often accompanies pain. Threat of the unknown and the inability to control the pain or the events surrounding it often augment the pain perception. Fatigue also reduces a person's ability to cope, thereby increasing pain perception. When pain interferes with sleep, fatigue and muscle tension often result and increase the pain; thus a cycle of pain, fatigue, pain develops.

The issue of control is central to pain management (Paradis 1992, p. 39). *Locus of control* refers to how individuals believe the events in their life are controlled. **Internal locus of control** refers to the belief that events in a person's life are self-controlled (internal orientation), whereas an **external locus of control** refers to an external control over events in life (external orientation). Clients who have an internal locus of control see themselves as having control over the events around them. People in pain who believe they can control their own pain are thought to have less pain than those who depend on others for relief. They are often relieved of the anxiety about whether they can obtain relief. Anxiety and pain are interrelated. Increasing anxiety makes pain less tolerable, just as increasing pain heightens anxiety (Paradis 1992, p. 39).

ASSESSING

To assess a client's pain, the nurse obtains a pain history and a daily diary (optional) and conducts a physical examination that focuses on the client's physiologic and behavioral responses to the pain.

Table 36–4 Age Variations in the Pain Experience

Age Group	Pain Perception and Behavior	Selected Nursing Interventions
Infant	Perceives pain. Responds to pain with increased sensitivity. Older infant tries to avoid pain; for example, turns away and physically resists.	Give a glucose pacifier. Use tactile stimulation. Play music or tapes of a heartbeat.
Toddler and preschooler	Develops the ability to describe pain and its intensity and location. Often responds with crying and anger because child perceives pain as a threat to security. Reasoning with a child at this stage is not always successful. May consider pain a punishment. Feels sad. May learn there are gender differences in pain expression. Tends to hold someone accountable for the pain.	Distract the child with toys, books, pictures. Involve the child in blowing bubbles as a way of "blowing away the pain." Appeal to the child's belief in magic by using a "magic" blanket or glove to take away pain. Hold the child to provide comfort. Explore misconceptions about pain.
School-age child	Tries to be brave when facing pain. Rationalizes in an attempt to explain the pain. Responsive to explanations. Can usually identify the location and describe the pain. With persistent pain, may regress to an earlier stage of development.	Use imagery to turn off "pain switches." Provide a behavioral rehearsal of what to expect and how it will look and feel. Provide support and nurturing.
Adolescent	May be slow to acknowledge pain. Recognizing pain or "giving in" may be considered weakness. Wants to appear brave in front of peers and not report pain.	Provide opportunities to discuss pain. Provide privacy. Present choices for dealing with pain. Encourage music or TV for distraction.
Adult	Behaviors exhibited when experiencing pain may be gender-based behaviors learned as a child. May ignore pain because to admit it is perceived as a sign of weakness or failure. May use pain for secondary gain, for example, to get attention. Fear of what pain means may prevent some adults from taking action.	Deal with any misconceptions about pain. Focus on the client's control in dealing with the pain. Allay fears and anxiety when possible.
Older adult	May perceive pain as part of the aging process. May have decreased sensations or perceptions of the pain. Lethargy, anorexia, and fatigue may be indicators of pain. May withhold complaints of pain because of fear of the treatment, of any life-style changes that may be involved, or of becoming dependent. May describe pain differently, that is, as "ache," "hurt," or "discomfort." May consider it unacceptable to admit or show pain. See also the box on page 985.	Spend time with the client, and listen carefully. Clarify misconceptions. Encourage independence whenever possible.

ASSESSMENT INTERVIEW

Pain History

- *Location:* Where is your pain?
- *Intensity:* On a scale of 0 to 10 (with 1 representing the least pain level), how would you rate the degree of discomfort you are having?
- *Quality:* Tell me what your pain feels like.
- *Pattern:*

  Time of onset: When did or does the pain start?

  Duration: How long have you had it, or how long does it usually last?

  Constancy: Do you have pain-free periods? When? And for how long?
- *Precipitating factors:* What triggers the pain or makes it worse?
- *Alleviating factors:* What measures or methods have you found helpful in lessening or relieving the pain? What pain medications do you use?
- *Associated symptoms:* Do you have any other symptoms (eg, nausea, dizziness, blurred vision, shortness of breath) before, during, or after your pain?
- *Effects on activities of daily living:* How does the pain affect your daily life (eg, eating, working, sleeping, social/recreational activities)?
- *Past pain experiences:* Tell me about past pain experiences you have had and the effectiveness of pain relief measures.
- *Meaning of pain:* How do you interpret your pain? What outcomes (implications) do you anticipate from this pain? What do you fear most about your pain?
- *Coping resources:* What do you usually do to help cope with pain?
- *Affective response:* How does the pain make you feel? Anxious? Depressed? Frightened? Tired? Burdensome?

PAIN HISTORY

While taking the pain histories, the nurse must provide an opportunity for clients to express in their own words how they view the pain and the situation. This will help the nurse understand what the pain means to the client and how the client is coping with it. Remember that each person's pain experience is unique and that the client is the best interpreter of the pain experience. This history should be geared to the specific client: for example, questions asked of an accident victim would be different from those asked of a postoperative client or one suffering from chronic pain. The initial pain assessment for someone in *severe acute pain* may consist of only a few questions (eg, pain location, intensity, and description) before intervention occurs. In addition, the nurse may focus on the following:

- Previous pain treatment and effectiveness
- When and what analgesics were last taken
- Other medications being taken
- Allergies to medications

For the person with *chronic pain*, the nurse may focus on the client's coping mechanisms, effectiveness of current pain management, and ways in which the pain has affected activities of daily living (ADLs).

Data that should be obtained in a comprehensive pain history include pain location, intensity, quality, patterns, precipitating factors, alleviating factors, associated symptoms, effect on ADLs, past pain experiences, meaning of the pain to the person, coping resources, and affective responses. Questions to elicit this data are shown in the box at the left.

Location Nurses need to ascertain where the client experiences pain. The various body landmarks for describing abdominal pain location are shown in Chapter 22, pages 532 and 534. In addition, the nurse needs to use such terms as *proximal*, *distal*, *medial*, *lateral*, and *diffuse* when describing the location of pain.

When assessing the location of a child's pain, the nurse needs to understand the child's vocabulary. For example, *tummy* might refer either to the abdomen or to part of the chest. Asking a child to point to the pain helps clarify the child's word usage to identify location. Parents, too, can help nurses interpret the meaning of a child's words.

A *pain chart* consisting of drawings of the body and body parts is another means of determining pain location (Figure 36–9, later in this chapter). The client marks the location of pain on the drawing. This tool can be especially effective with clients who have more than one source of pain.

Intensity Because pain is a subjective experience, the nurse must remember that the single most important indicator of the existence and intensity of pain is the client's report of the pain. Pain intensity rating scales are usually available in all health care agencies for all clients and caregivers to use. Such scales provide consistency for nurses to communicate with the client and with each other. One simple rating scale is shown in Figure 36–7.

The client is asked to indicate the scale point that best represents the client's pain intensity. It is very important to note and report any change in intensity and factors that may have caused this change. For example, the abrupt ces-

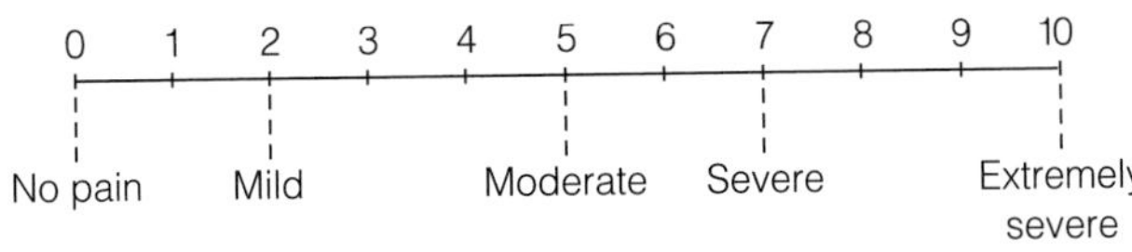

Figure 36–7 A pain intensity scale.

sation of acute abdominal pain may indicate a ruptured appendix. Several factors affect the perception of intensity. One is amount of distraction, or the client's concentration on another event; a second is the client's state of consciousness, and a third is the person's expectations. Beliefs of elderly clients that may interfere with their willingness to acknowledge and report pain are shown in the box at the right.

Nonverbal assessment tools can be used with children who are unable to communicate discomfort verbally or with elderly clients who manifest language or mental capacity difficulties. Two of these are the Wong/Baker Faces Rating Scale (Figure 36–8) and color tools. *Color tools* are used not only to help describe pain intensity, but also to locate it. The client selects colors that represent different levels of pain intensity and then, on a full body diagram, colors the body part or parts that hurt, using the color best representing the current pain.

For infants and preschoolers, the nurse must rely on observation of behavioral cues. See Physical Examination, later in this chapter.

Terms used to describe pain intensity are consistent across cultures. *Pain* is used for the most intense pain, *hurt* for less intense, and *ache* for least intense (Gaston-Johansson et al 1990, p. 99).

BELIEFS OF ELDERLY CLIENTS THAT MAY INTERFERE WITH WILLINGNESS TO ACKNOWLEDGE AND REPORT PAIN

- Pain is a normal component of aging and should be expected and tolerated.
- Pain and suffering are challenges with positive effects.
- Pain is a weakness.
- Pain is a punishment for some wrong deed.
- Reporting pain will cause the health care staff to label one a "bad patient."
- Nursing staff is "too busy" to hear complaints.
- Reporting pain may lead to further tests and expenses.
- Using drugs now will render the drug inefficient if or when the pain becomes worse.
- Use of opioids will lead to addiction.
- The side effects of drugs will make daily living more difficult or change one's behavior or personality.
- Use of drugs signals the nearness of death.

Source: SL Hofland, Elder beliefs: Blocks to pain management, *Journal of Gerontological Nursing*, June 1992, 18:19–24, 39–40.

Quality Descriptive adjectives help people communicate the quality of pain. A headache may be described as "hammerlike" or an abdominal pain as "piercing like a knife." Sometimes clients have difficulty describing pain because they have never experienced any sensation like it.

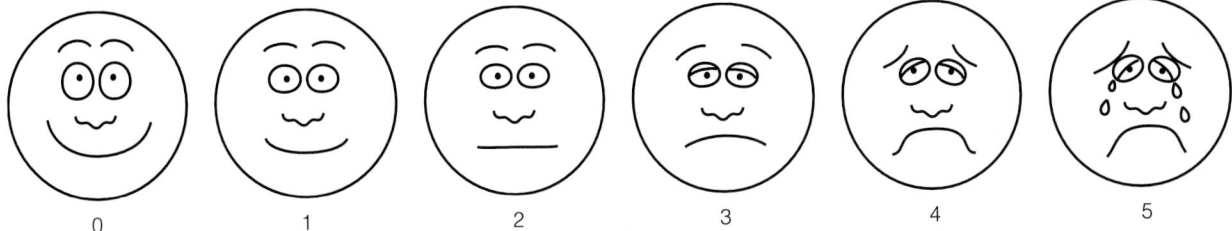

1. Explain to the child that each face represents either a person who feels happy because the person has no pain ("hurt," or whatever word the child uses) or a person who feels sad because the person has some or a lot of pain.
2. Point to the appropriate face and say, "This face . . .":
   0—"is very happy because he (or she) doesn't hurt at all."
   1—"hurts just a little bit."
   2—"hurts just a little more."
   3—"hurts even more."
   4—"hurts a whole lot."
   5—"hurts as much as you can imagine, although you don't have to be crying to feel this bad."
3. Ask the child to choose the face that best describes how the child feels. Be specific about which pain (eg, "shot" or incision) and what time (eg, now? Earlier, before lunch?).

Figure 36–8 The Wong/Baker Faces Rating Scale. **Source:** DL Wong, *Whaley and Wong's Essentials of Pediatric Nursing,* 4th ed. (St Louis: Mosby, 1993), p. 597. Reprinted with permission.

COMMONLY USED PAIN DESCRIPTORS

	Sensory Words	Affective Words		Sensory Words	Affective Words
Pain	searing	unbearable	Hurt	hurting	
	scalding	killing		pricking	
	sharp	intense		pressing	
	piercing	torturing		tender	
	drilling	agonizing	Ache	numb	annoying
	wrenching	terrifying		cold	nagging
	shooting	grueling		flickering	tiring
	splitting	suffocating		radiating	troublesome
	crushing	frightful		dull	
	penetrating	punishing		sore	
		miserable		aching	
				cramping	

Source: Reprinted by permission of Elsevier Science Inc. from F Gaston-Johansson, M Albert, E Fagen, and L Zimmerman, Similarities in pain descriptors of four different ethnic-cultural groups, *Journal of Pain and Symptom Management*, April 1990, 5:94–100. Copyright 1990 by the US Cancer Pain Relief Committee.

This is particularly true of children, and of adults who have pain originating within the nervous system. Some of the terms commonly used to describe pain are listed in the box above.

Nurses need to record the exact words clients use to describe pain. A client's words are more accurate and descriptive than an interpretation in the nurse's words.

Pattern The pattern of pain includes time of onset, duration, and persistence of or intervals without pain. The nurse therefore determines when the pain began; how long the pain lasts; whether it recurs and, if so, the length of the interval without pain; and when the pain last occurred.

Precipitating Factors Certain activities sometimes precede pain, for example, physical exertion may precede chest pain, or abdominal pain may occur after eating. These observations can help prevent pain and determine its cause.

Environmental factors such as extreme cold or heat and extremes of humidity can affect some types of pain. For example, sudden exercise on a hot day can cause muscle spasm.

Physical and emotional stressors can also precipitate pain. Emotional tension frequently brings on a migraine headache. Intense fear or physical exertion can cause angina.

Alleviating Factors Included in this area of assessment are analgesics taken, rest, and applications of heat or cold. The nurse should also explore how long such measures were employed before relief was obtained and whether they had any effect at all or even made the pain worse.

Associated Symptoms Also included in the clinical appraisal of pain are any other associated symptoms, such as nausea, vomiting, dizziness, and diarrhea. Sometimes clients experience such a symptom immediately prior to the pain.

Effect on Activities of Daily Living Knowing how activities of daily living (ADLs) are affected by chronic pain helps the nurse understand the client's perspective on the pain's severity. A number of tools have been developed to assist the nurse with this assessment, including a scale measuring the effects of pain on daily life. See Table 36–5.

Past Pain Experiences Previous pain experiences alter a client's sensitivity to pain. People who have personally experienced pain or who have been exposed to the suffering of someone close are often more threatened by anticipated pain than people without a pain experience. In addition, the success or lack of success of pain relief measures influence a person's expectations for relief. For example, a person who has tried several pain relief measures without success may have little hope about the helpfulness of nursing interventions.

Meaning of Pain Some clients may accept pain more readily than others, depending on the circumstances and the client's interpretation of its significance. A client who associates the pain with a positive outcome may withstand

Table 36–5 Scale for Assessing the Effects of Pain on Daily Life

On a scale of 0 (no pain) to 10 (maximum pain) the client should indicate the areas of life (listed below) currently affected and the severity of the interference. If the client's current level of pain is less than that usually felt, the client should be asked to rate the most pain ever experienced in these areas.

Sleep	Home activities
Appetite	Driving/walking
Concentration	Leisure activities
Work/school	Emotional status (mood, irritability, depression, anxiety)
Interpersonal relationships	
Marital relations/sex	

Source: E Matassarin-Jacobs, PhD, RN, OCN, Pain Assessment, unpublished presentation, Chicago, Illinois, May 1981. Used by permission. As cited in JP Bellack and PA Bamford, *Nursing Assessment: A Multi Dimensional Approach* (Monterey, CA: Wadsworth Health Sciences, 1984), p. 338.

the pain amazingly well. For example, a woman giving birth to a child or an athlete undergoing knee surgery to prolong his career may tolerate pain better because of the benefit associated with it. These clients may view the pain as a temporary inconvenience rather than a potential threat or disruption to daily life.

By contrast, clients with unrelenting chronic pain may suffer more intensely. They may respond with despair, anxiety, and depression, since they cannot attach a positive significance or purpose to the pain. In this situation, the pain may be looked upon as a threat to body image or life-style and as a sign of possible impending death.

Coping Resources Clients sometimes learn highly effective ways of coping with pain. These methods may modify the pain to such a degree that assessment of pain will be incomplete unless the nurse is aware of them. For example, Mr Green may tell the nurse that his abdominal pain lasted only a few minutes and neglect to say that he took an antacid when the pain started. People in pain often display coping strategies and styles learned in childhood. Some of these include distraction, withdrawal, and expectations of help from others.

Affective Responses Affective responses vary according to the situation, the degree and duration of pain, the interpretation of it, and many other factors. The nurse needs to explore the client's feelings, be they anxiety, fear, exhaustion, depression, or a sense of failure. Because many people with chronic pain become depressed and potentially suicidal, it may also be necessary to assess the client's suicide risk. In such situations, the nurse needs to ask the client, "Do you ever feel so bad that you want to die? Do you feel that way now?"

THE MCGILL-MELZACK PAIN QUESTIONNAIRE

Some pain centers ask clients to complete a comprehensive pain questionnaire. The McGill-Melzack Pain Questionnaire (MPQ) shown in Figure 36–9 incorporates 20 categories of pain descriptors grouped into (a) sensory components, (b) affective components, (c) one evaluative component, and (d) miscellaneous terms. In addition, a present pain intensity (PPI) rating scale of 0 to 5 enables clients to indicate the degree of pain they experience. The anterior and posterior figures of the human body allow the client to mark the location of the pain.

Although the MPQ is one of the most commonly known assessment tools for assessing a pain problem, it is complex, and time consuming. Some of the possible descriptors may be difficult for some clients to understand and the large list of choices may be overwhelming. This questionnaire may take some clients several sittings to complete.

DAILY PAIN DIARY

A daily diary may help the client and nurse identify certain factors associated with the pain, for example, factors that exacerbate or mediate the pain experience. The client records various information, such as time of onset of pain, activity before pain, pain-related positions or behaviors, pain intensity level, use of analgesics or other relief measures, duration of pain, time spent in relief activities, and so on. Recorded data can provide useful information to plan interventions. As a prerequisite to using this type of assessment tool, the nurse must first assess the client's fine motor skills and cognitive functioning.

PHYSICAL EXAMINATION

To determine the client's physiologic and behavioral responses to pain, the nurse assesses the client's vital signs and observes the client for skin color changes, skin dryness, diaphoresis, facial expression, and body gestures that reflect pain, discomfort, or anxiety. These findings provide valuable information about the severity of pain and how the client is coping with it.

Physiologic Responses Physiologic responses vary according to whether the pain is acute or chronic. Acute pain stimulates the sympathetic nervous system, resulting in increased blood pressure, pulse rate, respiratory rate, pallor, diaphoresis, and pupil dilation. With prolonged severe chronic pain or visceral pain, signs of parasympathetic stimulation may be observed: lowered blood

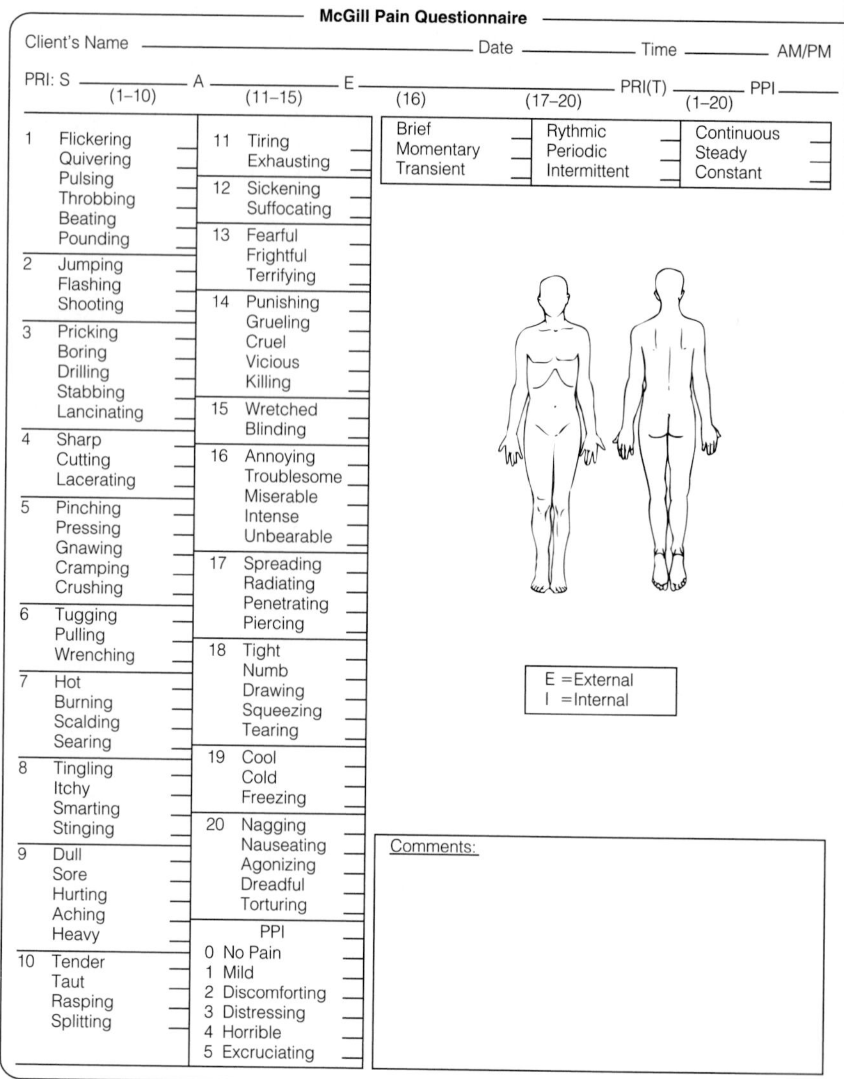

McGill Pain Questionnaire

Client's Name ______ Date ______ Time ______ AM/PM

PRI: S ______ (1–10) A ______ (11–15) E ______ (16) ______ (17–20) PRI(T) ______ (1–20) PPI ______

1 Flickering, Quivering, Pulsing, Throbbing, Beating, Pounding
2 Jumping, Flashing, Shooting
3 Pricking, Boring, Drilling, Stabbing, Lancinating
4 Sharp, Cutting, Lacerating
5 Pinching, Pressing, Gnawing, Cramping, Crushing
6 Tugging, Pulling, Wrenching
7 Hot, Burning, Scalding, Searing
8 Tingling, Itchy, Smarting, Stinging
9 Dull, Sore, Hurting, Aching, Heavy
10 Tender, Taut, Rasping, Splitting
11 Tiring, Exhausting
12 Sickening, Suffocating
13 Fearful, Frightful, Terrifying
14 Punishing, Grueling, Cruel, Vicious, Killing
15 Wretched, Blinding
16 Annoying, Troublesome, Miserable, Intense, Unbearable
17 Spreading, Radiating, Penetrating, Piercing
18 Tight, Numb, Drawing, Squeezing, Tearing
19 Cool, Cold, Freezing
20 Nagging, Nauseating, Agonizing, Dreadful, Torturing

PPI
0 No Pain
1 Mild
2 Discomforting
3 Distressing
4 Horrible
5 Excruciating

Brief	Rythmic	Continuous
Momentary	Periodic	Steady
Transient	Intermittent	Constant

E = External
I = Internal

Comments:

A

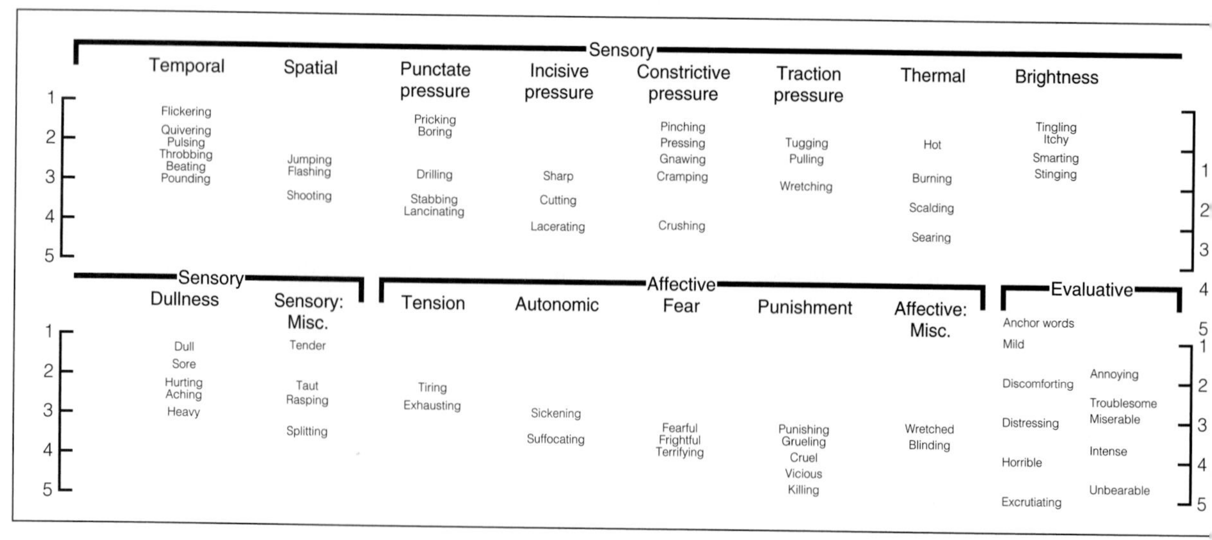

Figure 36–9 *A,* McGill Pain Questionnaire. The descriptors fall into four major groups: *sensory,* 1 to 10; *affective,* 11 to 15; *evaluative,* 16; and *miscellaneous,* 17 to 20. The rank value of each descriptor is based on its position in the word set. The sum of the rank values is the pain rating index (PRI). The present pain intensity (PPI) is based on a scale of 0 to 5. *B,* Spatial display of pain descriptors based on intensity ratings by clients. The intensity scale values range from 1 (mild) to 5 (excruciating).

Source: *A* and *B* reprinted with permission from R Melzack, *Pain Measurement and Assessment* (New York: Raven, 1983).

349036010 8/10/94 ss

pressure, lower pulse rate, pupil constriction, and warm, dry skin.

Behavioral Responses The very young, the aphasic, and confused or disoriented persons often communicate their experience of pain only nonverbally. Facial expression is often the first indication of pain and may be the only one. Clenched teeth, tightly shut eyes, open somber eyes, biting of the lower lip, and other facial grimaces are indicative of pain.

Immobilization of the body or a part of the body may also indicate pain. The client with chest pain often holds the left arm across the chest. A person with abdominal pain may assume the position of greatest comfort, often with the knees and hips flexed, and moves reluctantly.

Purposeless body movements can also indicate pain—for example, tossing and turning in bed or flinging the arms about. Involuntary movements such as a reflexive jerking away from a needle inserted through the skin indicate pain. An adult may be able to control this reflex; however, a child may be unable or unwilling to do so.

Rhythmic body movements or rubbing may indicate pain. An adult or child may assume a fetal position and rock back and forth when experiencing abdominal pain. During labor a woman may massage her abdomen rhythmically with her hands.

Speech and vocal pitch can also help the nurse assess pain. Rapid speech and elevated pitch often reflect anxiety, and slow speech and monotonous tone can signal intense pain. See the box at the right for some culturally oriented responses to pain.

SOME CULTURALLY ORIENTED RESPONSES TO PAIN

- Minimizes pain with significant others.
  or
  Uses pain to elicit sympathy and support from others.
- Carefully controls the expression of pain (is calm and unemotional).
  or
  Is vocal about pain (complains, cries, moans).
- Withdraws and wants to be alone when pain is severe.
  or
  Seeks the attention and presence of others.
- Willingly accepts pain-relief measures.
  or
  Avoids pain-relief measures in the belief that they indicate weakness.
- Wants and expects quick pain relief.
  or
  Accepts pain for long periods before requesting help.

DIAGNOSING

The nursing diagnoses given to clients experiencing pain are **Pain** (implying acute pain) and **Chronic pain.** When writing the diagnostic statement, the nurse may further specify the type or location of the pain (eg, postoperative, chest, abdominal, back). Etiologic factors and precipitating factors, when known, must be part of the diagnostic statement. These diagnoses, with definitions, defining characteristics and contributing factors, are shown in the box on page 990. Clinical applications of these diagnoses are shown in Table 36–6 on page 991.

Because the pain experience affects so many facets of human functioning, **Pain** itself may be the etiology of other nursing diagnoses. Example of such nursing diagnoses are also shown below.

- **Ineffective airway clearance** related to postoperative incisional chest pain
- **Anxiety** related to past experiences of poor control of pain and to anticipation of pain
- **Ineffective breathing pattern** related to postoperative abdominal pain
- **Ineffective individual coping** related to prolonged continuous back pain, ineffective pain management, and inadequate support systems
- **Fear** related to anticipated pain after surgery
- **Altered health maintenance** related to chronic pain and fatigue
- **Hopelessness** related to ineffective pain management strategies
- **Knowledge deficit** (pain control measures) related to lack of exposure to information resources
- **Impaired physical mobility** related to arthritic pain in knee and ankle joints
- **Self-care deficit: Bathing/hygiene, dressing/grooming, toileting** related to pain in the joints
- **Sleep pattern disturbance** related to increased pain perception at night

NURSING DIAGNOSES

CLIENTS EXPERIENCING PAIN

Nursing Diagnosis: Pain: The state in which an individual experiences and reports the presence of severe discomfort or an uncomfortable sensation

Defining Characteristics

- Communication of pain descriptors
- Guarded, protective behavior
- Self-focusing
- Narrowed focus
- Distraction behavior (moaning, crying, pacing, seeking out others or activities, restlessness)
- Altered muscle tone, ranging from listlessness to rigidity
- Facial mask of pain (eg, lusterless eyes, grimace, and/or "beaten look")
- Sympathetic nervous system responses (eg, elevated pulse and blood pressure, diaphoresis, pupil dilation, and increased or decreased respiratory rate)

Related Factors

Injurious agents: *biologic* (disease, inflammation, ischemia; *chemical* (noxious agents, cytotoxic agents, electrolyte imbalance, endocrine function); *physical* (trauma, surgery, and temperature extremes); *psychologic* (anxiety, distress, fear, stress, tension); knowledge deficit of pain management techniques.

Nursing Diagnosis: Chronic pain: The state in which an individual experiences pain that continues for more than 6 months

Defining Characteristics

- Verbal report or observed evidence of pain (eg, guarded movement or facial expression of discomfort) lasting more than 6 months
- Physical and social withdrawal
- Reduced ability to continue previous activities
- Anorexia
- Weight changes
- Sleep pattern changes

Related Factors

Chronic physical or psychosocial disability; fear of drug tolerance or addiction; knowledge deficit of pain management techniques.

Sources: LJ Carpenito, *Nursing Diagnosis: Application to Clinical Practice*, 4th ed. (Philadelphia: Lippincott, 1992), pp. 227, 237–38; M Gordon, *Manual of Nursing Diagnosis 1993–1994*, 6th ed. (St Louis: Mosby-Year Book, 1993), pp. 225, 227; MJ Kim, GK McFarland, and AM McLane, *Pocket Guide to Nursing Diagnoses*, 5th ed. (St Louis: Mosby-Year Book, 1993), p. 40; GK McFarland, and EA McFarlane, *Nursing Diagnosis and Intervention: Planning for Patient Care*, 2nd ed. (St Louis: Mosby, 1993), p. 426; North American Nursing Diagnosis Association, *NANDA Nursing Diagnoses: Definitions and Classsification 1992–1993*, (Philadelphia: NANDA, 1992), p. 71; and JR Lederer, GL Marculescu, B Mocnik, and N Seaby. *Care Planning Pocket Guide—A Nursing Diagnosis Approach*, 5th ed. (Redwood City, CA: Addison-Wesley Nursing, 1993), pp. 128, 132.

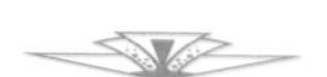

Planning

The nurse identifies nursing interventions that will assist the client in achieving the overall client goals of preventing, modifying, or eliminating pain so that the client is able partially or completely to resume usual daily activities and be able to cope more effectively with the pain experience. Examples of outcome criteria and nursing interventions with rationales are shown in the Care Planning Guide. Scheduling measures to *prevent* pain is far more supportive of the client than trying to deal with pain only once the client perceives it. Many postoperative clients need regularly administered analgesics as well as other nursing measures. In this way, the client's pain is anticipated and avoided, and recovery is often hastened.

When planning, nurses need to choose pain relief measures appropriate for the client. Nursing interventions may include a variety of pharmacologic and nonpharmacologic interventions. Selecting several strategies from both broad categories is usually most effective.

A critical pathway can also be useful for planning client care (see p. 1006).

Text continued on page 994

Table 36–6 Clinical Application: Assessment Data Clusters and Related Nursing Diagnoses for Clients Experiencing Pain

Data Cluster	Nursing Diagnoses
Mr Rodrigo Sanchez, a 73-year-old widower, has joint stiffness, swelling, and tenderness of the feet, knees, and hips. States pain gets worse when he walks to do his shopping and works in the garden all day. Weight is 25% above norm for height. States he eats mostly fried foods.	**Chronic pain** related to overactivity and excess weight secondary to rheumatoid arthritis
Mrs Rene Laurent, a frail 84-year-old, has osteoporosis and kidney disease. She rates her hip and back pain as an 8 on a scale of 0 (least intense) to 10. Is unable to sleep at night. Has tried various analgesics (prescribed and over-the-counter drugs) but because of kidney disease is unable to tolerate side effects (dizziness and nausea).	**Chronic pain** related to fatigue and ineffective pain management strategies secondary to osteoporosis
Mrs Lan Nguyen was diagnosed with breast cancer 3 years ago and had a metastatic lung tumor removed 4 months ago. Describes prolonged post thoracotomy pain as "unbearable." Sister says that although Lan loves sewing and needlepoint, Lan states she is too ill to perform previous hobbies.	**Chronic pain** related to fear of outcome, and inadequate coping method secondary to metastatic cancer
Mrs Robin Wilson, the mother of 2 children, recently separated from her husband. Works as bank clerk full time. Is worried about her finances and the responsibilities for her children. "Pounding" frontal headaches occur in the late afternoon and evening. At interview, held the palm of her hand across her forehead. Brow is furrowed, and facial muscle tense.	**Pain:** recurrent headaches related to emotional stress
Mary Anderson, 75 years old, fell and broke her hip while shopping. She had surgery yesterday to repair the fracture. She rates her pain in the surgical site as 9 on a 0 to 10 scale and states pain is "off the scale" when she is repositioned in bed. States the pain is slightly less if she lies very still. Says she has never had major surgery and has had little pain other than some stiffness in the mornings relieved by 1 or 2 aspirin capsules. She is receiving Demerol 75 mg q4–5h. Morphine 10 mg q4h prn is also ordered but has not been given. States, "I try to hold out as long as I can before asking for a pain killer; even after a shot, my pain is never less than a 4."	**Pain** related to surgical repair, movement, lack of knowledge about pain management, and possible inadequate analgesia (drug and dosing)

CARE PLANNING GUIDE
CLIENTS EXPERIENCING PAIN

NURSING DIAGNOSIS: Pain

Outcome Criteria	Nursing Interventions	Rationale
The client ▪ Verbalizes pain relief at a level of *(specify)*, or less, on a scale of 0 to 10; verbalizes feelings of reasonable comfort.	Assess, reassess, and document the client's verbal and nonverbal pain cues frequently (eg, every 2 hours for the first 24 hours postoperatively and thereafter every 3 to 4 hours until discharge.	Assessment enables the nurse to evaluate the effectiveness of prescribed analgesics. In addition, assessment and documentation are essential legal responsibilities.
	Administer analgesics or monitor patient-controlled analgesia (PCA) as prescribed (eg, q4h for 36 hours).	Scheduled analgesic administration prevents severe pain.
	Administer opioids with nonsteroidal anti-inflammatory drugs (NSAIDs) when both are ordered.	Analgesia is augmented when opioid analgesics are combined with NSAIDs. Opioids bind to opioid receptor sites in the central nervous system; NSAIDs act on peripheral tissues that receive painful stimuli (ie, the injury site).

PAIN CONTINUED

NURSING DIAGNOSIS: Pain *continued*

Outcome Criteria	Nursing Interventions	Rationale
	Provide nonpharmacologic alternatives for pain relief, such as position changes; back massage (see Procedure 35–1, page 965); or other various techniques as discussed in the text on pages 1002–1004.	Nonpharmacologic measures promote relaxation and supplement the effects of pharmacologic agents.
	Consult with the physician to modify orders for ineffective analgesics as required.	Ineffective analgesia increases client stress, decreases participation in required activities, and delays recovery.
▪ Demonstrates pain relief, as evidenced by (a) participation in required activities and (b) report of 3 to 4 hours or more (specify) of uninterrupted sleep at night.	Schedule and administer analgesics at least 30 minutes before painful procedures (eg, turning in bed, deep-breathing exercises and coughing, ambulating, physical therapy).	Peak blood levels of analgesics prevent severe pain and enable the client to perform activities that prevent complications from immobility and/or anesthesia.
	When variable drug dosages are prescribed (eg, morphine IM 5 to 15 mg 3 to 4 hours prn), adjust the prescribed drug dosage as needed according to the client's report of pain during and after activity.	Pain tolerance varies significantly among individuals. Dosage administered is based on client's report of pain.
	Assess the client's sleep pattern. Organize care at night to coincide with analgesic administration. Consider use of long-acting morphine if client's sleep is inadequate.	Appropriate pain interventions enable the client to sleep for intervals of at least 3 to 4 hours.

NURSING DIAGNOSIS: Chronic pain

Outcome Criteria	Nursing Interventions	Rationale
The client		
▪ Reduces or eliminates factors that precipitate or intensify the pain experience.	Explore with the client possible factors that precipitate or intensify the pain experience (eg, activity, emotional stress, environmental factors, inadequate pain medication, fear of addiction).	Identifying actual or potential precipitating factors helps the client avoid or minimize them.
▪ Reports relief or reduced level of pain (eg, 3 or less on a scale of 0 to 10) with pain control measures implemented.	Conduct a thorough pain assessment (see pp. 982–989), and establish a schedule for reassessing and evaluating the effectiveness of pain control measures used.	A complete assessment is essential to planning and implementing effective pain management.
	Encourage the client to keep a daily pain diary (see p. 987).	A diary helps to identify patterns or factors that increase or mediate the pain experienced as well as to evaluate the effectiveness of pain control measures used.

NURSING DIAGNOSIS: Chronic pain *continued*

Outcome Criteria	Nursing Interventions	Rationale
	Assess the client's desire and willingness to use particular interventions.	Knowledge of the client's conflicts or unwillingness to use certain therapies enables the nurse to correct misconceptions or avoid specific interventions.
	Teach the client to a. Use both pharmacologic and nonpharmacologic pain management techniques (see pp. 995 and 1002).	More effective pain relief can be achieved when several strategies are used; one method augments the action of another.
	b. Take analgesics *before* the client experiences severe pain (ie, as soon as pain is felt). *or* Take prescribed analgesics at times scheduled rather than waiting.	Scheduled dosages of analagesic maintain blood levels and prevent severe pain. Less dosage is often required to control the pain.
	c. Use a rescue analgesic dose for acute or break-through pain as required.	Chronic pain may have a stable pattern with occasional episodes of acute pain.
▪ Reports minimal or manageable side effects of pharmacologic agents used.	Identify side effects of drugs, and discuss with the client possible ways to prevent or manage them.	Many side effects can be prevented (eg, constipation from opioids and indigestion from nonnarcotic analgesics). Knowing how to manage side effects can facilitate the client's compliance with planned interventions.
▪ Reports decreased fear and anxiety about pain experience and/or analgesics required.	Establish a relationship that helps the client explore such fears as inadequate pain control, inability to tolerate or cope with increasing pain or painful death, loss of functional capacities and effects of the client's pain on family members or significant others.	Fear of increasing pain or what the pain might mean (eg, declining health) may cause depression and feelings of hopelessness.
	Explore any misconceptions or beliefs that may interfere with optimal pain control. Provide accurate information to reduce fears. Discuss the difference between drug tolerance and drug addiction.	Failure to clarify misconceptions can lead to values conflict and noncompliance with pain control strategies.
	Assist the family to respond to the client's pain experience in helping ways. a. Provide accurate information about the client's pain experience and therapy. b. Provide opportunities for support persons to discuss their fears and concerns.	Understanding the pain experience and therapy and participating in the implementation of nonpharmacologic therapy helps persons cope and provides support to the client.

PAIN CONTINUED

NURSING DIAGNOSIS: Chronic pain ***continued***

Outcome Criteria	Nursing Interventions	Rationale
	c. Include support persons in pain relief methods, such as massage and progressive relaxation.	
	Inform the client that all assessments and reassessments are being conducted to better understand the client's pain experience and the effectiveness of pain control measures—*not* to determine whether pain is present.	Fear of not being believed can lead to underreporting pain and anxiety.
▪ Reports increase in mobility and physical activity/quality of life.	Encourage diversional and physical activities unless the latter precipitates pain.	Diversion is distracting and reduces pain perception. Exercise decreases stress and promotes sleep. Both measures enhance psychosocial well-being.
	Help the client plan daily activities when pain is at lowest level.	

IMPLEMENTING

Pain management is the alleviation of pain or a reduction in pain to a level of comfort that is acceptable to the client (Herr & Mobily 1992, p. 357). It includes two basic types of nursing interventions: pharmacologic and nonpharmacologic interventions. Nursing management of pain consists of both independent and collaborative nursing actions. In general, noninvasive measures may be performed as an independent nursing function, whereas administration of analgesic medications requires a physician's order. However, the decision to administer the prescribed medication is frequently the nurse's, often requiring judgment as to the dose to be given and the time of administration.

Generally speaking, a combination of strategies is best for the client in pain. Sometimes strategies need to be tried and changed until the client obtains effective pain relief. See the box on page 995 for individualizing care for clients with pain.

GENERAL STRATEGIES FOR PAIN

Acknowledging the Client's Pain Basic to all strategies for reducing pain is that nurses convey to clients that they believe the client is having pain. Four ways of communicating this belief follow:

1. Verbally acknowledge the presence of the pain. "I understand your leg is very painful. How do you feel about the pain?"
2. Listen attentively to what the client says about the pain.
3. Convey that you are assessing the client's pain to understand it better, *not* to determine whether the pain is real, for example, "How does your pain feel now?" or "Tell me how it feels compared to an hour ago."
4. Attend to the client's needs promptly.

Assisting Support Persons Support persons often need assistance to respond positively to the client experiencing pain. Nurses can help by giving them accurate information about the pain and providing opportunities for them to discuss their emotional reactions, which may include anger, fear, frustration, and feelings of inadequacy. Enlisting the aid of support persons in the provision of pain relief to the client, such as massaging the client's back, may diminish their feelings of helplessness and foster a more positive attitude toward the client's pain experience. Support persons also may need the nurse's verbal recognition of their concern and participation in the client's care.

Reducing Misconceptions About Pain Reducing a client's misconceptions about the pain and its treatment will often avoid intensifying the pain. The nurse should

CLINICAL GUIDELINES

Individualizing Care for Clients with Pain

- *Establish a trusting relationship.* Convey your concern, and acknowledge that you believe that the client is experiencing pain. A trusting relationship promotes expression of the client's thoughts and feelings and enhances effectiveness of planned pain therapies.
- *Consider the client's ability and willingness to participate actively in pain relief measures.* Some clients who are excessively fatigued, are sedated, or have altered levels of consciousness are less able to participate actively. For example, a client with an altered level of consciousness or altered thought processes may not be able to deal with patient-controlled analgesia (PCA). In contrast, a fatigued client may express a willingness to use pain-relief measures that require little effort, such as listening to music or performing relaxation techniques.
- *Use a variety of pain relief measures.* It is thought that using more than one measure has an additive effect in relieving pain. Two measures that should always be part of any pain-relief plan are (a) establishing a client-nurse relationship and (b) client teaching. Because a client's pain may vary throughout a 24-hour period, different types of pain relief are often indicated during that time.
- *Provide measures to relieve pain before it becomes severe.* For example, providing an analgesic before the onset of pain is preferable to waiting for the client to complain of pain, when a larger dose may be required.
- *Use pain-relieving measures that the client believes are effective.* It has been recognized that clients are usually the authorities about their own pain. Thus, incorporating the client's measures into a pain relief plan is sensible unless they are harmful.
- *Base the choice of the pain relief measure on the client's report of the severity of the pain.* If a client reports mild pain, an analgesic such as aspirin may be indicated, whereas a client who reports severe pain often requires a more potent relief measure.
- *If a pain relief measure is ineffective, encourage the client to try it once or twice more before abandoning it.* Anxiety may diminish the effects of a pain measure, and some approaches, such as distraction strategies, require practice before they are effective.
- *Maintain an unbiased attitude (open mind) about what may relieve the pain.* New ways to relieve pain are being continually developed. It is not always possible to explain pain relief measures; however, measures should be supported unless they are harmful.
- *Keep trying.* Do *not* ignore a client because pain persists in spite of measures. In these circumstances, reassess the pain, and consider other relief measures.
- *Prevent harm to the client.* Pain therapy should not increase discomfort or harm the client. Some pain relief measures may have outward effects, such as fatigue, but they should not disable the client.
- *Educate the client and support persons about pain.* Clients and support persons need to be informed about possible causes of pain, precipitating and alleviating factors, and alternatives to drug therapy. Misconceptions also need to be corrected.

---

explain to the client that pain is a highly individual experience and that it is only the client who really experiences the pain, although others can understand and empathize. Misconceptions are also dealt with when nurse and client discuss why the pain has increased or decreased at certain times. For example, a client whose pain increases in the evening may mistakenly think this is the result of eating dinner rather than fatigue.

Reducing Fear and Anxiety It is important to help relieve the emotional component, that is, anxiety or fear, associated with the pain. When clients have no opportunity to talk about their pain and associated fears, their perceptions and reactions to the pain can be intensified. The client may become angry or complain about the nurse's care when the problem really is a belief that the pain is not being attended to. If the nurse is honest and sincere and promptly attends to the client's needs, the client is much more likely to know that the nurse does believe the client is in pain.

By providing accurate information, the nurse can also reduce many of the client's fears, such as a fear of addiction or a fear that the pain will always be present. It also helps many clients to have privacy when they are experiencing pain.

PHARMACOLOGIC PAIN MANAGEMENT

Pharmacologic pain management involves the use of opioids (narcotics), nonopioids/NSAIDs (nonsteroidal anti-inflammatory drugs), and adjuvants, or coanalgesic drugs. See the box on page 996.

Opioid Analgesics Opioid (narcotic) analgesics include opium derivatives, such as morphine and codeine.

CATEGORIES AND EXAMPLES OF ANALGESICS

Narcotic Analgesics

- Butorphanol (Stadol)
- Fentanyl citrate (Sublimaze)
- Hydromorphone hydrochloride (Dilaudid)
- Meperidine hydrochloride (Demerol)
- Methylmorphine phosphate (codeine, Tylenol 3, Empirin 3)
- Morphine sulfate (Morphine)
- Propoxyphene napsylate (Darvon-N, Darvocet-N)

Nonnarcotic Analgesics/NSAIDs

- Acetaminophen (Tylenol, Datril)
- Acetylsalicylic acid (aspirin)
- Choline magnesium trisalicylate (Trilisate)
- Diclofenac sodium (Voltaren)
- Ibuprofen (Motrin, Advil)
- Indomethacin sodium trihydrate (Indocin)
- Naproxen (Naprosyn)
- Naproxen sodium (Anaprox)
- Piroxicam (Feldene)
- Tolmetin sodium (Tolectin)

Adjuvant Analgesics

- Amitriptyline (Elavil)
- Chlorpromazine (Thorazine)
- Diazepam (Valium)
- Hydroxyzine (Vistaril)

Narcotics relieve pain and provide a sense of euphoria largely by binding to opiate receptors and activating endogenous pain suppression in the central nervous system. There are several types of opiate receptors, including mu, delta, and kappa receptors; however, it is not certain which receptors other than mu may be effective in relieving pain. Opiate analagesics currently used in clinical practice work primarily at the mu receptor (Watt-Watson & Donovan 1992, p. 132). Changes in mood and attitude and feelings of well-being make the person feel more comfortable even though the pain persists.

There are two primary types of opioids:

1. *Full agonists.* These pure opioid drugs bind tightly to mu receptor sites, producing maximum pain inhibition, an agonist effect. Full **agonist analgesics** include morphine, codeine, meperidine (Demerol), propoxyphene (Darvon), and hydromorphine (Dilaudid). There is no ceiling on the level of analgesia from these drugs; their dose can be steadily increased to relieve pain. There is also no maximum daily dose limit.
2. *Mixed agonists-antagonists.* **Agonist-antagonist analgesic** drugs can act like opioids and relieve pain (agonist effect) when given to a client who has not taken any pure opioids. However, they can block or inactivate other opioid analgesics when given to a client who has been taking pure opioids (antagonist effect). These drugs include buprenorphine (Buprenex), dezocine (Dalgan), pentazocine hydrochloride (Talwin), butorphanol tartrate (Stadol), and nalbuphine hydrochloride (Nubain). They block the mu receptor site and activate a kappa receptor site. If a client has been receiving a mu agonist, such as morphine, for pain, the administration of a mixed agonist-antagonist will result in the inactivation of the morphine effect and increase pain. These drugs also have a ceiling dose level. They are not recommended for use with terminally ill clients.

SEDATION RATING SCALE

S Sleeping, easy to rouse
1 Awake and alert
2 Occasionally drowsy, easy to rouse
3 Frequently drowsy, but rousable
4 Somnolent; hard to rouse, if at all

Source: CL Pasero, Pain control, *American Journal of Nursing,* February 1994, 94:23. Reprinted with permission.

When administering any analgesic, the nurse must review side effects. All opioids result in some initial drowsiness when first administered, but with regular administration, this side effect tends to decrease. Opioids also may cause nausea, vomiting, constipation, and respiratory depression. Opioids must be used cautiously in clients with respiratory problems.

If the client experiences significant respiratory depression (eg, a drop from 18 to 12) or is overly sedated, the dosage is excessive. *Before* administering narcotics, the nurse needs to assess a client's level of alertness and respiratory rate for baseline data. An increasing sedation level can be an early warning sign of impending respiratory depression (Pasero 1994, p. 23). See the sedation rating scale in the box above. Often clients will manifest an increase in sedation *before* they manifest a decrease in respiratory rate and depth. The nurse should assess and document the client's level of sedation at the same time that respiratory status is checked. Early recognition of an increasing level of sedation or respiratory depression will enable the nurse to implement appropriate measures promptly (eg, obtaining an order to decrease the opioid dosage). The accompanying box provides suggested measures to prevent side effects of opioid analgesics.

Another major concern of many clients is the tendency for opioids to become habit-forming. However, in a review of 12,000 records of clients taking these drugs for chronic medical pain, *fewer than 1%* were found to have significant addiction (Porter & Jick 1980, p. 123).

Elderly clients are particularly sensitive to the analgesic properties of opioids and often require less medication than younger clients. This sensitivity may be related to reduced excretion of the drug in elderly clients.

Nonopioids/NSAIDs Nonopioid (nonnarcotic analgesics) include **nonsteroidal anti-inflammatory drugs (NSAIDs)** such as aspirin, acetaminophen, and ibuprofen. These analgesics have anti-inflammatory, analgesic, and antipyretic effects. They relieve pain by acting on peripheral nerve endings at the injury site and decreasing the level of inflammatory mediators generated at the site of injury. They may also decrease prostaglandin release at the injury site (American Pain Society 1988, p. 817). In addition, several combinations of analgesic drugs are available, for example, a narcotic and nonnarcotic such as Tylenol #3, which combines acetaminophen with 30 mg of codeine.

Individual drugs in this category vary widely in their analgesic properties, metabolism, excretion, and side effects. In addition, the analgesic activity of these drugs has a *ceiling effect*—the level at which increasing the dose results in no further increase in analgesia (Ferrell & Ferrell 1990, p. 178).

The most common side effect of nonopioid analgesics is indigestion, which can be prevented by taking the medication with antacid or food. Stomach ulcers and gastric bleeding have also been reported. NSAIDs reduce the dose of opioids needed when the drugs are given together and provide better pain relief than use of either type separately. These drugs must be ordered by the physician; they all have a maximum daily dose limit.

Pharmacologic management of mild to moderate pain should begin with NSAIDs, unless there is a specific contraindication (AHCPR 1992a, p. 16). NSAIDs are contraindicated, for example, in clients with impaired blood clotting, gastrointestinal bleeding or ulcer risk, renal disease, thromobocytopenia, and possibly infection (because NSAIDs will obscure fever).

Adjuvant Analgesics Adjuvant analgesics are medications that were developed for uses other than analgesia but have been found to reduce certain types of chronic pain in addition to their primary action. For example, mild sedatives or tranquilizers, such as diazepam (Valium),

Common Opioid Side Effects and Preventive Measures

Constipation

- Increase fluid intake (eg, to 8 glasses daily).
- Increase fiber and bulk-forming agents to the diet (eg, fresh fruits and vegetables).
- Increase exercise regimen.
- If necessary, administer stool softeners and/or a mild laxative daily.

Nausea and Vomiting

- Inform client that tolerance to this emetic effect generally develops after several days of opiate therapy.
- Provide an antiemetic as required.
- Change the analgesic as indicated.

Sedation

- Inform client that tolerance usually develops over 3 to 5 days.
- Administer a stimulant, such as dextroamphetamine sulfate (Dexedrine) or methylphenidate hydrochloride (Ritalin) each morning to clients who receive opiate therapy for chronic pain and do not develop tolerance.

Respiratory Depression

- Administer an opioid antagonist, such as naloxone hydrochloride (Narcan) until respirations return to an acceptable rate. Administer the medication slowly by intravenous route with 10 mL of saline. Monitor the client, and repeat the procedure as required.
- If the client is receiving intravenous patient-controlled analgesia (PCA), stop or slow the infusion.

Pruritus

- Apply cool packs, lotion, and diversional activity.
- Administer an antihistamine (eg, diphenhydramine hydrochloride [Benadryl]).
- Inform the client that tolerance also develops to pruritus.

Urinary Retention

- May need to catheterize client.
- Administer narcotic antagonist (naloxone hydrochloride [Narcan]).

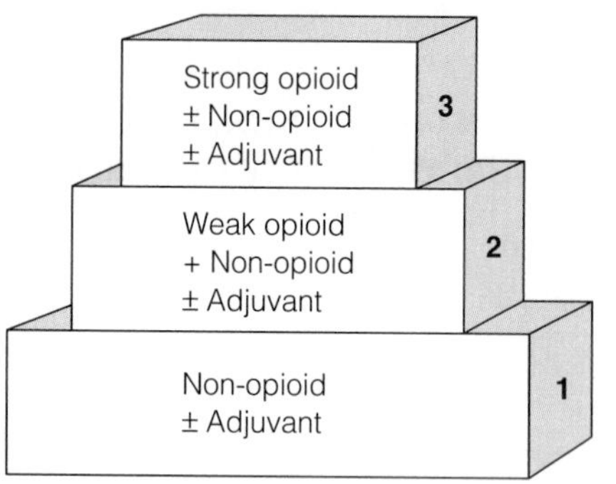

Figure 36–10 The analgesic ladder for cancer pain management proposed by the World Health Organization. **Source:** World Health Organization, *Cancer Pain Relief* (Geneva, Switzerland: WHO, 1986) and *Cancer Pain Relief and Palliative Care,* (Geneva, Switzerland: WHO, 1990).

may help reduce painful muscle spasms as well as reduce anxiety, stress, and tension so that the client can obtain a good night's sleep. Antidepressants, such as amitriptyline hydrochloride (Elavil), are used to treat underlying depression or mood disorders but may also enhance other pain strategies. Anticonvulsants, such as carbamazepine (Tegretol) and clonazepam (Klonopin), usually prescribed to treat seizures, can be useful in controlling painful neuropathies such as herpes zoster (shingles) and diabetic neuropathies.

WHO Three-Step Ladder Approach

The World Health Organization (WHO) recommends a sequential or three-step ladder approach to manage cancer pain (Figure 36–10). This approach may also apply to pain resulting from causes other than cancer. Therapy begins with a nonopioid/NSAID (step 1). If the client receives the maximum recommended dose of nonopioids and continues to experience pain, a weak opioid is given (step 2). The dose of the weak opioid is increased until the ceiling dose is reached. If the client continues to experience pain, a stronger opioid is given (step 3). Adjuvant drugs may also be given at any stage of therapy.

Routes for Opiate Delivery

Opioids have traditionally been administered by oral, subcutaneous, intramuscular, and intravenous routes. In addition, newer methods of delivering opiates have been developed to circumvent potential obstacles that occur with these traditional routes. Examples are transdermal drug therapy, continuous subcutaneous infusions, and intraspinal infusion.

Oral Oral administration of opiates remains the preferred route of delivery because of ease of administration. Because the duration of action of most opiates is approximately 4 hours, people with chronic pain have had to awaken several times during the night to medicate themselves for pain. To circumvent this problem, *long-acting* forms of morphine with a duration of 8 or more hours have been developed. Two examples of long-acting morphine are MS Contin and Oramorph SR. Clients receiving long-acting morphine also may need prn rescue doses of immediate-release analgesics (eg, short-acting morphine) for acute breakthrough pain.

Another new method of oral opiate delivery is high-concentration *liquid morphine.* This formulation enables clients who can swallow only small amounts to continue taking the drug orally.

Transdermal Transdermal drug therapy is advantageous in that it delivers a relatively stable plasma drug level and is noninvasive. Fentanyl (Duragesic) is the only opioid currently available as a skin patch with various dosages. It provides drug delivery for up to 72 hours.

Rectal Several opiates are now available in suppository form. The rectal route is particularly useful for clients who have dysphagia (difficulty swallowing) or nausea and vomiting. Oral analgesics, with the exception of sustained release analgesics, may be crushed, dissolved in water, and given rectally (McCaffery & Beebe 1989, p. 92).

Subcutaneous Although the subcutaneous (SC) route has been used extensively to deliver opioids, a new technique uses subcutaneous catheters and infusion pumps to provide *continuous subcutaneous infusion* (CSCI) of narcotics. CSCI is particularly helpful for clients (a) whose pain is poorly controlled by oral medications, (b) who are experiencing dysphagia or gastrointestinal obstruction, or (c) who have a need for prolonged use of parenteral narcotics. CSCI involves the use of a small, light, battery-operated pump that administers the drug through a 23- or 25-gauge butterfly needle. The needle can be inserted into the anterior chest, the subclavicular region, the abdominal wall, the outer aspects of the upper arms, or the thighs. Client mobility is maintained with the application of a shoulder bag or holster to hold the pump. The frequency of site change ranges from 3 to 7 days.

Because family caregivers must operate the pump and also change and care for the injection site, the nurse needs to provide appropriate instruction. Caregivers need to be able to

- Describe the basic parts and symbols of the system.
- Identify ways to determine whether the pump is working.

- Change the battery.
- Change the medication.
- Demonstrate stopping and starting the pump.
- Demonstrate tubing care, site care, and changing of the injection site.
- Identify signs indicating the need to change an injection site.
- Describe general care of the pump when the client is ambulatory, bathing, sleeping, or traveling.
- Identify actions to take to solve problems when the alarm signals.

Intramuscular The intramuscular (IM) route is the least desirable route for opioid administration because of variable absorption, pain involved with administration, and the need to repeat administration every 3 to 4 hours.

Intravenous The intravenous (IV) route provides rapid and effective pain relief with few side effects. The analgesic can be administered by IV bolus or by continuous infusion controlled by the client using a patient-controlled analgesia (PCA) machine at the bedside (see the discussion of PCA later in this chapter).

Intraspinal Another recent method of delivery is the infusion of opiates into the **epidural** or intrathecal (subarachnoid) space. Intraspinal analgesics act directly on opiate receptors in the dorsal horn of the spinal cord. Two commonly used medications are preservative-free morphine sulfate and fentanyl. The major benefit of intraspinal drug therapy is that it exerts a lesser sedative effect than do systemic opiates. The epidural space is most commonly used because the dura mater acts as a protective barrier against infection, including meningitis.

When the epidural space, rather than the intrathecal space, is used, a higher dosage of medication is required to achieve the same degree of analgesia. Because the intrathecal space contains cerebrospinal fluid (CSF) and directly surrounds the spinal cord, opiates act quickly on the dorsal horn. Very little drug is absorbed by blood vessels into the systemic circulation. In contrast, the epidural space is separated from the spinal cord by the dura mater, which acts as a barrier to drug diffusion. In addition, it is filled with fatty tissue and an extensive venous system. With this diffusion delay, some medication from the epidural space enters the systemic circulation via the venous plexus. Thus a higher dose of opiate is required to create the desired effect.

Intraspinal catheters, which are inserted by physicians, allow either intermittent bolus injections or continuous drug delivery when attached to electronic infusion pumps. Totally implanted systems are also available for clients with chronic pain.

Table 36–7 Nursing Interventions for Clients with an Epidural Catheter

Nursing Goals	Interventions
Maintain client safety.	Label the tubing, the infusion bag, and the front of the pump with tape marked "EPIDURAL" to prevent confusion with other similar-looking IV lines. Apply tape over all injection parts connected to the epidural line to avoid inadvertent injections of other substances intended for IV lines into the epidural space.
Maintain catheter placement.	Secure temporary catheters with tape. Limit the client's activity. Provide assistance in moving into and out of a bed or chair.
Maintain catheter patency.	Inspect the insertion or exit for signs of leakage, infection, and bleeding with each dose administered or at least every 12 hours.
Prevent infection.	Use strict aseptic technique when handling the catheter. Change tubing every 24 hours. Ensure that the insertion site is covered with a sterile, transparent occlusive dressing.
Maintain urinary and bowel function.	Monitor intake and output. Assess for bowel and bladder distention.
Prevent respiratory depression.	Assess sedation level and respiratory status q1h for the first 24 hours and thereafter q4h. Do not administer other opioids or central nervous system depressants unless ordered. Keep an ampule of naloxone hydrochloride (0.4 mg) at the bedside. Notify the clinician in charge if the respiratory rate falls below 8 per minute or if the client is difficult to rouse.

Temporary catheters are usually connected to tubing positioned along the spine and over the client's shoulder for the nurse to access. The entire catheter and tubing are taped securely to prevent dislodgement. Permanent catheters may be tunneled subcutaneously through the skin and exit at the client's side. Nursing care of clients with intraspinal infusions is summarized in Table 36–7.

PATIENT-CONTROLLED ANALGESIA

Patient-controlled analgesia (PCA) is the self-administration of an analgesic by a client properly instructed to do so (AHCPR 1992a, p. 97). The client controls the analgesic dose within safety limits set by the physician. It is monitored by the nurse. PCA can be effectively used for clients with short-term acute pain (eg, postoperative pain, post-injury pain, pain associated with labor and delivery), and for long-term chronic pain (eg, cancer pain). PCA enables the client to administer analgesics safely when they need them. Benefits include the following:

- Self-control over pain
- Lack of dependence on the nurse to provide pain relief
- Stable analgesic blood levels to provide continuous pain relief
- Tendency for the client to need less medication

The oral route for PCA has commonly been employed; however, the subcutaneous, intravenous, and epidural routes are increasingly being used. For example, the intravenous route for PCA is often used in lieu of intramuscular injections to control postoperative pain. A typical IV PCA order might read as follows (AHCPR 1992a, p. 20):

- Loading dose 3 to 5 mg morphine, repeated every 5 minutes until initial postoperative pain diminishes
- Basal infusion rate 0.5 to 1 mg/h
- Bolus dose (rescue dose for breakthrough pain) 1 mg morphine q6min
- Total hourly limit of 10 mg morphine

As with more traditional methods of pain control, the nurse is responsible for frequent assessments of the client and for recording the medication administered. The nurse is also responsible for setting up and maintaining the infusion pump system and for teaching the client how to operate the system. See Procedure 36–1.

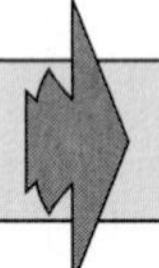

PROCEDURE 36–1 MANAGING PAIN WITH A PATIENT-CONTROLLED ANALGESIA (PCA) PUMP

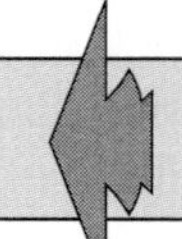

Before initiating PCA therapy, determine factors that may contraindicate use (eg, impaired mental status, impaired respiratory status), the amount of narcotic specified by the order, bolus and continuous infusion dosage parameters, and type of primary fluid. Calculate the following: (a) the initial bolus dose based on the number of milligrams of drug per milliliter of fluid, (b) the dose per intermittent bolus delivery, and (c) the 4-hour lockout drug limit. Confirm that the drug is premixed with the required amount of diluent.

PURPOSE

- To enhance pain control
- To decrease opioid requirements
- To facilitate client involvement in controlling pain

ASSESSMENT FOCUS

Pain (intensity, location, presence of radiation, associated factors, precipitating factors, and alleviating factors); client's allergies; baseline vital signs; client's understanding of the pump.

EQUIPMENT

- ☐ Gloves
- ☐ IV start kit
- ☐ IV catheter
- ☐ Primary line IV tubing
- ☐ Primary IV fluid (per orders)
- ☐ PCA pump and appropriate tubing
- ☐ Operational manual for specific pump to be used
- ☐ Premixed drug to be infused
- ☐ PCA flowsheet

INTERVENTION

1. Prepare the client.

- Explain the purpose and operation of the PCA.

2. Set up the primary IV line and fluid.

- Don gloves.
- Start the IV line. *This will secure venous access.*

3. Set up the PCA infusion line according to the manufacturer's instructions.

- Remove the protective caps from the injector (plunger) and premixed drug vial.

PROCEDURE 36–1 *continued*

- Connect (screw or twist) the injector into the drug vial.
- Remove excessive air from the vial by pushing the injector into the vial.
- Connect the PCA tubing to the injector.
- Prime the PCA tubing up to the point of the Y-connector.
- Clamp the tubing above the Y-connector. *This prevents accidental bolusing and flushing of the primary line with the narcotic.*
- Place the injector with attached vial in the PCA machine according to the operational instructions.

4. Connect the PCA infusion line to the primary fluid line.

- Connect the PCA tubing to the primary fluid line at the Y-connector site. (The clamps should still be closed on the primary IV line and the PCA line.)

5. Deliver the loading dose.

- Set the pump for a lockout time of zero minutes.
- Set the volume to be delivered based on calculated dosage volume for the loading dose.
- Inject the loading dose by pressing the loading dose control button.

6. Set the safety parameters for the infusion on the PCA pump according to the manufacturer's instructions. For example:

- Dose volume limits. *This will limit the amount of drug that the client can receive when the client pushes the control button.*
- Lockout interval between each dose. The lockout interval is generally between 5 and 12 minutes. *This sets the minimum time that must elapse before the client can receive another dose of the drug. Lockout time is based on the usual onset of the IV narcotic and the assessment of the client.*
- 4-hour limit. Set the 4-hour dosage limit as specified on the orders. *This is an additional safety feature to limit the amount of medication delivered over 4 hours.*

7. Lock the machine.

- Close the door on the pump.
- Look for any digital cues or alarms that may indicate the machine is not set, and make corrections as needed.
- Lock the machine with the key.

8. Begin the infusion.

- Release the clamp on the Y-connector, and press the start button to begin the infusion.
- Place the client control button within reach.

9. Monitor the client.

- Monitor the status of the client every 2 hours during the first 24 to 36 hours of infusion and regularly thereafter, depending on the client's health and agency protocol.

10. Monitor the infusion.

- Observe the IV site for signs of infiltration and phlebitis.
- Inspect the tubing for kinks that may occlude the line.
- Ascertain the total number of doses received and the total number of attempts by the client to activate a dose delivery.

11. Document all relevant information.

- Record the initiation of PCA, the dose setting, the doses received, pain intensity, and all assessments. See agency protocol.

EVALUATION FOCUS
Pain status; respiratory rate and character; amount of medication used and frequency of use.

The PCA device is a portable pump usually containing a chamber for the syringe (Figure 36–11, p. 1002). The pump delivers the medication either intravenously or subcutaneously. The most commonly prescribed analgesic is morphine. The client pushes a button attached to the infusion pump when pain medication is needed, whereupon a small preset dose of analgesic is administered. After each dose is administered, there is a programmable lockout interval (usually 10 to 15 minutes) during which the infusion pump cannot be reactivated. This allows time for the medication to take effect before the client receives another dose. There is also a mechanism for programming the maximum amount of medication to be administered within a given interval (usually 4 hours). Thus, the client typically receives the same amount of medication that would be given on a prn or atc (around the clock) schedule (and frequently less). The difference is that the client, rather than the nurse, decides when the medication is actually administered. Most pumps also have a locked safety system that is designed to prevent inadvertent triggering by the client, or other family members, or visitors.

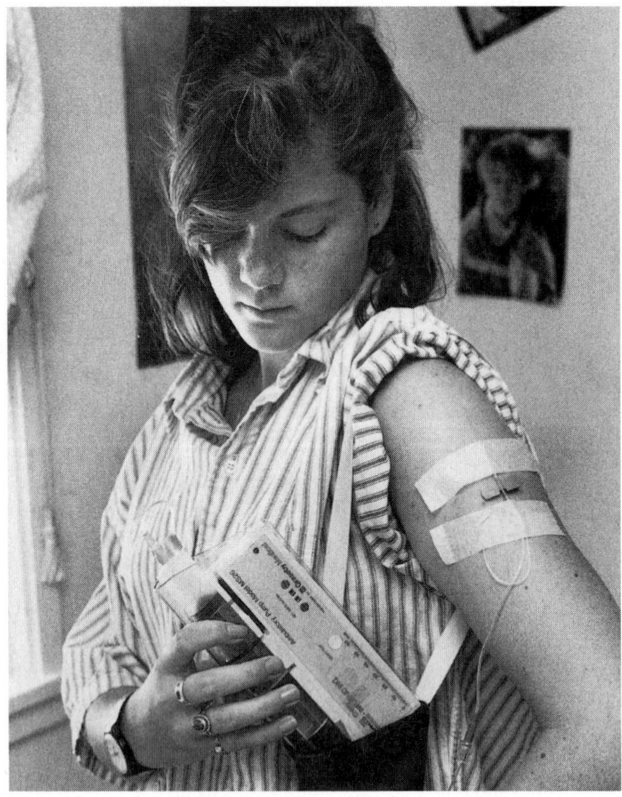

Figure 36–11 A patient-controlled analgesia (PCA) device.

NONPHARMACOLOGIC PAIN MANAGEMENT

Nonpharmacologic pain management consists of a variety of physical and cognitive-behavioral pain management strategies. Physical interventions include cutaneous stimulation, immobilization, transcutaneous electrical nerve stimulation (TENS), acupuncture, and administration of placebos. Cognitive-behavioral interventions include distraction activities, relaxation techniques, guided imagery, biofeedback, hypnosis, and therapeutic touch. Distraction is discussed below. For information about the other behavioral interventions, see Chapter 32.

Physical Interventions The goals of physical intervention are the following (AHCPR 1992a, p. 22):

- Provide comfort
- Correct physical dysfunction
- Alter physiologic responses
- Reduce fears associated with pain-related immobility or activity restriction

Cutaneous Stimulation Cutaneous stimulation can provide effective temporary pain relief. It distracts the client and focuses attention on the tactile stimuli, away from the painful sensations, thus reducing pain perception. Cutaneous stimulation is also believed to (a) create the release of **endorphins** that block pain stimuli transmission and (b) stimulate large-diameter A-beta sensory nerve fibers thus decreasing the transmission of pain impulses through the smaller A-delta and C fibers. Cutaneous stimulation techniques include the following:

- Massage
- Application of heat or cold
- Acupressure
- Contralateral stimulation

Cutaneous stimulation can be applied directly to the painful area, proximal to the pain, distal to the pain, and contralateral (opposite side) to the pain.

Massage Massage eases anxiety and muscle tension. Simple rubbing of a painful muscle or joint with an analgesic ointment or liniment containing menthol is a commonly used massage technique. *Analgesic ointments* containing menthol relieve pain, but the analgesic mechanism is unknown. These ointments produce immediate sensations of warmth that last for several hours, even longer if the body part is wrapped in plastic. They can be used to relieve joint or muscle pain. Moreover, menthol ointment rubbed into the neck, scalp, or forehead sometimes relieves tension headaches. Some cultures (eg, Filipino) use it on the abdomen to relieve gas pains or on the abdomen or lower back to relieve the pain of labor or delivery.

Counterirritants, such as mustard plasters, flaxseed poultices, and liniments, may be used to relieve the aching joint pain of rheumatoid arthritis and osteoarthritis. Counterirritants are thought to relieve pain by increasing circulation to the painful area.

The nurse can massage one body part or several. Various back massage techniques are discussed in Chapter 35. See Procedure 35–1, page 965.

Heat and Cold Applications A warm bath, heating pads, ice bags, ice massage, hot or cold compresses, and warm or cold sitz baths in general relieve pain and promote healing of injured tissues. Applications of heat or cold often require a physician's order. Some clinical facilities, however, have standing orders enabling the nurse to apply certain forms of heat or cold related to the client's condition. Care must be taken not to burn the client or seriously impair circulation to the tissues. Applications of heat and cold are discussed in detail in Chapter 44.

Acupressure Acupressure developed from the ancient Chinese healing system of acupuncture. The therapist applies finger pressure to points that correspond to many of the points used in acupuncture.

Acupressure is a simple, safe, inexpensive, and noninvasive technique that requires little time to learn or perform. As such, nurses familiar with the technique can use it in an attempt to reduce or alleviate pain. In addition, if the treatment proves effective, they can teach the specific technique to the client and/or support persons.

Contralateral Stimulation Contralateral stimulation can be accomplished by stimulating the skin in an area opposite to the painful area (eg, stimulating the left knee if the pain is in the right knee). The contralateral area may be scratched for itching, massaged for cramps, or treated with cold packs or analgesic ointments. This method is particularly useful when the painful area cannot be touched because it is hypersensitive, inaccessible by a cast or bandages, or when the pain is felt in a missing part (phantom pain).

Immobilization Immobilizing a painful body part (eg, an arthritic joint) in some instances provides pain relief. Static resting splints are applied particularly when contractures or muscle imbalances occur. The splints should be removed every 30 minutes for an exercise program in order to prevent additional disability.

Transcutaneous Electric Nerve Stimulation Transcutaneous electric nerve stimulation (TENS) is a noninvasive, nonanalgesic pain control technique that allows the client to assist in the management of acute and chronic pain. It provides an alternative or adjunct to some of the traditional therapies.

The TENS unit consists of a portable battery-operated unit, lead wires, and electrodes (Figure 36–12). It may be applied intermittently or worn discreetly by the client throughout the day. The placement of the electrodes depends on the location, nature, and origin of the pain. They may be placed along both sides of an incision, directly over identified pain areas, at an acupressure point, along peripheral nerve areas that innervate the pain area, or along the spinal column.

Many clients receive significant relief with TENS therapy. TENS units used near incision areas have been shown to provide partial relief of postoperative pain, thereby decreasing the amount of analgesia needed. One of the theories behind the development of the TENS unit is the gate control theory. Cutaneous stimulation from the electronic signals of the TENS unit activate large-diameter fibers to trigger central nervous centers to "close the gate" to signals given to small-diameter fibers. Another theory postulates that the electronic signals emitted by the TENS unit cause the release of endorphins from central nervous system centers. Adverse effects of TENS therapy are minimal.

Although TENS therapy may help decrease pain, the client may need adjunctive analgesic administration during more intense pain periods. The nurse should monitor the client closely to determine the level of pain relief and the need for adjunctive drug therapy.

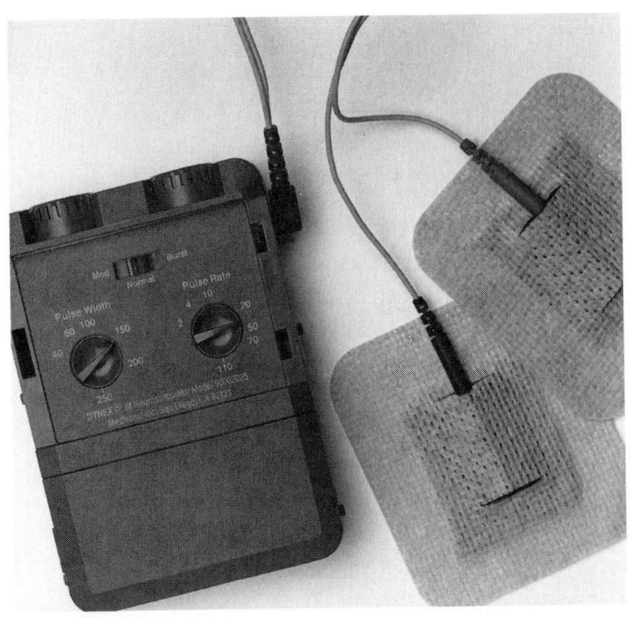

Figure 36–12 A transcutaneous electric nerve stimulator (TENS).

Acupuncture Acupuncture has been practiced for centuries in China and is receiving increasing attention in North America. It is currently being used selectively in North America to treat chronic pain. The acupuncturist inserts long, slender needles into the body at various sites, which are not necessarily near the body parts to be treated. The needles can be heated, attached to a mild electric current, or twirled continuously with the hand. It is believed that the insertion of the acupuncture needle closes the gate mechanism to pain or stimulates sites near pain fibers leading to the brain, thereby blocking the perception of pain.

Administration of Placebos A **placebo** is any form of treatment, such as medication or nursing intervention, that produces an effect in the client because of its intent rather than its physical or chemical properties (McCaffery & Beebe 1989, p. 16). Placebos usually contain sugar, normal saline, or water. They must be ordered by a physician. How placebos work or whether they really do affect pain is a controversial issue. McCaffery and Beebe (1989, p. 16) maintain that the only role for a placebo is in research where subjects know they may receive a placebo.

Cognitive-Behavioral Interventions The goals of cognitive-behavioral interventions are the following (AHCPR 1992a, p. 22):

- Alter pain perception
- Alter pain behavior
- Provide clients with greater sense of control over pain

TYPES OF DISTRACTION

Visual Distraction

- Reading or watching TV
- Watching a baseball game
- Guided imagery

Auditory Distraction

- Humor
- Listening to music

Tactile Distraction

- Slow, rhythmic breathing
- Massage
- Holding or stroking a pet or toy

Intellectual Distraction

- Crossword puzzles
- Card games (eg, bridge)
- Hobbies (eg, stamp collecting, writing a story)

Many cognitive-behavioral pain relief strategies are also used to relieve stress. Interventions such as progressive relaxation, guided imagery, therapeutic touch, and biofeedback are discussed in Chapter 32, page 846. Distraction activities and hypnosis are discussed below.

Distraction Distraction draws the person's attention away from the pain and lessens the perception of pain. In some instances, distraction can make a client completely unaware of pain. For example, a client recovering from surgery may feel no pain while watching a football game on television, yet feel pain again when the game is over. Different types of distractions are shown in the box at the top of this page.

The effectiveness of distraction in decreasing pain can be explained by the gate control theory. In the spinal cord, the peripheral pain stimuli are inhibited by stimuli from other peripheral nerve fibers carrying different stimuli. Because pain messages are slower than diversional messages, the gate in the spinal cord closes, and the client feels less pain. See the discussion of the gate control theory earlier in this chapter.

Distraction is most effective when pain is mild or moderate, but intense concentration on other subjects can also relieve acute pain. An example of the latter is an adolescent who feels pain from a fractured foot bone after she finishes playing a basketball game. However, certain distractions (eg, disturbing stimuli such as loud noises, bright lights, unpleasant odors, or an argumentative visitor), can increase pain perception. Therefore, the nurse needs to reduce disturbing stimuli. The following are five commonly used distraction activities:

- *Slow, rhythmic breathing.* Instruct the client to stare at an object and inhale slowly through the nose while counting from 1 to 4 and then exhale slowly through the mouth while counting to 4 again. Encourage the client to concentrate on the sensation of breathing and to picture a restful scene. Continue until a rhythmic pattern is established.
- *Massage and slow, rhythmic breathing.* Instruct the client to breathe rhythmically and at the same time massage a painful body part with stroking or circular movements.
- *Rhythmic singing and tapping.* Ask the client to select a well-liked song and concentrate attention on its words and rhythm. Encourage the client to mouth or sing the words and tap a finger or foot. Loud, fast songs are best for intense pain.
- *Active listening.* Have the client listen to music and concentrate on the rhythm by tapping a finger or foot.
- *Guided imagery.* Ask the client to close the eyes and imagine and describe something pleasurable. As the client describes the image, ask about the sights, sounds, and smells imagined, encouraging the client to provide details.

Hypnosis Hypnosis is an altered state of consciousness in which an individual's concentration is focused and distraction is minimized. Scientists do not understand exactly how hypnosis relieves pain; however, one theory is that it prevents pain stimuli in the brain from penetrating the conscious mind. Hypnosis requires a client's active participation; clients can even learn to invoke their own hypnotic state. Hypnosis does not take away a person's self-control; in fact, people under hypnosis cannot be made to do anything that they consider amoral or dangerous. In a hypnotic trance, the client does not fall asleep but does become so sharply focused that minor distractions are ignored. A number of hypnosis techniques are used for clients, depending on the type of pain, and the preference of the client and the therapist. One of the most commonly used is symptom suppression, in which the client's awareness of the pain is blocked and the client is distanced from the pain. The effectiveness of this type of hypnosis depends on the severity of the pain and the ability of the client to concentrate.

SURGICAL MANAGEMENT OF PAIN

In addition to pharmaceutical measures for pain, there are a number of surgical treatments for pain. A **nerve block** is a chemical interruption of a nerve pathway, effected by injecting a local anesthetic into the nerve. Nerve blocks

PAIN FLOW SHEET	DATE 5/31/95
PURPOSES: **1)** Record the patient's pain levels. **2)** Provide data to titrate the analgesic's dosage. **3)** Evaluate adverse reactions to the analgesic.	JOHN D. ELLIOT (Name) 1000 ELM STREET (Address) ALBERT, MICHIGAN
Patient's pain rating goal: 2 or less	RM. 301/DR. DIRK

DATE TIME INITIALS	ANALGESIC DOSE ROUTE	PAIN RATING 0 – 10 0 = No Pain 10 = Unbearable Pain	VITAL SIGNS R	VITAL SIGNS P	VITAL SIGNS BP	LEVEL OF AROUSAL/ ACTIVITY	MISCELLANEOUS: Adverse reactions, bowel function, other pain relief measures, care plan, and comments
5/31/95 TJ. 2P	MS 10 mg IM	8	14	90	130/80	Restless	Describes severe pain
TJ. 245P		6	14				
TJ. 4P		4					Describes moderate pain
RS 5p	M.S. 15 mg. IM	8		84	126/80		Describes increased pain
RS 615p		4	12		124/76		
RS 7 p		1	12			Relaxed, dozing	
RS 810p	M.S. 15 mg. IM	5			130/80		
RS 9 p		2					
RS 945p		1	12	84	120/80	Sitting up, reading	
RS 11 p	M.S. 15 mg. IM	2					
							pt. states pain
	continued	on M.S.					just about gone

Figure 36–13 Pain flowsheet. **Source:** T McCormick-Vandenbosch, How to use a pain flowsheet effectively, *Nursing88,* August 1988, 18:50. Used by permission from Springhouse Corporation, 1111 Bethlehem Pike, Springhouse, PA 19477.

are widely used during dental work. The injected drug blocks nerve pathways from the painful tooth, thus stopping the transmission of pain impulses to the brain. Nerve blocks are often used to relieve the pain of whiplash injury, low-back disorders, bursitis, and cancer. Sometimes alcohol blocks are used. These, however, destroy nerve fibers and as a result are generally used for peripheral blocks only, since peripheral nerve fibers regenerate.

Pain conduction pathways can be interrupted surgically. Because this disruption is permanent, surgery is performed only as a last resort, generally for intractable pain. Several surgical procedures may be performed. A **cordotomy** obliterates pain and temperature sensation below the level of the spinothalamic portion of the anterolateral tract severed, and is usually done for pain in the legs and trunk. **Rhizotomy** interrupts the anterior or posterior nerve root between the ganglion and the cord. Interruption of anterior *motor* nerve roots stops spasmodic movements that accompany paraplegia. Interruption of posterior *sensory* nerve roots eliminates pain in areas innervated by that specific nerve root. Rhizotomies are generally performed on cervical nerve roots to alleviate pain of the head and neck from cancer or neuralgia.

In **neurectomy,** peripheral or cranial nerves are interrupted to alleviate localized pain, such as pain in the lower leg or foot arising from a vascular occulsion. In a **sympathectomy,** pathways of the sympathetic division of the autonomic nervous system are severed. This procedure eliminates vasospasm, improves peripheral blood supply, and thus is effective in treating painful vascular disorders such as angina and Raynaud's disease.

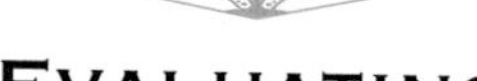

EVALUATING

Because pain is a subjective experience, most evaluative data collected are obtained by questioning the client about specific information taught; about level of comfort, level of energy, and sleep pattern; and whether modifications in activities or the use of noninvasive strategies were helpful. Some objective data may be obtained, particularly from clients with acute pain (eg, vital signs, behavioral postures and gestures).

To assist in the evaluation process, flowsheet records or a client diary may be helpful. See Figure 36–13 on page 1005 for an example of a flowsheet to evaluate the effectiveness of an analgesic. A weekly log or diary can be structured in a similar fashion for the individual client. For example, columns including day, time, onset of pain, activity before pain, pain relief measure, and duration of pain can be devised to help the client and nurse determine the effectiveness of pain relief strategies.

If client outcomes are not achieved, the nurse should explore the reasons. The following are some questions the nurse might consider:

- Were the client's beliefs and values about pain therapy considered?
- Did the client understate the pain experience for some reason?
- Were appropriate instructions provided to allay misconceptions about pain management?
- Did the client and support persons understand instructions provided about pain management techniques?
- Is the client receiving adequate support from significant others?
- Has the client's physical condition changed, necessitating modifications in interventions?
- Should selected intervention strategies be reevaluated?

See also the evaluation checklist in Table 8–3, page 158.

CRITICAL PATHWAY FOR LEE CHIN

ASSESSMENT DATA

Nursing Assessment
Mr Lee Chin is a 57-year-old Chinese businessman who was admitted yesterday morning to the surgical unit at the hospital for the treatment of a possible strangulated inguinal hernia. Yesterday afternoon he went to surgery, and a partial bowel resection was performed. This morning, Mr Chin is NPO. He has an intravenous infusion in the left arm, a nasogastric tube attached to low intermittent suction, and a clear dermal dressing applied to his large abdominal incision. He is in a dorsal recumbent (supine) position and is attempting to draw up his legs. Mr Chin appears to be somewhat restless and pale. He appears to be generally uncomfortable.

Physical Examination
Height: 162 cm (5′4″)
Weight: 72.5 kg (160 lb)
Temperature: 37 C (98.6 F)
Pulse rate: 90 bpm
Respirations: 24 per minute
Blood pressure: 158/82 mm Hg
Skin pale and moist
Midline abdominal incision—sutures dry and intact
Pupils dilated

Diagnostic Data
Chest X-ray film: negative
WBC: 12,000/μL
Urine: negative

CRITICAL PATHWAY FOR CLIENT FOLLOWING BOWEL RESECTION

Expected length of stay 5–6 days following surgery

	Date ________ Preoperative	Date ________ 1st Postoperative day	Date ________ 2d Postoperative day
Daily outcomes	Client ▪ verbalizes understanding of preoperative teaching including: turning, coughing, deep breathing, incentive spirometer, mobilization, possible tubes, pain management. ▪ verbalizes ability to cope.	Client will ▪ be afebrile. ▪ have a clean, dry wound with well-approximated edges, healing by first intention. ▪ recover from anesthesia as evidenced by: VS return to baseline, awake, alert, and oriented. ▪ verbalize understanding and demonstrate cooperation with turning, coughing, deep breathing, and splinting. ▪ demonstrate ability to use PCA. ▪ verbalize control of incisional pain. ▪ ambulate 4 times. ▪ verbalize ability to cope.	Client will ▪ be afebrile. ▪ have a clean, dry wound with well-approximated edges, healing by first intention. ▪ tolerate ordered diet without vomiting. ▪ demonstrate cooperation with turning, coughing, deep breathing, and splinting. ▪ ambulate 4–6 times. ▪ verbalize control of incisional pain. ▪ verbalize ability to cope. ▪ verbalize beginning understanding of home care instructions.
Tests and treatments	CBC. Urinalysis. Chest X-ray. Emergency surgery. Baseline physical assessment: with a focus on respiratory status and gastrointestinal function. IV fluids.	CBC. Electrolytes. Vital signs and O_2 saturation, neurovascular assessment, dressing and wound drainage assessment q15min × 4; q30min × 4; q1h × 4 and then q4h if stable. Assess respiratory status and gastrointestinal function q4h and prn. Incentive spirometer q2h. Intake and output q shift. Assess patency of NG tube q2h, noting volume q8h. Assess voiding—if unable to void try suggestive voiding techniques or catheterize q8h or prn if unable to void. IV antibiotics. IV fluids.	Vital signs and dressing and wound drainage assessment q4h. Assess respiratory status and gastrointestinal function q4h. Incentive spirometer q2h until fully ambulatory. Intake and output q shift. If still in place, assess patency and output of NG tube. Assess voiding pattern q shift. Using sterile asepsis change dressing: assess wound healing and wound drainage. IV antibiotics. IV fluids/Intermittent IV device.
Knowledge deficit	Orient to room and surroundings. Provide simple instructions.	Reorient to room and postoperative routine.	Reinforce earlier teaching regarding ongoing care.

➤

	Preoperative *continued*	**1st Postoperative day** *continued*	**2d Postoperative day** *continued*
Knowledge deficit *continued*	Review preoperative preparation including hospital and surgical routines. Discuss surgery and specific postoperative care: turning, coughing, deeep breathing, splinting incision, incentive spirometer, mobilization, possible tubes (Nasogastric tube [NG] and intravenous), pain management (PCA or prn medications).	Review plan of care and importance of early mobilization. Review importance of turning, coughing, deep breathing, splinting incision, incentive spirometer, mobilization, possible tubes (Nasogastric tube [NG] and intravenous), pain management (PCA or prn medications).	Begin discharge teaching regarding wound care/dressing change.
Psycho-social	Assess anxiety related to diagnosis and pending surgery. Assess fears of the unknown and surgery. Encourage verbalization of concerns. Provide information regarding surgical experience. Minimize external stimuli (eg, noise, movement).	Assess level of anxiety. Encourage verbalization of concerns. Provide information. Provide ongoing support and encouragement.	Encourage verbalization of concerns. Provide ongoing support and encouragement.
Diet	NPO Baseline nutritional assessment	NG tube until return of bowel sounds.	If NG tube removed, begin clear liquids to tolerance.
Activity	Provide safety precautions. Bedrest.	Provide safety precautions. Bathroom privileges with assistance. Ambulate 4 times with assistance.	Provide safety precautions. Ambulate 4–6 times with assistance.
Pain manage-ment	Assess and record the description, location, duration, and characteristics of client's pain q2–4h and prn. Encourage verbalization of pain and discomfort. Reduce or eliminate pain-producing factors (eg, fear, anxiety, lack of knowledge, a wet dressing, improper positioning). Employ distraction techniques (eg, slow rhythmic breathing and guided imagery) to produce pain relief.	Assess and record the description, location, duration, and characteristics of client's pain q2–4h and prn. Encourage verbalization of pain and discomfort. Reduce or eliminate pain-producing factors and employ distraction or relaxation techniques. Provide back rubs. Administer prescribed IM or IV/PCA analgesics and record response. Encourage client to request analgesic or use PCA before pain becomes severe.	Assess and record the description, location, duration and characteristics of client's pain q4h and prn. Reduce or eliminate pain-producing factors, employ distraction or relaxation techniques, and offer back rubs. Administer prescribed IM or IV/PCA analgesics and record response. Encourage client to request analgesic or use PCA before pain becomes severe.

	Preoperative *continued*	**1st Postoperative day** *continued*	**2d Postoperative day** *continued*
Pain management *continued*	Provide cutaneous stimulation prn (eg, back rub). Administer prescribed IM or IV analgesics and record response. Encourage client to request analgesic before pain becomes severe. Instruct in relaxation techniques (eg, tensing and relaxing muscle groups and rhythmic breathing).		
Transfer/ discharge plans	Assess discharge plans and support system.	Review progress toward discharge goals with client and significant other. Consult with social service re: projected needs for home health care (if any).	Review progress toward discharge goals with client and significant other.

	Date ________ **3d Postoperative day**	**Date ________** **4th Postoperative day**	**Date ________** **5th–6th Postoperative day**
Daily outcomes	Client will ▪ be afebrile. ▪ have a clean, dry wound with well-approximated edges, healing by first intention. ▪ tolerate ordered diet without nausea or vomiting. ▪ ambulate independently 4–6 times. ▪ verbalize control of incisional pain. ▪ verbalize ability to cope. ▪ verbalize beginning understanding of home care instructions.	Client will ▪ be afebrile. ▪ have a clean, dry wound with well-approximated edges, healing by first intention. ▪ tolerate ordered diet without nausea or vomiting. ▪ be fully ambulatory. ▪ verbalize control of incisional pain. ▪ verbalize ability to cope. ▪ verbalize beginning understanding of home care instructions.	Client ▪ is afebrile. ▪ has a dry, clean wound with well-approximated edges, healing by first intention. ▪ manages pain with non-pharmacologic measures. ▪ is independent in self-care. ▪ is fully ambulatory. ▪ has resumed preadmission urine and bowel elimination pattern. ▪ verbalizes home care instructions. ▪ tolerates usual diet. ▪ verbalizes ability to cope with ongoing stressors.
Tests and treatments	Vital signs and dressing and wound drainage assessment q4h. Incentive spirometer q2h until fully ambulatory. Intake and output q shift. Assess voiding pattern q shift.	Vital signs and dressing and wound drainage assessment q4h. Assess respiratory status and gastrointestinal function. Using sterile technique: change dressing and assess wound healing and drainage.	Vital signs and dressing and wound drainage assessment q4h. Assess respiratory status and gastrointestinal function. Remove dressing, assess wound healing

➤

	3d Postoperative day *continued*	**4th Postoperative day** *continued*	**5th–6th Postoperative day** *continued*
Tests and treatments *continued*	Assess respiratory status and gastrointestinal function. Using sterile asepsis change dressing: assess wound healing and wound drainage. Intermittent IV device.		
Knowledge deficit	Initiate discharge teaching regarding wound care, diet, and activity. Review written discharge instructions with client and significant other.	Continue discharge teaching regarding wound care, diet, signs and symptoms to report, medications, and activity. Review written discharge instructions with client and significant other.	Complete discharge teaching to include wound care, diet, follow-up care, signs and symptoms to report, activity, and medications: dose, frequency, route, and side effects. Provide client with written discharge instructions.
Psycho-social	Encourage verbalization of concerns. Provide ongoing support and encouragement.	Encourage verbalization of concerns. Provide ongoing support and encouragement.	Encourage verbalization of concerns. Provide ongoing support and encouragement.
Diet	If tolerating clear liquids, advance to full liquids as tolerated.	Advance diet to soft, regular diet to tolerance.	Regular diet as tolerated.
Activity	Ambulate independently at least 4 times.	Fully ambulatory.	Fully ambulatory.
Pain manage-ment	Assess and record description, location, duration, and characteristics of client's pain q4h and prn. Encourage client to employ distraction or relaxation techniques. Provide PO analgesics.	Assess and record description, location, duration, and characteristics of client's pain q4h and prn. Encourage client to employ distraction or relaxation techniques. Provide PO analgesics.	Assess and record description, location, duration, and characteristics of client's pain q4h and prn. Encourage client to employ distraction or relaxation techniques.
Transfer/ discharge plans	Continue to review progress toward discharge goals.	Finalize discharge plans. Continue to review progress toward discharge goals. Finalize plans for home care if needed.	Complete discharge instructions.

CHAPTER HIGHLIGHTS

- Pain is a subjective sensation to which no two people respond in the same way. It can directly impair health and prolong recovery from surgery, disease, and trauma.
- Pain can be categorized according to its origin as cutaneous, deep somatic, or visceral; or according to its cause as acute pain, chronic malignant pain, or chronic nonmalignant pain.
- Pain threshold is similar in all people, but pain tolerance and response vary considerably.
- For pain to be perceived, nociceptors must be stimulated. Three types of pain stimuli are mechanical, thermal, and chemical.
- The precise mechanism of pain transmission and perception is unknown. Type A-delta fibers are associated with fast, sharp, acute pain; type C fibers are associated with slow, chronic, aching pain.
- According to the gate control theory, peripheral nerve fibers carrying pain to the spinal cord can have their input modified at the spinal cord level before transmission to the brain. This theory is the basis of many pain intervention strategies. The body's analgesia system contains neuromodulators that release endogenous opioids to modulate pain transmission and perception. These endogenous opioids include enkephalins, endorphins, and dynorphins, which are morphinelike in their actions.
- Numerous factors influence a person's perception and reaction to pain: ethnic/cultural values, age, environment and support persons, and anxiety and stress.
- Assessment of a client who is experiencing pain should include a comprehensive pain history, a daily pain diary (optional), and physical examination focusing on autonomic nervous system responses and behavioral responses. Because pain is a subjective phenomenon, pain assessment is a complex process; however, tools are available to assist the nurse in this matter.
- Although the nursing diagnosis given to clients suffering pain is **Pain** or **Chronic pain,** the pain itself may be the etiology of many other nursing diagnoses.
- Overall client goals include preventing, modifying, or elminating pain so that the client is able partially or completely to resume usual daily activities and to cope more effectively with the pain experience.
- When planning, nurses need to choose pain relief measures appropriate for the client. Nursing interventions may include a variety of pharmacologic and nonpharmacologic interventions. Selecting several strategies from both broad categories is usually most effective.
- Scheduling measures to *prevent* pain is far more supportive of the client than trying to deal with pain once the client perceives it.
- Pain management includes two basic types of nursing interventions: pharmacologic and nonpharmacologic.
- Major nursing functions for all clients are to acknowledge and convey belief in the client's pain, assist support persons, reduce misconceptions about pain, and reduce fear and anxiety associated with the pain.
- Pharmacologic interventions, ordered by the physician, include the use of opioids, nonopioids/NSAIDs, and adjuvant drugs.
- The nurse assesses the client's pain needs, administers the ordered analgesics, and evaluates the client's response to analgesics provided.
- Analgesic medications can be delivered in several ways to meet the specific needs of individuals. More recent methods include long-acting and liquid morphine, transdermal preparations, continuous subcutaneous infusions, continuous intravenous infusions, and intraspinal infusion.
- Patient-controlled analgesia (PCA) enables the client to exercise control and minimize feelings of helplessness.
- Physical nonpharmacologic pain interventions include cutaneous stimulation, hot and cold applications, massage, acupressure, contralateral

stimulation, transcutaneous electrical nerve stimulation (TENS), and acupuncture.

- Cognitive-behavioral interventions include distraction techniques, relaxation techniques, guided imagery, biofeedback, therapeutic touch, and hypnosis.
- Evaluation of the client's pain therapy includes the response of the client, the changes in the pain, and the client's perceptions of the effectiveness of the therapy. Ongoing verbal or written feedback from the client and family is integral to this process.

READINGS AND REFERENCES

SUGGESTED READINGS

McCaffery, M and Ferrell, BR. Pain control vignettes. June 1991. Part I. How would you respond to these patients in pain? *Nursing91* 21:34–37; September 1991. Part II. Patient age: Does it affect your pain-control decisions? *Nursing91* 21:44–48; January 1992. Part III. How vital are vital signs? *Nursing92* 22:43–46; April 1992. Part IV. Does life-style affect your pain-control decisions? *Nursing92* 22:59–61.

This four-part series features patient vignettes to help nurses rate pain intensity, decide what actions to take, and consider factors involved in making decisions for interventions.

RELATED RESEARCH

Beyer, JE, Denyes, MJ, and Villarruel, AM. October 1992. The creation, validation, and continuing development of the Oucher: A measure of pain intensity in children. *Journal of Pediatric Nursing* 7:335–45.

McCaffery, M, Ferrell, B, O'Neil-Page, E, and Lester, M. February 1990. Nurse's knowledge of opioid analgesic drugs and psychological dependence. *Cancer Nursing* 13:21–27.

SELECTED REFERENCES

Agency for Health Care Policy and Research (AHCPR). 1992a. *Quick Reference Guide for Clinicians: Acute Pain Management in Adults: Operative Procedures.* US Department of Health and Human Services.

———. 1992b. *Quick Reference Guide for Clinicians: Acute Pain Management in Infants, Children, and Adolescents: Operative and Medical Procedures.* US Department of Health and Human Services.

———. February 1992. *Clinical Practice Guideline: Acute Pain Management: Operative or Medical Procedures and Trauma.* US Department of Health and Human Services.

American Pain Society. 1992. *Principles of Analgesic Use in the Treatment of Acute and Cancer Pain.* Skokie, IL: American Pain Society.

Bocchino, CA. May/June 1992. An interview with Daniel Carr and Ada Jacox. *Nursing Economics* 10:165–75.

Burckhardt, CS. December 1990. Chronic pain. *Nursing Clinics of North America* 25:863–70.

Cahill-Wright, C. December 1991. Managing postoperative pain. *Nursing91* 21:42–45.

Carpenito, LJ. 1992. *Nursing Diagnosis: Application to Clinical Practice.* 4th ed. Philadelphia: Lippincott.

Collier, M. March/April 1990. Controlling postoperative pain with patient-controlled analgesia. *Journal of Professional Nursing* 6(6):121–26.

Davis, R. January 1993. Phantom sensation, phantom pain and stump pain. *Archives of Physical Medicine and Rehabilitation* 74(1):79–91.

Donovan, MI. December 1990. Acute pain relief. *Nursing Clinics of North America* 25:851–61.

Dunajcik, L. January 1988. Controlling the dangers of epidural analgesia. *RN* 51:40–45.

East, E. September 30–October 6, 1992. How much does it hurt? *Nursing Times* 40:48–49.

Ferrell, BR. October 1991. Managing pain with long-acting morphine. *Nursing91* 21:34–39.

Ferrell, BR and Ferrell, BA. July/August 1990. Easing the pain. *Geriatric Nursing* 11:175–78.

Fitzgerald, JJ and Shammy, PG. July 1987. Let your patient control his analgesia. *Nursing87* 17:48–51.

Gaston-Johansson, F, Albert, M, Fagen, AM, and Zimmerman, L. April 1990. Similarities in descriptors of four different ethnic-cultural groups. *Journal of Pain and Symptom Management* 5:94–100.

Geach, B. Spring 1987. Pain and coping. *Image: Journal of Nursing Scholarship* 19:12–15.

Gordon, M. 1993. *Manual of Nursing Diagnosis 1993–1994.* 6th ed. St Louis: Mosby-Year Book.

Groft, J. August 1992. At home with pain. *Canadian Nurse* 88:36–37.

Guyton, A. 1991. *Textbook of Medical Physiology.* 8th ed. Philadelphia: WB Saunders.

Hansberry, JL, Bannick, KH, and Durkin, MJ. October 1990. Managing chronic pain with a permanent epidural catheter. *Nursing90* 20:53–55.

Herr, KA and Mobily, PR. April 1991. Complexities of pain assessment in the elderly: Clinical considerations. *Journal of Gerontological Nursing* 17:12–19.

———. June 1992. Interventions related to pain. *Nursing Clinics of North America* 27:347–69.

Hofland, SL. June 1992. Elder beliefs: Blocks to pain management. *Journal of Gerontological Nursing* 18:19–23.

Jacox, A, Ferrell, B, Heidrich, G, Hester, N, and Miaskowski, C. May 1992. A guideline for the nation: Managing acute pain. *American Journal of Nursing* 92:49–55.

Jones, L and Brooks, J. May 1990. The ABCs of PCA. *RN* 53:54–60.

Jordan, S. January 8–14, 1992. Drugs for severe pain. *Nursing Times* 88:24–27.

Kim, MJ, McFarland, GK, and McLane, AM. 1993. *Pocket Guide to Nursing Diagnoses.* 5th ed. St Louis: Mosby-Year Book.

Kresl, JS. September 1988. Patient-controlled analgesia: A new system for pain management. *AORN Journal* 48:481–82, 484, 486–87.

Lederer, JR, Marculescu, GL, Mocnik, B, and Seaby, N. 1993. *Care Planning Pocket Guide—A Nursing Diagnosis Approach.* 5th ed. Redwood City, CA: Addison-Wesley Nursing.

Leventhal, H, and Everhart, D. 1979. Emotion, pain and physical illness. In Izard, CE, editor. *Emotions and Psychopathology.* New York: Plenum Press.

Logan, M and Fothergill-Bourbonnais, F. April 1990. Continuous subcutaneous infusion of narcotics (CSCI). *Canadian Nurse* 86:31–32.

Lunse, CP and Price, P. April 1992. Pain and the critically ill. *Canadian Nurse* 88:22–25.

McCaffery, M. 1979. *Nursing Management of the Patient with Pain.* 2d ed. Philadelphia: Lippincott.

______. December 1980. Relieving pain with noninvasive techniques. *Nursing80* 10:55–57.

______. November 1987. Patient-controlled analgesia: More than a machine. *Nursing87* 17:63–64.

McCaffery, M and Beebe, A. 1989. *Pain: Clinical Manual for Nursing Practice.* St Louis: Mosby.

McCaffery, M and Ferrell, B. June 1990. Do you know a narcotic when you see one? *Nursing90* 20:62–63.

______. June 1991a. How would you respond to these patients in pain? *Nursing91* 21:34–37.

______. December 1991b. Patient age: Does it affect your pain control decisions? *Nursing91* 21:44–48.

______. January 1992. How vital are vital signs? *Nursing92* 22:43–46.

McCaffery, M, Ferrell, BR, and O'Neil-Page, E. April 1992. Does lifestyle affect your pain control decisions? *Nursing92* 22:58–61.

McFarland, GK and McFarlane, EA. 1993. *Nursing Diagnosis and Intervention: Planning for Patient Care.* 2d ed. St Louis: Mosby.

McGuire, L. April 1990. The power of non-narcotic pain relievers. *RN* 53:28–36.

McLaughlin-Hogan, M. July 1991. Continuous subcutanenous infusions: New use for an old route. *Nursing91* 21:58–59.

Maxwell, L and O'Flynn, I. August 1992. Working together to control postoperative pain. *Canadian Nurse* 88:42–44.

Meinhart, NT and McCaffery, M. 1983. *Pain: A nursing approach to assessment and analysis.* Norwalk, CT: Appleton-Century-Crofts.

Melzack, R and Wall, PD. November 19, 1965. Pain mechanisms: A new theory. *Science* 150:971–79.

______. 1982. *The Challenge of Pain.* New York: Penguin Books.

National Institutes of Health, Consensus Development Panel. November 30, 1986. New gains against pain, *Emergency Medicine* 18:143, 147, 151–53ff.

______. Winter 1987. The integrated approach to the management of pain. *Journal of Pain Symptom Management* 2:35–44.

Noah, VA. May 1990. Preop teaching is the key to PCA success. *RN* 53:60–64.

Nolan, MF. January/February 1990. Pain: The experience and its expression. *Clinical Management* 10:22–25.

North American Nursing Diagnosis Association. 1992. *NANDA Nursing Diagnoses: Definitions and Classification 1992–1993.* Philadelphia: NANDA.

Paice, JA. September 1987. New delivery systems in pain management. *Nursing Clinics of North America* 22:715–26.

Paradis, A. August 1992. Patient controlled analgesia. *Canadian Nurse* 88:39–41.

Parke, B. August 1992. Pain in the cognitively impaired elderly. *Canadian Nurse* 88:17–20.

Pasero, CL. February 1994. Pain control. *American Journal of Nursing* 94:22–23.

Pooler, C. August 1992. Pain and the critically ill. *Canadian Nurse* 88:22–25.

Porter, J and Jick, H. January 10, 1980. Addiction rare in patients treated with narcotics. *New England Journal of Medicine* 302:123.

Price, JA and Magolan, JM. June 1991. Intraspinal drug therapy. *Nursing Clinics of North America* 26:477–98.

Ray, L and Wilson, L. August 1992. Kids' pain: A collaborative approach. *Canadian Nurse* 88:26–28.

Romyn, D. June 1992. Pain management: Know the facts. *Canadian Nurse* 88:26–27.

St Marie, B. September/October 1991. Narcotic infusions: A changing scene. *Journal of Intravenous Nursing* 14:334–44.

Slack, J and Faut-Callahan, M. June 1991. Pain management. *Nursing Clinics of North America* 26:463–77.

Southern, JP. July 1990. How to access an epidural implanted port. *Nursing90* 20:48–51.

Stevens, B and Johnston, C. August 1992. Assessment and management of pain in infants. *Canadian Nurse* 88:31–34.

Taylor, AG, Skelton, JA, and Butcher, J. January/February 1984. Duration of pain condition and physical pathology as determinants of nurses' assessments of patients. *Nursing Research* 33:4–8.

US Department of Health and Human Services. February 1992. *Clinical Practice Guideline: Acute Pain Management: Operative or Medical Procedures and Trauma.* Rockville, MD: Public Health Service.

Walding, MF. April 1991. Pain, anxiety and powerlessness. *Journal of Advanced Nursing* 16:388–97.

Walker, M and Wong, DL. June 1991. A battle plan for patients in pain. *American Journal of Nursing* 91:33–36.

Watt-Watson, JH and Donovan, MI. 1992. *Pain Management: Nursing Perspective.* St Louis: Mosby-Year Book.

Weiler, K. October 1992. Pain management as a legal responsibility. *Journal of Gerontological Nursing* 18:46.

Whitaker, OC and Warfield, CA. Feburary 15, 1988. The measurement of pain. *Hospital Practice* 23:155–56, 159–62.

Wild, L and Coyne, C. April 1992. The basics and beyond: Epidural analgesia. *American Journal of Nursing* 92:26–34.

Willens, JS. February 1994. Giving fentanyl for pain outside the OR. *American Journal of Nursing* 94:24–28.

World Health Organization 1986. *Cancer Pain Relief.* Geneva, Switzerland: WHO.

37 Nutrition

Objectives

- Describe nutrition, metabolism, and energy requirements.
- Identify functions and food sources of selected nutrients and some clinical signs of deficiency and excess.
- Describe the use of daily food group guides in choosing a healthy diet.
- Identify potential nutritional problems of vegetarians and suggest ways to avoid them.
- Describe necessary dietary modifications for older adults.
- Identify clinical signs of inadequate nutritional status.
- Describe a format for nutritional assessment.
- Identify factors that influence a person's eating patterns.
- Identify nursing diagnoses and factors contributing to the client's nutritional status.
- Identify interventions to stimulate a client's appetite.
- Describe ways to assist clients with meals.
- Describe some aids that enable self-feeding.
- Discuss some special nutritional services available for selected subgroups of the population.
- Recognize characteristics of commonly prescribed diets.
- Identify nursing responsibilities in administering enteral and parenteral nutrition.

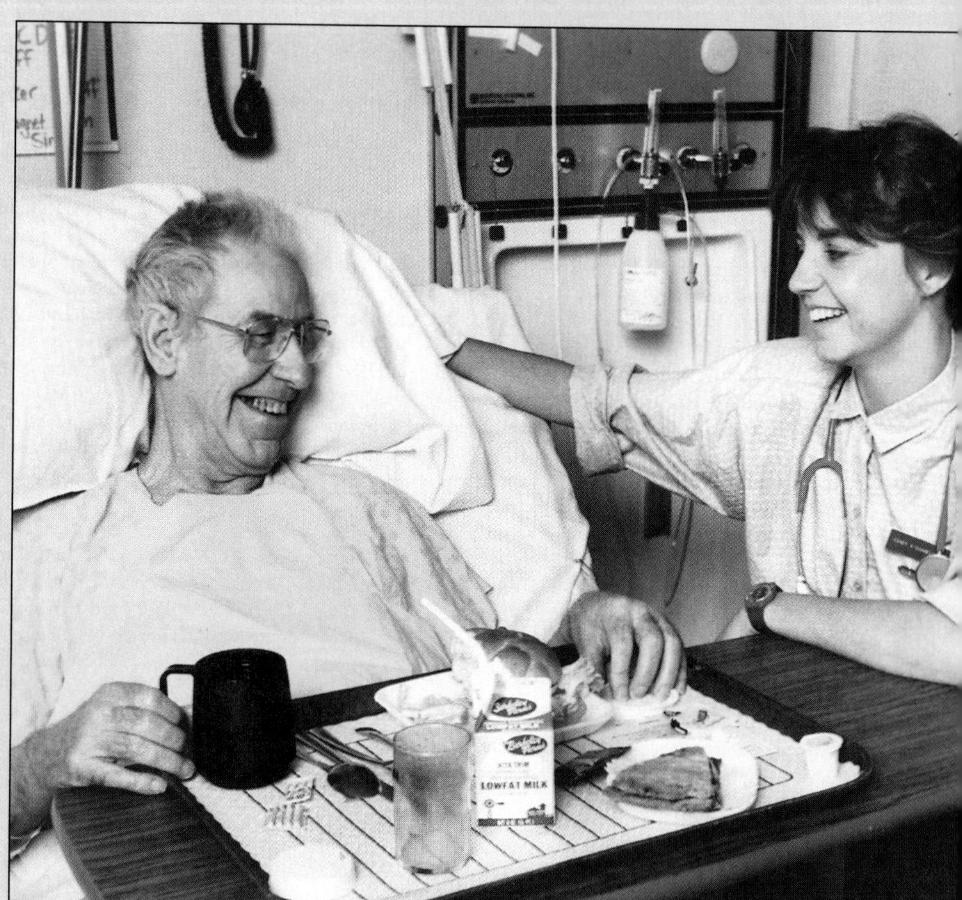

Nutrition is the sum of all the interactions between an organism and the food it consumes (Christian & Greger 1994, p. 3). In other words, nutrition is what a person eats and how the body uses it. **Nutrients** are the organic and inorganic substances found in foods and required for body functioning. People require the essential nutrients in food for the growth and maintenance of all body tissues and the normal functioning of all body processes.

An adequate food intake consists of a balance of essential nutrients: water, carbohydrates, proteins, fats, vitamins, and minerals. Foods differ greatly in their **nutritive value** (the nutrient content of a specified amount of food), and no one food provides all essential nutrients. Nutrients have three major functions: providing energy for body processes and movement, providing structural material for body tissues, and regulating body processes.

The amount of energy that nutrients or foods supply to the body is their **caloric value.** A **calorie** is a unit of heat energy. A **small calorie** is the amount of heat required to raise the temperature of 1 gram of water 1 degree C. A **large calorie (Calorie, kilocalorie [kcal])** is the amount of heat required to raise the temperature of 1 kilogram of water 1 degree C; it is the unit used in nutrition. The energy liberated from each gram of carbohydrate and protein after it is metabolized is about 4 kcal; from each gram of fat, about 9 kcal are liberated through metabolism. The average North American receives approximately 45% of energy from carbohydrates, 40% from fat, and 15% from protein (Guyton 1991, p. 777). In most other parts of the world, people derive far more energy from carbohydrates than from fats and proteins.

Metabolism refers to all biochemical and physiologic processes by which the body grows and maintains itself (Williams & Worthington-Roberts 1992, p. 15). Metabolic rate is normally expressed in terms of the rate of heat liberated during these chemical reactions. The **basal metabolic rate (BMR)** is the rate at which the body metabolizes food to maintain the energy requirements of a person who is awake and at rest. The energy in food maintains the basal metabolic rate of the body and provides energy for activities such as running and walking.

FACTORS AFFECTING CALORIC NEEDS

A person's energy requirements beyond the BMR are influenced by many factors, such as age, body size, activity, body temperature, environmental temperature, growth, sex, and emotional state.

Age and Growth During periods of growth, the body uses more energy. Rapid growth during the first 2 years of life, adolescence, and pregnancy increase the need for calories. The elderly usually require fewer calories. For example, an active adolescent body may need 3600 kcal daily, whereas a 70-year-old woman may require only 1800 kcal or fewer.

Gender Men usually have higher basal metabolic rates than women, a fact largely explained by the greater proportion of muscle in men's bodies.

Climate Climate affects heat production. Generally, people in cold climates have about a 20% higher metabolic rate than people in hot climates. This fact may be due to adaptation of the thyroid gland (increases thyroxin levels) in people who live in cold climates.

Sleep People need less energy during sleep, when the muscles are relaxed and physiologic processes are slowed. The metabolic rate drops about 10% to 15% during sleep.

Activity Muscular activity affects metabolic rate more than any other factor; the more strenuous the activity, the greater the stimulation of the metabolism. Mental activity, which requires only about 4 kcal per hour, provides very little metabolic stimulation.

When energy requirements are completely met by calories taken in as food, a person's weight does not change. When caloric intake exceeds energy needs, the person gains weight. When caloric intake fails to meet energy requirements, the person burns body fat and muscle for energy and loses weight. Energy requirements vary from day to day.

Fever Fever increases the metabolic rate because all chemical reactions in the body, as in the laboratory, occur faster as temperature rises.

Illness Illness often increases energy requirements because of stress and increased metabolic rate.

ESSENTIAL NUTRIENTS

The body's most basic nutrient need is water. Body fluids are discussed in Chapter 38. Because every cell requires a continuous supply of fuel, the most urgent nutritional need, after water, is for nutrients that provide fuel, or energy. The energy-providing nutrients are carbohydrates, fats, and proteins. These are called **macronutrients.** Hunger impels people to eat enough energy-providing nutrients to satisfy their energy needs, but no clear-cut body signals lead a person to ingest certain vitamins or minerals, both of which are often referred to as **micronutrients.**

CARBOHYDRATES

Carbohydrates are composed of the elements carbon (C), hydrogen (H), and oxygen (O) and are of two basic kinds: simple carbohydrates (sugars) and complex carbohydrates (starches and fiber).

Types of Carbohydrates

Sugars Sugars, the simplest of all carbohydrates, are water soluble and are produced naturally by both plants and animals. Sugars may be **monosaccharides** (single molecules) or **disaccharides** (double molecules). Of the three monosaccharides (glucose, fructose, and galactose) glucose is by far the most abundant.

Most sugars are produced naturally by plants, especially fruits, sugar cane, and sugar beet. However, lactose, a combination of glucose and galactose, is found in milk. Processed or refined sugars (eg, table sugar, molasses, and corn syrup) are those that have been extracted and concentrated from natural sources. Processed sugars are added to foods such as soft drinks, cookies, candy, ice cream, and some cereals.

Starches Starches are the insoluble, nonsweet forms of carbohydrate. They are **polysaccharides;** that is, they are composed of branched chains of dozens, sometimes hundreds, of glucose molecules. Like sugars, nearly all starches exist naturally in plants, such as grains, legumes, and potatoes. Starches are processed in various ways, for example, in making such foods as cereals, breads, flour, and puddings.

Fiber Fiber, a complex carbohydrate derived from plants, cannot be digested by humans but supplies roughage, or bulk, to the diet. This bulk satisfies the appetite and also helps the digestive tract to function effectively and to eliminate wastes.

Natural sources of carbohydrates also supply vital nutrients, such as protein, vitamins, minerals, and dietary fiber, that are not found in processed foods. Therefore, it is important that carbohydrate intake include natural as well as processed foods. Refined carbohydrate foods are relatively low in nutrients in relation to the large number of calories they contain and thus are often referred to as "empty calories."

Digestion The desired end products of carbohydrate digestion are monosaccharides (glucose, fructose, and galactose). Some simple sugars, therefore, require no digestion. Major enzymes of carbohydrate digestion include ptyalin (salivary amylase), pancreatic amylase, and the disaccharidases: maltase, sucrase, and lactase. **Enzymes** are biologic catalysts that speed up chemical reactions. Digestive enzymes, which break down nutrients chemically into smaller compounds by hydrolysis, are categorized according to the types of nutrients on which they act.

In healthy persons, essentially all digested carbohydrate is absorbed by the small intestine. Glucose transport through the cell membrane is augmented by insulin, a hormone secreted by the pancreas. Glucose metabolism is therefore controlled by the rate at which insulin is available from the pancreas.

Carbohydrate Metabolism Carbohydrate metabolism is a major source of body energy. After the body breaks carbohydrates down into glucose, some glucose continues to circulate in the blood to maintain blood glucose levels and to provide a readily available source of energy. The remainder is either used as energy or stored.

Storage and Conversion Carbohydrates are stored either as glycogen or as fat. **Glycogen** is a large polymer of glucose. The process of glycogen formation is called **glycogenesis.** All body cells are capable of storing glycogen; however, most is stored in the liver and skeletal muscles, where it is available for conversion back into glucose, either to maintain blood levels or to provide energy. Glucose that cannot be stored as glycogen is converted to fat.

Glycogenolysis is the breakdown of glycogen to reform glucose for use in the cells. Two hormones activate glycogenolysis: *glucagon* and *epinephrine.* When blood glucose concentrations fall, the alpha cells of the pancreas secrete glucagon, which stimulates glycogenolysis, mainly in the liver. The liver then delivers large amounts of glucose into the bloodstream, thus elevating the blood glucose level. When the sympathetic nervous system is stimulated, the adrenal medulla releases epinephrine. This stimulates glycogenolysis in both liver and muscle cells, thereby releasing energy needed by the body for action during sympathetic stimulation.

When body stores of carbohydrates fall below normal, some glucose forms from protein (amino acids) and fat reserves by **gluconeogenesis,** a process that occurs in the liver. Although not all amino acids can be converted, up to 60% of the body's protein can be changed into glucose. During periods of starvation, the body depletes first its fat and later its protein reserves.

Energy Production Once glucose enters the cell, a series of chemical reactions transforms it into energy in the form of **adenosine triphosphate (ATP).** ATP is a compound with high-energy bonds that stores energy for later use in cellular functions. There are two major pathways whereby energy is produced through the breakdown of glucose into the end products of carbon dioxide (CO_2) and water (H_2O):

1. Glycolysis and the formation of pyruvic acid
2. Citric acid cycle (Krebs cycle)

Glycolysis is the first stage in cellular production of energy from glucose. In this process, enzymes catalyze a succession of chemical reactions in which the cell **catabolizes** (breaks down) a glucose molecule into two molecules of pyruvic acid. As the end products of glycolysis are oxidized, energy is released in small packets to form ATP. The formation of pyruvic acid ends the glycolytic process, and provides the gateway to the next energy pathway, the citric acid cycle.

In the **citric acid cycle (Krebs cycle),** a sequence of biochemical reactions breaks down pyruvic acid (from glycolysis) into two molecules of acetyl coenzyme A (acetyl-CoA). The acetyl-CoA then combines with oxaloacetic acid to form citric acid, which gives this cycle its name. In the remainder of the cycle, a series of chemical reactions break down the acetyl portion of acetyl-CoA into carbon dioxide and hydrogen atoms. The hydrogen atoms are subsequently oxidized, thus releasing more energy to form ATP.

PROTEINS

Proteins are organic substances composed of amino acids. Like carbohydrates, proteins contain carbon, hydrogen, and oxygen, but proteins also contain nitrogen. Every cell in the body contains some protein, and about three-quarters of body solids are proteins.

Amino acids are categorized as essential or nonessential. **Essential amino acids** are those that cannot be manufactured in the body and must be supplied as part of the protein ingested in the diet. Nine essential amino acids, threonine, leucine, isoleucine, valine, lysine, methionine, phenylalanine, tryptophan, and histidine, are necessary for tissue growth and maintenance. Arginine is necessary during growth but not during adulthood (Christian & Greger, 1994, p. 211).

Nonessential amino acids are those that the body can manufacture. The body takes apart amino acids derived from the diet and reconstructs new ones from their basic elements (carbohydrates and nitrogen). Nonessential amino acids include glycine, alanine, aspartic acid, glutamic acid, proline, hydroxyproline, cystine, tyrosine, and serine.

Proteins may be complete or incomplete. **Complete proteins** contain all of the essential amino acids plus many nonessential ones. Most animal proteins, including meats, poultry, fish, dairy products, and eggs, are complete proteins. Some animal proteins, however, contain less than the required amount of one or more essential amino acids and therefore cannot alone support continued growth. These proteins are sometimes referred to as **partially complete proteins.** Examples are some fish, which have small amounts of methionine, and the milk protein casein, which has little arginine.

Incomplete proteins lack one or more essential amino acids (most commonly lysine, methionine, or tryptophan) and are usually derived from vegetables. If, however, an appropriate mixture of plant proteins is provided in the diet, a balanced ration of essential amino acids can be achieved. For example, a combination of corn (low in tryptophan and lysine) and beans (low in methionine) is a complete protein. Such combinations of two or more vegetables are called **complementary proteins.** Another way to take full advantage of vegetable proteins is to eat them with a small amount of animal protein. Examples are spaghetti with cheese, rice with pork, noodles with tuna, and cereal with milk. See also the discussion of vegetarian diets, later in this chapter.

Digestion Digestion of protein foods begins in the mouth, where the enzyme pepsin breaks protein down into smaller units. However, most protein is digested in the small intestine, where enzymes break it down into successively smaller molecules and finally into amino acids, the end products of protein digestion. The pancreas secretes the proteolytic enzymes trypsin, chymotrypsin, and carboxypeptidase; glands in the intestinal wall secrete aminopeptidase and dipeptidase.

Storage Amino acids are absorbed by active transport through the small intestine into the portal blood circulation. The liver uses some amino acids to synthesize specific proteins (eg, liver cells and the plasma proteins albumin, globulin, and fibrinogen). Plasma proteins are a labile storage medium that can rapidly be converted back into amino acids.

Other amino acids are transported to tissues and cells throughout the body, where they are used to make protein for cell structures. In a sense, protein is "stored" as body tissue. The body cannot actually store excess amino acids for future use. However, a limited amount is available in the "metabolic pool" that exists as a result of the constant breakdown and buildup of the protein in body tissues.

Protein Metabolism Protein metabolism includes three activities: **anabolism** (building tissue), **catabolism** (breaking down tissue), and balance.

Anabolism All body cells synthesize proteins from amino acids. The types of proteins formed depend on the characteristics of the cell and are controlled by its genes.

Catabolism Because a cell can accumulate only a limited amount of protein, excess amino acids are degraded for energy or converted to fat. Protein degradation occurs primarily in the liver. The process of **deamination**

removes the amino (NH_2) groups from the amino acids. Deaminated amino acids are further catabolized to release energy or converted into glucose or fatty acids. The body also catabolizes tissue proteins to supply amino acids during times of need (eg, during starvation). The balance of tissue and plasma proteins is regulated by hormones. Insulin, growth hormone, and thyroxine (in normal amounts) increase formation of tissue proteins; adrenocortical glucocorticoid hormones and thyroxine (in excess amounts) increase the concentration of plasma amino acids (Dudek 1993, p. 39).

Because nitrogen is the element that distinguishes protein from lipids and carbohydrates, nitrogen balance reflects the status of protein nutrition in the body. **Nitrogen balance** is a measure of the degree of protein anabolism and catabolism; it is the net result of intake and loss of nitrogen. When nitrogen intake equals nitrogen output, a state of nitrogen balance exists. Nitrogen balance is the "normal" state of healthy people who are not pregnant or growing and who are eating an adequate, balanced diet. Nearly all nitrogen is ingested in the form of protein; most nitrogen is lost from the body in the form of the end products of protein catabolism: urea, creatinine, uric acid, and ammonia salts.

Positive nitrogen balance exists when nitrogen intake exceeds output; that is, when protein anabolism exceeds protein catabolism. Positive nitrogen balance may exist under the following conditions:

- During periods of growth, such as
  a. Childhood and adolescence, when height and lean body mass increase
  b. Pregnancy, when new maternal and fetal tissues are forming
  c. Phases of physical exercise, when muscle mass increases
- During periods of tissue replacement, such as
  a. Convalescence from a protein-depleting illness, when body tissues are regenerated
  b. After fasting or inadequate intake of protein and calories, when body tissues are regenerated

Eating more protein than is necessary to meet body needs does not increase positive nitrogen balance or lean body mass in healthy adults. A surplus nitrogen intake is usually balanced by increased excretion of nitrogen as urea. Excess protein intake can lead to weight gain by adding excess calories to the diet.

Negative nitrogen balance exists when nitrogen output exceeds intake (when catabolism exceeds anabolism). This state usually occurs when a person (a) does not consume adequate essential amino acids and/or calories, (b) is immobilized, or (c) is exposed to unusual stress as a result of trauma. An obligatory loss of proteins occurs daily if a person eats no proteins. At the rate of 20 to 30 g per day, body proteins continue to be broken down into amino acids, then deaminated and oxidized. Thus, to prevent a net loss of protein, a person must ingest at least 20 to 30 g of protein each day (Guyton 1991, p. 769).

LIPIDS

Lipids are organic substances that are greasy and insoluble in water but soluble in alcohol or ether. **Fats** are lipids that are solid at room temperature; **oils** are lipids that are liquid at room temperature. In common use, the terms *fats* and *lipids* are used interchangeably. Lipids have the same elements (carbon, hydrogen, and oxygen) as carbohydrates, but they contain a higher proportion of hydrogen.

Fatty acids, made up of carbon chains and hydrogen, are the basic structural units of most lipids. Fatty acids are described as saturated or unsaturated, according to the relative number of hydrogen atoms they contain. **Saturated fatty acids** are those in which all carbon atoms are filled to capacity (ie, saturated) with hydrogen; an example is butyric acid, found in butter. An **unsaturated fatty acid** is one that could accommodate more hydrogen atoms than it currently does. It has at least two carbon atoms that are not attached to a hydrogen atom; instead, there is a double bond between the two carbon atoms. Fatty acids with one double bond are called **monounsaturated fatty acids;** those with more than one double bond (or many carbons not bonded to a hydrogen atom) are **polyunsaturated fatty acids.** An example of a polyunsaturated fatty acid is linoleic acid, found in vegetable oil.

On the basis of their chemical structure, lipids are classified as *simple* or *compound.* **Glycerides,** the *simple lipids,* are the most common form of lipids. They consist of a glycerol molecule with up to three fatty acids attached. **Triglycerides** (which have three fatty acids) account for over 90% of the lipids in food and in the body (Christian & Greger 1994, p. 160). Triglycerides may contain saturated or unsaturated fatty acids. Saturated triglycerides are found in animal products, such as butter, and are usually solid at room temperature. Unsaturated triglycerides are usually liquid at room temperature and are found in plant products, such as olive oil and corn oil.

Compound lipids are various combinations of triglycerides with other components. Two compound lipids important in nutrition are

1. *Phospholipids.* These resemble triglycerides, except that one of the fatty acids is replaced by a phosphoric acid. Because phospholipids can mix with both water and oil, their presence in cell membranes allow both water-soluble and fat-soluble materials to enter the cell.
2. *Sterols.* These are unlike triglycerides in structure. They consist of rings of carbon chains and may or may not have fatty acids attached. Even without fatty acids, sterols are classified as lipids because they are soluble

in ether and insoluble in water. Some important sterols are vitamin D, cholesterol, and certain hormones.

Cholesterol is a sterol that is both produced by the body and found in foods of animal origin. Most of the body's cholesterol is synthesized in the liver; however, some is absorbed from the diet (eg, from milk, egg yolk, and organ meats). Cholesterol is a precursor of bile acids and is necessary for the synthesis of steroid hormones. Along with phospholipids, large quantities of cholesterol are present in cell membranes as well as other cell structures.

Digestion Although chemical digestion of lipids begins in the stomach, they are digested mainly in the small intestine, primarily by bile, pancreatic lipase, and enteric lipase, an intestinal enzyme. The end products of lipid digestion are glycerol, fatty acids, and cholesterol. These are immediately reassembled inside the intestinal cells into triglycerides and cholesterol esters (cholesterol with a fatty acid attached to it), which are not water soluble. For these reassembled products to be transported and used, the small intestine and the liver must convert them into soluble compounds called lipoproteins. **Lipoproteins** are made up of various lipids and a protein. Lipoproteins made in the liver are classified as follows:

- High-density lipoproteins are those that contain the highest concentrations of protein (about 50%).
- Low-density lipoproteins contain few triglycerides but very high concentrations of cholesterol.
- Very-low-density lipoproteins contain little protein but high concentrations of triglycerides and moderate concentrations of phospholipids and cholesterol.

Lipid Transport and Storage Some end products of fat digestion (eg, glycerol and some free fatty acids) are absorbed into the portal blood system and carried to the liver. Others (eg, monoglycerides and cholesterol) are absorbed into the abdominal lacteals and transported through the lymphatic system to the thoracic duct, where they enter the blood through the left subclavian vein. Large quantities of lipids are stored in two major tissues: adipose tissue and the liver. Adipose tissue, referred to as the fat depot, has two functions: It (a) stores triglycerides until they are needed for energy, and (b) provides body insulation. The liver functions in lipid metabolism to degrade fatty acids into smaller compounds that can be used for energy, to synthesize triglycerides from carbohydrates and proteins, and to synthesize other lipids (eg, cholesterol and phospholipids) from fatty acids (Guyton 1991, p. 756).

MICRONUTRIENTS

A **vitamin** is an organic compound that cannot be manufactured by the body and is needed in small quantities to catalyze metabolic processes. Thus, when vitamins are lacking in the diet, metabolic deficits result. Vitamins are generally classified as fat soluble or water soluble. **Water-soluble vitamins** include C and the B-complex vitamins: B_1 (thiamine), B_2 (riboflavin), B_3 (niacin or nicotinic acid), B_6 (pyridoxine), B_9 (folic acid), B_{12} (cobalamin), pantothenic acid, and biotin. The body cannot store water-soluble vitamins; thus, people must get a daily supply in the diet. Water-soluble vitamins can be affected by food processing, storage, and preparation.

Fat-soluble vitamins include A, D, E, and K. The body can store these vitamins, although there is a limit to the amounts of vitamins E and K the body can store. Therefore, a daily supply of fat-soluble vitamins is not absolutely necessary. Vitamin content is highest in fresh foods that are consumed as soon as possible after harvest. The *Clinical Companion* has the usually recommended daily requirement of vitamins, food sources, functions, and signs of deficiencies and excesses.

Minerals are found in organic compounds, as inorganic compounds, and as free ions. On oxidation, minerals leave an ash, which can be acid or alkaline. Calcium and phosphorus make up 80% of all the mineral elements in the body. There are two categories of minerals; macrominerals and microminerals. **Macrominerals** are those that people require daily in amounts over 100 mg. They include calcium, phosphorus, sodium, potassium, magnesium, chloride, and sulfur. **Microminerals** are those that people require daily in amounts less than 100 mg. They include iron, zinc, manganese, iodine, fluoride, copper, cobalt, chromium, and selenium.

Common problems associated with the mineral nutrients are iron deficiency resulting in anemia, and osteoporosis resulting from loss of bone calcium. Key information about many essential minerals is shown in the *Clinical Companion*. Additional information about major minerals associated with the body's fluid and electrolyte balance is given in Chapter 38.

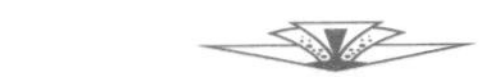

STANDARDS FOR A HEALTHY DIET

Various daily food guides have been developed to help healthy people meet the daily requirements of essential nutrients and to facilitate meal planning. Food group plans emphasize the general types or groups of foods rather than the specific foods, because related foods are similar in composition and often have similar nutrient values. For example, all grains, whether wheat, or oats, are significant sources of carbohydrate, iron, and the B vitamin thiamine. Daily food guides that are currently used include *Dietary Guidelines for Americans*, *The Food Guide Pyramid*, and *Canada's Food Guide to Healthy Eating*.

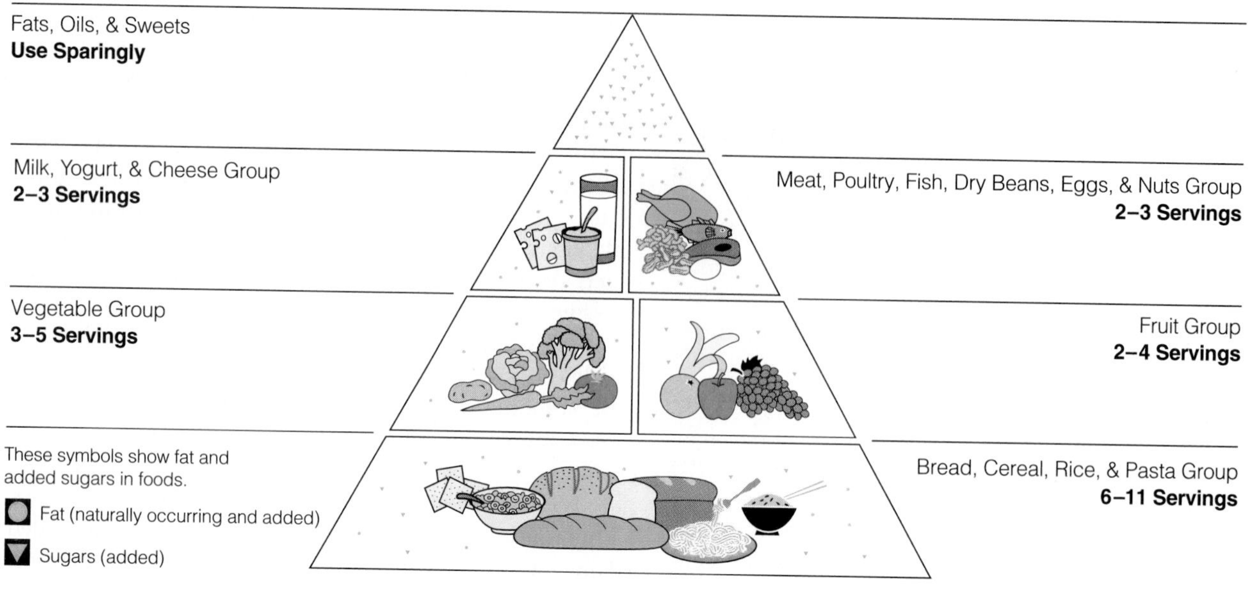

Figure 37–1 The Food Guide Pyramid. **Source:** US Department of Agriculture and US Department of Health and Human Services, *Nutrition and Your Health: Dietary Guidelines for Americans,* Home and Garden Bulletin No. 232 (Washington, DC: US Government Printing Office, 1980, 1985, 1990).

DIETARY GUIDELINES FOR AMERICANS

This guide was first published in 1980 by the United States Department of Agriculture (USDA) and the Department of Health and Human Services (DHHS). The 1990 revision contains recommendations for food choices to help promote health and prevent certain diseases. Key points of the *Dietary Guidelines* follow:

- Eat a variety of foods.
- Maintain a healthy weight.
- Eat a diet low in fat, saturated fat, and cholesterol.
- Eat plenty of vegetables, fruits, and grain products.
- Use sugars in moderation.
- Use salt and sodium in moderation.
- If you drink alcohol, do so in moderation.

These dietary recommendations are intended to help achieve the nutritional goals stated in *Healthy People 2000.* In that report, the US surgeon general identified 21 specific nutritional objectives, such as the following (1990, pp. 93–94):

- Reduce the incidence of overweight people by 23%.
- Reduce growth retardation among low-income children aged 5 and younger to less than 10%.
- Reduce coronary heart disease deaths to no more than 100 per 100,000 people.
- Reduce dietary fat intake to an average of 30% of calories.
- Decrease salt and sodium intake so that at least 60% of home meal preparers prepare foods without adding salt.
- Achieve useful and informative labeling for virtually all processed food.

THE FOOD GUIDE PYRAMID

The Food Guide Pyramid is a graphic aid that was developed by the USDA as a guide in making daily food choices (Figure 37–1). The Pyramid synthesizes the *Dietary Guidelines* and the old *Basic Four Food Guide.*

The Pyramid, like the *Basic Four*, suggests that people eat a variety of foods to obtain the nutrients they need. It divides foods into six groups, each rich in certain nutrients. The groups are assigned to blocks of different sizes; the foods needed in the largest amounts (ie, the bread, cereal, rice, and pasta group) appear in the largest block. In the smallest box, at the top of the Pyramid, are the fats, oils, and sweets group; these are labeled "Use Sparingly." Beside each block is the recommended number of daily servings. These are not listed as minimums, but as ranges to meet the nutrient needs of a variety of people. Because individuals differ in size, activity level, and so on, they need different amounts of food to meet their various nutrient needs. Numbers and sizes of servings are listed for each group in Table 37–1.

The Pyramid is designed to help people reduce their intake of fat and concentrated sugars. The small circles in the top box of the pyramid represent fat; the triangles represent concentrated sugars. The circles and triangles are

Table 37–1 Daily Food Guide

Food Groups and Servings	Foods and Sizes of Servings	Major Nutrients
Bread, Cereal, Rice and Pasta 6 to 11 servings, including several whole grains and enriched products. Limit fats and sugar (eg, pastries, cookies).	1 serving = 1 slice bread, 1 oz ready-to-eat cereal, or ½ cup of the following: cooked cereal, cornmeal, grits, spaghetti, macaroni, noodles, popcorn, tortillas, or rice.	Complex carbohydrate; thiamine; niacin; iron; some protein; fiber
Vegetable Group 3 to 5 servings, including	1 serving = 1 cup raw leafy vegetables; ½ cup other fresh, frozen, or canned vegetables; ¾ cup fresh, frozen, or canned juice; ¼ cup dried vegetables.	Carbohydrate; vitamin C; vitamin A; iron; folacin; calcium; fiber (naturally low in fat)
a. 1 to 2 servings of good sources of vitamin C.	Broccoli, brussels sprouts, green pepper, asparagus, cabbage, cauliflower, collards, potatoes, spinach, tomatoes.	
b. 1 good source of vitamin A at least every other day. (Choose dark green and orange vegetables often.)	Broccoli, carrots, chard, collards, kale, pumpkin, spinach, sweet potatoes, turnip greens, winter squash.	
Fruit Group 2 to 4 servings, including	1 serving = 1 medium apple, banana, or orange; ½ cup of raw, cooked, or canned fruit; ¾ cup of fruit juice; ¼ cup of dried fruit.	Vitamins A and C; potassium; folacin; fiber (naturally low in sodium)
a. 1 to 2 good sources of vitamin C	Grapefruit or grapefruit juice; orange or orange juice; cantaloupe; raw strawberries.	
b. Good sources of vitamin A. (Choose orange fruits often.)	Apricots, cantaloupe.	
Meat, Poultry, Fish, Beans, Eggs, and Nuts 2 to 3 servings. (Choose lean meat; poultry without skin; limit egg yolks, but not whites.)	1 serving = 1 egg; ½ cup cooked legumes (eg, garbanzo, kidney, lima, pinto, or navy beans; lentils, split peas); 3 oz tofu; 2 T peanut butter; ¼ cup nuts or seeds; 2 to 3 oz lean beef, pork, lamb, veal, poultry, or fish (no bone).	Protein; vitamin B; iron; zinc; niacin; fats (in meats, nuts, and seeds)
Milk, Yogurt, and Cheese Servings: Child under 9: 2 to 3; Child 9 to 12: 3 or more; Teenager: 4 or more; Adult: 2 or more; Pregnant: 3 or more; Lactating: 4 or more. (Choose skim and low-fat milk and yogurt often. Limit high-fat cheese and ice cream.)	1 serving = 1 cup (8 oz) milk or yogurt, 1½ oz natural cheese, 2 oz processed cheese food, 2 cups cottage cheese, 1 cup sauces or puddings, 1⅔ cups ice cream. (Servings are based on calcium content.)	Protein; fat; vitamins A and D; riboflavin; B_{12}; calcium; phosphorous
Fats, Oils, and Sweets Use sparingly	Butter, salad oils, margarine, lard.	Fat, carbohydrate (very high in calories)
	Table sugar, brown sugar, confectioner's sugar, honey, molasses, maple syrup, corn syrup, jams, jellies, colas, and soft drinks.	

Sources: Adapted from SG Dudek, *Nutrition Handbook for Nursing Practice*, 2d ed. (Philadelphia: Lippincott, 1993), pp. 182–85; DE Scholl, *Nutrition and Diet Therapy: A Handbook for Nurses*, (Oradell, NJ: Medical Economics Books, 1986), pp. 4–6; JL Christian and JL Greger, *Nutrition for Living*, 4th ed. (Redwood City, CA: Benjamin/Cummings, 1994), pp. 45–52; and *The Food Guide Pyramid*, (Washington, DC: US Department of Agriculture and US Department of Health and Human Services, 1990).

WELLNESS TEACHING

Reducing Dietary Fat

- Cook meat by grilling, baking, broiling, or microwaving rather than frying.
- Substitute popcorn or pretzels for such snacks as potato chips, cheese puffs, corn chips, and nuts.
- Read labels. Some crackers, for example, are high in fat; others are not.
- Limit desserts high in fat, such as candy, ice cream, cake, and cookies.
- Substitute hard candies for chocolate bars.
- Use skim or reduced-fat milk instead of whole milk, for drinking as well as in recipes.
- Use less butter or margarine on breads.
- Remove fat from meat and skin from chicken before cooking.
- Eat less meat; eat more fish.
- Use less dressing, or use low-fat dressings, on salads.
- Eat plant sources of protein (eg, kidney, lima, and navy beans).

shown in all boxes of the pyramid to indicate that fats and sugars are present in those groups as well. Widely scattered symbols indicate that the foods in that group are lower in fats and sugars (eg, the vegetable group contains less fat and sugar than the milk group). See also the box above for ways to reduce fat intake.

The Food Guide Pyramid does not address fluid intake or provide guidelines about combination foods (such as chili, which contains meat, beans, and a vegetable) or about convenience foods (such as hamburgers, milk shakes, and pizzas), which are an important part of the North American diet. Following this guide does not guarantee that a person will consume the necessary levels of all essential nutrients (for example, someone who chooses cooked and *low*-fiber fruits and vegetables might have an inadequate intake of dietary fiber even though the recommended number of servings is eaten). However, the food guide is easy to follow, and people who eat a variety of foods from each group, in the suggested amounts, are likely to come close to recommended nutrient levels.

CANADA'S FOOD GUIDE TO HEALTHY EATING

Canada's Food Guide to Healthy Eating (see Table 37–2) is a booklet of dietary guidelines for Canadians 4 years old and over. It stresses the need to choose a variety of foods from within each of its four groups. Foods selected according to the *Guide* supply 1000 to 1400 kilocalories. Those who need more calories or nutrients should increase the number and size of servings from the various groups and/or add other foods. Recommendations also include a decrease in fat consumption and limited use of salt, alcohol, and caffeine.

RECOMMENDED DIETARY ALLOWANCES

The Committee on Dietary Allowances of the Food and Nutrition Board of the National Academy of Sciences in Washington, DC, publishes lists of *recommended dietary allowances (RDAs)*. RDAs are the levels of intake, in grams and milligrams, of essential nutrients that, to the best available scientific knowledge, adequately meet the known nutritional needs of most healthy people (National Research Council 1989). RDAs are most appropriate for use by professionals, whereas the daily food guides are intended for widespread public use. The Canadian Department of National Health and Welfare also prepares standards, called the *recommended daily nutrient intakes*, for 15 different age groups, for each trimester of pregnancy, and for lactating women. RDAs for vitamins and minerals are found in the *Clinical Companion*. Separate recommendations are made for various subgroups defined by sex, age, pregnancy, and lactation. Recommended nutrient levels are usually set high enough to include the needs of 97.5% of the people in that group and to allow for some loss of the nutrient as it makes its way through the body. The effect of illness or injury (increasing the need for nutrients) and the variability among individuals within any given subgroup are not taken into account in the RDAs.

VEGETARIAN DIETS

People may become vegetarians for economic, health, religious, ethical, or ecologic reasons. There are two basic vegetarian diets: those that use only plant foods and those that include milk, eggs, and dairy products. Some people eat fish and poultry but not beef, lamb, or pork; others eat only fresh fruit, juices, and nuts; and still others eat plant foods and dairy products but not eggs. See Table 37–3 on page 1024 for additional types of vegetarian diets.

Vegetarian diets can be nutritionally sound if they include a wide variety of foods and if proper protein complementation and vitamin and mineral supplementation are provided. Because the proteins found in plant foods are incomplete proteins, vegetarians must eat complementary protein foods to obtain all the essential amino acids. A plant protein can be *complemented* by combining

Table 37–2 Canada's Food Guide to Healthy Eating (1992)

For people 4 years and over

Different People Need Different Amounts of Food

The amount of food you need every day from the four food groups and other foods depends on your age, body size, activity level, whether you are male or female, and whether you are pregnant or breast-feeding. That's why the Food Guide gives a lower and higher number of servings for each food group. For example, young children can choose the lower number of servings, whereas male teenagers can go to the higher number. Most other people can choose servings somewhere in between.

Food Group	Servings per Day	Examples of One Serving	Examples of Two Servings
Grain products	5 to 12	1 slice bread 30 g cold cereal 175 mL (3/4 cup) hot cereal	1 bagel, pita, or bun 250 mL (1 cup) pasta or rice
Vegetables and fruit	5 to 10	1 medium size vegetable or fruit 125 mL (1/2 cup) fresh, frozen, or canned vegetables or fruit 250 mL (1 cup) salad 125 mL (1/2 cup) juice	
Milk products	Children, 4 to 9: 2 to 3 Youth, 10 to 16: 3 to 4 Adults: 2 to 4 Pregnant and breastfeeding women: 3 to 4	250 mL (1 cup) milk 50 g (3″ × 1″ × 1″) cheese 50 g (2 slices) cheese 175 g (3/4 cup) yogurt	
Meat and alternatives	2 to 3	50 to 100 g meat, poultry, or fish 50 to 100 g (1/3 to 2/3 can) fish 1 to 2 eggs 125 to 250 mL beans 100 g (1/3 cup) tofu 30 mL (2 T) peanut butter	

Other Foods

Taste and enjoyment can also come from other foods and beverages that are not part of the four food groups. Some of these foods are higher in fat or calories, so use these foods in moderation.

Enjoy eating well, being active and feeling good about yourself. That's VITALITY®.

Sources: *Canada's Food Guide for Healthy Eating; Using the Food Guide* Catalog No. H39-252/1992E, (Ottawa: Health and Welfare Canada, 1992).

it with a different plant protein. The combination produces a complete protein. See the box on page 1024. Obtaining complete proteins is especially important for growing children and pregnant and lactating women, whose protein needs are high. Generally, legumes (starchy beans, peas, lentils) have complementary relationships with grains, nuts, and seeds. Complementary foods must be eaten in the same meal. Diets such as the fruitarian diet do not provide sufficient amounts of essential nutrients and are not recommended for long-term use.

Foods of animal origin are the best source of vitamin B_{12}. Therefore, vegans (strict vegetarians) need to obtain this vitamin from other sources: brewer's yeast, foods fortified with vitamin B_{12}, or a vitamin supplement. Because iron from plant sources is not absorbed as efficiently as iron from meat, vegans should eat iron-rich foods (eg, green leafy vegetables, whole grains, raisins, and molasses) and iron-enriched foods. They should eat a food rich in vitamin C at each meal to enhance iron absorption. Calcium deficiency is a concern only for strict vegetarians. It can be prevented by including in the diet soybean milk and tofu (soybean curd) fortified with calcium and leafy green vegetables. Table 37–4 on page 1024 shows a food guide for vegetarians. It includes specific vegetables to supplement any calcium, riboflavin, and vitamin D deficiencies.

Table 37–3 Types of Vegetarian Diets

Kind	Description
Vegans	Strict vegetarians; avoid all foods of animal origin
Lacto-ovo-vegetarians	Use dairy products and avoid eating flesh
Lacto-vegetarians	Use dairy products but avoid eating flesh and eggs
Ovo-vegetarians	Use eggs but avoid dairy products and flesh
Pesco-vegetarians	Use dairy products, eggs, and fish but avoid all other meat products
Partial vegetarians (semivegetarians)	Avoid selected meats (eg, red meat)
Fruitarians	Use only fresh (raw) fruits, juices, nuts, honey, and/or olive oil
Macrobiotic vegetarians	Progress through ten dietary stages from a widely inclusive selection to a restrictive selection

COMBINATIONS OF PLANT PROTEINS THAT PROVIDE COMPLETE PROTEINS

Grains plus legumes = complete protein.
Legumes plus nuts or seeds = complete protein.
Grains, legumes, nuts, or seeds plus milk or milk products (eg, cheese) = complete protein.

Grains	*Legumes*	*Nuts and Seeds*
brown rice	black beans	almonds
barley	kidney beans	Brazil nuts
corn meal	lima beans	cashews
millet	soybeans	pecans
oats/oatmeal	lentils	walnuts
rye	tofu	pumpkin seeds
whole wheat	black-eyed peas	sesame seeds
	split peas	sunflower seeds

Examples: black-eyed peas and rice
lentil soup and whole wheat bread
beans and tortillas
lima beans and sesame seeds

or

cereal with milk
macaroni with cheese

Table 37–4 Dietary Recommendations for Lacto-Vegetarians and Lacto-Ovo-Vegetarians Based on Food Guide Pyramid

Food Groups	Servings
Fats	0 to 4
Bread, rice, cereal, and pasta (include at least 4 servings of whole-grain bread or cereal)	6
Vegetables (at least 2 dark leafy vegetables per day and those rich in riboflavin and calcium, such as broccoli, rutabaga, avocado)	3 to 5
Fruits	2 to 4
Milk, yogurt, and cheese	2 (3 servings if under age 24)
Beans, eggs, and nuts (meats, poultry, fish not eaten)	1 serving of legumes 1 serving of nuts or seeds

- 4 to 6 daily servings of complementary protein should be included in the servings recommended above. Proteins are found in all except the fruit group; highest protein content is found in foods in the last two groups: milk/yogurt/cheese and beans/eggs/nuts.
- Eat a fruit or vegetable rich in vitamin C at each meal.
- Each of the following constitutes 1 serving:

1 egg	¼ to ½ cup nuts or seeds
½ to ¾ cup dried peas, beans, lentils (cooked)	½ cup cottage cheese
	1 oz cheddar cheese
2 T peanut butter	1 slice bread

Source: SG Dudek, *Nutrition Handbook for Nursing Practice*, 2d ed. (Philadelphia: Lippincott, 1993), pp. 45–50; DE Scholl, *Nutrition and Diet Therapy: A Handbook for Nurses* (Oradell, NJ: Medical Economics Books, 1986), pp. 21–23; SR Williams and BS Worthington-Roberts, editors, *Nutrition Throughout the Life Cycle*, (St Louis: Mosby, 1992), pp. 18–19; and JL Christian and JL Greger, *Nutrition for Living*, 4th ed. (Redwood City, CA: Benjamin/Cummings, 1994), pp. 43, 211.

Table 37–5 Problems Associated with Nutrition in the Elderly

Problems	Nursing Interventions
Difficulty chewing (may lead to a deficiency in vitamins A and C, minerals, and fiber)	Encourage regular visits to the dentist to have dentures repaired, refitted, or replaced.
	Chop fruits and vegetables finely; shred green, leafy vegetables; select ground meat, poultry, or fish.
Lowered glucose tolerance	Eat more complex carbohydrates (eg, breads, cereals, rice, pasta, potatoes, and legumes) rather than sugar-rich foods
Decreased social interaction, loneliness	Promote appropriate social interaction at meals, when possible.
	Encourage the client and spouse to take an interest in food preparation and serving, perhaps as an activity they can do together.
	If food preparation is not possible, suggest community resources, such as Meals-on-Wheels.
	Suggest picnics in the yard or inviting friends over for meals.
Loss of appetite and senses of smell and taste	Eat essential, nutrient-dense foods first; follow with desserts and low-nutrient-density foods.
	Review dietary restrictions, and find ways to make meals appealing within these guidelines.
	Eat small meals frequently instead of three large meals a day.
Limited income	Suggest using generic brands and coupons.
	Substitute milk, dairy products, and beans for meat
	Avoid convenience foods if able to cook. Buy foods that are on sale and freeze for future use.
	Suggest community resources and nutrition programs.
Difficulty sleeping at night	Have the major meal at noon instead of in the evening.
	Avoid tea, coffee, or other stimulants in the evening.

DIETARY MODIFICATIONS FOR OLDER ADULTS

Metabolic rates decrease with age, when physical activity usually slackens; therefore, elderly people require fewer calories than they required formerly. Some may need more carbohydrates for fiber and bulk, but most nutrient requirements remain relatively unchanged. Such physical changes as tooth loss and impaired sense of taste and smell may also affect eating habits. Decreased saliva and gastric juice secretion may also affect a person's nutrition (Williams & Worthington-Roberts 1992, pp. 348–54).

Psychosocial factors may also contribute to nutritional problems. Some elderly people who live alone do not want to cook for themselves or eat alone. As a result, they may adopt poor dietary habits. Loss of spouse, anxiety, depression, dependence on others, and lowered income all affect eating habits. See Table 37–5. Guidelines for the inclusion of high-nutrient foods that are compatible with the nutritional needs of older adults are summarized in the box on page 1026.

FACTORS INFLUENCING DIET

Before attempting to assess a client's nutritional status, the nurse needs to recognize factors that affect an individual's eating habits, such as ethnicity and culture, age, religion, economic status, peer group, personal preference, lifestyle, beliefs about health effects of food, alcohol abuse, advertising, psychologic factors, health status, therapy, and medications. These factors frequently occur in combination.

Ethnicity and Culture Ethnicity often determines food preferences. Traditional foods (eg, rice for Asians, pasta for Italians, curry for Indians) are eaten long after other customs are abandoned.

WELLNESS TEACHING

Nutrition for Older Adults

- *Include at least the minimal number of servings from each group on the Food Guide Pyramid:*

Bread, cereal, grains, and pasta	6 servings
Vegetables	3 servings
Fruits	2 servings
Milk, yogurt, and cheese	2 servings
Meat, poultry, fish, beans, eggs, and nuts	2 servings

- *Reduce caloric intake.* Caloric needs generally decrease in the elderly often because of decreased activity. Elderly people need to consume nutrient-dense foods and avoid foods that are high in calories but have few nutrients ("empty-calorie" foods).
- *Reduce fat consumption.* Use leaner cuts of meat, and limit portions to 4 to 6 oz per day. (But be sure intake of meat group is sufficient, because older people often consume inadequate amounts of these foods.) Broil, boil, or bake foods instead of frying them. Use low-fat milk and cheese; limit intake of butter, margarine, and salad dressings.
- *Reduce consumption of empty calories.* Substitute fruit or puddings made with low-fat milk in place of pastry, cookies, and rich desserts.
- *Reduce sodium consumption for clients who have hypertension or other cardiac problems.* Avoid canned soups, ketchup, mustard. Avoid salted, smoked, cured, and pickled meats (eg, ham and bacon), poultry, and fish. Do not add salt when cooking foods or at the table.
- *Ensure adequate calcium intake (at least 800 mg) to prevent bone loss.* Milk, cheese, yogurt, cream soups, puddings, and frozen milk products are good sources. See Table 37–6 for additional calcium-rich foods.
- *Ensure adequate vitamin D intake.* Vitamin D is essential to maintain calcium homeostasis. Include some milk, because other dairy products are not usually fortified with vitamin D. If milk cannot be tolerated because of a lactose deficiency, provide vitamin supplements.
- *Ensure adequate iron intake.* Iron intake in the elderly may be compromised by such factors as increased incidence of gastrointestinal disturbance, chronic diarrhea, regular aspirin use, and possible reduction in meat consumption. See Table 37–7 for iron-rich foods.
- *Consume fiber-rich foods to prevent constipation and minimize use of laxatives.* See Table 37–8 for examples of fiber-rich foods. Because fiber-rich foods provide bulk and a feeling of fullness, they help people control their appetites and lose weight.

Table 37–6 Major Food Sources of Calcium

Foods	Household Measure	Calcium (mg)
Dairy Products		
Milk, nonfat dry (reconstituted)	1 cup	240
Milk, skim (1% fat)	1 cup	296
Milk, whole	1 cup	288
Cheese, processed	1 oz (1 slice)	198
Cheese, cheddar	1 oz	213
Cheese, cottage, 4% milk fat	1 oz	27
Cheese, Swiss	1 oz	262
Custard	½ cup	148
Ice cream	½ cup	97
Yogurt	1 cup	295
Fish, Meat, and Poultry		
Salmon (canned)	1 oz	91
Sardines	1 oz	124
Shellfish	1 oz	35
Vegetables		
Broccoli (cooked)	1 medium stalk	158
Greens, collards	½ cup	179
Beet greens	½ cup	72
Okra	10 pods	98
Fruits		
Orange	1 medium	54
Blackberries	1 cup	46
Dates	10	45
Rhubarb (sweetened)	½ cup	105

Sources: AB Natow and J Heslin, *Nutritional Care of the Older Adult,* (New York: Macmillan, 1986), p. 212; and DE Scholl, *Nutrition and Diet Therapy: A Handbook for Nurses,* (Oradell, NJ: Medical Economics Books, 1986), p. 214.

Table 37–7 Major Food Sources of Iron

Foods	Household Measure	Iron (mg)
Meat, Fish, Poultry		
Beef (ground)	3 oz	3.2
Beef liver	3 oz	5.1
Beef heart	3½ oz	5.9
Beef kidneys	3½ oz	7.4
Chicken (breast)	3 oz	1.3
Oysters	5 to 8 medium	5.5
Scallops	3½ oz	3.0
Shrimp	3½ oz	3.1
Tuna (canned)	3 oz	1.5
Vegetables and Fruits		
Spinach		
raw	½ cup	2
cooked	½ cup	2.2
Beet greens	⅔ cup	1.9
Chick peas	½ cup	3
Kidney beans	½ cup	3
Soybeans	3½ oz	2.8
Dates (pitted)	½ cup	3
Prune juice	½ cup	4.1
Raisins	⅔ cup	3.5
Grain Products		
Bread		
white	1 slice	0.6
whole-wheat	1 slice	0.8
Enriched pasta	½ cup	2.0
Cereal (bran flakes)	1 oz	5.3
Cereal (oat flakes)	1 oz	5.4
Spaghetti (enriched)	½ cup	0.3
Other		
Tofu (soybean curd)	½ cup	1.9
Eggs	2 medium	2.3
Peanuts	⅔ cup	2.1
Corn syrup	⅓ cup	4.1
Molasses	1 T	0.9

Sources: JL Christian and JL Greger, *Nutrition for Living*, 4th ed. (Redwood City, CA: Benjamin/Cummings, 1994), pp. 384–85, 403; AB Natow and J Heslin, *Nutritional Care of the Older Adult*, (New York: Macmillan, 1986), p. 212; and SG Dudek, *Nutrition Handbook for Nursing Practice*, 2d ed. (Philadelphia: Lippincott, 1994), pp. 492–93.

Table 37–8 Fiber-Rich Foods

Food	Portion	Insoluble Dietary Fiber Content (g)
Apple	1 medium	3.3
Fresh pear	1 medium	4.2
Banana	1	2.1
Beans, green	½ cup	1.8 to 2.2
Broccoli	1 cup	4.8
Peas	1 cup	5.0
Cereal, All Bran	⅓ cup	7.8
Cereal, bran flakes	1 cup	6.8
Lima beans	½ cup	3.2
Kidney beans	½ cup	5.6

Source: Adapted from JL Christian and JL Greger, *Nutrition for Living*, 4th ed. (Redwood City, CA: Benjamin/Cummings, 1994), pp. 42–44.

Nurses should not use a "good food, bad food" approach, but rather should realize that variations of intake are acceptable under different circumstances. The only "universally" accepted guidelines are (a) to eat a wide variety of foods to furnish adequate nutrients, and (b) to eat moderately to maintain correct body weight (Herron 1991, p. 877). Food preference probably differs as much among individuals of the same cultural background as they do generally between cultures. Not all Italians like pepperoni, for example, and many undoubtedly eat tacos.

Age Throughout the life cycle, changes in activity, metabolism, and body composition change nutrient requirements. During periods of rapid growth (ie, during adolescence and pregnancy), the need for nutrients increases. People's needs stabilize during adulthood, although the elderly often require smaller quantities of food. For details about nourishment for each age group, see Chapters 24, 25, and 26.

Religion Religious practice also affects diet. Some Roman Catholics avoid meat on certain days, and some Protestant faiths prohibit meat, tea, coffee, or alcohol. Both Orthodox Judaism and Islam prohibit pork. Orthodox Jews observe kosher customs, eating certain foods only if they are inspected by a rabbi and prepared according to dietary laws. The nurse must be sensitive to such religious dietary practices.

Economic Status What, how much, and how often a person eats are frequently affected by economic status.

EXAMPLES OF FOOD FADS AND MYTHS

- Eating large amounts of yogurt and vitamin E retards aging.
- Honey is healthier than sugar, more readily digested, and a cure for the common cold.
- Cabbage and onions "turn" breast milk.
- Raw eggs, rare lean beef, and oysters increase sexual potency or fertility.
- Yogurt is more nutritious than milk.

For example, people with limited income, including some elderly people, may not be able to afford beef and fresh vegetables. In contrast, people with higher incomes may purchase more proteins and fats and fewer complex carbohydrates.

Peer Groups Peer groups distinguished by age, sex, occupation, or other interests also influence a person's food choices. For example, certain foods may become "in" with teenagers. Sexism may also influence food choices. Some men, for example, may not choose a salad as an entree because they perceive such a choice as feminine.

Personal Preference and Uniqueness People develop likes and dislikes based on associations with a typical food. A child who loves to visit his grandparents may love pickled crabapples because they are served in the grandparents' home. Another child who dislikes a very strict aunt grows up to dislike the chicken casserole she often prepares. People often carry such preferences into adulthood.

Individual likes and dislikes can also be related to familiarity. Children often say they dislike a food before they sample it. Some adults are very adventuresome and eager to try new foods. Others prefer to eat the same foods over and over again. Preferences in the tastes, smells, flavors (blends of taste and smell), temperatures, colors, shapes, and sizes of food influence a person's food choices. For example, some people may prefer sweet and sour tastes to bitter or salty tastes. Textures play a great role in food preferences. Some people prefer crisp food to limp food, firm to soft, tender to tough, smooth to lumpy, or dry to soggy.

Life-Style Certain life-styles are linked to food-related behaviors. People who are always in a hurry probably buy convenience grocery items or eat restaurant meals. People who spend many hours at home may take time to prepare more meals "from scratch." Individual differences also influence life-style patterns (eg, cooking skills, concern about health).

Beliefs About Health Effects of Food Beliefs about effects of foods on health and well-being can affect food choices. Many people acquire their beliefs about food from television, magazines, and other media. For example, some people are reducing their intake of animal fats in response to published evidence that excessive consumption of animal fats is a major risk factor in cardiovascular disease.

Food fads that involve nontraditional food practices are relatively common. A **fad** is a widespread but short-lived interest or a practice followed with considerable zeal. It may be based either on the belief that certain foods have special powers or on the notion that certain foods are harmful. Examples of some food fads are given in the accompanying box. Food fads typically appeal to the individual seeking a miracle cure for a disease or the person who desires superior health and wants to delay aging. Some fad diets are harmless, but others are potentially dangerous. Determining the needs a fad diet fills for the client enables the nurse both to support these needs and to suggest a more nutritious diet.

Alcohol Abuse Excessive alcohol use contributes to nutritional deficiencies in a number of ways. Alcohol may replace food in a person's diet, and it can also depress the appetite. Excessive alcohol can have a toxic effect on the intestinal mucosa, thereby decreasing the absorption of nutrients. The need for vitamin B increases, because it is used in alcohol metabolism.

Alcohol can impair the storage of nutrients and increase nutrient catabolism and excretion. Alcohol abuse is also associated with liver disease.

Advertising Food producers try to persuade people to change from the product they currently use to the brand of the producer. Often popular actors and actresses are used to influence television viewers' or radio listeners' choices. Advertising is thought to influence people's food choices and eating patterns to a certain extent. Of note is that such products as alcoholic beverages, cake and other dessert mixes, soups, tea, coffee, frozen dinners, and soft drinks are more heavily advertised than such products as milk, canned seafood, bread, cheese, poultry, vegetables, and fruits (Christian & Greger 1994, p. 10).

Psychologic Factors Although some people overeat when stressed, depressed, or lonely, others eat very little under the same conditions. Anorexia and weight loss can indicate severe stress or depression. Anorexia nervosa and bulimia are severe psychophysiologic conditions seen most frequently in female adolescents.

Health Status An individual's health status greatly affects eating habits and nutritional status. The lack of teeth, ill-fitting teeth, or a sore mouth makes chewing food difficult. Difficulty swallowing (dysphagia) due to a painfully inflamed throat or a stricture of the esophagus

Table 37–9 Selected Drug-Nutrient Interactions

Drug	Effect on Nutrition
Acetylsalicylic acid (aspirin)	Decreases serum folate and folacin nutrition
	Increases excretion of vitamin C, thiamine, potassium, amino acids, and glucose
	May cause nausea and gastritis
Antacids containing aluminum or magnesium hydroxide (Maalox)	Decrease absorption of phosphate and vitamin A
	Inactivate thiamine
	May cause deficiency of calcium and vitamin D
Thiazide diuretics (Diuril, HydroDIURIL)	Increase excretion of sodium, potassium, chloride, calcium, magnesium, zinc, and riboflavin
	May cause anorexia, nausea, vomiting, diarrhea, or constipation
Potassium chloride (Kaochlor, K-Lor, Slow-K)	Decreases absorption of vitamin B_{12}
	May cause diarrhea, nausea, or vomiting
	Increases excretion of potassium, magnesium, and calcium
	May cause anorexia, nausea, or vomiting
	Is incompatible with protein hydrolysates
Laxatives	May cause calcium and potassium depletion
	Mineral oil and phenolphthalein (Ex-Lax) decrease absorption of vitamins, A, D, E, and K.
Antihypertensives	Hydralazine (Apresoline) may cause anorexia, vomiting, nausea, and constipation
	Methyldopa (Aldomet) increases need for vitamin B_{12} and folate
	May cause dry mouth, nausea, vomiting, diarrhea, constipation
Antiinflammatory agents	Colchicine decreases absorption of vitamin B_{12}, carotene, fat, lactose, sodium, potassium, protein, and cholesterol
	Prednisone decreases absorption of calcium and phosphorus
Antidepressants	Amitriptyline (Elavil) increases food intake (large amounts may suppress intake)

Sources: AB Natow and J Heslin, *Nutritional Care of the Older Adult*, (New York: Macmillan, 1986), pp. 252–55; and D Raab and N Raab, Nutrition and the aging: An overview, *Canadian Nurse*, March 1985, 81:3.

can discourage a person from obtaining adequate nourishment. Disease processes and surgery of the gastrointestinal tract can affect digestion, absorption, metabolism, and excretion of essential nutrients. Gastrointestinal and other diseases also create anorexia, nausea, vomiting, and diarrhea, all of which can adversely affect a person's appetite and nutritional status. Gallstones, which can block the flow of bile, are a common cause of impaired lipid digestion. Metabolic processes can be impaired by diseases of the liver. Diseases of the pancreas can affect glucose metabolism or fat digestion.

Therapy Therapies (eg, chemotherapy and radiation) prescribed for certain diseases may also adversely affect eating patterns and nutrition. Normal cells of the bone marrow and the gastrointestinal mucosa are naturally very active and particularly susceptible to antineoplastic agents. Oral ulcers, intestinal bleeding, or diarrhea resulting from the toxicity of antineoplastics can diminish a person's nutritional status seriously.

The effects of radiotherapy depend on the area that is treated. For example, radiotherapy of the head and neck may cause decreased salivation, taste distortions, and swallowing difficulties; radiotherapy of the abdomen and pelvis may cause malabsorption, nausea, vomiting, and diarrhea. Many clients feel profound fatigue and anorexia.

Medications The effects of drugs on nutrition vary considerably. They may alter appetite, disturb taste perception, or interfere with nutrient absorption or excretion. Nurses need to be aware of the nutritional effects of specific drugs when evaluating a client for nutritional problems. The nursing history interview should include questions about the medications the client is taking. Conversely, nutrients can affect drug utilization. Some nutrients can decrease drug absorption; others enhance absorption. For example, the calcium in milk hinders absorption of the antibiotic tetracycline but enhances the absorption of the antibiotic erythromycin. Selected drug and nutrient interactions are shown in Table 37–9.

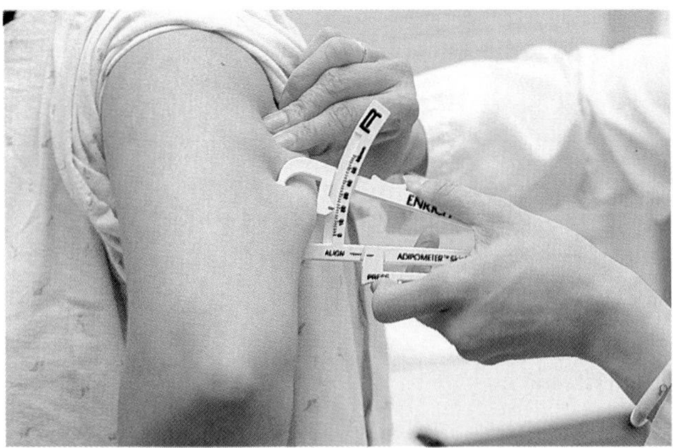

Figure 37–2 Measuring the triceps skinfold.

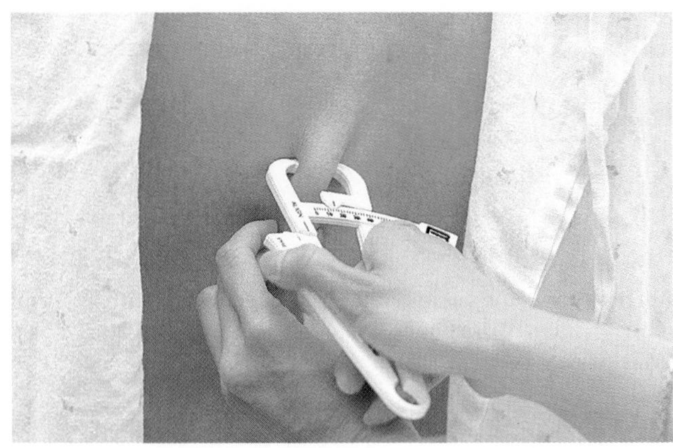

Figure 37–3 Measuring the subscapular skinfold.

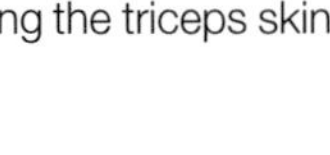

ASSESSING NUTRITIONAL STATUS

One method of assessing a client's nutritional status is to follow the "ABCD" approach:

A: Collect *anthropometric measurements*

B: Look at *biochemical data*

C: Examine the client for the *clinical signs* of nutritional status

D: Obtain a *dietary history*

ANTHROPOMETRIC MEASUREMENTS

Anthropometrics is a method of assessing nutritional status by using measurements of the human body. **Anthropometric measurements,** such as height, weight, skinfolds, and limb circumference, reflect the client's calorie-energy expenditure balance, muscle mass, body fat, and protein reserves. Assessment of height and weight is discussed in Chapter 22. Some measurements are made directly, and others are calculated mathematically.

Direct Measurements Direct measurements include skinfold measurements and mid-upper arm circumference (MAC). A **skinfold measurement** indicates the amount of body fat, the main form of stored energy. The fold of the skin measured includes the subcutaneous tissue but not the underlying muscle. The triceps, subscapular, biceps, and suprailiac skinfolds can be measured with special calipers. However, differences in calipers and in clinicians' methods and skill create wide variations in data obtained from skinfold measurements.

To measure the *triceps skinfold* (TSF), the nurse locates the midpoint of the upper arm, then grasps the skin on the back of the upper arm along the long axis of the humerus (Figure 37–2). Placing the calipers 1 cm (0.4 in) below the fingers, the nurse measures the thickness of the fold to the nearest millimeter. To measure the *subscapular skinfold,* the nurse picks up the skin below the scapula. Three fingers should be on top of the fold just below the scapula, the thumb below the fold, and the forefinger at the lower tip of the scapula. The skinfold should be angled about 45 degrees from the horizontal, upward medially and downward laterally (Figure 37–3). The nurse places the calipers about 1 cm (0.4 in) above or below the fingers and measures the skinfold.

Mid-upper arm circumference (MAC) is an index of skeletal muscle mass and therefore protein reserves. To measure the MAC, the nurse has the client sit or stand with arm hanging freely and the forearm flexed to horizontal. The nurse then locates the midpoint of the upper arm (halfway between the acromion process and the olecranon process). With the client's arm extended and hanging freely, the nurse measures the circumference at the midpoint of the arm, recording the measurement in centimeters, to the nearest millimeter (eg, 24.6 cm) (Figure 37–4). The average for adults aged 18 to 74 is 32.4 cm for men, 30.1 cm for women (National Center for Health Statistics 1987, p. 46, 47).

Calculated Measurements *Mid-upper arm muscle circumference* (MAMC) is an estimate of lean body mass, or skeletal muscle reserves. If tables are not available, the nurse uses the following formula to calculate the MAMC from the triceps skinfold and MAC direct measurements:

$$\text{MAMC (cm)} = \text{MAC (cm)} - \frac{3.14 \times \text{TSF (triceps skinfold) (mm)}}{10}$$

The *body mass index* (BMI) indicates whether the person's weight is appropriate for height and provides a useful estimate of obesity. A body mass index of 27 or greater is

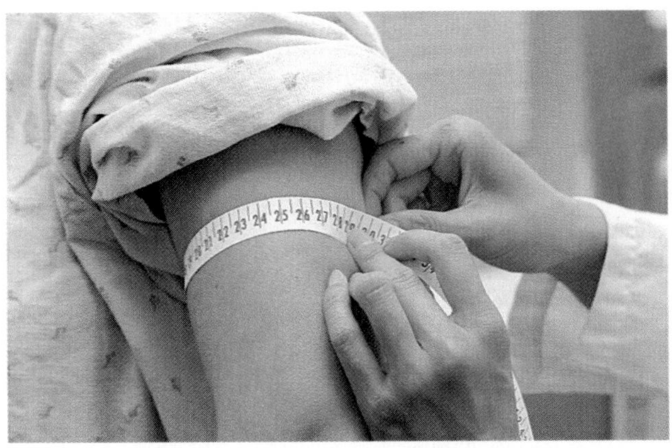

Figure 37–4 Measuring the mid-upper-arm circumference.

generally equated with obesity. Nutrition texts usually contain tables for these values; however, to calculate the BMI, the nurse can take the following steps:

1. Measure the person's height in meters (1 meter = 3.3 feet, or 39.6 in).
2. Multiply the height by itself (eg, 1.52 meters × 1.52 meters = 2.3 meters^2).
3. Measure the weight in kilograms (eg, 60 kg).
4. Calculate the BMI using the following formula and the above examples:

$$\text{BMI} = \frac{\text{Weight in kilograms}}{(\text{Height in meters})^2}$$

or

$$\frac{60 \text{ kilograms}}{1.5 \times 1.5 \text{ (meters}^2)} = 26.6$$

BIOCHEMICAL DATA

Biochemical tests can be used to detect malnutrition before anthropometric and clinical changes occur. Blood and urine samples are taken to measure **metabolites** (end products or enzymes) of particular nutrients. The laboratory studies most commonly used today to assess nutrition include hemoglobin and hematocrit, total lymphocyte count, albumin, transferrin, nitrogen balance, and creatinine excretion tests. Although less commonly used, other laboratory tests can be performed to assess vitamins, minerals, and trace elements. Because many factors can influence these laboratory tests, no single test can confirm a nutritional problem.

Hemoglobin and Hematocrit Indices A low hemoglobin level may be evidence of iron deficiency anemia. An elevated hematocrit may indicate dehydration. **Hematocrit** (Hct), or packed cell volume, is a measure of the percentage of a given volume of whole blood occupied by red blood cells. Thus, a hematocrit of 45% indicates that 45 mL of each deciliter of peripheral blood is composed of red blood cells.

Serum Albumin Albumin synthesis depends on healthy, functioning liver cells and on an appropriate supply of amino acids. Albumin, which accounts for over 50% of the total serum proteins, helps to maintain fluid and electrolyte balance and to transport many nutrients, hormones, and drugs.

Because there is so much albumin in the body and because it is not broken down very quickly, albumin concentrations change slowly. Thus, a low serum albumin level is a useful indicator of prolonged protein depletion. However, many conditions besides malnutrition can depress albumin concentration. Serum albumin level is therefore used as one indicator among several to determine protein status.

Transferrin Transferrin is a blood protein that binds with iron and transports it throughout the body. A transferrin level is a more sensitive indicator of protein malnutrition than albumin level, because it responds more promptly to changes in protein intake. Most transferrin is synthesized in the liver; levels are high when iron stores are low and low when iron stores are excessive. Certain diseases, such as liver disease, advanced kidney disease, and burns, also cause decreases in transferrin levels. An estimate of a client's transferrin level is sometimes obtained by measuring the total iron-binding capacity (TIBC), which is a more widely available test. The equation for converting the TIBC reading to a transferrin measurement is determined in the laboratory.

Total Lymphocyte Count Certain nutrient deficiencies and forms of protein-calorie malnutrition (PCM) can depress the immune system. The total number of lymphocytes decreases as protein depletion occurs.

Nitrogen Balance Nitrogen balance is discussed on page 1018. Nitrogen balance studies are useful in estimating the degree to which protein is being depleted or replaced in the body. Tests to measure nitrogen balance include the blood urea nitrogen (BUN) and the urine urea nitrogen (UUN). Urea, the chief end product of amino acid metabolism, is formed from ammonia detoxified by the liver and transported to the kidneys for excretion in urine. Urea concentrations in the blood and urine, therefore, directly reflect the intake and breakdown of dietary protein, the rate of urea production in the liver, and the rate of urea removal by the kidneys.

Decreased BUN levels may be caused by a low-protein diet. Elevated BUN levels may occur with starvation or excessive protein intake. Elevated BUN levels may also be caused by severe dehydration or general ill health and

Table 37–10 Clinical Signs Indicating Nutritional Status

Body Part or System	Normal Signs	Abnormal Signs
Hair	Shiny, neither dry nor oily	Oily, dry, dull, patchy in growth
Skin	Smooth, slightly moist, good turgor	Dry, oily, broken out in rash, scaly, rough, bruised
Eyes	Bright, clear	Dry, reddened
Tongue	Pink, moist	Reddened in patches, swollen
Mucous membranes	Reddish pink, moist	Reddened, dry, cracked
Cardiovascular	Heart rate and blood pressure within normal ranges, heart rhythm regular	Rapid heart rate, elevated blood pressure, irregular heart rhythm
Muscles	Firm, well developed	Poor in tone, soft, underdeveloped
Gastrointestinal	Appetite good, elimination regular and normal	Manifesting anorexia, indigestion, diarrhea, constipation
Neurologic	Reflexes normal, alert, good attention span, emotionally stable	Reflexes decreased, irritable, inattentive, confused, emotionally labile
Vitality	Vigorous, energetic, able to sleep well	Lacking energy, tired, apathetic, sleeping poorly
Weight	Normal for age, build, and height	Overweight, underweight

malnutrition; however, the most common cause is inadequate excretion of urea due to kidney disease or urinary obstruction.

Creatinine Excretion Creatinine is the chief end product of the creatine produced when energy is released during skeletal muscle metabolism. The rate of creatinine formation is directly proportional to the total muscle mass. Creatinine is removed from the bloodstream by the kidneys and excreted in the urine at a rate that closely parallels its formation. Creatinine excretion, therefore, reflects a person's total muscle mass. As skeletal muscle atrophies during malnutrition, creatinine excretion decreases. Standards for creatinine excretion are developed on the basis of sex and height.

CLINICAL SIGNS OF NUTRITIONAL STATUS

Because nutrition affects most body systems, an assessment of these systems can reveal nutritional problems. Table 37–10 lists some of the data that can be collected to assist nursing personnel in determining a client's nutritional status. This list is not exhaustive; for more detailed information, consult nutrition and assessment texts.

DIETARY HISTORY

A dietary history includes data about the client's usual eating patterns and habits, food preferences and restrictions, daily fluid intake, use of vitamin or mineral supplements, any dietary problems (eg, difficulty chewing or swallowing), physical activity, health history, and concerns related to food buying and preparation. See Figure 37–5 for an abbreviated nutritional history tool for an adult.

To obtain data about eating patterns and habits, the nurse elicits a typical 24-hour diet history. More detailed records of the client's food intake can be kept over a 3-day period, including 1 weekend day. The nurse also determines the client's perspective of the nutritional status. A question about what foods the client considers harmful or helpful to health is beneficial in eliciting cultural data. The client's medication intake is also important, especially in relation to mealtimes. Many medications are to be taken only before or after meals, so variations from the usual breakfast-lunch-dinner mealtimes need to be documented.

IDENTIFYING CLIENTS AT RISK FOR NUTRITIONAL PROBLEMS

After obtaining the dietary history, the nurse and the client can compare the data listed with recommended daily allowances to assess the nutritional balance of the diet.

Two commonly used approaches for analyzing the data involve using daily food group guides and food composition tables. Using daily food group guides, the nurse can quickly estimate the client's nutritional balance. The nurse simply determines whether the client is receiving the daily recommended servings of the basic food groups.

NUTRITIONAL HISTORY

Name __________
Age __________ Height __________

WEIGHT
Current Weight __________
Weight History (obesity, onset, fluctuations) __________
Percentage of
Overweight __________
Underweight __________

OTHER ANTHROPOMETRIC DATA
Triceps skin fold measurement __________
Arm muscle circumference __________

EATING PATTERNS AND HABITS

1. Typical day's food intake

Time	Item	Portion

2. Food likes __________
3. Food dislikes __________
4. Food allergies __________
5. Foods considered harmful or beneficial to health
   Harmful __________
   Benefical __________
6. Food restrictions
   Special diet __________
   Religious __________
   Cultural __________
7. Fluid intake
   Number of glasses of water per day __________
   Number of cups of tea or coffee per day __________
   Number of soft drinks per day __________
   Amount of alcohol or wine per day __________
8. Use of vitamins
   Kind __________
   Frequency __________
9. Use of minerals (eg, calcium, iron)
   Kind __________
   Frequency __________
10. Perception of diet
    Nutritionally balanced __________
    Not nutritionally balanced __________

DIETARY PROBLEMS

1. Describe appetite (usual, increased, decreased) __________
2. Foods causing indigestion, diarrhea, or gas __________
3. Difficulty following special diet
   Yes __________ No __________
   If yes, how __________
4. Chewing difficulties
   Number of teeth
   Upper __________ Lower __________
   Dentures
   Partial __________
   Complete __________
   Fit of dentures __________
5. Swallowing difficulties __________
6. Usual bowel movements __________

HEALTH HISTORY

1. Physical activity
   Type __________
   Frequency __________
2. Medication intake
   Name __________
   Time __________
3. History of diseases, surgical procedures, or weight problems

	Yes	No
Diabetes		
Heart Problems		
Surgery (specify) __________		
Cancer		
Kidney stones		
Gallstones		
Ulcers		
Intestinal disorder		
Allergies other than food (specify) __________		
Weight problems		

   Perception of general health
   Good __________
   Satisfactory __________
   Poor __________

FOOD BUYING AND PREPARATION

1. Ingredients used
   Salt __________
   Soy __________
   MSG __________
   Other __________
2. Methods most used
   Boil __________
   Bake __________
   Fry __________
   Broil __________
   Steam __________
   Other __________
3. Shopping/cooking capabilities
   Is able to shop __________
   Relies on others __________
   Is able to cook __________
   Relies on others __________
4. Living situation
   Number of family members __________
   Lives alone __________
5. Do food costs affect diet?
   Yes __________ No __________
   How? __________

Figure 37–5 A sample nutritional history.

SUMMARY OF RISK FACTORS FOR NUTRITIONAL PROBLEMS

Diet History

- Chewing or swallowing difficulties (including ill-fitting dentures, dental caries, and missing teeth)
- Inadequate food intake
- Restricted or fad diets
- No intake for 10 or more days
- Intravenous fluids (other than total parenteral nutrition for 10 or more days)
- Inadequate food budget
- Inadequate food preparation facilities
- Inadequate food storage facilities
- Physical disabilities
- Elderly living and eating alone

Medical History

- Weight 20% greater than ideal
- Weight 10% less than ideal
- Unintentional weight loss or gain of 10% within 6 months
- Recent major illness
- Recent major surgery
- Surgery of the gastrointestinal tract
- Anorexia
- Nausea
- Vomiting
- Diarrhea
- Alcoholism
- Cancer
- Liver disease
- Kidney disease
- Diabetes
- Thyroid or parathyroid disease
- Adrenal disease
- Mental disability
- Teenage pregnancy
- Multiple pregnancies
- Pancreatic insufficiency
- Radiation therapy

*Medication History**

- Aspirin
- Antacid
- Antidepressants
- Antihypertensives
- Anti-inflammatory agents
- Antineoplastic agents
- Digitalis
- Laxatives
- Diuretics (thiazides)
- Potassium chloride

* The potential effects of some medications on nutrition are shown in Table 37–9 on page 1029.

Food composition tables provide more specific data about specific nutrient intake, but these calculations take time. Fortunately, computerized nutrient data bases and diet analysis software have been developed to facilitate such analyses.

To identify clients at risk for nutritional problems, the nurse also considers data from the client's medication history and medical history. Any person who has a condition that interferes with the ability to ingest, digest, absorb, and metabolize nutrients can be considered at risk (see p. 1035). Clients who have an increased demand for nutrients to meet metabolic needs may also be at risk, for example, pregnant women, clients with hyperthyroidism, and those with cancer. Certain medical therapies, such as gastrointestinal tract surgery and radiation therapy, also place clients at risk. Medications, as noted earlier, can alter the absorption and metabolism of nutrients. See Table 37–9, earlier. A summary of risk factors for nutritional problems is shown in the box at the left.

DIAGNOSING

Nursing diagnoses that may apply to clients with or at risk for nutritional problems are broadly stated as **Altered nutrition: less than body requirements** (insufficient intake), **Altered nutrition: more than body requirements** (excessive intake), or **High risk for altered nutrition: more than body requirements.** *Intake* here is a relative term that depends on the client's energy expenditures. For example, a person who eats an apparently balanced and adequate diet but who performs frequent, rigorous physical activity may have a nutritional deficit. Similarly, an apparently "normal" intake may, in fact, be excessive for a person who has a minimal activity level. When using the label **Altered nutrition: less than body requirements,** the nurse should state the specific deficit (inadequate intake of protein, iron, or vitamin C). Indications of nutritional deficits of specific vitamins are outlined in the *Clinical Companion.*

Altered nutrition: more than body requirements is the condition in which calorie intake exceeds metabolic need. People become obese by eating too much food or eating too many foods of high caloric density. *Obesity* is present when the weight is 20% greater than the ideal for height and frame. Currently one of the most prevalent health problems in North America, obesity is associated with hypertension, cardiovascular disease, and diabetes. *Overweight* refers to weight 10% greater than the ideal for height and frame. Excessive intake is also manifested when the triceps skinfold is greater than 15 mm in men and 25 mm in women (Carpenito 1993, p. 535).

Definitions, defining characteristics, and related factors are shown in the accompanying box. Clinical

NURSING DIAGNOSES

CLIENTS WITH NUTRITIONAL PROBLEMS

Nursing Diagnosis: Altered nutrition: less than body requirements: The state in which a person experiences an intake of nutrients insufficient to meet metabolic needs

Defining Characteristics

- Body weight 20% or more under ideal
- Weight loss (with or without adequate intake)
- Reported inadequate food intake (less than RDA)
- Reported or evidenced lack of food
- Lack of interest in food
- Skinfold < 60% of standard measurement
- Reduced energy level
- Weakness of muscles involved in swallowing or masticating food
- Perceived inability to ingest food
- Aversion to eating
- Poor muscle tone
- Pale conjunctive and mucous membranes
- Abdominal cramping; pain; hyperactive bowel sounds
- Satiety immediately after ingesting food

Related Factors

Inability to ingest or digest food secondary to biologic factors (eg, buccal cavity discomfort/pain) or psychologic factors (eg, fatigue, grieving, depression); inability to absorb nutrients secondary to biologic or psychologic factors (eg, malabsorption condition, severe stress and anxiety); inability to procure food secondary to economic, biologic, or physical factors (eg, inadequate finances, lack of transportation, physical disability); lack of knowledge (eg, of vitamin or mineral requirements); food faddism; dieting practices.

Nursing Diagnosis: Altered nutrition: more than body requirements: The state in which an individual experiences an intake of nutrients that exceeds metabolic needs

Defining Characteristics

- Weight 10–20% over ideal for height and frame
- Triceps skinfold greater than 15 mm in men or greater than 25 mm in women
- Reported or observed dysfunctional eating patterns, such as pairing food with other activities, concentrating food intake at end of day, or eating in response to cues other than hunger (eg, anxiety)

Related Factors

Ingesting calories in excess of metabolic needs; hereditary predisposition; use of food as reward or comfort measure; low self-esteem; eating in response to cues other than hunger (eg, anxiety); sedentary life-style; inadequate financial resources (selection of low-cost–high-calorie foods); lack of knowledge of caloric requirements and/or nutrient content of foods.

Nursing Diagnosis: Altered nutrition: high risk for more than body requirements: The state in which an individual is at risk of experiencing an intake of nutrients that exceeds metabolic needs

Defining Characteristics/Risk Factors

- Reported or observed obesity in one or both parents; hereditary predisposition
- Rapid transition across growth percentiles in infants or children
- Reported use of solid food as major food source before 5 months of age
- Reported or observed higher baseline weight at beginning or end of pregnancy
- Use of food as a reward or comfort measure
- Dysfunctional eating patterns
- Low self-esteem
- Sedentary life-style
- Inadequate financial resources (selection of low-cost–high-calorie foods)

Sources: LJ Carpenito, *Nursing Diagnosis: Application to Clinical Practice*, 4th ed. (Philadelphia: Lippincott, 1992), pp. 584–85; 610; 614; M Gordon, *Manual of Nursing Diagnosis 1993–1994*, (St Louis: Mosby-Year Book, 1993), pp. 87–93; MJ Kim, GK McFarland, and AM McLane, *Pocket Guide to Nursing Diagnoses*, 5th ed. (St Louis: Mosby-Year Book, 1993), pp. 37–39; GK McFarland and EA McFarlane, *Nursing Diagnosis and Intervention: Planning for Patient Care*, 2d ed. (St Louis: Mosby, 1993), pp. 92–98; North American Nursing Diagnosis Association, *NANDA Nursing Diagnoses: Definitions and Classification 1992–1993*, (Philadelphia: NANDA, 1992), pp. 11–12; and JR Lederer, GL Marculescu, B Mocnik, and N Seaby, *Care Planning Pocket Guide—A Nursing Diagnosis Approach*, 5th ed. (Redwood City, CA: Addison-Wesley Nursing, 1993), pp. 118–24.

Table 37–11 Clinical Application: Assessment Data Clusters and Related Nursing Diagnoses

Data Cluster	Nursing Diagnosis
Mark Malakoff, 71 years old, has chronic obstructive lung disease. His wife died 2 years ago. He says, "I'm not interested in food. Even if I were, I don't have the energy to buy food. It's too much bother to fix meals for just me." He is 5′10″ (178 cm) tall and weighs 135 lbs (61.2 kg). His triceps skinfold measurement is 9.2 mm; arm muscle circumference is 20.4 mm. Dietary assessment indicates that he eats mostly bread, cereal, whole milk, and canned fish and meats. He eats almost no fruits and vegetables.	**Altered nutrition: less than body requirements** related to anorexia and physical and psychologic inability to procure and prepare food
Rose Rosenthal, a 27-year-old taxi dispatcher, says that her parents, who are both pastry cooks, are "fat." "I love Dad's doughnuts and often bring some to work to munch on through the day. I hate exercise, but at this rate, I'm going to have to do something, or I'll end up looking like Mum and Dad." Height, 5′1″ (155 cm); weight 130 lb (58.5 kg).	**Altered nutrition: high risk for more than body requirements** related to inappropriate eating patterns, family background, and sedentary life-style
Warren Ames, 55 years old, has had rheumatoid arthritis for over a year. He is 5′10″ (178 cm) tall and weighs 190 lb (85.5 kg). He says, "When I get up in the morning, I'm so stiff that I have to sit on the bed for 10 minutes before I can walk across the room. And my knees hurt too bad to walk much during the day." Mr Ames admits that he "doesn't do much except watch TV and eat junk food." His wife says he has been depressed since he "finally realized he has an incurable disease" and "I know I shouldn't cook high-calorie foods for him, but he doesn't get much other enjoyment out of life, and I can't bear to be mean to him."	**Altered nutrition: more than body requirements** (for calories) related to lack of exercise secondary to pain, excess intake of high-calorie foods and eating in response to boredom and depression

examples of assessment data clusters and related nursing diagnoses are shown in Table 37–11.

Because the focus of treatment is often behavior modification and change in life-style, the nursing diagnostic label **Altered health maintenance** related to excessive intake for metabolic requirements may be more relevant than **Altered nutrition** for some individuals (Carpenito 1993, p. 535).

Many other NANDA nursing diagnoses may apply to certain individuals, because nutritional problems often affect other areas of human functioning. In this case, the nutritional diagnostic label may be used as the *etiology* of other diagnoses. Examples are **Activity intolerance** related to inadequate intake of iron-rich foods, resulting in iron deficiency anemia; **Constipation** related to inadequate fluid and fiber intake; **Diarrhea** related to excessive intake of alcohol, sugar, or fiber; **Self-esteem disturbance** related to obesity; and **High risk for impaired skin integrity** (pressure sores) related to insufficient intake of tissue-building nutrients.

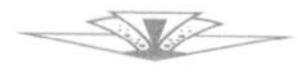

PLANNING

Broad client outcomes for persons with nutritional problems include maintaining, improving, or restoring nutritional status and preventing nutritional problems. The nurse writes specific outcome criteria that will indicate resolution of the particular problem identified. For example, if the problem is **Altered nutrition: more than body requirements (caloric intake),** the outcome criterion might be "Limits caloric intake to less than 1200 calories per day" or "Will lose 2 lb by August 27." The nurse and client choose interventions that are most likely to achieve client outcomes, given the etiology of the client's problem. For example, if the client's diagnosis is **Altered nutrition: more than body requirements (caloric intake),** the interventions for an etiology of sedentary life-style would be different from those for an etiology of knowledge deficit. The accompanying Care Planning Guide provides examples of outcome criteria, associated nursing interventions, and rationales for the three broad NANDA nutritional problem labels.

A critical pathway can also be useful for planning client care (see p. 1056).

IMPLEMENTING

Teaching is an important aspect of nursing intervention for clients with nutritional problems. Depending on clients' learning needs, specific information concerning a prescribed diet or general nutrition counseling may be planned. Clients with problems involving the actual intake of nutrients are assisted by nurses to attain the specific nutrients required.

CARE PLANNING GUIDE

CLIENTS WITH NUTRITIONAL PROBLEMS

NURSING DIAGNOSIS: Altered nutrition: less than body requirements

Outcome Criteria	Nursing Interventions	Rationale
The client		
▪ Identifies factors contributing to inadequate nutritional intake.	Discuss with the client factors contributing to inadequate nutrition (see the box on page 1035).	This enables the nurse to focus on information the client requires and to identify misinformation.
▪ Identifies necessary dietary alterations and foods high in needed nutrients (eg, calcium, iron, protein, total calories).	Instruct client and significant others about (a) content of a balanced diet based on the Food Guide Pyramid and/or (b) newly prescribed diet and/or (c) foods high in specific nutrient(s) required.	This fulfills a knowledge deficit and provides client with information for self-care.
	Confer with the dietitian as needed.	The dietitian can establish specific calorie, protein, and other requirements for the client.
▪ Consumes a well-balanced diet to restore deficient nutrients.	Monitor food and fluid intake, daily calorie counts, appropriate laboratory values (eg, electrolytes, transferrin, serum albumin)	Assessment of these parameters provides necessary data to evaluate food/fluid intake.
	Schedule procedures so that they do not conflict with meals. Administer ordered medications for pain or nausea.	Procedures, pain, and nausea inhibit appetite.
	Provide a rest period before meals as required.	Rest enables the client to conserve energy for self-feeding.
	Provide or assist the client with oral hygiene before meals.	Oral hygiene moistens and cleans oral mucous membranes, stimulates salivation, and helps to enhance the sense of taste.
	Encourage support persons to bring appropriate foods from home.	Home-prepared foods often stimulate appetite.
	Encourage/allow the client to choose foods and plan meal schedules.	Client's appetite may improve if preferred foods are offered. Client participation also provides an opportunity for required teaching and promotes self-care and self-esteem.
	Offer small, frequent feedings.	Three large meals may overwhelm the client; small meals are less fatiguing.
	Feed or assist the client to eat with self-feeding aids as needed.	Assistance may be necessary to ensure an adequate intake.
	Administer and/or teach clients about alternative feeding methods via nasogastric tube or gastrostomy or jejunostomy stomas.	Some clients' conditions are severe enough to require tube feedings.
	Give frequent positive reinforcement for increased intake, better food choices, life-style changes, weight gain, and so on.	Positive reinforcement provides encouragement and motivation to continue efforts to improve nutrition.

➤

NUTRITIONAL PROBLEMS CONTINUED

Outcome Criteria	Nursing Interventions	Rationale
▪ Demonstrates decrease (or absence) of signs of malnutrition, as evidenced by		
a. Specified weight gain of pounds per week. b. Normal skinfold measurements or 80% of the standard measurement. c. Reports of increased energy. d. Other signs (specify).	Weigh client daily at same time with same clothing; measure skinfold measurements weekly; observe client for signs of malnutrition cited in the client's defining characteristics.	Weighing at the same time and in the same clothes increased reliability of measurement. Other assessments determine the effectiveness of interventions.

NURSING DIAGNOSIS: Altered nutrition: more than body requirements, or **High risk for more than body requirements**

Outcome Criteria	Nursing Interventions	Rationale
The client		
▪ Identifies factors contributing to excess weight (or risk of excess weight).	Explore with the client physiologic, psychologic, and life-style factors that predispose to weight gain.	This helps the nurse and client focus on causative or risk factors that suggest appropriate interventions.
▪ Monitors eating habits for specified period (eg, 1 week) and identifies behaviors that need to be modified to lose weight (or prevent weight gain).	Have client keep a daily log of foods eaten.	Keeping a log provides continued awareness and information for problem solving throughout the weight-loss or maintenance program.
	Review the client's weekly dietary intake and eating times. Help the client identify dysfunctional eating patterns.	The review provides information needed to recognize the cause of the problem and helps the client begin to make changes.
▪ Chooses and ingests a diet that reduces daily caloric intake (eg, reduces calories by 500 per day for each pound of weight loss desired per week).	Provide information about normal weight range, recommended caloric intake, high- and low-calorie foods, and use of food exchanges. Confer with the dietitian as needed.	Knowledge helps the client choose appropriate foods that enhance weight loss.
	Encourage intake of low-calorie, caffeine-free beverages and plenty of water.	This keeps the stomach from being empty and helps prevent hunger. Caffeine may stimulate appetite.
▪ Loses prescribed amount of weight (specify) or maintains weight within prescribed standards.	Teach the client ▪ Principles of a well-balanced diet (see Food Pyramid or other food guides, page 1020)	A knowledge of these principles helps discourage the client from undertaking severe dietary measures and diminishes the risk of inadequate nutrition.
	▪ To adapt eating practices by using smaller plates, smaller servings, chewing each bit a specified number of times, and putting fork down between bites.	These practices help the client begin to modify behaviors.

Outcome Criteria	Nursing Interventions	Rationale
	▪ To control the desire to eat by taking a walk, drinking a glass of water, or doing slow deep-breathing exercises.	These measures enable the client to gain control and to substitute positive coping behaviors in response to cues that previously triggered eating.
	▪ Stress-reduction techniques.	These techniques help prevent eating in response to internal cues such as stress, anxiety, and depression and help the client develop alternative coping strategies.
	Positively reinforce each successful behavior change (eg, weight loss, improved eating behavior).	Positive reinforcement increases self-esteem and motivation to succeed.
▪ Establishes a physical activity program of 20 to 30 minutes' duration at least 3 times per week.	Help client plan an exercise program (eg, start a walking program and then gradually increase distance).	Exercise increases metabolism and helps burn calories ingested as food. It also enhances a feeling of well-being.
	Encourage the client to walk to destinations and to use stairs instead of elevators.	
▪ Verbalizes improvement in feelings about self and satisfaction with support provided.	Explore ways in which significant others can be supportive.	Involvement of significant others enables them to be supportive of the client and reinforce change.
	Provide information about available community resources (eg, weight-loss groups, dietary counseling, exercise programs, self-help groups).	Hearing the experiences of others and getting their encouragement help the client make (and maintain) life-style changes.

CLINICAL ALERT

Criteria and nursing strategies must be individualized for each client, taking into consideration the contributing factors, health beliefs, and preferences specific to the client.

COUNSELING ABOUT NUTRITION

Nutrition counseling involves more than simply providing information. The nurse must help clients integrate diet changes into their life-styles and provide strategies to motivate them to change their eating habits. Counseling can be likened to the teaching-learning process discussed in Chapter 19. Because it is the client's responsibility to make the necessary dietary changes and to change eating behavior, the nurse's major role is to support and encourage the client.

TEACHING ABOUT SPECIAL DIETS

Assisting clients and support persons with special or therapeutic diets prescribed by the physician is a function shared by the dietitian and the nurse. The dietitian informs the client and support persons about the specific foods allowed and not allowed and assists the client with meal planning. The nurse reinforces this instruction, assists the client to make changes, and evaluates the client's responses.

A *special* or *therapeutic diet* is one in which the amount of food, the kind of food, or the frequency of eating is prescribed. Special diets are used to treat a disease process, for example, a low-salt diet for high blood pressure; to prepare for a special examination or surgery; and to promote health, for example, a low-calorie diet for an overweight client.

Some diets are temporary, observed perhaps for one meal or 1 week, but some clients must follow certain diets

CRITICAL THINKING CHALLENGE

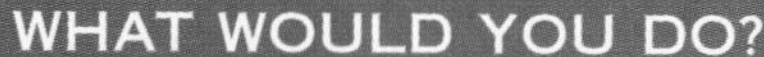

WHAT WOULD YOU DO?

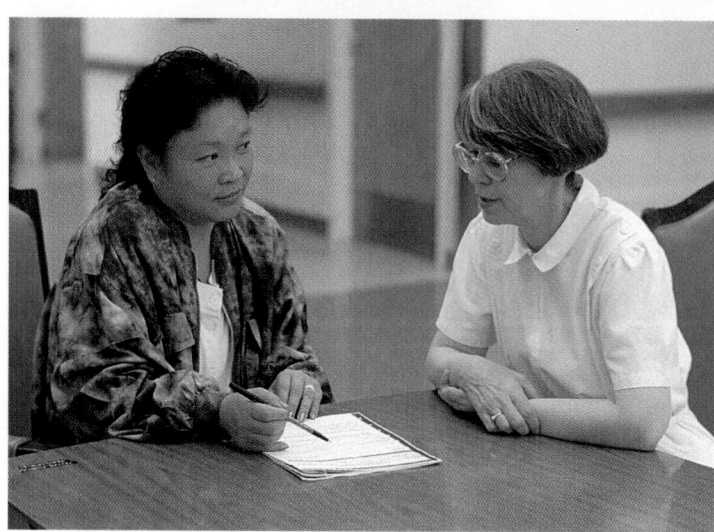

Ellen Tica is a 42-year-old female undergoing outpatient treatment for gallbladder disease. Her physician has ordered a low-fat diet and has given her a diet instruction sheet. After reviewing the instruction sheet, Ms Tica confides in you that she doesn't see any foods she likes, and asks if she can eat her usual foods.

What would you do?

(eg, the diabetic diet) for a lifetime. If the diet is long term, the client must not only understand the diet but also develop a healthy, positive attitude toward it.

Progressive hospital diets (eg, postoperative dietary protocols) are often unique to institutions, and nurses need to be familiar with the diets prescribed in their agencies. Clients who do not have special needs eat the **regular diet,** in which the quantity and content are designed to meet the needs of most clients. In some agencies, the regular diet is referred to as the normal, house, or standard diet. Some agencies offer clients a daily menu from which to select their meals for the next day; others provide standard meals to each client on the general diet. Certain foods (eg, cabbage, which tends to produce flatus, and highly seasoned and fried foods, which are difficult for some people to digest) are usually omitted from the regular diet.

A variation of the regular diet is the **light diet,** designed for postoperative and other clients who are not ready for the regular diet. Foods in the light diet are plainly cooked. Foods containing large amounts of fat are usually omitted, as are bran and foods containing a great deal of fiber. Not all agencies provide a light diet.

A **soft diet** is easily chewed and digested. It is often ordered for clients who have difficulty chewing and swallowing. It is a low-residue (low-fiber) diet containing very few uncooked foods; however, restrictions vary among agencies and according to individual tolerance. Examples of foods that can be included in a soft or semisoft diet are shown in the box on page 1041. The **pureed diet** is a modification of the soft diet. Liquid may be added to the food, which is then blended to a semisolid consistency.

A **full liquid diet** contains only liquids or foods that turn to liquid at body temperature, such as ice cream. Full liquid diets are eaten by clients who have gastrointestinal disturbances or are otherwise unable to tolerate solid or semisolid foods. This diet is not recommended for long-term use because it is low in iron, protein, and calories. In addition, its cholesterol content is high because of the amount of milk offered. Clients who must receive only liquids for long periods are usually given a nutritionally balanced oral supplement, such as Sustacal. The full liquid diet is monotonous and difficult for clients to accept. Planning six or more feedings per day may encourage a more adequate intake.

The **clear liquid diet** is limited to water, tea, coffee, clear broths, ginger ale or other carbonated beverages, strained and clear fruit juices, plain gelatin, sugar, and hard candy. This diet provides the client with fluid and carbohydrate (in the form of sugar) but does not supply adequate protein, fat, vitamins, minerals, or calories (no more than 600 kcal/day). It is a short-term diet (24 to 36 hours) provided for clients after certain surgery or in the acute stages of infection, particularly of the gastrointestinal tract. The major objectives of this diet are to relieve thirst, prevent dehydration, and minimize stimulation of the gastrointestinal tract. Examples of foods allowed in clear liquid, full liquid, and soft diets are shown in the box on page 1041.

There are many other special diets, sometimes especially devised for individual clients. Details about these diets are provided in nutrition and medical/surgical nursing textbooks. Common special diets are reducing, diabetic, low-salt, low-fat, and allergy diets.

EXAMPLES OF FOODS FOR CLEAR LIQUID, FULL LIQUID, AND SOFT DIETS

Clear Liquid	*Full Liquid*	*Soft*
Coffee, regular and decaffeinated Tea Carbonated beverages Bouillon, fat-free broth Clear fruit juices (apple, cranberry, grape) Other fruit juices, strained Popsicles Gelatin Sugar, honey Hard candy	All foods on clear liquid diet, plus: Milk and milk drinks Puddings, custards Ice cream, sherbet Vegetable juices Refined or strained cereals (eg, cream of rice) Cream, butter, margarine Eggs (in custard and pudding) Smooth peanut butter Yogurt	All foods on full and clear liquid diets, plus: *Meat:* All lean, tender meat, fish, or poultry (chopped, shredded); spaghetti sauce with ground meat, over pasta *Meat alternatives:* Scrambled eggs, omelet, poached eggs; cottage cheese and other mild cheese *Vegetables:* Mashed potatoes, sweet potatoes, or squash; vegetables in cream or cheese sauce; other cooked vegetables as tolerated (eg, spinach, cauliflower, asparagus tips), chopped and mashed as needed; avocado *Fruits:* Cooked or canned fruits; bananas, grapefruit and orange sections without membranes, applesauce *Breads and cereals:* Enriched rice, barley, pasta; all breads; cooked cereals (eg, oatmeal) *Desserts:* Soft cake, bread pudding

Clients often need assistance in adapting special diets to their cultural, religious, ethnic, and economic patterns. Most diets in North America are devised for the Anglo-American taste and omit many otherwise acceptable ethnic foods. Such a diet may be unfamiliar or unpalatable to some clients. Nutritionists and dietitians can often help nurses adapt a diet to suit a person's life-style or economic status. Often, less costly foods can be substituted for recommended foods, such as powdered milk for fresh milk.

Information can be a motivating force. Clients are more likely to change their eating patterns if they understand the relationship between the diet and their disease, and if they know the benefits of the special diet and the consequences of choosing not to follow it. Even highly motivated clients, however, can follow a diet only if they have the knowledge to do so. Clients need specific facts about foods they can and cannot have. For example, a client may understand that sugar in coffee is not allowed on a low-calorie diet but may not understand that bread also contains sugar and is also restricted. An elderly woman may understand that she is not to add salt to foods when cooking but she still salts her food at the table.

STIMULATING THE APPETITE

Physical illness, unfamiliar or unpalatable food, environmental and psychologic factors, and physical discomfort or pain, may depress the appetites of many hospitalized clients. A short-term decrease in food intake usually is not a problem for adults; over time, however, it leads to weight loss, decreased strength and stamina, and other nutritional problems. A decreased food intake is often accompanied by a decrease in fluid intake, which may cause fluid and electrolyte problems. See Chapter 38 for further information. Stimulating a person's appetite requires the nurse to determine the reason for the lack of appetite and then deal with the problem. Some interventions for improving the client's appetite are summarized in the box above.

IMPROVING APPETITE

- Relieve illness symptoms that depress appetite prior to mealtime; for example, give an analgesic for pain or an antipyretic for a fever or allow rest for fatigue.
- Provide familiar food that the person likes. Often the relatives of clients are pleased to bring food from home but may need some guidance about special diet requirements.
- Select small portions so as not to discourage the anorexic client.
- Avoid unpleasant or uncomfortable treatments immediately before or after a meal.
- Provide a tidy, clean environment that is free of unpleasant sights and odors. A soiled dressing, a used bedpan, an uncovered irrigation set, or even used dishes can destroy appetite.
- Encourage or provide oral hygiene before mealtime. This improves the client's ability to taste.
- Reduce psychologic stress. A lack of understanding of therapy, the anticipation of an operation, and fear of the unknown can cause anorexia. Often, the nurse can help by discussing feelings with the client, giving information and assistance, and allaying fears.

PROVIDING CLIENT MEALS

- Check the client's chart or Kardex for the diet order and to determine whether the client is fasting for laboratory tests or surgery or whether the physician has ordered "nothing by mouth" (NPO). For clients who are fasting or on NPO, ensure that the appropriate signs are placed on either the room door or the client's bed, according to agency practice.
- If there is a change in the type of food the client is to receive, notify the dietary staff.
- Assist the client to the bathroom or onto a bedpan or commode if the client needs to urinate.
- Offer the client assistance with hand washing and oral hygiene prior to a meal.
- Most people sit during a meal; if it is permitted, assist the client to a comfortable position in bed (Figure 37–6) or in a chair, whichever is appropriate.
- Clear the overbed table so that there is space for the tray. If the client must remain in a lying position in bed, arrange the overbed table close to the bedside, so that the client can see the food.
- Check each tray for the client's name, the type of diet, and completeness. If the diet does not seem to be correct, check it against the client's chart. Confirm the client's name by checking the wristband before leaving the tray. Do *not* leave an incorrect diet for a client to eat.
- Assist the client as required, for example, in removing the food covers, buttering the bread, pouring the tea, and cutting the meat.
- For a blind person, identify the placement of the food as you would describe the time on a clock (Figure 37–7). For instance, the nurse may say, "The potatoes are at eight o'clock; the chicken at 12 o'clock; and the green beans at 4 o'clock."
- After the client has completed the meal, replace the food covers, and note how much and what the client has eaten and the amount of fluid taken. Record fluid intake and calorie count as required.
- If the client is on a special diet or is having problems eating, record the amount of food eaten and any pain, fatigue, or nausea experienced.
- If the client is not eating, notify the nurse in charge so that the diet can be changed or other nursing measures can be taken, such as rescheduling the meals, providing smaller, more frequent meals, or obtaining special self-feeding aids.

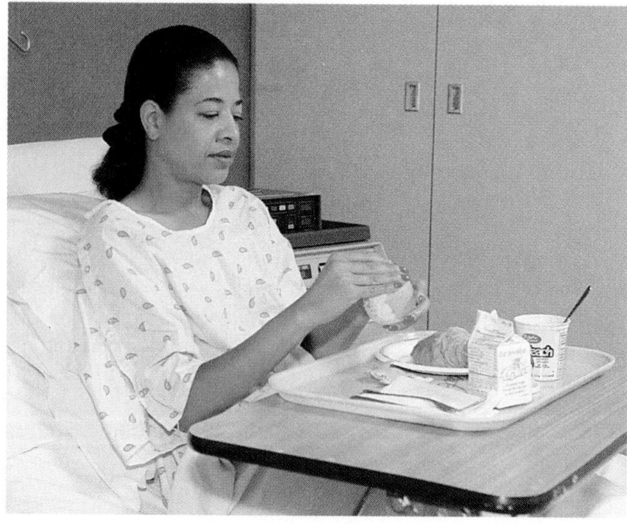

Figure 37–6 A supported sitting position contributes to a client's comfort while eating.

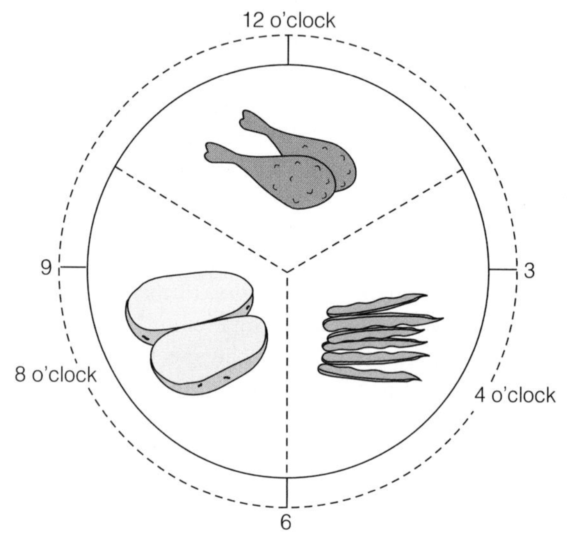

Figure 37–7 For a client who is blind, the nurse can use the clock system to describe the location of food on the plate.

ASSISTING CLIENTS WITH MEALS

Because clients in acute-care hospitals are frequently confined to their beds, most hospitals have meals brought to the client. Often the client receives a tray that has been assembled in a central hospital kitchen or a kitchen adjacent to the nursing unit. Nursing personnel may be responsible for giving out and collecting the trays; in some settings this is done by special dietary personnel. Long-term care facilities and some hospitals serve meals to ambulatory clients in a special dining area, and the clients are expected to go there to eat. Other agencies have a coffee shop for food or machines from which clients can obtain sandwiches and beverages. Guidelines for providing meals to clients are summarized in the box on page 1042.

ASSISTING CLIENTS WITH FEEDING

The need for assistance with eating depends on the physical and mental limitations of the client. Two groups of people frequently require help: the elderly, who are weakened and quickly fatigued when they are ill; and the handicapped, such as blind clients, those who must remain in a back-lying position, or those who cannot use their hands. The client's nursing care plan will indicate that assistance is required with meals.

The nurse must be sensitive to clients' feelings of embarrassment, resentment, and loss of autonomy. Whenever possible, the nurse should help incapacitated clients feed themselves rather than feed them. Some clients become depressed because they require help and because they believe they are burdensome to busy nursing personnel. Although feeding a client is time consuming, nurses should try to appear unhurried and convey that they have ample time. Sitting at the bedside is one way to convey this impression.

When feeding a client, the nurse asks in which order the client would like to eat the food. If the client cannot see, the nurse tells the client which food is being given. The nurse must always allow ample time for the client to chew and swallow the food before offering more. Also, the nurse provides fluids as requested, or, if the client is unable to communicate, the nurse offers fluids after every three of four mouthfuls of solid food. It is important to make the time a pleasant one, choosing topics of conversation that are of interest to clients who want to talk.

Although normal utensils should be used whenever possible, the nurse may need to use special utensils to assist a client to eat. For clients who have difficulty drinking from a cup or glass, a straw often permits them to obtain liquids with less effort and less spillage. Special drinking cups are also available. One model has a spout; another is specially designed to permit drinking with less tipping of the cup than is normally required.

Many adaptive feeding aids are available to help clients maintain independence. A standard eating utensil with a built-up or widened handle helps clients who cannot grasp objects easily. Utensils with wide handles can be purchased, or a regular eating utensil can be modified by taping foam around the handle. The foam increases friction and thus steadies the client's grasp. Handles may be bent or angled to compensate for limited motion. Collars or bands that prevent the utensil from being dropped can be attached to the end of the handle and fit over the client's hand. Clients requiring pureed or liquid diets are sometimes fed with a feeding syringe.

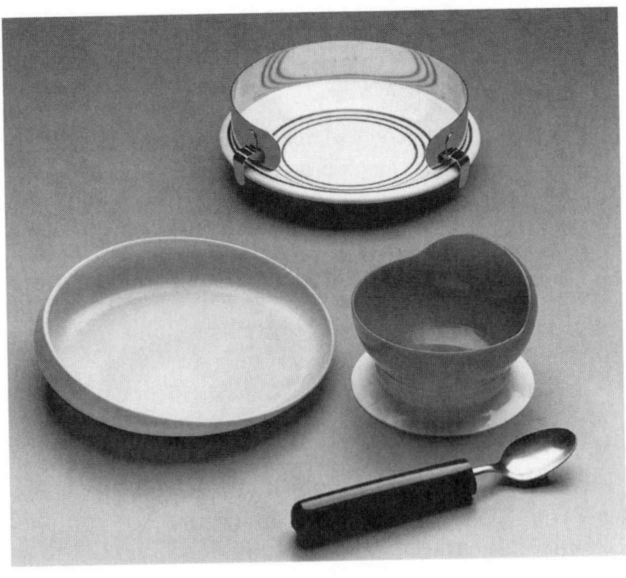

Figure 37–8 Clockwise from top: dinner plate with guard attached; bowl with stable base and lip; wide-handled spoon; lipped plate.

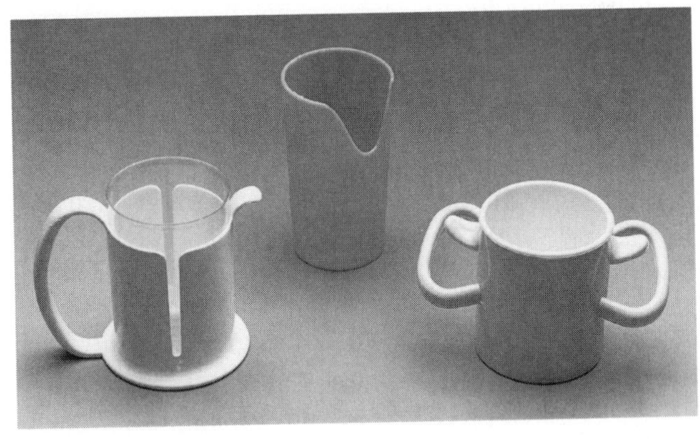

Figure 37–9 Left to right: glass holder, cup with hole for nose, two-handled cup with thumb tabs.

Plates with rims and plastic or metal plate guards enable the client to pick up the food by first pushing it against this raised edge. A suction cup or damp sponge or cloth may be place under the dish to keep it from moving while the client is eating. No-spill mugs and two-handled drinking cups are especially useful for persons with impaired hand coordination. Stretch terry cloth and knitted or crocheted glass covers enable the client to keep a secure grasp on a glass. Lidded tip-proof glasses are also available. Figures 37–8 and 37–9 show some of these aids.

SPECIAL COMMUNITY NUTRITIONAL SERVICES

In many areas, community programs have been developed to help special subgroups of the population meet their nutritional needs. For the elderly who cannot prepare meals or leave their homes, ready-to-eat meals or frozen dinners are delivered to the home by local organizations. Meals-on-Wheels is one such well-known organization. For people who can prepare meals but are physically handicapped and unable to shop for groceries, some organizations provide grocery delivery services.

For the impoverished, the US Department of Agriculture funds a food stamp program. People with low incomes can use stamps to purchase food at any approved grocery store. The value of the food stamps provided depends on the size and income of the family.

Other programs include

- The Commodity Supplemental Food Program provides food to a targeted poor population and to women with children up to age 6. The Agriculture Department contracts, through state human services agencies, with nonprofit church and other social service groups to distribute food packages containing approved groceries such as iron-fortified infant formula, rice, cereal, canned juice, evaporated milk or nonfat dry milk, canned vegetables or fruits, peanut butter, and dry beans.
- The Emergency Food Assistance Program (TEFAP) distributes food commodities and cash subsidies free of charge to soup kitchens, hunger centers, food banks and similar nonprofit food-distribution centers whose goal is to relieve situations of emergency and distress.
- The Supplemental Food Program for Women, Infants, and Children (WIC) provides food stamps and vouchers for pregnant and lactating women and children under age 5.

Some industries have established health maintenance programs for their employees. These programs generally include exercise facilities, education, stress management, and nutritional counseling. In some companies, the food service departments make a special effort to adhere to the recommendations of food guides. Such programs are thought to be cost effective; illness is reduced, less time is lost from work, and employee satisfaction increases work productivity.

ALTERNATIVE FEEDING METHODS

Alternative feeding methods to ensure adequate nutrition include both **enteral** (through the gastrointestinal system) and **parenteral** (intravenous) methods. The more common enteral feedings are administered through nasogastric and small-bore feeding tubes or through gastrostomy or jejunostomy tubes. Total parenteral nutrition (TPN), administered through the intravenous route, is discussed in Chapter 38, page 1114.

Nasogastric/Nasointestinal Feedings A **nasogastric feeding (gastric gavage)** or small intestine tube feeding is the instillation of specially prepared nutrients into the digestive tract through a tube that is inserted through one of the nostrils, down the nasopharynx, and into the alimentary tract. In some instances, the tube is passed through the mouth and pharynx, although this route may be more uncomfortable for the adult client and cause gagging. This approach is often used for infants who are obligatory nose breathers (who must breathe through the nose), and premature infants who have no gag reflex.

Traditional firm *large-bore* nasogastric tubes (ie, those larger than 12 Fr. in diameter) are placed in the stomach. Examples are the *Levin tube*, a flexible, rubber or plastic, single-lumen tube with holes near the tip, or the *Salem sump tube*, with a double lumen. The larger tube of the Salem sump tube drains gastric contents; the smaller tube allows for an inflow of atmospheric air which prevents a vacuum if the gastric tube adheres to the wall of the stomach. Irritation of the gastric mucosa is thereby avoided. Newer, softer, more flexible and less irritating *small-bore* tubes (smaller than 12 Fr. in diameter) can be placed in either the stomach or the upper small intestine (ie, duodenum or jejunum). Clients at risk for pulmonary aspiration (eg, those with altered pharyngeal reflexes and/or unconsciousness) should be fed via the small intestine rather than the stomach (Metheny 1988, p. 324).

Generally, the position of small-bore pliable tubes is confirmed by radiography before feedings are introduced. The nurse is responsible, however, for verifying tube placement (ie, gastrointestinal placement versus respiratory placement) before each intermittent feeding and at regular intervals (eg, at least once per shift) when continuous feedings are being administered. Traditionally, placement of *large-bore* tubes has been verified by the following methods, none of which alone guarantees that the tube is correctly positioned. In addition, most methods do not apply to small-bore tubes. For additional information about how to aspirate fluid from small-bore feeding tubes, see Metheny et al 1993 in Suggested Readings.

1. *Aspirate gastrointestinal secretions.* Gastrointestinal secretions are aspirated more readily through large-bore tubes than through small-bore tubes. Failure to obtain aspirate even with large-bore tubes may or may not indicate that the tube is malpositioned. For example, the tubing parts may be obstructed by the stomach mucosa. Failure to obtain fluid from a small-bore tube may indicate that the walls of the tube collapsed on syringe application. Several authors (Theodore et al 1984; and Hand et al 1984) have reported instances in

which pleural fluid was aspirated from small-bore tubes inadvertently placed in the pleural space or lung. This straw-colored, clear fluid closely resembles gastric fluid and can be erroneously mistaken for gastric fluid.

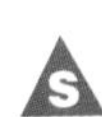

2. *Measure the pH of aspirated fluid.* An acidic pH generally indicates gastric fluid. Values within the acidic range may be as low as 0.8 (with hydrochloric acid secretion) and as high as 5, with a usual pH of 2 to 3 (Guyton 1991, p. 727). If the client is taking a medication altering the pH, some secretions may even become alkaline. Intestinal fluids have a slightly alkaline pH in the range of 7.5 to 8.0 (Guyton 1991, p. 724). Because normal pleural fluid has a pH of 7.4 (Byrne et al 1986, p. 468), this test to determine placement of small-bore intestinal tubes is not effective in differentiating intestinal from pleural fluid. However, it is effective in differentiating gastric from intestinal fluid.
3. *Inject 5 to 20 mL of air through the feeding tube while auscultating the epigastrum or left upper abdominal quadrant and listening for a whooshing, gurgling, or bubbling sound.* Because of the difficulty encountered in aspirating gastrointestinal secretions through small-bore tubes, many nurses use this method to test tube placement. Air injected in the stomach should be heard immediately. However, it is difficult to differentiate esophageal, gastric, distal duodenal, and proximal jejunal placement because of the proximity of these sites. Several authors also report "pseudoconfirmatory gurgling" sounds heard when the tube is malpositioned in the pharynx, esophagus, and respiratory tract (Hand et al 1984; Miller et al 1985; and Metheny et al 1988). Further research may indicate more precise differentiation of sounds using a Doppler stethoscope.
4. *Ask the client to speak or hum.* It is generally assumed that large-bore tubes placed in the trachea will interfere with the client's ability to speak. However, clients with small-bore tubes may be able to speak since the vocal cords may not be sufficiently separated to affect phonation. In one study, all clients with small-bore tubes were able to speak unless they were comatose, aphasic, or intubated (Metheny et al 1988, p. 376).
5. *Observe the client for coughing and choking.* Coughing and choking are likely to occur when large-bore tubes enter the respiratory tract but are less likely to occur with the use of small-bore tubes. These responses, however, may be absent with either type of tube in clients with decreased tracheal irritability or an altered level of consciousness.

Currently, the most effective method appears to be radiographic verification of tube placement. Repeated X-ray studies, however, are not feasible in terms of cost and radiation risk. More research is required to devise effective alternatives, especially for placement of small-bore tubes. In the meantime, nurses should (a) ensure initial radiographic verification of small-bore tubes, (b) aspirate contents when possible and check their acidity, (c) auscultate air insufflation, (d) closely observe the client for signs of obvious distress, and (e) suspect tube dislodgement after episodes of coughing, sneezing, and vomiting.

Tube feedings are indicated for clients who cannot eat by mouth or swallow a sufficient diet without aspirating food or fluid into the lungs. Feedings may be given continuously over a 24-hour period or at prescribed intervals, for example, four times per day. Liquid feeding mixtures are available commercially or may be prepared by the dietary department in accordance with the physician's orders. A standard formula provides 1 kcal per milliliter of solution with protein, fat, carbohydrate, minerals, and vitamins in specified proportions.

The frequency of feedings and amounts to be administered are ordered by the physician. An adult often requires 300 to 500 mL of mixture per feeding.

Before administering a tube feeding, the nurse must determine any food allergies of the client and assess tolerance to previous feedings. See Table 37–12 on page 1046 for essential assessments to conduct before administering tube feedings. The nurse must also check the expiration date on a commercially prepared formula or the preparation date and time of agency-prepared solution, discarding any formula that has passed the expiration date or solution more than 24 hours old.

Feedings are usually administered at room temperature unless the order specifies otherwise. The nurse warms the specified amount of solution in a basin of warm water or leaves it to stand for a while until it reaches room temperature. Continuous feeding should be kept cold; excessive heat coagulates feedings of milk and egg, and hot liquids can irritate the mucous membranes. However, excessively cold feedings can reduce the flow of digestive juices by causing vasoconstriction and may cause cramps. Commercially prepared feedings are available in cans and bottles ready for administration. Some containers are designed so that ice chips can be placed in an outer section to keep the formula cooled.

A feeding pump can be used with a prefilled tube-feeding set to regulate the exact amount of feeding for the client (Figure 37–10, p. 1046). The pump is often used to administer the feeding in instances when smaller-bore gastric tubes are used or when gravity flow is insufficient to instill the feeding. Because the feeding is administered over a long time period, a formula that is warmed can grow microorganisms. It should not hang longer than the manufacturer recommends, for example, 3 to 4 hours. If it will hang longer, it should be kept cool with ice chips.

Although the focus of this chapter is nutrition, *nasogastric tubes* may be inserted for reasons other than providing a route for feeding the client. These include

Table 37–12 Assessing Clients Receiving Tube Feedings

Assessments	Rationale
Allergies to any food in the feeding	Common allergenic foods include milk, sugar, water, eggs, and vegetable oil.
Bowel sounds prior to each feeding or, for continuous feedings, every 4 to 8 hours	To determine intestinal activity.
Abdominal distention, at least daily. Measure abdominal girth at the umbilicus	Abdominal distention may indicate intolerance to a previous feeding.
Correct placement of tube, before feedings	To prevent aspiration of feedings.
Presence of regurgitation and feelings of fullness after feedings	May indicate delayed gastric emptying, need to decrease quantity or rate of the feeding, or high fat content of the formula.
Dumping syndrome: nausea, vomiting, diarrhea, cramps, pallor, sweating, heart palpitations, increased pulse rate, and fainting after a feeding	Jejunostomy clients may experience these symptoms, which result when hypertonic foods and liquids suddenly distend the jejunum. To make the intestinal contents isotonic, body fluids shift rapidly from the client's vascular system.
Diarrhea, constipation, or flatulence	The lack of bulk in liquid feedings may cause constipation. The presence of hypertonic or concentrated ingredients may cause diarrhea and flatulence.
Urine for sugar and acetone	Hyperglycemia may occur if the sugar content is too high.
Hematocrit and urine specific gravity	Both increase as a result of dehydration.
Serum BUN and sodium levels	Feeding formula may have a high protein content. If a high protein intake is combined with an inadequate fluid intake, the kidneys may not be able to excrete nitrogenous wastes adequately.

1. To prevent nausea, vomiting, and gastric distention following surgery. In this case, the tube is attached to a suction source.
2. To remove stomach contents for laboratory analysis.

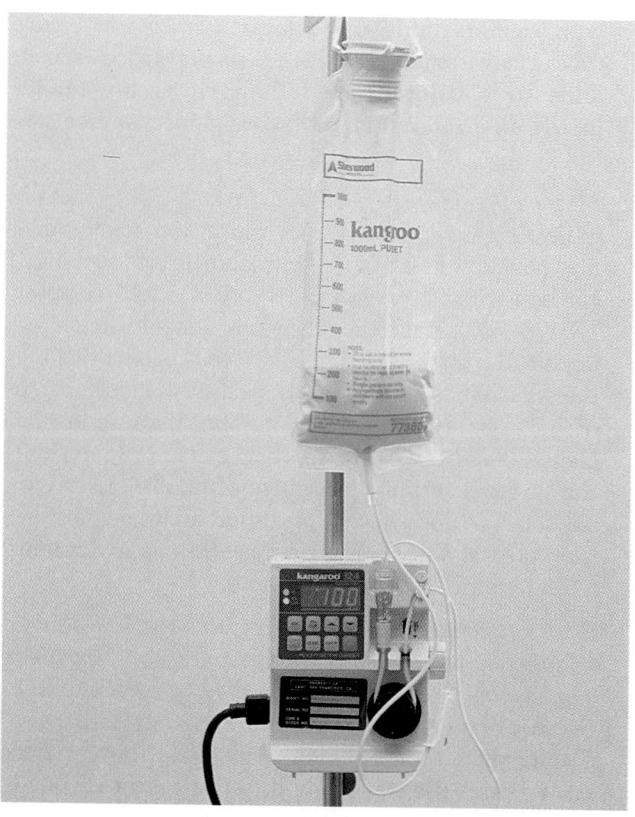

Figure 37–10 A feeding pump.

3. To lavage (wash) the stomach in cases of poisoning or overdose of medications.

Procedure 37–1 provides guidelines for inserting a nasogastric or nasointestinal tube. Procedure 37–2 on page 1050 provides the essential steps involved in administering a tube feeding, and Procedure 37–3 on page 1053 indicates the steps involved in removing a nasogastric tube.

Gastrostomy/Jejunostomy Feedings A **gastrostomy feeding** is the instillation of liquid nourishment through a tube that enters a surgical opening (called a gastrostomy) through the abdominal wall into the stomach. A **jejunostomy feeding** is the instillation of liquid nourishment through a tube that enters a surgical opening (a jejunostomy) through the abdominal wall into the jejunum. These feedings are usually temporary measures. When there is an obstruction in the esophagus, they may become permanent, for example, after removal of the esophagus.

Increasingly, **percutaneous endoscopic gastrostomy (PEG)** is being used. This procedure does not require general anesthesia or the use of an operating room. PEG is usually performed in the endoscopy suite but may also be done in the client's room. Using an endoscope to

Text continued on page 1052

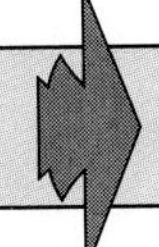

PROCEDURE 37–1 INSERTING A NASOGASTRIC TUBE

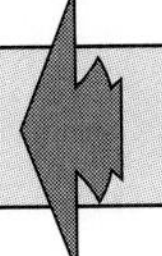

Before inserting a nasogastric tube, determine the size of tube to be inserted and whether or not the tube is to be attached to a suction.

PURPOSES

- To administer tube feedings and medications to clients unable to eat by mouth or swallow a sufficient diet without aspirating food or fluids into the lungs
- To establish a means for suctioning stomach contents to prevent gastric distention, nausea, and vomiting
- To remove stomach contents for laboratory analysis
- To lavage (wash) the stomach in case of poisoning or overdose of medications

ASSESSMENT FOCUS
Patency of nares and intactness of nasal tissues (note especially history of nasal surgery or deviated septum); presence of gag reflex; mental status or ability to cooperate with procedure.

EQUIPMENT

- ☐ Large- or small-bore tube (plastic or rubber)
- ☐ Solution basin filled with warm water (if a plastic tube is being used) or ice (if a rubber tube is being used)
- ☐ Nonallergenic adhesive tape, 2.5 cm (1 in) wide
- ☐ Disposable gloves
- ☐ Water-soluble lubricant
- ☐ Facial tissues
- ☐ Glass of water and drinking straw or medicine cup with water
- ☐ 20- to 50-mL syringe with an adapter
- ☐ Basin
- ☐ Stethoscope
- ☐ Clamp (optional)
- ☐ Suction apparatus if required
- ☐ Gauze square or plastic specimen bag and elastic band
- ☐ Safety pin and elastic band
- ☐ Infant seat, towel, or pillow
- ☐ Restraint or hand mitts (for infants or small children)
- ☐ 5-mL or 12-mL syringe

INTERVENTION

1. Prepare the client.

- Explain to the client what you plan to do. The passage of a gastric tube is not painful, but it is unpleasant because the gag reflex is activated during insertion.
- Assist the client to a high-Fowler's position if health permits, and support the head on a pillow. *It is often easier to swallow in this position, and gravity helps the passage of the tube.*
- Place the infant in an infant seat, or position the infant with a rolled towel or pillow under the head and shoulders.
- Place the towel across the chest. A bib or diaper can be used for an infant.

2. Assess the client's nares.

- Ask the client to hyperextend the head, and, using a flashlight, observe the intactness of the tissues of the nostrils, including any irritations or abrasions.
- Examine the nares for any obstructions or deformities by asking the client to breathe through one nostril while occluding the other.
- Select the nostril that has the greater airflow.
- Obstruct one of the infant's nares, and feel for air passage from the other.

3. Prepare the tube.

- If a rubber tube is being used, place it on ice. *This stiffens the tube, facilitating insertion.* If a plastic tube is being used, place it in warm water. *This makes the tube more flexible, facilitating insertion.*

4. Determine how far to insert the tube.

- Use the tube to mark off the distance from the tip of the client's nose to the tip of the earlobe and then from the tip of the earlobe to the tip of the sternum (Figure 37–11, p. 1048). *This length approximates the distance from the nares to the stomach. This distance varies among individuals.*
- For infants and young children, measure from the nose to the tip of the earlobe and then to the point midway between the umbilicus and the xiphoid process (Speer & Swann 1993, p. 266).

PROCEDURE 37–1 INSERTING A NASOGASTRIC TUBE *continued*

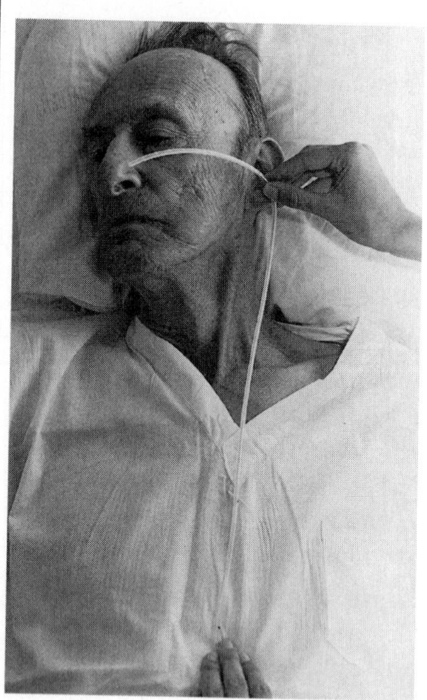

Figure 37–11 Measuring the appropriate length to insert a nasogastric tube.

- Mark this length with adhesive tape if the tube does not have markings.

5. Insert the tube.

- Don gloves.
- Lubricate the tip of the tube well with water-soluble lubricant or water to ease insertion. *A water-soluble lubricant dissolves if the tube accidentally enters the lungs. An oil-based lubricant, such as petroleum jelly, will not dissolve and could cause respiratory complications if it enters the lungs.*
- Insert the tube, with its natural curve toward the client, into the selected nostril. Ask the client to hyperextend the neck, and gently advance the tube toward the nasopharynx. *Hyperextension of the neck reduces the curvature of the nasopharyngeal junction.*
- Do not hyperextend or hyperflex an infant's neck. *Hyperextension or hyperflexion of the neck could occlude the airway* (Oberc 1991).
- Direct the tube along the floor of the nostril and toward the ear on that side. *Directing the tube along the floor avoids the projections (turbinates) along the lateral wall.*
- Slight pressure is sometimes required to pass the tube into the nasopharynx, and some clients' eyes may water at this point. Tears are a natural body response. Provide the client with tissues as needed.
- If the tube meets resistance, withdraw it, relubricate it, and insert it in the other nostril. *The tube should never be forced against resistance, because of the danger of injury.*

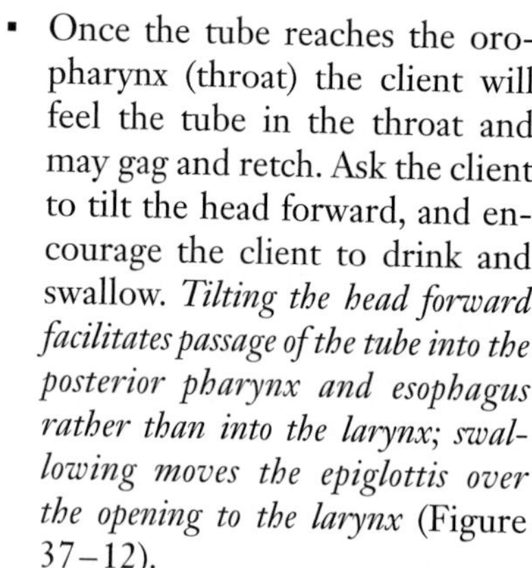

- Once the tube reaches the oropharynx (throat) the client will feel the tube in the throat and may gag and retch. Ask the client to tilt the head forward, and encourage the client to drink and swallow. *Tilting the head forward facilitates passage of the tube into the posterior pharynx and esophagus rather than into the larynx; swallowing moves the epiglottis over the opening to the larynx* (Figure 37–12).
- If the client gags, stop passing the tube momentarily. Have the client rest, take a few breaths, and take sips of water to calm the gag reflex.
- In cooperation with the client, pass the tube 5 to 10 cm (2 to 4 in) with each swallow, until the indicated length is inserted.
- If the client continues to gag and the tube does not advance with each swallow, withdraw it slightly, and inspect the throat by looking through the mouth. *The tube may be coiled in the throat.* If so, withdraw it until it is straight, and try again to insert it.

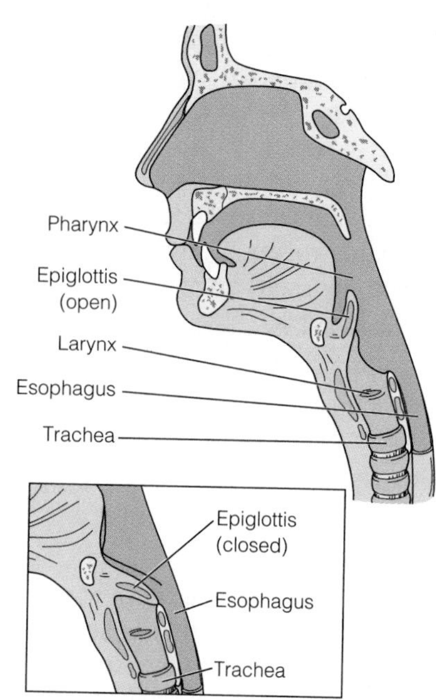

Figure 37–12 Swallowing closes the epiglottis.

6. Ascertain correct placement of the tube.

- Aspirate stomach contents, and check their acidity.
- Auscultate air insufflation.
- Use other methods in accordance with agency protocol (see p. 1045).
- If the signs do not indicate placement in the stomach, advance the tube 5 cm (2 in), and repeat the tests.
- For tubes that are to be placed into the duodenum or jejunum, advance the tube 5 to 7.5 cm (2 to 3 in) per hour until X-ray study confirms its placement.

7. Secure the tube by taping it to the bridge of the client's nose.

- If the client has oily skin, wipe the nose first with alcohol.

Procedure 37–1 *continued*

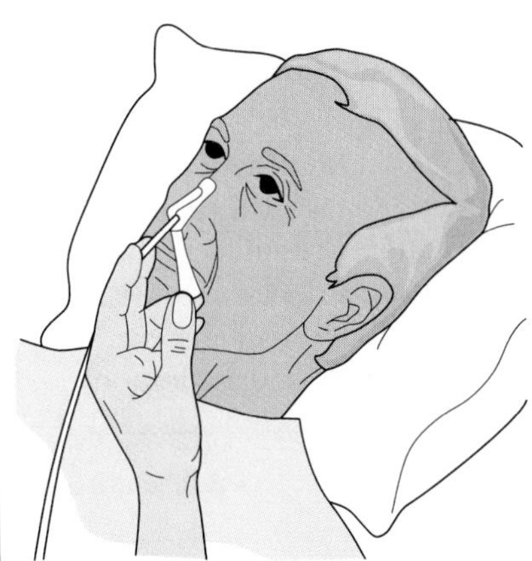

Figure 37–13 Taping a nasogastric tube to the bridge of the nose.

- Cut 7.5 cm (3 in) of tape, and split it lengthwise at one end, leaving a 2.5-cm (1-in) tab at the end.
- Place the tape over the bridge of the client's nose, and bring the split ends under the tubing and back up over the nose (Figure 37–13). *Taping in this manner prevents the tube from pressing against and irritating the edge of the nostril.* For infants or small children, tape the tube to the area between the end of the nares and the upper lip, as well as to the cheek.

8. Attach the tube to a suction source or feeding apparatus as ordered, or clamp the end of the tubing.

- The tube, if inserted preoperatively, is usually clamped; or it may be covered with a gauze square or plastic specimen bag and an elastic band.

9. Secure the tube to the client's gown.

- Loop an elastic band around the end of the tubing, and attach the elastic band to the gown with a safety pin.

  or

  Attach a piece of adhesive tape to the tube, and pin the tape to the gown. *The tube is attached to prevent it from dangling and pulling.*
- For infants and young children, restraints may be necessary during tube insertion and throughout therapy. *Restraints will prevent accidental dislodging of the tube.*

10. Document relevant information.

- Document the insertion of the tube, means by which correct placement was determined, and client responses (eg, discomfort or abdominal distention).

11. Establish a plan for providing daily nasogastric tube care.

- Inspect the nostril for discharge and irritation.
- Clean the nostril and tube with moistened, cotton-tipped applicators.
- Apply water-soluble lubricant to the nostril if it appears dry or encrusted.
- Change the adhesive tape as required.
- Give frequent mouth care. *The client may breathe through the mouth and cannot drink.*

12. If suction is applied, ensure that the patency of both the nasogastric and suction tubes is maintained.

- Irrigations of the tube with 30 mL of normal saline may be required at regular intervals. For infants or small children, use 1 to 10 mL of saline. In some agencies, irrigations must be ordered by the physician. Managing gastrointestinal suction and irrigating a nasogastric tube are discussed in Procedure 45–2, page 1417.
- Keep accurate records of the client's fluid intake and output, and record the amount and characteristics of the drainage.

13. Document all relevant information.

- Document the type of tube inserted, date and time of tube insertion, type of suction used, color and amount of gastric contents, and the client's tolerance of the procedure.

Variation: Inserting an Orogastric Tube

If the nasal passageway is very small or is obstructed, an orogastric tube may be more appropriate.

- Measure from the tip of the earlobe to the corner of the mouth to the xiphoid process.
- Open the mouth of an infant or comatose client, or ask an older child or adult to open the mouth wide.
- Advance the tube to the back of the throat along the side of the tongue. Withdraw the tube if the client gags.
- Stimulate swallowing with sips of water, and advance the tube with each swallow.
- Check tube placement.
- Tape tubing to the cheek.

Evaluation Focus

Degree of client comfort; client tolerance of tube; correct placement of nasogastric tube in stomach; client understanding of restrictions; color and amount of gastric contents, if attached to suction or contents aspirated.

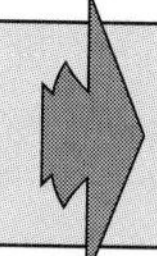

PROCEDURE 37–2 ADMINISTERING A TUBE FEEDING THROUGH AN ESTABLISHED FEEDING TUBE

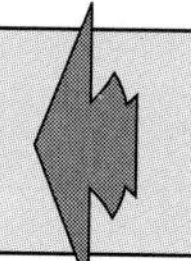

Before commencing a nasogastric or orogastric feeding determine the type, amount, and frequency of feedings and tolerance of previous feedings.

PURPOSES

- To restore or maintain nutritional status
- To administer medications

ASSESSMENT FOCUS

Clinical signs of malnutrition or dehydration (see Table 37–10 and Chapter 38, page 1071); allergies to any food in the feeding; presence of bowel sounds; any problems that suggest lack of tolerance of previous feedings (eg, abdominal distention, dumping syndrome, constipation, or dehydration).

EQUIPMENT

- ☐ Correct amount of feeding solution
- ☐ Pacifier
- ☐ 20- to 50-mL syringe with an adapter
- ☐ Emesis basin
- ☐ Bulb syringe (for an intermittent feeding)
  or
- ☐ Calibrated plastic feeding bag and a drip chamber, which can be attached to the tubing
  or
- ☐ Prefilled bottle with a drip chamber, tubing, and a flow-regulator clamp
- ☐ Measuring container from which to pour the feeding (if using bulb syringe)
- ☐ Water (60 mL unless otherwise specified) at room temperature
- ☐ Feeding pump (optional)

INTERVENTION

1. Prepare the client and the feeding.

- Explain to the client that the feeding should not cause any discomfort but may cause a feeling of fullness. For an adult, the usual intermittent feeding will take about 30 minutes; the exact length of time depends largely on the volume of the feeding.
- Provide privacy for this procedure if the client desires it. *Nasogastric feedings are embarrassing to some people.*
- Assist the client to a Fowler's position in bed or a sitting position in a chair, the normal position for eating. If a sitting position is contraindicated, a slightly elevated right side-lying position is acceptable. *These positions enhance the gravitational flow of the solution and prevent aspiration of fluid into the lungs.*
- Position a small child or infant in your lap, and provide a pacifier during feeding. *This promotes comfort, supports the normal sucking instinct of the infant, and facilitates digestion.*

2. Assess tube placement.

- Attach the syringe to the open end of the tube, aspirate alimentary secretions. Check the pH. See p. 1045 for other methods.

3. Assess residual feeding contents.

- Aspirate all the stomach contents, and measure the amount prior to administering the feeding. *This is done to evaluate absorption of the last feeding, that is, whether undigested formula from a previous feeding remains.*
- If 50 mL or more of undigested formula is withdrawn in adults, or 10 mL or more in infants, check with the nurse in charge before proceeding. The precise amount is usually determined by the physician's order or by agency policy. *At some agencies, a feeding is withheld when the specified amount or more of formula remains in the stomach. In other agencies, the amount withdrawn is subtracted from the total feeding and that volume (less the undigested portion) is administered slowly.*
  or
  Reinstill the gastric contents into the stomach if this is the agency or physician's practice. Remove the syringe bulb or plunger, and pour the gastric contents via the syringe into the nasogastric tube. *Removal of the contents could disturb the client's electrolyte balance.*

PROCEDURE 37–2 *continued*

4. Administer the feeding.

- Before administering feeding:
  a. Check the expiration date of the feeding.
  b. Warm the feeding to room temperature. *An excessively cold feeding may cause cramps.*

Bulb Syringe

- Remove the bulb from the syringe, and connect the syringe to a pinched or clamped nasogastric tube. *Pinching or clamping the tube prevents excess air from entering the stomach and causing distention.*
- Add the feeding to the syringe barrel (Figure 37–14).

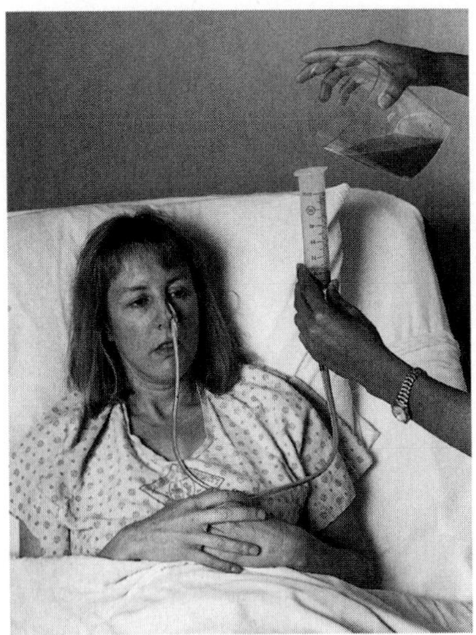

Figure 37–14 Using a bulb syringe to administer a tube feeding.

- Permit the feeding to flow in slowly at the prescribed rate. Raise or lower the syringe to adjust the flow as needed. Pinch or clamp the tubing to stop the flow for a minute if the client experiences discomfort. *Quickly administered feedings can cause flatus, crampy pain, and/or reflux vomiting.*

Feeding Bag

- Hang the bag from an infusion pole about 30 cm (12 in) above the tube's point of insertion into the client.
- Clamp the tubing, and add the formula to the bag, if it is not prefilled.
- Open the clamp, run the formula through the tubing, and reclamp the tube. *The formula will displace the air in the tubing, thus preventing the instillation of excess air into the client's stomach or intestine.*
- Attach the bag to the nasogastric tube (Figure 37–15), and regulate the drip by adjusting the clamp to drop factor on bag (eg, 20 drops/mL).

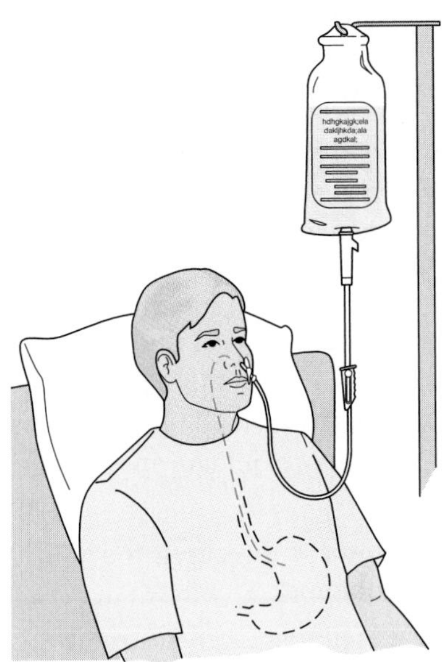

Figure 37–15 Using a calibrated plastic bag to administer a tube feeding.

Prefilled Bottle with Drip Chamber

- Remove the sealed cap from the container, and replace it with the screw-on cap to which the drip chamber and tubing are attached (Figure 37–16).

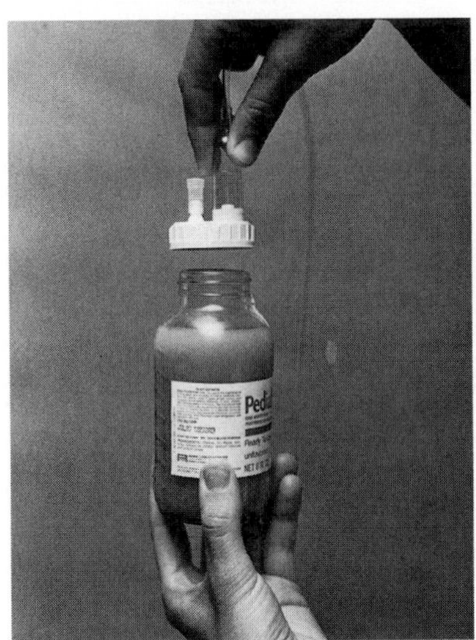

Figure 37–16 A prefilled bottle with drip chamber.

- Close the clamp on the tubing.
- Hang the container on an intravenous pole about 30 cm (12 in) above the tube's insertion point into the client. *At this height the formula should run at a safe rate into the stomach or intestine.*
- Squeeze the drip chamber to fill it to one-third to one-half of its capacity.
- Open the tubing clamp, run the formula through the tubing, and reclamp the tube. *The formula will displace the air in the tubing, thus preventing the installation of excess air.*
- Attach the feeding set tubing to the feeding tube, and regulate the drip rate to deliver the feeding over the desired length of time. Some prefilled tube-feeding sets can be attached to a feeding pump.

5. Rinse the feeding tube immediately before all of the formula has run through the tubing.

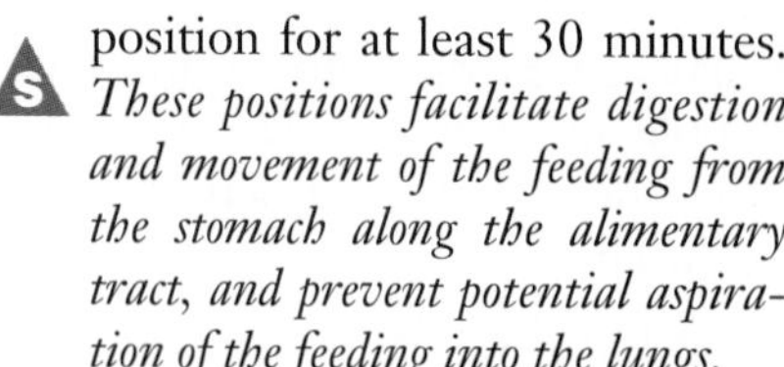

PROCEDURE 37–2 ADMINISTERING A TUBE FEEDING THROUGH AN ESTABLISHED FEEDING TUBE *continued*

- Instill 60 mL of water through the feeding tube. *Water cleans the lumen of the tube, preventing future blockage by sticky formula.*
- Be sure to add the water before the feeding solution has drained from the neck of a bulb syringe or from the tubing of an administration set. Before adding water to a feeding bag or prefilled tubing set, first clamp and disconnect both feeding and administration tubes. *Adding the water before the syringe or tubing is empty prevents the instillation of air into the stomach or intestine and thus prevents unnecessary distention.*

6. Clamp and cover the feeding tube.

- Clamp the feeding tube before all of the water is instilled. *Clamping prevents leakage and air from entering the tube if done before water is instilled.*
- Cover the end of the feeding tube with gauze held by an elastic band. *Covering the tube end prevents leakage from it.*

7. Ensure client comfort and safety.

- Pin the tubing to the client's gown. *This minimizes pulling of the tube, thus preventing discomfort and dislodgement.*
- Ask the client to remain sitting upright in Fowler's position or in a slightly elevated right lateral position for at least 30 minutes. *These positions facilitate digestion and movement of the feeding from the stomach along the alimentary tract, and prevent potential aspiration of the feeding into the lungs.*
- Check the agency's policy on the frequency of changing the nasogastric tube and the use of smaller-lumen tubes if a large-bore tube is in place. *These measures prevent irritation and erosion of the pharyngeal and esophageal mucous membranes.*

8. Dispose of equipment appropriately.

- If the equipment is to be reused, wash it thoroughly with soap and water so that it is ready for reuse.
- Change the equipment every 24 hours or according to agency policy.

9. Document all relevant information.

- Document the feeding, including amount and kind of solution taken, duration of the feeding, and assessments of the client.
- Record the volume of the feeding and water administered on the client's intake and output record.

10. Monitor the client for possible problems.

- Carefully assess clients receiving tube feedings for problems.
- To prevent dehydration, give the client supplemental water in addition to the prescribed tube feeding as ordered.

Variation: Continuous-Drip Feeding

If the feeding is a continuous-drip tube feeding, clamp the tubing at least every 4 to 6 hours or as indicated by agency protocol or the manufacturer, and aspirate and measure the gastric contents. Then flush the tubing with 30 to 50 mL of water. Determine agency protocol regarding withholding a feeding. Many agencies withhold the feeding if more than 75 to 100 mL of feeding is aspirated. To prevent spoilage, the same solution should not be hung longer than 3 to 4 hours at a time or the manufacturer's recommended time. *This determines adequate absorption and verifies correct placement of the tube. If placement of a small bore tube is questionable, a repeat X ray should be done.*

EVALUATION FOCUS

Tolerance of feeding; regurgitation and feelings of fullness after feedings; weight gain or loss; fecal elimination pattern (eg, diarrhea, flatulence, constipation); skin turgor; urine output; glucose and acetone in urine.

visualize the inside of the stomach, the physician makes a puncture through the skin and subcutaneous tissues of the abdomen into the stomach and inserts the PEG catheter through the puncture. The catheter has internal and external bumpers and an inflatable retention balloon to maintain placement. Once the opening has healed, replacement tubes can be inserted without the use of endoscopy.

Long-term use of PEG feedings is preferable to gastric or small intestine feedings; there are fewer risks of aspiration, and it is psychologically more acceptable. Clients initially receive feedings continuously but advance to intermittent feedings after a few days of uncomplicated continuous feedings. The feeding tube is not visible except when in use. PEG tubes often have small lumens, so care must be taken to avoid clogging the tube. Use liquid med-

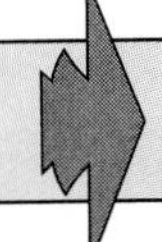

Procedure 37–3 Removing a Nasogastric Tube

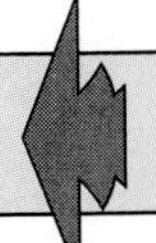

Assessment Focus
Presence of bowel sounds; absence of nausea or vomiting when tube is clamped.

Equipment

- ☐ Disposable pad
- ☐ Tissues
- ☐ Clean disposable gloves
- ☐ 50-mL syringe (optional)
- ☐ Plastic disposable bag

INTERVENTION

1. Confirm the physician's order to remove the tube.

2. Prepare the client.

- Explain that the procedure will cause no discomfort.
- Assist the client to a sitting position if health permits.
- Place the disposable pad across the client's chest to collect any spillage of mucous and gastric secretions from the tube.
- Provide tissues to the client to wipe the nose and mouth after tube removal.

3. Detach the tube.

- Disconnect the nasogastric tube from the suction apparatus, if present.
- Unpin the tube from the client's gown.
- Remove the adhesive tape securing the tube to the nose.

4. Remove the tube.

- Put on disposable gloves.
- (Optional). Instill 50 mL of air into the tube. *This clears the tube of any contents such as feeding or gastric drainage.*
- Ask the client to take a deep breath and to hold it. *This closes the glottis, thereby preventing accidental aspiration of any gastric contents.*
- Pinch the tube with the gloved hand. *Pinching the tube prevents any contents inside the tube from draining into the client's throat.*
- Quickly and smoothly withdraw the tube.
- Place the tube in the plastic bag. *Placing the tube immediately into the bag prevents the transference of microorganisms from the tube to other articles or people.*
- Observe the intactness of the tube.

5. Ensure client comfort.

- Provide mouthwash if desired.
- Assist the client as required to blow the nose. *Excessive secretions may have accumulated in the nasal passages.*

6. Dispose of the equipment appropriately.

- Place the pad, bag with tube, and gloves in the receptacle designated by the agency. *Correct disposal prevents the transmission of microorganisms.*

7. Assess the nasogastric drainage if suction was used.

- Measure the amount of gastric drainage, and record it on the client's fluid output record.
- Inspect the drainage for appearance and consistency.

8. Document all relevant information.

- Record the removal of the tube, the amount and appearance of any drainage if connected to suction, and any relevant assessments of the client.

Evaluation Focus
Presence of bowel sounds; absence of nausea or vomiting when tube is removed; intactness of tissues of the nares.

ications when possible. If liquid preparations are not available, finely crush tablets and dissolve them with water before inserting; flush the tube with water afterward. Crushing interferes with the action of some medications; the nurse should check with a pharmacist or consult a drug formulary beforehand.

For conventional gastrostomies and jejunostomies, a surgeon inserts a plastic or rubber tube or catheter into either the stomach or the jejunum. The surgical opening is sutured tightly around the tube or catheter to prevent leakage. Care of this opening before it heals requires surgical asepsis. When the incision heals (10 to 14 days), the tube or catheter can be removed and reinserted for each feeding. Between feedings, a prosthesis may be used to close the ostomy opening. It consists of a shaft 3 to 5 cm (1½ to 2 in) long, with internal and external flanges and a screw cap.

Gastrostomy and jejunostomy feedings allow clients greater mobility than gastric or duodenal tube feedings and enable clients to feed themselves. Similar principles for administration and assessment are appropriate. Procedure 37–4 provides the steps in administering a gastrostomy or jejunostomy feeding. The amount of solution is gradually increased with each feeding, from 200 to 800 mL. Commercially prepared formulas that are past the manufacturer's expiration date and agency-prepared solutions older than 24 hours must be discarded.

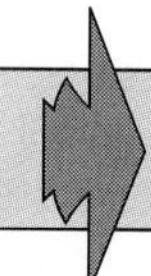

PROCEDURE 37–4 ADMINISTERING A GASTROSTOMY OR JEJUNOSTOMY FEEDING

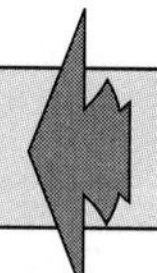

Before commencing a gastrostomy or jejunostomy feeding determine the type and amount of feeding to be instilled, frequency of feedings, and any pertinent information about previous feedings (eg, the position in which the client best tolerates the feeding).

PURPOSES

- To improve or maintain nutritional status
- To administer medications

ASSESSMENT FOCUS

See Procedure 37–2 on page 1050.

EQUIPMENT

- ☐ Correct amount of feeding solution
- ☐ Graduated container to hold the feeding
- ☐ Large bulb syringe
- ☐ Graduated container with 60 mL of water to flush the tubing
- ☐ Graduated container to measure residual formula

For a Tube Sutured in Place

- ☐ 4 × 4 gauze squares to cover the end of the tube
- ☐ Elastic band

For Tube Insertion

- ☐ Clean disposable gloves
- ☐ Moistureproof bag
- ☐ Water-soluble lubricant
- ☐ #18 Fr. whistle-tip catheter or other feeding tube
- ☐ Tubing clamp

For Cleaning the Peristomal Skin and Dressing the Stoma

- ☐ Mild soap and water
- ☐ Petrolatum, zinc oxide ointment, or other skin protectant
- ☐ Precut 4 × 4 gauze squares
- ☐ Uncut 4 × 4 gauze squares
- ☐ Abdominal pads
- ☐ Abdominal binder or Montgomery straps

INTERVENTION

1. Assess and prepare the client.

- See Procedure 37–1 on page 1047.

2. Insert a feeding tube, if one is not already in place.

- Wearing gloves, remove the ostomy dressing. Then discard the dressing and gloves in the moistureproof bag.

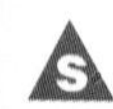

- Lubricate the end of the tube, and insert it into the ostomy opening 10 to 15 cm (4 to 6 in).

3. Check the patency of a tube that is sutured in place.

- Determine placement of the tube. See page 1044.
- Pour 15 to 30 mL of water into the syringe, remove the tube clamp, and allow the water to flow into the tube. *This determines the patency of the tube. If water flows freely, the tube is patent.*
- If the water does not flow freely, notify the nurse in charge and/or physician.

4. Check for residual formula.

- Attach the bulb to the syringe, and compress the bulb. *Compressing the bulb before the syringe is attached to the feeding tube prevents the instillation of air into the stomach or jejunum.*
- Attach the syringe to the end of the feeding tube, and withdraw and measure the stomach or jejunal contents.
- Follow agency practice if there is no more than 50 mL of undi-

PROCEDURE 37–4 *continued*

gested formula. Hold the feeding if there is more than 150 mL, and recheck in 3 to 4 hours. Notify the physician if a large residual still remains.

- For continuous feedings, check the residual every 4 to 6 hours, and hold feedings if there is a 2-hour volume. Then recheck in 2 hours, and restart unless the residual remains large; the physician should be notified if a large residual persists.

5. Administer the feeding.

- Position infant comfortably in your lap, and provide a pacifier.
- Hold the syringe 7 to 15 cm (3 to 6 in) above the ostomy opening.
- Slowly pour the solution into the syringe, and allow it to flow through the tube by gravity.
- Just before all the formula has run through and the syringe is empty, add 30 mL of water. *Water rinses the tube and preserves its patency.*
- If the tube is sutured in place, hold it upright, remove the syringe, and then clamp the tube to prevent leakage. Cover the end of the tube with a 4 by 4 gauze, and secure the gauze with a rubber band.
- If a catheter was inserted for the feeding, remove it.

6. Ensure client comfort and safety.

- After the feeding, ask the client to remain in the sitting position or a slightly elevated right lateral position for at least 30 minutes. *This minimizes the risk of aspiration.*
- Assess status of peristomal skin. *Gastric or jejunal drainage contains digestive enzymes that can irritate the skin.* Document any redness and broken skin areas.
- Check orders about cleaning the peristomal skin, applying a skin protectant, and applying appropriate dressings. Generally, the peristomal skin is washed with mild soap and water at least once daily. Petrolatum, zinc oxide ointment, or other skin protectant may be applied around the stoma, and precut 4 by 4 gauze squares may be placed around the tube. The precut squares are then covered with regular 4 by 4 gauze squares, and the tube is coiled over them. The coiled tube is covered with abdominal pads and secured with either an abdominal binder or Montgomery straps.
- Observe for common complications of enteral feedings: aspiration, hyperglycemia, abdominal distention, diarrhea, and fecal impaction. Report findings to physician. Often a change in formula or rate of administration can correct problems.
- When appropriate, teach the client how to administer feedings and when to notify the physician or nurse practitioner concerning problems.

7. Document all assessments and interventions.

EVALUATION FOCUS
See Procedure 37–2, page 1052.

EVALUATING

Depending on the outcome criteria established in the planning phase, the nurse may perform the following evaluative activities: (a) taking anthropometric measurements, (b) observing the client for changes in signs of malnutrition, (c) questioning the client about dietary alterations required or listening to the client's reports of dietary alterations achieved, (d) reviewing and discussing a dietary log or plan of a balanced meal, (e) weighing the client, and (f) checking laboratory data for desired changes or assessing the client for complications of enteral feedings.

If the outcomes are not achieved, the nurse should explore the reasons. The nurse might consider the following questions:

- Was the cause of the problem correctly identified?
- Was the family included in the teaching plan? Are they supportive?
- Is the client experiencing symptoms that cause loss of appetite (eg, pain, nausea, fatigue)?
- Were the outcomes unrealistic for this person?
- Were the client's food preferences considered?
- Is anything interfering with digestion or absorption of nutrients (eg, diarrhea)?

See also the evaluation checklist in Chapter 8, page 158.

CRITICAL PATHWAY FOR ROSE SANDUSKI

ASSESSMENT DATA

Nursing Assessment

Mrs Rose Sanduski, a 59-year-old homemaker, is admitted to the hospital by her personal medical doctor, Dr Peters. When she was recently at the office she complained of frequent urination and thirst. Her fasting blood sugar the next morning was 425 mg/dL. Dr Peters has admitted her for uncontrolled diabetes and teaching about her diabetic regimen. Mrs Sanduski is a recent widow, who tells the admitting nurse, Ms Pamela Norris, that since the death of her husband 9 months ago, she has lost interest in many of her usual physical and social activities. She no longer attends the YMCA exercise and swimming sessions and has lost contact with many friends. She reports a 40-pound weight gain in the last year. She tends to snack a great deal while watching TV and rarely prepares a complete meal.

Physical Examination

Height: 162.6 cm (5′6″)
Weight: 75 kg (165 lb)
Temperature: 37 C (98.6 F)
Pulse rate: 76 bpm
Respirations: 16 per minute at rest
Blood pressure: 144/84 mm Hg
Triceps skin fold 33 mm
Small frame, weight in excess of 10% over ideal for height and frame

Diagnostic Studies

CBC: normal
Urine: 4+ glucose
Chest X-ray film: negative
Thyroid profile: within normal limits
Blood sugar: 375 mg/dL

CRITICAL PATHWAY FOR CLIENT WITH TYPE II DIABETES

Expected length of stay 5 days

	Date ________ Day 1	Date ________ Day 2	Date ________ Day 3
Daily outcomes	Client will ▪ have stable vital signs. ▪ verbalize understanding and importance of diet compliance and regular blood sugar testing. ▪ have episodes of hypo- or hyperglycemia detected early. ▪ verbalize ability to cope.	Client will ▪ have stable vital signs. ▪ verbalize understanding and importance of diet compliance and regular blood sugar testing. ▪ have weight loss of ½ pound. ▪ have episodes of hypo- or hyperglycemia detected early. ▪ verbalize ability to cope. ▪ verbalize beginning understanding of home care instructions.	Client will ▪ have stable vital signs and unlabored respirations at rest. ▪ verbalize understanding and importance of diet compliance and regular blood sugar testing. ▪ have weight loss of ½ pound. ▪ have episodes of hypo- or hyperglycemia detected early. ▪ verbalize ability to cope. ▪ verbalize willingness to participate in a regular exercise program. ▪ identify eating behaviors that lead to weight gain.

	Day 1 *continued*	Day 2 *continued*	Day 3 *continued*
Daily outcomes *continued*			▪ demonstrate ability to self-administer insulin and perform self-monitoring of blood glucose safely and correctly with minimal supervision. ▪ verbalize beginning understanding of home care instructions.
Tests and treatments	CBC. Fasting blood sugar. Vital signs q4h if stable. Fingerstick blood sugar ac, hs, and prn. Monitor for signs and symptoms of hypo- and hyperglycemia. Follow hypoglycemia protocol if symptoms occur. Intake and output q shift.	Fasting blood sugar. Vital signs q4h if stable. Fingerstick blood sugar ac, hs, and prn. Monitor for signs and symptoms of hypo- and hyperglycemia. Follow hypoglycemia protocol if symptoms occur. Intake and output q shift.	Fasting blood sugar. Vital signs q4h if stable. Fingerstick blood sugar ac, hs, and prn. Monitor for signs and symptoms of hypo- and hyperglycemia. Follow hypoglycemia protocol if symptoms occur. Intake and output q shift.
Knowledge deficit	Orient to room and hospital routine. Review plan of care. Review steps of insulin administration and provide written instruction sheets. Review steps of self-monitoring of blood glucose (SMBG). Consult with diabetic nurse educator. Consult with registered dietician for instruction in diet and exchange lists.	Reorient to room and hospital routine. Review plan of care. Review steps of insulin administration and SMBG. Allow client to practice with related equipment. Show client and significant other videotapes related to Type II diabetes and self-care practices.	Reorient to room and hospital routine. Review plan of care. Supervise client in self-administration of insulin and performing SMBG. Client attends classes on general health care rules and foot care and watch video related to identifying and managing hypo- and hyperglycemia.
Psycho-social	Assess level of anxiety. Encourage verbalization of concerns. Provide information. Provide ongoing support and encouragement.	Assess level of anxiety. Encourage verbalization of concerns. Provide information. Provide ongoing support and encouragement.	Encourage verbalization of concerns. Provide ongoing support and encouragement.
Diet	Daily weight. 1200 calorie ADA diet. Encourage fluid intake of 2000 mL/day. Assess for causes of excessive weight gain.	Daily weight. 1200 calorie ADA diet. Encourage fluid intake of 2000 mL/day. Encourage client to identify activities and food that contribute to excessive intake.	Daily weight. 1200 calorie ADA diet. Encourage fluid intake of 2000 mL/day. Encourage client to identify activities and food that contribute to excessive intake.

➤

	Day 1 *continued*	**Day 2** *continued*	**Day 3** *continued*
Diet *continued*	Encourage client to identify activities and food that contribute to excessive intake.	Discuss with client strategies such as knitting or sewing instead of eating when watching TV. Identify behavior modification strategies (eg, drink 8 oz of water before each meal, eat slowly, and chew thoroughly) to assist in weight loss.	Encourage client to utilize behavior modification strategies. Explain the relationship between regular physical exercise and weight loss and control. Encourage client to establish regular exercise program.
Activity	Provide safety precautions. Bathroom privileges. OOB ad lib in room. Provide rest periods.	Provide safety precautions. OOB ad lib. Encourage rest periods.	Provide safety precautions. Ambulate ad lib. Encourage rest periods.
Medications	Regular insulin to scale ac and hs.	Regular insulin to scale ac and hs. NPH insulin per order AM and PM.	Regular insulin to scale ac and hs. NPH insulin per order AM and PM.
Transfer/ discharge plans	Review discharge goals with client and significant others. Consult with social service re: projected needs for home health care (if any).	Review progress towards discharge goals with client and significant other.	Review progress toward discharge goals with client and significant other. Refer to Diabetic Support group. Refer to diabetic nurse educator for continued teaching after discharge.

	Date ________ **Day 4**	**Date ________** **Day 5**
Daily outcomes	Client will ▪ have stable vital signs. ▪ verbalize understanding and importance of diet compliance and regular blood sugar testing. ▪ have weight loss of ½ pound. ▪ verbalize responsibility for weight loss. ▪ have episodes of hypo- or hyperglycemia detected early. ▪ verbalize ability to cope. ▪ verbalize understanding of home care instructions.	Client ▪ is afebrile and has stable vital signs. ▪ has normal blood sugar. ▪ is independent in self-care ▪ is fully ambulatory. ▪ verbalizes responsibility for weight loss. ▪ verbalizes plan to exercise 15–20 min 3–4 times/week. ▪ has resumed preadmission urine and bowel elimination pattern. ▪ verbalizes home care instructions including aspects of diabetic care: (1) diet control, (2) SMBG, (3) insulin care and administration, (4) foot care, (5) general health care rules, and (6) S & S of hypo- and hyperglycemia and management of those problems.

	Day 4 *continued*	Day 5 *continued*
Daily outcomes *continued*		▪ verbalizes importance of on-going nursing and medical care. ▪ tolerates ordered diet and has fluid intake of 2000 mL/day. ▪ verbalizes ability to cope with ongoing stressors.
Tests and treatments	Fasting blood sugar. Vital signs q4h if stable. Fingerstick blood sugar ac, hs, and prn. Monitor for signs and symptoms of hypo- and hyperglycemia. Follow hypoglycemia protocol if symptoms occur. D/C intake and output if stable.	Fasting blood sugar. Vital signs q4h if stable. Fingerstick blood sugar ac, hs, and prn. Monitor for signs and symptoms of hypo- and hyperglycemia. Follow hypoglycemia protocol if symptoms occur.
Knowledge deficit	Reinforce earlier teaching regarding ongoing care. Review written discharge instructions with client and significant other. Attend diabetic classes per diabetic nurse educator.	Reinforce earlier teaching regarding ongoing care. Complete discharge teaching to include diet, follow-up care, signs and symptoms to report, activity, and medications: dose, frequency, route, and side effects. Provide client with written discharge instructions specific to care and management of diabetes.
Psycho-social	Encourage verbalization of concerns. Provide ongoing support and encouragement.	Encourage verbalization of concerns. Provide ongoing support and encouragement.
Diet	Daily weight. 1200 calorie ADA diet. Encourage fluid intake of 2000 mL/day. Encourage client to utilize behavior modification strategies. Encourage client to establish regular exercise program following discharge.	Daily weight. 1200 calorie ADA diet. Encourage fluid intake of 2000 mL/day. Encourage client to utilize behavior modification strategies. Encourage client to establish regular exercise program after discharge.
Activity	Fully ambulatory.	Fully ambulatory.
Medications	Regular insulin to scale ac and hs. NPH insulin per order AM and PM.	Regular insulin to scale ac and hs. NPH insulin per order AM and PM.
Transfer/ discharge plans	Continue to review progress toward discharge goals. Finalize discharge plans.	Finalize plans for home care if needed. Complete discharge teaching.

CHAPTER HIGHLIGHTS

- Nutrition is the sum total of all interactions between an organism and the food it consumes.
- Although people are continually bombarded with information about what to eat and what not to eat, each person is responsible for selecting foods that provide essential nutrients.
- Nurses can assist people to evaluate the information they receive about nutrients.
- Essential nutrients are grouped into six categories: water, carbohydrates, fats, proteins, vitamins, and minerals.
- Nutrients serve three basic purposes: forming body structures (such as bones and blood), providing energy, and helping to regulate the body's biochemical reactions.
- Both inadequate and excessive intakes of nutrients result in malnutrition.
- The effects of malnutrition can be general or specific, depending on which nutrients and what level of deficiency or excess are involved.
- Some of the long-range effects of certain nutrient excesses are among the many factors involved in certain diseases, such as coronary artery disease and cancer.
- Nutritional needs vary considerably according to age, growth, and energy requirements.
- Adolescents have high energy requirements due to their rapid growth; a diet plentiful in milk, meats, green and yellow vegetables, and fresh fruits is required.
- Middle-aged adults and older adults often need to reduce their caloric intake because of decreases in metabolic rate and activity levels. Fats, sugary foods, and sodium must often be limited.
- To assess the nutritional status of a person, the nurse follows the ABCD approach: anthropometric measurements are taken, biochemical data are assessed, clinical signs of nutritional status are assessed, and a dietary history is obtained.
- During the assessment stage and when planning nursing interventions to help clients reach nutritional goals, nurses must consider the many factors that influence a person's dietary patterns.
- Nursing diagnoses for clients with nutritional problems are broadly stated as **Altered nutrition: less than body requirements, more than body requirements,** or **high risk for more than body requirements.**
- Obesity is a common nutritional problem of North Americans. Nurses can assist obese clients by recommending increased activity and intake of foods that have a low caloric density.
- Counseling about nutrition can be likened to the teaching-learning process, which includes assessing specific learning needs, setting goals, planning strategies to meet goals, and establishing outcome criteria to evaluate goal achievement.
- Assisting clients and support persons with therapeutic diets is a function shared by the nurse and the dietitian. The nurse reinforces the dietitian's instructions, assists the client to make beneficial changes, and evaluates the client's response to planned changes.
- Because many hospitalized clients have poor appetites, a major responsibility of the nurse is to provide nursing interventions that stimulate their appetites.
- Whenever possible, the nurse should help incapacitated clients to feed themselves; a number of self-feeding aids help clients who have difficulty handling regular utensils.
- The nurse can refer clients to various community programs that help special subgroups of the population meet their nutritional needs.
- The administration of enteral and parenteral feedings to clients unable to ingest sufficient intake to maintain nutritional balance requires skill to prevent aspiration of the feeding.

READINGS AND REFERENCES

SUGGESTED READINGS

Cerrato, PL. December 1992. Goodbye four food groups. *RN* 55: 61–62.

This article provides a brief background of the development of the Food Guide Pyramid; compares the Pyramid to the previous standard for nutrition, the Basic Four Food Groups; and explains the advantages of the new approach.

Metheney, N, Reed, L, Worseck, M, and Clark, J. May 1993. How to aspirate fluid from small-bore feeding tubes. *American Journal of Nursing* 93:86–88.

Small-bore flexible feeding tubes are difficult to aspirate; nevertheless, the nurse must frequently assess placement. This article identifies the most common obstacles to aspiration and describes nursing interventions and rationale for each.

RELATED RESEARCH

Smith, CE, Moushey, L, Ross, JA, and Gieffer, C. June 1993. Responsibilities and reactions of family caregivers of patients dependent on total parenteral nutrition at home. *Public Health Nursing* 10:122–28.

Wilson, DM. 1992. Ethical concerns in a long-term tube feeding study. *Image: Journal of Nursing Scholarship* 3:195–99.

SELECTED REFERENCES

Breslow, RA, Hallfrisch, J, Guy, DG, Crawley, B, and Goldberg, AP. 1993. The importance of dietary protein in healing pressure ulcers. *Journal of the American Geriatrics Society* 41:357–62.

Byrne, CJ, Saxton, DF, Pelikan, PK, and Nugent, PM. 1986. *Laboratory Tests: Implications for Nursing Care*. 2d ed. Menlo Park, CA: Addison-Wesley Nursing.

Canada's Food Guide to Healthy Eating. Catalog No. H39-252/1992E. Ottawa, Ontario: Health and Welfare Canada.

Carpenito, LJ. 1993. *Nursing Diagnosis: Application to Clinical Practice*. 5th ed. Philadelphia: Lippincott.

Cerrato, PL. August 1991. Nutrition support: Surgery, stress, and metabolism. *RN* 54:63–65.

———. April 1992. The patient's eating—why is he losing weight? *RN* 55:77–80.

———. July 1992. Don't overlook this mineral deficiency. *RN* 55:61–62.

Christian, JL and Greger, JL 1994. *Nutrition for Living*. 4th ed. Redwood City, CA: Benjamin/Cummings.

Cox, HC, Hinz, MD, Lubno, MA, Newfield, SA, Ridenour, NA, Slater, MM, and Sridaromont, K. 1993. *Clinical Applications of Nursing Diagnosis*. Philadelphia: FA Davis.

Dudek, SG. 1993. *Nutrition Handbook for Nursing Practice*. 2d ed. Philadelphia: Lippincott.

Gizis, FC. December 1992. Nutrition in women across the life span. *Nursing Clinics of North America*, 27:971–82.

Gordon, M. 1993. *Manual of Nursing Diagnosis 1993–1994*. 6th ed. St Louis: Mosby-Year Book.

Grant, JA and Kennedy-Caldwell, C. 1988. *Nutritional Support in Nursing*. New York: Grune and Stratton.

Guyton, AC. 1991. *Textbook of Medical Physiology*. 8th ed. Philadelphia: WB Saunders.

Hand, R, Kempster, M, Levy, J, Rogol, R, and Spirn, P. 1984. Inadvertent transbronchial insertion of narrow-bore feeding tubes. *Journal of the American Medical Association* 251:2396–87.

Herron, DG. December 1991. Strategies for promoting a healthy dietary intake. *Nursing Clinics of North America* 26:875–84.

Jarvis, C. 1992. *Physical Examination and Health Assessment*. Philadelphia: WB Saunders.

Kim, MJ, McFarland, GK, and McLane, AM. 1993. *Pocket Guide to Nursing Diagnoses*. 5th ed. St Louis: Mosby.

McCloskey, JC and Bulechek, GM, editors. 1992. *Nursing Interventions Classification (NIC)*. St Louis: Mosby.

McFarland, GK and McFarlane, EA. 1993. *Nursing Diagnosis and Intervention: Planning for Patient Care*. 2d ed. St. Louis: Mosby.

Metheny, N. November/December 1988. Measures to test placement of nasogastric and nasointestinal feeding tubes: A review. *Nursing Research* 37:324–29.

Metheny, NA, Spies, MA, and Eisenberg, P. August 1988. Measures to test placement of nasoenteral feeding tubes. *Western Journal of Nursing Research* 10:367–83.

Miller, K, Tomlinson, J, and Sahn, S. August 1985. Pleuropulmonary complications of enteral tube feeding. *Chest* 88:230–33.

Nagy, M. November 1991. Nutritional status of institutionalized older Americans. *Journal of Gerontological Nursing* 17:44–47.

National Center for Health Statistics. October 1987. *Health and Nutrition Examination Survey of 1976 to 1980*. Vital and Health Statistics Series of Reports, Series 11, No. 238. DHHS Publication No. (PHS) 87-1688. Hyattsville, MD.

National Research Council, Committee on Dietary Allowances: Food and Nutrition Board. 1989. *Recommended Dietary Allowances*. 10th ed. Washington, DC: National Academy of Sciences.

North American Nursing Diagnosis Association. 1992. *NANDA Nursing Diagnoses: Definitions and Classification 1992–1993*. Philadelphia: NANDA.

Oberc, MC. 1991. Inserting and maintaining a gastric or jejunal tube. In Smith, DA, editor. pp.418–28. *Comprehensive Child and Family Nursing Skills*. St Louis: Mosby.

Osak, MP. Spring 1993. Nutrition and would helaing. *Plastic Surgery Nursing 13:29–36.*

Osato, EE, Stone, JT, Phillips, SL, and Winne, DM. August 1993. Clinical manifestations: Failure to thrive in the elderly. *Journal of Gerontological Nursing* 19:28–34.

Rhodes, VA. December 1990. Nausea, vomiting, and retching. *Nursing Clinics of North America* 25:885–900.

Sparks, SM and Taylor, CM. 1991. *Nursing Diagnosis Reference Manual*. Springhouse, PA: Springhouse.

Speer, KM and Swann, CL. 1993. *The Addison-Wesley Manual of Pediatric Nursing Procedures*. Redwood City, CA: Addison-Wesley Nursing.

Theodore, A, Frank, J, Ende, J, Snider, G, and Beer, D. 1984. Errant placement of nasogastric feeding tubes: A hazard in obtunded patients. *Chest* 86:931–33.

US Department of Agriculture and US Department of Health and Human Services. 1980, 1985, 1990. *Nutrition and Your Health: Dietary Guidelines for Americans*. Home and Garden Bulletin No. 232. Washington, DC: US Government Printing Office.

US Department of Health and Human Services, Public Health Service. *Healthy People 2000: National Health Promotion and Disease Prevention Objectives*. Washington, DC: US Government Printing Office.

Using the Food Guide. Catalog No. H39-253/1992E. Ottawa, Ontario: Health and Welfare Canada.

Vhymeister, IA, Register, UD, and Sonnenberg, LM. February 1977. Safe vegetarian diets for children. *Pediatric Clinics of North America* 24:207.

Williams, SR and Worthington-Roberts, BS, editors. 1992. *Nutrition Throughout the Life Cycle*. St Louis: Mosby.

Wong, DL. 1993. *Whaley and Wong's Essentials of Pediatric Nursing*. 4th ed. St Louis: Mosby.

38

Fluid, Electrolyte, and Acid-Base Balance

Objectives

Describe factors affecting the proportion of the body weight that is fluid.

Identify the major electrolytes of the intracellular and extracellular fluid compartments and body secretions.

Describe how fluids and electrolytes move through the body.

Explain how the osmotic and hydrostatic pressures influence movement of fluid through membranes.

List factors that influence fluid and electrolyte balance.

Describe how body mechanisms regulate fluid and electrolyte balance.

Identify information to obtain in a health history to assess fluid and electrolyte balance.

Describe the significance of diagnostic tests used to monitor fluid, electrolyte, and acid-base balance.

Identify the causes of selected fluid, electrolyte, and acid-base imbalances.

Recognize clinical signs and laboratory findings of selected fluid and electrolyte imbalances.

Describe the role of the lungs and kidneys in regulating acid-base balance.

Describe four primary acid-base disturbances.

List examples of nursing diagnoses related to fluid, electrolyte, and acid-base balance.

State outcome criteria for evaluating the client's responses to strategies implemented to promote fluid and electrolyte balance.

Assist clients to modify their fluid intake.

Monitor and regulate intravenous infusions.

Describe how to change intravenous containers and tubing.

Give guidelines for discontinuing an intravenous infusion.

Identify potential problems and risks of blood transfusions.

Explain basic purposes of and sites used for total parenteral nutrition.

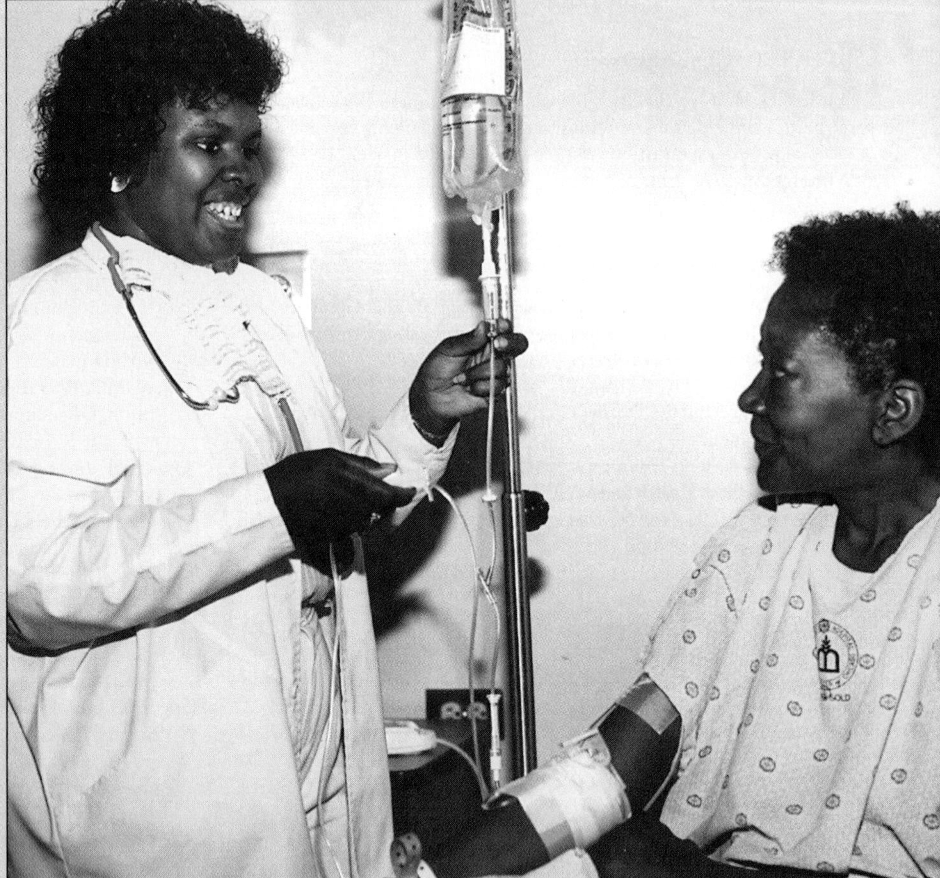

Fluids and electrolytes are necessary to maintain good health, and their relative amounts in the body must be maintained within a narrow range. The balance of fluids and electrolytes in the body is a part of physiologic homeostastis (see Chapter 14).

This delicate balance is maintained in health by the body's physiologic processes. Almost every illness, however, threatens the balance. Even in normal daily living, excessive temperatures or excessive activity can disturb the balance if adequate water and salt intake is not maintained. Some therapeutic measures for clients, such as the use of diuretics, can also disturb the body's homeostasis unless water and electrolytes are replaced.

The body's fluid is divided into two major reservoirs, intracellular and extracellular. The **intracellular fluid (ICF),** also referred to as the **cellular fluid,** is found within the cells of the body. It constitutes two-thirds to three-quarters of the total body fluid. In adults, the **extracellular fluid (ECF)** is found outside the cells; it is subdivided into three compartments, **intravascular fluid** (plasma), **interstitial fluid,** and **transcellular fluid. Plasma** is fluid found within the vascular system; interstitial fluid is fluid that surrounds the cells, and it includes lymph. Transcellular fluid is secreted primarily by the epithelial cells. Its ionic composition is different from that of plasma and interstitial fluid. Cerebrospinal, pleural, peritoneal, and synovial fluids, are examples of transcellular fluids. According to Metheny (1992, p. 3), transcellular fluid is an extracellular fluid; others, however, consider it distinct from intracellular and extracellular fluids (Figure 38–1).

Extracellular fluid is in constant motion throughout the body. Although it is the smaller of the two compartments, it is the transport system that carries nutrients to and waste products from the cells. For example, plasma carries oxygen in the hemoglobin of red blood cells from the lungs and glucose from the gastrointestinal tract to the capillaries of the vascular system. From there, the oxygen and glucose move across the capillary membranes into the interstitial spaces and then across the cellular membranes into the cells. The opposite route is taken for waste products, such as carbon dioxide going from the cells to the lungs and metabolic acid wastes going eventually to the kidneys. Interstitial fluid transports wastes from the cells by way of the lymph system as well as directly into the blood plasma through capillaries. Lymph circulation ultimately enters the vascular circulation through the thoracic duct into the venous system.

Interstitial fluid comprises three-quarters of extracellular fluid. Normal body functioning requires that the volume of each fluid compartment remain relatively constant. Regulating mechanisms are discussed later in this chapter.

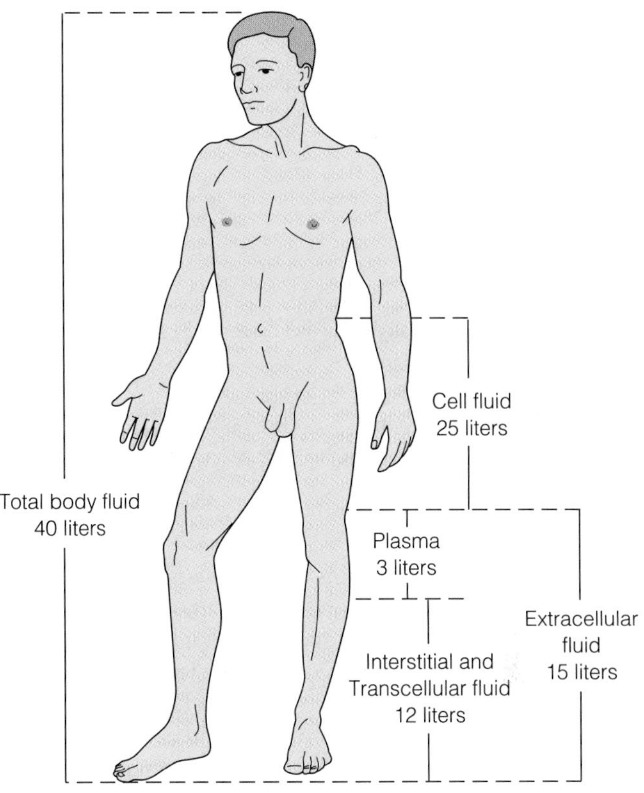

Figure 38–1 Total body fluid represents 40 liters in an adult male weighing 70 kilograms (154 lb).

Secretions and excretions are also part of the body's total fluid volume and serve essential functions. They are part of the extracellular fluid. A **secretion** is the product of a gland; for example, the salivary glands secrete saliva, the gastric glands secrete gastric juices, and the choroid plexuses of the ventricles in the brain secrete cerebrospinal fluid. An **excretion** is waste produced by the cells of the body. Just as balances exist between cellular and extracellular compartments, special balances exist between plasma and secretions and excretions. Most of the fluid and electrolytes that are secreted into the gastrointestinal tract are reabsorbed from the large intestine back into the blood stream.

Proportions of Body Fluid

The proportion of the human body composed of fluid is surprisingly large, considering that the external appearance suggests mostly solid tissue such as muscle and bone. Fluid constitutes about 47% to 55% of the average healthy adult's weight. In health, this volume (about 40

Table 38–1 Fluid as Percentage of Body Weight (by Age)

Age	Percentage of Fluid*
Full-term newborn	70 to 80
1 year	64
Puberty to 39 years	52 to 60
40 to 60 years	47 to 55
Over 60 years	46 to 52

* Generally, men have a slightly higher percentage of fluid than women.

Source: Adapted from NM Metheny, *Fluid and Electrolyte Balance: Nursing Considerations*, (Philadelphia: Lippincott, 1992), p. 5.

Table 38–2 Secretions of the Adult Alimentary Tract

Secretion	Volume (mL/day)
Saliva	1000
Gastric secretion	1500
Pancreatic secretion	1000
Bile	1000
Small-intestine secretion	1800
Brunner's gland secretion	200
Large-intestine secretion	200
Total	6700

Source: Adapted from AC Guyton, *Textbook of Medical Physiology*, 8th ed. (Philadelphia: WB Saunders, 1991), p. 711. Reprinted with permission.

liters) of body fluid remains relatively constant. In fact, a healthy person's weight varies less than 0.2 kg (0.5 lb) in 24 hours, regardless of the amount of fluid ingested. Some diseases cause serious excesses or deficiencies of body fluid. For example, a client with heart failure can retain fluid in the tissues and may suffer a fluid excess. A person with kidney disease may not be able to excrete the required amount of urine and also suffer a fluid excess. Another person with a mouth injury may not be able to drink and may suffer a fluid loss.

The percentage of total body fluid varies according to the individual's age, body fat, and sex. See Table 38–1. Infants have the highest proportion of fluid; fluid constitutes 70% to 80% of their body weight (Metheny 1992, p. 3). As people grow older, the proportion decreases. Body fat is essentially free of fluid; the less body fat present, the greater the proportion of body fluid. For example, a thin man's body may be 70% fluid, whereas an obese man's may be only 53%. This variable, body fat, also accounts for the difference in total body fluid between the sexes. After adolescence, women have proportionately more fat than men. Thus, they have a smaller percentage of fluid in relation to total body weight than do men.

Large volumes of fluid also carry dissolved waste materials through the kidneys and through the gastrointestinal tract. However, in both instances, most of this fluid is reabsorbed into the vascular spaces and reused by the body. For example, of 6700 mL produced in the alimentary tract, only 100mL is usually excreted in the feces, just enough to keep the feces lubricated. Of 180 liters of glomerular filtrate that filters through the kidneys per day, only 1.4 liters are excreted from the body under normal conditions.

Nurses need to be aware of abnormal amounts of secretions and excretions. Excessive losses can seriously deplete first the extracellular fluid volume and then the intracellular fluid volume. See Table 38–2 for alimentary tract secretions.

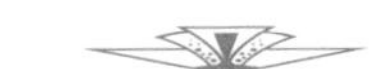

BODY ELECTROLYTES

Extracellular and intracellular fluids are similar in their content of electrolytes and other substances. These fluids contain oxygen from the lungs; dissolved nutrients, from the gastrointestinal tract; excretory products of metabolism, of which carbon dioxide is the most abundant; and particles called **ions.**

Many salts dissociate in water, that is, break up into electrically charged ions. The salt sodium chloride breaks up into one ion of sodium (Na^+) and one ion of chloride (Cl^-). These charged particles are called **electrolytes** because they are capable of conducting electricity. Ions that carry a positive charge are called **cations,** and ions carrying a negative charge are called **anions.** Examples of cations are sodium (Na^+), potassium (K^+), calcium (Ca^{2+}), and magnesium (Mg^{2+}). Anions include chloride (Cl^-), bicarbonate (HCO_3^-), monohydrogen phosphate (HPO_4^{2-}), and sulfate (SO_4^{2-}).

COMPOSITION OF BODY FLUIDS

The composition of fluids varies from one body compartment to another. Principal ions of extracellular fluid are sodium and chloride; principal ions of intracellular fluid are potassium and phosphate. The ion composition of the two extracellular fluid reservoirs (intravascular and interstitial) is similar; the main difference is that intravascular

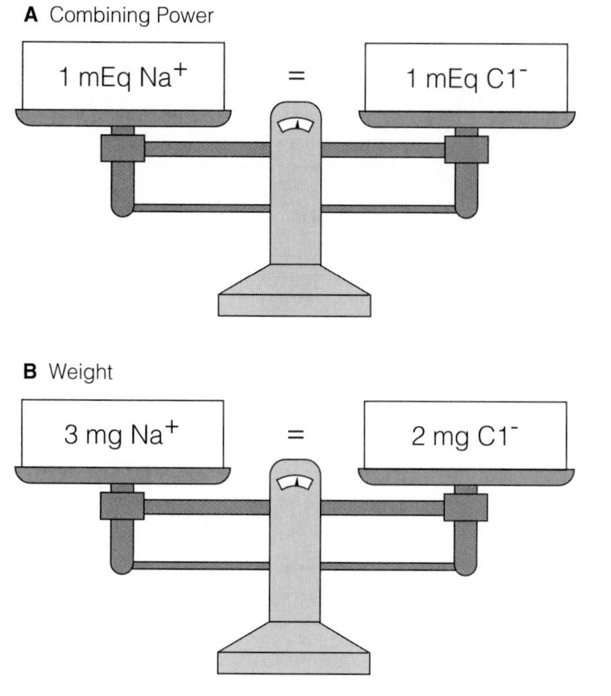

Figure 38–2 Relating sodium (Na^+) and chloride (Cl^-) *A*, by combining power; *B*, by weight.

fluid (plasma) has a greater quantity of protein (eg, red blood cells) than interstitial fluid does. This is because large particles of protein have difficulty passing through the vascular (capillary) membranes into the interstitial fluid. All other electrolytes move readily between these two extracellular compartments.

Just as fluid volumes must be maintained within compartments, so must the electrolyte composition of the various compartments. Balances of electrolytes are maintained in proportion to the quantities of fluid in the compartments. Although the specific numbers of cations and anions may differ in the fluid compartments, in a state of homeostasis the total number of cations equals the number of anions within each compartment.

Body secretions and excretions also contain electrolytes. This is of particular concern when excretions are abnormally increased or decreased or when a secretion is lost from the body (for example, in severe vomiting or diarrhea, or when gastric suction removes the gastric secretions). Fluid and electrolyte imbalance can result from prolonged loss through these routes.

Measurement of Electrolytes Electrolytes are measured in milliequivalents per liter of water (mEq/L) or milligrams per 100 milliliters (mg/100 mL). The term **milliequivalent** means one thousandth of an equivalent; equivalent refers to the *chemical combining power* of a substance, or the capacity of cations to unite with anions to form molecules. This chemical combining activity is measured in relation to the chemical combining activity of the hydrogen ion (H^+). One mEq equals the chemical combining capacity of 1 mg of hydrogen. Thus, 1 mEq of any anion equals 1mEq of any cation. For example, sodium and chloride ions are equivalent, since they combine equally: 1mEq of Na^+ equals 1mEq of Cl^-. However, these cations and anions are not equal in weight: 1 mg of Na^+ does not equal 1 mg of Cl^-; rather, 3 mg of Na^+ equals 2 mg of Cl^- (Figure 38–2).

Clinically, the milliequivalent system is commonly used. However, nurses need to be aware of the different systems of measurement when interpreting laboratory results. It is also important to realize that a laboratory examination usually indicates the findings of blood plasma, since intracellular fluid is not easily accessible for examination. Examination of extracellular fluid (plasma) can frequently reflect the state of the intracellular fluid, though not always precisely.

MOVEMENT OF BODY FLUIDS AND ELECTROLYTES

Movement of fluid and substances such as ions occurs in three phases. During the first phase, blood plasma moves around the body within the circulatory system, and nutrients and fluids are picked up from the lungs and the gastrointestinal tract. In the second phase, interstitial fluid and its components move between the blood capillaries and the cells. Finally, during the third phase, fluid and substances move from the interstitial fluid into the cells. In the reverse direction, fluid and its components move back from the cells to the interstitial spaces and then to the intravascular compartment. The intravascular fluid then flows to the kidneys, where the metabolic by-products of the cells are excreted.

Capillary and cellular membranes in the body are described as **selectively permeable** because not all substances move with the same ease across the membranes. Compounds such as proteins and glycogen do not readily cross capillary and cellular membranes. Organic compounds such as glucose and amino acids move freely across capillary walls, although they often require active transport.

The methods by which body fluids and electrolytes move are diffusion, filtration, osmosis, and active transport.

Diffusion Diffusion is the continual intermingling of molecules in liquids, gases, or solids brought about by the random movement of the molecules. For example, two

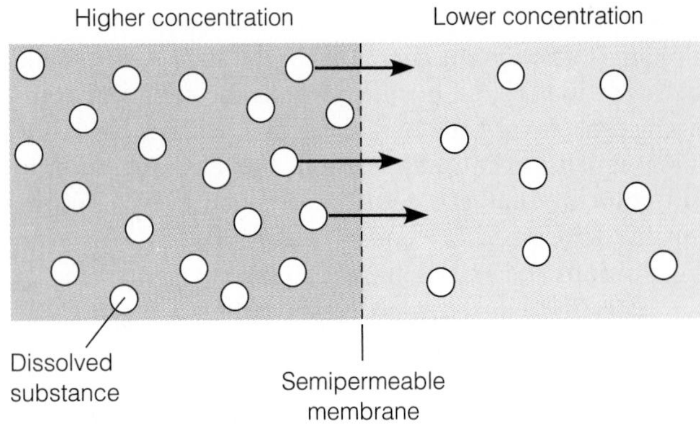

Figure 38–3 Diffusion: The movement of molecules through a semipermeable membrane from an area of higher concentration to an area of lower concentration.

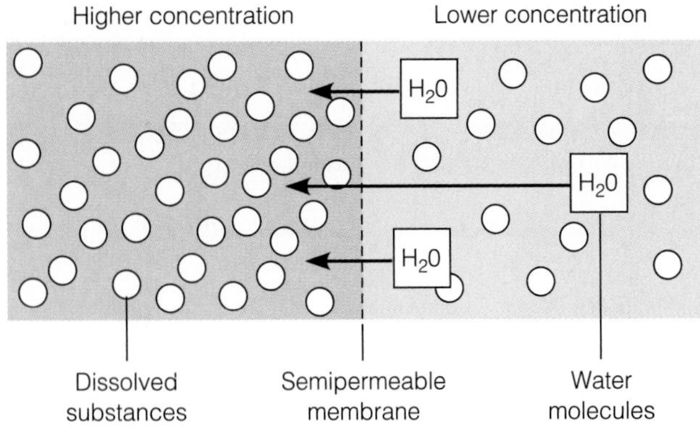

Figure 38–5 Osmosis: Water molecules move from the less concentrated area to the more concentrated area in an attempt to equalize the concentration of solutions on two sides of a membrane.

gases become mixed by the incessant motion of their molecules. The process of diffusion occurs even when two substances are separated by a thin membrane. In the body, diffusion of *water, electrolytes*, and *other substances* occurs through the "slit pores" of capillary membranes.

The rate of diffusion of substances varies according to (a) size of the molecules, (b) concentration of the solution, and (c) temperature of the solution. Larger molecules move less quickly than smaller ones, because they require more energy to move about. With diffusion, the molecules move from a solution of higher concentration to a solution of lower concentration (Figure 38–3). Increases in temperature increase the rate of motion of molecules and therefore the rate of diffusion.

Filtration Filtration is a process whereby fluid and solutes move together across a membrane from one compartment to another. The movement is from an area of higher pressure to one of lower pressure. An example of filtration is the movement of fluid and nutrients from the capillaries of the arteries to the interstitial fluid around the cells. The pressure in the compartment which results in the movement of the fluid and substances dissolved in fluid out of the compartment is called *filtration pressure*. **Hydrostatic pressure** is the pressure exerted by a fluid within a closed system on the walls of a container in which it is contained. The hydrostatic pressure of blood is the force exerted by blood against the vascular walls (eg, the artery walls). The principle involved in hydrostatic pressure is that fluids move from the area of greater pressure to the area of lesser pressure. Using the example of the blood vessels, the plasma proteins in the blood exert a colloid osmotic pressure (see the following section) that opposes the hydrostatic pressure and holds the fluid. When the hydrostatic pressure is greater than the osmotic pressure, the fluid filters out of the blood vessels. The *filtration pressure* in this example is the difference between the hydrostatic pressure and the osmotic pressure (Figure 38–4).

Osmosis Osmosis is the movement of pure solvent (eg, water) across cell membranes, from the less concentrated solution to the more concentrated solution (Figure 38–5). In other words, water moves toward the higher concentration of solute.

Solutes are substances dissolved in a liquid. For example, when sugar is added to coffee, the sugar is the sol-

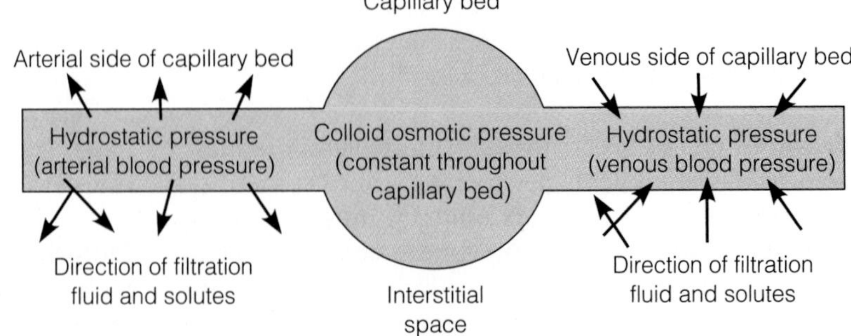

Figure 38–4 Schematic of filtration pressure changes within a capillary bed. On the arterial side, arterial blood pressure exceeds colloid osmotic pressure, so that water and dissolved substances move out of the capillary into the interstitial space. On the venous side, venous blood pressure is less than colloid osmotic pressure, so that water and dissolved substances move into the capillary.

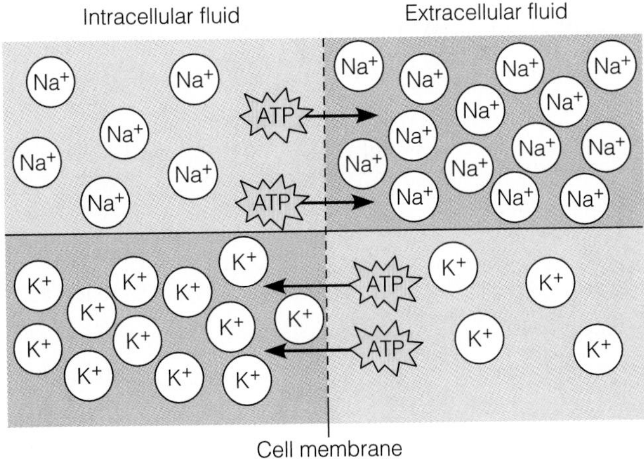

Figure 38–6 An example of active transport. Energy (ATP) is used to move sodium molecules and potassium molecules across a semipermeable membrane against sodium's and potassium's concentration gradients (ie, from areas of lesser concentration to areas of greater concentration).

ute. Solutes may be **crystalloids** (salts that dissolve readily into true solutions) or **colloids** (substances such as large protein molecules that do not readily dissolve into true solutions). A **solvent** is the component of a solution that can dissolve a solute. In the previous example, coffee is the solvent for the sugar. In a salt solution, water is the solvent, and sodium chloride (NaCl) is the solute. Osmosis is important in maintaining proper balance in the volumes of extracellular and intracellular fluid.

The number of particles in a unit of water determines the concentration of the solution. It can be expressed as *osmolality* or *osmolarity*. *Osmolality* refers to the number of *osmols* per kilogram of solution, that is, the weight of the solution. An *osmol* is the standard unit of osmotic pressure. Osmolarity uses volume (liters); it refers to the number of osmols per liter of solution. It is expressed as mOsm/L (milliosmols of solute per liter of fluid).

Osmotic pressure is the drawing power of a solvent such as water. It is exerted through a semipermeable membrane and depends on the number of molecules in the solution. A solution with a large number of molecules has a high osmotic pressure; one with few molecules has a low osmotic pressure. The solvent can pass freely through the semipermeable membrane, but the large molecules cannot. This pressure occurs when the solvent flows from an area of lesser solute concentration to an area of greater solute concentration.

Active Transport Substances can move across cell membranes from a less concentrated solution to a more concentrated one by active transport (Figure 38–6). This process differs from diffusion and osmosis in that metabolic energy is expended. In active transport, the substance combines with a carrier on the outside surface of the cell membrane, and they move to the inside surface of the cell membrane. Once inside, they separate, and the substance is released to the inside of the cell. A specific carrier is required for each substance, and enzymes are required for active transport.

This process is of particular importance in maintaining the differences in sodium and potassium ion concentrations of extracellular and intracellular fluid. Under normal conditions, sodium concentrations are higher in the extracellular fluid, while potassium concentrations are higher inside the cells. To maintain these proportions, the active transport mechanism (the **sodium-potassium pump**) is activated, moving sodium from the cells and potassium into the cells.

REGULATING BODY FLUID VOLUMES

In a healthy person, the fluid volumes and chemical composition of the fluid compartments stay within narrow safe limits. Normally, a person's fluid intake is counterbalanced by fluid loss. Illness can upset this balance so that the body has too little or too much fluid.

Obligatory loss is the essential fluid loss required to maintain body functioning. Water lost as vapor in expired air, and as vapor from the skin, a minimum volume of about 500 mL from the kidneys, and the fluid required to excrete the solid metabolic wastes produced daily are the obligatory losses, totaling about 1300 mL per day.

Since the vaporized losses are not readily measured, the measured obligatory kidney loss become of prime importance in critical illness. An adult hourly urine volume of less than 30 mL or daily volume under 500 mL is serious. Clients with inadequate output require immediate attention, and such a finding by the nurse must therefore be reported promptly. Although losses from the skin, lungs, and intestines in health account for approximately half of the daily loss, they can account for a much larger percentage of loss from a client who has a fever or accelerated respiration. Increases in respiratory rate, fever, **diaphoresis** (sweating), and diarrhea can magnify fluid loss from the normal routes immensely. Other routes of loss, such as from the stomach through emesis or suction or from abnormal body openings such as fistulas or surgically implanted drainage tubes, often account for significant losses, all of which require intake replacements.

FLUID INTAKE

During periods of moderate activity at moderate temperature, the average adult drinks about 1500 mL per day but

RESEARCH NOTE

Do You Know How Much Fluid Your Elderly Client Consumes?

The purpose of this study was to describe and analyze the fluid intake of 57 male and female institutionalized elders. Clients were derived from psychogeriatric, long-term care, and geriatric admission units. The sample consisted of individuals with a wide range of cognitive and physical activities. Fluids consumed by each client were directly observed and recorded by a research associate for a period of 72 hours.

All of the 57 clients received considerably less than the recommended 2000–2500 mL per day; however, clients who were cognitively impaired, dependent upon staff for assistance with activities of daily living, or incontinent received the least amount of fluid. Clients without these impediments consumed higher volumes of fluid but still did not consume the recommended amount.

As part of the research and analysis, 47 nurses working on the same three units completed a self-administered questionnaire on the fluid needs of the elderly. The questionnaire revealed that nurses on each of the units had knowledge deficits related to signs and complications of dehydration and the fluid requirements of the elderly.

Implications: Although the authors conclude that small sample size prohibits general conclusions, the results suggest that nurses must be more fastidious in providing fluids to dependent clients.

Source: CA Armstrong-Esther, KD Browne, DC Armstrong-Esther, and L Sander, The institutionalized elderly: Dry to the bone!, *International Journal of Nursing Studies*, December 1996, 33(6):619–28.

needs 2500 mL per day, an additional 1000 mL. This added volume is acquired from foods (referred to as preformed water) and from the oxidation of these foods during metabolic processes. Interestingly, the water content of food is relatively large, contributing about 750 mL per day. The water content of fresh vegetables is approximately 90%, of fresh fruits about 85%, and of lean meats around 60%.

Oxidative water, which is formed as a by-product of the body's oxidation of food, accounts for most of the remaining fluid volume required. This quantity ranges from 150 to 250 mL per day for the average adult (Guyton 1991, p. 274).

Table 38–3 Average Daily Fluid Requirements by Age and Weight

Age	Approximate Body Weight (kg)	mL/24 Hours
3 days	3.0	250 to 300
1 year	9.5	1150 to 1300
2 years	11.8	1350 to 1500
6 years	20.0	1800 to 2000
10 years	28.7	2000 to 2500
14 years	45.0	2200 to 2700
18 years (adult)	54.0	2200 to 2700

Source: RE Behrman, *Nelson Textbook of Pediatrics*, (Philadelphia: WB Saunders, 1992), p. 107. Reproduced with permission.

The primary regulator of fluid intake is the body's thirst mechanism. The thirst center is located in the brain. A number of stimuli trigger this center: intracellular dehydration, excess angiotensin II (a hormone released into the blood in response to very low blood pressure) in the body fluids, and hemorrhage, resulting in lowered blood volume. Angiotensin II is a potent vasoconstrictor.

Dryness of the mouth is often associated with thirst but can occur independently (for example, when a person's salivary glands do not secrete saliva). Thirst is normally relieved immediately after drinking a small amount of fluid, even before it is absorbed from the gastrointestinal tract. However, this relief is only temporary, and the thirst returns in about 15 minutes. The thirst is again temporarily relieved after the ingested fluid distends the upper gastrointestinal tract. These mechanisms protect the individual from drinking too much, because it takes from 30 minutes to 1 hour for the fluid to be absorbed and distributed throughout the body. If a person continued to drink during that time, the fluid ingested would overdilute the body fluids. See Table 38–3 for average fluid requirements.

FLUID OUTPUT

Fluid losses from the body counterbalance the adult's 2500-mL average daily intake of fluid. See Table 38–4. There are four routes of fluid output:

1. Urine
2. Insensible loss through the skin as perspiration and through the lungs as water vapor in the expired air
3. Noticeable loss through the skin as sweat
4. Loss through the intestines in feces

Table 38–4 Average Daily Fluid Output for an Adult

Route	Amount (mL)
Urine	1400 to 1500
Insensible losses	
Lungs	350 to 400
Skin	350 to 400
Sweat	100
Feces	100 to 200
Total	2300 to 2600

Urine The formation of urine by the kidneys and its excretion from the urinary bladder is the major avenue of fluid output. Normal urine output is 1400 to 1500 mL per 24 hours, or at least 30 to 50 mL per hour, for an adult. In healthy people, urine output may vary noticeably from day to day. For example, sweat gland activity often increases when the environmental temperature increases. Urine volume automatically increases as fluid intake increases. If fluid loss from the skin is large, however, the urine volume may decrease to maintain fluid balance in the body. For further information about urine formation, see Chapter 41, page 1223, and Chapter 14 for information about homeostatic mechanisms.

Insensible Losses Insensible fluid loss occurs through the skin and lungs. It is called *insensible* because it is usually not noticeable. The insensible loss through the skin is by diffusion. It is normally controlled by the outer layer of the epidermis, the stratum corneum. However, when the skin layers are destroyed by burns and abrasions, fluid loss can increase considerably.

Another type of insensible loss is the water in exhaled air. In an adult, this is normally 300 to 400 mL per day. When respiratory rate accelerates, for example, due to exercise or an elevated body temperature, this loss can increase.

Sweat Sweating occurs when the body becomes overheated. The sweat glands secrete large quantities of sweat onto the surface of the body to provide cooling by evaporation. Sweating occurs in response to stimulation of the preoptic area in the anterior hypothalamus. Impulses are transmitted to the spinal cord and via the sympathetic nervous system to the skin.

Large amounts of sweat contain large amounts of sodium chloride, whereas small amounts of sweat contain lower concentrations of sodium chloride. Sweat also contains urea, lactic acid, and potassium ions.

Feces The chyme that passes from the small intestine into the large intestine contains water and electrolytes. The volume of chyme that passes through the ileocecal valve into the cecum in an adult is normally about 1500 mL per day (Guyton 1991, p. 705). Of this amount, all but about 100 mL is reabsorbed in the proximal half of the large intestine. Sodium and chloride ions are also actively reabsorbed, and bicarbonate ions are secreted by the mucosa of the large intestine. The bicarbonate helps to neutralize the acidic end products of bacterial action in the colon. For further information about the composition of feces, see Chapter 40, page 1183.

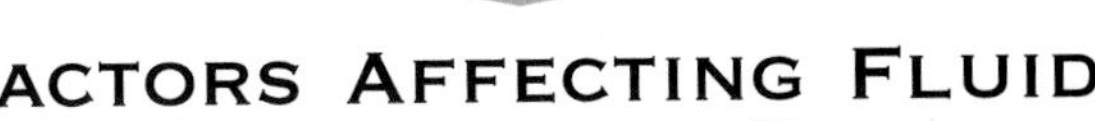

FACTORS AFFECTING FLUID AND ELECTROLYTE BALANCE

Age Fluid intake requirements vary with age. Intake requirements have been determined for various ages in relation to body surface area, metabolic requirements, and body weight.

Infants and growing children have much greater fluid turnover than adults, that is, greater water needs and greater water losses. This is due to their greater metabolic rate, which increases fluid loss through the kidneys. Because immature kidneys are less efficient than adult kidneys, infants lose more fluid through the kidneys. Infant losses from both the lungs and the skin are also greater in proportion to body weight, essentially because respirations are more rapid and the body surface area is proportionately greater. The more rapid turnover of fluid plus the losses produced by disease can create critical fluid imbalances in children much more rapidly than in adults. See Table 38–3, earlier, for approximate fluid requirements at different ages according to body weight.

In elderly people, fluid and electrolyte imbalances are often associated with kidney or cardiac problems. Because the kidneys are less able to concentrate urine, elderly persons may need to take in additional fluid to meet their fluid needs.

Climate People in an environment of high heat and low humidity have an increased loss of body fluid and electrolytes through sweating. A person who exercises in a hot environment can lose as much as 5 L of fluid in one day as well as excessive amounts of salt. A nonacclimatized person in a hot environment can lose 700 mL of sweat per hour; an acclimatized person can lose 2 L per hour (Guyton 1991, p. 801).

Diet A person's diet obviously affects the intake of fluids and electrolytes. When nutritional intake is inadequate or unbalanced, the body tries to preserve stored protein by breaking down glycogen and fat. Once these resources are gone, the body draws on protein stores, and the serum albumin level decreases. Serum albumin plays an important role in drawing fluid from the interstitial body compartment into the blood through osmosis. When fluid is not drawn normally into the bloodstream, it remains in the interstitial space, causing edema.

Stress Stress affects a person's fluid and electrolyte balance. Stress can increase cellular metabolism, blood glucose concentration, and muscle glycolysis. These mechanisms can lead to sodium and water retention. In addition, stress can increase production of the antidiuretic hormone, which in turn decreases urine production. The overall response to the body to stress is to increase the blood volume. See Chapter 32, page 833, for additional information.

Illness Tissue trauma can cause the loss of fluid and electrolytes from within the damaged cells. An example of such trauma is severe burns. The burned person loses plasma and interstitial fluid as exudate. (An **exudate** is material that has escaped from the blood vessels and is deposited in the tissues or on the tissue surfaces.) Also, water vapor is lost from the burn site, blood leaks from damaged capillaries, and water and sodium move into the tissue cells.

Cardiac and renal disorders also affect the body's fluid and electrolyte balance. For example, impaired heart function can decrease blood flow to the kidneys and thus hinder the elimination of the waste products of metabolism. When urine output decreases, the body retains sodium, and circulatory overload (hypervolemia) can result. Fluid retention can also lead to pulmonary edema (fluid in the lungs).

The client's level of consciousness (LOC) affects the ability to take in fluids and respond independently to the sensation of thirst. Any client with an altered level of consciousness should be considered at risk for inadequate fluid intake. Clients may also be confused and unable to communicate needs or to respond appropriately to caregivers asking about fluid intake or thirst. In addition, some clients may have difficulty swallowing thus impairing their fluid intake.

Medical treatments Many medical treatments have a secondary effect on the body's fluid and electrolytes. Gastric and intestinal suctioning can result in depletions similar to those resulting from persistent vomiting. Frequently, intravenous solutions are given to counteract the losses by suction.

Medications The excessive use of medications such as diuretics and laxatives can cause the excessive loss of fluid from the body, thereby producing a fluid deficit. Some diuretics can cause an excessive loss of potassium from the body, whereas others can result in elevated serum potassium levels in the blood. Another group of medications that can alter the body's fluid and electrolyte balance is the corticosteroids. Their ingestion can result in the retention of excessive sodium and water.

Surgery Clients having surgery are at risk of fluid imbalances. Some clients experience considerable blood loss during surgery, which can affect fluid and electrolyte balance. Other clients experience fluid overload due to large volumes of intravenous fluids administered during surgery or to secretion of the antidiuretic hormone (ADH) in response to stress or anesthetic agents.

DISTURBANCES IN FLUID AND ELECTROLYTE BALANCE

Fluid balance disturbances occur when the body's compensating mechanisms are unable to maintain physiologic homeostasis. Usually the person is unaware of the adjustments the body makes to maintain these balances; however, when these adjustments fail, the person may experience unpleasant sensations, the severity of which depends on the severity of the imbalance.

FLUID IMBALANCES

Fluid imbalances are of two basic types: isotonic and osmolar. Isotonic imbalances occur when water and electrolytes are lost or gained in equal proportions. Osmolar imbalances involve the loss or gain of *only* water, so that the concentration, or osmolality, of the serum is altered. Thus four categories of fluid imbalances may occur: (a) an isotonic loss of water and electrolytes (b) an osmolar loss of only water (c) an isotonic gain of water and electrolytes and (d) osmolar gain of only water. These are referred to respectively as fluid volume deficit, dehydration (hyperosmolar imbalance), fluid volume excess, and overhydration (hypo-osmolar imbalance).

Fluid Volume Deficit Fluid volume deficit (FVD) occurs when the body loses both water and electrolytes from the ECF in similar proportions (isotonic deficit), for example, a 25% water loss and a 25% electrolyte loss. This state is commonly referred to as **hypovolemia.** In FVD, fluid is initially lost from the intravascular compartment. Then fluid is drawn from the interstitial compartment into the intravascular compartment, depleting the interstitial compartment. To compensate for the decreased interstitial volume, the body then draws intracellular fluid out of the cells.

Table 38–5 Fluid Volume Deficit (FVD)*

Risk Factors	Clinical Signs	Nursing Interventions
1. Excessive losses from ▪ Vomiting ▪ Diarrhea ▪ Suction (eg, gastric) ▪ Drainage of secretions (eg, from fistula) ▪ Extreme sweating 2. Insufficient fluid intake due to ▪ Anorexia ▪ Nausea, vomiting ▪ Inability to swallow ▪ Unavailability of fluids ▪ Confusion, depression 3. Laboratory values ▪ Increased hematocrit ▪ Increased hemoglobin ▪ Increased blood urea nitrogen (BUN) ▪ Decreased central venous pressure (CVP)	Weight loss (possible weight gain with third-spacing) ▪ 2% loss—mild ▪ 5% loss—moderate ▪ 8% loss—severe Decreased tissue turgor Weak and rapid pulse Decreased blood pressure Postural hypotension (drop in blood pressure when moving from lying to standing position) Decreased blood volume Clear breath sounds Fluid intake less than fluid output Decreased urine volume (often less than 30mL/h); may increase with regulatory mechanism failure Increased urine specific gravity (more than 1.030); may decrease with regulatory mechanism failure Dry mucous membranes, sunken eyeballs, decreased tearing and salivation Flat neck veins Slow filling of hand veins (eg, 5 seconds) when hand dependent Reports of weakness and thirst	Assess changes in clinical signs of FVD. Administer oral fluids as indicated. Provide prn medications for nausea as required. Monitor vital signs and weight. Assess tissue turgor. Assess breath sounds. Monitor fluid intake and output. Implement measures to prevent skin breakdown (see Chapter 30, p. 791). Monitor laboratory findings.

* See also the Care Planning Guide for Fluid Volume Deficit on page 1086.

FVD generally occurs as a result of (a) abnormal losses through the skin, gastrointestinal tract, or kidney; (b) decreased intake of fluid; (c) bleeding; or (d) movement of fluid into a **third space.** Third-spacing refers to "a shift of fluid from the intra-vascular space into a portion of the body from which it is not easily exchanged with the rest of the ECF" (Metheney 1992, p. 46). Fluids can shift from the intravascular space into potential body spaces, such as the pleural, peritoneal, pericardial, or joint cavities. It may also become trapped in the bowel by obstruction; in the interstitial space as edema after burns or other trauma; or in inflamed tissue, as in peritonitis or pancreatitis.

Third-space fluids are essentially unavailable for functional use. Treatment of a third-space fluid shift is directed toward correcting the cause of the shift.

For the risk factors, clinical signs, and nursing interventions related to fluid volume deficit, see Table 38–5.

Dehydration Dehydration, also called **hyperosmolar imbalance,** results from water loss *without* the proportionate loss of electrolytes, particularly sodium. Loss of only water results in an increased serum sodium level and concentration (osmolality) and subsequent intracellular dehydration. Water is drawn out of the cells and interstitial compartments and into the blood (intravascular compartment). Eventually this causes impaired cellular function and collapse of the circulation.

People at risk for dehydration include the elderly and infirm clients who have a decreased response to thirst or whose kidneys have a decreased ability to concentrate urine. In addition, elderly clients who have a higher proportion of body fat have more limited reserves when there is a water deficit (Aaronson & Seaman 1989, p. 30). Clients who have diabetes insipidus, a decrease in antidiuretic hormone (ADH) secretion, often have severe fluid losses resulting in a hyperosmolar imbalance. The administration of hypertonic solutions also increases the number of solutes in the blood stream.

Fluid Volume Excess Fluid volume excess (FVE) occurs when the body retains both water and electrolytes in the ECF in similar proportions. This state is commonly referred to as **hypervolemia** (increased blood volume or circulatory overload). Because there is isotonic retention of both substances, the serum sodium concentration remains essentially normal. FVE is always secondary to an increase in the total body sodium content (Metheney 1992, p. 48). FVE occurs when a client is overloaded with fluids or when a client has diminished function of homeostatic mechanisms responsible for regulating fluid balance. Specific causes are (a) excessive intake of sodium chloride; (b) too rapid administration of sodium-containing infusions, particularly to clients with impaired regulatory mechanisms; (c) disease processes that alter regulatory mechanisms, such as congestive heart failure, renal failure, cirrhosis of the liver, and Cushing's syndrome; and (d) steroid excess.

In FVE, the excessive water and sodium in the ECF increases its osmotic pressure. Fluid is pulled out of the cells, resulting in **edema,** excessive fluid in the interstitial space. Normally, the interstitial fluid compartment is not bogged with water; rather, it is compact, elastic, and expandable, with just enough fluid to fill the crevices between tissues. This compact state facilitates diffusion of nutrients from the intravascular fluid to the cells. Edema is most frequently observed around the eyes, and in the feet and hands. *Dependent edema* is found in the lowest body parts, such as in the feet and legs or in the sacrum of the sitting client. Edema can be localized or generalized in the body and can account for an increase in weight of at least 4.5 kg (10 lb) in an adult.

Edema can develop whenever there is increased formation of interstitial fluid or impaired removal of interstitial fluid. This commonly occurs when (a) the capillary permeability increases (eg, due to burns, allergy), resulting in increased movement of fluid from the capillaries into the interstitial space or (b) the hydrostatic pressure in the capillaries increases (eg, due to blood hypervolemia, venous blood circulation obstruction). As a result of the hypervolemia, more fluid is pushed out of the arterial capillary bed into the interstitial space. Venous obstruction results in an increased pressure in the venous capillaries, impeding the flow of fluid from the interstitial spaces into the venous capillaries. Edema can also occur when (c) removal of fluid from the interstitial space is decreased (eg, due to lymphatic blockage).

Pitting edema is edema that leaves a small depression or pit after finger pressure is applied to the swollen area. The pit is caused by movement of fluid to adjacent tissue, away from the point of pressure. Within 10 to 30 seconds, the pit normally disappears. Edema related to sodium retention is usually pitting edema, whereas edema related only to water retention is **nonpitting edema** (Metheney, 1992, p. 22).

For the clinical signs, risk factors and nursing intervention related to fluid volume excess, see Table 38–6.

Overhydration Overhydration, also called *hypo-osmolar imbalance*, results from water gain without the proportionate gain of electrolytes, particularly sodium. Gains of only water result in a decreased serum sodium level and concentration (osmolality) and subsequent movement of water into the cells. Because brain cells are particularly sensitive, level of consciousness can decrease if this situation leads to cerebral edema. Overhydration occurs when there is (a) an excessive intake of water (polydipsia), or (b) excessive ADH secretion, commonly referred to as the syndrome of inappropriate antidiuretic hormone (SIADH). SIADH can result from disorders such as head injuries, malignancies, and certain drugs, such as amitriptyline hydrochloride (Elavil).

ELECTROLYTE IMBALANCES

Sodium (Na^+) Normal serum sodium ranges from 135 to 145 mEq/L. It is the most abundant cation (positively charged electrolyte) in the extracellular fluid. Normal sodium concentrations in the extracellular fluid are regulated by ADH and aldosterone. Aldosterone, a hormone produced by the adrenal cortex, acts to maintain sodium concentrations, although its action can be overridden by ADH and the thirst mechanism described earlier.

Sodium not only moves into and out of the body but also moves in careful balance among the three fluid compartments. It is found in most body secretions, for example, saliva, gastric and intestinal secretions, bile, and pancreatic fluid. Therefore, continuous excretion of any of these fluids, such as via intestinal suction, can result in a sodium deficit.

Sodium ions function largely in the control and regulation of the body fluids (ie, water balance). When sodium is reabsorbed into the blood from the tubules of the kidney glomeruli, chloride and water are reabsorbed with it. The combined reabsorption increases the fluid held in the body. Sodium also helps maintain blood volume and interstitial fluid volume through this mechanism. With potassium, sodium helps maintain the electrolyte balance of intracellular and extracellular fluids by means of the active transport mechanism, the sodium-potassium pump. Sodium is also involved in transmitting nerve impulses and contracting muscles.

Sodium is found in many foods, such as bacon, ham, processed cheese, and table salt. Excess sodium is chiefly excreted in the urine; small amounts are lost in perspiration and feces.

Table 38–6 Fluid Volume Excess (FVE)

Risk Factors	Clinical Signs	Nursing Interventions
1. Excessive intake of sodium-containing fluids from intravenous therapy 2. Excessive ingestion of sodium salts in diet or drugs (eg, Alka-Seltzer or hypertonic enemas) 3. Disturbed regulation of fluid balance, as in ▪ Heart failure ▪ Renal failure ▪ Cirrhosis of the liver 4. Laboratory values ▪ Decreased hematocrit ▪ Decreased hemoglobin ▪ Decreased BUN ▪ Increased CVP	Weight gain ▪ 2% gain—mild ▪ 5% gain—moderate ▪ 8% gain—severe Peripheral edema Full, bounding pulse; increased pulse rate Increased blood pressure and central venous pressure Moist breath sounds (rales); dyspnea; shortness of breath Fluid intake greater than fluid output Possible oliguria and decreased urine gravity (less than 1.003) Moist mucous membranes Distended neck and peripheral veins Slow emptying of hand veins (eg, 5 seconds) when hand elevated Mental confusion	Assess changes in clinical signs of FVE. Encourage intake of low-sodium food and fluid as ordered. Monitor fluid intake and output. Administer diuretics as ordered. Employ measures to prevent skin breakdown (see Chapter 30, p. 791).

Hyponatremia is a sodium deficit in the blood plasma. Hyponatremia causes water to move out of the vascular space into the interstitial space and then into the intracellular space (Figure 38–7, *A*). Water retention in the brain cells accounts for many of the clinical signs of hyponatremia (eg, confusion). A typical sign of hyponatremia is pitting edema over the bony prominences, such as the ankles. Hypovolemia accounts for other clinical signs.

Hypernatremia is excess sodium in the blood plasma. Because of the increased extracellular osmotic pressure, fluid moves out of the cells into the extracellular fluid (Figure 38–7, *B*). As a result, the cells have insufficient fluid and become dehydrated. See Table 38–7 on page 1074 for risk factors, clinical signs, and nursing interventions for hyponatremia and hypernatremia.

Cell swells as water is pulled in from ECF

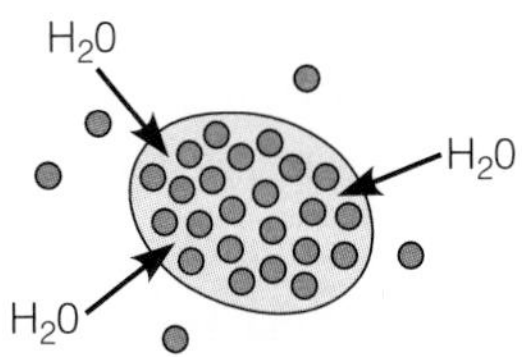

Hyponatremia: Na less than 130 mEq/L

Cell shrinks as water is pulled out into ECF

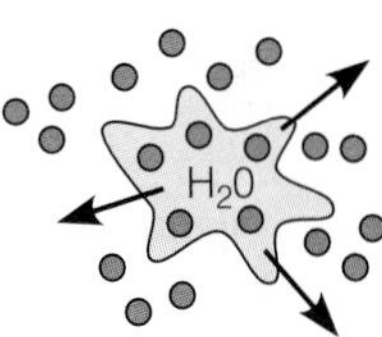

Hypernatremia: Na greater than 150 mEq/L

Figure 38–7 The extracellular sodium level affects cell size. In hyponatremia, cells swell; in hypernatremia, cells shrink in size.

Chloride (Cl^-) Chloride is the major anion (negatively charged electrolyte) of extracellular fluid. A very small amount is found in intracellular fluid. Normal serum chloride of an adult is 95 to 105 mEq/L. Chloride is essential for the production of hydrochloric acid (HCl) in the stomach.

Chloride functions as sodium does to maintain the osmotic pressure of the blood. Its reabsorption in the kidney is secondary to that of sodium; that is, each sodium ion reabsorbed is accompanied by the chloride or bicarbonate ion. Because aldosterone controls the reabsorption of sodium, it controls the reabsorption of chloride indirectly. Chloride is also involved in regulating the acid-base balance in the body. It also has an important buffering function in the exchange of oxygen and carbon dioxide in the red blood cells.

Chloride intake is usually similar to sodium intake. Chloride is found in foods high in sodium, such as table

Table 38–7 Disturbances in Sodium Balance

Risk Factors	Clinical Signs	Nursing Interventions
Hyponatremia		
1. Excessive losses of sodium through ▪ Gastrointestinal fluids (eg, diarrhea) ▪ Sweating ▪ Use of diuretics 2. Excessive gains of water through ▪ Hypotonic tube feedings ▪ Drinking water 3. Conditions such as ▪ Head injury ▪ Stroke	Feelings of apprehension Lethargy Muscle cramps Abdominal cramps Anorexia, nausea, vomiting Postural hypotension Seizures, coma *Laboratory findings:* Serum sodium below 135 mEq/L Serum osmolality below 285 mOsm/kg Urine sodium less than 20 mEq/L and urine specific gravity less than 1.010; however, these vary according to the cause	Monitor fluid intake and output. Assess clinical signs. Monitor laboratory data (eg, serum sodium). Encourage food and fluid high in sodium if permitted (eg, table salt, bacon, ham, processed cheese). Assess client closely if administering hypertonic saline solutions.
Hypernatremia		
1. Excessive loss of fluids through ▪ Insensible water loss through hyperventilation ▪ Diarrhea 2. Deprivation of water 3. Excessive salt intake through ▪ Parenteral administration of sodium ▪ Hypertonic tube feedings without adequate water 4. Conditions such as ▪ Diabetes insipidus ▪ Heat stroke ▪ Excessive use of table salt (1 tsp contains 2300 mg of sodium)	Extreme thirst Dry, sticky mucous membranes Tongue red, dry, swollen Severe hypernatremia: ▪ Agitated behavior ▪ Fatigue ▪ Restlessness ▪ Disorientation ▪ Hallucinations *Laboratory findings:* Serum sodium above 145 mEq/L Serum osmolality above 295 mOsm/kg Urine specific gravity less than 1.015	Monitor fluid intake and output. Monitor behavior changes, (eg, restlessness, disorientation). Monitor laboratory findings (eg, serum sodium). Encourage fluids as ordered. Monitor diet as ordered (eg, restrict intake of salt and foods high in sodium).

salt, ham, and bacon. Chloride is absorbed in the intestines and excreted through the kidneys.

Hypochloremia (a deficit in serum chloride) and **hyperchloremia** (an excess serum chloride) usually develop along with sodium disturbances.

Potassium (K^+) Potassium is the major cation of intracellular fluid. The normal adult's serum potassium range is 3.5 to 5.0 mEq/L. Potassium balance is regulated in the kidneys by two mechanisms: exchange with sodium ions in the kidney tubules and secretion of aldosterone. Aldosterone is extremely important in controlling potassium concentrations in extracellular fluids.

Potassium affects the functions of most body systems, including the cardiovascular system, the gastrointestinal system, the neuromuscular system, and the respiratory system. Potassium also plays a role in the acid-base bal ance of the body. Of particular importance is potassium's role in transmitting electrical impulses to the heart and other muscles, to lung tissues, and to intestinal tissues. Clients having surgery usually have their potassium levels assessed because abnormal levels can cause heart arrhyth-

POTASSIUM-RICH FOODS

Vegetables	Fruits	Beverages
Avocado	Dried fruits (eg, raisins and dates)	Milk
Raw carrot	Bananas	Orange juice
Baked potato	Apricots	Apricot nectar
Raw tomato	Cantaloupe	
	Orange	

mias. Most of the body's potassium is found inside the cells. A small amount is found in the plasma and interstitial fluids.

Potassium is usually excreted by the kidneys. However, the kidneys do not regulate potassium excretion as effectively as they do sodium excretion. Therefore, an acute potassium deficiency can develop rapidly. Of the body's secretions, the gastrointestinal secretions are high in potassium.

Like other electrolytes, potassium moves continually into and out of the cells. This movement from the interstitial fluid, which has less potassium, to the intracellular fluid, which has a greater concentration, is influenced by the presence of insulin, adrenal steroids, testosterone, pH changes, glycogen formation, and hyponatremia. If tissues are damaged, the body can lose potassium quickly.

Potassium is found in many fruits and vegetables. See the box above.

Hypokalemia is a potassium deficit in the blood plasma. Hypokalemia can develop quickly in people who are starving. The combined effects of inadequate potassium intake and excessive potassium loss due to prolonged diarrhea can deplete potassium stores acutely. A common cause of hypokalemia is the use of potassium-wasting diuretics, such as thiazide diuretics or loop diuretics (eg, furosemide). **Hyperkalemia** is a potassium excess in the blood plasma. See Table 38–8 on page 1076 for the risk factors, clinical signs, and nursing interventions for hypokalemia and hyperkalemia.

Calcium (Ca^{2+}) The normal total serum calcium in an adult is 4.5 to 5.5 mEq/L. This value includes the sum of ionized calcium (56%) and nonionized calcium (44%) (Metheney 1992, p. 16). Many agencies now measure only the ionized calcium, which is physiologically active and clinically significant. The normal serum ionized calcium level is approximately 2.5 mEq/L.

Calcium functions in bone formation and in the transmission of nerve impulses, muscle contraction, blood coagulation, and activation of certain enzymes, such as pancreatic lipase and phospholipase. It is also required for Vitamin B_{12} absorption. Only 1% of the body's calcium is found in ECF. The richest sources of calcium are milk and milk products. Drinking water in some parts of the country also contains an absorbable calcium. Major food sources of calcium are shown in Table 37–6, page 1026.

Calcium is excreted in urine, feces, bile, digestive secretions and sweat. The concentration of body calcium is controlled indirectly by the effect of parathyroid hormone on bone reabsorption. When calcium levels in extracellular fluid fall too low, the parathyroid glands are stimulated to increase parathyroid hormone (parathormone, PTH) secretion. This hormone acts directly on the bones to increase the release of calcium into the blood. When the bones run out of calcium, parathyroid hormone acts on both the kidney tubules and the intestinal mucosa to increase the reabsorption of calcium from the kidneys and the intestine.

Another hormone, *calcitonin*, has an effect nearly opposite that of the parathyroid hormone. Calcitonin reduces the concentration of calcium ions in the blood. Calcitonin, which is secreted by the thyroid gland, stimulates the deposition of calcium in bone and depresses the formation of osteoclasts in the bone.

Older postmenopausal women may experience accelerated bone loss because of decreased calcium absorption from the intestines and increased calcium loss in the urine.

Hypocalcemia is a calcium deficit in the blood plasma. Severe depletion of calcium can cause **tetany** (muscle spasms, sharp flexion of the wrists and ankles, cramps), which can lead to convulsions. Clients at risk for hypocalcemia include those who have hypomagnesemia (low serum magnesium levels). The magnesium deficiency suppresses the secretion of parathyroid hormone necessary for the release of calcium from the bone to the blood. Chronic alcohol abuse can cause hypocalcemia as a result of intestinal malabsorption of calcium and hypomagnesia. Many drugs also predispose to hypocalcemia: loop diuretics (furosemide), anticonvulsants (phenytoin [Dilantin], phenobarbital), phosphates given orally, intravenously, or by enema, and drugs that lower serum magnesium level (eg, cisplatin, gentamicin).

Hypercalcemia is an excess of calcium in the blood plasma. See Table 38–9 on page 1077 for the risk factors, clinical signs, and nursing interventions related to hypocalcemia and hypercalcemia.

Magnesium (Mg^{2+}) Magnesium is important for maintaining neuromuscular activity, for the metabolism of carbohydrates and proteins, and for activating many intracellular enzyme systems. Next to potassium, magnesium is the most abundant intracellular cation. Many of

Table 38–8 Disturbances in Potassium Balance

Risk Factors	Clinical Signs	Nursing Interventions
Hypokalemia		
1. Excessive losses of potassium through ▪ Vomiting and gastric suction ▪ Urine ▪ Diarrhea ▪ Heavy perspiration 2. Prolonged use of potassium-losing drugs (eg, diuretics) 3. Poor intake of potassium (as with debilitated clients, alcoholics, anorexia nervosa) 4. Hyperaldosteronism	Muscle weakness, leg cramps Fatigue Anorexia, nausea, vomiting Decreased bowel sounds, decreased bowel motility Cardiac arrythmias Depressed deep-tendon reflexes *Laboratory findings:* Serum potassium below 3.5 mEq/L Arterial blood gases (ABGs) may show increased pH and HCO_3^- (alkalosis results with a pH above 7.45) Electrocardiogram may show flattening of the T waves and depression of the ST segment	Monitor clients receiving digitalis closely, because hypokalemia enhances digitalis toxicity. Administer oral potassium as ordered with food or fluid to prevent gastric irritation. Monitor heart rate and rhythm. Teach client about potassium-rich foods. Closely monitor clients receiving intravenous potassium. Teach clients how to prevent excessive loss of potassium (eg, through abuse of diuretics and laxatives).
Hyperkalemia		
1. Decreased loss of potassium through the kidneys due to ▪ Renal failure ▪ Hypoaldosteronism ▪ Intake of potassium-conserving diuretics 2. High potassium intake through ▪ Excessive use of potassium-containing salt substitutes ▪ Excessive or rapid IV infusion of potassium 3. Conditions in which potassium moves out of the tissue cells into the plasma (eg, infections, burns)	Gastrointestinal hyperactivity, diarrhea Irritability, apathy, confusion Cardiac arrhythmia, bradycardia, cardiac arrest Muscle weakness, areflexia (absence of reflexes) Paresthesias and numbness in extremities *Laboratory findings:* Serum potassium above 5.0 mEq/L ECG abnormalities	Closely monitor clients receiving diuretics. Before administering intravenous potassium, determine serum potassium level and follow protocols for administration carefully. K^+ is always well diluted when given intravenously. Teach clients to avoid foods high in potassium. Draw blood specimens carefully to avoid false hyperkalemia reports: ▪ Apply tourniquet for short periods only. ▪ Rest the extremity immediately before taking the specimen. ▪ Do not take a specimen from a site near an IV insertion.

the same factors that regulate calcium also regulate magnesium; for example, magnesium is affected by the parathyroid hormone and is absorbed from the intestinal tract. The magnesium content of the body is also affected by the potassium concentration. If magnesium is deficient, the kidneys tend to excrete more potassium. Normal serum magnesium for an adult is 1.5 to 2.5 mEq/L (Guyton 1991, p. 786). Low extracellular fluid levels are referred to as **hypomagnesemia;** elevated levels are **hypermagnesemia.** See Table 38–10 on page 1078 for risk factors, clinical signs, and nursing interventions for magnesium imbalances.

Phosphate (PO_4^-) The phosphate anion is found both in intracellular and extracellular fluid. Most of the phosphorus (P^+) in the body exists as PO_4^-. Normal serum phosphate levels range from 1.8 to 2.6 mEq/L.

Table 38–9 Disturbances in Calcium Balance

Risk Factors	Clinical Signs	Nursing Interventions
Hypocalcemia		
1. Conditions such as ▪ Hypoparathyroidism ▪ Acute pancreatitis ▪ Hyperphosphatemia ▪ Thyroid carcinoma 2. Inadequate intake of vitamin D 3. Excessive loss of intestinal secretions 4. Alcohol abuse	Numbness, tingling of the extremities and around the mouth Muscle tremors, cramps; if severe can progress to tetany and convulsions Cardiac arrhythmias; decreased stroke volume and ventricular contractions Positive Trousseau's and Chvostek's signs (see p. 1083) *Laboratory findings:* Serum calcium less than 4.0 mEq/L (total)	Monitor the clients' breathing closely because of possible laryngeal stridor. Take precautions to protect a confused client. Teach postmenopausal women about ▪ Food sources of calcium. See Chapter 37, page 1026. ▪ Calcium supplements as ordered. ▪ Value of regular exercise.
Hypercalcemia		
1. Prolonged immobilization 2. Conditions such as ▪ Hyperparathyroidism ▪ Malignancy of the bone ▪ Paget's disease	Flank pain secondary to urinary calculi Lethargy, weakness Reduced muscle tone Anorexia, nausea, vomiting Depressed deep-tendon reflexes Constipation Polyuria Cardiac arrest may occur in hypercalcemia crisis *Laboratory findings:* Serum calcium greater than 5.5 mEq/L (total)	Increase client movement and exercise. Encourage oral fluids as permitted to maintain a dilute urine. Teach clients to limit intake of food and fluid high in calcium (see Chapter 37). Encourage ingestion of fiber to prevent constipation. Protect a confused client. Encourage intake of acid-ash fluids (eg, prune or cranberry juice) to counteract deposits of calcium salts in the urine. A urinary pH of more than 6.5 predisposes to calcium deposits.

Together with calcium, phosphate is involved in bone and tooth formation. Phosphate is involved in many chemical actions of the cell; it is essential for functioning of muscles, nerves, and red blood cells. It is also involved in the metabolism of protein, fat, and carbohydrate.

Phosphate is absorbed exceedingly well from the intestine, and it is excreted in the urine. Phosphate is a threshold substance; that is, none is lost in urine when blood plasma concentrations fall below a critical level. When the concentration is above the critical level, however, phosphate is excreted in proportion to the increase. Thus, the kidneys regulate the concentration of phosphate in the extracellular fluid. In addition, phosphate excretion is regulated by the parathyroid hormone. See Table 38–11 on page 1079 for risk factors, clinical signs, and nursing interventions for **hypophosphatemia** (phosphate deficit) and **hyperphosphatemia** (phosphate excess).

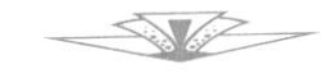

ASSESSING

Assessment of clients with or at risk for developing fluid and electrolyte disturbances includes (a) taking a nursing history; (b) obtaining clinical measurements, such as daily weights, vital signs, and fluid intake and output; (c) assessing skin turgor and neuromuscular irritability; (d) performing a physical examination; and (e) reviewing results of laboratory tests performed to evaluate fluid and electrolyte balance.

NURSING HISTORY

Fluid and electrolyte disturbances are characterized by numerous signs and symptoms that affect many areas of

Table 38–10 Disturbances in Magnesium Balances

Risk Factors	Clinical Signs	Nursing Interventions
Hypomagnesemia		
1. Excessive loss from the gastrointestinal tract, (eg, from nasogastric suction, diarrhea, fistula drainage) 2. Long-term use of certain drugs (eg, diuretics, cisplatin) 3. Conditions such as ▪ Chronic alcoholism ▪ Renal disease ▪ Pancreatitis ▪ Burns	Neuromuscular irritability with tremors Increased reflexes, tremors, convulsions Positive Chvostek's and Trousseau's signs (see p. 1083) Tachycardia, elevated blood pressure, arrythmias Disorientation and confusion Vertigo *Laboratory findings:* Serum magnesium below 1.5 mEq/L	Assess clients receiving digitalis closely for digitalis toxicity. Hypomagnesemia predisposes to toxicity. Take protective measures when there is a possibility of seizures. Encourage clients to eat magnesium-rich foods if permitted (eg, whole grains, meat, seafood, and green leafy vegetables). Monitor clients closely for laryngeal stridor. If the client uses excessive laxatives or diuretics, teach healthy use of these medications.
Hypermagnesemia		
1. Abnormal retention of magnesium, as in ▪ Advanced renal failure ▪ Adrenal insufficiency 2. Treatment with magnesium salts	Peripheral vasodilatation Lethargy, drowsiness Coma Impaired respirations, breaths below 10 to 12 per minute Nausea, vomiting Muscle weakness, paralysis Hypotension, bradycardia Depressed deep-tendon reflexes Respiratory and cardiac arrest if hypermagnesemia is severe *Laboratory findings:* Serum magnesium above 2.5 mEq/L Electrocardiogram showing prolonged QT interval; an atrioventricular (AV) block may occur	Monitor vital signs when clients are at risk. If patellar reflexes are absent, notify the physician. Advise clients who have renal disease to determine the magnesium content of over-the-counter drugs.

body function and are often interrelated. The nurse therefore needs to elicit specific data about many aspects of the client's needs and functional health patterns. Although each specific imbalance is manifested as a unique syndrome, the history must not be focused on any one specific problem from the start. Data must be obtained about the client's fluid and food intake; fluid output; recent fluid losses; signs of fluid deficit or excess; common signs of electrolyte problems; long-term and recent disease processes, and medications and treatments that alter fluid and electrolyte balance. Examples of interview questions to elicit this information are shown in the box on page 1080.

CLINICAL MEASUREMENTS

Three simple clinical measurements that the nurse can initiate without a physician's order are daily weights, vital signs, and fluid intake and output.

Daily Weights Daily weight measurements can provide a relatively accurate assessment of a client's fluid

Table 38–11 Disturbances in Phosphate Balances

Risk Factors	Clinical Signs	Nursing Interventions
Hypophosphatemia		
1. Excessive ingestion of glucose, as, for example, in ▪ Parenteral administration of glucose ▪ Administration of calories to clients who are severely malnourished ▪ Hyperalimentation 2. Respiratory alkalosis 3. Conditions such as ▪ Burns ▪ Diabetes ▪ Chronic alcoholism	*Acute hypophosphatemia:* Confusion, seizures, coma Muscle pain Decreased muscle strength Positive Chvostek's sign (see p. 1083) *Chronic hypophosphatemia:* Memory loss Fatigue Bone pain and joint stiffness Respiratory failure *Laboratory findings:* Serum phosphate below 1.8 mEq/L Decreased cardiac function, heart muscle damage Decreased oxygen saturation of blood	Monitor malnourished clients closely. Administer IV phosphate well diluted and slowly. Do not infuse it together with calcium. Assess clients taking oral phosphorus supplements for diarrhea. Employ precautions to prevent infections. Teach clients to eat foods high in phosphorus: milk, cheese, fish products, whole grains.
Hyperphosphatemia		
1. Conditions such as ▪ Renal failure ▪ Hypoparathyroidism 2. Chemotherapy 3. Excessive ingestion of phosphorus by ▪ Mouth (eg, laxatives) ▪ Phosphorus-based enemas ▪ Oral phosphorus	Tetany Circumoral (around or near the mouth) paresthesias Anorexia, nausea, and vomiting Hyperreflexia Tachycardia *Laboratory findings:* Serum phosphate level above 2.6 mEq/L Electrocardiogram showing shortened ST segment and QT interval Low serum calcium	Monitor for neuromuscular irritability. Administer calcium supplements as ordered. Teach client to avoid foods high in phosphorus: milk, cheese, meat, poultry, whole grains Teach client to avoid excessive use of phosphorus-containing laxatives and enemas.

status. Notable changes in weight are indicative of *acute* fluid changes. Each kilogram (2.2 lb) of weight gained or lost is equivalent to one liter of fluid gained or lost. Such fluid gains or losses indicate total body fluid volume changes in all of the fluid compartments rather than in any specific compartment, such as the intravascular compartment. Rapid losses or gains of 5% to 8% of total body weight indicate moderate to severe fluid volume deficits or excesses.

To obtain accurate weight measurements, the nurse should balance the scale before each use and weigh the client (a) at the same time each day (eg, before breakfast and after the first void), (b) wearing the same or similar clothing, and (c) on the same scale. The type of scale (ie, standing, bed, chair) should be documented.

Vital Signs Changes in the vital signs may indicate fluid, electrolyte, and acid-base imbalances or compensating mechanisms for maintaining balance. Elevations in body temperatures may be a result of dehydration or a cause of fluid balance problems. Fever causes further increases in loss of body fluids.

Tachycardia is one of the first signs of hypovolemia associated with FVD. Pulse volume decreases in FVD and increases in FVE. Irregular pulse rates may occur with potassium imbalances. Changes in respiratory rates and

ASSESSMENT INTERVIEW

Fluid and Electrolyte Balance

Fluid and Food Intake

- What amount and type of fluids do you drink each day?
- What types of food do you eat each day? (The nurse may focus on protein, sodium, and potassium-rich foods.)
- Have there been any recent changes in food or fluid intake, for example, as a result of taking part in a weight-loss program?
- Have you experienced any nausea, pain, or loss of appetite that has altered your intake?

Fluid Output

- Have you noticed any recent changes in the frequency or amount of urine output?

Fluid Imbalances

- Are you losing body fluids in any major way (eg, vomiting, diarrhea, excessive perspiration, or other route)?
- Have you noticed any signs that indicate your body is experiencing too little hydration (eg, excessive thirst, dry skin, dry mucous membranes, concentrated urine, reduced urine output)?
- Have you had any signs indicating that your body is experiencing too much hydration (swollen ankles, difficulty breathing, weight gain)?

Electrolyte Balance

- Have you noticed any of the following signs that might indicate an electrolyte imbalance: loss of mental alertness; disorientation; faintness; muscle weakness, twitching, cramps, fatigue, pain, or spasm; abnormal sensations, such as burning, prickling, tingling; abdominal cramps or distention; heart palpitations?

Disease Processes

- Have you experienced any long-term or recent disease processes that might disrupt fluid or electrolyte balance, such as kidney disease, heart disease, high blood pressure, diabetes insipidus, thyroid or parathyroid disorders, severe trauma, or other chronic disease states (eg, cancer, colitis, ileitis)?

Medications

- Are you taking any of the following medications that could affect your fluid and electrolyte balance: diuretics, steroids, potassium supplements, salt substitutes, antacids, aldosterone inhibitor agents?

Treatments

- Have you recently had any treatments such as dialysis, total parenteral nutrition, tube drainages (eg, nasogastric or intestinal suction), or tube feedings?

depth may cause respiratory acid-base imbalances or act as a compensatory mechanism in metabolic acidosis or alkalosis. (See the discussion of acid-base imbalances, later in this chapter).

Blood pressure, a sensitive measure to detect blood volume changes, may fall significantly with FVD and hypovolemia or increase with FVE. Orthostatic hypotension may also occur with FVD and hypovolemia.

Fluid Intake and Output (I & O) The measurement and recording of all fluid intake and output during a 24-hour period provides important data about the client's fluid and electrolyte balance. Generally, intake and output are measured for at-risk clients (see the box on page 1081).

The unit used to measure intake and output is the milliliter (mL) or cubic centimeter (cc); these are equivalent metric units of measurement. In household measures, 30 mL is roughly equivalent to 1 fluid ounce, 500 mL is about 1 pint, and 1000 mL is about 1 quart. To measure fluid intake, nurses must convert household measures such as a glass, cup, or soup bowl to metric units. Most agencies provide conversion tables, since the sizes of dishes vary from agency to agency. Such a table is often provided on or with the bedside I & O record. Examples of equivalents are given in the box on page 1081.

Most agencies have a form for recording I & O, usually a bedside record on which the nurse lists all items measured and their quantities per shift (Figure 38–8, p. 1082). Some agencies have another form for recording the specifics of intravenous fluids, such as the type of solution, additives, time started, amounts absorbed, and amounts remaining per shift.

Nurses must inform clients, family members, and all caregivers that accurate measurements of the client's fluid intake and output are required, explaining why and emphasizing the need to use a bedpan or urinal or commode (unless a urinary drainage system is in place). If a bedpan is used, instruct the client not to put toilet tissue in the bedpan. Clients who wish to be involved in recording

Clients at Risk for Fluid and Electrolyte Imbalances

- Clients dependent on others to meet their food and fluid needs—for example, elderly, very young, handicapped
- Clients who have gained or lost more than 5 lb in a week
- Clients who are permitted nothing by mouth (NPO)
- Clients with intravenous infusions.
- Clients with retention catheters and urinary drainage systems
- Clients with special drainages or suctions, such as a nasogastric suction
- Clients receiving diuretics
- Clients experiencing excessive fluid losses and requiring increased intake
- Clients who retain fluids
- Clients with fluid restrictions
- Postoperative clients
- Clients with severe trauma or burns
- Clients with chronic diseases such as congestive heart failure, diabetes, chronic obstructive lung disease, and cancer
- Confused clients or those with altered level of consciousness who may not be able to communicate needs or respond to thirst

Commonly Used Fluid Containers and Their Volumes

Water glass	200mL
Juice glass	120 mL
Cup	180 mL
Soup bowl mL	
Adult	180 mL
Child	100 mL
Teapot	240 mL
Creamer	
Large	90 mL
Small	30 mL
Water pitcher	1000 mL
Jello, custard dish	100 mL
Ice cream dish	120 mL
Paper cup	
Large	200 mL
Small	120 mL

fluid intake measurements need to be taught how to compute the values and what foods are considered fluids.

To measure *fluid intake*, the nurse records on the I & O form each fluid item taken (if the client has not already done so), specifying the time and type of fluid. All of the following fluids need to be recorded:

- *Oral fluids.* Water, milk, juice, soft drinks, coffee, tea, cream, soup, sherry, and wine. Include water taken with medications. To assess the amount of water taken from a water pitcher, measure what remains and subtract this amount from the volume of the full pitcher. Then refill the pitcher.
- *Ice chips.* Record these as fluids at approximately one-half their volume.
- *Foods that are or tend to become liquid at room temperature.* These include ice cream, sherbert, custard, and gelatin (Jello). Do *not* measure foods that are pureed, because purees are simply solid foods prepared in a different form.
- *Tube feedings.* Remember to include the 30- to 60-mL water rinse at the end of intermittent feedings or during continuous feedings.
- *Parenteral fluids.* The exact amount of intravenous fluid administered is to be recorded, since some fluid containers may be overfilled. Blood transfusions are included.
- *Intravenous medications.* Intravenous medications that are prepared with solutions such as normal saline (NS) and are added to an infusion, for example, must also be included (eg, tobramycin sulfate 80 mg in 50 mL of sterile water). Most intravenous medications are mixed in 50 to 100 mL of solution.
- *Catheter or tube irrigants.* Fluid used to irrigate urinary catheters, nasogastric tubes, and intestinal tubes must be measured and recorded.

To measure *fluid output*, the nurse must wear gloves and measure the following fluids:

- *Urinary output.* Following each voiding, pour the urine into a measuring container, observe the amount, and record it and the time of voiding on the bedside I & O form. For clients with retention catheters, note and record the amount of urine at the end of the shift, and then empty the drainage bag. Drainage bags are usually calibrated to indicate the amount of urine. If there is any doubt about the amount in the drainage bag,

EL CAMINO HOSPITAL

INTAKE AND OUTPUT RECORD

PATIENT LABEL

PATIENT NAME ______________________

PATIENT # ______________________

PHYSICIAN ______________________

INTAKE							OUTPUT					
TOTAL IV	INTRAVENOUS			TUBE FEED	ORAL	TIME	URINE	NG	EMESIS	BM	MISC.
					Date:						
						6-2					
						2-10					
						10-6					
						24°					
					Date:						
						6-2					
						2-10					
						10-6					
						24°					

Figure 38–8 A sample 24-hour fluid intake and output record. **Source:** Courtesy of El Camino Hospital, Mountain View, California.

empty it into an accurate measuring container. In critical care areas, the urine ideally is measured hourly.

If the client is incontinent of urine or is extremely diaphoretic, estimate and record these outputs. For example, for an incontinent client the nurse might record "Incontinent × 3" or "Drawsheet soaked in 12-in diameter." A more accurate estimate of the urine of incontinent clients may be obtained by first weighing diapers or incontinent pads that are dry, and then subtracting this weight from the weight of the soiled items. Each gram of weight left after subtracting is equal to 1 mL of urine. If urine is frequently soiled with feces the nurse can record the number of voidings rather than the volume of urine.

- *Vomitus and liquid feces.* The type of fluid and time need to be specified.
- *Diaphoresis.* For a diaphoretic client, record "Perspiring profusely [or ++++]. Gown and drawsheet changed × 2." Follow agency protocol in this regard.
- *Tube drainage,* such as gastric or intestinal drainage.
- *Wound drainage* and *draining fistulas.* Wound drainage may be recorded by documenting the type and number of dressings or linen saturated with drainage or by measuring the exact amount of drainage collected in a vacuum drainage (eg, Hemovac) or gravity drainage system.
- *Rapid, deep respiratory rate.* Because hyperventilation can contribute to insensible fluid loss, the rate and depth of respirations in such clients should be recorded.

Fluid intake and output measurements are totaled at the end of the shift (every 8 or 12 hours), and the totals are transferred to the correct column on the client's permanent record. In some critical care areas, the nurse may need to record intake and output hourly. Usually the staff on night shift totals the amounts of I & O recorded for each shift and records the 24-hour total on the client's graphic sheet.

To determine whether the fluid output is proportional to fluid intake or whether there are any changes in the client's fluid status, the nurse (a) compares the total 24-hour fluid output measurement with the total fluid intake measurement and (b) compares both to previous measurements. Urinary output is normally equivalent to the amount of fluids ingested; the usual range is 1500 to 2000 mL in 24 hours, or 40 to 80 mL in 1 hour. Clients whose output substantially exceeds intake are at risk for fluid volume deficit. By contrast, clients whose intake substantially exceeds output are at risk for fluid volume excess. Inadequate intakes and outputs need to be reported to the nurse in charge. In adults, for example, a urine output of less than 500 mL in 24 hours or less than 30 mL per hour is considered inadequate.

PHYSICAL EXAMINATION

The client is examined for clinical signs of fluid, electrolyte, and acid-base imbalances. The nurse needs a knowledge of significant signs as well as the normal clinical picture presented by the client. Tables 38–5 to 38–11 in this chapter describe some common clinical signs of fluid, electrolyte, and acid-base imbalances.

The physical examination for assessing a client's fluid and electrolyte status is focused on the skin, the oral cavity, the eyes, the jugular veins, the veins of the hand, and the neurologic system. Data from this physical examination expand and verify information obtained during the nursing history. Skin turgor and neuromuscular irritability are discussed here.

Skin Turgor Skin turgor is an indication of interstitial fluid volume and skin elasticity. Decreased skin turgor is associated with a fluid volume deficit. Normally, when the skin is pinched it immediately springs back to its normal position when released. In a person with FVD, the skin flattens more slowly after being released and may remain elevated or tented for several seconds. In adults, skin turgor is best measured over the sternum, forehead, or inner aspects of the thigh. In children, it may be assessed over the abdominal area or medial aspects of the thigh. Because tissue turgor normally decreases in people older than 55 to 60 years of age and in people with recent weight loss, other signs of FVD should always be considered along with tissue turgor.

Neuromuscular Irritability When imbalances of calcium and magnesium are suspected, the nurse may assess the client for increased or decreased neuromuscular irritability. Assessments include checking for Chvostek's sign and Trousseau's sign and observing deep-tendon reflexes. Deep-tendon reflexes are discussed in detail in Chapter 22, page 544.

To assess **Chvostek's sign,** the nurse percusses (taps) the facial nerve about 2 cm anterior to the earlobe. A positive response, that is, unilateral twitching of the facial muscles, including the eyelids and lips, may occur in some clients with hypocalcemia or hypomagnesemia.

To assess **Trousseau's sign,** the nurse places a blood pressure cuff on the area and inflates the cuff above the systolic pressure for 2 to 3 minutes to occlude the blood supply. The development of carpal spasm or tetany indicates a positive reaction and possible hypocalcemia or hypomagnesemia.

LABORATORY TESTS

Many laboratory studies are conducted to determine the existence of fluid, electrolyte, and acid-base imbalances. Some of the more common tests are discussed here.

NORMAL ELECTROLYTE VALUES OF ADULTS*

Venous Blood	
Sodium	135 to 145 mEq/L
Potassium	3.5 to 5.0 mEq/L
Chloride	95 to 105 mEq/L
Calcium (total)	4.0 to 5.5 mEq/L
(ionized)	56% of total calcium
Magnesium	1.5 to 2.5 mEq/L
Phosphate (phosphorus)	1.8 to 2.6 mEq/L
Serum osmolality	280 to 300 mOsm/kg water

*Normal laboratory values vary from agency to agency.

Serum Electrolytes Serum electrolyte levels are often routinely ordered for any client admitted to hospital as a screening test for electrolyte and acid-base imbalances. The most commonly ordered serum tests are for sodium, potassium, chloride, and bicarbonate ions. Normal values of commonly measured electrolytes are shown in the box above.

Complete Blood Count (CBC) The complete blood count, another basic screening test, includes information about the hematocrit (Hct) and hemoglobin (Hgb) levels. The **hematocrit** measures the volume (percentage) of whole blood that is composed of red blood cells (RBCs). Because the hematocrit is a measure of the volume of cells in relation to plasma, it is affected by changes in plasma volume. Thus, the hematocrit increases with severe dehydration and hypovolemic shock and decreases with severe overhydration. Normal hematocrit values are 40% to 54% (males) and 37% to 47% (females).

An increase in hemoglobin levels may accompany an increase in hematocrit levels. Decreased levels of hemoglobin are found with severe hemorrhage. Normal adult values are 95% to 98% by electrophoresis or 12 to 18 g/100 mL of blood. Men tend to have higher Hgb values than women.

Osmolality Osmolality is an indicator of the concentration or number of particles dissolved in serum and urine. It is reported as milliosmols of solute per kilogram of fluid (mOsm/kg). For clarification, Figure 38–9 compares milliosmols and milliequivalents. Milliosmols measure *osmotic activity* as a total of the number of particles *present* in solution (eg, serum). In Figure 38–9, *A*, the total number of particles is 10. In contrast, milliequivalents measure *chemical activity* as a total of the number of available electrovalent bonds. In Figure 38–9, *B*, the total number of electrovalent bonds is 20, because each of the

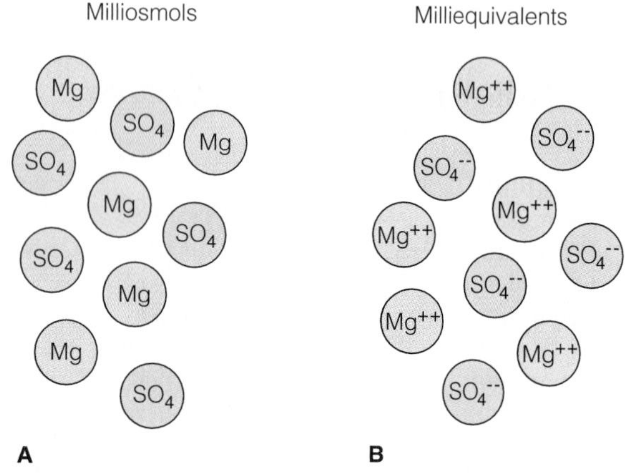

Figure 38–9 Comparison of milliosmols and milliequivalents. *A*, Milliosmols measure osmotic activity as a total of the number of particles present—in this case 10. *B*, Milliequivalents measure the chemical activity as a total of the number of available electrovalent bonds (− −, + +)—in this case, 20.

five SO_4^{2-} particles and each of the five Mg^{2+} particles has two available electrovalent bonds. *Serum osmolality* is a measure of the solute concentration of the blood. The particles included are sodium ions, glucose, and urea (blood urea nitrogen, or BUN). Serum osmolality can be estimated by doubling the serum sodium, because sodium and its associated chloride ions are the major determinants of serum osmolality. Serum osmolality levels are the major regulator of antidiuretic hormone (ADH) release, which, in turn, controls the rate of water reabsorption by the kidneys and therefore urine osmolality. An increased plasma osmolality level stimulates ADH secretion, which causes the reabsorption of water from the renal tubules and thus increases the concentration and osmolality of urine. Serum osmolality values are used primarily to measure the extent of dehydration, because they reflect the balance of osmotic pressure between tissue cells and body fluids. Normal values are 280 to 300 mOsm/kg. An increase in serum osmolality indicates a fluid volume deficit; a decrease reflects a fluid volume excess.

Urine osmolality is a measure of the solute concentration of urine. The particles included are nitrogenous wastes, such as creatinine, urea, and uric acid. Normal values are 500 to 800 mOsm/kg (Metheney 1992, p. 34). An increased urine osmolality indicates a fluid volume deficit; a decreased urine osmolality reflects a fluid volume excess.

Urine pH Measurement of urine pH may be obtained by laboratory analysis or by using a dipstick on a freshly voided specimen. See Chapter 41, page 1236. Since the kidneys play a critical role in regulating acid-base balance, assessment of urine pH can be useful in determining whether the kidneys are responding appropriately to metabolic acid-base imbalances. See Acid-Base Balance on page 1115. Normally, the pH of the urine is relatively acidic, averaging about 6.0, but a range of 4.6 to 8.0 is considered normal. In metabolic acidosis, urine pH should decrease, indicating that the kidneys are responding appropriately; in metabolic alkalosis, the pH should increase. Increases of the pH in metabolic acidosis or decreases of the pH in metabolic alkalosis are abnormal.

Urine Specific Gravity Specific gravity is discussed in detail in Chapter 41, page 1236. Although it is a less reliable indicator of concentration than urine osmolality, the test can be performed quickly and easily by nursing personnel. Specific gravity is affected by both the number and weight of solutes. Therefore, the presence of a few large solutes such as protein or glucose can cause a deceptively high specific gravity. Other substances that may also

Table 38–12 Clinical Application: Assessment Data Clusters and Related Nursing Diagnoses

Data Cluster	Nursing Diagnoses
Merlyn Chapman, a 27-year-old sales clerk, reported generalized weakness, malaise, and symptoms of flu for 3 to 4 days. She was unable to tolerate fluids even though thirsty because of nausea and vomiting and had liquid stools 2 to 4 times per day. Physical findings indicated dry oral mucosa, furrowed tongue, cracked lips, mild fever (38.6 C) and scanty concentrated urine output (specific gravity: 1.035).	**Fluid volume deficit** related to poor fluid intake, vomiting, and diarrhea for 3 to 4 days
Luella Fisher, a frail 93-year-old with congestive heart failure, uses a daily diuretic (furosemide). She has recently had a stroke that impairs her swallowing. A nasogastric tube and urinary catheter are in place. Appetite is poor.	**High risk for fluid volume deficit** related to inadequate fluid intake, loss of fluid through nasogastric tube, urinary catheter, and diuretic therapy
Tom Bricker, a 67-year-old pensioner who has a history of heart disease, has experienced a weight gain of 4 to 5 kg (9 to 11 lb) over the past month. He states his rings are too tight to remove, his ankles are swollen, his heart pounds at times, he gets breathless with exertion, and feels bloated. Physical findings reveal jugular vein distension above 3 cm, delayed emptying of hand veins, bounding pulse (86), pitting edema in feet, ankles, and lower legs, and moist lung sounds (rales).	**Altered tissue perfusion** related to fluid volume excess secondary to decreased cardiac output

NURSING DIAGNOSES

CLIENTS WITH FLUID/ELECTROLYTE PROBLEMS

NURSING DIAGNOSIS: Fluid volume deficit: The state in which an individual experiences vascular, interstitial, or intracellular dehydration

Defining Characteristics

See Table 38–5 on page 1071.

Related Factors

Active fluid volume loss related to excessive diaphoresis, vomiting, diarrhea, hemorrhage, wound drainage, indwelling tubes, or suction; failure of regulatory mechanisms related to neurohypophyseal impairment (diabetes insipidus), adrenal insufficiency (Addison's disease), or pancreatic impairment (diabetes mellitus).

NURSING DIAGNOSIS: High risk for fluid volume deficit: The state in which an individual is *at risk* of experiencing vascular, interstitial, or intracellular dehydration due to active or regulatory losses of body water in excess of needs

Risk Factors

Extremes of age or weight; excessive fluid losses through normal routes (eg, diarrhea, vomiting); loss of fluid through abnormal routes; diuretic medications, disorders affecting access to fluids or intake or absorption of fluids; presence of factors such as a hot environment or hypermetabolic state that influences fluid requirements.

NURSING DIAGNOSIS: Fluid volume excess: The state in which an individual experiences increased fluid retention and edema

Defining Characteristics

See Table 38–6 on page 1073.

Related Factors

Excessive fluid intake (eg, excessive intravenous infusions); excessive sodium intake; compromised regulatory mechanism; increased loss or decreased intake of protein; specific drug therapies.

Sources: LJ Carpenito, *Nursing Diagnosis: Application to Clinical Practice*, 4th ed. (Philadelphia: Lippincott, 1992), pp. 379–90; M Gordon, *Manual of Nursing Diagnosis 1993–1994*, 6th ed. (St Louis: Mosby-Year Book, 1993), pp. 111–13; MJ Kim, GK McFarland, and AM McLane, *Pocket Guide to Nursing Diagnoses*, 5th ed. (St Louis: Mosby-Year Book, 1993), pp. 23–29; GK McFarland and EA McFarlane, *Nursing Diagnosis and Intervention: Planning for Patient Care*, 2d ed. (St Louis: Mosby, 1993), pp. 151–52; North American Nursing Diagnosis Association, *NANDA Nursing Diagnoses: Definitions and Classification 1992–1993*, (Philadelphia: NANDA, 1992), pp. 23–24; and JR Lederer, GL Marculescu, B Mocnik, and N Seaby, *Care Planning Pocket Guide—A Nursing Diagnosis Approach*, 5th ed. (Redwood City, CA: Addison-Wesley Nursing, 1993), pp. 76–80.

---

give a falsely high specific gravity include dextran, radiographic contrast material, and some medications. Normal specific gravity ranges from 1.005 to 1.030 (usually 1.010 to 1.025).

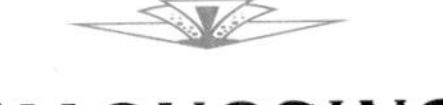

DIAGNOSING

NANDA nursing diagnoses that relate to fluid and electrolyte imbalances include the following:

- **Fluid volume deficit**
- **High risk for fluid volume deficit**
- **Fluid volume excess**

These diagnoses, with definitions, contributing factors, and defining characteristics, are shown in the box above. Clinical applications of these diagnoses are shown in Table 38–12 on the previous page.

Fluid and electrolyte imbalances affect many other body areas and as a consequence may be the etiology of many other nursing diagnoses. Examples follow:

- **Altered oral mucous membrane** related to fluid volume deficit
- **Impaired skin integrity** related to dehydration and/or edema
- **Decreased cardiac output** related to hypovolemia
- **Altered tissue perfusion** related to decreased cardiac output secondary to fluid volume deficit
- **Altered tissue perfusion** related to edema
- **Decreased cardiac output** related to cardiac dysrhythmias secondary to electrolyte imbalance (K^+)

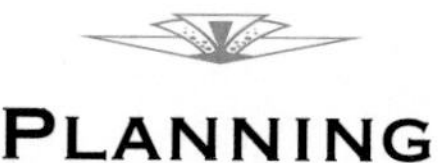

PLANNING

The major outcomes for clients with actual or potential fluid and electrolyte imbalances are to regain adequate fluid and electrolyte balance and to avoid potential associated risks, such as skin breakdown, loss of tissue integrity, and decreased cardiac output. Specific outcome criteria, nursing interventions, and rationales are presented in the accompanying Care Planning Guide.

A critical pathway can also be useful for planning client care (see p. 1122).

CARE PLANNING GUIDE
CLIENTS WITH FLUID/ELECTROLYTE PROBLEMS*

NURSING DIAGNOSIS: Fluid volume deficit or High risk for fluid volume deficit

Outcome Criteria	Nursing Interventions	Rationale
The client		
▪ Experiences a reduction or alleviation of the causative fluid loss factor, as evidenced by decrease in amount of or absence of emeses, diarrhea, or wound drainage.	Assess and document amount, color, and characteristics of vomitus, diarrhea, and drainage from wounds or tubes.	Accurate assessment enables the nurse to develop appropriate plans for fluid replacement therapy.
	Assess vital signs, weight, and skin turgor.	
	Administer medications as ordered to prevent further fluid loss.	Medications such as antiemetics or antidiarrheals may be necessary to reduce or eliminate fluid losses.
▪ Has a balanced fluid intake and output (averaging 2500 mL per day) for 3 days.	Measure and document fluid intake and output.	Measuring intake and output allows the nurse to determine fluid balance or extent of imbalance.
	Encourage oral fluid intake as permitted. Schedule amounts to be ingested during each shift (see page 1089).	Scheduling specific amounts for each shift helps the client achieve short-term goals.
	Provide at the bedside oral fluids that the client prefers.	Fluid intake may be greater when desired fluids are provided.
	Report and document an output under 30 to 60 mL/h.	This rate of output may not be sufficient to excrete required metabolic wastes and to sustain life. It may reflect decreased blood volume and decreased blood flow to the kidneys.
▪ Manifests clinical signs of adequate hydration: a. Normal vital signs for age, sex, and health status.	Monitor vital signs every 1 to 2 hours or as the client's condition indicates.	Hypotension and an increased pulse rate are indicative of intravascular fluid deficit.
b. Good skin turgor and color. c. Moist mucous membranes. d. Absence of thirst.	Assess skin and mucous membrane moisture, skin color and turgor, presence of thirst, and mental status.	Poor skin turgor, tissue dryness, and the presence of thirst are indications of dehydration.

*Criteria and nursing strategies must be individualized for each client, taking into consideration the client's health beliefs and preferences.

NURSING DIAGNOSIS: Fluid volume deficit or High risk for fluid volume deficit *continued*

Outcome Criteria	Nursing Interventions	Rationale
e. Orientation to time, place, and person.		
f. Normal urine color, characteristics, and specific gravity (1.010 to 1.025).	Measure specific gravity of urine q2h or as the client's condition indicates.	Dark concentrated urine and an elevated specific gravity are indicative of a fluid deficit with increased osmolality of body fluids, which releases antidiuretic hormone (ADH).
	If fluid loss is related to failure of a regulatory mechanism, assess urine for sugar and acetone, and monitor serum glucose and plasma volumes as indicated.	These parameters measure the extent of regulatory mechanism failure (in this case, pancreatic function associated with diabetes mellitus).
g. Stable weight.	Weigh the client at the same time each day with the same amount of clothing.	A stable body weight is a measure of body fluid balance.
▪ Has serum osmolality, hemoglobin, and hematocrit within normal limits.	Monitor serum osmolality, hemoglobin, and hematocrit levels.	An increased serum osmolality and an elevated hemoglobin and hematocrit are indicative of intravascular fluid volume deficit.
▪ Identifies reasons for fluid deficit and the amounts and type of food and fluids to consume to prevent a recurrence.	Assess knowledge base of client/family. Provide information about causes of fluid volume deficit, reasons for prescribed therapy, and prevention of recurrences.	Client's understanding of condition and preventive measures may facilitate necessary follow-up care.

NURSING DIAGNOSIS: Fluid volume excess

Outcome Criteria	Nursing Interventions	Rationale
The client		
▪ Has a balanced fluid intake and output (averaging 2500 mL/day) for 3 days.	Measure and document fluid intake and output.	Measuring intake and output enables the nurse to determine fluid balance or the extent of imbalance.
	Restrict fluid intake as ordered (see page 1089).	Restricting intake prevents an increase in signs associated with fluid retention (eg, dyspnea, and circulatory overload).
	Administer diuretics as ordered.	Diuretics are given to promote urine output and fluid loss.
▪ Loses specified amount of body weight within 1 week and then maintains stable body weight.	Weigh the client daily at the same time with the same amount of clothing.	A gradual loss in weight accompanies a reduction in fluid retention.
▪ Regains normal hydration status, as manifested by		
a. Hemodynamic status within normal limits for the client (blood pressure, central venous pressure, and absence of jugular vein distention).	Monitor hemodynamic status every 1 or 2 hours or as the client's condition warrants.	This allows the nurse to determine desired changes (decreases) in blood pressure, central venous pressure, and jugular vein distention.

➤

FLUID/ELECTROLYTE PROBLEMS CONTINUED

NURSING DIAGNOSIS: Fluid volume excess *continued*

Outcome Criteria	Nursing Interventions	Rationale
b. Clear breath sounds, respiratory rate within normal limits, regular rhythm, and freedom from dyspnea or shortness of breath.	Auscultate the lungs, ask client about dyspnea and shortness of breath, observe the respiratory rate rhythm and depth, and note the position client assumes for ease of breathing.	Abnormal lung sounds, shortness of breath, and orthopnea are indicative of excess fluid in the lungs.
c. Gradual reduction in edema.	Inspect and palpate areas of edema (periorbital, sacral, peripheral).	Accurate assessment and documentation of edema are essential to evaluate effects of therapy.
	Measure circumference of ankle edema.	
	Document location and degree of edema on a scale of +1 to +4 (see Chapter 22, p. 476).	
▪ Maintains skin integrity over edematous areas.	Provide pillow supports to edematous extremities, and elevate edematous extremities above heart level whenever possible.	Pillow supports reduce pressure on edematous skin. Elevation promotes venous circulation and reduces edema.
	Provide proper skin care to edematous areas (use soap sparingly, thoroughly rinse soap from skin, and apply lotions to skin).	Soap has a drying effect. Lotion moistens the skin and maintains its resiliency.
	Inspect the skin for redness and blanching.	These signs indicate impaired blood circulation.
▪ Has electrolyte levels within normal limits.	Monitor serum electrolytes, hemoglobin and hematocrit.	A decreased hemoglobin and hematocrit may indicate intravascular fluid volume excess. An elevated sodium level supports fluid retention. Serum sodium may be decreased with excessive fluid retention.
▪ Identifies reasons for fluid excess and the amounts and types of food and fluid to consume to prevent a recurrence.	Assess knowledge of condition.	Client's understanding of condition and preventive measures may facilitate necessary follow-up care.
	Provide information about causes of volume excess, reasons for prescribed therapy, and how to prevent recurrence (eg, by eating a low-salt diet), and side effects of medications.	

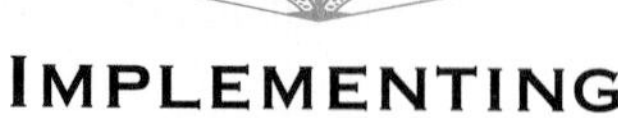

IMPLEMENTING

ORAL FLUIDS AND ELECTROLYTES

Fluids and electrolytes can be provided orally in the home and hospital if the client's health permits, that is, if the client is not vomiting, has not experienced an excessive fluid loss, and has an intact gastrointestinal tract. Some clients who are unable to ingest solid foods are often able to ingest fluids.

Fluids *Increased* fluids (ordered as "push fluids") are often prescribed for clients with actual or potential fluid volume deficits arising, for example, from mild diarrhea or mild to moderate fevers. Clients recovering from anesthesia and certain types of surgery (eg, bladder surgery)

CLINICAL GUIDELINES

Facilitating Fluid Intake

- Explain to the client the reason for the required intake and the specific amount needed. This gives the client a rationale for the requirement and promotes compliance.
- Establish a 24-hour plan for ingesting the fluids. Generally, half of the total volume is ingested during the day shift, and the other half is divided between the evening and night shifts, with the majority ingested during the evening shift. For example, if 2500 mL is to be ingested in 24 hours, the plan may specify 7–3 (1500 mL); 3–11 (700 mL); and 11–7 (300 mL. Try to avoid the ingestion of large amounts of fluid immediately before bedtime to prevent the need to urinate during sleeping hours.
- Set short-term outcomes that the client can realistically meet. Examples include ingesting a glass of fluid every hour while awake or a pitcher of water by 12 noon.
- Identify fluids or fluidlike substances the client likes and make available a variety of those items, including fruit juices, tea, coffee, and milk (if allowed).
- Help clients to select foods that tend to become liquid at room temperature (eg, gelatin, ice cream, sherbert, custard), if these are allowed.
- For clients who are confined to bed, supply appropriate cups, glasses, and straws to facilitate appropriate fluid intake and keep the fluids within easy reach.
- Make sure fluids are served at the appropriate temperature: hot fluids hot and cold fluids iced and cold.
- Encourage clients when possible to participate in maintaining the fluid intake record. This assists them to evaluate the achievement of preestablished outcomes.
- Be alert for the cultural implications of food and fluids. Some cultures may restrict certain foods and fluids and view others as having healing properties.

are also commonly given only clear liquids initially and then, if these are tolerated, are advanced to a regular diet. Guidelines for helping clients increase fluid intake are shown in the box above.

Restricted fluids may be necessary for clients who have fluid retention (fluid volume excess) as a result of renal failure, congestive heart failure, syndrome of inappropriate antidiuretic hormone (SIADH), or other disease processes. Fluid restrictions vary from "nothing by mouth" to a precise amount ordered by a physician. In addition, the client may be limited to only clear fluids (see Chapter 37, p. 1040). The restriction of fluids can be difficult for some clients, particularly if they are experiencing thirst. Guidelines for helping clients restrict fluid intake are shown in the box at the right.

CLINICAL GUIDELINES

Helping Clients Restrict Fluid Intake

- Explain the reason for the restricted intake and how much and what types of fluids are permitted orally. Many clients need to be informed that ice chips, gelatin, and ice cream, for example, are considered fluid.
- Help the client decide the amount of fluid to be taken with each meal, between meals, before bedtime, and with medications. Generally, half the total volume is scheduled during the day shift, when the client is most active, receives two meals, and often most oral medications. A large part of the remainder is scheduled for the evening shift to permit fluids with meals and evening visitors.
- Identify fluids or fluidlike substances the client likes and make sure that these are provided, unless contraindicated. A client who is allowed only 200 mL of fluid for breakfast, for example, should receive the type of fluid the client favors.
- Set short-term goals that make the fluid restriction more tolerable. For example, schedule a specified amount of fluid at one or two hourly intervals between meals. Some clients may prefer fluids between meals only since the food provided at mealtime may help relieve feelings of thirst.
- Provide the client with small fluid containers that make the container appear to contain more fluid than it actually does.
- Periodically offer the client ice chips as an alternative to water, since ice chips when melted are approximately one-half of the frozen volume.
- Help clients to rinse their mouths with water if they can do so without swallowing the fluid.
- Ensure meticulous oral care.
- Instruct the client to avoid ingesting or chewing salty or sweet foods (hard candy or gum), since these foods tend to produce thirst. Sugarless gum may be an alternative for some clients.
- Encourage the client when possible to participate in maintaining the fluid intake record.

Foods Specific fluid and electrolyte imbalances may require simple dietary changes. For example, clients receiving potassium-depleting diuretics are commonly given potassium supplements. In addition, the client needs to be informed about foods with a high potassium content (eg, bananas, oranges, and leafy greens). Some clients with fluid retention due to hypernatremia need to avoid foods high in sodium. Most healthy clients can benefit from foods high in calcium. Nurses can often help clients by

Table 38–13 Selected Intravenous Solutions

Type/Example	Nursing Interventions
Isotonic	
Normal (0.9%) saline D5W (acts as a hypotonic solution in the body) Lactated Ringer's solution	Isotonic solutions expand the intravascular compartment. Monitor clients for fluid overload. Avoid D5W if client is at risk of increased intracranial pressure (ICP) because it moves from the intravascular to the intracellular compartment (ie, into the brain cells).
Hypotonic	
0.33% saline 0.45% saline 2.5 % dextrose	Monitor the client carefully. These solutions shift fluid from the intravascular compartment into the cells. Hypotonic solutions are contraindicated for clients with increased intracranial pressure because of fluid shift into the brain cells. Hypotonic solutions are contraindicated for clients at risk of third-space fluid shifts (movement of fluid into the interstitial compartments or body cavities).
Hypertonic	
5% dextrose in 0.45% saline 5% dextrose in normal saline 5% dextrose in lactated Ringer's	Monitor clients closely for circulatory overload, because these solutions expand the intravascular compartment. These solutions are contraindicated for clients who have kidney and heart problems. These solutions are contraindicated for clients who are dehydrated because the solutions draw fluid from the cells to the intravascular compartment.

Source: Adapted from L Gasparis, EB Murray, and P Ursomanno, IV solutions—which one's right for your patient? *Nursing89*, April 1989,

giving them a list of foods and fluids high in the electrolytes they require or need to avoid.

INTRAVENOUS INFUSIONS

Intravenous (IV) fluid therapy is a common practice. It is an efficient and effective method of supplying fluids directly into the intravascular fluid compartment. Intravenous fluid therapy is usually ordered by the physician. The nurse is responsible for administering and maintaining the therapy and for teaching the client and significant others how to continue the therapy at home.

INTRAVENOUS SOLUTIONS

Intravenous solutions can be classified as isotonic, hypotonic, or hypertonic. Most IV solutions are **isotonic,** having the same concentration of solutes (osmolarity) as blood plasma. This prevents sudden shifts of fluids and electrolytes in the body. In some instances, however, hypertonic or hypotonic solutions are infused intravascularly. **Hypertonic** solutions have a greater concentration of solutes than plasma; **hypotonic** solutions have a lesser concentration of solutes. An example of hypertonic solution is 5% dextrose in normal saline (D5NS). See Table 38–13 for selected IV solutions.

IV solutions can also be categorized according to their purpose. *Nutrient solutions* contain some form of carbohydrate (eg dextrose, glucose, or levulose) and water. Water is supplied for fluid requirements and carbohydrate for calories and energy. For example, 1 liter of 5% dextrose provides 170 calories. Nutrient solutions are useful in preventing dehydration and ketosis but do not provide sufficient calories to promote wound healing, weight gain, or normal growth in children. Common nutrient solutions are 5% dextrose in water (D5W) and 5% dextrose in 0.45% sodium chloride (dextrose in half-strength saline).

Electrolyte solutions contain varying amounts of cations and anions. Commonly used solutions are normal saline (0.9% sodium chloride solution), Ringer's solution (which contains sodium, chloride, potassium, and calcium), and lactated Ringer's solution (which contains sodium, chloride, potassium, calcium, and lactate). Lactate is a salt of lactic acid that is metabolized in the liver to form bicarbonate (HCO_3^-). Saline solutions are frequently used as initial hydrating solutions. Multiple electrolyte solutions approximate the ionic profile of plasma and are used to prevent dehydration or to restore or correct fluid and electrolyte imbalances.

Alkalizing solutions are administered to counteract metabolic acidosis. One commonly used solution is lactated Ringer's solution. *Acidifying solutions*, in contrast, are administered to counteract metabolic alkalosis. Examples of acidifying solutions are 5% dextrose in 0.45% sodium chloride and 0.9% sodium chloride solution.

Blood volume expanders are used to increase the volume of blood following severe loss of blood (eg, from hemorrhage) or loss of plasma (eg, from severe burns, which draw large amounts of plasma from the bloodstream to the burn site). Common blood volume expanders are dextran, plasma, and human serum albumin.

PERIPHERAL VENIPUNCTURE SITES

The site chosen for venipuncture varies with the client's age, the length of time the infusion is to run, the type of solution used, and the condition of veins. For adults, veins in the arm are commonly used; for infants, veins in the scalp and dorsal foot veins are often used. The larger veins of the forearm are preferred to the metacarpal veins of the hand for infusions that need to be given rapidly and for solutions that could be irritating (eg, certain medications).

The most convenient veins for venipuncture in the adult are the basilic and median cubital veins in the crease of the elbow, that is, the antecubital space (Figure 38–10, *A*). Technicians often withdraw blood for examination from these large superficial veins. Unfortunately, use of these veins for prolonged infusions limits arm mobility, because a splint is needed to stabilize the elbow joint. For prolonged therapy and when repeated venipunctures will be required, the veins on the back of the hand and on the forearm are preferred. The metacarpal, basilic, and cephalic veins are commonly used (Figure 38–10, *B*). The ulna and radius act as natural splints at these sites, and the client has greater freedom of arm movements for activities such as eating. If an infusion is to be maintained for a long period, veins in the back of the hand or the dorsum of the foot are used (Figure 38–10, *C*). See the box on page 1092 for clinical guidelines for vein selection.

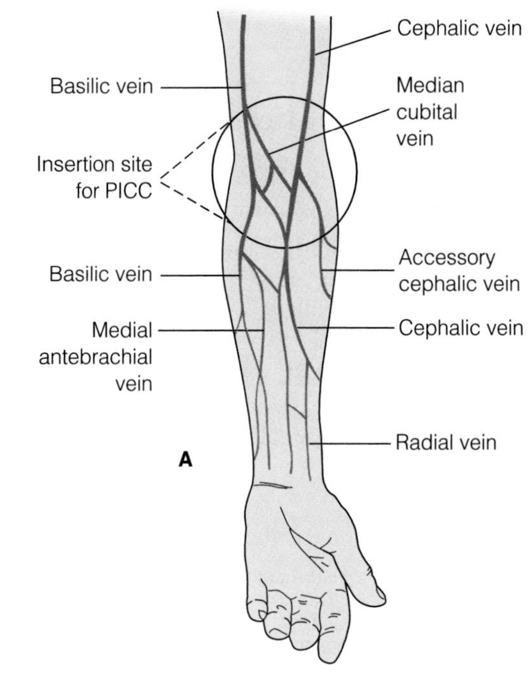

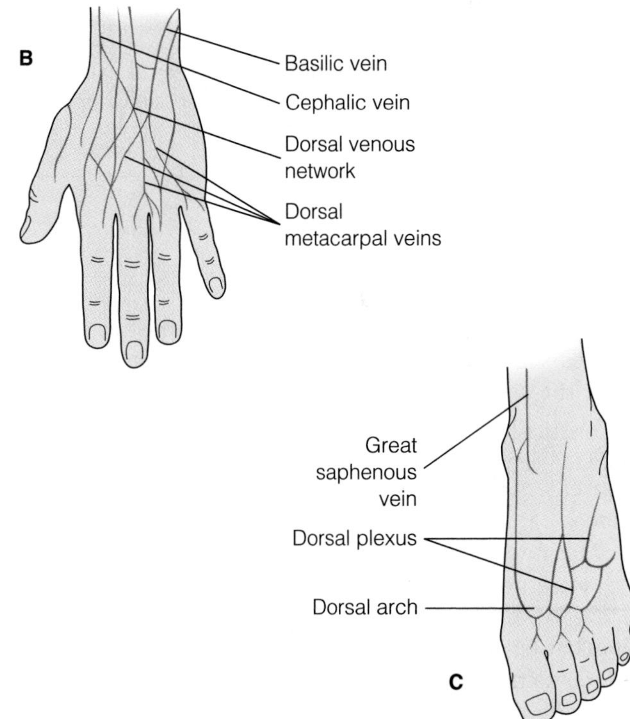

Figure 38–10 Commonly used venipuncture sites of the *A*, arm; *B*, hand; *C*, foot. *A* shows also the site used for a peripherally inserted central catheter (PICC).

INTRAVENOUS EQUIPMENT

Because equipment varies according to the manufacturer, the nurse must become familiar with the equipment used in each particular agency.

Solution containers are available in various sizes (50, 100, 250, 500, or 1000 mL); the smaller containers are often used to administer medications. Most solutions are currently dispensed in plastic bags (Figure 38–11, p. 1092). However, glass containers may need to be used if the administered medications are incompatible with plastic. Glass containers require an air vent so that air can replace the fluid that enters the client's vein. Some have a tube inside the bottle that serves as a vent; other containers

CLINICAL GUIDELINES

Vein Selection

- Use distal veins of the arm first.
- Use the client's nondominant arm whenever possible.
- Use veins in the feet and legs only when arm veins are inaccessible, since they are more prone to thrombus formation and subsequent emboli.
- Select a vein that:
  a. Is easily palpated and feels soft and full.
  b. Is naturally splinted by bone.
  c. Is large enough to allow adequate circulation around the catheter.

Avoid using the following veins:

- Those in areas of flexion (eg, the antecubital fossa).
- Those that are highly visible, since they tend to roll away from the needle.
- Those damaged by previous use, phlebitis, infiltration, or sclerosis.
- Those continually distended with blood or that have become knotted or tortuous.
- Veins of a surgically compromised or injured extremity (eg, following a mastectomy) because of possible impaired circulation and discomfort for the client.

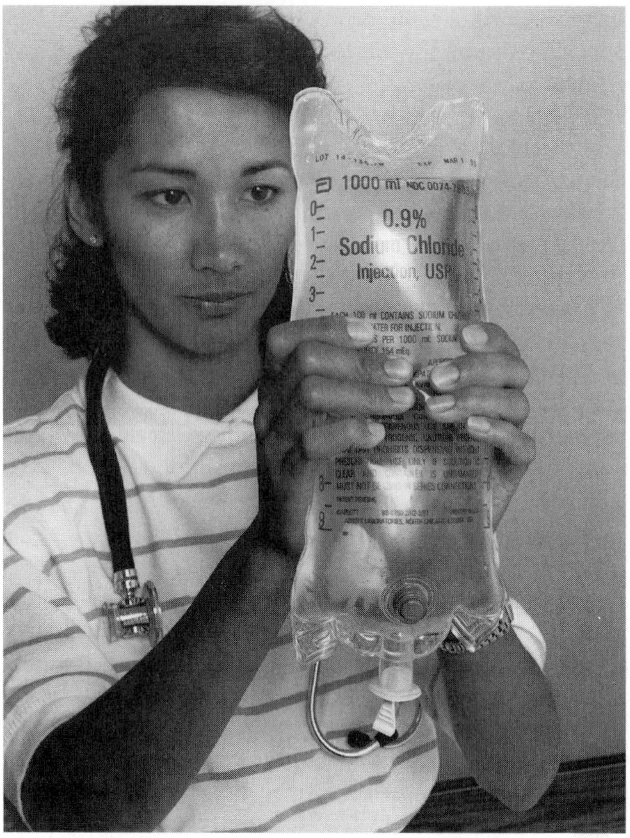

Figure 38–11 A plastic intravenous fluid container.

without air vents require a vent on the administration set. Air vents usually have filters to remove any contamination from the air that enters the container. Air vents are not required for plastic solution containers, because plastic bags collapse under atmospheric pressure when the solution enters the vein. See Figures 43–44 and 43–46 on page 1335.

The nurse should avoid selecting a container whose volume is greater than the volume ordered. For example, if 750 mL D5NS (750 mL of 5% dextrose in normal saline) has been ordered, the nurse should obtain one 500-mL container and one 250-mL container, which total 750 mL. The nurse should not obtain a 1000-mL container with the intention of stopping the solution after 750 mL has been administered. Too often, the incorrect amount can be instilled unless an electronic device is used to regulate the volume. If a 1000-mL solution container *must* be used, the nurse should remove 250 mL before starting the infusion. Note that some agencies use abbreviations to describe commonly used solutions, for example, NS (normal saline), D5W (5% dextrose in water), D5NS (5% dextrose in normal saline). The nurse should therefore become familiar with the abbreviations used by the agency.

It is essential that the solution be sterile and in good condition, that is, clear. Cloudiness, evidence that the container has been opened previously, or leaks indicate possible contamination. The nurse should also check the expiration date on the label and squeeze and inspect plastic solution bags for leaks or hairline cracks. The nurse must return any unsatisfactory container to the central supply or distributing department, indicating the reason for the return.

Infusion sets usually include an insertion spike, a drip chamber, a roller valve or screw clamp, tubing, and a protective cap over the needle adapter (Figure 38–12). The insertion spike is kept sterile and inserted into the solution container when the equipment is set up and ready to start. The drip chamber permits a predictable amount of fluid to be delivered. A commonly used drip chamber is the macrodrip, which delivers 10 to 20 drops per milliliter of solution. This information is found on the package. There are also microdrip sets, which deliver 60 drops per milliliter of solution. The roller valve or screw clamp, which compresses the lumen of the tubing, controls the rate of the flow. The protective cap over the needle adapter maintains the sterility of the end of the tubing so that it can be attached to a sterile needle inserted in the client's vein.

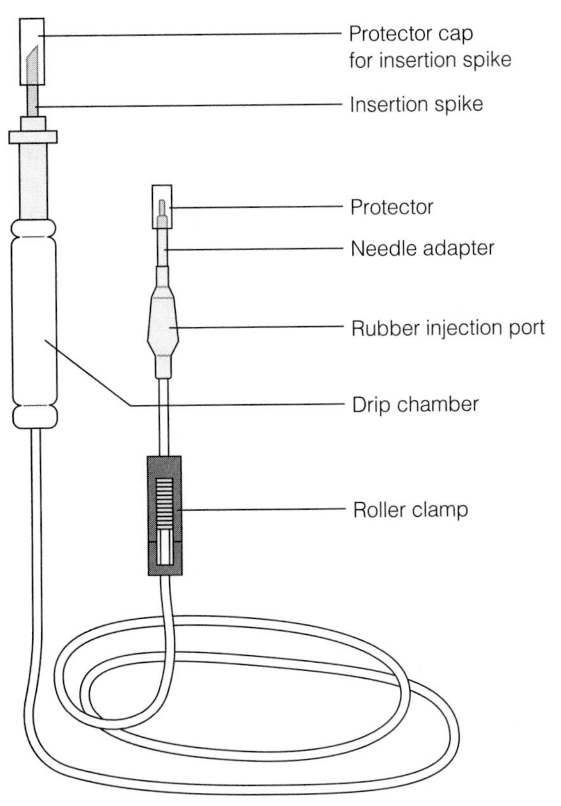

Figure 38–12 Schematic of a standard infusion set.

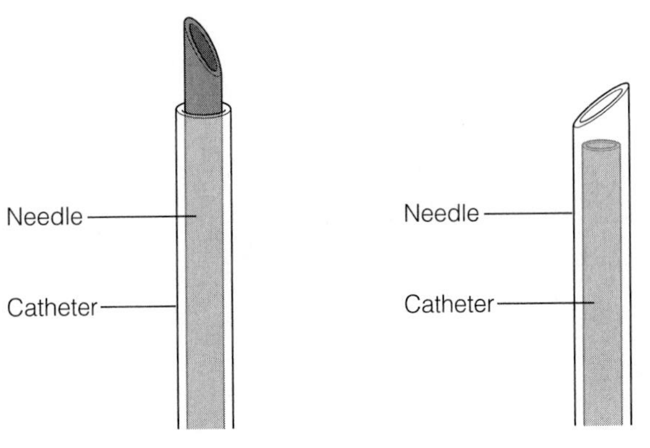

Figure 38–13 Schematic of an over-the-needle catheter and an inside-the-needle catheter.

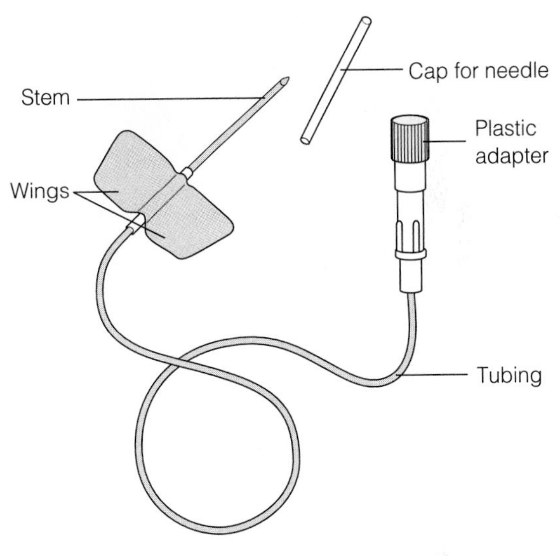

Figure 38–14 Schematic of a butterfly needle with adapter.

A **sterile injection cap** can be attached to an existing intravenous catheter to keep the venous access available for the administration of intermittent or emergency medication when a continuous infusion is not required. The device is commonly referred to as an intravenous lock (a *heparin* or *saline lock*). Heparin or saline is usually injected periodically to keep blood from coagulating within the tubing. The lock consists of small plastic tubing with one self-sealing end into which medications can be injected. The other end is inserted into the intravenous catheter. See Chapter 43, page 1333.

When selecting an appropriate administration set, the nurse must consider several factors:

- *Vents.* Tubing appropriate for either the rigid or flexible container should be selected.
- *Drop size.* For accurate regulation, a *microdrip* set is usually required if the fluid is to be administered at a rate of 50 to 70 mL/h or less; a *macrodrip* should be selected when large quantities of solution or fast rates are required.
- *IV ports.* Ports are required to administer secondary infusions and medications.
- *Volumetric chamber.* This will be required if small doses of medications or fluid are to be delivered over an extended period of time.

Catheters and *needles* are commonly used for intravenous infusions. An intravenous catheter (intracath) is a plastic tube inserted into the vein. Some catheters fit over a needle during insertion, whereas others fit inside a needle (Figure 38–13). An *angiocatheter* has a metal stylet (needle) which pierces the skin and vein and is then withdrawn, leaving the catheter in place.

Butterfly, or wing-tipped, *needles* with plastic flaps attached to the shaft are sometimes used (Figure 38–14). The flaps are held tightly together to hold the needle securely during insertion; after insertion, they are flattened against the skin and secured with tape.

A *vein finder* can be used to locate hard-to-find veins. For example, the Landry Vein Light uses a bright light that comes from two fiberoptic arms to reveal the client's vein (Figure 38–15, p. 1094). The light is strapped to the client's arm, and the room light is dimmed. The light on the finder is turned to its brightest setting, and the finder is moved along the arm below the tourniquet to search for

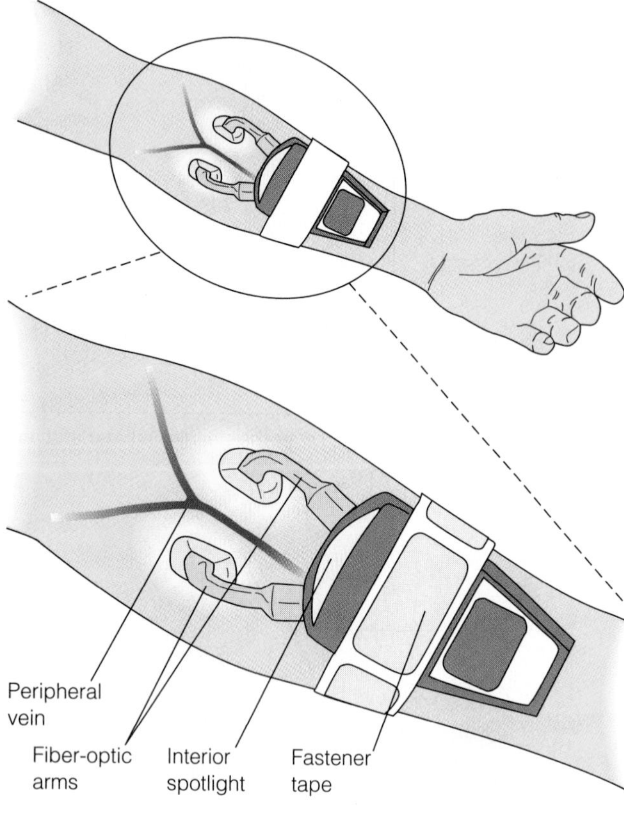

Figure 38–15 A vein finder.

a vein. The vein will appear as a dark line between the arms of the finder.

IV filters are increasingly being used to remove air, particulate matter, and microbes from intravenous infusions and to reduce the risk of contamination and complications such as, infusion-related **phlebitis** associated with routine intravenous therapies. In addition, most agencies advise use of a filter if the infusion contains potassium chloride (KCl) or if the site is to be used for medication administration. Although all clients may benefit from the use of filters, the Intravenous Nurse Society (INS) recommends them for clients at risk (eg, those receiving longterm infusion therapy, total parenteral nutrition [discussed later in this chapter] and intra-arterial infusion chemotherapy). Further research to prove the value of filters in preventing clinical infection is needed.

Most IV filters in current use consist of membrane (pore size of 0.22 μm, although sizes vary). Ideally, the filter should be located within the intravenous line as close to the venipuncture site as possible (Crow 1987, p. 101).

IV poles (rods) are needed to hang the solution container. Some poles are attached to hospital beds; others stand on the floor or hang from the ceiling. Still others are floor models with casters that can be pushed along when a client is up and walking. The height of most poles is adjustable. The higher the solution container, the greater the force of the solution as it enters the client and the faster the rate of flow.

STARTING AN INTRAVENOUS INFUSION

Agency practices vary about which nurses perform venipunctures and start intravenous infusions. In many settings, nurses must be supervised and certified before they are permitted to start infusions on their own. Some agencies have teams of specially prepared nurses who initiate all intravenous infusions. Before starting an infusion, the nurse must determine the following:

- The exact orders.
- Whether the client has any allergies, for example, to tape or povidone-iodine.
- The agency protocol about shaving the area before a venipuncture. Some agencies advise against shaving because of the possibility of nicking the skin and subsequent infection.

To perform venipuncture and start an intravenous infusion, see Procedure 38–1.

Text continued on page 1099

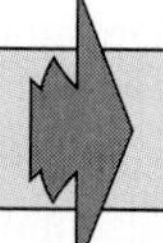

PROCEDURE 38–1 STARTING AN INTRAVENOUS INFUSION

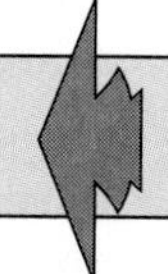

Before preparing the infusion, the nurse first verifies the physician's order indicating the type of solution; the amount to be administered; the rate of flow of the infusion; and any client allergies (eg, to tape or povidone-iodine).

PURPOSES

- To supply fluid when clients are unable to take in an adequate volume of fluids by mouth
- To provide salts needed to maintain electrolyte balance

PROCEDURE 38–1 *continued*

- To provide glucose (dextrose), the main fuel for metabolism
- To provide water-soluble vitamins and medications
- To establish a lifeline for rapidly needed medications

ASSESSMENT FOCUS
Vital signs (pulse, respiratory rate, and blood pressure) for baseline data; skin turgor; allergy to tape or iodine; bleeding tendencies; disease or injury to extremities and status of veins to determine appropriate venipuncture site.

EQUIPMENT

- ☐ Infusion set
- ☐ Container of sterile parenteral solution
- ☐ IV pole
- ☐ Adhesive or nonallergenic tape
- ☐ Clean gloves
- ☐ Tourniquet
- ☐ Antiseptic swabs
- ☐ Antiseptic ointment, such as povidone-iodine (Betadine)
- ☐ Intravenous catheter (over-the-needle catheter, through-the-needle catheter, angiocatheter). See Variation at end of this procedure for butterfly (winged-tip) needle
- ☐ Gauze squares or other appropriate dressings
- ☐ Arm splint, if required
- ☐ Towel or pad
- ☐ Electronic infusion device or pump, as ordered

INTERVENTION

1. Prepare the client.

- Explain the procedure to the client. A venipuncture can cause discomfort for a few seconds, but there should be no discomfort while the solution is flowing. Use a doll to demonstrate for children, and explain the procedure to the parents. Clients often want to know how long the process will last. The physician's order may specify the length of time of the infusion, for example, 3000 mL over 24 hours.
- Provide any scheduled care before establishing the infusion to minimize movement of the affected limb during the procedure. *Moving the limb after the infusion has been established could dislodge the needle.*
- Make sure that the client's gown can be removed over the IV apparatus if necessary. Some agencies provide special gowns that open over the shoulder and down the sleeve for easy removal.
- Wash hands.

2. Open and prepare the infusion set.

- Remove tubing from the container, and straighten it out.
- Slide the tubing clamp along the tubing until it is just below the drip chamber to facilitate its access.
- Close the clamp.
- Leave the ends of the tubing covered with the plastic caps until the infusion is started. *This will maintain the sterility of the ends of the tubing.*

3. Spike the solution container.

- Remove the protective cover from the entry site of the bag.

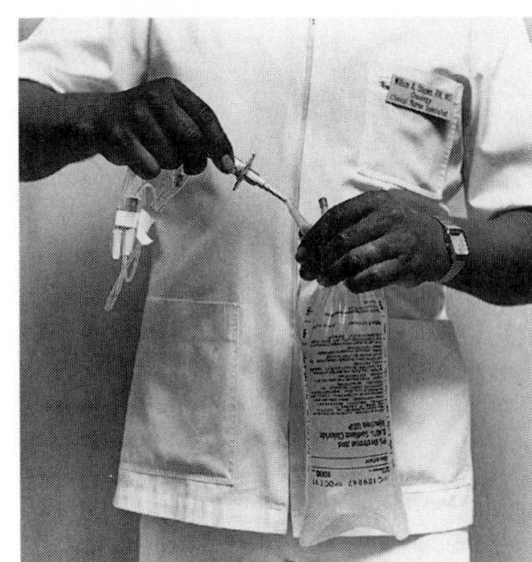

Figure 38–16 Inserting the spike.

- Remove the cap from the spike, and insert the spike into the insertion site of the bag or bottle (Figure 38–16). Follow manufacturer's instructions.
- See Procedure 43–6 for adding medications to an intravenous fluid container, p. 1333.

PROCEDURE 38–1 STARTING AN INTRAVENOUS INFUSION *continued*

4. Hang the solution container on the pole.

- Adjust the pole so that the container is suspended about 1 m (3 ft) above the client's head. *This height is needed to enable gravity to overcome venous pressure and facilitate flow of the solution into the vein.*

5. Partially fill the drip chamber with solution.

For a Flexible Drip Chamber

- Squeeze the chamber gently until it is half full of solution (Figure 38–17).

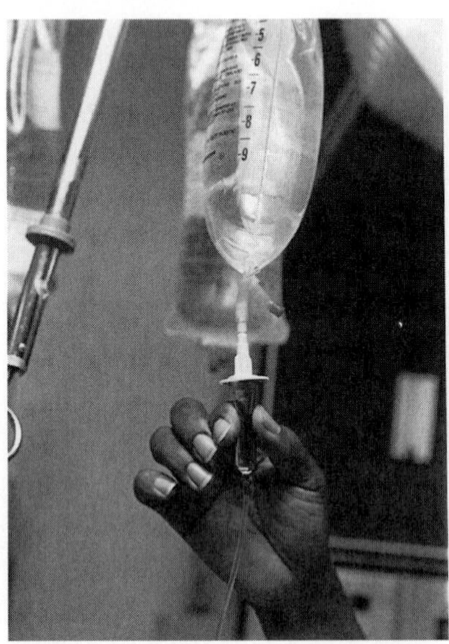

Figure 38–17 Squeezing the drip chamber.

For a Firm Drip Chamber

- The chamber will usually fill automatically. *The drip chamber is partly filled with solution to prevent air from moving down the tubing.*

6. Prime the tubing.

- Remove the protective cap, and hold the tubing over a container. Maintain the sterility of the end of the tubing and the cap.
- Release the clamp, and let the fluid run through the tubing until all bubbles are removed. Tap the tubing if necessary with your fingers to help the bubbles move. *The tubing is primed to prevent the introduction of air into the client. Air bubbles in large amounts (eg, 10 mL) can act as emboli in the bloodstream. Air bubbles smaller than 0.5 mL usually do not cause problems in peripheral lines* (Millam 1991, p. 75).
- Reclamp the tubing, and replace the tubing cap, maintaining sterile technique.
- For caps with air vents, do not remove the cap when priming this tubing. The flow of solution through the tubing will cease when the cap is moist with one drop of solution.
- If an infusion control pump, electronic device, or controller is being used, follow the manufacturer's directions for inserting the tubing and setting the infusion rate.

7. Apply appropriate labels to the solution container. Include the client's name, date, and note time infusion started.

- In many agencies, medications and labels are applied in the pharmacy; if they are not, apply the label upside down on the container (see Figure 43–42 on p. 1334). *The label is applied upside down so it can be read easily when the container is hanging up.*

8. Apply a timing label on the solution container.

- The timing label may be applied at the time the infusion is started. Follow agency practice. See discussion of regulating infusion flow rates and Figure 38–23 on page 1099.

9. Wash hands.

10. Select and prepare the venipuncture site.

- Starting at the distal end of the vein, select a site by palpating accessible veins. Veins can become sclerotic from irritation by the infusion or the needle. Sclerosis may then interfere with venous flow. If so, use more proximal parts of the veins.
- Check agency protocol about shaving if tape is to be applied on skin that has a great deal of hair.

11. Dilate the vein.

- Place the extremity in a dependent position (lower than the client's heart). *Gravity slows venous return and distends the veins. Distending the veins makes it easier to insert the needle properly.*
- Apply a tourniquet firmly 15 to 20 cm (6 to 8 in) above the venipuncture site. (Figure 38–18). For children, explain that the tourniquet will feel tight. The tourniquet must be tight enough to obstruct venous flow but not so tight that it occludes arterial flow. *Obstructing arterial flow inhibits venous filling.* If a radial pulse can be palpated, the arterial flow is not obstructed.

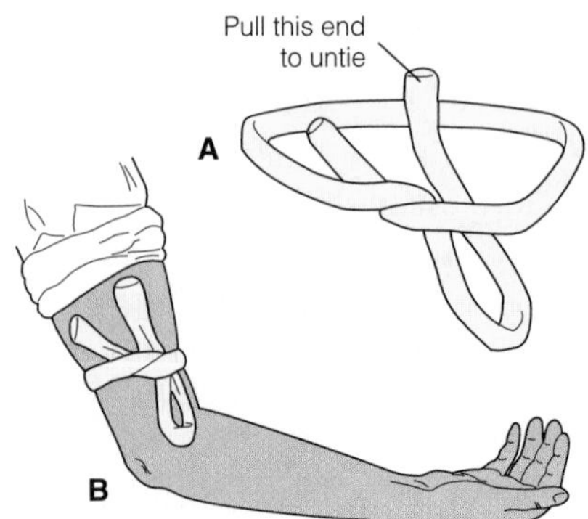

Figure 38–18 Applying a tourniquet.

PROCEDURE 38–1 *continued*

- If the vein is not sufficiently dilated,
  a. Massage or stroke the vein distal to the site and in the direction of venous flow toward the heart. *This action helps fill the vein.*
  b. Encourage the client to clench and unclench the fist rapidly. *Contracting the muscles compresses the distal veins, forcing blood along the veins and distending them.*
  c. Lightly tap the vein with your fingertips. *Tapping may distend the vein.*

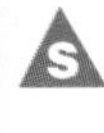

- If the above steps fail to distend the vein so that it is palpable, remove the tourniquet, and apply heat to the entire extremity for 10 to 15 minutes. *Heat dilates superficial blood vessels, causing them to fill.* Then repeat the steps above.

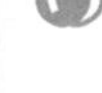

12. Don clean gloves, and clean the venipuncture site. *Gloves protect the nurse from contamination by the client's blood.*

- Clean the skin at the site of entry with a topical antiseptic swab, (eg, alcohol) and then an anti-infective solution such as povidone-iodine (Betadine).
- Use a circular motion, moving from the center outwards for several inches. *This motion carries microorganisms away from the site of entry.*
- Permit the solution to dry on the skin. *Povidine-iodine should be in contact with the skin for 1 minute to be effective.*

13. Insert the catheter, and initiate the infusion.

- Use one thumb to pull the skin taut below the entry site. *This stabilizes the vein and makes the skin taut for needle entry. It can also make initial tissue penetration less painful.*
- Insert the catheter by the direct or indirect method. The direct method is preferred for large veins and the indirect method for smaller veins (Peck 1985, p. 40). For the *direct method,* hold the over-the-needle catheter with bevel up, at a 15- to 30-degree angle, and insert the catheter through the skin and into the vein in one thrust. For the *indirect method,* hold the needle at a 30°- to 40-degree angle, pierce the skin, then reduce the angle until it is almost parallel to the skin and advance the needle into the vein. Sudden lack of resistance is felt as the needle enters the vein.
- Once blood appears in the lumen of the needle or you feel the lack of resistance, then advance the needle so that it is inserted 2.5 cm (1 in). *The catheter is advanced to ensure that it, and not just the metal needle, is in the vein.* The exact technique depends on the type of catheter used.
- Release the tourniquet.
- Remove the protective cap from the distal end of the tubing, and hold it ready to attach to the catheter, maintaining the sterility of the end.
- Attach the end of the infusion tubing to the catheter hub.
- Initiate the infusion.

14. Tape the catheter.

- Place a small-gauze dressing under the hub. *This will support the catheter in position.*
- Tape the catheter by the "U" method or according to manufacturer's instructions. Using three strips of adhesive tape, each about 7.5 cm (3 in) long:
  a. Place one strip, sticky side up, under the catheter's hub.
  b. Fold each end over so that the sticky sides are against the skin (Figure 38–19).
  c. Place second strip, sticky side down, over catheter hub.
  d. Place third strip, sticky side down, over tubing hub.

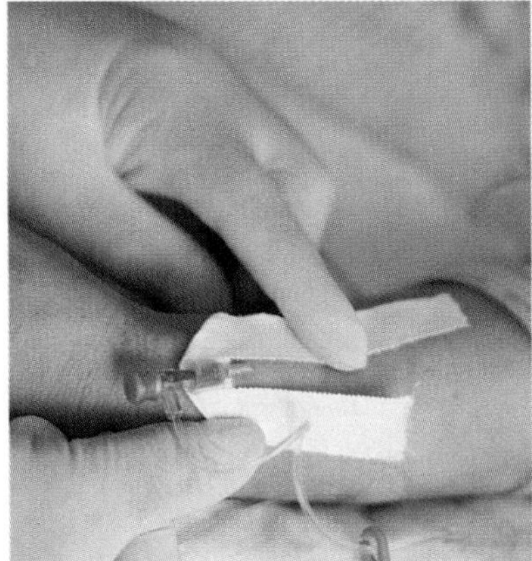

Figure 38–19 Taping an intravenous catheter by the "U" method.

15. Dress and label the venipuncture site and tubing according to agency policy.

- In some agencies, the nurse puts a small amount of antiseptic ointment, such as povidone-iodine, over the venipuncture site, then a gauze square. In other agencies, a sterile transparent occlusive dressing is applied after the ointment. This permits assessment of the site without disturbing the dressing. This type of dressing can be left on for 72 hours, then changed.
- Remove soiled gloves, and discard appropriately.
- Loop the tubing, and secure it to the dressing with tape. *Looping and securing the tubing prevent the*

PROCEDURE 38–1 STARTING AN INTRAVENOUS INFUSION *continued*

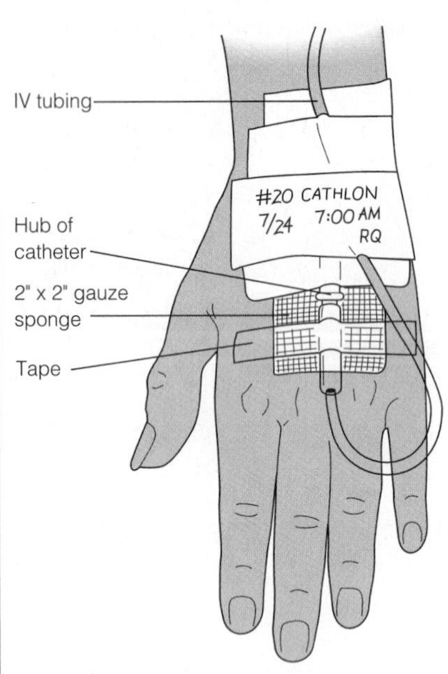

Figure 38–20 Labeled tape for a venipuncture dressing.

weight of the tubing or any movement from pulling on the needle or catheter.

- Label a piece of tape with the date and time of insertion, type and gauge of needle or catheter used, and your initials. Apply the tape label over the venipuncture dressing (Figure 38–20).

16. Ensure appropriate infusion flow.

- Apply a padded arm board (folded towel on a board) to splint the elbow or wrist joint, as needed.
- Adjust the infusion rate of flow according to the order.

17. Label the IV tubing.

- Label tubing with date; time of attachment, and initials (Figure 38–21). This labeling may also be done when the infusion is started. *The tubing is labeled to ensure that it is changed at regular intervals* (ie, every 24 to 72 hours according to agency policy).

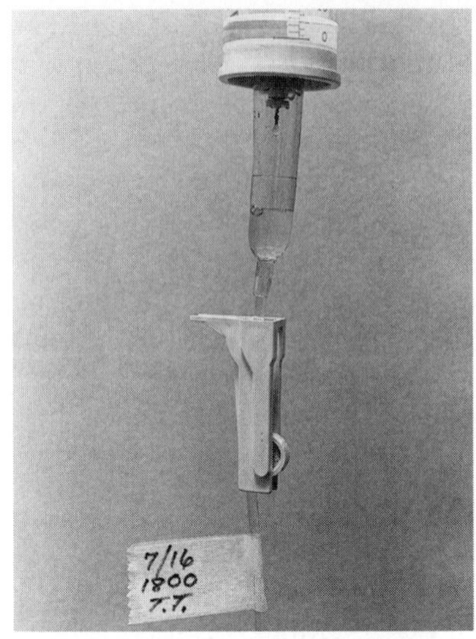

I.V. SET–72 HRS.–ONLY
START DATE 9/11 HR. 0800
DISCARD DATE 9/14 HR. 0800
R.N. INITIAL LA

Figure 38–21 Tubing labeled with date, time of attachment, and nurse's initials. Also shown is a preprinted label.

18. Document relevant data, including assessments.

- Record the start of the infusion on the client's chart. Some agencies provide a special form for this purpose. Include the date and time of the venipuncture; amount and type of solution used, including any additives (eg, kind and amount of medications); absorption time; container number; drip rate, type and gauge of the needle or catheter; venipuncture site; and client's general response.

Variation: Inserting a Butterfly (Winged-Tip) Needle

- Hold the needle, pointed in the direction of the blood flow, at a 30-degree angle, with the bevel up, and pierce the skin beside the vein about 1 cm (1/2 in) below the site planned for piercing the vein.
- Once the needle is through the skin, lower the needle so that it is almost parallel with the skin. *Lowering the needle reduces the chances of puncturing both sides of the vein.* Follow the course of the vein, and pierce one side of the vein.
- When blood flows back into the needle tubing, insert the needle farther up the vein 2 to 2.5 cm. (3/4 to 1 in) or to the hub of the butterfly needle. Sudden lack of resistance can be felt as blood enters the needle.
- Release the tourniquet, attach the infusion, and initiate flow as quickly as possible. *Attaching the tubing quickly prevents blood from clotting and obstructing the needle.*

Securing a Butterfly Needle

- Tape the butterfly needle securely by the crisscross (chevron) method (Figure 38–22). Place a

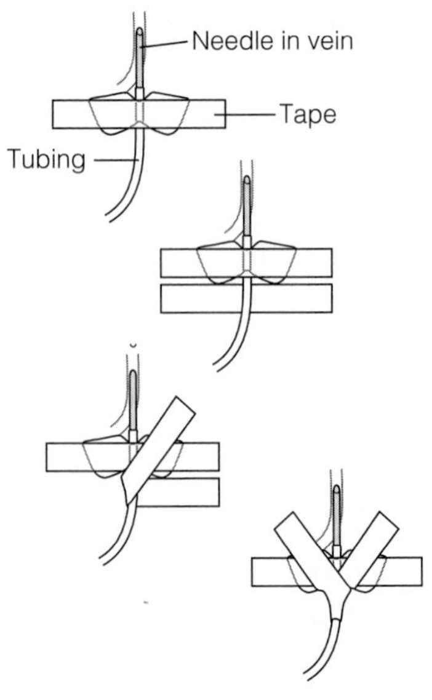

Figure 38–22 Taping the butterfly needle by the crisscross (chevron) method.

PROCEDURE 38–1 *continued*

cotton ball or small gauze square under the needle, if required. *The gauze keeps the needle in position in the vein.*

EVALUATION FOCUS
Skin status at IV site (warm temperature and absence of pain, redness, and swelling); status of dressing; IV flow rate consistent with that ordered; ability to perform self-care activities; understanding of any mobility limitations; vital signs compared to baseline level.

REGULATING INTRAVENOUS FLOW RATES

An important nursing function is to regulate the flow rate of an intravenous infusion. The physician usually describes in the order how long an infusion should last. The order may take several forms: "3000 mL over 24 hours"; "1000 mL over 8 hours × 3 bags"; "125 mL/h until po is adequate." The latter order means that the infusions are to continue until the client takes adequate fluid by mouth without problems. It is a nursing responsibility to calculate the correct flow rate and regulate the infusion. Problems that can result from incorrectly regulated infusions include hypervolemia and hypovolemia. Unless a regulating device (ie, a controller, infusion pump, or electronic infusion device) is being used, the nurse administering the intravenous solution must regulate the drops per minute manually by using the roller clamp to ensure that the prescribed amount of solution will be infused in the correct time span.

There are a number of commercially prepared infusion sets, each with its own type of drip chamber; so, it is important to know the number of drops per milliliter of solution for a particular drip chamber before calculating a drip rate. This rate, called the **drop** or **drip factor,** is printed on most commercially prepared packages. Common drop factors are 10, 15, and 20 for macrodrips (regular infusion sets) and 60 for microdrips (minidrip infusion sets).

To calculate flow rates, the nurse must know the volume of fluid to be infused and the specific time for the infusion. Two commonly used methods of indicating flow rates are designating the number of milliliters to be administered in 1 hour (mL/h) and the number of drops to be given in 1 minute (gtt/min). Since 1 milliliter of fluid displaces 1 cubic centimeter of space, the volume to be infused in the first method may also be designated as cubic centimeters per hour (cc/h).

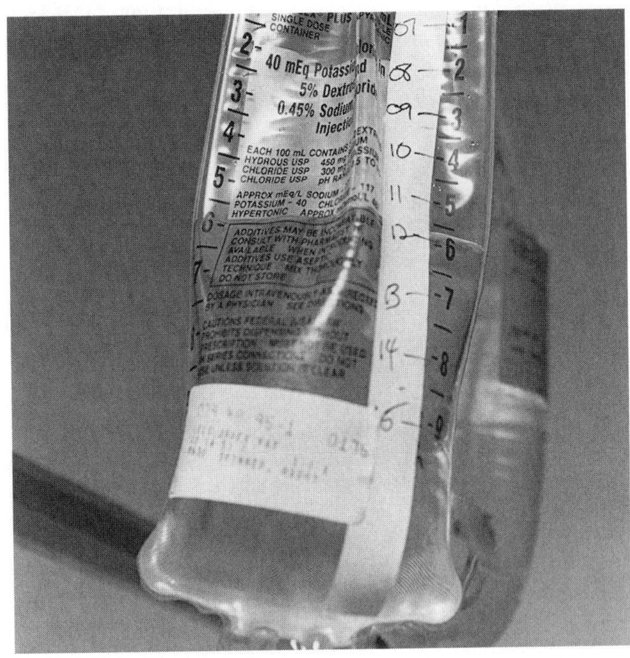

Figure 38–23 Timing label on an intravenous container. The first time marked (0700 hours) would be correct for a bag hung at 0600 hours with a rate of 100 mL per hour.

Milliliters per Hour Hourly rates of infusion can be calculated by dividing the total infusion volume by the total infusion time in hours. For example, if 3000 mL is infused in 24 hours, the number of milliliters per hour is

$$\frac{3000 \text{ mL (total infusion volume)}}{24 \text{ h (total infusion time)}} = 125 \text{ mL/h}$$

Nurses need to check infusions at least every hour to ensure that the indicated milliliters per hour have infused. A strip of adhesive marking the exact time and/or amount to be infused may be taped to the solution container. Some agencies make premarked labels available (Figure 38–23).

FACTORS INFLUENCING FLOW RATES

- *The position of the forearm.* Sometimes a change in the position of the client's arm decreases flow. Slight pronation, supination, extension, or elevation of the forearm on a pillow can increase flow.
- *The position and patency of the tubing.* Not infrequently, the tubing is obstructed by the client's weight, a kink, or a clamp closed too tightly. The flow rate also diminishes when part of the tubing dangles below the puncture site.
- *The height of the infusion bottle.* Elevating the height of the infusion bottle a few inches can speed the flow by creating more pressure.

- *Possible infiltration or fluid leakage.* Swelling, a feeling of coldness, and tenderness at the venipuncture site may indicate infiltration.
- *Relationship of the size of the angiocatheter to the vein.* A catheter that is too large may impede the infusion flow.

Drops per Minute The nurse who begins an infusion must regulate the drops per minute to ensure that the prescribed amount of solution will infuse. Drops per minute are calculated by the following formula:

$$\text{Drops per minute} = \frac{\text{Total infusion volume} \times \text{drops/mL (or drop factor)}}{\text{Total time of infusion in } \textit{minutes}}$$

If the requirements are 1000 mL in 8 hours (480 minutes) and the drip factor is 20 drops/mL, the drops per minute should be

$$\frac{1000 \text{ mL} \times 20 \text{ drops/mL}}{480 \text{ min}} = 41 \text{ drops/min}$$

Approximating this rate as 40 drops/min, the nurse must then regulate the drops per minute by tightening or releasing the intravenous tubing clamp and counting the drops the same way a pulse is counted.

A number of factors influence flow rate. See the box above.

Devices to Control Infusions There are a number of devices that are used to control the rate of an infusion. *Electronic infusion devices* (EIDs) regulate the infusion rate at present limits. They also have an alarm that is triggered when the solution in the IV bag is low, when there is air in the tubing, or when the tubing is low. The *Dial-A-Flow* in-line device (Figure 38–24) is a regulator that controls the amount of fluid to be administered. It is preset at the

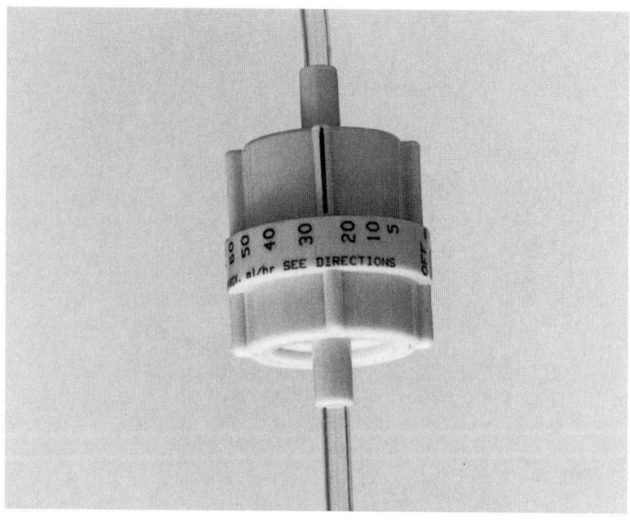

Figure 38–24 The Dial-A-Flo in-line device.

volume to be infused and can be attached at the time the infusion is set up or when the tubing is changed. Another variation is a *volume-control set*, which is used if the volume of fluid administered is to be carefully controlled. The set is attached below the solution container, and the drip chamber is placed below the set. Volume-control sets are frequently used in pediatric settings, where the volume administered is critical. See Figure 43–51 on page 1340.

An infusion *pump* (Figure 38–25) delivers fluids intravenously by exerting positive pressure on the tubing or on the fluid. In situations where the fluid flow is unrestricted, the pump pressure is comparable to that of gravity flow. However, if restrictions develop (increased venous resistance), the pump can maintain the fluid flow by increasing the pressure applied to the fluid.

A *controller*, by contrast, operates solely by gravitational force. The delivery pressure depends on the height of the container in relation to the venipuncture site. The container must be at least 76 cm (30 in) above the venipuncture site for a controller to work. A controller does not have the ability to add pressure to the line and to overcome resistances to fluid flow.

ALTERNATIVE VENOUS ACCESS DEVICES

There are several other ways to access the venous circulation. Two of the most common are the implantable venous access device and the central venous catheter.

Implantable Venous Access Devices Implantable venous access devices or ports are used in the management of clients with chronic illness who require long-term intravenous therapy (eg, intermittent medications such as chemotherapy, total parenteral nutrition, and frequent

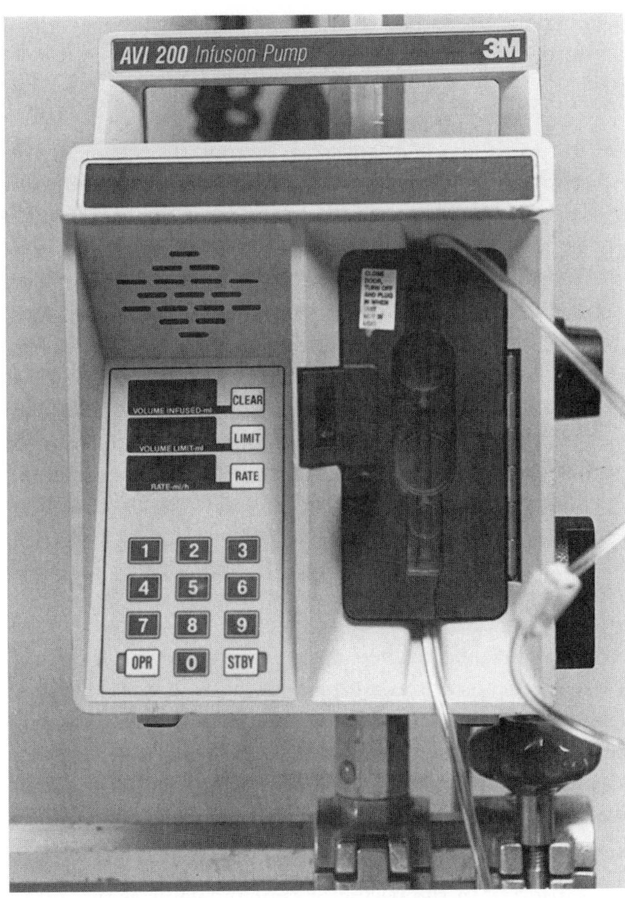

Figure 38–25 An intravenous infusion pump.

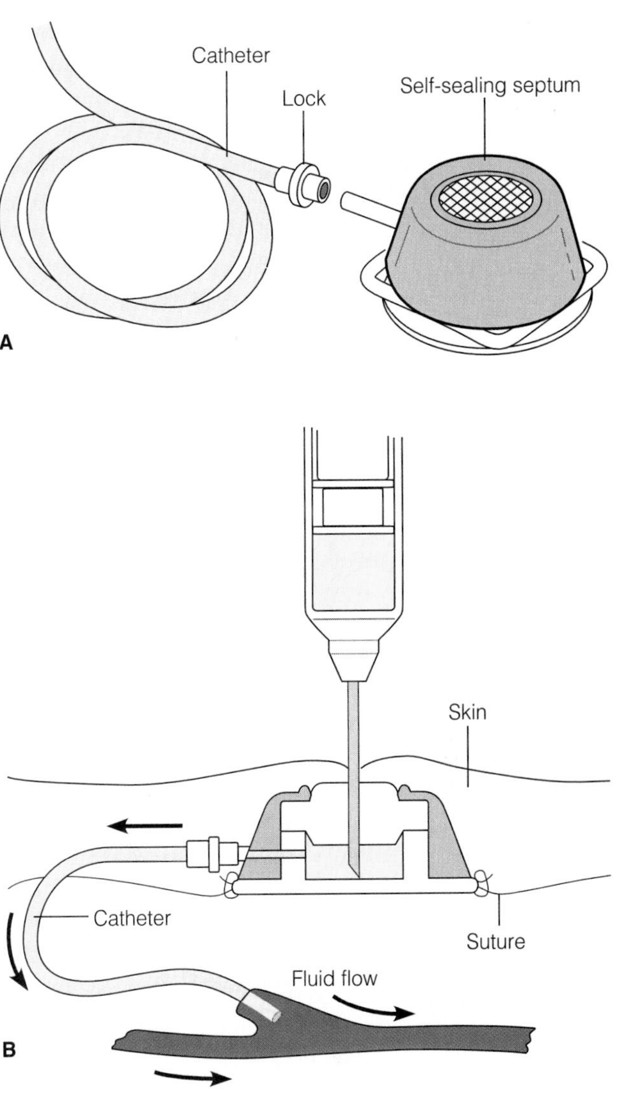

Figure 38–26 An implantable venous access device: *A,* components; *B,* the device in place.

blood samples). The device is designed to provide repeated access to the central venous system, hence avoiding the trauma and complications of multiple venipunctures.

The device consists of a radiopaque silicone catheter and a plastic or stainless steel injection port with a self-sealing silicone-rubber septum (Figure 38–26). Current brand names of the implantable ports are Port-a-Cath, Infuse-A-Port, Mediport, and Chemo-Port. Manufacturers guarantee the septum for a specific number of punctures (eg, 1000 to 2000). Implantable ports are surgically placed into a small subcutaneous pocket, using local anesthesia, usually over the third or fourth rib lateral to the sternum. The distal end of the catheter is inserted into the desired central venous blood vessel (see the discussion of central venous sites, in the next section); the proximal end is routed through a subcutaneous tunnel to the injection portal. These ports can be used immediately after placement. However, a special angled needle, the *Huber needle,* must be used to access the port. The delivery opening of this needle is on the side rather than the tip. The needle is inserted at a 90-degree angle. The site of the port is located by palpation. Agency protocol must be followed

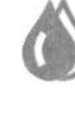

when accessing these devices. Before use, aseptic skin preparation is required; after every use, the port must be flushed with heparinized saline to maintain catheter patency.

Central Venous Catheter A central venous line is a catheter inserted into a large vein located centrally in the body. The tip of the catheter may terminate in the vein, for example, the superior vena cava, or in the right atrium of the heart (Figure 38–27, p. 1102). The catheters are radiopaque so that they will show up on fluoroscopy or X-ray films. Correct placement of the catheter is confirmed by X-ray film.

Central venous lines can be inserted surgically or nonsurgically. In the nonsurgical procedure, three insertion

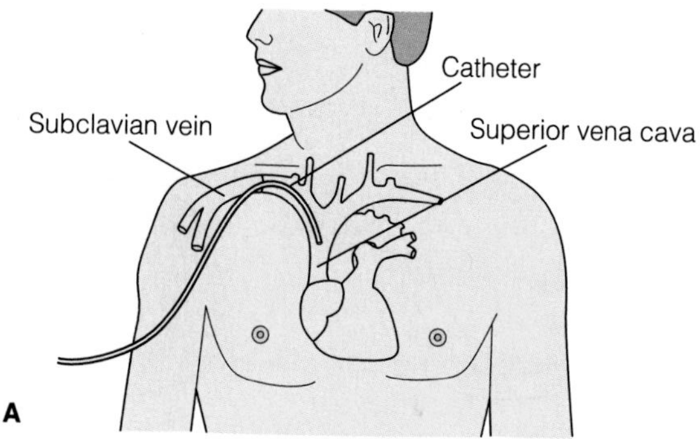

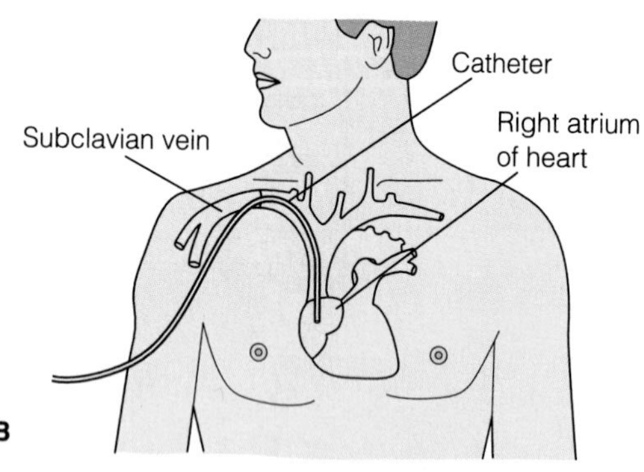

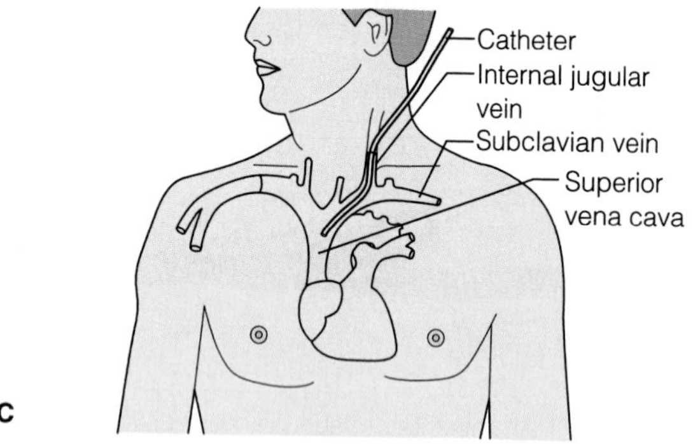

Figure 38–27 Central venous lines with *A,* the catheter tip in the superior vena cava; *B,* the catheter tip in the right atrium of the heart; and *C,* left jugular insertion and catheter tip placement in the superior vena cava.

sites may be used: The subclavian vein, the internal jugular vein, or a peripheral vein.

Subclavian Vein Two approaches may be used:

1. The *infraclavicular approach* (below the clavicle), in which the catheter is inserted into the right or left subclavian vein. The tip of the catheter remains in the subclavian vein or the superior vena cava (Figure 38–27, *A*); that is, a short line is used. The catheter tip can also be extended into the atrium of the heart (Figure 38–27, *B*), that is, a long line can be used. This site permits freedom of movement for ambulation, but a pneumothorax can occur during insertion. Clinical signs include sudden, sharp chest pain; cough; sudden shortness of breath; hypotension; weak, rapid pulse, pallor or cyanosis; and anxiety.
2. The *supraclavicular approach* (above the clavicle), in which the catheter also enters the subclavian vein.

Internal Jugular Vein The right or left internal jugular vein may be approached anteriorly, posteriorly, or between the heads of the sternocleidomastoid muscles. This site hinders head and neck movement somewhat but provides a straight line to the subclavian vein (and superior vena cava; Figure 38–27, *C*). This site is also difficult to dress and tape securely.

Peripheral Vein In the peripheral approach, the catheter is inserted in the basilic or cephalic veins at the antecubital fossa of the right arm. The tip of the catheter may be placed in either the brachiocephalic vein or the superior vena cava. The median basilic vein is the preferred site because the basilic vein offers the most direct route to the central venous system. The exit of this catheter (at the antecubital fossa) looks like that of an intravenous line. It is important for nurses to know that the catheter extends farther into the vein and that its purpose and care differ.

MONITORING AN INTRAVENOUS INFUSION

Intravenous infusions are monitored so that the correct solution is infused at the correct rate and any problems are prevented. See Procedure 38–2.

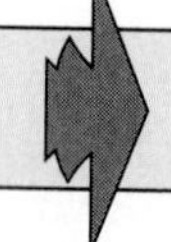

PROCEDURE 38–2 MONITORING AN INTRAVENOUS INFUSION

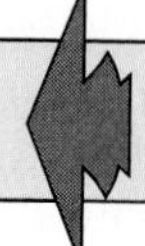

PURPOSES

- To maintain the prescribed flow rate
- To prevent complications associated with IV therapy

ASSESSMENT FOCUS

Appearance of infusion site; patency of system; type of fluid being infused and rate of flow; any adverse response of the client.

PROCEDURE 38–2 *continued*

INTERVENTION

1. Gather the pertinent data.

- From the physician's order, determine the type and sequence of solutions to be infused.
- Determine the rate of flow and infusion schedule.

2. Ensure that the correct solution is being infused.

- If the solution is incorrect, slow the rate of flow to a minimum to maintain the patency of the catheter. *If the infusion is terminated, the client will have to have another venipuncture before the new solution is administered.*
- Report the error to the nurse in charge, and change the solution to the correct one. Note that agencies have different policies about how and to whom to report an incident.

3. Observe the rate of flow every hour.

- Compare the rate of flow regularly, for example, every hour, against the infusion schedule. *Infusions that are off schedule can be harmful to a client.*

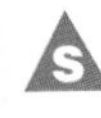

- If the rate is *too fast*, slow it so that the infusion will be completed at the planned time. *Solution administered too quickly may cause a significant increase in circulating blood volume (which is about 6 liters in an adult). Hypervolemia may result in pulmonary edema and cardiac failure.* The clinical signs of cardiac failure are dyspnea, reduced urine output, edema, weak and rapid pulse, and shallow, rapid respirations. The clinical signs of pulmonary edema are dyspnea, coughing, frothy sputum, and rales on lung ascultation.
- If the rate is *too slow*, check agency practice. Some agencies permit nursing personnel to adjust a rate of flow 3 mL/min or less. Adjustments above 3 mL/min may require a physician's order. *Solution that is administered too slowly can supply insufficient fluid, electrolytes, or medication for a client's needs.*

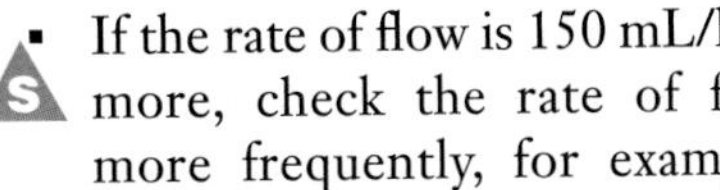

- If the rate of flow is 150 mL/h or more, check the rate of flow more frequently, for example, every 15 to 30 minutes.

4. Inspect the patency of the IV tubing and needle.

- Inspect the tubing for pinches or kinds or obstructions to flow. Arrange the tubing so that it is lightly coiled and under no pressure. Sometimes the tubing becomes caught under the client's arm and the weight of the arm blocks the flow.
- Observe the position of the tubing. If it is dangling below the venipuncture, coil it carefully on the surface of the bed. *The solution cannot flow upward into the vein against the force of gravity.*
- Open the drip regulator, and observe for a rapid flow of fluid from the solution container into the drip chamber. Then partially close the drip chamber to reestablish the prescribed rate of flow. *Rapid flow of fluid into the drip chamber indicates patency of the IV line. Closing the drip chamber to the prescribed rate of flow prevents fluid overload.*
- Lower the solution container below the level of the infusion site, and observe for a return flow of blood from the vein. *A return flow of blood indicates that the needle is patent and in the vein. Blood returns in this instance because venous pressure is greater than the fluid pressure in the IV tubing. Absence of blood return may indicate that the needle is no longer in the vein.*
- Observe the position of the solution container. If it is less than 1 m (3 ft) above the IV site, readjust it to the correct height of the pole. *If the container is too low, the solution may not flow into the vein because there is insufficient gravitational pressure to overcome the pressure of the blood within the vein.*
- Observe the drip chamber. If it is less than half full, squeeze the chamber to allow the correct amount of fluid to flow in (Figure 38–17, earlier).
- Determine whether the bevel of the catheter is blocked against the wall of the vein. If it is blocked, pull back gently, turn it slightly, or carefully raise or lower the angle of insertion slightly, using a sterile gauze pad underneath to protect the skin and change the position of the catheter bevel.
- If there is leakage, locate the source. If the leak is at the catheter connection, tighten the tubing into the catheter. If the leak cannot be stopped, slow the infusion as much as possible without stopping it, and replace the tubing with a new sterile set. Estimate the amount of solution lost, if it was substantial.

5. Inspect the insertion site for fluid infiltration.

- The escape of intravenous fluid into the interstitial tissues, usually near the intravenous site, often causes swelling. In such a case the needle becomes dislodged from the vein, and the intravenous fluid flows into the

PROCEDURE 38–2 MONITORING AN INTRAVENOUS INFUSION *continued*

subcutaneous tissue. The clinical signs are swelling, coolness, pain, pallor at the site, and discomfort.

- To ascertain the presence of infiltration:
  a. Palpate the surrounding tissue for edema.
  b. Feel the surrounding skin for changes in temperature.

6. If infiltration is not evident but the infusion is not flowing, determine whether the needle is dislodged from the vein.

- Gently pinch the IV tubing adjacent to the needle site. *This will cause blood to flow (flash back) into the tubing if the needle is in the vein.*
- Use a sterile syringe of saline to withdraw fluid from the rubber at the end of the tubing near the venipuncture site. If blood does not return, discontinue the intravenous solution.

7. Inspect the insertion site for phlebitis (inflammation of a vein).

- Inspect and palpate the site every 8 hours (Lonsway 1987, p. 107). Phlebitis can occur as a result of injury to a vein, for example, because of mechanical trauma or chemical irritation. Chemical injury to a vein can occur from intravenous electrolytes (especially potassium and magnesium) and medications. The clinical signs are redness, warmth, and swelling at the intravenous site and burning pain along the course of a vein.

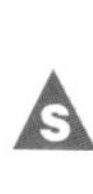

- If phlebitis is detected, discontinue the infusion, and apply warm compresses to the venipuncture site. Do not use this injured vein for further infusions.

8. Inspect the intravenous site for bleeding.

- Oozing or bleeding into the surrounding tissues can occur while the infusion is freely flowing but is more likely to occur after the needle has been removed from the vein.
- Observation of the venipuncture site is extremely important for clients who bleed readily, such as those receiving anticoagulants.

9. Teach the client ways to maintain the infusion system, for example:

- Call for assistance if the solution stops dripping or the venipuncture site becomes swollen.
- Avoid sudden twisting or turning movements of the arm with the needle or catheter.
- Avoid stretching or placing tension on the tubing.
- Try to keep the tubing from dangling below the level of the needle.
- Notify a nurse if:
  a. There is a sudden change in the flow rate or if the solution stops dripping.
  b. The solution container is nearly empty.
  c. There is blood in the IV tubing.
  d. Discomfort or swelling is experienced at the IV site.

10. Document all relevant information.

EVALUATION FOCUS

Amount of fluid infused according to the schedule; intactness of IV system; appearance of IV site (eg, dry, tissue infiltration, discomfort); urinary output compared to urinary intake; tissue turgor; specific gravity of urine; vital signs compared to baseline data.

CHANGING INTRAVENOUS CONTAINERS AND TUBING

Intravenous solution containers are changed when only a small amount of fluid remains in the neck of the container and fluid still remains in the drip chamber. The Centers for Disease Control and Prevention (CDC) recommend that tubing be changed every 48 hours to decrease the incidence of phlebitis and infection. However, some studies indicate that 72-hour intervals may be appropriate (Josephson et al 1985, p. 367; Snydman et al 1987, p. 116). Tubing is changed most easily when a new container is added. All IV bags should be changed every 24 hours regardless of how much solution remains (Holder 1990, p. 46). Procedure 38–3 provides guidelines for changing an intravenous container and tubing.

CHANGING AN INTRAVENOUS DRESSING

The dressing over the IV site is changed according to hospital protocol, generally every 48 to 72 hours. Gauze or transparent dressings may be used, but the latter are often preferred because they allow the nurse to inspect the

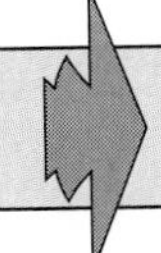

PROCEDURE 38–3 CHANGING AN INTRAVENOUS CONTAINER AND TUBING

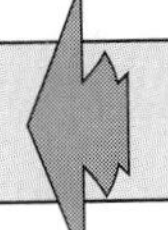

PURPOSES

- To maintain the flow of required fluids
- To maintain sterility of the IV system and decrease the incidence of phlebitis and infection
- To maintain patency of the IV tubing

ASSESSMENT FOCUS

Presence of fluid infiltration, bleeding, or phlebitis at IV site; allergy to tape or iodine; infusion rate and amount absorbed; blockages in IV system.

EQUIPMENT

- ☐ Container with the correct kind and amount of sterile solution
- ☐ Administration set, including sterile tubing and drip chamber
- ☐ Timing label
- ☐ Clean gloves
- ☐ Sterile swabs
- ☐ Receptacle (eg, a basin) for discarded fluid
- ☐ Antiseptic solution and/or ointment for the cleaning site (check agency practice)
- ☐ Tape
- ☐ Sterile gauze square for positioning the needle

INTERVENTION

1. Obtain the correct solution container.

- Verify the physician's order.
- Read the label of the new container.
- Verify correct solution, correct client, correct additives (if any), and correct dose (number of bags or total volume ordered).

2. Set up the intravenous equipment with the new container, and label them.

- See Procedure 38–1, earlier.
- Apply a timing label to the container.
- Prime the tubing.
- Label the tubing as shown in Figure 38–21, earlier.

3. Remove the venipuncture dressing to expose the needle or catheter hub.

- Loosen the tape at the venipuncture site.
- Don clean gloves to prevent exposure to the client's secretions.

- Remove the tape and the dressing from around the needle or catheter, taking care not to dislodge the needle or catheter from the vein.

4. Disconnect the used tubing.

- Place a sterile swab under the hub of the catheter. *This absorbs any leakage that might occur when the tubing is disconnected.*
- Holding the hub of the catheter with the nondominant hand, loosen the tubing with the dominant hand, using a twisting, pulling motion. *Holding the catheter firmly but gently maintains its position in the vein.*
- Clamp and remove the used IV tubing.
- Place the end of the tubing in the basin or other receptacle.

5. Connect the new tubing, and reestablish the infusion.

- Continue to hold the catheter, and grasp the new tubing with the dominant hand.
- Remove the protective tubing cap, and, maintaining sterility, insert the tubing end securely into the needle hub. Twist it to secure it.
- Open the clamp to start the solution flowing.

6. Clean the venipuncture site, and apply a sterile dressing with label.

- Clean the venipuncture site, working from the insertion point outward in a circular manner. Iodine or ethyl alcohol is frequently used. Some agencies also place water-soluble iodine ointment, such as Betadine, at the site.
- Tape the catheter in place. See Procedure 38–1.
- Apply a sterile dressing over the site.
- Remove gloves.
- Apply a labeled tape over the dressing. The label should include (a) the date and time the dressing is applied; (b) the original date and time of the venipuncture; (c) the size of the catheter or needle; and (d) your initials, as the nurse who changed the dressing.

7. Regulate the rate of flow of the solution according to the order on the chart.

➤

PROCEDURE 38–3 CHANGING AN INTRAVENOUS CONTAINER AND TUBING *continued*

8. Document all relevant information.

- Record the change of the solution container and/or tubing in the appropriate place on the client's chart. Also record the fluid intake according to agency practice. Record the number of the container if the containers are numbered at the agency. Also record your assessments.

EVALUATION FOCUS
Skin integrity around IV insertion site; absence of signs of infection, circulatory overload, infiltration, or phlebitis.

venipuncture site. When possible, the nurse changes the dressing at the same time as replacing IV fluid and tubing. Procedure 38–4 describes how to change an IV dressing.

DISCONTINUING AN INTRAVENOUS INFUSION

Discontinuing an infusion is not uncomfortable; in fact, it is usually a relief for the client and takes only a couple of minutes. Infusions are usually discontinued for one of three reasons:

1. The client's oral fluid intake and hydration status are satisfactory, so that no further intravenous solutions are ordered.
2. There is a problem with the infusion that cannot be fixed.
3. The medications administered by the intravenous route (eg, antibiotics) are no longer required.

Before removing a catheter or needle from the vein, determine whether a sterile injection cap (heparin or saline lock) should be attached to the catheter so that intravenous medications can be administered intermittently. See Procedure 38–5 for discontinuing an IV infusion.

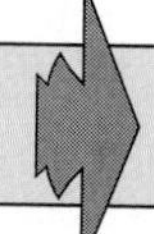

PROCEDURE 38–4 CHANGING AN INTRAVENOUS DRESSING

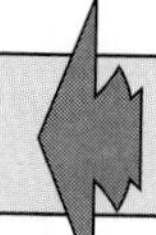

PURPOSES

- To prevent infection at the IV site and the introduction of microorganisms into the blood stream

ASSESSMENT FOCUS
Appearance of the dressing for integrity, moisture, and need for change; the date and the time of the previous dressing change.

EQUIPMENT

- ☐ Sterile 2 × 2 or 4 × 4 gauze or transparent dressing
- ☐ Povidone-iodine (Betadine) swabs
- ☐ Adhesive remover
- ☐ Antiseptic ointment or solution (eg, povidone-iodine or other recommended by the agency)
- ☐ Alcohol swabs
- ☐ Tape
- ☐ Towel
- ☐ Clean disposable gloves

INTERVENTION

1. Prepare the equipment.

- Prepare strips of tape as needed for the type of needle or catheter. For the butterfly needle, two or three strips of 1.25 cm (1/2 in) tape are needed. For a catheter, three strips of 1.25 cm (1/2 in) tape are needed. *These will be used later to secure the needle or catheter without covering the insertion site.*
- Hang the pieces of tape from the edge of a table. *This places the tape in readiness for use without disrupting the adhesive.*
- Open all equipment: povidone-iodine solution or swabs, alcohol

Procedure 38–4 *continued*

swabs, dressing and adhesive bandage, and ointment. *This facilitates access to supplies after gloves are donned.*

- Place a towel under the extremity. *This prevents soiling of bed linens.*
- Don gloves. *Gloves reduce the risk of contact with blood and secretions.*

2. Remove the soiled dressing and all tape, except the tape holding the catheter or IV needle in place.

- Remove tape and gauze from the old dressing one layer at a time. *This prevents dislodgement of the catheter or needle in case tubing becomes entangled between layers of dressing.*
- Remove adhesive dressings in the direction of the client's hair growth when possible. *This minimizes discomfort when adhesive is removed from the skin.*
- Discard the used dressing materials in the appropriate container.

3. Assess the IV site.

- Inspect the IV site for the presence of infiltration or inflammation. *Inflammation and infiltration necessitates removal of the IV needle or catheter to avoid further trauma to the tissues.*
- Go to step 4, or discontinue and relocate the IV site if indicated. See Procedures 38–5 and 38–1.

4. Remove the tape securing the needle or catheter.

- When removing this tape, stabilize the needle or catheter hub with one hand. *This prevents inadvertent dislodgement of the needle or catheter.*

5. Clean the IV site.

- Start with adhesive remover to remove adhesive residue. *Removal of adhesive residue facilitates adherence of the new dressing.*
- Then, using alcohol swabs and povidone-iodine swabs, clean the site, beginning at the catheter or needle and cleaning outward in a 2-inch diameter. *Cleaning in this manner prevents contamination of the IV site from bacteria on the peripheral skin areas. Antiseptics reduce the number of microorganisms present at the site, thus reducing the risk of infection.*
- Follow agency protocol about cleaning procedures. Some agencies recommend cleaning with alcohol before the povidone-iodine swabs; others recommend the reverse.

6. Retape the needle or catheter.

- For a *butterfly needle,* apply strips of tape to the wings of the butterfly using the crisscross (chevron) method (see p. 1098).
- For a *catheter,* apply to tape using the "U" method; see step 14 on page 1097.

7. Apply antiseptic ointment or solution if indicated and apply the dressing.

- Place povidone-iodine ointment or solution at the entry site in accordance with agency protocol. *This reduces skin bacteria and risk of infection.* Solution is preferred to ointment when transparent dressings are used because the former facilitates the dressing's adherence. However, solution can traumatize the skin.
- Apply a sterile gauze or transparent dressing over the site.
- Remove gloves.

8. Label the dressing, and secure IV tubing.

- Place date and time of dressing change and initials either on label provided or directly over the top of the dressing.
- Secure IV tubing with additional tape as required.

9. Document all relevant information.

Evaluation Focus
Status of IV site; patency of IV system; accuracy of flow.

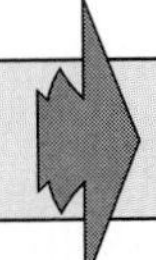

Procedure 38–5 Discontinuing an Intravenous Infusion

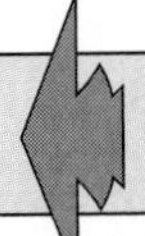

Assessment Focus
Appearance of the venipuncture site; any bleeding from the infusion site; amount of fluid infused.

PROCEDURE 38–5 DISCONTINUING AN INTRAVENOUS INFUSION *continued*

EQUIPMENT

- ☐ Clean gloves
- ☐ Dry or antiseptic-soaked swabs, according to agency practice
- ☐ Small sterile dressing and tape.

INTERVENTION

1. Prepare the equipment.

- Clamp the infusion tubing. *Clamping the tubing prevents the fluid from flowing out of the needle onto the client or bed.*
- Loosen the tape at the venipuncture site while holding the needle firmly and applying countertraction to the skin. *Movement of the needle can injure the vein and cause discomfort to the client. Countertraction prevents pulling the skin and causing discomfort.*

- Don clean gloves, and hold a sterile gauze above the venipuncture site. *Gloves prevent direct contact with the client's blood.*

2. Withdraw the needle or catheter from the vein.

- Withdraw the needle or catheter by pulling it out along the line of the vein. *Pulling out in line with the vein avoids injury to the vein.*
- Immediately apply firm pressure to the site, using sterile gauze, for 2 to 3 minutes. *Pressure helps stop the bleeding and prevents hematoma formation.*
- Hold the client's arm or leg above the body if any bleeding persists. *Raising the limb decreases blood flow to the area.*

3. Examine the catheter removed from the client.

- Check the catheter to make sure it is intact. *If a piece of tubing remains in the client's vein it could move centrally (toward the heart or lungs) and cause serious problems.*
- Report a broken catheter to the nurse in charge or physician immediately.
- If the broken piece can be palpated, apply a tourniquet above the insertion site. *Application of a tourniquet decreases the possibility of the piece moving until a physician is notified.*

4. Cover the venipuncture site.

- Apply the sterile dressing. *The dressing continues the pressure and covers the open area in the skin, preventing infection.*
- Discard the IV solution container, if infusions are being discontinued, and discard the used supplies appropriately.

5. Document all relevant information.

- Record the amount of fluid infused on the intake and output record and on the chart, according to agency practice. Include the container number, type of solution used, time of discontinuing the infusion, and the client's response.

EVALUATION FOCUS

Appearance of the venipuncture site; the pulse; respirations, skin color, edema, sputum, cough, and urine output; and how the person feels physically and psychologically.

EVALUATING

Using data collected during the implementing phase, such as skin turgor assessment, fluid intake and output, vital signs, and body weight measurements, the nurse judges whether client outcomes have been achieved.

If outcomes are not achieved, the nurse should explore why they are not, asking, for example, the following questions:

- Why are fluid intake and output not in balance?
- What reason does the client give?
- Is the client not able to ingest enough fluids orally?
- Did the nurse fail to help the client establish an appropriate schedule for ingesting the fluids?
- Is the client feeling nauseated?
- Are abnormal sources of fluid loss persisting?
- Are ordered medications affecting fluid intake or output?

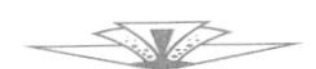

BLOOD TRANSFUSIONS

A **blood transfusion** is the introduction of whole blood or components of the blood (eg, plasma or erythrocytes) into the venous circulation.

Blood Groups Human blood is classified into four main groups (A, B, AB, and O) on the basis of polysaccharide antigens on the erythrocyte (red blood cell) surface. See Table 38–14. These antigens, type A and type B, commonly cause antibody reactions and are called **agglutinogens.** In other words, group A blood contains type A agglutinogen, group B blood contains type B agglutinogen, group AB blood contains both A and B agglutinogens, and group O blood contains neither agglutinogen. Types A and O are the most common.

In addition to agglutinogens on the erythrocytes, **agglutinins** (antibodies) are present in the blood plasma. No individual can have agglutinins and agglutinogens of the same type; that person's system would attack its own cells. They do, however, have agglutinins to the red cell antigens they lack. Thus, group A blood does not contain agglutinin A but does contain agglutinin B. Group B blood does not contain agglutinin B but does contain agglutinin A. Group AB blood contains neither agglutinin, and Group O contains both A and B agglutinins. Blood transfusions must be matched to the client's blood type in terms of compatible agglutinogens. Mismatched blood will cause a hemolytic reaction.

Rhesus (Rh) Factor There are six common types of Rh antigens (C, D, E, c, d, e), each of which is called an **Rh factor.** The type D antigen is considerably more antigenic than the others. Therefore, any person who has D antigen is said to be Rh positive; those who do not are referred to as Rh negative.

Table 38–14 The Blood Groups with Their Constituent Agglutinogens and Agglutinins

Blood Types	Agglutinogens	Agglutinins
O	—	A and B
A	A	B
B	B	A
AB	A and B	—

Unlike the A and B agglutinogens, the Rh factor cannot cause **hemolysis** of red blood cells (hemolytic reaction) on the first exposure to mismatched blood, because the Rh antibody is *not* normally present in the plasma of Rh-negative persons. However, on subsequent transfusions with Rh positive blood, a hemolytic reaction may occur.

Transfusion Reactions Transfusion reactions can be categorized as hemolytic, febrile, allergic, hypervolemic, and septic. The nurse must assess a client closely for reactions. See Table 38–15 on page 1110.

Blood Administration Blood is usually provided in plastic bags by the blood bank. One unit of whole blood is 500 mL of blood in a container. No more than one blood component or unit is obtained for the client at a time. See Table 38–16 on page 1111 for information about blood and blood products.

There are two types of blood administration sets: the Y-set (Figure 38–28, p. 1111) and the straight-line set. The Y-set is often used to administer packed red blood cells (RBCs). This enables the nurse to add normal saline solution to the packed cells to decrease their viscosity—provided that the client can tolerate the added fluid volume. When a straight-line set is used, the nurse sets up a primary infusion of normal saline and piggybacks the blood to the established straight-line tubing. Piggybacking however, increases the risk of microorganisms entering the tubing when the blood line is attached to the established line. Normal saline is used to prime the IV set before blood administration and to maintain tube patency between separate administrations of blood units. Saline is used because it simulates plasma isotonicity. Other solutions, such as dextrose, Ringer's solution, medications and other additives, are incompatible and may cause hemolysis and clumping of RBCs. In most agencies, new tubing is used with each unit of blood.

Because both whole blood and packed RBCs contain cellular debris, blood administration sets are equipped with filters to filter out this debris. Filters may be of either mesh or microaggregate type. The latter is preferred, particularly when multiple units of blood are to be transfused. Leukocyte (white blood cell) removal filters are also available for use in transfusing whole blood and packed RBCs; these filters delay a sensitivity response to transfusion therapy.

Blood transfusions are administered through a #18 or #19 needle or catheter. When blood is to be administered quickly, a #15 needle or large catheter, for example #14, is often used. Large-gauge needles prevent damage to RBCs. Children and other clients with small or thin-walled veins may require needles as small as #23 gauge. The smaller the gauge, the slower the infusion rate.

Table 38–15 Transfusion Reactions

Reaction/Cause	Clinical Signs	Nursing Intervention*
Hemolytic reaction: Client's blood and blood transfusion are incompatible	Chills, fever, headache, backache, dyspnea, cyanosis, chest pain, tachycardia, hypotension	1. Discontinue the transfusion immediately. 2. Keep the vein open with normal saline, or according to agency protocol. 3. Send the remaining blood and a sample of the client's blood to the laboratory for repeat cross-matching and typing. 4. Notify the physician immediately. 5. Monitor vital signs. 6. Monitor fluid intake and output.
Febrile reaction: Sensitivity of the client's blood to white blood cells, platelets, or plasma proteins	Fever; chills; warm, flushed skin; headache; anxiety, muscle pain	1. Discontinue the transfusion immediately. 2. Give antipyretics as ordered. 3. Notify the physician.
Allergic reaction (mild): Sensitivity to infused plasma proteins	Flushing, itching, urticaria, bronchial wheezing	1. Slow or stop the transfusion, depending on agency protocol. 2. Notify the physician. 3. Administer medication (antihistamines) as ordered.
Allergic reaction (severe): Antibody-antigen reaction	Dyspnea, chest pain, circulatory collapse, cardiac arrest	1. Stop the transfusion. 2. Keep the vein open with normal saline. 3. Notify the physician immediately. 4. Monitor vital signs. Administer cardiopulmonary resuscitation (CPR) if needed. 5. Administer medications and/or oxygen as ordered.
Hypervolemia: Blood is administered faster than the circulation can accommodate	Cough, dyspnea, pulmonary congestion (rales), distended neck veins, tachycardia, hypertension	1. Place the client upright, with feet dependent. 2. Administer diuretics and oxygen as ordered. 3. Notify the physician. 4. Slow the transfusion.
Sepsis: Contaminated blood administered	High fever, chills, vomiting, diarrhea, hypotension	1. Stop the transfusion. 2. Send the remaining blood to laboratory. 3. Notify the physician. 4. Obtain a blood specimen from the client for culture. 5. Administer IV fluids, antibiotics.

* Nurses should follow agency's protocol regarding interventions. These may vary among agencies.

Table 38–16 Blood and Blood Products

Product (Volume)	General Information
Citrated whole human blood (500 mL)	Contains RBCs and plasma and anticoagulation preservative Replenishes both the intravascular volume and the oxygen-carrying capacity of the blood. Has a hematocrit of 35–40%.
Red blood cells (packed cells) (250 mL)	Has a hematocrit of approximately 75%. 80% of the plasma is removed. Restores only the oxygen-carrying capacity. Some are prepared with a preservative solution. Should raise hematocrit and hemoglobin; 1 unit will raise Hct approximately 3% and Hgb by 1g/dL (American Journal of Nursing 1991, p. 45).
Platelet concentrates (30 mL)	Used to treat or prevent bleeding. Administer rapidly through a filter.
Granulocyte concentrates	Used to treat infections. Administer through a filter. Requires pretransfusion RBC compatibility testing.
Plasma (200 mL)	Provides coagulation factors. Can transmit infections. Transfuse with a filter.
Cryoprecipitate (10 to 20 mL)	Blood product containing high concentrations of fibrinogen and antihemophilic factor (factor VIII). May transmit infections. Transfuse with a filter.
Albumin (50 mL)	Expands blood volume rapidly. Increases plasma albumin level. Does not transmit infection.
Plasma protein fraction (Plasmanate)	Expands blood volume rapidly. Does not transmit infection.
Clotting factors (Fibrinogen) (10 mL)	Used to prevent or treat bleeding. Monitor blood volume.
Immune globulins, gamma-globulin, hepatitis B globulin	Used to treat exposure to hepatitis A or B. Administer intramuscularly, intravenously.

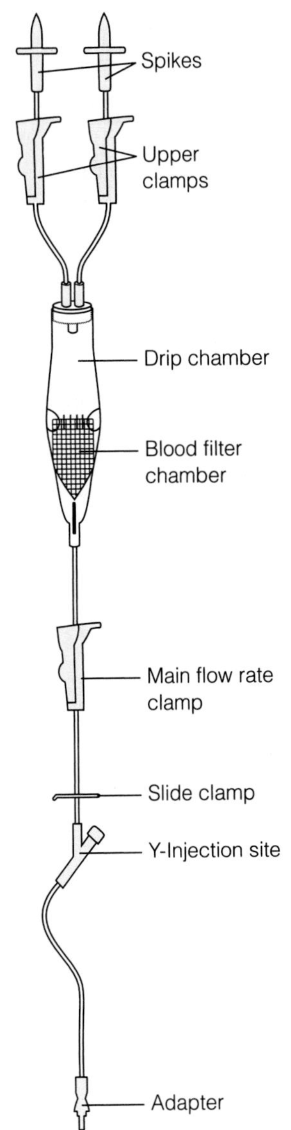

Figure 38–28 Schematic of a Y-set for blood administration.

To decrease the risk of bacterial growth, a blood transfusion should be started within 30 minutes after it is received from the blood bank. RBCs deteriorate when stored at room temperature. The maximum time for infusing a unit of blood is usually 4 hours. Determine agency protocol. The potential for bacterial growth increases if the blood is allowed to hang for a longer period of time.

To start, maintain, and terminate a blood transfusion, see Procedure 38–6.

Text continued on page 1114

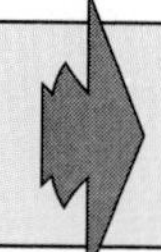

PROCEDURE 38–6 INITIATING, MAINTAINING, AND TERMINATING A BLOOD TRANSFUSION USING A Y-SET

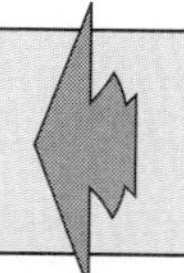

Before commencing a blood transfusion, determine (a) baseline data regarding blood pressure, temperature, pulse, and respirations; (b) any previous reactions to a blood transfusion; (c) the appropriate consent form has been completed.

PURPOSES

- To restore blood volume after severe hemorrhage
- To restore the capacity of the blood to carry oxygen
- To provide plasma factors, such as antihemophilic factor (AHF) or factor VIII, or platelet concentrates, which prevent or treat bleeding

ASSESSMENT FOCUS

Clinical signs of reaction (eg, sudden chills, fever, nausea, itching, rash, low back pain, dyspnea); status of infusion site; any unusual symptoms.

EQUIPMENT

- ☐ Unit of whole blood or packed RBCs
- ☐ Blood administration set
- ☐ Container of normal saline solution
- ☐ IV pole
- ☐ Venipuncture set containing a #18 or #19 needle or catheter (if one is not already in place) or, if blood is to be administered quickly, a #15 needle or a larger catheter (eg, #14)
- ☐ Alcohol swabs
- ☐ Tape
- ☐ Gloves to protect the nurse from contamination by the client's blood

INTERVENTION

1. Verify client consent and obtain baseline data before the transfusion.

- Verify that signed consent form was obtained if required.
- Assess vital signs for baseline data.
- 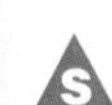 Determine any known allergies or previous adverse reactions to blood.
- Note specific signs related to the client's pathology and reason for transfusion. For example, for an anemic client, note the hemoglobin level.

2. Prepare the client.

- Explain the procedure and its purpose to the client. Instruct the client to report promptly any sudden chills, nausea, itching, rash, dyspnea, or other unusual symptoms.
- If the client has an intravenous solution infusing, check whether the needle and solution are appropriate to administer blood. The needle should be #18 or #19 gauge, and the solution must be normal saline. If the infusing solution is not compatible, remove it and dispose of it according to agency policy. Dextrose, which causes lysis of RBCs, Ringer's solution, medications and other additives, and hyperalimentation solutions are incompatible.
- If the client does not have an intravenous solution infusing, check agency policies. In some agencies an infusion must be running before the blood is obtained from the blood bank. In this case, you will need to perform a venipuncture on a suitable vein (see Procedure 38–1), and start an IV infusion of normal saline.

3. Obtain the correct blood component for the client.

- Check the physician's order with the requisition.
-  Check the requisition form and the blood bag label with a laboratory technician or according to agency policy. Specifically, check the client's name, identification number, blood type (A, B, AB, or O) and Rh group, the blood donor number, and the expiration date of the blood. Observe the blood for abnormal color, RBC clumping, gas bubbles, and extraneous material. Return outdated or abnormal blood to the blood bank.
- 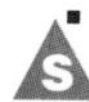 With another nurse (the agency may require an RN), compare the laboratory blood type record with
  a. The client's name and identification number. Ask the client to state the full name as a double check.
  b. The number on the blood bag label.
  c. The ABO group and Rh type on the blood bag label.

PROCEDURE 38–6 *continued*

- If any of the information does not match *exactly*, notify the charge nurse and the blood bank. Do not administer blood until discrepancies are corrected or clarified.
- Sign the appropriate form with the other nurse according to agency policy.

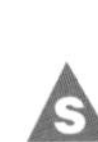

- Make sure that the blood is left at room temperature for no more than 30 minutes before starting the transfusion. *RBCs deteriorate and lose their effectiveness after 2 hours at room temperature. Lysis of RBCs releases potassium into the bloodstream, causing hyperkalemia.* Agencies may designate different times at which the blood must be returned to the blood bank if it has not been started. *As blood components warm, the risk of bacterial growth also increases.*

4. Verify the client's identity.

- Ask the client's full name.

- Check the client's arm band. Do not administer blood to a client without an arm band.

5. Set up the infusion equipment.

- Ensure that the blood filter inside the drip chamber is suitable for whole blood or the blood components to be transfused. Blood filters have a surface area large enough to allow the blood components through easily but are designed also to trap clots.

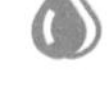

- Put on gloves.
- Close all the clamps on the Y-set: the main flow rate clamp and both Y-line clamps.
- Insert one Y-set piercing pin with twisting motion (spike) into a container of 0.9% saline solution.
- Hang the container on the IV pole about 1 m (36 in) above the planned venipuncture site.

6. Prime the tubing.

- Open the upper clamp on the normal saline tubing, and squeeze the drip chamber until it covers the filter and one-third of the drip chamber above the filter.
- Tap filter chamber to expel any residual air in the filter.
- Remove the adapter cover at the tip of the blood administration set.
- Open the main flow-rate clamp, and prime the tubing with saline.
- Close both clamps.

7. Start the saline solution.

- Attach the IV tubing to the venipuncture device.
- Open the clamps and adjust the flow rate. Use only the main flow-rate clamp to adjust the rate.
- Allow a small amount of solution to infuse to make sure there are no problems with the flow or with the venipuncture site.

8. Prepare the blood bag.

- Invert the blood bag gently several times to mix the cells with the plasma. *Rough handling can damage the cells.*
- Expose the port on the blood bag by pulling back the tabs (Figure 38–29).
- Insert the remaining Y-set spike into the blood bag.
- Suspend the blood bag.

9. Establish the blood transfusion.

- Close upper clamp below IV solution container. Open upper clamp below blood bag. The blood will run into the saline filled drip chamber. If necessary, squeeze drip chamber to re-establish liquid level with drip chamber one-third full. (Tap filter to expel any residual air within the filter.)

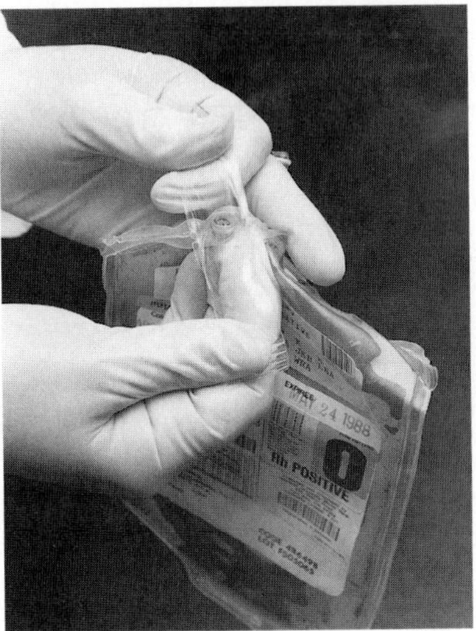

Figure 38–29 Exposing the port on the blood bag by pulling back the tabs.

- Readjust flow rate with the main clamp.

10. Observe the client closely for the first 5 to 10 minutes.

- Run the blood slowly for the first 15 minutes at 20 drops per minute.
- Note adverse reactions, such as chilling, nausea, vomiting, skin rash, or tachycardia. *The earlier a transfusion reaction occurs, the more severe it tends to be. Identifying such reactions promptly helps to minimize the consequences.*
- Remind the client to call a nurse immediately if any unusual symptoms are felt during the transfusion.
- If any of these reactions occur, report these to the nurse in charge, and take appropriate nursing action. See Table 38–15 on page 1110.

PROCEDURE 38–6 INITIATING, MAINTAINING, AND TERMINATING A BLOOD TRANSFUSION USING A Y-SET *continued*

11. Document relevant data.

- Record starting the blood, including vital signs, type of blood, blood unit number, sequence number (eg, no. 1 of three ordered units), site of the venipuncture, size of the needle, and drip rate.

12. Monitor the client.

- Fifteen minutes after initiating the transfusion, check the vital signs of the client. If there are no signs of a reaction, establish the required flow rate. Most adults can tolerate receiving one unit of blood in 1½ to 2 hours. Do not transfuse a unit of blood for longer than 4 hours.
- Assess the client every 30 minutes or more often, depending on the health status, including vital signs until 1 hour post transfusion. If the client has a reaction and the blood is discontinued, send the blood bag to the laboratory for investigation of the blood.

13. Terminate the transfusion.

- Don clean gloves.
- If no infusion is to follow, clamp the blood tubing and remove the needle.
- If the primary IV is to be continued, flush the maintenance line with saline solution. Disconnect the blood tubing system from the primary system. Adjust the drip to the desired rate. *Often a normal saline or other solution is kept running in case of a delayed reaction to the blood.*
- Discard the administration set according to agency practice. Needles should be placed in a labeled, puncture-resistant container designed for such disposal. Blood bags and administration sets should be bagged and labeled before being sent for decontamination and processing. See agency policy. Some agencies keep the used blood bags for a specified time period for analysis of the blood if the client has a delayed reaction.
- Remove gloves.
- Again monitor vital signs.

14. Follow agency protocol for appropriate disposition of the blood bag.

- On the requisition attached to the blood unit, fill in the time the transfusion was completed and the amount transfused.
- Attach one copy of the requisition to the client's record and another to the empty blood bag.
- Return the blood bag and requisition to the blood bank.

15. Document relevant data.

- Record completion of the transfusion, the amount of blood absorbed, the blood unit number, and the vital signs. If the primary intravenous infusion was continued, record connecting it. Also record the transfusion on the IV flow sheet and I & O record.

EVALUATION FOCUS
Changes in vital signs or health status; presence of chills, nausea, vomiting, or skin rash.

TOTAL PARENTERAL NUTRITION

Total parenteral nutrition (TPN), also referred to as **intravenous hyperalimentation (IVH),** is the parenteral administration of solutions of dextrose, water, fat, proteins, electrolytes, vitamins, and trace elements; it is the provision of all needed calories. Because TPN solutions are *hypertonic* (highly concentrated in comparison to the solute concentration of blood), they are injected only into high-flow central veins, where they are diluted by the client's blood.

TPN is a means of achieving an anabolic state in clients who are unable to maintain a normal nitrogen balance. Such clients may include those with severe malnutrition, severe burns, bowel disease disorders (eg, ulcerative colitis or enteric fistula), acute renal failure, hepatic failure, metastatic cancer, or major surgeries where nothing may be taken by mouth for more than 5 days.

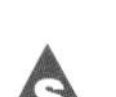

Infection control is of utmost importance during TPN therapy. The nurse must always observe surgical aseptic technique when changing solutions, tubing, dressings, and filters.

TPN solutions are a mixture of 10% to 50% dextrose in water, amino acids, and special additives such as vitamins (eg, B complex, C, D, K), minerals (eg, potassium, sodium, chloride, calcium, phosphate, magnesium), and trace elements (eg, cobalt, zinc, manganese). Additives are adapted to each client's nutritional needs. Fat emulsions

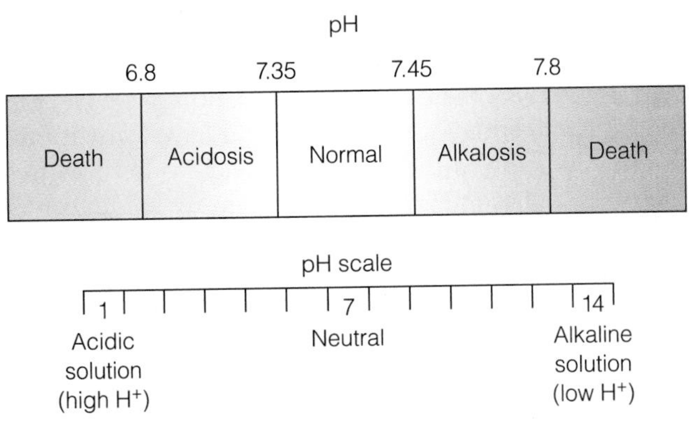

Figure 38–30 Body fluids are normally slightly alkaline, between a pH of 7.35 and 7.45.

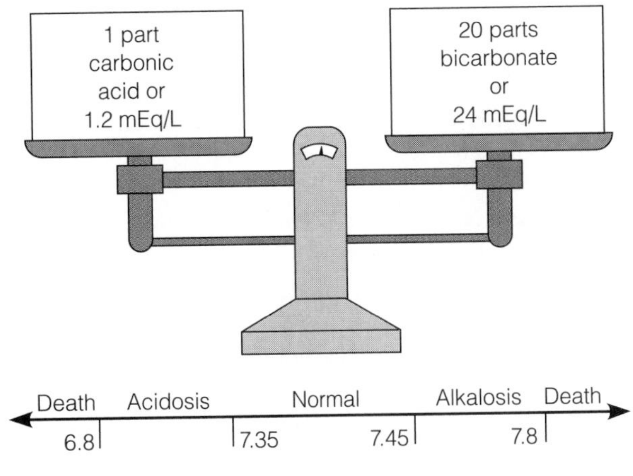

Figure 38–31 Carbonic acid–bicarbonate ratio and pH.

may be given to provide essential fatty acids to correct and/or prevent essential fatty acid deficiency or to supplement the calories for clients who, for example, have high calorie needs or cannot tolerate glucose as the only calorie source.

Because TPN solutions are high in glucose, infusions are started gradually to prevent hyperglycemia. The client needs to adapt to TPN therapy by increasing insulin output from the pancreas. For example, an adult client may be given 1 liter (40 mL/h) of TPN solution the first day, if the infusion is tolerated; the amount may be increased to 2 liters (80 mL/h) for 24 to 48 hours, and then to 3 liters (120 mL/h) within 3 to 5 days. Glucose levels are monitored during the infusion.

When TPN therapy is to be discontinued, the TPN infusion rates are decreased slowly to prevent hyperinsulinemia and hypoglycemia. Weaning a client from TPN may take up to 48 hours but can occur in 6 hours as long as the client receives adequate carbohydrates either orally or intravenously.

ACID-BASE BALANCE

The body's cellular activity requires an alkaline medium. Alkalinity and its opposite, acidity, are measured in terms of hydrogen ion concentration, expressed on a scale called **pH.** A pH of 7 is neutral; above 7 is alkaline; below 7 is acid. An *acid* is a substance that contains hydrogen ions that can be released. An *alkali,* also called a **base,** is a substance that can accept hydrogen ions. For example, carbonic acid releases hydrogen ions:

H_2CO_3	$\rightarrow$	H^+	+	HCO_3^-
carbonic acid		hydrogen (ion)		bicarbonate (base)

Bicarbonate accepts hydrogen ions:

HCO_3^-	+	H^+	$\rightarrow$	H_2CO_3
bicarbonate (base)		hydrogen (ion)		carbonic acid

Body fluids are normally maintained at a pH of about 7.4. Alterations of pH or even a few tenths can be incompatible with cellular activity. The normal pH range of extracellular fluid is 7.35 to 7.45 (Figure 38–30). The lower pH limit at which a person can live more than a few hours is about 6.8, and the upper limit approximately 8.0 (Guyton 1991, p. 331). This precise balance is maintained as long as the ratio of 1 carbonic acid molecule to 20 bicarbonate ions is maintained in the extracellular fluid. The ratio, rather than the specific amount of each, is important (Figure 38–31).

Opposing the body's alkalinity are cellular chemical processes that are constantly producing large amounts of acid as by-products of metabolism. Fortunately, precise control mechanisms maintain the pH of body fluids within a very narrow range. The pH is controlled by buffer systems in all body fluids and by respiratory and kidney regulatory systems.

BUFFER SYSTEMS

A **buffer** system resists change in the pH of a fluid by chemically binding excess hydrogen ions to prevent an increase in pH or by releasing hydrogen ions to prevent a decrease in the pH. Buffers do not neutralize, but they prevent body fluids from becoming strongly acidic or strongly alkaline, so that the pH of the body fluid falls or rises only slightly.

There are three main buffer systems in the body: the bicarbonate–carbonic acid buffer, the phosphate buffer, and the protein buffer. The *bicarbonate–carbonic acid buffer* system, the body's major buffer system is discussed below. The *phosphate buffer* system is important in controlling the intracellular fluids of the body. *Protein buffers* include the globin of hemoglobin in the red blood cells and histone proteins and nucleic acids inside the cells.

Bicarbonate–Carbonic Acid Buffer System The bicarbonate (HCO_3^-)–carbonic acid (H_2CO_3) buffer system is important in controlling the pH of *extracellular* fluids of the body. It consists of sodium bicarbonate ($NaHCO_3$) or potassium bicarbonate ($KHCO_3$) and carbonic acid (H_2CO_3) in the same solution.

If a strong acid, such as hydrochloric acid (HCl) is introduced into an unbuffered system, such as a glass of water, the pH of the fluid drops significantly to 1 or 2. However, if a bicarbonate buffer system is present in the water, the HCl quickly combines with the buffer, producing a weaker acid (carbonic acid), and the pH drops only slightly. This is the reaction:

HCl	$+ NaHCO_3 \rightarrow$	H_2CO_3	$+ NaCl$
hydrochloric acid	sodium bicarbonate	carbonic acid	sodium chloride
(strong acid)	(buffer)	(weak acid)	(salt)

A strong acid is a compound that completely releases its hydrogen ions; for example, HCl yields H^+ and Cl^-. A weak acid frees only some of its hydrogen ions; for example, H_2CO_3 (carbonic acid) yields H^+ and HCO_3^-. One hydrogen ion is free; the other is not.

Alkalis (bases) undergo a similar change. When a strong base such as sodium hydroxide is added to body fluids, it combines with carbonic acid to form a weaker base, sodium bicarbonate:

$NaOH$	$+ H_2CO_3 \rightarrow$	$NaHCO_3$	$+ H_2O$
sodium hydroxide	carbonic acid	sodium bicarbonate	water
(strong base)	(buffer)	(weaker base)	

Although the bicarbonate buffer system is not the strongest buffer system in the body (the most powerful and plentiful one consists of the proteins of plasma and cells), it is important, because the concentration of sodium bicarbonate is regulated by the kidneys and the concentration of carbonic acid by the respiratory system.

RESPIRATORY REGULATION

Elimination of carbon dioxide by the lungs also regulates acid-base balance. The carbon dioxide that a person exhales comes from carbonic acid as follows:

H_2CO_3	$\rightarrow$	CO_2	$+$	H_2O
(carbonic acid)		(carbon dioxide)		(water)

The more CO_2 exhaled, the more H_2CO_3 is removed from the blood, thus elevating the blood pH to a more alkaline level. Hyperventilation is an example of a mechanism by which respiratory regulation of acid-base balance is achieved. Increasing the ventilation rate raises the pH by eliminating CO_2, which would have formed carbonic acid if still in the body. As the acid is lost, the pH increases (ie, becomes alkaline). By contrast, holding one's breath, or hypoventilating, causes the body to retain CO_2, which is then available to form carbonic acid. This reduces the pH and acidifies body fluids. Respiratory alterations, therefore, change the pH of body fluids significantly and rapidly.

Carbonic acid levels are measured by the $Paco_2$ value of the blood. **$Paco_2$** is the partial pressure of carbon dioxide in arterial blood. The *P* stands for partial pressure—here, the pressure exerted by CO_2—and the *a* stands for arterial blood. The normal $Paco_2$ is 35 to 45 mm Hg. An acute rise in the $Paco_2$ is a powerful stimulant to respiration.

The **Pao_2** (partial pressure of oxygen dissolved in the plasma) also influences respiration, but its effect is much less influential than that of the $Paco_2$. This oxygen is separate from the oxygen carried by the hemoglobin of the erythrocytes. The Pao_2 has no major role in acid-base regulation if it is within normal limits. The normal Pao_2 is 80 to 100 mm Hg. The Pao_2 must fall to a very low level (eg, 40 mm Hg) before it significantly increases alveolar ventilation (Metheny 1992, p. 133).

RENAL REGULATION

The kidney's role in maintaining acid-base balance is complex. A simplified account of the process follows. The kidneys excrete hydrogen ions and form bicarbonate ions (HCO_3^-) in specific amounts as indicated by the pH of the blood. When the plasma pH drops (becomes more acidic), hydrogen ions (acid) are excreted, and bicarbonate ions (base) are formed and retained. Conversely, when the plasma pH rises (becomes more alkaline), hydrogen ions are retained in the body, and bicarbonate ions are excreted. Normal values of serum bicarbonate are 22 to 26 mEq/L. Renal compensation for imbalances is slow (ie, several hours or days).

ACID-BASE IMBALANCES

Imbalances in pH can result in either acidosis or alkalosis. **Acidosis** (blood pH below 7.35) occurs with increases in blood carbonic acid or with decreases in blood bicarbonate. It is also referred to as **acidemia.** **Alkalosis** (blood pH above 7.45) occurs with increases in blood bicarbonate or decreases in blood carbonic acid. It is also referred to as **alkalemia.** A client will not become acidotic or alkalotic, however, unless the normal ratio of 1 carbonic acid molecule to 20 bicarbonate ions is altered.

The primary general cause or origin of a pH imbalance is indicated by the terms *metabolic* or *respiratory*. Metabolic acidosis and metabolic alkalosis are imbalances brought about by changes in bicarbonate levels as a result of metabolic alterations. Respiratory acidosis and respiratory alkalosis are imbalances brought about by changes in carbonic acid levels as a result of respiratory alterations.

In all acid-base imbalances, there is a corrective body response by both the kidneys and the lungs called **compensation.** Any given acid-base imbalance can be described as compensated until body reserves are used up. Then the condition is described as uncompensated. In compensated acidosis or alkalosis, the kidneys and lungs are able to restore the altered ratio of 1 carbonic acid molecule to 20 bicarbonate ions, thereby maintaining a normal pH. For example in (compensated) respiratory acidosis, the plasma pH is maintained at normal even though there is an increase in the carbonic acid because the kidneys retain bicarbonate.

Respiratory Acidosis (Carbonic Acid Excess) Respiratory acidosis occurs when exhalation of carbon dioxide is inhibited, creating a carbonic acid excess in the body. As a result, the pH of the blood falls below 7.35, if not compensated. Hypoventilation is its general cause. Two major conditions that cause hypoventilation are central nervous system depression and obstructive lung disease. Morphine overdose and anesthesia are examples of central nervous system depression, whereas asthma and emphysema are obstructive lung diseases.

Respiratory Alkalosis (Carbonic Acid Deficit) Respiratory alkalosis occurs when exhalation of carbon dioxide is excessive, resulting in a carbonic acid deficit. As a result, the blood pH rises above 7.45. The root cause is hyperventilation, which can occur as a result of fever, anxiety, or pulmonary infections. A hyperventilating client blows off abundant carbon dioxide, resulting in lowered carbonic acid blood levels.

Metabolic Acidosis (Base Bicarbonate Deficit) Metabolic acidosis occurs when levels of base bicarbonate are low in relation to carbonic acid blood levels. The kidneys normally retain bicarbonate (HCO_3^-) or excrete hydrogen ions (H^+) in response to altered blood pH. Starvation, renal impairment, and diabetes mellitus are among the conditions that deluge the plasma with acid metabolites. With renal impairment, related electrolyte imbalances may develop. Prolonged diarrhea can decrease bicarbonate.

Metabolic Alkalosis (Bicarbonate Excess) Metabolic alkalosis occurs when the level of base bicarbonate is high. Metabolic alkalosis may be due to excess intake of baking soda and other alkalis, prolonged vomiting, and other conditions that flood plasma with the bicarbonate anion. Prolonged vomiting causes the body to lose chloride (Cl^-) and hydrogen (H^+) ions. Loss of chloride ions causes a proportionate increase of bicarbonate in the blood. Related electrolyte imbalances account for some of the clinical signs.

See Table 38–17 on page 1118 for risk factors, clinical signs, and nursing interventions for acid-base imbalances.

NORMAL VALUES OF ARTERIAL BLOOD GASES (ABGS)*

pH	7.35 to 7.45
$Paco_2$	35 to 45 mm Hg
HCO_3^-	22 to 26 mEq/L
Base excess	−2 to +2 mEq/L
Pao_2	80 to 100 mm Hg
O_2 saturation	95% to 98%

*Some normal values will vary according to the kind of test carried out in the laboratory. Nurses are advised to use the normal values issued by the agency when interpreting laboratory results.

ASSESSING ARTERIAL BLOOD GASES (ABGS)

To determine the adequacy of alveolar gas exchange and evaluate the ability of the lungs and kidneys to maintain the acid-base balance of body fluids, specimens of arterial blood are taken. Arterial blood gases (ABGs) taken routinely include pH, $Paco_2$ (carbonic acid concentration), bicarbonate (HCO_3^-), Pao_2, BE (base excess), and O_2 saturation. The pH, $Paco_2$, Pao_2, and bicarbonate are discussed earlier, on page 1116. Normal values are summarized in the box above.

Base excess (BE), like serum bicarbonate, reflects the metabolic (kidney-regulated) component of acid-base balance, but it adjusts for the client's hemoglobin level, which affects the buffering ability of blood. Low hemoglobin decreases the blood's ability to buffer H^+ ions. The normal values of BE range from −2 to 2 mEq/L.

Oxygen saturation (O_2 Sat) is a measure of the degree to which hemoglobin is saturated with oxygen. Normal values are 95% to 98% in arterial blood and 60% to 85% in venous blood. Oxygen saturation provides some indication of the efficiency of the client's lung ventilation. Hemoglobin is also important in maintaining acid-base balance in the blood. A low hemoglobin reduces the blood's ability to buffer H^+ ions.

To interpret a client's blood gases (ABGs), the nurse follows these steps:

1. *Start with the pH.* This indicates the primary problem of the client:
   a. *If the pH is below 7.35,* the problem is acidosis.

Table 38–17 Acid-Base Imbalances

Risk Factors	Clinical Signs	Nursing Interventions
Respiratory Acidosis (H_2CO_3 excess) 1. Acute lung conditions that alter O_2 or CO_2 alveolar gas exchange (eg, pneumonia, acute pulmonary edema, aspiration of foreign body, drowning) 2. Chronic lung disease (eg, asthma, cystic fibrosis, or emphysema) 3. Overdose of narcotics or sedatives that depress respiratory rate and depth. 4. Brain injury that affects the respiratory center.	***Acute:*** Increased pulse and respiratory rates Shallow respirations Dyspnea Dizziness Confusion Convulsions Lethargy *Laboratory findings:* Plasma pH below 7.35 $Paco_2$ above 45 mm Hg HCO_3^- normal or slightly elevated ***Chronic:*** Weakness Headache Symptoms of underlying disease process pH less than 7.35, or within lower limit of normal if compensation has occurred $Paco_2$ above 45 Hg HCO_3^- above 26mEq/L (compensatory)	Improve respiratory ventilation (eg, administer bronchial dilators, antibiotics, oxygen, as ordered). Maintain adequate hydration (2 to 3 L of fluid per day) Carefully regulate mechanical ventilator, if used. Monitor fluid intake and output, vital signs, arterial blood gases (ABGs), and pH.
Respiratory Alkalosis (H_2CO_3 deficit) 1. Conditions that produce excessive exhalation of carbon dioxide, resulting in a carbonic acid deficit, such as ▪ Extreme anxiety ▪ Elevated body temperature ▪ Overventilation with a mechanical ventilator ▪ Hypoxia ▪ Salicylate overdose	Hyperventilation (ie, deep, rapid respirations) Difficulty concentrating Positive Trousseau's sign (see p. 1083) *Laboratory findings (in uncompensated respiratory alkalosis):* Arterial blood pH above 7.45 $Paco_2$ less than 35 mm Hg	Monitor vital signs and ABGs. Assist client to breath more slowly. Administer CO_2 inhalations, or help client breathe in a paper bag (to inhale CO_2).

b. *If the pH is above 7.45,* the problem is alkalosis.

2. *Next, look at the $Paco_2$.* This value relates to respirations.

   a. *If the $Paco_2$ is below 35 mm Hg,* respiratory alkalosis is present. A low value indicates too little CO_2 (ie, too little carbonic acid), which results in alkalosis. This happens when the person exhales too much CO_2 (ie, when the person hyperventilates).

   b. *If the $Paco_2$ is above 45 mm Hg,* respiratory acidosis is present. A high value indicates too much CO_2 (ie, too much carbonic acid), which causes acidosis. This happens when respirations are depressed and are very slow and often shallow, or when the lungs are diseased and gas exchange is compromised. Carbon dioxide builds up in the body because the lungs are not eliminating it at the usual rate.

Table 38–17 ***continued***

Risk Factors	Clinical Signs	Nursing Interventions
Metabolic Acidosis (HCO_3^- deficit)		
1. Conditions that deluge the plasma with acid metabolites (eg, renal impairment, diabetes mellitus, starvation) 2. Conditions that decrease bicarbonate (eg, prolonged diarrhea) 3. Excessive infusion of chloride fluids (eg, NaCl)	Fruity breath Kussmauls' respirations (deep, rapid respirations) Lethargy Headache Weakness Disorientation *Laboratory findings:* Plasma pH below 7.35, or normal (in compensated metabolic acidosis) Normal Pa_{CO_2}, or low (if compensated in an attempt by the lungs to blow off more acid) Low plasma bicarbonate (below 21 mEq/L in adults, below 20 mEq/L in children) Low urine pH (below 6)	Monitor ABG values. Administer IV sodium bicarbonate carefully if ordered. Correct underlying problem as ordered.
Metabolic Alkalosis (HCO_3^- excess)		
1. Excessive losses of acids in the body due to ▪ Vomiting ▪ Gastric suction ▪ Excessive use of potassium-losing diuretics 2. Conditions of regulatory organs such as ▪ Cushing's syndrome ▪ Hyperaldosteronism 3. Excessive bicarbonate intake from ▪ Antacids ▪ Parenteral $NaHCO_3$	Decreased respiratory rate and depth Dizziness Hypertonic muscles Nausea, vomiting Tetany Irritability Mental dullness *Laboratory findings:* High plasma pH (above 7.45) Normal or high Pa_{CO_2} (above 45 mm Hg) as a compensatory elevation High plasma bicarbonate (above 28 mEq/L in adults, above 25 mEq/L in children) High urine pH (above 7)	Monitor client's fluid losses closely. Monitor vital signs, especially respirations. Administer ordered IV fluids carefully. Reverse underlying problem.

3. *Evaluate the metabolic indicators, HCO_3^- and BE.* These reflect the kidney's ability to maintain acid-base balance and indicate the metabolic causes of imbalances.
   a. *If HCO_3^- is below 22 mEq/L,* metabolic acidosis is present. *If BE is below −2 mEq/L,* metabolic acidosis is present. These two values will usually both be low, indicating that the amount of base is inadequate to balance the acid.
   b. *If HCO_3^- is above 26 mEq/L,* metabolic alkalosis is present. *If BE is above +2 mEq/L,* metabolic alkalosis is present. These two values will usually both be elevated, indicating an excess of base in relation to the amount of acid in the body.
4. If both values described in 2 and 3 above are abnormal, (ie, the Pa_{CO_2} and the HCO_3 and BE), with one indicating acidosis and the other indicating alkalosis, the

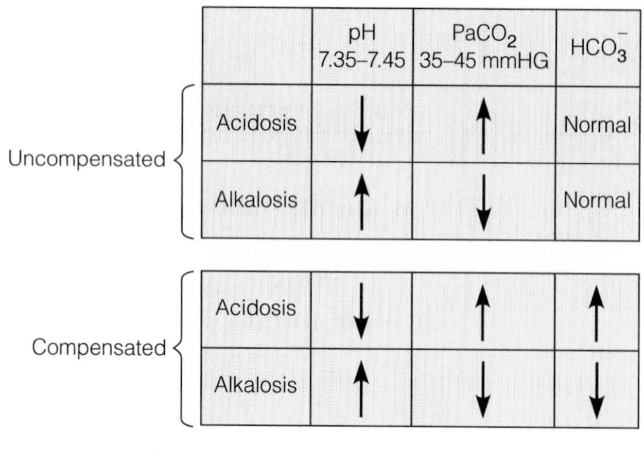

		pH 7.35–7.45	$PaCO_2$ 35–45 mmHG	HCO_3^-
Uncompensated	Acidosis	↓	↑	Normal
	Alkalosis	↑	↓	Normal
Compensated	Acidosis	↓	↑	↑
	Alkalosis	↑	↓	↓

Figure 38–32 Arterial blood gas values for uncompensated and compensated respiratory acidosis and alkalosis.

Table 38–18 Clinical Application: Assessment Data Clusters and Related Nursing Diagnoses

Data Cluster	Nursing Diagnoses
Fred Boysniak was admitted to emergency after being found with an empty bottle of codeine tablets by his bed. He appears very lethargic and stuporous; pulse is 120, respirations 12 and very shallow. Blood gases reveal pH of 7.1, $Paco_2$ 49 mm Hg, and HCO_3^- 29 mEq/L.	**Impaired gas exchange** related to hypoventilation secondary to overdose of respiratory depressant drug

body is compensating and attempting to reestablish acid-base balance. However, the pH indicates the primary problem; therefore, the nurse identifies whichever values are normal and compatible with the pH—that is, the primary problem. The other abnormal values indicate compensation.

5. *Establish the amount of hypoxemia present from the* Pao_2 *and* O_2 *Sat.* If these are below the normal, some degree of hypoxemia is present.
   a. *If the* Pao_2 *is 60 to 80 mm Hg,* mild hypoxemia is present.
   b. *If the* Pao_2 *is 40 to 60 mm Hg,* moderate hypoxemia is present.
   c. *If the* Pao_2 *is below 40 mm Hg,* severe hypoxemia is present.

When hypoxemia is present, the client usually requires oxygen. However, care should be taken when administering oxygen to a client with chronic obstructive pulmonary disease (COPD), because elevating the Pao_2 into a normal range may stop breathing. Whereas an increase in $Paco_2$ stimulates respirations in most people, it is the hypoxemia itself that stimulates respirations in clients with COPD. Figures 38–32 and 38–33 show laboratory values for uncompensated and compensated respiratory and metabolic acidosis and alkalosis.

DIAGNOSING

The NANDA diagnosis that relates to acid-base imbalances is **Impaired gas exchange.** Its definition, defining characteristics, and related factors are shown in the upper box on page 1121. A clinical example of assessment data clusters and related nursing diagnoses is shown in Table 38–18.

PLANNING AND IMPLEMENTING

The major outcome for clients with acid-base imbalances is to maintain adequate ventilation and oxygen status. Specific outcome criteria, nursing interventions, and rationales are shown in the accompanying Care Planning Guide.

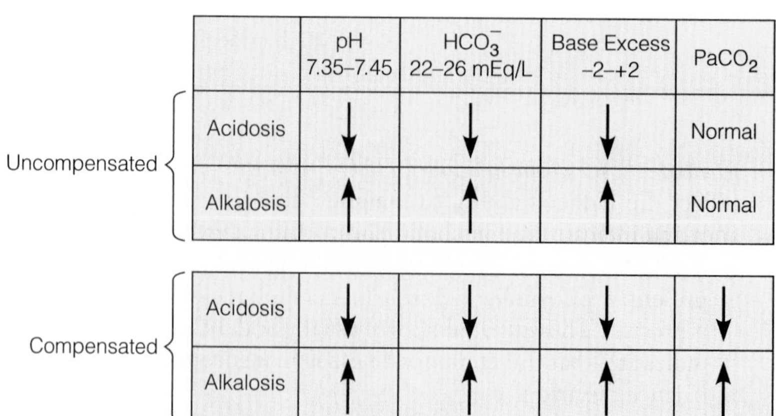

		pH 7.35–7.45	HCO_3^- 22–26 mEq/L	Base Excess −2–+2	$PaCO_2$
Uncompensated	Acidosis	↓	↓	↓	Normal
	Alkalosis	↑	↑	↑	Normal
Compensated	Acidosis	↓	↓	↓	↓
	Alkalosis	↑	↑	↑	↑

Figure 38–33 Arterial blood gas values for uncompensated and compensated metabolic acidosis and alkalosis.

NURSING DIAGNOSES
CLIENTS WITH ACID-BASE IMBALANCE

NURSING DIAGNOSIS: Impaired gas exchange: The state in which an individual experiences a decreased passage of oxygen and/or carbon dioxide between the alveoli of the lungs and the vascular system

Defining Characteristics

- Confusion
- Restlessness
- Irritability
- Somnolence
- Hypoxia
- Hypercapnia
- Inability to move secretions

Related Factors

Altered oxygen supply; altered pulmonary blood flow; altered oxygen-carrying capacity of the blood; changes in the alveolar capillary membrane; ventilation-perfusion imbalance.

Sources: M Gordon, *Manual of Nursing Diagnosis 1993–1994*, 6th ed. (St Louis: Mosby-Year Book, 1993), pp. 203; MJ Kim, GK McFarland, and AM McLane, *Pocket Guide to Nursing Diagnoses*, 5th ed. (St Louis: Mosby-Year Book, 1993), pp. 25–26; GK McFarland and EA McFarlane, *Nursing Diagnosis and Intervention: Planning for Patient Care*, 2d ed. (St Louis: Mosby, 1993), p. 362: North American Nursing Diagnosis Association, *NANDA Nursing Diagnoses: Definitions and Classification 1992–1993*, (Philadelphia: NANDA, 1992), p. 25; and JR Lederer, GL Marculescu, B Mocnik, and N Seaby, *Care Planning Pocket Guide—A Nursing Diagnosis Approach*, 5th ed. (Redwood City, CA: Addison-Wesley Nursing, 1993), p. 82.

CARE PLANNING GUIDE
CLIENTS WITH ACID-BASE IMBALANCE

NURSING DIAGNOSIS: Impaired gas exchange

Outcome Criteria	Nursing Interventions	Rationale
The client		
▪ Experiences maximal pulmonary ventilation and adequate gas exchange, as evidenced by a. Arterial blood gases within normal limits. b. Absence of hypoxia.	Monitor the client's blood gas levels and oxygenation status. Observe the client for signs of hypoxia (eg, tachycardia, anxiety, cyanosis). Use a pulse oximeter if available (see p. 1138).	This allows the nurse to determine desired changes and evaluate the effects of therapy.
	Administer prescribed therapies, such as oxygen, medications (bronchodilators, inhalants, expectorants, antibiotics).	This helps increase the PaO_2, promote ventilation depth, and clear air passages for adequate gas exchange.
	Auscultate lung sounds, monitor vital signs (note especially respiratory pattern and pulse rate), inspect sputum, and assess mental status for mental disorientation or agitation.	This allows the nurse to evaluate effects of therapy.
	Pace activities to the client's tolerance, and offer support during periods of respiratory distress or anxiety.	This minimizes shortness of breath and fatigue.
	Position the client in semi- or high-Fowler's position as indicated.	This maximizes pulmonary ventilation.
	Encourage deep-breathing exercises and coughing as indicated.	This helps maintain a patent airway.
▪ Identifies reasons for impaired pulmonary function, and necessary self care techniques.	Provide instruction about (a) breathing and relaxation techniques to enhance breathing pattern, (b) medications, (c) activity allowed, (d) supportive equipment (eg, oxygen device and safety precautions), (e) reportable signs and symptoms, and (f) available community resources.	Client's understanding of condition and preventive measures may facilitate necessary follow-up care.

CRITICAL PATHWAY FOR JOAN O'BRIEN

ASSESSMENT DATA

Nursing Assessment

Ms Joan O'Brien is a 22-year-old waitress who was admitted for a 3-day history of diarrhea and vomiting, dehydration, and evaluation of diarrhea. Ms O'Brien lives alone and tells the admitting nurse, Janet Clark, that she was too sick to try to eat or take fluids. She called her personal medical doctor on the 3d day of this current illness, and he recommended admission. She is NPO and receiving intravenous infusion at an 8-hour rate. Her skin and mucous membranes are dry.

Physical Examination

Height: 160 cm (5′3″)
Weight: 66.2 kg (146 lb)
Temperature: 38.1 C (100.6 F)
Pulse rate: 96 bpm
Respirations: 28 per minute
Blood pressure: 110/70 mm Hg
Skin turgor poor
Skin dry and mucous membranes dry and sticky
Dark amber urine

Diagnostic Data

Serum sodium: 155 mEq/L
Serum osmolarity: 298 mOsm/kg
Serum potassium: 3.2 mEq/L
Serum bicarbonate: 33 mEq/L
Plasma pH: 7.48

CRITICAL PATHWAY FOR CLIENT WITH DIARRHEA AND DEHYDRATION

Expected length of stay 5 days

	Date ________ Day 1	Date ________ Day 2	Date ________ Day 3
Daily outcomes	Client will ▪ have stable vital signs. ▪ have an intake of 2000 mL/day (IV). ▪ remain free of nausea and vomiting. ▪ verbalize understanding of ongoing care. ▪ have a soft, non-distended abdomen. ▪ verbalize ability to cope.	Client will ▪ have stable vital signs. ▪ have an intake of 2000 mL/day (IV). ▪ remain free of nausea and vomiting. ▪ verbalize understanding of ongoing care. ▪ have moist mucous membranes and skin. ▪ have a urine output of at least 30 mL/h. ▪ have a soft, non-distended abdomen. ▪ vebalize ability to cope.	Client will ▪ have stable vital signs. ▪ have an intake of 2000 mL/day (IV/PO). ▪ verbalize understanding of ongoing care. ▪ have a soft, non-distended abdomen, active bowel sounds. ▪ tolerate clear liquids without nausea and vomiting. ▪ have balanced fluid and electrolyte status. ▪ have urine output of at least 30 mL/h. ▪ verbalize ability to cope. ▪ vebalize beginning understanding of home care instructions.

	Day 1 *continued*	**Day 2** *continued*	***Day 3*** *continued*
Tests and treatments	CBC with differential. Electrolytes. Abdominal X-rays. Blood culture × 2 if temp over 38.3C (101 F). Vital signs q4h if stable. Assess gastrointestinal status q4h and prn. Intake and output q shift. Daily weight. Monitor diagnostic studies. Assess mental status q shift. Assist with/provide perianal care p each loose stool. Stool cultures as ordered. Assess usual bowel elimination pattern. Report worsening abdominal pain, nausea, vomiting, diarrhea, or increasing abdominal distention.	Electrolytes. Blood culture × 2 if temp over 38.3C (101 F). Vital signs q4h if stable Assess gastrointestinal status q4h and prn. Intake and output q shift. Daily weight. Monitor diagnostic studies. Assess mental status q shift. Assist with/provide perianal care p each loose stool. Report worsening abdominal pain, nausea, vomiting, diarrhea, or increasing abdominal distention.	Electrolytes. Blood culture × 2 if temp over 38.3C (101 F). Vital signs q4h if stable. Assess gastrointestinal status q4h and prn. Intake and output q shift. Daily weight. Monitor diagnostic studies. Assess mental status q shift. Assist with/provide perianal care p each loose stool. Report worsening abdominal pain, nausea, vomiting, diarrhea or increasing abdominal distention.
Knowledge deficit	Orient to room and hospital routine. Review plan of care and importance of bowel rest, bedrest, and emotional rest.	Review plan of care and continued importance of bowel rest, bedrest, and emotional rest.	Reinforce earlier teaching regarding ongoing care. Begin discharge teaching regarding rest, activity, and diet.
Psycho-social	Assess level of anxiety. Encourage verbalization of concerns. Provide information. Provide ongoing support and encouragement.	Assess level of anxiety. Encourage verbalization of concerns. Provide information. Provide ongoing support and encouragement.	Encourage verbalization of concerns. Provide ongoing support and encouragement.
Diet	NPO. Mouth care prn. NG to low suction with persistent vomiting.	NPO. Mouth care prn. D/C NG if no vomiting and active BS.	Begin clear liquids to tolerance.
Activity	Provide safety precautions. Bedrest with commode privileges. Provide rest periods. Assist with ADLs.	Provide safety precautions. Bathroom privileges with assistance. Provide rest periods. Assist with ADLs.	Provide safety precautions. Up to chair ad lib. Provide rest periods. Assist with ADLs.

	Day 1 *continued*	**Day 2** *continued*	**Day 3** *continued*
Medications	IV fluids with electrolyte replacement as ordered. Antidiarrheal drugs as ordered. Tylenol 650 mg q4h PO for temp over 38.3C (101 F).	IV fluids and electrolyte replacement. Antidiarrheal drugs as ordered. Tylenol 650 mg q4h PO for temp over 38.3C (101 F). If indicated, initiate treatment based on stool cultures.	IV fluids and electrolyte replacement. Antidiarrheal drugs as ordered. Tylenol 650 mg q4h PO for temp over 38.3C (101 F).
Fluid volume deficit	Accurate intake and output. Assess client for dry skin, dry mucous membranes, and poor skin turgor. If NG in place, irrigate with normal saline. Assess volume of diarrhea stools.	Accurate intake and output. Assess client for dry skin, dry mucous membranes and poor skin turgor. If NG in place, irrigate with normal saline. Assess volume of diarrhea stools.	Accurate intake and output. Assess client for dry skin, dry mucous membranes, and poor skin turgor. If NG in place, irrigate with normal saline. Assess volume of diarrhea stools.
Transfer/ discharge plans	Review discharge goals with client and significant other. Consult with social service re: projected needs for home health care (if any).	Review progress towards discharge goals with client and significant other.	Review progress toward discharge goals with client and significant other.

	Date __________ **Day 4**	**Date __________** **Day 5**	
Daily outcomes	Client will ▪ have stable vital signs. ▪ have an intake of 2000 mL/ day (IV). ▪ remain free of nausea and vomiting. ▪ verbalize understanding of ongoing care. ▪ have a soft, non-distended abdomen, active bowel sounds, passing soft, brown stools. ▪ tolerate ordered diet without nausea and vomiting. ▪ verbalize ability to cope. ▪ verbalize beginning understanding of home care instructions.	Client ▪ is afebrile and has a stable vital signs. ▪ has a soft, non-distended abdomen and passing soft, brown stools each day. ▪ is independent is self-care. ▪ is fully ambulatory. ▪ has resumed preadmission urine elimination pattern. ▪ verbalizes home care instructions. ▪ tolerates ordered diet and has an intake of 2000 mL/ day. ▪ verbalizes ability to cope with ongoing stressors.	

	Day 4 *continued*	**Day 5** *continued*	
Tests and treatments	Blood culture × 2 if temp over 101 F. Vital signs q 4h if stable. Electrolytes. Daily weight. Assess gastrointestinal status q4h and prn. Intake and output q shift. Report worsening abdominal pain, nausea, vomiting, diarrhea, or increasing abdominal distention. Discuss need to eat 3 to 4 regularly scheduled meals. Teach client signs and symptoms requiring follow-up: worsening abdominal pain, nausea, vomiting, change in bowel habits, and/or fever.	Blood culture × 2 if temp over 38.3 C (101 F). Daily weight. Vital signs q4h if stable. Assess gastrointestinal status q4h and prn. Intake and output q shift.	
Knowledge deficit	Reinforce earlier teaching regarding ongoing care. Review written discharge instructions with client and significant other.	Reinforce earlier teaching regarding ongoing care. Complete discharge teaching to include diet, follow-up care, signs and symptoms to report, activity, and medications: dose, frequency, route, and side effects. Provide client with written discharge instructions.	
Psycho-social	Encourage verbalization of concerns. Provide ongoing support and encouragement.	Encourage verbalization of concerns. Provide ongoing support and encouragement.	
Diet	Full liquids to soft diet as tolerated, providing small, frequent, nutritious feedings. Encourage fluid intake of 2000 mL/day.	Soft diet as tolerated, providing small, frequent, nutritious feedings. Encourage fluid intake of 2000 mL/day.	
Activity	Self-care. Ambulate independently at least 4 times.	Self-care. Fully ambulatory.	
Medications	D/C if PO intake > 2000 mL/day. Tylenol 650 mg q4h PO for temp over 38.3 C (101F).	PO antibiotics. Tylenol 650 mg q4h PO for temp over 38.3 C (101F).	

	Day 4 *continued*	**Day 5** *continued*	
Fluid volume deficit	Accurate intake and output. Assess client for dry skin, dry mucous membranes, and poor skin turgor. If NG in place, irrigate with normal saline. Assess volume of diarrhea stools.	Accurate intake and output. Assess client for dry skin, dry mucous membranes, and poor skin turgor. If NG in place, irrigate with normal saline. Assess volume of diarrhea stools.	
Transfer/ discharge plans	Continue to review progress toward discharge goals. Finalize discharge plans.	Finalize plans for home care if needed. Complete discharge teaching.	

CHAPTER HIGHLIGHTS

- A balance of both fluids and electrolytes in the body is necessary for health and life.
- The body fluid is divided into two major reservoirs: the intracellular fluid (ICF) inside the cells and extracellular fluid (ECF) outside the cells.
- Extracellular fluid is subdivided into two compartments: intravascular (plasma) and interstitial. It constitutes about one-fourth to one-third of total body fluid.
- ECF is in constant motion throughout the body. It is the transport system that carries nutrients to and waste products from the cells.
- Secretions and excretions, also part of the body's total fluid volume, are part of the ECF.
- The percentage of total body fluids varies according to the individual's age, body fat, and sex. The younger the person, the higher the proportion of water in the body. The less body fat present, the greater the proportion of body fluid. Postadolescent females have a smaller percentage of fluid in relation to total body weight than do men.
- There are two types of body electrolytes (ions): positively charged ions (cations) and negatively charged ions (anions).
- The principal ions of ECF are sodium and chloride; the principal ions of ICF are potassium and phosphate.
- Fluids and electrolytes move among the body compartments by diffusion, filtration, osmosis, and active transport.
- The major fluid pressures exerted as part of the movement of fluid and electrolytes from one compartment to another are oncotic pressure and hydrostatic pressure.
- The three sources of body fluid are fluids taken orally, food ingested, and the oxidation of food. Fluid intake is regulated by the thirst mechanism.
- Fluid output occurs chiefly through excretion of urine, although body fluid is also lost through sweat, feces, and insensible vapor loss.
- In healthy adults, measurable fluid intake and output should balance (about 1500 mL per day). The output of urine normally approximates the oral intake of fluids. Water from food and oxidation is balanced by fluid loss through the skin, respiratory process, and feces.
- Fluid imbalances include
  a. Fluid volume deficit (FVD), also referred to as hypovolemia.
  b. Dehydration, a deficit in water only.
  c. Fluid volume excess (FVE), also referred to as hypervolemia.
  d. Overhydration, an excess of water only.

- The most common electrolyte imbalances are deficits or excesses in sodium, potassium, and calcium.
- Fluid and electrolyte imbalance is most accurately determined through laboratory examination of blood plasma.
- Assessment relative to fluid and electrolyte balance includes (a) a nursing history; (b) measurement of body weight, vital signs, and fluid intake and output; (c) physical examination of the skin, oral cavity, eyes, jugular vein, veins of the hand, and the neurologic system; and (d) various diagnostic studies of blood and urine.
- A nursing history includes data about the client's fluid and food intake; fluid output; signs of fluid, electrolyte, and acid-base imbalances; and medications, therapies, or disease processes that may disrupt these balances.
- NANDA approved nursing diagnoses that relate specifically to fluid and electrolyte imbalances include **Fluid volume deficit, High risk for fluid volume deficit,** and **Fluid volume excess.** Other diagnoses that may be relevant are **Altered oral mucous membrane, Impaired skin integrity, Decreased cardiac output,** and **Altered tissue perfusion.**
- In many instances, fluids and electrolytes can be provided orally to clients who are experiencing or at risk of developing fluid deficits. The nurse needs to establish with the client a 24-hour plan for ingesting the necessary fluids and to respect the client's fluid preferences.
- For clients with fluid retention, fluids may need to be restricted; a schedule and short-term outcomes that make the fluid restriction more tolerable need to be developed.
- For clients experiencing excessive fluid losses, the administration of fluids and electrolytes intravenously is necessary. Meticulous aseptic technique is required when caring for clients with intravenous infusions.
- Preventing complications such as infiltration, phlebitis, hypervolemia (circulatory overload), and infection are an important aspect of intravenous therapy.
- The administration of blood transfusions involves accurately matching and identifying the blood for the individual, correctly identifying the recipient, and monitoring the client throughout the procedure for transfusion reactions.
- The hypertonic solutions used in total parenteral nutrition are infused in a central vein and are given to achieve a positive nitrogen balance and weight gain.
- The acid-base balance (pH range) of body fluids is maintained within a precise range of 7.35 to 7.45, controlled by buffer systems in all body fluids (bicarbonate, phosphate, and protein) and by respiratory and kidney regulating systems.
- Acid-base imbalance occurs when the body fluids are higher or lower than the normal pH range. Imbalances may result in respiratory or metabolic disturbances; either can result in acidosis or alkalosis.
- The normal pH range for extracellular fluids is 7.35 to 7.45.
- The body has buffer systems which maintain body fluids within a normal range.

READINGS AND REFERENCES

SUGGESTED READINGS

Anderson, S. August 1990. ABGs—Six easy steps to interpreting blood gases. *American Journal of Nursing* 90:42–45.

This article reviews basic acid-base balance and uses three examples to help the reader apply the six suggested steps in interpreting common blood gas values.

Gasparis, L, Murray, EB, and Ursomanno, P. April 1989. IV solutions—which one's right for your patient? *Nursing89* 19:62–64.

This article reviews hypotonic, isotonic, and hypertonic IV solutions and presents factors that nurses need to know when administering them. The nurse is asked to decide whether the physicians' IV orders are in the client's best interest or whether the client's fluid and electrolyte status indicates the orders should be questioned.

RELATED RESEARCH

Adams, F. July/August 1988. How much do elders drink? *Geriatric Nursing* 9:218–21.

Gaspar, PM. July/August 1988. What determines how much patients drink? *Geriatric Nursing* 9:221–24.

SELECTED REFERENCES

Aaronson, L and Seaman, LP. July 1989. Managing hypernatremia in fluid deficient elderly. *Journal of Gerontological Nursing* 15:29–36.

American Association of Blood Banks, American Red Cross, and Council of Community Blood Centers. 1991. *Circular of Information for the Use of Human Blood and Blood Components.* Arlington, VA: American Association of Blood Banks.

Anderson, S. August 1990. ABGs—Six easy steps to interpreting blood gases. *American Journal of Nursing* 90:42–45.

Boykoff, SL, Boxwell, AO, and Boxwell, JJ. February 1988. Six ways to clear air from an IV line. *Nursing88:* 46–48.

Bryan, CS. June 1987. "CDC says . . .": The case of IV tubing replacement. *Infection Control* 8:255–56.

Byrne, CJ, Saxton, DF, Pelikan, PK, and Nugent, PM. 1986. *Laboratory Tests: Implications for Nursing Care.* 2d ed. Redwood City, CA: Addison-Wesley Nursing.

Carpenito, LJ. 1992. *Nursing Diagnosis: Application to Clinical Practice.* 4th ed. Philadelphia: Lippincott.

Chenevey, B. December 1987. Overview of fluids and electrolytes. *Nursing Clinics of North America* 22:749–59.

Cohen, MR and Davis, NM. June 1993. Recognizing the dangers of free flow from an E.I.D. *Nursing93* 23:56–59.

Crow, S. March/April 1987. Infection risks in IV therapy. *Journal of the National Intravenous Therapy Association* 10:101–5.

Dick, MJ, Maree, SM, and Gray, J. June 1992. How to boost the odds of a painless IV start. *American Journal of Nursing* 92:49–50.

Gaspar, PM. July/August 1988. What determines how much patients drink? *Geriatric Nursing* 9:221–24.

Gasparis, L, Murray, EB, and Ursomanno, P. April 1989. IV solutions—which one's right for your patient? *Nursing89* 19:62–64.

Goodinson, SM. February 1990. The risks of I.V. therapy. *Professional Nurse* 5:235–36.

Guyton, AC. 1991. *Textbook of Medical Physiology.* 8th ed. Philadelphia: WB Saunders.

Holder, C. February 1990. A new and improved guide to IV therapy. *American Journal of Nursing* 90:43–47.

Holder, C and Alexander, J. February 1990. A new and improved guide to I.V. therapy . . . protocols for intravenous therapy. *American Journal of Nursing* 90:43–47.

Horne, MM and Swearington, PL, editors. 1989. *Pocket Guide to Fluids and Electrolytes.* St Louis: Mosby.

Janusek, LW. July 1990. Metabolic acidosis: Pathophysiology, signs and symptoms. *Nursing90* 20:52–53.

Josephson, A, Gombert, ME, Sierra, MF, Karanfil, LV, and Tansino, GF. September 1985. The relationship between intravenous fluid contamination and the frequency of tubing replacement. *Infection Control* 6:637–70.

Kim, MJ, McFarland, GK, and McLane, AM 1993. *Pocket Guide to Nursing Diagnoses.* 5th ed. St Louis: Mosby-Year Book.

Larkin, M. May/June 1987. Home I.V. therapy. *Journal of the National Intravenous Therapy Association* 10:171.

LaRocca, JC and Otto, SE. 1989. *Pocket Guide to Intravenous Therapy.* St Louis: Mosby.

Lederer, JR, Marculescu, GL, Mocnik, B, and Seaby, N. 1993. *Care Planning Pocket Guide—A Nursing Diagnostic Approach.* 5th ed. Redwood City, CA: Addison-Wesley Nursing.

Lenox, AC. March 1990. I.V. therapy: Reducing the risk of infection. *Nursing90* 20:60–61.

Lonsway, RA. March/April 1987. Research, standards, and infection control: The impact of I.V. nursing. *Journal of the National Intravenous Therapy Association* 10:106–9.

McFarland, GK, and McFarlane, EA. 1993. *Nursing Diagnosis and Intervention: Planning for Patient Care.* 2d ed. St Louis: Mosby.

McMullen, A, Fioravanti, ID, Pollack, V, Rideout, K, and Sciera, M. March/April 1993. Heparinized saline or normal saline as a flush solution in intermittent intravenous lines in infants and children. *American Journal of Maternal/Child Nursing* 18:78–85.

Marieb, EN. 1992. *Human Anatomy and Physiology.* 2d ed. Redwood City, CA: Benjamin/Cummings.

Mathewson, M. February 1989. Intravenous therapy. *Critical Care Nurse* 9:21–23, 26–28, 30–36.

Metheny, NM. June 1990. Why worry about I.V. fluids? *American Journal of Nursing* 90:50–55.

———. 1992. *Fluid and Electrolyte Balance.* 2d ed. Philadelphia: Lippincott.

Millam, DA. March 1988. Managing complications of IV therapy. *Nursing88* 18:34–43.

———. May 1991. Myths and facts . . . about IV therapy. *Nursing* 21:75–76.

———. July 1993. How to teach good venipuncture technique. *American Journal of Nursing* 93:38–41.

National Blood Resource Education Program's Nursing Education Working Group. June 1991. Transfusion nursing: Trends and practices for the '90s. Choosing blood components and equipment. *American Journal of Nursing* 91:42–46.

North American Nursing Diagnosis Association. 1992. *NANDA Nursing diagnoses: Definitions and Classification 1992–1993.* Philadelphia: NANDA.

Peck, N. May, June, and July 1985. Perfecting your IV therapy techniques. (3 parts.) *Nursing85* 15:38–43; 48–51; 32–35.

Snydman, DR, Donnelly-Reidy, M, Perry, LK, and Martin, JW. March 1987. Intravenous tubing containing burettes can be safely changed at 72-hour intervals. *Infection Control* 8:113–16.

Townend, M. January/March 1990. The importance of developing and using standards of practice for IV therapy. *CINA Journal* 6:4.

Weinstein, S. May 1987. Intravenous filters. *Infection Control* 8:113–16.

Winskunas, CA. March/April 1990. A creative approach to comprehensive I.V. therapy documentation. *Journal of Intravenous Nursing* 13:115–18.

Wiseman, M. April 1985. Setting standards for home IV therapy. *American Journal of Nursing* 85:421–23.

Wittig, P and Semmler-Bertanzi, DJ. July 1983. Pumps and controllers: A nurse's assessment guide. *American Journal of Nursing* 83:1022–25.

Young, ME and Flynn, KT. August 1988. Third-spacing: When the body conceals fluid loss. *RN* 51:46–48.

39 Oxygenation

Objectives

- Explain the three phases of respiration.
- Describe the basic mechanics of breathing.
- Explain mechanisms regulating the respiratory process.
- Explain how oxygen is transported to the tissues and how carbon dioxide is transported from the tissues.
- Identify factors influencing respiratory and circulatory function.
- Describe clinical signs of hypoxia.
- Describe common altered breathing patterns.
- List the signs of an obstructed airway.
- Identify common responses to alterations in respiratory and circulatory status.
- Explain pulse oximetry.
- Describe how to promote healthy breathing.
- Explain the importance of hydration in promoting adequate oxygenation.
- Explain selected medications for respiratory function.
- Describe the use of selected inhalation therapy devices and practices.
- Explain deep breathing and coughing.
- Explain oropharyngeal and nasopharyngeal suctioning.
- Describe various methods to administer oxygen.
- Compare administering oxygen therapy by nasal cannula, face mask, and face tent.
- State outcome criteria for evaluating client responses to implemented measures to promote adequate oxygenation.
- Explain artificial airways.
- Describe essential care related to chest drainage.
- Monitor clients with chest drainage effectively.

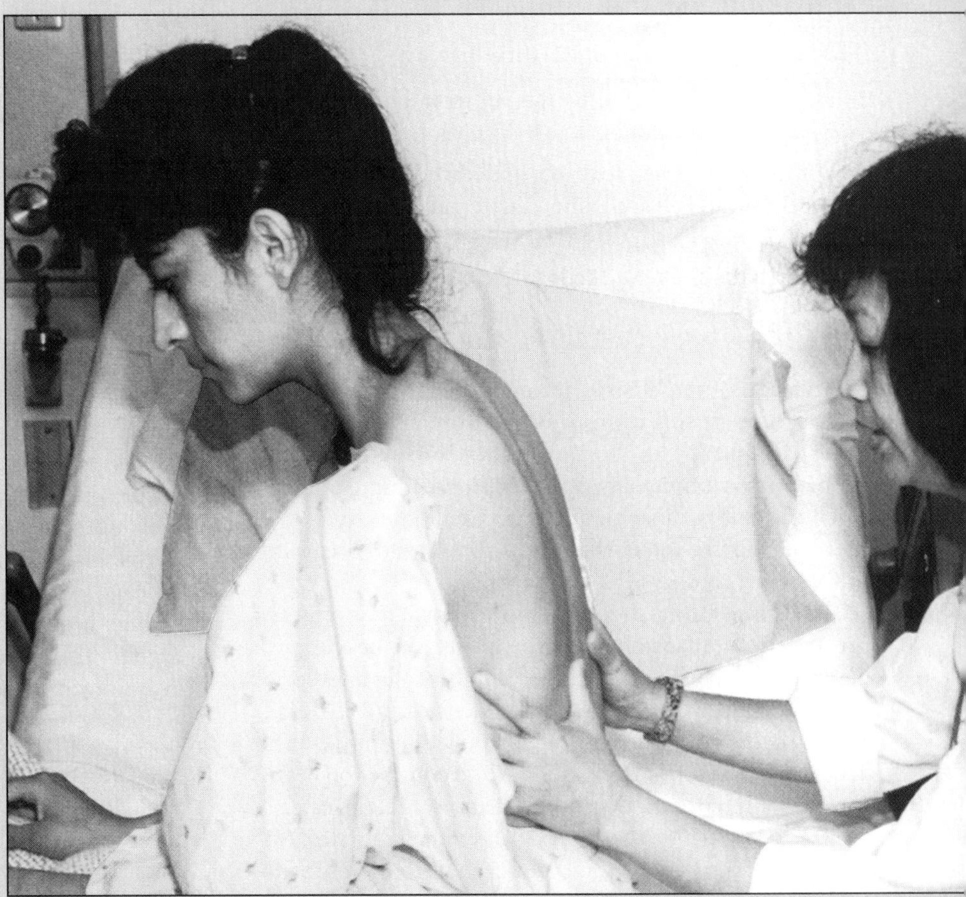

Respiration is the process of gaseous exchange between the individual and the environment. Respiration is necessary for life, but people take their breathing for granted until they encounter problems breathing. Because oxygen is necessary for all living cells, the absence of oxygen can lead to death.

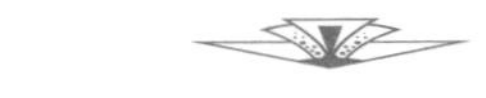

Physiology of Respiration

The process of respiration has three parts:

1. Pulmonary ventilation, or the inflow and outflow of air between the atmosphere and the alveoli of the lungs
2. Diffusion of gases (oxygen and carbon dioxide) between the alveoli and pulmonary capillaries
3. Transport of oxygen and carbon dioxide via the blood to and from the tissue cells

Pulmonary Ventilation

Ventilation of the lungs is accomplished through the act of breathing **(inspiration** or **inhalation,** and **expiration** or **exhalation).** The degree of chest expansion during ventilation is minimal with normal breathing but can reach maximum capacities during strenuous activity. See the discussion of the mechanics and control of breathing in Chapter 21, page 445.

Breathing during strenuous exercise or illness requires greater chest expansion and effort. The greater chest expansion of heavy breathing is accomplished by intercostal and other muscles that elevate or depress the rib cage. During inspiration, the rib cage is pulled upward by the action of the anterior neck muscles and contraction of the external intercostals. During expiration, the rib cage is pulled downward by the anterior abdominal muscles. Active use of these muscles and noticeable effort in breathing are seen in clients with obstructive respiratory disease.

Pulmonary Volumes The volume to which the lungs expand during ventilation depends on whether breathing is normal and whether maximum inspiration and expiration occur. The normal volume of air inspired and expired is referred to as the **tidal volume.** In young adults, the tidal volume is about 500 mL in males and 400 mL in females. Volumes may be smaller in small persons or greater in large or athletic persons. There are three other volumes: the **inspiratory reserve volume,** the **expiratory reserve volume,** and the **residual volume.** These three volumes added to the tidal volume yield the **total lung capacity,** which is the maximum volume to which the lungs can expand. See Table 39–1.

Pulmonary Capacities Pulmonary volumes are often grouped in combinations of two or more. These combined volumes are referred to as the **pulmonary capacities** and include total lung capacity plus the **inspiratory capacity,** the **functional residual capacity,** and the **vital capacity.** See Table 39–1. The residual volume is normally about 20% of the total lung capacity.

Pulmonary Pressures Breathing produces changes in **intrapulmonic pressure** (pressure within the lungs) and in **intrapleural pressure** (pressure outside or around the lungs). These pressure changes are related to the changes in the lung volumes in accordance with *Boyle's law,* which states that the volume of a gas at constant temperature varies inversely with its pressure. On inspiration, the volume of the lungs increases, and thus the intrapulmonic pressure decreases. This decreased pressure allows atmospheric air to enter, since its pressure is greater. Conversely, on expiration the volume of the lungs decreases, and the intrapulmonic pressure increases. This allows the air to escape to the atmosphere, where the pressure is lower than that in the lungs.

Unless the chest cavity is damaged or opened, the intrapleural pressure is always negative. This negative pressure is essential because it creates the suction that holds the visceral pleura and the parietal pleura together as the chest cage expands and contracts. The recoil tendency of the lungs is a major factor responsible for this negative pressure. The fluid in the intrapleural space, however, provides even more negative pressure. Intrapleural fluid causes the pleura to adhere together, much as a film of water can cause two glass slides to adhere together.

Ventilation of the lungs depends on four factors:

1. Adequate atmospheric oxygen
2. Clear air passages
3. Adequate pulmonary compliance and recoil
4. Regulation of respiration

The presence of atmospheric oxygen in adequate concentration is basic to adequate respirations. Concentrations of oxygen are lower at high altitudes than at sea level. In some instances, people at very high altitudes need supplementary oxygen.

During inspiration, air passes through the nose, pharynx, larynx, trachea, bronchi, and bronchioles to the alveoli, and expiration reverses that course. The nose performs three important functions. It warms, moistens, and filters the air. Large particles in the air are filtered by the

Table 39–1 Summary of Pulmonary Volumes and Capacities

Measurement	Adult Male Average Value (mL)*	Description
Respiratory Volumes		
Tidal volume (TV)	500	Amount of air inhaled or exhaled with each breath under resting conditions
Inspiratory reserve volume (IRV)	3100	Amount of air that can be forcefully inhaled after a normal tidal volume inhalation
Expiratory reserve volume (ERV)	1200	Amount of air that can be forcefully exhaled after a normal tidal volume exhalation
Residual volume (RV)	1200	Amount of air remaining in the lungs after a forced exhalation
Respiratory Capacities		
Total lung capacity (TLC)	6000	Maximum amount of air contained in lungs after a maximum inspiratory effort: TLC = TV + IRV + ERV + RV
Vital capacity (VC)	4800	Maxmimum amount of air that can be expired after a maximum inspiratory effort: VC = TV + IRV + ERV (should be 80% TLC)
Inspiratory capacity (IC)	3600	Maximum amount of air that can be inspired after a normal expiration: IC = TV + IRV
Functional residual capacity (FRC)	2400	Volume of air remaining in the lungs after a normal tidal volume expiration: FRC = ERV + RV

* Female values are 20% to 25% smaller.

Source: EN Marieb, *Human Anatomy and Physiology*, 2d ed. (Redwood City, CA: Benjamin/Cummings, 1992), p. 742. Used with permission.

hairs at the entrance of the nares, and smaller particles are filtered by nasal turbulence. Each time air contacts the nasal turbinates or nasal septum it must change direction, and in the process small particles are trapped.

Air passages are cleared by the mucous membrane lining, which contains **cilia** (hairlike projections of the respiratory mucous membrane). Mucus entraps organisms or other small foreign material while the cilia move the trapped material. The cilia beat continually at a rate of 10 to 20 times per second, directed toward the pharynx. Thus the cilia in the lower respiratory passageways (eg, the bronchi) beat upward, and the cilia in the nose beat downward. Material can be moved as much as 1 cm per minute along the trachea (Guyton 1991, p. 411).

The **cough** reflex and the sneeze reflex are also essential cleaning mechanisms. The *cough reflex* is triggered by irritants that send nerve impulses through the vagus nerve to the medulla. Any foreign matter in the larynx, trachea, or bronchi initiates the cough reflex. A particularly sensitive area is the **carina,** the ridge or junction where the main bronchi meet at the trachea. The cough reflex process is described in the box on page 1132. The *sneeze reflex* is to the nasal passages as the cough is to lower respiratory passages. Sneezing is initiated when irritating impulses pass by way of the fifth cranial nerve to the medulla. Sneezing involves a series of reactions similar to the cough reflex; however, the uvula is depressed so that a large volume of air passes rapidly through the nose as well as the mouth, thus helping to clear the nasal passages.

Lung compliance is lung expansibility or stretchability. It generally includes expansibility of both the lungs and the thorax but sometimes denotes compliance of the lungs alone.

In contrast to lung compliance is **lung recoil.** The lungs have a continual tendency to collapse away from the chest wall. Two factors are responsible for this recoil tendency: (a) elastic fibers present in lung tissue and (b) surface tension of the fluid lining the alveoli. The latter accounts for two-thirds of the recoil phenomenon. Counterbalancing this surface tension in the alveoli is a lipoprotein mixture called **surfactant.** When surfactant is absent, lung expansion is exceedingly difficult and the lungs collapse. Normally, the secretion of surfactant by the alveoli is stimulated several times each hour by yawning, sighing, or deep breaths. Surfactant stimulation is important for clients on automatic ventilation. The alveoli must be stretched several times every hour by a sigh mechanism on the respirator.

THE COUGH REFLEX PROCESS

1. 2.5 liters of air is inspired.
2. The epiglottis closes.
3. The vocal cords shut tightly to entrap air in the lungs.
4. The abdominal muscles contract forcefully, pushing against the diaphragm.
5. Simultaneously, the thoracic expiratory muscles—for example, the internal intercostal muscles—contract forcefully.
6. As a result, the pressure in the lungs rises to as high as 100 mm Hg or more.
7. The vocal cords and epiglottis open suddenly.
8. The pressure in the lungs explodes outward, sometimes at a velocity as high as 75 to 100 mph.
9. The compression of the lungs collapses the bronchi and trachea, causing their non-cartilaginous parts to invaginate inward, and the exploding air therefore passes through bronchial and tracheal slits.

Source: AC Guyton, *Textbook of Medical Physiology*, 8th ed. (Philadelphia: WB Saunders, 1991), pp. 411–12.

DIFFUSION OF GASES

After the alveoli are ventilated, the second phase of the respiratory process—*the diffusion of oxygen from the alveoli and into the pulmonary blood vessels*—begins. **Diffusion** is the movement of gases or other particles from an area of greater pressure or concentration to an area of lower pressure or concentration. Because the alveolar walls are very thin and are surrounded by a closely intertwined network of blood capillaries, these membranes together are often referred to as the **respiratory membrane.**

Pressure differences in the gases on each side of the respiratory membrane obviously affect diffusion. When the pressure of oxygen is greater in the alveoli than in the blood, oxygen diffuses into the blood. Normally the oxygen pressure gradient between the alveoli and the blood entering the pulmonary capillaries is about 40 mm Hg. The **partial pressure** (the pressure exerted by each individual gas in a mixture according to its concentration in the mixture) of oxygen (**PaO_2**) in the alveoli is about 100 mm Hg, whereas the PaO_2 in the entering venous blood of the pulmonary arteries is about 60 mm Hg. These pressures equalize very rapidly, however, so that the arterial pressure also reaches about 100 mm Hg. By contrast, carbon dioxide in the venous blood entering the pulmonary capillaries has a partial pressure of about 45 mm Hg (**$PaCO_2$**), whereas that in the alveoli has a partial pressure of about 40 mm Hg. These partial pressures frequently are used diagnostically to assess deficiencies or excesses of oxygen and carbon dioxide in persons with pulmonary disease.

TRANSPORT OF OXYGEN AND CARBON DIOXIDE

The third part of the respiratory process involves the transport of respiratory gases. Oxygen needs to be transported from the lungs to the tissues, and carbon dioxide must be transported from the tissues back to the lungs. Normally, most of the oxygen (97%) combines loosely with the **hemoglobin** (oxygen-carrying red pigment) in the red blood cells and is carried to the tissues as **oxyhemoglobin** (the compound of oxygen and hemoglobin). The remaining oxygen is dissolved and transported in the fluid of the plasma and cells.

Several factors affect the rate of oxygen transport from the lungs to the tissues:

1. Cardiac output
2. Number of erythrocytes
3. Exercise
4. Blood hematocrit

Normal **cardiac output** (amount of blood pumped by the heart) is approximately 5 liters per minute. Any pathologic condition that decreases cardiac output (eg damage to the heart muscle, blood loss, or pooling of blood in the peripheral blood vessels) diminishes the amount of oxygen delivered to the tissues. Generally, the heart compensates for inadequate output by increasing its pumping rate. Normally, compensatory cardiac output can increase the oxygen transport fivefold; but when disease conditions exist, this is not possible.

The second factor influencing oxygen transport is the number of **erythrocytes** (red blood cells, or RBCs). In men the number of circulating erythrocytes normally averages about 5 million per cubic milliliter of blood, and in women, about 4½ million per cubic milliliter. Reductions in these normal values can be brought about by anemia of any cause.

Exercise also has a direct influence on oxygen transport. In well-trained athletes, oxygen transport can be increased up to 20 times normal, due in part to an increased cardiac output and to increased utilization of oxygen by the cells (utilization coefficient).

The **hematocrit** is the percentage of the blood that is erythrocytes. It is also referred to as the packed cell volume per 100 mL. Normally this ratio is about 40% to 54% in men and 37% to 47% in women. Excessive increases in the blood hematocrit increase the blood viscosity, reduce the cardiac output, and therefore reduce oxygen transport. Excessive reductions in the blood hematocrit, such as occur in anemia, also reduce oxygen transport.

A moderate amount of carbon dioxide (30%) is transported by reduced hemoglobin (which is able to combine with carbon dioxide to form **carbaminohemoglobin**). The largest amount (about 65%) is carried in the form of bicarbonate (HCO_3^-) inside the red blood cells. Smaller amounts (5%) are transported in solution in the plasma and as **carbonic acid** (the compound formed when CO_2 combines with water).

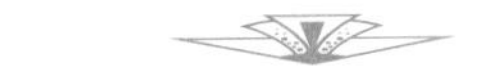

REGULATION OF RESPIRATION

Respiratory regulation of oxygen, carbon dioxide, and hydrogen ions in body fluids includes both neural and chemical controls. Respiratory control basically functions to maintain the correct concentrations. The nervous system of the body adjusts the rate of alveolar ventilations to meet the needs of the body so that Pa_{O_2} and Pa_{CO_2} remain relatively constant. The body's "respiratory center" is actually a number of groups of neurons located in the medulla oblongata and pons of the brain.

A **chemosensitive** center in the medulla oblongata is highly responsive to increases in blood CO_2 or hydrogen ion concentration. By influencing other respiratory centers, this center can increase the activity of the inspiratory center, the rate of respirations, and the rate and depth of inspirations. In addition to direct chemical stimulation of the respiratory center in the brain, there are special receptors sensitive to decreases in O_2 concentration located outside the central nervous system, in the carotid bodies (just above the bifurcation of the common carotid arteries) and aortic bodies. Impulses from these **chemoreceptors** travel along Hering's nerves to the glossopharyngeal nerves and then to the dorsal respiratory area in the medulla. Decreases in arterial oxygen concentrations stimulate the chemoreceptors in the aortic and carotid bodies, and they, in turn, stimulate the respiratory center to increase ventilation. Of the three blood gases (hydrogen, oxygen, and carbon dioxide) that can trigger chemoreceptors, increased carbon dioxide concentration stimulates respiration most strongly.

In clients with certain lung ailments, such as **emphysema,** however, oxygen concentrations, *not carbon dioxide concentrations*, play a major role in regulating respiration. For such clients, decreased oxygen concentrations are the main stimuli for respiration. This is sometimes called the *hypoxic drive*. Increasing the concentration of oxygen depresses the respiratory rate. Thus, only low concentrations of supplemental oxygen are administered to these clients.

FACTORS AFFECTING RESPIRATORY FUNCTION

Factors that influence oxygenation affect the cardiovascular system as well as the respiratory system. These factors include development, environment, life-style, health status, and narcotics (opioids).

Development At birth a major respiratory change occurs: The lungs, which had been filled with fluid, become filled with air. Infants have a small chest and short airways. The latter predisposes to aspiration of foreign objects that can block the airways. During infancy, the respiratory rate is more rapid than at any other time in life. See Table 21–7, page 448.

In infants, the chest is rounded; in children, the diameter from front to back decreases in proportion to the transverse diameter. In adults, the thorax assumes an oval shape. See Chapter 22, page 510. The elderly also experience changes in the thorax and breathing patterns. See the box on page 518.

Environment Altitude, heat, cold, and air pollution affect oxygenation. The higher the *altitude*, the lower the partial pressure of the oxygen (Pa_{O_2}) an individual breathes. As a result, the person at high altitudes has increased respiratory and cardiac rates and increased respiratory depth, which usually become most apparent when the individual exercises.

In response to *heat*, the peripheral blood vessels dilate; consequently, blood flows to the skin, increasing the amount of heat lost from the body surface. With vasodilation, the lumens of blood vessels enlarge, thus decreasing the resistance to the blood flow. In response, the heart increases output to maintain blood pressure. The increased cardiac output requires additional oxygen, which is acquired through increased rate and depth of breathing. In a *cold* environment, by contrast, the peripheral blood vessels constrict, raising the blood pressure, which decreases cardiac action, thereby reducing the need for oxygen.

Healthy people exposed to *air pollution*, such as smog, often experience stinging of the eyes, headache, dizziness, coughing, and choking. Persons who have a history of existing lung disease and altered respiratory function experience varying degrees of respiratory difficulty in a polluted environment. Some are unable to maintain self-care activities in such an environment.

Life-Style Physical exercise or activity increases the rate and depth of respirations and the heart rate and hence the supply of oxygen in the body. Cigarette smoking and certain occupations predispose an individual to lung disease. For example, silicosis is seen more often in sandstone blasters and potters than in the rest of the population; asbestosis in asbestos workers; anthracosis in coal miners; and organic dust disease in farmers and agricultural employees who work with moldy hay. Activity patterns are also a factor. Sedentary persons lack the alveolar expansion and deep breathing patterns of persons who exercise on a routine basis and are therefore less able to respond effectively to respiratory stressors.

Health Status In the healthy person, the cardiovascular and respiratory systems can provide sufficient oxygen to meet the body needs. However, diseases of the cardiovascular system often affect the delivery of oxygen to the cells of the body. In addition, diseases of the respiratory system can adversely affect the oxygenation of the blood.

One cardiovascular condition that affects oxygenation is **anemia.** Because hemoglobin carries oxygen and carbon dioxide, as explained earlier, anemia can affect the delivery of these gases to and from the body cells.

Narcotics (Opioids) Narcotics such as morphine and meperidine hydrochloride (Demerol) decrease the rate and depth of respirations by depressing the respiratory center in the medulla. When administering narcotic analgesics, the nurse must monitor respiratory rates and depths.

TERMS RELATED TO HYPOXIA

- *Respiratory insufficiency*—inability of the lungs to maintain normal arterial blood gas levels when the individual is breathing 21% oxygen (at sea level)
- *Hyperpnea*—excessively high rate of alveolar ventilation
- *Hypopnea*—low rate of alveolar ventilation, that is, underrespiration
- *Hypocarbia (hypocapnia)*—depressed blood carbon dioxide level
- *Acapnia*—absence of carbon dioxide in the blood (this state is incompatible with life)

SIGNS OF HYPOXIA

- Increased rapid pulse
- Rapid, shallow respirations and dyspnea
- Increased restlessness or lightheadedness
- Flaring of the nares
- Substernal or intercostal retractions
- Cyanosis

ALTERATIONS IN RESPIRATORY FUNCTION

Respiratory function can be altered by conditions that affect three areas of function:

1. The movement of air into or out of the lungs
2. The diffusion of oxygen and carbon dioxide between the alveoli and the pulmonary capillaries
3. The transport of oxygen and carbon dioxide via the blood to and from the tissue cells

Three major alterations in respiration are hypoxia, altered breathing pattern, and obstructed or partially obstructed airway.

HYPOXIA

Hypoxia is a condition of insufficient oxygen anywhere in the body, from the inspired gas to the tissues. It can be related to any of the three parts of respiration: ventilation, diffusion of gases, or transport of gases by the blood, and can be caused by any condition that alters one or more parts of the process.

Another cause of hypoxia is **hypoventilation,** that is, inadequate alveolar ventilation due to decreased tidal volume. Whatever the reason for a decreased tidal volume (for example, diseases of the respiratory muscles, drugs, or anesthesia), carbon dioxide often accumulates in the blood. This condition is called **hypercarbia (hypercapnia).** Additional terms relating to hypoxia are given in the box above.

Hypoxia can also develop when the lungs' ability to diffuse oxygen into the arterial blood decreases, as with pulmonary edema, or can result from problems in the delivery of oxygen to the tissues (eg, anemia, cardiac failure, and embolism). The term **hypoxemia** refers to reduced oxygen in the blood and is characterized by a low partial pressure of oxygen in arterial blood or a low saturation of oxyhemoglobin. See the second box above for the signs of hypoxia.

Cyanosis (bluish discoloration of the skin, nail beds, and mucous membranes, due to reduced oxygen levels of hemoglobin) may also be present. Cyanosis requires these two conditions: the blood must contain about 5 g or more of unoxygenated hemoglobin per 100 mL of blood, and the surface blood capillaries must be dilated. Any factors that interfere with either of these conditions (eg, severe anemia or the administration of adrenaline) will eliminate cyanosis as a sign even if the client is experiencing hypoxia.

Adequate oxygenation is essential for cerebral functioning. The cerebral cortex can tolerate hypoxia for only 3 to 5 minutes before permanent damage occurs. The face of the acutely hypoxic person usually appears anxious, tired, and drawn. The person usually assumes a sitting position, often leaning forward slightly to permit greater expansion of the thoracic cavity. The hypoxic client may or may not experience pain on breathing. Although lung tissue lacks pain receptors, pain can arise from the pleura, chest wall, or upper respiratory tract.

With *chronic* hypoxia, the client often appears fatigued and is lethargic. The client's fingers may be clubbed as a result of long-term lack of oxygen in the arterial blood supply to the fingers. With clubbing, the base of the nail becomes swollen and the ends of the fingers and toes increase in size. The angle between the nail and the base of the nail increases to more than 180 degrees. See Figure 22–5, *D*, page 479.

ALTERED BREATHING PATTERNS

Breathing patterns refer to the rate, volume, rhythm, and relative ease or effort of respiration. Normal respiration **(eupnea)** is quiet, rhythmic, and effortless. **Tachypnea** (rapid rate) is seen with fevers, metabolic acidosis, and pain and with hypercapnia (elevated blood CO_2) or **anoxemia** (decreased oxygen in the blood). **Bradypnea** is an abnormally slow respiratory rate, which may be seen in clients who have taken drugs such as morphine sulphate (a respiratory depressant), who have metabolic acidosis, or who have increased intracranial pressure (eg, from brain injuries).

Hyperventilation is an excessive amount of air in the lungs. It is often called **alveolar hyperventilation** because the amount of air in the alveoli exceeds the body's metabolic requirements; that is, more CO_2 is eliminated than is produced. Hyperventilation usually results from an increase in the rate and depth of respirations. One particular type of hyperventilation that accompanies metabolic acidosis is **Kussmaul's breathing,** by which the body attempts to compensate (give off excess body acids) by blowing off the carbon dioxide through deep and rapid breathing. Hyperventilation can also occur after the administration of amphetamines because of the increased metabolic rate such drugs induce.

Hypoventilation is inadequate alveolar ventilation, that is, ventilation that does not meet the body's requirements. As a result, carbon dioxide is retained in the bloodstream. Hypoventilation can occur as a result of collapse of the alveoli, leaving too few functioning alveoli to meet the body's ventilation needs; or it may result from airway obstruction or the side effects of some drugs.

Abnormal respiratory *rhythms* create an irregular breathing pattern. Three abnormal respiratory rhythms are described in the box above.

ABNORMAL RESPIRATORY RHYTHMS

- **Cheyne-Stokes breathing.** Marked rhythmic waxing and waning of respirations from very deep to very shallow breathing and temporary apnea (cessation of breathing); common causes include congestive heart failure, increased intracranial pressure, and drug overdose.
- **Apneustic breathing.** Prolonged gasping inspiration followed by a very short, usually inefficient, expiration; associated with central nervous system disorders.
- **Biot's breathing.** Shallow breaths interrupted by apnea; may be seen in healthy people and in clients with central nervous system disorders.

Normal breathing is effortless, and respirations are evenly spaced and vary little in depth. Difficult or labored breathing is called **dyspnea.** The dyspneic person often appears anxious and may say, "I can't catch my breath." Often the nostrils are flared because of the increased effort of inspiration. The skin may appear dusky; heart rate is increased. **Orthopnea** is the inability to breathe except in an upright sitting or standing position.

OBSTRUCTED AIRWAY

A complete or partially obstructed airway can occur anywhere along the upper or lower respiratory passageways. An upper airway obstruction—that is, in the nose, pharynx, larynx, or trachea—can arise because of a foreign object, such as food; because the tongue falls back into the oropharynx when a person is unconscious; or when secretions collect in the passageways. In the latter instance, the respirations will sound gurgly or bubbly as the air attempts to pass through the secretions. Lower airway obstruction involves partial or complete occlusion of the passageways in the bronchi and lungs.

Maintaining an open (patent) airway is a frequent nursing intervention, one that often requires immediate action. Partial obstruction of the upper airway passages is indicated by a low-pitched snoring sound during inhalation. Complete obstruction is indicated by extreme inspiratory effort that produces no chest movement. Such a

ASSESSMENT INTERVIEW

Oxygenation

Current Respiratory Problems

- Have you noticed any changes in your breathing pattern (eg, shortness of breath, difficulty in breathing, need to be in upright position to breathe, or rapid and shallow breathing)? See below for cough, sputum, and pain.
- Which of your activities might cause the above symptom(s) to occur?

History of Respiratory Disease

- Have you had colds, allergies, croup, asthma, tuberculosis, bronchitis, pneumonia, or emphysema?
- How frequently have these occurred? How long did they last? And how were they treated?
- Have you been exposed to any pollutants?

Current or Past Cardiovascular Problems

- Do you have a history of cardiac or blood circulation problems (eg, anemia, hypertension, heart disease)?

Life-Style

- Do you smoke? If so, how much? If not, did you smoke previously, and when did you stop?
- Does any member of your family smoke?
- Are there smokers or other pollutants (eg, fumes, dust, coal, asbestos) in your workplace?

Presence of Cough

- How often and how much do you cough?
- Is it *productive*, that is, accompanied by sputum, or *non-productive*, that is, dry?
- Does the cough occur during certain activity or at certain times of the day?

Description of Sputum

- When is the sputum produced?
- What is the amount, color, thickness, odor?
- Is it ever tinged with blood?

Presence of Chest Pain

- Do you experience any pain with breathing or activity?
- Where is the pain located?
- Describe the pain. How does it feel?
- Does it occur when you breathe in or out?
- How long does it last, and how does it affect your breathing?
- What activities precede your pain?
- What do you do to relieve the pain?

Presence of Risk Factors

- Do you have a family history of lung cancer, cardiovascular disease (including strokes), or tuberculosis?
- The nurse should also note the client's weight, activity pattern, and dietary assessment. In addition to smoking, risk factors include obesity, sedentary life-style, and diet high in saturated fats.

Medication History

- Have you taken or do you take any over-the-counter or prescription medications for heart, blood pressure, or breathing (eg, bronchodilator, inhalant, narcotic)?
- Which ones? And what are the dosages, times taken, and results, including side effects?

client, in an effort to obtain air, may also exhibit marked sternal and intercostal retractions. Lower airway obstruction is not always as easy to observe. The client may have altered arterial blood gas levels, restlessness, dyspnea, and **adventitious breath sounds** (abnormal breath sounds). See Table 22–8, page 512.

ASSESSING

Nursing assessment of oxygenation status includes a history, physical examination, pulse oximetry, and review of relevant diagnostic data.

NURSING HISTORY

A comprehensive nursing history relevant to oxygenation status should include data about current and past respiratory and cardiovascular problems; life-style; presence of cough, sputum, pain, medications for heart, blood pressure, or breathing; and presence of risk factors for impaired oxygenation status. Examples of interview questions to elicit this information are shown in the box above.

PHYSICAL EXAMINATION

In assessing a client's oxygenation status the nurse uses all four physical examination techniques: inspection, palpation, percussion, and auscultation. The nurse first observes the rate, depth, rhythm, and quality of respirations, noting the position the client assumes for breathing. Some clients with chronic respiratory problems prefer to bend forward at the waist to ease breathing or to sit leaning over a table because these positions permit greater lung expansion. Lying on the back or on either side restricts expansion of part of the thorax (the underlying portion). This relatively small increase in expansion may be important to a dyspneic client. Chapter 21 provides additional information on assessing respirations.

Variations in the shape of the thorax may indicate adaptation to chronic respiratory conditions. For example, clients with emphysema frequently develop a *barrel chest.* See Figure 22–41, on page 511, for an illustration of variations in the shape of the chest. The lungs and heart should be assessed very carefully. See Chapter 22. Terms commonly used in recording physical assessment findings related to respiratory function are shown in the box on page 449.

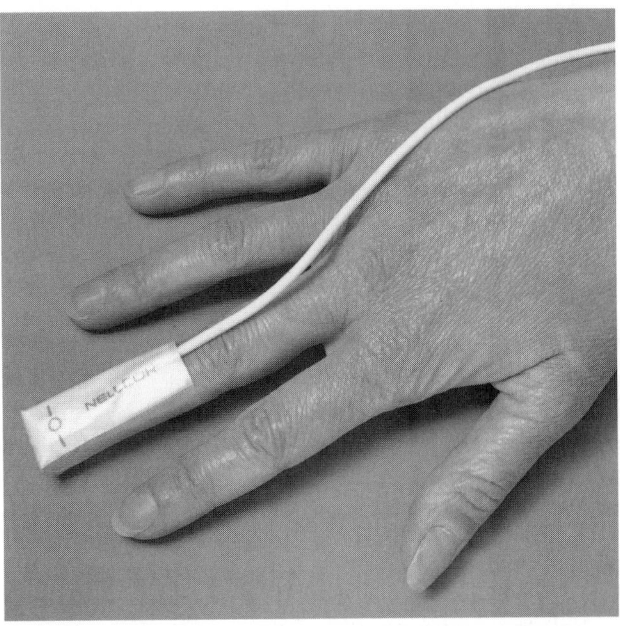

Figure 39–1 A finger clip pulse oximeter sensor.

PULSE OXIMETRY

A **pulse oximeter** is a noninvasive device that measures a client's arterial blood oxygen saturation (SaO_2, or O_2 Sat) by means of a sensor attached to the client's finger (Figure 39–1), toe, nose, earlobe, or forehead (or around the hand or foot of a neonate). The pulse oximeter can detect hypoxemia before clinical signs and symptoms, such as dusky skin color and dusky nailbeds color develop.

The pulse oximeter's *sensor* has two parts: (a) two light-emitting diodes (LEDs)—one red, the other infrared—that transmit light through nails, tissue, venous blood, and arterial blood; and (b) a photodetector placed directly opposite the LEDs (eg, the other side of the finger, toe, or nose). The photodetector receives red and infrared light. By a process known as **spectrophotometry,** the photodetector measures the amount of red and infrared light absorbed by oxygenated and deoxygenated hemoglobin in arterial blood: Oxygenated hemoglobin absorbs more infrared light; deoxygenated hemoglobin, more red light. The SaO_2 is computed on the basis of the amount of light (red and infrared) that reaches the photodetector. Normal SaO_2 is 95% to 100%. An SaO_2 below 70% is life-threatening.

Because pulse oximetry measures only the **functional hemoglobin** (the ratio of oxygen bound to hemoglobin compared to the amount of hemoglobin that is available for binding), it can create misleading results if the client's hemoglobin is bound to another substance, such as carbon monoxide. Pulse oximetry doesn't account for hemoglobin bound to carbon monoxide.

The *oximeter unit* consists of an inlet connection for the sensor cable, a faceplate that indicates (a) the oxygen saturation measurement (expressed as a percentage) and (b) the pulse rate. A preset alarm system signals high and low SaO_2 measurements and a high and low pulse rate. The high and low SaO_2 levels for adults are generally preset at 100% and 85%, respectively (95% and 80% for neonates). The high and low pulse rates for adults are usually preset at 140 and 50 beats per minute (200 and 100 for neonates). These alarm limits can, however, be changed according to the manufacturer's directions. Procedure 39–1 on page 1138 explains how to set up and use a pulse oximeter.

DIAGNOSTIC STUDIES

The physician may order various diagnostic tests to assess respiratory status, function, and oxygenation. Included are sputum specimens, throat cultures, venous and arterial blood specimens, pulmonary function tests, visual inspection procedures, and thoracocentesis (thoracentesis). Often it is the nurse who collects specimens to be sent to the laboratory for analysis.

Specimens **Sputum** is the mucous secretion from the lungs, bronchi, and trachea. It is important to differentiate it from *saliva,* the clear liquid secreted by the salivary glands in the mouth, sometimes referred to as "spit." Healthy individuals do not produce sputum. Clients need to cough to bring sputum up from the lungs, bronchi, and trachea into the mouth in order to expectorate it into a collecting container. Sputum specimens are usually collected for one or more of the following reasons:

- For *culture and sensitivity* to identify a specific microorganism and its drug sensitivities.

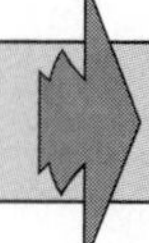

PROCEDURE 39–1 USING A PULSE OXIMETER

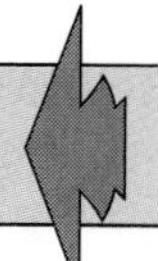

PURPOSES

- To measure the arterial blood oxygen saturation (SaO_2)
- To detect the presence of hypoxemia before visible signs develop

ASSESSMENT FOCUS

Risk factors for development of hypoxemia (eg, respiratory or cardiac disease); vital signs and skin and nailbed color as baseline data; allergy to adhesive; tissue perfusion of extremities; hemoglobin level.

EQUIPMENT

- ☐ Pulse oximeter
- ☐ Alcohol wipe
- ☐ Nail polish remover as needed
- ☐ Sheet or towel

INTERVENTION

1. Select an appropriate sensor.

- Choose a sensor appropriate for the client's weight and size. Because weight limits of infant, pediatric, and adult sensors overlap, a neonatal sensor could be used for an infant or a pediatric sensor for a small adult. See the manufacturer's directions for weight limits.
- If the client is allergic to adhesive, use a clip or reflectance sensor without adhesive.

2. Select an appropriate site.

- Use a location appropriate for the type of sensor.
- If using an extremity, assess the proximal pulse and capillary refill at the point closest to the site. *Decreased circulation can alter the SaO_2 measurements.*
- If the client has low tissue perfusion due to peripheral vascular disease or therapy using vasoconstrictive medications, use a nasal sensor or a reflectance sensor on the forehead.
- Avoid using lower extremities that have a compromised circulation and extremities that are used for infusions or other invasive monitoring.

3. Prepare the site.

- Clean the site with an alcohol wipe before applying the sensor.
- Remove a female client's nail polish or acrylic nails. *These items can interfere with accurate measurements.*

4. Apply the sensor, and connect it to the pulse oximeter.

- Make sure the LED and photodetector are accurately aligned, that is, opposite each other on either side of the finger, toe, nose, or earlobe. Many sensors have markings to facilitate correct alignment of the LEDs and photodetector. *Correct alignment is essential for accurate SaO_2 measurement.*
- Attach the sensor cable to the connection outlet on the oximeter. Appropriate connection will be confirmed by an audible beep indicating each arterial pulsation. Turn on the machine according to the manufacturer's directions. Some devices have a wheel that can be turned clockwise to increase the pulse volume and counterclockwise to decrease it.
- Ensure that the bar of light or waveform on the face of the oximeter fluctuates with each pulsation and reflects the pulse volume or strength. *A signal that is too weak will not produce an accurate SaO_2 measurement.*

5. Set and turn on the alarm.

- Check the preset alarm limits for high and low oxygen saturation and high and low pulse rates.
- Change these alarm limits according to the manufacturer's directions as indicated.
- Ensure that the audio and visual alarms are on before you leave the client. A tone will be heard and a number will blink on the faceplate.

6. Ensure client safety.

- Inspect and/or move or change the location of an adhesive toe or finger sensor every 4 hours and a spring-tension sensor every 2 hours. *Movement prevents tissue necrosis due to prolonged pressure.*
- Inspect the sensor site tissues for irritation from adhesive sensors.

7. Ensure the accuracy of measurement.

- Minimize motion artifacts by using an adhesive sensor, or immobilize the client's monitoring site. *Movement of the client's finger or toe may be misinterpreted by the oximeter as arterial pulsations.*

PROCEDURE 39–1 *continued*

- Cover a sensor with a sheet or towel to block large amounts of light from external sources (eg, sunlight, procedure lamps, or bilirubin lights in the nursery). *Large amounts of outside light may be sensed by the photodetector and alter the SaO_2 value.*
- Verify that the client's hemoglobin level is normal. *An SaO_2 measurement may register normal when the client's hemoglobin is low because the available hemoglobin to carry oxygen is fully saturated.*

8. Document all relevant information.

- Record the application of the pulse oximeter, its type and size, and all nursing assessments.

EVALUATION FOCUS
Oxygen saturation level; pulse rate and other vital signs; tissue response to the sensor.

- For *cytology* to identify the origin, structure, function, and pathology of cells. Specimens for **cytology** often require serial collection of three early morning specimens and are tested to identify cancer in the lung and its specific cell type.
- For *acid-fast bacillus* (AFB), which also require serial collection, often for 3 consecutive days, to identify the presence of tuberculosis (TB). Some agencies use a special glass container when the presence of AFB is suspected.
- To assess the *effectiveness of therapy.*

Sputum specimens are often collected in the morning. Upon awakening, the client can cough up the secretions that have accumulated during the night. Sometimes specimens are collected during postural drainage, when the client can usually produce sputum. When a client cannot cough, the nurse must sometimes use pharyngeal suctioning to obtain a specimen.

To collect a sputum specimen, the nurse follows these steps:

- Offer mouth care so that the specimen will not be contaminated with microorganisms from the mouth.
- Ask the client to breathe deeply and then cough up 1 to 2 tablespoons, or 15 to 30 mL (4 to 8 fluid drams) of sputum.
- Wear gloves to avoid direct contact with the sputum, particularly if hemoptysis (blood in the sputum) is present.
- Ask the client to **expectorate** (spit out) the sputum into the specimen container. Make sure the sputum does not contact the outside of the container (Figure 39–2). If the container does become contaminated, wash it with a disinfectant.
- Following sputum collection, offer mouthwash to remove any unpleasant taste.

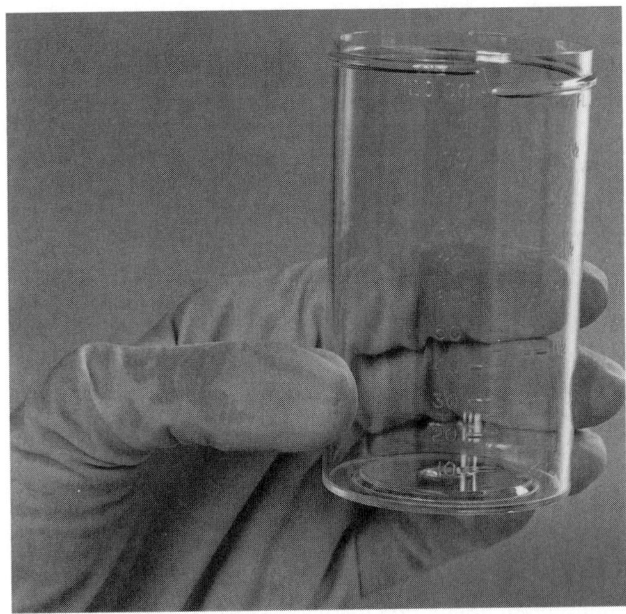

Figure 39–2 Sputum specimen container.

- Document amount of sputum collected, color, odor, consistency (thick, tenacious, watery), and presence of hemoptysis.

A **throat culture** sample is collected from the mucosa of the oropharynx and tonsillar regions using a culture swab. The sample is then cultured and examined for the presence of disease-producing microorganisms. To obtain a throat culture specimen, the nurse inserts the swab into the oropharynx and runs the swab along the tonsils and areas on the pharynx that are reddened or contain exudate. The gag reflex, active in some clients, may be decreased by having the client sit upright if health permits,

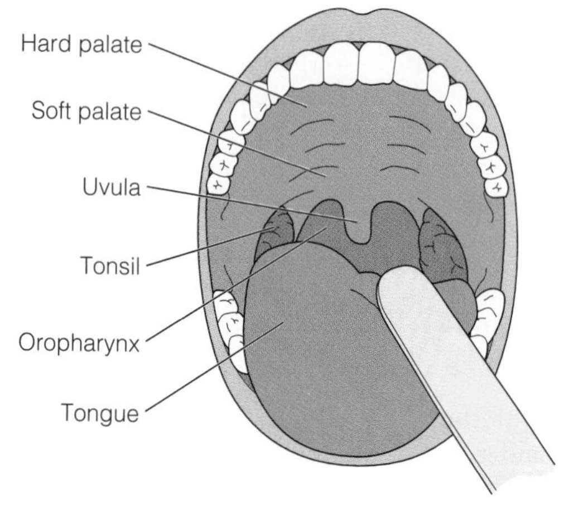

Figure 39–3 Depressing the tongue to view the pharynx.

open the mouth, extend the tongue and say "ah," and by taking the specimen quickly. The sitting position and extension of the tongue help expose the pharynx; saying "ah" relaxes the throat muscles and helps minimize contraction of the constrictor muscle of the pharynx (the gag reflex). If the posterior pharynx cannot be seen, use a light, and depress the tongue with a tongue blade (Figure 39–3).

Blood Specimens Specimens of venous blood are taken for a *complete blood count* (CBC), which includes hemoglobin and hematocrit measurements, erythrocyte (RBC) count, leukocyte (WBC) count, and a differential red cell and white cell count.

The hematocrit is the packed cell volume. It denotes the percent of a given volume of whole blood occupied by erythrocytes (RBCs). Therefore, a hematocrit level of 25% indicates that erythrocytes make up 25% of the total volume of whole blood. *Erythrocyte counts* show the number of red blood cells in 1 μL or 1 mm^3 of whole blood. The level of red blood cells is regulated by their rate of formation in the bone marrow. The rate of red blood cell formation normally remains relatively constant; however, in clients with hypoxia, **erythropoiesis** (the formation of red blood cells) is stimulated.

A *white blood cell count* determines the number of circulating leukocytes (white blood cells) in 1 μL or 1 mm^3 of whole blood. Above-normal WBC counts indicate increased production of leukocytes by the bone marrow, often in response to the presence of bacterial pathogens in the body. Decreased WBC levels, by contrast, are due to decreased production of leukocytes, often because of the presence of viruses or toxic chemicals in the body.

Differential leukocyte and erythrocyte counts enumerate the different kinds of white and red blood cells in the blood specimen. A number of white blood cells are identified and classified according to their *morphology* (their form and structure). The percentage distribution of the different kinds of white blood cells can assist in diagnosis because characteristic patterns of distribution are consistent with certain disorders. Red blood cells are examined for their size, shape, color, maturation, and content.

Measurement of *arterial blood gases* is another important diagnostic procedure (see Chapter 38, p. 1117). Specimens of arterial blood are normally taken by specialty nurses or medical technicians. Blood for these tests is taken from the radial, brachial, or femoral arteries. Because of the relatively great pressure of the blood in these arteries, it is important to prevent hemorrhaging by applying pressure to the puncture site for about 5 minutes after removing the needle.

Pulmonary Function Tests *Pulmonary function tests* measure lung volume and capacity. Clients undergoing pulmonary function tests, which are usually carried out by a respiratory therapist, do not require an anesthetic. The client breathes into a machine. The tests are painless, but the client's cooperation is essential. Nurses need to explain the tests to people beforehand and help clients to get rest afterward, because the tests are often tiring. See Table 39–1, page 1131, for a description of the measurements taken and the normal adult values.

Visualization Procedures A number of visualization procedures can be done to view parts of the respiratory tract. Roentgengraphy, lung scan, and endoscopy (bronchoscopy and laryngoscopy) are a few. Nursing interventions related to these examinations are shown in the *Clinical Companion* accompanying this book.

X-ray examination of the lung and chest cavity is done both to diagnose disease and to assess the progress of a disease. For an X-ray examination, the nurse needs to inform the client that jewelry and clothing from the waist up must be removed.

A **lung scan** records on a photographic plate the emissions of radioactive waves from a substance injected intravenously as it circulates through the lung. Lung scan usually involves a perfusion and ventilation scan. The *perfusion scan* (Q scan) measures the integrity of the blood vessels and evaluates blood flow abnormalities (eg, emboli). The *ventilation scan* (V scan), performed after the perfusion scan, detects ventilation abnormalities, particularly in clients with emphysema. For this scan, the client inhales a radioactive gas through a mask and then exhales it into room air. The client needs to be informed that the injected and inhaled radioactive isotopes disintegrate and are removed from the circulation within 8 hours. The scan may take 20 to 40 minutes.

Laryngoscopy and **bronchoscopy** are sterile procedures using a laryngoscope and bronchoscope, respectively. Tissue samples may also be taken for biopsy. A general or local anesthetic may be given before the examination. If a general anesthetic is given, routine preoperative care is given. See Chapter 45. A local anesthetic, if given, is sprayed on the client's pharynx to prevent gagging; alternatively, the client gargles with an anesthetic to anesthetize the throat. The bronchoscope is then inserted to visualize the larynx or bronchi. Informed consent is required for this procedure.

Thoracocentesis (Thoracentesis) Thoracocentesis is the withdrawal of fluid or air from the pleural cavity. Normally there is only enough fluid to lubricate the pleura so that they can move freely. However, excessive fluid or air can accumulate in the pleural cavity as a result of injury or disease. Pleural fluid is removed for both diagnostic and therapeutic purposes. Aspiration of air or fluid may be indicated to relieve pain, dyspnea, and other symptoms of pleural pressure. A thoracocentesis is also performed to introduce chemotherapeutic drugs intrapleurally.

Informed consent is required for this procedure. Clients need to be informed that (a) a local anesthetic will be given so that only pressure, not pain, is felt when the needle/catheter is inserted; (b) the procedure takes only a few minutes, depending primarily on the time it takes the fluid to drain from the pleural cavity; (c) a small dressing will be placed over the puncture site when the needle/catheter is removed, and (d) a chest X-ray examination may be done following the procedure.

Before the procedure, the nurse should assess (a) vital signs (body temperature, pulse, respirations, and blood pressure) to obtain baseline data, if these are not already available; (b) respiratory depth and the movement of both sides of the chest during inspiration, to note differences between the two sides; (c) complaints of chest pain; (d) breath sounds; (e) dyspnea; (f) type and frequency of cough, if present; and (g) character and amount of sputum. After the procedure, the nurse assesses the client's blood pressure, pulse, respiration rate, and skin color, because a shift in the mediastinum (heart and large blood vessels) can occur with removal of large amounts of fluid. The nurse also observes any changes in the client's cough, sputum, respiration depth, breath sounds, and chest pain.

DIAGNOSING

NANDA nursing diagnoses that relate to respiratory problems include **Ineffective airway clearance, Ineffective breathing pattern,** and **Impaired gas exchange.** The first two diagnoses, with definitions, defining characteristics, and contributing factors, are shown in the box on page 1142. Clinical applications of these diagnoses are shown in Table 39–2. **Impaired gas exchange** is discussed in Chapter 38 on page 1121.

Table 39–2 Clinical Application: Assessment Data Clusters and Related Nursing Diagnoses

Data Cluster	Nursing Diagnosis
Barry Galloway reports recent flu with malaise, diaphoresis, headache, nausea, and vomiting. Now has fever and chills, chest pain, and painful nonproductive cough. Rhonchi (gurgles) auscultated anteriorly over bronchi.	**Ineffective airway clearance** related to inflammatory process and dehydration
Mr Michael Parry has shortness of breath, moist cough, and fatigue. His lips and nail beds are cyanotic. Respirations are 32 and shallow. Uses pursed-lip breathing and accessory muscles (intercostal and supraclavicular) to exhale. Blood gases indicate elevated $PaCO_2$. Has history of COPD. Is most comfortable sitting in orthopneic position.	**Impaired gas exchange** related to alveolar-capillary membrane changes
Gloria Way, 32 years old, reports severe upper abdominal pain and abdominal distention on her first postoperative day following cholecystectomy. Is reluctant to perform deep breathing and coughing exercises. Respirations are 18 but shallow.	**Ineffective breathing pattern** related to upper abdominal incisional pain

Ineffective airway clearance and **Ineffective breathing pattern** may also be the etiology of several other nursing diagnoses. Examples follow:

- **Anxiety** related to ineffective airway clearance and feeling of suffocation
- **Activity intolerance** related to ineffective breathing pattern (shortness of breath)
- **Fatigue** related to ineffective breathing pattern and impaired gas exchange
- **Fear** related to chronic disabling respiratory illness
- **Powerlessness** related to inability to maintain independence in self-care activities associated with chronic obstructive pulmonary disease (COPD)
- **Sleep pattern disturbance** related to orthopnea and required O_2 therapy.
- **Social isolation** related to inability to travel to usual social activities

NURSING DIAGNOSES

CLIENTS WITH RESPIRATORY PROBLEMS

NURSING DIAGNOSIS: Ineffective airway clearance: The state in which one is unable to clear secretions or obstructions from the respiratory tract to maintain airway patency

Defining Characteristics

- Abnormal breath sounds (crackles, wheezes)
- Change in respiratory rate and/or depth
- Tachypnea
- Dyspnea
- Cyanosis
- Cough with or without sputum

Related Factors

Tracheobronchial infection and obstruction; excessive, thick tracheobronchial secretions; decreased energy; fatigue; trauma; pain.

NURSING DIAGNOSIS: Ineffective breathing pattern: The state in which one's inhalation and/or exhalation pattern does not allow adequate pulmonary inflation or deflation

Defining Characteristics

- Respiratory depth changes
- Pursed-lip breathing and prolonged expiratory phase
- Dyspnea, shortness of breath
- Use of accessory muscles
- Tachypnea
- Cyanosis
- Abnormal arterial blood gases
- Altered chest excursion
- Increased anteroposterior diameter

Related Factors

Anxiety; neuromuscular or musculoskeletal impairment; pain; decreased energy; fatigue.

Sources: LJ Carpenito, *Nursing Diagnosis: Application to Clinical Practice*, 4th ed. (Philadelphia: Lippincott, 1992), pp. 675–78; M Gordon, *Manual of Nursing Diagnosis 1993–1994*, 6th ed. (St Louis: Mosby-Year Book, 1993), pp. 199–201; MJ Kim, GK McFarland, and AM McLane, *Pocket Guide to Nursing Diagnoses*, 5th ed. (St Louis: Mosby-Year Book, 1993), pp. 3, 8–9; GK McFarland and EA McFarlane, *Nursing Diagnosis and Intervention: Planning for Patient Care*, 2d ed. (St Louis: Mosby, 1993), pp. 349–50, 354–57; North American Nursing Diagnosis Association, *NANDA Nursing Diagnoses: Definitions and Classification 1992–1993*, (Philadelphia: NANDA, 1992), pp. 25–26; and JR Lederer, GL Marculescu, B Mocnik, and N Seaby, *Care Planning Pocket Guide—A Nursing Diagnosis Approach*, 5th ed. (Redwood City, CA: Addison-Wesley Nursing, 1993), p. 8, 28.

PLANNING

Planning for a client's oxygenation problems involves facilitating pulmonary ventilation, the diffusion of gases, and the transport of oxygen and carbon dioxide. *Facilitating pulmonary ventilation* may include ensuring a patent airway, positioning, encouraging deep breathing and coughing, and ensuring adequate hydration. Other nursing interventions helpful to ventilation are suctioning, lung inflation techniques, administration of analgesics before deep breathing and coughing, postural drainage, and percussion and vibration. Nursing strategies to *facilitate the diffusion of gases* through the alveolar membrane include encouraging coughing, deep breathing, and suitable activity. To *promote the transport of oxygen and carbon dioxide*, the nurse can optimize cardiac output by reducing stress, planning appropriate activities, and positioning the client for improved vascular blood flow. A client's nursing care plan should also include appropriate dependent nursing interventions such as oxygen therapy, tracheostomy care, and maintenance of a chest tube.

Overall client outcomes for individuals with oxygenation problems are to maintain airway patency, to maintain adequate ventilation, to maintain adequate cardiac output, to reduce cardiac workload, and to maintain tissue perfusion and cellular oxygenation. Specific outcome criteria, nursing interventions, and rationales are shown in the accompanying Care Planning Guide.

A critical pathway can also be useful for planning client care (see p. 1172).

CARE PLANNING GUIDE

CLIENTS WITH RESPIRATORY PROBLEMS

NURSING DIAGNOSIS: Ineffective airway clearance

Outcome Criteria	Nursing Interventions	Rationale
The client ▪ Maintains a patent airway, as evidenced by a. Normal respiratory rate, rhythm, and depth. b. Clear breath sounds bilaterally. c. Skin, nails, lips, and earlobes of pink color for light-skinned clients or of normal (usual) color for dark-skinned clients. d. Effective expectoration (or removal) of secretions. e. Effective performance of deep-breathing exercises and coughing as instructed every 2 hours.	Assess and document the client's respiratory status. Include respiratory rate and rhythm; breath sounds; chest expansion; use of accessory muscles; pursed-lip breathing; skin color; color, consistency, and amount of sputum; arterial blood gases; and pulse oximetry.	Assessment of respiratory status provides baseline data to evaluate the efficacy of nursing interventions.
	Monitor the client's respiratory status at least every 4 hours.	Monitoring respiratory status facilitates early detection of complications.
	Encourage the client to drink at least 2000 mL of fluid daily if not contraindicated by cardiac or renal disease.	Adequate fluids hydrate the pulmonary mucous membranes and decrease the viscosity (thickness) of secretions, thus facilitating expectoration or removal by suction.
	Maintain adequate humidity of inspired air. Use a room or oxygen humidifier as indicated.	Adequate humidity prevents drying of the respiratory tract and aggravation of the problem.
	Encourage physical activity as much as possible.	Activity promotes the movement of secretions.
	Demonstrate diaphragmatic breathing techniques and controlled coughing (see the box on page 1146).	Deep breathing expands lung tissue and moves secretions.
	Provide analgesics for pain as indicated before breathing and coughing activities.	Control of pain allows for maximum participation in, and effectiveness of, activities.
	Splint incisions, if present, during deep breathing and coughing.	Splinting provides support and minimizes pain, thus facilitating deeper breathing and coughing.
	Assist the client to assume an appropriate breathing and cough position (eg, high-Fowler's).	High-Fowler's position allows maximal chest expansion for ventilation.
	Confer with the physician and/or respiratory therapist as indicated about the need for adjunctive therapy, such as percussion, postural drainage, and/or supportive equipment (eg, oxygen, suction, incentive spirometer, nebulization, IPPB). Explain procedures appropriately to the client.	Adjunctive therapy may be necessary to mobilize secretions. Providing appropriate client education before initiating procedures decreases anxiety and increases the client's sense of control.
▪ Verbalizes and demonstrates understanding of self-care activities required for follow-up care.	Instruct the client and family in plans for care at home (medications hydration, nebulization, equipment, postural drainage, signs and symptoms of complications, community resources).	Appropriate instruction enables the client to follow accurately the required regimen at home.

➤

RESPIRATORY PROBLEMS CONTINUED

NURSING DIAGNOSIS: Ineffective breathing pattern

Outcome Criteria	Nursing Interventions	Rationale
The client ▪ Establishes a normal effective respiratory pattern, as evidenced by a. Respiratory rate of 12 to 20 per minute. b. Effortless breathing (no use of accessory muscles). c. Symmetric chest expansion on inhalation. d. Absence of cyanosis. e. Normal arterial blood gases. f. Performance of activities of daily living (ADLs) without shortness of breath.	Assess the client's respiratory patterns (see previous page for **Ineffective airway clearance**).	Assessment of the client's respiratory pattern provides baseline data to gauge the efficacy of nursing interventions.
	Explore causative factors (eg, anxiety, pain, decreased energy, fatigue, neuromuscular or musculoskeletal impairment).	Knowledge of the causative factors influences the selection of nursing interventions.
	Instruct client to notify the nurse at the onset of ineffective breathing.	Having a nurse present provides reassurance and support during periods of respiratory distress.
	Implement measures to alleviate contributing factors:	
	▪ If pain is present, a. Administer analgesics according to a schedule (specify). b. Reposition the client. c. Provide other appropriate comfort measures.	Pain and improper positions may cause hypoventilation. Scheduled analgesics promote an optional respiratory pattern. Repositioning moves secretions and facilitates maximum lung inflation.
	▪ If anxiety or fear is present, a. Remain with the client. b. Encourage the client to express concerns. c. Demonstrate conscious controlled slow abdominal breathing for use during periods of anxiety. d. Instruct the client in relaxation techniques.	Anxiety and fear can cause the client to hyperventilate. Conscious controlled breathing and relaxation techniques can lower anxiety, increase sense of control, and improve breathing pattern. Expressing concerns may reduce anxiety.
	▪ If neuromuscular or musculoskeletal impairment is present, consult with the physician and/or respiratory therapist about adjunctive respiratory therapy (see previous page for **Ineffective airway clearance**).	As previous page for **Ineffective airway clearance.**
	Administer medications as ordered (eg, expectorants, bronchodilators, antibiotics, steroids).	Medications can increase ventilation and air flow.
	Assess the client's activity tolerance and ability to perform ADLs; provide assistance as indicated.	Ineffective breathing patterns often alter the client's activity tolerance.
	Plan care to allow for adequate rest periods.	Rest periods help conserve the client's energy.

IMPLEMENTING

PROMOTING HEALTHY RESPIRATIONS

Normally, adequate ventilation is maintained by frequent changes of position, ambulation, and exercise. See the box at the right for promoting healthy breathing. When persons become ill, however, their respiratory functions may be inhibited, for such reasons as pain and immobility.

Shallow respirations inhibit both diaphragmatic excursion and lung distensibility. The result of inadequate chest expansion is stasis and pooling of respiratory secretions, which ultimately harbor microorganisms and promote infection. This situation is often compounded by giving narcotics for pain, because narcotics further depress the rate and depth of respiration.

Interventions by the nurse to maintain the normal respirations of clients include

- Positioning the client to allow for maximum chest expansion.
- Encouraging or providing frequent changes in position.
- Encouraging ambulation.
- Implementing measures that promote comfort, such as giving pain medications.

The semi-Fowler's or high-Fowler's position allows maximum chest expansion in bed-confined clients, particularly dyspneic clients. The nurse also encourages clients to turn from side to side frequently, so that alternate sides of the chest are permitted maximum expansion. Dyspneic clients often sit in bed and lean over their overbed tables (which are raised to a suitable height), usually with a pillow for support. This *orthopneic position* is an adaptation of the high-Fowler's position. It has a further advantage in that, unlike in high-Fowler's, the abdominal organs are not pressing on the diaphragm. Also, a client in the orthopneic position can press the lower part of the chest against the table to help in exhaling.

DEEP BREATHING AND COUGHING

The nurse can facilitate respiratory functioning by encouraging deep breathing exercises and coughing to remove secretions. Breathing exercises are frequently indicated for clients with restricted chest expansion, such as people with chronic obstructive pulmonary disease (COPD) or clients recovering from thoracic surgery. Commonly employed breathing exercises are abdominal (diaphragmatic) and pursed-lip breathing, apical expansion, and basal expansion exercises. *Abdominal (diaphragmatic) breathing* permits deep full breaths with little effort.

Pursed-lip breathing helps the client develop control over breathing. The pursed lips create a resistance to the air flowing out of the lungs, thereby prolonging exhalation.

The client purses the lips as if about to whistle and breathes out slowly and gently, tightening the abdominal muscles to exhale more effectively. The client usually inhales to a count of 3 and exhales to a count of 7. The box on page 1146 provides instructions to perform abdominal (diaphragmatic) and pursed-lip breathing.

Apical or *basal expansion exercises* are often required for clients who restrict their upper or lower chest movement because of pain from a severe respiratory disease, chest surgery, or upper abdominal surgery.

To assist the client with *apical* expansion exercises, which (a) reexpand lung tissue, (b) move secretions to promote effective elimination, and (c) minimize flattening of the upper chest wall from disuse, the nurse follows these steps:

- Place hands below the clavicles, exerting moderate pressure (Figure 39–4, p. 1146)
- Ask the client to
  - Concentrate on expanding the upper chest forward and upward while inhaling to aerate apical lobes of the lung.
  - Hold the breath for 3 to 4 seconds to promote aeration of the alveoli.
  - Exhale passively and slowly through the mouth or nose.
- Repeat this exercise for 5 respirations four times a day.

WELLNESS TEACHING

Promoting Healthy Breathing

- Assume a posture that permits full lung expansion.
- Exercise regularly.
- Breathe through the nose.
- Breathe in so as to expand the chest fully.
- Do not smoke cigarettes, cigars, or pipes.
- Eliminate or reduce the use of household pesticides and irritating chemical substances.
- Do not incinerate garbage in the house.
- Avoid exposure to second-hand smoke.
- Use building materials that do not emit vapors.
- Make sure furnaces, ovens, and wood stoves are correctly ventilated.
- Support a pollution-free environment.

CLIENT TEACHING

Abdominal (Diaphragmatic) and Pursed-Lip Breathing and Coughing

- Assume a comfortable semi-sitting position in bed or chair *or* a lying position in bed with one pillow.
- Flex your knees to relax the muscles of the abdomen.
- Place one or both hands on your abdomen, just below the ribs.
- Breathe in deeply through the nose, keeping the mouth closed.
- Concentrate on feeling your abdomen rise as far as possible; stay relaxed, and avoid arching your back. If you have difficulty raising your abdomen, take a quick, forceful breath through the nose.
- Then purse your lips as if about to whistle, and breathe out slowly and gently, making a slow "whooshing" sound without puffing out the cheeks. This *pursed-lip breathing* creates a resistance to air flowing out of the lungs, increases pressure within the bronchi (main air passages), and minimizes collapse of smaller airways, a common problem for people with chronic obstructive pulmonary disease.
- Concentrate on feeling the abdomen fall or sink and tighten (contract) the abdominal muscles while breathing out to enhance effective exhalation. Count to seven during exhalation.
- If indicated, cough two or more times during exhalation.
- Use this exercise whenever feeling short of breath, and increase gradually to 5 to 10 minutes four times a day. Regular practice will help you do this type of breathing without conscious effort. The exercise, once learned, can be performed when sitting upright, standing, and walking.

For *basal* expansion exercises, the client follows these steps:

- Place the palms of the hands on the lower ribs along the midaxillary lines, and exert moderate pressure.
- Concentrate on moving the lower chest outward on inhalation.
- Exhale slowly, quietly, and passively.

HYDRATION

Adequate hydration maintains the moisture of the respiratory mucous membranes. Normally, respiratory tract secretions are thin and therefore moved readily by ciliary action. However, when the client is dehydrated or when the environment has a low humidity, the respiratory secretions can become thick and tenacious. Fluid intake should be as great as the client can tolerate. See Chapter 38 for normal daily fluid intake.

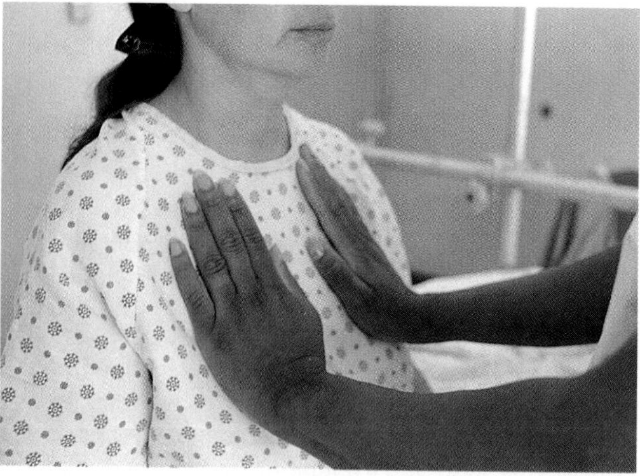

Figure 39–4 Assisting the client to carry out apical expansion exercises.

Humidifiers are devices that add water vapor to inspired air. Their purposes are to prevent mucous membranes from drying and becoming irritated and to loosen secretions for easier expectoration.

A *room humidifier* can provide either cool mist or steam. Some types can be used with gas lines, such as oxygen, to provide moistened air directly to the client (see p. 1154). Steam vaporizers must be used carefully to prevent burns. A cool-mist humidifier, however, presents no possibility of burning the client. 

MEDICATIONS

Sometimes medications are given to help remove excessive secretions from the lungs. Lungs that have these secretions are referred to as congested. When a person coughs but produces no secretions, the cough is called a **nonproductive cough.** A cough that produces secretions is called a **productive cough.** Respiratory secretions that are thick and tenacious are often referred to as phlegm. The cough mechanism was discussed on page 1132.

Two types of medications commonly prescribed are cough suppressants and expectorants. A *cough suppressant* is a medication that suppresses or stops the cough reflex. Codeine is a common constituent of these medications. *Expectorants* are medications that decrease the viscosity of the secretions, thereby making them easier to cough up. In some instances, a nonproductive cough can become productive with the use of expectorants. See the box on page 1147 for client teaching about cough medications.

Another type of medication delivery frequently used for coughs is the lozenge. A lozenge is usually a tablet that is held in the mouth while it dissolves. Some lozenges contain a local anesthetic that acts on the sensory nerve

CLIENT TEACHING

Using Cough Medications

- Do not take cough medications in excessive amounts because of adverse side effects.
- If you have diabetes mellitus, avoid cough syrups that contain sugar or alcohol; these can disturb metabolism.
- When a cough medicine does not act as expected, consult a health care professional.
- Be aware of side effects (eg, drowsiness) that can make the operation of machinery dangerous.

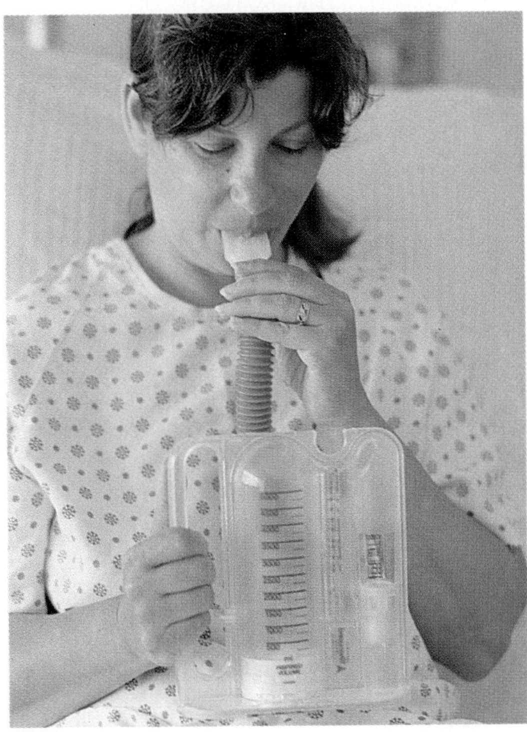

Figure 39–5 Plastic disposable volume-oriented incentive spirometer, or SMI.

endings in the throat, thus stopping the irritation that causes coughing. Medications can also be delivered in a fine spray that is inhaled. See Nebulizers in Chapter 43, page 1351.

LUNG INFLATION DEVICES

Lung inflation devices are used to

- Improve pulmonary ventilation
- Counteract the effects of anesthesia and/or hypoventilation
- Loosen respiratory secretions
- Facilitate respiratory gaseous exchange
- Expand collapsed alveoli

Incentive spirometers, also referred to as *sustained maximal inspiration devices* (SMIs), measure the flow of air inhaled through the mouthpiece. They therefore offer an incentive to improve *inhalation* (Figure 39–5).

The client should be assisted preferably to an upright sitting position in bed or in a chair when using any of these devices. This position facilitates maximum ventilation. The box above lists instructions for clients in the use of incentive spirometers.

CLIENT TEACHING

Using an Incentive Spirometer

- Hold or place the spirometer in an upright position. A tilted *flow-oriented* device requires less effort to raise the balls or discs; a volume-oriented device will not function correctly unless upright.
- Exhale normally.
- Seal the lips tightly around the mouthpiece.
- Take in a *slow, deep breath* to elevate the balls or cylinder, and then hold the breath for 2 seconds initially, increasing to 6 seconds (optimum), to keep the balls or cylinder elevated if possible.
- For a flow-oriented device, avoid brisk, low-volume breaths that snap the balls to the top of the chamber. Greater lung expansion is achieved with a very slow inspiration than with a brisk, shallow breath, even though it may not elevate the balls or keep them elevated while you hold your breath. Sustained elevation of the balls or cylinder ensures adequate ventilation of the alveoli (lung air sacs).
- If you have difficulty breathing only through the mouth, a nose clip can be used.
- Remove the mouthpiece, and exhale normally.
- Cough after the incentive effort. Deep ventilation may loosen secretions, and coughing can facilitate their removal.
- Relax, and take several normal breaths before using the spirometer again.
- Repeat the procedure several times and then four or five times hourly. Practice increases inspiratory volume, maintains alveolar ventilation, and prevents atelectasis (collapse of the air sacs).
- Clean the mouthpiece with water and shake it dry. Change disposable mouthpieces every 24 hours.

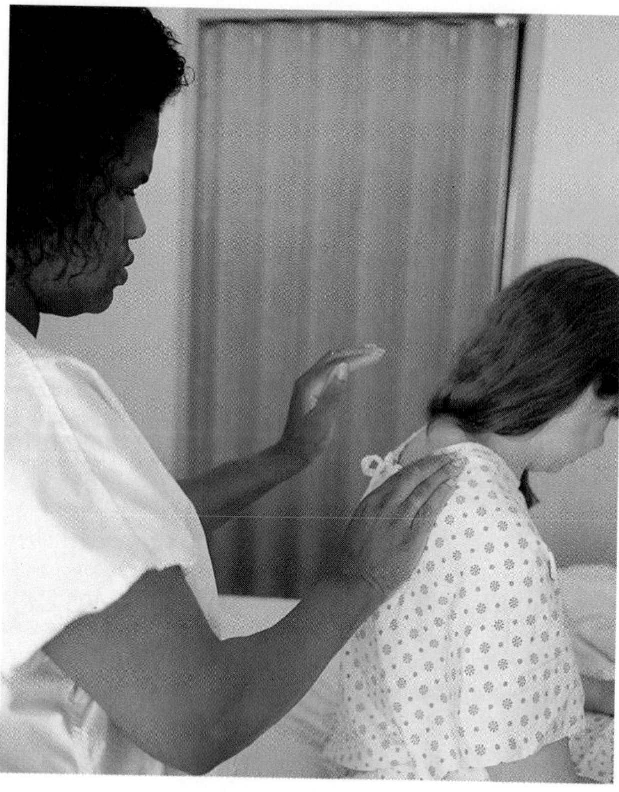

Figure 39–6 Percussing the upper posterior chest.

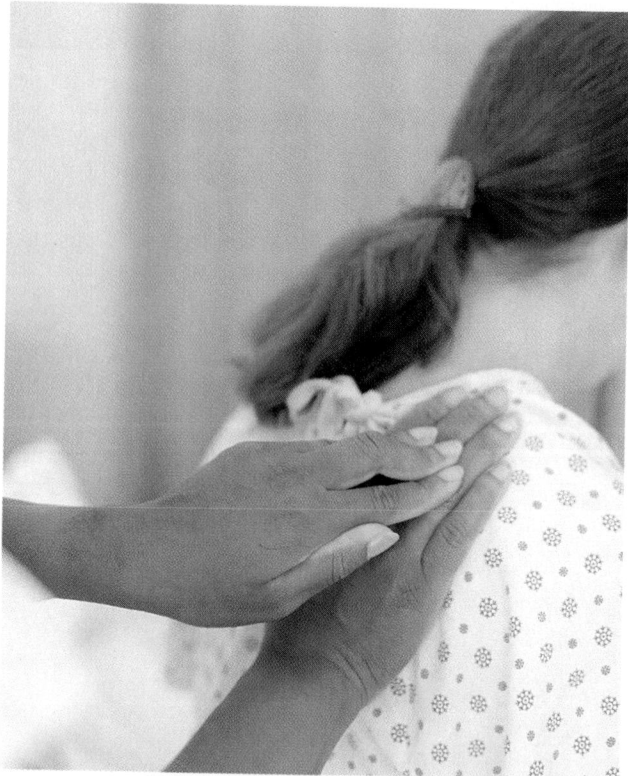

Figure 39–7 Vibrating the upper posterior chest.

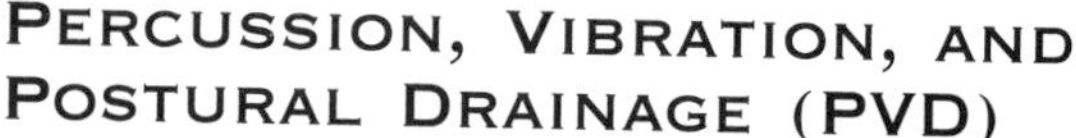

Percussion, Vibration, and Postural Drainage (PVD)

Percussion, vibration, and postural drainage (PVD) are dependent nursing functions performed according to a physician's order. **Percussion,** sometimes called *clapping,* is forceful striking of the skin with cupped hands. Mechanical percussion cups and vibrators are also available. When the hands are used, the fingers and thumb are held together and flexed slightly to form a cup, as one would to scoop up water. Percussion over congested lung areas can mechanically dislodge tenacious secretions from the bronchial walls. Cupped hands trap the air against the chest. The trapped air sets up vibrations through the chest wall to the secretions.

To percuss a client's chest, the nurse follows these steps:

- Cover the area with a towel or gown to reduce discomfort.
- Ask the client to breathe slowly and deeply to promote relaxation.
- Alternately flex and extend the wrists rapidly to slap the chest (Figure 39–6).
- Percuss each affected lung segment for 1 to 2 minutes.

When done correctly, the percussion action should produce a hollow, popping sound. Percussion is avoided over certain easily injured structures, such as the breasts, sternum, spinal column, and kidneys.

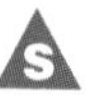

Vibration is a series of vigorous quiverings produced by hands that are placed flat against the client's chest wall. Vibration is used after percussion to increase the turbulence of the exhaled air and thus loosen thick secretions. It is often done alternately with percussion.

To vibrate, the nurse follows these steps:

- Place hands, palms down, on the chest area to be drained, one hand over the other with the fingers together and extended (Figure 39–7). Alternatively, the hands may be placed side by side.
- Ask the client to inhale deeply and exhale slowly through the nose or pursed lips.
- During the exhalation, tense all the hand and arm muscles, and, using mostly the heel of the hand, vibrate (shake) the hands, moving them downward. Stop the vibrating when the client inhales.
- Vibrate during 5 exhalations over one affected lung segment.
- After each vibration, encourage the client to cough and expectorate secretions into the sputum container.

Postural drainage is the drainage, by gravity, of secretions from various lung segments. Secretions that remain in the lungs or respiratory airways promote bacterial growth and subsequent infection. They also can obstruct the smaller airways and cause **atelectasis** (collapse of lung tissue). Secretions in the major airways, such as the trachea and the right and left main bronchi, are usually coughed into the pharynx, where they can be expectorated, swallowed, or effectively removed by suctioning.

A wide variety of positions is necessary to drain all segments of the lungs, but not all positions are required for every client. Only those positions that drain specific affected areas are used. The lower lobes require drainage most frequently because the upper lobes drain during normal daily activities. Prior to postural drainage, the client may be given a bronchodilator medication or nebulization therapy to loosen secretions. Frequently, postural drainage treatments are scheduled two or three times daily, depending on the degree of lung congestion. The best times include before breakfast, before lunch, in the late afternoon, and before bedtime. It is best to avoid hours shortly after meals because postural drainage at these times can be tiring and can induce vomiting.

The nurse needs to evaluate the client's tolerance of postural drainage by assessing the stability of the client's vital signs, particularly the pulse and respiratory rates, and by noting signs of intolerance, such as pallor, diaphoresis, dyspnea, and fatigue. Some clients do not react well to certain drainage positions, and the nurse must make appropriate adjustments. For example, some become dyspneic in Trendelenburg's position and require only a moderate tilt or a shorter time in those positions.

The sequence for PVD is usually as follows: positioning, percussion, vibration, and removal of secretions by coughing or suction. Each position is usually assumed for 10 to 15 minutes, although beginning treatments may start with shorter times and gradually increase. Usually, the entire treatment, including preparatory nebulization and deep breathing as well as all postures, takes 30 minutes. Postural drainage position and percussion areas for specific lung segments are shown in the *Procedures Supplement* that accompanies this book.

Following PVD, the nurse should auscultate the client's lungs, compare the findings to the baseline data, and document the amount, color, and character of expectorated secretions.

OROPHARYNGEAL AND NASOPHARYNGEAL SUCTIONING

The nurse must sometimes apply suction to the oropharynx and nasal passages of clients who have difficulty swallowing or expectorating secretions. **Suctioning** is the aspiration of secretions, often through a rubber or polyethylene catheter connected to a suction machine or wall outlet. It is recommended that sterile technique be used for all suctioning, so that microorganisms are not introduced into the pharynx, where they can multiply and move into the trachea and bronchi. This is particularly important for debilitated clients, who are more susceptible to infection.

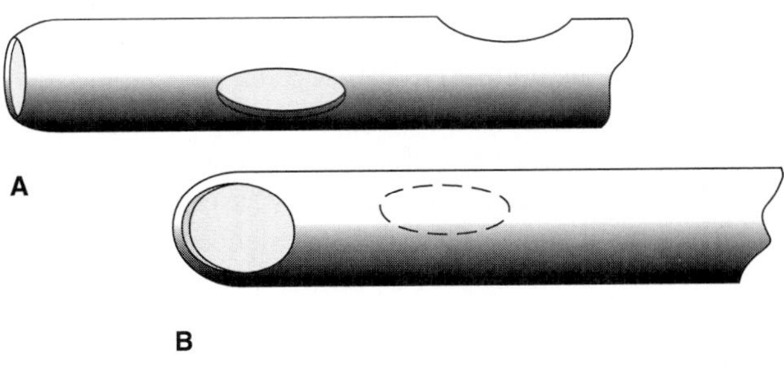

Figure 39–8 Types of pharyngeal suction catheters: *A*, open-tipped; *B*, whistle-tipped.

Several types of catheters are available for suctioning. The open-tipped catheter has an opening at the end and several openings along the sides to distribute the negative pressure of the suction over a wide area, thus preventing excessive irritation of any one area of the respiratory mucous membrane (Figure 39–8, *A*). It is effective for thick mucus plugs, but it can irritate tissue. The whistle-tipped catheter has a slanted opening at the tip (Figure 39–8, *B*). Most catheters have a thumb port on the side, which is used to control the suction.

The suction apparatus includes a collection bottle, a tubing system connected to the suction catheter, and a gauge that registers the degree of suction. These apparatus are either portable or wall mounted (Figure 39–9).

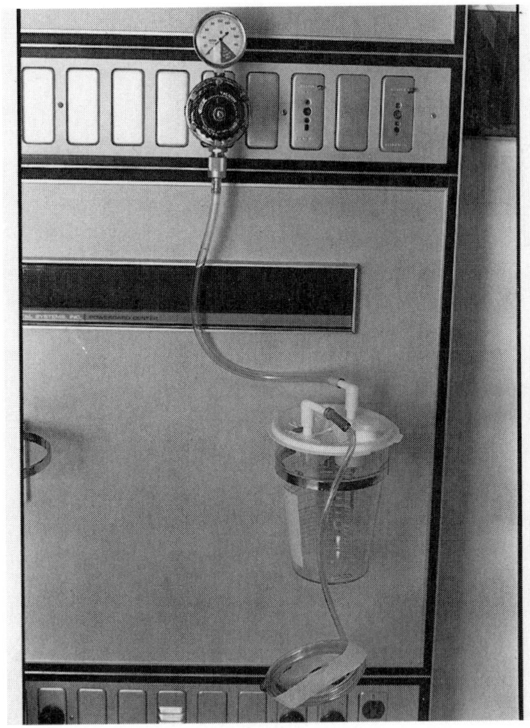

Figure 39–9 A wall suction unit.

Oropharyngeal or *nasopharyngeal suctioning* removes secretions from the upper respiratory tract. Deeper suctioning, called *endotracheal suctioning*, removes secretions from the trachea and the bronchi. Deep suctioning requires considerably more skill and is usually carried out by a critical-care nursing specialist or an experienced nurse.

Suctioning of the upper respiratory airways is indicated when the client (a) is unable to expectorate coughed secretions, (b) is unable to swallow, and (c) makes light bubbling or rattling breath sounds that signal the accumulation of secretions. The client may also be dyspneic or appear cyanotic. Whether and how often to suction are decisions that require judgment on the part of the nurse. Irritation of the mucous membranes by the suction catheter can increase secretions. Suctioning can also cause some hypoxia. Guidelines for oropharyngeal and nasopharyngeal suctioning are described in Procedure 39–2.

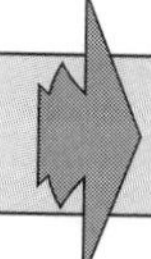

PROCEDURE 39–2 SUCTIONING OROPHARYNGEAL AND NASOPHARYNGEAL CAVITIES

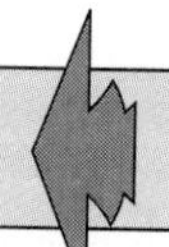

PURPOSES

- To remove secretions that obstruct the airway
- To facilitate respiratory ventilation
- To obtain secretions for diagnostic purposes
- To prevent infection that may result from accumulated secretions

ASSESSMENT FOCUS
Clinical signs indicating the need for suctioning: restlessness; gurgling sounds during respiration; adventitious breath sounds when the chest is auscultated; change in mental status, skin color, rate and pattern of respirations, and pulse rate and rhythm.

EQUIPMENT

- ☐ Towel or moisture-resistant pad
- ☐ Portable or wall suction machine with tubing and collection receptacle
- ☐ Sterile disposable container for fluids
- ☐ Sterile normal saline or water
- ☐ Sterile gloves
- ☐ Sterile suction catheter (#12 to #18 Fr. for adults; #8 to #10 Fr. for children, and #5 to #8 Fr. for infants); if both the oropharynx and the nasopharynx are to be suctioned, one sterile catheter is required for each
- ☐ Water-soluble lubricant (optional)
- ☐ Y-connector
- ☐ Sterile gauzes
- ☐ Moisture-resistant disposal bag
- ☐ Sputum trap, if specimen is to be collected

INTERVENTION

1. Prepare the client.

- Explain to the client that suctioning will relieve breathing difficulty and that the procedure is painless but may stimulate the cough, gag, or sneeze reflex. *Knowing that the procedure will relieve breathing problems is often reassuring and enlists the client's cooperation.*
- Position a *conscious* person who has a functional gag reflex in the semi-Fowler's position with the head turned to one side for oral suctioning or with the neck hyperextended for nasal suctioning. *These positions facilitate the insertion of the catheter and help prevent aspiration of secretions.*

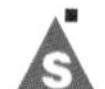

- Position an *unconscious* client in the lateral position, facing you. *This position allows the tongue to fall forward, so that it will not obstruct the catheter on insertion. Lateral position also facilitates drainage of secretions from the pharynx and prevents the possibility of aspiration.*
- Place the towel or moisture-resistant pad over the pillow or under the chin.

2. Prepare the equipment.

- Set the pressure on the suction gauge, and turn on the suction. Many suction devices are calibrated to three pressure ranges:

Wall unit

Adult: 100 to 120 mm Hg
Child: 95 to 110 mm Hg
Infant: 50 to 95 mm Hg

Portable unit

Adult: 10 to 15 mm Hg
Child: 5 to 10 mm Hg
Infant: 2 to 5 mm Hg

- Open the sterile suction package.
  a. Set up the cup or container, touching only its outside.

PROCEDURE 39–2 *continued*

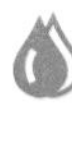

b. Pour sterile water or saline into the container.

c. Don the sterile gloves, or don a nonsterile glove on the nondominant hand and then a sterile glove on the dominant hand. *The sterile gloved hand maintains the sterility of the suction catheter, and the unsterile glove prevents the transmission of the microorganisms to the nurse.*

- With your sterile gloved hand, pick up the catheter, and attach it to the suction unit (Figure 39–10).
- Open the lubricant if performing nasopharyngeal suctioning.

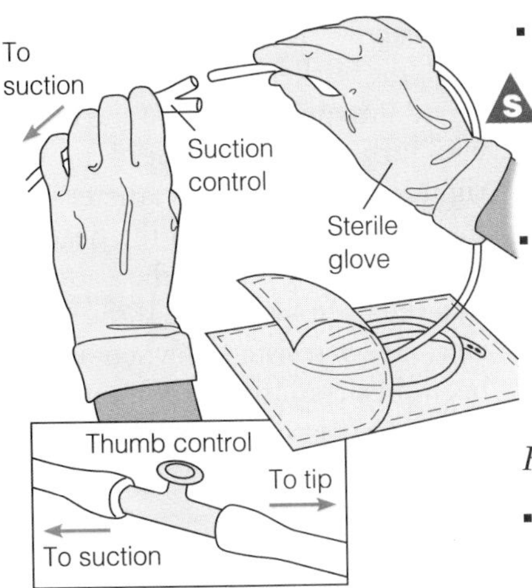

Figure 39–10 Attaching the catheter to the suction unit.

3. Make an approximate measure of the depth for the insertion of the catheter and test the equipment.

- Measure the distance between the tip of the client's nose and the earlobe, or about 13 cm (5 in) for an adult.
- Mark the position on the tube with the fingers of the sterile gloved hand.
- Test the pressure of the suction and the patency of the catheter by applying your sterile gloved finger or thumb to the port or open branch of the Y-connector (the suction control) to create suction.

4. Lubricate and introduce the catheter.

- For nasopharyngeal suction, lubricate the catheter tip with sterile water, saline, or water-soluble lubricant; for oropharyngeal suction, moisten the tip with sterile water or saline. *This reduces friction and eases insertion.*

For an Oropharyngeal Suction

- Pull the tongue forward, if necessary, using gauze.
- Do not apply suction (that is, leave your finger off the port) during insertion. *Applying suction during insertion causes trauma to the mucous membrane.*
- Advance the catheter about 10 to 15 cm (4 to 6 in) along one side of the mouth into the oropharynx. *Directing the catheter along the side prevents gagging.*

For a Nasopharyngeal Suction

- Without applying suction, insert the catheter the premeasured or recommended distance into either naris, and advance it along the floor of the nasal cavity. *This avoids the nasal turbinates.*
- Never force the catheter against an obstruction. If one nostril is obstructed, try the other.

5. Perform suctioning.

- Apply your finger to the suction control port to start suction, and gently rotate the catheter. *Gentle rotation of the catheter ensures that all surfaces are reached and prevents trauma to any one area of the respiratory mucosa due to prolonged suction.*
- Apply intermittent suction for 5 to 10 seconds; rotate catheter; then remove your finger from the control, and remove the catheter.
- A suction attempt should last only 10 to 15 seconds. During this time, the catheter is inserted, the suction applied and discontinued, and the catheter removed.
- It may be necessary during oropharyngeal suctioning to apply suction to secretions that collect in the vestibule of the mouth and beneath the tongue.

6. Clean the catheter, and repeat suctioning as above.

- Wipe off the catheter with sterile gauze if it is thickly coated with secretions. Dispose of the used gauze in a moisture-resistant bag.
- Flush the catheter with sterile water or saline.
- Relubricate the catheter, and repeat suctioning until the air passage is clear.
- Allow 20- to 30-second intervals between each suction, and limit suction to 5 minutes in total. *Applying suction for too long may cause secretions to increase or decrease the client's oxygen supply.*
- Alternate nares for repeat suctionings.

7. Encourage the client to breathe deeply and to cough between suctions. *Coughing and deep breathing help carry secretions from the trachea and bronchi into the pharynx, where they can be reached with the suction catheter.*

8. Obtain a specimen if required. Use a sputum trap (Figure 39–11) as follows:

PROCEDURE 39–2 SUCTIONING OROPHARYNGEAL AND NASOPHARYNGEAL CAVITIES *continued*

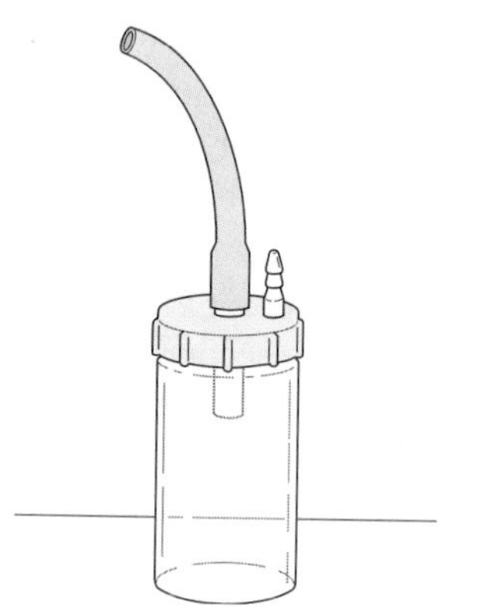

Figure 39–11 A sputum collection trap.

- Attach the suction catheter to the rubber tubing of the sputum trap.
- Attach the suction tubing to the sputum trap air vent.
- Suction the client's nasopharynx or oropharynx. The sputum trap will collect the mucus during suctioning.
- Remove the catheter from the client. Disconnect the sputum trap rubber tubing from the suction catheter. Remove the suction tubing from the trap air vent.
- Connect the rubber tubing of the sputum trap to the air vent. *This retains any microorganisms in the sputum trap.*
- Flush the catheter to remove secretions from the tubing.

9. Promote client comfort.

- Offer to assist the client with oral or nasal hygiene.
- Assist the client to a position that facilitates breathing.

10. Dispose of equipment and ensure availability for the next suction.

- Dispose of the catheter, gloves, water, and waste container. Wrap the catheter around your sterile glove and roll it inside the glove for disposal.
- To ensure that equipment is available for the next suctioning, change suction collection bottles and tubing daily or more frequently as necessary.

11. Assess the effectiveness of suctioning.

- Auscultate the client's breathing sounds to ensure they are clear of secretions. Observe skin color, dyspnea, and level of anxiety.

12. Document relevant data.

- Record the procedure: the amount, consistency, color, and odor of sputum (eg, foamy, white mucus; thick, green-tinged mucus; or blood-flecked mucus) and the client's breathing status before and after the procedure.
- If the technique is carried out frequently, for example, every hour, it may be appropriate to record only once, at the end of the shift; however, the frequency of the suctioning must be recorded.

Variation: Endotracheal suctioning

Endotracheal suctioning is similar to pharyngeal suctioning; the main difference is that the suction catheter is inserted farther into the client's trachea and/or bronchi. For an adult, it is usually inserted 20 cm (8 in). To ascertain the correct length to insert the catheter for nasal tracheal suctioning, measure the distance from the tip of the nose to the earlobe and then along the side of the neck to the thyroid cartilage (Adam's apple). For oral tracheal suctioning, measure from the mouth to the midsternum. To prevent unnecessary trauma to the tracheal mucosa, always premeasure the correct length for catheter insertion prior to suctioning a child.

Having the client inhale while you insert the catheter facilitates its entry into the trachea because the epiglottis is open during inhalation. Hyperextending the head and extending the tongue with the mouth open places the glottis in line with the trachea, thereby easing entry into the trachea rather than into the esophagus.

If the catheter needs to be inserted into one or both of the bronchi, turn the client's head to the right to help direct the catheter into the left bronchus. Turn the head to the left to help direct the catheter into the right bronchus. If the catheter meets resistance when it has been inserted the recommended distance, it is probably against the carina. In this instance, pull the catheter back about 1 cm (0.4 in) before applying suction or advancing it farther.

Tracheal and bronchial suctioning should be done intermittently, and the catheter should remain in the client no more than 10 seconds to avoid hypoxemia and cardiopulmonary complications. Once the client coughs, secretions are frequently dislodged to the upper airway, requiring pharyngeal suctioning.

EVALUATION FOCUS

Appearance of secretions suctioned; breath sounds; respiratory rate, rhythm, and depth; pulse rate and rhythm; skin color.

OXYGEN THERAPY FOR CLIENTS WITH COPD

Low-flow oxygen systems are essential for clients with COPD. A high carbon dioxide level in the blood is the normal stimulus to breathe. However, people with COPD may already have a high carbon dioxide level, and their stimulus to breathe is hypoxemia. Low flows of oxygen (2 L/min) stimulate breathing for such persons by maintaining slight hypoxemia. This depends on the client's inspiratory flow and normal ventilation. During continuous oxygen administration, levels of oxygen (Pa_{O_2}) and carbon dioxide (Pa_{CO_2}) in arterial blood are measured periodically to monitor hypoxemia and adjust the liter flow as needed. Pa_{O_2} is normally 80 to 100 mm Hg; Pa_{CO_2} is normally 35 to 45 mm Hg.

OXYGEN THERAPY SAFETY PRECAUTIONS

- Place cautionary signs reading "No Smoking: Oxygen in Use" on the client's door, at the foot or head of the bed, and on the oxygen equipment.
- Instruct the client and visitors about the hazard of smoking with oxygen in use.
- Request other clients in the room and visitors to smoke in areas provided elsewhere in the hospital.
- Make sure that electrical devices (such as razors, hearing aids, radios, televisions, and heating pads) are in good working order to prevent the occurrence of short-circuit sparks.
- Avoid materials that generate static electricity, such as woolen blankets and synthetic fabrics. Cotton blankets should be used, and nurses are advised to wear cotton fabrics.
- Avoid the use of volatile, flammable materials, such as oils, greases, alcohol, and ether, near clients receiving oxygen. Avoid alcohol back rubs and take nail polish removers or the like away from the immediate vicinity.
- Ground electric monitoring equipment, suction machines, and portable diagnostic machines.
- Make known the location of fire extinguishers, and make sure personnel are trained in their use.

OXYGEN THERAPY

Additional oxygen is indicated for numerous clients who have hypoxemia, for example, people who have reduced lung diffusion of oxygen through the respiratory membrane, heart failure leading to inadequate transport of oxygen, or substantial loss of lung tissue due to tumors or surgery. Oxygen therapy is prescribed by the physician, who specifies the specific concentration, method, and liter flow per minute. The concentration is of more importance than the liter flow per minute. When the administration of oxygen is an emergency measure, the nurse may 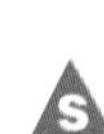 initiate the therapy. For clients who have chronic obstructive pulmonary disease (COPD), a *low*-flow oxygen system is essential. See the box above.

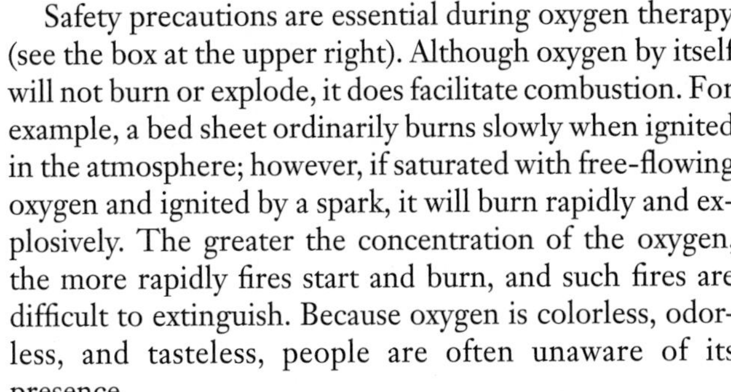

Safety precautions are essential during oxygen therapy (see the box at the upper right). Although oxygen by itself will not burn or explode, it does facilitate combustion. For example, a bed sheet ordinarily burns slowly when ignited in the atmosphere; however, if saturated with free-flowing oxygen and ignited by a spark, it will burn rapidly and explosively. The greater the concentration of the oxygen, the more rapidly fires start and burn, and such fires are difficult to extinguish. Because oxygen is colorless, odorless, and tasteless, people are often unaware of its presence.

Oxygen is supplied in hospitals in two ways: by liquid portable systems (cylinders) and from wall outlets. Oxygen cylinders are made of steel. Large ones contain 244 cubic feet of oxygen stored at a pressure of 2200 pounds per square inch (psi). Smaller cylinders are available for emergency and ambulatory use. Piped-in oxygen is stored at much lower pressure, usually 50 to 60 psi.

Oxygen administered from a cylinder or wall-outlet system is dry. Dry gases dehydrate the respiratory mucous membranes. Humidifying devices that add water vapor to inspired air are thus an essential adjunct of oxygen therapy, particularly for liter flows over 2 liters per minute (Figure 39–12, p. 1154). These devices provide 20% to 40% humidity. The oxygen passes through sterile distilled water or tap water (see the Research Note on p. 1154) and then along a line to the device through which the moistened oxygen is inhaled (eg, a cannula, nasal catheter, or oxygen mask).

Humidifiers prevent mucous membranes from drying and becoming irritated and loosen secretions for easier expectoration. Oxygen passing through water picks up water vapor before it reaches the client. The more bubbles created during this process, the more water vapor is produced. Very low liter flows (eg, 1 to 2 liters per minute by nasal cannula) do not require humidification.

Oxygen cylinders need to be handled and stored with caution and strapped securely in wheeled transport devices or stands to prevent possible falls and outlet breakages. They should be placed away from traffic areas and heaters.

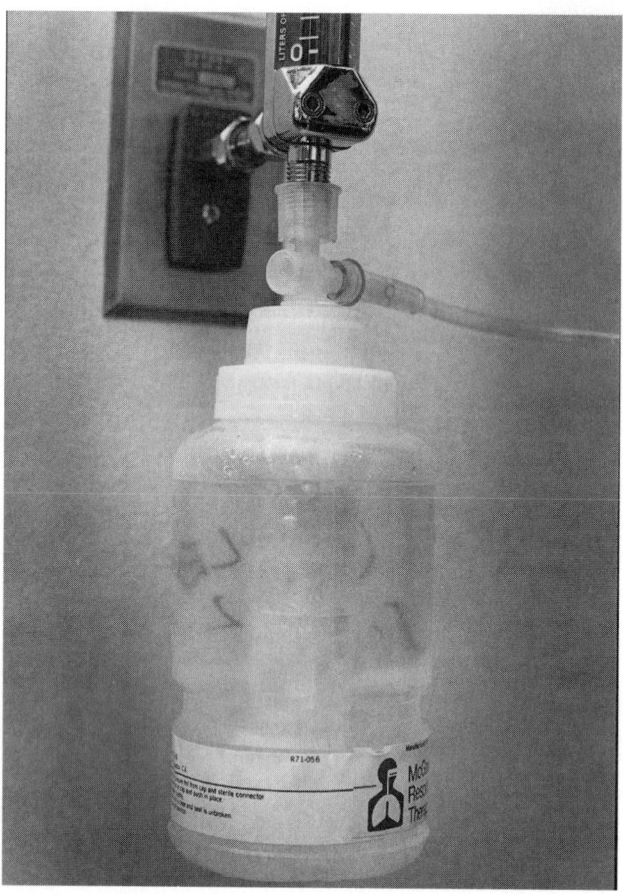

Figure 39–12 An oxygen humidifier.

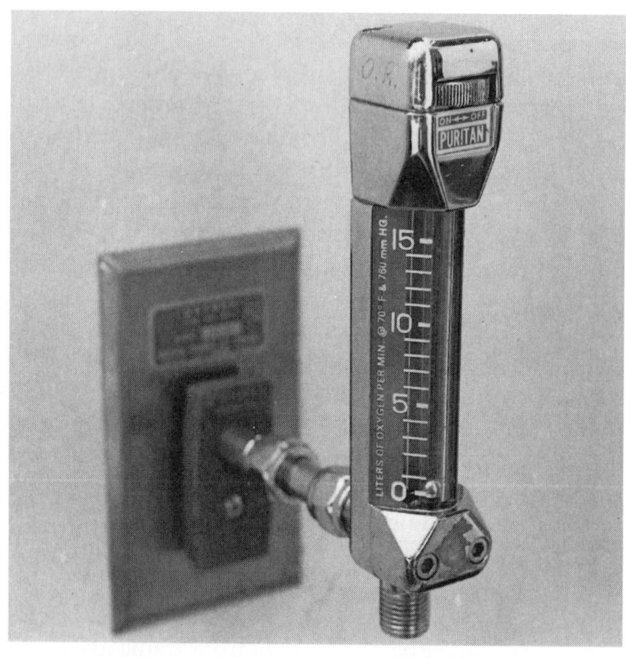

Figure 39–13 An oxygen flow meter attached to a wall outlet.

RESEARCH NOTE

Is Sterile Water Necessary for Humidification in Low-Flow Oxygen Therapy?

This study compared the bacterial contamination of tap water with that of sterile water used to fill clean (nonsterile) disposable oxygen humidifier reservoirs. Disposable oxygen humidification reservoirs were assembled weekly according to standard protocol and regulated to deliver oxygen, 4 to 6 L/min, continuously for 5 consecutive days. Each of 48 reservoirs was filled daily with either tap water (24) or sterile water (24) and cultured daily. The total number of reservoirs used over the 5-day period was 240.

Bacterial growth was observed from 54 (45.0%) of 120 sterile water reservoir cultures and from 38 (31.7%) of 120 tap water reservoir cultures. The microorganisms identified from the sterile water reservoirs included *Enterobacter agglomerans* and species of the genus *Serratia* and the genus *Bacillus.* The findings of this study demonstrate (a) that bacterial contamination of both sterile water and tap water used in clean disposable humidifier oxygen reservoirs does occur; (b) that the use of tap water for low-flow oxygen humidification was determined to be safe at the hospital under study; and (c) that this procedural change contributed approximately $9000 to the cost-reduction efforts of the respiratory therapy department.

Implications: Tap water may safely be used in disposable oxygen humidification reservoirs. However, it is recommended that any facility considering the use of tap water in low-flow oxygen humidifier reservoirs culture the tap water to determine its bacterial load in the particular geographic location.

Source: K Cahill and J Heath. Sterile water used for humidification in low-flow oxygen therapy: Is it necessary? *American Journal of Infection Control,* February 1990, 18:13–17.

To use an oxygen wall outlet, the nurse carries out these steps:

- Attach the flow meter to the wall outlet, exerting firm pressure. The flow meter should be in the OFF position (Figure 39–13).
- Fill the humidifier bottle with distilled or tap water in accordance with agency protocol. (This can be done before coming to the bedside.)
- Attach the humidifier bottle to the base of the flow meter (Figure 39–12).
- Attach the prescribed oxygen tubing and delivery device to the humidifier.
- Regulate the flow meter to the prescribed level.

OXYGEN DELIVERY

Oxygen is administered by either low-flow or high-flow systems. In *low-flow systems*, gas is delivered via small bore tubing at a rate shown on the flowmeter. Because room air is also inhaled along with oxygen, the fraction of inspired oxygen (FiO_2) will vary depending on the respiratory rate, tidal volume, and liter flow. Low-flow systems are generally used for clients who have a respiratory rate below 25 per minute and a regular and consistent respiratory pattern. They are contraindicated for clients who require carefully monitored concentrations of oxygen. Low-flow administration devices include the nasal cannula, simple face mask, partial rebreathing mask, humidity tent, and oxygen tent.

High-flow systems supply all of the gas required during ventilation in precise amounts, regardless of the client's respiratory status. The ratio of room air to oxygen is regulated and does not vary with the client's respirations. Thus it is a precise and consistent method for controlling the client's FiO_2. In high-flow systems, gas is delivered via a Venturi device and large-bore tubing placed near the client. The Venturi mask is an example of a high-flow administration device.

Some devices can be used for both low- and high-flow administration, for example, the face tent and the oxygen hood. Both low-flow and high-flow systems can deliver a variety of oxygen concentrations.

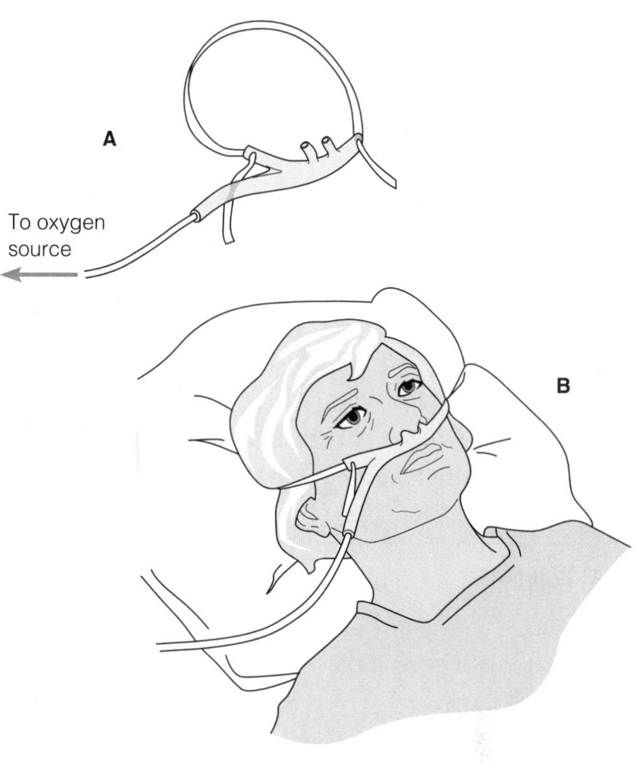

Figure 39–14 *A,* nasal cannula; *B,* the cannula in place.

Cannula The nasal cannula (nasal prongs) is the most common inexpensive low-flow device used to administer oxygen. It consists of a rubber or plastic tube that extends around the face, with 0.6- to 1.3-cm (¼- to ½-in) curved prongs that fit into the nostrils. One side of the tube connects to the oxygen tubing and oxygen supply. The cannula is often held in place by an elastic band that fits around the client's head or under the chin (Figure 39–14). For clients who are confused or particularly active, it may be helpful to secure the cannula in place with small pieces of tape on each side of the face.

The nasal cannula is easy to apply and does not interfere with the client's ability to eat or talk. It also is relatively comfortable, permits some freedom of movement, and is well tolerated by the client. It delivers a relatively low concentration of oxygen (24% to 45%) at flow rates of 2 to 6 liters per minute. Higher concentrations and flow rates can be administered; however, above 6 liters per minute there is a tendency for the client to swallow air and for the nasal and pharyngeal mucosa to become irritated In addition, the FiO_2 is *not* increased.

Administering oxygen by cannula is detailed in Procedure 39–3.

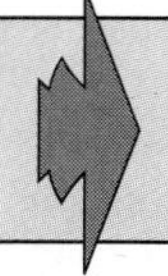

PROCEDURE 39–3 ADMINISTERING OXYGEN BY CANNULA, FACE MASK, OR FACE TENT

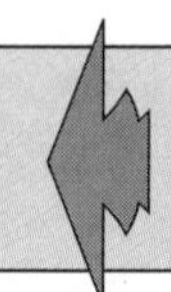

Before administering oxygen, determine (a) whether the client has COPD; (b) the levels of oxygen (PaO_2) and carbon dioxide ($PaCO_2$) in the client's arterial blood (PaO_2 is normally 80 to 100 mm Hg; $PaCO_2$ is normally 35 to 45 mm Hg); and (c) the order for oxygen, including the administering device and the liter flow rate (L/min) or the percentage of oxygen.

PURPOSES

Cannula

- To deliver a relatively low concentration of oxygen when only minimal O_2 support is required
- To allow uninterrupted delivery of oxygen while the client ingests food or fluids

PROCEDURE 39–3 ADMINISTERING OXYGEN BY CANNULA, FACE MASK, OR FACE TENT *continued*

Face Mask

- To provide moderate O_2 support and a higher concentration of oxygen and/or humidity than is provided by cannula

Face Tent

- To provide high humidity
- To provide oxygen when a mask is poorly tolerated
- To provide a high flow of O_2 when attached to a Venturi system

ASSESSMENT FOCUS

Vital signs; arterial blood gas levels; signs of hypoxia (eg, tachycardia, tachypnea, dyspnea); signs of hypercarbia (eg, restlessness, hypertension, headache); lung sounds; patency of nares (if nasal cannula is to be used); mental status; signs of oxygen toxicity (eg, tracheal irritation, cough, decreased pulmonary ventilation).

EQUIPMENT

Cannula

- ☐ Oxygen supply with a flow meter
- ☐ Humidifier with sterile, distilled water or tap water according to agency protocol
- ☐ Nasal cannula and tubing
- ☐ Tape
- ☐ Gauzes

Face Mask

- ☐ Oxygen supply with a flow meter
- ☐ Humidifier with sterile distilled or tap water
- ☐ Prescribed face mask of the appropriate size
- ☐ Padding for the elastic band

Face Tent

- ☐ Oxygen supply with a flow meter
- ☐ Humidifier with sterile distilled or tap water
- ☐ Face tent of the appropriate size

INTERVENTION

1. Determine the need for oxygen therapy, and verify the order for the therapy.

- Perform a respiratory assessment to determine the need for O_2 therapy and to develop baseline data if not already available.

2. Prepare the client and support persons.

- Assist the client to a semi-Fowler's position if possible. *This position permits easier chest expansion and hence easier breathing.*
- Explain that oxygen is not dangerous when safety precautions are observed and that it will ease the discomfort of dyspnea. Inform the client and support persons about the safety precautions connected with oxygen use.

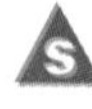

3. Set up the oxygen equipment and the humidifier. See p. 1154.

4. Turn on the oxygen at the prescribed rate, and ensure proper functioning.

- Check that the oxygen is flowing freely through the tubing. There should be no kinks in the tubing, and the connections should be airtight. There should be bubbles in the humidifier as the oxygen flows through the water. You should feel the oxygen at the outlets of the cannula.
- Set the oxygen at the flow rate ordered, for example, 2 to 6 liters per minute.

5. Apply the appropriate oxygen cannula delivery device.

Cannula

- Put the cannula over the client's face, with the outlet prongs fitting into the nares and the elastic band around the head. Some models have a strap to adjust under the chin.
- If the cannula will not stay in place, tape it at the sides of the face.
- Slip gauze pads under the tubing over the cheekbones to prevent skin irritation as necessary.

Face Mask

- Guide the mask toward the client's face, and apply it from the nose downward.
- Fit the mask to the contours of the client's face. *The mask should mold to the face, so that very little oxygen escapes into the eyes or around the cheeks and chin.*

PROCEDURE 39–3 *continued*

- Secure the elastic band around the client's head so that the mask is comfortable but snug.
- Pad the band behind the ears and over bony prominences. *Padding will prevent irritation from the mask.*

Face Tent

- Place the tent over the client's face, and secure the ties around the head.
- Turn on the oxygen at the prescribed flow rate.

6. Assess the client regularly.

- Assess the client's level of anxiety, color, and ease of respirations, and provide support while the client adjusts to the cannula.
- Assess the client in 15 to 30 minutes, depending on the client's condition, and regularly thereafter. Assess vital signs, color, breathing patterns, and chest movements.
- Assess the client regularly for clinical signs of hypoxia, tachycardia, confusion, dyspnea, restlessness, and cyanosis. Obtain arterial blood gas results, if they are available.

Nasal Cannula

- Assess the client's nares for encrustations and irritation. Apply a water-soluble lubricant as required to soothe the mucous membranes.

Face Mask or Tent

- Inspect the facial skin frequently for dampness or chafing, and dry and treat it as needed.

7. Inspect the equipment on a regular basis.

- Check the liter flow and the level of water in the humidifier in 30 minutes and whenever providing care to the client.
- Maintain the level of water in the humidifier.
- Make sure that safety precautions are being followed.

8. Document relevant data.

- Record the initiation of the therapy and all nursing assessments.

EVALUATION FOCUS

Vital signs; signs of hypoxia, hypercarbia; bilateral lung sounds; blood gas levels; color of skin, nails, lips, and earlobes; activity tolerance; level of anxiety.

Face Mask Face masks that cover the client's nose and mouth may be used for oxygen inhalation. Most masks are made of clear, pliable plastic or rubber that can be molded to fit the face. They are held to the client's head with elastic bands. Some have a metal clip that can be bent over the bridge of the nose for a snug fit. There are several holes in the sides of the mask (exhalation ports) to allow the escape of exhaled carbon dioxide.

Some masks have reservoir bags, which provide higher oxygen concentrations to the client. A portion of the client's expired air is directed into the bag. Because this air comes from the upper respiratory passages (eg, the trachea and bronchi), where it does not take part in gaseous exchange, its oxygen concentration remains the same as that of inspired air.

A variety of oxygen masks are marketed:

- The *simple face mask* (low-flow system) delivers oxygen concentrations from 40% to 60% at liter flows of 5 to 8 liters per minute respectively (Figure 39–15).

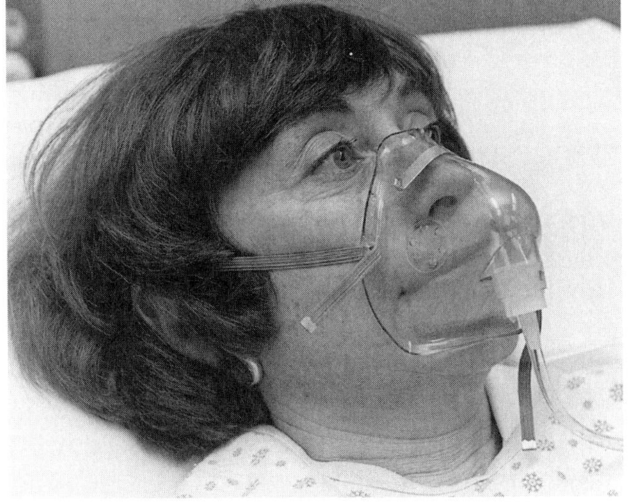

Figure 39–15 A simple face mask for a low-flow oxygen system.

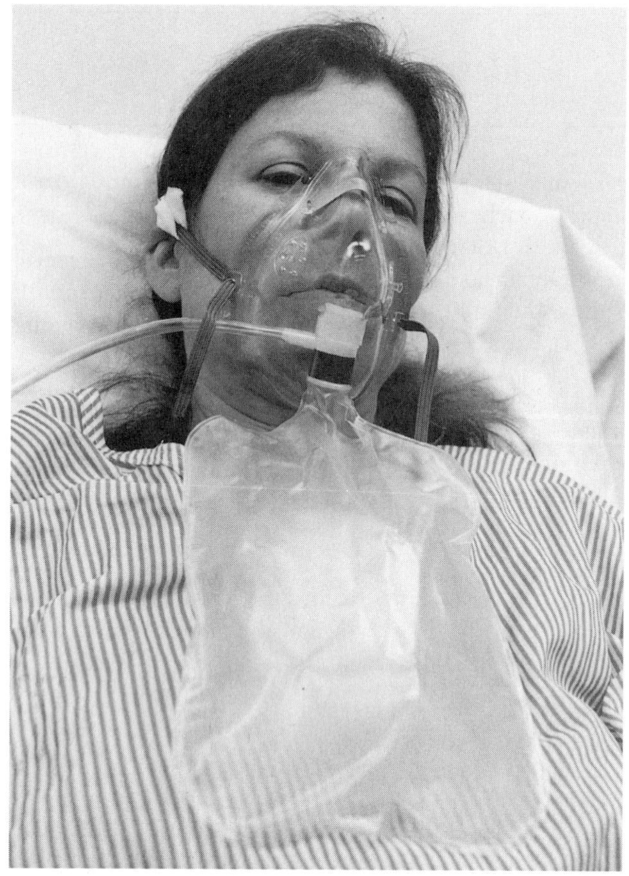

Figure 39–16 A partial rebreather mask for a low-flow oxygen system.

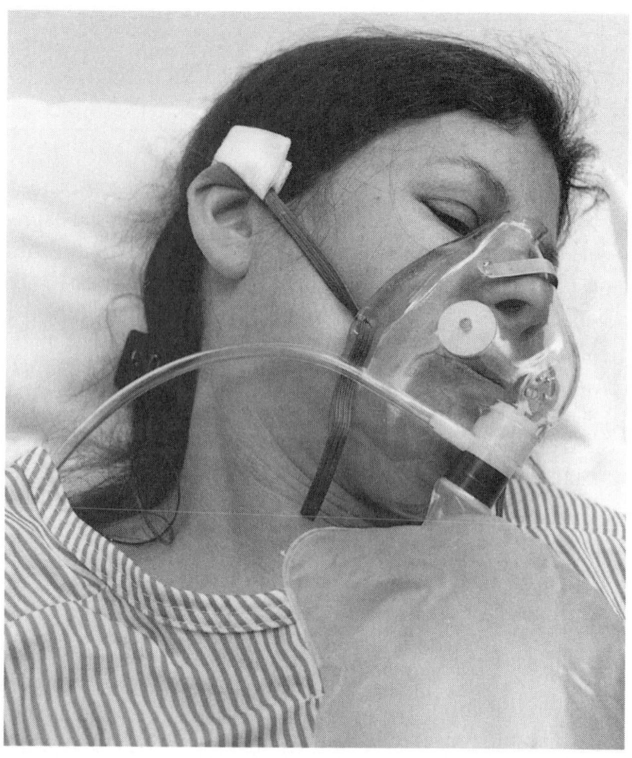

Figure 39–17 A nonrebreather mask for a low-flow or a high-flow oxygen system.

- The *partial rebreather mask* (low-flow system) delivers oxygen concentrations of 60% to 90% at liter flows of 6 to 10 liters per minute respectively. The oxygen reservoir bag that is attached allows the client to rebreathe about the first third of the exhaled air in conjunction with oxygen (Figure 39–16). Thus it increases the FiO_2 by recycling expired oxygen. The partial rebreather bag must not totally deflate during inspiration to avoid carbon dioxide buildup. If this problem occurs, the nurse increases the liter flow of oxygen.
- The *nonrebreather mask* (low-flow system) delivers the highest oxygen concentration possible—that is, 95% to 100%—by means other than intubation or mechanical ventilation, at liter flows of 10 to 15 liters per minute. Using a nonrebreather mask, the client breathes only the source gas from the bag. One-way valves on the mask and between the reservoir bag and the mask prevent the room air and the client's exhaled air from entering the bag (Figure 39–17). To prevent carbon dioxide buildup, the nonrebreather bag must not totally deflate during inspiration. If it does, the nurse can correct this problem by increasing the liter flow of oxygen.
- The *Venturi mask* (high-flow system) delivers oxygen concentrations precise to within 1% and is often used for clients with COPD (Figure 39–18). Oxygen concentrations vary from 24% to 40% or 50%, depending on the brand, at liter flows of 4 to 10 liters per minute. The Venturi mask is designed with wide-bore tubing and various color-coded jet adapters. Each color code corresponds to a precise oxygen concentration and a specific liter flow. For example, a blue adapter delivers a 24% concentration of oxygen at 4 liters per minute, and a green adapter delivers a 35% concentration of oxygen at 8 liters per minute. Optional humidification adapters are also available for clients who require them, such as those receiving oxygen concentrations in excess of 30%.

Initiating oxygen by mask is much the same as initiating oxygen by cannula, except that the nurse must find a mask of appropriate size. Smaller sizes are available for children. Administering oxygen by mask is detailed in Procedure 39–3 on page 1155.

Face Tent Face tents (Figure 39–19) can replace oxygen masks when masks are poorly tolerated by clients. When a face tent alone is used to supply oxygen, the concentration of oxygen varies; therefore, it is often used

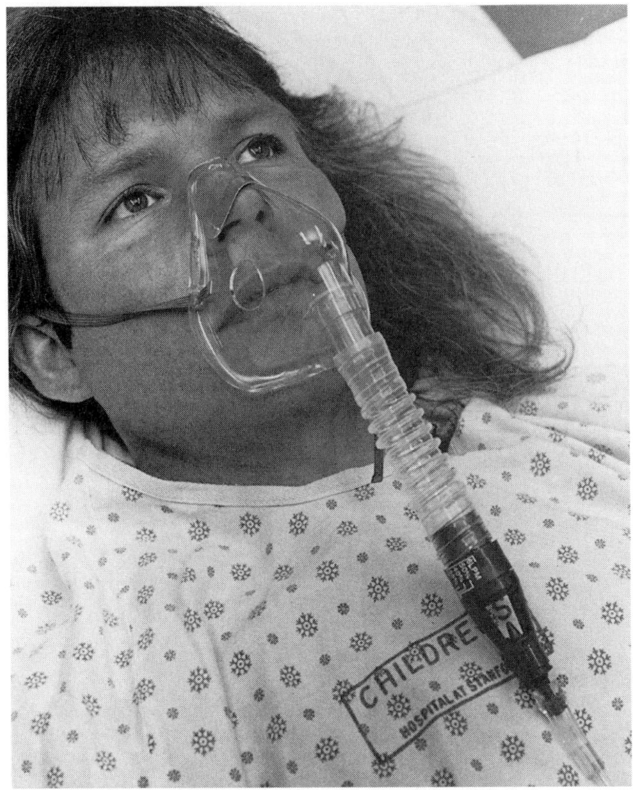

Figure 39–18 A Venturi mask for a high-flow oxygen system.

in conjunction with a Venturi system. Face tents provide varying concentrations of oxygen, for example, 30% to 50% concentration of oxygen at 4 to 8 liters per minute. Frequently inspect the client's facial skin for dampness or chafing, and dry and treat as needed. As with face masks, the client's facial skin must be kept dry. Administering oxygen by face tent is detailed in Procedure 39–3 on page 1155.

Oxygen Analyzer Oxygen analyzers (Figure 39–20) measure the concentration of oxygen being received by the client. The analyzer is first used to measure the concentration of oxygen in the room. It should register 0.21 (21%). If it does not, the nurse adjusts the dial to this calibration. The nurse then places the sample tube next to the client's nose, monitors the reading on the analyzer, and adjusts the oxygen flow rate to obtain the desired fraction of inspired oxygen (FiO_2).

Transtracheal Oxygen Delivery Home delivery devices are now available to clients who require continuous oxygen therapy at home. *Transtracheal oxygen delivery* refers to oxygen given through a small, narrow plastic cannula that is inserted through the skin at the base of the neck directly into the trachea (Figure 39–21). A chain around the neck holds the catheter in place.

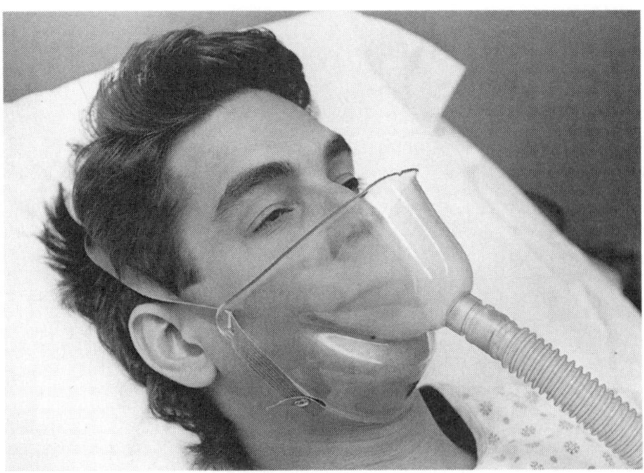

Figure 39–19 An oxygen face tent.

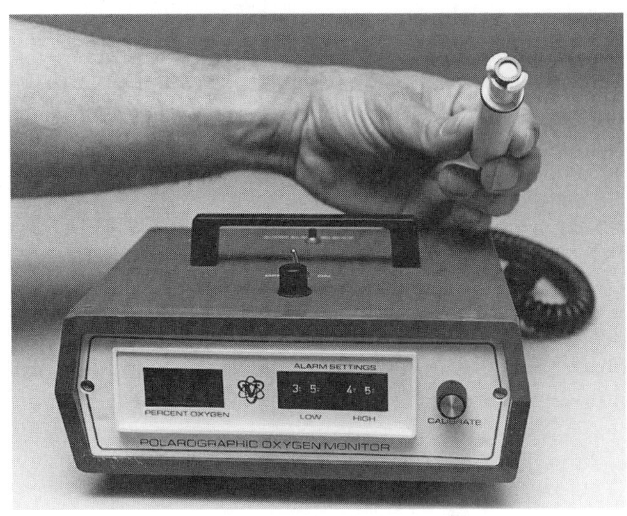

Figure 39–20 An oxygen analyzer.

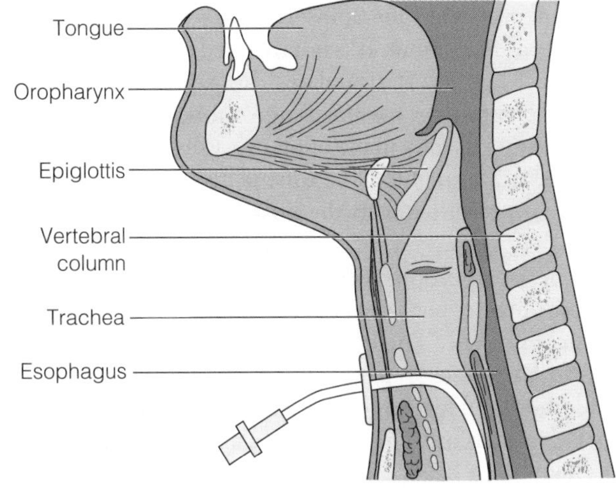

Figure 39–21 A transtracheal oxygen catheter in place.

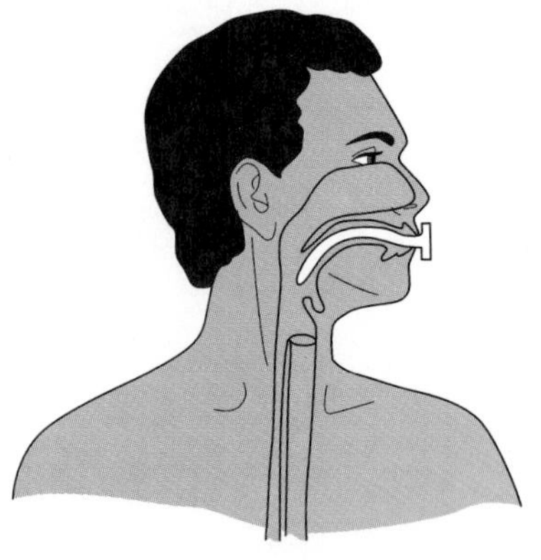

Figure 39–22 An oropharyngeal tube in place.

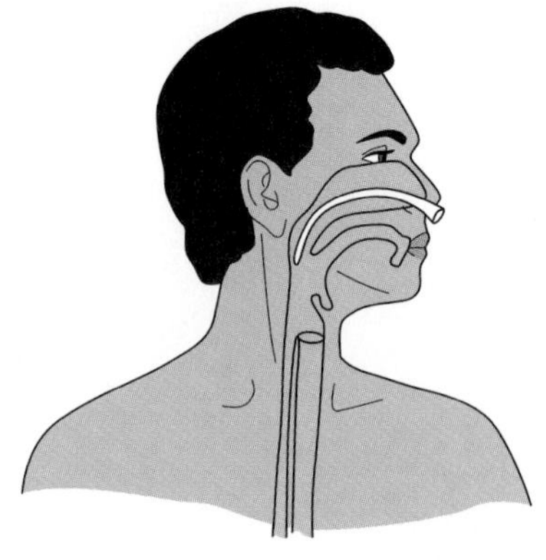

Figure 39–23 A nasopharyngeal tube in place.

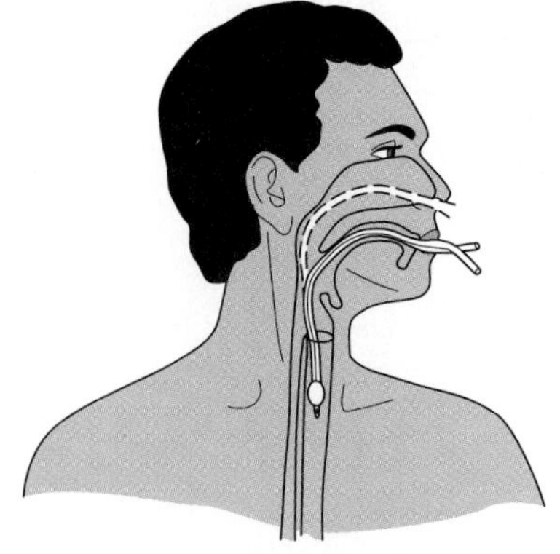

Figure 39–24 An endotracheal tube in place.

With this delivery system, the client requires less oxygen because all of the flow delivered enters the lungs. The nurse keeps the catheter patent by injecting 1.5 mL of normal saline into it, moving a cleaning rod in and out of it and then injecting another 1.5 mL of saline solution. This is done two or three times a day.

ARTIFICIAL AIRWAYS

Artificial airways are inserted to maintain a patent air passage for clients whose airway has become or may become obstructed. A patent airway is necessary so that air can flow to and from the lungs. Four of the more common types of intubation are oropharyngeal, nasopharyngeal, endotracheal, and tracheostomy.

Oropharyngeal Intubation Oropharyngeal intubation is done most frequently for clients who have had general anesthesia and for those who are semiconscious and are likely to obstruct their own airways with their tongues. An oropharyngeal tube is inserted in some instances for pharyngeal suctioning. It is not inserted in clients who are conscious, because it stimulates the gag reflex and thus can cause vomiting. Oropharyngeal tubes are somewhat S-shaped and usually made of plastic. Adult, child, and infant sizes are available. The tube is inserted through the mouth and terminates in the posterior pharynx. (Figure 39–22).

To insert an oropharyngeal airway, the nurse dons disposable gloves, opens the client's mouth, and removes any dentures present. The client should be in a supine position, with the neck hyperextended or with a pillow placed under the shoulders so that the tongue cannot fall back to block the pharynx. This position may be contraindicated for clients with head, neck, or back injuries. Before insertion lubricate the airway with a water-soluble lubricant and advance the airway sideways along the roof of the mouth until the flange touches the lips. While observing the position of the tongue in the mouth, rotate the airway when introducing it over the tongue to the pharynx. If necessary, tape the airway in position and suction secretions as necessary.

Nursing interventions for intubated clients include the following:

- Maintain the client in a lateral or semiprone position so that blood, vomitus, and mucus will drain out of the mouth and not be aspirated.
- Remove the airway once the client has regained consciousness and has the swallow, gag, and cough reflexes.

Nasopharyngeal Intubation Nasopharyngeal intubation is carried out if the oropharyngeal route is contraindicated, for example, following oral surgery, or to protect the nasal and pharyngeal mucosa during nasopharyngeal or nasotracheal suctioning. The nasopharyngeal tube is inserted through a nostril and terminates in the pharynx, below the upper edge of the epiglottis (Figure 39–23). Tubes vary in size for adults, children, and infants and are usually made of latex rubber.

To insert a nasopharyngeal tube, lubricate the entire tube with a topical anesthetic (if ordered) to prevent irritation of the nasopharyngeal mucosa and undue discomfort. Then hold the airway by the wide end and insert the narrow end into the naris, applying gentle inward and downward pressure when advancing the airway to follow the natural course of the nasal structures. Remove excess lubricant from the client's face and nares before securing the tube in place with tape.

Nursing interventions for clients with nasopharyngeal tubes include the following:

- Remove the tube, and insert it in the other nostril at least every 8 hours, or as ordered by the physician, or more often to prevent irritation of the mucosa.

CLINICAL GUIDELINES

Nursing Interventions for Clients with Endotracheal Tubes

- Maintain the client in a lateral or semiprone position so that blood, vomitus, or secretions can drain from the mouth and are not aspirated.
- Provide oral or nasal hygiene every 3 hours or as needed.
- For an oral insertion, provide a bite block so that the client cannot bite the tube and occlude the airway.
- Assess the condition of the nasal or oral mucosa for irritation, and notify the physician should the need to change a nasal endotracheal tube arise; reposition an oral endotracheal tube from one side of the mouth to the other every 8 hours or as required.
- Closely monitor the air pressure in the endotracheal cuff. If it is greater than 20 mm Hg, necrosis of the tracheal tissues can result.
- Tape the airway in place to prevent accidental slippage or extubation.

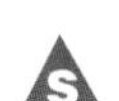

- Change the tape daily, and position the tube on the opposite side of the mouth at each change.
- Provide continuous humidification or aerosol therapy to prevent undue drying and irritation of the mucous membranes, if the tube is left in for more than a short time (eg, for days or weeks).
- Deflate and reinflate the cuff according to the manufacturer's directions.
- Communicate frequently with the client, and provide a notepad or other means for the client to communicate. Most clients cannot speak with an inflated cuff, because no air can pass over the vocal chords.

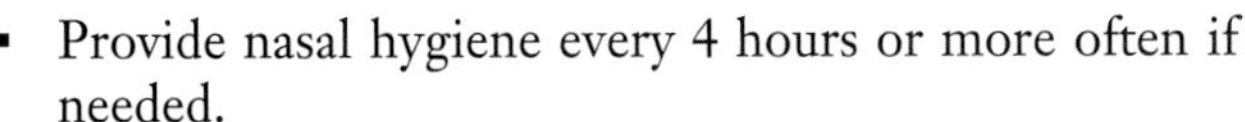

- Provide nasal hygiene every 4 hours or more often if needed.

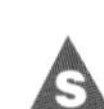

- Monitor the client closely for stimulation of the vagus nerve if nasotracheal suctioning is carried out. Vagal stimulation can lead to cardiac arrest.

Endotracheal Tubes Endotracheal tubes are most commonly inserted for clients who have had general anesthetics or for those in emergency situations where mechanical ventilation is required. An endotracheal tube is a curved polyvinylchloride tube that is inserted through either the mouth or the nose and into the trachea with the guide of a laryngoscope (Figure 39–24). The tube terminates just superior to the bifurcation of the trachea into the bronchi. Because an endotracheal tube passes through the epiglottis and splits it open, an inflated cuff is needed to close the system. Nursing interventions for clients with endotracheal tubes are shown in the box at the left.

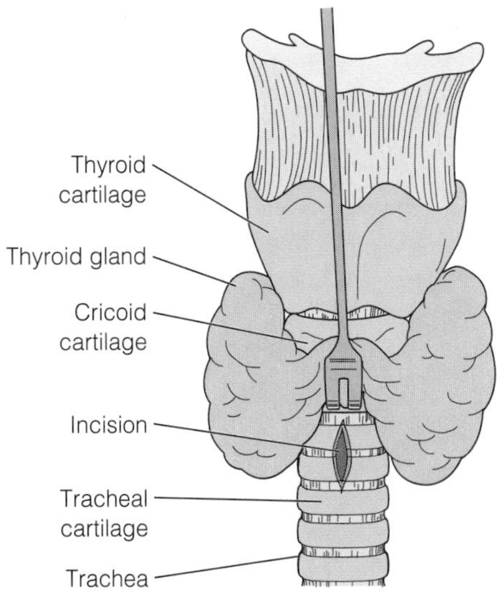

Figure 39–25 Site of a tracheostomy incision.

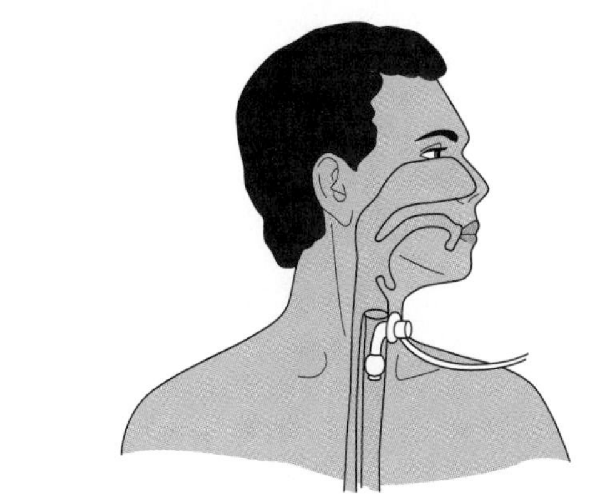

Figure 39–26 A tracheostomy tube in place.

Note: Only nurses with special preparation perform endotracheal intubation.

Tracheostomy Tubes Tracheostomy tubes are inserted to provide and maintain a patent airway, to remove tracheobronchial secretions from clients unable to cough, to replace endotracheal tubes, to permit the use of positive pressure ventilation, and to prevent unconscious clients from aspirating secretions.

A tracheostomy tube is a curved tube that is inserted into a tracheostomy, a surgical incision in the trachea just below the first or second tracheal cartilage (Figure 39–25). The tube extends through the tracheostomy stoma into the trachea (Figure 39–26). Tracheostomy tubes come in different sizes and may be made of metal, plastic, or foam. Plastic tubes are increasingly popular, because they are lightweight, their parts are interchangeable, and crusting from the tissues rarely forms on plastic materials.

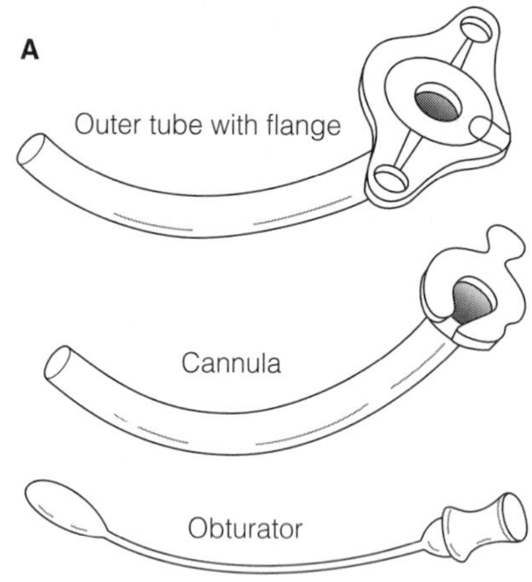

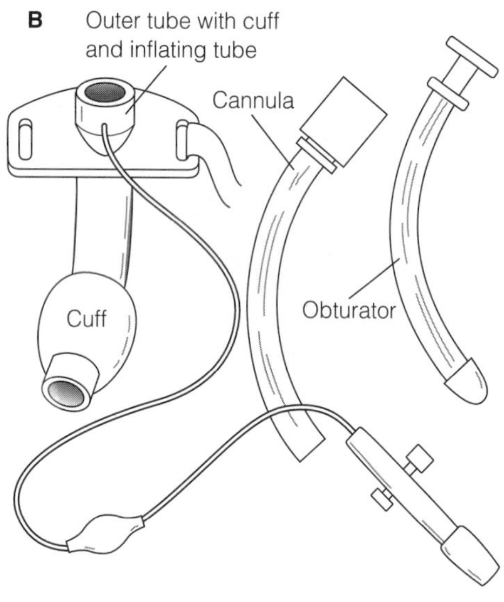

Figure 39–27 Two types of tracheostomy sets: *A*, noncuffed; *B*, cuffed.

The main parts of a tracheostomy set are the outer tube, the inner tube or inner cannula, and the obturator (Figure 39–27). The obturator is used only to insert the outer tube. It is removed once the outer tube is in place. The outer tube usually has ties to secure it around the client's neck, although many plastic tubes are cuffed with a soft balloon that can be inflated to hold the tube in place (Figure 39–27, *B*). Fitted inside the outer tube is an inner cannula. (Some plastic sets do not have this, because it is unnecessary to change the tube. They are called *single-cannula tubes.*) In double-cannula sets, the inner cannula is inserted and locked in place after the obturator is removed; it acts as a removable liner for the more permanent, outer cannula. The inner tube is withdrawn only for brief periods to be cleaned.

Cuffed tracheostomy tubes are surrounded by an inflatable cuff that produces an airtight seal between the tube and the trachea. This seal prevents aspiration of oropharyngeal secretions and air leakage between the tube and the trachea. Cuffed tubes are often used immediately after a tracheostomy in adults and infants and are essential when ventilating a tracheostomy client with a ventilator. Children do not require cuffed tubes, because their tracheas are resilient enough to seal the air space around the tube.

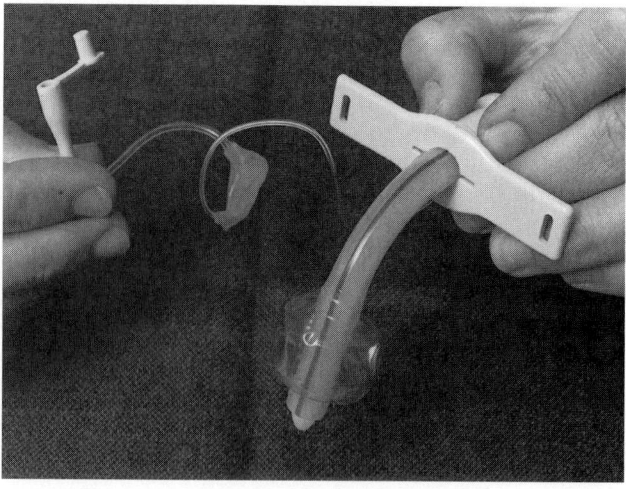

Figure 39–28 A tracheostomy tube with a foam cuff.

Some tubes have high-pressure cuffs; others have low-pressure cuffs. Some high-pressure tubes are double-cuffed; these can be inflated alternately to alter the pressure points on the trachea and prevent tracheal irritation and tissue damage. Alternate inflation also allows uninterrupted respirator function for people using ventilators. Commercially prepared cuffs are available for use on cuffless tracheostomy tubes.

Different cuffed tubes have different advantages and disadvantages. Cuffs that are bonded to the tracheostomy tube eliminate the risk of accidental detachment inside the trachea. Low-pressure cuffs, which are more costly than others, distribute a low, even pressure against the trachea, thus decreasing the risk of tracheal tissue necrosis. They do not need to be deflated periodically to reduce pressure on the tracheal wall. Double-cuffed high-pressure tubes may reduce the risk of tissue necrosis with alternate inflation of cuffs, but *only* if there is rigid adherence to the alternate inflation schedule. If tracheal damage does occur, a larger area of the trachea is involved with double-cuffed tubes.

A variation of the cuffed tube is the foam cuff. It does not require injected air; instead, when the port is opened, ambient air enters the balloon, which then conforms to the client's trachea (Figure 39–28). The physician removes air from the cuff prior to insertion or removal of the tube.

ENDOTRACHEAL SUCTIONING

Following a tracheostomy, the trachea and surrounding respiratory tissues are irritated and react by producing excessive secretions. Suctioning is necessary to remove these secretions and maintain a patent airway. The frequency of suctioning depends on the client's health and how recently the tracheostomy was done.

Suctioning is associated with several complications: hypoxemia, trauma to the airway, nosocomial infection, and cardiac dysrhythmia, which is related to the hypoxemia. Suctioning also stimulates the cough reflex and stimulates cells in the bronchi to secrete more mucus (Noll et al 1990, p. 318). Suctioning should therefore be done only when breath sounds indicate that the need is present, or according to the physician's routine orders.

Several techniques that minimize or decrease these complications have evolved over the past decade:

- *Hyperinflation.* This involves giving the client breaths that are 1 to 1.5 times the tidal volume set on the ventilator through the ventilator circuit or via a manual resuscitation bag. Three to five quick breaths are delivered before and after each pass of the suction catheter.
- *Hyperoxygenation.* This can be done with a manual resuscitation bag or through the ventilator and is performed by increasing the oxygen flow (usually to 100%) before suctioning and between suction attempts.
- *Oxygen insufflation suction catheter.* A double-lumen catheter system has been developed that allows oxygen insufflation during the suctioning procedure *except* during the suctioning phase. This 22-inch, #14 Fr. catheter has a second lumen of oxygen insufflation (Bodai et al 1987, p. 39). The suction port is equivalent to a regular #12 Fr. suction catheter. The oxygen port has five side holes to allow oxygen dispersal within the trachea. This port accommodates a flow rate of 15 liters per minute. The end of the catheter has a fingertip control valve. When the valve tabs are compressed, suction is applied, and the oxygen circuit is occluded. Oxygen is thus administered before suction is applied.

For tracheostomy and endotracheal suctioning, the diameter of the suction catheter should be about half the inside diameter of the tracheostomy tube so that hypoxia can be prevented. The nurse uses sterile technique to prevent infection of the respiratory tract.

If the client's secretions are thick, the nurse performs *tracheal lavage* before suctioning. This is the insertion of sterile normal saline through the tracheostomy tube into the trachea. See Procedure 39–4. To clean a double-cannula tracheostomy tube, see Procedure 39–5 on page 1166.

Text continued on page 1167

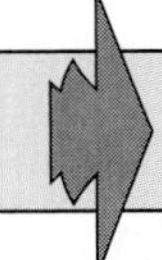

PROCEDURE 39–4 SUCTIONING A TRACHEOSTOMY OR ENDOTRACHEAL TUBE

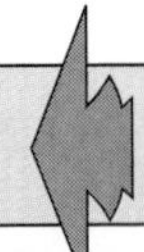

PURPOSES

- To maintain a patent airway and prevent airway obstructions
- To promote respiratory function (optimal exchange of oxygen and carbon dioxide into and out of the lungs)
- To prevent pneumonia that may result from accumulated secretions

ASSESSMENT FOCUS

Presence of congestion on auscultation of the thorax; client's inability to remove the secretions through coughing.

EQUIPMENT

- ☐ Resuscitation bag (Ambu bag) connected to 100% oxygen
- ☐ Sterile towel
- ☐ Sterile 2- to 10-mL syringe and sterile normal saline
- ☐ Equipment for suctioning the oropharyngeal cavity (see Procedure 39–2, page 1150).
- ☐ Goggles and mask if necessary
- ☐ Gown (if necessary)
- ☐ Sterile gloves
- ☐ Moisture-resistant bag

PROCEDURE 39–4 SUCTIONING A TRACHEOSTOMY OR ENDOTRACHEAL TUBE *continued*

INTERVENTION

1. Prepare the client.

- Inform the client that suctioning usually causes some intermittent coughing and that this assists in removing the secretions.
- If not contraindicated because of health, place the client in semi-Fowler's position to promote deep breathing, maximum lung expansion, and productive coughing. *Deep breathing oxygenates the lungs, counteracts the hypoxic effects of suctioning, and may induce coughing. Coughing helps to loosen and move secretions.*

2. Prepare the equipment.

- Attach the resuscitation apparatus to the oxygen source (Figure 39–29). Adjust the oxygen flow to "100% flush."
- Open the sterile supplies in readiness for use.
- Place the sterile towel, if used, across the client's chest, below the tracheostomy.

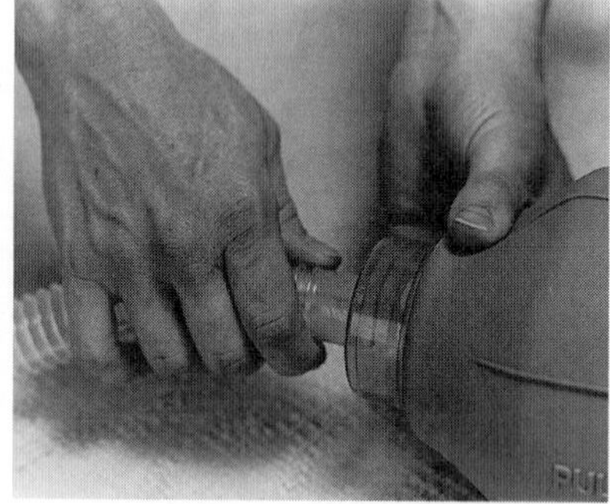

Figure 39–29 Attaching the resuscitation apparatus to the oxygen source.

- Prepare the saline for instillation by opening the ampules and drawing up the saline in a syringe.
- Turn on the suction, and set the pressure in accordance with agency policy. For a wall unit, pressure of about 100 to 120 mm Hg is normally used for adults, 50 to 95 mm Hg for infants and children.

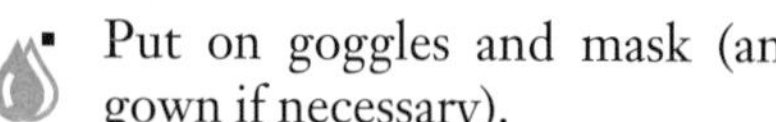

- Put on goggles and mask (and gown if necessary).
- Put on sterile gloves. Some agencies recommend putting a sterile glove on the dominant hand and an unsterile glove on the nondominant hand to protect the nurse.
- Holding the catheter in the dominant hand and the connector in the nondominant hand, attach the catheter to the Y-connector or straight connector (see Figure 39–10 on page 1151).

3. Flush and lubricate the catheter.

- Using the dominant hand, place the catheter tip in the sterile saline solution.
- Using the thumb of the nondominant hand, occlude the thumb control, and suction a small amount of the sterile solution through the catheter. *This determines that the suction equipment is working properly and lubricates the outside and the lumen of the catheter. Lubrication eases insertion and reduces tissue trauma during insertion. Lubricating the lumen also helps prevent secretions from sticking to the inside of the catheter.*

4. If the client does *not* have copious secretions, hyperventilate the lungs with a resuscitation bag before suctioning.

- Summon an assistant, if one is available, for this step.
- Using your nondominant hand, turn on the oxygen to 12 to 15 liters per minute.

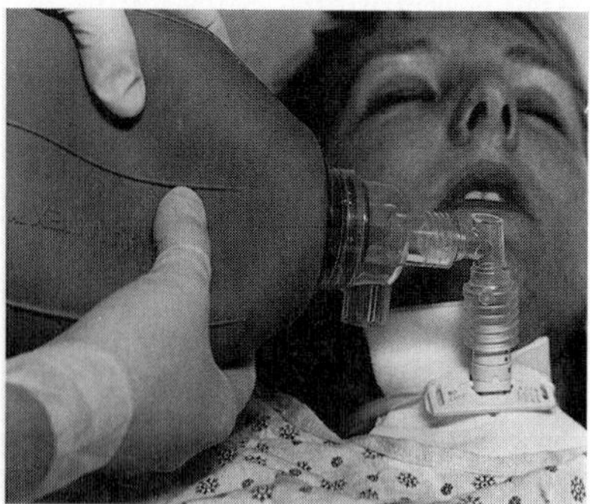

Figure 39–30 Attaching the resuscitator to the tracheostomy.

- If the client is receiving oxygen, disconnect the oxygen source from the tracheostomy tube using your nondominant hand.
- Attach the resuscitator to the tracheostomy or endotracheal tube (Figure 39–30).
- Compress the Ambu bag three to five times as the client *inhales*. This is best done by a second person, who can use both hands to compress the bag, providing a greater inflation volume.
- Observe the rise and fall of the client's chest to assess the adequacy of each ventilation.
- Remove the resuscitation device, and place it on the bed or the client's chest with the connector facing up.

5. If the client has copious secretions, do *not* hyperventilate with a resuscitator. Instead:

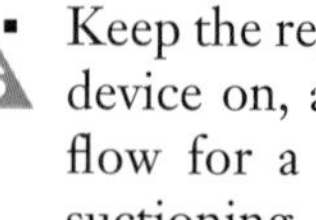

- Keep the regular oxygen delivery device on, and increase the liter flow for a few minutes before suctioning. *Hyperventilating a client who has copious secretions can force the secretions deeper into the respiratory tract.*

6. Quickly, but gently, insert the catheter without applying any suction.

PROCEDURE 39–4 *continued*

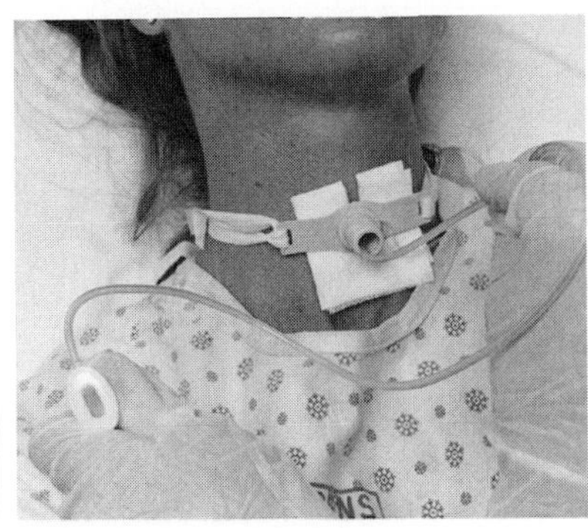

Figure 39–31 Inserting the catheter into the trachea through the tracheostomy tube.

- With your nondominant thumb off the suction port, quickly but gently insert the catheter into the trachea through the tracheostomy tube (Figure 39–31). *To prevent tissue trauma and oxygen loss, suction is not applied during insertion of the catheter.*

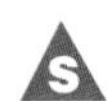

- Insert the catheter about 12.5 cm (6 in) for adults, less for children, or until the client coughs or you feel resistance. Resistance usually means that the catheter tip has reached the bifurcation of the trachea. To prevent damaging the mucous membranes at the bifurcation, withdraw the catheter about 1 to 2 cm (0.4 to 0.8 in) before applying suction.

7. Perform suctioning.

- Apply intermittent suction for 5 to 10 seconds by placing the nondominant thumb over the thumb port. *Suction time is restricted to 10 seconds or less to minimize oxygen loss.*
- Rotate the catheter by rolling it between your thumb and forefinger while slowly withdrawing it. *This prevents tissue trauma by minimizing the suction time against any part of the trachea.*
- Withdraw the catheter completely, and release the suction.
- Hyperventilate the client.

8. If secretions are thick, flush the catheter and perform tracheal lavage according to agency protocol.

- Flush the catheter with sterile water or saline.
- For adults, insert 2 to 5 mL of sterile saline solution through the tracheostomy tube into the trachea. For infants, use 0.5 to 1 mL; for children, use 2 mL. *This liquefies tenacious secretions so that they are more easily suctioned out.*
- Then suction again.

9. Reassess the client's oxygenation status, and repeat suctioning as above.

- Observe the client's respirations and skin color. With your clean hand, check the client's pulse if necessary.
- Encourage the client to breathe deeply and to cough between suctions.
- Allow 2 to 3 minutes between suctions when possible. *This provides an opportunity for reoxygenation of the lungs.*
- Flush the catheter, and repeat suctioning until the air passage is clear and the breathing is relatively effortless and quiet.
- After each suction, pick up the resuscitation bag with your clean hand, and ventilate the client with five breaths.

10. Dispose of equipment and ensure availability for the next suction.

- Flush the catheter and suction tubing.
- Turn off the suction, and disconnect the catheter from the suction tubing.
- Wrap the catheter around your sterile hand, and peel the glove off, so that it turns inside out over the catheter.
- Discard the glove and the catheter in the moisture-resistant bag.
- Replenish the sterile fluid and supplies so that the suction is ready to be used again. *Clients who require suctioning often require it quickly, so it is essential to leave the equipment at the bedside ready for use.*

11. Provide for client comfort and safety.

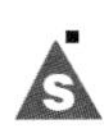

- Assist the client to a comfortable, safe position that aids breathing. If the person is conscious, a semi-Fowler's position is frequently indicated. If the person is unconscious, Sims' position can assist the drainage of secretions from the mouth.

12. Document relevant data.

- Record the suctioning, including the amount and description of suction returns, the amount of sterile saline instilled, and any other relevant assessments.

EVALUATION FOCUS

Respiratory rate, depth, and character after suctioning; tracheal breath sounds; color of skin and nail beds; character and amount of secretions suctioned; changes in vital signs.

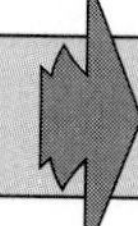

PROCEDURE 39–5 CLEANING A DOUBLE-CANNULA TRACHEOSTOMY TUBE

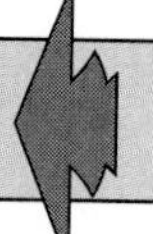

Double-cannula tracheostomy tubes are cleaned whenever necessary, but at least once per shift.

PURPOSES

- To maintain cleanliness and prevent infection at the tracheostomy site
- To maintain airway patency
- To prevent skin breakdown around the tracheostomy stoma

ASSESSMENT FOCUS

Presence of excessive peristomal secretions, excessive tube secretions, or soiled tracheostomy dressing or ties; labored breathing indicating diminished air flow through tracheostomy tube.

EQUIPMENT

- ☐ Sterile bowls
- ☐ Hydrogen peroxide and sterile normal saline
- ☐ Sterile gloves (1 pair and 1 glove or 2 pairs)
- ☐ Clean (nonsterile) glove
- ☐ Sterile nylon brush or pipe cleaners
- ☐ Sterile gauze squares or sterile cotton-tipped applicator sticks

INTERVENTION

1. Don gloves, and suction the tracheostomy tube.

- Put a nonsterile glove on the nondominant hand and a sterile glove on your dominant hand.
- Suction the entire length of the inner cannula prior to its removal to remove secretions and ensure a patent airway. (See Procedure 39–4).

2. Remove and soak the inner cannula.

- With the nondominant hand, unlock the inner cannula by turning the lock about 90 degrees counterclockwise. *The nondominant hand is used to handle the flange of the cannula, which is not sterile.*
- With the nondominant hand, remove the inner cannula by gently pulling it out toward you in line with its curvature.
- Soak the inner cannula in the hydrogen peroxide solution for several minutes. *This moistens and loosens dried secretions.*
- Suction the outer cannula. *This removes accumulated secretions.*

3. Change gloves, and clean the cannula.

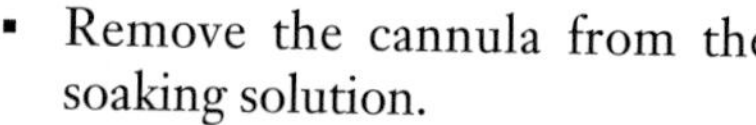

- Remove the gloves, and replace them with sterile gloves on both hands. Both hands are needed to clean the tube. *To maintain sterile technique, both hands must be gloved.*
- Remove the cannula from the soaking solution.
- Clean the lumen and entire inner cannula thoroughly, using the pipe cleaners or brush moistened with sterile saline (Figure 39–32).
- Agitate the cannula for several seconds in the sterile saline. *This thoroughly rinses the cannula and provides a thin film of moisture to lubricate for insertion.*
- Inspect the cannula for cleanliness by holding it at eye level and looking through it into the light. If encrustations are evident, repeat above steps.

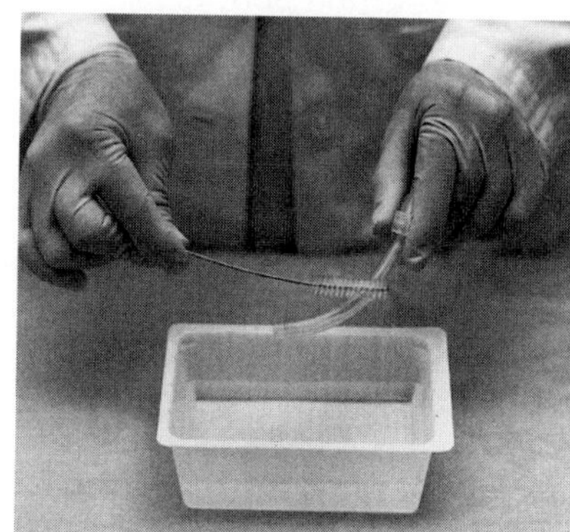

Figure 39–32 Cleaning the inner cannula with a brush.

- After rinsing the cannula, gently tap it against the inside edge of the sterile solution bowl. *This removes excess liquid from the cannula and prevents possible aspiration of it by the client.*

4. Dry the *inside* of the cannula.

- Use two or three pipe cleaners twisted together to dry the inside of the cannula. Do not dry the outer surface. *A thin film of moisture on the outer surface acts as a lubricant for insertion.*

PROCEDURE 39–5 *continued*

5. Suction the outer cannula if secretions are excessive. *Secretions must be removed to prevent adherence of the two tubes when the inner cannula is inserted.*

6. Insert the clean inner cannula, and secure it.

- Grasp the outer flange of the inner cannula, and insert the cannula in the direction of its curvature.
- Lock the inner cannula in place by turning the lock clockwise about 90° to an upright position.
- Gently pull on the inner cannula to ensure that the position is secure.

7. Clean the flange of the outer cannula if necessary.

- Use clean cotton-tipped applicators or gauze squares moistened with sterile saline to clean the flange.

8. Document relevant data.

- On the client's chart record the removal, cleaning, and reinsertion of the cannula and all assessments.

EVALUATION FOCUS
Character and amount of the secretions; client's respiration status compared to baseline data; tracheal breath sounds.

Changing a Tracheostomy Dressing and Tie Tapes

A tracheostomy dressing and the tie tapes need to be changed whenever they become soiled. Soiled dressings harbor microorganisms and can be a potential source of skin excoriation, breakdown, and infection. Usually, the dressing is changed after the cannula is cleaned, but a more frequent dressing change may be necessary. The dressing technique is described in Chapter 44.

Before applying a new dressing, the nurse needs to check any special orders or agency protocol (eg, the application of antibiotic ointment to the stoma after cleaning it). Noncotton-filled squares are used to clean the wound because cotton fibers can pull off and remain in the wound, where they encourage bacterial growth and contamination. Procedure 39–6 describes how to change a tracheostomy dressing and tie tapes.

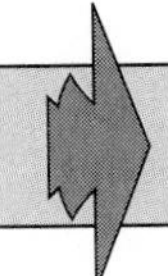

PROCEDURE 39–6 CHANGING A TRACHEOSTOMY DRESSING AND TIE TAPES

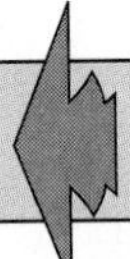

PURPOSES

- To prevent skin excoriation and infection of the tracheostomy site
- To provide comfort

ASSESSMENT FOCUS
Character of secretions from the tracheostomy site; clinical signs of infection at the tracheostomy site (eg, inflammation, purulent discharge, odor); pulse and respiratory rates.

EQUIPMENT

- ☐ Disposable gloves
- ☐ Moistureproof bag
- ☐ Sterile gloves
- ☐ Cleaning solutions (eg, sterile normal saline and hydrogen peroxide)
- ☐ Sterile containers
- ☐ Sterile noncotton-filled gauze squares and sterile cotton-tipped applicator sticks
- ☐ Antibiotic ointment if ordered or recommended by agency policy
- ☐ Commercially prepared dressing or sterile 4 × 4 gauze square
- ☐ Cotton twill tape
- ☐ Gauze square and tape

➤

PROCEDURE 39-6 CHANGING A TRACHEOSTOMY DRESSING AND TIE TAPES *continued*

INTERVENTION

1. Prepare the client and the equipment.

- Assist the client to a semi-Fowler's position to promote lung expansion.
- While wearing a disposable glove, remove the tracheostomy dressing. Discard the dressing and glove in the moistureproof bag.
- Inspect the tracheostomy wound and drainage.
- Open the sterile equipment, and put on the sterile gloves.

2. Clean the incision site and tube flange.

- Clean around the incision site with gauze squares or applicator sticks dampened with sterile normal saline (Figure 39–33). If encrustations are difficult to remove, use hydrogen peroxide at the ordered strength, for example, 50% hydrogen peroxide and 50% sterile saline.

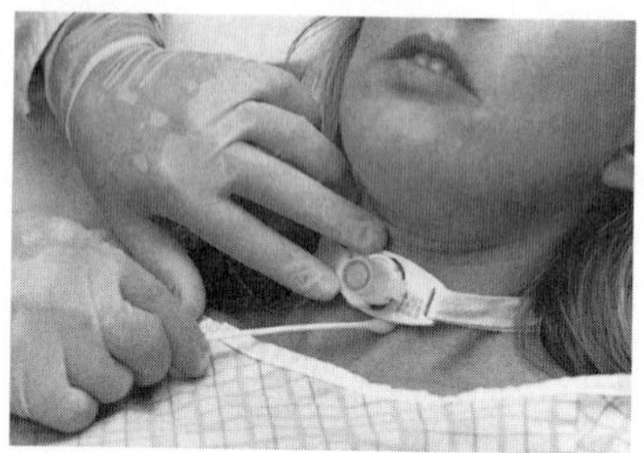

Figure 39–33 Using an applicator stick to clean the tracheostomy site.

- Wipe only once with each gauze square, and then discard it. *This avoids contaminating a clean area with a soiled gauze square.*
- Thoroughly rinse the cleaned area, using gauze squares moistened with sterile normal saline. *Hydrogen peroxide can be irritating to the skin.*
- Clean the flange of the tube in the same manner.
- Thoroughly dry the client's skin and tube flanges with dry gauze squares.

3. Apply a sterile dressing.

- Use an applicator stick to apply antibiotic ointment around the incision site if ordered or recommended by agency policy.
- For the insertion site, use a commercially prepared tracheostomy dressing of nonraveling material, if available.

  or

  Open and refold a 4 × 4 gauze as shown in Figure 39–34, *A* to *D*.
- Place the gauze as shown in Figure 39–34, *E*.
- Avoid using cotton-filled gauze squares, and avoid cutting the 4 × 4 gauze. *The client might aspirate cotton lint or frayed fibers, which could subsequently create a tracheal abscess.*
- While applying the dressing, ensure that the tracheostomy tube is securely supported. *Excessive movement of the tracheostomy tube irritates the trachea.*

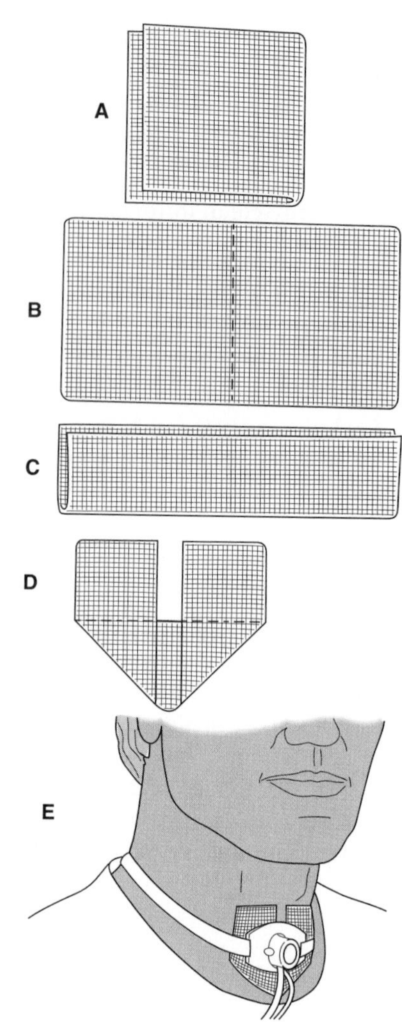

Figure 39–34 Folding a 4 × 4 gauze to make a tracheostomy dressing.

4. Change the tie tapes.

Two-Strip Method

- Cut two strips of cotton twill tape, one about 25 cm (10 in) long and the other 50 cm (20 in) long. *When one tape is longer than the other, they can be fastened at the side of the client's neck for easy access. A knot at the back of the neck could create pressure and irritate the skin.*
- Cut a 1-cm (0.5-in) slit approximately 2.5 cm (1 in) from one end of each strip. This is best achieved by folding the end of the tape back onto itself about 2.5 cm and then cutting a slit in the middle of the tape from its folded edge.
- Have an assistant put on a sterile glove and hold the tracheostomy tube in place while you change the ties. If an assistant is not available, fasten the clean ties before removing the soiled ties. *Holding the tube prevents accidental expulsion of it if the client coughs or moves.*

PROCEDURE 39–6 *continued*

- Detach and remove the soiled tapes from the client. The ties can be cut or untied.
- Thread the slit end of one clean tape through the eye of the tracheostomy faceplate from the bottom side; then thread the other end of the tie through the slit of the tape, pulling it taut until it is securely fastened to the faceplate. *This method avoids the use of knots, which produce pressure, discomfort, and skin irritation.*
- Repeat the above step for the second tie.
- Ask the client to flex the neck, and have the assistant place one or two fingers under the tapes while you tie the tapes together at the side of the client's neck (Figure 39–35). *Flexion of the neck increases neck circumference the way coughing does. The client's neck flexion and the assistant's finger placement prevent the nurse from making the ties too tight, which could cause choking or pressure on the jugular veins.*
- Tie the tapes using two square knots. Cut off any long ends. *Two square knots will prevent slippage and loosening, allowing the tube to dislodge.*

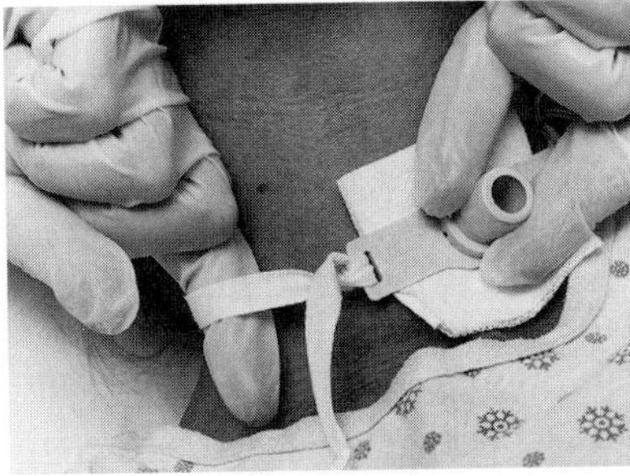

Figure 39–35 Placing a finger underneath the tie tape before tying it.

One-Strip Method

- Determine the length of twill tape required:
  a. Hold one end of the tape at the slot on one side of the tracheostomy faceplate.
  b. Pull the tape around the back of the client's neck to the slot on the other side.
  c. Multiply this length by 2.5.
- Apply the tie as follows:
  a. Thread one end of the tape into the upper half of the slot on one side.
  b. Bring both ends of the tape together, and take them around the client's neck, keeping them flat and untwisted.
  c. Thread the piece of tape closest to the client's neck from back to front through the other slot.
  d. Tie square knots with the loose tape ends as described above.

5. Pad the tie tape knot.

- Place a folded 4 × 4 gauze square under the tie where it is knotted, and apply tape over the knot. *Gauze under the knot prevents skin irritation. Taping over the knot prevents confusing the dressing ties with the client's gown ties.*

6. Check the tautness of the tracheostomy tie.

- Frequently check the tautness of the tracheostomy tie, particularly for clients whose neck diameter may increase from swelling (eg, those with radical neck surgery, neck trauma, or cardiac failure) or for clients who are restless and may loosen their ties.

7. Document all relevant information.

- Record the dressing change, the application of any ointments, and your assessments.

EVALUATION FOCUS
Character of secretions from tracheostomy site; appearance of tracheostomy wound; pulse and respiratory rates compared to baseline data; complaints of pain or discomfort at tracheostomy site.

Plugging a Tracheostomy Tube A tracheostomy plug is usually inserted into a tracheostomy tube for specified lengths of time before the tube is removed. While the tube is plugged, the client is carefully monitored for signs of respiratory distress. Often the length of time the tube is plugged is increased over a number of days if the person tolerates the procedure well. The nurse must check the physician's orders to determine the length of time the tracheostomy tube should remain plugged. To plug a tracheostomy tube, the nurse follows these steps:

- Assist the client to a semi-Fowler's position if not contraindicated. This position enhances lung expansion and may decrease fears about not being able to breathe.
- Suction the client's nasopharynx if there are any secretions present.

- Change suction catheters, and suction the tracheostomy. If there are excessive secretions, report this finding to the nurse in charge or physician to determine whether to proceed with the procedure.
- Using sterile gloves, fit the tracheostomy plug into either the inner or the outer cannula, depending on whether the tracheostomy tube has a double or single cannula.
- Monitor the client closely for 10 minutes for signs of respiratory distress, for example, noisy and/or rapid respirations and use of accessory muscles for breathing. At the first signs of distress, remove the tracheostomy plug, and suction the tracheostomy if necessary.
- Clean the inner cannula, if it was removed, so that it is ready to be reinserted.
- Remove the plug at the designated time.
- After removing the plug, suction the tracheostomy if indicated, and replace the inner cannula if removed.

CHEST TUBES AND DRAINAGE SYSTEMS

Chest tubes are usually inserted through an intercostal space into the pleural cavity. They are used following chest surgery or trauma and for pneumothorax and/or hemothorax. A **pneumothorax** is a collection of air or other gas in the pleural space that causes the lung to collapse (atalectasis). A **hemothorax** is the accumulation of blood and fluid in the pleural cavity usually as a result of trauma or surgery.

Chest tubes that are used to remove air are usually inserted superiorly (ie, through the second intercostal space) and anteriorly because air tends to rise in the pleural cavity. Tubes used to drain fluids are inserted more inferiorly, often in the eighth or ninth intercostal space, and more posteriorly. Sometimes a tube used to drain air is inserted inferiorly and threaded superiorly in the pleural space. When a client requires drainage of both fluid and air, two chest tubes may be inserted. These are sometimes joined externally by a Y-connector.

Because the pleural cavity normally has negative pressure, which allows lung expansion, any drainage system connected to it must be sealed so that air or liquid cannot enter. Such a drainage system is called a water-sealed (underwater) drainage or a disposable pleural drainage system. In water-sealed drainage, fluid in the bottom of the container prevents air from entering the chest tube and thus entering the pleural cavity. *The system must be kept below the level of the client's chest so that the fluid in the container is not drawn into the pleural cavity by gravity.* It is also very important to maintain the patency of the tubing.

Drainage systems use three mechanisms to drain fluid and air from the pleural cavity; positive expiratory pressure, gravity, and suction. When the pleural cavity contains some air or fluid, a positive pressure develops during expiration. This positive pressure is abnormal, but it does help expel the air and, to some extent, fluid from the space. Placing the tubing so that it descends from the insertion site to the drainage receptacle allows gravity to act as an evacuation force. Suction is used in conjunction with the other two forces in some drainage systems.

There are several kinds of water-sealed drainage systems: one- and two-bottle gravity systems; two- and three-bottle suction systems, and disposable unit systems.

In a *one-bottle (water-seal) system*, a single receptacle receives both the fluid and/or air from the client and seals the system (Figure 39–36, *A*). The air or fluid enters through the collection inlet, which terminates under sterile water. The air then exits through the water and through the air vent; the fluid remains in the bottle. The fluid in this bottle then is a combination of fluid from the client and sterile water—it forms the water seal. The one-bottle system depends on gravity and positive expiratory pressure for drainage.

A *two-bottle system* uses one bottle to receive the fluid or air from the client and the second bottle to create the water seal (Figure 39–36, *B*). The air or fluid from the pleural cavity is received into bottle 1. The air from bottle 1 is passed into bottle 2. The air then passes through the sterile water and exits from bottle 2 through the air vent. The fluid from the pleural cavity remains in bottle 1. This system uses gravity and positive expiratory pressure for drainage.

The *three-bottle system* has a collection bottle (1), a water-seal bottle (2), and a suction-control bottle (3) (Figure 39–36, *C*). Fluid from the pleural cavity collects in bottle 1, which is connected to a tube in bottle 2 that terminates below the fluid level. Bottle 2 is then connected to bottle 3 by a short tube. Bottle 3 also has a manometer tube submerged in sterile water. The depth to which this tube is submerged determines the amount of suction exerted in the pleural cavity. The suction-control bottle has another inlet, for suction. This system uses positive expiratory pressure, gravity, and suction for drainage. Several types of disposable unit systems are also available commercially. See Figure 39–37.

Nursing responsibilities regarding drainage systems include

- Assisting with the insertion and removal of the tube.
- Maintaining the water seal and patency of the drainage system.
- Assessing the client's vital signs, cardiovascular status, and respiratory status.
- Monitoring the patency and integrity of the drainage system.
- Keeping chest forceps and rubber-tipped clamps near the client. The chest tube will need to be clamped

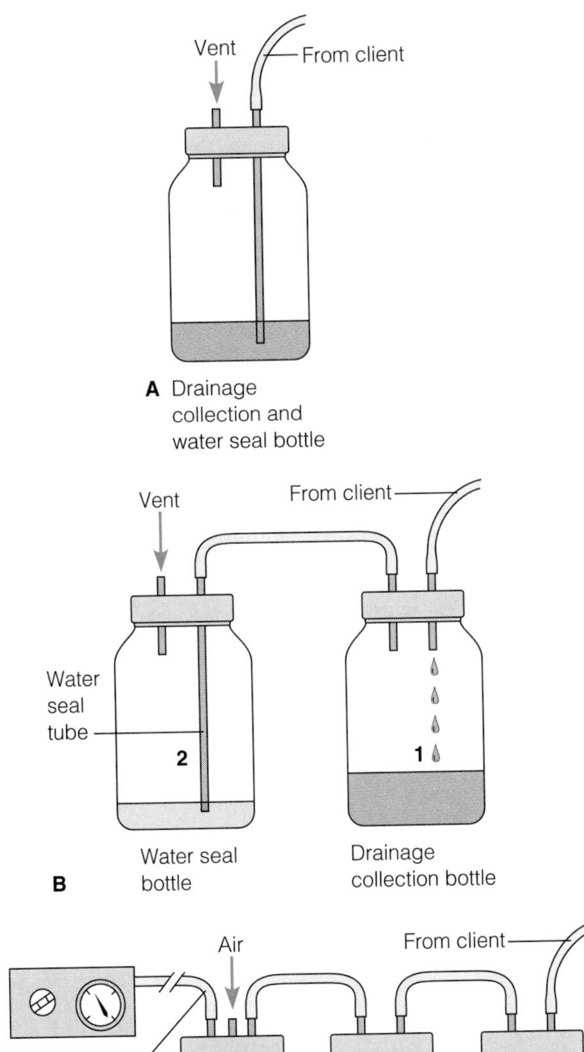

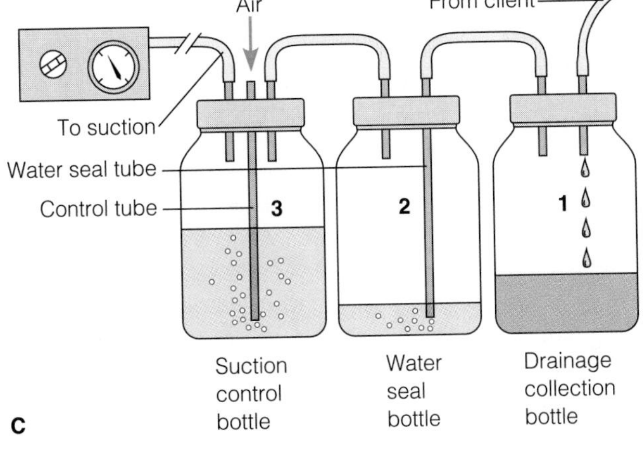

Figure 39–36 Drainage systems for chest tubes: *A,* one-bottle system; *B,* two-bottle system; *C,* three-bottle system.

quickly, close to the insertion site, if an air leak develops in the drainage system.

CARDIOPULMONARY RESUSCITATION

Cardiopulmonary resuscitation (CPR) is a combination of oral **resuscitation** (mouth-to-mouth breathing), which supplies oxygen to the lungs, and **external cardiac massage** (chest compression), which is intended to reestablish cardiac function and blood circulation. CPR is also referred to as **basic life support (BLS).**

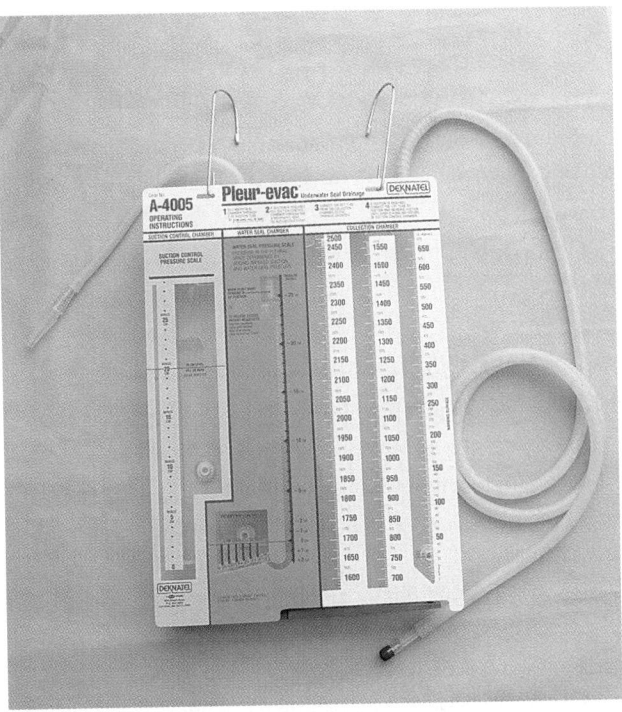

Figure 39–37 Disposable, commercial chest drainage system.

A **cardiac arrest** is the cessation of cardiac function; the heart stops beating. Often a cardiac arrest is unexpected and sudden. When it occurs, the heart no longer pumps blood to any of the organs of the body. Breathing then stops, and the person becomes unconscious and limp. Within 20 to 40 seconds of a cardiac arrest, the victim is clinically dead. After 4 to 6 minutes, the lack of oxygen supply to the brain causes permanent and extensive damage.

The three cardinal signs of a cardiac arrest are **apnea,** absence of a carotid or femoral pulse, and dilated pupils. The person's skin appears pale or grayish and feels cool. Cyanosis is evident when respiratory function fails prior to heart failure.

A **respiratory arrest** (pulmonary arrest) is the cessation of breathing. It often occurs as a result of a blocked airway, but it can occur following a cardiac arrest and for other reasons. A respiratory arrest is preceded by short, shallow breathing. The breathing becomes increasingly labored. Then the person becomes flushed and disoriented and experiences feelings of suffocation.

Most health care agencies have established practices and policies governing CPR. For instructions in how to perform CPR, see the *Procedures Supplement.*

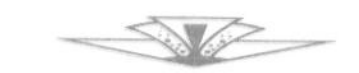

EVALUATING

To evaluate whether client goals have been achieved, the nurse collects data pertaining to the established outcome criteria. Evaluation activities may include the following:

- Observing rate, depth, and character of respirations
- Observing chest movements and symmetry of expansion
- Observing ability to expectorate secretions
- Auscultating breath sounds
- Assessing pulse rate, volume, and rhythm
- Assessing peripheral pulse volume
- Inspecting color of skin, mucous membranes, lips, and earlobes
- Observing the client demonstrating deep-breathing exercises as taught
- Reviewing recent laboratory data, eg, blood gas results
- Asking the client about ability to perform activities of daily living without shortness of breath
- Asking the client to describe purposes and side-effects of medications or to explain home care treatments

If client outcomes are not achieved, the nurse should ask questions such as the following to determine why:

- Were contributing or risk factors identified correctly?
- Has the client's mental or physical condition changed?
- Were adequate fluids ingested to hydrate the pulmonary mucous membranes?
- Was the client encouraged to be as physically active as possible to promote movement of respiratory secretions?
- Did the client fail to perform deep breathing exercises as instructed?
- Were adequate rest periods scheduled to conserve the client's energy?
- Was the client's pain controlled adequately to allow maximum participation in activities?
- Was the client's position appropriate to encourage maximal chest expansion?
- Did anxiety or fear interfere with the client's breathing pattern?
- Were the needs for home care assistance and available community resources correctly identified or selected?

CRITICAL PATHWAY FOR ANGELA MARTINELLI

ASSESSMENT DATA

Nursing Assessment

Ms Angela Martinelli is a 59-year-old secretary who was admitted to the hospital yesterday with an elevated temperature, a productive cough, and rapid, labored respirations. In taking a nursing history, Nurse Hayes finds that Ms Martinelli had a "bad cold" for several weeks that just wouldn't go away. She has been dieting for several months and skipping meals in order to decrease her caloric intake. Ms Martinelli mentions that in addition to her full-time job as a secretary, she is attending college classes 2 evenings a week. Ms Martinelli, who is a smoker, states she has been unable to smoke for several days because of her cough and cold.

Physical Examination

Height: 167.6 cm (5′6″)
Weight: 54.4 kg (120 lb)
Temperature: 39.4 C (103 F)
Pulse rate: 28 bpm
Blood pressure: 118/70 mm Hg
Skin pale, cheeks flushed, chills
Nasal flaring
Use of accessory muscles
Inspiratory rales with diminished breath sounds right base

Diagnostic Data

Chest X-ray film: R lobar infiltration
WBC: 14,000/μL

CRITICAL PATHWAY FOR CLIENT WITH PNEUMONIA

Expected length of stay 5 days

	Date ________ Day 1	**Date ________ Day 2**	**Date ________ Day 3**
Daily outcomes	Client will ▪ have stable vital signs and unlabored respirations at rest. ▪ verbalize understanding and demonstrate cooperation with turning and splinting. ▪ cough and deep breathe purposefully q1–2h during day. ▪ have a productive cough. ▪ have an intake of 3000 mL/ day (IV/PO). ▪ verbalize ability to cope.	Client will ▪ have stable vital signs and unlabored respirations at rest. ▪ verbalize understanding and demonstrate cooperation with turning and splinting. ▪ cough and deep breathe purposefully q1–2h during day. ▪ have a productive cough. ▪ have an intake of 3000 mL/ day (IV/PO). ▪ verbalize ability to cope.	Client will ▪ be afebrile, have stable vital signs and unlabored respirations with activity. ▪ verbalize understanding and demonstrate cooperation with turning and splinting. ▪ cough and deep breathe purposefully q1–2h during day. ▪ have a productive cough. ▪ have an intake of 3000 mL/ day (PO). ▪ verbalize ability to cope. ▪ verbalize beginning understanding of home care instructions.
Tests and treatments	CBC with differential PA and lateral chest X-ray ABGs Blood culture × 2, if temp over 38.3 C (101 F) Sputum for Gram stain and C & S Vital signs and O_2 saturation q4h if stable Assess respiratory status q4h and prn Incentive spirometer q2h Intake and output q shift	Vital signs and O_2 saturation q4h if stable Assess respiratory status q4h and prn Incentive spirometer q2h Intake and output q shift	Vital signs and O_2 saturation q4h if stable Assess respiratory status q4h and prn Incentive spirometer q2h Intake and output q shift
Knowledge deficit	Orient to room and hospital routine. Review plan of care and importance of increased fluids, activity, turning, coughing, deep breathing, and incentive spirometer.	Review plan of care and continued importance of increased fluids, activity, turning, coughing, deep breathing, and incentive spirometer.	Reinforce earlier teaching regarding ongoing care. Begin discharge teaching regarding rest, activity, and diet.

➤

	Day 1 *continued*	**Day 2** *continued*	**Day 3** *continued*
Psycho-social	Assess level of anxiety. Encourage verbalization of concerns. Provide information. Provide ongoing support and encouragement.	Assess level of anxiety. Encourage verbalization of concerns. Provide information. Provide ongoing support and encouragement.	Encourage verbalization of concerns. Provide ongoing support and encouragement.
Diet	Diet as tolerated, providing small, frequent, nutritious feedings. Encourage fluid intake of 2000 mL/day.	Diet as tolerated, providing small, frequent, nutritious feedings. Encourage fluid intake of 2000 mL/day.	Diet as tolerated, providing small, frequent, nutritious feedings. Encourage fluid intake of 2000 mL/day.
Activity	Provide safety precautions. Bathroom privileges with assistance. Provide rest periods.	Provide safety precautions. Bathroom privileges with assistance. Provide rest periods.	Provide safety precautions. Ambulate 4–6 times with assistance. Provide rest periods.
Medications	IV fluids IV antibiotics Bronchodilators Tylenol 650 mg q4h PO for temp over 38.3 C (101 F)	IV fluids/intermittent IV device IV antibiotics Bronchodilators Tylenol 650 mg q4h PO for temp over 38.3 C (101 F)	Intermittent IV device; D/C if IV antibiotics D/C IV/PO antibiotics Bronchodilators Tylenol 650 mg q4h PO for temp over 38.3 C (101 F)
Airway and respiratory manage-ment	Assess respirations and respiratory movements q4h and prn. Encourage coughing and deep breathing q1–2h. Demonstrate effective coughing while splinting client's chest. Position client in semi-Fowler's or high-Fowler's position. Assist with postural drainage 3 times daily. Assist with IPPB and/or nebulizer treatments. Maintain oxygen per nasal cannula at 5L. Assist with ADLs. Monitor ABGs/pulse oximeter.	Assess respirations and respiratory movements q4h and prn. Encourage coughing and deep breathing q1–2h. Demonstrate effective coughing while splinting client's chest. Position client in semi-Fowler's or high-Fowler's position. Assist with postural drainage 3 times daily. Assist with IPPB and/or nebulizer treatments. Maintain oxygen per nasal cannula at 5L. Assist with ADLs. Monitor pulse oximeter.	Assess respirations and respiratory movements q4h and prn. Encourage coughing and deep breathing q1–2h. Position client in semi-Fowler's or high-Fowler's position. Assist with postural drainage 3 times daily. Assist with IPPB and/or nebulizer treatments. Maintain oxygen per nasal cannula at 2 to 5L to maintain pulse oximeter at 98%. Assist with ADLs.
Transfer/ discharge plans	Review discharge goals with client and significant other. Consult with social services re: projected needs for home health care (if any).	Review progress towards discharge goals with client and significant other.	Review progress toward discharge goals with client and significant other.

	Date ______ Day 4	Date ______ Day 5	
Daily outcomes	Client will ▪ be afebrile and have stable vital signs and unlabored respirations with activity. ▪ verbalize understanding and demonstrate cooperation with turning and splinting. ▪ cough and deep breathe purposefully q1–2h during day. ▪ have an intake of 3000 mL/day (PO). ▪ verbalize ability to cope. ▪ verbalize understanding of home care instructions.	Client ▪ is afebrile and has stable vital signs. ▪ has unlabored respirations, and lungs are clear to auscultation. ▪ is independent in self-care. ▪ is fully ambulatory. ▪ has resumed preadmission urine and bowel elimination pattern. ▪ verbalizes home care instructions. ▪ tolerates usual diet and has a fluid intake of 3000 mL/day. ▪ verbalizes ability to cope with ongoing stressors.	
Test and treatments	Vital signs and O_2 saturation q4h if stable Assess respiratory status q4h and prn Incentive spirometer q2h Intake and output q shift	Vital signs and O_2 saturation q4h if stable Assess respiratory status q4h and prn Incentive spirometer q2h Intake and output q shift	
Knowledge deficit	Reinforce earlier teaching regarding ongoing care. Review written discharge instructions with client and significant other.	Reinforce earlier teaching regarding ongoing care. Complete discharge teaching to include diet, follow-up care, signs and symptoms to report, activity, and medications: dose, frequency, route, and side effects. Provide client with written discharge instructions.	
Psycho-social	Encourage verbalization of concerns. Provide ongoing support and encouragement.	Encourage verbalization of concerns. Provide ongoing support and encouragement.	
Diet	Diet as tolerated, providing small, frequent, nutritious feedings. Encourage fluid intake of 3000 mL/day.	Diet as tolerated, providing small, frequent, nutritious feedings. Encourage fluid intake of 3000 mL/day.	

	Day 4 *continued*	**Day 5** *continued*	
Medications	PO antibiotics Bronchodilators Tylenol 650 mg q4h PO for temp over 38.3 C (101 F)	PO antibiotics Bronchodilators Tylenol 650 mg q4h PO for temp over 38.3 C (101 F)	
Airway and respiratory management	Assess respirations and respiratory movements q4h and prn. Encourage coughing and deep breathing q1–2h. Position client in semi-Fowler's or high-Fowler's position. Assist with postural drainage 3 times daily. Assist with IPPB and/or nebulizer treatments. D/C oxygen if pulse oximeter 98% on room air.	Assess respirations and respiratory movements q4h and prn. Encourage coughing and deep breathing q1–2h. Position client in semi-Fowler's or high-Fowler's position.	
Transfer/ discharge plans	Continue to review progress toward discharge goals. Finalize discharge plans.	Finalize plans for home care if needed. Complete discharge teaching.	

CHAPTER HIGHLIGHTS

- Respiration, the process of gaseous exchange between the individual and the atmosphere, involves pulmonary ventilation, diffusion of gases, and transport of oxygen and carbon dioxide to and from the body's cells.
- Pulmonary ventilation, the inflow and outflow of air between the atmosphere and the alveoli of the lungs, is accomplished through the mechanical act of breathing (inspiration and expiration).
- The volume to which the lungs expand during ventilation depends on the pattern of breathing, the size and position of the individual, medical or surgical conditions affecting the thorax, and developmental variations in the shape of the chest.
- Ventilation depends upon adequate atmospheric oxygen, clear air passages, adequate pulmonary compliance and recoil, and neurochemical regulation of respiration.
- Diffusion of oxygen and carbon dioxide is the movement of the gases from areas of greater pressure or concentration to areas of lower pressure or concentration.
- Factors affecting the rate of oxygen transport include cardiac output, the number of erythrocytes present in the blood, exercise, and blood hematocrit.
- In healthy individuals, increased concentration of carbon dioxide in the blood stimulates respiration. Clients with respiratory disorders such as COPD have what is called a *hypoxic drive;* that is, decreased levels of blood oxygen stimulate respiration.
- Factors that influence oxygenation of the body's tissues include development, environment (eg, altitude, air pollution), life-style, health status, and narcotics (opioids).

- Respiratory function may be altered by any condition that affects the movement of air into or out of the lungs, changes in the diffusion rate of oxygen and carbon dioxide between the alveoli and the pulmonary capillaries, or alterations in the transport of oxygen and carbon dioxide via the blood to and from the tissue cells.
- Hypoxia is insufficient oxygenation of body tissues.
- Clinical signs of hypoxia may be early (increased heart and respiratory rates and slight rise in systolic blood pressure) or late (decreased pulse and systolic blood pressure, dyspnea, cough, and hemoptysis). Cyanosis is not a reliable sign.
- Normal respiration (eupnea) is quiet, rhythmic, and effortless. Common altered breathing patterns include tachypnea, bradypnea, dyspnea, orthopnea, hyperventilation, and hypoventilation.
- The signs of airway obstruction include: labored noisy respirations, extreme inspiratory effort without chest movement, sternal or intercostal retractions, altered arterial blood gas values, restlessness, dyspnea, and abnormal or absent breath sounds.
- To assess respiratory function, the nurse conducts a nursing history, performs a complete physical assessment of the client, and reviews relevant diagnostic data.
- The nursing history should be structured to obtain data about the client's present respiratory problem, history, current or past cardiovascular problems, life-style, presence of cough, smoking and other risk factors, and medications.
- Pulse oximetry is a noninvasive measure of arterial blood oxygen saturation.
- Physical assessment should include general assessment and specific attention to cardiopulmonary status.
- The nurse is responsible for obtaining specimens for diagnostic tests, preparing the client and support persons for diagnostic procedures, monitoring the client after selected procedures, and reviewing records and reports of diagnostic tests.
- Nursing diagnoses for clients with respiratory problems include categories specific to respiration: **Impaired gas exchange, Ineffective airway clearance,** and **Ineffective breathing patterns.** The latter two can also be the etiology of several other nursing diagnoses, including **Anxiety, Activity intolerance, Fatigue, Fear, Powerlessness, Sleep pattern disturbance,** and **Social isolation.**
- Planning care for clients with respiratory problems includes identifying strategies to facilitate pulmonary ventilation and diffusion and the transport of oxygen and carbon dioxide.
- Interventions for clients with respiratory problems include promoting healthy breathing, deep breathing and coughing, hydration, implementing measures to clear secretions (eg, percussion, vibration, postural drainage, and suctioning), administering medications, using lung inflation devices, managing artificial airways, monitoring oxygen therapy and chest drainage systems, and tracheostomy care.

READINGS AND REFERENCES

SUGGESTED READINGS

Spyr, J and Preach, MA. May 1990. Pulse oximetry: Understanding the concept, knowing the limits. *RN* 53:38–45.

Pulse oximetry permits continuous, noninvasive monitoring of arterial oxygen saturation (SaO_2) in contrast to arterial blood gas analysis, which reflects the client's oxygenation status at only one moment in time. This article includes basic principles of oxygen transport, evaluation of pulse oximetry readings, technical limitations of pulse oximetry, and information to help the nurse choose the right oximeter.

Yeaw, EMJ. March 1992. How position affects oxygenation: Good lung down? *American Journal of Nursing* 92:27–32.

This article helps the nurse (a) distinguish between clients with unilateral lung disease who should be positioned on the affected side versus those who should not; (b) assess the impact of position on cardiopulmonary status of a client with lung disease; (c) describe how the ventilatory/perfusion ratio changes within the normal lung; and (d) explain the rationale for positioning a client with bilateral lung disease on the right side.

RELATED RESEARCH

Cahill, CK and Heath, J. February 1990. Sterile water used for humidification in low-flow oxygen therapy: Is it necessary? *American Journal of Infection Control* 18:13–17.

Stone, KS, Bell, SD, and Preusser, BA. November 1991. The effect of repeated endotracheal suctioning on arterial blood pressure. *Applied Nursing Research* 4:152–58.

SELECTED REFERENCES

Bodai, BI, Walton, CB, Briggs, S, and Goldstein, M. January 1987. A clinical evaluation of an oxygen insufflation/suction catheter. *Heart and Lung* 16:39–46.

Bolgiano, C. June 1990. Administering oxygen therapy: What you need to know. *Nursing90* 20:47–51.

Cahill, K and Heath, J. February 1990. Sterile water used for humidification in low-flow oxygen therapy: Is it necessary? *American Journal of Infection Control,* 18:13–17.

Carpenito, LJ. 1992. *Nursing Diagnosis: Application to Clinical Practice.* 4th ed. Philadelphia: Lippincott.

Caruana, S. June 1990. Myths and facts about tracheal tubes. *Nursing90* 20:30.

Carroll, PF. May 1988. Lowering the risks of endotracheal suctioning. *Nursing88* 18:46–50.

———. September 1989. Safe suctioning. *Nursing89* 18:48–51.

———. May 1991. What's new in chest tube management? *RN* 54:34–40.

Ellstrom, K. November 1990. What's causing your patient's respiratory distress? *Nursing90* 20:57–61.

Erickson, R. May 1989a. Mastering the ins and outs of chest drainage. Part I. *Nursing89* 18:36–43.

———. June 1989b. Mastering the ins and outs of chest drainage. Part II. *Nursing89* 18:46–49.

Finesilver, C. February 1992. Perfecting the art: Respiratory assessment. *RN* 55:22–29.

Gift, A. December 1990. Dyspnea. *Nursing Clinics of North America* 25:955–63.

Gordon, M. 1993. *Manual of Nursing Diagnosis 1993–1994.* 6th ed. St Louis: Mosby-Year Book.

Guyton, AC. 1991. *Textbook of Medical Physiology.* 8th ed. Philadelphia: WB Saunders.

Hayden, RA. December 1992. What keeps oxygenation on track? *American Journal of Nursing* 92:32–42.

Kim, MJ, McFarland, GK, and McLane, AM. 1993. *Pocket Guide to Nursing Diagnoses.* 5th ed. St Louis: Mosby-Year Book.

Lederer, JR, Marculescu, GL, Mocnik, B, and Seaby, N. 1993. *Care Planning Pocket Guide—A Nursing Diagnosis Approach.* 5th ed. Redwood City, CA: Addison-Wesley Nursing.

Mapp, C. July 1988. Trach care: Are you aware of all the dangers? *Nursing88* 17:34–42.

Mathews, PJ. January 1992a. Artificial airways: Resuscitation guidelines you can follow. *Nursing92* 22:53–59.

———. February 1992b. Airway monitoring and ventilation: What the future holds. *Nursing92* 22:48–51.

McConnell, E. November 1991. Minimizing respiratory problems. *Nursing91* 21:34–39.

McFarland, GK and McFarlane, EA. 1993. *Nursing Diagnosis and Intervention: Planning for Patient Care.* 2d ed. St Louis: Mosby.

Miller, KS. February 1987. Chest tubes: Indications, techniques, management and complications. *Chest* 91:258–64.

Miracle, V and Allnutt, D. April 1990. How to perform basic airway management. *Nursing90* 20:55–60.

North American Nursing Diagnosis Association. 1992. *NANDA Nursing Diagnoses: Definitions and Classification 1992–1993.* Philadelphia: NANDA.

Noll, ML, Hix, CD, and Scott, G. August 1990. Closed tracheal suction system: Effectiveness and nursing implications. *AACN Clinical Issues in Critical Care Nursing* 1:318–28.

Palau, D and Jones, S. October 1986. Test your skill at trouble shooting chest tubes. *RN* 49:43–45.

Quinn, A. September 1986. Thora-Drain III: Closed chest drainage made simpler and safer. *Nursing86* 16:46–51.

Schnapp, LM and Cohen, NH. November 1990. Pulse oximetry: Uses and abuses. *Chest* 98:1244–50.

Somerson, SW, Kozole, A, Andrea, J, and Sheehy, SB. November/December 1990. Suctioning a neonate: Nose or mouth first? *Journal of Emergency Nursing* 16:378.

Sonnesso, G. August 1991. Are you ready for pulse oximetry? *Nursing91* 21:60–64.

Spearing, C and Cornell, D. September 1987. Inspiring your patient to breathe deeply. *Nursing87* 17:50–51.

Spyr, J and Preach, M. May 1990. Pulse oximetry. *RN* 53:38–45.

Stevens, S and Becker, K. January 1988. How to perform picture-perfect respiratory assessment. *Nursing88* 18:57–63.

Transtracheal oxygen: The nose knows the difference. April 1987. *American Journal of Nursing* 87:421–22.

Wesmiller, S, Hoffman, L, and Wiseman, M. December 1989. Understanding transtracheal oxygen delivery. *Nursing89* 18:43–47.

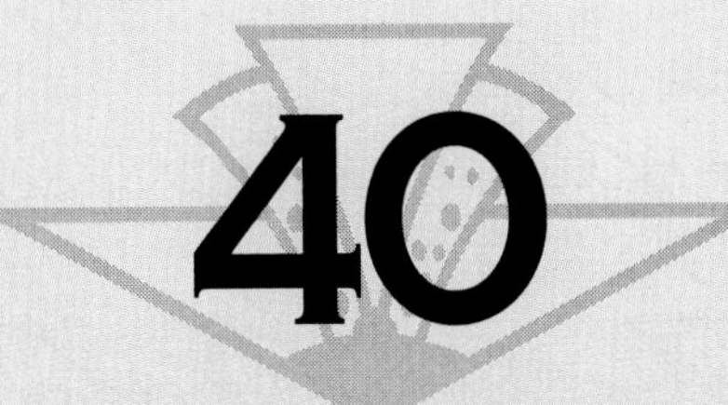

40 Fecal Elimination

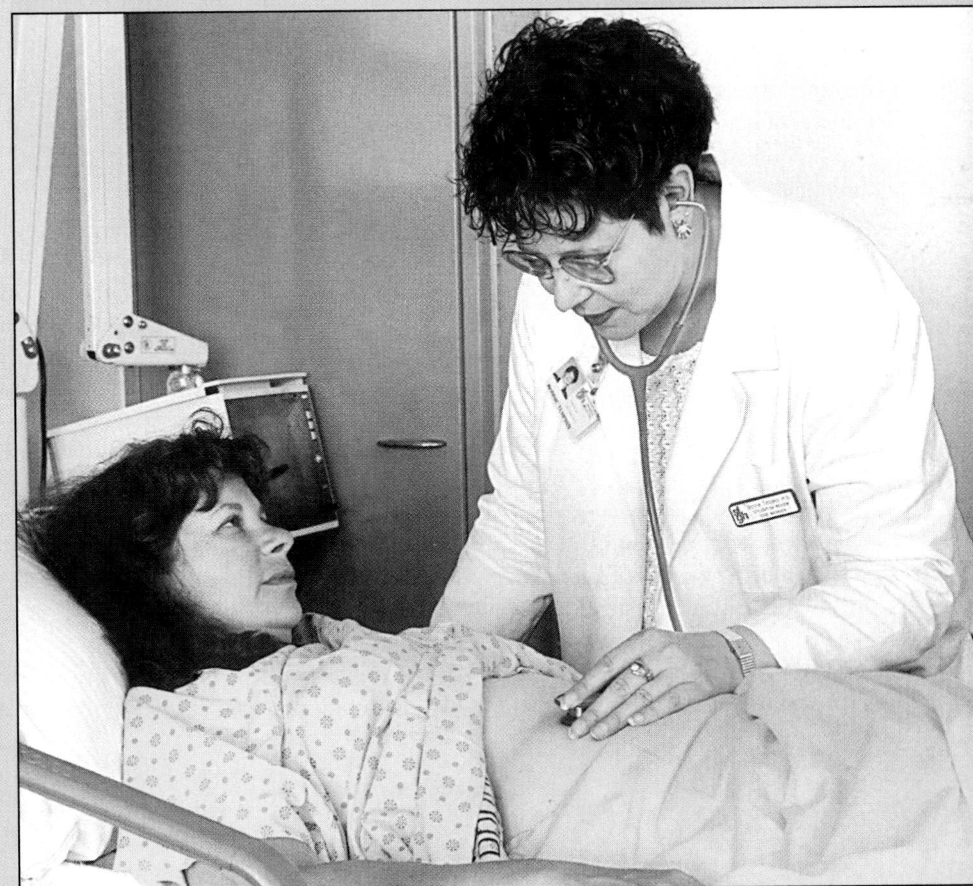

Objectives

Describe the functions of the lower intestinal tract.

Identify factors that influence fecal elimination and patterns of defecation.

Distinguish normal from abnormal characteristics and constituents of feces.

Describe methods used to assess the intestinal tract.

Differentiate among specific common fecal elimination problems.

Identify common causes and effects of selected fecal elimination problems.

Identify measures that maintain normal fecal elimination patterns.

Relate common interventions to specific fecal elimination problems.

Give reasons for selected nursing interventions.

Describe modifications for clients with ostomies.

State outcome criteria essential for evaluating the client's progress.

The elimination of feces is a prominent public topic in North America. Laxative advertisements, describing such feelings as tiredness due to irregularity, keep the subject in the public consciousness. Some elderly people are preoccupied with their bowels. Often elimination is a matter of great concern to them when they are hospitalized. People who have had a bowel movement once a day for 75 years can view missing 1 day as a serious problem, even though they may not have eaten anything for 2 days and thus have little fecal matter to eliminate.

Nurses frequently are consulted or involved in assisting clients with elimination problems. These problems are often embarrassing and can cause considerable discomfort. An understanding, competent nurse can provide information and assistance, thereby relieving discomfort.

Physiology of Defecation

Elimination of the waste products of digestion from the body is essential to health. The excreted waste products are referred to as **feces** or **stool.**

Large Intestine

The large intestine extends from the ileocecal (ileocolic) valve, which lies between the small and large intestines, to the anus. The colon (large intestine) in the adult is generally about 125 to 150 cm (50 to 60 in) long. It has seven parts: the cecum; ascending, transverse, and descending colons; sigmoid colon; rectum; and anus or external orifice (Figure 40–1).

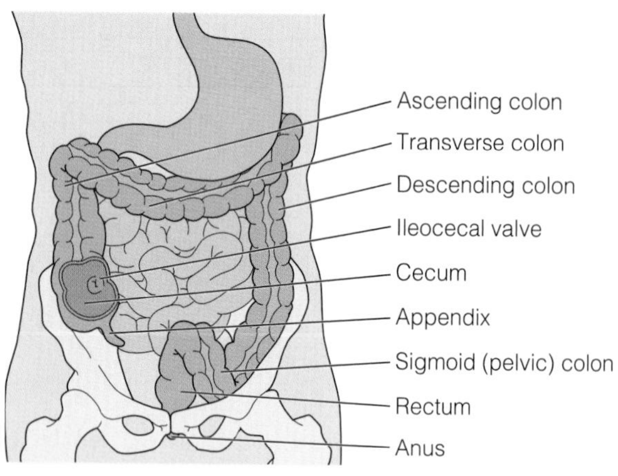

Figure 40–1 The large intestine and rectum.

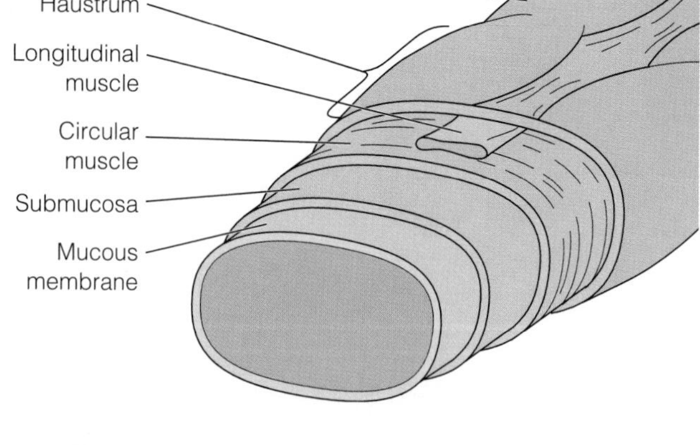

Figure 40–2 The layers of the wall of the large intestine.

The large intestine is a muscular tube lined with mucous membrane (Figure 40–2). The muscle fibers are both circular and longitudinal, thus permitting the intestine to enlarge and contract in both width and length. The longitudinal muscles are shorter than the colon and therefore cause the large intestine to form pouches, or **haustra.**

The colon's main functions are the absorption of water and nutrients, the mucal protection of the intestinal wall, and fecal elimination. The contents of the colon normally represent foods ingested over the previous 4 days, although most of the waste products are excreted within 48 hours of **ingestion** (the act of taking food). The waste products leaving the stomach through the small intestine and then passing through the ileocecal valve are called **chyme.** The colon absorbs water and significant amounts of sodium and chloride as food passes along it. As much as 1500 mL of chyme passes into the large intestine daily, and all but about 100 mL is absorbed in the proximal half of the colon. The 100 mL of fluid is excreted in the feces (Guyton 1991, p. 734).

The colon also serves a protective function in that it secretes mucus. This mucus contains large amounts of bicarbonate ions. The mucus secretion is stimulated by excitation of parasympathetic nerves. Therefore, during extreme stimulation—for example, as a result of emotions—large amounts of mucus are secreted, resulting in the passage of stringy mucus as often as every 30 minutes with little or no feces (Guyton 1991, p. 740). Mucus serves to protect the wall of the large intestine from trauma by the acids formed in the feces, and it serves as an adherent for holding the fecal material together. Mucus also protects the intestinal wall from bacterial activity.

The colon acts to transport along its lumen the products of digestion, which are eventually eliminated through

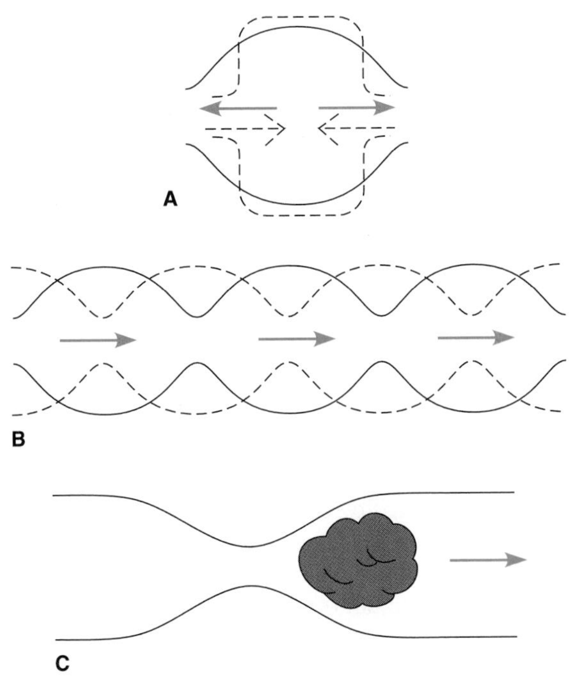

Figure 40–3 Three types of intestinal movements: *A,* haustral churning; *B,* peristalsis; *C,* mass peristalsis.

the anal canal. These products are flatus and feces. Flatus is largely air and the by-products of the digestion of carbohydrates. Three types of movements occur in the large intestine: haustral churning, colon peristalsis, and mass peristalsis (Figure 40–3). **Haustral churning** or **shuffling** involves movement of the chyme back and forth within the haustra. In addition to mixing the contents, this action aids in the absorption of water and moves the contents forward to the next haustra. **Peristalsis** is wavelike movement produced by the circular and longitudinal muscle fibers of the intestinal walls; it propels the intestinal contents forward. Colon peristalsis is very sluggish and is thought to move the chyme very little along the large intestine. **Mass peristalsis,** the third type of colonic movement, involves a wave of powerful muscular contraction that moves over large areas of the colon. Usually mass peristalsis occurs after eating, stimulated by the presence of food in the stomach and small intestine. In adults, mass peristaltic waves occur only a few times a day.

RECTUM AND ANAL CANAL

The rectum in the adult is usually 10 to 15 cm (4 to 6 in) long; the most distal portion, 2.5 to 5 cm (1 to 2 in) long, is the anal canal. In the rectum are three folds of tissue that extend across the rectum and several folds that extend vertically. Each of the vertical folds contains a vein and an artery. It is believed that these folds help retain feces within the rectum. When the veins become distended, as

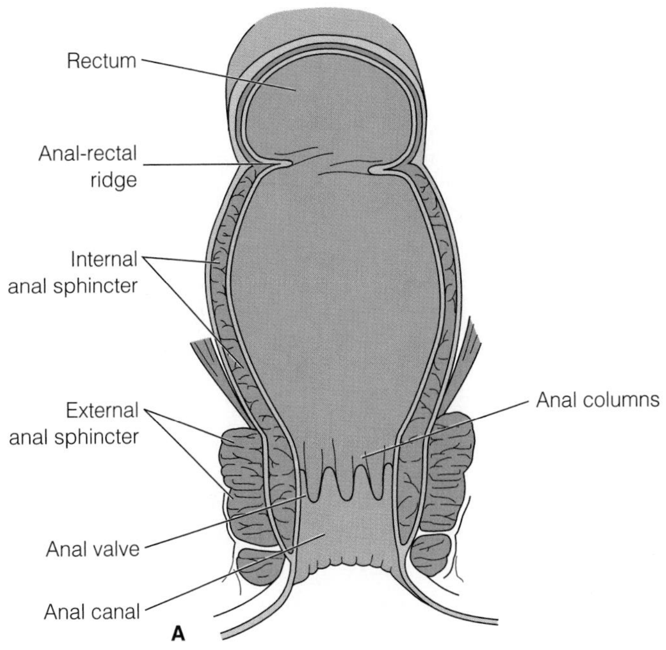

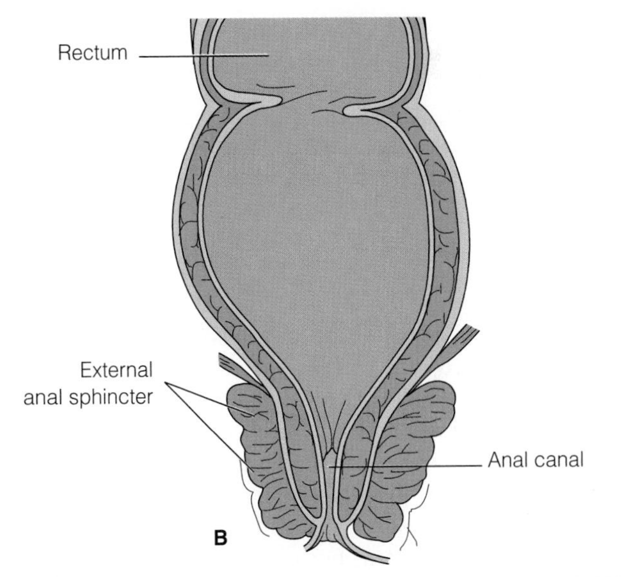

Figure 40–4 The rectum, anal canal, and anal sphincters: *A,* open; *B,* closed.

can occur with repeated pressure, a condition known as **hemorrhoids** occurs.

The anal canal is bounded by an internal and an external sphincter muscle (Figure 40–4). The *internal sphincter* is under involuntary control, and the *external sphincter* normally is voluntarily controlled. The external sphincter's action is augmented by the levator ani muscles of the pelvic floor. The internal sphincter muscle is innervated by the autonomic nervous system; the external sphincter is innervated by the somatic nervous system.

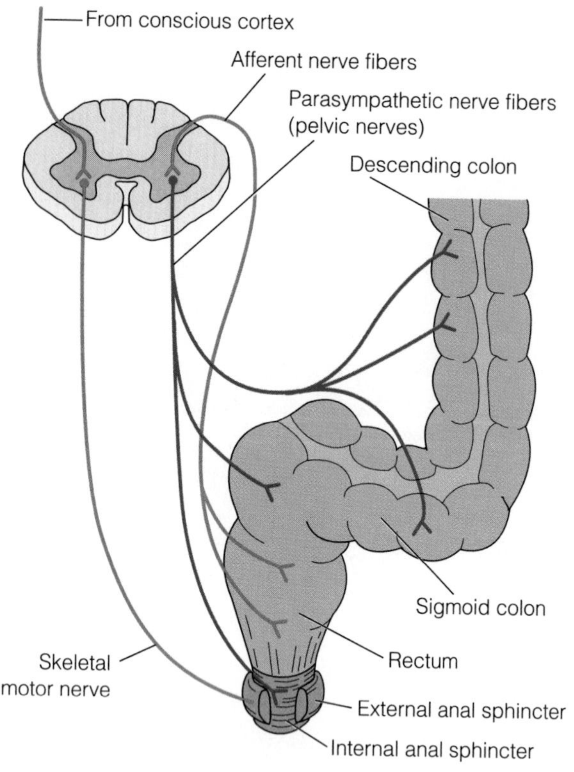

Figure 40–5 The afferent and efferent pathways of the parasympathetic nervous system for stimulating defecation.

DEFECATION

Defecation is the expulsion of feces from the anus and rectum. It is also called a *bowel movement.* The frequency of defecation is highly individual, varying from several times per day to two or three times per week. The amount defecated also varies from person to person. When peristaltic waves move the feces into the sigmoid colon and the rectum, the sensory nerves in the rectum are stimulated and the individual becomes aware of the need to defecate.

Defecation is normally initiated by two defecation reflexes (Figure 40–5). When feces enter the rectum, distention of the rectal walls intiates a signal that spreads through the mesenteric plexus to initiate peristaltic waves in the descending and sigmoid colons and in the rectum. These waves force the feces toward the anus. As the peristaltic waves approach the anus, the internal anal sphincter becomes inhibited from closing and, if the external sphincter is relaxed, defecation occurs. This is called the *intrinsic defecation reflex.*

The second reflex, called the *parasympathetic defecation reflex,* is also actively involved in defecation. When nerve fibers in the rectum are stimulated, signals are transmitted to the spinal cord and then back to the descending and sigmoid colons and the rectum. These parasympathetic signals intensify the peristaltic waves, relax the internal anal sphincter, and intensify the intrinsic defecation reflex.

The *internal* anal sphincter relaxes, and feces move into the anal canal. After the individual is seated on a toilet or bedpan, the *external* anal sphincter is relaxed voluntarily. Expulsion of the feces is assisted by contraction of the abdominal muscles and the diaphragm, which increases abdominal pressure, and by contraction of the levator ani muscles of the pelvic floor, which moves the feces through the anal canal. Normal defecation is facilitated by (a) thigh flexion, which increases the pressure within the abdomen, and (b) a sitting position, which increases the downward pressure on the rectum.

If the defecation reflex is ignored, or if defecation is consciously inhibited by contracting the external sphincter muscle, the urge to defecate normally disappears for a few hours before occurring again. Repeated inhibition of the urge to defecate can result in expansion of the rectum to accommodate accumulated feces and eventual loss of sensitivity to the need to defecate. Constipation can be the ultimate result.

Normal feces are made of about 75% water and 25% solid materials. They are soft but formed. If the feces are propelled very quickly along the large intestine, so that there is not time for most of the water in the chyme to be reabsorbed, the feces will be more fluid, perhaps containing 95% water. Normal feces require a normal fluid intake; feces that contain less water may be hard and difficult to expel.

Feces are normally brown, chiefly due to the presence of stercobilin and urobilin, which are derived from **bilirubin** (a red pigment in bile). Another factor that affects fecal color is the action of bacteria such as *Escherichia coli* or staphylococci, which are normally present in the large intestine. The action of microorganisms on the chyme is also responsible for the odor of feces. See Table 40–1 for characteristics of normal and abnormal feces.

An adult usually forms 7 to 10 liters of flatus (gas) in the large intestine every 24 hours. The gases include carbon dioxide, methane, hydrogen, oxygen, and nitrogen. Some are swallowed with food and fluids taken by mouth; others are formed through the action of bacteria on the chyme in the large intestine, and other gas diffuses from the blood into the gastrointestinal tract (Guyton 1991, p. 742).

FACTORS THAT AFFECT DEFECATION

Age and Development Some control of defecation starts at 1½ to 2 years of age. By this time, children have learned to walk, and the nervous and muscular systems are

Table 40–1 Characteristics of Normal and Abnormal Feces

Characteristic	Normal	Abnormal	Possible Cause
Color	Adult: brown Infant: yellow	Clay or white	Absence of bile pigment (bile obstruction): diagnostic study using barium
		Black or tarry	Drug (eg, iron); bleeding from upper gastrointestinal tract (eg, stomach, small intestine); diet high in red meat and dark green vegetables (eg, spinach)
		Red	Bleeding from lower gastrointestinal tract (eg, rectum); some foods (eg, beets)
		Pale	Malabsorption of fats; diet high in milk and milk products and low in meat
		Orange or green	Intestinal infection
Consistency	Formed, soft, semisolid, moist	Hard, dry, constipated stool	Dehydration; decreased intestinal motility resulting from lack of fiber in diet, lack of exercise, emotional upset, laxative abuse
		Diarrhea	Increased intestinal motility (eg, irritation of the colon by bacteria)
Shape	Cylindrical (contour of rectum) about 2.5 cm (1 in) in diameter in adults	Narrow, pencil-shaped, or stringlike stool	Obstructive condition of the rectum
Amount	Varies with diet (about 100 to 400 g per day)		
Odor	Aromatic: affected by ingested food and person's own bacterial flora	Pungent	Infection, blood
Constituents	Small amounts of undigested roughage; sloughed dead bacteria and epithedial cells; fat; protein; dried constituents of digestive juices (eg, bile pigments); inorganic matter (calcium, phosphates)	Pus	Bacterial infection
		Mucus	Inflammatory condition
		Parasites	
		Blood	Gastrointestinal bleeding
		Large quantities of fat	Malabsorption
		Foreign objects	Accidental ingestion

sufficiently well developed to permit bowel control. A desire to control daytime bowel movements and to use the toilet generally starts when the child becomes aware of (a) the discomfort caused by a soiled diaper and (b) the sensation that indicates the need for a bowel movement. Daytime control is normally attained by age 2½, after a process of toilet training.

Nurses may become directly or indirectly involved in the bowel training of children. Direct involvement may occur when a young child is admitted to a health care agency and the staff continues a bowel training program established at home. In this situation, it is important for nurses to know what words and gestures the child uses to indicate a need and the child's usual routine for defecation. Indirect involvement often includes providing information to parents about ways to facilitate the toilet training process. The following measures are helpful to assist a child with toilet training:

- Provide clothing that the child can remove independently.
- Give the child a personal toilet seat—either a portable toilet or a special seat for the regular toilet. In the latter instance, provide a step so that the toddler can reach the toilet.
- Allow sufficient time, and provide a consistent, relaxed routine.

- Offer praise for successful behavior, but avoid excessive praise.
- Avoid punishment or disapproval when the child is unsuccessful. Children generally wish to please adults but cannot always be successful.
- Initiate toilet training during nonstressful periods of the child's life. For example, avoid beginning at the time a move to a new house is occurring or on admission to a hospital.

The elderly also experience changes that can affect bowel evacuation. Two of these are **atony** (lack of normal muscle tone) of the smooth muscle of the colon, which can result in a slower peristalsis and thus hardened (drier) feces, and decreased tone of the abdominal muscles, which also decreases the pressure that can be exerted during bowel evacuation. Some elderly people also have decreased control of the anal sphincter muscles, which can result in an urgency to defecate.

Diet Sufficient bulk (cellulose, fiber) in the diet is necessary to provide fecal volume. Certain foods are difficult or impossible for some people to digest. This inability results in digestive upsets and, in some instances, the passage of watery stools. Irregular eating can also impair regular defecation. Individuals who eat at the same times every day have a regularly timed, physiologic response to the food intake and a regular pattern of peristaltic activity in the colon.

Spicy foods can produce diarrhea and flatus in some individuals. Other foods that may also influence bowel elimination include the following:

- Gas-producing foods, such as cabbage, onions, cauliflower, bananas, and apples
- Laxative-producing foods, such as bran, prunes, figs, chocolate, and alcohol
- Constipation-producing foods, such as cheese, pasta, eggs, and lean meat

Fluid When fluid intake is inadequate or output (urine or vomitus, for example) is excessive for some reason, the body continues to reabsorb fluid from the chyme as it passes along the colon. As a result the chyme becomes drier than normal, resulting in hard feces. In addition, reduced fluid intake slows the chyme's passage along the intestines, further increasing the reabsorption of fluid from the chyme. Healthy fecal elimination usually requires a daily fluid intake of 2000 to 3000 mL. If chyme moves abnormally quickly through the large intestine, however, there is less time for fluid to be absorbed into the blood; as a result, the feces are soft or even watery.

Activity Activity also stimulates peristalsis, thus facilitating the movement of chyme along the colon. Weak abdominal and pelvic muscles are often ineffective in increasing the intra-abdominal pressure during defecation or in controlling defecation. Weak muscles can result from lack of exercise, immobility, or impaired neurologic functioning.

Psychologic Factors Certan diseases that involve severe diarrhea, such as ulcerative colitis, may have a psychologic component. It is also known that some people who are anxious or angry experience increased peristaltic activity and subsequent diarrhea. In addition, people who are depressed may experience slower intestinal motility, resulting in constipation.

Life-Style Early bowel training may establish the habit of defecating at a regular time. Many people defecate after breakfast, when the gastrocolic and duodenocolic reflexes cause mass peristaltic waves in the large intestine. If a person ignores this urge to defecate, water continues to be reabsorbed, making the feces hard and difficult to expel.

During defecation, people usually assume a sitting position, with the hips flexed and torso leaning slightly forward. This position increases the downward pressure on the rectum and increases intra-abdominal pressure. Many people find it difficult to defecate in another position necessitated by illness, such as a back-lying position.

The availability of toilet facilities, embarrassment about odors, and the need for privacy also affect fecal elimination patterns. A client who shares a room in a hospital may be unwilling to use a bedpan because of the lack of privacy.

Medications Some drugs have side effects that can interfere with normal elimination. Some cause diarrhea; others, such as large doses of certain tranquilizers and repeated administration of morphine and codeine, cause constipation.

Some medications directly affect elimination. **Laxatives** are medications that stimulate bowel activity and so assist fecal elimination. There are medications that soften stool, facilitating defecation. Certain medications, such as dicyclomine hydrochloride (Bentyl), suppress peristaltic activity and sometimes are used to treat diarrhea.

Diagnostic Procedures Before certain diagnostic procedures, such as visualization of the sigmoid colon (sigmoidoscopy), the client is allowed no food or fluid after midnight preceding the examination. Often the client is given a cleansing enema prior to the examination. In these instances the client will not usually defecate normally until eating has been resumed.

Barium (used in radiologic exams) presents a further problem. It hardens if allowed to remain in the colon, producing constipation and sometimes an impaction.

Anesthesia and Surgery General anesthetics cause the normal colonic movements to cease or slow down by blocking parasympathetic stimulation to the muscles of the colon. Clients who have regional or spinal anesthesia are less likely to experience this problem.

Surgery that involves direct handling of the intestines can cause temporary cessation of intestinal movement. This condition, called *paralytic ileus*, usually lasts 24 to 48 hours. Listening for bowel sounds that reflect intestinal motility is an important nursing assessment following surgery. See Chapter 22, page 536, for assessment of bowel sounds.

Pathologic Conditions Spinal cord injuries and head injuries, for example, can decrease the sensory stimulation for defecation. Impaired mobility may limit the client's ability to respond to the urge to defecate when the client is unable to reach a toilet or summon assistance. As a result, the client may experience constipation. Or a client may experience fecal incontinence because of poorly functioning anal sphincters (see p. 1187).

Irritants Spicy foods, bacterial toxins, and poisons can irritate the intestinal tract and produce diarrhea and often large amounts of flatus.

Pain Clients who experience discomfort when defecating (eg, following hemorrhoid surgery) often suppress the urge to defecate to avoid the pain. Such clients can experience constipation as a result.

COMMON FECAL ELIMINATION PROBLEMS

There are six common problems related to fecal elimination: constipation, fecal impaction, diarrhea, fecal incontinence, flatulence, and helminths.

CONSTIPATION

Constipation refers to the passage of small, dry, hard stool or the passage of no stool for a period of time. It occurs when the movement of feces through the large intestine is slow, thus allowing time for additional reabsorption of fluid from the large intestine. Associated with constipation are difficult evacuation of stool and increased effort or straining of the voluntary muscles of defecation. It is important to define constipation in relation to the person's regular elimination pattern. Some people normally defecate only a few times a week and therefore are not necessarily constipated when they fail to defecate every day. Other people defecate more than once a day; to them, a movement only once a day can indicate constipation. Careful assessment of the person's habits is necessary before a diagnosis of constipation is made. See the box on page 1192 for defining characteristics of constipation.

Many causes and factors contribute to constipation. Among them are the following:

- *Irregular defecation habits.* When the normal defecation reflexes are inhibited or ignored, these conditioned reflexes tend to be progressively weakened. When habitually ignored, the urge to defecate is ultimately lost. Children at play may ignore these reflexes; adults ignore them because of the pressures of time or work. Hospitalized clients may suppress the urge because of embarrassment about using a bedpan or because defecation is too uncomfortable.
- *Overuse of laxatives.* Overuse of laxatives has the same effect as ignoring the urge to defecate—natural defecation reflexes are inhibited. The habitual user of laxatives eventually requires larger or stronger doses, because they have a progressively reduced effect with continual use.
- *Increased psychologic stress.* Strong emotion is thought to cause constipation by inhibiting intestinal peristalsis through the action of epinephrine and the sympathetic nervous system. Stress can also cause a spastic bowel (spastic or hypertonic constipation or an irritable colon). Associated with this type of constipation are abdominal cramps, increased amounts of mucus, and alternating periods of constipation and diarrhea.
- *Inappropriate diet.* Bland diets and low-fiber diets are lacking in bulk and therefore create insufficient residue of waste products to stimulate the reflex for defecation. Low-residue foods, such as rice, eggs, and lean meats, move more slowly through the intestinal tract. Increasing fluid intake with such foods increases their rate of movement. A change in diet can also contribute to constipation.
- *Insufficient fluid.* An insufficient fluid intake reduces the amount of fluid in the chyme, which enters the large intestine. This lack of fluid in turn results in drier, harder feces.
- *Medications.* Some drugs, such as morphine or codeine as well as adrenergic and anticholinergic drugs, slow the motility of the colon through their action on the central nervous system, thus causing constipation. Others, such as iron tablets, have an astringent effect and act more locally on the bowel mucosa to cause constipation. Iron also has an irritating effect and can cause diarrhea in some people.
- *Insufficient exercise.* In clients on prolonged bed rest, generalized muscle weakness extends to the muscles of the abdomen, diaphragm, and pelvic floor, which are used in defecation. Indirectly associated with lack of

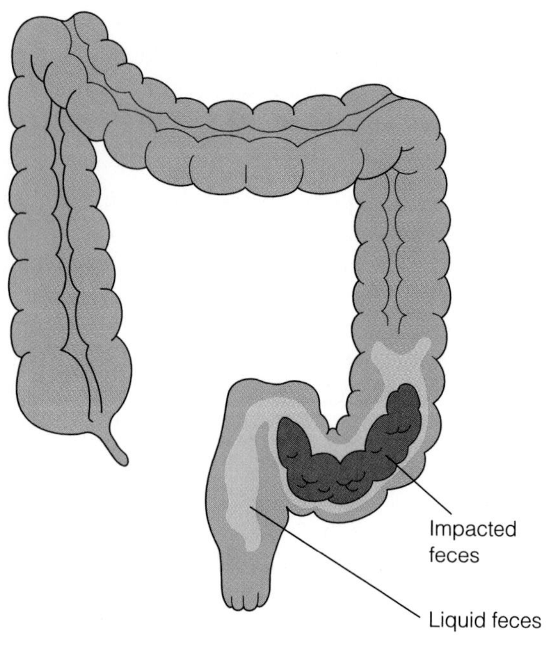

Figure 40–6 A fecal impaction with liquid feces passing around the impaction.

exercise is lack of appetite and possible subsequent lack of fiber.

- *Age.* The muscle weakness and poor sphincter tone that occur in some elderly people contribute to constipation. In addition, the decrease in mucus and intestinal secretions contributes to this problem.
- *Disease processes.* Several diseases produce constipation, such as bowel obstruction; paralysis, which inhibits the client's ability to bear down; and pelvic inflammatory conditions, which create paralysis or atony of the bowel.

Constipation can be hazardous to clients. Straining in order to defecate can place stress on abdominal or perineal sutures, rupturing them if the pressure is sufficiently great. In addition, straining often is accompanied by holding the breath. This Valsalva maneuver can present serious problems to people with heart disease, brain injuries, or respiratory disease. Holding the breath increases the intrathoracic and the intracranial pressures. To some degree this pressure can be reduced if the person exhales through the mouth while straining. However, avoiding straining altogether is the best precaution.

FECAL IMPACTION

Fecal impaction is a mass or collection of hardened, puttylike feces in the folds of the rectum. Impaction results from prolonged retention and accumulation of fecal material. In severe impactions the feces accumulate and extend well up into the sigmoid colon and beyond. Fecal impaction is recognized by the passage of liquid fecal seepage (diarrhea) and no normal stool. The liquid portion of the feces seeps out around the impacted mass (Figure 40–6). Impaction can also be assessed by digital examination of the rectum, during which the hardened mass can often be palpated.

Along with fecal seepage and constipation, symptoms include frequent but nonproductive desire to defecate and rectal pain. A generalized feeling of illness results; the client becomes anorexic, the abdomen becomes distended, and nausea and vomiting may occur.

The causes of fecal impaction are usually poor defecation habits and constipation. Certain medications (see page 1184) also contribute to impactions. The barium used in radiologic examinations of the upper and lower gastrointestinal tracts can be a causative factor. Therefore, after these examinations, measures are usually taken to ensure removal of the barium. In the elderly, a combination of factors contribute to impactions: poor fluid intake, insufficient bulk in the diet, lack of activity, and weakened muscle tone.

An impaction can sometimes be palpated through the client's abdomen. Digital examination of the impaction through the rectum should be done gently and carefully because stimulation of the vagus nerve in the rectal wall can slow the client's heart. Some nurses advise against digital rectal examination without a physician's order. 

Although fecal impaction can generally be prevented, digital removal of impacted feces is sometimes necessary. When fecal impaction is suspected, the client is often given an oil retention enema, a cleansing enema 2 to 4 hours later, and daily additional cleansing enemas, suppositories, or stool softeners. If these measures fail, manual removal is often necessary.

DIARRHEA

Diarrhea refers to the passage of liquid feces and an increased frequency of defecation. It is the opposite of constipation and results from rapid movement of fecal contents through the large intestine. Rapid passage of chyme reduces the time available for the large intestine to reabsorb water and electrolytes. Some people pass stool with increased frequency, but diarrhea is not present unless the stool is relatively unformed and excessively liquid. The person with diarrhea finds it difficult or impossible to control the urge to defecate for very long. Diarrhea and the threat of incontinence are sources of concern and embarrassment. Often, spasmodic and piercing abdominal cramps are associated with diarrhea. Sometimes the client passes blood and excessive mucus; nausea and vomiting may also occur. With persistent diarrhea, irritation of the anal region extending to the perineum and buttocks gen-

CRITICAL THINKING CHALLENGE

WHAT WOULD YOU DO?

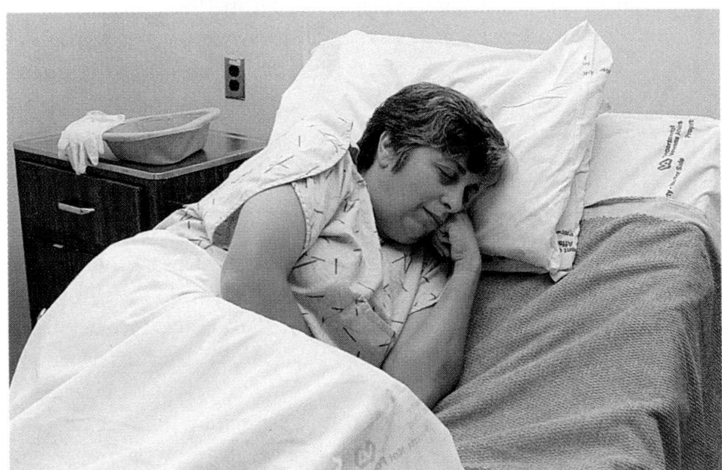

Doreen Harris is a 53-year old female who has a fecal impaction in the lower bowel. The physician has ordered that the impaction be digitally removed. As you are assembling the equipment needed to remove the fecal impaction, Ms Harris tells you she doesn't want the procedure done.

What would you do?

erally results. Fatigue, weakness, malaise, and emaciation are the results of prolonged diarrhea.

When the cause of diarrhea is irritants in the intestinal tract, diarrhea is thought to be a protective flushing mechanism. It can create serious fluid and electrolyte losses in the body, however, that can develop within frighteningly short periods of time, particularly in infants and small children. Table 40–2 lists some of the major causes of diarrhea and the physiologic responses of the body. Client teaching to manage diarrhea is shown in the accompanying box on page 1188.

FECAL INCONTINENCE

Fecal incontinence refers to loss of voluntary ability to control fecal and gaseous discharges through the anal sphincter. The incontinence may occur at specific times, such as after meals, or it may occur irregularly. Two types of fecal incontinence are described: partial and major. *Partial incontinence* is the inability to control flatus or to prevent minor soiling. *Major incontinence* is the inability to control feces of normal consistency (Hanauer 1988, p. 107).

Fecal incontinence is generally associated with impaired functioning of the anal sphincter or its nerve supply, such as in some neuromuscular diseases, spinal cord trauma, and tumors of the external anal sphincter muscle. It is estimated that 60% of the elderly may be affected by fecal incontinence at some time (Hanauer 1988, p.105).

Fecal incontinence is an emotionally distressing problem that can ultimately lead to social isolation. Afflicted

Table 40–2 Major Causes of Diarrhea

Cause	Physiologic Response
Psychologic stress, (eg, anxiety)	Increased intestinal motility and mucus secretion
Medications	
Antibiotics	Inflammation and infection of mucosa due to overgrowth of pathogenic intestinal microorganisms
Iron	Irritation of intestinal mucosa
Cathartics	Irritation of intestinal mucosa
Allergy to food, fluid/drugs	Incomplete digestion of food or fluid
Intolerance of food or fluid	Increased intestinal motility and mucus secretion
Diseases of the colon	
Malabsorption syndrome	Reduced absorption of fluids
Crohn's disease	Inflammation of the mucosa often leading to ulcer formation
Others	
Surgical operations	
Imbalance of intestinal flora	Use of antibiotics destroys normal flora

CLIENT TEACHING

Managing Diarrhea

- Drink at least 8 glasses of water per day to prevent dehydration.
- Avoid alcohol, beverages with caffeine, and excessively cold fluids, which aggravate the problem.
- Ingest foods with sodium and potassium. Most foods contain sodium. Potassium is found in dairy products, meats, and many vegetables and fruits, especially tomatoes, potatoes, bananas, peaches, and apricots.
- Limit foods containing insoluble fiber, such as whole-wheat and whole-grain breads and cereals, and raw fruits and vegetables.
- Increase foods containing soluble fiber, such as oatmeal and skinless fruits and potatoes.
- Limit fatty foods (eg, dairy products and packaged processed meats).
- Use soft toilet tissue or cotton balls for wiping if the perianal area is irritated.
- Thoroughly clean and dry the perianal area after passing stool to prevent skin irritation and breakdown. Use soft cotton balls to clean and dry the area. Apply a moisture-barrier cream or ointment, such as zinc oxide or petrolatum, as needed.
- Discontinue medications or foods that cause diarrhea.
- When diarrhea has stopped, reestablish normal bowel flora by taking fermented dairy products, such as yogurt or buttermilk.

---

persons withdraw into their homes or, if in the hospital, the confines of their room to minimize the embarrassment associated with soiling. Such people may come to prefer easily washable night garments to street clothes. Incontinent feces are acidic and contain digestive enzymes that are highly irritating to skin. Therefore, the area around the anal region should be kept clean and dry and be protected with zinc oxide or other ointment.

More recently, a fecal collector has been used. This pouch is applied to the skin after the application of a protective barrier. The pouch, which is made of an odor-barrier film and has a drainage outlet, can be attached to a bedside receptacle when there is a high volume of loose feces (Mowlam et al 1986, p. 59). See page 1208 for details.

FLATULENCE

Air or gas in the gastrointestinal tract is called **flatus.** There are three primary causes of flatus: (a) action of bacteria on the chyme in the large intestine, (b) swallowed air, and (c) gas that diffuses from the bloodstream into the intestine. Normally all but 0.6 liters of this gas is absorbed into the intestinal capillaries (Guyton 1991, p. 742).

Flatulence is the presence of *excessive* flatus in the intestines and leads to stretching and inflation of the intestines (*intestinal distention*). This condition is also referred to as **tympanites.** Large amounts of air and other gases can accumulate in the stomach, resulting in gastric distention.

Most gases that are swallowed are expelled through the mouth by **eructation** (belching). The gases formed in the large intestine are chiefly absorbed, through the intestinal capillaries, into the circulation. Flatulence can occur in the colon, however, from a variety of causes, such as abdominal surgery, anesthetics, or narcotics. If this gas cannot be expelled through the anus, it may be necessary to insert a rectal tube or provide a return flow enema to remove it.

Common causes of flatulence and distention are constipation; codeine, barbiturates, and other medications that decrease intestinal motility; and states of anxiety, during which large amounts of air are swallowed. Postoperative distention after abdominal surgery is commonly seen in hospitals. This type of distention generally occurs on about the third postoperative day and is caused by the effects of anesthetics, narcotics, dietary changes, and reduction in activity.

HELMINTHS

Common *parasitic worms*, or *helminths*, that infest the intestine in North America are the hookworm, roundworm, pinworm, and tapeworm. They cause faulty digestion, intestinal inflammation, intestinal obstruction, and anemia. Medications used against worms are called *anthelmintics*. *Hookworms* are transmitted by soil contaminated with the larvae that comes in contact with the skin (eg, when a person walks barefoot), or by contaminated food or water that is ingested. Hookworms are small, less than 1 cm (0.3 in) long, but they have teeth that hook the head into the mucosa and enable it to gain nourishment from the blood. *Roundworms* are longer, 25 cm (10 in), with a cylindrically shaped body. They also enter the body by means of contaminated food or drink. *Pinworms*, which are 1.2 cm (0.5 in) long, are the most common worm parasites in North America, generally infesting children. The female pinworm moves through the anal opening at night and deposits ova in the surrounding area, causing the anal region to itch. This leads to scratching, contamination of the fingernails, and ultimately reinfection by mouth. *Tapeworms* are flat, segmented, large worms, up to 10 m (30 ft) long, with small heads that are equipped with suckers. The suckers embed the head into the intestinal mucosa. Common tapeworms are those transmitted by uncooked beef or pork.

Worms can be treated by an oral medication, such as mebendazole 100 mg bid for 3 days for an adult. The exact medication prescribed depends on the kind of worm that has infested the intestine.

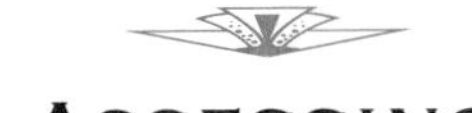

ASSESSING

Assessment of fecal elimination includes taking a nursing history; performing a physical examination of the abdomen, rectum, and anus; and inspecting the feces. The nurse also should review any data obtained from relevant diagnostic tests.

NURSING HISTORY

A nursing history for fecal elimination helps the nurse ascertain the client's normal pattern. The nurse elicits a description of usual feces and any recent changes and collects information about any past or current problems with elimination, the presence of an ostomy, and factors influencing the elimination pattern.

Examples of interview questions to elicit this information are shown in the accompanying box. The number of questions to ask is adapted to the individual client, according to the client's responses in the first three categories. For example, questions about factors influencing elimination are addressed perhaps only to clients who are experiencing problems.

When eliciting data about the client's defecation pattern, the nurse needs to understand that the time of defecation and the amount of feces expelled are as individual as the frequency of defecation. Often, the patterns individuals follow depend largely on early training and on convenience. Most people develop the habit of defecating after breakfast, when the gastrocolic and duodenocolic reflexes cause mass movements in the large intestine.

PHYSICAL EXAMINATION

Physical examination of the abdomen, rectum, and anus is discussed in Chapter 22. Physical examination of the abdomen in relation to fecal elimination problems includes inspection, auscultation, percussion, and palpation with specific reference to the intestinal tract. Auscultation precedes palpation, since palpation can alter peristalsis. Examination of the rectum and anus includes inspection and palpation.

CHARACTERISTICS OF FECES

The client's stool is inspected for color, consistency, shape, amount, odor, and the presence of abnormal constituents. See Table 40–1, earlier, for a summary of normal and abnormal characteristics of stool and possible causes.

ASSESSMENT INTERVIEW

Fecal Elimination

Defecation Pattern

- What is the frequency and time of day of defecation?
- Has this pattern changed recently?

Description of Feces and Any Changes

- How would you describe your stool in terms of color, texture (hard, soft, watery), shape, odor?
- Have you noticed any changes in your stool recently?

Fecal Elimination Problems

- What problems have you had or do you now have with your bowel movements (constipation? diarrhea? excessive flatulence? seepage or incontinence?)
- When and how often does it occur?
- What causes it (food, fluids, exercise, emotions, medications, disease, surgery)?
- What methods have you used to remedy the problem, and how effective were they?

Presence and Management of Ostomy

- What is your usual routine with your colostomy/ileostomy?
- What problems, if any, do you have with it?
- How can the nurses help you manage colostomy/ileostomy?

Factors Influencing Elimination

- *Use of elimination aids.* What routines do you follow to maintain your usual defecation pattern? Do you use natural aids such as specific foods or fluids (eg, a glass of hot lemon juice before breakfast), laxatives, or enemas to maintain elimination?
- *Diet.* What foods do you believe affect defecation? What foods do you typically eat? What food do you always avoid? Do you take meals at regular times?
- *Fluid.* What amount and kind of fluid do you take each day (eg, 6 glasses of water, 5 cups of coffee)?
- *Exercise.* What is your usual daily exercise pattern? (Obtain specifics about exercise rather than asking whether it is sufficient; ideas of what is sufficient vary among individuals.)
- *Medications.* Have you taken any medications that could affect the gastrointestinal tract (eg, iron, antibiotics)?
- *Stress.* Are you experiencing any long-term or short-term stressors? If so, what are these? Do you think these affect your defecation pattern? How?

DIAGNOSTIC STUDIES

Diagnostic studies of the gastrointestinal tract include direct visualization techniques, indirect visualization techniques, and laboratory tests for abnormal constituents.

Visualization Studies *Direct visualization techniques* include **anoscopy,** the viewing of the anal canal; **proctoscopy,** the viewing of the rectum; **proctosigmoidoscopy,** the viewing of the rectum and sigmoid colon; and **colonoscopy,** the viewing of the large intestine. *Indirect visualization* of the gastrointestinal tract is achieved by roentgenography. Roentgenography of the large intestine requires the introduction into the colon of barium, a radiopaque substance. Barium permits the viewing of the outline of the colon by either fluoroscopy or roentgenography. See the *Clinical Companion* accompanying this book for client preparation and follow-up care for diagnostic studies.

Collecting Stool Specimens The nurse is responsible for collecting stool specimens ordered for laboratory analysis. Before obtaining a specimen, the nurse needs to determine the reason for collecting the stool specimen and the correct method of obtaining and handling it (ie, how much stool to obtain, whether a preservative needs to be added to the stool, and whether it needs to be sent immediately to the laboratory). It may be necessary to confirm this information by checking with the agency laboratory. In many situations, only a single specimen is required; in others, timed specimens are necessary, and every stool passed is collected within a designated time period.

Nurses need to give clients the following instructions:

- Defecate in a clean bedpan or bedside commode.
- Do not contaminate the specimen, if possible, by urine or menstrual discharge. Void before the specimen collection.
- Do not place toilet tissue in the bedpan after defecation. Contents of the paper can affect the laboratory analysis.
- Notify the nurse as soon as possible after defecation, particularly for specimens that need to be sent to the laboratory immediately.

To secure a stool specimen from a baby or young child who is not toilet trained, the nurse obtains newly passed feces from the diaper.

When obtaining stool samples, that is, when handling the client's bedpan, when transferring the stool sample to a specimen container, and when disposing of the bedpan contents, the nurse follows medical aseptic technique meticulously. Wear disposable gloves to prevent hand contamination and take care not to contaminate the outside of the specimen container. Use one or two clean tongue blades to transfer the specimen to the container and then wrap them in a paper towel before disposing of them in the waste container. This practice lessens the chance of contact with other articles and the spread of microorganisms. The amount of stool to be sent depends on the purpose for which the specimen is collected. Usually about 2.5 cm (1 in) of formed stool or 15 to 30 mL of liquid stool is adequate. For some timed specimens, however, the entire stool passed may need to be sent. Visible pus, mucus, or blood should be included in sample specimens. For a stool culture, the nurse dips a sterile swab into the specimen, preferably where purulent fecal matter is present, and, using sterile technique, places the swab in a sterile test tube.

Because fresh specimens provide the most accurate results, the nurse sends the specimen to the laboratory immediately. If this is not possible, the nurse follows the directions on the specimen container. In some instances refrigeration is indicated, because bacteriologic changes take place in stool specimens left at room temperature.

Testing Feces for Occult Blood Several test products are available to test stool specimens for occult blood: the guaiac test, Hematest, and Hemoccult slide. Because results of occult blood tests may be positive if the client has eaten meat within 3 days, the client may need to refrain from eating red meat for 3 days before the test. Oral iron preparations may also be discontinued because, if partially undigested, they may mask the presence of occult blood in the stool. Before the test, the nurse should assess the client for hemorrhoids that may bleed. This is particularly important for clients who are constipated, because constipated stool can aggravate existing hemorrhoids. Any bleeding can affect test results.

To perform the test, the nurse obtains a stool specimen, selects a test product, puts on gloves, and follows the manufacturer's directions:

- For a guaiac test, smear a thin layer of feces on a paper towel or filter paper with a tongue blade, and drop reagents onto the smear as directed.

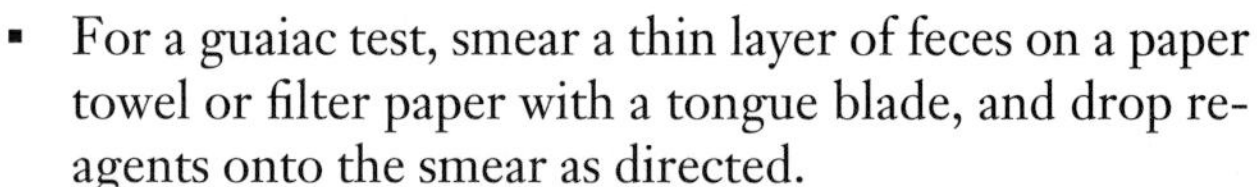

- For a Hematest, smear a thin layer of feces on filter paper, place a tablet in the middle of the specimen, and add two drops of water as directed.
- For a Hemoccult slide, smear a thin layer of feces over the circle inside the envelope, and drop reagent solution onto the smear.

For all tests, a blue color indicates a positive result, that is, the presence of occult blood.

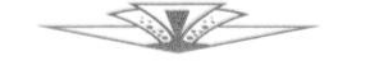

DIAGNOSING

NANDA nursing diagnoses that relate to fecal elimination problems include **Bowel incontinence, Constipa-**

tion, Colonic constipation, Perceived constipation, and **Diarrhea.** These diagnoses, with definitions, defining characteristics, and contributing factors, are shown in the box on page 1192. Clinical applications of these diagnoses are shown in Table 40–3. The diagnosis **Knowledge deficit** may be used when alterations in bowel elimination require new self-care behaviors (eg, ostomy care).

Fecal elimination problems may affect many other areas of human functioning and as a consequence may be the etiology of other NANDA diagnoses. Examples follow:

- **High risk for fluid volume deficit** related to
  a. Prolonged diarrhea
  b. Abnormal fluid loss through ostomy
- **High risk for impaired skin integrity** related to
  a. Prolonged diarrhea
  b. Bowel incontinence
  c. Bowel diversion ostomy
- **Self-esteem disturbance** related to
  a. Ostomy
  b. Fecal incontinence
  c. Need for assistance with toileting
- **Altered growth and development** related to parent's misconceptions about bowel and bladder training
- **Knowledge deficit** (bowel training, ostomy management) related to lack of previous experience
- **Ineffective individual coping** related to
  a. Inability to accept ostomy
  b. Inability to carry out toileting independently
- **Anxiety** related to
  a. Lack of control of fecal elimination secondary to ostomy
  b. Response of others to ostomy

Table 40–3 Clinical Application: Assessment Data Clusters and Related Nursing Diagnoses

Data Cluster	Nursing Diagnosis
Mrs Amy Ballaster states she feels fullness in her rectum and wants to move her bowels but cannot, even with straining. Her last bowel movement was 3 days ago. She lives alone and tends to eat only tea, toast, and noodle soup. Because of arthritis, her activities (gardening and walking) have decreased. Bowel sounds are decreased.	**Constipation** related to inadequate physical activity and insufficient fiber in diet
Marvin Lombardi reports having loose, liquid, light brown stools for 2 days. Passage of stools is associated with cramping abdominal pain. Bowel sounds are increased. Temperature is 38 C (100.4 F). Has not taken any medications but reports a feeling of general malaise. States he "ate at a fast-food restaurant 2 nights ago."	**Diarrhea** of unknown etiology, possibly related to spoiled food
Mary Kuoko has had involuntary leakage of stool. States her clothing is soiled several times a day. Says she is too embarrassed to go out with her friends because of the fecal odor. Last bowel movement was more than 3 days ago. Digital examination reveals impaction.	**Bowel incontinence** related to fecal impaction
Mr John Deer had a bowel diversion ostomy 2 days ago. Effluent is continuous and liquid. Peristomal skin is intact. Disposable colostomy device was applied.	**High risk for impaired skin integrity** related to discharge from bowel diversion ostomy

PLANNING

The overall client outcome for persons with fecal elimination problems is to maintain or restore a regular elimination pattern. For clients who have prolonged diarrhea, maintenance of fluid balance is also an essential goal.

Appropriate nursing interventions and outcome criteria that relate to these broad goals must be identified. Preventive and corrective interventions need to be included. Among the strategies the nurse should consider are the following:

- Implementing measures that promote normal defecation in hospitalized clients
- Implementing medically prescribed therapies, such as cathartics, antidiarrheal preparations, and enemas
- Checking for and digitally removing an impaction
- Teaching clients about appropriate life-style changes, such as increasing fluid intake, exercise, and intake of dietary fiber
- Providing special care for clients with bowel diversion ostomies and teaching them about ostomy management

Specific outcome criteria, nursing interventions, and rationales are shown in the Care Planning Guide on page 1193.

A critical pathway can also be useful for planning client care (see p. 1216).

Text continued on page 1196

NURSING DIAGNOSES
CLIENTS WITH BOWEL ELIMINATION PROBLEMS

NURSING DIAGNOSIS: Constipation: The state in which one experiences a change in normal bowel habits characterized by a decrease in frequency and/or passage of hard, dry stools. Not associated with a pathological state *or* **Colonic constipation:** Constipation that results from a delay in passage of food residue

Defining Characteristics

- Decreased frequency of defecation
- Hard, dry, formed stools
- Straining at stool; painful defecation
- Palpable mass
- Reports of rectal fullness or pressure or incomplete bowel evacuation
- Abdominal pain, cramps, and/or distention
- Use of laxatives
- Decreased appetite

Related Factors

Low-roughage diet; less than adequate fluid intake; decreased activity level; change in daily routine; dietary changes; routine use of enemas or laxatives; use of other medications affecting bowel function (eg, narcotic analgesics).

NURSING DIAGNOSIS: Perceived constipation: The state in which one makes a self-diagnosis of constipation and ensures a daily bowel movement through abuse of laxatives, enemas, and/or suppositories

Defining Characteristics

- Expected passage of stool at the same time every day
- Overuse of laxatives, enemas, and/or suppositories

Related Factors

Cultural/family health beliefs; faulty appraisal of normal bowel function; impaired thought processes.

NURSING DIAGNOSIS: Diarrhea: The state in which one experiences a frequent passage of loose, fluid, unformed stools

Defining Characteristics

- Loose, liquid stools
- Abdominal discomfort (cramps, pain)
- Urgency to defecate
- Frequent bowel movements
- Increased bowel sounds
- Change in color of stool

Related Factors

Dietary changes; food intolerance; stress and anxiety; medications; medical therapy (eg, radiation).

NURSING DIAGNOSIS: Bowel incontinence: The state in which one experiences involuntary passage of stool

Defining Characteristics

- Involuntary passage of stool

Related Factors

Decreased awareness of need to defecate; loss of sphincter control secondary to neuromuscular impairment.

Sources: LJ Carpenito, *Nursing Diagnosis: Application to Clinical Practice*, 4th ed. (Philadelphia: Lippincott, 1992), pp. 173–196; M Gordon, *Manual of Nursing Diagnosis 1993–1994*, 6th ed. (St Louis: Mosby-Year Book, 1993), pp. 133–141; MJ Kim, GK McFarland, and AM McLane, *Pocket Guide to Nursing Diagnoses*, 5th ed. (St Louis: Mosby-Year Book, 1993), pp. 6, 12–14, 19; GK McFarland and EA McFarlane, *Nursing Diagnosis and Intervention: Planning for Patient Care*, 2d ed. (St Louis: Mosby, 1993), pp. 216–27; North American Nursing Diagnosis Association, *NANDA Nursing Diagnoses: Definitions and Classification 1992–1993* (Philadelphia: NANDA, 1992), pp. 16–18; and JR Lederer, GL Marculescu, B Mocnik, and N Seaby, *Care Planning Pocket Guide—A Nursing Diagnosis Approach*, 5th ed. (Redwood City, CA: Addison-Wesley Nursing, 1993), pp. 18, 38–42, 58.

CARE PLANNING GUIDE

CLIENTS WITH BOWEL ELIMINATION PROBLEMS

NURSING DIAGNOSIS: Colonic constipation

Outcome Criteria	Nursing Interventions	Rationale
The client		
▪ Identifies usual pattern of bowel elimination.	Explore with the client the usual pattern of bowel elimination. Encourage the client to keep a diary as indicated.	Identifying the usual or normal pattern provides the client and nurse with baseline data to establish goals and gauge efficacy of interventions.
	Explain that wide variations in bowel elimination (eg, 1 to 3 days) occur among individuals.	Knowledge of what is "normal" may reduce anxiety about perceived bowel elimination problems.
▪ Identifies factors that alter bowel function.	Discuss the effects of fluid, fiber, exercise, daily activity changes, laxatives, and other medications on bowel function.	Awareness of personal factors affecting bowel function may result in behavior changes to alleviate problems.
▪ Alters diet to include adequate amounts of fluid and fiber, as evidenced by a. Drinking 8 glasses of water daily. b. Eating two high-fiber vegetables or fruit and at least one bran muffin or high-fiber bread or cereal daily.	Explore the client's dietary pattern, and recommend necessary dietary changes. Have the client record all intake for 48 hours. Teach the client to	Recording intake helps the nurse determine adequacy of fluid and fiber intake.
	▪ Drink 8 glasses of water daily if no cardiac or renal disease exists.	Adequate amounts of fluid promote normal bowel elimination and are essential with a high-fiber diet.
	▪ Avoid coffee, tea, or grapefruit juice.	These fluids act as diuretics.
	▪ Eat foods high in fiber (eg, whole-grain cereals, fresh fruits and vegetables).	Fiber absorbs water and increases stool bulk, which stimulates peristalsis and bowel evacuation.
	▪ Avoid highly refined breads and cereals (eg, pasta, pastries).	
	▪ Avoid overuse of bran.	Too much bran causes cramping and flatus.
	▪ Consider taking a fiber supplement once a day if taking constipating medications.	
▪ Walks for at least 15 to 20 minutes daily and exercises abdominal muscles three times daily.	Explain the relationship of exercise and intestinal motility.	Exercise increases peristalsis, thus promoting bowel evacuation.
	Encourage the client to walk at least 15 to 20 minutes daily, and teach abdominal strengthening exercises.	Exercise maintains tone of abdominal and pelvic floor muscles used in defecation.
▪ Achieves previously identified "normal" elimination pattern, as evidenced by	Monitor the client's bowel elimination pattern and stool consistency.	Regular assessment provides data to evaluate the effectiveness of nursing interventions.
a. Bowel movement at least every 3 days. b. Regular time for defecation.	Encourage the client to respond immediately to the urge to defecate.	Immediate response to the urge to defecate prevents retention of stool and subsequent hardness and drying of the stool.
c. Easy passage of stool. d. Normal consistency of stool.	Assess the client's self-care abilities related to toileting, and provide assistance as needed.	Many older clients have mobility problems due to a major neurologic deficit, arthritis, or fracture.

➤

BOWEL ELIMINATION PROBLEMS CONTINUED

NURSING DIAGNOSIS: Colonic constipation *continued*

Outcome Criteria	Nursing Interventions	Rationale
e. Absence of abdominal distention, discomfort, and feeling of incomplete bowel evacuation.	Encourage the client to establish a regular time to defecate, preferably 20 to 30 minutes after a meal.	The presence of food in stomach initiates the gastrocolic reflex.
	Discuss the problems associated with straining at stool and overuse of laxatives.	Straining at stool elicits the Valsalva maneuver, which may aggravate hemorrhoids and anal fissures, increase cardiac pressure, and rupture abdominal or perineal sutures.
	Obtain an order for a stool softener as indicated to prevent straining at defecation.	Chronic use of laxatives inhibits natural defecation reflexes, causing constipation.

NURSING DIAGNOSIS: Perceived constipation

Outcome Criteria	Nursing Interventions	Rationale
The client		
▪ Verbalizes (a) understanding of need to decrease use of laxatives, enemas, and suppositories; and (b) accepts as normal an interval of 2 to 3 days between bowel movements.	Explore the client's perceptions of and method of maintaining healthy bowel elimination.	Knowledge of the client's perceptions and regular practices enables the nurse to identify misinformation and focus on information the client requires.
▪ Alters diet and exercise pattern to include adequate daily amounts of fiber, fluids, and exercise (see above for **Colonic constipation**).	Monitor the client's pattern of bowel elimination, diet, and exercise.	
▪ Reports decreased use of laxative or suppository (eg, only once per week)	Discuss use of alternatives to laxatives, enemas, and suppositories (eg, Metamucil).	Fiber substances such as Metamucil supplement natural fiber in the diet.
	Establish a plan for gradual withdrawal of laxative use (eg, gradually reduce the dose or change to a milder product while increasing fiber and fluid intake).	A gradual increase in fiber prevents excessive flatulence in persons who rarely eat high-roughage foods.

NURSING DIAGNOSIS: Diarrhea

Outcome Criteria	Nursing Interventions	Rationale
The client		
▪ Has stools of normal consistency, experiences decreased frequency of bowel evacuation (eg, no more than two bowel movements per day), and is free of abdominal pain.	Determine etiologic factors (see page 1187).	Identifying etiologic factors provides data needed to plan appropriate nursing intervention.
	Obtain stool for culture and sensitivity as ordered.	Testing is done to determine causative infectious agent and verify appropriate therapy.

Outcome Criteria	Nursing Interventions	Rationale
	Determine side effects of all medications the client is receiving.	Gastrointestinal side effects of certain medications can aggravate or cause diarrhea.
	Inform the client about actions and side effects of prescribed antidiarrheal medications.	Knowledge of prescribed drugs enhances appropriate use of medications.
	Monitor and record the color, consistency, volume, frequency, and odor of stools; or ask the client to keep a record of this information.	Ongoing assessment provides data to evaluate the effectiveness of interventions.
	Teach the client to avoid foods and fluids containing substances that stimulate or irritate the bowel. See the box on page 1188.	Avoiding such substances prevents aggravation of the problem.
▪ Maintains fluid and electrolyte balance, as evidenced by a. Serum electrolyte values of: ▪ Sodium 135 to 145 mEq/L ▪ Potassium 3.5 to 5.0 mEq/L ▪ Chloride 95 to 105 mEq/L ▪ Bicarbonate 21 to 28 mEq/L b. Normal or baseline body weight or (weight gain) c. Normal skin turgor.	Encourage adequate oral intake of liquids (eg, 2500 mL of fluid per day) Provide high-calorie drinks as needed. Encourage ingestion of foods high in sodium and potassium as indicated. Monitor and record the fluid intake, skin turgor, body weight, and serum electrolytes daily.	This helps prevent dehydration. This increases caloric intake and helps maintain body weight. This helps maintain electrolyte balance. This allows the nurse to evaluate the client's progress toward goal achievement.
▪ Maintains perianal skin integrity, as evidenced by absence of redness or breakdown.	Inspect the skin after each bowel movement.	Skin inspection enables the nurse to compare skin status with baseline data.
	Provide appropriate skin care with mild soap and water, or use mineral oil or perianal spray cleanser to cleanse the skin.	Mild cleaning agents prevent skin irritation.
	Apply protective paste or ointment (eg, zinc oxide) to the skin as needed.	A skin barrier prevents skin erosion.
	Ensure that the bedside commode is easily accessible.	Accessibility to a commode prevents accidental soiling of skin and clothing and subsequent embarrassment.

NURSING DIAGNOSIS: Bowel incontinence

Outcome Criteria	Nursing Interventions	Rationale
The client ▪ Has fewer episodes of incontinence and soiling.	Assess and document each episode of incontinence (ie, time, amount, stool consistency).	This enables the nurse to determine the pattern of incontinence.
	Determine etiologic factors (eg, diarrhea, fecal impaction, antibiotic chemotherapy, excessive use of laxatives, neuromuscular impairment).	Knowledge of contributing factors influences the planning of nursing interventions.

BOWEL ELIMINATION PROBLEMS CONTINUED

NURSING DIAGNOSIS: Bowel incontinence *continued*

Outcome Criteria	Nursing Interventions	Rationale
	Select appropriate measures to reduce episodes of incontinence:	
	▪ Note when incontinence occurs, and assist the client with toileting at those times; or, plan a schedule of providing assistance every 1 or 2 hours, including times after meals.	These measures help establish regularity and may prevent incontinent episodes.
	▪ Instruct the client about pelvic floor exercises (see p. 1246).	Pelvic floor exercises strengthen anal sphincters and may reduce episodes of incontinence.
	▪ Apply a fecal incontinence pouch if incontinence is continuous or of a large volume (see p. 1208).	A pouch protects the perianal skin.
▪ Maintains perianal skin integrity, as evidenced by absence of redness or breakdown, and is free of perianal odor.	Provide meticulous skin care after each incontinent episode, and apply protective skin barriers as indicated. See specific interventions above for **Diarrhea.**	Skin care measures help prevent skin irritation and breakdown and odors that are embarrassing to the client.
▪ Demonstrates effective coping skills, as evidenced by a. Ability to meet self-care needs and use protective aids.	Acknowledge the client's feelings about incontinence episodes. Explore coping mechanisms, and assist the client to identify those that decrease anxiety.	Fecal incontinence induces anxiety and feelings of embarrassment and low self-esteem.
b. Reports of participation in social activities once or twice per week.	Explore previous social activities and encourage a return to them.	Social interaction enhances self-esteem.

IMPLEMENTING

PROMOTING REGULAR DEFECATION

The nurse can help the client achieve regular defecation by attending to (a) the provision of privacy, (b) timing, (c) nutrition and fluids, (d) exercise, and (e) positioning. See the accompanying box for wellness teaching related bowel elimination.

Privacy Privacy during defecation is extremely important to many people. The nurse should therefore provide as much privacy as possible for such clients. Some clients also prefer to wipe, wash, and dry themselves after defecating. A nurse may need to provide water and a washcloth and towel for this purpose.

WELLNESS TEACHING

Defecation

- Establish a regular exercise regimen.
- Include high-fiber foods, such as vegetables, fruits, and whole grains, in the diet.
- Maintain fluid intake of 2000 to 3000 mL/day
- Do not ignore the urge to defecate.
- Allow time to defecate, preferably the same time each day.
- Avoid over-the-counter medications to treat constipation and diarrhea.

Timing A client should be encouraged to defecate when the urge to defecate is recognized. To establish regular bowel elimination, the client and nurse can discuss when mass peristalsis normally occurs and provide time for defecation. Many people have well-established times and routines for defecation that should be part of the client's schedule. Other activities, such as bathing and ambulating, should not interfere with the defecation time. Also, clients should not be hurried but given adequate time to defecate.

Nutrition and Fluids The diet a client needs for regular normal elimination varies, depending on the kind of feces the client currently has, the frequency of defecation, and the types of foods that the client finds assist normal defecation.

For the client who is constipated:

- Increase daily fluid intake, and instruct the client to drink hot liquids and fruit juices, especially prune juice.
- Include fiber in the diet, that is, foods such as prunes, raw fruit, bran products, and whole-grain cereals and bread.

For the client who has diarrhea, encourage oral intake of fluids and food. Because ingestion of foods and fluids stimulates the gastrocolic and duodenocolic reflexes, thus inducing more stool, the client may be reluctant to eat or drink. Eating small amounts of bland foods can be helpful because they are more easily absorbed. Diarrhea can lead to great potassium losses, and the ingestion of food or fluids containing potassium should be encouraged. See the discussion of hypokalemia in Chapter 38. Excessively hot or cold fluids should be avoided, because they stimulate peristalsis. In addition, highly spiced foods and high-fiber foods can aggravate diarrhea. See the box on page 1188 for details about managing diarrhea.

For the client who has flatulence the nurse should limit carbonated beverages, the use of drinking straws, and chewing gum—all of which increase the ingestion of air. Gas-forming foods, such as cabbage, beans, onions, and cauliflower, should also be avoided.

Exercise Regular exercise helps clients develop a regular defecation pattern and normal feces. Walking and swimming, for example, help stimulate normal motility of the intestines. Postsurgical clients often are encouraged to ambulate, with regaining normal intestinal motility as one of the reasons.

A client with weak abdominal and pelvic muscles (which impede normal defecation) may be able to strengthen them with the following isometric exercises.

- In a supine position, the client tightens the abdominal muscles as though pulling them inward, holding them for about 10 seconds and then relaxing them. This should be repeated five to ten times, four times a day, depending on the client's health.
- Again in a supine position, the client can contract the thigh muscles and hold them contracted for about 10 seconds, repeating the exercise five to ten times, four times a day. This helps the client confined to bed gain strength in the thigh muscles, thereby making it easier to use a bedpan.

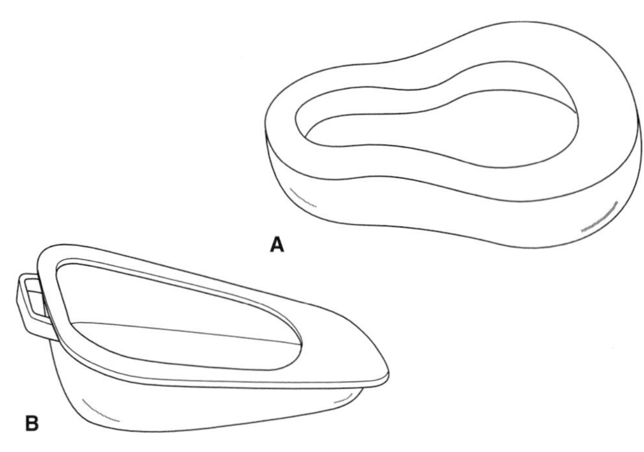

Figure 40–7 Two types of bedpans: *A,* the high-back, or regular pan; *B,* the slipper, or fracture, pan.

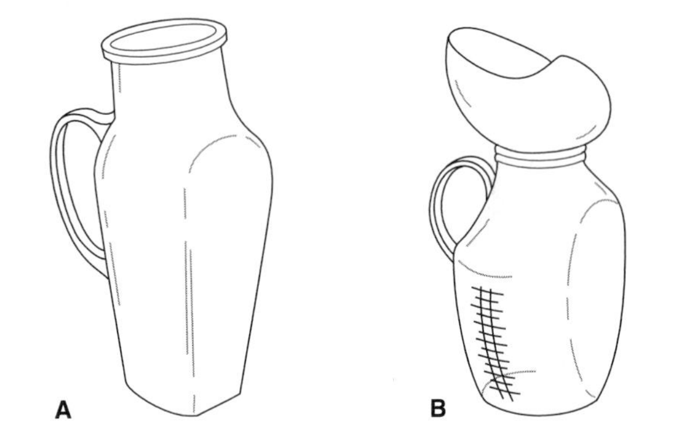

Figure 40–8 Two types of urinals: *A,* male urinal; *B,* female urinal.

Positioning Clients who are confined to bed may need assistance to sit on a bedpan. There are two main types of bedpans, the regular high-back pan (Figure 40–7, *A*) and the slipper, or fracture, pan (Figure 40–7, *B*). The slipper pan has a low back and is used for clients unable to raise their buttocks because of physical problems or therapy that contraindicates such movement. Female clients use a bedpan for both urine and feces; male clients use a bedpan for feces and a urinal for urine. A urinal is a receptacle for urine only. Several designs are available: one is used for males (Figure 40–8, *A*) and another for females (Figure 40–8, *B*).

A *commode* is sometimes used instead of a bedpan when the client can get out of bed but is unable to go to a bathroom. A commode is like an armchair with an open, toiletlike seat and a receptacle underneath for receiving the urine and feces. The receptacle may be specially fitted to the commode or simply a bedpan that fits under the toiletlike seat. A commode may or may not be on wheels and freely movable. Some commodes have an additional plain seat, thus doubling as a regular chair.

For clients who have difficulty in raising themselves from the toilet, an elevated toilet seat can be attached to a regular toilet. Clients then do not have to lower themselves as far onto the seat and do not have to lift as far off the seat.

A client confined to bed may require assistance getting on and off a bedpan. The nurse should bear in mind that clients using bedpans should not exert themselves unduly and therefore provide support while the client is seated on the bedpan to avoid muscle strain.

Many people confined to bed are able to use a bedpan or urinal independently, provided the equipment is placed within safe and easy reach. Some, however, require varying degrees of assistance from a nurse. The nurse has to determine the individual's needs and provide the appropriate assistance.

Using a bedpan or urinal can be embarrassing to many people. For the elderly, physically impaired, or critically ill people, it can also be a tiring procedure. Most male clients will be familiar with a male urinal. Some female clients, however, may not be familiar with female urinals and may require instruction about their use. Note that some female clients find it easier to void using a bedpan rather than a urinal. Procedure 40–1 describes how to give and remove a bedpan and urinal.

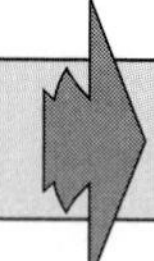

PROCEDURE 40–1 GIVING AND REMOVING A BEDPAN AND URINAL

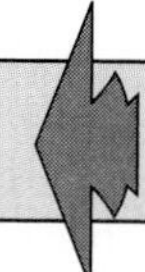

PURPOSES

- To provide a receptacle for elimination of waste material for clients confined to bed
- To obtain a specimen of urine or stool for laboratory examination
- To obtain an accurate measurement or assessment of the client's urine or stool

ASSESSMENT FOCUS

Color, odor, amount, clarity, and consistency of urine; color, odor, amount, and consistency of feces; redness or excoriation of the perineal area; method client uses to indicate need to defecate or urinate.

EQUIPMENT

- ☐ Clean bedpan or urinal and cover or cap
- ☐ Basin of water, soap, washcloth, and towel
- ☐ Disposable gloves
- ☐ Toilet tissue
- ☐ Aerosol freshener (optional)
- ☐ Equipment for a specimen as required

INTERVENTION

Giving a Bedpan

1. Prepare the equipment.

- Don disposable gloves.
- Warm the bedpan, if it is metal, by running water inside the rim of the pan or over the pan. Dry the outside of the pan, and place it on the foot of the bed or on an adjacent chair. *A cold bedpan may make a person tense and thus hinder elimination.* When warming a

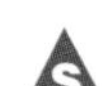

metal pan, which retains heat, take care not to burn the client.

2. Prepare the client.

- For clients who can assist by raising their buttocks, fold down the top bed linen on the near side to expose the hip, and adjust the gown so that it will not fall into the bedpan. *A pie fold of the top bedclothes exposes the client minimally and facilitates placement of the bedpan.*
- For helpless clients who cannot raise their buttocks onto and off a bedpan, fold the top bedclothes down to the hips.

3. Give the bedpan.

- For the client who can assist
  a. Ask the client to flex the knees, rest the weight on the back and the heels, and then raise the buttocks. Assist the client to lift the buttocks by placing the hand nearest the

PROCEDURE 40–1 *continued*

person's head palm up under the lower back, resting the elbow on the mattress, and using the forearm as a lever. *Use of appropriate body mechanics by both client and nurse prevents unnecessary muscle strain and exertion.*

b. Place a regular bedpan under the buttocks with the narrow end toward the foot of the bed and the buttocks resting on the smooth, rounded rim. Place a slipper (fracture) pan with the flat, low end under the client's buttocks. *Improper placement of the bedpan can cause skin abrasion to the sacral area and spillage of the bedpan's contents.*

c. Replace the top bed linen and the side rail as needed.

- For the client who cannot assist
  a. Assist the person to a side-lying position facing toward you (Figure 40–9).
  b. Place the bedpan against the buttocks with the open rim toward the foot of the bed.
  c. Hold the far hip with one hand and the bedpan with the other. Smoothly roll the client away from you and onto the back with the bedpan in place. Assume a wide stance, and move weight from the back leg to the front leg when moving the client. *Use of appropriate body mechanics prevents undue muscle exertion and strain.*

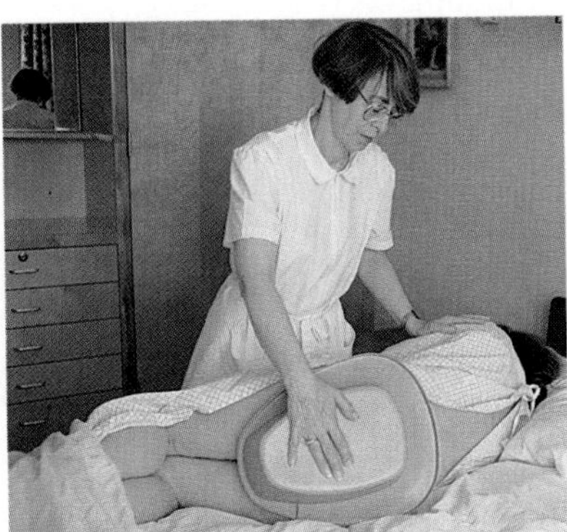

Figure 40–9 Placing a bedpan against a client's buttocks.

- For all clients
  a. Elevate the head of the bed to a semi-Fowler's position, if permitted. *This position relieves strain on the client's back and permits a more normal position for elimination.*
  b. Provide the client with toilet tissue, and ensure that the call light is readily accessible. Ask the client to signal when finished. Leave only when, in your judgment, it is safe to do so. *Having necessary items within reach prevents falls.*
  c. Place the client in a semi-Fowler's position if health permits, or help the client to another comfortable position.
  d. Ensure that the call light is within reach.
  e. Remove gloves.

5. Remove the bedpan.

- Don disposable gloves.
- For the client who can assist
  a. Return the bed to the position used when giving the bedpan.
  b. Ask the client to raise the buttocks, and then remove the bedpan.
  c. Hold the bedpan steady to avoid spilling the contents.
  d. Cover the bedpan, and place it on the adjacent chair. *Covering the bedpan reduces offensive odors and the client's embarrassment.*
- For the client who cannot assist
  a. Return the bed to the flat position, if health permits.
  b. Fold the top bed linen down to the thighs.
  c. Gently roll the client to a side-lying position facing either toward or away from you while holding the bedpan securely with one hand. If you are alone, it is safer and easier to roll the client toward you rather than away from you. If you are planning to turn the client away from you, raise the side rail on the far side, or have another nurse present to prevent a fall.
  d. Remove and cover the bedpan, and place it safely on an adjacent chair or at the foot of the bed.
  e. Clean the perineal area as described below.
  f. Offer the client materials to wash and dry the hands.

6. Assist the client with any needed hygienic measures.

- Wrap toilet tissue several times around the hand, and wipe the person from the pubic area to the anal area, using one stroke for each piece of tissue. *Cleaning in this direction—from the less soiled area to the more soiled area—helps prevent the spread of microorganisms.*
- Turn the client on the side, spread the buttocks, and clean the anal area in the same manner as above.
- Place the soiled tissue in the bedpan unless a specimen is required. If a specimen is required, place the soiled tissue in a moisture resistant receptacle.
- Wash the anal area with soap and water as indicated, and thoroughly dry the area. *Adequate washing and drying prevents skin*

PROCEDURE 40–1 GIVING AND REMOVING A BEDPAN AND URINAL *continued*

abrasion and excessive accumulation of microorganisms.

- Replace the drawsheet if it is soiled.
- Offer the client materials to wash and dry the hands. *Hand washing following elimination is a practice that helps prevent the spread of microorganisms.*

7. Attend to any unpleasant odors in the environment.

- Spray the air with an air freshener, unless contraindicated because of respiratory problems or because it is offensive. *Elimination odor can be embarrassing to clients and visitors alike. However, sprays may be harmful to people with respiratory problems, and some perfume sprays are offensive to some people.*

8. Attend to the used bedpan.

- Acquire a specimen if required. Place it in the appropriately labeled container.
- Empty and clean the bedpan. Provide a clean bedpan cover or cap, if necessary, before returning it to the client's unit.
- Go to step 13.

Giving a Urinal

9. Assist the client to an appropriate position.

- Both males and females confined to bed may prefer a semi-Fowler's position, or the male may prefer a standing position at the side of the bed if health permits.

10. Assist the client with using the urinal.

- Offer the urinal so that the client can position it independently.
  or
  Place the urinal between the client's legs with the handle uppermost so that urine will flow into it.
- Leave the signal cord within reach of the person. *The client can then call for assistance if required.*
- Leave for 2 to 3 minutes or until the client signals.
  or
  Remain if the client needs support to stand at the bedside or other assistance.

Removing the Urinal

11. Assist the client as needed.

- Don gloves.
- Remove and recap or cover the urinal, or place it in a urinal bag.
- If wet, wipe the area around the urethral orifice with a tissue.
- Make sure the perineum is dry.
- Offer a dampened washcloth or water, soap, and a towel to wash and dry hands.
- Change the drawsheet if it is wet.

12. Attend to the urine as required.

- Measure the urine if the client is on monitored intake and output, and provide a specimen if required.
- Empty and rinse out the urinal, and return it to the bedside unit.
- Remove gloves.

13. Document all relevant information.

- Record the defecation results and all assessments.
- Record the amount of urine, if it was measured, and all assessment data (eg, cloudy urine, reddened perineum).

EVALUATION FOCUS

Urine: amount, color, clarity, and odor; presence of abnormal constituents. Feces: amount, color, consistency, and odor; presence of abnormalities. Urine and feces: condition of perineum.

ADMINISTERING PRESCRIBED MEDICATIONS

Cathartics Cathartics, frequently referred to as *laxatives*, are drugs that induce defecation. They vary in their degree and method of action. Cathartics can have a laxative effect or a purgative effect. A laxative effect is mild in comparison to a purgative effect, which produces frequent movements of the bowel, soft liquid stools, and sometimes abdominal cramps. Different cathartics have different effects, but even the same cathartic may have either a purgative or laxative effect depending on the dosage taken. A large dose of a cathartic may have a purgative effect, whereas a small dose of the same cathartic may have a laxative effect and produce a normal bowel movement. Table 40–4 describes the different types of cathartics.

The administration of cathartics is prescribed with caution by the physician. Constipation is not the only reason for prescribing cathartics. For example, cathartics are prescribed in preparation for radiologic examinations or surgery.

Table 40–4 Types of Cathartics

Type	Action	Examples	Pertinent Teaching Information
Bulk-forming	Increases the fluid, gaseous, or solid bulk in the intestines	Psyllium hydrophilic mucilloid (Metamucil)	May take 12 or more hours to act. Sufficient fluid must be taken.
Lubricant or emollient	Softens and delays the drying of the feces	Mineral oil, Haley's M-O	Refrigerated oil has less odor. Mixing with fruit juice decreases unpleasant taste. Prolonged use inhibits the absorption of some fat-soluble vitamins.
Wetting agents	Lower the surface tension of the feces, thus helping water to penetrate the feces	Docusate sodium (Colace, Disonate)	Slow-acting, may take several days.
Chemical (stimulant) irritant	Irritates the intestinal mucosa, causing rapid propulsion of the contents.	Castor oil, cascara sagrada, Bisacodyl	Fluid is passed with the feces. May cause cramps. Prolonged use may cause fluid and electrolyte imbalance.
Saline	Salts are not absorbed in the intestine; therefore, fluid bulk is increased because fluid absorption is decreased. Also, may lubricate the feces.	Epsom salts, magnesium hydroxide (Milk of Magnesia), magnesium citrate	May be rapid-acting. Can cause fluid and electrolyte imbalance, particularly in elderly people and children with cardiac and renal disease.

Laxative abuse is thought to be a common problem. The elderly, in particular, often use laxatives improperly. Research shows that the elderly spend millions of dollars on products to relieve constipation. Persistent self-administration of laxatives, however, can result in chronic constipation. There is a trend toward the "natural laxative" approach, that is, the use of increased dietary fiber such as that found in fruits and vegetables to obtain a laxative effect. Unfortunately, the desired laxative effect may not persist. In the elderly, laxatives should always be used secondarily to dietary and life-style changes. Fluid intake should also be at least 1500 mL per day.

Cathartics are contraindicated in the client who has nausea, cramps, colic, vomiting, or undiagnosed abdominal pain. Clients at home should be aware of the dangers of laxative use. The first step is to eliminate laxative use and then to increase dietary fiber and regular exercise. In addition, the medication regimen should be examined, because it may adversely affect normal bowel activity. Sometimes medication can be changed to reduce undesirable side effects, such as constipation.

Suppositories Some cathartics are given in the form of suppositories. These act in various ways: by softening the feces, by releasing gases such as carbon dioxide to distend the rectum, or by stimulating the nerve endings in the rectal mucosa. Suppositories need to be inserted beyond the internal anal sphincter.

Generally, suppositories are effective within 30 minutes. The best results can be obtained by inserting the suppository 30 minutes before the client's usual defecation time or when the peristaltic action is greatest, such as after breakfast. See Chapter 43, page 1355.

Antidiarrheal Medications Clients who have diarrhea may require antidiarrhetics. Some of these mechanically coat the irritated bowel and act as protectives (**demulcents**). Others absorb gas or toxic substances from the bowel (**adsorbents**) or shrink swollen and inflamed tissues (**astringents**). In certain situations, sedatives and antispasmodics may also be required. The box on page 1202 provides guidelines for using antidiarrheal medications.

ADMINISTERING ENEMAS

An **enema** is a solution introduced into the rectum and sigmoid colon. Its function is to remove feces and/or flatus. Enemas are classified into four groups, according to their action: cleansing, carminative, retention, or return flow.

A *cleansing enema* stimulates peristalsis by irritating the colon and rectum and/or by distending the intestine with

RESEARCH NOTE

How Can the Use of Laxatives, Suppositories, and Enemas Be Reduced to Control Constipation?

A two-phase, 16-week clinical study was conducted to determine whether the use of laxatives, suppositories, and enemas could be reduced through the use of a controlled bran supplement in clients already receiving a high-fiber diet. The study was conducted in an extended care facility, using a random sample of 50 subjects. Twenty-five subjects were assigned to the experimental group; the other 25 were assigned to a control group.

The first 3 weeks of the study (Phase 1) focused on assessment. Data collected on *all* subjects included (a) factors relevant to the development of constipation; (b) frequency, amount, and consistency of bowel movements; (c) 24-hour intake of foods and fluids; and (d) a count of the total daily laxatives, enemas, and suppositories given each week. No significant differences were found between the two groups on any of these variables.

In the remaining 13 weeks of the study (Phase II), subjects in the experimental group were given natural bran mixed in applesauce for breakfast every day. The bran was gradually increased from 1 tablespoon each day for 3 weeks, to 2 tablespoons each day for the next 3 weeks, and 3 tablespoons each day for the remaining weeks.

Findings indicated (a) a greater decline in laxative use in the experimental group than in the control group and (b) increased bowel regularity in the experimental group, 47%, compared to 15% in the control group. A major outcome of the study was a more precise understanding of the diagnosis and management process for dealing with constipation.

Implications: Accurate assessment data were critical in monitoring the results of this study. Practitioners can use the research procedures in this study to make relevant observations of functional patterns and the efficacy of nursing interventions and to make sound clinical decisions.

Source: J Mantle, Research and serendipitous secondary findings. *Canadian Nurse*, January 1992, 88:15–18.

GUIDELINES FOR USING ANTIDIARRHEAL MEDICATIONS

- If the diarrhea persists over 3 or 4 days, determine the underlying cause. Using medications such as opiates when the cause is an infection can prolong the diarrhea.
- Long-term use of over-the-counter medications, for example, loperamide hydrochloride (Imodium), can produce dependence.
- Some antidiarrheal agents can cause drowsiness, for example, diphenoxylate HCL (Lomotil), and should not be used when driving an automobile or running machinery.
- Chronic diarrhea (lasting 3 to 4 weeks) usually requires fluid and electrolyte replacement as well as pharmacologic intervention. Some causes are chemotherapy, laxative or alcohol abuse, surgery, and radiation.
- Opiates and their derivatives are the most effective antidiarrheal medications. The dose requirements are usually smaller than those required to treat pain.

the volume of fluid introduced. Two kinds of cleansing enemas are the high enema and the low enema. The *high enema* is given to clean as much of the colon as possible. It is often used before diagnostic studies. Often about 1000 mL (1 liter) of solution is administered to an adult. The client changes from the left lateral to the dorsal recumbent position and then to the right lateral position during the administration so that the fluid can follow the large intestine (Figure 40–1, earlier). The fluid is administered at a higher pressure than for a low enema; that is, the container of solution is held higher. Cleansing enemas are most effective if held for 5 to 10 minutes. The *low enema* is used to clean the rectum and the sigmoid colon only. About 500 mL (0.5 liters) of solution is administered to an adult, and the client maintains the left side-lying position during its administration.

A *carminative enema* is given primarily to expel flatus. The solution instilled into the rectum releases gas, which in turn distends the rectum and the colon, thus stimulating peristalsis. For an adult, 60 to 180 mL of fluid is instilled.

A *retention enema* introduces oil into the rectum and sigmoid colon. The oil is retained for a relatively long period of time (eg, 1 to 3 hours). It acts to soften the feces and to lubricate the rectum and anal canal, thus facilitating passage of the feces.

A *return flow enema*, sometimes referred to as the *Harris flush* or *colonic irrigation*, is used to expel flatus. Alternating flow of 100 to 200 mL of fluid into and out of the large intestine stimulates peristalsis and the expulsion of feces.

Various solutions are used for enemas. The specific solution may be ordered by the physician or indicated by agency protocol. Table 40–5 lists some of these solutions, giving the quantity and proportions frequently used.

Table 40–5 Types of Enemas for Adults

Solution	Constituents	Action	Time to Take Effect	Adverse Effects
Hypertonic	90 to 120 mL of solution (eg, sodium phosphate)	Distends colon, irritates mucosa	5 to 10 min	Retention of sodium
Hypotonic	500 to 1000 mL of tap water	Distends colon, stimulates peristalsis, and softens feces	15 to 20 min	Fluid and electrolyte imbalance; water intoxication
Isotonic	500 to 1000 mL of normal saline (9 mL NaCl to 1000 mL water)	Distends colon, stimulates peristalsis, and softens feces	15 to 20 min	Possible sodium retention
Soap	500 to 1000 mL (3 to 5 mL soap to 1000 mL of water)	Irritates mucosa, distends colon	10 to 15 min	Irritates and may damage mucosa
Oil (Mineral, olive, cottonseed)	90 to 120 mL	Lubricates the feces and the colonic mucosa	30 to 60 min	

Some agencies use commercially prepared disposable enemas. It is important that the nurse be aware that prepackaged enemas have their own instructions, which should be followed unless there are other instructions from the physician or the agency.

Clinical Guidelines for Administering Enemas Enemas for adults are usually given at 40 to 43 C (105 to 110 F); those for children are given at 37.7 C (100 F), unless otherwise specified. Some oil retention enemas are given at 33 C (91 F). High temperatures can be injurious to the bowel mucosa; cold temperatures are uncomfortable for the client and may trigger a spasm of the sphincter muscles.

The amount of solution to be administered depends on the kind of enema, the age of the person, and the person's ability to retain the solution. The following are approximate amounts:

Age	*Volume*
18 months	50 to 200 mL
18 months to 5 years	200 to 300 mL
5 to 12 years	300 to 500 mL
12 years and older	500 to 1000 mL

The rectal tube needs to be of an appropriate size:

Age	*Size*
Infant/small child	#10 to 12 Fr.
Toddler	#14 to 16 Fr.
School-age child	#16 to 18 Fr.
Adults	#22 to 30 Fr.

The force of flow of the solution is governed by the (a) height of the solution container, (b) size of the tubing, (c) viscosity of the fluid, and (d) resistance of the rectum. The higher the solution container is held above the rectum, the faster the flow and the greater the force (pressure) in the rectum. During most adult enemas, the solution container should be no higher than 30 cm (12 in) above the rectum. During a high cleansing enema, the solution container is usually held 30 to 45 cm (12 to 18 in) above the rectum, because the fluid is instilled farther to clean the entire bowel. For an infant, the solution container is held no more than 7.5 cm (3 in) above the rectum.

The time it takes to administer an enema largely depends on the amount of fluid to be instilled and the client's tolerance. Large volumes, such as 1000 mL, may take 10 to 15 minutes to instill; small volumes require less time.

The amount of time the client retains the enema solution depends on the purpose of the enema and the client's ability to contract the external sphincter to retain the solution. Oil retention enemas are usually retained 1 to 3 hours. Other enemas are normally retained 5 to 10 minutes.

Many children require an enema prior to undergoing gastrointestinal procedures; the procedure for giving an enema to an infant or child is similar to that for an adult. The enema solution should be isotonic (usually normal saline). If prepared saline is not available, the nurse can prepare it by mixing one teaspoon of table salt in 500 mL of tap water. Plain water is hypotonic and can therefore create a rapid fluid shift and fluid overload. Some hypertonic commercial solutions (eg, Fleet enema) can lead to hypovolemia and electrolyte imbalances. In addition, the osmotic effect of the Fleet enema may produce diarrhea and subsequent metabolic acidosis.

Infants and small children do not exhibit sphincter control and need to be assisted in retaining the enema. The nurse administers the enema while the infant or child is lying with the buttocks over the bedpan, and the nurse firmly presses the buttocks together to prevent the immediate expulsion of the solution. Older children can usually hold the solution if they understand what to do and are not required to hold it for too long a period. It may be necessary to ensure that the bathroom is available for an ambulatory child before starting the procedure or to have a bedpan ready.

Procedure 40–2 describes how to administer an enema.

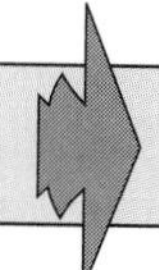

PROCEDURE 40–2 ADMINISTERING AN ENEMA

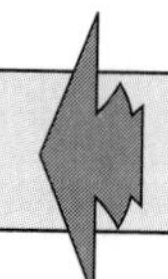

Before administering an enema, determine whether a physician's order is required. At some agencies, a physician must order the kind of enema and the time to give it, for example, the evening before surgery or the morning of the examination. When the client has rectal disease, the physician may also specify the size of the rectal tube to use. At other agencies, enemas are given at the nurses' discretion (ie, as necessary on a prn order). In addition, determine the presence of kidney or cardiac disease that contraindicates the use of a hypotonic solution.

PURPOSES

- To stimulate peristalsis and remove feces or flatus
- To soften feces and lubricate the rectum and colon
- To clean the rectum and colon in preparation for an examination
- To remove feces prior to a surgical procedure or a delivery, thereby preventing inadvertent defecation and subsequent contamination

ASSESSMENT FOCUS

When the client last had a bowel movement and the amount, color, and consistency of the feces; presence of abdominal distention (the distended abdomen appears swollen and feels firm rather than soft when palpated); whether the client has sphincter control; whether the client can use a toilet or commode or must remain in bed and use a bedpan.

EQUIPMENT

- ☐ Moistureproof absorbent pad
- ☐ Bath blanket
- ☐ Bedpan or commode if the client is unable to reach the bathroom
- ☐ Disposable enema unit with instructions for use

or

- ☐ Enema set containing:
  a. Container to hold the solution
  b. Tubing
  c. Clamp
  d. Rectal tube of the correct size
- ☐ Lubricant
- ☐ Thermometer to measure temperature of solution
- ☐ Prescribed amount of solution at the correct temperature
- ☐ Disposable gloves
- ☐ Disposable towel

INTERVENTION

1. Prepare the client.

- Explain the procedure to the client. Indicate that the client may experience a feeling of fullness while the solution is being administered. Careful explanation is especially important for the preschool child. *An enema is an intrusive procedure and therefore threatening.*
- Assist the adult client to a left lateral position, with the right leg as acutely flexed as possible (Figure 40–10). *This position facilitates the flow of solution by gravity into the sigmoid and descending colon, which are on the left side. Having the right leg acutely flexed provides for adequate exposure of the anus.*
- During a high cleansing enema, have the client change position from left lateral to dorsal recumbent and then to right lateral. *In this way the entire colon is reached by the fluid.*

PROCEDURE 40–2 *continued*

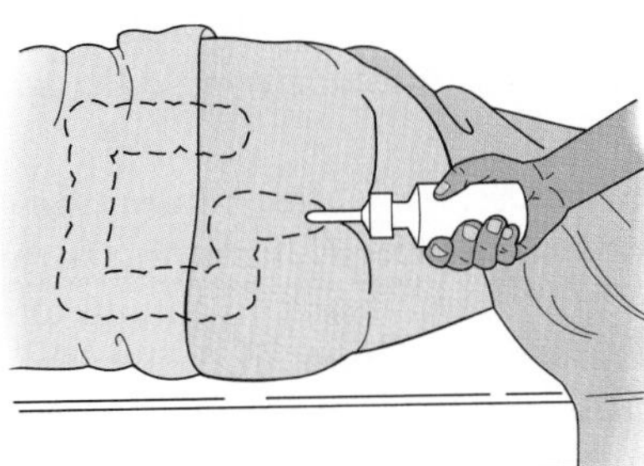

Figure 40–10 Assuming a left lateral position for an enema. Note the commercially prepared enema.

For infants and small children, the dorsal recumbent position is frequently used. Position them on a small padded bedpan with support for the back and head. Secure the legs by placing a diaper under the bedpan and then over and around the thighs.

- Place the waterproof pad under the client's buttocks to protect the bed linen, and drape the client with the bath blanket.

2. Prepare the equipment.

- Lubricate about 5 cm (2 in) of the rectal tube (some commercially prepared enema sets already have lubricated nozzles). *Lubrication facilitates insertion through the sphincters and minimizes trauma.*
- Open the clamp, and run some solution through the connecting tubing and the rectal tube to expel any air in the tubing; then close the clamp. *Air instilled into the rectum, although not harmful, causes unnecessary distention.*

3. Don gloves, and insert the rectal tube.

- For clients in the left lateral position, lift the upper buttock to ensure good visualization of the anus.

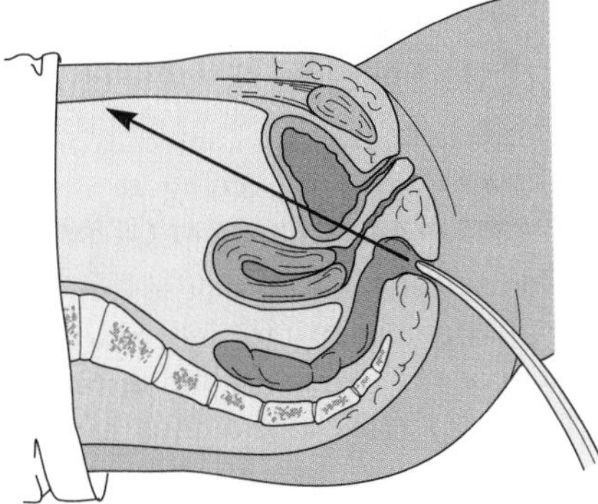

Figure 40–11 Inserting the rectal tube following the direction of the rectum.

- Insert the tube smoothly and slowly into the rectum, directing it toward the umbilicus (Figure 40–11). *The angle follows the normal contour of the rectum. Slow insertion prevents spasm of the sphincter.*
- Insert the tube 7 to 10 cm (3 to 4 in) in an adult. *Since the anal canal is about 2.5 to 5 cm (1 to 2 in) long in the adult, insertion to this point places the tip of the tube beyond the anal sphincter into the rectum.* Insert the tube 5 to 7.5 cm (2 to 3 in) in the child and only 2.5 to 3.75 cm (1 to 1.5 in) in the infant.
- If resistance is encountered at the internal sphincter, ask the client to take a deep breath, then run a small amount of solution through the tube to relax the internal anal sphincter.
- Never force tube entry. If resistance persists, withdraw the tube, and report the resistance to the nurse in charge.

4. Slowly administer the enema solution.

- Raise the solution container, and open the clamp to allow fluid flow.

  or

  Compress a pliable container by hand.
- During most adult low enemas, hold the solution container no higher than 30 cm (12 in) above the rectum. *The higher the solution container is held above the rectum, the faster the flow and the greater the force (pressure) in the rectum.* During a high enema, hold the solution container a little higher (eg, 45 cm [18 in]). *The fluid must be instilled farther to clean the entire bowel.* For children, lower the height of the solution container appropriately for the age of the child. See agency protocol.
- Administer the fluid slowly. If the client complains of fullness or pain, use the clamp to stop the flow for 30 seconds, and then restart the flow at a slower rate. *Administering the enema slowly and stopping the flow momentarily decrease the likelihood of intestinal spasm and premature ejection of the solution.*
- If you are using a plastic commercial container, roll it up as the fluid is instilled. *This prevents subsequent suctioning of the solution.*
- After all of the solution has been instilled or when the client cannot hold any more and wants to defecate (the urge to defecate usually indicates that sufficient fluid has been administered), close the clamp, and remove the rectal tube from the anus.
- Place the rectal tube in a disposable towel as you withdraw it.

5. Encourage the client to retain the enema.

- Ask the client to remain lying down. *It is easier for the client to retain the enema when lying down than when sitting or standing, because gravity promotes drainage and peristalsis.*

PROCEDURE 40–2 ADMINISTERING AN ENEMA *continued*

- To assist a small child in retaining the solution, apply firm pressure over the anus with tissue wipes, or firmly press the buttocks together.
- Ensure that the client retains the solution for the appropriate amount of time, for example, 5 to 10 minutes for a cleansing enema or at least 30 minutes for a retention enema.

6. Assist the client to defecate.

- Assist the client to a sitting position on the bedpan, commode, or toilet. *A sitting position facilitates the act of defecation.*
- Ask the client who is using the toilet not to flush it. *The nurse needs to observe the feces.*
- If a specimen of feces is required, ask the client to use a bedpan or commode.

7. Record and report relevant data.

- Record administration of the enema; type of solution; length of time solution was retained; the amount, color, and consistency of the returns; and the relief of flatus and abdominal distention.

Variation: Administering an Enema to an Incontinent Client

Occasionally a nurse needs to administer an enema to a client who is unable to control the external sphincter muscle and thus cannot retain the enema solution for even a few minutes. In that case, the client assumes a supine position on a bedpan. The head of the bed can be elevated slightly, to 30 degrees if necessary, and the client's head and back are supported by pillows. Pressing the buttocks together may help the client to retain the solution. The nurse wears gloves to prevent direct contact with the solution and feces that are expelled over the hand into the bedpan during the administration of the enema.

Variation: Administering a Return Flow Enema

Administering the return flow enema (the Harris flush, or colonic irrigation) is similar to administering and siphoning an enema. Initially, the solution (100 to 200 mL for an adult) is instilled into the client's rectum and sigmoid colon. Then the solution container is lowered so that the fluid flows back out through the rectal tube into the container. The inflow-outflow process is repeated five or six times (to stimulate peristalsis and the expulsion of flatus), and the solution is replaced several times during the procedure as it becomes thick with feces. A total of about 100 mL of solution is usually used for an adult.

EVALUATION FOCUS
Amount, color, and consistency of returns; relief of flatus or abdominal distention; any problems encountered (eg, resistance at the external or internal sphincter when inserting the rectal tube).

Siphoning an Enema In some instances, a client may be unable to expel the solution after administration of an enema. The solution must then be siphoned off. In siphoning, the nurse uses the force of gravity to draw the fluid out of the rectum and colon.

The equipment required is a bedpan, a disposable large plastic volume enema container, rectal tube, lubricant, and a container of water at 40 C (105 F). During siphoning, the client assumes a *right* side-lying position so that the sigmoid colon is uppermost, thus facilitating drainage of the solution from the rectum and the colon. The client lies on the bed with hips close to the side of the bed. The nurse places a bedpan on a chair at the side of the bed near the client's hips. The chair must be lower than the bed. The rectal tube is lubricated and attached to the partially filled enema set. The tube is filled with solution, then pinched and gently inserted into the rectum as for an enema. The nurse holds the enema container about 10 cm (4 in) above the anus, releases the pinched rectal tube, and quickly lowers the enema container. This action should draw the fluid from the colon and rectum, permitting it to flow through the rectal tube into the solution container. The nurse then notes the amount of fluid siphoned off, as well as the color, odor, and presence of any feces or abnormal constituents, such as blood or mucus.

DIGITAL REMOVAL OF A FECAL IMPACTION

Digital removal involves breaking up the fecal mass digitally and removing it in portions. Because the bowel mucosa can be injured during this procedure, some agencies restrict and specify the personnel permitted to conduct digital disimpactions. Rectal stimulation is also contraindicated for some people because it may cause an excessive vagal response resulting in cardiac arrhythmia. After a disimpaction, the nurse can use various interventions to remove remaining feces, such as a cleansing enema or the insertion of a suppository.

For digital removal of a fecal impaction, the nurse takes the following steps:

1. The client assumes a side-lying position, with the knees flexed and the back toward the nurse. Although some clients may prefer to stand by a toilet, the bed position is advised because disimpaction can be exhausting.
2. Place a waterproof bedpad under the client's buttocks and a bedpan nearby to receive stool.
3. Put on a pair of gloves, and liberally lubricate the index finger to be inserted.
4. Gently insert the index finger into the rectum, and move the finger toward the client's umbilicus, along the length of the rectum.
5. Loosen and dislodge stool by gently massaging around it. Break up stool by working the finger into the hardened mass, taking care to avoid injury to the mucosa of the rectum.
6. Carefully work stool downward to the end of the rectum and remove it in small pieces. Continue to remove as much fecal material as possible. Periodically assess the client for signs of fatigue, such as facial pallor, diaphoresis, or change in pulse rate. Manual stimulation should be minimal, since excessive vagal nerve stimulation could result in cardiac arrhythmia.
7. Following disimpaction, assist the client to clean the anal area and buttocks. Then assist the client onto a bedpan or commode for a short time, because digital stimulation of the rectum often induces the urge to defecate.

DECREASING FLATULENCE

There are several ways to reduce or prevent flatulence: not providing gas-producing foods, encouraging exercise, and repositioning clients are recommended. Encouraging ambulation is an effective means of reducing flatulence, since the motility stimulates reabsorption of gases in intestinal capillaries. A method of treating flatulence is to insert a rectal tube into the rectum and leave it there for varying lengths of time (generally no longer than 30 minutes, to prevent undue irritation to the rectal lining). The tube can then be reinserted, as needed, every 2 to 3 hours. Some nurses advocate connecting the open end of the rectal tube, via another tube, to a collecting receptacle. The passage of flatus is confirmed by noting bubbles in the water. The equipment required for relieving flatulence is shown in the accompanying box.

EQUIPMENT FOR RELIEVING FLATULENCE

- A rectal tube (#22 to #30 Fr for adults; #14 to #18 Fr for children, according to their age)
- Lubricant for the tip of the rectal tube
- A container in which to carry the lubricant and rectal tube to the bedside
- Tape to attach the rectal tube to the buttock (optional)
- Either a waterproof absorbent pad (eg, an abdominal or incontinence pad) to wrap around the open end of the rectal tube, or a connecting tube and a receptacle containing water

BOWEL TRAINING PROGRAMS

For clients who have chronic constipation, frequent impactions, or fecal incontinence, *bowel training programs* may be helpful. The program is based on factors within the client's control and is designed to help the client establish normal defecation. Such matters as food and fluid intake, exercise, and defecation habits are all considered. Before beginning such a program, clients must understand it and want to be involved. The major phases of the program are as follows:

- Determine the client's usual bowel habits and factors that help and hinder normal defecation.
- Design a plan with the client that includes the following:
  a. Fluid intake of about 2500 mL to 3000 mL per day
  b. Increase in fiber in the diet
  c. Intake of hot drinks, especially just before the usual defecation time
  d. Increase in exercise
- Maintain the following daily routine for 2 to 3 weeks:
  a. Administer a cathartic suppository (eg, Dulcolax) 30 minutes before the client's defecation time.
  b. When the client experiences the urge to defecate, assist the client to the toilet or commode or onto a bedpan. Note the length of time between the insertion of the suppository and the urge to defecate.
  c. Provide the client with privacy for defecation and a time limit; 30 to 40 minutes is usually sufficient.
  d. Teach the client to lean forward at the hips, apply pressure on the abdomen with the hands, and to bear down for defecation. These measures increase

pressure on the colon. Straining should be avoided, however, because it can cause hemorrhoids.

- Provide positive feedback when the client successfully defecates. Refrain from negative feedback if the client fails to defecate.
- Offer encouragement to the client, and convey that patience is often required. Many clients require weeks or months of training to achieve success.

FECAL INCONTINENCE POUCH

To collect and contain large volumes of feces, the nurse may place a fecal incontinence pouch (rectal pouch) around the anal area. The purpose of the pouch is to prevent progressive perianal skin irritation and breakdown and frequent linen changes necessitated by incontinence. In many agencies, the pouch is replacing the traditional approach to this problem, that is, inserting a large Foley catheter into the client's rectum and inflating the balloon to keep it in place—a practice that may damage the rectal sphincter and rectal mucosa. Some nurses also believe that a rectal catheter increases peristalsis and increases incontinence by stimulating sensory nerve fibers in the rectum.

A rectal pouch is secured around the anal opening and may or may not be attached to drainage. Pouches are best applied before the perianal skin becomes excoriated. If perianal skin excoriation is present, the nurse either (a) applies a moisture barrier cream to the skin to protect it from feces until it heals, and then applies the pouch (Freedman 1991, p. 105); or (b) applies a protective powder, skin barrier, or hydrocolloid wafer such as Duoderm (see Table 44–3, p. 1370) underneath the pouch to achieve the best possible seal. To apply a pouch, the nurse follows these steps:

- Position the client on one side, with the knees drawn up to expose the anal area. For maximal exposure, have an assistant retract the buttocks.
- Clean and dry the skin thoroughly.
- Shave excessive perianal hair within the pouch area that may prevent a secure seal with the pouch wafer.
- Apply a protective skin sealant (eg, Prep Site) to the skin, and let it air dry.
- Cut the opening of the fecal pouch slightly larger than the anus (eg, about 6.6 cm, or ¼ inch, larger than the anal opening).
- Remove the paper backing from the pouch and apply the pouch, following the manufacturer's instructions.
- Hold and press the wafer against the skin for at least 30 seconds to enhance adherence.
- Seal the edges of the wafer with waterproof tape (optional).
- Connect the pouch to a drainage bag, or, if stool is thick, cut off the port at the base of the pouch and use a clamp to close the pouch.

Nursing responsibilities for clients with a rectal pouch include (a) regular assessment and documentation of the perianal skin status; (b) changing the bag every 72 hours or sooner if there is leakage; (c) maintaining the drainage system; and (d) providing explanations and support to the client and support persons.

ABDOMINAL MASSAGE

Abdominal massage may be used to stimulate peristalsis and manage chronic constipation in clients with major neuromusculoskeletal disabilities (Emly 1993, p. 34). Because these clients have decreased muscle tone and minimal functional movement or ambulation, immobility is a major factor contributing to their constipation. Abdominal massage negates the need for regular suppositories and enemas and is less invasive. It may be performed by a physiotherapist or nurse with specialized training. The procedure takes about 15 to 20 minutes. The abdomen is massaged along the line of the colon, beginning in the right iliac fossa and moving along the ascending, transverse, and descending colons. More research is required to obtain a deeper understanding of this approach to manage constipation and to determine which clients would benefit most.

BOWEL DIVERSION OSTOMIES

An **ostomy** is an opening on the abdominal wall for the elimination of feces or urine. There are many types of ostomies. A **gastrostomy** is an opening through the abdominal wall into the stomach. A **jejunostomy** is an opening through the abdominal wall into the jejunum. An **ileostomy** is an opening into the ileum (small bowel). A **colostomy** is an opening into the colon (large bowel). A **ureterostomy** is an opening into the ureter. Gastrostomies and jejunostomies are generally performed to provide an alternate feeding route. The purpose of bowel and urinary ostomies is to divert and drain fecal or urinary material. Urinary diversion ostomies are discussed in Chapter 41 on page 1263. **Bowel diversion ostomies** are often classified according to (a) their status as permanent or temporary, (b) their anatomic location, and (c) the construction of the **stoma,** the opening created in the abdominal wall by the ostomy.

Permanence Colostomies can be either temporary or permanent. Temporary colostomies are generally performed for traumatic injuries or inflammatory conditions of the bowel. They allow the distal diseased portion of the bowel to rest and heal. Permanent colostomies are performed to provide a means of elimination when the rec-

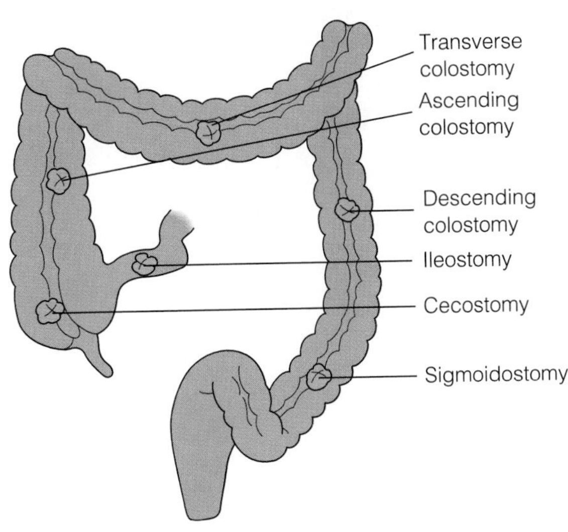

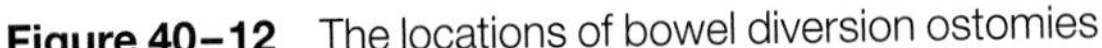

Figure 40–12 The locations of bowel diversion ostomies.

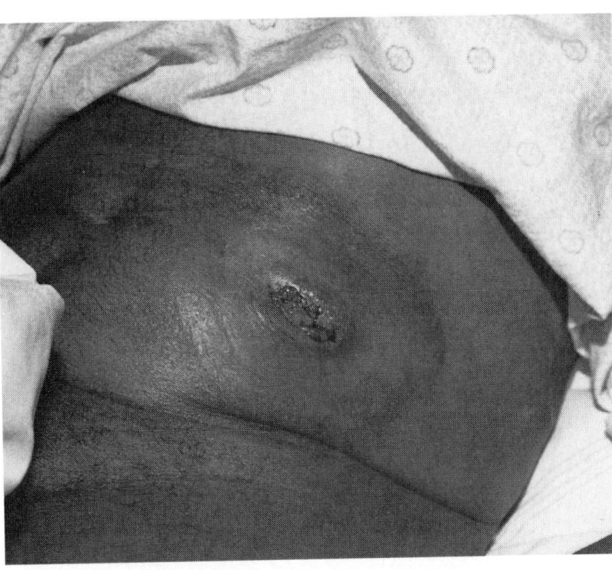

Figure 40–13 A colostomy stoma.

tum or anus is nonfunctional as a result of a birth defect or a disease such as cancer of the bowel. The diseased portion may or may not be removed.

Anatomic Location An ileostomy generally empties from the distal end of the small intestine. A cecostomy empties from the cecum (the first part of the ascending colon). An ascending colostomy empties from the ascending colon. A transverse colostomy empties from the transverse colon. A descending colostomy empties from the descending colon. A sigmoidostomy empties from the sigmoid colon (Figure 40–12).

The location of the ostomy influences the character and management of the fecal drainage. The farther along the bowel, the more formed the stool, because the large bowel reabsorbs water from the fecal mass. In addition, more control over the frequency of stomal discharge can be established. For example:

- An ileostomy produces liquid fecal drainage. Drainage is constant and cannot be regulated. Ileostomy drainage contains some digestive enzymes, which are damaging to the skin. For this reason, ileostomy clients must wear an appliance continuously and take special precautions to prevent skin breakdown. Compared to colostomies, however, odor is minimal because fewer bacteria are present.
- An ascending colostomy is similar to an ileostomy in that the drainage is liquid and cannot be regulated, and digestive enzymes are present. Odor, however, is a problem requiring control (eg, a deodorant inside the appliance).
- A transverse colostomy produces a malodorous, mushy drainage because some of the liquid has been reabsorbed. There is usually no control.
- A descending colostomy produces increasingly solid fecal drainage. Stools from a sigmoidostomy are of normal or formed consistency, and the frequency of discharge can be regulated. People with a sigmoidostomy may not have to wear an appliance at all times, and odors can usually be controlled.

The length of time that an ostomy is in place also helps to determine the consistency of the stool, particularly with transverse and descending colostomies. Over time, the stool becomes more formed because the remaining functioning portions of the colon tend to compensate by increasing water reabsorption.

Stoma and Skin Care Care of the stoma (Figure 40–13) and skin is important for all clients who have ostomies. The fecal material from a colostomy or ileostomy is irritating to the peristomal skin. This is particularly true of ileal effluent, which contains digestive enzymes. It is important to assess the peristomal skin for irritation each time the appliance is changed. See the box on page 1210 for assessing a stoma. Any irritation or skin breakdown needs to be treated immediately. The skin is kept clean by washing off any excretion and then dried thoroughly. A barrier such as karaya is applied over the skin around the stoma to prevent contact with any excretion. An appliance (bag) is then fitted to the stoma so that there is no leakage around it. It is exceedingly important to dry the skin before attaching the appliance. The pouch will not adhere

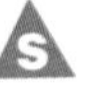

ASSESSING A STOMA

- *Stoma color:* The stoma should appear red, similar in color to the mucosal lining of the inner cheek. Very pale or darker-colored stomas with a bluish or purplish hue indicate impaired blood circulation to the area.
- *Stoma size and shape:* Most stomas protrude slightly from the abdomen. New stomas normally appear swollen, but swelling generally decreases over 2 or 3 weeks or for as long as 6 weeks. Failure of swelling to recede may indicate a problem, such as blockage.
- *Stomal bleeding:* Slight bleeding initially when the stoma is touched is normal, but other bleeding should be reported.
- *Status of peristomal skin:* Any redness and irritation of the peristomal skin—the 5 to 13 cm (2 to 5 in) of skin surrounding the stoma—should be noted. Transient redness after removal of adhesive is normal.
- *Amount and type of feces:* For ileal effluent and feces (colostomy effluent), assess the amount, color, odor, and consistency. Inspect for abnormalities, such as pus or blood. For a urinary diversion ostomy, assess the amount, color, clarity, and odor of the urine.
- *Complaints:* Complaints of burning sensation under the faceplate may indicate skin breakdown. The presence of abdominal discomfort and/or distention also needs to be determined.

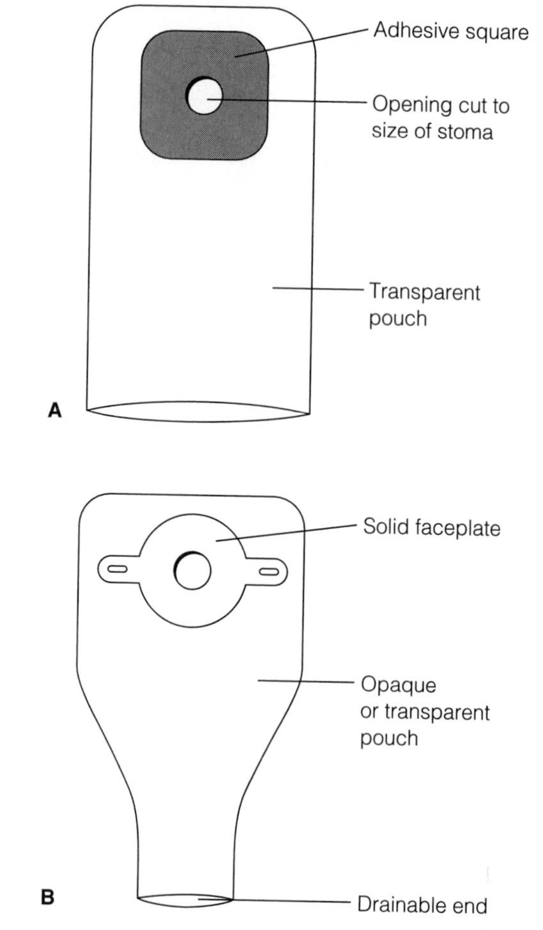

Figure 40–14 Ostomy appliances: *A,* temporary, disposable; *B,* permanent, resuable.

to moist skin, causing effluent to leak onto the skin. Numerous pouch systems are commercially available. All appliances have three features in common: a pouch to collect the effluent, an outlet at the bottom for easy emptying, and a faceplate. Temporary, disposable pouches are made of transparent plastic and have a peel-off adhesive square into which a hole the size of the stoma is cut. Permanent pouches may be clear or opaque, rubber or vinyl, and have a solid ring faceplate that fits around the stoma (Figure 40–14).

Odor control is essential to clients' self-esteem. As soon as clients are ambulatory, they can learn to work with the ostomy in the bathroom to avoid odors at the bedside. Selecting the appropriate kind of appliance promotes odor control. An intact appliance contains odors. The appliance should be rinsed thoroughly when it is emptied. Deodorizers can be placed in the pouch of the appliance, or pouches with charcoal filter discs are available. Some recommend oral intake of charcoal or bismuth subcarbonate, which should be taken only with the physician's approval. Many agencies employ an enterostomal therapy nurse who can assist in selecting the appliance.

Disposable ostomy appliances can be applied for up to 7 days. They need to be changed whenever the effluent leaks onto the peristomal skin or when it cannot be rinsed completely away. Many people prefer to change them daily or whenever they become soiled, but this practice can be detrimental to the integrity of the peristomal skin and is expensive. Check agency practice in this regard. Erickson (1987, p. 314) recommends removing the pouch and skin barrier twice a week to clean and inspect the peristomal skin. If the peristomal skin is erythematous, Broadwell (1987, p. 331) recommends removing and changing the system every 48 to 72 hours; if the skin is eroded, denuded, or ulcerated, it should be changed every 24 to 48 hours to allow appropriate treatment of the skin. More frequent changes are recommended if the client complains of pain or discomfort. Procedure 40–3 explains how to change a bowel diversion ostomy appliance.

Text continued on page 1215

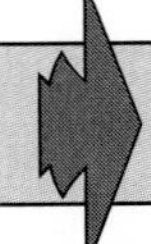

PROCEDURE 40-3 CHANGING A BOWEL DIVERSION OSTOMY APPLIANCE

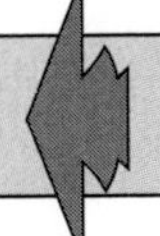

Before changing a bowel diversion ostomy appliance, determine the kind of ostomy and its placement on the abdomen. It is important to confirm which is the functioning stoma and any orders about the care of the stomas.

PURPOSES

- To assess and care for the persistomal skin
- To collect effluent for assessment of the amount and type of output
- To minimize odors for the client's comfort and self-esteem

ASSESSMENT FOCUS
Stoma size and shape; color of stoma; presence of swelling; status of peristomal skin; amount and type of effluent; allergy to tape; type and size of appliance currently used; complaints of discomfort; client and support persons learning needs; client's emotional status.

EQUIPMENT

- ☐ Disposable gloves
- ☐ Electric or safety razor
- ☐ Bedpan
- ☐ Solvent (presaturated sponges or liquid)
- ☐ Moistureproof bag (for disposable pouches)
- ☐ Cleaning materials, including tissues, warm water, mild soap (optional), washcloth or cotton balls, towel
- ☐ Tissue or gauze pad
- ☐ Peristomal skin paste or powder
- ☐ Skin barrier (liquid protective covering or peristomal skin barrier)
- ☐ Measuring guide
- ☐ Pen or pencil
- ☐ Scissors
- ☐ Cardboard or heavy paper with which to create a template of the stoma pattern (for solid wafer or disc skin barrier)
- ☐ Clean ostomy appliance,with optional belt
- ☐ Tail closure or elastic band
- ☐ Special adhesive and brush, if needed
- ☐ Stoma guidestrip, if needed
- ☐ Deodorant (liquid or tablet) for a nonodorproof colostomy bag
- ☐ Tape for securing a detachable faceplate as necessary

INTERVENTION

1. Determine the need for appliance change.

- Assess the used appliance for leakage of effluent. *Effluent can irritate the peristomal skin.*
- Ask the client about any discomfort at or around the stoma. *A burning sensation may indicate breakdown beneath the faceplate of the pouch.*
- Assess the fullness of the pouch. Pouches need to be emptied when they are one-third to one-half full. *The weight of an overly full bag may loosen the faceplate and separate it from the skin, causing the effluent to leak and irritate the peristomal skin.*
- If there is pouch leakage or discomfort at or around the stoma, change the appliance.

2. Select an appropriate time.

- Avoid times close to meal or visiting hours. *Ostomy odor and effluent may reduce appetite or embarrass the client.*
- Avoid times immediately after the administration of any medications that may stimulate bowel evacuation. *It is best to change the pouch when drainage is least likely to occur.*

3. Prepare the client and support persons.

- Explain the procedure to the client and support persons. Changing an ostomy appliance should not cause discomfort, but it may be distasteful to the client. *Support persons are often more supportive if properly informed.*
- Communicate acceptance and support to the client. It is important to change the appliance competently and quickly and not to convey disgust.
- Provide privacy, preferably in the bathroom, where clients can learn to deal with the ostomy as they would at home.
- Assist the client to a comfortable sitting or lying position in bed or preferably a sitting or standing position in the bathroom. *Lying or standing positions may facilitate*

PROCEDURE 40–3 CHANGING A BOWEL DIVERSION OSTOMY APPLIANCE *continued*

smoother pouch application, that is, avoid wrinkles.

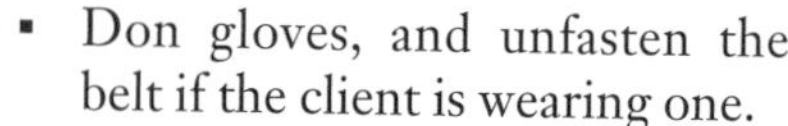

- Don gloves, and unfasten the belt if the client is wearing one.

4. Shave the peristomal skin of well-established ostomies as needed.

- Use an electric or safety razor on a regular basis to remove excessive hair. *Hair follicles can become irritated or infected by repeated pulling out of hairs during removal of the appliance and skin barrier.*

5. Empty and remove the ostomy appliance.

- Empty the contents of the pouch through the bottom opening into a bedpan. *Emptying before removing the pouch prevents spillage of effluent onto the client's skin.*
- Assess the consistency and the amount of effluent.
- If needed, apply an adhesive solvent to remove the appliance. This is not needed in most cases and should be used only when absolutely necessary.
- Peel the bag off slowly while holding the client's skin taut. *Holding the skin taut minimizes client discomfort and prevents abrasion of the skin.*
- If the appliance is disposable, discard it in a moistureproof bag.

6. Clean and dry the peristomal skin and stoma.

- Use toilet tissue to remove excess stool.
- Use warm water, mild soap (optional), and cotton balls or a washcloth and towel to clean the skin and stoma. Check agency practice on the use of soap. *Soap is sometimes not advised because it can be irritating to the skin.*

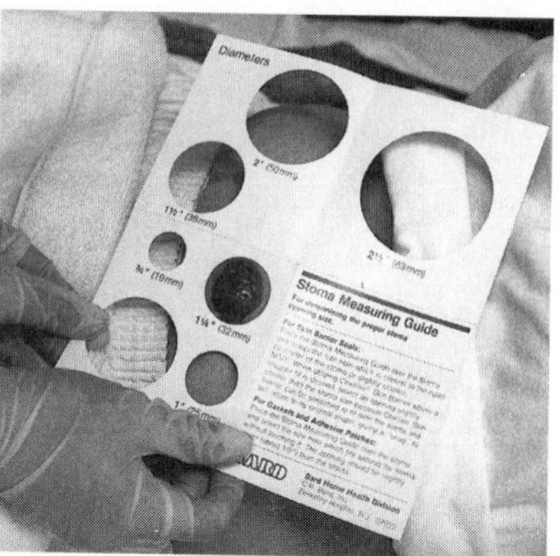

Figure 40–15 A guide for measuring the stoma.

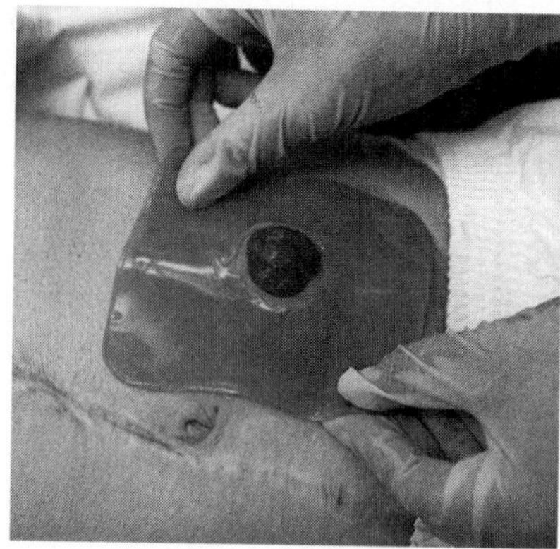

Figure 40–16 Centering the skin barrier over the stoma.

- Use a special skin cleanser to remove dried, hard stool. *This emulsifies the stool, making removal less damaging to the skin.*
- Dry the area thoroughly by patting with a towel or cotton swabs. *Excess rubbing can abrade the skin.*

7. Assess the stoma and peristomal skin.

- Inspect the stoma for color, size, shape, and bleeding.
- Inspect the peristomal skin for any redness, ulceration, or irritation. Transient redness *after the removal of adhesive* is normal.
- Place a piece of tissue or gauze pad over the stoma, and change it as needed. *This absorbs any seepage from the stoma.*

8. Apply paste-type skin barrier if needed.

- Fill in abdominal creases or dimples with paste. *This establishes a smooth surface for application of the skin barrier and pouch.*
- Allow the paste to dry for 1 to 2 minutes or as recommended by the manufacturer.

9. Prepare and apply the skin barrier (peristomal seal).

For a Solid Wafer or Disc Skin Barrier

- Use the guide (Figure 40–15) to measure the size of the stoma.
- On the backing of the skin barrier, trace a circle the same size as the stomal opening.
- Make a template (mold) out of cardboard or heavy paper of the stoma pattern. Keep this template for future use. *A template aids other nurses and the client with future appliance changes.* However, the template will need to be adjusted as the stoma size decreases.
- Cut out the traced stoma pattern to make an opening in the skin barrier.
- Remove the backing to expose the sticky adhesive side.
- Center the skin barrier over the stoma, and gently press it onto the client's skin, smoothing out any wrinkles or bubbles (Figure 40–16).

For Liquid Skin Sealant

- Cover the stoma with a gauze pad. *This prevents contact with the skin sealant.*

PROCEDURE 40–3 *continued*

- Either wipe the product evenly around the peristomal skin, or use a brush to apply a thin layer of the liquid plastic coating to the same area.
- Allow the skin barrier to dry until it no longer feels tacky.

10. Fill in any exposed skin around an irregularly shaped stoma.

- Apply paste to any exposed skin areas. Use a nonalcohol-based product if the skin is excoriated. *Alcohol may cause stinging and burning.*
  or
- Sprinkle peristomal powder on the skin, wipe off the excess, and dab the powder with a slightly moist gauze or an applicator moistened with a liquid skin barrier. *This creates a barrier or seal.*

11. Prepare and apply the clean appliance.

- Remove the tissue over the stoma before applying the pouch.

For a Disposable Pouch with Adhesive Square

- If the appliance does not have a precut opening, trace a circle 0.3 to 0.4 cm (1/8 to 1/6 in) larger than the stoma size on the appliance's adhesive square. *The opening is made slightly larger than the stoma to prevent rubbing, cutting, or trauma to the stoma.*
- Cut out a circle in the adhesive. Take care not to cut any portion of the pouch.
- Peel off the backing from the adhesive seal.
- Center the opening of the pouch over the client's stoma, and apply it directly onto the skin barrier (Figure 40–17).

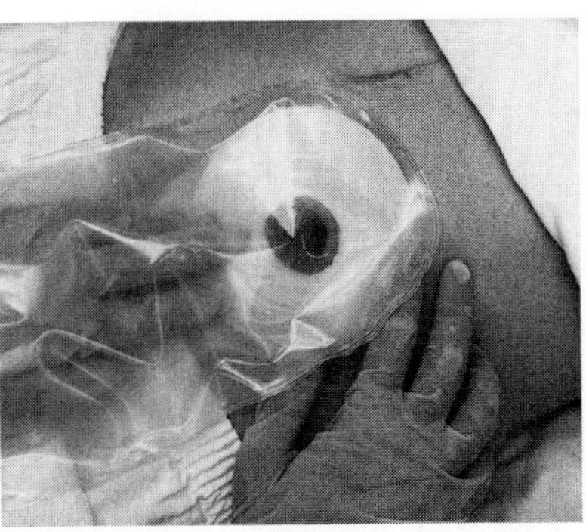

Figure 40–17 Applying the disposable pouch.

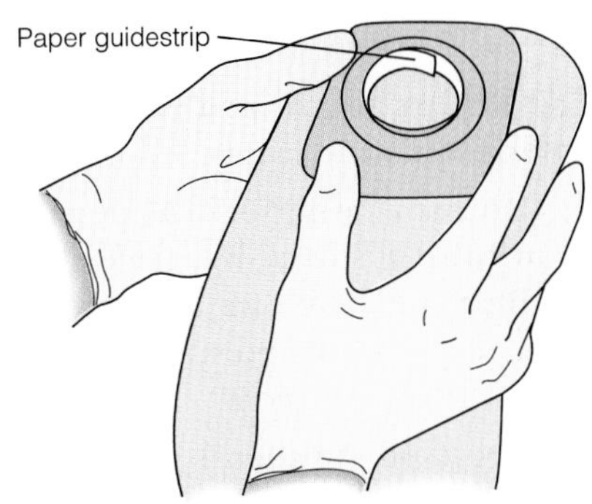

Figure 40–18 The coiled paper guidestrip in the faceplate opening.

- Gently press the adhesive backing onto the skin and smooth out any wrinkles, working from the stoma outward. *Wrinkles allow seepage of effluent, which can irritate the skin or soil clothing.*
- Remove the air from the pouch. *Removing the air helps the pouch lie flat against the abdomen.*
- Place a deodorant in the pouch (optional).
- Close the pouch by turning up the bottom a few times, fanfolding its end lengthwise and securing it with a rubber band or tail closure clamp.

For a Reusable Pouch with Faceplate Attached

- Apply either adhesive cement or a double-faced adhesive disc to the faceplate of the appliance, depending on the type of appliance being used. Follow the manufacturer's directions.
- Insert a coiled paper guidestrip (15-cm [6-in] strip of 1.3-cm [1/2-in] wide paper) into the faceplate opening (Figure 40–18). The strip should protrude slightly from the opening and expand to fit it. *The guidestrip helps the nurse center the appliance over the stoma and prevents pressure or irritation to the stoma due to an ill-fitting appliance.*
- Using the guidestrip, center the faceplate over the stoma.
- Firmly press the adhesive seal to the peristomal skin. The guidestrip will fall into the pouch; commercially prepared guidestrips will dissolve in the pouch.
- Place a deodorant in the bag if the bag is not odorproof. Most pouches are odorproof.
- Close the end of the pouch with the designated clamp.
- Attach the pouch belt, and fasten it around the client's waist (optional).

12. Dispose of equipment, or clean reusable equipment.

- Discard disposable bags in plastic bags before placing in the waste container.
- If feces is liquid, measure its volume before emptying the feces into a toilet or hopper.
- Wash reusable bags with cool water and mild soap, rinse, and dry.
- Wash a soiled belt with warm water and mild soap, rinse, and dry.

➤

PROCEDURE 40–3 CHANGING A BOWEL DIVERSION OSTOMY APPLIANCE *continued*

- Remove and discard gloves.

13. Report and record pertinent assessments and interventions.

- Report to the nurse in charge any increase in stoma size, change in color indicative of circulatory impairment, and presence of skin irritation or erosion.
- Record on the client's chart discoloration of the stoma; the appearance of the peristomal skin; the amount and type of drainage; the client's fatigue, discomfort, and significant behavior about the ostomy; and skills learned.
- Adjust the teaching plan and nursing care plan as needed. Include on the teaching plan the equipment and procedure used. *Client learning is facilitated by consistent nursing interventions.*

Variation: Applying a Reusable Pouch with Detachable Faceplate

- Note allergies and the results of tape patch test performed before surgery.
- Some nurses recommend applying a skin sealant (eg, Skin Prep) to the faceplate before attaching the adhesive disc. *This makes it easier to remove the adhesive disc from the faceplate.*
- Remove the protective paper strip from one side of the double-faced adhesive disc.
- Apply the sticky side to the back of the faceplate.
- Remove the remaining protective paper strip from the other side of the adhesive disc.
- Center the faceplate over the stoma and skin barrier, then press and hold the faceplate against the client's skin for a few minutes to secure the seal.

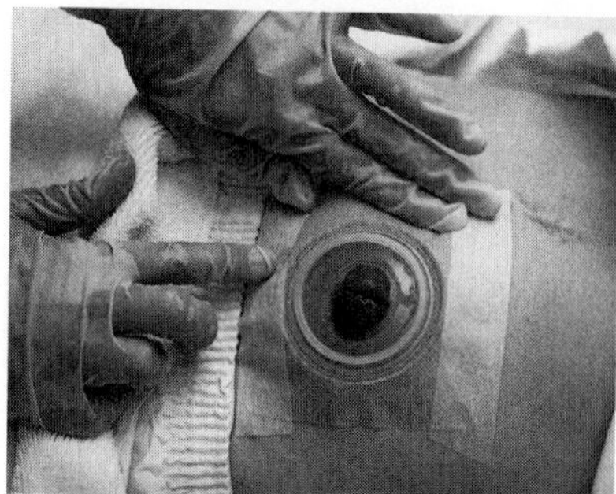

Figure 40–19 Taping the faceplate to the client's abdomen.

- Press the adhesive around the circumference of the adhesive disc.
- Tape the faceplate to the client's abdomen using four or eight 7.5-cm (3-in) strips of hypoallergenic tape. Place the strips around the faceplate in a "picture-framing" manner, one strip down each side, one across the top, and one across the bottom (Figure 40–19). The additional four strips can be placed diagonally over the other tapes to secure the seal.
- Stretch the opening on the back of the pouch, and position it over the base of the faceplate. Ease it over the faceplate flange.
- Place the lock ring between the pouch and the faceplate flange (Figure 40–20) to seal the pouch against the faceplate.
- Close the base of the pouch with the appropriate clamp.
- Attach the pouch belt, and fasten it around the client's waist (optional).

Variation: Applying the Skin Barrier and Appliance as One Unit

If a disc- or wafer-type skin barrier is used, the skin barrier and appliance can be applied as one unit. Applying the skin barrier and the appliance together not only is quicker but also is thought to reduce the chance of wrinkles. It also is easier for the client to apply without help.

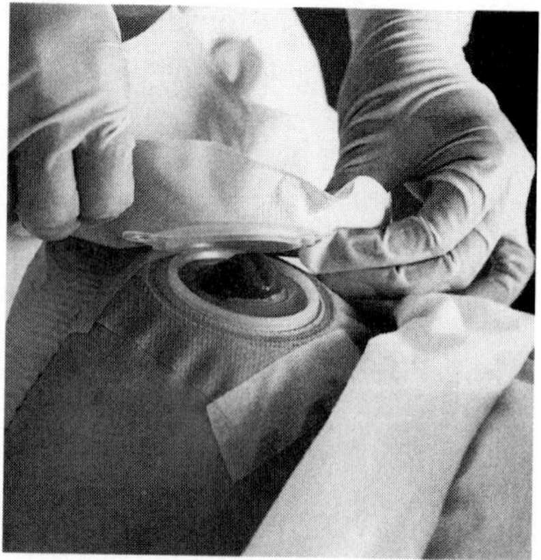

Figure 40–20 Sealing the pouch against the faceplate.

- Prepare the skin barrier by measuring the size of the stoma, tracing a circle on the backing of the skin barrier, and cutting out the traced stoma pattern to make an opening in the skin barrier.
- Prepare the appliance by cutting an opening 0.3 to 0.4 cm (1/8 to 1/6 in) larger than the stoma size (if not already present) and peeling off the backing from the adhesive seal.
- Center the opening of the pouch over the skin barrier.
- Remove the skin barrier backing to expose the sticky adhesive side.
- Center the skin barrier and appliance over the stoma, and press it onto the client's skin.

EVALUATION FOCUS
Color and size of stoma; amount, color, and consistency of feces; status of peristomal skin; client responses.

Colostomy Irrigation A colostomy irrigation, similar to an enema, is a form of stoma management used only for clients who have a sigmoid or descending colostomy. It is not done for ileostomies, because the feces are usually liquid. The purpose of irrigation is to distend the bowel sufficiently to stimulate peristalsis, which stimulates evacuation. When a regular evacuation pattern is achieved, the wearing of a colostomy pouch is unnecessary.

Routine daily irrigations for control of the time of elimination ultimately become the client's decision. Some clients prefer to control the time of elimination through rigid dietary regulation and not be bothered with irrigations, which can take up to an hour to complete. When regulation by irrigation is chosen, it should be done at the same time each day. Control by irrigations also necessitates some control of the diet. For example, laxative foods that might cause an unexpected evacuation need to be avoided.

For most clients, a relatively small amount of fluid (300 to 500 mL) stimulates evacuation. For others, up to 1000 mL may be needed, because a colostomy has no sphincter and the fluid tends to return as it is instilled. This problem is reduced by the use of a cone on the irrigating catheter. The cone helps to hold the fluid within the bowel during the irrigation.

Before starting an irrigation, assess the client's readiness to select and use the equipment. Because many types of irrigation sets are available, clients should begin with a "starter set" until they are familiar with the colostomy and the problems of irrigating it. Later, with the help of an enterostomal therapy nurse or a qualified person from a surgical supply house, the client can select the set most appropriate for the client's needs.

If the client has had a colostomy for a long time, the irrigation needs to be given at the time the client has established, or the pattern of regularity will be disrupted. For a newly established colostomy, select a time based on the client's previous bowel habits and one that will allow the client to participate in usual daily activities. Encourage the client to select the time and to maintain it.

For colostomy irrigation, see the *Procedures Manual* accompanying this text.

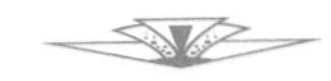

EVALUATING

Evaluation activities may include the following:

- Observing the character of stool
- Recording the frequency of defecation
- Measuring the client's fluid intake and output
- Inspecting the anal, perianal, or peristomal skin
- Palpating the abdomen for distention
- Auscultating the abdomen for bowel sounds
- Asking the client about flatulence, feelings of rectal fullness, abdominal discomfort before or during defecation, straining at defecation, or urgency
- Observing the client demonstrate self-care skills for ostomy managment
- Questioning the client about dietary intake, daily exercise, or other measures implemented to relieve or eliminate contributing factors

If outcomes are not achieved, the nurse should explore the reasons. The nurse might consider the following questions:

- Were baseline data complete and validated?
- Were contributing factors of nursing diagnoses identified correctly?
- Were all factors affecting the client's bowel elimination pattern considered?
- Was enough time allowed for goal achievement?
- Did the client fail to comply with dietary alterations or other planned interventions?
- Were all appropriate measures implemented to prevent skin breakdown?
- Did the client misinterpret health instructions?
- Were sufficient physical and emotional support provided?

CRITICAL PATHWAY FOR EMMA BROWN

ASSESSMENT DATA

Nursing Assessment

Mrs Emma Brown is a 78-year-old widow of 9 months. She lives alone in a low-income housing complex for the elderly. Her two children live with their families in a city approximately 150 miles away. She has always enjoyed cooking for her family in the past; however, now that she is alone, she does not enjoy cooking for herself. As a result, she has developed irregular eating patterns and tends to prepare soup-and-toast meals. She does not walk or exercise very much. She has bouts of insomnia since her husband's death. Lately, Mrs Brown has been having a problem with constipation. She has a bowel movement approximately every 3 or 4 days, and her stools are hard and painful to excrete. Mrs Brown has noticed increasing abdominal discomfort, anorexia, and a low-grade fever in the last week. She tells the county public health nurse about these symptoms and reports that her bowels have not moved in 5 days. The nurse refers Mrs Brown to her personal medical doctor, who diagnoses acute diverticulitis and admits her to the hospital for bowel rest, IV fluids, and antibiotics.

Physical Examination

Height: 162 cm (5′6″)
Weight: 65 kg (143 lb)
Temperature: 36.2 C (97.2 F)
Pulse rate: 82 bpm
Respirations: 20 per minute at rest
Blood pressure: 128/74 mm Hg
Active bowel sounds
Abdomen slightly distended

Diagnostic Data

WBC: 12,000/μL
Hgb: 12.4 g/dL
Urine: negative

CRITICAL PATHWAY FOR CLIENT WITH DIVERTICULITIS AND CONSTIPATION

Expected length of stay 5 to 6 days

	Date ________ Day 1	Date ________ Day 2	Date ________ Day 3
Daily outcomes	Client will ▪ have stable vital signs. ▪ have an intake of 2000 mL/day (IV). ▪ remain free of nausea and vomiting. ▪ state control of pain. ▪ verbalize understanding of ongoing care. ▪ have a soft, non-distended abdomen. ▪ verbalize ability to cope.	Client will ▪ have stable vital signs. ▪ have an intake of 2000 mL/day (IV). ▪ remain free of nausea and vomiting. ▪ state control of pain. ▪ verbalize understanding of ongoing care. ▪ have a soft, non-distended abdomen. ▪ verbalize ability to cope.	Client will ▪ have stable vital signs. ▪ have an intake of 2000 mL/day (IV/PO). ▪ state control of pain. ▪ verbalize understanding of ongoing care. ▪ have a soft, non-distended abdomen, active bowel sounds. ▪ tolerate clear liquids without nausea and vomiting. ▪ verbalize ability to cope. ▪ verbalize beginning understanding of home care instructions.
Tests and treatments	CBC with differential. Electrolytes. Abdominal X-ray studies.	Blood culture × 2, if temp over 38.3 C (101 F). Vital signs q4h if stable.	Blood culture × 2, if temp over 38.3 C (101 F). Vital signs q4h if stable.

	Day 1 *continued*	Day 2 *continued*	Day 3 *continued*
Tests and treatments *continued*	Blood culture × 2, if temp over 38.3 C (101 F). Vital signs q4h if stable. Assess gastrointestinal status q4h and prn. Intake and output q shift.	Assess gastrointestinal status q4h and prn. Intake and output q shift.	Assess gastrointestinal status q4h and prn. Intake and output q shift.
Knowledge deficit	Orient to room and hospital routine. Review plan of care and importance of bowel rest, bed rest, and emotional rest.	Review plan of care and continued importance of bowel rest, bed rest, and emotional rest.	Reinforce earlier teaching regarding ongoing care. Begin discharge, teaching regarding rest, activity, and diet.
Psycho-social	Assess level of anxiety. Encourage verbalization of concerns. Provide information. Provide ongoing support and encouragement.	Assess level of anxiety. Encourage verbalization of concerns. Provide information. Provide ongoing support and encouragement.	Encourage verbalization of concerns. Provide ongoing support and encouragement.
Diet	NPO. Mouth care prn.	NPO. Mouth care prn.	Begin warm, clear liquids to tolerance.
Activity	Provide safety precautions. Bed rest with commode privileges. Provide rest periods. Assist with ADLs.	Provide safety precautions. Bathroom privileges with assistance. Provide rest periods. Assist with ADLs.	Provide safety precautions. Up to chair ad lib. Provide rest periods Assist with ADLs.
Medications	IV fluids. IV antibiotics. IM/IV analgesics. Tylenol 650 mg q4h PO for temp over 38.3 C (101 F).	IV fluids. IV antibiotics. IM/IV analgesics. Tylenol 650 mg q4h PO for temp over 38.3 C (101 F).	IV fluids. IV antibiotics. IM analgesics. Tylenol 650 mg q4h PO for temp over 38.3 C (101 F).
Bowel manage-ment	Assess usual bowel elimination pattern. Assess gastrointestinal status q4h and prn. Report worsening abdominal pain, nausea, vomiting, or increasing abdominal distention.	Assess gastrointestinal status q4h and prn. Report worsening abdominal pain, nausea, vomiting, or increasing abdominal distention.	Assess gastrointestinal status q4h and prn. Report worsening abdominal pain, nausea, vomiting, or increasing abdominal distention.
Transfer/ discharge plans	Review discharge goals with client and significant other. Consult with social service re: projected needs for home health care (if any).	Review progress towards discharge goals with client and significant other.	Review progress toward discharge goals with client and significant other.

	Date ________ Day 4	Date ________ Day 5/6	
Daily outcomes	Client will ▪ have stable vital signs. ▪ have an intake of 2000 mL/day (IV). ▪ remain free of nausea and vomiting. ▪ state control of pain. ▪ verbalize understanding of ongoing care. ▪ have a soft, non-distended abdomen, active bowel sounds, passing soft, brown stools. ▪ tolerate ordered diet without nausea and vomiting. ▪ verbalize ability to cope. ▪ verbalize beginning understanding of home care instructions.	Client ▪ is afebrile and has a stable vital signs. ▪ has a soft, non-distended abdomen and passing soft, brown stools each day. ▪ is independent in self-care. ▪ is fully ambulatory. ▪ has resumed preadmission urine elimination pattern. ▪ verbalizes home care instructions. ▪ tolerates ordered diet and has a fluid intake of 2000 mL/day. ▪ verbalizes ability to cope with ongoing stressors.	
Tests and treatments	Blood culture × 2, if temp over 38.3 C (101 F). Vital signs q4h if stable. Assess gastrointestinal status q4h and prn. Intake and output q shift.	Blood culture × 2, if temp over 38.3 C (101 F). Vital signs q4h if stable. Assess gastrointestinal status q4h and prn. Intake and output q shift.	
Knowledge deficit	Reinforce earlier teaching regarding ongoing care. Review written discharge instructions with client and significant other.	Reinforce earlier teaching regarding ongoing care. Complete discharge teaching to include diet, follow-up care, signs and symptoms to report, activity, and medications: dose, frequency, route and side effects. Provide client with written discharge instructions.	
Psycho-social	Encourage verbalization of concerns. Provide ongoing support and encouragement.	Encourage verbalization of concerns. Provide ongoing support and encouragement.	
Diet	Full liquids to soft diet as tolerated, providing small, frequent, nutritious feedings. Encourage fluid intake of 2000 mL/day.	Soft diet as tolerated, providing small, frequent, nutritious feedings. Encourage fluid intake of 2000 mL/day.	

	Day 4 *continued*	Day 5/6 *continued*	
Activity	Self-care. Ambulate independently at least 4 times.	Self-care. Fully ambulatory.	
Medications	D/C IV if PO intake > 2000 mL/day. PO antibiotics. PO analgesics. Tylenol 650 mg q4h PO for temp over 38.3 C (101 F).	PO antibiotics. Tylenol 650 mg q4h PO for temp over 38.3 C (101 F).	
Bowel management	Assess gastrointestinal status q4h and prn. Report worsening abdominal pain, nausea, vomiting, or increasing abdominal distention. Offer warm liquids early each morning. Discuss need to eat 3 to 4 regularly scheduled meals. Encourage increased physical activity. Teach client signs and symptoms requiring follow-up: worsening abdominal pain, nausea, vomiting, change in bowel habits, and/or fever. Encourage client to eat a well-balanced diet, including all food groups after this acute episode. Instruct client regarding the importance of increasing fiber intake by consuming whole grains, fruits, and vegetables while avoiding nuts, seeds, and berries. Encourage client to avoid straining for a BM and to avoid constipation by using a hydrophilic colloid laxative. Instruct client to avoid strong laxatives and enemas and any activities that increase intra-abdominal pressure (lifting, bending, and coughing), constipation, or restrictive clothing.	Assess gastrointestinal status q4h and prn. Report worsening abdominal pain, nausea, vomiting, or increasing abdominal distention. Offer warm liquids early each morning. Reinforce the following instructions: (a) need to eat 3 to 4 regularly scheduled meals; (b) importance of increasing physical activity. Review signs and symptoms requiring follow-up: worsening abdominal pain, nausea, vomiting, change in bowel habits, and/or fever. Reinforce importance of eating a well-balanced diet and increasing fiber from whole grains, fruits, and vegetables while avoiding nuts, seeds, and berries.	
Transfer/ discharge plans	Continue to review progress toward discharge goals. Finalize discharge plans.	Finalize plans for home care if needed. Complete discharge teaching.	

CHAPTER HIGHLIGHTS

- Primary functions of the large bowel are the excretion of digestive waste products and the maintenance of fluid balance.
- Patterns of fecal elimination vary greatly among people, but a regular pattern of fecal elimination with formed, soft stools is essential to health and a sense of well-being.
- A variety of factors affect defecation: age, diet, fluid intake, activity/exercise, psychologic stress, life-style, medications, diagnostic procedures, anesthesia, and pathologic conditions.
- Common fecal elimination problems include constipation, fecal impaction, diarrhea, fecal incontinence, flatulence. Each has specific defining characteristics and contributing causes that often relate to or are identical to the factors that affect defecation.
- Assessment relative to fecal elimination includes a nursing history; physical examination of the abdomen, rectum, and anus; and, in some situations, visualization studies and inspection and analysis of stool for abnormal constituents such as blood.
- A nursing history includes data about the client's defecating pattern, description of feces and any changes, problems associated with elimination, and data about possible factors altering bowel elimination.
- Physical examination of the abdomen includes methods of inspection, auscultation, percussion, and palpation. Physical examination of the rectum and anus includes inspection and palpation.
- When inspecting the client's stool, the nurse must observe its color, consistency, shape, amount, odor, and the presence of abnormal constituents.
- A major function of the nurse is to assist clients with endoscopic and radiographic studies of the large intestine. Client assistance for visualization involves diet and bowel preparation before the study and appropriate follow-up care after the study.
- Clients also often need assistance to obtain stool specimens for laboratory analysis. In many agencies, nurses test the stool for occult blood.
- NANDA approved nursing diagnoses that relate specifically to altered bowel elimination include **Constipation, Colonic constipation, Perceived constipation, Diarrhea,** and **Bowel incontinence.** However, because altered elimination patterns affect several areas of human functioning, diagnoses such as **High risk for fluid volume deficit, Body image disturbance,** and **High risk for impaired skin integrity** may also apply.
- Constipation can be categorized as rectal, colonic, or perceived. Clients with perceived constipation often require education because overuse of laxatives can itself cause constipation.
- Lack of exercise, irregular defecation habits, stress, and bland diets are all thought to contribute to constipation. Sufficient fluid and fiber intake are required to keep feces soft.
- An adverse effect of constipation is straining during defecation, during which the Valsalva maneuver may be used. Cardiac problems may ensue.
- An adverse effect of prolonged diarrhea is fluid and electrolyte imbalance.
- Digital removal of an impaction should be carried out gently because of vagal nerve stimulation and subsequent depressed cardiac rate. An order is often necessary.
- Normal defecation is often facilitated in both well and ill clients by providing privacy, teaching clients to attend to defecation urges promptly, assisting clients whenever possible to normal sitting positions, encouraging appropriate food and fluid intake, and scheduling regular exercise.
- Additional nursing strategies include administering cathartics and antidiarrheals; administering cleansing, carminative, or retention enemas; removing an impaction digitally; inserting rectal tubes to decrease flatulence; applying protective skin agents; monitoring fluid and electrolyte balance; and instructing clients in ways to promote normal defecation.
- Clients who have bowel diversion ostomies require special care, with attention to psychologic adjustment, diet, and stoma and skin care. A variety of stomal management methods are available to these clients, depending on the type and position of the ostomy.

READINGS AND REFERENCES

SUGGESTED READINGS

Hogstel, MO and Nelson, M. January/February 1992. Anticipation and early detection can reduce bowel elimination complications. *Geriatric Nursing* 13:28–33.

This article focuses on bowel elimination problems of frail older adults. The author discusses essentials of initial assessment, documentation of daily assessments, nursing diagnoses of constipation and fecal incontinence, contributing factors common to frail older adults, nursing interventions related to the contributing factors, and client/family teaching for self-care.

Kemp, GK. September/October 1990. Trouble-shooting ostomy problems. *Geriatric Nursing* 11:233–38.

This continuing education article includes nursing interventions required to manage ostomy problems related to skin erosion, candidiasis, hyperplasia, and product sensitivities.

RELATED RESEARCH

Beverly, L and Travis, I. October 1992. Constipation: Proposed natural laxative mixtures. *Journal of Gerontological Nursing* 18:5–12.

Schmelzer, M. November/December 1990. Effectiveness of wheat bran in preventing constipation of hospitalized orthopaedic surgery patients. *Orthopaedic Nursing* 9:55–59.

SELECTED REFERENCES

Alterescu, KB. June 1987. Colostomy. *Nursing Clinics of North America.* 22:281–89.

Anastasi, JK. August 1993. AIDS update: Caring for patients with diarrhea. *Nursing93* 23:68–70.

Broadwell, DC. June 1987. Peristomal skin integrity. *Nursing Clinics of North America* 22:321–32.

Carpenito, LJ. 1992. *Nursing Diagnosis: Application to Clinical Practice.* 4th ed. Philadelphia: Lippincott.

Cerrato, PL. May 1989. Nutritionist on call: Is America really constipated? *RN* 52:81–86.

Doughty, D. May/June 1991. Maintaining normal bowel function in the patient with cancer. *Journal of Enterostomal Nursing* 18:90–94.

Ellickson, EB. January 1988. Bowel management plan for the homebound elderly. *Journal of Gerontological Nursing* 14:16–19.

Emly, M. January 20–26, 1993. Abdominal massage. *Nursing Times* 89:34–36.

Erickson, PJ. June 1987. Ostomies: The art of pouching. *Nursing Clinics of North America* 23:311–20.

Fifield, MY. July 1991. Relieving constipation and pain in the terminally ill. *American Journal of Nursing* 91:18–19.

Freedman, P. May 1991. The rectal pouch: A safer alternative to rectal tubes. *American Journal of Nursing* 91:105–6.

Gordon, M. 1993. *Manual of Nursing Diagnosis 1993–1994.* 6th ed. St Louis: Mosby-Year Book.

Guyton, AC. 1991. *Textbook of Medical Physiology.* 8th ed. Philadelphia: WB Saunders.

Hanauer, S.B. March 30, 1988. Fecal incontinence in the elderly. *Hospital Practice* 23:105–8.

Hogstel, MO and Nelson, M. January/February 1992. Anticipation and early detection can reduce bowel elimination complications. *Geriatric Nursing* 13:28–33.

Kemp, MG. September/October 1990. Trouble-shooting ostomy problems. *Geriatric Nursing* 11: 233–38.

Kim, MJ, McFarland, GK, and McLane, AM. 1993. *Pocket Guide to Nursing Diagnoses.* 5th ed. St Louis: Mosby-Year Book.

Lederer, JR, Marculescu, GL, Mocnik, B, and Seaby, N. 1993. *Care Planning Pocket Guide—A Nursing Diagnosis Approach.* 5th ed. Redwood City, CA: Addison-Wesley Nursing.

Lincoln, R, and Roberts, R. September 1989. Continence issues in acute care. *Nursing Clinics of North America* 24:741–54.

McCann JAS. March 1990. A guide to colostomies. *Nursing90* 20:32.

McFarland, GK and McFarlane, EA. 1993. *Nursing Diagnosis and Intervention: Planning for Patient Care.* 2nd ed. St Louis: Mosby.

McShane, RE and McLane, AM. April 1988. Constipation: Impact of etiological factors. *Journal of Gerontological Nursing* 14:31–34.

Mowlam V, North, K, and Myers, C. November 26–December 2, 1986. Continence: Managing fecal incontinence. *Nursing Times* 82:55, 57, 59.

North American Nursing Diagnosis Association. 1992. *NANDA Nursing Diagnoses: Definitions and Classification 1992–1993.* Philadelphia: NANDA.

Practice briefs. April 1992. Constipation: Removing an impaction. *Nursing92* 22:73.

Rolstad, BS. June 1987. Innovative surgical procedures and stoma care in the future. *Nursing Clinics of North America* 22:341–56.

Salter, M. May 2–8, 1990. Overcoming the stigma . . . irrigation and continent pouches. *Nursing Times* 86:67–69, 71.

Shipes, E. June 1987. Psychosocial issues: The person with an ostomy. *Nursing Clinics of North America* 22:291–302.

Wadle, KR. December 1990. Diarrhea. *Nursing Clinics of North America* 25:901–8.

41 Urinary Elimination

Objectives

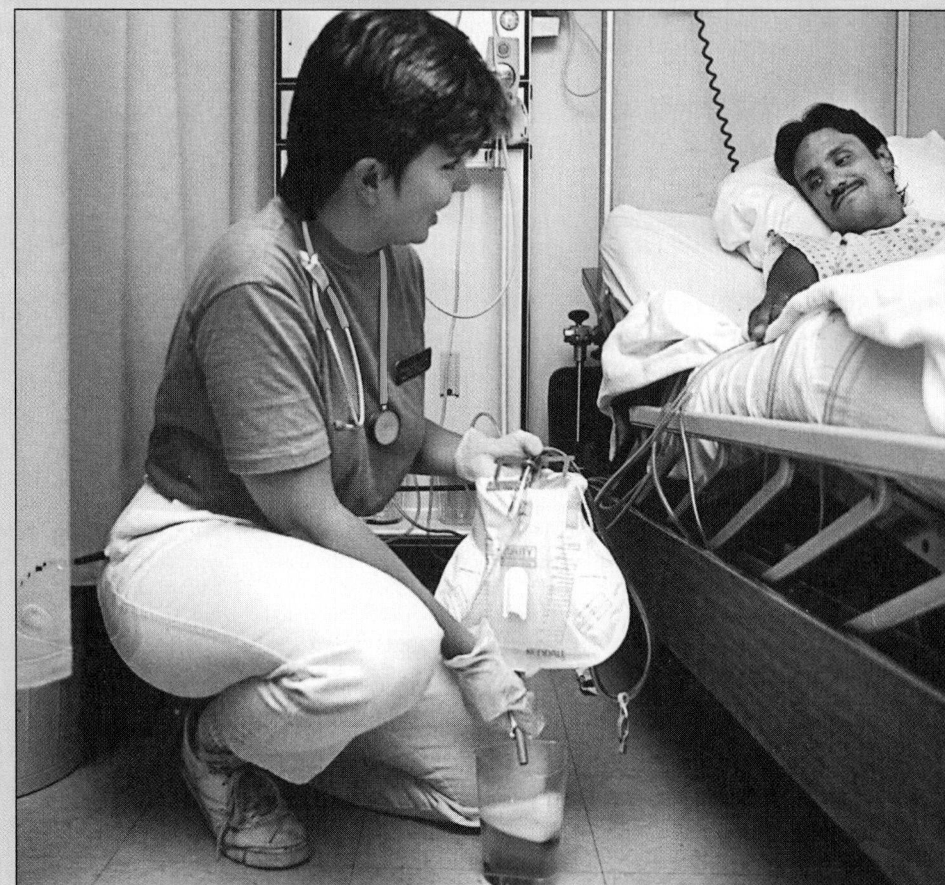

- Describe the process of micturition.
- Identify factors that influence urinary elimination.
- Describe common alterations in urinary elimination.
- Identify common causes of selected urinary problems.
- Identify essential components of a urinary elimination nursing history.
- Describe physical examination methods used to identify urinary elimination problems.
- Explain how to collect urine specimens and perform simple tests.
- Identify normal and abnormal characteristics and constituents of urine.
- Identify purposes of measuring residual urine.
- Describe diagnostic measures to assess kidney function and urinary tract abnormalities.
- Develop nursing diagnoses related to urinary elimination.
- Develop outcome criteria for clients with nursing diagnoses related to urinary elimation.
- Describe interventions to maintain normal urinary elimination and to assist clients with urinary incontinence and retention.
- Identify ways to prevent urinary infection.
- Identify interventions required for clients with retention catheters.
- Describe two urinary diversion ostomies.
- Identify essential aspects of suprapubic catheter care.

Elimination from the urinary tract is generally taken for granted by most people. It is only when a problem arises that people usually become aware of their urinary habits and any associated symptoms.

A person's urinary habits depend on both social culture and personal habit. In North America, most people are accustomed to privacy and clean (even decorative) surroundings while they urinate. The lack of privacy that is normal in many European and Far Eastern countries surprises and frequently disturbs North Americans traveling there.

Personal habits regarding urination are affected by the social propriety of leaving to urinate, the availability of a private clean facility, and initial bladder training. Urinary elimination is essential to health, and voiding can be postponed for only so long before the urge normally becomes too great to control.

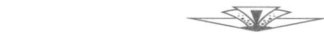

Physiology of Urinary Elimination

Urinary elimination depends on effective functioning of four urinary tract organs: kidneys, ureters, bladder, and urethra.

Kidneys

The kidneys filter from the blood any products for which the body has no use. Each kidney has one *renal artery* that originates from the abdominal aorta and enters the kidney at the hilum (Figure 41–1). The renal vein exits through the hilum and joins the inferior vena cava. It is estimated that, in the average adult, 1200 mL of blood passes through the kidneys every minute. This figure represents about 21% of the cardiac output (5600 mL per minute). The body's total blood supply circulates through the kidneys approximately 12 times per hour.

From this blood, the **nephron,** the functional unit of the kidney (Figure 41–2), forms a fluid called **glomerular filtrate** (about 180 liters daily, or 25 mL per minute). This volume-time ratio is referred to as the *glomerular filtration rate (GFR).* The **glomerulus** is a tuft or cluster of blood vessels surrounded by Bowman's capsule. The pores of the glomerulus are large enough for water and some solutes to pass through but are too small for large molecules, such as protein and formed elements in the blood, to filter through. The glomerular filtrate is chemically almost the same as **plasma** but has only minute quantities of protein (0.03%) compared to the amount found in plasma (7%). **Proteinuria** (the presence of protein in the urine) is a sign of glomerular injury. Glomerular filtrate consists of water,

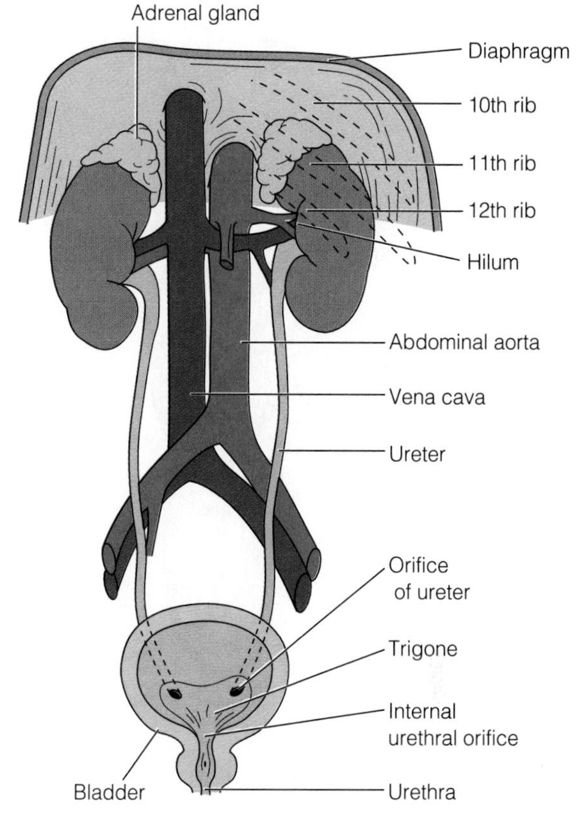

Figure 41–1 Anatomic structures of the urinary tract.

electrolytes, creatinine, glucose, urea, amino acids, uric acid, bicarbonate, and other electrolytes.

After the filtrate enters Bowman's capsule, it passes into the tubular system, where about 99% of it is reabsorbed into the bloodstream. The remaining 1% forms the urine to be excreted from the body (Guyton 1991, p. 286). Thus, the function of the nephron is to return the majority of glomerular filtrate to the circulation. The kidneys are therefore the most important organs in regulating body fluid balance.

Ureters

Once the urine is formed in the kidneys, it enters the ureters via collecting ducts and then passes on to the bladder (Figure 41–1). The ureters are from 25 to 30 cm (10 to 12 in) long in the adult and about 1.25 cm (0.5 in) in diameter. The upper end of each ureter is funnel-shaped as it enters the kidney, forming what is referred to as the *renal pelvis.* The lower ends of the ureters enter the bladder at the posterior corners of the floor of the bladder. At this junction between the ureter and the bladder there is a flaplike fold of mucous membrane that acts as a valve to

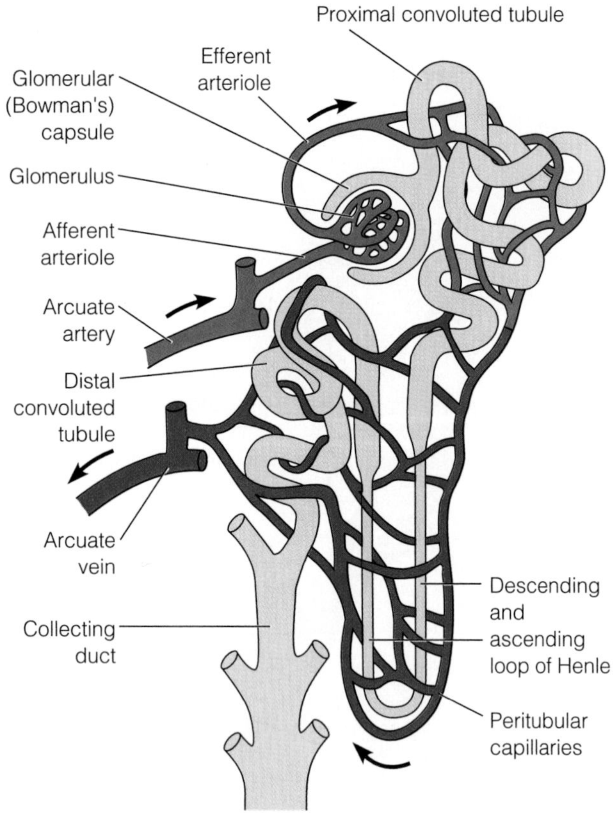

Figure 41–2 The nephrons of the kidney are composed of five parts: Bowman's capsule, proximal convoluted tubule, loop of Henle, distal convoluted tubule, and collecting duct.

prevent **reflux** (backflow) of urine up the ureters to the kidneys.

BLADDER

The urinary bladder is a hollow, muscular organ that serves as a reservoir for urine and as the organ of excretion. When empty, it lies behind the symphysis pubis. In the male, the bladder lies in front of the rectum and above the prostate gland (Figure 41–3); in the female, it lies in front of the uterus and vagina (Figure 41–4). The wall of the bladder is made up of four layers: (a) an inner mucous layer that is continuous with that of the ureters and the urethra; (b) a submucous connective tissue layer; (c) a muscular layer consisting of three layers of smooth muscle fibers, some of which extend lengthwise, some obliquely, and some more or less circularly; and (d) an outer serous layer. The smooth muscle layers are collectively called the **detrusor muscle.** The base of the bladder, called the **trigone,** is a triangular area marked by the ureter openings at the posterior corners forming the base and the opening of the urethra at the anterior inferior corner forming the apex. Urine exits from the bladder through the urethra.

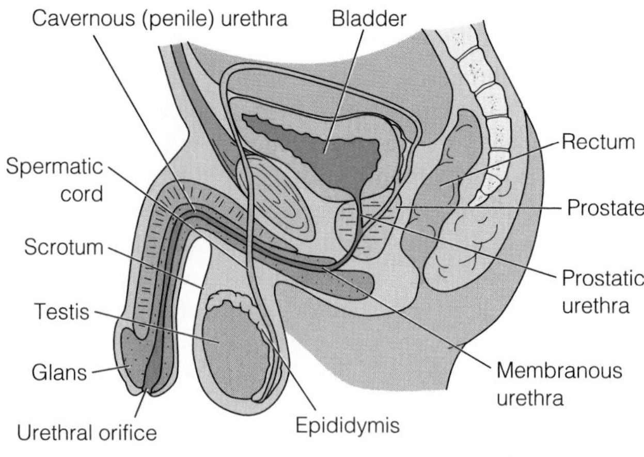

Figure 41–3 The male urogenital system.

The amount of urine normally stored in the bladder varies to some degree among individuals and with age. For an adult, the desire to void is normally experienced when the bladder contains between 250 and 450 mL of urine. Normal output of urine for an adult is about 1500 mL/day.

The bladder is capable of considerable distention because of *rugae* (folds) in the mucous membrane lining and because of the elasticity of its walls. When full, the dome of the bladder may extend above the symphysis pubis; in extreme situations it may extend as high as the umbilicus.

URETHRA

The urethra extends from the bladder to the urinary **meatus** (opening, or passage) and is the exit passageway for the urine. It is lined with mucous membrane. In the adult male, the urethra functions as a passageway for reproduction fluid (semen) as well as urine (Figure 41–3).

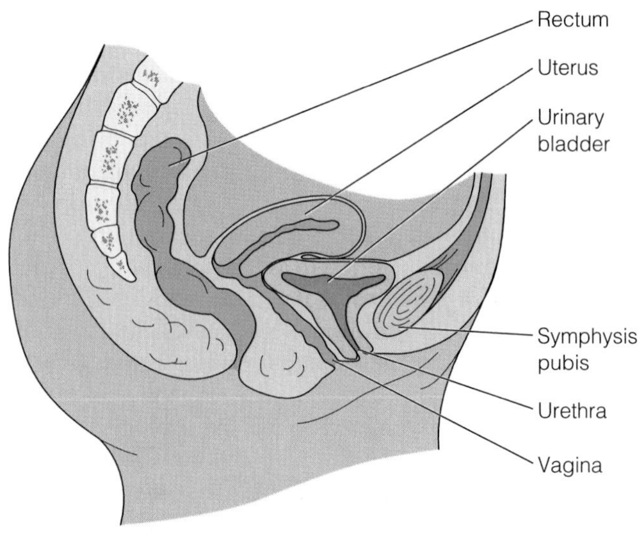

Figure 41–4 The female urogenital system.

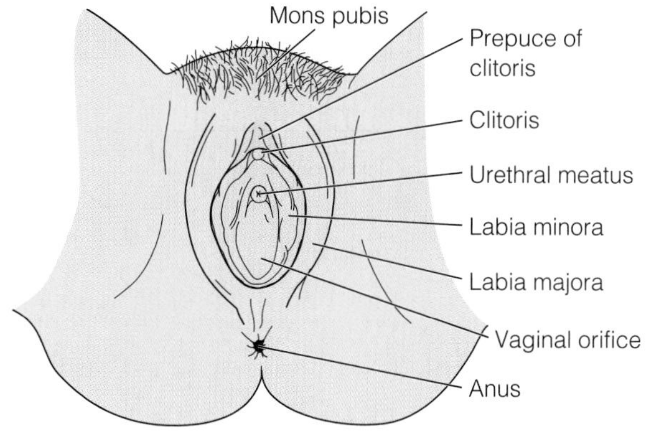

Figure 41–5 Location of the female urinary meatus in relation to surrounding structures.

Table 41–1 Average Daily Excretion of Urine by Age

Age	Amount (mL)
1 to 2 days	15 to 60
3 to 10 days	100 to 300
10 days to 2 months	250 to 450
2 months to 1 year	400 to 500
1 to 3 years	500 to 600
3 to 5 years	600 to 700
5 to 8 years	700 to 1000
8 to 14 years	800 to 1400
14 years through adulthood	1500
Older adulthood	1500 or less

In the adult female, the urethra lies directly behind the symphysis pubis, anterior to the vagina, and is about 3.7 cm (1.5 inches) in length (Figure 41–4). The urethra serves only as a passageway for the elimination of urine. The urinary meatus is located between the labia minora, in front of the vagina and below the clitoris (Figure 41–5); in the male, it is located at the distal end of the penis. The male urethra is about 20 cm (8 inches) long.

In both the male and female, the urethra has two **sphincter** muscles. The internal sphincter muscle is situated at the base of the urinary bladder and is involuntary. The second sphincter muscle is under voluntary control. In the female it is situated at about the midpoint of the urethra; in the male it is distal to the prostatic portion of the urethra.

In both males and females, the urethra has a mucous membrane lining that is continuous with the bladder and the ureters. Thus, an infection of the urethra can readily extend through the urinary tract to the kidneys. Women are particularly prone to urinary tract infections because of the shortness of their urethras.

URINATION

Micturition, voiding, and **urination** all refer to the process of emptying the urinary bladder. Urine collects in the bladder until pressure stimulates special sensory nerve endings in the bladder wall called *stretch receptors.* This occurs when the adult bladder contains between 250 and 450 mL of urine. In children, a considerably smaller volume, 50 to 200 mL, stimulates these nerves. See Table 41–1 for average urine output at various ages.

Once excited, the stretch receptors transmit impulses to the spinal cord, specifically to the voiding reflex center located at the level of the second to fourth sacral vertebrae. Some impulses continue up the spinal cord to the voiding control center in the cerebral cortex. If the time is appropriate to void, the brain then sends impulses through the spinal cord to the motor neurons in the sacral area, causing stimulation of the parasympathetic nerves. As a result, urine can be released from the bladder, but it is still impeded by the external urinary sphincter. If the time and place are appropriate for urination, the conscious portion of the brain relaxes the external urethral sphincter muscle, and urination takes place. If the time and place are inappropriate, the micturition reflex usually subsides until the bladder becomes more filled and the reflex is stimulated again. The sympathetic nervous system also innervates the bladder, causing it to relax.

Voluntary control of urination is possible only if the nerves supplying the bladder and urethra, the neural tracts of the cord and brain, and the motor area of the cerebrum are all intact.The individual must be able to sense that the bladder is full. Injury to any of these parts of the nervous system—by, for example, a cerebral hemorrhage or spinal cord injury above the level of the sacral region—results in intermittent involuntary emptying of the bladder. Elderly people whose cognition is impaired may not be aware of bladder fullness. Involuntary micturation is called **urinary incontinence.** When there is damage to the spinal cord above the sacral vertebrae, the micturition reflex may remain intact and urination may occur reflexively. This situation is referred to as an *automatic bladder.*

Occasionally a person is unable to void even though the bladder contains an excessive amount of urine. This condition is known as **retention.** Catheterization (introduction of a tube—known as a **catheter**—through the urethra into the bladder to remove urine) relieves the discomfort that accompanies retention. A more serious complication, which is also characterized by the inability to void, is called **urinary suppression.** In this situation the person cannot void because the kidneys are not secreting any urine; the bladder is empty.

Table 41–2 Changes in Urinary Elimination through the Life Cycle

Stage	Variations
Fetus	The fetal kidney begins to excrete urine between the 11th and 12th week of development.
	Fetal urine is hypotonic to plasma.
	The placenta serves as a pseudo-kidney in regulating fetal fluid and electrolyte balance.
	The kidney does not function independently until after birth.
Infant	Ability to concentrate urine is minimal; therefore, urine appears light yellow.
	Voluntary urinary control is absent.
Children	Kidney function reaches maturity between the first and second year of life; urine is concentrated effectively and appears a normal amber color.
	Voluntary control of urine begins at 18 to 24 months of age, when the child starts to recognize bladder fullness, holds urine beyond the urge to void, and communicates the urge to void.
	Full urinary control is not gained until age 4 or 5 years; daytime control is usually achieved by age 2 years.
	Boys are slower than girls in gaining control.
	The kidneys grow in proportion to overall body growth.
Adults	The kidneys reach maxmium size between 35 and 40 years of age.
	After age 50 the kidneys begin to diminish in size and function. Most shrinkage occurs in the cortex of the kidney, due primarily to the loss of glomeruli.
Elderly adults	There is an estimated 30% loss of glomeruli by age 80.
	Renal blood flow decreases because of vascular changes and a decrease in cardiac output.
	Urine concentratability declines.
	Excessive urination at night and increased frequency of urination occur because of loss of concentratability and diminished bladder muscle tone.
	Residual urine may increase due to diminished bladder muscle tone and contractability, which increases the risk of bacterial growth and infection and increases voiding frequency.
	Urinary incontinence may occur due to mobility problems or neurologic impairments.

FACTORS AFFECTING VOIDING

Numerous factors affect the volume of urine formed and the process of voiding.

Growth and Development Voiding changes throughout the life cycle. See Table 41–2.

Psychosocial Factors For many people, a set of conditions helps stimulate the micturition reflex. These conditions include privacy, normal position, sufficient time, and, occasionally, running water. Circumstances that counter the client's accustomed conditions may produce anxiety and muscle tension. As a result, the person is unable to relax abdominal and perineal muscles and the external urethral sphincter. Voiding may be incomplete and result in urinary retention.

Fluid and Food Intake The healthy body maintains a sensitive balance between the amount of fluid ingested and the amount of fluid eliminated. When the amount of fluid intake increases, therefore, the output normally increases. Certain fluids, such as alcohol, increase fluid output by inhibiting the production of antidiuretic hormone. Fluids that contain caffeine (eg, coffee, tea, and cola drinks) also increase urine production. Foods that are high in fluid content (eg, iceberg lettuce, milk, and cooked cereal) also increase fluid output. By contrast, food and fluids high in sodium can cause fluid retention.

Some foods and fluids can change the color of urine. For example, beets and blackberries can cause urine to appear red; foods containing carotene can cause the urine to appear yellower than usual.

Medications Many medications interfere with the normal urination process and may cause retention. See the box on page 1228. Diuretics (eg, chlorothiazide, furosemide, and ethacrynic acid) increase urine formation by preventing the reabsorption of water and electrolytes from the tubules of the kidney into the blood stream. Diuretics are commonly taken for hypertension and cardiac disease.

Muscle Tone and Activity People who exercise regularly will likely have good muscle tone, increased body metabolism, and good urine production. Poor muscle tone can lead to impaired bladder muscle contraction and poor control of the external urethral sphincter and thus poor urination control. The presence of an indwelling catheter can also lead to poor bladder muscle tone; the bladder does not fill and stretch, and the external sphincter does not completely close. When the catheter is removed, therefore, the client may have difficulty in regaining urinary control.

Pathologic Conditions Specific pathologic conditions affect the formation and/or excretion of urine. Endocrine disorders such as diabetes insipidus increase urine formation. Diseases that impair blood flow to the kidneys (eg, atherosclerosis) can decrease urine formation. Diseases of the kidneys themselves can reduce kidney function and perhaps eventually result in renal failure.

Any process that impairs the flow of the urine from the kidneys to the urethra can impair urine excretion. Hypertrophy of the prostate gland, which commonly occurs in older men, can interfere with the ability to empty the bladder. Febrile conditions can interfere with urine formation: Because the body loses excessive fluid through perspiration, less urine is formed in the kidneys to maintain the fluid and electrolyte balance. The urine formed under such circumstances is normally highly concentrated so that the waste products of metabolism are still excreted.

Surgical and Diagnostic Procedures Some surgical and diagnostic procedures can affect the passage of urine and the urine itself. The urethra may swell following a cystoscopy, and surgical procedures on any part of the urinary tract may result in some postoperative bleeding; as a result, the urine may be red- or pink-tinged for a time.

Spinal anesthetics can also affect the passage of urine, because they decrease the client's awareness of the need to void. Other anesthetic agents can decrease blood pressure and glomerular filtration, thereby decreasing urine formation. Surgery on structures adjacent to the urinary tract (eg, the uterus) can also affect voiding because of swelling in the lower abdomen and often necessitates the use of a retention catheter for a short time.

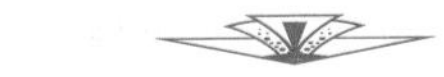

ALTERED URINE PRODUCTION

Although people's patterns of urination are highly individual, most people void about five or more times a day. People usually void when they first awaken in the morning, before they go to bed, and around mealtimes. Most people void about 70% of their daily urine during the waking hours and do not need to void during the night.

Polyuria Polyuria, or **diuresis,** refers to the production of abnormally large amounts of urine by the kidneys, such as 2500 mL/day for an adult. Polyuria can be the result of (a) excessive fluid intake, (b) the ingestion of substances containing caffeine and alcohol, (c) diabetes mellitus, (d) hormone imbalances (eg, deficiency of antidiuretic hormone [ADH]), or (e) chronic kidney disease. Other signs often associated with diuresis are **polydipsia** (intense thirst), dehydration, and weight loss.

Oliguria and Anuria Oliguria refers to voiding scant amounts of urine, such as less than 500 mL in 24 hours. Anuria refers to an adult's voiding less than 100 mL/day. The terms *complete kidney shutdown*, *renal failure*, and *urinary suppression* have the same meaning. Oliguria may result from an extremely low fluid intake but may also follow disease. Both anuria and oliguria can result from kidney disease, severe heart failure, burns, and shock. These clinical signs can be fatal if some other means—such as an artificial kidney—is not used to remove body wastes. Oliguria may also normally accompany fever and heavy perspiration. Because of excessive fluid losses via the skin, urine production is decreased.

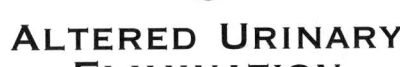

ALTERED URINARY ELIMINATION

Frequency and Nocturia **Frequency** is generally considered voiding at frequent intervals, that is, more often than usual. Normally with an increased intake of fluid there is some increase in the frequency with which a person voids. Frequency without an increase in fluid intake may be the result of *cystitis* (an acutely inflamed bladder), stress, or pressure on the bladder (because of pregnancy, for example).

With frequency, the total amount of urine voided may be normal, because the amounts voided each time are small, such as 50 to 100 mL.

Nocturia, or **nycturia,** is increased frequency at night that is not a result of an increase in fluid intake. Like frequency, it is usually expressed in terms of the number of times the person gets out of bed to void, for example, "nocturia × 4."

Urgency Urgency is the feeling that the person *must* void. There may or may not be a great deal of urine in the bladder, but the person feels a need to void immediately. Often the person hurries to the toilet with the fear of

MEDICATIONS CAUSING URINARY RETENTION

- Anticholinergic/antispasmodic medications, such as atropine, belladonna, Donnatal (containing atropine), and papaverine
- Antidepressant/antipsychotic agents, such as phenothiazines and MAO inhibitors
- Antiparkinsonism drugs, such as levodopa, trihexyphenidyl (Artane), and benztropine mesylate (Cogentin)
- Antihistamine preparations, such as Actifed and Sudafed
- Beta-adrenergic blockers, such as propanolol (Inderal)
- Antihypertensives, such as hydralazine (Apresoline) and methyldopate (Aldomet)

being incontinent. Urgency accompanies psychologic stress and irritation of the trigone and urethra. It is also common in young children who have poor external sphincter control.

Dysuria Dysuria means voiding that is either painful or difficult. It can accompany a **stricture** (decrease in caliber) of the urethra, urinary infections, and injury to the bladder and/or urethra. Often clients will say they have to push to void or that burning accompanies or follows voiding. Burning during micturition is often due to an irritated urethra; burning following urination may be the result of a bladder infection when the irritated rugae (ridges) of the trigone rub together. The burning may be described as severe, like a hot poker, or more subdued, like a sunburn. Often, **urinary hesitancy** (a delay and difficulty in initiating voiding) is associated.

Enuresis Enuresis is defined as repeated involuntary urination in children beyond the age when voluntary bladder control is normally acquired, usually 4 or 5 years of age.

Enuresis can also be described as *primary*, meaning there has never been a long, dry, symptom-free period, or *secondary (acquired)*, meaning the enuresis occurs after a dry period of at least a year. It is also described as *nocturnal* (nighttime), *diurnal* (daytime), or both. There are many reasons for enuresis; several causes or contributing factors may exist in each individual situation.

Urinary Incontinence Incontinence is a symptom, not a disease. Figures range from 10% to 47% (Turner & Plymat 1988, p. 133). There are different types of incontinence: total, stress, urge, functional, and reflex incontinence. See page 1239 for descriptions and definitions.

Urinary retention with overflow is a dribbling incontinence that results when the bladder is greatly distended with urine because of an obstruction, such as an enlarged prostate gland. The client voids small amounts of urine frequently, or dribbles urine, while the bladder remains distended. The term **neurogenic bladder** describes any voiding problem relating to neurologic impairment or dysfunction. The client is unaware of bladder filling; the bladder walls become overstretched and atonic. Urine "overflows" or dribbles when the pressure increases in the bladder to a point where it surpasses the urethral sphincter's resistance to urine. This is also called *reflex incontinence.*

Retention Urinary retention is the accumulation of urine in the bladder with associated inability of the bladder to empty itself. Because urine production continues, retention distends the bladder. An adult urinary bladder normally holds 250 to 450 mL of urine when the micturition reflex is triggered. With urinary retention, some adult bladders may distend to hold 3000 mL of urine. Prolonged retention leads to **stasis** (a slowing of the flow of urine) and stagnation of urine, which increase the possibility of urinary tract infection. Clinical signs of retention are listed on page 1240. Retention is distinguished from oliguria or anuria by the bladder distention. Bladder distention can be assessed by palpation and percussion above the symphysis pubis. Percussion of the suprapubic area produces a "kettle-drum" or dull sound when the bladder is full. The most common type of retention is postoperative retention.

Many medications interfere with the normal urination process and may cause retention. Examples are listed in the accompanying box.

Certain psychosocial factors may be associated with retention. Many people have developed a set of behaviors that help stimulate the micturition reflex; these are discussed earlier.

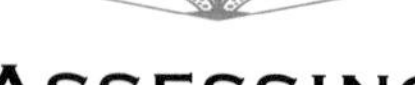

ASSESSING

A complete assessment of a client's urinary function includes the following:

- Nursing history, including
  a. Data about voiding patterns and habits, any problems voiding, and past or present problems involving the urinary system
  b. Data about any problems that may affect urination (eg, problems with mobility)

ASSESSMENT INTERVIEW

Urinary Elimination

Voiding Pattern

- How many times do you void during a 24-hour period?
- Has this pattern changed recently?
- Do you need to get out of bed to void at night? How often?

Description of Urine and Any Changes

- How would you describe your urine in terms of color, clarity (clear, transparent, or cloudy), and odor (faint or strong)?

Urinary Elimination Problems

What problems have you had or do you now have with passing your urine?

- Passage of large amounts of urine?
- Passage of small amounts of urine?
- Voiding at more frequent intervals?
- Trouble getting to the bathroom in time or feeling of urgency to void?
- Painful voiding?
- Difficulty starting urine stream?
- Frequent dribbling of urine or feeling of bladder fullness associated with voiding small amounts of urine?
- Reduced force of stream?
- Accidental leakage of urine? If so, when does this occur (eg, when coughing, laughing, or sneezing; at night; during the day)?
- Past urinary tract illness such as urinary tract infection of the kidney, bladder, or urethra; urinary calculi; urinary tract surgery of kidney, ureters or bladder?

Presence and Management of Urinary Diversion Ostomy

- What is your usual routine with your ostomy?
- What problems, if any, do you have with it?
- How can the nurse help you manage it?

Factors Influencing Urinary Elimination

- *Medications.* Have you taken any medications that could increase urinary output (eg, diuretic) or cause retention of urine (eg, anticholinergic-antispasmodic, antidepressant-antipsychotic, antiparkinsonism drugs, antihistamines, antihypertensives)? Note specific medication and dosage.
- *Fluid intake.* What amount and kind of fluid do you take each day (eg, 6 glasses of water, 5 cups of coffee, 3 cola drinks with or without caffeine)?
- *Environmental factors.* Do you have any problems with toileting (mobility, dexterity with clothing, toilet seat too low, facility without grab bar)?
- *Presence of long-term catheter.* How do you care for your catheter? Do you have any discomfort with it or other problems? How can the nurse help you manage it?
- *Stress.* Are you experiencing any long-term or short-term stress? If so, what are the stressors? Do you think these affect your urinary pattern?
- *Disease.* Have you had or do you have any illnesses other than urinary tract disease that may affect urinary function, such as hypertension, heart disease, neurologic disease (eg, multiple sclerosis), cancer, prostatic enlargement, diabetes mellitus, or diabetes insipidus?
- *Diagnostic procedures.* Have you recently had a cystoscopy or spinal anesthetic?

- Physical assessment of the kidneys, bladder, urethral meatus, integrity of the skin surrounding the meatus, hydration status, and examination of the urine
- Relating the above data to the results of any diagnostic tests and procedures

NURSING HISTORY

The nurse determines the client's normal voiding pattern and frequency, appearance of the urine and any recent changes, any past or current problems with urination, the presence of an ostomy, and factors influencing the elimination pattern.

Examples of interview questions to elicit this information are shown in the accompanying box. The number of questions asked depends on the individual and the responses to the first three categories. Table 41–3 summarizes factors related to altered urinary elimination patterns.

Table 41–3 Selected Factors Associated with Altered Urinary Elimination Patterns

Altered Pattern	Selected Influencing and Associated Factors to Be Determined
Polyuria	Increase in fluid intake and ingestion of fluids containing caffeine or alcohol
	Prescribed diuretic
	Presence of thirst, dehydration, and weight loss
	Presence of or familial history of diabetes insipidus or kidney disease
Oliguria, anuria	Decrease in fluid intake
	Signs of dehydration (see Chapter 38)
	Presence of known kidney disease or familial history of kidney disease
	Signs of renal failure, such as the presence of uremic frost (urea crystals) on the skin, an elevated BUN, and an aromatic odor to the skin; and signs of fluid and electrolyte imbalances (see Chapter 38)
	Presence of febrile condition
Frequency or nocturia	Pregnancy
	Increase in fluid intake
	Presence of known urinary tract inflammation or infection
	Any known contributing or initiating causes, such as stress
Urgency	Presence of psychologic stress
	Presence of known urinary tract inflammation or infection
Dysuria	Presence of known urinary tract inflammation, infection, or injury
	Presence of other signs that may accompany dysuria, such as hesitancy, hematuria, pyuria, and frequency
Enuresis	Family history of enuresis
	Difficult access to toilet facilities
	Home stresses
	Strict bladder-training methods
Incontinence	Presence of known bladder inflammation or other disease
	Difficulties in independent toileting (mobility impairment)
	Leakage when coughing, laughing, sneezing
	Cognitive impairment
Retention	Presence of distended bladder on palpation and percussion
	Associated signs, such as pubic discomfort, restlessness, frequency, and small urine volume
	Low fluid intake
	Recent anesthesia
	Recent perineal surgery
	Presence of perineal swelling
	Medications prescribed
	Lack of privacy or other factors that initiate micturition

PHYSICAL ASSESSMENT

Complete physical assessment of the urinary tract usually includes percussion of the kidneys to detect areas of tenderness and palpation for contour, size, tenderness, and lumps. Palpation and percussion of the bladder are performed also. See Chapter 22, page 538. These aspects of physical assessment are included in the ongoing assessment of the client as well and are routinely performed by the assigned nurse. During examination of the genitals, the urethral meatus of both male and female clients is inspected for swelling, discharge, and inflammation.

Because problems with urination can affect the elimination of wastes from the body, it is important that the nurse assess the skin for color, texture, and tissue turgor as well as the presence of any waste products (eg, crystals on the skin). In addition, the skin of the perineum should be inspected for irritation because contact with urine can excoriate the skin. This is particularly evident in the incontinent client.

COLLECTING URINE SPECIMENS

The nurse is responsible for collecting urine specimens for a number of tests: clean voided specimens for routine

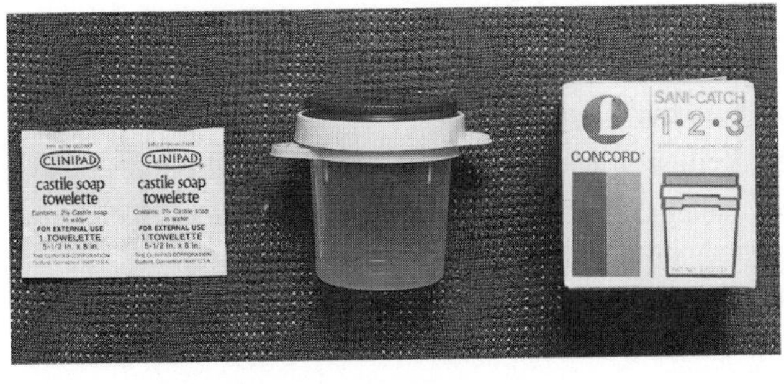

Figure 41–6 A commercially prepared disposable clean-catch kit.

urinalysis, *clean-catch* or *midstream urine specimens* for urine culture, and timed urine specimens for a variety of tests that depend on the client's specific health problem. Procedure 40–1 on page 1198 describes how to give and remove a bedpan and urinal. A clear voided specimen is usually adequate for routine examination; a clean-catch specimen is needed for bacteriologic culture.

Clean-catch or midstream specimens must be as free as possible from external contamination by microorganisms near the urethral opening. Sterile specimen containers and lids are used for those specimens. Commercially prepared disposable clean-catch kits are available (Figure 41–6).

Several urine tests require timed specimens. Urine specimens are collected at timed intervals, for short periods (1 to 2 hours) or long periods (12 to 24 hours). All timed urine specimens should be refrigerated to prevent bacterial growth and decomposition of the urine components, unless a special preservative has been added. Each voiding of urine is collected in a small, clean container and then emptied immediately into the large refrigerated bottle or carton.

Clients need varying degrees of instruction and assistance to provide clean voided specimens. Many clients are able to provide the specimen independently. Male clients generally have little difficulty voiding directly into the specimen container, but female clients usually need to stand over a toilet bowl and hold the container between their legs during the process of voiding. About 120 mL (4 oz) of urine is generally required. Clients who are seriously ill, physically incapacitated, or disoriented may need to use a bedpan or urinal in bed; others may require supervision and/or assistance in the bathroom. Whatever the situation, explicit directions are required:

- The specimen must be free of fecal contamination, so voiding needs to occur at a different time from defecation.
- Female clients should discard the toilet tissue in the toilet or in a waste bag rather than in the bedpan, since tissue in the specimen makes laboratory analysis more difficult.
- Put the lid tightly on the container to prevent spillage of the urine and contamination of other objects.
- If the outside of the container has been contaminated by urine, clean it with a disinfectant.

The nurse must (a) make sure that the specimen label and the laboratory requisition carry the correct information and (b) attach them securely to the specimen. Inappropriate identification of the specimen can lead to errors of diagnosis or therapy for the client.

Collecting a Timed Urine Specimen Timed urine specimen containers are usually obtained from the laboratory and kept in the client's bathroom. To collect a timed urine specimen, the nurse follows these steps:

- Place alert signs about the specimen collection at the client's bedside or bathroom.
- Label specimen containers to include date and time of each voiding as well as the usual client identification data. Containers may be numbered sequentially (eg, 1st specimen, 2nd specimen, and so on).
- Explain to the client the purpose of the test, when it begins, and what to do with the urine. Agencies usually have protocols for different tests.
- Ensure that urine is free of feces.

Collecting a Specimen from a Foley Catheter Sterile urine specimens can be obtained from closed drainage systems by inserting a sterile needle attached to a 3-mL syringe through a drainage port in the tubing. Aspiration of urine from catheters can be done only with self-sealing rubber catheters—not plastic, silicone, or silastic catheters. When self-sealing rubber catheters are used, the needle is inserted just above the place where the catheter is attached to the drainage tubing. The area from which to obtain urine may be marked by a patch on the catheter.

To collect a specimen from a Foley (retention) catheter or a drainage tube, the nurse follows these steps:

- Don disposable gloves.
- Wipe the area where the needle will be inserted with a disinfectant swab. The site should be remote from the tube leading to the balloon to avoid puncturing this tube. Disinfecting the needle insertion site removes or destroys any microorganisms on the surface of the catheter thereby avoiding contamination of the needle and the entrance of microorganisms into the catheter.
- If there is no urine in the catheter, clamp the drainage tubing for about 30 minutes. This allows fresh urine to collect in the catheter.

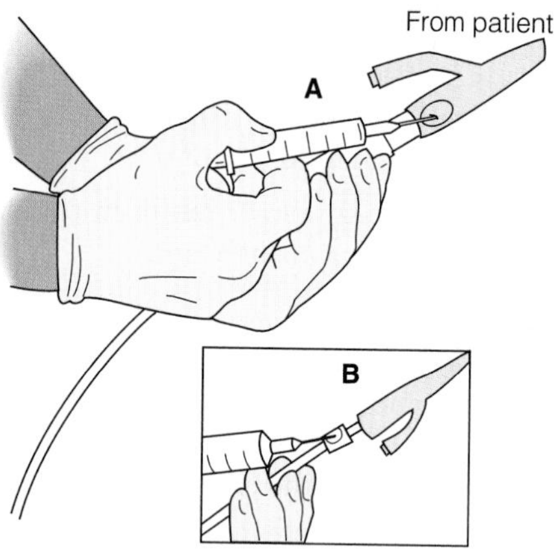

Figure 41–7 Obtaining a urine specimen from a retention catheter: *A,* from a specific area, sometimes designated by a patch, near the end of the catheter; *B,* from a drainage port in the tubing.

- Unclamp the catheter.
- Insert the needle at a 30- to 45-degree angle (Figure 41–7). This angle of entrance facilitates self-sealing of the rubber.
- Withdraw the required amount of urine, for example, 3 mL for a urine culture or 30 mL for a routine urinalysis.
- Transfer the urine to the specimen container. Make sure the needle does not touch the outside of the container, if a sterile culture tube is used.
- Cap the container.
- Remove gloves and discard appropriately.
- Label the container, and send the urine to the laboratory immediately for analysis or refrigeration.
- Record collection of the specimen and any pertinent observations of the urine on the appropriate records.

Collecting a Specimen by Clean-Catch or Midstream Clean-catch or midstream specimens must be as free as possible from external contamination by microorganisms near the urethral opening. Sterile specimen containers and lids are used for those specimens. Procedure 41–1 describes the steps involved in obtaining these specimens.

Urine culture and sensitivity tests are done to identify specific causative microorganisms of urinary tract infections and appropriate antimicrobial agents. The nurse's role in bacteriologic urine culture tests is to obtain a clean-catch specimen, also referred to as a clean voided midstream urine (CVMS). In the past, catheterization was the preferred method for acquiring uncontaminated culture specimens, particularly from females. Today, even though the clean-catch specimen may be somewhat contaminated by skin bacteria, it is considered better to have a contaminated specimen than to risk causing infection of the client's urinary tract by introducing microorganisms

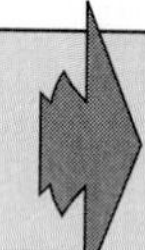

PROCEDURE 41–1 COLLECTING A URINE SPECIMEN FOR CULTURE AND SENSITIVITY BY CLEAN CATCH

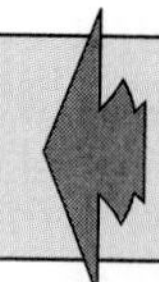

PURPOSE

- To determine the presence of microorganisms, the type of organism(s), and the antibiotics to which the organisms are sensitive.

ASSESSMENT FOCUS

Ability of the client to provide the specimen; color, odor, and consistency of the urine; presence of clinical signs of urinary tract infection (eg, frequency, urgency, dysuria, hematuria, flank pain, cloudy urine with foul odor).

EQUIPMENT

Equipment used varies greatly from agency to agency. Some agencies use commercially prepared disposable clean-catch kits. Others are agency-prepared sterile trays. Both prepared trays and kits generally contain the following items:

- ☐ Disposable or sterile gloves
- ☐ Antiseptic, such as povidone-iodine
- ☐ Sterile cotton balls or 2 × 2 gauze pads
- ☐ Sterile specimen container
- ☐ Specimen identification label
- ☐ Completed laboratory requisition form
- ☐ Urine receptacle, if the client is not ambulatory

PROCEDURE 41-1 *continued*

INTERVENTION

1. Instruct and assist the client appropriately.

- Inform the client that a urine specimen is required; give the reason, and explain the method to be used to collect it.
- Ask an *ambulatory* client to wash and dry the genitals and perineum thoroughly with soap and water. *A clean perineum is essential to reduce the number of skin bacteria and to minimize contamination of the specimen.*
- Assist the *ambulatory* client to the bathroom. The preferred method to collect specimens from ambulatory clients is to have them provide the specimen while standing over the toilet in the bathroom. See step 4.
- Assist *nonambulatory* clients to an upright sitting position on a urine receptacle. Provide appropriate covers for the client: Drape the client, exposing only the perineal area.
- Assist the *female* client to spread the legs enough to ensure that the urine does not touch the legs.

2. Prepare the equipment, and implement body fluid precautions.

- Open the sterile kit or tray, using sterile technique. *Sterile technique is essential to maintain the sterility of the specimen container.*

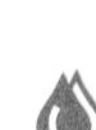

- Put on the sterile gloves or clean gloves as long as the inside of the container is kept sterile.
- Pour the antiseptic solution over the cotton balls.

3. Clean the area at the external urinary meatus with the antiseptic. *The antiseptic reduces the number of bacteria near the urethral opening and minimizes contamination of the urine specimen.*

For Female Clients

- Swab the labia minora from front to back, using one swab for each wipe. *Swabbing from front to back cleans the area of least contamination to the area of greatest contamination.*
- Spread the labia minora well apart, using the thumb and another finger (eg, the third finger) of one hand.
- Swab between the labia minora over the urethra from front to back. *The urethra is considered less contaminated than the vagina and anus.*

For Male Clients

- Hold the penis with one hand, and clean the urinary meatus using a circular motion: First retract the foreskin of an uncircumcised male.
- Wash outward from the meatus in a circular motion, using one swab for each wipe and moving down the shaft of the penis a few inches. *This cleans from the area of least contamination to the area of greatest contamination.*

4. Collect the specimen.

- Ask the client to start voiding. *Initial voiding clears additional external contaminations at the urethral opening.*
- After the client has begun to void, place the specimen container under the stream of urine near to, but not touching, the meatus.
- Collect 30 to 60 mL of midstream urine.
- Handle only the outside of the container. *This protects the sterility of the inside.*

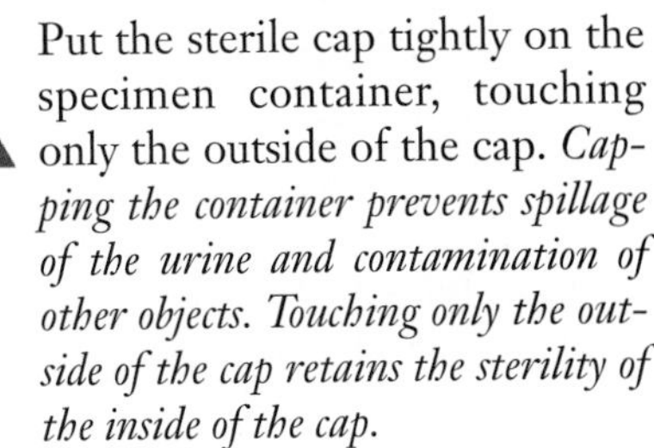

- Put the sterile cap tightly on the specimen container, touching only the outside of the cap. *Capping the container prevents spillage of the urine and contamination of other objects. Touching only the outside of the cap retains the sterility of the inside of the cap.*

- If spillage occurs on the outside of the container, clean the outer surface with a disinfectant. *This prevents the transfer of microorganisms to others.*
- Remove gloves and wash hands.

5. Label and transport the specimen to the laboratory.

- Ensure that the specimen label and the laboratory requisition carry the correct information. Attach them securely to the specimen. *Inaccurate identification and/or information on the specimen container can lead to errors of diagnosis or therapy.*
- Arrange for the specimen to be sent to the laboratory immediately. *Bacterial cultures must be started immediately, before any contaminating organisms can grow, multiply, and produce false results.*

6. Document pertinent data.

- Record collection of the specimen, any pertinent observations of the urine in terms of color, odor, or consistency, and any difficulty in voiding that the client experienced.

EVALUATION FOCUS
Appearance and odor of urine; amount voided, if output is being assessed.

RESEARCH NOTE

Do Nurse-Prepared Multistix Tests Compare Favorably with Laboratory Urinalysis?

For this study, the authors taught six nurse researchers to use nitrite and leukocyte esterase dipsticks to test urine. Both the *leukocyte* and nitrite tests are appropriate for rapid screening for urinary tract infection. The *leukocyte esterase* test screens the urine for pyuria (pus in the urine), a possible indication of infection; by contrast, the nitrite test, when positive, provides stronger evidence of infection.

These nurses obtained early morning clean-catch or catheter-aspirated urine specimens on 37 male subjects in a 2-week period. Working in the nursing area utility room, the researchers performed the dipstick test on the fresh urine and then sent the specimen to the laboratory for culture.

Comparisons of the nurse-conducted leukocyte esterase dipstick test to the laboratory culture revealed that 30 of the 37 (81%) gave the same result.

Comparisons of the nurse-prepared nitrite tests to the laboratory prepared tests revealed that 36 of the 37 (97%) gave the same result. When the results of the nurse-conducted nitrite tests were compared to those of the laboratory culture, once again 30 of the 37 (81%) were found to be the same. A comparison of the laboratory nitrite tests to laboratory culture results showed only 28 of the 37 (76%) to be the same. The fact that the nurses had fresher urine may have accounted for their slightly better result.

Implications: The results of this small study suggest that nurse-prepared nitrite tests could be considered for assisting community extended care facilities with earlier detection of urinary tract infection. A negative result may also be used as a criterion for dispensing with laboratory testing. The cost of multistix testing was estimated at 17 cents per client, compared to the much more costly laboratory analyses.

Source: V Pritchard and J Levernier, Multistix versus laboratory urinalysis in the detection of urinary tract infection, *Journal of Gerontological Nursing*, August 1991, 17:39–42.

through catheterization. If a client has an indwelling catheter, the aspiration method is used.

ASSESSING URINE

Normal urine consists of 96% water and 4% solutes. Organic solutes include urea, ammonia, creatinine, and uric acid. Urea is the chief organic solute. Inorganic solutes include sodium, chloride, potassium, sulfate, magnesium, and phosphorus. Sodium chloride is the most abundant inorganic salt. Characteristics of normal and abnormal urine are shown in Table 41–4.

Measuring Urinary Output Urine volume depends on fluid intake, the amount of solutes to be excreted, loss of fluid in perspiration and exhaled air, the cardiac status and renal status of the client, hormonal influences, and the amount of fluid ingested. Normally, the kidneys produce urine continuously at the rate of 60 to 120 mL per hour (720 to 1440 mL per day) in the adult, but the rate may be as high as 2000 mL per day if fluid intake is high. Fluid balance and measurement of all fluid intake and output are discussed in Chapter 38. Urine outputs below 30 mL per hour may indicate kidney malfunction and must be reported. Urine production of more than 2000 mL per day or 55 mL per hr constitutes polyuria. In children, normal values for urine volumes are 300 to 1500 mL per day.

To measure fluid output, the nurse follows these steps:

- Wear disposable gloves to prevent contact with microorganisms or blood in urine.
- Ask the client to void in a urinal or bedpan.
- If the client needs to defecate, collect the specimen separately or, for a female client who uses a bedpan, collect it at another time.
- Pour the voided urine into a calibrated container.
- Holding the container at eye level, read the amount in the container. Containers usually have a measuring scale on the inside.
- If a specimen is required, pour some urine into the specimen container and discard the remainder unless all urine is to be saved.
- Record the amount on the fluid intake and output sheet, which may be at the bedside or in the bathroom.
- Remove gloves, and wash hands.
- Total and document the amount of output at the end of each shift and at the end of 24 hours on the client's chart.

Many clients can measure and record their own urine output when it is explained to them.

When measuring urine from a client who has an indwelling catheter, the nurse follows these steps:

- Don disposable gloves.
- Take the calibrated container to the bedside.
- Place the container under the urine collection bag so that the spout of the bag is above the container but not touching it. The calibrated container is not sterile, but the inside of the collection bag is sterile.
- Open the spout and permit the urine to flow into the container.
- Close the spout, then proceed as above.

Table 41–4 Characteristics of Normal and Abnormal Urine

Characteristic	Normal	Abnormal	Nursing Considerations
Amount in 24 hours (adult)	1200 to 1500 mL	Under 1200 mL Over 1500 mL	Decreased output is usual with decreased intake. Increased output is usual with increased intake.
Color	Straw, amber Transparent	Dark amber Cloudy Dark orange Red or dark brown	Concentrated urine is darker in color. Excessive urine output is lighter in color (less concentrated). Certain drugs color urine (eg, phenacetin, sulfonamides). Certain foods change urine color (eg, beets, rhubarb).
Clarity	Clear liquid	Mucus plugs, viscid, thick	Cloudiness in urine may be due to the presence of red blood cells, white blood cells, bacteria, prostatic fluid, sperm, or vaginal discharge.
Odor	Faint aromatic	Offensive	Some foods (eg, asparagus) cause a musty odor; infected urine can have a fetid odor; urine high in glucose has a sweet odor.
Sterility	No microorganisms present	Microorganisms present	
pH	4.5 to 8	Under 4.5 Over 8	High-protein foods cause an acid urine; other foods (eg, citrus fruit, dairy products) cause an alkaline urine. Cranberry juice produces an acidic urine. Some medications influence pH; for example, potassium citrate and sodium bicarbonate produce an alkaline urine, ammoniun chlorite an acidic urine. Freshly voided urine is normally acidic. Urine that stands for several hours can become alkaline as a result of bacterial action.
Specific gravity	1.010 to 1.025	Under 1.010 Over 1.025	Concentrated urine has a higher specific gravity; diluted urine has a lower specific gravity. A high specific gravity can reflect dehydration; a low specific gravity, overhydration.
Glucose	Not present	Present	Ingestion of a large amount of glucose can result in glucose in the urine, even in a healthy person.
Ketone bodies (acetone)	Not present	Present	Ketones, the end product of the breakdown of fatty acids, are not normally present in the urine. They may be present in the urine of clients who are dehydrated or who have ingested excessive amounts of aspirin.
Blood	Not present	Occult Bright red	Blood may be present in the urine of clients who have kidney disease or bleeding from the urinary tract.

Measuring Residual Urine **Residual urine** (urine remaining in the bladder following the voiding) is normally not present in the bladder or consists of only a few milliliters. However, whenever there is a bladder outlet obstruction (eg, enlargement of the prostate gland) or loss of bladder muscle tone, there can be large amounts of residual urine. Incomplete emptying of the bladder may be suspected when the client experiences frequency and when only small amounts of urine are voided at a time (eg, 100 mL in an adult). The consequence of incomplete emptying of the bladder is urinary stasis and, ultimately, infection. The purposes of measuring the residual urine are (a) to determine the degree to which the bladder is emptying and (b) to assess the need to establish therapy that will empty the bladder (eg, insertion of a retention catheter).

To measure the residual urine, the nurse asks the client to void and then immediately catheterizes the client. Both the amount of urine voided and the amount of residual urine are measured and recorded. Generally, an indwelling catheter is inserted when the residual urine exceeds a certain amount. Check agency protocol.

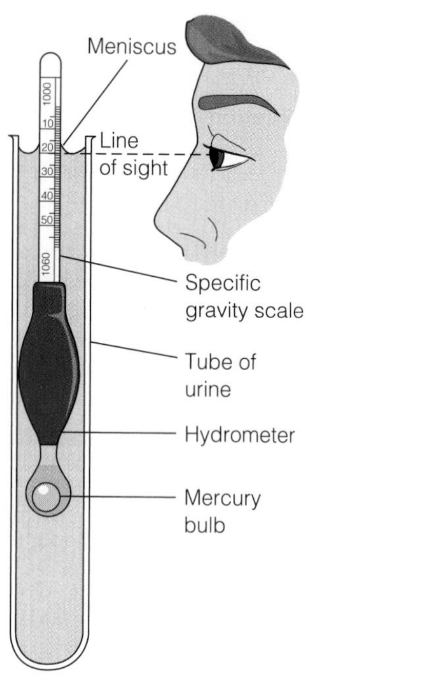

Figure 41–8 A urinometer measurement of the specific gravity of the urine is taken at the base of the meniscus.

URINE TESTING

Several simple urine tests are often done by nurses on the nursing units or are taught to clients, who perform them independently. Tests commonly performed on urine include those for specific gravity, pH, and presence of glucose and occult blood.

Specific Gravity Specific gravity is the weight or degree of concentration of a substance compared with that of an equal volume of another, such as distilled water, taken as a standard. The specific gravity of distilled water is 1.00 g/mL (in other words, 1 mL of water weights 1g).

The specific gravity of urine can be measured by a urinometer, or **hydrometer,** calibrated in units of 0.001. The instrument is placed in a glass cylinder containing the urine (Figure 41–8). The scale on the urinometer progresses from 1.000 at the top to 1.060 at the bottom. The specific gravity of urine is normally about 1.010 to 1.025 g/mL. A low specific gravity is often the result of overhydration or a disease that affects the kidneys' ability to concentrate solutes in urine. A high specific gravity may indicate dehydration or a disease that increases water reabsorption by the kidneys, causing concentrated urine. False positive results are caused by drugs such as dextran and radiopaque materials used in X-ray examination of the urinary tract.

Urinary pH Urinary pH is a measurement of the concentration of hydrogen ions in the client's urine, which indicates its acidity or alkalinity. Discrete measurements of pH are made on a scale of 1 to 14, in which the value 7 is neutral, below 7 is acid, and above 7 is alkaline (base). Such quantitative measurements, however, are conducted in the agency laboratory, where specific reactive agents are used. Nurses can make less discrete measurements of urinary pH using litmus paper (ie, to determine whether the urine is acidic or alkaline).

Glucose Urine is tested for glucose to screen clients for diabetes mellitus or to follow the progress of a known diabetic. Normally, the amount of glucose in the urine is negligible, although individuals who have ingested large amounts of sugar may show small amounts of glucose in their urine.

Several commercial products are commonly used to test for the presence of glucose, for example, Clinitest tablets and Clinistix, Diastix, and Tes-Tape reagent strips. Each uses a color scale to measure the quantity of glucose in the urine, but the scales are not interchangeable from one product to the other. The scales grade the results as negative, trace, one plus (1+, or +), two plus (2+, or ++), three plus (3+, or +++), and so on. Each grade reflects a specific percentage of glucose, which varies from one testing product to another. For example, a 2+ result from a Clinitest reaction indicates 75% glucose in the urine, whereas a 2+ result from a Tes-Tape strip indicates 25% glucose.

False readings can arise from medications a client is receiving, depending on the type of chemical product used to test the urine for glucose. For example, tetracycline and large doses of ascorbic acid and chloral hydrate can generate false positive results from Clinitest tablets. For this reason, many agencies stock more than one testing product. Nurses need to compare the medications a client is receiving with the literature about each product and choose the appropriate product for the test.

Ketone Bodies Ketone bodies are products of incomplete fat metabolism and appear in the urine in instances of fasting, very low intake of carbohydrates, and uncontrolled diabetes mellitus. Usually, the urine is tested for ketone bodies at the same time it is tested for glucose. Tablets or reagent strips are used.

Occult Blood Normal urine is free from blood. When blood is present, it may be clearly visible or not visible **(occult)**. Commercial reagent strips are used to test for occult blood in the urine.

Procedure 41–2 describes how to test urine for specific gravity, pH, glucose, ketones, and occult blood.

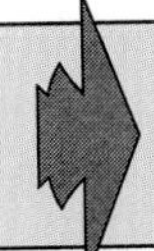

PROCEDURE 41–2 TESTING URINE FOR SPECIFIC GRAVITY, pH, GLUCOSE, KETONES, AND OCCULT BLOOD

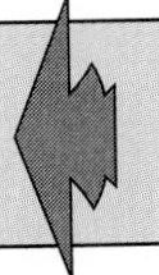

PURPOSES

- To determine the client's hydration status from a specific gravity measurement
- To determine the acidity or alkalinity of the client's urine
- To determine the presence of glucose and ketone bodies in the urine
- To determine the presence of occult blood in the urine

EQUIPMENT

For All Tests

- ☐ Gloves

For Specific Gravity

- ☐ Urinometer (hydrometer) and a glass cylinder
  or
- ☐ Spectrometer or refractometer

For Urine pH

- ☐ Litmus paper (red or blue)

For Glucose

- ☐ Reagent tablet or reagent test strip
- ☐ Appropriate color scale
- ☐ Clean test tube and a dropper, if a tablet is used

For Ketone Bodies

- ☐ Reagent tablet or test strip

For Occult Blood

- ☐ Reagent strip

INTERVENTION

1. To measure specific gravity:

- If a controlled specimen is ordered, ask the client to withhold fluids for the specified time, such as 8 to 12 hours. When routine specific gravity measurements are being taken (eg, for clients with burns), fluids are not withheld.
- To measure with a *urinometer:*

  a. Don gloves, and pour at least 20 mL of a fresh urine sample in the glass cylinder, or fill the cylinder three-quarters full.
  b. Place the urinometer into the cylinder, and give it a gentle spin to prevent it from adhering to the sides of the cylinder.
  c. Hold the urinometer at eye level, and read the measurement at the base of the meniscus at the surface of the urine (Figure 41–8, earlier). *The concentration of the urine affects the degree to which the urinometer will float. The depth to which it sinks indicates the specific gravity.*
- To measure with a *spectrometer* or *refractometer:*
  a. Be sure to follow the manufacturer's directions.

  b. Don gloves, and place one or two drops of urine on the slide.
  c. Turn on the instrument light, and look into the instrument. The specific gravity will appear on a scope.
  d. Write down the number, then turn off the instrument.
  e. Remove the urine with a damp towel or gauze.

2. To measure pH:

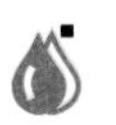

- Put on a glove, and dip a strip of either red or blue litmus paper into the urine specimen.
- Observe the color of the litmus paper, and compare it to a standardized color chart on the bottle. The blue litmus paper, more commonly used, remains blue if the urine is alkaline and turns red if it is acidic. The red litmus paper remains red in the presence of acidic urine and turns blue if the urine is alkaline. Whichever litmus strip is used, red always indicates acidic urine, and blue always indicates alkaline urine.

3. To test for glucose:

- Obtain a freshly voided specimen. Most agencies require a *second-voided specimen:* Ask the client to void, and in 30 minutes to void again, providing a specimen for the test this time. *A second-voided specimen more accurately reflects the present condition of the body. Urine that has accumulated in the bladder (eg, overnight) reflects the condition of the body at the time the urine was produced* (eg, 0300 hours).
- Select the appropriate equipment and testing product for the client. If Clinitest tablets are used, obtain a clean test tube and dropper.

PROCEDURE 41–2 TESTING URINE FOR SPECIFIC GRAVITY, pH, GLUCOSE, KETONES, AND OCCULT BLOOD *continued*

- To carry out the test, put on gloves and follow the directions specified by the manufacturer. If Clinitest tablets are used, be careful not to touch the bottom of the test tube because it becomes extremely hot when the tablet boils in the presence of urine and water.
- Compare the results with the appropriate color chart, and record them on the client's chart. (Most agencies now record the findings as a percentage of glucose in the urine rather than as 2+ or 3+.)

4. **To test for ketone bodies:**

- Put on a glove, and place one or two drops of urine on a reagent tablet (eg, an Acetest tablet) or dip a reagent test strip (eg, Ketostix) into the urine.
- Observe and compare the results with the appropriate color chart to determine the quantity of ketones present.
- Record the results in accordance with the product used and agency practice. The results may be graded as negative, small, moderate, or large amounts or as negative, positive, or strongly positive amounts.

5. **To test for occult blood:**

- Don a glove, and dip the reagent strip (eg, Hemastix) into a sample of urine.
- Compare the color change with a color chart in the same manner as with other reagent strips.

6. **For all tests:**

- Discard the urine following the tests. Clean the equipment with soap and water. Remove gloves.
- Document the results of the test on the client's record.

DIAGNOSTIC TESTS

Two blood tests commonly conducted to examine renal function are the **blood urea nitrogen (BUN)** clearance test and the **creatinine clearance** test. These measure how effectively the kidneys are excreting the respective substances.

Various diagnostic procedures are performed in the operating room. A **cytoscopy** permits direct visualization of the bladder, the ureteral orifices in the bladder, and the urethra. A *cytoscope* is a lighted instrument that is inserted through the urethra. A **intravenous pyelogram** (IVP) or **excretory pyelogram** involves the injection of dyes into the venous system and subsequent X-ray examination of the kidneys, bladder, and urethra. A **retrograde pyelogram** is the injection of dye through a ureteral catheter that is inserted through the urethra, bladder, and ureters into the pelvis of the kidneys. X-ray studies are taken following the injection of the dye. Nurses are responsible for preparing clients before these studies and for follow-up care. An IVP is described in the *Clinical Companion.*

Computerized axial tomography (CAT or **CT)** is a painless, noninvasive X-ray procedure with the unique capability of distinguishing minor differences in the radiodensity of soft tissues. Dense substances appear white; low-density substances appear dark. The organ to be studied gives the scan its name, for example, kidney scan.

Ultrasonography (ultrasound), another noninvasive technique, uses high-frequency sound waves well above the upper limit of human hearing. During this procedure, which has no known harmful effects, acoustic densities of tissues are measured. In contrast to usual radiography, ultrasound reveals the depth of a structure below the skin and the anteroposterior dimension of masses. Sound waves travel at different speeds, depending on the density of the structures through which they pass. The kidneys may be examined by ultrasound.

DIAGNOSING

Nursing diagnoses that are related to urinary elimination problems include **Incontinence, Altered urinary elimination,** and **Urinary retention.** The North American Nursing Diagnosis Association subcategorizes the diagnosis of **Incontinence** as follows:

- **Functional incontinence**
- **Reflex incontinence**
- **Stress incontinence**
- **Total incontinence**
- **Urge incontinence**

These diagnoses, with definitions, defining characteristics, and contributing factors, are shown in the box at the right. Clinical examples of assessment data clusters and related nursing diagnoses are in Table 41–5 (p. 1241).

NURSING DIAGNOSES
CLIENTS WITH URINARY ELIMINATION PROBLEMS

NURSING DIAGNOSIS: Functional incontinence: The state in which one experiences an involuntary, unpredictable passage of urine

Defining Characteristics

- Urge to void or bladder contractions sufficiently strong to result in loss of urine before reaching an appropriate receptacle.

Related Factors

Impaired physical mobility; cognitive impairment; disorientation; altered environment (eg, poor lighting, inability to locate toilet), reluctance to use call light or bedpan).

NURSING DIAGNOSIS: Reflex incontinence: The state in which one experiences an involuntary loss of urine occurring at somewhat predictable intervals when a specific bladder volume is reached

Defining Characteristics

- No awareness of bladder filling
- No urge to void or feelings of bladder fullness
- Uninhibited bladder contraction/spasm at regular intervals

Related Factors

Neurologic impairment (eg, spinal cord lesion)

NURSING DIAGNOSIS: Stress incontinence: The state in which one experiences a loss of urine of less than 50 mL occurring with increased intra-abdominal pressure

Defining Characteristics

- Reported or observed dribbling with increased intra-abdominal pressure
- Urinary urgency
- Urinary frequency (more often than every 2 hours)

Related Factors

Age-related degenerative changes in pelvic muscles and structural supports, or weakened muscles and structures; high intra-abdominal pressure associated with obesity, gravid uterus; incontinent bladder outlet; overdistention between voidings.

NURSING DIAGNOSIS: Total incontinence: The state in which one experiences a continuous and unpredictable loss of urine

Defining Characteristics

- Constant flow of urine at unpredictable times without distention or uninhibited bladder contractions/spasms
- Unsuccessful refractory treatments
- Nocturia
- Lack of perineal or bladder filling awareness
- Lack of awareness of incontinence

Related Factors

Neuropathy preventing transmission of reflex indicating bladder fullness; neurologic dysfunction causing triggering of micturition at unpredictable times; independent contraction of detrusor reflex due to surgery; trauma or disease affecting spinal cord nerves; anatomic disorder (fistula).

➤

URINARY ELIMINATION PROBLEMS CONTINUED

NURSING DIAGNOSIS: Urge incontinence: The state in which one experiences involuntary passage of urine occurring soon after a strong sense of urgency to void

Defining Characteristics

- Urinary urgency
- Frequency (voiding more often than every 2 hours)
- Bladder contraction/spasm
- Nocturia (more than 2 times per night)
- Voiding in small amounts (less than 100 mL) or in large amounts (more than 500 mL).
- Inability to reach toilet in time

Related Factors

Decreased bladder capacity (eg, history of pelvic inflammatory disease, abdominal surgery, indwelling urinary catheter); irritation of bladder stretch receptors, causing spasm (eg, due to bladder infection); alcohol intake; caffeine intake; increased fluid intake; increased urine concentration; overdistention of bladder.

NURSING DIAGNOSIS: Altered urinary elimination: The state in which one experiences a disturbance in urine elimination (see also **Incontinence** and **Urinary retention**)

Defining Characteristics

- Dysuria
- Frequency
- Hesitancy
- Nocturia
- Retention
- Urgency
- Incontinence

Related Factors

Sensory motor impairment; neuromuscular impairment; mechanical trauma; urinary infection.

NURSING DIAGNOSIS: Urinary retention: The state in which one experiences incomplete emptying of the bladder

Defining Characteristics

- Bladder distention
- Small, frequent voiding or absence of urine output
- Sensation of bladder fullness
- Dribbling
- Overflow incontinence
- Residual urine

Related Factors

High urethral pressure caused by weak detrusor; inhibition of reflex arc; strong sphincter; blockage of urine.

Sources: LJ Carpenito, *Nursing Diagnosis: Application to Clinical Practice*, 4th ed. (Philadelphia: Lippincott, 1992), pp. 908–30; M Gordon, *Manual of Nursing Diagnosis 1993–1994*, 6th ed. (St Louis: Mosby-Year Book, 1993) pp. 143–55; MJ Kim, GK McFarland, and AM McLane, *Pocket Guide to Nursing Diagnoses*, 5th ed. (St Louis; Mosby-Year Book, 1993), pp. 31–33, 64–65; GK McFarland and EA McFarlane, *Nursing Diagnosis and Intervention: Planning for Patient Care*, 2d ed. (St Louis: Mosby, 1993), pp. 243–53; North American Nursing Diagnosis Association, *NANDA Nursing Diagnoses: Definitions and Classification 1992–1993*. (Philadelphia: NANDA, 1992), pp. 18–21; and JR Lederer, GL Marculescu, B Mocnik, and N Seaby, *Care Planning Pocket Guide—A Nursing Diagnosis Approach*, 5th ed. (Redwood City, CA: Addison-Wesley Nursing, 1993), pp. 224–36.

Table 41–5 Clinical Application: Assessment Data Clusters and Related Nursing Diagnoses

Data Cluster	Nursing Diagnosis
Mrs Amy Brown, 75 years old, reports accidental loss of urine before she is able to reach the toilet. She is aware of the urge to void but "because of my stroke I sometimes can't get there soon enough."	**Functional incontinence** related to mobility deficit
Anthony Cherry, a teenaged victim of a spinal cord injury, has no awareness of bladder filling, the urge to void, or feelings of bladder fullness. He reports loss of urine at fairly regular intervals.	**Reflex incontinence** related to neurologic impairment (spinal cord lesion)
Tammy Tyndale reports dribbling whenever she laughs, coughs, or sneezes. She is 8 months pregnant.	**Stress incontinence** related to high intra-abdominal pressure associated with pregnancy
Mr Gino Mingo is wheelchair-bound from the effects of multiple sclerosis. He has a constant flow of urine at unpredictable times, including nocturia. He is unaware of bladder filling and of incontinence.	**Total incontinence** related to neurologic impairment
Mrs Gail Brady reports urinary urgency, difficulty in getting to the bathroom in time, frequency (more often than every 2 hours), and leakage of urine when unable to reach the toilet in time.	**Urge incontinence** related to unknown etiology

Other diagnoses, depending on the data obtained, may arise:

- **High risk for infection** if the client has urinary retention or undergoes an invasive procedure such as catheterization or cystoscopic examination.
- **Self-esteem disturbance** if the client is incontinent. Incontinence can be physically and emotionally distressing to clients because it is considered socially unacceptable. Often the client is embarrassed about dribbling or having an accident and may restrict normal activities for this reason.
- **High risk for impaired skin integrity** if the client is incontinent. Bed linens and clothes saturated with urine irritate and excoriate the skin. Prolonged skin dampness leads to dermatitis (inflammation of the skin) and subsequent formation of decubitus ulcers.
- **Social isolation** if the client is incontinent (see also **Self-esteem disturbance**).
- **Self-care deficit: Toileting** if the client has functional incontinence.
- **High risk for fluid volume deficit** or **Fluid volume excess** if the client has impaired urinary function associated with a disease process.
- **Body image disturbance** if the client has a urinary diversion ostomy.
- **Knowledge deficit** if the client requires self-care skills to manage, for example, a new urinary diversion ostomy.

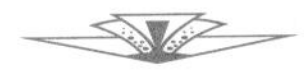

PLANNING

The overall outcomes for clients with urinary elimination problems are to maintain or restore the client's normal urinary elimination pattern and to prevent associated risks such as infection, skin breakdown, fluid and electrolyte imbalance, and lowered self-esteem. Specific outcome criteria, nursing interventions, and rationales associated with **Urinary incontinence** and **Urinary retention** are shown in the Care Planning Guide on page 1242.

A critical pathway can also be useful for planning client care (see p. 1265).

IMPLEMENTING

MAINTAINING NORMAL URINARY ELIMINATION

Most interventions to maintain normal urinary elimination are independent nursing functions. These include promoting adequate fluid intake, maintaining normal voiding habits, and assisting with toileting. See also the Wellness Teaching box on page 1245.

Promoting Fluid Intake Increasing fluid intake increases urine production, which in turn stimulates the micturition reflex. A normal, average daily intake of 1200 to 1500 mL of measurable fluids is adequate for most clients. Additional amounts are required for clients whose fluid demands are great, such as those who have abnormal fluid losses from other routes (eg, excessive perspiration, vomiting, or diarrhea).

Text continued on page 1244

CARE PLANNING GUIDE

CLIENTS WITH URINARY ELIMINATION PROBLEMS

NURSING DIAGNOSIS: Urinary incontinence

Outcome Criteria	Nursing Interventions	Rationale
The client		
▪ Has a decrease in episodes of incontinence to fewer than ______ times a week (specify).	Assess the client's pattern of incontinence. Use a voiding record or diary as indicated.	Knowledge of the client's current pattern serves as a baseline to gauge the severity of the problem and efficacy of therapy.
	Implement appropriate bladder management techniques (see page 1245):	Interventions vary according to the client's type of incontinence and related factors.
	▪ Scheduled toileting and prompted voiding: Encourage voiding every 1 to 2 hours and gradually increase to 3 to 4 hours.	Scheduling assists the client to delay voiding. Prompted voiding is a reminder to use the toilet and to void.
	▪ Instruction in relaxation techniques to use when first feeling the urge to void (ie, a deep breath through the nose held briefly followed by exhalation through the mouth).	The urge to void may subside momentarily with relaxation, giving the client time to use a bedpan or to walk to the toilet.
	▪ Kegel's exercises **(Functional incontinence** and **Stress incontinence).**	Kegel's exercises strengthen pelvic support muscles to enable the client to control the start and stoppage of urine flow.
	▪ Clean intermittent self-catheterization **(Reflex incontinence)** with schedule (eg, every 4 to 6 hours).	CISC helps clients with bladder dysfunction or urinary incontinence establish bladder control.
	▪ Positive feedback for success	
	Discourage the use of caffeine, alcohol, citrus juices, carbonated drinks, cigarettes, and certain spicy foods.	These act as bladder irritants and some as diuretics, which aggravate the incontinence problem.
	▪ Monitor and document the client's urinary elimination pattern.	This enables the nurse to evaluate the effectiveness of therapy.
▪ Alters environment and clothing as instructed to accommodate needs and to facilitate toileting and continence.	Identify needs to facilitate toileting and continence: (a) grab bars in bathroom; (b) raised toilet seat; (c) improved lighting to reach bathroom; (d) provision of commode, bedpan, or urinal; (e) mobility aids, such as a walker; (f) adjustment to garments to make disrobing easier; (g) instruction in transfer techniques.	A comprehensive assessment of self-care abilities affecting toileting enables the nurse to focus on appropriate interventions for the client or to obtain appropriate referral resources.

Outcome Criteria	Nursing Interventions	Rationale
▪ Maintains fluid intake of 1500 to 2000 mL per day and establishes and adheres to schedule for fluid intake.	Encourage the client to drink 6 to 8 glasses of water per day.	Many clients decrease their fluid intake to control incontinence episodes and may become dehydrated. Without adequate fluid intake, urine may become more concentrated, irritate the bladder mucosa, and increase the urge to urinate. Fluids also help to distend the bladder to its normal capacity.
	Establish a written plan for fluid intake (eg, 200 mL every 2 hours between 0800 and 1800 hours).	A written plan facilitates achievement and evaluation of goals.
	Decrease fluid intake several hours before bedtime.	This helps decrease the need to void at night.
▪ Has intact perineal skin.	Clean and dry the skin immediately after an incontinence episode. Use protective skin barriers as needed for clients with total incontinence.	Ammonia in the urine can quickly irritate the skin and predispose the client to skin breakdown.
	Monitor the skin for areas of redness and breakdown after each voiding.	Early recognition of problems facilitates prompt intervention to deal with the problem.
	Use continence aids such as an external urinary device for male clients or absorbent pads and protective clothing for female clients.	These items collect drainage and prevent soiling of clothing and subsequent embarrassment.
▪ Reports reestablishment of short social contacts twice per week, (eg, 1- to 2-hour visits two times per week) and gradually returns to usual activities.	Explore the client's previous activities, and help the client plan short trips away from home. Advise using continence aids to protect clothing.	Use of continence aids reduces the client's anxiety and prevents soiling.
	Actively listen to the client's concerns and feelings about incontinence episodes.	Active listening conveys caring and sensitivity to the client's feelings.
	Inform the client about different products that absorb urine and where they can be purchased.	Use of appropriate absorbent products can reassure the client and prevent soilage of clothing.

NURSING DIAGNOSIS: Urinary retention

Outcome Criteria	Nursing Interventions	Rationale
The client		
▪ Voids sufficient amounts with no bladder distention and no overflow dribbling.	Identify and document the client's urinary elimination pattern.	Knowledge of the client's elimination pattern provides baseline data that will serve to gauge the effectiveness of therapy.
	Palpate the bladder every 4 hours or at preestablished frequency (specify).	Palpation allows the nurse to determine the presence of bladder distention.

➤

URINARY ELIMINATION PROBLEMS CONTINUED

NURSING DIAGNOSIS: Urinary retention *continued*

Outcome Criteria	Nursing Interventions	Rationale
	Implement techniques that encourage voiding (see positioning and relaxation techniques in the box on page 1245).	These measures may initiate the voiding reflex.
	Consider using Credé's maneuver if there is no obstruction (see page 1248).	Manual pressure on the bladder may force urine through the urinary sphincters.
	Establish a bladder-evacuation program.	
	Plan schedule for fluid intake (eg, ____ mL for daytime; ____ mL for evenings; and ____ mL for nights).	Following a schedule ensures adequate fluid intake without overdistending the bladder.
▪ Has past void residual (PVR) volume of less than 50 mL.	If voiding is successful, assess PVR urine volume.	A PVR of less than 50 mL is considered adequate bladder emptying; over 200 mL is considered inadequate.
	If voiding is repeatedly unsuccessful or the PVR is inadequate, catheterize the client, wait for bladder filling, and then repeat the above measures. A physician's order for catheterization may be required.	Catheterization is used as a last resort because of the danger of urinary tract infection (UTI).
	If independent nursing actions fail to produce bladder emptying, consult a physician about administering a parasympathomimetic agent, such as bethanechol hydrochloride (Urecholine).	Parasympathomimetic agents stimulate micturition.
▪ Demonstrates no signs of urinary tract infection.	Instruct the client in reportable signs/symptoms of urinary tract infection (fever, chills, flank pain, hematuria, change in consistency and odor of urine).	Early recognition of infection facilitates prompt intervention to alleviate the problem.

Immobilized clients who are susceptible to calculi (kidney stone) formation require daily intakes of 2000 to 3000 mL per day (unless medically contraindicated). Dilute urine helps prevent urinary tract stones and infection. Increased fluid intakes are contraindicated in clients who require fluid restrictions, such as those with renal impairment or congestive heart failure. Fluid intake can also be increased by encouraging the client to eat plenty of raw fruits and vegetables, which have a high water content.

Maintaining Normal Voiding Habits Hospital routines and prescribed medical therapies often interfere with a client's normal voiding habits. When a client's urinary elimination pattern is adequate, the nurse helps the client adhere to normal voiding habits as much as possible. Clinical guidelines are in the box at the far right.

Assisting with Toileting Clients who are weakened by a disease process or impaired physically require assistance to toilet. The nurse should assist these clients to the bathroom and remain with them if the client is at high risk for falling. The bathroom should contain an easily accessible call signal to summon help if needed. Clients also need to be encouraged to use hand rails placed near the toilet.

For clients unable to use bathroom facilities, the nurse provides urinary equipment close to the bedside (eg, urinal, bedpan, commode) and provides the necessary assistance to use them.

WELLNESS TEACHING

Urinary Elimination

- Respond as soon as possible to the urge to void.
- Drink eight to ten 8-oz glasses of water a day.
- After urination, females should wipe from the urinary meatus toward the anus.
- Maintain perineal-genital cleanliness.
- Avoid foods and fluids that contain excessive sodium, which can lead to fluid retention.
- Empty the bladder completely at each voiding.
- Obtain medical assistance if burning accompanies voiding or if the urine changes in color, clarity, odor, or amount.

Assisting to use bedpans and urinals is discussed in Chapter 40 on page 1198. Effective methods to transfer a client from bed to commode (or wheelchair) are discussed in Chapter 34, page 924.

MANAGING URINARY INCONTINENCE (UI)

Independent nursing interventions for clients with urinary incontinence (UI) include (a) a behavior-oriented continence training program that may consist of bladder training, habit training, prompted voiding, pelvic muscle exercises, and positive reinforcement; (b) meticulous skin care; and (c) for males, application of an external drainage device (condom). The physician may order urinary catheterization for clients unable to control micturition. Nursing interventions for catheterized clients are discussed later in the chapter.

Continence (Bladder) Training A continence training program requires the involvement of the nurse, the client, and support persons. Clients must be alert and physically able to follow a program. The goal of training is to decrease the frequency of UI. A bladder training program generally consists of the following (McCormick, Newman, et al 1992, p. 78):

- Education of the client and support persons.
- **Bladder training,** which requires that the client postpone voiding, resist or inhibit the sensation of urgency, and void according to a timetable rather than according to the urge to void. The goals are to gradually lengthen the intervals between urination to correct the client's habit of frequent urination, to stabilize the bladder, and to diminish urgency. This form of training may be used for clients who have bladder instability

CLINICAL GUIDELINES

Maintaining Normal Voiding Habits

Positioning

- Assist the client to a normal position for voiding; standing for males; for females, squatting or leaning slightly forward when sitting. These positions enhance movement of urine through the tract by gravity.
- Use bedside commodes as necessary for females and urinals for males standing at the bedside.
- Encourage the client to push over the pubic area with the hands or to lean forward to increase intra-abdominal pressure and external pressure on the bladder.

Relaxation

- Provide privacy for the client. Many people cannot void in the presence of another person.
- Allow the client sufficient time to void.
- Suggest the client read or listen to music.
- Provide sensory stimuli that may help the client relax. Pour warm water over the perineum of a female or have the client sit in a warm bath to promote muscle relaxation. Applying a hot-water bottle to the lower abdomen of both men and women may also foster muscle relaxation.
- Turn on running water within hearing distance of the client to mask the sound of voiding for persons who find this embarrassing.
- Relieve physical and emotional discomfort to decrease muscle tension and encourage the mental concentration that may be needed for micturition. Make sure to provide ordered analgesics and emotional support.

Timing

- Assist clients who have the urge to void immediately. Delays only increase the difficulty in starting to void, and the desire to void may pass.
- Offer toileting assistance to the client at usual times of voiding, for example, on awakening, before or after meals, and at bedtime.

For Bed-Confined Clients

- Warm the bed pan. A cold bedpan may prompt contraction of the perineal muscles and inhibit voiding.
- Elevate the head of the client's bed to Fowler's position, place a small pillow or rolled towel at the small of the back to increase physical support and comfort, and have the client flex the hips and knees. This position simulates the normal voiding position as closely as possible.

CLIENT TEACHING

Routine for Kegel's Exercises

- First, sit or stand with the legs apart.
- Pull your rectum, urethra, and vagina up inside, and hold for a count of 3 to 5 seconds. The pull should be felt at the cleft of your buttocks.
- Initially perform each contraction ten times, five times daily.
- Develop a schedule that will help remind you to do these exercises, for example, while driving to work, when working at the kitchen sink, or at scheduled times (eg, 0700, 1000, 1300, 1600, and 1900 hours).
- Try to start and stop your stream of urine.
- To control episodes of stress incontinence, brace the muscles and use the Kegel maneuver when doing any activity that increases intra-abdominal pressure, such as coughing, laughing, sneezing, or lifting.

and stress incontinence. Delayed voiding provides larger voided volumes and longer intervals between voiding. Initially, voiding may be encouraged every 2 to 3 hours except during sleep and then every 4 to 6 hours. A vital component of bladder training is inhibiting the urge-to-void sensation. To do this, the nurse instructs the client to practice deep, slow breathing until the urge diminishes or disappears. This is performed every time the client has a premature urge to void.

- **Habit training,** also referred to as timed voiding or scheduled toileting, attempts to keep clients dry by having them void at *regular* intervals. With habit training, there is no attempt to motivate the client to delay voiding, if the urge occurs.
- **Prompted voiding** supplements habit training by encouraging the client to try to use the toilet (prompting) and reminding the client when to void.

Pelvic Muscle Exercises (PME) Pelvic muscle exercises, referred to as perineal muscle tightening or *Kegel's exercises,* strengthen pubococcygeal muscles and can increase the incontinent female's ability to start and stop the stream of urine. The client can feel the perineal muscle group to be exercised by stopping urination midstream. The following technique is sometimes used to teach Kegel's exercises. Ask the client to think of her perineal muscles as an elevator. When the client relaxes, the elevator is on the first floor. To perform the exercise, contract the perineal muscles, bringing the elevator to the second, third, and fourth floors. Keep the elevator on the fourth floor for a few seconds, and then gradually relax the area. When the exercise is properly performed, contraction of the muscles of the buttocks and thighs is avoided.

Kegel's exercises can be performed anytime, anywhere, sitting or standing—even when voiding. Specific client instructions for performing Kegel's exercises suggested by Kuhns-Hastings (1988, p. 82) are summarized in the box at the left above.

CLINICAL GUIDELINES

Bladder Retraining

- Determine the client's voiding pattern and encourage voiding at those times, or establish a regular voiding schedule and help the client to maintain it, whether the client feels the urge or not (eg, on awakening, every 1 or 2 hours during the day and evening, before retiring at night, every 4 hours at night). The stretching-relaxing sequence of such a schedule tends to increase bladder muscle tone and promote more voluntary control.
- When the client finds that voiding can be controlled, the intervals between voiding can be lengthened slightly without loss of continence.
- Regulate fluid intake, particularly before the client retires, to help reduce the need to void during the night.
- Encourage fluids about half an hour before the voiding time between the hours of 0600 and 1800, or allow 2 hours between the last fluid and bedtime. Large amounts of fruit juices and carbonated beverages should be avoided, since fruit juice alkalinizes the urine and soft drinks cause bladder irritation.
- Stimulants (eg, tea, coffee, and alcoholic beverages) should be avoided at bedtime to decrease the possibility of nocturia.
- Schedule diuretics early in the morning.
- Explain to clients that adequate fluid intake is required to ensure adequate urine production to stimulate the micturition reflex. Clients who have fluid restrictions due to a medical condition may be maintained on 1500 mL per day.
- Apply protector pads to keep the bed linen dry, and provide specially made waterproof underwear to contain the urine and decrease the client's embarrassment. Avoid using diapers, which are demeaning and also suggest that incontinence is permissible.
- Assist the client with an exercise program to increase the tone of abdominal and pelvic muscles.
- Provide a system of positive and negative reinforcements to encourage continence. Such systems are commonly referred to as *behavior modification* and require the cooperation of all persons involved in the client's care.

To help clients identify the pelvic muscles, including the anal sphincter, the nurse explains that it is the muscle they would use to hold a bowel movement. To ensure that the client properly identifies and adequately tightens the sphincter, the nurse can insert a gloved finger into the client's rectum and ask the client to squeeze the nurse's finger (Scheve et al 1991, p. 124).

Positive Reinforcement Positive reinforcement is used in conjunction with all continence measures the nurse implements. Clients are praised for attempting to toilet and for maintaining continence.

Clinical guidelines for bladder retraining are summarized in the box on the previous page.

Maintaining Skin Integrity Skin that is continually moist becomes macerated. Over a period of time urine that accumulates on the skin is converted to ammonia, which is very irritating to the skin. Because both skin irritation and maceration predispose the client to skin breakdown and decubitus ulcers, the incontinent person requires meticulous skin care. To prevent alterations in skin integrity, the nurse washes the client's perineal area with soap and water after periods of incontinence, rinses it thoroughly, dries it thoroughly, and provides clean, dry clothing or bed linen. If the skin is irritated, the nurse applies barrier creams such as zinc oxide ointment to protect it from contact with urine. If it is necessary to pad the client's clothes for protection, the nurse should use products that absorb wetness and leave a dry surface in contact with the skin.

Specially designed *incontinence drawsheets* that provide significant advantages over standard drawsheets for bedridden incontinent clients have been introduced in North American and Great Britain (Cefalu 1987; Pottle 1986). These sheets are like a drawsheet but are double layered, with a colored (eg, yellow or pink) quilted upper nylon or polyester surface and an absorbent viscose rayon layer below. The rayon soaker layer generally has a waterproof backing on its underside. Fluid (ie, urine) passes through the upper quilted layer and is absorbed and dispersed by the viscose rayon, leaving the quilted surface dry to the touch. This absorbent sheet helps maintain skin integrity; it does not stick to the skin when wet, decreases the risk of bedsores, and reduces odor.

Applying External Urinary Devices The application of a **condom,** also referred to as a *urinary sheath* or *external catheter,* and attachment of its base to a urinary drainage system are commonly prescribed for incontinent males. Use of a condom appliance is preferable to insertion of a retention catheter, because it avoids entrance into the urethra and bladder and minimizes the risk of urethral or bladder infection.

Methods of applying condoms vary according to the length of time the condom is to be worn. Condoms that are to be worn for short periods are generally applied with elastic tape only; if the condom is to be worn for longer periods (eg, a few days), additional measures are required to protect the foreskin and to ensure secure attachment. The nurse needs to follow manufacturer's instructions when applying a condom. Before applying the condom, the nurse determines when the client experiences incontinence. Some clients may require a condom appliance at night only, others continuously. Procedure 41–3 describes how to apply and remove a drainage condom.

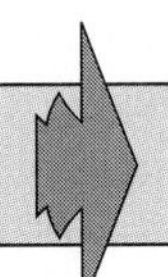

PROCEDURE 41–3 APPLYING A DRAINAGE CONDOM

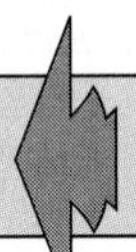

PURPOSES

- To collect urine and control urinary incontinence
- To permit the client physical activity without fear of embarrassment because of leaking urine
- To prevent skin irritation as a result of urine incontinence

ASSESSMENT FOCUS

Times of urinary incontinence; amount of urine passed (eg, large, dribble); skin irritation, excoriation, swelling, and discoloration of penis.

EQUIPMENT

- ☐ Leg drainage bag with tubing or urinary drainage bag with tubing
- ☐ Condom sheath
- ☐ Bath blanket
- ☐ Disposable gloves
- ☐ Basin of warm water and soap
- ☐ Washcloth and towel
- ☐ Elastic tape or Velcro strap

PROCEDURE 41-3 APPLYING A DRAINAGE CONDOM *continued*

INTERVENTION

1. Prepare the equipment.

- Assemble the leg drainage bag or urinary drainage bag for attachment to the condom sheath.
- Roll the condom outward onto itself to facilitate easier application. On some models an inner flap will be exposed. *This flap is applied around the urinary meatus to prevent the reflux of urine* (Figure 41–9).

2. Position and drape the client.

- Position the client in either a supine or a bed-sitting position.
- Drape the client appropriately with the bath blanket, exposing only the penis.

3. Inspect and clean the penis.

- Don gloves.
- Inspect the penis for skin irritation (contact dermatitis), excoriation, swelling, or discoloration. *The nurse needs to obtain baseline data.*
- Clean the genital area, and dry it thoroughly. *This minimizes skin irritation and excoriation after the condom is applied.*

4. Apply and secure the condom.

- Roll the condom smoothly over the penis, leaving 2.5 cm. (1 in) between the end of the penis and the rubber or plastic connecting tube (Figure 41–10). *This space prevents irritation of the tip of the penis and provides for full drainage of urine.*

- Secure the condom firmly, but not too tightly, to the penis by wrapping a strip of elastic tape or Velcro around the base of the penis over the condom. *Ordinary tape is contraindicated because it is*

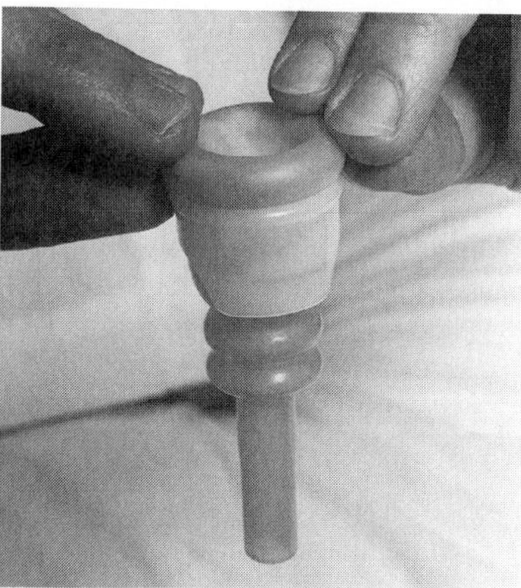

Figure 41–9 Before application, roll the condom outward onto itself.

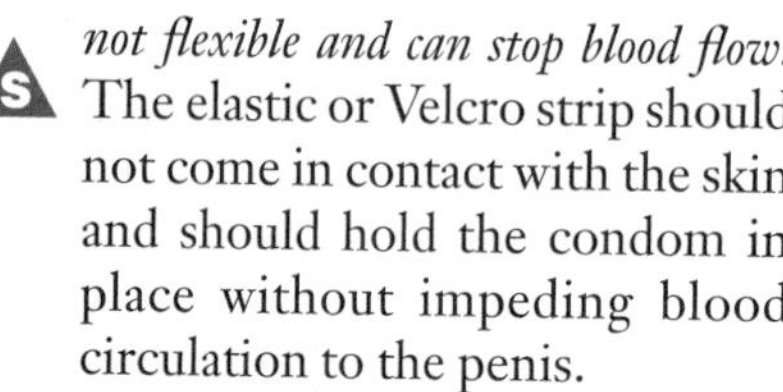

not flexible and can stop blood flow. The elastic or Velcro strip should not come in contact with the skin and should hold the condom in place without impeding blood circulation to the penis.

5. Securely attach the urinary drainage system.

- Make sure that the tip of the penis is not touching the condom and that the condom is not twisted. *A twisted condom could obstruct the flow of urine.*
- Attach the urinary drainage system to the condom.
- Remove gloves.

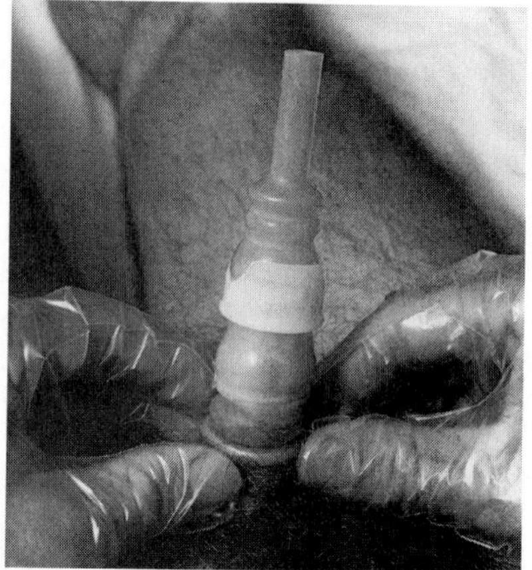

Figure 41–10 Rolling the condom over the penis.

- If the client is to remain in bed, attach the urinary drainage bag to the bed frame.
- If the client is ambulatory, attach the bag to the client's leg (Figure 41–11). *Attaching the drainage bag to the leg helps control the movement of the tubing and prevents twisting of the thin material of the condom appliance at the tip of the penis.*

6. Teach the client about the drainage system.

- Instruct the client to keep the drainage bag below the level of the condom and to avoid loops or kinks in the tubing.

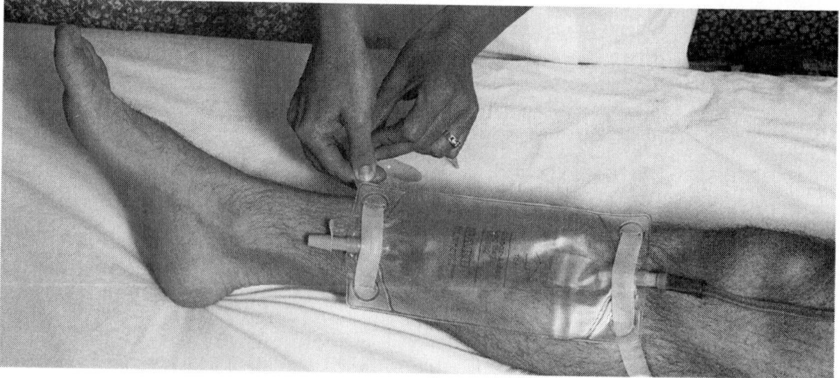

Figure 41–11 Attaching the urinary drainage bag to the leg.

PROCEDURE 41–3 *continued*

7. Document pertinent data.

- Record the application of the condom, the time, and pertinent observations, such as irritated areas on the penis.

8. Inspect the penis 30 minutes following the condom application, and check urine flow.

- Assess the penis for swelling and  discoloration, which indicates that the condom is too tight.
- Assess urine flow. Normally, some urine is present in the tube if the flow is not obstructed.

9. Change the condom daily, and provide skin care.

- Remove the elastic or Velcro strip and roll off the condom.
- Wash the penis with soapy water, rinse, and dry it thoroughly.
- Assess the foreskin for signs of irritation, swelling, and discoloration.

EVALUATION FOCUS
Penis swelling and discoloration; urine flow; skin irritation.

MANAGING URINARY RETENTION (UR)

Interventions that assist the client to maintain a normal voiding pattern, discussed earlier, are applicable when dealing with urinary retention. If these actions are unsuccessful, the physician may order a cholinergic drug such as bethanecol chloride (Urecholine) to stimulate bladder contraction and facilitate voiding. For clients who have bladder **flaccidity** (weak, soft, and lax bladder muscles), manual exertion of pressure on the bladder may be necessary to force urine out. This is known as **Credé's maneuver** or *Credé's method.* It is not advised without a physician's order and is used only for clients who have lost and are not expected to regain voluntary bladder control. For clients who are expected to regain control, this maneuver does not promote increased bladder muscle tone and may cause damage to the urethral sphincters. When all measures fail to initiate voiding, urinary catheterization may be ordered. When the client's postvoid residual urine is 500mL or more, an indwelling Foley catheter may be inserted until the underlying cause is treated; alternatively, intermittent straight catheterization may be performed every 6 to 8 hours (Williams et al 1993, p. 10). Check agency protocol.

URINARY CATHETERIZATION

Urinary catheterization is the introduction of a catheter through the urethra into the urinary bladder. This is usually performed only when absolutely necessary, because the procedure incurs certain hazards. Because the urinary structures are normally sterile except at the end of the urethra, the danger exists of introducing microorganisms into the bladder. This hazard is greatest for clients who have lowered resistance due to disease processes. Once an infection is introduced into the bladder, it can ascend the ureters and eventually involve the kidneys. Even after the catheter has been inserted and left in place for a time, the hazard of infection remains, because microorganisms can be introduced through the catheter lumen. Thus, strict sterile technique is used for catheterization.

Another hazard is trauma, particularly in the male client, whose urethra is longer and more tortuous. It is important to insert a catheter along the normal contour of the urethra. Damage to the urethra can occur if the catheter is forced through strictures or at an incorrect angle. In females, the urethra lies posteriorly, then takes a slightly anterior direction toward the bladder (Figure 41–4, earlier). In males, the urethra is normally curved (Figure 41–3, earlier), but it can be straightened by elevating the penis to a position perpendicular to the body.

Catheters are tubes commonly made of rubber or plastics, although certain types are made of woven silk or metal. *Urethral catheters* are inserted through the urethra into the urinary bladder. Two categories of urethral catheters are straight catheters and retention catheters. The *straight*, or *Robinson, catheter* is a single-lumen tube with a small eye or opening about 1¼ cm (½ in) from the insertion tip (Figure 41–12, *A*, p. 1250).

The *retention*, or *Foley, catheter* contains a second, smaller tube throughout its length on the inside. This tube is connected to a balloon near the insertion tip. After catheter insertion, the balloon is inflated to hold the catheter in place within the bladder. The outside end of the retention catheter is bifurcated; that is, it has two openings, one to drain the urine, the other to inflate the balloon (Figure 41–12, *B*).

Another type of straight catheter is the *coudé* (elbowed) *catheter*, which has a curved tip (Figure 41–13). This is sometimes used for elderly men who have a hypertrophied prostate, because its passage is often less traumatic

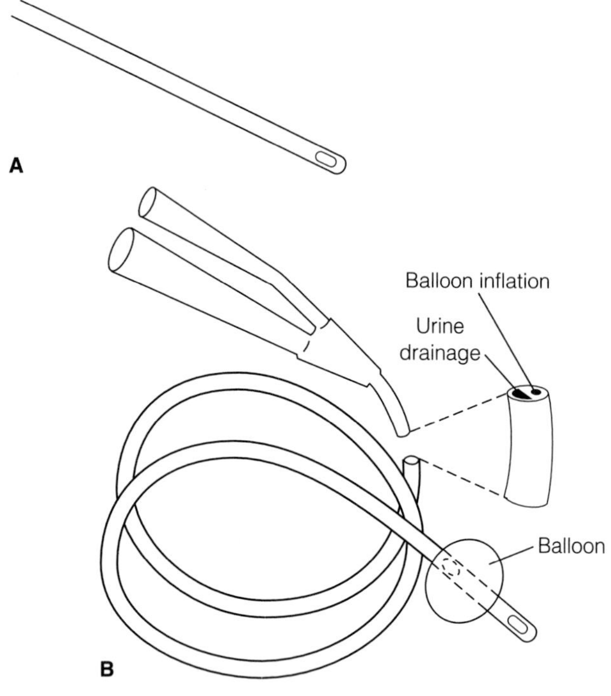

Figure 41–12 Two types of commonly used catheters: *A,* a straight (Robinson) catheter; *B,* a retention (Foley) catheter with the balloon inflated.

to the gland than the passage of a straight catheter. It is somewhat stiff and is more readily controlled.

There are several other types of retention catheters. One that is frequently used for a client requiring continual or periodic bladder irrigations is the *three-way Foley catheter* (Figure 41–14). It is similar to the two-way Foley catheter described earlier, except that it has a third channel through which sterile fluid can flow into the urinary bladder. From the bladder, the fluid then flows through a second channel into a receptacle.

Catheters are made of various types of materials: plastic, latex, silicone, and polyvinylchloride (PVC). They are sized by the diameter of the lumen and are graded on a French scale of numbers; the larger the number, the larger the lumen.

The balloons of retention catheters are sized by the volume of fluid or air used to inflate them. The two commonly used sizes are 5 mL and 30 mL balloons. The size of the balloon is indicated on the catheter along with the diameter, for example, "#18 Fr.—5 mL." The accompanying box provides guidelines for catheter selection.

The procedure for inserting a urinary retention catheter is similar to the basic catheterization procedure, with differences occurring primarily after the catheter is in-

SELECTING AN APPROPRIATE CATHETER

- Select the type of material in accordance with the estimated length of the catheterization period.
  a. Use *plastic* catheters for short periods only (eg, 1 week or less), because they are inflexible.
  b. Use a *latex* or *rubber* catheter for periods of 2 or 3 weeks.
  c. Use *silicone* catheters for long-term use (eg, 2 to 3 months), because they create less encrustation at the urethral meatus. However, they are expensive.
  d. Use *PVC* catheters for 4- to 6-week periods. They soften at body temperature and conform to the urethra.
- Determine appropriate catheter length by the client's gender. For adult females, use a 22-cm catheter; for adult males, a 40-cm catheter.
- Determine appropriate catheter size by the size of the urethral canal. Use sizes such as #8 or #10 for children, #14 or #16 for adults. Men frequently require a larger size than women, for example, #18.
- Select the appropriate balloon size. For adults, use a 5-mL balloon to facilitate optimal urine drainage. The drainage tips of smaller balloons lie closer to the urethra and lower in the bladder than those of large balloons, thereby allowing more complete bladder emptying. However, 30-mL balloons or larger are commonly used to achieve hemostasis of the prostatic area following a prostatectomy. Use small 3-mL balloons for children.

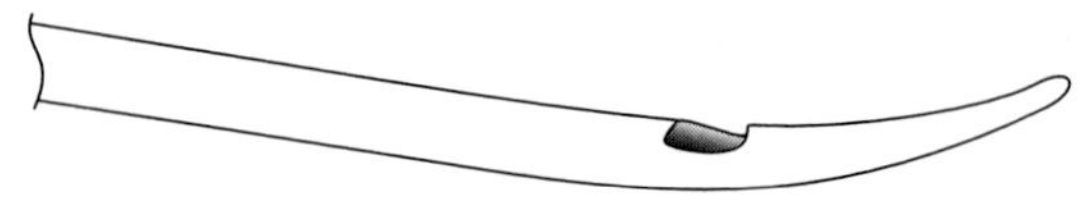

Figure 41–13 The coudé catheter, a urethral catheter with a curved tip.

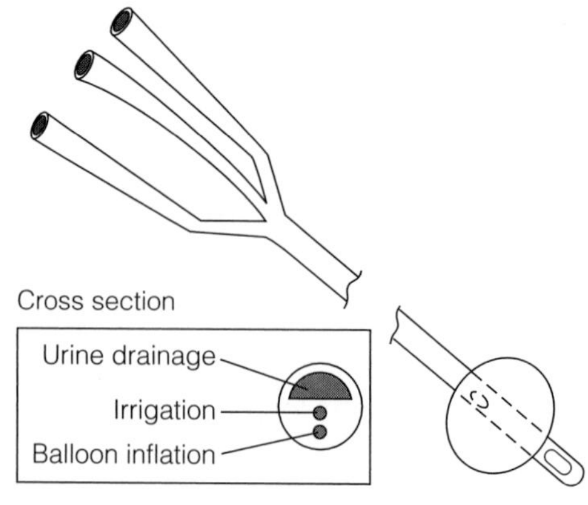

Figure 41–14 A three-way Foley catheter.

serted. Prior to insertion of the catheter, the nurse tests the balloon of the retention catheter to see that it is intact and, following the insertion, inflates the balloon and attaches a urinary drainage system.

A simple urinary drainage system consists of a retention catheter, tubing, and a receptacle (collecting bag) for the urine. This is called a straight drainage system, and it depends on the force of gravity to move the urine from the urinary bladder to the collecting bag. When this system is not or cannot be opened anywhere along it from the catheter to the bag, it is referred to as a closed system.  Closed systems are being used increasingly because of the danger of microorganisms entering the urinary tract whenever the system is opened. The more traditional type of system is the open system, in which the tubing may be separated from the catheter.

Catheterization of females and males, using straight catheters, is described in Procedures 41–4 and 41–5, respectively. Procedure 41–6 outlines how to insert a retention catheter.

Text continued on page 1258

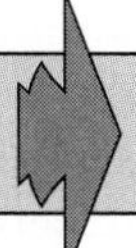

PROCEDURE 41–4 FEMALE URINARY CATHETERIZATION USING A STRAIGHT CATHETER

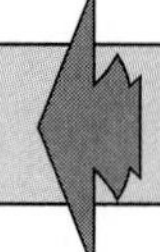

Before inserting a urinary catheter, determine (a) the order for the catheterization; (b) whether the order specifies a maximum amount of urine to be removed during the catheterization (if the client is retaining urine); usually no more than 750 mL is removed at one time, to avoid redirection of the blood supply to the pelvic blood vessels, leading to hypovolemic shock; and (c) any direction on the client's chart about the type or size of catheter to use.

PURPOSES

- To relieve discomfort due to bladder distention and/or to provide gradual decompression of a distended bladder
- To assess the amount of residual urine if the bladder empties incompletely
- To obtain a urine specimen
- To empty the bladder completely prior to surgery

ASSESSMENT FOCUS

When the client last voided and amount; presence of urinary retention; symptoms of urinary infection; voiding pattern; ability to maintain position during catheterization.

EQUIPMENT

- ☐ Flashlight or lamp
- ☐ Mask, if required by agency policy
- ☐ Bath blanket or drape
- ☐ Soap, a basin of warm water, a washcloth, and a towel
- ☐ Disposable gloves
- ☐ A sterile catheterization kit containing
  - Water-soluble lubricant
  - Sterile gloves
    Sterile drapes, fenestrated drape (optional) to place over the perineum
  - Antiseptic solution
  - Cotton balls or gauze squares
  - Forceps
  - Basin for urine (base of kit can be used)
- ☐ Sterile catheter of appropriate size (eg, for an adult #14 or #16 is often used)
- ☐ Specimen container as required
- ☐ Bag or receptacle for disposal of the cotton balls

INTERVENTION

1. Percuss and palpate the bladder to assess for urinary retention.

- To percuss the bladder, place the middle finger of one hand against the skin, and strike it sharply with the middle finger of the other hand. When the bladder is full, the resulting sound will be duller than normal.
- To palpate the bladder, indent the skin more than 1.3 cm (0.5 in) just above the pubic symphysis by pressing the fingers of one hand on the fingers of the other. *This increases the pressure for palpation.*

2. Prepare the client.

- Explain the catheterization to the client, and provide privacy. *Exposure of the genitals is embarrassing to most clients.* Some people fear that the procedure will

PROCEDURE 41–4 FEMALE URINARY CATHETERIZATION USING A STRAIGHT CATHETER *continued*

be painful; explain that normally a catheterization is painless and that there may be a sensation of pressure. *Relieving the client's tension can facilitate insertion of the catheter, because the urinary sphincters are more likely to be relaxed.*

- Assist the client to a supine position, with knees flexed and thighs externally rotated. Pillows can be used to support the knees and to elevate the buttocks. *Raising the client's pelvis gives the nurse a better view of the urinary meatus and reduces the risk of contaminating the catheter.*
- Drape the client. *This maintains comfort and prevents unnecessary exposure.* Cover the client's chest and abdomen with a bath blanket. Pull the client's gown up over her hips. Cover her legs and feet as for perineal care. See Figure 29–3 on page 743.
- Don disposable gloves.
- Wash the perineal–genital area with warm water and soap. Wear disposable gloves. *Cleaning reduces the number of microorganisms around the urinary meatus and the possibility of introducing microorganisms with the catheter.*
- Rinse and dry the area well. *Rinsing removes soap that could inhibit the action of the antiseptic later.*
- Remove disposable gloves.
- Obtain assistance if the client requires help in maintaining the required position. *The client must remain still throughout the procedure to maintain a clear view of the urinary meatus and prevent contamination of the sterile field.*

3. Prepare the equipment.

- Adjust the light to view the urinary meatus. It may be necessary to use a flashlight or to place a gooseneck lamp at the foot of the bed, so that it focuses on the perineal area.
- Put on a mask, gown, and/or cap if required by agency policy.

4. Create a sterile field

- At the client's bedside, open a sterile kit and the catheter, if it is packaged separately, and put on the sterile gloves (see Procedure 27–3, p. 698).
- Drape the client with the sterile drapes, being careful to protect the sterility of the drapes and your gloves. Use the first drape as an underpad, and place it under the buttocks. Keep the underpad edges cuffed over your gloves. *This prevents contamination of the gloves against the client's buttocks.* If the other drape is fenestrated, place it over the perineal area, exposing only the labia. If a fenestrated drape is not available, place the two thigh drapes so that they overlap between the client's thighs. Place the thigh drapes from the side farthest to the side nearest you. *This prevents reaching across a sterile field and possible contamination of the new drape.*
- Place the sterile kit on the drape between the client's thighs. *This facilitates access to supplies.*
- Pour the antiseptic solution over the cotton balls, if they are not already prepared.
- Lubricate the insertion tip of the catheter liberally, and place it in the sterile container ready for use. *Water-soluble lubricant facilitates insertion of the catheter by reducing friction. Lubrication is done at this point because the nurse will subsequently have only one sterile hand available.*
- Open the urine specimen container, and keep the top sterile. *This prepares the container for specimen collection.*

5. Clean the meatus (if recommended by agency).

- There is controversy regarding the value of meatal cleansing using antiseptics before catheterization. Prospective trials have been unable to demonstrate any reduction in the rate of bacteriuria when various methods of cleansing are used (Burke et al 1983, p. 334; Conti & Eutropius 1987, p. 308). Check agency protocol about cleansing methods.
- With the nondominant hand, separate the labia majora with the thumb and finger, and clean the labia minora on each side, using forceps and cotton balls soaked in antiseptic. Use a new swab for each stroke. *This prevents the transfer of microorganisms.* Move downward from the pubic area to the anus (Figure 41–15). *Cleaning from anterior to*

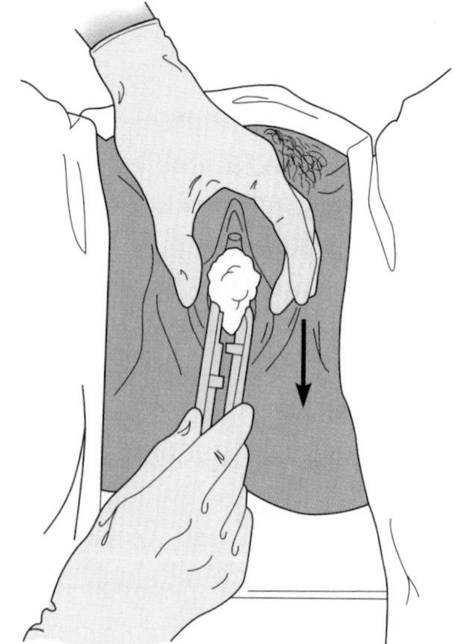

Figure 41–15 When cleaning the labia minora, move the swab downward.

PROCEDURE 41–4 *continued*

posterior cleans from the area of least contamination to the area of greatest contamination.

- Then, separate the labia minora with two other fingers, still using the nondominant hand (Figure 41–16).

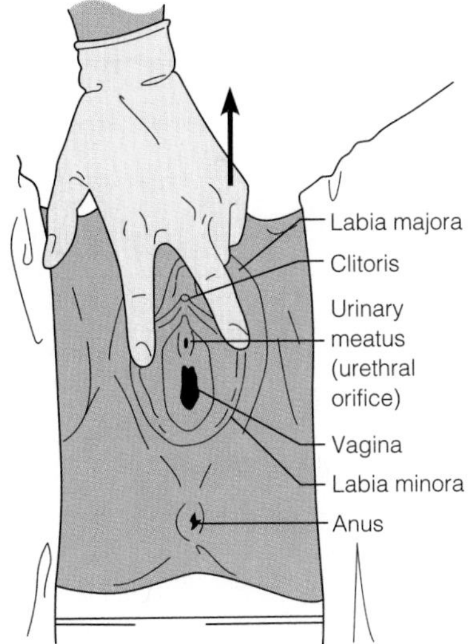

Figure 41–16 To expose the urinary meatus, separate the labia minora and retract the tissue upward.

- Expose the urinary meatus adequately by retracting the tissue of the labia minora in an upward (anterior) direction (Figure 41–16). Clean first from the meatus downward and then on either side, using a new swab for each stroke. Once the meatus is cleaned, do not allow the labia to close over it. *Keeping the labia apart prevents the risk of contaminating the urinary meatus. Note:* The hand that touches the client becomes unsterile. It remains in position exposing the urinary meatus, while the other hand remains sterile holding the sterile forceps.

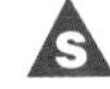

or

- Clean the urinary meatus first and then work outward to clean the labia.

6. Inspect the meatus.

- Assess any signs, such as excoriation of the tissues surrounding the urinary meatus, swelling of the urinary meatus, or the presence of discharge around the urinary meatus. *This assessment provides baseline data.* If any discharge is present, refer to the nurse in charge for a culture order.

7. Insert the catheter until urine flows.

- Place the drainage end of the catheter in the urine receptacle. Pick up the insertion end of the catheter with your uncontaminated, sterile, gloved hand, holding it about 5 cm (2 in) from the insertion tip. *Because the adult female urethra is approximately 4 cm (1.5 in) long, the catheter is held far enough from the end to allow full insertion into the bladder and to maintain control of the tip of the catheter so it will not accidentally become contaminated.*
- Gently insert the catheter into the urinary meatus until urine flows. Insert the catheter in the direction of the urethra. If the catheter meets resistance during insertion, do not force it. *Forceful pressure exerted against the urethra can produce trauma.* Ask the client to take deep breaths. *This helps relax the external sphincter.* If this does not relieve the resistance, discontinue the procedure, and report the problem to the nurse in charge. Exercise caution to prevent the catheter tip from becoming contaminated. If it becomes contaminated, discard it.
- When the urine flows, transfer your hand from the labia to the catheter to hold it in place 2 cm from the meatus. *This prevents its expulsion by a possible bladder contraction.*

8. Collect a urine specimen.

- Pinch the catheter, and transfer the drainage end of it into the sterile specimen bottle. Usually, 30 mL of urine is sufficient for a specimen. Securely place the top on the specimen container, and set it aside for labeling later.

9. Empty or partially drain the bladder, and then remove the catheter.

- For adults experiencing urinary retention, some orders limit the amount of urine drained to 700 to 1000 mL. Whether to limit the amount of urine drained has been a controversial issue. *Rapid removal of large amounts of urine is thought to induce engorgement of the pelvic blood vessels and hypovolemic shock. However, retained urine may serve as a reservoir for microorganisms to multiply.* Usually, agency policy or the physician indicates the amount to be removed and times at which the remaining urine is to be withdrawn. Bristol et al (1989, p. 345) concluded from research that *complete* drainage of a distended bladder is likely to be more comfortable and certainly seems as safe as threshold clamping.
- Pinch the catheter. *This prevents leakage of urine.* Remove the catheter slowly.

10. Promote client comfort.

- Dry the client's perineum with a towel or drape. *Excess lubricant*

PROCEDURE 41–4 FEMALE URINARY CATHETERIZATION USING A STRAIGHT CATHETER *continued*

and solution in the area can irritate the skin.

11. Assess the urine.

- Inspect the urine for color, clarity, odor, and the presence of any abnormal constituents, such as blood.
- Measure the amount of urine.

12. Document the catheterization.

- Include assessments before and after the procedure, type and size of catheter inserted; time; characteristics and amount of urine obtained; whether a specimen was sent to the laboratory; and client response to the procedure.

EVALUATION FOCUS
Signs of urinary infection; discomfort; bladder distention; amount, color, and clarity of urine.

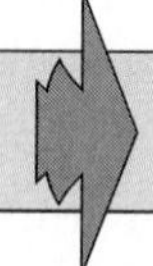

PROCEDURE 41–5 MALE URINARY CATHETERIZATION USING A STRAIGHT CATHETER

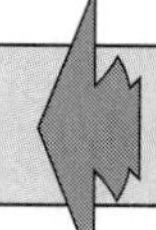

PURPOSES

- See Procedure 41–4, page 1251.

ASSESSMENT FOCUS
See Procedure 41–4, page 1251.

EQUIPMENT

See Procedure 41–4. A #16 or #18 catheter is often used for an adult male

INTERVENTION

1. Percuss and palpate the bladder as in Procedure 41–4, step 1, page 1251.

2. Prepare the client.

- Explain the catheterization, as in Procedure 41–4.
- Assist the client to a supine position, with the knees slightly flexed and the thighs slightly apart. *This allows greater relaxation of the abdominal and perineal muscles and permits easier insertion of the catheter.*
- Drape the client by folding the top bedclothes down so that the penis is exposed and the thighs are covered. Use a bath blanket to cover the client's chest and abdomen.
- Wash the perineal area, as in Procedure 41–4.

3. Create a sterile field.

- Open the sterile tray, and don the sterile gloves (see Procedure 27–3, p. 698).
- Place a drape under the penis and a second drape above the penis over the pubic area. If a fenestrated drape is available, place it over the penis and pubic area, exposing only the penis.
- Place the sterile kit on the sterile drape over the client's thighs or next to the thigh.
- Pour the antiseptic solution over the cotton balls, if they are not already prepared.
- Lubricate the insertion tip of the catheter liberally for about 5 to 7 cm (2 to 3 in). Place it in the sterile container ready for insertion. *Water-soluble lubricant facilitates insertion of the catheter by reducing friction. This step is done before cleaning because the nurse will subsequently have only one sterile hand available.*

4. Clean the urinary meatus.

- Grasp the penis firmly behind the glans with the nondominant hand, and spread the meatus between the thumb and forefinger. Retract the foreskin of an uncircumcised male. The hand holding the penis is now considered contaminated. *Firmly grasp the penis to avoid stimulating an erection.*
- With the dominant hand, use sterile forceps to pick up a swab.

PROCEDURE 41–5 *continued*

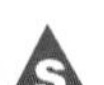

Clean the meatus first, and then wipe the tissue surrounding the meatus in a circular motion. Discard each swab after only one wipe. *Using forceps maintains the sterility of your gloves.*

5. Insert the catheter.

- Place the drainage end of the catheter in the urine receptacle. Then, pick up the insertion end of the catheter with your uncontaminated, sterile, gloved hand, holding it about 8 to 10 cm (3 to 4 in) from the insertion tip for an adult or about 2.5 cm (1 in) for a baby or small boy. In some agencies, the catheter is picked up with forceps. *The male urethra is approximately 20 cm (8 in) long. Holding the catheter far enough from the end to maintain control of the tip of the catheter avoids accidental contamination.*
- Lift the penis to a position perpendicular to the body (90 degree angle), and exert slight traction (pulling or tension upward). Insert the catheter steadily about 20 cm (8 in) or until urine begins to flow. *Lifting the penis so that it is perpendicular to the body straightens the downward curvature of the urethra.*
- To bypass slight resistance at the sphincters, twist the catheter, or wait until the sphincter relaxes. Ask the client to take deep breaths or try to void. If difficult resistance is met, discontinue the 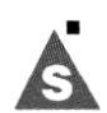 procedure, and report the problem to the nurse in charge. *Slight resistance is normally encountered at the external and internal urethral sphincters. Deep breathing can help to relax the external sphincter. Forceful pressure exerted against a major resistance can traumatize the urethra.*
- While the urine flows, lower the penis, and transfer your hand to hold the catheter in place at the meatus.

6. Drain the urine from the bladder.

- Collect a urine specimen (if required) after the urine has flowed for a few seconds. Pinch the catheter, and transfer the drainage end of the catheter into the sterile specimen bottle taking care not to contaminate the specimen container. Usually, 30 mL of urine is sufficient for a specimen.
- Empty the bladder, or drain the amount of urine specified in the order. See Procedure 41–4, step 9.

7. Make the client comfortable.

- Dry the penis with a towel or drape.
- Replace the foreskin. *This prevents a mechanical phimosis (constriction), which may compromise circulation to the glans.*

8. Assess the client and the urine, as in Procedure 41–4, and document the procedure and the assessments.

EVALUATION FOCUS
See Procedure 41–4, page 1254.

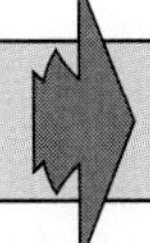

PROCEDURE 41–6 INSERTING A RETENTION (INDWELLING) CATHETER

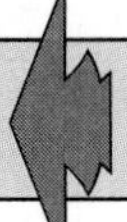

PURPOSES

- To manage incontinence when other measures have failed
- To provide for intermittent or continuous bladder drainage and irrigation
- To prevent urine from contacting an incision after perineal surgery
- To facilitate accurate measurement of urinary output for critically ill clients whose output needs to be monitored hourly

ASSESSMENT FOCUS
Distention of urinary bladder; signs of urinary infection; voiding pattern; ability to maintain position during catheterization.

PROCEDURE 41-6 INSERTING A RETENTION (INDWELLING) CATHETER *continued*

EQUIPMENT

In addition to the equipment used for a straight catheterization, the following equipment is needed:

- ☐ Sterile retention catheter (#14 or #16 for adults, #8 or #10 for children is often used)
- ☐ Prefilled syringe (sterile water is often used)
- ☐ Nonallergenic tape or Velcro
- ☐ Safety pin or clip
- ☐ Urine collection bag and tubing (the tubing may be attached to the retention catheter if a closed drainage system is used)

INTERVENTION

1. Prepare the client and the equipment.

- Explain to the client why the retention catheter is to be inserted, how long it will be in place, and how the urinary drainage equipment needs to be handled to maintain and facilitate the drainage of urine. Reassure the client that the procedure is painless. Some clients fear spillage of urine when they experience the urge to void during insertion of the catheter and for a short period of time after the catheter is in place. Reassure these clients that the catheter drains the urine and that the urge to void will disappear.
- Follow procedure as for straight catheterization up to and including draping the client with a sterile drape.

2. Test the catheter balloon.

- Attach the prefilled syringe to the balloon valve, and inject the fluid. *Sterile water rather than sterile saline should be used because the saline can crystallize and prevent complete deflation of the balloon.* The balloon should inflate appropriately and not leak. Withdraw the fluid, and set aside the catheter with the syringe attached for later use. If the balloon leaks or does not inflate adequately, replace the catheter. In such a case, withdraw the fluid, and detach the syringe for later use. Ask another nurse to obtain a second catheter and open the package for you, then test the new balloon.

  or

  Remove the equipment, and obtain another catheter. Then begin again with the new sterile equipment.

3. Follow steps as for straight catheterization.

- Lubricate the insertion tip of the catheter.
- Remove the sterile cap from the specimen container.
- Expose and clean the urinary meatus and surrounding tissues.
- Insert the catheter and inflate the balloon.
- Collect a urine specimen as required.

4. Move the catheter farther into the bladder, and inflate the balloon.

- Insert the catheter an additional 2.5 to 5 cm (1 to 2 in) beyond the point at which urine began to flow. The balloon of the catheter is located behind the opening at the insertion tip, and sufficient space needs to be provided to inflate the balloon. *This ensures that*

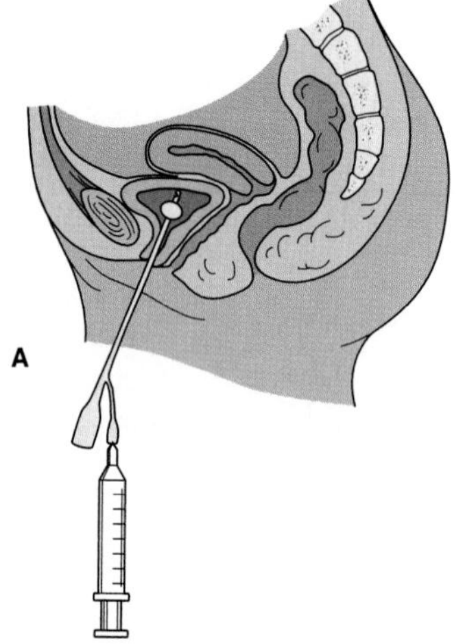

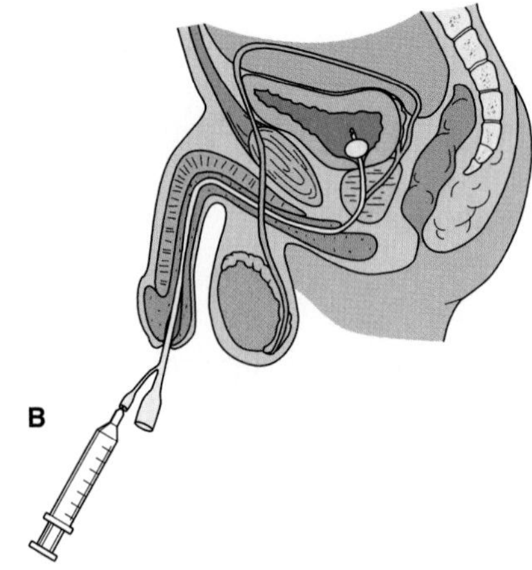

Figure 41-17 Placement of retention catheter and inflated balloon in *A,* female client; and *B,* male client.

PROCEDURE 41–6 *continued*

the balloon is inflated inside the bladder and not in the urethra, where it could produce trauma.

- Inflate the balloon by injecting the contents of the prefilled syringe into the valve of the catheter (Figure 41–17, *A*). Placement of the catheter and balloon in a male client is shown in Figure 41–17, *B*. If the client complains of discomfort or pain during the balloon inflation, withdraw the fluid, insert the catheter a little farther, and inflate the balloon again. Insert no more fluid than the balloon size indicates (eg, 5 mL or 30 mL), and remove the syringe. A special valve prevents backflow of the fluid out of the catheter.
- Follow agency policy when using a 30-mL balloon. Some agency policies state that only 15 mL of fluid is injected for inflation.

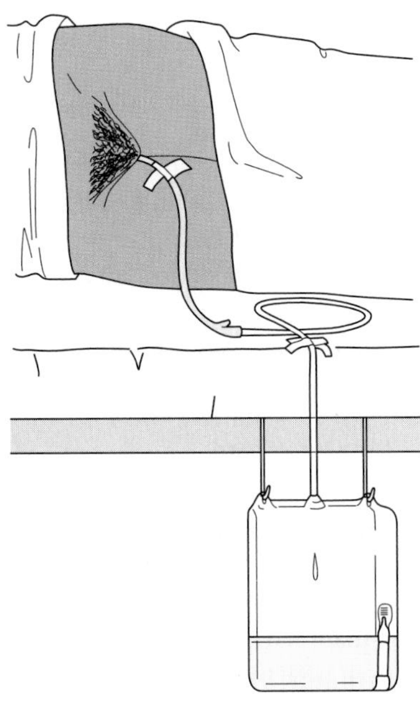

Figure 41–18 Tape the catheter to the inside of a female's thigh.

5. Ensure effective balloon inflation.

- When the balloon is safely inflated, apply slight tension on the catheter until you feel resistance. *Resistance indicates that the catheter balloon is inflated appropriately, and that the catheter is well anchored in the bladder.*
- Then, release the resistance on the catheter. This keeps the balloon from exerting undue pressure on the neck of the bladder.

6. Anchor the catheter.

- Tape the catheter with nonallergenic tape to the inside of a female's thigh or to the thigh or abdomen of a male client (Figure 41–18 and 41–19). Some nurses prefer taping the catheter to the abdomen whenever there is increased risk of penile scrotal excoriation. *Taping restricts the movement of the catheter, thus reducing friction and irritation in the urethra when the client moves. It also prevents skin excoriation at the penile-scrotal junction in the male.*

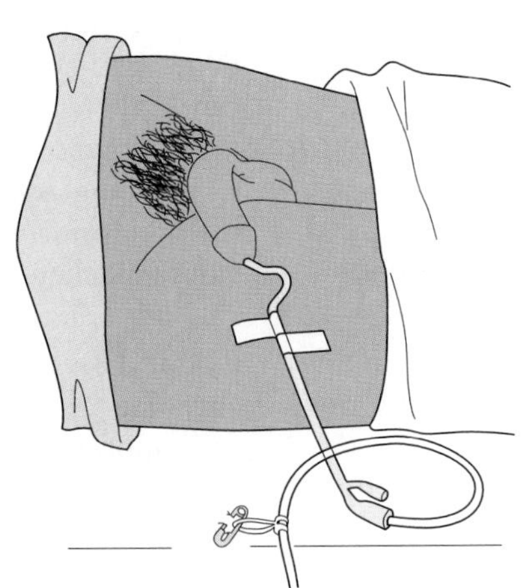

Figure 41–19 Tape the catheter to the thigh or abdomen of a male client.

7. Establish effective drainage.

- Ensure that the emptying base of the drainage bag is closed.
- Secure the drainage bag to the bed frame, using the hook or strap provided. Suspend the bag off the floor, but keep it below the level of the client's bladder (Figure 41–18). *Urine flows by gravity from the bladder to the drainage bag. The bag should be off the floor so that the emptying spout does not become grossly contaminated.*
- Coil the drainage tubing loosely beside the client, so that the remaining tubing runs in a straight line down to the drainage bag. Fasten the vertical tubing to the bedclothes with tape, a tubing clamp, or a safety pin and elastic band (Figures 41–18 and 41–19). *The drainage tubing should not loop below its entry into the drainage bag, because this impedes the flow of urine by gravity.*

8. Document pertinent data.

- Record the time and date of the catheterization; type and size of catheter; the reason; number of mL of fluid used to inflate the balloon; assessments before and after the procedure, including amount, color, and clarity of urine obtained; whether a specimen was taken and sent to the laboratory; whether all urine was emptied from the bladder; and the client's response.

EVALUATION FOCUS
Amount, color, and clarity of urine; any discomfort; fluid intake, palpable bladder.

NURSING INTERVENTIONS FOR CLIENTS WITH RETENTION CATHETERS

Nursing care of the client with an indwelling catheter and continuous drainage is largely directed toward preventing infection of the urinary tract and encouraging urinary flow through the drainage system. It includes encouraging large amounts of fluid intake, accurate recording of the fluid intake and output, changing the retention catheter and tubing, maintaining the patency of the drainage system, preventing contamination of the drainage system, and teaching these measures to the client.

Fluids and Fluid Balance An appropriate fluid balance is essential for the client with a retention catheter to minimize the risk of infection. The client should drink up to 3000 mL per day if permitted. Large amounts of fluid ensure a large urine output, which keeps the bladder flushed out and decreases the likelihood of urinary statis and subsequent infection. Large volumes of urine also minimize the risk of sediment or other particles obstructing the drainage tubing. Accurate recording of fluid intake and output is discussed in Chapter 38.

Dietary Measures Many agencies implement prophylactic measures to acidify the client's urine to prevent urinary infection. By changing the composition of the diet, the urine can be made either acid or alkaline. Most vegetables and fruits yield an alkaline urine, whereas meat, fish, fowl, eggs, and cereals yield an acid urine. Alkalinization of the urine may be warranted to soothe an irritated bladder. See Table 41–4 on page 1235.

Perineal Care Neither daily cleaning of the perineum with soap and water nor twice-daily cleaning with povidone-iodine solution has been shown to reduce the incidence of catheter-associated infections (Epstein 1985, p. 273). No special cleaning other than routine hygienic care is therefore officially recommended at this time. Nor is special meatal care recommended. Some studies have shown no improvement in catheter-associated infections and in fact a higher incidence of bacteriuria in groups of people receiving routine meatal care (Epstein 1985, p. 273). Agency practices regarding catheter care vary considerably. The nurse should check agency practice in this regard.

Changing the Catheter and Tubing According to the CDC, "changing indwelling catheters at arbitrary fixed intervals" is not cost-effective and should not be performed (Epstein 1985, p. 274). Furthermore, the closed system should be maintained and the catheter and tubing not disconnected unless absolutely necessary. Clients should therefore be catheterized only when absolutely necessary and the retention catheter removed as soon as possible.

Agency policies may specify the frequency of catheter and tubing changes. Some agencies advocate that both be changed when sediment accumulates at the distal end. Sediment is present if sandy particles are felt when the end of the catheter is rolled between the thumb and fingers. The drainage bag and tubing are generally changed along with the catheter but need to be changed more frequently if sediment accumulates, if leakage occurs, or if a strong odor is evident. Recommendations for changes are made on the basis of reducing the incidence of infection and preventing unpleasant odors.

During tubing changes, strict surgical asepsis is essential to prevent contamination of the distal lumen of the catheter.

To change tubing, the nurse follows these steps:

- Obtain a new sterile drainage bag and tubing, a sterile towel or sterile gauzes, clamp, and antiseptic solution.
- Wash hands thoroughly, and don gloves.
- Set up a sterile field.
- Remove the protective cap from the drainage tube, and place the open end of the tubing on the sterile field.
- Clamp the catheter above the tubing connector, and clean the catheter tubing junction with an antiseptic solution.
- Disconnect the catheter from the old tubing, being careful not to contaminate the end of the catheter, and connect the catheter to the new tubing.
- Unclamp the catheter, and establish drainage by securing the tubing and drainage receptacle to the bed at an appropriate level.

Some agencies recommend instillation of hydrogen peroxide in the drainage bag of open systems to prevent the growth of microorganisms in the bag and to reduce odor. Agency policies vary, however. Guidelines to prevent catheter-associated urinary tract infections are given in the first box on page 1259.

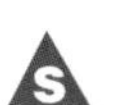

Ongoing assessment of clients with retention catheters is a high priority. The right hand box on page 1259 provides guidelines.

Client Teaching Usually nurses need to teach the client some principles about the gravity drainage system and the importance of maintaining a closed system. The client has to understand that the drainage tubing and drainage bag need to be kept lower than the bladder at all times. The client also needs to know how to prevent tension on the catheter tubing, to prevent loops or kinks in the drainage tubing, and to avoid lying on the tubing. Understanding how to manipulate the system when ambulating can give the client a sense of independence. Some clients also

CLINICAL GUIDELINES

Preventing Catheter-Associated Urinary Infections

- Have an established infection control program.
- Catheterize clients only when necessary, by using aseptic technique, sterile equipment, and trained personnel.
- Maintain a sterile closed-drainage system.
- Do not disconnect the catheter and drainage tubing unless absolutely necessary.
- Remove the catheter as soon as possible.
- Follow and reinforce good handwashing technique.
- Changing indwelling catheters at arbitrary, fixed intervals and regular bacteriologic monitoring of catheterized clients are not cost-effective practices and should not be performed.
- Avoid other measures until further data are available. New products that appear to be questionable or gimmicky probably should be avoided.
- Although instillation of H_2O_2 into the outlet tube of the drainage set or into the drainage bags has been associated with a reduction in bag contamination, studies indicate no difference in the rate of bag-source infection in clients with the suggested instillation of H_2O_2 into the drainage bag when compared with clients who had conventional closed-drainage systems (Epstein 1985).

ONGOING ASSESSMENT OF CLIENTS WITH RETENTION CATHETERS

- Ensure that there are no obstructions in the drainage. Check that there are no kinks in the tubing, the client is not lying on the tubing, and the tubing is not clogged with mucus or blood.
- Check that there is no tension on the catheter or tubing, that the catheter is securely taped to the thigh or abdomen, and that the tubing is fastened appropriately to the bedclothes.
- Ensure that gravity drainage is maintained. Make sure there are no loops in the tubing below its entry to the drainage receptacle and that the drainage receptacle is below the level of the client's bladder.
- Ensure that the drainage system is well sealed or closed. Check that there are no leaks at the connection sites in open systems. Apply waterproof tape around the connection site of the catheter and tubing.
- Observe the flow of the urine every 2 or 3 hours, and note color, odor, and any abnormal constituents. If blood clots are present, check the catheter more frequently to ascertain whether it is plugged.

benefit from instruction about fluid intake measurement and perineal care. Clients who wish to be involved in recording fluid intake measurements need information about how to compute these values and which foods are considered fluids.

Removing Retention Catheters Retention catheters are removed after their purpose has been achieved, usually on the order of the physician. Clients who have had retention catheters for a prolonged period may lose some bladder muscle tone because the bladder remains relatively empty and thus is never stretched to its capacity. When a muscle is not stretched regularly, atrophy develops. When a catheter is removed, the client may have difficulty in regaining urinary control. Another potential problem is urine retention due to urethral swelling. Therefore, the nurse palpates the bladder for urinary retention following a retention catheter removal (see Chapter 22 for the technique).

A few days prior to removal the catheter may be clamped for specified periods of time (eg, 2 to 4 hours) and then released. This causes some distention of the bladder and stimulation of the bladder musculature and may be ordered as "bladder training." This procedure must be ordered at most agencies. There is some evidence that clamping following short-term catheterization (up to 6 days) is beneficial to regaining continence (Row 1990b, p. 67).

To remove a retention catheter, the nurse follows these steps:

- Obtain a receptacle for the catheter (eg, a disposable basin); a clean, disposable towel; disposable gloves; and a sterile syringe and needle to deflate the balloon. The syringe should be large enough to withdraw *all* the solution in the catheter balloon. The size of the balloon is indicated on the label at the end of the catheter.
- Ask the client to assume a back-lying position as for a catheterization.
- Optional: Obtain a sterile specimen before removing the catheter. Check agency protocol.
- Remove the tape attaching the catheter to the client, don gloves, and then place the towel between the legs of the female client or over the thighs of the male.
- Insert the syringe into the injection port of the catheter, and withdraw the fluid from the balloon. If not all the fluid can be removed, report this fact to the nurse in charge before proceeding.

CLIENT TEACHING

Clean Intermittent Self-Catheterization (CISC)

- Catheterize as often as needed to maintain a residual urine volume specified by your physician or nurse. At first, catheterization may be necessary every 2 to 3 hours and then increased to 4 to 6 hours.
- Attempt to void before catheterization; then insert the catheter to remove residual urine.
- Assemble all needed supplies ahead of time. Good lighting is essential, especially for females.
- If female, remove a tampon before carrying out CISC. A tampon can inhibit catheterization.
- Wash your hands.
- Clean the urinary meatus with either a towelette or soapy washcloth, then rinse with a wet washcloth. If female, clean the area from front to back.
- Assume a position that is comfortable and that facilitates passage of the catheter, such as a semireclining position in bed or sitting on a chair or the toilet. Men may prefer to stand over the toilet; women may prefer to stand with one foot on the side of the bathtub.
- Apply lubricant to the catheter tip (1 inch for women; 2 inches for men).
- Insert the catheter until urine flows through.
  a. If *female*, locate the meatus using a mirror or other aid, or use the "touch" technique as follows:
    - Place the index finger of your nondominant on your clitoris.
    - Place the third and fourth fingers at the vagina.
    - Locate the meatus between the index and third fingers.
    - Separate the labia with your dominant hand.
    - Direct the catheter through the meatus and then upward and forward toward the umbilicus.

  b. If *male*, lift the penis to a 60 degree angle to straighten the urethra before inserting the catheter. Return the penis to its natural position after catheter insertion when urine starts to flow.
- Hold the catheter in place until all urine is drained.
- Withdraw the catheter *slowly* to ensure complete drainage of urine.
- Clean and store the catheter according to the manufacturer's directions. Replace the catheter with a new one every week, or sooner if it becomes difficult to clean.
- Contact your physician if your urine appears cloudy or contains sediment; if you have bleeding, difficulty, or pain when passing the catheter; or if you have fever.
- Drink at least 1500 mL of fluid a day to ensure adequate bladder filling and flushing. To keep your urine acidic and reduce the risk of bladder infections, drink cranberry and prune juices.

Sources: Adapted from JE Webber-Jones, Performing clean, intermittent self-catheterization. *Nursing91*, August 1991, 21:56–59; and A Winder, Catheters: Intermittent self-catheterization, *Nursing Times*, October 24–30, 86:63–64.

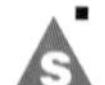

- Do *not* pull the catheter while the balloon is inflated, because the urethra may be injured. Puncturing the balloon using sterile technique is a procedure usually performed by a physician. A sterile wire stylet is inserted up the lumen of the catheter, and the balloon is punctured. This permits the fluid to flow out of the balloon (Mocsny 1980, p. 88).
- After all the fluid is withdrawn from the balloon, gently withdraw the catheter, and place it in the waste receptacle.
- Dry the perineal area with a towel.
- Remove gloves
- Measure the urine in the drainage bag, and record the removal of the catheter. Include in the recording (a) the time the catheter was removed; (b) the amount, color, and clarity of the urine, (c) the intactness of the catheter; and (d) instructions given to the client.
- Following removal of the catheter, determine the time of the first voiding and the amount voided over the first 8 hours. Compare this output to the client's intake.

CLEAN INTERMITTENT SELF-CATHETERIZATION

Clean intermittent self-catheterization (CISC) is performed by many clients who have some form of neurogenic bladder dysfunction. Clean or medical aseptic technique is used. CISC provides several benefits to the client (Winder 1990, p. 64; Webber-Jones 1991, p. 56): It

- Enables the client to retain independence and gain control of the bladder.
- Reduces incidence of urinary tract infection.
- Protects the upper urinary tract from reflux.
- Allows normal sexual relationship without incontinence.
- Reduces the use of aids and appliances.
- Frees the client from embarrassing dribbling.
- Enables some clients to return to work.

The procedure for self-catheterization is similar to that used by the nurse to catheterize a client. Essential steps are outlined in the box at the left. Because the procedure requires great motivation and thorough physical and mental preparation, client assessment is important. Selection criteria include the following (Winder 1990, p. 64):

- Sufficient manual dexterity to manipulate a catheter
- Sufficient mental ability
- Motivation and acceptability
- For females, reasonable agility to access the urethra
- Bladder capacity not less than 100 mL

Before teaching CISC, the nurse should establish the client's voiding patterns, the volume voided, fluid intake, and residual amounts. CISC is easier for males to learn because of the visibility of the urinary meatus. Females need to learn initially with the aid of a mirror but eventually should perform the procedure by using only the sense of touch (see the box at the left).

URINARY IRRIGATIONS

An **irrigation** is a flushing or washing-out with a specified solution. A *bladder irrigation* is carried out on a physician's order, usually to wash out the bladder and/or apply an antiseptic solution to the bladder lining to treat a bladder infection. Sterile technique is used. *Catheter irrigations* are usually carried out to maintain or restore the patency of a catheter, for example, to remove pus or blood clots that have formed in the bladder and are blocking the catheter. A physician's order may or may not be required, depending on agency protocol.

There are three ways of irrigating a catheter or bladder: (a) maintaining the closed system and injecting the solution through an aspiration port (closed intermittent irrigation), (b) irrigating through a three-way catheter (closed intermittent or continuous irrigation), and (c) irrigating through a catheter after separating the catheter and tubing (open intermittent system). Although the open system may be used in some agencies, closed sterile drainage systems are recommended.

In the usual bladder irrigation, a two-way Foley catheter is usually in place. For a bladder irrigation, the frequency and the type, amount, and strength of solution to be used are ordered by the physician. If the physician has not specified these on the client's chart, the nurse checks agency policies. Some agencies recommend the use of sterile normal saline at room temperature for both catheter and bladder irrigations. To irrigate an adult bladder, 1000 mL is commonly used for the entire irrigation; for a catheter irrigation, 200 mL is normally required.

Irrigations performed via straight gravity drainage are referred to as *plain irrigations*. A variation of the plain irrigation is the *intermittent irrigation*, in which one lumen of a three-way catheter is connected by tubing to a drip chamber and then to a container of sterile solution. The second lumen is attached to tubing and then to a urine

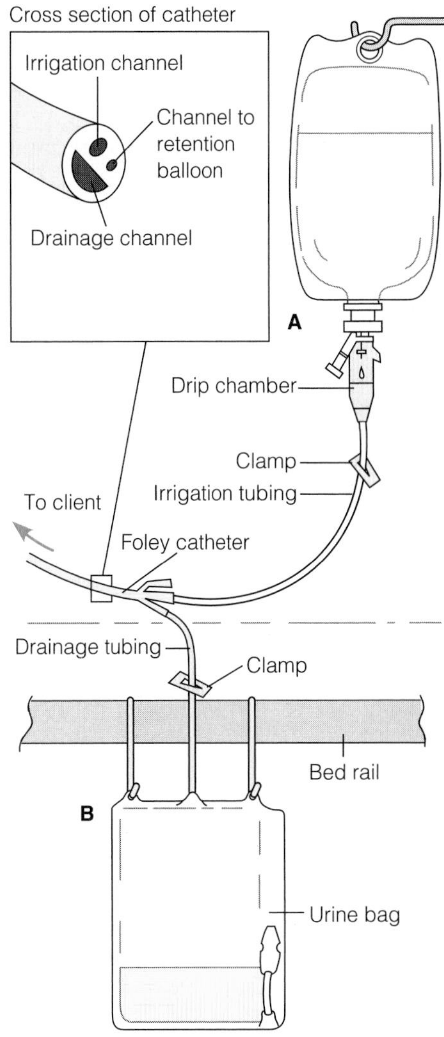

Figure 41–20 An intermittent bladder irrigation: *A*, solution container; *B*, urine bag.

receptacle (Figure 41–20). There are clamps on both tubes. The clamp from the solution container (*A*) is released while the clamp to the urine bag (*B*) is closed. The fluid enters and remains in the bladder. The nurse then reclamps the container tubing and unclamps the urine receptacle tubing, permitting the solution to flow out of the bladder. This process is carried out regularly. The nurse can use the same system for continuous irrigations by carefully regulating the flow of fluid, leaving the solution container and permitting the solution to flow freely out of the bladder into the urine bag.

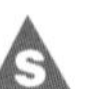

There are several variations of this irrigation system. One requires a specific fluid pressure to build up in the urinary bladder before the irrigation system "trips," allowing the solution to flow out of the bladder into a receptacle. These systems are usually set up by a physician and monitored by nurses.

Procedure 41–7 outlines the steps in irrigating a catheter or bladder (closed system).

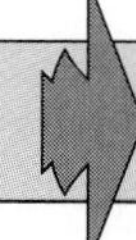

PROCEDURE 41–7 IRRIGATING A CATHETER OR BLADDER (CLOSED SYSTEM)

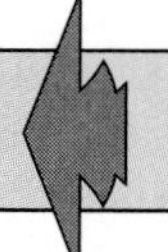

Before irrigating a catheter or bladder, determine (a) the order for a bladder irrigation (in most agencies, a physician's order is required); and (b) the type of sterile solution, amount, and strength to be used. If these are not specified on the client's chart, check agency protocol.

PURPOSES

- To maintain the patency of a urinary catheter and tubing (continuous irrigation)
- To free a blockage in a urinary catheter or tubing (intermittent irrigation)

ASSESSMENT FOCUS

Amount, clarity, and color of urine; comparison of fluid intake to output; presence of bladder distention; level of discomfort.

EQUIPMENT

- ☐ Disposable gloves
- ☐ Disposable, water-resistant sterile towel
- ☐ Sterile 30- or 50-mL syringe with a #19 to #23 needle
- ☐ Sterile antiseptic swabs
- ☐ Sterile receptacle
- ☐ Sterile irrigating solution as ordered or according to agency practice

For irrigating an open system

- ☐ Sterile protector (cover) for the end of the tubing
- ☐ Sterile asepto or Toomey syringe (see Figure 43–56, p. 1345)

INTERVENTION

1. Determine that the catheter and tubing are indeed blocked.

- Palpate the client's bladder to assess for urine retention.
- Compare the amount of urine in the bag with the drainage on the previous shift or with the client's fluid intake.
- If urine does not appear to be running freely, "milk" the catheter and tubing, working from the client toward the drainage bag. *This can dislodge an obstruction, avoiding the necessity of an irrigation to remove it. "Milk" away from the client so that the obstruction (eg, a blood clot) is forced into the drainage bag and not into the urinary bladder.*

2. Prepare the client.

- Explain the procedure to the client. A bladder or catheter irrigation should not be painful, although solution that is not at body temperature may be uncomfortable to the client.
- Assist the client to a dorsal recumbent position. *This position facilitates the flow of the irrigating fluid into the bladder.*
- Fold back the top bedclothes to expose the retention catheter. Place a bath blanket across the client's chest and abdomen if they are exposed.
- Determine the amount of urine in the drainage bag. *This amount has to be deducted from subsequent measurements of the irrigating fluid returns.*

3. Prepare the equipment.

- Open the sterile set beside or between the client's thighs, using sterile technique.
- Don gloves.
- Place the sterile towel under the end of the catheter.
- For a bladder irrigation, clamp the drainage tubing distal to the irrigation port. *Clamping prevents the urine and solution from draining into the drainage bag.* For a catheter irrigation, leave the tubing unclamped.
- Remove the cap from the needle, and draw the irrigation solution into the syringe, maintaining the sterility of the syringe and the solution.
- Using the antiseptic swab, wipe the place on the catheter lumen or the port on the drainage tubing through which the solution is to be instilled. The correct place on the catheter lumen is usually marked.

4. Instill the fluid into the catheter.

- Insert the needle into the port (Figure 41–7, p. 1232).

- Infuse the solution gently into the catheter. For each catheter infusion, instill about 30 to 40 mL of fluid for an adult; for each bladder infusion, instill about 100 to 200 mL. Use smaller amounts for children. *Gentle instillation avoids injury to the lining of the bladder and bladder spasms.*

PROCEDURE 41–7 *continued*

- Remove the needle from the port.

5. Drain the fluid.

- For a catheter irrigation, immediately lower the catheter so that the fluid will run toward the distal end of the catheter into the drainage tubing.
  or
  For a bladder irrigation, unclamp the drainage tubing so that the solution will run out of the bladder through the catheter and tubing.
- Repeat the process outlined in steps 4 and 5 until all of the solution has been used or until the purpose of the irrigation has been accomplished.

6. Calculate the amount of urine drained.

- Empty the urine bag and subtract the amount of solution used from the volume of fluid in the bag.

7. Assess both the client and the drainage.

- Note any change in discomfort.
- Assess the drainage for color, clarity, and presence of abnormal constituents.
- Assess the flow of urine in the catheter and tubing.

8. Document the irrigation.

- Include assessments before and after the irrigation.

Variation: Continuous Irrigation Using a Three-Way Foley Catheter

1. Assemble the equipment.

- Expell air from the tubing connected to the irrigation bag.
- Connect one port of the three-way catheter to the irrigation tubing which in turn is connected to the irrigation solution in a bag. Connect the second port of the catheter to the drainage tubing and bag, and the third port to the catheter balloon (Figure 41–20, p. 1261).

2. Irrigate the bladder.

- Open the flow clamp on the drainage tubing.
- Adjust the flow rate, using the clamp on the irrigation tubing, as specified by the physician. If the order does not specify, the rate should be 40 to 60 drops per minute or according to agency protocol.
- Inspect the fluid returns for amount, color, and clarity. The amount of returning fluid should correspond to the amount of fluid entering the bladder.

3. Document the assessments as above.

Variation: Irrigating a Catheter or Bladder Using the Open System

- Don sterile gloves.
- After disinfecting the ends, separate the catheter from the drainage tubing, and place the sterile tubing protector over the end of the tubing. Hold the catheter and the tubing at least 2.5 cm (1 in) from their ends. *By maintaining this distance, the nurse avoids contaminating the ends of the catheter and tubing.*
- Draw the fluid into the syringe, then gently inject it into the catheter, maintaining the sterility of the end of the catheter, the syringe, and the solution. Remove the syringe, and allow the fluid to return through the catheter into the drainage receptacle. Repeat until the catheter is running freely or until the purpose of the irrigation has been accomplished.
- Reattach the catheter to the tubing, maintaining the sterility of the ends of the tubing and the catheter.
- Coil the drainage tubing carefully on the bed so that the urine can flow through it freely.
- Remove gloves.
- Make assessments as for irrigating using a closed system.

EVALUATION FOCUS
Catheter patency; amount, color, and clarity of drainage; any discomfort.

URINARY DIVERSIONS

A urinary diversion is the surgical rerouting of the urine formed in the kidneys to a site other than the bladder. These operations are often necessary when the urine flow is obstructed by, for example, a malignancy of the bladder. A *urinary stoma* is an artificial opening in the abdominal wall through which urine can be excreted. Ureterostomies are small compared to colostomies (about 0.5 mm, or ¼ in, in diameter) and drain continuously.

The **ileal (ileo) conduit** (Figure 41–21), also referred to as *ileal (ileo) loop*, *ileal (ileo) bladder*, *ureteroileostomy*, or *Bricker's loop*, is one of the most commonly used urinary diversion procedures. In this procedure, a segment of the

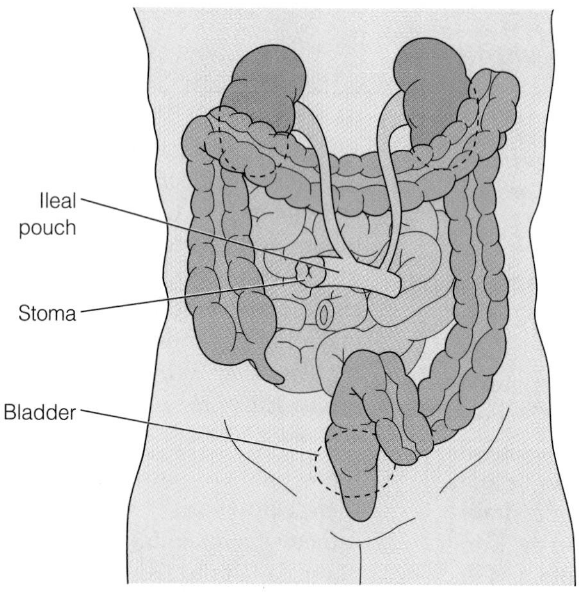

Figure 41–21 An ileal conduit.

ileum is removed and the intestinal ends are reattached. One end of the portion removed is closed with sutures to create an ileal pouch, and the other end is brought out through the abdominal wall to create a stoma. The ureters are implanted into the ileal pouch, and the bladder is usually removed. The advantages of this procedure over ureterostomies are that the ileal stoma is larger and more readily fitted with an appliance; there is less chance of an ascending kidney infection, since the mucous membrane lining of the ileum acts as a barrier to microorganisms; and the stoma is less likely to stenose, a major problem with ureterostomy stomas.

Clients with urinary diversions usually are required to wear an external pouch to collect the urine. An exception is the person with a Kock pouch, who needs a small dressing over the stoma to protect the clothing from mucous drainage. The **Kock pouch,** also called a *continent vesicostomy,* is formed by the bladder wall sutured to the abdominial wall (Figure 41–22).

The external appliances are made of either soft rubber or plastic and may be reusable or disposable. The appliance must be emptied several times a day before it becomes too heavy. Clients with urinary diversions may experience problems with their body image and may require assistance in coping with these changes and managing the stoma. Most clients are able to resume their normal activities and life-style.

SUPRAPUBIC CATHETER CARE

A **suprapubic** catheter is inserted through the abdominal wall above the symphysis pubis into the urinary bladder (Figure 41–23). The physician inserts the catheter using

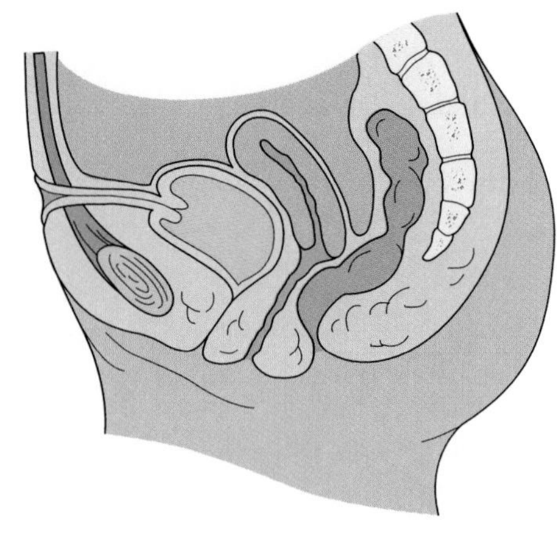

Figure 41–22 A continent vesicostomy (Kock pouch).

local anesthesia (in the client's bed unit) or using general anesthesia in conjunction with bladder or vaginal surgery (in the operating room). The catheter may be secured in place with sutures, with a commercial retention body seal, or with both sutures and a body seal. The catheter is then attached to a closed drainage system.

Care of clients with suprapubic catheter includes regular assessments of the client's urine, fluid intake, and comfort; maintenance of a patent drainage system; skin care around the insertion site; periodic clamping of the catheter preparatory to removing it; and measurement of residual urine. Orders generally include leaving the catheter open to drainage for 48 to 72 hours, then clamping the catheter for 3- to 4-hour periods during the day until the client can void satisfactory amounts. Satisfactory void-

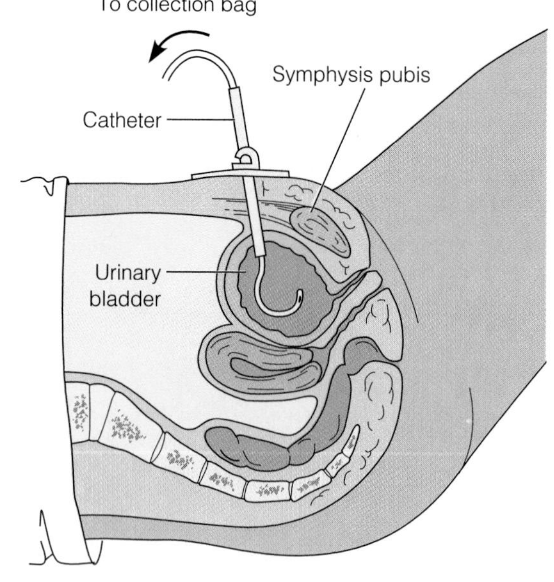

Figure 41–23 A suprapubic catheter in place.

ing is determined by measuring the client's residual urine after voiding.

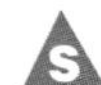
Care of the catheter insertion site involves sterile technique. Dressings around the suprapubic catheter are changed whenever they are soiled with drainage to prevent bacterial growth around the insertion site and reduce the potential for infection. A small amount of povidone-iodine ointment is frequently applied around the insertion site and the site covered with gauze dressings. Procedures for cleaning wounds and changing dressings are discussed in Chapter 44. Any redness and discharge at the skin around the insertion site must be reported.

EVALUATING

To evaluate the achievement of client outcomes, the nurse collects data pertaining to the established outcome criteria at specified intervals. Evaluation activities may include the following:

- Observing the character of urine
- Recording the frequency of urination
- Measuring the client's fluid intake and output
- Inspecting the skin around the urinary meatus, perineum, and sacral area
- Percussing or palpating the bladder for distention
- Asking the client about dysuria, frequency, incontinence episodes (including overflow dribbling), time intervals between urge and involuntary loss of urine, methods used to prevent incontinence, and frequency of performing Kegel's exercises
- Observing the client demonstrate self-care skills for retention catheter, external urinary device, or urinary diversion stoma
- Measuring residual urine
- Measuring urine pH
- Determining results of urine cultures or other urinary function tests

If outcomes are not achieved, the nurse should explore the reasons. The nurse might consider the following questions:

- Has the client's mental or physical condition changed?
- Were baseline data complete and validated?
- Were outcome criteria realistic?
- Was enough time allowed for outcome achievement?
- Was sufficient physical and emotional support provided for bladder retraining or other interventions?
- Was the client's fluid intake adequate?
- Did the client misinterpret self-care instructions?
- Were appropriate support services for home care obtained?

CRITICAL PATHWAY FOR TORWALD WILLIAMSON

ASSESSMENT DATA

Nursing Assessment

Mr Torwald Williamson is a 68-year-old shopkeeper who was admitted to the hospital early this morning because he has been unable to void since 7 o'clock last evening. Mrs Fran Whittmer, the nurse, gathers the following information when taking a nursing history. He states he has noticed that for the past few weeks he has had to go to the bathroom more frequently during the day and that he doesn't always feel he has emptied his bladder after voiding. He has also noticed that he must get up a few times during the night to urinate. As of the past few days, he has noted some problems in starting urination and then dribbling urine afterward. He states that this is very embarrassing to him because he must deal with his customers during the day. Mr Williamson is seen by the urologist, who recommends a transuretheral resection of the prostate (TURP) for benign prostatic hypertrophy. Mr Williamson consents to surgery, which is scheduled for the following day.

Physical Examination

Height: 185.4 cm (6′1″)
Weight: 85.7 kg (189 lb)
Temperature: 37 C (98.6 F)
Pulse rate: 78 bpm
Respirations: 20 per minute
Blood pressure: 146/86 mm Hg
Retention catheter to closed drainage bag draining 800 mL amber urine

Diagnostic Data

CBC: within normal range
Urine: amber, clear, pH 7.5, specific gravity 1.025, negative for glucose, protein, ketone, RBC, and bacteria
IVP: evidence of enlarged prostate gland

CRITICAL PATHWAY FOR CLIENT FOLLOWING TRANSURETHRAL RESECTION OF THE PROSTATE

Expected length of stay 3 days following surgery

	Date ________ **Preoperative day**	**Date ________** **1st 24 hours postoperative**
Daily outcomes	Client ▪ verbalizes understanding of preoperative teaching, including turning, coughing, deep breathing, incentive spirometer, mobilization, tubes (Foley catheter, continuous bladder irrigation, and intravenous), pain management (prn medications). ▪ verbalizes ability to cope.	Client will ▪ be afebrile. ▪ recover from anesthesia, as evidenced by VS return to baseline; awake, alert, and oriented; clear lungs. ▪ verbalize understanding and demonstrate cooperation with turning, coughing, and deep breathing. ▪ have a patent Foley catheter. ▪ tolerate ordered diet without nausea and vomiting. ▪ verbalize control of bladder spasms. ▪ verbalize ability to cope.
Tests and treatments	CBC Urinalysis Baseline physical assessment with a focus on respiratory status.	Hct/Hgb Vital signs and O_2 saturation, neurovascular assessment q15min × 4; q30min × 4; q1h × 4 and then q4h if stable. Assess respiratory status and urinary function q4h and prn. Incentive spirometer q2h. Intake and output q shift.
Knowledge deficit	Orient to room and surroundings. Provide simple, brief instructions. Review preoperative preparation, including hospital and surgical routines. Discuss surgery and specific postoperative care: turning, coughing, deep breathing, incentive spirometer, mobilization, possible tubes (Foley catheter, continuous bladder irrigations, and intravenous), pain management (prn medications).	Reorient to room and postoperative routine. Review plan of care and importance of early mobilization. Begin discharge teaching signs and symptoms to report following discharge.
Elimination	Observe amount, color, and character of urine output. Maintain accurate intake and output. Maintain patency of retention catheter. Provide catheter care. Tape retention catheter to lower abdomen. Maintain drainage receptacle below level of client's bladder. Observe bowel elimination pattern. Fleet enema if ordered.	3-way Foley catheter: assess patency, color, and amount of urine, and presence of clots and character of urine output q15min × 4; q30min × 4; q1h × 4, and then q2h × 24 hours unless bleeding. Continuous bladder irrigation (CBI): regulate flow so that urine is free flowing and pink in color for 12–24 hours. Instruct client to avoid straining for BM. Irrigate catheter prn.

	Preoperative day *continued*	**1st 24 hours postoperative** *continued*
Elimination *continued*		Provide catheter care q shift and prn. Explain the importance of reporting bladder spasms. Maintain accurate intake and output. Tape retention catheter to lower abdomen. Maintain drainage receptacle below level of client's bladder
Psycho-social	Assess anxiety related to diagnosis and pending surgery. Assess fears of the unknown and surgery. Encourage verbalization of concerns. Provide information regarding surgical experience. Minimize external stimuli (eg, noise, movement).	Assess level of anxiety. Encourage verbalization of concerns. Provide information. Provide ongoing support and encouragement.
Diet	Regular diet. Encourage fluid intake of 2000 mL per day. Encourage fluids, such as cranberry juice, that acidify urine. Baseline nutritional assessment.	Advance from clear liquids to regular diet as tolerated. Encourage fluid intake to tolerance. Encourage fluids, such as cranberry juice, that acidify urine.
Activity	Provide safety precautions. OOB ad lib until premedicated.	Provide safety precautions. Reposition q2h and prn. Bed rest for 12 to 24 hours, and if free of bleeding then up with assistance. Avoid prolonged sitting.
Medications	Laxatives as ordered	IM or PO muscle relaxants IV antibiotics IV fluid or intermittent IV device Stool softener
Transfer/ discharge plans	Assess discharge plans and support system.	Determine needs at time of discharge. Begin home care teaching.

	Date ________ **2d Postoperative day**	**Date ________** **3d Postoperative day**
Daily outcomes	Client will ▪ be afebrile and have clear lungs. ▪ demonstrate cooperation with turning, coughing, and deep breathing. ▪ tolerate ordered diet without nausea and vomiting. ▪ ambulate 4 times per day.	Client ▪ is afebrile and has stable vital signs and clear lungs. ▪ manages pain with nonpharmacologic measures. ▪ is independent in self-care. ▪ is fully ambulatory.

➤

	2d Postoperative day *continued*	**3d Postoperative day** *continued*
Daily outcomes *continued*	▪ verbalize control of bladder spasms. ▪ have a patent Foley catheter. ▪ verbalize ability to cope. ▪ verbalize beginning understanding of home care instructions.	▪ has resumed preadmission bowel elimination pattern; is passing soft stools without straining. ▪ is voiding in sufficient amounts. ▪ verbalizes home care instructions. ▪ tolerates usual diet. ▪ verbalizes ability to cope with ongoing stressors.
Tests and treatments	Vital signs q4h. Assess respiratory status and urinary function q shift and prn. Incentive spirometer q2h until fully ambulatory. Intake and output q shift.	Vital signs assessment q4h. Assess respiratory status and urinary function.
Knowledge deficit	Initiate discharge teaching regarding diet, bowel management, and activity. Review written discharge instructions.	When Foley catheter is removed, instruct client to void in urinal and notify nurse with each voiding. Complete discharge teaching to include diet, follow-up care, signs and symptoms to report, activity, and medications: dose, frequency, route and side effects. Provide client with written discharge instructions that address (a) avoiding straining or lifting, (b) adequate fluid intake, (c) the importance of reporting heavy bleeding, (d) avoiding aspirin, and (e) avoiding prolonged sitting or car rides.
Elimination	3-way Foley catheter: assess patency, color and amount of urine, and presence of clots and character of urine q2–4h × 24 hours unless bleeding. D/C continuous bladder irrigation (CBI). Instruct client to avoid straining for BM. Irrigate catheter prn. Provide catheter care q shift and prn. Explain the importance of reporting bladder spasms. Maintain accurate intake and output. Maintain patency of retention catheter. Tape retention catheter to lower abdomen. Maintain drainage receptacle below level of client's bladder.	Remove Foley catheter; monitor time and amount of voiding and record on intake and output. Observe amount, color, and character of urine output. Assess bowel elimination pattern.
Psycho-social	Encourage verbalization of concerns. Provide ongoing support and encouragement.	Encourage verbalization of concerns. Provide ongoing support and encouragement.

	2d Postoperative day *continued*	**3d Postoperative day** *continued*
Diet	Regular diet to tolerance. Encourage fluid intake of 2000 mL per day when IV fluids D/C. Encourage fluids, such as cranberry juice, that acidify urine.	Regular diet as tolerated. Encourage fluids to 2000 mL per 24 hours unless contraindicated. Offer fluids, such as cranberry juice, that acidify urine.
Activity	Provide safety precautions. Ambulate independently at least 4 times. Avoid prolonged sitting.	Fully ambulatory. Avoid prolonged sitting.
Medications	PO analgesics IV or oral antibiotics Intermittent IV device Stool softener Laxative if no BM in 48 h	PO analgesics Stool softener D/C intermittent IV device
Transfer/ discharge plans	Complete discharge plans. Continue home care instructions.	Complete discharge instructions. Discharge when voiding in sufficient amounts without difficulty.

CHAPTER HIGHLIGHTS

- Urinary elimination depends on normal functioning of the urinary, cardiovascular, and nervous systems.
- The normal process of micturition includes sufficient accumulation of urine in the bladder to stimulate the sensory stretch nerves in the bladder wall. Impulses from these stretch receptors then travel to the spinal cord, to the voiding reflex center and to the voiding control center in the cerebral cortex, where conscious control of micturition is regulated.
- In the adult, micturition generally occurs after 250 to 450 mL of urine has collected in the bladder.
- Many factors influence a person's urinary elimination including fluid intake, stress, activity, medications, and various diseases.
- Alterations in urinary elimination include polyuria, oliguria, anuria, frequency, nocturia, urgency, dysuria, enuresis, hematuria, incontinence, and retention. Each has various influencing and associated factors that need to be identified.
- A comprehensive assessment of a client's urinary function includes (a) a nursing history that identifies normal voiding patterns, usual urine and recent changes, past and current problems with urination, and factors influencing the elimination pattern; (b) a physical assessment of the kidneys, bladder, and urethral meatus; (c) inspection of the urine for amount, color, clarity, and odor, and, if indicated, (d) testing of urine for specific gravity, pH, and the presence of glucose, ketone bodies, and occult blood.
- Many NANDA approved nursing diagnoses may be applicable to clients with altered urinary elimination patterns, for example, **High risk for infection.**
- Incontinence can be physically and emotionally distressing to clients because it is considered socially unacceptable.

- Bladder-training programs can effectively reduce the incidence of incontinence episodes.
- Clients with urinary retention not only experience discomfort but also are at risk of urinary tract infection.
- The most common cause of urinary tract infection are invasive procedures such as catheterization and cystoscopic examination. Females in particular are prone to ascending urinary tract infections because of their short urethras.
- Nursing interventions related to urinary elimination are generally directed toward facilitating the normal functioning of the urinary system or toward assisting the client with particular problems.
- Interventions include (a) assisting the client to maintain an appropriate fluid intake, (b) assisting the client to maintain normal voiding patterns, (c) monitoring the client's daily fluid intake and output, and (d) maintaining cleanliness of the genital area.
- Urinary catheterization is frequently required for clients with urinary retention but is only performed when all other measures to facilitate voiding fail. Sterile technique is essential to prevent ascending urinary infections.
- Care of clients with indwelling catheters is directed toward preventing infection of the urinary tract and encouraging urinary flow through the drainage system.

READINGS AND REFERENCES

SUGGESTED READINGS

McCormick, KA, Newman, DK, Colling, J, and Pearson, BD. October 1992. Clinical guidelines: Urinary incontinence in adults. *American Journal of Nursing* 92:75–88.

These clinical guidelines for urinary incontinence (UI) in adults were released by the Agency for Health Care Policy and Research (AHCPR) in March 1992. The guidelines include causes and types of UI, basic evaluation of UI with recommended supplementary assessments, behavioral treatment, pharmacologic treatments, and surgical treatments.

Williams, MP, Wallhagen, M, and Dowling, G. February 1993. Urinary retention in hospitalized elderly women. *Journal of Gerontological Nursing* 19:7–14.

These authors suggest that urinary retention (UR) may be an underrecognized or overlooked clinical phenomenon in elderly hospitalized women. The article includes a definition of UR, complications, factors influencing urinary retention, recognition and assessment, and immediate management and treatment.

RELATED RESEARCH

McKeever, MP. October 1990. An investigation of recognized incontinence within a health authority. *Journal of Advanced Nursing* 15:1197–1207.

Thomas, AM and Morse, JM. June 1991. Managing urinary incontinence with self-care practices. *Journal of Gerontological Nursing* 17:9–14.

SELECTED REFERENCES

Agency for Health Care Policy and Research, Urinary Incontinence Guideline Panel. *Urinary Incontinence in Adults: Guideline Report* Rockville, MD: USDHHS. (AHCPR Publication No. 92 0039.)

Black, PA. April 1990. Urinary incontinence: A many faceted problem. *Professional Nurse* 5:378, 380, 392.

Bristol, SL, Fadden, T, Fehring, RJ, Rohde, L, Prue, KS, and Wohlitz, BA. March 1989. The mythical danger of rapid urinary drainage. *American Journal of Nursing* 89:344–45.

Brogna, L and Lakaszawski, ML. February 1986. The continent urostomy . . . the Kock pouch. *American Journal of Nursing* 86:160–63.

Burke, JP, Jacobsen, JA, Garibaldi, RA, Conti, M, and Alling, DW. February 1983. Evaluation of daily meatal care with polyantibiotic ointment in prevention of urinary catheter-associated bacteriuria. *Journal of Urology* 129:331–34.

Carpenito, LJ. 1992. *Nursing Diagnosis: Application to Clinical Practice.* 4th ed. Philadelphia: Lippincott.

Cefalu, CA. June 1987. Management of the bedridden patient with irreversible urinary incontinence. *Hospital Medicine* 23:183–87.

Clancy, B and Malone-Lee, J. February 1991. Reducing leakage of body-worn incontinence pads. *Journal of Advanced Nursing* 16:187–93.

Colley, W. February 13–19, 1991. Continence: The Colley Model. *Nursing Times* 87:61–63.

Conti, MT and Eutropius, L. March 1987. Preventing UTIs: What works? *American Journal of Nursing* 87:307–9.

Cooper, C. August 1993. What color is that urine specimen? *American Journal of Nursing* 93:37.

Epstein, SE. December 1985. Cost-effective application of the Centers for Disease Control Guidelines for prevention of catheter-associated urinary tract infections. *American Journal of Infection Control* 13:272–75.

Gordon, M. 1993. *Manual of Nursing Diagnosis 1993–1994.* 6th ed. St Louis: Mosby-Year Book.

Gray, M and Dougherty, MC. July/August, 1987. Urinary incontinence: Pathophysiology and treatment. *Journal of Enterostomal Therapy* 14:152–62.

Guyton, AC. 1991. *Textbook of Medical Physiology.* 8th ed. Philadelphia: WB Saunders.

Kim, MJ, McFarland, GK, and McLane, AM. 1993. *Pocket Guide to Nursing Diagnoses.* 5th ed. St Louis: Mosby-Year Book.

Kohler-Ockmare, J. January 13–19, 1993. Catheter concerns. *Nursing Times* 89:34–36.

Kuhns-Hastings, J. February 1988. Management of female incontinence with Kegel exercises. *American Association of Occupational Health Nurses Journal* 36:78–83.

Laycock, J. July 10, 1987. Graded exercises for the pelvic floor muscles in the treatment of urinary incontinence. *Physiotherapy* 73:371–73.

Lederer, JR, Marculescu, GL, Mocnik, B, and Seaby, N. 1993. *Care Planning Pocket Guide—A Nursing Diagnosis Approach.* 5th ed. Redwood City, CA: Addison-Wesley Nursing.

McConnell, EA. October 1991. Clinical do's and dont's. How to use a urinometer. *Nursing 91* 21:28.

McCormick, KA. March 1988. Urinary incontinence in the elderly. *Nursing Clinics of North America* 23:135–37.

McCormick, KA, Burgio, LD, Engel, BT, Scheve, A, and Leahy, E. March 1992. Urinary incontinence: An augmented prompted void approach. *Journal of Gerontological Nursing* 18:3–10.

McCormick, KA, Newman, DK, Colling, J, and Pearson, BD. October 1992. Clinical guidelines: Urinary incontinence in adults. *American Journal of Nursing* 92:75–88.

McCormick, KA, Scheve, AAS, and Leahy, E. March 1988. Nursing management of urinary incontinence in geriatric inpatients. *Nursing Clinics of North America* 23:231–64.

McFarland, GK and McFarlane, EA. 1993. *Nursing Diagnosis and Intervention: Planning for Patient Care.* 2d ed. St Louis: Mosby.

McKeever, MP. October 1990. An investigation of recognized incontinence within a health authority. *Journal of Advanced Nursing* 15:1197–1207.

Mocsny, N. March 1980. Puncturing catheter balloons. *Nursing80* 10:88.

Newman, DK, Lynch, K, Smith, DA, and Cell, P. January 1991. Restoring urinary continence. *American Journal of Nursing* 91: 28–34.

North American Nursing Diagnosis Association. 1992. *NANDA Nursing Diagnoses: Definitions and Classification 1992–1993.* Philadelphia: NANDA.

Palmer, MH. December 1990. Urinary incontinence. *Nursing Clinics of North America* 25:919–34.

Pomfret, I. February 24–March 2, 1993. Men only. *Nursing Times* 89:55–56, 58.

Pottle, B. November 26–December 2, 1986. When the sheets were changed . . . absorbent sheets designed for incontinent patients. *Nursing Times* 82:64, 66.

Powers, I and Williams, D. December 1992. Urinary incontinence: Helping a patient regain control. *Nursing92* 22:46–47.

Pritchard, V and Levernier, J. August 1991. Multistix versus laboratory urinalysis in the detection of urinary tract infection. *Journal of Gerontological Nursing* 17:39–42.

Roe, BH. February 1990a. Study of the effects of education on patient's knowledge of their indwelling urethral catheters. *Journal of Advanced Nursing* 15:223–31.

———. October 23–30, 1990b. Do we need to clamp catheters? *Nursing Times* 86:66–67.

Scheve, A, Engel, BT, McCormick, K, and Leahy, EG. May/June 1991. Exercise in continence. *Geriatric Nursing* 12:124.

Stark, JL. July 1988. A quick guide to urinary tract assessment. *Nursing88* 18:56–58.

Thomas, AM and Morse, JM. June 1991. Managing urinary incontinence with self-care practices. *Journal of Gerontological Nursing* 17:9–14.

Thompson, J. November 14–16, 1990. Managing continence systematically. *Nursing Times* 86:60–62.

Tulloch, GJ. January/February 1989. The incontinency taboo. *Geriatric Nursing* 10:19.

Turner, SL and Plymat, KR. May/June 1988. As women age: Perspectives on urinary incontinence. *Rehabilitation Nursing* 13:132–35.

Webber-Jones, JE. August 1991. Performing clean, intermittent self-catheterization. *Nursing91* 21:56–59.

Williams, MP, Wallhagen, M, and Dowling, G. February 1993. Urinary retention in hospitalized elderly women. *Journal of Gerontological Nursing* 19:7–14.

Winder, A. October 24–30, 1990. Catheters: Intermittent self-catheterization. *Nursing Times* 86:63–64.

Woodtli, MA. January/February 1993. Assessing urge incontinence in elderly women. *Geriatric Nursing* 14:19–22.

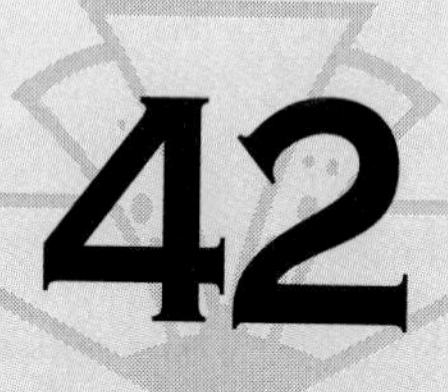

42 Sensory Perception and Cognition

Objectives

- Describe structural and physiologic components of the sensory/perceptual process.
- Identify causes and signs of sensory deprivation and sensory overload.
- Describe factors influencing sensory function.
- Identify clients at risk of sensory disturbances.
- Identify essential information required to assess a client's sensory/perceptual function and cognition.
- Develop nursing diagnoses and outcome criteria for clients with impaired sensory and cognitive function.
- Describe nursing interventions to promote and maintain sensory stimulation.
- Identify interventions to prevent sensory overload.
- Identify interventions that help the client adapt to altered sensory function and maximize the use of existing senses.
- Identify measures to enhance a confused client's orientation to time, place, person, and situation.

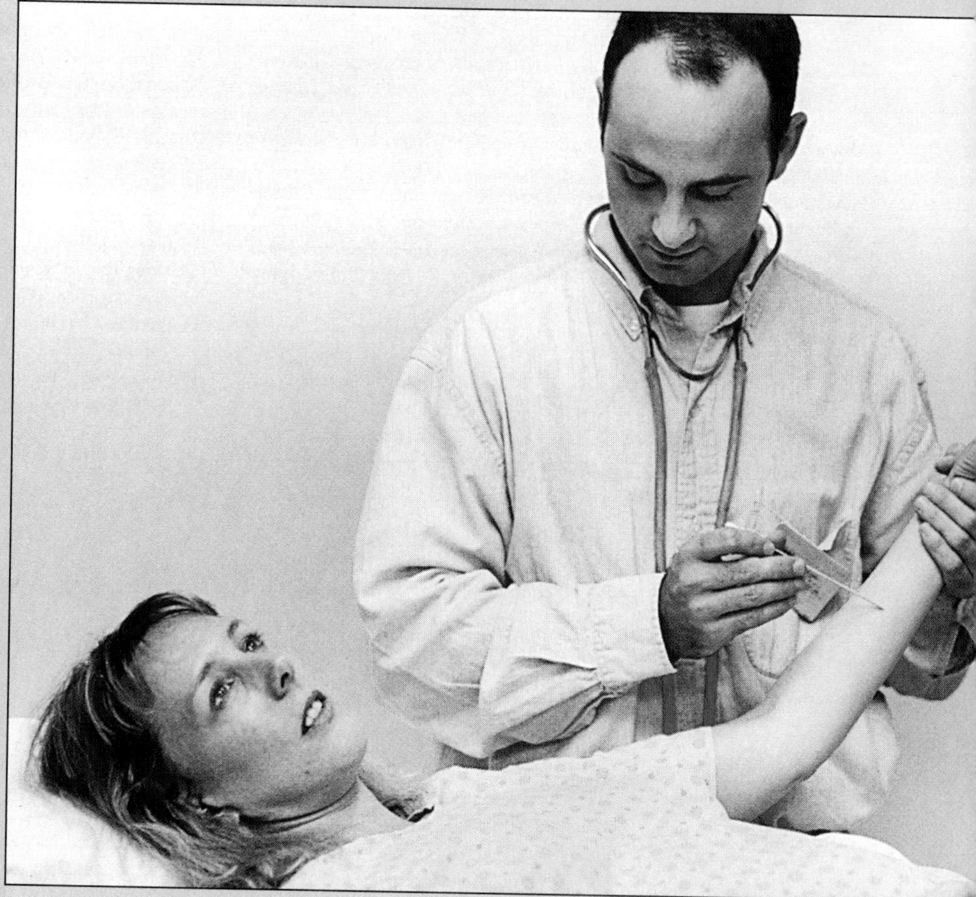

The sensory process involves two components: reception and perception. **Sensory reception** is the process of receiving stimuli or data. These stimuli are either external or internal to the body. External stimuli are **visual** (sight), **auditory** (hearing), **olfactory** (smell), **tactile** (touch), and **gustatory** (taste). Gustatory stimuli can be internal as well. Other types of internal stimuli are kinesthetic or visceral. **Kinesthetic** refers to awareness of the position and movement of body parts. For example, a man walking is aware of which leg is forward. **Stereognosis** is the awareness of an object's size, shape, and texture. For example, a person holding a tennis ball is aware of its size, round shape, and soft surface without seeing it. **Visceral** refers to any large organ within the body. Visceral organs may produce stimuli which make a person aware of them (ie, fullness). **Sensory perception** involves the conscious organization and translation of the data or stimuli into meaningful information.

Associated with these senses is the ability to speak. Use of only the senses enables people to be aware of their environments; speech enables people to interact with others in the environment.

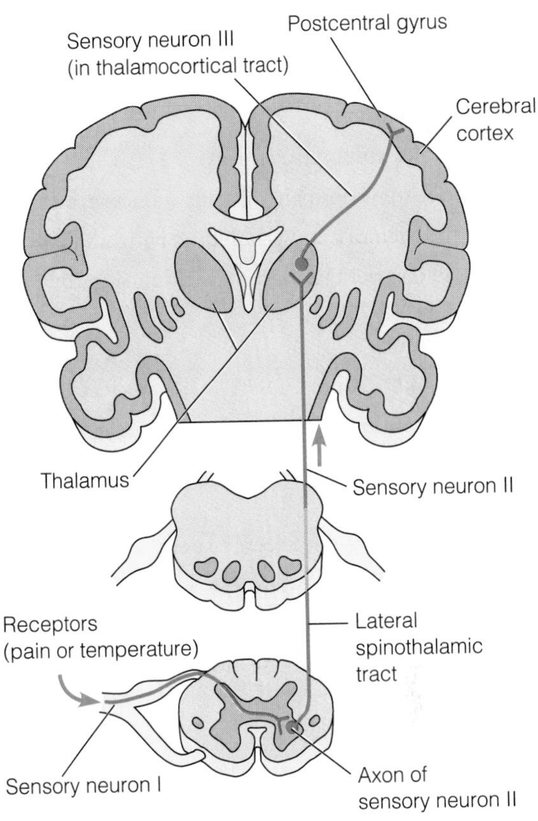

Figure 42–1 The lateral spinothalamic tract transmits sensory impulses up the spinal cord to the thalamus. The thalamocortical tract transmits impulses from the thalamus to the somatosensory area of the parietal lobe.

Components of the Sensory Experience

Sensory reception and perception are the two components of the sensory experience. They are controlled by the nervous system. Normally the nervous system continually receives hundreds of stimuli. Once a stimulus triggers a sensory receptor, the stimulus travels along a sensory neuron I, to the central nervous system. From the spinal cord or brain stem, the impulses travel along sensory neuron II to the thalamus. These neurons synapse with sensory neurons III, which conduct the impulses from the thalamus to the somatosensory area of the postcentral gyrus of the parietal lobe of the brain, also called the primary sensory area (Figure 42–1). In most instances, sensory pathways **decussate** (cross over) and register sensations from the opposite side of the body. Usually, decussation takes place at the level of sensory neuron II.

The awareness of the stimuli takes place in the cerebral cortex, where the stimuli are perceived and interpreted. For the person to receive and interpret these stimuli, the brain must be alert. The *reticular activating system* (RAS) in the brain stem is thought to mediate the arousal mechanism. See Figure 36–4, page 979. People have their own zone of optimum arousal, at which the person feels comfortable. *Sensoristasis* is the term used to describe when a person is in optimum arousal. Beyond this comfort zone people must adapt to the increased or decreased sensory stimuli. An absence of stimuli from the RAS to the cerebrum results in the brain's becoming inactive or useless. The level of activity of the RAS depends largely on receiving sensory stimuli. Pain, in particular, increases the activity of the RAS. Once the sensory stimuli reach the RAS, they are passed along to the cerebral cortex. The role of the cortex is to process, interpret, use, and store the incoming data in an organized manner. The thalamus acts as the distribution center for signals, and signals go back and forth between the cerebral cortex and the thalamus.

Another area that performs an important role in brain activity is the *reticular inhibitory area* (RIA) located in the medulla. This area can reduce the number of nerve signals descending through the spinal cord to the muscles and decrease the activity of the higher brain centers.

The brain has the capacity to adapt to sensory stimuli. For example, a person living in a city may not notice the noise of traffic, which someone from a rural area may find loud and disturbing. Not all sensory stimuli are acted on;

CLINICAL SIGNS OF SENSORY DEPRIVATION AND OVERLOAD

Sensory Deprivation

- Excessive yawning; drowsiness
- Reduced attention span; difficulty concentrating
- Impaired memory and problem-solving ability
- Periodic disorientation, general confusion, or nocturnal confusion
- Hallucinations
- Feelings of boredom
- Apathy, emotional lability, depression, annoyance about small matters

Sensory Overload

- Complaints of fatigue, sleeplessness
- Irritability, anxiety, restlessness
- Periodic or general disorientation
- Reduced problem-solving ability and task performance
- Increased muscle tension

some are stored by the memory to be used at a later date. *Cognition* is cerebral functioning. It involves such processes as conscious thought, reality orientation, problem solving, judgment, and comprehension.

Awareness is the ability to perceive environmental stimuli and body reactions and to respond appropriately through thought and action. The normal, alert person can assimilate many kinds of information at one time. The restaurant patron, for example, appreciates odors, tastes, conversation, and company at the same time. The normal person perceives reality accurately and acts on these perceptions.

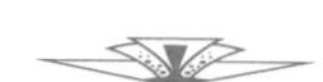

SENSORY ALTERATIONS

People become accustomed to certain sensory stimuli, and when these change markedly, the individual may experience discomfort. For example, when clients enter a hospital they usually experience many differences in the quantity and quality of the stimuli. These clients may become confused and disoriented. *Confusion* is a mental state in which the individual becomes bewildered and may make inappropriate statements. *Disorientation* is a state of mental confusion in which the individual may be confused about time, place, and person; that is, clients may not know the time or day of the week or year, where they are (place), or who their support persons are.

Nurses in hospitals are aware of the behaviors that often result from different stimuli. More attention is now paid to color, sound, privacy, and social interaction for hospital clients so that the stimuli more resemble those in the home environment. As a result, behavioral changes in hospitalized clients have been reduced. Factors that contribute to sensory alterations in behavior include sensory deprivation, sensory overload, and sensory deficits, which are discussed next. Sleep deprivation is discussed in Chapter 35. Social deprivation and cultural deprivation should also be considered by nurses when assessing clients' needs.

SENSORY DEPRIVATION

Sensory deprivation is generally thought of as a decrease in or lack of meaningful stimuli. When a person experiences sensory deprivation, the balance of the reticular activating system (RAS) is disturbed. The RAS is unable to maintain normal stimulation to the cerebral cortex. Because of this reduced stimulation, a person becomes more acutely aware of the remaining stimuli and often perceives these in a distorted manner. Thus the person often experiences alterations in perception, cognition, and emotion. See the accompanying box for the clinical signs of sensory deprivation.

Factors that place a client at risk of sensory deprivation include the following:

- A nonstimulating or monotonous environment; for example, a person confined to the bedroom in the home or a client who is on bed rest or confined to a hospital room.
- Inability to process environmental stimuli; for example, a client who has brain damage or who is taking drugs that affect the central nervous system.
- Inability to receive environmental stimuli; for example, clients who have impaired vision or hearing or who have emotional disorders and withdraw within themselves.

Figure 42–2 shows an elderly person who is isolated and is experiencing sensory deprivation.

SENSORY OVERLOAD

Sensory overload generally occurs when an individual is unable to process or manage the amount or intensity of sensory stimuli.

Three factors contribute to sensory overload:

1. Increased quantity or quality of internal stimuli, for example, pain, intravenous lines, catheters, endotracheal tubes

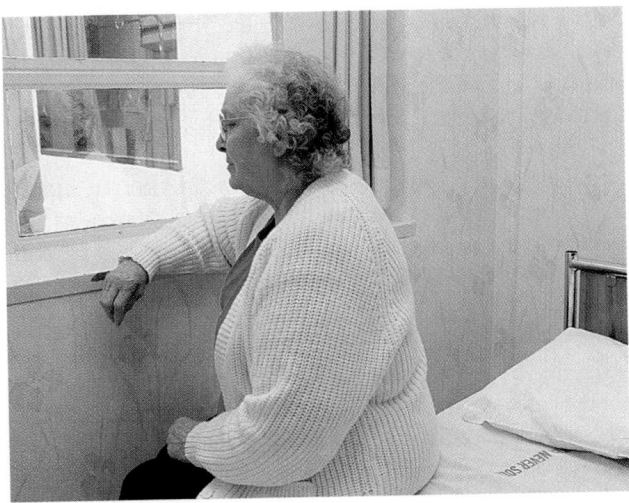

Figure 42–2 An elderly woman who is alone lacks sensory stimulation.

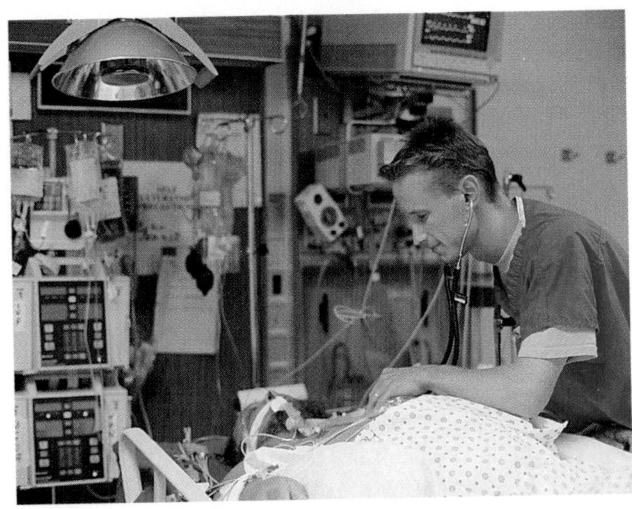

Figure 42–3 A client experiencing sensory overload in an intensive care unit (ICU).

2. Increased quantity or quality of external stimuli, for example, from busy health care setting, presence of strangers, intrusive procedures (eg, diagnostic tests)
3. Inability to disregard stimuli selectively, for example, as a result of nervous system disturbances or medications that stimulate the arousal mechanism

The person usually feels overwhelmed and does not feel in control. Hospitalized clients exposed to bright lights, noise, unfamiliar machinery, and too many visitors, including health personnel, may suffer sensory overload. It is important for nurses to remember that the sights and sounds that are familiar to them often represent overload to clients. People who have sensory overload often appear fatigued. See the box on page 1274 for clinical signs of sensory overload. They often cannot internalize new information and experience cognitive overload as a result of everything that has happened to them. Such factors as pain, lack of sleep, and worry can also contribute to sensory overload. Two cognitive problems that may appear are hallucinations and illusions. **Hallucinations** are perceptions of external stimuli in the absence of such stimuli, for example, hearing voices when there are none. **Illusions** are misinterpretations of external stimuli; for example, a person interprets a shadow as a person.

People at risk of sensory overload include the following:

- Clients who have pain
- Clients who are acutely ill and have been admitted to an acute care facility
- Clients who are being closely monitored, such as in an ICU unit (Figure 42–3)
- Clients who have central nervous system disturbances

Sensory Deficits

A *sensory deficit* is impaired function of sensory reception or perception. Blindness and deafness are sensory deficits. When only one sense is affected, other senses may become more acute to compensate for the loss. However, sudden loss of eyesight can result in total disorientation.

When there is gradual loss of sensory function, individuals often develop behaviors to compensate for the loss; sometimes these behaviors are unconscious. For example, a person with gradual hearing loss in the right ear may unconsciously turn the left ear toward a speaker. When the loss is sudden, however, compensatory behavior often takes days or weeks to develop.

Some neurologic diseases cause changes in the kinesthetic sense and tactile perceptions. Diseases of the inner ear, for example, can cause loss of kinesthetic sense. Spinal cord injuries and cerebrovascular accidents (CVAs) can cause paralysis and loss of tactile perception.

Clients with sensory deficits are at risk of both sensory deprivation and sensory overload. Persons with visual problems may be unable to read, watch television, or recognize nurses by sight. An unfamiliar environment can add to their confusion. The blind often have highly structured home environments, and the diversity and unfamiliarity of the hospital environment can create sensory overload. At the same time, impaired vision often leads to the inability to move around readily or socialize with others. Deaf persons who cannot lip-read also may feel isolated.

Social Deprivation

Social deprivation is the lack of meaningful interaction with people. The client who is confined to bed may be socially isolated. Elderly people can become socially deprived for a number of reasons: limited mobility, death of a spouse, or changed living arrangements. Prolonged social deprivation can be a major cause of sensory deprivation.

CULTURAL DEPRIVATION

Cultural deprivation or cultural care deprivation is "a lack of culturally assistive, supportive or facilitative acts" (Kloosterman 1991, p. 121). It is important that nurses be sensitive to what stimulation is culturally acceptable to a client. For example, in some cultures touching is comforting, whereas in others it is offensive. Some clients may find the presence of cultural or religious symbols reassuring and their absence a source of anxiety. Nurses should encourage clients to have culturally related symbols present and to follow practices with which they are comfortable, provided that these practices do not endanger health.

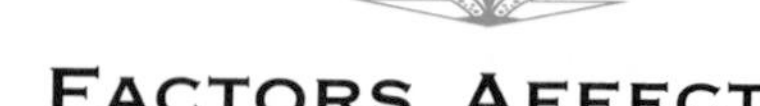

FACTORS AFFECTING SENSORY STIMULATION

A number of factors affect the amount and quality of sensory stimulation, including a person's developmental stage, culture, level of stress, medications, illness, and life-style.

Developmental Stage Perception of sensation is critical to the intellectual, social, and physical development of infants and children. As children grow, they learn that certain sensations provide cues for behavior already learned, for example, stopping and looking both ways before crossing a street. Adults have many learned responses to sensory cues. Loss or impairment of any sense, therefore, has profound effects on both the child and young adult. The gradual diminishing of sensory perception that often comes with age does not have as profound an effect.

Culture An individual's culture often determines the amount of stimulation that a person considers usual or "normal." For example, a child raised in a large, active Mexican-American family may be accustomed to more stimulation than an only child raised in an Anglo-American family. In addition, the normal amount of stimulation associated with ethnic origin, religious affiliation, and income level, for example, also affects the amount of stimulation an individual desires and believes to be meaningful.

Stress During times of increased stress, people may find their senses already overloaded and thus seek to decrease sensory stimulation. For example, a client dealing with physical illness, pain, hospitalization, and diagnostic tests may wish to have only close support persons visit. In addition, the client may need the nurse's help to decrease unnecessary stimuli (eg, noise) as much as possible.

Medications Certain medications can alter an individual's awareness of environmental stimuli. Narcotics and sedatives, for example, can decrease awareness of stimuli. Some antidepressants can alter perceptions of stimuli.

Illness Certain diseases, such as atherosclerosis, restrict blood flow to the receptor organ and the brain, thereby decreasing awareness and slowing responses. Uncontrolled diabetes mellitus can impair vision. Some central nervous system diseases cause varying degrees of paralysis and sensory loss.

Life-Style and Personality Life-style influences the quality and quantity of stimulation to which an individual is accustomed. A client who is employed in a large company may be accustomed to many diverse stimuli, whereas a client who is self-employed and works in the home is exposed to fewer, less diverse stimuli. People's personalities also differ in terms of the quantity and quality of stimuli with which they are comfortable. Some people delight in constantly changing stimuli and excitement, whereas others prefer a more structured life with few changes.

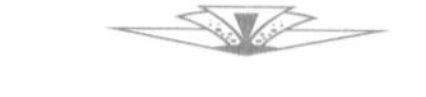

ASSESSING

When assessing the client for sensory/perceptual and cognitive alterations, nurses should take a health history, examine the client for signs of sensory disturbance, perform required physical examinations, and identify clients at risk.

NURSING HISTORY

The nursing history includes the client's sensory deficits, present sensory perceptions, usual functioning, and potential problems. In some instances, significant others can provide data the person cannot. For example, a woman may detect her partner's hearing loss long before the partner is aware of it. Examples of interview questions to elicit data about the client's sensory/perceptual functioning are shown in the box on page 1277.

PHYSICAL EXAMINATION

The nurse assesses vision, hearing, and olfactory, gustatory, tactile, and kinesthetic status. Physical assessment, in particular, should reveal the client's specific visual and hearing abilities; perception of heat, cold, light touch, and pain in the limbs; and awareness of the position of the body parts. See Chapter 22, page 550, for details about assessing sensory function.

The nurse should also determine whether the client uses sensory adaptive devices such as eyeglasses or hearing aids and whether they are functioning properly.

MENTAL STATUS

Assessment of mental status is critical to any evaluation of the sensory/perceptual process. The nurse obtains considerable data about mental status during history taking, during physical examination, and while providing care. In many instances, a separate examination is not always indicated. Details about assessing orientation, memory, attention span, and calculation are discussed in Chapter 22, page 543.

ADAPTATIONS TO SENSORY ALTERATIONS

Sensory alteration can lower the quality of a person's life, particularly in the area of communication. The nurse needs to explore

- How the client perceives the sensory loss, asking, for example, "How has your life changed since you experienced your (hearing, visual, speech) loss?" See also the discussion of self-care ability and safety earlier.
- What adjustments the person has made to modify the loss, asking for example, "What have you done to adjust to your (hearing, visual, speech) loss?"

Clients with sensory deficits develop or need to develop alternative ways of communicating. For example, hearing-impaired clients may listen with the help of a hearing aid, read lips, use sign language, write and read notes, and increase their use of vision to observe body language. A visually impaired person, who cannot observe facial expressions and other nonverbal behaviors that often clarify the content of verbal communication, often relies on voice tones and changes in inflection to determine the emotional tone of communication. Some visually impaired clients also learn to read Braille.

Temporary or permanent loss of the ability to speak produces extreme anxiety. The nurse needs to establish alternative means of communication, such as writing notes or using a communication board. However, before implementing alternative communication methods, the nurse needs to understand the nature of the communication problem. For example, **expressive aphasia** is the inability to verbalize simple ideas in words or writing or to name objects, even though the person understands what is said. **Sensory** or **receptive aphasia** is the inability to understand written or spoken language. **Global aphasia** is the inability to understand language and communicate verbally.

ASSESSMENT INTERVIEW

Sensory/Perceptual Functioning

Auditory

- Do you have any difficulty hearing, or have you had any recent changes in hearing?
- Do you wear a hearing aid? If so, when did you obtain it, and how well does it work for you?
- Can you locate the direction of sounds and distinguish various voices? (Persons with hearing aids often have difficulties in these areas.)
- Have you ever experienced a humming, ringing, buzzing, or crackling noise in the ears?

Visual

- Do you have any difficulty seeing near or far objects?
- Do you wear eyeglasses or contact lenses?
- Have you ever experienced any visual disturbances, such as blurred or double vision, rainbows or halos around lights or objects, blind spots, flashing lights, light sensitivity, troublesome spots or floaters?
- Have you or anyone in your family ever had glaucoma, cataracts, retinal detachment, or other eye problems?
- When did you last visit an eye doctor?

Gustatory

- Have you noticed any changes in your ability to taste (eg, difficulty in differentiating sweet, sour, salty, and bitter tastes)?
- Do you find certain foods unpalatable? Which ones?

Olfactory

- Have you noticed any changes in your ability to smell (eg, can you distinguish foods by their odors and tell when something is burning)?

Tactile

- Have you noticed any unusual sensations, such as "pins and needles" in your legs or arms?
- Have you ever had difficulty in perceiving heat, cold, or pain in your limbs? Have you had problems that alter your ability to do so?

Kinesthetic

- Have you ever noticed any difficulty in perceiving the position of parts of your body?

CRITICAL THINKING CHALLENGE

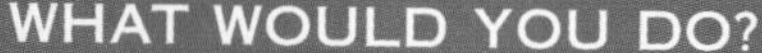

WHAT WOULD YOU DO?

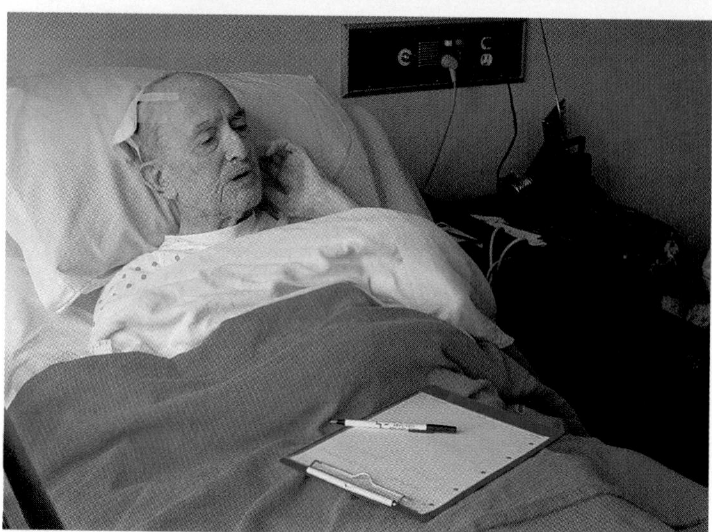

Martin McClanahan, a 74-year-old male, was recently admitted to your unit following a stroke (cerebrovascular accident), resulting in expressive aphasia. His speech therapist has provided a pen and paper, but most of the time Mr McClanahan refuses to use them and responds to your questions with unintelligible speech.

What would you do?

THE CLIENT'S ENVIRONMENT

The nurse assesses the quantity, quality, and type of stimuli within the health care and/or home environment. The client's environment may produce insufficient stimuli, placing the client at risk for sensory deprivation, or excessive stimuli, placing the client at risk for sensory overload. Nonstimulating environments include those that (a) severely restrict physical activity, such as isolation units, incubators, the use of body casts or traction, or prescribed bed rest; and (b) limit social contact with family and friends. People who have limited social contact include those who are institutionalized, homebound, chronically ill, or discredited because of mental illness, retardation, or physical handicap. Elderly people are particularly susceptible to sensory deprivation because of social isolation and a restricted environment. The elderly person can become socially isolated for a number of reasons, including limited physical mobility, death of a spouse and/or friends, and changed living arrangements.

Excessively stimulating environments (eg, intensive care units) are overloaded with sensory stimuli that are meaningless to the client. These environments also affect sensory perception and may cause sensory distortions, disorientation, or hallucinations. People who normally live alone and have little contact with others can also experience sensory overload. This is particularly true of the elderly and of people who work at home alone. Because appropriate or meaningful stimuli decrease the incidence of sensory deprivation, the nurse must consider the client's health care environment for the presence of the following stimuli:

- Radio or other auditory device (eg, cassette recorder), television
- Clock or calendar
- Reading material (or toys for children)
- Number and compatibility of roommates
- Number of visitors

In the client's home, the nurse may also note the presence of a videocassette recorder, pets, bright colors, adequacy of lighting, and so on.

To assess a health care environment that produces excessive stimuli, the nurse considers the presence of the following:

- Bright lighting
- Noise from electrical monitors, equipment, elevators, doors, staff
- Odors (eg, of body fluids)
- Therapeutic measures (eg, tubes, dressings)
- Pain
- Frequent assessments and procedures

CLINICAL SIGNS OF SENSORY DEPRIVATION AND OVERLOAD

In addition to assessing the client for sensory deficits, the nurse observes clients for signs of sensory deprivation and sensory overload:

- *Changes in attention span*, such as decreased concentration (inability to follow the flow of conversation), increased distractibility, restlessness, and daydreaming. Persons who are daydreaming appear absorbed in their own thoughts and may talk and laugh to themselves. It may be difficult to engage such a person in conversation. These persons may confuse a daydream with reality and imagine a conversation that did not take place.

- *Changes in thought processes*, such as confusion about time, place, or person; disordered sequencing of time or events (eg, the person may start a sentence on one subject and end it with an unrelated subject); difficulty in remembering what one was saying; difficulty in grasping ideas; slowness in communicating; indecision; bizarre thinking; illusions (eg, interpreting a shadow as a man with a knife); and hallucinations.
- *Emotional lability*, such as rapid mood swings, irritability, exaggerated responses; apathy; ambivalence; emotional detachment; inappropriate reaction (eg, laughing at bad news); anger; depression; anxiety, fear.
- *Changes in usual routines*, such as altered sleeping pattern (difficulty staying awake or difficulty sleeping) and altered eating pattern (eg, loss of appetite). People tolerate the amount of environmental stimuli differently. For example, a mother of six active, noisy children may hardly notice the noise of her environment, whereas another person may find the noise bothersome. People whose developmental levels are characterized by short attention spans, a need for physical activity, and dependence on others for amusement are often more susceptible to sensory deprivation than people who are more self-reliant and contemplative. Likewise, persons who are stressed and anxious may have more difficulty in coping with sensory deprivation.

SELF-CARE ABILITY AND SAFETY

Clients with sensory/perceptual alterations may have difficulty performing activities of daily living (ADLs) and maintaining a safe, comfortable, and clean home environment. The nurse assesses the client's self-care abilities in the areas of feeding, dressing, grooming, toileting, bathing, driving, reading, writing, and so on. Visually impaired clients are particularly at risk for self-care deficits. Community resources and support may be needed to help the client with physical care, home maintenance management, shopping, banking, paying bills, and obtaining medications. See also Chapter 28 for a home hazard appraisal and required safety measures.

SOCIAL SUPPORT NETWORK

The degree of isolation a person feels is significantly influenced by the quality and quantity of support from family members and friends. The nurse assesses (a) whether the client lives alone; (b) who and when support people visit; (c) presence of signs indicating social deprivation, such as withdrawal from contact with others to avoid embarrassment or dependence on others, negative self image, reports of lack of meaningful communication with others, absence of opportunities to discuss fears or concerns that facilitate coping mechanisms, and so on.

DIAGNOSING

NANDA nursing diagnosis labels that relate to sensory/perceptual and cognitive alterations include the following:

- **Sensory/perceptual alterations,** which must be specified as **visual, auditory, kinesthetic, gustatory, tactile,** or **olfactory**
- **Social isolation**
- **Altered thought processes**
- **Impaired home maintenance management**

The definitions, contributing factors, and defining characteristics of **Sensory/perceptual alterations** and **Social isolation** are shown in the box on page 1280. Clinical examples of assessment data clusters and related nursing diagnoses are shown in Table 42–1 on page 1281. Because the etiologies of **Sensory/perceptual alterations** and **Altered thought processes** are often the result of a disease process or permanent physiologic change, the nurse may find that focusing on the client's *response* to the sensory or thought process alteration may be more appropriate (Carpenito 1993, p. 696). For example, for a diagnosis of **Sensory/perceptual alterations: visual** related to cataracts, there are no independent (nonmedical) nursing interventions that will relieve the etiology, cataracts. In addition, expected outcomes must demonstrate alleviation of the problem, which in this case is poor vision. The nurse cannot actually improve the client's vision, so it is not reasonable to write as an outcome, "Vision will improve." In this situation, it is more appropriate to use the NANDA label **Sensory/perceptual alteration: visual** as the etiology of other nursing diagnoses, for example, **High risk for injury (falls)** related to **Visual sensory/perceptual alteration (specify).** This diagnosis focuses on the client's *responses* and suggests an expected outcome that is achievable by nursing actions (eg, "Avoids personal injury from falling") as well as independent nursing interventions. See Chapter 28 for details about the diagnosis **High risk for injury.**

Examples of nursing diagnoses for which **Sensory/perceptual alterations** is the etiology include the following:

NURSING DIAGNOSES

CLIENTS WITH SENSORY/PERCEPTUAL AND COGNITIVE PROBLEMS

NURSING DIAGNOSIS: Sensory/perceptual alteration (specify): A state in which an individual experiences a change in the amount or intepretation of internal or external stimuli (auditory, gustatory, kinesthetic, olfactory, tactile, visual), accompanied by absent, diminished, exaggerated, distorted, or impaired response to such stimuli; these altered responses are a change from the individual's usual response to stimuli and are not a result of mental or personality disorders

Defining Characters

Major

- Anxiety
- Apathy
- Altered abstraction or conceptualization
- Change in problem-solving abilities
- Reported or measured change in sensory acuity
- Change in usual response to stimuli
- Body image alteration
- Disorientation to time, place, persons, or situation
- Change in behavior patterns
- Restlessness, irritability
- Altered communication pattern

Minor

- Complaints of fatigue
- Changes in posture, muscle tension
- Inappropriate responses
- Hallucinations

Related Factors

Excessive, altered, or insufficient environmental stimuli, either exogenous (eg, alcohol, substance abuse) or endogenous (eg, electrolyte imbalance); altered sensory reception, transmission, and/or integration secondary to cerebrovascular accident (CVA), brain trauma, increased intracranial pressure; psychologic stress; sensory deficit; sensory overload.

NURSING DIAGNOSIS: Social isolation: Aloneness experienced by an individual and perceived as a negative or threatened state imposed by others

Defining Characteristics

Major

- Expressed feelings of rejection or of aloneness imposed by others
- Absence of supportive others (family, friends)
- Inability to meet expectations of others
- Uncommunicative, withdrawn, lack of eye contact
- Inappropriate or immature interests/activities for developmental age/stage

Minor

- Expressed anger, feelings of indifference from others, or feelings of insecurity in public
- Preoccupation with own thoughts
- Shows behavior unaccepted by dominant cultural group
- Repetitive, meaningless actions
- Projection of hostility in voice, behavior
- Desire to be alone, existence in subculture

Related Factors

Absence of satisfying personal relationships; delay in accomplishing developmental tasks; immature interests; impaired mobility; body image disturbance; chemical dependence; psychologic impairment; medical condition or treatment-imposed isolation; alterations in physical appearance, mental status, life-style, or state of wellness; inadequate or community resources and/or unaccepted social values.

Sources: LJ Carpenito, *Nursing Diagnosis: Application to Clinical Practice*, 4th ed. (Philadelphia: Lippincott, 1992), pp. 407–10, 695–97, 731–32, 763–64; MJ Kim, GK McFarland, and AM McLane, *Pocket Guide to Nursing Diagnosis*, 5th ed. (St Louis: Mosby, 1993), pp. 195–97, 302–3, 325–27, 336–37; JR Lederer, GL Marculescu, B Mocnik, and N Seaby, *Care Planning Pocket Guide: A Nursing Diagnosis Approach*, 5th ed. (Redwood City, CA: Addison-Wesley Nursing, 1993), pp. 94–95, 176–77, 194–97, 211–13; North American Nursing Diagnosis Association, *NANDA Nursing Diagnoses: Definitions and Classification 1992–1993* (Philadelphia: NANDA, 1992), pp. 37, 57–58, 67–68, 70; and JM Wilkinson, *Nursing Process in Action: A Critical Thinking Approach* (Redwood City, CA: Addison-Wesley Nursing, 1992), pp. 353–54, 365–69.

Table 42–1 Clinical Application: Assessment Data Clusters and Related Nursing Diagnoses for Clients with Sensory/Perceptual Alterations

Data Cluster	Nursing Diagnosis
Ralph Roberts, a 93-year-old widower, lives alone in his condominium. He can hear clearly spoken words close to the left ear but cannot hear any sounds with the right ear. He says he spends his time listening to the TV and radio (set at loud volumes). He tends to speak loudly and shout when talking with others, and he nods and smiles when others speak. His daughter, who visits, says he refuses to wear a hearing aid (he says, "It increases all the background sounds and doesn't help"). She has noticed recently that he has become withdrawn, appears absorbed in his own thoughts, and talks and laughs to himself.	**Social isolation** related to declining auditory function associated with aging
Tony Brown, a 52-year-old lawyer, has multiple sclerosis. Muscle strength in hands, arms, and legs has declined over the past 2 years. He uses a three-wheeled motorized wheelchair to move about. Reports loss of sensation in lower limbs and inability to discern temperature differences. Wife assists with bathing/grooming hygiene care.	**High risk for injury** related to decreased tactile sensation secondary to neurologic impairment

- **High risk for injury** related to sensory/perceptual alterations (specify). For example:
  a. Visual impairment (eg, decreased depth perception)
  b. Reduced tactile sensation secondary to neurologic or circulatory alterations
  c. Decreased sense of smell
  d. Decreased kinesthetic sense
- **Impaired home maintenance management** related to sensory/perceptual alterations (declining visual abilities)
- **High risk for impaired skin integrity** related to sensory/perceptual alterations (reduced tactile sensation)
- **Impaired verbal communication** related to sensory/perceptual alterations (specify). For example:
  a. Altered level of consciousness
  b. Hearing impairment
  c. Sensory overload
  d. Sensory deprivation
- **Self-care deficit: bathing/hygiene** related to sensory/perceptual alterations (specify). For example:
  a. Visual impairment
  b. Diminished kinesthetic sense
- **Social isolation** related to sensory/perceptual alterations (specify). For example:
  a. Impaired vision
  b. Impaired hearing

Examples of nursing diagnoses for which **Altered thought processes** is the etiology include the following:

- **High risk for injury (eg, falls, burns)** related to altered thought processes (eg, confusion, decreased alertness)
- **Impaired home maintenance management** related to altered thought processes (eg, memory loss)

Gordon (1993, pp. 233–35) categorizes sensory/perceptual alterations as follows:

- **Sensory/perceptual alteration: input deficit or sensory deprivation,** defined as "reduced environmental and social stimuli relative to habitual (or basic orienting) level"
- **Sensory/perceptual alteration: input excess or sensory overload,** defined as "environmental stimuli greater than habitual level of input and/or monotonous environmental stimuli."

Defining characteristics and etiologies for these diagnoses are provided on page 1280.

PLANNING

Overall client outcomes for persons with sensory/perceptual or cognitive alterations include (a) maintaining or promoting the function of existing senses, (b) decreasing or eliminating signs of altered function, (c) preventing injury, (d) maintaining or improving communication, (e) maintaining or restoring ability to function in the environment safely, and (f) achieving self-care. The client's nursing diagnoses determine which outcomes are appropriate. Specific outcome criteria must be written to guide evaluation of client progress. Examples of outcome criteria, along with nursing interventions to achieve the outcomes, are shown in the Care Planning Guide on page 1282.

A critical pathway can also be useful for planning client care (see p. 1287).

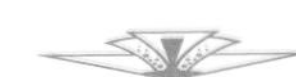

IMPLEMENTING

Nurses can take a number of actions to prevent or modify sensory deprivation, sensory overload, and sensory deficits.

Text continued on page 1284

CARE PLANNING GUIDE

CLIENTS WITH SENSORY/PERCEPTUAL AND COGNITIVE PROBLEMS

NURSING DIAGNOSIS: Sensory/perceptual alterations

Outcome Criteria	Nursing Interventions	Rationale
The client:		
▪ Remains free of injury.	Identify and implement appropriate safety precautions: side rails up, bed wheels locked, call bell and assistive devices within reach. See also the Care Planning Guide: High Risk for Injury on page 714.	Appropriate safety precautions prevent potential accident hazards.
▪ Demonstrates improved orientation to time, place, person, and situation.	With each interaction, orient the client to time, place, person, and situation (see the box on page 1286).	Providing frequent information helps allay confusion and anxiety.
	Acknowledge the client's limitations as indicated.	Acknowledging the client's frustration can communicate understanding and acceptance.
▪ Demonstrates decreased signs/symptoms of *sensory overload*, as evidenced by a. A 3- to 4-hour uninterrupted sleep period in 24 hours. b. Orientation to time, place, and person. c. Reports of increased energy and reduced feelings of anxiety.	Reduce the number of environmental stimuli to achieve appropriate sensory input (see the box on page 1284). Assess orientation to time, place, and person. Ask the client about feelings of fatigue or anxiety and satisfaction with sleep.	Reducing environmental stimuli helps decrease sensory overload and allows the client to focus on sensory input that can be cognitively handled. Clients in institutions are bombarded with unfamiliar, sometimes unpleasant, sensations that exceed their cognitive capabilities to handle.
or		
▪ Demonstrates decreased signs/symptoms of *sensory deprivation*, as evidenced by a. Orientation to time, place, person, and situation. b. Reports of decreased boredom and depression. c. Increased attention span. d. Appropriate emotional responses.	Increase the number of environmental stimuli to achieve appropriate sensory input. See the box on page 1284.	Increasing environmental stimuli helps counteract sensory deprivation. The client's usual, familiar stimuli are missing from the hospital environment.
	Assess orientation to time, place, person, and situation.	Disorientation and confusion may occur with sensory deprivation.
	Observe the client's response to questions, stimuli, and events. Actively listen to the client.	Observation of client response helps the nurse evaluate the client's progress toward outcome achievement.
▪ Uses appropriate assistive devices/methods and maximizes use of unimpaired senses to compensate for sensory deficits.	Ensure access to and use of assistive devices such as hearing aid, glasses.	Assistive devices must be within reach of the client.
	Promote the use and function of existing senses. See page 1285.	Using existing senses prevents sensory alterations.
▪ Expresses thoughts and feelings about sensory deficits or unusual sensory experiences.	Listen; use a calm, patient, reassuring approach; give prompt replies.	Active, helpful listening can minimize the client's frustration.
	Ask family members to help interpret the client's communication as necessary.	Family members are familiar with the client's usual communication patterns and can often interpret more accurately.
	Provide meaningful communication, for example, through touch, one-way conversation, use of paper or pencil, or other method as indicated.	

Outcome Criteria	Nursing Interventions	Rationale
▪ Identifies community support services.	Provide information about social services, occupational therapy, and other appropriate agencies (eg, senior centers and church groups).	Information may be needed for problem solving, home maintenance management, or stimulation.

NURSING DIAGNOSIS: Social isolation

Outcome Criteria	Nursing Interventions	Rationale
The client:		
▪ Identifies factors/behaviors that produce social isolation.	Discuss with the client possible reasons for feelings of social isolation.	Identifying causes enables the nurse and client to focus on relevant interventions.
	Actively listen to the client.	Active listening facilitates expression of thoughts and feelings.
▪ Formulates a plan to become more involved with others and reduce social isolation.	Encourage involvement in existing relationships; reinforce efforts by the client and significant others to establish interactions.	Companionship is essential for physical and emotional well-being. Significant others help the client try out new methods of communication and decrease feelings of isolation.
	Suggest that the client form relationships with those who have common interests and goals.	Common interests and goals provide a basis on which to build a relationship.
	Encourage patience in developing relationships.	So that client does not become discouraged.
	Help the client become aware of strengths and limitations in communicating with others.	This knowledge enables the client to make use of strengths and work on limitations if realistic.
	Encourage the sharing of common problems and honesty in presenting self to others.	Failure to share self honestly may be a barrier in forming relationships.
	Give positive feedback when the client reaches out to others.	The nurse should encourage the client to make the effort, especially if the client perceives interactions as risky.
	Help the client distinguish reality from perceptions.	Past isolation may have contributed to inability to interpret situations clearly.
	Schedule time to interact with the client.	Interacting with the client provides support and stimulation. The client may regard the nurse as a safe person with whom to communicate and interact.
▪ Identifies community resources that will assist in decreasing social isolation.	Discuss possibility of becoming involved in social and community activities. Provide information on community resources.	Becoming involved in these activities can offer a less personal, perhaps less threatening way to create a support system.
	Explore with the client the possibility of becoming involved in new interests and/or changing environment.	These discussions may provide stimulation and incentive to work on developing new relationships.

Nursing Interventions for Clients with Sensory Deprivation

- Encourage the client to use aids such as eyeglasses and hearing aids.
- Address the client by name, and touch the client while speaking if this is not culturally offensive.
- Communicate frequently with the client, and maintain meaningful interactions (eg, discuss current events).
- Provide a radio and/or TV, clock, and calendar.
- Adjust the environment to provide meaningful stimulation (eg, enable the client to look through a window).
- Encourage social interaction.

Sensory Deprivation

Interventions for the understimulated client should address the etiology of the deprivation, such as inadequate stimuli, inability to receive stimuli, or inability to process stimuli.

Inadequate Stimuli Providing the client with a variety of stimuli appropriate for that person is important; for example, newspapers, books, and television can stimulate the visual and auditory senses. Providing objects that are pleasant to touch, such as a pet to stroke, can provide tactile and interactive stimulation. Clocks that differentiate night from day by color can help orient a client to time.

For the client who is inadequately stimulated, the nurse can arrange for people to visit and talk with the client regularly. Many church and community groups provide visitors to "shut-ins," that is, people who are confined to their homes or who reside in nursing homes.

Inability to Receive Stimuli For the client who cannot receive all stimuli, such as a client who is blind, the nurse should make extra effort to provide stimuli for the other senses, for example, touch, hearing, and taste. See the discussion of sensory deficits later in this chapter.

Inability to Process Stimuli For clients who cannot process stimuli, the nurse can provide suitable explanations and perhaps written notes to help them know what to expect. For example, the man who cannot remember to take his pills may be able to take them at the right time from a pill compartment that is labeled with the date and time. See the box at the top of this column for nursing interventions for clients with sensory deprivation.

Nursing Interventions to Reduce Sensory Overload

- Minimize unnecessary light, noise, and distraction.
- Control pain as indicated.
- Describe any tests and procedures to the client beforehand.
- Plan care to allow for uninterrupted periods for rest or sleep.
- Support accurate perceptions.
- Provide orienting cues, such as clocks, calendars, equipment, and furniture in the room.
- Introduce self by name and address the client by name.
- Provide new information gradually.
- Speak in a low tone of voice and in an unhurried manner.
- Provide a private room.
- Limit visitors.
- Take time to discuss the client's problems and correct misinterpretations.
- Assist the client with stress-reducing techniques.
- When providing information, ask the client to repeat it so that there are no misunderstandings.

Sensory Overload

For clients who are at risk of overstimulation, nurses should reduce the number and type of environmental stimuli. The nurse can counteract sensory overload by blocking stimuli and by helping the client organize the stimuli and alter responses to the stimuli.

Dark glasses can partially block light rays, and a window shade or drape can reduce visual stimulation. Ear plugs reduce auditory stimuli, as do soft background music and earphones. The odor from a draining wound can be minimized by keeping the dressing dry and clean and applying a liquid deodorant on a gauze near the wound.

Another method of blocking stimuli is to reduce novelty and surprise and provide rest intervals free of interruptions. Sometimes the number of visitors and the length of visits must be restricted. If the nurse carries out several nursing measures together, the client can have a scheduled quiet period before the next activity.

By explaining sounds in the environment, the nurse can help the client organize them mentally: A bell signals a change of shift; a buzzer, a change of IV. When clients understand their meaning, stimuli are frequently less con-

SUPPORTING VISUAL FUNCTION

Strengthening Visual Stimuli

- Arrange for suitable lighting, including night lights.
- Obtain reading material with large print.
- Obtain a magnifying glass and a phone dialer and wrist watch with large numbers.
- Use two side mirrors on a car to increase the visual field.
- Use contrasting colors to highlight material to be seen.
- Use colored rims on dishes.
- Color-code dials on stoves, washer, and so on.
- Provide the client with eyeglasses of the correct prescription.

Increasing Use of Other Senses

- Provide materials that can be identified by other senses, that is, materials of various textures and odors.
- Point out odors, shapes, and so on.
- Encourage handling of articles.
- Announce who you are when entering the room of a visually impaired person.

Establishing a Meaningful Environment

- Minimize glare by using soft, diffuse lighting.
- Use sunglasses and shades on windows.
- Keep furniture in its usual places.

CLINICAL GUIDELINES

Caring for the Hearing Impaired

- Talk at a moderate rate and in a normal tone of voice. Shouting does not make your voice more distinct and, in some instances, makes understanding more difficult.
- Address the person directly. Do not turn away in the middle of a remark or story. Make sure the person can see your face easily and that it is well lighted.
- Avoid talking when you have something in your mouth, such as a pipe, cigar, cigarette, or chewing gum. Avoid covering your mouth with your hand.
- Keep your voice at about the same volume throughout each sentence, without dropping the voice at the end of each sentence.
- Always speak as clearly and accurately as possible. Articulate consonants with particular care.
- Do not "overarticulate"; mouthing or overdoing articulation is just as troublesome as mumbling.
- Use longer phrases, which tend to be easier to understand than short ones. For example, "Will you get me a drink of water?" presents much less difficulty than "Will you get me a drink?" Word choice is important here: "Fifteen cents" and "fifty cents" may be confused, but "half a dollar" is clear.
- Pronounce every name with care. Make a reference to the name for easier understanding, for example, "Joan, the girl from the office" or "Sears, the big downtown store."
- Change to a new subject at a slower rate, making sure that the person follows the change to the new subject. A key word or two at the beginning of a new topic is a good indicator.

fusing and more easily ignored. People can also learn to alter their responses to the stimuli. Clients can employ relaxation techniques to reduce anxiety and stress despite continual sensory stimulation. See Chapter 32 for additional information. See the box on page 1284 for nursing measures for clients with sensory overload.

SENSORY DEFICITS

Vision Because visual problems are commonly due to refractive errors, children and adults may need encouragement to undergo visual screening. To promote existing visual function, the nurse can teach the client to strengthen visual stimuli, use other senses to supplement sight, and establish a meaningful environment. See the box above.

Hearing The following measures can help maximize a person's residual hearing:

- Encouraging the client to have a hearing test
- Obtaining a telephone with an amplified ring and speaker
- Maintaining a hearing aid in good order
- Reducing background noise
- Keeping conversational groups small

The nurse communicates appropriately to the hearing-impaired client to convey respect, enhance the person's self-esteem, and ensure the exchange of correct information. The hearing-impaired person has to concentrate more than the unimpaired person and therefore tires more readily. Fatigue compounded by an illness can seriously alter the person's ability to hear. See the box above for guidelines of care for the hearing impaired.

PROMOTING ORIENTATION TO TIME, PLACE, PERSON, AND SITUATION

- Wear a readable name tag.
- Address the person by name and introduce yourself frequently: "Good morning Mr. Richards. I am Betty Brown. I will be your nurse today."
- Identify time and place as indicated: "Today is December 5, and it is 8:00 in the morning."
- Ask the client, "Where are you?" and orient the client to place (eg, nursing home) if indicated.
- Place a calendar and clock in the client's room. Mark holidays with ribbons, pins, or other means.
- Speak clearly and calmly to the client, allowing time for your words to be processed and for the client to give a response.
- Provide frequent face-to-face contact.
- Provide clear, concise explanations of each treatment procedure or task.
- Reinforce reality by interpreting unfamiliar sounds, sights, and smells; clarify misconceptions of events or situations.
- Schedule activities (eg, meals, bath, activity/rest periods, treatments) at the same time each day to provide a sense of security. If possible, assign the same caregivers.
- Keep familiar items in the client's environment (eg, photographs), and keep the environment uncluttered. A disorganized, cluttered environment increases confusion.
- Encourage the client to wear familiar or personal clothing and to arrange personal hygiene articles in order of use as needed.
- Encourage participation in familiar activities/hobbies to emphasize the client's strengths rather than problems.
- Tell the client when you are leaving and when you will return.

Taste Maintaining good oral hygiene and hydration enhances the sense of taste. Foods need to be well seasoned, hot foods served hot, and cold foods served cold. Foods should also provide a variety of textures and be eaten separately. The nurse can experiment with different tastes to find the ones the client likes best.

Smell Nurses can encourage clients to use the sense of smell. The aroma of fragrant flowers or cologne can make the environment more attractive. Nurses can eliminate unpleasant odors by ensuring adequate ventilation and by removing soiled dressings and equipment. Nurses and support persons can assist the client by refraining from wearing heavy perfumes. Encourage clients to remember pleasant or familiar odors, such as freshly brewed coffee and the perfume of sweet peas.

Touch Clients with an impaired sense of touch must take protective measures to prevent injury. They may not be aware of hot temperatures, which can cause burns, or pressure on bony prominences, which can produce pressure ulcers. Nurses can also provide the client with a variety of textures to enhance the remaining tactile sense. It is important to respect the client's desire to be touched or not touched.

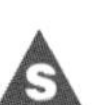

THE CONFUSED CLIENT

There are certain predictors of a client developing a state of confusion. If these predictors are identified early, the confusion can in many instances be prevented. Confusion is most often seen in elderly people who are suddenly removed from their homes and taken to hospitals for therapy, such as an elderly woman who fractures her femur and is admitted for a fracture repair. The following are some of the predictors of a state of confusion (Wolanin & Holloway 1980):

- Loss of sense of self (depersonalization)
- Loss of continuity of life
- Distortion of time and space cues (as occurs with hospitalization)
- Loss of control over events affecting self
- Immobilization
- Physiologic problems, such as hypoxia and dehydration, which can interfere with cerebral blood supply
- Physiologic reaction to certain medications

Often, clients who are confused know something is wrong and want help. See the accompanying box for nursing interventions to help orient the confused person to time, place, person, and situation.

THE UNCONSCIOUS CLIENT

The person who is unconscious and unable to respond to the spoken word nevertheless can often hear what is spoken. It is therefore important that nurses talk to the client as though they were understood, using a normal tone of voice and speaking before touching the client. Nurses should also try to keep the environmental noises at a minimum so that the client can focus on words. The following are some additional measures nurses can take in caring for the unconscious client:

- Orient the unconscious client to self, time, and place.
- Listen carefully to the support person's concerns. Often they simply want to express them.
- Maintain the same schedule each day. Routine gives the client a sense of security.
- Touch and stroke the unconscious client.
- To the support persons, explain what is happening, and encourage them to talk to and touch the client as though the client were conscious. This auditory and tactile stimulation supports the client and may restore some degree of consciousness.
- Always address the client by name, and explain beforehand the care to be provided. Unconscious clients require bathing, skin care, turning, feeding, and assistance with elimination needs.

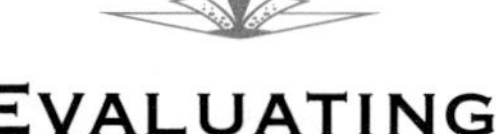

EVALUATING

Evaluative activities depend on the outcome criteria set in the planning phase. For example, if the outcome is for the client to remain free of injury, the nurse simply asks or observes the client for verification of this. If the outcomeis for the client to maintain a usual communication pattern, the nurse may need to determine whether the client responds to questions appropriately and initiates conversation with others.

If outcomes are not achieved, the nurse should explore the reasons, considering questions such as the following:

- Were nursing diagnoses and contributing or risk factors identified correctly?
- Were appropriate measures implemented to *stimulate* the client's functioning senses and prevent sensory deprivation or social isolation?

or

- Were all measures to *reduce* stimuli considered and provided?
- Were adaptive aids for hearing functioning properly?
- Were alternative communication methods appropriate?
- What other adaptive aids can be considered?
- Were arrangements for people to visit and talk with the client fulfilled?
- Were needs for home care assistance and available community resources correctly identified or selected?
- Were routines and activities structured as much as possible to prevent confusion and promote rest?

CRITICAL PATHWAY FOR JULIA GRABOWSKI

ASSESSMENT DATA

Nursing Assessment

Mrs Julia Grabowski, an 80-year-old widow, is admitted to ambulatory surgery for removal of a cataract in her right eye. She has also has been experiencing some problems with her hearing, but refuses to purchase hearing aids. She has reportedly told her family, "They are too expensive." Mrs Grabowski lives alone in her home and cares for herself independently. Her children, who live nearby, check on her daily.

Physical Examination

Height: 160 cm (5′3″)
Weight: 55.3 kg (122 lb)
Temperature: 37 C (98.6 F)
Pulse rate: 72 bpm
Respirations: 18 per minute
Blood pressure: 128/74 mm Hg
Rinne test: negative

Diagnostic Data

CBC: negative
Urine: negative

➤

CRITICAL PATHWAY FOR CLIENT FOLLOWING CATARACT SURGERY

Expected length of stay less than 6 hours

	Date ________ **Preoperative day**	**Date ________** **By discharge**
Daily outcomes	Client ▪ is prepared for eye surgery including instillation of eye drops, presurgical scrub, NPO per order, IV infusion, and empty bladder. ▪ verbalizes ability to cope with fear and anxiety regarding surgery and potential loss of vision. ▪ verbalizes understanding of preoperative teaching including preoperative routine, intraoperative experience, and postoperative care. ▪ remains oriented to time, place, person, and situation. ▪ demonstrates the ability to compensate for sensory deficits.	Client ▪ is afebrile. ▪ is independent in self-care. ▪ is fully ambulatory. ▪ has resumed preadmission urine elimination pattern. ▪ verbalizes/demonstrates home care instruction including (1) signs and symptoms of infection and hemorrhage, (2) instillation of eye drops, (3) avoiding activities that increase intraocular pressure, (4) maintaining eye shield, (5) aseptic technique when caring for eyes, and (6) follow-up care. ▪ verbalizes control of pain with oral analgesics or nonpharmacologic pain relief measures such as relaxation techniques. ▪ tolerates usual diet. ▪ verbalizes ability to cope with ongoing stressors. ▪ demonstrates the ability to compensate for sensory deficits.
Tests and treatments	CBC. Urinalysis. Baseline physical assessment with a focus on mental status and sensory-perceptual needs. Anesthesia consult. Assess use of anticoagulants, aspirin, or nonsteroidal anti-inflammatory medications.	Vital signs and O_2 saturation, neurovascular assessment, dressing q15min × 4; q30min × 4; q1h × 4; and then q4h if stable. Monitor for complaints of sudden pain in eye accompanied by nausea, diaphoresis, or increased pulse rate and report immediately. Assess voiding—if unable to void, try suggestive voiding techniques or catheterize prn.
Knowledge deficit	Orient to room and surroundings. Provide simple, brief instructions. Review preoperative preparation including hospital and surgical routines. Reinforce preoperative teaching regarding specific postoperative care: lying on the nonoperative side, avoiding bending at the waist, requesting assistance with ambulation.	Reorient to room and postoperative routine. Review plan of care. Complete discharge teaching using standardized teaching sheet and provide client with large print copy.

	Preoperative day *continued*	**By discharge** *continued*
Sensory perceptual	Assess level of consciousness on admission and prn. Use dim lights, limit visitors, and provide rest periods. Introduce self upon entering room. Speak clearly and distinctly facing the client and assess client's understanding. Use large print teaching materials on off-white paper. Minimize extraneous noise.	Assess level of consciousness prn and prior to discharge. Use dim lights, limit visitors, and provide rest periods. Introduce self upon entering room. Speak clearly and distinctly and assess client's understanding. Use large print teaching materials on off-white paper.
Psycho-social	Assess anxiety related to pending surgery. Assess fears of the unknown and surgery. Encourage verbalization of concerns. Provide information regarding surgical experience.	Assess level of anxiety. Encourage verbalization of concerns. Provide information and ongoing support and encouragement.
Diet	NPO. Baseline nutritional assessment.	Offer liquids ad lib, if tolerated advance to usual diet.
Activity	OOB ad lib with assistance until premedicated for surgery. Protect from injury by removing any potential hazards.	Provide safety precautions. Bathroom privileges with assistance after surgery and begin progressive ambulation with assistance to tolerance until fully ambulatory.
Medications	NPO except ordered medications.	PO analgesics. IV fluids until adequate PO intake.
Transfer/ discharge plans	Assess discharge plans and support system. Assist client and family to plan for home care for first 2 weeks following surgery. Encourage family to remove hazards from home environment, such as throw rugs, low furniture, and electrical cords.	Probable discharge within 2 to 6 hours of surgery. Complete discharge home care teaching when fully awake and oriented and before discharge. Include family/significant other in discharge teaching. Provide a written copy of discharge instructions.

CHAPTER HIGHLIGHTS

- The sensory experience consists of two components: sensory reception and sensory perception.
- Sensory stimuli can be either external or internal. Visual, auditory, olfactory, tactile, and gustatory stimuli orient a person to the *external* environment. Kinesthetic and visceral stimuli orient the person to the *internal* environment. Kinesthetic stimuli make the person aware of the position and movement of body parts.
- Sensory perception involves the organization and translation of stimuli into meaningful information. This process occurs in the cerebral cortex.

- In most instances, sensory pathways decussate and register sensations from the opposite side of the body.
- The reticular activating system (RAS), with its many ascending and descending connections to other areas of the brain, monitors and regulates incoming stimuli. The RAS maintains, enhances, or inhibits critical arousal.
- The normal alert person can assimilate many kinds of information at one time and respond appropriately through thought and action.
- Sensory deprivation occurs when a person receives decreased sensory input or monotonous or meaningless sensory input.
- Sensory overload occurs when a person experiences excessive sensory input and is unable to process or manage the stimuli. The person feels overwhelmed and not in control.
- Responses to both sensory deprivation and sensory overload include perceptual changes (eg, mild distortions or hallucinations), cognitive changes (eg, decreased concentration and problem-solving ability), and affective changes (eg, apathy, anxiety, anger, depression, and rapid mood swings).
- Clients at risk for sensory deprivation include (a) those who are homebound or institutionalized, (b) those on bed rest or isolation precautions, (c) those with sensory deficits, (d) those who come from a different culture, (e) those with certain affective disorders or disturbances of the nervous system, and (f) those on certain medications that affect the central nervous system.
- Clients at risk for sensory overload include (a) those in pain, (b) those in critical care settings, (c) those with intrusive and uncomfortable monitoring or treatment equipment, and (d) those with disturbances of the nervous system.
- Factors affecting sensory stimulation include developmental stage, culture, stress, medications, illness, and life-style and personality.
- Assessment for sensory/perceptual alterations includes (a) a nursing history to identify sensory deficits; (b) physical examinations to determine sensory functioning; (c) mental status; (d) adaptations to sensory alterations; (e) immediate environment; (f) presence of clinical signs of sensory deprivation or overload; and (g) self-care ability and safety, and support network.
- NANDA nursing diagnoses related to a client's sensory/perceptual impairments are **Sensory/perceptual alterations: visual, auditory, gustatory, olfactory, tactile, kinesthetic; Altered thought processes; Social isolation; Impaired home maintenance management**; and **High risk for injury.**
- Overall client outcomes for persons with sensory/perceptual or cognitive alterations include (a) maintaining or promoting the function of existing senses, (b) decreasing or eliminating signs of altered function, (c) preventing injury, (d) maintaining or improving communication, (e) maintaining or restoring ability to function in the environment safely, and (f) achieving self-care.
- Interventions to prevent or modify sensory deprivation, sensory overload, and sensory deficits include (a) providing sufficient stimuli (for sensory deprivation); (b) ensuring use of aids, such as hearing aids; (c) reducing stimuli (for sensory overload); (d) communicating appropriately or establishing an adequate means for the client to communicate; (e) ensuring client safety; and (f) providing measures that promote orientation to time, place, person, and situation.

READINGS AND REFERENCES

SUGGESTED READINGS

Chovaz, C. March 1989. Nursing the hearing impaired patient. *Canadian Nurse* 85:34–36.

This article presents a unique perspective on hearing loss. The client in this article is the nurse-author. She describes the meaning of her hearing loss, her reactions to this loss, and the problems she encountered. She also provides three suggestions to help allay the anxiety of the hearing-impaired person.

Hahn, K. February 1989. Think twice about sensory loss. *Nursing89* 19:97–99.

The article describes the meaning of sensory impairment to an elderly female client with both impaired vision requiring cataract surgery and presbycusis. The article provides tips for the use of hearing aids and addresses the implications of taste impairment and touch deprivation.

RELATED RESEARCH

Abraham, IL, Neundorfer, MM, and Currie, LJ. July/August 1992. Effects of group interventions on cognition and depression in nursing home residents. *Nursing Research* 41:196–202.

Stewart, NJ. Fall 1986. Perceptual and behavioral effects of immobility and social isolation in hospitalized orthopedic patients. *Nursing Papers* 18:59–74.

SELECTED REFERENCES

Alberti, PW, Ginsberg, IA, and Goode, RL. February 15, 1988. Managing adult hearing loss. *Patient Care* 22:54–58, 63, 67.

Andresen, GP. July 1992. How to assess the older mind. *RN* 55:34–41.

Bentz, L. September 1987. Caring for and communicating with blind and visually impaired elderly persons. *Journal of Visual Impairment and Blindness* 81:326–27.

Carpenito, LJ. November 1985. Altered thoughts or altered perceptions? *American Journal of Nursing* 85:1283.

______. 1992. *Nursing Diagnosis: Application to Clinical Practice.* 4th ed. Philadelphia: Lippincott.

Chodil, J and Williams, B. September 1970. The concept of sensory deprivation. *Nursing Clinics of North America* 5:544–48.

Daly, MR. November/December 1990. Sensory supports for the visually impaired. *Journal of Ophthalmic Nursing and Technology* 9:243–44.

Downs, FS. March 1974. Bed rest and sensory disturbances. *American Journal of Nursing* 74:434–38.

Foreman, MD. May/June 1990. Complexities of acute confusion. *Geriatric Nursing* 11:136–39.

Gordon, M. 1993. *Manual of Nursing Diagnosis 1993–1994.* 6th ed. St Louis: Mosby-Year Book.

Hahn, K. February 1989. Think twice about sensory loss. *Nursing89* 19:97–99.

Kim, MJ, McFarland, GK, and McLane, AM. 1993. *Pocket Guide to Nursing Diagnoses.* 5th ed. St Louis: Mosby.

Kloosterman, ND. Fall 1991. Cultural care: The missing link in severe sensory alteration. *Nursing Science Quarterly* 4:119–22.

Lederer, JR, Marculescu, GL, Mocnik, B, and Seaby, N. 1993. *Care Planning Pocket Guide—A Nursing Diagnosis Approach.* 5th ed. Redwood City, CA: Addison-Wesley Nursing.

McFarland, GK and McFarlane, EA. 1993. *Nursing Diagnosis and Intervention: Planning for Patient Care.* 2d ed. St Louis: Mosby.

Moore, T. February 6–12, 1991. Making sense of . . . sensory deprivation. *Nursing Times* 87:36–38.

Murphy, K. February 1987. Problems of impaired hearing. *Geriatric Nursing and Home Care* 7:9–11.

North American Nursing Diagnosis Association. 1992. *NANDA Nursing Diagnoses: Definitions and Classification 1992–1993.* Philadelphia: NANDA.

Pace, K and Emerich, M. June 1990. Keeping track of confused patients. *Nursing90* 20:64.

Perron, DM. June 1974. Deprived of sound. *American Journal of Nursing* 74:1057–59.

Ravish, T. October 1985. Prevent social isolation before it starts. *Journal of Gerontological Nursing* 11:10–13.

Sullivan, N. April 1983. Vision in the elderly. Declining visual function in old age. Parts 1 and 2. *Journal of Gerontological Nursing* 9:228–35.

Taylor, KS. March/April 1993. Geriatric hearing loss: Management strategies for nurses. *Geriatric Nursing* 14:74–76.

Wolanin, MO and Holloway, J. 1980. Relocation confusion: Intervention for prevention. In Burnside, IM, editor. 1980. *Psychosocial Aspects of Nursing.* 2d ed. New York: McGraw-Hill.

UNIT

11

Implementing Special Nursing Measures

STUDENT PROFILE

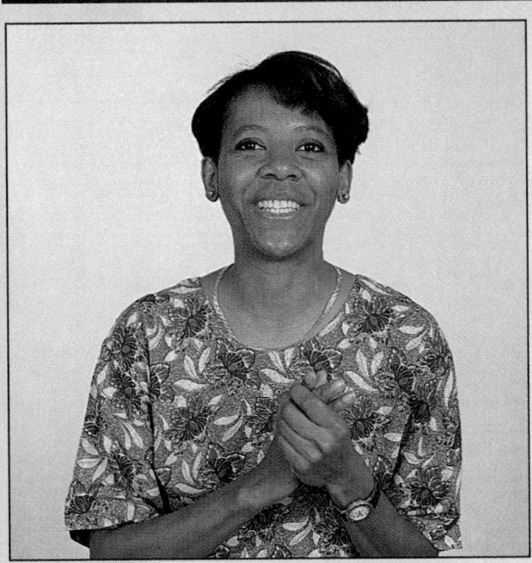

Name	Merilyn Francis
School of Nursing	University of District of Columbia
Hometown	Washington, District of Columbia

Why did you enter the field of nursing?
I've been in the field of clinical research and I became interested in doing my own clinical research.

Why do you think this is a good time to be in nursing?
I want diversity in my career, the chance to do things differently. There is greater flexibility in today's nursing roles. There is more opportunity to do things outside of the hospital and to deliver quality care.

What qualities do you think are necessary to be a good nurse?
Organization, empathy, open-mindedness, flexibility, and creativity.

What has been your most gratifying moment as a student nurse?
I worked with a patient who was 97 years old; he was anxious to get well so he could go home to be with this wife of 75 years. I taught him how to do things for himself to the extent that he was able to live at home.

What advice would you give a new student?
Study hard and take each situation (especially the rough times) as a learning experience.

43 Medications

Objectives

Define selected terms related to the administration of medications.

Describe legal aspects of administering drugs.

Identify physiologic factors and individual variables affecting drug action.

Describe various routes of drug administration.

Identify essential parts of a drug order.

Give examples of various types of medication orders.

Recognize abbreviations commonly used in medication orders.

List five essential steps to follow when administering drugs.

Describe physiologic changes in elderly persons that alter drug administration and effectiveness.

Outline steps required to administer oral medications safely.

Identify equipment required for parenteral medications.

Describe how to mix selected drugs from vials and ampules.

Identify sites used for subcutaneous, intramuscular, and intradermal injections.

Describe essential steps for safely administering parenteral medications by intradermal, subcutaneous, intramuscular, and intravenous routes.

Describe essential steps in safely administering topical medications: dermatologic, ophthalmic, otic, nasal, vaginal, and rectal preparations.

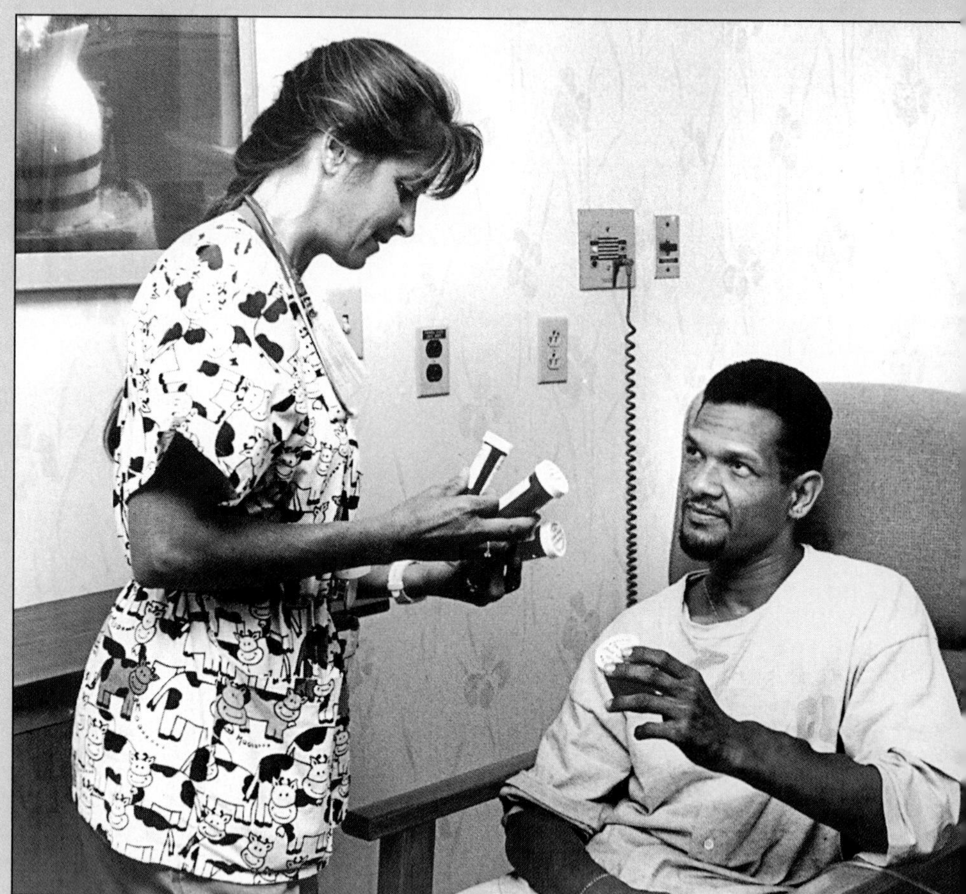

A **medication** is a substance administered for the diagnosis, cure, treatment, mitigation (relief), or prevention of disease. In the health care context, the words *medication* and *drug* are generally used interchangeably. The term **drug** also has the connotation of an illicitly obtained substance such as heroin, cocaine, or amphetamines. Medications have been known and used since antiquity. Crude drugs, such as opium, castor oil, and vinegar, were used in ancient times. Over the centuries the number of drugs available has increased greatly, and knowledge about these drugs has become correspondingly more accurate and detailed.

In the United States and Canada, medications are usually dispensed on the order of physicians and dentists. In some US states, specially qualified nurse-practitioners and physicians' assistants may prescribe drugs. The written direction for the preparation and administration of a drug is called a **prescription.** One drug can have as many as four kinds of names: its generic name, official name, chemical name, and trademark or brand name. The **generic name** is given before a drug becomes official. The **official name** is the name under which it is listed in one of the official publications (eg, the *United States Pharmacopeia*). The **chemical name** is the name by which a chemist knows it; this name describes the constituents of the drug precisely. The **trademark,** or **brand name,** is the name given by the drug manufacturer. Because one drug may be manufactured by several companies, it can have several trade names; for example, the drug hydrochlorothiazide (official name) is known by the trade names Esidrix and Hydro-Diuril. Medications are often available in a variety of forms. Common types of drug preparations are described in Table 43–1 on page 1296.

Pharmacology is the study of the effect of drugs on living organisms. Drugs are prepared by a **pharmacist,** a person licensed to prepare and dispense drugs and to make up prescriptions. A **clinical pharmicist** is a specialist who often guides the physician in prescribing drugs. A **pharmacy assistant** is a member of the health team who in some states administers drugs to clients. **Pharmacy** is the art of preparing, compounding, and dispensing drugs. The word also refers to the place where drugs are prepared and dispensed.

Drug Standards

Drugs may have natural (eg, plant, mineral, and animal) sources, or they may be synthesized in the laboratory. For example, digitalis and opium are plant derived, iron and sodium chloride are minerals, insulin and vaccines have animal or human sources, and the sulfonamides and propoxyphene hydrochloride (the analgesic Darvon) are the products of laboratory synthesis. Early drugs were derived from the three natural sources only. During the past 45 years, however, more and more drugs have been produced synthetically.

Drugs vary in strength and activity. Drugs derived from plants, for example, vary in strength according to the age of the plant, the variety, the place in which it is grown, and the method by which it is preserved. Drugs must be pure and of uniform strength if drug dosages are to be predictable in their effect. Drug standards have therefore been developed to ensure uniform quality. In the United States, official drugs are those so designated by the Federal Food, Drug, and Cosmetic Act. These drugs are officially listed in the *United States Pharmacopeia (USP)* and described according to their source, physical and chemical properties, tests for purity and identity, method of storage, assay, category, and normal dosages. In Canada, the *British Pharmacopoeia* is used for the same purpose, although some drugs used in Canada conform to the *USP* because they are obtained from the United States.

A **pharmacopoeia** is a book containing a list of products used in medicine, with descriptions of the product, chemical tests for determining identity and purity, and formulas for certain mixtures. A **formulary** is a collection of formulas and prescriptions. The United States' *National Formulary* lists drugs and their therapeutic value and can include drugs that may still be used but not listed in the *USP.* The *Canadian Formulary* lists drugs used extensively in Canada but not necessarily listed in the *British Pharmacopoeia.*

Pharmacopoeias and formularies are invaluable reference sources for nurses and nursing students. Nurses not only administer thousands of medications but also are responsible for assessing their effectiveness and recognizing unfavorable reactions to drugs. Since it is impossible to commit to memory all pertinent information about a very large number of drugs, nurses must have a reliable reference readily available.

Legal Aspects of Drug Administration

The administration of drugs in both the United States and Canada is controlled by law. In the United States the major federal acts controlling drugs are the Food, Drug, and Cosmetic Act (1938), its amendments, and the

Table 43–1 Types of Drug Preparations

Type	Description
Aqueous solution	One or more drugs dissolved in water
Aerosol spray or foam	A liquid, powder, or foam deposited in a thin layer on the skin by air pressure
Aqueous suspension	One or more drugs finely divided in a liquid such as water
Capsule	A gelatinous container to hold a drug in powder, liquid, or oil form
Cream	A nongreasy, semisolid preparation used on the skin
Elixir	A sweetened and aromatic solution of alcohol used as a vehicle for medicinal agents
Extract	A concentrated form of a drug made from vegetables or animals
Fluid extract	An alcoholic solution of a drug from a vegetable source; the most concentrated of all fluid preparations
Gel or jelly	A clear or translucent semisolid that liquefies when applied to the skin
Liniment	An oily liquid used on the skin
Lotion	An emollient liquid that may be a clear solution, suspension, or emulsion used on the skin
Lozenge (troche)	A flat, round, or oval preparation that dissolves and releases a drug when held in the mouth
Ointment	A semisolid preparation of one or more drugs used for application to the skin and mucous membrane
Paste	A preparation like an ointment, but thicker and stiffer, that penetrates the skin less than an ointment
Pill	One or more drugs mixed with a cohesive material, in oval, round, or flattened shapes
Powder	A finely ground drug or drugs; some are used internally, other externally
Spirit	A concentrated alcoholic solution of a volatile substance
Suppository	One or several drugs mixed with a firm base such as gelatin and shaped for insertion into the body; the base dissolves gradually at body temperature, releasing the drug
Syrup	An aqueous solution of sugar often used to disguise unpleasant-tasting drugs
Tablet	A powdered drug compressed into a hard small disc; some are readily broken along a scored line; others are enteric-coated to prevent them from dissolving in the stomach
Tincture	An alcoholic or water-and-alcohol solution prepared from drugs derived from plants
Transdermal patch	A semipermeable membrane shaped in the form of a disk or patch that contains a drug to be absorbed through the skin over a lengthy period of time

Comprehensive Drug Abuse Prevention and Control Act (1970) (Controlled Substances Act). In Canada, three federal acts control drugs: The Food and Drugs Act (1953), the Proprietary or Patent Medicine Act (1908), and the Narcotics Control Act (1961). See Table 43–2 for a summary of US drug legislation. Table 43–3 provides a summary of Canadian drug legislation.

Nurses need to (a) know how nursing practice acts in their areas define and limit their functions and (b) be able to recognize the limits of their own knowledge and skill. To function beyond the limits of nursing practice acts or one's ability is to endanger clients' lives and leave oneself open to malpractice suits. Under the law, nurses are responsible for their own actions regardless of whether there is a written order. If a physician writes an incorrect order (eg, Demerol 500 mg instead of Demerol 50 mg), a nurse who administers the written incorrect dosage is responsible for the error. Therefore, nurses should question any order that appears unreasonable and refuse to give the medication until the order is clarified.

Another aspect of nursing practice governed by law is the use of controlled substances. In hospitals, controlled substances are kept in a locked drawer, cupboard, medication cart, or computer-controlled dispensing system. Agencies have special forms for recording the use of controlled substances. The information required usually includes the name of the client, the date and time of administration, the name of the drug, the dosage, and the

Table 43–2 United States Drug Legislation

Legislation	Content
Food, Drug, and Cosmetic Act (1938)	Implemented by Food and Drug Administration (FDA); requires that labels be accurate and that all drugs be tested for harmful effects.
Durkham-Humphrey Amendment (1952)	Differentiates clearly drugs that can be sold only with a prescription, those that can be sold without a prescription, and those that should not be refilled without a new prescription.
Kefauver-Harris Amendment (1962)	Requires proof of safety and efficacy of a drug for approval.
Comprehensive Drug Abuse Prevention and Control Act (1970) (Controlled Substances Act)	Categorizes controlled substances and limits how often a prescription can be filled; established government-funded programs to prevent and treat drug dependence.

Table 43–3 Canadian Drug Legislation

Legislation	Content
Proprietary or Patent Medicine Act (1908)	Protects the public against unsafe and ineffective over-the-counter drugs.
Canada Food and Drugs Act (1953)	Prohibits advertising any food, drug, cosmetic, or device as a cure for certain specified diseases. Prohibits the sale of certain drugs unless approved by the federal government.
Canadian Narcotic Control Act (1961)	Allows only authorized people to possess narcotics. Specifies records about narcotics that must be kept.

signature of the person who prepared and gave the drug. The name of the physician who ordered the drug may also be part of the record.

Included on the record are the controlled substances wasted during preparation. In most agencies, counts of controlled substances are taken at the end of each shift. The count total should tally with the total at the end of the last shift minus the number used. If the totals do not tally, the discrepancy must be reported immediately. In facilities that use a computerized dispensing system, manual counts are not required, because the dispensing system runs a continuous count.

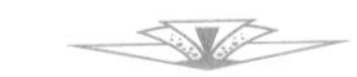

EFFECTS OF DRUGS

The **therapeutic effect** of a drug, also referred to as the *desired effect*, is the primary effect intended, that is, the reason the drug is prescribed. For example, the therapeutic effect of morphine sulphate is analgesia, and the therapeutic effect of diazepam is relief of anxiety. See Table 43–4 on page 1298 for kinds of therapeutic actions.

A **side effect,** or secondary effect, of a drug is one that is unintended. Side effects are usually predictable and may be either harmless or potentially harmful. For example, digitalis increases the strength of myocardial contractions (desired effect), but it can have the side effect of inducing nausea and vomiting. Some side effects are tolerated for the drug's therapeutic effect; hazardous side effects justify the discontinuation of a drug.

Drug toxicity (deleterious effects of a drug on an organism or tissue) results from overdosage, ingestion of a drug intended for external use, and buildup of the drug in the blood because of impaired metabolism or excretion (cumulative effect). Some toxic effects are apparent immediately; some are not apparent for weeks or months. Fortunately, most drug toxicity is avoidable if careful attention is paid to dosage and monitoring for toxicity. An example of a toxic effect is respiratory depression due to the cumulative effect of morphine sulfate in the body.

A **drug allergy** is an immunologic reaction to a drug. When a client is first exposed to a foreign substance (antigen), the body may react by producing antibodies. A client can react to a drug as to an antigen and thus develop symptoms of an allergic reaction.

Allergic reactions can be either mild or severe. A mild reaction has a variety of symptoms, from skin rashes to diarrhea. See Table 43–5 on page 1298. An allergic reaction can occur anytime from a few minutes to 2 weeks after the administration of the drug. A severe allergic reaction usually occurs immediately after the administration of the drug; it is called an **anaphylactic reaction.** This response can be fatal if the symptoms are not noticed immediately and treatment is not obtained promptly. The earliest symptoms are acute shortness of breath, acute hypotension, and tachycardia.

Drug tolerance exists in a person who has unusually low physiologic activity in response to a drug and who requires increases in the dosage to maintain a given therapeutic effect. Drugs that commonly produce tolerance are opiates, barbiturates, ethyl alcohol, and tobacco. A **cumulative effect** is the increasing response to repeated

Table 43–4 Therapeutic Actions of Drugs

Drug Type	Description	Examples
Palliative	Relieves the symptoms of a disease but does not affect the disease itself	Morphine sulfate, aspirin for pain
Curative	Cures a disease or condition	Penicillin for infection
Supportive	Supports body functions until other treatment or the body's response can take over	Norepinephrine bitartrate for low blood pressure; aspirin for high body temperature
Substitutive	Replaces body fluids or substances	Thyroxine for hypothyroidism; insulin for diabetes mellitus
Chemotherapeutic	Destroys malignant cells	Busulfan for leukemia
Restorative	Returns the body to health	Vitamin, mineral supplements

Table 43–5 Common Mild Allergic Responses

Symptom	Description/Rationale
Skin rash	Either an intraepidermal vesicle rash or a rash typified by an urticarial wheal or macular eruption; rash is usually generalized over the body
Pruritus	Itching of the skin with or without a rash
Angioedema	Edema due to increased permeability of the blood capillaries
Rhinitis	Excessive watery discharge from the nose
Lacrimal tearing	Excessive tearing
Nausea, vomiting	Stimulation of these centers in the brain
Wheezing and dyspnea	Shortness of breath and wheezing upon inhalation and exhalation due to accumulated fluids and swelling of the respiratory tissues
Diarrhea	Irritation of the mucosa of the large intestine

doses of a drug that occurs when the rate of administration exceeds the rate of metabolism or excretion. As a result, the amount of the drug builds up in the client's body unless the dosage is adjusted. Toxic symptoms may occur. An **idiosyncratic effect** is unexpected and individual. Underresponse and overresponse to a drug may be idiosyncratic. Also, the drug may have a completely different effect from the normal one or cause unpredictable and unexplainable symptoms in a particular client.

A **drug interaction** occurs when the administration of one drug before, at the same time as, or after another drug alters the effect of one or both drugs. The effect of one or both drugs may be either increased *(potentiating effect)* or decreased *(inhibiting effect).* Drug interactions may be beneficial or harmful. For example, probenecid, which blocks the excretion of penicillin, is often given with penicillin to increase blood levels of the penicillin for longer periods (potentiating effect). Two analgesics, such as aspirin and codeine, are often given together because together they provide greater pain relief (additive effect).

Iatrogenic disease (disease caused unintentionally by medical therapy) can be due to drug therapy. Hepatic toxicity resulting in biliary obstruction, renal damage, and malformations of the fetus as a result of drugs taken during pregnancy are examples.

DRUG MISUSE

Drug misuse is the improper use of common medications in ways that lead to acute and chronic toxicity. both over-the-counter drugs and prescription drugs may be misused. Laxatives, antacids, vitamins, headache remedies, and cough and cold medications are often self-prescribed and overused. Most people suffer no harmful effects from these drugs, but some people do. A persistent cough may go undiagnosed until the underlying problem becomes serious and advanced.

Drug abuse is inappropriate intake of a substance, either continually or periodically. By definition, drug use is abusive when society considers it abusive. For example, the intake of alcohol at work may be considered alcohol abuse, but intake at a social gathering may not. Drug abuse has two main facets, drug dependence and habituation. **Drug dependence** is a person's reliance on or need to take a drug or substance. The two types of dependence, physiologic and psychologic, may occur separately or together. **Physiologic dependence** is due to biochemical changes in body tissues, especially the nervous system. These tissues come to require the substance for normal functioning. A dependent person who stops using the drug experiences withdrawal symptoms. **Psychologic dependence** is emotional reliance on a drug to maintain a sense of well-being, accompanied by feelings of need or cravings for that drug. There are varying degrees of psychologic dependence, ranging from mild desire to craving and compulsive use of the drug. In severe cases, the dependent person gives up other goals and satisfactions to satisfy the dependence. For example, a man highly dependent on tobacco may give up his job and increase a health problem rather than stop smoking.

Drug habituation denotes a mild form of psychologic dependence. The individual develops the habit of taking the substance and feels better after taking it. The habituated individual tends to continue the habit even though it may be injurious to health.

Illicit drugs, also called *street drugs,* are those sold illegally. Illicit drugs are of two types: (a) drugs unavailable for purchase under any circumstances, such as heroin (in the United States), and (b) drugs normally available with a prescription that are being obtained through illegal channels. Illicit drugs often are taken because of their mood-altering effect; that is, they make the person feel happy or relaxed.

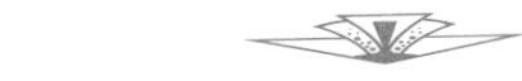

ACTIONS OF DRUGS ON THE BODY

The action of a drug in the body can be described in terms of its **half-life,** the time interval required for the body's elimination processes to reduce the concentration of the drug in the body by one-half. For example, if a drug's half-life is 8 hours, then the amount of drug in the body is as follows:

Initially: 100%

After 8 hours: 50%

After 16 hours: 25%

After 24 hours: 12.5%

After 32 hours: 6.25%

Because the purpose of most drug therapy is to maintain a constant drug level in the body, repeated doses are required to maintain that level. When an orally adminis-

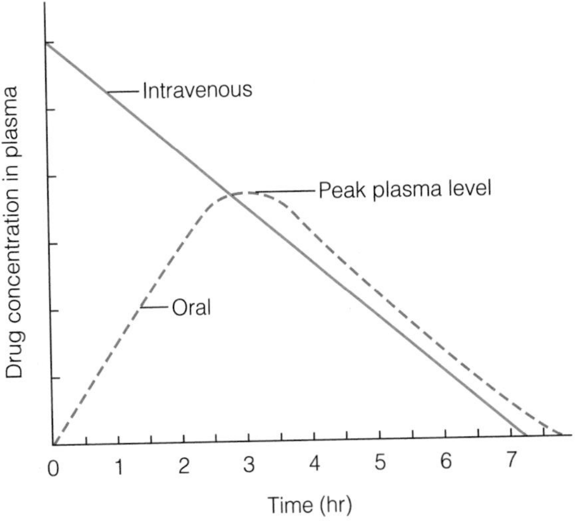

Figure 43–1 A graphic plot of drug concentration in the blood plasma following a single dose.

tered drug is absorbed from the gastrointestinal tract into the blood plasma, its concentration in the plasma increases until the elimination rate equals the rate of absorption. This point is known as the **peak plasma level** (Figure 43–1). Unless the client receives another dose of the drug, the concentration steadily decreases. Key terms related to drug actions are listed and described in the box below.

A drug that interacts with a receptor to produce a response is known as an **agonist.** Drugs that have no special pharmacologic action of their own but that inhibit or prevent the action of an agonist are called **specific antagonists.** Drugs may also produce a response by stimulating enzyme activity or hormone production.

KEY TERMS RELATED TO DRUG ACTION

- *Onset of action:* The time after administration when the body initially responds to the drug
- *Peak plasma level:* The highest plasma level achieved by a single dose when the elimination rate of a drug equals the absorption rate
- *Drug half-life (elimination half-life):* The time required for the elimination process to reduce the concentration of the drug to one-half what it was at initial administration
- *Plateau:* A maintained concentration of a drug in the plasma during a series of scheduled doses

PHARMACOKINETICS

Pharmacokinetics is the study of the absorption, distribution, biotransformation, and excretion of drugs. **Absorption** is the process by which a drug passes into the bloodstream. Unless the drug is administered directly into the bloodstream, absorption is the first step in the movement of the drug through the body. For absorption to occur, the correct form of the drug must be given by the route intended.

The rate of absorption of a drug in the stomach is variable. Food, for example, can delay the dissolution and absorption of some drugs as well as their passage into the small intestine, where most drug absorption occurs. Food can also combine with molecules of certain drugs, thereby changing their molecular structure and subsequently inhibiting or preventing their absorption. Another factor that affects the absorption of some drugs is the acid medium in the stomach. Acidity can vary according to the time of day, foods ingested, and the age of the client. Some drugs do not dissolve or have limited ability to dissolve in the gastrointestinal fluids, decreasing their absorption into the bloodstream. Some drugs are absorbed by tissues before they reach the stomach. For example, nitroglycerin is administered under the tongue, where it is absorbed into the blood vessels that carry it directly to the heart, the intended site of action. If swallowed, this drug will be absorbed into the bloodstream and carried to the liver, where it will be destroyed.

A drug administered directly into the bloodstream, that is, intravenously, is immediately in the vascular system without having to be absorbed. This, then, is the route of choice for rapid action. Because subcutaneous tissue has a poorer blood supply than muscle tissue, absorption from subcutaneous tissue is slower. The rate of absorption of a drug can be accelerated by the application of heat, which increases blood flow to the area; conversely, absorption can be slowed by the application of cold. In addition, the injection of a vasoconstrictor drug such as epinephrine into the tissue can slow absorption of other drugs. Some drugs intended to be absorbed slowly are suspended in a low-solubility medium, such as oil. The absorption of drugs from the rectum into the bloodstream tends to be unpredictable. Therefore, this route is normally used when other routes are unavailable or when the intended action is localized to the rectum or sigmoid colon.

Distribution is the transportation of a drug from its site of absorption to its site of action. When a drug enters the bloodstream, it is carried to the most vascular organs—that is, liver, kidneys, and brain. Body areas with lower blood supply—that is, skin and muscles—receive the drug later. The chemical and physical properties of a drug largely determine the area of the body to which the drug will be attracted. For example, fat-soluble drugs will accumulate in fatty tissue, whereas other drugs may bind with plasma proteins.

Biotransformation, also called **detoxification,** is a process by which a drug is converted to a less active form. Most biotransformation takes place in the liver, where many drug-metabolizing enzymes in the cells detoxify the drugs. The products of this process are called **metabolites.** There are two types of metabolites: active and inactive. An *active metabolite* has a pharmacologic action itself, whereas an *inactive metabolite* does not.

The biotransformation capability of a client's liver may be impaired. For example, an elderly client, just like a client with hepatic damage, may have a decreased ability to metabolize drugs. In these situations, nurses must be alert to the accumulation of the active drug in the client and to subsequent toxicity.

Excretion is the process by which metabolites and drugs are eliminated from the body. Most metabolites are eliminated by the kidneys in the urine; however, some are excreted in the feces, the breath, perspiration, saliva, and breast milk. Certain drugs, such as general anesthetic agents, are excreted in an unchanged form via the respiratory tract. In addition to metabolites, alcohol is eliminated, unchanged, through the lungs. The efficiency with which the kidneys excrete drugs and metabolites diminishes with age. Elderly people may require smaller doses of a drug because the drug and its metabolites may accumulate in the body. Also, kidney disease can impair excretion of drugs and metabolites.

FACTORS INFLUENCING DRUG ACTION

A number of factors influence the actions of drugs on the body. Among them are age, weight, sex, genetic and psychologic factors, illness and disease, time of administration, and environment. *Age* is a factor in that very young people and elderly people often are highly responsive to drugs and thus require lower doses. Immature liver and kidney function as well as diminished renal functioning due to aging can affect the action of a drug. *Body weight* also directly affects drug action; the greater the body weight, the greater the dosage required.

Sex-linked differences in the way men and women respond to drugs are chiefly due to two factors: differences in distribution of fat and water and hormonal differences. Because women usually weigh less than men, equal drug dosages are likely to affect women more than men. Women usually have more fatty pads than men, and men have more body fluid than women. Some drugs may be more soluble in fat, whereas others are more soluble in water. Thus, some drugs are more readily absorbed in men than in women, whereas others are more readily absorbed in women.

Individuals may react differently to drugs as a result of *genetic factors.* A client may be abnormally sensitive to a drug or may metabolize a drug differently than most people because of genetic influences. Sometimes these reactions are mistaken for allergic reactions. *Psychologic factors* influence how one feels about a drug and what one believes it can do. For example, a woman who has joint pain is prescribed Ibuprofen. However, her friend, who also has pain tried Ibuprofen and said it didn't work. So the client believes it will not relieve her pain.

Illness and *disease* can also affect the action of drugs. For example, aspirin can reduce the body temperature of a feverish client but has no effect on the body temperature of a client without fever. Drug action is altered in clients with circulatory, liver, or kidney dysfunction. Diabetics need larger doses of insulin with fever or infection.

The *time of administration* of oral medications affects the relative speed with which they act. Orally administered medications are absorbed more quickly if the stomach is empty. Thus, oral medications taken 2 hours before meals act faster than those taken after meals. However, some medications, for example, iron preparations, irritate the gastrointestinal tract and need to be given after a meal, when they will be better tolerated. A client's sleep-wake rhythm may affect the action of a drug. Circadian variations in urine output and blood circulation, for example, may affect a client's response to a drug.

The client's *environment* can affect the action of drugs, particularly those used to alter behavior and mood. Therefore, nurses assessing the effects of a drug need to consider the drug itself as well as the client's personality and milieu. Environmental temperature may also affect drug activity. When environmental temperature is high, the peripheral blood vessels dilate, thus intensifying the action of vasodilators. In contrast, a cold environment and the consequent vasoconstriction inhibit the action of vasodilators but enhance the action of vasoconstrictors.

Recent research has indicated *ethnicity* and *culture* may contribute to differences in responses to medications. The rates of drug metabolism are known to vary considerably (Kudzma 1992, p. 49).

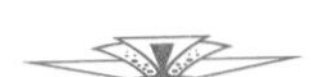

ROUTES OF ADMINISTRATION

Pharmaceutical preparations are generally designed for one or two specific routes of administration. See Table 43–6 on page 1302. The route of administration should be indicated when the drug is ordered. When administering a drug, the nurse should ensure that the pharmaceutical preparation is appropriate for the route specified.

Oral Oral administration is the most common, least expensive, and most convenient route for most clients. Because the skin is not broken as it is for an injection, oral administration is also a safe method.

The major disadvantages are possible unpleasant taste of the drugs, irritation of the gastric mucosa, irregular absorption from the gastrointestinal tract, slow absorption, and, in some cases, harm to the client's teeth. For example, hydrochloric acid can damage the enamel of teeth.

Sublingual In sublingual administration, a drug is placed under the tongue, where it dissolves (Figure 43–2, p. 1303). In a relatively short time, the drug is largely absorbed into the blood vessels on the underside of the tongue. The medication should not be swallowed. Nitroglycerin is one example of drugs commonly given in this manner.

Buccal Buccal means "pertaining to the cheek." In buccal administration, a medication (eg, a tablet) is held in the mouth against the mucous membranes of the cheek until the drug dissolves (Figure 43–3, p. 1303). The drug may act locally on the mucous membranes of the mouth or systemically when it is swallowed in the saliva.

Parenteral Parenteral administration is administration other than through the alimentary tract, that is, by needle. The following are some of the more common routes for parenteral administration:

- *Subcutaneous (hypodermic)*—into the subcutaneous tissue, just below the skin
- *Intramuscular*—into a muscle
- *Intradermal*—under the epidermis (into the dermis)
- *Intravenous*—into a vein

Some of the less commonly used routes for parenteral administration are **intra-arterial** (into an artery), **intracardiac** (into the heart muscle), **intraosseous** (into a bone), and **intrathecal** or **intraspinal** (into the spinal canal). These less common injections are normally administered by physicians. Sterile equipment and sterile drug solution are essential for all parenteral therapy. The main advantage is fast absorption.

Topical Topical applications are those applied to a circumscribed surface area of the body. They affect only the area to which they are applied. Topical applications include the following:

Table 43–6 Routes of Administration

Route	Advantages	Disadvantages
Oral	Most convenient Usually least expensive Safe, does not break skin barrier Administration usually does not cause stress	Inappropriate for clients with nausea or vomiting Drug may have unpleasant taste or odor Inappropriate when gastrointestinal tract has reduced motility Inappropriate if client cannot swallow or is unconscious Cannot be used before certain diagnostic tests or surgical procedures Drug may discolor teeth, harm tooth enamel Drug may irritate gastric mucosa Drug can be aspirated by seriously ill clients
Sublingual	Same as for oral, *plus:* Drug can be administered for local effect Drug is rapidly absorbed into the bloodstream Ensures greater potency because drug directly enters the blood and bypasses the liver	If swallowed, drug may be inactivated by gastric juice Drug must remain under tongue until dissolved and absorbed
Buccal	Same as for sublingual	Same as for sublingual
Rectal	Can be used when drug has objectionable taste or odor Drug released at slow, steady rate	Dose absorbed is unpredictable
Vaginal	Provides local therapeutic effect	Limited use
Topical	Provides a local effect Few side effects	May be messy and may soil clothes Drug can rapidly enter body through abrasions and cause systemic effects
Transdermal	Prolonged systemic effect Few side effects Avoids gastrointestinal absorption problems	Leaves residue on the skin that may soil clothes
Subcutaneous	Onset of drug action faster than oral	Must involve sterile technique because breaks skin barrier More expensive than oral Can administer only small volume Slower than intramuscular administration Some drugs can irritate tissues and cause pain Can be anxiety-producing
Intramuscular	Pain from irritating drugs is minimized Can administer larger volume than subcutaneous Drug is rapidly absorbed	Breaks skin barrier Can be anxiety-producing
Intradermal	Absorption is slow (this is an advantage in testing for allergies)	Amount of drug administered must be small Breaks skin barrier
Intravenous	Rapid effect	Limited to highly soluble drugs Drug distribution inhibited by poor circulation
Inhalation	Introduces drug throughout the respiratory tract Rapid localized relief Drug can be administered with unconscious client	Drug intended for localized effect can have systemic effect Of use only for the respiratory system

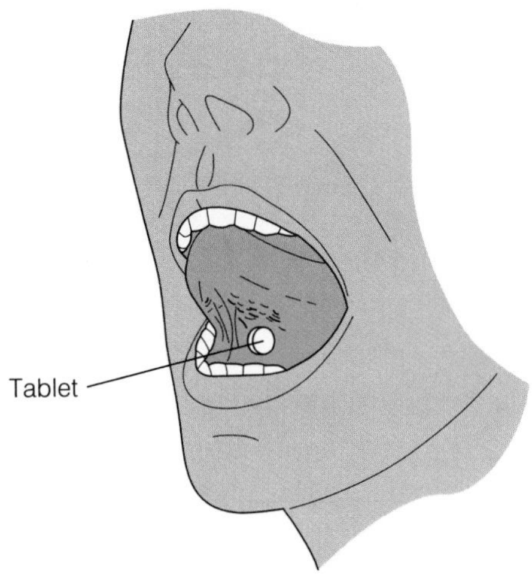

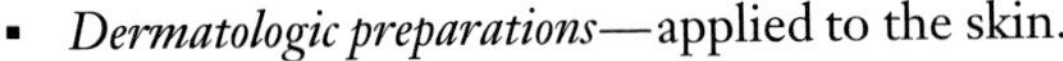

Figure 43–2 Sublingual administration of a tablet.

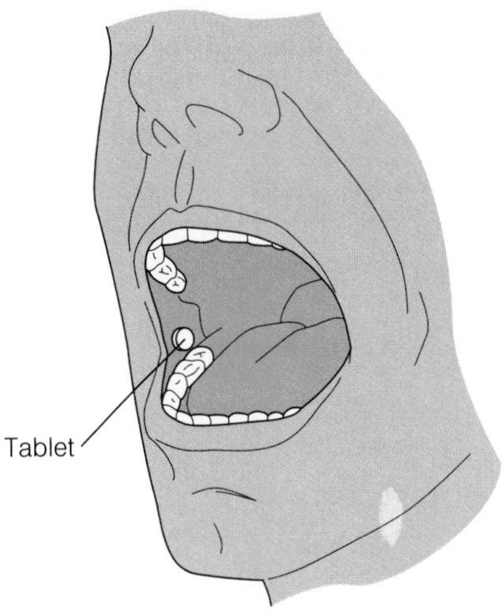

Figure 43–3 Buccal administration of a tablet.

- *Dermatologic preparations*—applied to the skin.
- *Instillations and irrigations*—applied into body cavities or orifices, such as the urinary bladder, eyes, ears, nose, rectum, or vagina.
- *Inhalations*—administered into the respiratory tract by nebulizers or positive pressure breathing apparatuses. Air, oxygen, and vapor are generally used to carry the drug into the lungs. See Chapter 39.

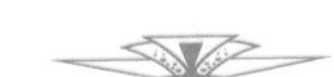

MEDICATION ORDERS

A physician usually determines the clients' medications needs and orders medications, although in some settings nurse-practitioners and physicians' assistants now order some drugs. Usually, the order is written, although telephone and verbal orders are acceptable in a number of agencies. Nursing students need to know the agency policies about medication orders. In some hospitals, for example, only licensed nurses are permitted to accept telephone and verbal orders.

Policies about physicians' orders vary considerably from agency to agency. For example, a client's orders are frequently automatically canceled after surgery or an examination involving an anesthetic agent. New orders must then be written. Most agencies also have lists of abbreviations officially accepted for use in the agency. Both nurses and physicians may need to refer to these lists if they have been working in a different agency. These abbreviations can be used on legal documents, such as clients' charts. See Table 43–7 on page 1304.

TYPES OF MEDICATION ORDERS

Four common medication orders are the stat order, the single order, the standing order, and the prn order.

1. A **stat order** indicates that the medication is to be given immediately and only once (eg, Demerol 100 mg IM stat).
2. The **single order** is for a medication to be given once at a specified time (eg, Seconal 100 mg hs before surgery).
3. The **standing order** may or may not have a termination date. A standing order may be carried out indefinitely (eg, multiple vitamins daily) until an order is written to cancel it, or it may be carried out for a specified number of days (eg, Demerol 100 mg IM q4h × 5 days). In some agencies, standing orders are automatically canceled after a specified number of days and must be reordered.
4. A **prn order** permits the nurse to give a medication when, in the nurse's judgment, the client requires it (eg, Amphojel 15 mL prn). The nurse must use good judgment about when the medication is needed and when it can be safely administered.

ESSENTIAL PARTS OF A DRUG ORDER

The drug order has six essential parts, as listed in the box on page 1305. In addition, unless it is a standing order, the order should state the number of doses or the number of days the drug is to be administered.

Table 43–7 Common Abbreviations Used in Medication Orders

Abbreviation	Explanation	Example of Administration Time
ac	before meals	0700, 1100, and 1700 hours
ad lib	freely, as desired	
agit	shake, stir	
aq	water	
aq dest	distilled water	
bid	twice a day	0900 and 2100 hours
$\bar{c}$	with	
cap	capsule	
comp	compound	
dil	dissolve, dilute	
elix	elixir	
f℥	fluid ounce	
g, gm, or Gm	gram	
gr	grain	
gtt	drop	
h	an hour	
hs	at bedtime	
IM	intramuscular	
IV	intravenous	
kg or Kg	kilogram	
l or L	liter	
M or m	mix	
mcg or μg	microgram	
mg	milligram	
no.	number	
non rep	do not repeat	
OD	right eye	
OS or ol	left eye	
OU	both eyes	
pc	after meals	0900, 1300, and 1900 hours
po	by mouth	
prn	when needed	
q	every	
qAM (om)	every morning	1000 hours
qh (q1h)	every hour	
q2h	every 2 hours	0800, 1000, 1200 hours, and so on
q3h	every 3 hours	0900, 1200, 1500 hours, and so on
q4h	every 4 hours	1000, 1400, 1800 hours, and so on
q6h	every 6 hours	0600, 1200, 1800, 2400 hours
qhs	every night at bedtime	
qid	four times a day	1000, 1400, 1800, 2200 hours
qod	every other day	0900 hours on odd dates
qs	sufficient quantity	
rept	may be repeated	
Rx	take	
$\bar{s}$	without	
sc	subcutaneous	
Sig or S	label	
sos	if it is needed	
ss or $\overline{ss}$	one half	
stat	at once	
sup or supp	suppository	
susp	suspension	
tid	three times a day	1000, 1400, and 1800 hours
Tr or tinct	tincture	

The *client's full name,* that is, the first and last names and middle initials or names, should always be used to avoid confusion between two clients who have the same last names. In some agencies, the client's admission number is put on the order as further identification. Some hospitals imprint the client's name and hospital number on all forms. This imprinter is on the nursing unit; it is much like a credit card imprinter.

In addition to *the day, the month, and the year* the order was written, some agencies also require that the *time of day* be written. Writing the time of day on the order can eliminate errors when the nursing shifts change and makes

ESSENTIAL PARTS OF A DRUG ORDER

- Full name of the client
- Date the order is written
- Name of the drug to be administered
- Dosage of the drug
- Method of administration
- Signature of the physician or nurse practitioner

PARTS OF A PRESCRIPTION

- Descriptive information about the client: name, address, and, sometimes, age
- Date on which the prescription was written
- The Rx symbol, meaning "take thou"
- Medication name, dosage, and strength
- Route of administration
- Dispensing instructions for the pharmacist, for example, "Dispense 30 capsules"
- Directions for administration to be given to the client, for example, "Sig. Tab ī tid with meals"
- Refill and/or special labeling, for example, "Refill × 1"
- Prescriber's signature

clear when certain orders automatically terminate. For example, in some settings, narcotics can be ordered only for 48 hours after surgery. Therefore, a drug that is ordered at 1600 hours November 1, 1995, is automatically canceled at 1600 hours November 3, 1995. Many health agencies use the 24-hour clock, which eliminates confusion between morning and afternoon times. Time with the 24-hour clock starts at midnight, which is 0000 hours. See Chapter 9, page 176.

The *name of the drug* to be administered must be clearly written. In some settings, only generic names are permitted; however, trade names are widely used in hospitals and health agencies.

The *dosage of the drug* includes the amount, the times or frequency of administration, and in many instances the strength; for example, tetracycline *250 mg* (amount) *four times a day* (frequency); hydrochloric acid *10%* (strength) *5 mL* (amount) *three times a day with meals* (time and frequency). Dosages can be written in apothecaries' or metric systems.

Also included in the order is the *method of administering* the drug. This part of the order, like other parts, is frequently abbreviated. See Table 43–7 for abbreviations of routes of administration. It is not unusual for a drug to have several possible routes of administration; therefore, it is important that the route be included in the order.

The *signature* of the ordering physician or nurse makes the drug order a legal request. An unsigned order has no validity, and the ordering physician or nurse needs to be notified if the order is unsigned.

In agencies where telephone orders are taken, the nurse usually indicates the name of the person who phoned in the order. The nurse signs the order, but usually the person who ordered the drug must also sign at a later date. Some hospitals have policies that those who give orders by telephone must sign those orders within a certain time, for example, 48 hours after they have communicated the order.

When a physician writes a prescription for a client, the prescription also includes information for the pharmacist. Therefore, a prescription's content differs from that of a medication order in a hospital. Compare the parts of a prescription listed in the box above with those shown in Figure 43–4.

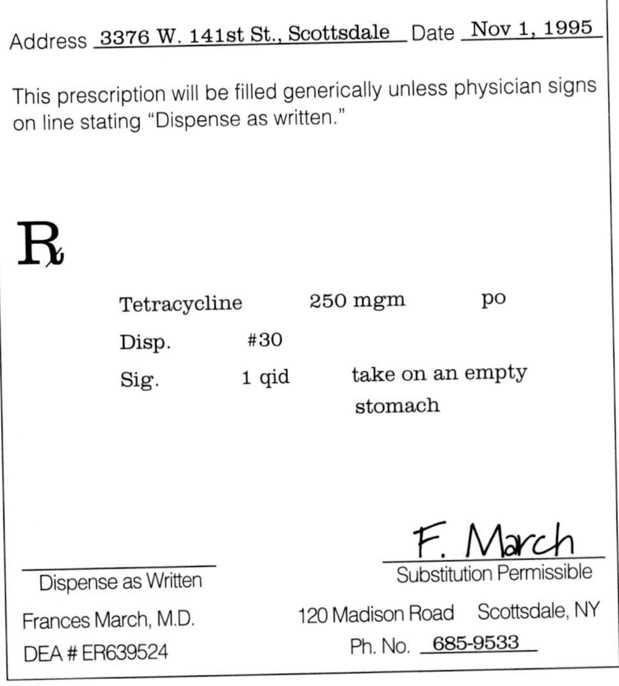

Name Jane Cleary Age 36

Address 3376 W. 141st St., Scottsdale Date Nov 1, 1995

This prescription will be filled generically unless physician signs on line stating "Dispense as written."

℞

Tetracycline 250 mgm po

Disp. #30

Sig. 1 qid take on an empty stomach

F. March

Dispense as Written Substitution Permissible

Frances March, M.D. 120 Madison Road Scottsdale, NY

DEA # ER639524 Ph. No. 685-9533

Figure 43–4 A prescription filled out by a physician.

WEST BAY
MEDICAL CENTER

Division of Nursing
Redmond, California 94000

Administration
0400 05/03/95 to 0359 05/04/95

MEDICATIONS	Checked By	0400	0500	0600	0700	0800	0900	1000	1100	1200	1300	1400	1500	1600	1700	1800	1900	2000	2100	2200	2300	2400	0100	0200	0300
CEFAZOLIN SODIU 1GM 5 ML ANCEF 30 MIN Q8H MD REQUESTED TIMES SRT: 04/28 STP: 05/05 IV 02,08,18						X	DC									X								X	
RANITIDINE HCL 150MG ZANTAC ORAL <150MG > BID SRT: 04/30 STP: 08,20	W					X 08 LS												X Ec							
ASPIRIN 325MG ECOTRIN ORAL <325 MG > QD SRT: 04/29 STP: 08	W					X 08 LS																			
FERROUS GLUCONATE ORAL <325 MG > TID SRT: 4/30 STP: 08/14/22 ORDER: 31	W					X LS						X 14 LS								X Ec					
MAGNESIUM HYDROXIDE MILK OF MAGNESIA ORAL <30ML > AM SRT: 05/01 STP: 08	W					X 08 LS																			

INIT.	SIGNATURE	INIT.	SIGNATURE	INIT.	SIGNATURE
EC	EClarianshin RN	LS	LSoho RN		

DIAGNOSIS:
MULTI CONTUSIONS CEREBRAL CON

ALLERGIES:
ADR:NKA

COMMENTS:

INJECTION SITE LEGEND

A- LUOQ
B- RUOQ
C- L VENTROGLUTEAL
D- R VENTROGLUTEAL
E- L THIGH
F- R THIGH
G- L DELTOID
H- R DELTOID
I- ABDOMEN
NN- OTHER - SEE NURSES' NOTES

PAGE: 1

5518-A STS

ACCT # : 0871421
ADMITTED : 04/24/95
PHYSICIAN : Brenna, Jane

AGE: 35Y
SEX: F

Medication Administration Record

Figure 43–5 A computerized medication administration record.

COMMUNICATING A MEDICATION ORDER

A drug order is written on the client's chart by a physician or by a nurse receiving a telephone or verbal order from a physician. Most agencies have a specified time frame (eg, 24 or 48 hours) in which the physician issuing the telephone or verbal order must cosign the order written by the nurse. The medication order is then copied by a nurse or clerk to a Kardex or medication administration record (MAR). Increasingly, nurses are being provided with computer printouts of a client's medications instead of copying the physician's order. This method avoids errors of copying and saves nursing time.

Medication administration records (Figure 43–5) vary in form, but all include the client's name, room, and bed number; drug name and dose; and times and method of administration. In some agencies, the date the order was prescribed and the date the order expires are also included.

SYSTEMS OF MEASUREMENT

Three systems of measurement are used in North America: the metric system, the apothecaries' system, and the household system, which is similar to the apothecaries' system.

METRIC SYSTEM

The metric system, devised by the French in the latter part of the 18th century, is the system prescribed by law in most European countries and in Canada. The metric system is logically organized into units of ten; it is a decimal system. Basic units can be multiplied or divided by ten to form secondary units. Multiples are calculated by moving the decimal point to the right, and divisions by moving the decimal point to the left.

Basic units of measurement are the meter, the liter, and the gram. Prefixes derived from Latin designate subdivisions of the basic unit: *deci* (1/10 or 0.1), *centi* (1/100 or 0.01), and *milli* (1/1000 or 0.001). Multiples of the basic unit are designated by prefixes derived from Greek: *deka* (10), *hecto* (100), and *kilo* (1000). Only the measurements of volume (the liter) and of weight (the gram) are discussed in this chapter. These are the measures used in medication administration (Figure 43–6). In nursing practice, the kilogram (kg) is the only multiple of the gram used, and the milligram (mg) and microgram (mcg or μg) are subdivisions. Fractional parts of the liter are usually expressed in milliliters (mL), for example, 600 mL; multiples of the liter are usually expressed as liters or milliliters, for example, 2.5 liters or 2500 mL.

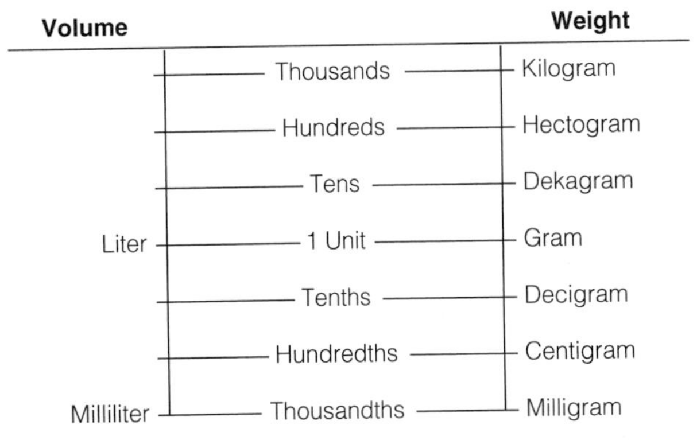

Figure 43–6 Basic metric measurements of volume and weight.

APOTHECARIES' SYSTEM

The apothecaries' system, older than the metric system, was brought to the United States from England during the colonial period. The basic unit of weight in the apothecaries' system is the grain (gr) likened to a grain of wheat, and the basic unit of volume is the **minim,** a volume of water equal in weight to a grain of wheat. The word *minim* means "the least." In ascending order, the other units of weight are the scruple, the dram, the ounce, and the pound. Today, the scruple (scr) is seldom used. The units of volume are, in ascending order, the fluid dram, the fluid ounce, the pint, the quart, and the gallon.

Quantities in the apothecaries' system are often expressed by lowercase Roman numerals, particularly when the unit of measure is abbreviated. The Roman numeral follows rather than precedes the unit of measure. For example, a fluid ounce is abbreviated as f℥. Two fluid ounces are written as f℥ii, and 4 fluid ounces are written as f℥iv. Quantities less than 1 are expressed as a fraction, for example, gr 1/6. See Chapter 9, Table 9–4, page 179.

HOUSEHOLD SYSTEM

Household measures may be used when more accurate systems of measure are not required. Included in household measures are drops, teaspoons, tablespoons, cups, and glasses. Although pints and quarts are often found in the home, they are defined as apothecaries' measures. Equivalent units of the household system are listed in the *Clinical Companion.*

CONVERTING UNITS OF WEIGHT AND MEASURE

Sometimes drugs are dispensed from the pharmacy in grams when the order specifies milligrams, or they are dispensed in milligrams though ordered in grains. For example, a physician orders morphine gr ¼. The medication is available only in milligrams. The nurse knows that 1 mg = 1⁄60 gr or 60 mg = 1 grain. To convert the ordered dose to milligrams, the nurse calculates as follows:

$$\text{If } 60 \text{ mg} = 1 \text{ gr}$$
$$\text{Then } x \text{ mg} = \frac{1}{4} \text{ gr } (0.25 \text{ gr})$$
$$x = \left(\frac{60 \times 0.25}{1}\right)$$
$$x = 15 \text{ mg}$$

Converting Weights within the Metric System It is relatively simple to arrive at equivalent units of weight within the metric system, because the system is based on units of ten. Only three metric units of weight are used for drug dosages, the gram (g), milligram (mg), and microgram (mcg or μg): 1000 mg or 1,000,000 mcg equals 1 g. Equivalents are computed by dividing or multiplying; for example, to change milligrams to grams, the nurse divides the number of milligrams by 1000. The simplest way to divide by 1000 is to move the decimal point three places to the left:

500 mg = ? g
Move the decimal point three places to the *left*
Answer = 0.5 g

Conversely, to convert grams to milligrams, multiply the number of grams by 1000, or move the decimal point three places to the right:

0.006 g = ? mg
Move the decimal point three places to the *right*
Answer = 6 mg

Converting Weights and Measures between Systems When preparing client medications, a nurse may need to convert weights or volumes from one system to another. As an example, the pharmacy may dispense milligrams or grams of chloral hydrate, yet the nurse must administer an order that reads "chloral hydrate gr $\overline{\text{viiss}}$." To prepare the correct dose, the nurse must convert from the apothecaries' to the metric system. To give clients a useful, realistic measure for home use, the nurse may have to convert from the apothecaries' or metric system to the household system. All conversions are approximate, that is, not totally precise.

Converting Units of Volume Commonly used approximate equivalents are shown in Table 43–8.

By learning these equivalents, the nurse can make many conversions readily. For example, 15 minims = approximately 15 drops (gtt); therefore, 1 minim is approximately 1 drop. Similarly, 1 quart approximates 1000 mL, and 1 gallon approximates 4000 mL; therefore 4 quarts is approximately 1 gallon.

Table 43–8 Approximate Volume Equivalents: Metric, Apothecaries', and Household Systems

Metric		Apothecaries'		Household
1 mL	=	15 minims (min or m)	=	15 drops (gtt)
15 mL	=	4 fluid drams (fʒ)	=	1 tablespoon (Tbsp)
30 mL	=	1 fluid ounce (f℥)	=	same
500 mL	=	1 pint (pt)	=	same
1000 mL	=	1 quart (qt)	=	same
4000 mL	=	1 gallon (gal)	=	same

The following are some situations in which nurses need to apply a knowledge of volume conversion.

1. Milliliter dosages may need to be fractionalized. The nurse can fractionalize milliliter dosages by remembering that 1 mL contains 15 drops or minims.
2. Fluid drams and ounces are commonly used in prescribing liquid medications, such as cough syrups, laxatives, antacids, and antibiotics for children. The fluid ounce is frequently converted to milliliters when measuring a client's fluid intake or output.
3. Liters and milliliters are the volumes commonly used in preparing solutions for enemas, irrigating solutions for douches, bladder irrigations, and solutions for cleaning open wounds. In some situations, the nurse needs to convert the volumes of such solutions.

Converting Units of Weight The units of weight most commonly used in nursing practice are the gram, milligram, and kilogram and the grain and the pound. Household units of weight are generally not applicable.

Table 43–9 shows metric and apothecaries' approximate equivalents. Learning these equivalents helps the nurse make weight conversions readily, as, for example, in the following situations.

1. Converting grams and milligrams to grains and vice versa, for example, when preparing medications.
2. Converting pounds to kilograms and vice versa, for example, a person's weight.

When converting units of weight from the metric system to the apothecaries' system, the nurse should keep in mind that a milligram is smaller than a grain (1 mg = 1⁄60 grain and 1 grain = 60 mg). The result of converting a smaller unit (milligram) to a larger unit (grain) is a smaller number. Thus, the nurse must divide (by 60 if converting

Table 43–9 Approximate Weight Equivalents: Metric and Apothecaries' Systems

Metric		Apothecaries'
1 mg	=	1/60 grain
60 mg	=	1 grain
1 g	=	15 grains
4 g	=	1 dram
30 g	=	1 ounce
500 g	=	1.1 pound (lb)
1000 g (1 kg)	=	2.2 lb

from milligrams to grains). Conversely, when converting from a larger unit to a smaller unit, the nurse multiplies (by 60 if converting from grains to milligrams), and the product is a larger number. In other words:

Small units (mg) to large units (grains) = a smaller number

Large units (grains) to small units (mg) = a larger number

$$\frac{3000 \text{ mg}}{60} = 50 \text{ grains}$$

$$50 \text{ grains} \times 60 = 3000 \text{ mg}$$

When converting pounds to kilograms, the nurse applies the same rule. The pound is a smaller unit than the kilogram, and the nurse converts by dividing or multiplying by 2.2:

$$2.2 \text{ lb} = 1 \text{ kg}$$

$$110 \text{ lb} = x \text{ kg}$$

$$x = \frac{110 \times 1}{2.2}$$

$$= 50 \text{ kg}$$

or

$$50 \text{ kg} = x \text{ lb}$$

$$1 \text{ kg} = 2.2 \text{ lb}$$

$$x = \frac{2.2 \times 50}{1}$$

$$= 110 \text{ lb}$$

The conversion of milligrams to grams was previously discussed. The decimal point is moved three spaces to the left:

$$3000 \text{ mg} = 3\text{g}$$

CALCULATING DOSAGES

There are several formulas that can be used to calculate drug dosages. One formula uses ratios:

$$\frac{\text{dose on hand}}{\text{quantity on hand}} = \frac{\text{desired dose}}{\text{quantity desired } (x)}$$

For example, erythromycin 500 mg is ordered. It is supplied in a liquid form containing 250 mg in 5 mL. To calculate the dosage, the nurse uses the formula

$$\frac{\text{dose on hand (250 mg)}}{\text{quantity on hand (5 mL)}} = \frac{\text{desired dose (500 mg)}}{\text{quantity desired } (x)}$$

Then, the nurse cross-multiplies:

$$250\,x = 5 \text{ mL} \times 500 \text{ mg}$$

$$x = \frac{5 \text{ mL} \times 500 \text{ mg}}{250 \text{ mg}}$$

$$x = 10 \text{ mL}$$

Therefore, the dose ordered is 10 mL.

The nurse can also use this formula to calculate dosages:

$$\text{amount to administer } (x) = \frac{\text{desired dose}}{\text{dose on hand}} \times \text{quantity on hand}$$

For example, heparin is often distributed in large vials and prepared dilutions of 10,000 units per mL. If the order calls for 5000 units, the nurse can calculate using the formula above:

$$x = \frac{5000}{10{,}000} \times 1$$

$$x = \frac{1}{2} \text{ mL}$$

Therefore, the nurse injects 0.5 mL for a 5000-unit dose.

Dosages for Children Although dosage is stated in the medication order, nurses must understand something about the safe dosage for children. Unlike adult dosages, children's dosages are not always standard. Body size significantly affects dosage.

Body Surface Area Body surface area is determined by using a nomogram and the child's height and weight. This is considered to be the most accurate method of calculating a child's dose. Standard nomograms give a child's body surface area according to weight and height (Figure 43–7, p. 1310). The formula is the ratio of the child's body surface area to the surface area of an average adult (1.7 square meters, or 1.7 m^2), multiplied by the normal adult dose of the drug:

$$\text{Child's dose} = \frac{\text{Surface area of child } (m^2)}{1.7 \text{ m}^2} \times \text{normal adult dose}$$

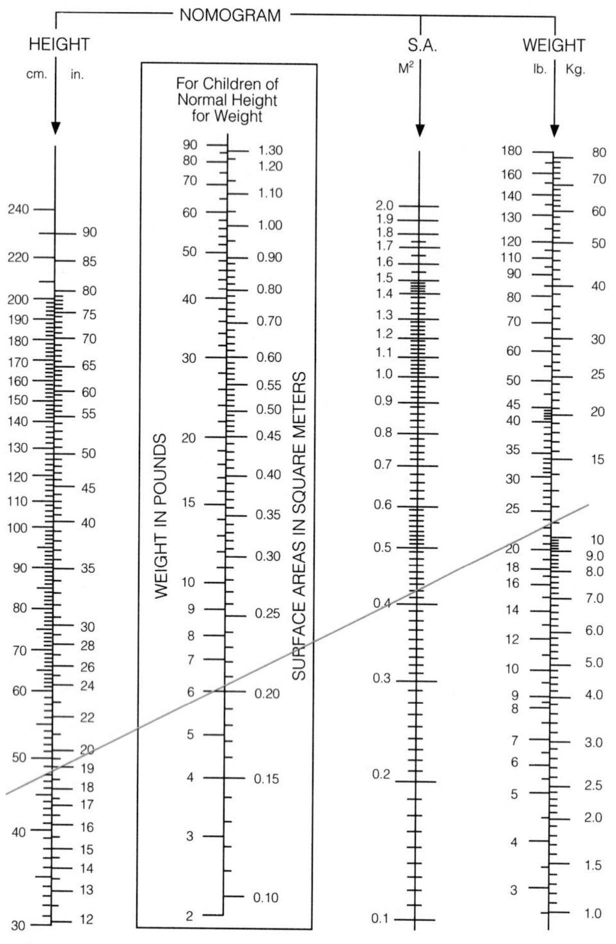

Figure 43–7 Nomogram with estimated body surface area. A straight line is drawn between the child's height (on the left) and the child's weight (on the right). The point at which the line intersects the surface area column is the estimated body surface area.

For example, a child who weights 10 kg and is 50 cm tall has a body surface area of 0.4 m^2. Therefore, the child's dose of tetracycline corresponding to an adult dose of 250 mg would be as follows:

$$\text{Child's dose} = \frac{0.4\ \text{m}^2}{1.7\ \text{m}^2} \times 250\ \text{mg}$$

$$= 0.23 \times 250 = 58.82\ \text{mg}$$

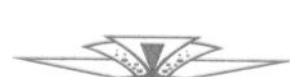

ADMINISTERING MEDICATIONS SAFELY

The nurse should always assess a client's physical status prior to giving *any* medication. The extent of the assessment depends on the client's illness or current condition, the intended drug and route of administration. For example, the nurse assesses a dyspneic client's respirations carefully before administering any medication that might affect breathing. In general, the nurse assesses the client *prior* to administering any medication to obtain baseline data by which to evaluate the effectiveness of the medication. Clinical guidelines for administering medications are given in the box on page 1311.

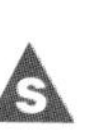

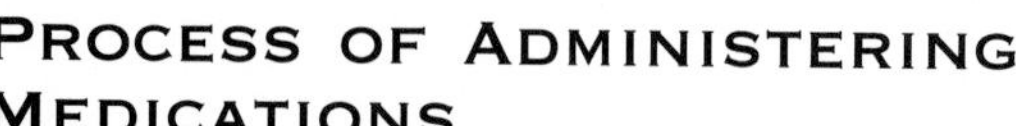

PROCESS OF ADMINISTERING MEDICATIONS

When administering any drug, regardless of the route of administration, the nurse must do the following:

1. *Identify the client.* Errors can and do occur, usually because one client gets a drug intended for another. In hospitals, most clients wear some sort of identification, such as a wristband with name and hospital identification number. Before giving the client any drug, check the identification band with the medication administration record (MAR). As a double check, ask the client's name or ask another nurse to identify the client before administering any medication.
2. *Administer the drug.* Read medication orders and records carefully and check against the name on the medication envelope or on the drawer in which the client's medications are kept if a medication cart is used. Then administer the medication in the prescribed dosage, by the route ordered, at the correct time.
3. *Provide adjunctive interventions as indicated.* Clients may need help when receiving medications. They may require physical assistance, for instance, in assuming positions for intramuscular injections, or they may need explanations about the medications and guidance about measures to enhance drug effectiveness and prevent complications, such as drinking fluids. Some clients convey fear about their medications. The nurse can allay fears by listening carefully to clients' concerns and giving correct information.
4. *Record the drug administered.* The facts recorded in the chart, in ink or by computer printout, are name of the drug, dosage, method of administration, specific relevant data such as pulse rate (taken in most settings prior to the administration of digitalis), and any other pertinent information. The record should also include the exact time of administration and the signature of the nurse providing the medication. Many medication records are designed so that the nurse signs once on the page and initials each medication administered. Often, medications that are given regularly are recorded on a special flow record, and prn or stat medications are recorded separately.

CLINICAL GUIDELINES

Administering Medications

- Nurses who administer medications are responsible for their own actions. Question any order that you consider incorrect.
- Be knowledgeable about medications that you administer.
- Federal laws govern the uses of narcotics and barbiturates. Keep these medications in a locked place.
- Use only medications that are in a clearly labeled container.
- Return liquid medications that are cloudy or have changed color to the pharmacy.
- Before administering a medication, identify the client correctly using the appropriate means of identification, such as checking the identification bracelet and/or asking clients to state their names.
- Do not leave medication at the bedside, with certain exceptions (eg, nitroglycerin, cough syrup). Determine agency policy.
- If a client vomits after taking an oral medication, report this to the nurse in charge and/or physician.
- Take special precautions when administering certain medications; for example, have another nurse check the dosages of anticoagulants, insulin, and certain IV preparations.
- Most hospital policies require new orders from the physician for the client's postsurgery care.
- When a medication is omitted for any reason, record the fact together with the reason.
- When a medication error is made, report it immediately to the nurse in charge and/or physician.

5. *Evaluate the client's response to the drug.* The kinds of behavior that reflect the action or lack of action of a drug and its untoward effects (both minor and major) are as variable as the purposes of the drugs themselves. The anxious client may show the desired effects of a tranquilizer by behavior that reflects a lowered stress level (eg, slower speech or fewer random movements). The effectiveness of a sedative can often be measured by how well a client slept; the effectiveness of an antispasmodic, by how much pain the client feels. In all nursing activities, nurses need to be aware of the medications that a client is taking and record their effectiveness as assessed by the client and the nurse on the client's chart. The nurse may also report the client's response directly to the senior nurse and physician.

See the accompanying box for the five "rights" to accurate drug administration.

DEVELOPMENTAL CONSIDERATIONS

Knowledge of growth and development is essential for the nurse administering medications to children. Oral medications for children are usually prepared in sweetened liquid form to make them more palatable. The parents may provide suggestions about what method is best for their child. Necessary foods such as milk or orange juice should not be used to mask the taste of medications, because the child may develop unpleasant associations and refuse that food in the future.

Children tend to fear any procedure in which a needle is used because they anticipate pain or because the procedure is unfamiliar and threatening. The nurse needs to acknowledge that the child will feel some pain; denying this fact only deepens the child's distrust. After the injection, the nurse (or the parent) can cuddle and speak softly to the infant and give the child a toy to dispel the child's association of the nurse only with pain.

An older person can present special problems, most of which are related to physiologic changes, to past experiences, and to established attitudes toward medications. The physiologic changes in elderly persons that may affect the administration and effectiveness of medications are included in the box on page 1312.

Many of these changes enhance the possibility of cumulative effects and toxicity. For example, impaired circulation delays the action of medications given intramuscularly or subcutaneously. Digitalis, which is frequently taken by elderly people, can accumulate to toxic levels and be lethal. It is not uncommon for elderly clients to take several different medications daily. The possibility of error increases with the number of medications taken, whether self-administered at home or administered by nurses in a hospital. The greater number of medications also compounds the problem of drug interactions, because much is yet to be learned about the effects of drugs given in combinations. A general rule to follow is that elderly clients should take as few medications as possible.

Elderly persons usually require smaller dosages of drugs, especially sedatives and other central nervous system depressants. Reactions of the elderly to medications,

FIVE "RIGHTS" OF DRUG ADMINISTRATION

- Right drug
- Right dose
- Right time
- Right route
- Right client

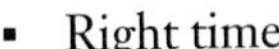

Physiologic Changes Associated with Aging that Influence Medication Administration and Effectiveness

- Altered memory
- Less acute vision
- Decrease in renal function, resulting in slower elimination of drugs and higher drug concentrations in the bloodstream for longer periods
- Less complete and slower absorption from the gastrointestinal tract
- Increased proportion of fat to lean body mass, which facilitates retention of fat-soluble drugs and increases potential for toxicity
- Decreased liver function, which hinders biotransformation of drugs
- Decreased organ sensitivity, which means that the response to the same drug concentration in the vicinity of the target organ is less in older people than in the young
- Altered quality of organ responsiveness, resulting in adverse effects becoming pronounced before therapeutic effects are achieved.

particularly sedatives, are unpredictable and often bizarre. It is not uncommon to see irritability, confusion, disorientation, restlessness, and incontinence as a result of sedatives. Nurses therefore need to observe clients carefully for untoward reactions. The use of alcohol (eg, brandy) as a bedtime relaxant and as an appetizer before meals is becoming more common. The moderate use of alcohol by people who are accustomed to it can contribute to a sense of well-being.

Attitudes of elderly people toward medical care and medications vary. Elderly people tend to believe in the wisdom of the physician more readily than younger people. Some older people are bewildered by the prescription of several medications and may passively accept their medications from nurses but not swallow them, spitting out tablets or capsules after the nurse leaves the room. For this reason, the nurse is advised to stay with clients until they have taken the medications. Others may be suspicious of medications and actively refuse them.

Elderly people are mature adults capable of reasoning. Therefore, the nurse needs to explain the reasons for and effects of medications. This education can prevent clients from taking a medication long after there is a need for it or discontinuing a drug too quickly. For example, clients should know that diuretics will cause them to urinate more frequently and may reduce ankle edema. Instructions about medications need to be given to all clients prior to discharge from a hospital. These instructions should include when to take the drugs, what effects to expect, and when to consult a physician.

Because some clients are required to take several medications daily and because visual acuity and memory may be impaired, the nurse needs to develop simple, realistic plans for clients to follow at home. For example, remembering to take drugs can be difficult for most persons, including the elderly. If medications are scheduled to be taken with meals or at bedtime, clients are not as likely to forget. Some clients may take their medications and then an hour later not remember whether they took them. One solution to forgetfulness is to use a special container or glass strictly for medications. An empty glass or container indicates that the person took the pills. Loss of visual acuity presents problems that can be overcome by writing out the plan in block letters large enough to be read. In some situations the help of a spouse, son, or daughter can be enlisted.

Medication History

The medication history includes information about the drugs the client is taking currently or has taken recently. This includes prescription drugs, over-the-counter drugs such as antacids, alcohol and tobacco, and nonsanctioned drugs such as marijuana. Sometimes one or more of these drugs may affect the choice of another, different medication, since they may be incompatible.

An important part of the history is clients' knowledge of their drug allergies. Some clients can tell a nurse, "I am allergic to penicillin, adhesive tape, and curry." Other clients may not be sure about allergic reactions. An illness occurring after a drug was taken may not be identified as an allergy, but the client may associate the drug with an illness or unusual reaction. The client's physician can often give information about allergies. During the history, the nurse tries to elicit information about drug dependencies. The frequency with which drugs are taken and the client's perceived need for them are measures of dependence.

Also included in the history are the client's normal eating habits. Sometimes the medication schedule needs to be coordinated with mealtimes or the ingestion of foods. Where a medication must be taken with food on a specified schedule, clients can often adjust their mealtime or have a snack (eg, with a bedtime medication). In addition, certain foods are incompatible with certain medications; for example, milk is incompatible with tetracycline.

Any problems the client may have in self-administering a medication must also be identified. A client with poor eyesight, for example, may require special labels for the medication container; elderly clients with unsteady hands may not be able to hold a syringe or to inject themselves or another person.

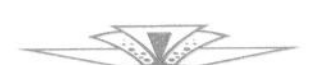

ORAL MEDICATIONS

The oral route is the most common route by which medications are given. As long as a client can swallow and retain the drug in the stomach, this is the route of choice. See Procedure 43–1. Oral medications are contraindicated when a client is vomiting, has gastric or intestinal suction, or is unconscious and unable to swallow. Such clients in a hospital usually are on orders "nothing by mouth" (NPO).

PARENTERAL MEDICATIONS

Parenteral medications are given intradermally, subcutaneously, intramuscularly, or intravenously. Because these medications are absorbed more quickly than oral medications and are irretrievable once injected, the nurse must prepare and administer them carefully and accurately. Administering parenteral drugs requires the same nursing knowledge as for oral and topical drugs, plus considerable manual dexterity and the use of sterile technique.

Text continued on page 1316

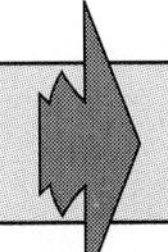

PROCEDURE 43–1 ADMINISTERING ORAL MEDICATIONS

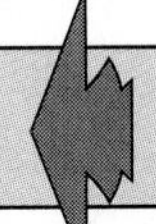

PURPOSE

- To provide a medication that has systemic effects and/or local effects on the gastrointestinal tract (see specific drug action)

ASSESSMENT FOCUS

Allergies to medication(s); client's ability to swallow the medication; presence of vomiting or diarrhea that would interfere with the ability to absorb the medication; specific drug action; side effects and adverse reactions; client's knowledge of and learning needs about the medication.

EQUIPMENT

- ☐ Medication tray or cart
- ☐ Disposable medication cups: small paper or plastic cups for tablets and capsules, waxed or plastic calibrated medication cups for liquids
- ☐ Medication administration record (MAR) or computer printout
- ☐ Pill crusher
  or
  Syringe of appropriate size for child's mouth and medication amount
- ☐ Straws to administer medications that may discolor the teeth or to facilitate the ingestion of liquid medication for certain clients

INTERVENTION

1. Organize the supplies.

- Assemble the medication tray and cups in the medicine room, or place the medication cart outside the client's room.
- Assemble the medication cards or records for each client together so that medications can be prepared for one client at a time. *Organization of supplies saves time and reduces the chance of error.*

2. Verify the client's ability to take medication orally.

- Determine whether the client can swallow, is on NPO, is nauseated or vomiting, has gastric suction, or has diminished or absent bowel sounds.

3. Verify the order for accuracy.

- Check the accuracy of the MAR, or printout with the physician's written order. It should contain the following information: (a) client's name, (b) drug name and dosage, (c) time for administration, and (d) route of administration.
- Check the expiration date.
- Report any discrepancies in the order to the nurse in charge or the physician, as agency policy dictates.

4. Obtain appropriate medication.

- Read the MAR, and take the appropriate medication from the

PROCEDURE 43-1 ADMINISTERING ORAL MEDICATIONS *continued*

shelf, drawer, or refrigerator. The medication may be dispensed in the bottle, box, or unit-dose package.

- Compare the label of the medication container or unit-dose package against the order on the MAR. If these are not identical, recheck the client's chart. If there is still a discrepancy, check with the nurse in charge and/or the pharmacist.

5. Prepare the medication.

- Prepare the correct amount of medication for the required dose, without contaminating the medication. *Aseptic technique maintains drug cleanliness.*

- While preparing the medication, recheck each MAR with the prepared drug and container. *This second check reduces the chance of error.*

Tablets or Capsules from a Bottle

- Pour the required number into the bottle cap, and then transfer the medication to the disposable cup without touching the tablets (Figure 43–8). Usually, all tablets or capsules to be given to the client are placed in the same cup.
- Keep medications that require specific assessments, such as pulse measurements, respiratory rate or depth, or blood pressure, separate from the others. *This enables the nurse to withhold the medication if indicated.*

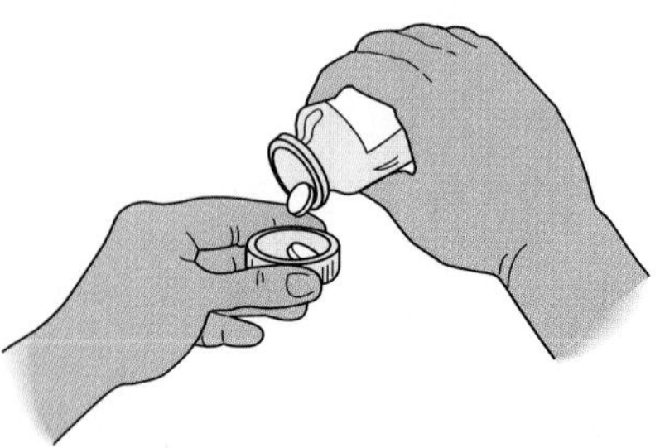

Figure 43–8 Pouring a tablet into the container lid.

- If the client has difficulty swallowing, crush the tablets to a fine powder with a pill crusher or between two medication cups or spoons. Then, mix the powder with a small amount of soft food (eg, custard, applesauce). *Note:* Check with pharmacy before crushing tablets. Sustained-action, enteric-coated, buccal, or sublingual tablets should not be crushed.

Liquid Medication

- Remove the cap, and place it upside down on the countertop to avoid contaminating it.
- Hold the bottle with the label next to your palm, and pour the medication away from the label (Figure 43–9). *This prevents the label from becoming soiled and illegible as a result of spilled liquids.*

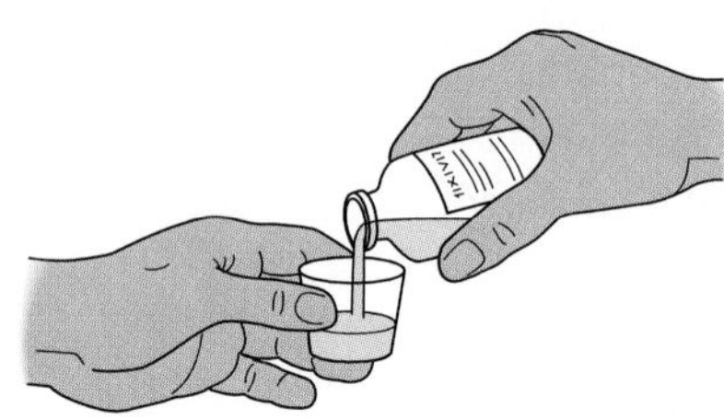

Figure 43–9 Pouring a liquid medication from a bottle.

- Hold the medication cup at eye level, and fill it to the desired level, using the bottom of the **meniscus** (crescent-shaped upper surface of a column of liquid) as the measurement guide (Figure 43–10). *This method ensures accuracy of measurement.*
- Before capping the bottle, wipe the lip with a paper towel. *This prevents the cap from sticking.*

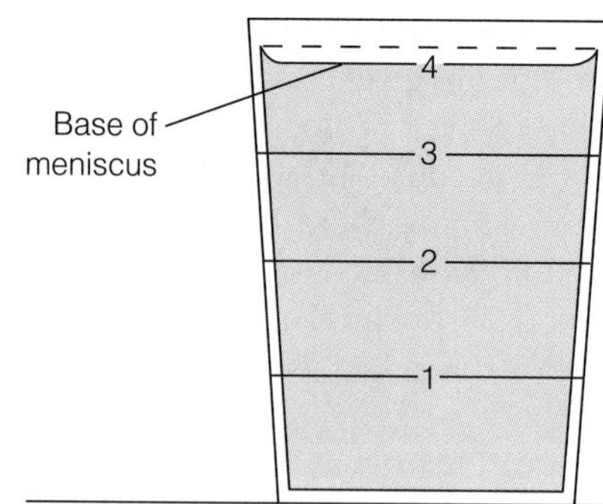

Figure 43–10 The bottom of the meniscus is the measuring guide.

Oral Narcotics

- If an agency uses a manual recording system for controlled substances, check the narcotic record for the previous drug count, and compare it with the supply available. Some medications including narcotics are kept in plastic containers that are sectioned and numbered (Figure 43–11).

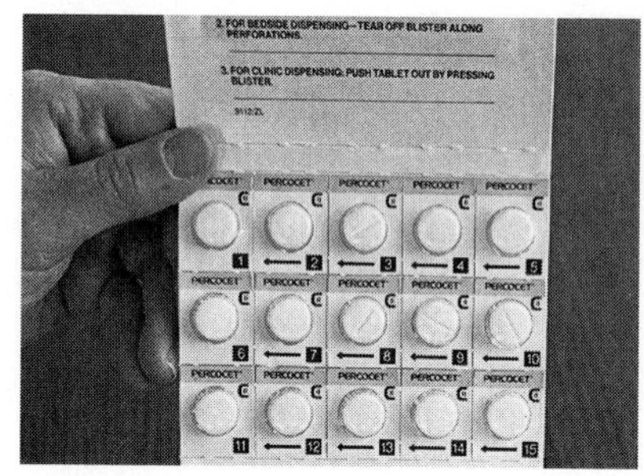

Figure 43–11 Commercially packaged controlled substances.

- Remove the next available tablet, and drop it in the medicine cup.
- After removing a tablet, record the necessary information on the appropriate narcotic control record, and sign it.

Note: Computer-controlled dispensing systems allow access only to the selected drug and automatically record its use.

PROCEDURE 43–1 *continued*

Unit-Dose Medication

- Place the *unwrapped* unit-dose medications directly into the medicine cup. *The wrapper keeps the medication clean and facilitates identification.*

All Medications

- Place the prepared medication and MAR together on the tray or cart.

- Return the bottle, box, or envelope to its storage place, and recheck the label on the container. *This third check further reduces the risk of error.*

- Avoid leaving prepared medications unattended. *Accidental disarrangement of the medication could occur.*

6. Administer the medication at the correct time.

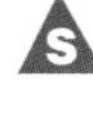

- Identify the client by comparing the name on the medication record or list with the name on the client's identification bracelet and by asking the client's name. *Accurate identification is essential to prevent error.*
- Explain the purpose of the medication and how it will help, using language that the client can understand. Include relevant information about effects; for example, tell the client receiving a diuretic to expect an increase in urine. *Information facilitates acceptance of and compliance with the therapy.*

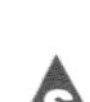

- Assist the client to a sitting position or, if not possible, to a lateral position. *These positions facilitate swallowing and prevent aspiration.*
- Take the required assessment measures, such as pulse and respiratory rates or blood pressure. Take the apical pulse rate before administering digitalis preparations. Take blood pressure before giving hypotensive drugs. Take the respiratory rate prior to administering narcotics. *Narcotics depress the respiratory center.* If any of the findings are above or below the predetermined parameters, consult the physician before administering the medication.
- Give the client sufficient water or preferred juice to swallow the medication. *Fluids ease swallowing and facilitate absorption from the gastrointestinal tract.* Liquid medications other than antacids or cough preparations are generally diluted with 15 mL (½ oz) of water to facilitate absorption.
- If the client is unable to hold the pill cup, use the pill cup to introduce the medication into the client's mouth, and give only one tablet or capsule at a time. *Putting the cup to the client's mouth maintains the cleanliness of the nurse's hands. Giving one medication at a time eases swallowing.*
- If an older child or adult has difficulty swallowing, ask the client to place the medication on the back of the tongue before taking the water. *Stimulation of the back of the tongue produces the swallowing reflex.*
- If the medication has an objectionable taste, ask the client to suck a few ice chips beforehand, or give the medication with juice, applesauce, or bread. *The cold will desensitize the taste buds, and juices or bread can mask the taste of the medication.*
- If the client says that the medication you are about to give is different from what the client has been receiving, do not give the medication without checking the original order. Most clients are familiar with the appearance of medications taken previously. *Unfamiliar drugs may signal a possible error.*
- Stay with the client until all medications have been swallowed. *The nurse must see the client swallow the medication before the drug administration can be recorded.* A physician's order or agency policy is required for medications left at the bedside.

7. Document each medication given.

- Record the medication given, dosage, time, any complaints or assessments of the client, and your signature.
- If medication was refused or omitted, record this fact on the appropriate record; document the reason, when possible, and the nurse's actions.

8. Dispose of all supplies appropriately.

- Return the medication records to the appropriate file for the next administration time.
- Replenish stock (eg, medication cups) and return cart to medicine room.
- Discard used disposable supplies.

9. Evaluate the effects of the medication.

- Return to the client when the medication is expected to take effect (usually 30 minutes) to evaluate the effects of the medication on the client.

Variation: Giving Oral Medications to Infants and Children

- Select an appropriate vehicle to measure and administer the medication, for example, plastic disposable cup, plastic syringe

PROCEDURE 43-1 ADMINISTERING ORAL MEDICATIONS *continued*

without needle, or tuberculin syringe (see page p. 1317). For young infants, a plastic syringe is usually used. For older infants who can drink from a cup, a medicine cup can be used.

- Dilute the oral medication, if indicated, with a *small* amount of water. *Many oral medications are readily swallowed if they are diluted with a small amount of water. If large quantities of water are used, the child may refuse to drink the entire amount and receive only a portion of the medication.*
- Crush medications not supplied in liquid form and mix them with substances available on most pediatric units, such as honey, flavored syrup, jam, or a fruit puree. Note: When selecting a substance to mix with a medication, *avoid essential food items* such as milk, cereal, and orange juice. *If essential food items are used, the child may become intolerant of them and refuse these foods in the diet.*

- Disguise disagreeable-tasting medications with sweet-tasting substances mentioned above. However, present any altered medication to the child honestly and not as a food or treat.
- To prevent nausea, pour a carbonated beverage over finely crushed ice and give it before or immediately after the medication is administered.
- To prevent aspiration and choking, position infants in a semireclining position, and administer the medication slowly in divided doses by spoon or a plastic syringe.
- If using a spoon, retrieve and refeed medication that is thrust outward by the infant's tongue.
- If using a syringe, place it along the side of the infant's tongue. *This position prevents gagging and expulsion of the medication.*
- A child's parents or guardians may be able to provide valuable information on how best to give the child medications. However, a nurse may need to partially restrain a child who refuses to cooperate or consistently resists despite explanation, encouragement, and attempts to determine the reason for the behavior.
  a. Place the child in your lap with the right arm behind you.
  b. Grasp the child's left hand firmly by your left hand.
  c. Secure the head between your arm and body.
- Follow all medication with a drink of water, juice, a soft drink, or a Popsicle or frozen juice bar. *This removes any unpleasant aftertaste.*
- For children who take sweetened medications on a long term basis, follow the medication administration with oral hygiene. *These children are at high risk for dental caries.*

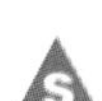

EVALUATION FOCUS
Desired effect (eg, relief of pain or decrease in body temperature); any adverse effects or side effects (eg, nausea, vomiting, skin rash, change in vital signs).

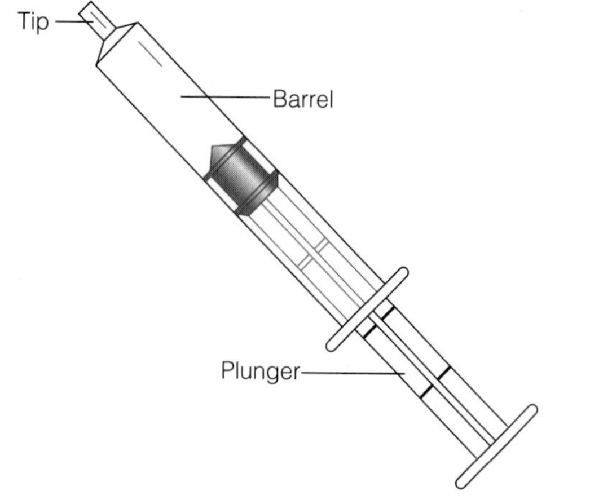

Figure 43–12 The three parts of a syringe.

EQUIPMENT

Syringes To administer parenteral medications, nurses use injectable equipment (ie, syringes, needles, vials, and ampules). Syringes have three parts: the tip, which connects with the needle; the barrel, or outside part, on which the scales are printed; and the plunger, which fits inside the barrel (Figure 43–12). When handling a syringe, the nurse may touch the outside of the barrel and the handle of the plunger; however, the nurse must avoid letting any unsterile object contact the tip or inside of the barrel, the shaft of the plunger, or the shaft or tip of the needle. Most syringes used today are made of plastic and are individually packaged for sterility in a paper wrapper or a rigid

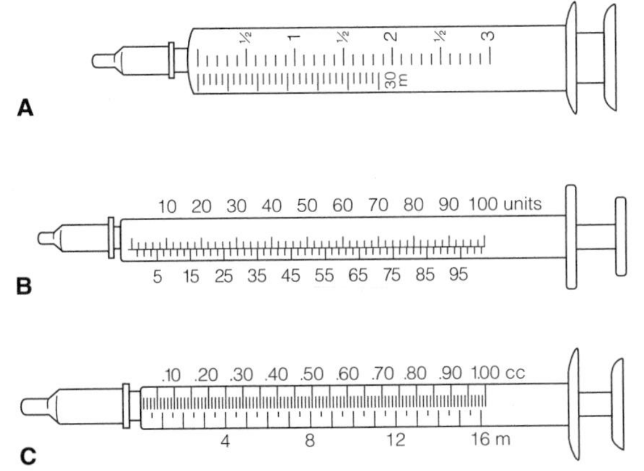

Figure 43–13 Three kinds of syringes: *A,* hypodermic; *B,* insulin; *C,* tuberculin.

plastic container. Glass syringes are used when the medication is incompatible with plastic.

There are several kinds of syringes, differing in size, shape, and material. The three most commonly used types are the standard hypodermic syringe, the insulin syringe, and the tuberculin syringe (Figure 43–13). *Hypodermic syringes* come in 2-, 2.5-, and 3-mL sizes. They usually have two scales marked on them: the minim and the milliliter. The milliliter scale is the one normally used; the minim scale is used for very small dosages.

Insulin syringes are similar to hypodermic syringes, but they have a scale specially designed for insulin: a 100-unit calibrated scale intended for use with U-100 insulin. Several low-dose insulin syringes are also available and frequently have a nonremovable needle. All insulin syringes are calibrated on the 100-unit scale. The correct choice of syringe is based on the amount of insulin required.

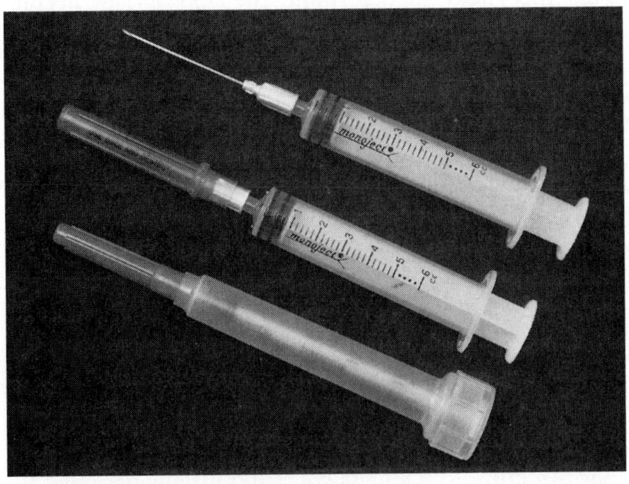

Figure 43–14 Disposable plastic syringes and needles: *top,* with syringe and needle exposed; *middle,* with plastic cup over the needle; *bottom,* with plastic case over the needle and syringe.

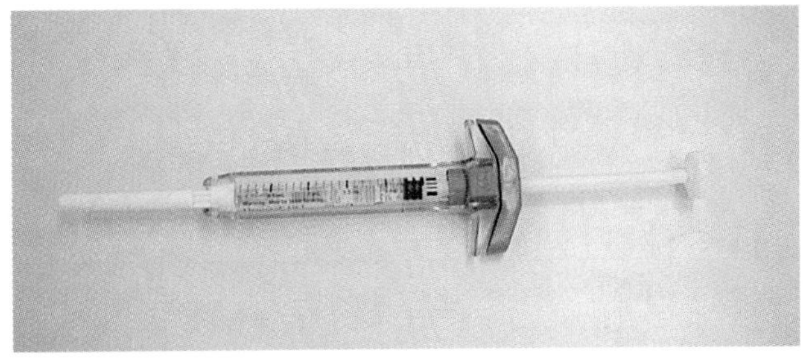

Figure 43–15 A cartridge holder and prefilled medication cartridge with needle.

The *tuberculin syringe* was originally designed to administer tuberculin. It is a narrow syringe, calibrated in tenths and hundredths of a milliliter (up to 1 mL) on one scale and in sixteenths of a minim (up to 1 minim) on the other scale. This type of syringe can also be useful in administering other drugs, particularly when small or precise measurement is indicated (eg, pediatric dosages). Syringes are made in other sizes as well, for example, 5, 10, 20, and 50 mL. These are not generally used to administer drugs directly but can be useful for adding medications to intravenous solutions or for irrigating wounds.

The *disposable plastic syringe* (Figure 43–14) is most frequently used today. The syringe is supplied with a needle, which may have a plastic cap over it. The syringe and needle may be packaged together or separately.

Injectable medications are frequently supplied in *prefilled unit-dose syringes* with needles or cartridge-needle units (Figure 43–15). These prefilled syringes and cartridge-needle units are disposable. The cartridge-needle units, however, require special metal or plastic cartridge holders or syringes for administration. These syringes and cartridges come with manufacturer's directions for use.

Needles Needles are made of stainless steel, and most are disposable. Reusable needles (eg, for special procedures) need to be sharpened periodically before resterilization, because the points become dull with use and are occasionally damaged or acquire burrs on the tips. A dull or damaged needle should *never* be used.

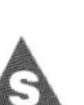

A needle has three discernible parts: the hub, which fits onto the syringe; the cannula, or shaft, which is attached to the hub; and the bevel, which is the slanted part at the tip of the needle (Figure 43–16, p. 1318). A disposable needle has a plastic hub. Needles used for injections have three variable characteristics:

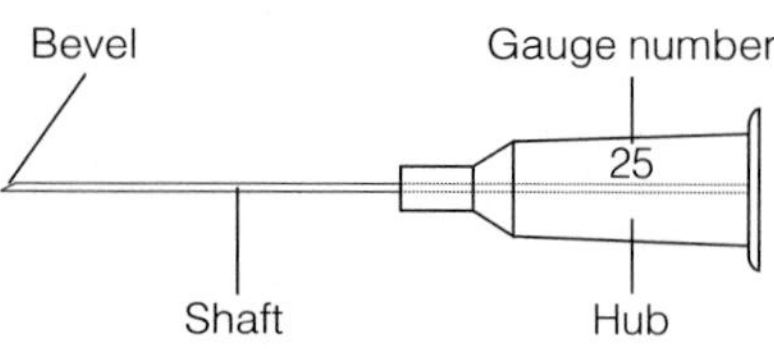

Figure 43–16 The parts of a needle.

1. *Slant or length of the bevel.* The bevel of the needle may be short or long. Longer bevels provide the sharpest needles and cause less discomfort and are commonly used for subcutaneous and intramuscular injections. Short bevels are used for intradermal and intravenous injections, because a long bevel can become occluded if it rests against the side of a blood vessel.
2. *Length of the shaft.* The shaft length of commonly used needles varies from ¼ to 5 inches. The appropriate needle length is chosen according to the client's muscle development, the client's weight, and the type of injection.
3. *Gauge (or diameter) of the shaft.* The gauge varies from #14 to #28. The larger the gauge number, the smaller the diameter of the shaft. Smaller gauges produce less tissue trauma, but larger gauges are necessary for viscous medications, such as penicillin.

For an adult requiring a subcutaneous injection, it is usual to use a needle of #24 to #26 gauge and ⅜ to ⅝ in long. Obese clients may require a 1-in needle. For intramuscular injections, a longer needle (eg, 1 to 1½ in) with a larger gauge (eg, gauge #20 to #22) is used. Slender adults and children usually require a shorter needle. The nurse must assess the client to determine the appropriate needle length.

AVOIDING PUNCTURE INJURIES

- Use appropriate sharps disposal containers. DO NOT throw sharps into wastebaskets.
- Contaminated sharps must not be purposely bent, broken, sheared, resheathed, or removed from disposable syringes by hand unless agency can demonstrate that no alternative is feasible or that failure to do so is required by the medical procedure (ie, procedures such as obtaining blood cultures or blood gases).
- If needles must be recapped or removed, a safety mechanical device or a one-handed technique should be used.
- Sharps or any items that can cut or puncture skin include:
  - Needles
  - Surgical blades
  - Lancets
  - Razors
  - Broken glass
  - Broken capillary pipettes
  - Exposed dental wires
  - Reusable items (eg, large bore needles, hooks, rasps, drill points)
  - ANY SHARP INSTRUMENT!
- Remember that all of the work practice controls must be used consistently to ensure safety.

Source: LM Bruning. The bloodborne pathogens final rule: Understanding the regulation. *AORN Journal* February 1993, 57:437, 439, 441+.

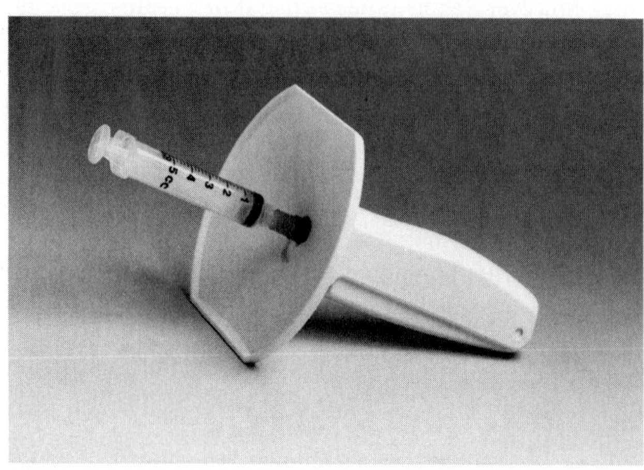

Figure 43–17 A device to prevent accidental needle sticks.

Needle Recappers New devices, such as the On • Gard Recapper™ (Figure 43–17), allow the nurse to uncap and recap any needle safely and effectively, without changing current technique or needle brand. To use the On • Gard Recapper, the nurse inserts the entire syringe in the center hole of the shield. The Recapper firmly grips the needle cap and holds it in place until it is ready to recap. See methods for preventing puncture injuries in the box above.

Ampules and Vials *Ampules* and *vials* (Figure 43–18) are frequently used to package sterile parenteral medications. An **ampule** is a glass container usually designed to hold a single dose of a drug. It is made of clear glass and has a distinctive shape with a constricted neck. A **vial** is a small glass bottle with a sealed rubber cap. Most ampule necks have colored marks around them, indicating where

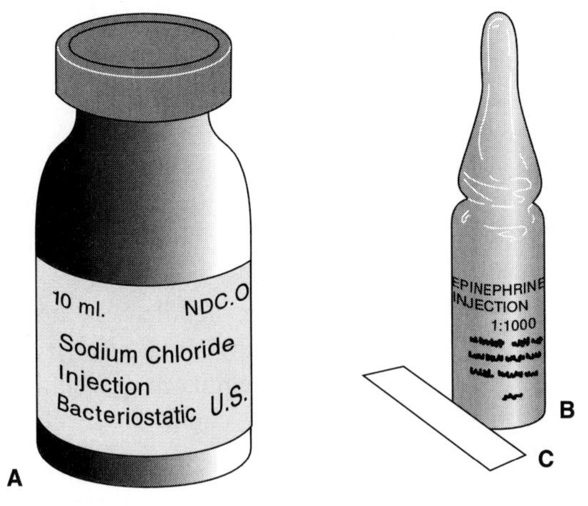

Figure 43–18 *A,* vial; *B,* ampule; *C,* ampule file.

they are prescored for easy opening. If the neck is not scored, it should be filed with a small file, then broken off at the neck. Vials come in different sizes, from single to multidose vials. They usually have a metal or plastic cap that protects the rubber seal.

Several drugs (eg, penicillin) are dispensed as powders in vials. A liquid (solvent or diluent) must be added to a powdered medication before it can be injected. The technique of adding a solvent to a powdered drug to prepare it for administration is called **reconstitution.** Powdered drugs usually have printed instructions (enclosed with each packaged vial) that describe the amount and kind of solvent to be added. Commonly used solvents are sterile water or sterile normal saline. Some preparations are supplied in individual-dose vials; others come in multidose vials. The following are two examples of the preparation of powdered drugs:

1. *Single-dose vial:* Instructions for preparing a single-dose vial direct that 1.5 mL of sterile water be added to the sterile dry powder, thus providing a single dose of 2 mL. The volume of the drug powder was 0.5 mL. Therefore, the 1.5 mL of water plus the 0.5 mL of powder results in 2 mL of solution. In other instances, the addition of a solution does *not* increase the volume. Therefore, it is important to follow the manufacturers' directions.
2. *Multidose vial:* A dose of 750 mg of a certain drug is ordered for a client. On hand is a 10-g multidose vial. The directions for preparation read: "Add 8.5 mL of sterile water, and each milliliter will contain 1.0 g or 1000 mg." To determine the amount to inject, the nurse calculates as follows:

$$1 \text{ mL} = 1000 \text{ mg}$$

$$x \text{ mL} = 750 \text{ mg}$$

(cross multiply)

$$x = \frac{750 \times 1}{1000}$$

$$x = 0.75$$

The nurse will give 0.75 mL of the medication.

Procedure 43–2 describes how to prepare medications from ampules and vials.

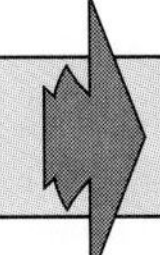

Procedure 43–2 Preparing Medications from Ampules and Vials

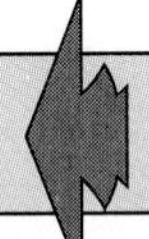

Equipment

- ☐ MAR or computer printout
- ☐ Vial or ampule of sterile medication
- ☐ File (if ampule is not scored) and small gauze square
- ☐ Antiseptic wipe
- ☐ Needle and syringe
- ☐ Special filter needle (optional) for withdrawing premixed liquid medications from multidose vials or for filtering out glass slivers from ampules
- ☐ Sterile water or normal saline, if drug is in powdered form

Intervention

1. Ensure the accuracy of the order and drug administration.

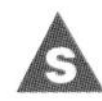

- Check the label on the ampule or vial carefully against the MAR or client's chart to make sure that the correct medication is being prepared.
- Check the expiration date. Follow the three checks for administering medications. Read the label on the medication (a) before it is taken off the shelf, (b) before withdrawing the medication, and (c) after placing it back on the shelf.

2. Prepare the medication ampule or vial for drug withdrawal.

PROCEDURE 43–2 PREPARING MEDICATIONS FROM AMPULES AND VIALS *continued*

Ampules

- Flick the upper stem of the ampule several times with a fingernail or, holding the upper stem of the ampule, make a large circle with the arm extended. *This will bring all the medication down to the main portion of the ampule.*
- Partially file the neck of the ampule, if necessary, to start a clean break.
- Place a piece of sterile gauze between your thumb and the ampule neck or around the ampule neck, and break off the top by bending it toward you (Figure 43–19). *The sterile gauze protects the fingers from the broken glass and any glass fragments will spray away from the nurse.*
  or
  Place the antiseptic wipe packet over the top of the ampule before breaking off the top. *This method ensures that all the glass fragments fall into the packet and reduces the risk of cuts.*
- Dispose of the top of the ampule in the sharps container.

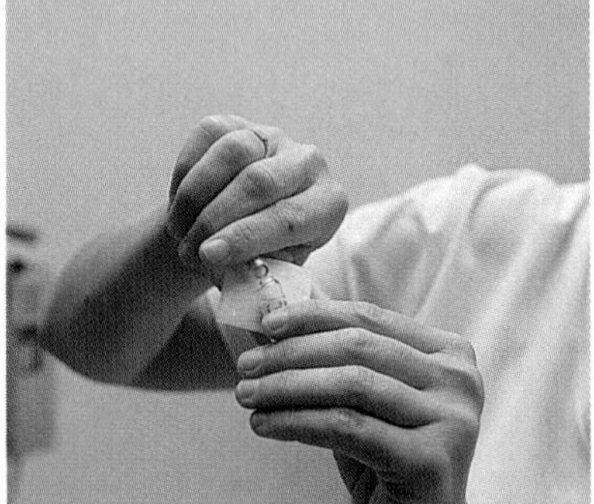

Figure 43–19 Breaking the neck of an ampule.

Vials

- Mix the solution, if necessary, by rotating the vial between the palms of the hands, not by shaking. *Some vials contain aqueous suspensions, which settle when they stand. In some instances shaking is contraindicated because it may cause the mixture to foam.*
- Remove the protective metal cap, and clean the rubber cap with an antiseptic wipe, by rubbing in a circular motion. *The antiseptic cleans the cap so that the needle will remain sterile when it is inserted.*

3. Withdraw the medication.

Ampules

- Some nurses recommend using a needle with a filter to withdraw the medication in case there is any broken glass from the ampule in the medication. In this case, disconnect the regular needle, leaving its cap on, and attach the filter needle to the syringe.
- Remove the cap from the needle, and insert the needle into the ampule. Either hold the ampule with the bottom higher than the top or place it on a flat surface. Insert the needle into the center of the ampule. Do not touch the rim of the ampule with the needle tip or shaft. *This will keep the needle sterile.* Withdraw the amount of drug required for the dosage (Figure 43–20).

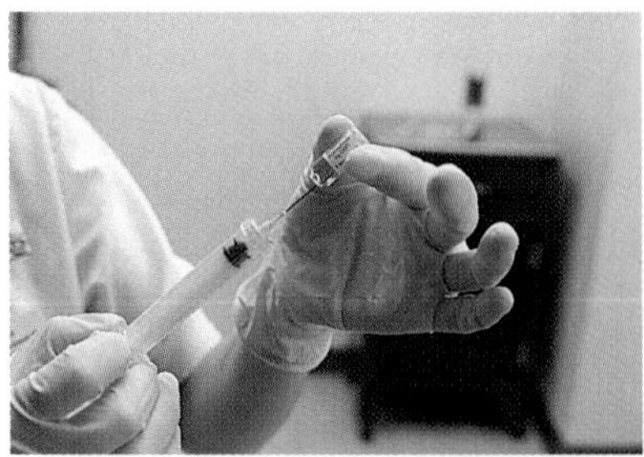

Figure 43–20 Withdrawing a medication from an ampule.

- With a single-dose ampule, hold the ampule slightly on its side, if necessary, to obtain all the medication.
- If a filter needle was used to withdraw the medication, replace it with a regular needle before injecting the client.
- If a filter needle was not used, recap the needle and tighten the cap at the hub of the needle.

Vials

- Attach a special filter needle as agency practice dictates to draw up premixed liquid medications from multidose vials. *The filter prevents any solid material from being drawn up through the needle.*
- Remove the cap from the needle; then draw up into the syringe the amount of air equal to the volume of the medication to be withdrawn.
- Carefully insert the needle into the upright vial through the center of the rubber cap, maintaining the sterility of the needle.
- Inject the air into the vial, keeping the bevel of the needle above the surface of the medication (Figure 43–21). *The air will allow the medication to be drawn out easily, because negative pressure is not created inside the vial. The bevel is kept above the medication to avoid creating bubbles in the medication.*
- Invert the vial to withdraw medication, and hold it vertically at eye level to determine the correct dosage of the drug into the syringe (Figure 43–22). *Holding the vial in a vertical position at eye level ensures correct measurement.*
- If necessary, tap the syringe barrel to dislodge any air bubbles present in the syringe. *The tapping motion will cause the air bubbles to rise to the top of the syringe.*

PROCEDURE 43–2 *continued*

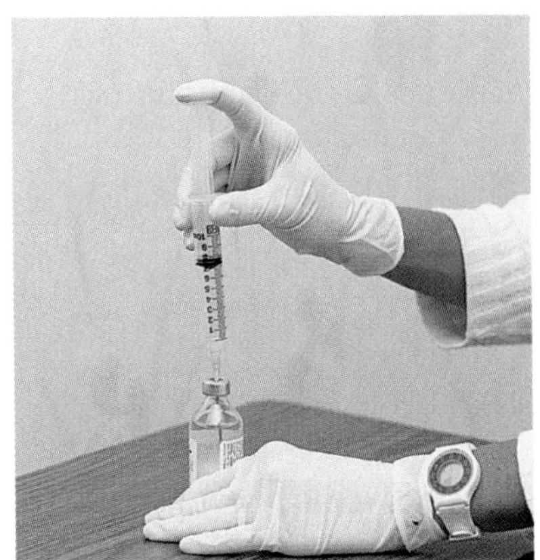

Figure 43–21 Injecting air into a vial.

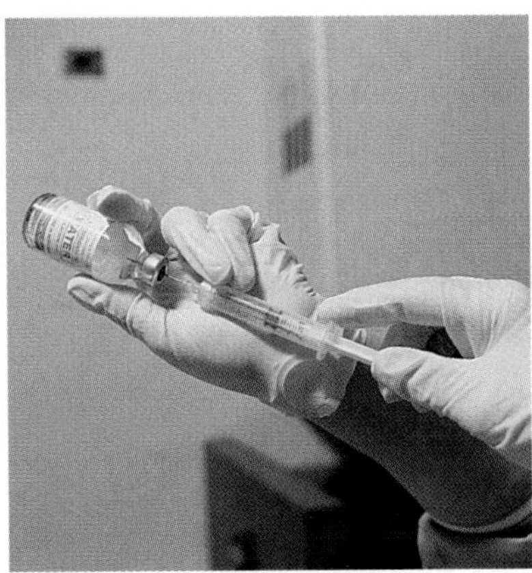

Figure 43–22 Withdrawing a medication from a vial.

This air can be ejected into the vial.

- When the correct volume of medication is obtained, withdraw the needle from the vial, and replace the cap over the needle, thus maintaining its sterility.
  or
  Replace the filter needle with the regular needle.

Variation: Preparing Powdered Drugs

- Read the manufacturer's directions.
- Withdraw an equivalent amount of air from the vial before adding the solvent, unless otherwise indicated by the directions.
- Add the amount of sterile water or saline indicated in the directions.
- If a multidose vial is reconstituted, label the vial with the date, time it was prepared, the amount of drug contained in each milliliter of solution, and your initials. *Time is an important factor to consider in the expiration of these medications.*
- Once reconstituted, store the medication in the vial in a refrigerator or as recommended by the manufacturer.

MIXING MEDICATIONS IN ONE SYRINGE

Frequently, clients need more than one drug injected at the same time. To spare the client the experience of being injected twice, two drugs (if compatible) are often mixed together in one syringe and given as one injection. It is common, for instance, to combine two types of insulin in this manner or to combine injectable preoperative medications such as morphine or meperidine (Demerol) with atropine or scopolamine. Drugs can also be mixed in intravenous solutions. When uncertain about drug compatibilities, the nurse should consult a pharmacist or check a compatibility chart before mixing the drugs.

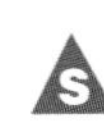

The nurse must also exercise caution when mixing short- and long-acting insulins, because they vary in content. Chemically, insulin is a protein that, when hydrolyzed in the body, yields a number of amino acids. Some insulin preparations contain an additional modifying protein, such as globulin or protamine, that slows absorption. This fact is particularly relevant to mixing two insulin preparations for injection because many insulin syringes have needles that cannot be changed. A vial of insulin that does *not* have the added protein should never be contaminated with insulin that does have the added protein. For example, a vial of regular insulin should never be entered with a needle that had been previously used to withdraw Lente, or isophane (NPH) insulins, all of which have added protein (see Figure 43–23, p. 1323).

Procedure 43–3 describes how to mix medications in one syringe.

INTRADERMAL INJECTIONS

An intradermal injection is the administration of a drug into the dermal layer of the skin just beneath the epidermis. Usually only a small amount of liquid is used, for example, 0.1 mL. This method of administration is frequently indicated for allergy and tuberculin tests and for vaccinations. Common sites for intradermal injections are the inner lower arm, the upper chest, and the back beneath the scapulae (Figure 43–24, p. 1323). Commonly the left arm is used for tuberculin tests and the right arm is used for all other tests.

The equipment normally used is a 1-mL syringe calibrated into hundredths of a milliliter. The needle is short

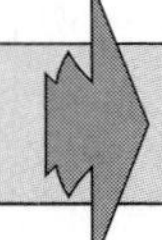

Procedure 43–3 Mixing Medications Using One Syringe

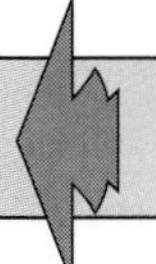

Equipment

- ☐ Computer printout or chart
- ☐ Two vials of medication, or one vial and one ampule, or two ampules, or one vial and one cartridge
- ☐ Sterile antiseptic-soaked swabs
- ☐ Sterile hypodermic or insulin syringe and needle (if insulin is being given, use a small-gauge hypodermic needle, eg, #26 gauge).
- ☐ Additional sterile subcutaneous or intramuscular needle (optional)

INTERVENTION

1. Verify the order for accuracy.

- Check the label on the ampule or vial carefully against the MAR or client's chart to make sure that the correct medication is being prepared.

- Follow the three checks for administering medications. Read the label on the medication (a) before it is taken off the shelf, (b) before withdrawing the medication, and (c) after placing it back on the shelf.
- Before preparing and combining the medications, ensure that the total volume of the injection is appropriate for the injection site.

2. Prepare the medication ampule or vial for drug withdrawal.

- See Procedure 43–2, step 2.
- Inspect the appearance of the medication for clarity. Some medications are always cloudy. *Preparations that have changed in appearance should be discarded.*
- If using insulin, thoroughly mix the solution in each vial prior to administration. Rotate the vials between the palms of the hands and invert the vials. *Mixing ensures an adequate concentration and thus an accurate dose. Shaking insulin vials can make the medication frothy, making precise measurement difficult.*
- Clean the tops of the vials with disinfectant swabs.

3. Withdraw the medications.

Mixing Medications from Two Vials

- Withdraw a volume of air equal to the volume of medications to be withdrawn from vials A and B.
- Inject a volume of air equal to the volume of medication to be withdrawn into vial A.
- Withdraw the needle from vial A, and inject the remaining air into vial B.
- Withdraw the required amount of medication from vial B. *The same needle is used to inject air into and withdraw medication from the second vial. It must not be contaminated with the medication in vial A.*
- Using a newly attached sterile needle, withdraw the required amount of medication from vial A. If using a syringe with a fused needle, withdraw the medication from vial A. The syringe now contains a mixture of medications from vials A and B. *With this method, neither vial is contaminated by microorganisms or by medication from the other vial.*
- See also the Variation below.

Mixing Medications from One Vial and One Ampule

- First prepare and withdraw the medication from the vial. *Ampules do not require the addition of air prior to withdrawal of the drug.*
- Then withdraw the required amount of medication from the ampule.

Mixing Medications from One Cartridge and One Vial or Ampule

- First ensure that the correct dose of the medication is in the cartridge. Discard any excess medication and air.
- Draw up the required medication from a vial or ampule into the cartridge. Note that when withdrawing medication from a vial, an equal amount of air must first be injected into the vial.
- If the total volume to be injected exceeds the capacity of the cartridge, use a syringe with sufficient capacity to withdraw the desired amount of medication from the vial/ampule, and transfer the required amount from the cartridge to the syringe.

Variation: Mixing Insulins

The following is an example of mixing 10 units of regular and 30 units of NPH insulin, which contains protamine.

- Inject 30 units of air into the NPH vial, and withdraw the needle. (There should be no insulin in the needle.) The needle

PROCEDURE 43-3 *continued*

should not touch the insulin (Figure 43–23, step 1).

- Inject 10 units of air into the Regular insulin vial, and immediately withdraw 10 units of Regular insulin (Figure 43–23, steps 2 and 3).
- Reinsert the needle into the NPH insulin vial, and withdraw 30 units of NPH insulin (Figure 43–23, step 4). (The air was previously injected into the vial.)

By using this method, you avoid adding NPH insulin to the regular insulin.

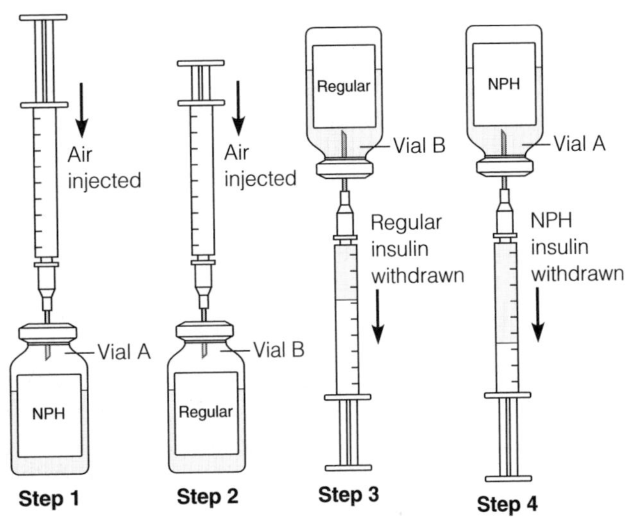

Figure 43–23 Mixing two types of insulin together.

and fine, frequently a #25, #26, or #27 gauge, ¼- to ⅝-inch long. After the site is cleaned, the skin is held tautly, and the syringe is held at about a 15-degree angle to the skin, with the bevel of the needle upward. The needle is then inserted through the epidermis into the dermis, and the fluid is injected. The drug produces a small bleb just under the skin (Figure 43–25, p. 1324). The needle is then withdrawn quickly, and the site is very lightly wiped with an antiseptic swab. The area is not massaged because the medication may disperse into the tissue or out through the needle insertion site. Intradermal injections are absorbed slowly through blood capillaries in the area.

SUBCUTANEOUS INJECTIONS

Among the many kinds of drugs administered subcutaneously are vaccines, preoperative medications, narcotics, insulin, and heparin. Common sites for subcutaneous injections are the outer aspect of the upper arms and the anterior aspect of the thighs. These areas are convenient and normally have good blood circulation. Other areas that can be used are the abdomen, the scapular areas of the upper back, and the upper ventrogluteal and dorsogluteal areas (Figure 43–26, p. 1324). Only small doses (0.5 to 1.5 mL) of medication should be injected via the subcutaneous route. Determine agency policy.

Subcutaneous injection sites need to be rotated in an orderly fashion to minimize tissue damage, aid absorption, and avoid discomfort. This is especially important for clients who must receive repeated injections, such as diabetics. The effect of rotating injection sites is actively being studied in clinical research. As the location of the injection site changes, so does the rate at which the medication is absorbed. For example, insulin is absorbed from the abdomen much more rapidly than from limb sites. To

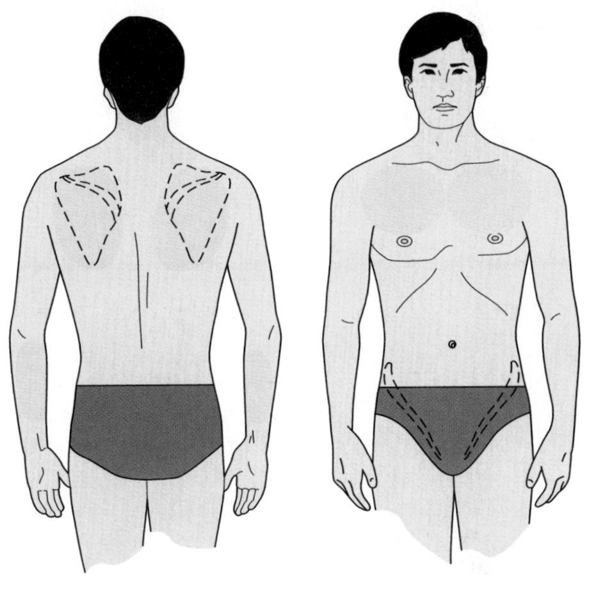

Figure 43–24 Body sites commonly used for intradermal injections.

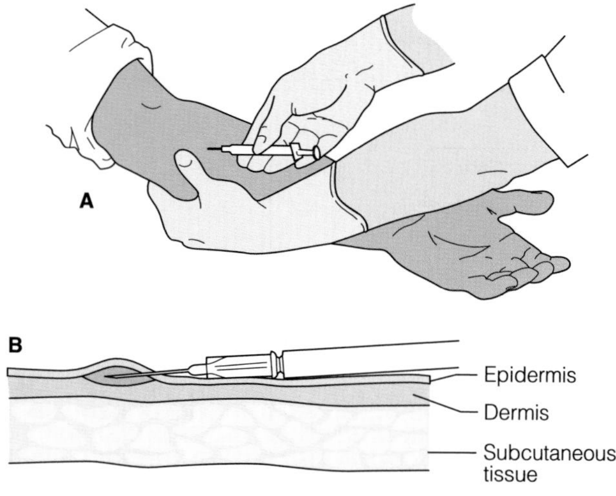

Figure 43–25 For an intradermal injection: *A*, the needle enters the skin at a 15-degree angle; and *B*, the medication forms a bleb under the epidermis.

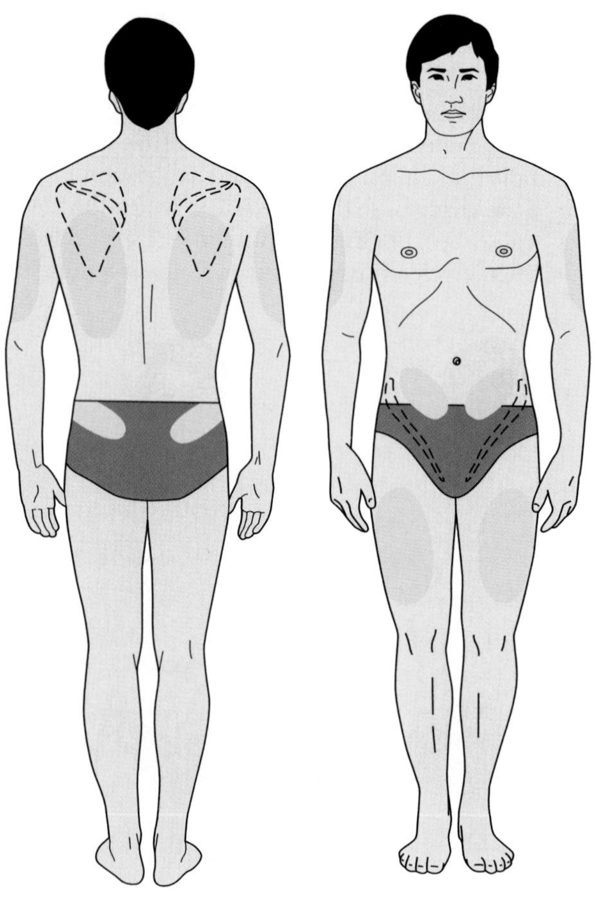

Figure 43–26 Body sites commonly used for subcutaneous injections.

maintain consistent blood glucose levels, diabetics should be encouraged to rotate sites within an injection zone. A diabetic who self-administers insulin once per day needs to learn to use one area consistently (the abdomen) and rotate sites within that injection zone. If a diabetic requires both a morning and an evening injection, the morning dose should always be injected in the same area. The site for the evening injection may differ from the morning site, but each evening injection should be administered in the same injection zone.

Generally, a 2-mL syringe and a #25 gauge needle are used for subcutaneous injections. The length of the needle depends on the amount of adipose tissue at the site and the angle used to administer the injection. Generally, a ⅝-inch needle is used for adults when the injection is administered at a 45-degree angle; a ½-inch needle is used at a 90-degree angle. Shorter needles (eg, ⅜ in) may be used for children, and longer ones (eg, 1 in) may be necessary for very obese adults. To determine the appropriate length of the needle for a 90-degree angle injection, the nurse pinches a fold of skin between the thumb and forefinger at the injection site, then measures the width of the skinfold by placing a needle that will not be used for the injection against the skin surface. The appropriate needle length is one-half the width of the skinfold (Pitel 1971, p. 78). When this method of measuring is used, the needle is inserted without pinching the skin.

The steps for administering a subcutaneous injection are described in Procedure 43–4.

INTRAMUSCULAR INJECTIONS

The intramuscular (IM) injection route is ordered for the following reasons:

- The speed of absorption by the intramuscular route is faster than by the subcutaneous route because the blood supply to the body muscles is greater.
- Muscles can usually take a larger volume of fluid without discomfort than subcutaneous tissues can, although the amount varies among individuals, chiefly with muscle size and condition. An adult of average size can usually safely tolerate up to 3 mL of medication in the large dorsogluteal or vastus lateralis muscle. As the size of the muscle decreases, the maximum amount of medication that can be safely injected also decreases.
- Medications that irritate subcutaneous tissue may safely be given by intramuscular injection.

Usually, a 2- to 5-mL syringe is needed. Some medications, such as paraldehyde, require a glass syringe because the medication interacts with plastic. The standard prepackaged intramuscular needle is 1½ inches and #21 or #22 gauge. However several factors indicate the size and length of the needle to be used: the muscle, the type

Text continued on page 1327

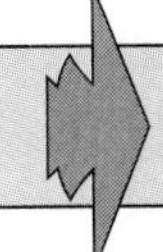

PROCEDURE 43-4 ADMINISTERING A SUBCUTANEOUS INJECTION

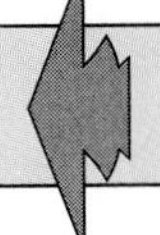

PURPOSES

- To provide a medication the client requires (see specific drug action)
- To allow slower absorption of a medication compared with either the intramuscular or intravenous route

ASSESSMENT FOCUS

Allergies to medication; specific drug action; side effects and adverse reactions; client's knowledge and learning needs about the medication; status and appearance of subcutaneous site for lesions, erythema, swelling, ecchymosis, inflammation, and tissue damage from previous injections; ability to cooperate during the injection; and previous injection sites used.

EQUIPMENT

- ☐ Client's MAR or computer printout
- ☐ Vial or ampule of the correct sterile medication
- ☐ Sterile syringe and needle (eg, 2-mL syringe, #25 gauge ⅝- or ½-in needle)
- ☐ Sterile antiseptic-soaked swabs
- ☐ Dry sterile gauze for opening an ampule (optional)
- ☐ Gloves

INTERVENTION

1. Verify the medication order for accuracy.

- See Procedure 43–2, step 1.

2. Prepare the medication from the vial or ampule.

- See Procedure 43–2, steps 2 and 3.

3. Identify the client, and assist the client to a comfortable position.

- Check the client's arm band, and ask the client's name.
- Assist the client to a position in which the arm, leg, or abdomen can be relaxed, depending on the site to be used. *A relaxed muscle at the site minimizes discomfort.*
- Obtain assistance in holding an uncooperative client or small child. *This prevents injury due to sudden movement after needle insertion.*

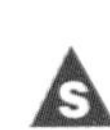

4. Select and clean the site.

- Select a site free of tenderness, hardness, swelling, scarring, itching, burning, or localized inflammation. Select a site that has not been used frequently. *These conditions could hinder the absorption of the medication and also increase the likelihood of an infection at the injection site.*
- Don gloves.
- As agency protocol indicates, clean the site with an antiseptic swab. Start at the center of the site and clean in a widening circle to about 5 cm (2 in). Allow the area to dry thoroughly. *The mechanical action of swabbing removes skin secretions, which contain microorganisms.*
- Discard the swab appropriately.

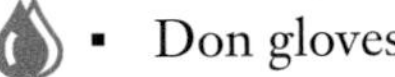

5. Prepare the syringe for injection.

- Remove the needle cap while waiting for the antiseptic to dry. Pull the cap straight off to avoid contaminating the needle by the outside edge of the cap. *The needle will become contaminated if it touches anything but the inside of the cap, which is sterile.*
- Confirm that the medication and the dosage are both correct.

6. Inject the medication.

- Grasp the syringe in your dominant hand by holding it between your thumb and fingers. With palm facing to the side or upward for a 45-degree angle insertion, or with the palm downward for a 90-degree angle insertion, prepare to inject. (Figure 43–27).
- Using the nondominant hand, pinch or spread the skin at the site, and insert the needle, using

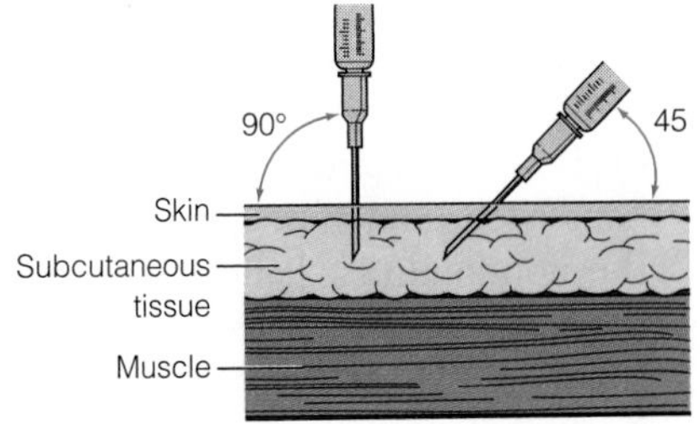

Figure 43–27 Inserting a needle into the subcutaneous tissue using 90- and 45-degree angles.

PROCEDURE 43–4 ADMINISTERING A SUBCUTANEOUS INJECTION *continued*

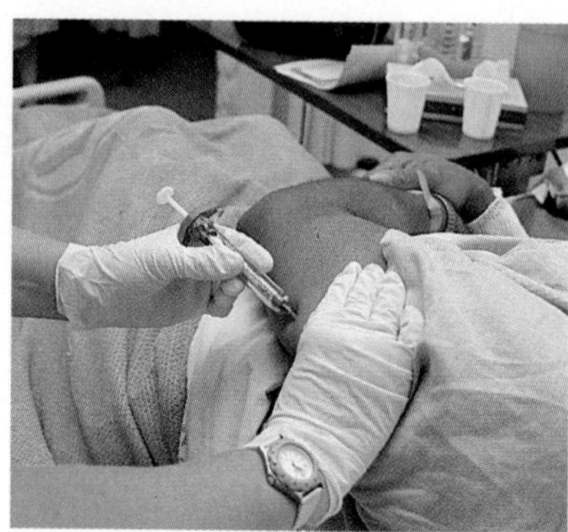

Figure 43–28 Administering a subcutaneous injection.

the dominant hand and a firm steady push (Figure 43–28). The nondominant hand can be used to immobilize the extremity of an infant or a young child as the needle is inserted. Recommendations vary about whether to pinch or spread the skin. *Pinching the skin is thought to desensitize the area somewhat and thus lessen the sensation of needle insertion. Spreading the skin can make it firmer and facilitate needle insertion.* Some recommend neither pinching nor spreading the skin (Pitel 1971, p. 79). The nurse needs to judge which method to use, depending on the client's tissue firmness.

- When the needle is inserted, move your nondominant hand to the end of the plunger. Some nurses find it easier to move the nondominant hand to the barrel of the syringe and the dominant hand to the end of the plunger. If the nondominant hand is holding the extremity of an infant or small child, use the dominant hand to aspirate and inject the medication.
- Aspirate by pulling back on the plunger. If blood appears in the syringe, withdraw the needle, discard the syringe, and prepare a new injection. If blood does not appear, continue to administer the medication. *This allows the nurse to determine whether the needle has entered a blood vessel. Subcutaneous medications may be dangerous if placed directly into the bloodstream; they are intended for the subcutaneous tissues, where the absorption time is greater.* See variation for administering a heparin injection.
- Inject the medication by holding the syringe steady and depressing the plunger with a slow, even pressure. *Holding the syringe steady and injecting the medication at an even pressure minimizes discomfort for the client.*

7. Remove the needle, and massage the site.

- Remove the needle quickly, pulling along the line of insertion while depressing the skin with your nondominant hand. *Depressing the skin places countertraction on it and minimizes the client's discomfort when the needle is withdrawn.*
- Massage the site lightly with a sterile antiseptic-soaked swab, or apply slight pressure. *Massage is thought to disperse the medication in the tissues and facilitate its absorption. Massaging is omitted with heparin and insulin injections or when contraindicated by the drug manufacturer.*
- If bleeding occurs, apply pressure to the site with a dry sterile gauze until it stops. Bleeding rarely occurs after subcutaneous injection.

8. Dispose of supplies appropriately.

- Discard the uncapped needle and attached syringe into designated receptacles. *Proper disposal protects*

the nurse and others from injury and contamination. The CDC recommends not capping the needle before disposal to reduce the risk of needle-prick injuries.
- Remove gloves. Wash hands.

9. Document all relevant information.

- Document the medication given, dosage, time, route, any assessments, and add your signature.
- Many agencies prefer that medication administration be recorded on the medication record. The nurse's notes are used when prn medications are given or when there is a special problem.

10. Assess the effectiveness of the medication when it is expected to act.

Variation: Administering a Heparin Injection

The subcutaneous administration of heparin requires special precautions because of the drug's anticoagulant properties.

- Select a site on the abdomen away from the umbilicus and above the level of the iliac crests. *These areas are away from major muscles and are not involved in muscular activity, as the arms and legs are; thus, the possibility of hematoma is reduced. In addition, muscular activity increases the absorption of the drug.*
- Use a ½-inch #25 or #26 gauge needle, and insert it at a 90-degree angle. Draw 0.1 mL of air into the syringe when preparing the heparin, and inject it after the heparin. *This step fills the needle with air and prevents any leakage of heparin into the intradermal layers when the needle is inserted and when the needle is withdrawn.*

PROCEDURE 43–4 *continued*

- Do not aspirate when giving heparin by subcutaneous injection. *Aspiration can cause the needle to move, possibly damaging tissue and rupturing small blood vessels and causing bleeding as well as severe bruising.*
- Do not massage the site after the injection. *Massaging could cause*

bleeding and ecchymoses and hasten drug absorption.

- Alternate sites of subsequent injections.

EVALUATION FOCUS

Desired effect (eg, relief of pain, sedation, lowered blood sugar or decreased urine glucose, a prothrombin time within preestablished limits); any adverse effects (eg, nausea, vomiting, skin rash); clinical signs of side effects.

of solution, the amount of adipose tissue covering the muscle, and the age of the client. A large muscle, such as the gluteus medius, usually requires a #20 or #23 gauge needle, 1½ to 3 inches long, whereas the deltoid muscle requires a smaller, #23 to #25 gauge needle, ⅝ to 1 inch long. Oily solutions such as paraldehyde require a thicker needle, such as #21 gauge instead of #23 gauge. Also, the greater the amount of adipose tissue over the muscle, the longer the needle must be to reach the muscle. Therefore, 3-inch needles may be needed for obese clients, whereas ½-inch needles are used for thinner people. Infants and young children usually require smaller, shorter needles (#22 to #25 gauge, ⅝ to 1 inch long).

To decrease the pain of an intramuscular injection, Murphy (1991, p. 35) suggests the following:

1. Clean the insertion site with an alcohol sponge using a circular motion and covering an area of about 10 cm (4 inches). Allow 15 seconds for the alcohol to dry so it can't be tracked into the subcutaneous tissues.
2. Inject the medication slowly (ie, 20 seconds) to allow the tissues to accommodate the volume.
3. Use the Z-track method and add an air bubble to clear the needle before withdrawal.
4. Use the correct needle length to reach the intended muscle.

A number of body sites are used for intramuscular injections. Frequently used sites are the ventrogluteal, dorsogluteal, vastus lateralis, rectus femoris, and deltoid muscles. Only healthy muscles should be used for injections.

Ventrogluteal Site The ventrogluteal site, also known as von Hochsteter's site, is in the gluteus medius muscle, which lies over the gluteus minimus (Figure 43–29). The ventrogluteal site is the preferred site for intramuscular injections because the area contains no large nerves or blood vessels and less fat than the buttock area. It is also farther from the rectal area and tends to be less contaminated. These considerations are important when giving injections to incontinent adults.

This site is suitable for infants, children, and adults. It is particularly suitable for immobilized clients, whose dorsogluteal muscles may be atrophying. The client position for the injection can be a back- or side-lying position with the knee and hip flexed to relax the gluteal muscles. To establish the exact site, the nurse places the heel of the hand on the client's greater trochanter, with the fingers pointing toward the client's head. The right hand is used for the left hip, and the left hand for the right hip. With the index finger on the client's anterior superior iliac spine, the nurse stretches the middle finger dorsally, palpating the crest of the ilium and then pressing below it.

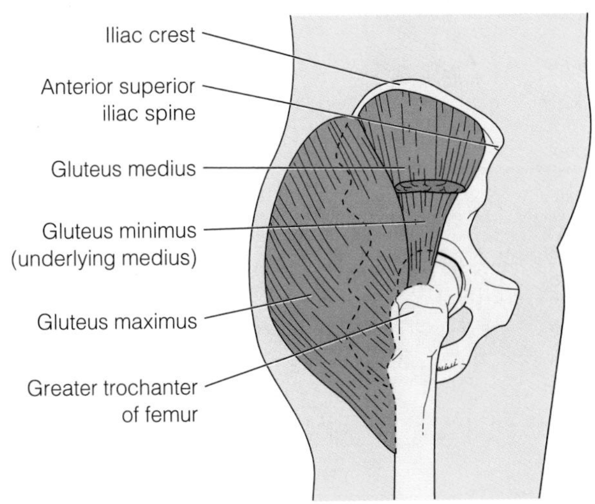

Figure 43–29 Lateral view of the right buttock showing the three gluteal muscles used for intramuscular injections.

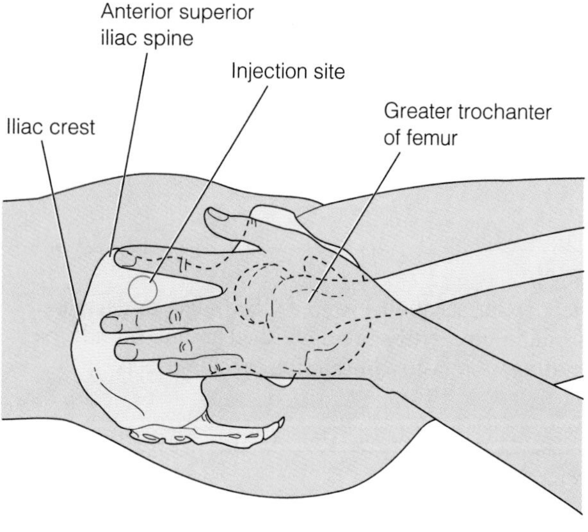

Figure 43–30 The ventrogluteal site for an intramuscular injection.

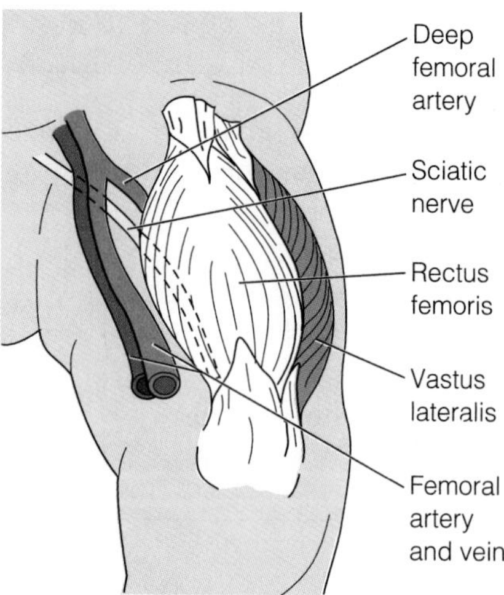

Figure 43–32 The vastus lateralis muscle of the upper thigh, used for intramuscular injections.

The triangle formed by the index finger, the third finger, and the crest of the ilium is the injection site (Figure 43–30).

Dorsogluteal Site The dorsogluteal site is composed of the thick gluteal muscles of the buttocks (Figure 43–29). The dorsogluteal site can be used for adults and for children with well-developed gluteal muscles. Because these muscles are developed by walking, this site should not be used for children under 3 years unless the child has been walking for at least 1 year. The nurse must choose the injection site carefully to avoid striking the sciatic nerve, major blood vessels, or bone.

The nurse palpates the posterior superior iliac spine, then draws an imaginary line to the greater trochanter of the femur. This line is lateral to and parallel to the sciatic nerve. The injection site is, then, lateral and superior to this line (Figure 43–31). Palpating the ilium and the trochanter is important; visual calculations alone can result in an injection that is placed too low and injures other structures.

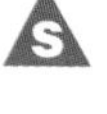

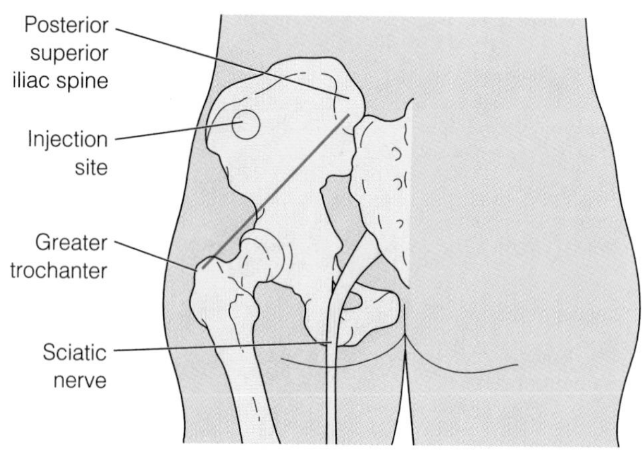

Figure 43–31 The dorsogluteal site for an intramuscular injection.

Vastus Lateralis Site The vastus lateralis muscle is usually thick and well developed in both adults and children. It is increasingly recommended as the site of choice for intramuscular injections for infants because there are no major blood vessels or nerves in the area. It is situated on the anterior lateral aspect of the thigh (Figure 43–32). The middle third of the muscle is suggested as the site. It is established by dividing the area between the greater trochanter of the femur and the lateral femoral condyle into thirds and selecting the middle third (Figure 43–33). The client can assume a back-lying or a sitting position for an injection into this site.

Rectus Femoris Site The rectus femoris muscle, which belongs to the quadriceps muscle group, can also be used for intramuscular injections. It is situated on the anterior aspect of the thigh (Figure 43–34). This site can

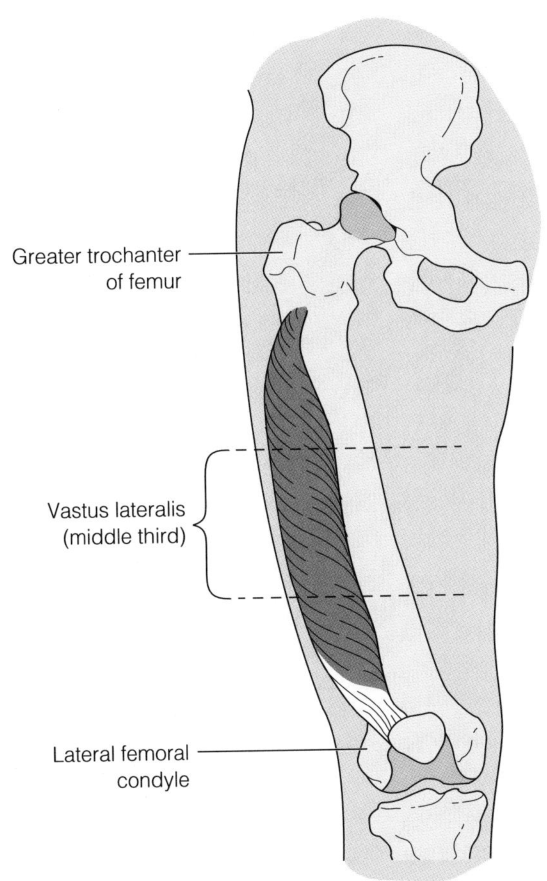

Figure 43–33 The vastus lateralis site of the right thigh, used for an intramuscular injection.

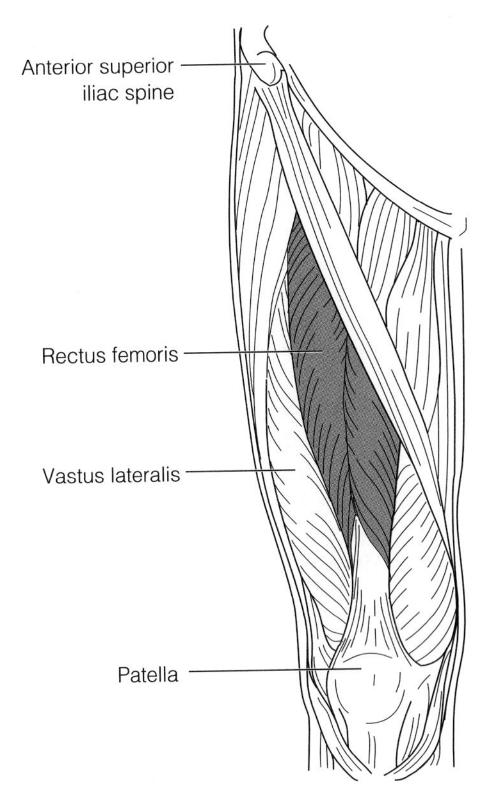

Figure 43–34 The rectus femoris muscle of the upper right thigh, used for intramuscular injections.

be used for occasional injections for infants and children and for adults when other sites are contraindicated. Its chief advantage is that clients who administer their own injections can reach this site easily. Its main disadvantage is that an injection here may cause considerable discomfort for some people. The client assumes a sitting or back-lying position for an injection at this site.

Deltoid Site The deltoid muscle is found on the lateral aspect of the upper arm. It is not used often for intramuscular injections because it is a relatively small muscle and is very close to the radial nerve and radial artery. It is sometimes considered for use in adults and children over 18 months of age because of rapid absorption from the deltoid area.

To locate the densest part of the muscle, the nurse palpates the lower edge of the acromion and the midpoint on the lateral aspect of the arm that is in line with the axilla. A triangle within these boundaries indicates the deltoid muscle about 5 cm (2 in) below the acromion process (Figure 43–35). Another method of establishing the

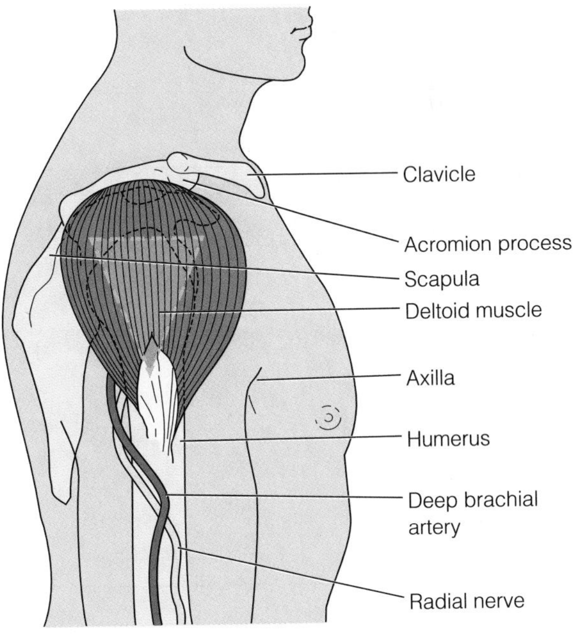

Figure 43–35 The deltoid muscle of the upper arm, used for intramuscular injections.

RESEARCH NOTE

Can Needle-Stick Injuries Be Prevented?

This research focused on the effectiveness of recent measures instituted to protect health care workers from needle-stick injuries. The objective of the study was to reduce the number of needle sticks among health care workers. Reported needle-stick injuries from 1986 to 1990 were investigated at a 388-bed county teaching hospital in San Jose, California. The review revealed that more measures had been implemented in the hospital in 1987 from April to December. Protective needle disposal containers were strategically placed in as many client care areas of the hospital as possible. The containers were placed within close proximity of the areas of work use. Extensive educational programs for the staff were also started. Needle sticks decreased significantly. In 1986, 259 total needle stick injuries were reported. By 1988, needle-stick injuries had decreased by 45%. In 1989, injuries decreased another 6% from 1988. In 1990, there was a 23% decrease from 1989. By 1990, the total number of needle sticks had decreased by 60% from 1990. The number of injuries from recapping needles from 1986 to 1990 had decreased by 81 to 89%.

Implications: This study suggests that safety hazard programs focusing on educating health care workers and providing supportive equipment necessary for those measures to be taken will reduce occupational injury due to needle sticks.

Source: DJ Haiduven, TM DeMaio, and DA Stevens, A five-year study of needlestick injuries. *Infection Control and Hospital Epidemiology,* May 1992, 13:265–71.

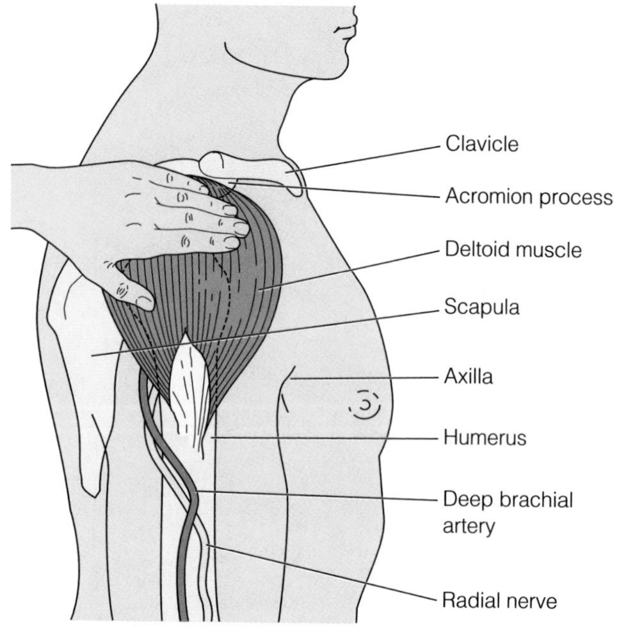

Figure 43–36 A method of establishing the deltoid muscle site for an intramuscular injection.

deltoid site is to place four fingers across the deltoid muscle, with the first finger on the acromion process; the site is three finger breadths below the acromion process (Figure 43–36).

Procedure 43–5 describes how to administer an intramuscular injection.

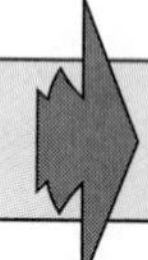

PROCEDURE 43–5 ADMINISTERING AN INTRAMUSCULAR INJECTION

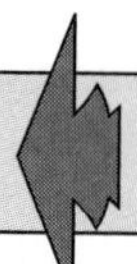

PURPOSE

- To provide a medication the client requires (see specific drug action)

ASSESSMENT FOCUS

Allergies to medication(s); specific drug action, side effects, and adverse reactions; client's knowledge of and learning needs about the medication; tissue integrity of the selected site; client's age and weight to determine site and needle size; client's ability or willingness to cooperate.

EQUIPMENT

- ☐ MAR or computer printout
- ☐ Sterile medication (usually provided in an ampule or vial)
- ☐ Sterile syringe and needle of a size appropriate for the amount of solution to be administered
- ☐ Swab saturated in an antiseptic solution
- ☐ Gloves

PROCEDURE 43–5 *continued*

INTERVENTION

1. Verify the medication order for accuracy.

- See Procedure 43–2, step 1.

2. Prepare the medication from the vial or ampule.

- See Procedure 43–2, step 2.
- If the medication is particularly irritating to subcutaneous tissue, change the needle on the syringe before the injection. *Because the outside of the new needle is free of medication, it does not irritate subcutaneous tissues as it passes into the muscle.*
- Invert the syringe, and expel excess air, leaving only 0.2 mL of air. *This technique, referred to as the air-lock or air-bubble technique, prevents tracking of the medication through sensitive subcutaneous tissues in two ways: (a) it keeps the needle clean of medication on insertion; and (b) because the air bubble moves to the end of the plunger when the needle is pointed downward, the air bubble is injected behind the medication into the tissues* (Figure 43–37). *This provides a seal at the point of insertion, and prevents tracking of the medication. It is particularly helpful when injecting a medication that is irritating to the skin and subcutaneous tissue.*

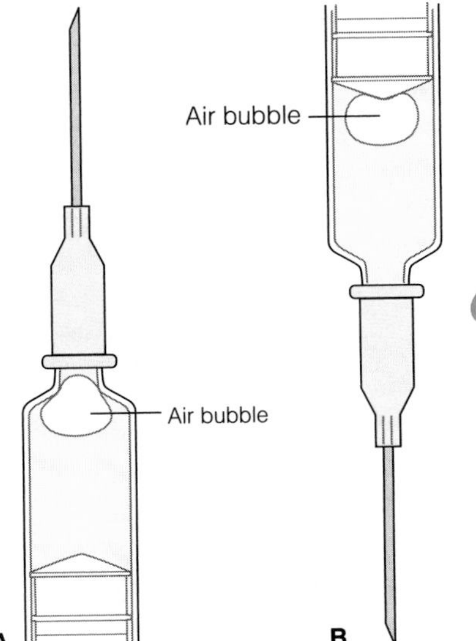

Figure 43–37 An air bubble in the medication in the syringe: *A,* needle pointed up; *B,* needle pointed down.

3. Identify the client, and assist the client to a comfortable position.

- Check the client's arm band, and ask the client to tell you his or her name.
- Assist the client to a supine, lateral, prone, or sitting position, depending on the chosen site.

- Obtain assistance to immobilize an infant or young child. The parent may hold the infant or young child. *This prevents accidental injury during the procedure.*

4. Select, locate, and clean the site.

- Wash hands.
- Select a site free of skin lesions, tenderness, swelling, hardness, or localized inflammation and one that has not been used frequently.
- If injections are to be frequent, alternate sites. If necessary, discuss with the prescribing physician an alternative method of providing the medication.
- Determine whether the size of the muscle is appropriate to the amount of medication to be injected. An average adult's deltoid muscle can usually absorb 0.5 mL of medication, although some authorities believe 2 mL can be absorbed by a well-developed deltoid muscle. The gluteus medius muscle can often absorb 1 to 5 mL, although 5 mL may be very painful.
- Locate the exact site for the injection. See the discussion of sites, earlier in this chapter.
- Don gloves.
- Clean the site with an antiseptic swab. Using a circular motion, start at the center and move outward about 5 cm (2 in).
- Discard the swab appropriately. Allow skin to dry prior to injecting medication.

5. Prepare the syringe for injection.

- Remove the needle cover without contaminating the needle.
- Confirm that the medication and the dose are both correct.
- Ensure appropriate air lock.

6. Inject the medication.

- Use the nondominant hand to spread the skin at the site. Under some circumstances, such as for an emaciated client or an infant, the muscle may be pinched. *Spreading the skin or pinching the muscle makes it firmer and facilitates needle insertion.*
- Holding the syringe between the thumb and forefinger (as if holding a pencil), pierce the skin quickly at a 90-degree angle (Figure 43–38), and insert the needle into the muscle (Figure 43–39). *Using a quick motion lessens the client's discomfort.*
- Aspirate by holding the barrel of the syringe steady with your nondominant hand and by pulling back on the plunger with

Procedure 43–5 Administering a Intramuscular Injection *continued*

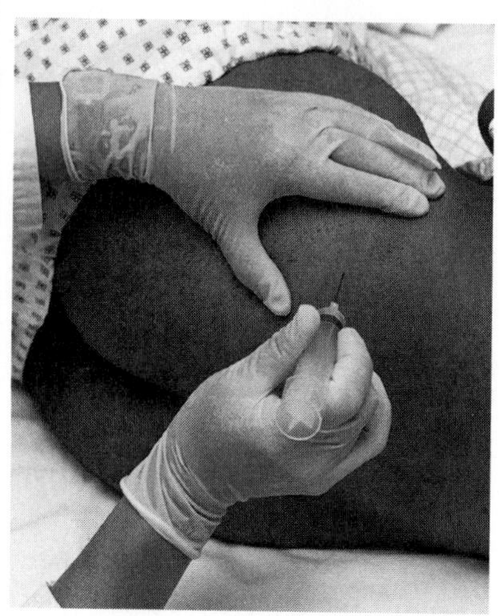

Figure 43–38 Administering an intramuscular injection.

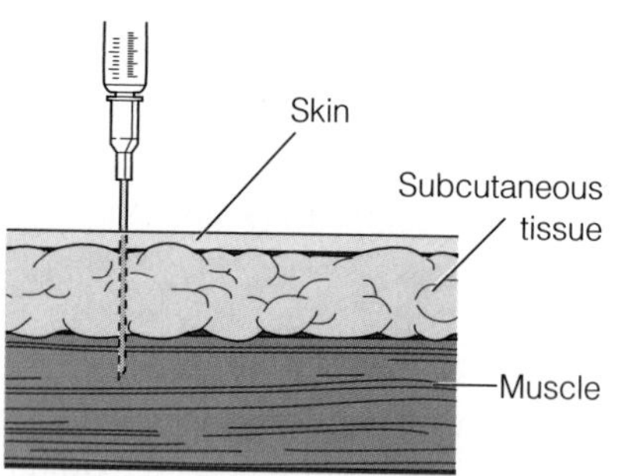

Figure 43–39 An intramuscular needle inserted into the muscle layer.

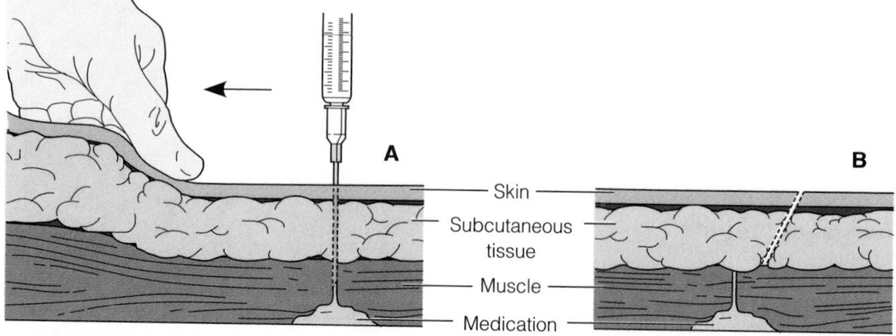

Figure 43–40 Inserting the needle using the Z-tract method: *A,* skin pulled to the side, *B,* skin released.

your dominant hand. If blood appears in the syringe, withdraw the needle, discard the syringe, and prepare a new injection. *This step determines whether the needle has been inserted into a blood vessel.*

- If blood does not appear, inject the medication steadily and slowly, holding the syringe steady. *Injecting medication slowly permits it to disperse into the muscle tissue, thus decreasing the client's discomfort. Holding the syringe steady minimizes discomfort.*

7. Withdraw the needle quickly, and massage the site.

- See Procedure 43–4, step 7, page 1326.

8. Discard the uncapped needle and attached syringe into the proper receptacle.

- Remove gloves. Wash hands.

9. Document all relevant information.

- Include the time of administration, drug name, dose, route, and the client's reactions.

10. Assess effectiveness of the medication when it is expected to act.

Variation: Administering a Z-Tract Injection

This variation of the standard intramuscular technique is used to administer intramuscular medications that are highly irritating to subcutaneous and skin tissues.

- Follow steps 1 through 4 earlier.
- Attach a new sterile needle to the syringe. *A new needle will not have any medication adhering to the outside that could be irritating to tissues.*
- Prepare an air lock (see step 2, earlier).
- With the nondominant hand, pull the skin and subcutaneous tissue about 2.5 to 3.5 cm (1 to 1¼ in) to one side at the injection site (Figure 43–40).
- Insert the syringe, aspirate, and inject the medication as in step 6.
- Maintain the traction for 10 seconds before withdrawing the needle, and then permit the skin to return to its normal position. *This provides a seal over the injected medication, thus preventing tracking to subcutaneous tissues.*
- Do not massage the site. *This can lead to tissue irritation.*

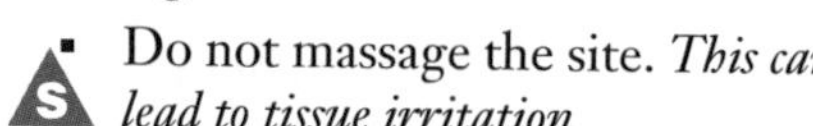

Evaluation Focus

Desired effect (eg, relief of pain or vomiting, reduction in body temperature); any adverse reactions or side effects.

INTRAVENOUS MEDICATIONS

Because intravenous (IV) medications enter the client's bloodstream directly, they are appropriate when a rapid effect is required (eg, in a life-threatening situation such as cardiac arrest). This route is also appropriate when medications are too irritating to tissues to be given by other routes. When an intravenous line is already established, this route is desirable because it avoids the discomfort of other parenteral routes. Medications are administered intravenously by the following methods:

- Intravenous fluid container (continuous infusion)
- Additional container (intermittent infusion by piggyback [IVPB] or partial fill [IVPF])
- Volume-control administration set (often used for children)
- Intravenous push (IVP or bolus)

Other IV drug delivery systems are shown in Table 43–10 on page 1337.

There are potential hazards in giving intravenous medications: infection, rapid severe reactions to the medication, and fluid volume overload. The nurse must dilute medication in the smallest possible volume, particularly when administering medication and fluid to infants, small children, elderly clients, or clients with renal failure or heart disease.

Medications administered by continuous infusion are given slowly over a long period. The nurse must monitor the client for possible adverse effects at least every hour.

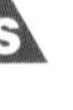

To prevent infection, the nurse uses sterile technique during all aspects of administering intravenous medication. To safeguard the client against severe reactions, the nurse must administer the drug slowly, following the manufacturer's recommendations. The nurse assesses the client closely during the administration and discontinues the medication immediately if an untoward reaction occurs.

Adding Medications to Intravenous Fluid Containers
Medications can be added to a fluid container that is already attached and running, or they can be added to a fluid container before it is hung and infusing. Electrolytes (eg, potassium chloride) and vitamins (eg, Solu-B) are commonly administered by this method. Before administering any intravenous medication, the nurse (a) inspects and palpates the intravenous insertion site for signs of infection, infiltration, or a dislocated catheter; (b) inspects the surrounding skin for redness, pallor, or swelling; and (c) palpates the surrounding tissues for coldness and presence of edema, which could indicate leakage of the IV fluid into the tissues. The nurse then takes the vital signs for baseline data and makes sure that the drug and solutions are compatible. A nurse may need to consult a pharmacist for this information. An **incompatibility** is an undesired chemical or physical reaction between a drug and an infusion solution, between two or more drugs, or between a drug and the container or tubing (eg, the incompatibility of some medications with plastic containers or syringes).

Procedure 43–6 describes how to add medications to intravenous fluid containers.

Text continued on page 1338

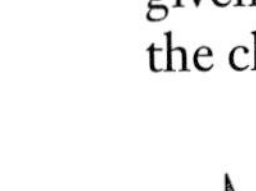

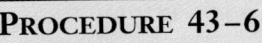

PROCEDURE 43–6 ADDING MEDICATIONS TO INFUSING INTRAVENOUS FLUID CONTAINERS

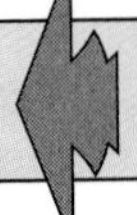

PURPOSES

- To provide and maintain a constant level of a medication in the blood
- To administer well-diluted medications at a continuous and slow rate

ASSESSMENT FOCUS
Signs of infiltration, infection, or a dislodged needle at the infusion site: redness, pallor, swelling, coldness or edema of the surrounding tissues; vital signs for baseline data; allergies to medications; compatibility of medication(s) and IV fluid.

EQUIPMENT

- ☐ MAR or computer printout
- ☐ Correct sterile medication
- ☐ Diluent for medication in powdered form (see manufacturer's instructions)
- ☐ Correct solution container, if a new one is to be attached
- ☐ Antiseptic swabs
- ☐ Sterile syringe of appropriate size (eg, 5 or 10 mL) and a 1- to 1½-inch, #20 or #21 gauge sterile needle
- ☐ Medication label

PROCEDURE 43–6 ADDING MEDICATIONS TO INFUSING INTRAVENOUS FLUID CONTAINERS *continued*

INTERVENTION

1. Verify the medication order for accuracy, and confirm the compatibility of the drugs and solutions being mixed.

- Check the physician's orders carefully for the medication, dosage, and route. Verify which infusions are to be used with the medication. For example, the order may say to infuse the medication with 1000 mL of 5% dextrose and water rather than with normal saline.
- Consult a pharmacist, if required, to confirm compatibility of the drugs and solutions being mixed.

2. Prepare the medication from a vial or ampule.

- See Procedure 43–2, step 2.
- Check the agency's practice for using a special filter needle to withdraw premixed liquid medications from multidose vials or ampules.

3. Confirm the sterility of the solution container (if a new one is to be attached), and locate and clean the injection port.

- Be sure that the solution container has no leaks, that the fluid is not discolored or has visible particles, that the seal is undamaged, and that the date on the container has not expired.
- Locate the separate, self-sealing, soft rubber injection port.
- Clean the injection port with an antiseptic swab, and allow it to dry completely. *This reduces the risk of introducing microorganisms into the container when the needle is inserted.*

4. Inject the medication into the container.

- Make sure there is sufficient solution in the container to ensure proper dilution of the drug. *Undiluted medication can produce a severe reaction.*
- Close the IV flow clamp. *Closing the clamp is essential to prevent the medication from infusing to the client before it is properly diluted with the solution.*
- Remove the needle cover from the medication syringe.
- While supporting and stabilizing the bag with your thumb and forefinger, carefully insert the syringe needle through the port, and inject the medication (Figure 43–41). *The bag is supported during the injection of the medication to avoid punctures.*

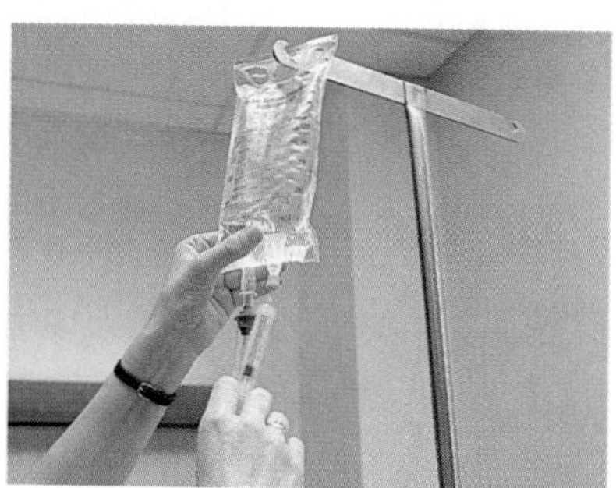

Figure 43–41 Instilling a medication into an intravenous fluid container.

- Withdraw the needle. The port is self-sealing.
- Gently lift and rotate the container to mix the solution and medication.

5. Attach a medication label.

- Apply the medication label to the fluid container so it can be easily read when the container is hanging.
- See Figure 43–42 for the information to be included on the medication label.

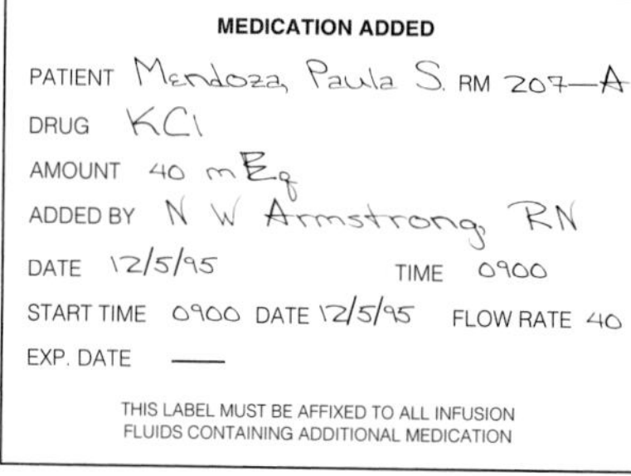

MEDICATION ADDED

PATIENT Mendoza, Paula S. RM 207–A
DRUG KCl
AMOUNT 40 mEq
ADDED BY N W Armstrong RN
DATE 12/5/95 TIME 0900
START TIME 0900 DATE 12/5/95 FLOW RATE 40
EXP. DATE —

THIS LABEL MUST BE AFFIXED TO ALL INFUSION FLUIDS CONTAINING ADDITIONAL MEDICATION

Figure 43–42 A medication label for an intravenous infusion.

6. Establish the infusion.

- Regulate the flow rate according to the dosage required. *This prevents rapid infusion of the medication and fluid and subsequent complications.*

7. Document all relevant information.

- Record the type and amount of solution, medication and dose added, and times of starting and completing the infusion. Some agencies have a special parenteral fluid form for this purpose.
- Record fluid volume on the intake and output record.

8. Monitor the client and the infusion.

- During the administration, observe the client at least hourly for signs of an adverse reaction, such as noisy respirations, changes in pulse rate, chills, nausea, or headache. If any adverse sign occurs, follow agency policy (ie,

PROCEDURE 43–6 *continued*

slow rate or stop flow), and notify the physician or nurse in charge. Also monitor the client for signs of the intended action of the medication.

- Carefully monitor the infusion to maintain delivery of the medication and fluid at the specified rate.

Variation: Using a Transfer Needle

A special transfer needle (Figure 43–43). can be used to put medications in vials into a *plastic* IV container, provided the entire amount of medication is to be transferred to the IV container. After cleaning the top of the medication vial and the medication port on the IV bag with an antiseptic sponge, insert the small end of the transfer needle into the medication vial and the large end into the port of the IV container. To mix the medication and solution:

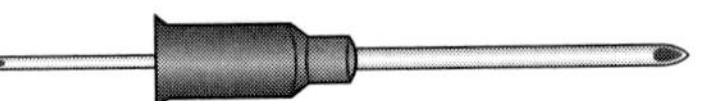

Figure 43–43 A transfer needle.

- Invert the bag, so that the medication bottle is on top.
- Gently squeeze the bag to transmit some air from the bag into the medication vial.
- Release the pressure on the bag to allow medication to drain into the bag.
- Repeat squeezing and releasing pressure until all the medication is transferred into the IV solution. The transfer needle may need to be pulled down so that all the medication is obtained from the vial.
- Remove the needle, and gently rotate the bag to disperse the medication.

Variation: Using Glass Containers to Administer IV Medications

For medications that are incompatible with the commonly used plastic solution containers, a glass infusion bottle must be used. Some glass containers are vented (ie, they have a tube inside the bottle that acts as an air vent). Air replaces the solution as it runs out of the bottle (Figure 43–44).

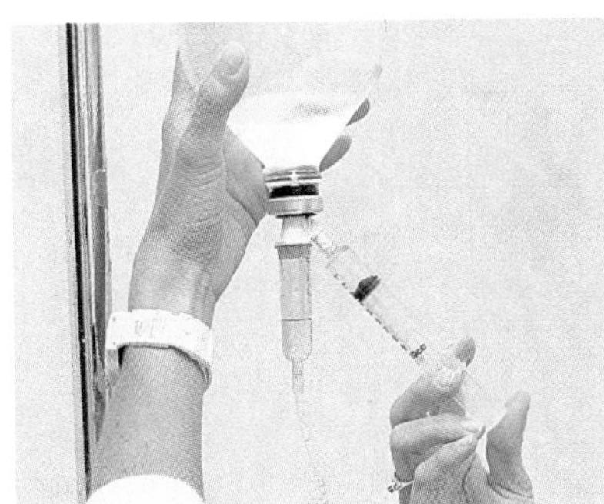

Figure 43–44 An intravenous fluid container with an inside air vent.

Adding Medication to a Vented Glass Container

- Remove the metal cap and the rubber disc to locate the injection port. An injection port may be designated in several ways (eg, by a triangle, cross, or circle). Do *not* inject medication through the port for the administration spike or through an air vent port if there is an injection port.
- Clean the injection port with an antiseptic swab.
- Inject the medication through the port (Figure 43–45).

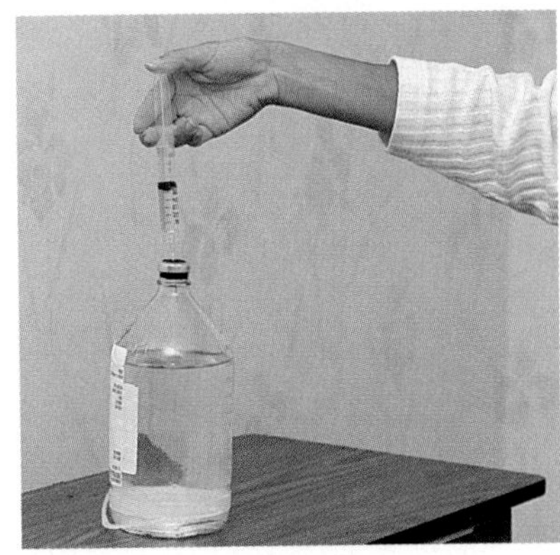

Figure 43–45 Inserting a medication into an intravenous fluid bottle.

- Cover the top immediately with either (a) an antiseptic swab with the metal IV cap taped over it, or (b) the special sterile cap provided by the manufacturer. *An open tubing port increases the risk of fluid contamination by microorganisms.*
- Immediately attach an infusion set and administer the solution.

Adding Medication to a Nonvented Glass Container

Glass IV containers with a vent require a vented infusion set (Figure 43–46).

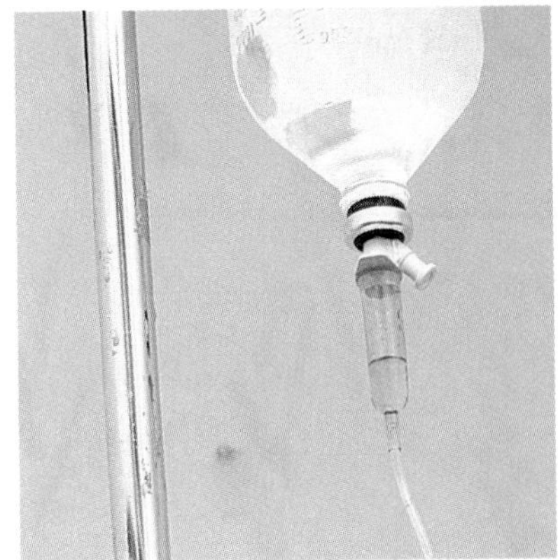

Figure 43–46 A nonvented intravenous fluid container. Note the air vent on administration tubing.

Procedure 43-6 Adding Medications to Infusing Intravenous Fluid Containers *continued*

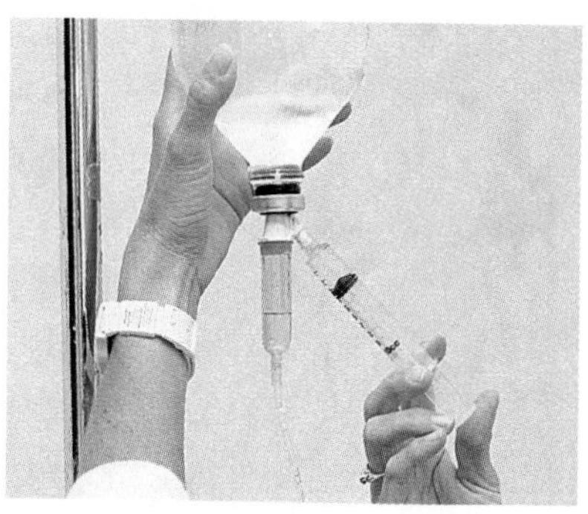

Figure 43-47 Instilling a medication into a hanging intravenous fluid bottle.

- Detach the air vent cap, taking care not to contaminate the end.
- Insert the tip of the medication syringe, *without the needle*, into the air vent port (Figure 43-47).
- Instill the medication.
- Reattach the air vent.

Evaluation Focus
Desired effect of the medication; any adverse reactions or side effects; change in vital signs; status of the IV site; patency of the IV infusion.

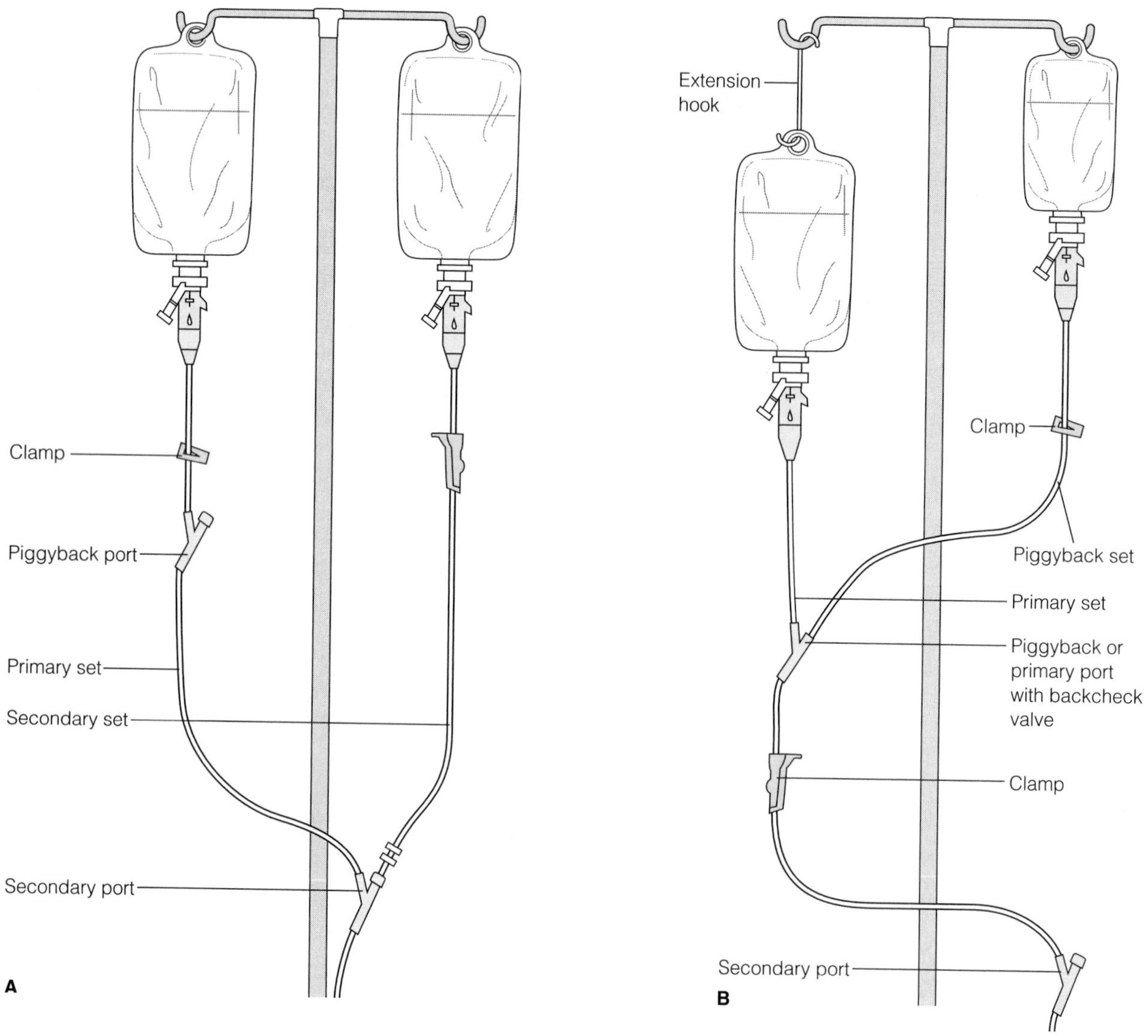

Clamp
Piggyback port
Primary set
Secondary set
Secondary port
A

Extension hook
Clamp
Piggyback set
Primary set
Piggyback or primary port with backcheck valve
Clamp
Secondary port
B

Figure 43-48 Secondary intravenous lines: *A,* a tandem intravenous alignment; *B,* an intravenous piggyback (IVPB) alignment.

Table 43–10 IV Drug Delivery Systems*

System	Description
Minibag	A reconstituted drug is added to a small plastic bag containing diluent. 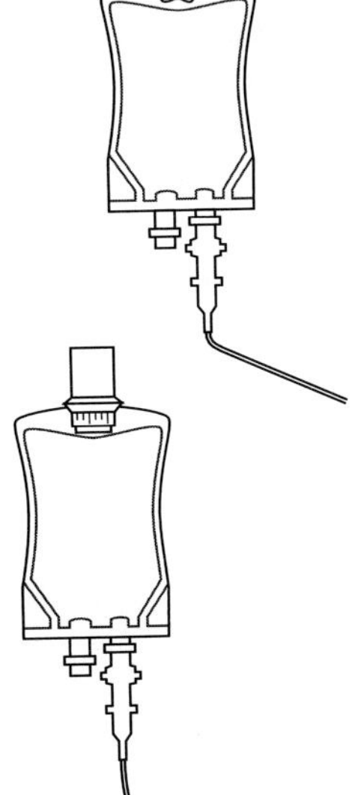
ADD-Vantage	A vial containing the medication is attached to a partially filled IV bag. Immediately before administering the medication, the nurse must break an internal seal that separates the drug from the fluid and mix the drug and diluent.
Ready-to-use (RTU) premix	The drug and diluent are premixed in a plastic bag. Less stable drugs may be frozen and must be thawed before use. 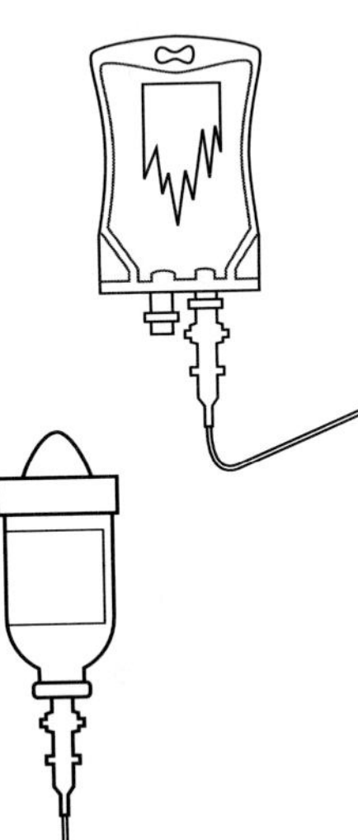
Drug manufacturer's piggyback (DMPB)	The container is prefilled with a single dose of medication to which diluent must be added. 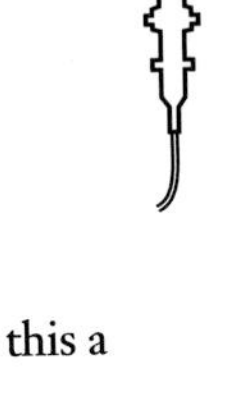
CRIS adapter	A two-position valve is placed in the primary IV line below the IV container. To this a vial of reconstituted drug is directly attached. 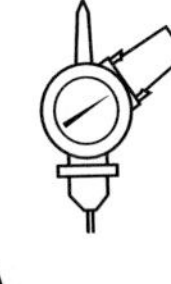
Minisyringe pump	The reconstituted drug is withdrawn into a syringe. Medication is delivered by mechanical pressure on the syringe plunger. 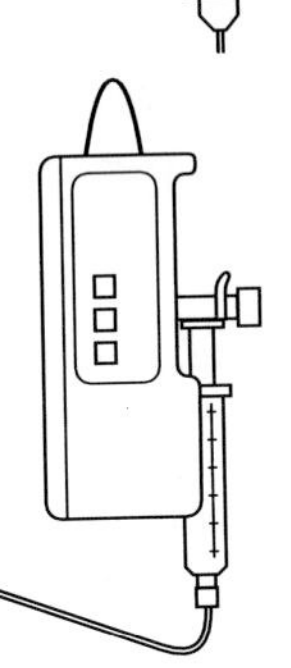

* All systems are attached to a check valve Y-site on the primary IV line, *except* the CRIS adapter, which is attached between the IV container and drip chamber.

Using Additional Containers/Additive Sets Two setups are used to deliver IV medications: the tandem setup and the piggyback setup. In a *tandem setup*, a second container is attached to the line of the first container at the lower, secondary port (Figure 43–48, *A*, p. 1336). It permits medications to be administered intermittently or simultaneously with the first solution.

In the *piggyback alignment*, a second set connects the second container to the tubing of the first at the upper port (Figure 43–48, *B*). This setup is used solely for intermittent drug administration. Various manufacturers describe these sets differently, so the nurse must check the manufacturer's labeling and directions carefully.

Traditionally, the tubing of additive sets has been attached to ports of the primary infusion tubing by inserting a needle through the port and taping it in place (Figure 43–49, in Procedure 43–7). New systems, referred to as needleless systems, are now available. These systems use threaded-lock or lever-lock cannulae to connect the additive set to the primary ports (Figure 43–50, in Procedure 43–7). Because the systems are needleless, accidental needle-stick injuries are prevented. The design also prevents touch contamination at the IV connection site. Procedure 43–7 describes how to use additive sets to administer intravenous medications.

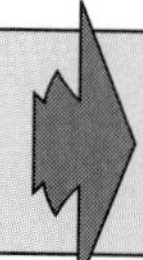

PROCEDURE 43–7 USING ADDITIVE SETS TO ADMINISTER INTRAVENOUS MEDICATIONS

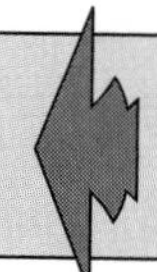

PURPOSES

- To administer intermittently IV drugs that cannot be mixed with the primary solution for reasons of incompatibility
- To administer different IV drugs at different times
- To maintain peak levels of a medication in the client's bloodstream by simultaneous infusion

ASSESSMENT FOCUS

See Assessment Focus for Procedure 43–6 on page 1333.

EQUIPMENT

- ☐ Physician's order or MAR
- ☐ Medication label
- ☐ Antiseptic swab
- ☐ Sterile needle, syringe, and saline, if medication is incompatible with the primary infusion
- ☐ Adhesive tape

Piggyback

- ☐ 50- to 100-mL infusion bag with medication (most piggybacks are prepared by the pharmacist)
- ☐ Microdrip or macrodrip infusion set
- ☐ Needle (1-in, #21 or #23 gauge)
- ☐ Extension hook

Tandem Setup

- ☐ Solution container with medication added
- ☐ Long secondary tubing set

INTERVENTION

1. Verify the medication order for accuracy, and confirm the compatibility of the medication.

- See Procedure 43–6, step 1.

2. Add the medication to the additive set, if required.

- Prepare the medication from an ampule or vial. See Procedure 43–2, step 2.
- Add the medication to the additional container. See Procedure 43–6, step 4.
- Apply the medication label.

3. Assemble the secondary infusion.

- Spike the secondary infusion container.
- Hang the secondary container at or above the level of the primary infusion. Use the extension hook to lower the primary infusion if a piggyback setup is required.
- Attach the 1-inch needle to the tubing, prime the tubing, and close the clamp.

4. Attach the secondary infusion to the primary infusion.

- Clean the Y-port on the primary IV line with an antiseptic swab. Clean the *primary port* (that furthest from the client) for a piggy-

Procedure 43–7 *continued*

back alignment and the *secondary port* (that closest to the client) for a tandem setup.

- If the medication is *not* compatible with the primary infusion, flush the primary line with a sterile saline solution before attaching the secondary set. To flush the line, wipe the port with an antiseptic swab, clamp the primary line, and, using a sterile needle and syringe, instill a few milliliters of sterile saline solution through the port to wash any primary infusion fluid out of the infusion tubing.
- Insert the needle of the secondary line through the injection port of the primary line (Figure 43–49).

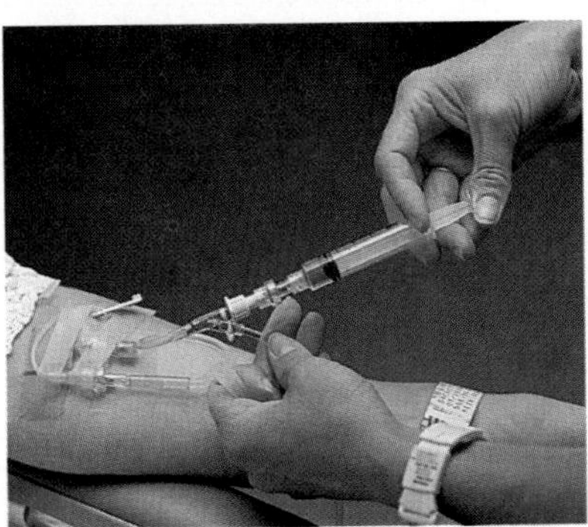

Figure 43–49 Inserting needle into secondary port.

- Secure the needle with adhesive tape. *Tape prevents needle dislodgment.* Some agencies recommend that a needle guard be taped alongside the needle to support the needle placement and keep the needle guard handy for use when discontinuing the secondary attachment.

or

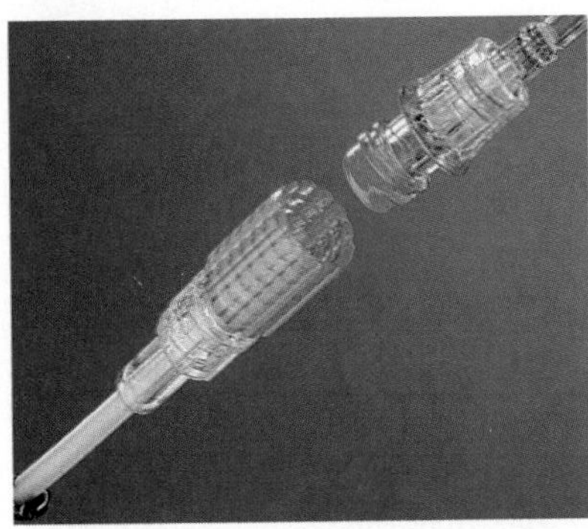

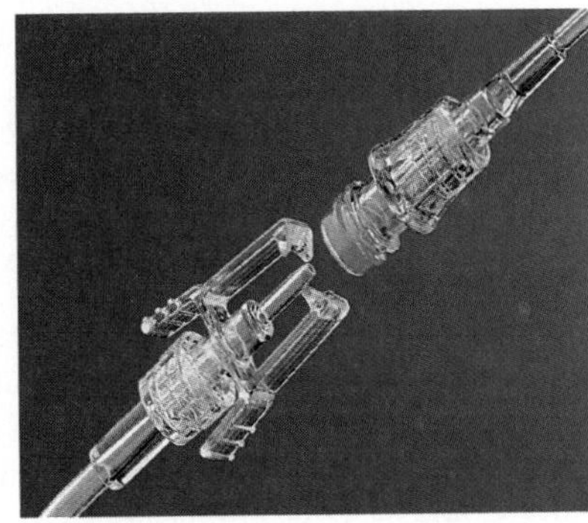

Figure 43–50 Cannulae used to connect the tubing of additive sets to primary infusions: *A,* threaded-lock cannula; *B,* lever-lock cannula.

- Attach a needleless cannula system (Figure 43–50) according to the manufacturer's directions.
- Attach appropriate label to the tubing.

5. Administer the medication.

Piggyback

- Ensure that the primary line is unclamped if the port has a backcheck valve. *The valve automatically stops the flow of the primary infusion while the additive set infuses and automatically starts it running after the piggyback solution has been administered.*
- Open the clamp on the piggyback line, and regulate it in accordance with the recommended rate for that medication. Usually, medications are administered in 30 to 60 minutes.

Tandem Infusion

- Open the clamp on the secondary line, and regulate its flow.
- For a *continuous* infusion, set the secondary solution to the appropriate drip rate for the medication, and then adjust the primary solution to achieve the desired total infusion flow.
- For *intermittent* infusion, clamp the primary line, and adjust the secondary drip rate. After the secondary solution is completed, clamp the secondary line and reestablish the primary line infusion rate.

6. Document relevant data.

- Record the date, time, medication, dose, route, and solution; assessments of IV site, if appropriate; and client response.
- Enter fluid intake according to agency protocol.

Evaluation Focus

See Evaluation Focus for Procedure on page 1336.

Volume-Control Sets Intermittent medications may also be administered by **volume-control sets** such as Buretrol, Soluset, Volutrol, and Pediatrol (Figure 43–51). They are small fluid containers (100 to 150 mL in size) attached below the primary infusion container. Volume-control sets are frequently used to infuse solutions into children and elderly clients when the volume administered is critical and must be carefully monitored.

Procedure 43–8 describes how to use volume-control sets to administer intravenous medications.

Intravenous Push An intravenous push (**IVP** or **bolus**) is the intravenous administration of a medication that cannot be diluted or that is needed in an emergency. Also, certain drugs are administered this way to achieve maximum effect. It is important to remember that the rapid administration of an IVP could be dangerous for the client. An IVP can be administered directly into a vein through venipuncture, into an existing intravenous apparatus through an injection port (Figure 43–53 in Proce-

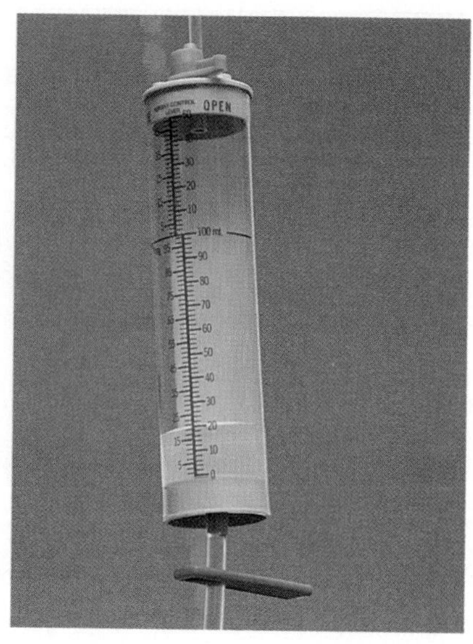

Figure 43–51 A volume-control set above the drip chamber of an intravenous infusion.

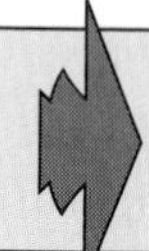

PROCEDURE 43–8 ADMINISTERING INTRAVENOUS MEDICATIONS BY VOLUME-CONTROL ADMINISTRATION SETS

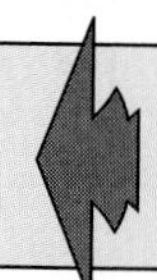

PURPOSES

- To administer intravenous medications (such as some antibiotics) that do not remain stable for the length of time it takes an entire solution container to infuse
- To administer medications intermittently
- To avoid mixing medications that are incompatible
- To dilute a drug so that it is less irritating to the veins than if given by direct intravenous push
- To deliver medications diluted in precise amounts of fluid

ASSESSMENT FOCUS
See Procedure 43–6 on page 1333.

EQUIPMENT

- ☐ Physician's order or MAR
- ☐ Correct sterile medication
- ☐ Antiseptic swabs
- ☐ Sterile syringe of appropriate size (eg, 5 or 10 mL)
- ☐ 1- to 1½-inch, #20 or #21 gauge, sterile needle
- ☐ Sterile filter needle if needed to withdraw the medication
- ☐ Volume-control administration set
- ☐ Correct solution container
- ☐ Medication label for the volume-control set

INTERVENTION

1. Verify the medication order, and confirm the compatibility of the medication.

- See Procedure 43–2, step 1.

2. Prepare the medication from an ampule or vial.

- See Procedure 43–2, step 2.

3. Attach the volume-control set to the infusion container.

PROCEDURE 43–8 *continued*

- Insert the spike of the volume-control set into the solution container, and hang the container on the pole.
- Open the air vent clamp on the volume-control set.
- Position the lower clamp on the tubing below the drip chamber, and clamp it.

4. Fill the volume-control device, and prime the tubing.

Set with a Stationary Membrane Filter

- Open the upper clamp, and allow the fluid chamber to fill with about 30 mL of solution, then close this clamp.
- Open the lower clamp, and flatten the drip chamber with two fingers and the thumb of your opposite hand. *The membrane filter can be damaged if the drip chamber is squeezed while the lower clamp is closed.*
- While keeping the drip chamber flattened, close the lower clamp. *These actions create a vacuum, so that solution from the fluid chamber will then flow into the drip chamber.*
- Release your pressure on the drip chamber, and reshape it until it becomes about half full.
- Repeat the above steps as necessary.
- Open the lower clamp, prime the tubing, and close the clamp.

Set with a Floating Valve Filter

- Open the upper clamp, and squeeze the fluid chamber until it is filled with about 30 mL of solution.
- Close the clamp, and again gently squeeze the drip chamber until it is about half full.
- Open the lower clamp, prime the tubing, and close the clamp.

5. Administer the medication.

- Ensure that there is sufficient fluid in the volume-control fluid chamber to dilute the medication. Generally, 50 to 100 mL of fluid is used. Check the directions from the drug manufacturer or consult the pharmacist.
- Close the inflow to the fluid chamber by adjusting the upper roller or slide clamp above the fluid chamber; also ensure that the clamp on the air vent of the chamber is open.
- Clean the medication port on the volume-control fluid chamber with an antiseptic swab.
- Insert the needle of the medication syringe into the port (Figure 43–52).
- Inject the medication.

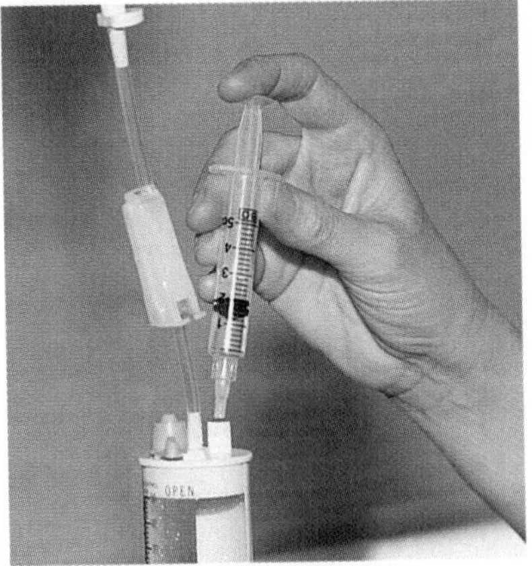

Figure 43–52 Adding medication to the port of a volume-control administration set.

- Gently rotate the fluid chamber until the fluid is well mixed.
- Open the line's upper clamp, and regulate the flow by adjusting the lower roller or slide clamp below the fluid chamber.

6. Attach a medication label to the volume-control fluid chamber.

7. Document relevant data, and monitor the client and the infusion.

- See Procedure 43–6, steps 7 and 8.

EVALUATION FOCUS
See Procedure 43–6 on page 1336.

dure 43–9), or through an intermittent infusion set (IV lock, also referred to as a heparin or saline lock) when the client does not have an IV running but does have an IV lock in place. The IV lock (Figure 43–54 in Procedure 43–9), also called a male adapter plug (MAP), is used primarily for clients who require regular intermittent intravenous medications but not the fluid volume of an intravenous infusion. The set usually consists of an indwelling catheter attached to a plastic tube with a sealed injection tip. Small amounts of heparin or saline are injected into the catheter to maintain its patency. After administering an IVP, the nurse discards the used syringe and needle in a designated container without recapping the needle, as for any other type of injection. See Procedure 43–9.

Text continued on page 1344

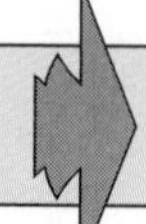

PROCEDURE 43-9 ADMINISTERING INTRAVENOUS MEDICATIONS USING IV PUSH

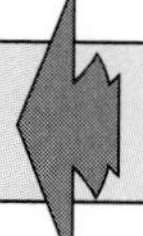

PURPOSE

- To achieve immediate and maximum effects of a medication

ASSESSMENT FOCUS

Signs of infiltration or infection at the infusion site or IV lock insertion site: redness, pallor, or swelling of the surrounding skin, coldness and edema of the surrounding tissues; vital signs for baseline data; allergies to medications; compatibility of medication(s) and IV fluid; specific drug action; side effects; normal dosage; recommended administration time; time of peak of action.

EQUIPMENT

- ☐ Physician's order or MAR
- ☐ Correct sterile medication
- ☐ Sterile syringe of the appropriate size for the volume of medication
- ☐ Gloves
- ☐ Antiseptic swabs
- ☐ Sterile 2.5-cm (1-in) #25 gauge needle to prevent large puncture holes in the injection port

In Addition, for an IV Lock

- ☐ One or two syringes and needles, each with 2 mL (or amount prescribed by the agency) of normal saline
- ☐ Sterile syringe and needle with a heparin flush solution (optional)

INTERVENTION

1. Verify the medication order.

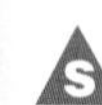

- Check the physician's order carefully for the medication, dosage, route, and rate of administration. Medication rate may also come from the agency, pharmacy, or manufacturer's insert. *A medication that is injected too rapidly can create toxic concentrations in the blood plasma.*

2. Prepare the medication and heparin and/or saline as required.

- Prepare the medication according to Procedure 43–2. Label the syringe with the name of the medication and the dosage.
- For IV locks maintained by heparin injection, prepare the heparin solution according to agency practice. Many hospital protocols include the use of 100 units/mL of solution, and 0.5 mL or 1.0 mL is injected. Label this syringe. A prepackaged heparin syringe may be used.
- Prepare two 2-mL saline flushes. Label these syringes.

3. Administer the medication.

- Check the client's identification band, and ask the client's name.

To Administer Medication into an Existing Line

- Don gloves.
- Inspect the injection site for any signs of infiltration, then identify an injection port nearest the client. Some ports have a circle indicating the site for the needle insertion. *An injection port must be used because it is self-sealing. Any puncture to the plastic tubing will leak.*
- Clean the port with an antiseptic swab.

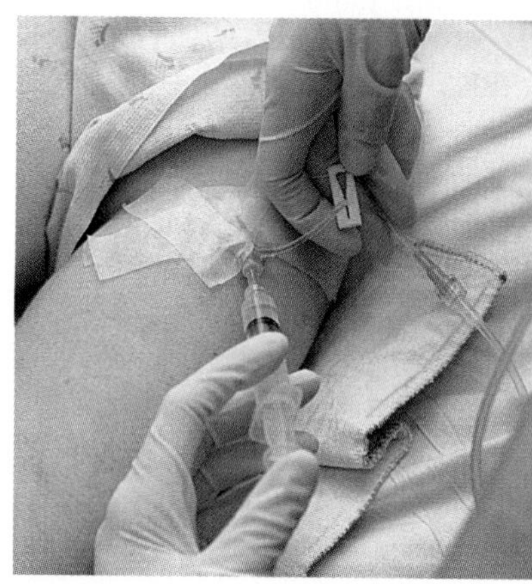

Figure 43–53 Administering medication through an injection port of an existing IV apparatus.

- Stop the IV flow by closing the clamp or pinching the tubing above the injection port (Figure 43–53).
- While holding the port steady, insert the needle into the port.

PROCEDURE 43–9 *continued*

- Draw back on the plunger to withdraw some blood into the IV tubing (not into the syringe) *This shows that the needle or catheter is in the vein.*
- Inject the medication at the ordered rate, withdraw the needle, reopen the clamp, and reestablish the intravenous infusion at the correct rate. If the medication is particularly irritating to the veins, run the IV rapidly for about a minute to dilute the medication, and then adjust the rate.

To Administer Medication into an Intermittent Infusion Set (IV Lock)

- Swab the injection port with an antiseptic swab and permit it to dry.
- Insert the needle attached to the normal saline syringe into the port, and aspirate for blood return (Figure 43–54). *This confirms that the IV lock catheter is in the vein. In some situations, blood will not return even though the IV lock is patent.*

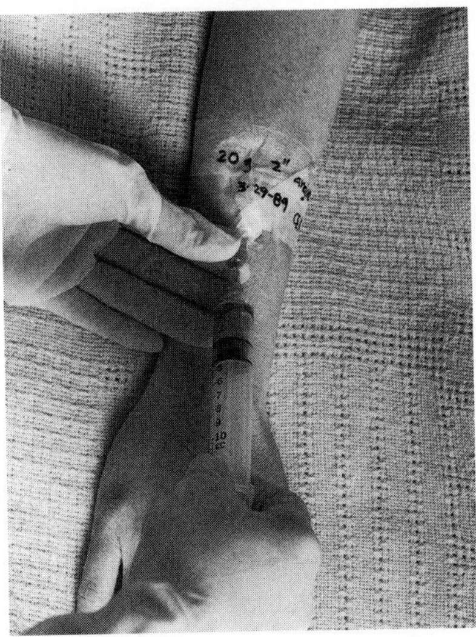

Figure 43–54 Administering medication through an intermittent infusion set (IV Lock).

- Inject ½ to 2 mL of normal saline. This step is *optional.* Check agency practice. *This is done to flush the catheter and to verify patency of the vein.* If the client experiences a burning or stinging sensation, this may be normal, or it may indicate that the needle or catheter is not in the vein and the fluid is infiltrating the tissue. In this case, withhold the medication until the IV lock is replaced.
- Remove the saline syringe.
- Insert the needle attached to the medication syringe into the injection port.
- Inject the medication slowly at the recommended rate of infusion. Observe the client closely for adverse reactions. Remove the needle and syringe when all medication is administered.
- Attach the second saline syringe, and inject the recommended amount of saline. *The saline injection flushes the medication through the catheter and prepares the lock for heparin if this medication is used. Heparin is incompatible with many medications.*
- If heparin is to be used, insert the heparin syringe, and inject the heparin slowly into the set (Figure 43–55).
- Check the patency of the IV lock at least every 8 hours or according to agency practice.
  a. Aspirate for return blood flow.
  b. Flush the catheter with ½ to 2 mL of normal saline.

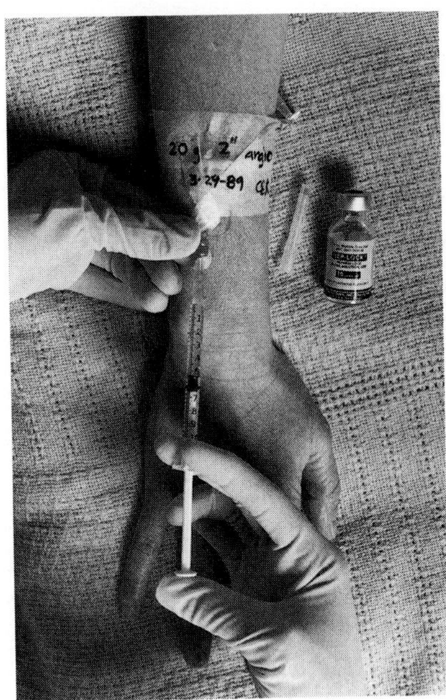

Figure 43–55 Injecting heparin into an intermittent infusion set (IV Lock).

  c. Refill the IV lock with saline or heparin as per agency policy.

- Check agency practice about recommended times for changing the IV lock. Some agencies advocate a change every 48 to 72 hours.

4. Document all relevant information.

- Record the date, time, drug, dose, and route; client response; and assessments of infusion or heparin lock site if appropriate.

EVALUATION FOCUS
Desired effect of medication; any adverse reactions or side effects; change in vital signs; status of IV lock site; patency of IV infusion, if running.

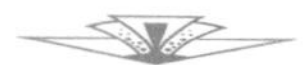

TOPICAL MEDICATIONS

Topical medications include dermatologic medications and irrigations and instillations. Irrigations may or may not be medicated. *Dermatologic medications* are commonly applied for one of the following reasons:

- To decrease itching (pruritus)
- To lubricate and soften the skin
- To cause local vasoconstriction or vasodilation
- To increase or decrease secretions from the skin
- To provide a protective coating to the skin
- To apply an antibiotic or antiseptic to treat or prevent infection

In addition, some medications that are routinely administered by other routes may also be available for use transdermally by applying a "patch" to provide sustained action. Examples of these are nitroglycerin patches and anti–motion sickness preparations. Absorption is facilitated by washing the area well before the application. Dermatologic preparations include lotions, liniments, ointments, pastes, and powders. See Table 43–1, earlier in the chapter.

Unless contraindicated by a specific order, the nurse washes and carefully dries the area, using a patting motion, before applying a dermatologic preparation. Skin encrustations and discharges harbor microorganisms and cause local infections. They can also prevent the medication from coming in contact with the area to be treated. Nurses should always use surgical asepsis when an open wound is present. If a client has lesions, the nurse must wear gloves or use tongue depressors. In this way, the nurse's hand will not come in direct contact with microorganisms in and around the lesions. See Table 43–11 for general guidelines for applying topical medications.

An **irrigation (lavage)** is the washing out of a body cavity by a stream of water or other fluid. An **instillation** is the insertion of a medication into a body cavity. Irrigation is performed for one or more of the following reasons:

- To clean the area, that is, to remove a foreign object or discharge
- To apply heat or cold
- To apply a medication, such as an antiseptic
- To prepare an area for surgery, such as the eye

Surgical asepsis is required when there is a break in the skin (eg, in a wound irrigation), or whenever a sterile body cavity (eg, the bladder) is entered. Some irrigations (eg, an eye irrigation to remove foreign material; or a vaginal, rectal, or gastric irrigation) are often safely conducted using medical asepsis.

Table 43–11 Topical Applications

Medication	Application
Lotion	Shake before use to distribute suspended particles. Pour onto sterile gauze, and pat onto affected area. To avoid aggravating affected area, do not rub.
Liniment	Pour onto hands, and rub into client's skin with long, smooth strokes.
Ointment and paste	Usually applied with a tongue blade or with gloves. Some (eg, cortisone) must be applied thinly over the area. Sterile dressing may be applied over ointment. If a corticosteroid is applied, avoid using an occlusive dressing or plastic-covered diaper. Occlusive materials increase the percutaneous absorption of corticosteroids thus increasing the possibility of systemic absorption and effects.
Powder	Sprinkle over the surface.

Different kinds of syringes are used for irrigations. The most common are the Asepto, the rubber bulb, the Toomey, and the Pomeroy. The syringes are often calibrated, permitting the nurse to determine the amount of irrigant being delivered at any given time. The *Asepto syringe* is a plastic (or glass) syringe with a rubber bulb (Figure 43–56, *A*). Squeezing the air out of the bulb produces negative pressure, and fluid can be sucked into the syringe. When the bulb is squeezed again, the fluid is ejected from the syringe. Asepto syringes come in several sizes, including 30 mL (1 oz), 60 mL (2 oz), and 120 mL (4 oz).

The *rubber bulb syringe* is often used for irrigating the ears (Figure 43–56, *B*). Like the Asepto syringe, the rubber bulb syringe comes in a range of sizes. The *Toomey syringe*, which is made of plastic or glass, is also calibrated (Figure 43–56, *C*). This syringe has a removable tip of metal or plastic that can fit into the end of tubing, such as a catheter. Toomey syringes are used for deep-wound irrigations that require a catheter and for some types of bladder irrigations. The *Pomeroy syringe* is a metal syringe commonly used for ear irrigations. A shield near the tip prevents the solution from spraying outward (Figure 43–56, *D*).

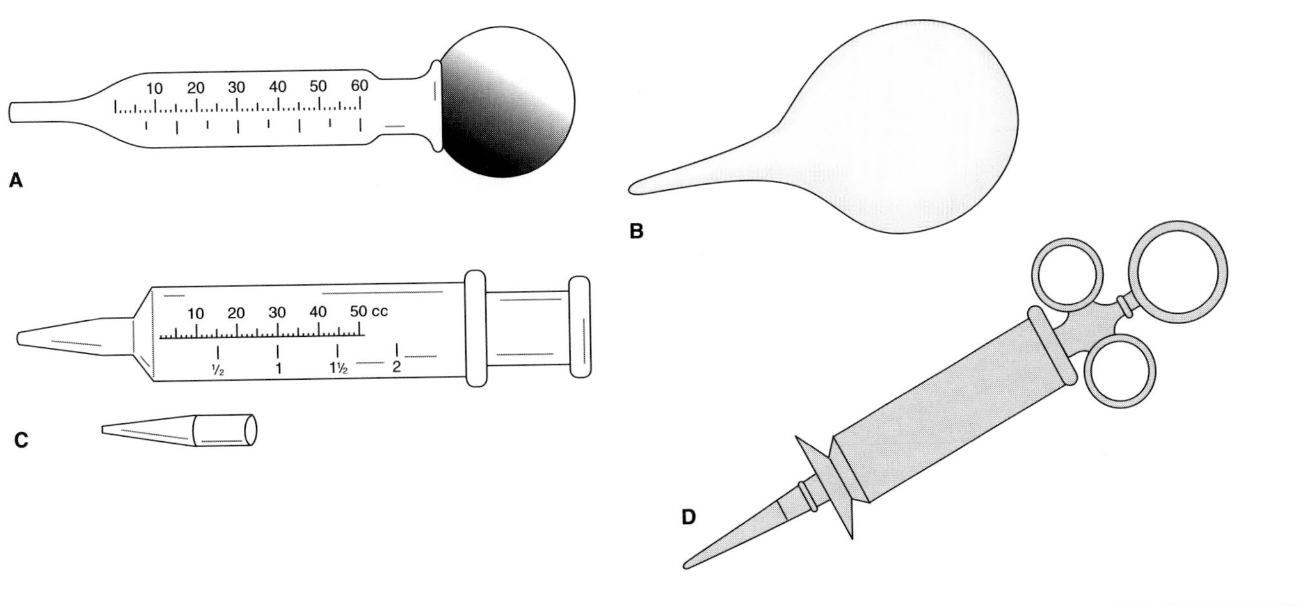

Figure 43–56 Four types of syringes commonly used for irrigations: *A,* Asepto; *B,* rubber bulb; *C,* Toomey with adapter tip to fit into tubing; *D,* Pomeroy.

OPHTHALMIC INSTILLATIONS AND IRRIGATIONS

An eye irrigation is administered to wash out the conjunctival sac of the eye. In a hospital, sterile equipment is usually used. Medications for the eyes are instilled in the form of liquids or ointments. Eye drops are packaged in monodrip plastic containers that are used to administer the preparation. Ointments are usually supplied in small tubes. All containers must state that the medication is for ophthalmic use. Sterile preparations and sterile technique are indicated. Prescribed liquids are usually dilute, for example, less than 1% strength. Procedure 43–10 illustrates how to administer ophthalmic instillations and irrigations.

Text continued on page 1348

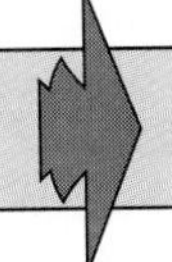

PROCEDURE 43–10 ADMINISTERING OPHTHALMIC INSTILLATIONS AND IRRIGATIONS

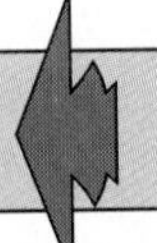

PURPOSES

Instillation

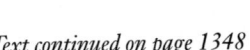

- To provide an eye medication the client requires (eg, an antibiotic) to treat an infection or for other reasons (see specific drug action)

Irrigation

- To clear the eye of noxious or other foreign material or excessive secretions or in preparation for surgery

ASSESSMENT FOCUS

Allergy to medication; appearance of eye and surrounding structures for lesions, exudate, erythema, or swelling; the location and nature of any discharge; lacrimation, and swelling of the eyelids or of the lacrimal gland; client complaints (eg, itching, burning, pain, blurred vision, and photophobia); client behavior (eg, squinting, blinking excessively, frowning, or rubbing the eyes); client's level of consciousness and ability or willingness to cooperate (eg, restlessness, disorientation); specific drug action and side effects; client's knowledge about the medication.

PROCEDURE 43–10 ADMINISTERING OPHTHALMIC INSTILLATIONS AND IRRIGATIONS *continued*

EQUIPMENT

Instillation

- ☐ Sterile gloves
- ☐ Sterile absorbent sponges soaked in sterile normal saline
- ☐ Medication
- ☐ Dry sterile absorbent sponges
- ☐ Sterile eye dressing (pad) as needed and paper eye tape to secure it

Irrigation

- ☐ Moistureproof drape
- ☐ Sterile kidney basin
- ☐ Sterile gloves
- ☐ Sterile cotton balls
- ☐ Sterile normal saline (optional)
- ☐ Sterile container for the irrigating solution
- ☐ Irrigating solution [usually 60 to 240 mL (2 to 8 oz) of solution at 37 C (98.6 F) is appropriate]
- ☐ Sterile eye syringe or eye irrigator (eyedropper can be used if only small amounts of solution are required)

INTERVENTION

1. Verify the medication or irrigation order.

Instillation

- Check the physician's order for the preparation, strength, and number of drops. Also confirm the prescribed frequency of the instillation and which eye is to be treated. Abbreviations are frequently used to identify the eye: OD (right eye), OS (left eye), OU (both eyes).
- Check the expiration date and ensure that the medication is clearly labeled.

Irrigation

- Check the type, amount, temperature, and strength of the solution and the frequency of the irrigation.

2. Prepare the client.

- Check the client's identification band, and ask the client's name.
- Explain the technique to the client or to the parents of an infant or child. The administration of an ophthalmic irrigating solution or medication is not usually painful. Ointments are often soothing to the eye, but some liquid preparations may sting initially.
- For a young child, use a doll to demonstrate the procedure. *This facilitates cooperation and decreases anxiety.*
- Assist the client to a comfortable position, either sitting or lying. For an irrigation, tilt the client's head toward the affected eye, and ensure that the light source does not shine into the person's eyes. *The head is tilted so that the irrigating or cleaning solution will run from the eye to the basin at the side, not to the other eye. The light source is directed slightly away from the eye, particularly if the person is photophobic.*
- For a young child or infant, enlist assistance to immobilize the arms and head. The parent may hold the infant or young child. *This prevents accidental injury during medication administration.*
- For an irrigation, place the drape to protect the client and the bedclothes, and position the basin against the cheek below the eye on the affected side.

3. Clean the eyelid and the eyelashes.

- Don sterile gloves.
- Use sterile cotton balls moistened with sterile irrigating solution or sterile normal saline, and wipe from the inner canthus to the outer canthus: *If not removed, material on the eyelid and lashes can be washed into the eye. Cleaning toward the outer canthus prevents contamination of the other eye and the lacrimal duct.*

4. Administer the eye medication or irrigation.

Instillation

- Check the ophthalmic preparation for the name, strength, and number of drops if a liquid is used. Draw the correct number of drops into the shaft of the dropper if a dropper is used. If ointment is used, discard the first bead. *Checking medication data is essential to prevent a medication error. The first bead of ointment from a tube is considered to be contaminated.*
- Instruct the client to look up to the ceiling. Give the client a dry sterile absorbent sponge. *The person is less likely to blink if looking up. While the client looks up, the cornea is partially protected by the top eyelid. A sponge is needed to press on the nasolacrimal duct after a liquid instillation or to wipe excess ointment from the eyelashes after an ointment is instilled.*

PROCEDURE 43–10 *continued*

- Expose the lower conjunctival sac by placing the thumb or fingers of your nondominant hand on the client's cheekbone just below the eye and gently drawing down the skin on the cheek. If the tissues are edematous, handle the tissues carefully to avoid damaging them. *Placing the fingers on the cheekbone minimizes the possibility of touching the cornea, avoids putting any pressure on the eyeball, and prevents the person from blinking or squinting.*

- Approach the eye from the side and instill the correct number of drops onto the outer third of the lower conjunctival sac. Hold the dropper 1 to 2 cm (0.4 to 0.8 in) above the sac (Figure 43–57). *The client is less likely to blink if a side approach is used. When instilled into the conjunctival sac, drops will not harm the cornea as they might if dropped directly on it. The dropper must not touch the sac or the cornea.*

or

- Holding the tube above the lower conjunctival sac, squeeze 2 cm (0.8 in) of ointment from the tube into the lower conjunctival sac from the inner canthus outward (Figure 43–58).

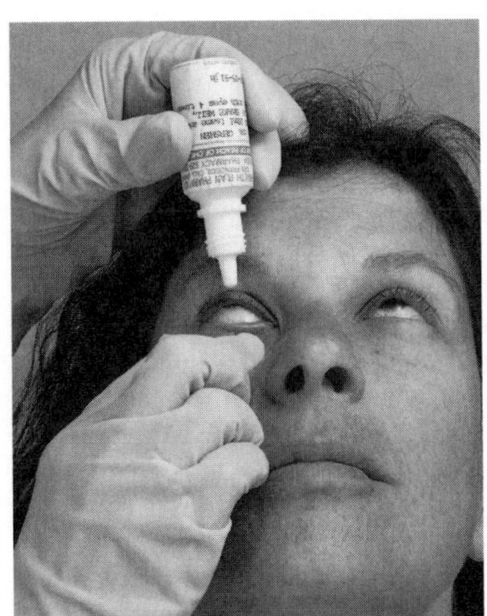

Figure 43–57 Instilling an eye drop into the lower conjuctival sac.

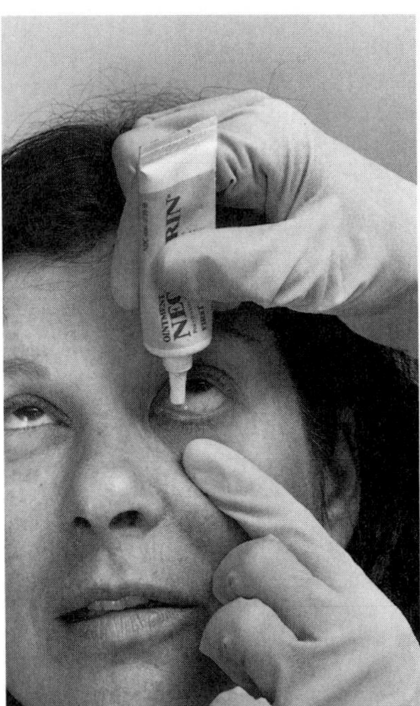

Figure 43–58 Instilling an eye ointment into the lower conjunctival sac.

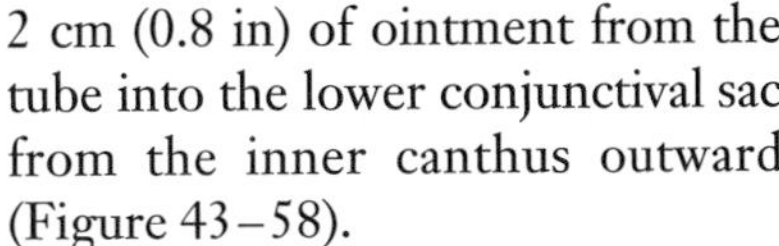

- Instruct the client to close the eyelids but not to squeeze them shut. *Closing the eye spreads the medication over the eyeball. Squeezing can injure the eye and push out the medication.*
- For liquid medications, press firmly or have the client press firmly on the nasolacrimal duct for at least 30 seconds (Figure 43–59). Check agency practice. *Pressing on the nasolacrimal duct prevents the medication from running out of the eye and down the duct.*

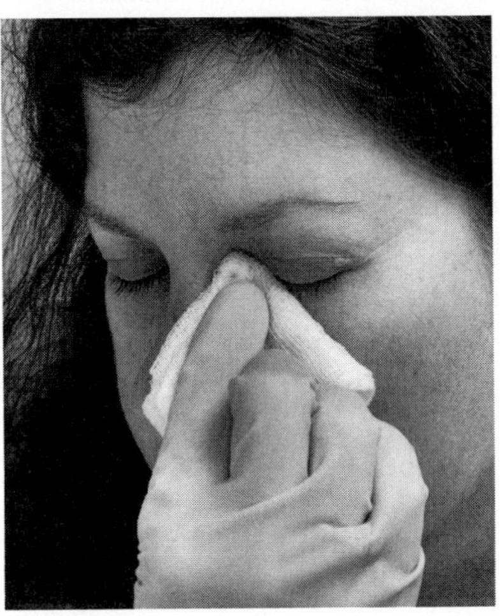

Figure 43–59 Pressing on the nasolacrimal duct.

Irrigation

- Expose the lower conjunctival sac by separating the lids with the thumb and forefinger (Figure 43–60). Or, to irrigate in stages, first hold the lower lid down, then hold the upper lid up. Exert pressure on the bony prominences of the cheekbone and beneath the eyebrow when holding the eyelids. *Separating the lids prevents reflex blinking. Exerting pressure on the bony prominences minimizes the possibility of pressing the eyeball and causing discomfort.*

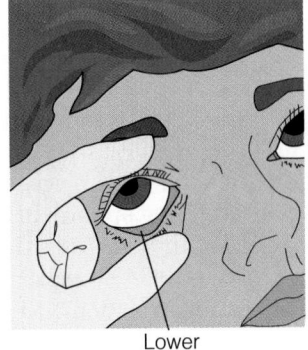

Figure 43–60 Exposing the lower conjunctival sac.

PROCEDURE 43–10 ADMINISTERING OPHTHALMIC INSTILLATIONS AND IRRIGATIONS *continued*

- Fill and hold the eye irrigator about 2.5 cm (1 in) above the eye. *At this height the pressure of the solution will not damage eye tissue, and the irrigator will not touch the eye.*
- Irrigate the eye, directing the solution onto the lower conjunctival sac and from the inner canthus to the outer canthus. *Directing the solution in this way prevents possible injury to the cornea and prevents fluid and contaminants from flowing down the nasolacrimal duct.*

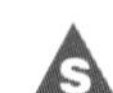

- Irrigate until the solution leaving the eye is clear (no discharge is present) or until all the solution has been used.
- Instruct the client to close and move the eye periodically. *Eye closure and movement help to move secretions from the upper to the lower conjunctival sac.*
- Dry around the eye with cotton balls.

5. Clean the eyelids as needed. Wipe the eyelids gently from the inner to the outer canthus to collect excess medication.

6. Apply an eye pad if needed, and secure it with paper eye tape.

7. Assess the client's response.

- Assess responses immediately after the instillation or irrigation and again after the medication should have acted.

8. Document all relevant information.

- Record nursing assessments and interventions relative to the instillation or irrigation. Include the name of the drug, the strength, the number of drops if a liquid, the time, and the response of the client.

EVALUATION FOCUS

Relief of complaints; change in appearance of eye in accordance with drug action; amount and character of exudate; character of irrigation returns; adverse reactions or side effects of medication.

OTIC INSTILLATIONS AND IRRIGATIONS

Irrigations of the external auditory canal are generally carried out for cleaning purposes, although applications of heat and of antiseptic solutions are sometimes prescribed. Irrigations are usually performed in a hospital, using sterile supplies and equipment so that microorganisms will not be introduced into the ear. Normal saline at body temperature (37.0 C, or 98.6 F) is frequently used to irrigate the ear. The nurse uses a thermometer to ensure that the temperature of the solution is appropriate. Medical aseptic technique is used to instill medications to the ear unless the tympanic membrane is damaged, in which case sterile technique is used. The position of the external auditory canal varies with age. In the child under 3 years of age, it is directed upward. In the adult, the external auditory canal is an S-shaped structure about 2.5 cm (1 in) long. Procedure 43–11 explains how to administer otic instillations and irrigations.

NASAL INSTILLATIONS

Nasal instillations (nose drops) usually are instilled for their astringent effect (to shrink swollen mucous membranes), to loosen secretions and facilitate drainage, or to treat infections of the nasal cavity or sinuses. Nasal decongestants are the most common nasal instillations. Many of these products are available over-the-counter. Clients need to be taught to use these agents with caution. Chronic use of nasal decongestants may lead to a rebound effect, that is, an increase in nasal congestion.

Prior to a nasal instillation, the nurse should instruct the client to blow the nose to clear the nasal passages. Instilling nose drops requires that the client assume a back-lying position. A pillow is placed under the shoulders thus allowing the head to fall over the edge of the pillow (Figure 43–63, p. 1351).

To facilitate insertion of the drops, the nurse elevates the nares slightly by pressing the thumb against the tip of the client's nose. The nurse holds the dropper just above the client's nostril and directs the drops toward the midline of the superior concha of the ethmoid bone as the client breathes through the mouth. If the drops are directed toward the base of the nasal cavity, they will run down the eustachian tube. The nurse avoids touching the mucous membranes of the nostrils to avoid injury to tissue and contamination of the dropper. The nurse asks the client to (a) inhale slowly and deeply through the nose; (b) hold the breath for several seconds and then exhale slowly; and (c) remain in a back-lying position for 1 minute so that the solution will come into contact with all of

Text continued on page 1351

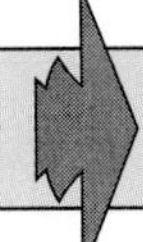

PROCEDURE 43–11 ADMINISTERING OTIC INSTILLATIONS AND IRRIGATIONS

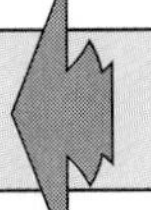

PURPOSES

Instillation

- To soften earwax so that it can be readily removed at a later time
- To provide local therapy to reduce inflammation and/or destroy infective organisms in the external ear canal
- To relieve pain

Irrigation

- To clean the canal, for example, to remove cerumen or pus
- To apply heat
- To remove a foreign object, such as an insect

ASSESSMENT FOCUS

Allergy to medication; the pinna of the ear and meatus for signs of redness and abrasions; the type and amount of any discharge; complaints of discomfort; intactness and appearance of the tympanic membrane and presence of foreign bodies in the ear canal (an irrigation is contraindicated if the membrane is not intact or a foreign body is present); ability to cooperate during the procedure; specific drug action and side effects; client's knowledge about the medication to be used.

EQUIPMENT

Instillation

- ☐ Gloves (optional)
- ☐ Cotton-tipped applicator
- ☐ Correct medication bottle with a dropper
- ☐ Flexible rubber tip (optional) for the end of the dropper, which prevents injury from sudden motion, for example, by a child or disoriented client
- ☐ Cotton fluff

Irrigation

- ☐ Moisture-resistant towel
- ☐ Basin (eg, kidney basin)
- ☐ Gloves (optional)
- ☐ Applicator swabs
- ☐ Irrigating solution at the appropriate temperature, about 500 mL (16 oz) or as ordered
- ☐ Container for the irrigating solution
- ☐ Syringe (rubber bulb or Asepto syringe is frequently used)
- ☐ Absorbent cotton balls

INTERVENTION

1. Verify the medication or irrigation order.

- Check the physician's order for the kind of medication or irrigation; the time, amount, and dosage (if it is an instillation) or strength (if it is an irrigation); the temperature (if it is an irrigation); and which ear is to be treated.

2. Prepare the client.

- Check the client's identification band, and ask the client's name.

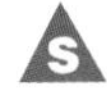

- Obtain assistance to immobilize an infant or young child. *This prevents accidental injury due to sudden movement during the procedure or medication administration.*

Instillation

- Assist the client to a side-lying position with the ear being treated uppermost (Figure 43–61).

Irrigation

- Explain that the client may experience a feeling of fullness, warmth, and, occasionally, discomfort when the fluid comes in contact with the tympanic membrane.
- Assist the client to a sitting or lying position with head turned toward the affected ear. *The solution can then flow from the ear canal to a basin.*

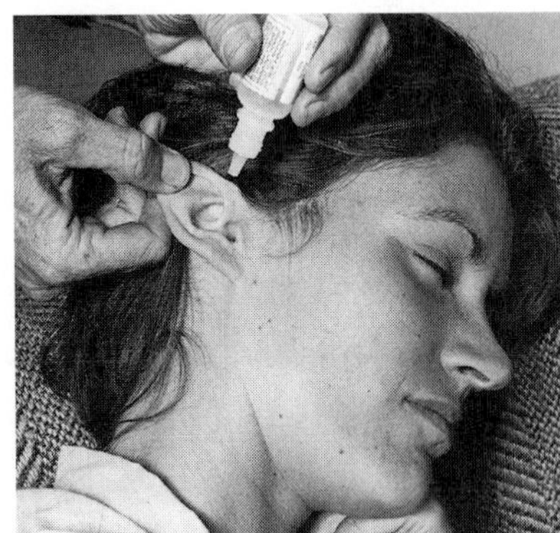

Figure 43–61 Instilling ear drops.

- Place the moisture-resistant towel around the client's shoul-

PROCEDURE 43-11 ADMINISTERING OTIC INSTILLATIONS AND IRRIGATIONS *continued*

der under the ear to be irrigated, and place the basin under the ear to be irrigated.

3. Clean the pinna of the ear and the meatus of the ear canal.

- Don gloves if infection is suspected.

- Use cotton-tipped applicators and solution to wipe the pinna and auditory meatus. *Any discharge is removed so that it will not be washed into the ear canal during an irrigation. It is cleaned before an instillation to remove any drainage.*

4. If doing an irrigation, prepare the equipment. (Omit this step for an instillation.)

- Fill the syringe with solution.
  or
  Hang up the irrigating container, and run solution through the tubing and the nozzle. *Solution is run through to remove air from the tubing and nozzle.*

5. Administer the ear medication or irrigation.

Instillation

- Warm the medication container in your hand, or place it in warm water for a short time. *This promotes client comfort.*
- Partially fill the ear dropper with medication.
- Straighten the auditory canal. For an infant, gently pull the pinna down and back (Figure 43–62). For an adult or a child older than 3 years of age, pull the pinna upward and backward. See Figure 22–19, page 493. *The auditory canal is straightened so that the solution can flow the entire length of the canal.*

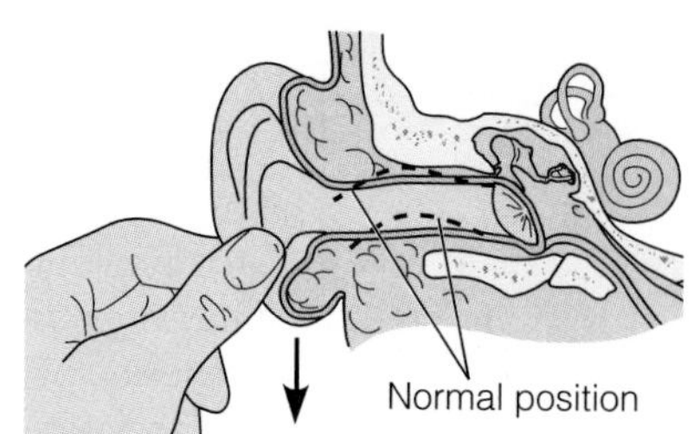

Figure 43–62 Straightening the ear canal of a child by pulling the pinna down and back.

- Instill the correct number of drops along the side of the ear canal.
- Press gently but firmly a few times on the tragus of the ear. *Pressing on the tragus assists the flow of medication into the ear canal.*
- Ask the client to remain in the side-lying position for about 5 minutes. *This prevents the drops from escaping and allows the medication to reach all sides of the canal cavity.*
- Insert a small piece of cotton fluff loosely at the meatus of the auditory canal for 15 to 20 minutes. Do not press it into the canal. *The cotton helps retain the medication when the client is up. If pressed tightly into the canal, the cotton would interfere with the action of the drug and the outward movement of normal secretions.*

Irrigation

- Straighten the ear canal.
- Insert the tip of the syringe into the auditory meatus, and direct the solution gently upward against the top of the canal. *The solution will flow around the entire canal and out at the bottom. The solution is instilled gently because*

strong pressure from the fluid can cause discomfort and damage the tympanic membrane.

- Continue instilling the fluid until all the solution is used or until the canal is cleaned, depending on the purpose of the irrigation. Take care not to block the outward flow of the solution with the syringe.
- Dry the outside of the ear with absorbent cotton balls. Place a cotton fluff in the auditory meatus to absorb the excess fluid.
- Assist the client to a side-lying position on the affected side. *Lying with the affected side down helps drain the excess fluid by gravity.*

6. Assess the client's response.

Instillation

- Assess the character and amount of discharge, appearance of the canal, discomfort, and so on, immediately after the instillation and again when the medication is expected to act. Inspect the cotton ball for any drainage.

Irrigation

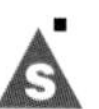

- Assess the client for any discomfort and the appearance and odor of the fluid returns.

7. Document all relevant information.

- Document all nursing assessments and interventions relative to the procedure.

Instillation

- Include the time, the dose, and any complaints of pain. Many agencies use flowsheets; others may require that a notation be made on the nurse's notes.

PROCEDURE 43-11 *continued*

Irrigation

- Include the type, concentration, amount, and temperature of the solution used; the appearance of the returns; and the presence of any discomfort.

EVALUATION FOCUS
Relief of complaints; change in appearance of ear in accordance with drug action; amount and character of discharge; appearance of tympanic membrane; character of irrigation returns; presence of adverse reactions or side effects of medication.

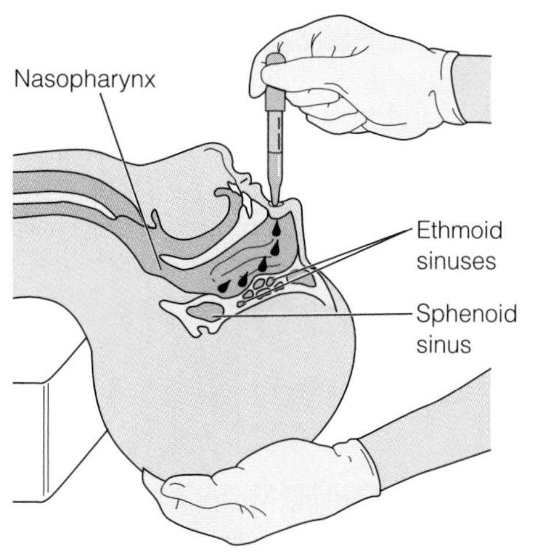

Figure 43-63 Position to instill drops into the nostrils.

the nasal surface. The nurse discards any medication remaining in the dropper before returning the dropper to the bottle.

NEBULIZERS

A **nebulizer** is used to deliver a fine spray of medication or moisture to a client. **Nebulization** is the production of a fog or mist.

There are two kinds of nebulization: atomization and aerosolization. In *atomization*, a device called an *atomizer* produces rather large droplets for inhalation. In *aerosolization*, or **inhalation therapy,** the droplets are suspended in a gas, such as oxygen. The smaller the droplets, the further they can be inhaled into the respiratory tract. When a medication is intended for the nasal mucosa, it is inhaled through the nose; when it is intended for the trachea, bronchi, and/or lungs, it is inhaled through the mouth.

A *large-volume nebulizer* can provide a heated or cool mist. It is used for long-term therapy, such as that following a tracheostomy. These nebulizers have a 250-mL capacity and deliver oxygen or room air. The *ultrasonic nebulizer* provides 100% humidity and can provide particles small enough to be inhaled deeply into the respiratory tract. There are two types of ultrasonic nebulizers: one has a cup filled with sterile distilled water; the other requires a continuous supply of sterile distilled water from a bag connected by tubing to the nebulizer bottle.

The *hand (metered-dose) nebulizer* (Figure 43-64) is a container of medication that can be compressed by hand to release the medication through a nosepiece or mouthpiece. The force with which the air moves through the nebulizer causes the large particles of medicated solution to break up into finer particles, forming a mist or fine spray. Aerosol inhalers must be used properly to ensure

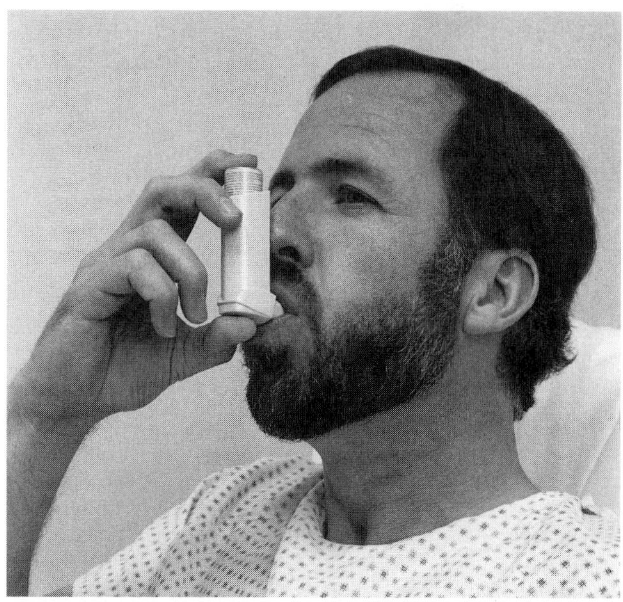

Figure 43-64 A hand nebulizer, or metered-dose inhaler.

correct delivery of the prescribed medication. See the box below for instructions on teaching a client to use a hand nebulizer. The *mininebulizer* is used with oxygen or a pressurized gas source, such as air. With this device, the client inhales and exhales independently. Medication is administered during inhalation. A *side-stream nebulizer* provides a medication to a client on a ventilator or receiving intermittent positive pressure breathing (IPPB) therapy. The gas (eg, oxygen) passes through a device containing the medicated solution and then into the ventilator and to the client.

Vaginal Instillations and Irrigations

A vaginal irrigation (douche) is the washing of the vagina by a liquid at a low pressure. It is similar to the irrigation of the external auditory canal in that the fluid returns immediately after being inserted. Vaginal irrigations are not necessary for ordinary female hygiene but are used to prevent infection by applying an antimicrobial solution that discourages the growth of microorganisms, to remove an offensive or irritating discharge, and to reduce inflammation or prevent hemorrhage by the application of heat or cold. Commonly a povidone-iodine solution is prescribed.

In hospitals, sterile supplies and equipment are used; in a home, sterility is not usually necessary because people are accustomed to the microorganisms in their environments. Sterile technique is indicated if there is an open wound. Usually, 1000 to 2000 mL of irrigating solution at 40.5 C (105 F) is required. Check agency protocol. Normal saline, tap water, sodium bicarbonate solution (8 mL of sodium bicarbonate to 1000 mL of water), and vinegar solution (8 mL of vinegar to 1000 mL of water) are commonly used. Before taking the equipment to the client, the nurse uses a thermometer to check the temperature of the solution.

Vaginal medications, or instillations, are inserted as creams, jellies, foams, or suppositories to relieve infection or to relieve vaginal discomfort, for example, itching or pain. Medical aseptic technique is usually used. Vaginal creams, jellies, and foams are applied by using a tubular applicator with a plunger. Suppositories are inserted with the index finger of a gloved hand. Suppositories are designed to melt at body temperature, so they are generally stored in the refrigerator to keep them firm for insertion. See Procedure 43–12 for administering vaginal instillations and irrigations.

CLIENT TEACHING

Using a Hand Nebulizer

- Make sure the canister is firmly and fully inserted into the outer shell or actuator. Press the canister firmly into the actuator with a twisting motion, and rotate back and forth several times.
- Remove the cap from the mouthpiece. Hold the inhaler in the hand and shake by inverting it several times.
- Breathe out slowly until no more air can be expelled from the lungs, then immediately *(for the next step there are two alternatives, depending on the technique preferred by the physician)*:
- Place the mouthpiece over the tongue and well into the mouth. Close the lips tightly around the mouthpiece. Press the top of the canister firmly between forefinger and thumb, while inhaling deeply and slowly,

  or

  Place the inhaler directly in front of the mouth. Begin a slow inward breath through the wide open mouth, at the same time pressing the canister down firmly into the inhaler.
- Continue inhaling to carry the spray deep into the lungs. Hold the breath for as long as is comfortable.
- Release the pressure on the canister. Remove the inhaler away from mouth and breathe out gently.
- *Before the second puff,* wait for at least 30 seconds for the valve pressure to rebuild. Then rotate the canister back and forth, and again shake several times before reusing.

Common Problems in Using an Inhaler

- Not taking the medication as prescribed, but taking either too much or too little.
- Incorrect activation. This usually occurs through pressing the canister before taking a breath. Both should be done simultaneously so that the drug can be carried down to the lungs with the breath.
- Forgetting to shake the inhaler. Because the drug is in a suspension, particles may settle. If the inhaler is not shaken, it may not deliver the correct dose of the drug.
- Not waiting long enough (30 seconds) between puffs. The whole process should be repeated to take the second puff; otherwise, the dose may be incorrect, or the drug may not penetrate the lungs.

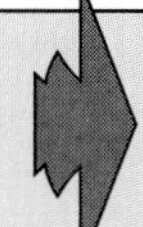

PROCEDURE 43–12 ADMINISTERING VAGINAL INSTILLATIONS AND IRRIGATIONS

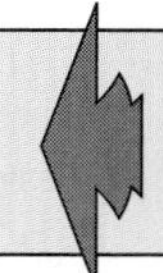

PURPOSES

- To treat or prevent infection
- To remove an offensive or irritating discharge
- To reduce inflammation
- To relieve vaginal discomfort

ASSESSMENT FOCUS

Allergy to medications or irrigating fluid; vaginal orifice for inflammation; amount, character, and odor of vaginal discharge; complaints of vaginal discomfort (eg, burning or itching).

EQUIPMENT

Vaginal Instillation

- ☐ Drape
- ☐ Correct vaginal suppository or cream
- ☐ Applicator for vaginal cream
- ☐ Disposable gloves
- ☐ Lubricant for a suppository
- ☐ Disposable towel
- ☐ Clean perineal pad and T-binder or sanitary belt

Vaginal Irrigation

- ☐ Bedpan
- ☐ Roll or pillow
- ☐ Moistureproof pad
- ☐ Moisture-resistant drape
- ☐ Vaginal irrigation set (these are often disposable) containing a nozzle, tubing and a clamp, and a container for the solution
- ☐ IV pole
- ☐ Irrigating solution
- ☐ Gloves
- ☐ Tissues
- ☐ Clean perineal pad and T-binder or sanitary belt

INTERVENTION

1. Verify the medication or irrigation order.

- Carefully check the physician's order for the specific medication or solution ordered, its dosage, and the time of administration.

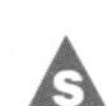

- Check the client's identification band, and ask the client's name.

2. Prepare the client.

- Explain to the client that a vaginal irrigation or instillation is normally a painless procedure and, in fact, may bring relief from itching and burning if an infection is present. An irrigation usually takes about 10 minutes. Many people feel embarrassed about these procedures, and some may prefer to perform the procedure themselves if instruction is provided.
- Provide privacy, and ask the client to void. *If the bladder is empty, the client will have less discomfort during the treatment, and the possibility of injuring the vaginal lining is decreased.*

3. Position and drape the client appropriately.

Instillation

- Assist the client to a back-lying position with the knees flexed and the hips rotated laterally.
- Drape the client appropriately so that only the perineal area is exposed.

Irrigation

- Assist the client to a back-lying position with the hips higher than the shoulders so that the solution will flow into the posterior fornix of the vagina. Position the client on a bedpan, and provide comfortable support for the lumbar region of the back with a roll or pillow.
- Place the waterproof pad under the bedpan to protect the bedding.
- Provide a drape for the legs so that only the perineal area is exposed.

4. Prepare the equipment.

Instillation

- Unwrap the suppository, and put it on the opened wrapper.
  or
  Fill the applicator with the prescribed cream, jelly, or foam. Directions are provided with the manufacturer's applicator.

Irrigation

- Clamp the tubing. Hang the irrigating container on the IV pole so that the base is about 30 cm (12 in) above the vagina. *At this*

PROCEDURE 43-12 ADMINISTERING VAGINAL INSTILLATIONS AND IRRIGATIONS *continued*

height, the pressure of the solution should not be great enough to injure the vaginal lining.

- Run fluid through the tubing and nozzle into the bedpan. *Fluid is run through the tubing to remove air and to moisten the nozzle.*

5. Assess and clean the perineal area.

- Don gloves. *Gloves prevent contamination of the nurse's hands from vaginal and perineal microorganisms.*
- Inspect the vaginal orifice, note any odor or discharge from the vagina, and ask about any vaginal discomfort. (See Assessment Focus, earlier.)
- Provide perineal care to remove microorganisms. *This decreases the chance of moving microorganisms into the vagina.*

6. Administer the vaginal suppository, cream, foam, jelly, or irrigation.

Suppository

- Lubricate the rounded (smooth) end of the suppository, which is inserted first. *Lubrication facilitates insertion.*
- Lubricate your gloved index finger.
- Expose the vaginal orifice by separating the labia with your nondominant hand.
- Insert the suppository about 8 to 10 cm (3 to 4 in) along the posterior wall of the vagina, or as far as it will go (Figure 43–65). The posterior wall of the vagina is about 2.5 cm (1 in) longer than the anterior wall because the cervix protrudes into the uppermost portion of the anterior wall. The anterior wall is usually about 6 to 7.5 cm (2½ to 3 in).

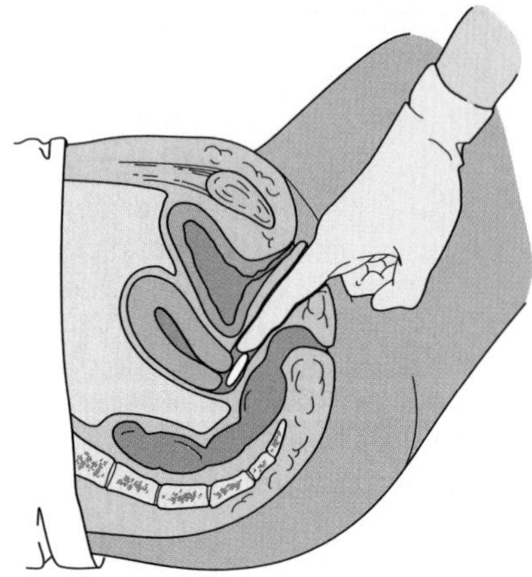

Figure 43–65 Instilling a vaginal suppository.

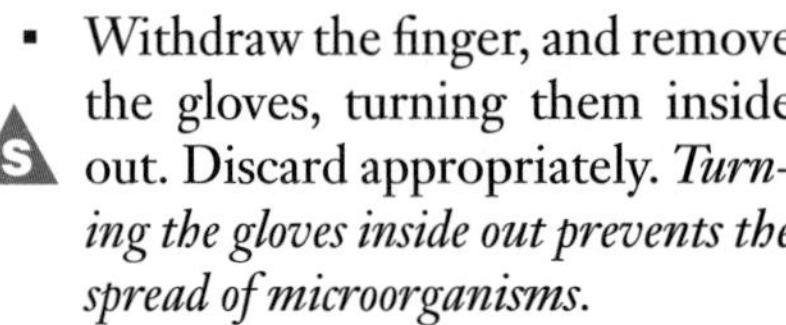

- Withdraw the finger, and remove the gloves, turning them inside out. Discard appropriately. *Turning the gloves inside out prevents the spread of microorganisms.*
- Ask the client to remain lying in the supine position for 5 to 10 minutes following insertion. The hips may also be elevated on a pillow. *This position allows the medication to flow into the posterior fornix after it has melted.*

Vaginal Cream, Jelly, or Foam

- Gently insert the applicator about 5 cm (2 in).
- Slowly push the plunger until the applicator is empty (Figure 43–66).
- Remove the applicator, and place it on the towel. *The applicator is put on the towel to prevent the spread of microorganisms.*
- Discard the applicator if disposable or clean it according to the manufacturer's directions.
- Remove the gloves, turning them inside out. Discard appropriately.
- Ask the client to remain in bed in the supine position for 5 to 10 minutes following the instillation.

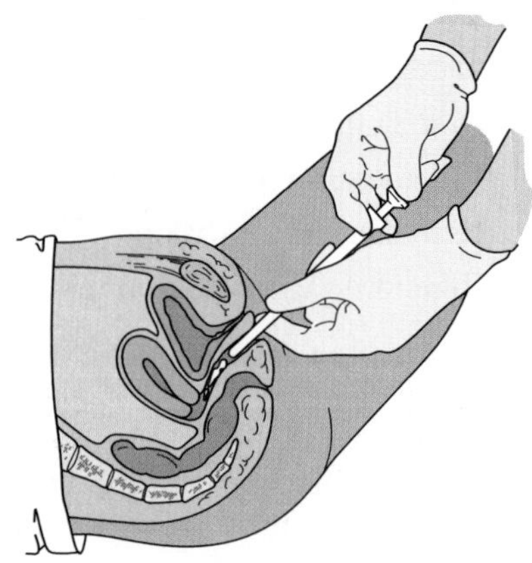

Figure 43–66 Using an applicator to instill a vaginal cream.

Irrigation

- Run some fluid over the perineal area, then insert the nozzle carefully into the vagina. Direct the nozzle toward the sacrum, following the direction of the vagina.
- Insert the nozzle about 7 to 10 cm (3 to 4 in), start the flow, and rotate the nozzle several times. *Rotating the nozzle irrigates all parts of the vagina.*
- Use all the irrigating solution, permitting it to flow out freely into the bedpan. *Obstructing the flow of the returns could result in injury to the tissues from pressure.*
- Remove the nozzle from the vagina.
- Assist the client to a sitting position on the bedpan. *Sitting on the bedpan will help drain the remaining fluid by gravity.*

7. Ensure client comfort.

- Dry the perineum with tissues as required.

PROCEDURE 43–12 *continued*

- Remove the bedpan, if used.
- Remove the moisture-resistant pad and the drape.
- Apply a clean perineal pad and a T-binder if there is excessive drainage.

8. Document all relevant information.

- Record the instillation and assessments as for other medications and instillations.
- To record the administration of the irrigation, note when it was administered; the amount, type, strength, and temperature of the irrigating solution; and all nursing assessments.

9. Assess the client's response.

EVALUATION FOCUS
Relief of complaints; amount, character, and odor of discharge; appearance of vaginal orifice to compare to baseline data; character of irrigation returns; adverse reactions or side effects of medication.

RECTAL INSTILLATIONS

Insertion of medications into the rectum in the form of suppositories is a frequent practice. Rectal administration is a convenient and safe method of giving certain medications. Advantages include the following:

- It avoids irritation of the upper gastrointestinal tract in clients who encounter this problem.
- It is advantageous when the medication has an objectionable taste or odor.
- The drug is released at a slow but steady rate.
- Rectal suppositories are thought to provide higher bloodstream levels (titers) of medication, because the venous blood from the lower rectum is not transported through the liver.

To insert a rectal suppository

- Assist the client to a left lateral position, with the upper leg flexed.
- Fold back the top bedclothes to expose the buttocks.
- Don a glove on the hand used to insert the suppository.
- Unwrap the suppository and lubricate the smooth rounded end, or see manufacturer's instructions. The rounded end is usually inserted first and lubricant reduces irritation of the mucosa.
- Lubricate the gloved index finger.
- Encourage the client to relax by breathing through the mouth.
- Insert the suppository gently into the anal canal, rounded end first (or according to manufacturer's instructions), along the rectal wall using the gloved index finger (see Figure 43–67). For an adult, insert the suppository beyond the internal sphincter (ie, 10 cm [4 inches]); for a child or infant, insert it 5 cm (2 inches) or less.
- Avoid embedding the suppository in feces.
- Press the client's buttocks together for a few minutes.
- Ask the client to remain in the left lateral or supine position for at least 5 minutes to help retain the suppository. The suppository should be retained for at least 30 to 40 minutes or according to manufacturer's instructions.

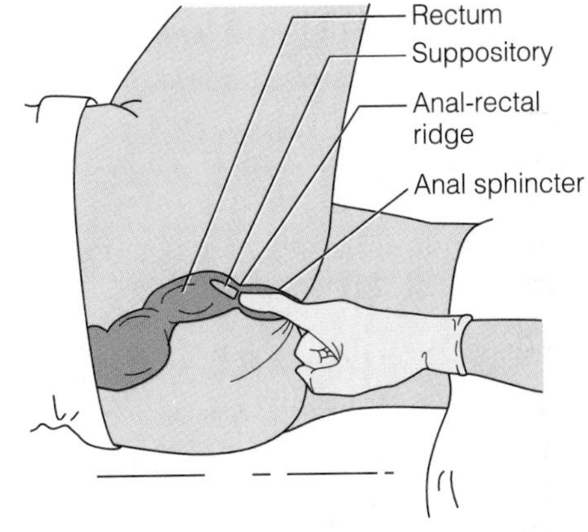

Figure 43–67 Inserting a rectal suppository beyond the internal sphincter and along the rectal wall.

CRITICAL THINKING CHALLENGE

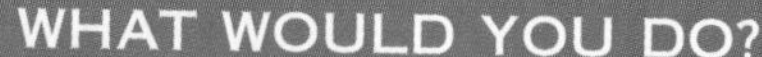

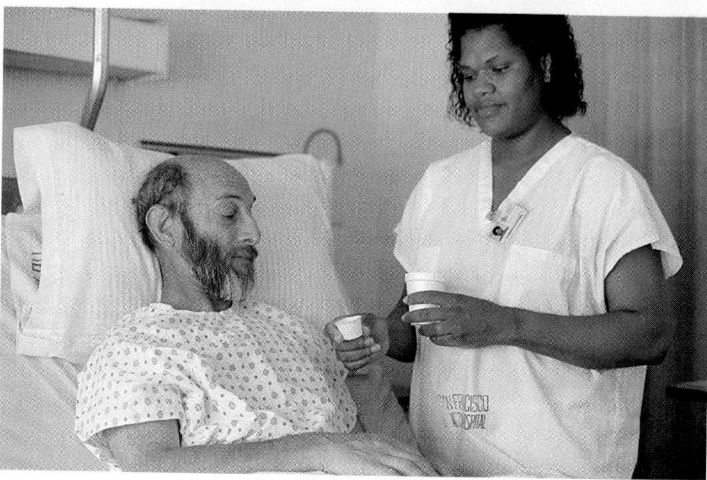

Rich Horowitz, a 55-year-old male on your medical unit, refuses to take his medication. He tells you that it makes him extremely thirsty, and leaves a metallic taste in his mouth.

What would you do?

CHAPTER HIGHLIGHTS

- Federal drug legislation in the United States and Canada regulates the production, prescription, distribution, and administration of drugs.
- Nursing practice acts define limits on the nurse's responsibilities regarding medications.
- Drugs are classified according to their overall action in the body.
- Primary actions of drugs in the body are stimulation and inhibition of tissue or organ functions.
- A drug may be incompatible with another drug or a particular food or an intravenous solution.
- Repeated doses of a drug will achieve a sustained level in the bloodstream.
- Obese clients require a larger dose of a drug than thin clients.
- Drugs given parenterally act more quickly than drugs given orally or topically.
- The five "rights" help ensure accurate administration of a drug.
- Parenteral administration of medications employs sterile technique.
- Clients receiving a series of injections should have the injection sites rotated.
- Administered drugs must be recorded immediately after they have been given.
- Medications should be given at the time they are ordered.
- Drug errors must be reported immediately upon occurrence.
- Nurses must always consider client safety and universal precautions when administering medications.
- All clients should be monitored for therapeutic effects and side effects of medications.
- The Z-track method of intramuscular injections protects subcutaneous tissues from medications that are irritating.

READINGS AND REFERENCES

Suggested Readings

Cohen, MR, Senders, J, and Davis, NM. February 1994. 12 ways to prevent medication errors. *Nursing94* 24:34–42.

Cohen, Senders, and Davis provide an overview of how, when, and why medication errors occur. With an emphasis on safety, the authors also present 12 techniques that may be used by staff nurses and students alike to prevent medication errors.

Wiggins, MS and Sesin, P. April 1990. Guidelines for administering I.V. drugs. *Nursing90* 20:145–52.

Wiggins and Sesin provide an easy-to-follow chart offering guidelines for administering common intravenous drugs by various methods: IV push, intermittent infusion, and continuous infusion. Developed by staff members at Boston's New England Deaconess Hospital, the chart also includes a column designating which intravenous solutions are compatible with the designated drug.

Related Research

Strong, A, Wolff, H, Kinder, S, and Lubischer, A. January 1991. Drug administration in relation to meals in the institutional setting. *Heart and Lung* 20:39–44.

Walters, JA. May 1992. Nurses' perceptions of reportable medication errors and factors that contribute to their occurrence. *Applied Nursing Research* 92:86–88.

Selected References

American Diabetic Association. April 1992. Clinical practice recommendations (1991–92): Continuous subcutaneous insulin infusion. *Diabetes Care* 15 (suppl 2):34–35.

Berlin, CM. 1989. Advances in pediatric pharmacology and toxicology. *Advanced Pediatrics* 36:431–59.

Bindler, R and Bayne, T. Winter 1991. Medication calculation ability of registered nurses. *Image: Journal of Nursing Scholarship* 23:221–24.

Bruning, LM. February 1993. The bloodborne pathogens final rule: Understanding the regulation. *AORN Journal* 57:437, 439, 441+.

Byington, KC. 1991. Your guide to pediatric drug administration. *Nursing91*, 21:82, 84, 86–89.

Canadian Pharmaceutical Association. 1993. *Compendium of Pharmaceuticals and Specialties*, 27th ed. Ottawa: Canadian Pharmaceutical Association.

Cobb, MD. March 1990. Dealing fairly with medication errors. *Nursing90* 20:42–43.

Cohen, MR. January 1990. Better way to transcribe orders. *Nursing90* 20:9.

Cohen, MR, Senders, J, and Davis, NM. February 1994. 12 ways to prevent medication errors. *Nursing94* 24:34–42.

Cooper, JW. December 1989. Reviewing geriatric concerns with commonly used drugs. *Geriatrics* 44:79–86.

Cyganski, JM, Donahue, JM, and Heaton, JS. June 1987. The case for the heparin flush. *American Journal of Nursing* 87:796–97.

Davis, NM and Cohen, MR. March 1982. Learning from mistakes: 20 tips for avoiding medication errors. *Nursing82* 12:65–72. Canadian ed. 12:23–30.

Hahn, AB, Oestreich, SJK, and Barkin, RL. 1986. *Pharmacology in Nursing*, 16th ed. St Louis: Mosby.

Handbook of Nonprescription Drugs, 10th ed. 1992. Washington, DC: American Pharmaceutical Association.

Hussar, DA. August 1986. Drug interactions: Another good reason for checking and rechecking before you administer medications. *Nursing86* 16:34–40.

Keen, MF. July/August 1986. Comparison of intramuscular injection techniques to reduce site discomfort and lesions. *Nursing Research* 35:207–10.

Kudzma, EC. December 1992. Drug response: All bodies are not created equal. *American Journal of Nursing* 92:48–50.

LeSage, J. February 1991. Polypharmacy in geriatric patients. *Nursing Clinics of North America* 26:273–90.

Lund, VE and Frank, DI. July 1991. Helping the medicine go down: Nurse's and patient's perceptions about medication compliance. *Journal of Psychosocial Nursing and Mental Health Service* 29:6–9.

McConnell, EA. March 1991. How to irrigate the eye. *Nursing91* 21:28.

McGovern, K. March 1992. 10 golden rules for administering drugs safely. *Nursing92* 22:49–56.

Mahoney, DF. January/February 1992. Nurse practitioners as prescribers: Past research trends and future study needs. *Nurse Practitioner* 17:44–51.

Murphy, JI. July/August 1991. Reducing the pain of intramuscular (IM) injections. *Advancing Clinical Care* 6:35.

O'Donnell, J. August 1992. Understanding adverse drug reactions. *Nursing92* 22:34–39.

Pitel, M. January 1971. The subcutaneous injection. *American Journal of Nursing* 71:76–79.

Schwertz, DW. February 1991. Basic principles of pharmacologic action. *Nursing Clinics of North America* 26:242–62.

Shlafer, M. 1993. *The Nurse, Pharmacology, and Drug Therapy: A Prototype Approach*, 2d ed. Redwood City, CA: Addison-Wesley Nursing.

Smith, AJ and Johnson, JY. 1990. *Nurse's Guide to Clinical Procedures.* Philadelphia: Lippincott.

Wiggins, MS and Sesin, P. April 1990. Guidelines for administering I.V. drugs. *Nursing90* 20:145–52.

Williams, PJ. January 1989. How do you keep medicine from clogging feeding tubes? *American Journal of Nursing* 89:181.

Zehrer, C, Hansen, R, and Bantle, J. June 1990. Reducing blood glucose variability by use of abdominal insulin injection sites. *Diabetes Educator* 16:474–77.

44 Wound Care

Objectives

Identify terms commonly used to describe wounds.

Describe the three phases of wound healing.

Differentiate primary, secondary, and tertiary wound healing.

Identify three major types of exudate.

Describe factors that affect wound healing.

Identify the main complications of wound healing.

Identify assessment data pertinent to wounds.

Describe nursing strategies to promote wound healing and prevent complications of wound healing.

Identify purposes of commonly used dressing materials and binders.

Identify physiologic responses to heat and cold and purposes of heat and cold.

Describe methods of applying dry and moist heat and cold.

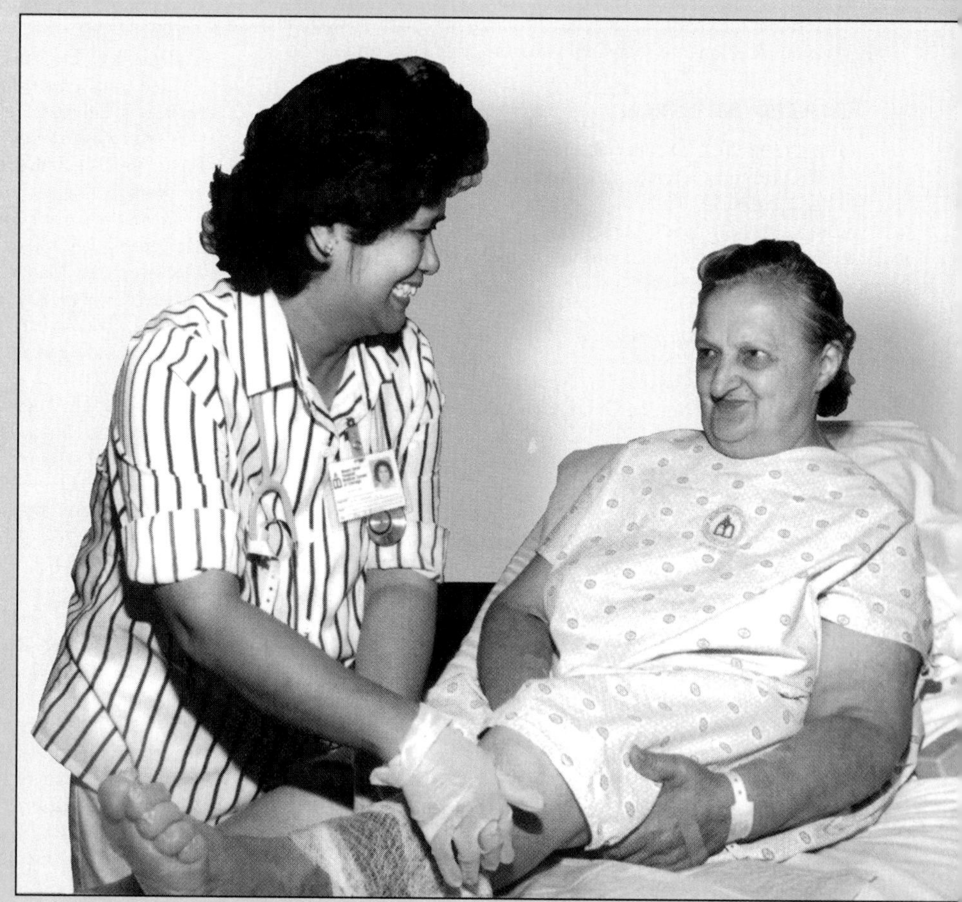

Although the body is remarkably protected from **traumas** (injury) by the skin and by the subcutaneous and adipose tissues, trauma does occur intentionally and unintentionally. Trauma frequently results in a body wound, that is, a break in the continuity of the skin, mucous membranes, bone, or any body organ.

A major component of nursing is the management of both acute and chronic wounds. To manage wounds effectively, the nurse must understand the physiology of wound healing and specific measures that promote it. Such measures include preventing or controlling infection, enhancing the client's nutritional status, and providing topical therapies that provide an optimal healing environment.

TYPES OF WOUNDS

Body wounds are either intentional or unintentional. *Intentional* traumas occur during therapy. Examples are operations, venipunctures, or radiation burns. Although removing a tumor, for example, is therapeutic, the surgeon must cut into body tissues, thus traumatizing them. *Unintentional* wounds are accidental; for example, a person may fracture an arm in an automobile collision. If the tissues are traumatized without a break in the skin, the wound is *closed.* The wound is *open* when the skin or mucous membrane surface is broken.

Wounds are frequently described according to how they are acquired. See Table 44–1. They also can be described according to the likelihood and degree of wound contamination (Garner 1986, p. 73).

- *Clean wounds* are uninfected wounds in which no inflammation is encountered and the respiratory, alimentary, genital, and urinary tracts are not entered. Clean wounds are primarily closed wounds; or, if necessary, they are drained with closed drainage.
- *Clean-contaminated wounds* are surgical wounds in which the respiratory, alimentary, genital or urinary tract has been entered. Such wounds show no evidence of infection.
- *Contaminated wounds* include open, fresh, accidental wounds and surgical wounds involving a major break in sterile technique or a large amount of spillage from the gastrointestinal tract. Contaminated wounds show evidence of inflammation.
- *Dirty or infected wounds* include old, accidental wounds containing dead tissue and wounds with evidence of a clinical infection, such as purulent drainage.

Table 44–1 Types of Wounds

Type	Cause	Description and Characteristics
Incision	Sharp instrument (eg, knife or scalpel)	Open wound; painful
Contusion	Blow from a blunt instrument	Closed wound, skin appears ecchymotic (bruised) because of damaged blood vessels
Abrasion	Surface scrape, either unintentional (eg, scraped knee from a fall) or intentional (eg, dermal abrasion to remove pockmarks)	Open wound involving the skin; painful
Puncture	Penetration of the skin and, often, the underlying tissues from a sharp instrument	Open wound; can be intentional or unintentional
Laceration	Tissues torn apart, often from accidents (eg, machinery)	Open wound; edges are often jagged
Penetrating wound	Penetration of the skin and the underlying tissues	Open wound; usually accidental (eg, from a bullet or metal fragments)

Wounds are also classified by depth, that is, the tissue layers involved in the wound. See the box below. Partial-thickness wounds heal by regeneration, whereas full-thickness wounds require connective tissue repair.

CLASSIFYING WOUNDS BY DEPTH

- *Partial-thickness:* Confined to the skin, that is, the dermis and epidermis
- *Full-thickness:* Involving the dermis, epidermis, subcutaneous tissue, and possibly muscle and bone

WOUND HEALING

Healing is a quality of living tissue; it is also referred to as **regeneration** (renewal) of tissues. It can be broken down into three phases: inflammatory, proliferative, and maturation. The healing process for a surgical wound is described below.

Inflammatory Phase The *inflammatory phase* is initiated immediately after injury and lasts 3 to 4 days. Two major processes occur during this phase: hemostasis and phagocytosis.

Hemostasis (the cessation of bleeding) results from vasoconstriction of the larger blood vessels in the affected area, retraction (drawing back) of injured blood vessels, the deposition of **fibrin** (connective tissue), and the formation of blood clots in the area. The blood clots, formed from blood platelets, provide a matrix of fibrin that becomes the framework for cell repair. A scab also forms on the surface of the wound. Consisting of clots and dead and dying tissue, this scab serves to aid hemostasis and inhibit contamination of the wound by microorganisms. Below the scab, epithelial cells migrate into the wound from the edges. The epithelial cells serve as a barrier between the body and the environment, preventing the entry of microorganisms.

The inflammatory phase also involves vascular and cellular responses intended to remove any foreign substances and dead and dying tissues. The blood supply to the wound increases, bringing with it substances and nutrients needed in the healing process. The area appears reddened and edematous as a result.

During cell migration, leukocytes (specifically, neutrophils) move into the interstitial space. These are replaced about 24 hours after injury by macrophages, which arise from the blood monocytes. These macrophages engulf microorganisms and cellular debris by a process known as **phagocytosis.** The macrophages also secrete an angiogenesis factor (AGF), which stimulates the formation of epithelial buds at the end of injured blood vessels. The microcirculatory network that results sustains the healing process and the wound during its life. Macrophages and AGF are now considered essential to the healing process, (Cooper 1990a, p. 171). This inflammatory response is essential to healing, and measures that impair inflammation, such as administering steroid medications, can place the healing process at risk. Also during this stage, a thin wall of epithelial cells develops across the wound.

Proliferative Phase The *proliferative phase*, second phase in healing, extends from day 3 or 4 to about day 21 post injury. Fibroblasts (connective tissue cells), which migrate into the wound starting about 24 hours after injury, begin to synthesize collagen and a ground substance called proteoglycan about day 5 post injury. **Collagen** is a whitish protein substance that adds tensile strength to the wound. As the amount of collagen increases, so does the strength of the wound; thus, the chance that the wound will open progressively decreases. During this time, a raised "healing ridge" appears under the intact suture line. In a wound that is not sutured, the new collagen is often visible.

Capillaries grow across the wound, increasing the blood supply, which brings with it oxygen and nutrients needed for healing. Fibroblasts move from the blood stream into the wound, depositing fibrin. As the capillary network develops, the tissue becomes a translucent red color. This tissue, called **granulation tissue,** is fragile and bleeds easily.

When the skin edges of a wound are not sutured, the area must be filled in with granulation tissue. (See the discussion of secondary intention healing, below). When the granulation tissue matures, marginal epithelial cells migrate to it, proliferating over this connective tissue base to fill the wound. If the wound does not close by epithelialization, the area becomes covered with dried plasma proteins and dead cells. This is called **eschar.** Initially, wounds healing by secondary intention seep serosanguineous drainage. Later, if they are not covered by epithelial cells, they become covered with thick, gray, fibrinous tissue that is eventually converted into dense scar tissue.

Maturation Phase The *maturation phase* begins about day 21 and can extend 1 or 2 years after the injury. Fibroblasts continue to synthesize collagen. The collagen fibers themselves, which were initially laid in a haphazard fashion, reorganize into a more orderly structure. The scar becomes a thin, less elastic, white line.

TYPES OF HEALING

There are three types of healing, distinguished by the amount of tissue loss. **Primary intention healing** occurs where the tissue surfaces have been **approximated** (closed) and there is minimal or no tissue loss; it is characterized by the formation of minimal granulation tissue and scarring. It is also called *primary union* or *first intention healing.* An example of wound healing by primary intention is a surgical incision.

A wound that is extensive and involves considerable tissue loss, and in which the edges cannot be approximated, heals by **secondary intention healing.** An example of wound healing by secondary intention is a pressure ulcer. Secondary intention healing differs from primary intention healing in three ways: (a) the repair time is longer; (b) the scarring is greater; and (c) the susceptibility to infection is greater.

Tertiary intention healing, also known as *delayed* or *secondary closure*, is indicated when there is a reason to delay suturing a wound, for example, where there is poor circulation in the area. These wounds are sutured later, after the initial stage of deposition of granulation tissue. Wounds that heal by tertiary intention require more connective tissue (scar tissue) than wounds that heal by primary intention but less than those that heal by secondary intention. An example of wound healing by tertiary intention is an abdominal wound that is initially left open for drainage but is later closed (Bryant 1992, p. 33).

KINDS OF WOUND DRAINAGE

Exudate is material, such as fluid and cells, that has escaped from blood vessels during the inflammatory process and is deposited in tissue or on tissue surfaces. The nature and amount of exudate vary according to the tissue involved, the intensity and duration of the inflammation, and the presence of microorganisms.

There are three major types of exudate: serous, purulent, and sanguineous (hemorrhagic). A **serous exudate** consists chiefly of serum (the clear portion of the blood) derived from the blood and serous membranes of the body, such as the peritoneum. It is watery in appearance and has few cells. An example is the fluid in a blister from a burn.

A **purulent exudate** is thicker than serous exudate because of the presence of **pus.** It consists of leukocytes, liquefied dead tissue debris, and dead and living bacteria. The process of pus formation is referred to as **suppuration,** and the bacteria that produce pus are called **pyogenic bacteria.** Not all microorganisms are pyogenic. Purulent exudates vary in color, some acquiring tinges of blue, green, or yellow. The color may depend on the causative organism.

A **sanguineous (hemorrhagic) exudate** consists of large amounts of red blood cells, indicating damage to capillaries that is severe enough to allow the escape of red blood cells from plasma. This type of exudate is frequently seen in open wounds. Nurses often need to distinguish whether the sanguineous exudate is dark or bright. A bright sanguineous exudate indicates fresh bleeding, whereas dark sanguineous exudate denotes older bleeding.

Mixed types of exudates are often observed. A serosanguineous (consisting of clear and blood-tinged drainage) exudate is commonly seen in surgical incisions. A purosanguineous discharge (consisting of pus and blood) is often seen in a new wound that is infected.

FACTORS AFFECTING WOUND HEALING

Developmental Considerations Healthy children and adults often heal more quickly than the elderly. Elderly people are more likely to have chronic diseases, for example, peripheral vascular disease, which impairs blood flow (Jones & Millman 1990, p. 271). Reduced liver function can impair the synthesis of blood clotting factors. See the box above for factors inhibiting wound healing in the elderly.

FACTORS INHIBITING WOUND HEALING IN THE ELDERLY

- Vascular changes associated with aging, such as atherosclerosis and atrophy of capillaries in the skin, can impair blood flow to the wound.
- Collagen tissue is less flexible.
- Changes in the immune system may reduce the formation of antibodies and monocytes necessary for wound healing.
- Nutrition deficiencies may reduce the numbers of red blood cells and leukocytes, thus impeding the delivery of oxygen and the inflammatory response essential for wound healing. Oxygen is needed for the synthesis of collagen and the formation of new epithelial cells.
- Scar tissue is less elastic.

Nutrition Wound healing places additional demands on the body. Clients require a diet rich in protein, carbohydrates, lipids, vitamins A and C, and minerals, such as iron, zinc, and copper. Malnourished clients may require time to improve their nutritional status before surgery, if this is possible. Obese clients are at increased risk of wound infection and slower healing because adipose tissue usually has an inadequate blood supply.

Life-Style People who exercise regularly tend to have a good circulation and are therefore more likely to heal quickly, because blood brings oxygen and nourishment to the wound. Smoking reduces the amount of functional hemoglobin in the blood, thus limiting the oxygen-carrying capacity of the blood. Smoking is also thought to increase platelet aggregation and hence the formation of blood clots in the circulatory system.

Medications Anti-inflammatory drugs (eg, steroids and aspirin), heparin, and antineoplastic agents interfere with healing (Kloth et al 1990, p. 24). Prolonged use of antibiotics may make a person susceptible to a wound infection (Kloth et al 1990, p. 60).

Infection A wound infection slows healing. Bacteria, either from endogenous (within the client) or exogenous (outside the client) sources cause wound infections.

Clients who have acquired immune deficiency syndrome (AIDS) are already immunocompromised. This state affects fibroblast function, collagen synthesis, and phagocytic action, all of which are required for wound healing. These clients are very vulnerable to microorganisms found in hospitals, which can infect a wound and then spread systemically.

The Centers for Disease Control recommend the following (Garner 1986, p. 77) to control some of the external (environmental) factors that affect wound healing:

- Bacterial infections should be treated before surgery.
- The preoperative hospital stay should be as short as possible.
- Malnourished clients should receive enteral or parenteral nutrition preoperatively if the surgery is not urgent.
- Clients having elective surgery should bathe with an antimicrobial soap the night before surgery.
- Hair near the operative site should not be removed unless absolutely necessary.
- If hair must be removed, it should be clipped or removed with a depilatory, rather than shaved.

The preoperative use of antibiotics is recommended where there is a high risk of infection. The timing and dosage of the antibiotics are important factors in preventing postoperative infections in high-risk clients. Nichols (1982, p. 34) recommends administering parenteral antibiotics within 1 hour of surgery and continuing for 24 to 72 hours. This practice allows time for drugs to reach therapeutic levels in the tissues but does not permit bacterial resistance to develop.

COMPLICATIONS OF WOUND HEALING

Hemorrhage Some escape of blood from a wound is normal intraoperatively and postoperatively. **Hemorrhage** (persistent bleeding), however, is abnormal. It may be caused by a dislodged clot, a slipped ligature, or erosion of a blood vessel, for example.

Internal hemorrhage may often be detected by swelling or distention in the area of the wound and, possibly, sanguineous drainage from a surgical drain. Other signs of internal hemorrhage reflect *hypovolemic shock* (ie, fall in blood pressure); rapid, thready pulse; increased rate of respirations; diaphoresis; restlessness; and cold, clammy skin. Some clients will have a **hematoma,** a localized collection of blood underneath the skin. A hematoma may appear as a swelling that is reddish-blue in color. A large hematoma may be dangerous in that it places pressure on blood vessels and can thus obstruct blood flow.

External hemorrhage is often easily identified from the blood that either appears under the dressing or escapes from the dressing and pools under the client. The risk of hemorrhage is greatest during the first 48 hours after surgery. Hemorrhage is an emergency; the nurse should apply extra sterile pressure dressings to the area and monitor the client's vital signs. In many instances, the client must return immediately to the operating room for surgical intervention.

Infection A wound can be infected with microorganisms at the time of injury, during surgery, or postoperatively. Wounds that occur as a result of injury (eg, bullet and knife wounds) are most likely to be contaminated at the time of injury. Surgery involving the intestines can also result in infection from the microorganisms inside the intestine. Infection is most likely to become apparent 2 to 11 days postoperatively.

Dehiscence with Possible Evisceration **Dehiscence** is the partial or total rupturing of a wound. Dehiscence often involves an abdominal wound in which the layers below the skin also separate. **Evisceration** is the protrusion of the internal viscera through an incision. A number of factors, including obesity, poor nutrition, multiple trauma, failure of suturing, excessive coughing, vomiting, and dehydration, heighten a client's risk of wound dehiscence. Wound dehiscence is more likely to occur 4 to 5 days postoperatively before extensive collagen is deposited in the wound.

An increase in the flow of serosanguineous drainage into the wound dressing can indicate an impending dehiscence (Schumann 1979, p. 683). Dehiscence may also be preceded by sudden straining, such as coughing or sneezing. It is not unusual for a client to feel that "something has given way." When dehiscence or evisceration occurs, the wound should be quickly supported by large sterile dressings soaked in sterile normal saline. The surgeon should be notified immediately and the client prepared for immediate surgical repair of the area.

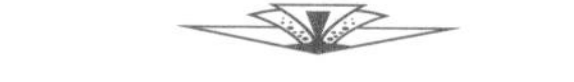

ASSESSING WOUNDS

Nurses commonly assess both untreated and treated wounds. *Untreated wounds* usually are seen shortly after an injury (eg, at the scene of an accident or in an emergency center). Assessment for these wounds is shown in the left hand box on page 1363. Guidelines for care follow.

- Control severe bleeding by (a) applying direct pressure over the wound and (b) elevating the involved extremity.
- Prevent infection by (a) cleaning or flushing abrasions or lacerations with water and (b) covering the wound with a clean dressing, if possible (a sterile dressing is

CLINICAL GUIDELINES

Assessing Untreated Wounds

- Assess client's condition. Determine the presence of a clear airway, adequacy of breathing, and presence of a carotid pulse.
- Assess the size and severity of the wound. If severe, have someone call an ambulance or, if in an emergency center, inform the physician.
- Inspect the wound for bleeding. The amount of bleeding varies according to the type of wound and location. Penetrating wounds may cause internal bleeding.
- Inspect the wound for foreign bodies (soil, broken glass, shreds of cloth, or other foreign substances).
- Assess associated injuries such as fractures, internal bleeding, spinal cord injuries, or head trauma.
- If the wound is contaminated with foreign material, determine when the client last had a tetanus toxoid injection. A tetanus antitoxin will be necessary if 5 years have elapsed.

preferred). When applying a dressing, wrap the wound tightly enough to apply pressure and approximate the wound edges, if possible. If the first layer of dressing becomes saturated with blood, apply a second layer. Do so without removing the first layer of dressing, because blood clots might be disturbed, resulting in more bleeding.

- Control swelling and pain by applying ice over the wound and surrounding tissues.
- If bleeding is severe or if internal bleeding is suspected, and if emergency equipment is available, assess the client for signs of shock (see Table 45–2, p. 1413).

Treated wounds, or *sutured wounds*, are usually assessed to determine the progress of healing. These wounds may be inspected during a dressing change unless a transparent dressing has been applied. If the wound itself cannot be directly inspected, the dressing is inspected and other data regarding the wound (eg, the presence of pain) are assessed. Many treated wounds are covered with a transparent occlusive dressing that permits observation of the wound without exposure to the air.

CLINICAL ASSESSMENT OF TREATED WOUNDS

Nurses assess wounds by visual inspection, palpation, and the sense of smell, noting the wound's appearance and any drainage, swelling, odor, dehiscence, and pain. See the box at the right.

The nurse can expect the following sequential signs of healing for a surgical incision:

1. *Absence of bleeding and the appearance of a clot binding the wound edges.* The wound edges are well approximated and bound by fibrin in the clot within the first few hours after surgical closure.
2. *Inflammation (redness and swelling) at the wound edges for 1 to 3 days.*
3. *Reduction in inflammation when the clot diminishes*, as granulation tissue starts to bridge the area. The wound is bridged and closed within 7 to 10 days. Increased inflammation associated with fever and drainage is indicative of wound infection; the wound edges then appear brightly inflamed and swollen.
4. *Scar formation.* Collagen synthesis starts 4 days after injury and continues for 6 months or longer.
5. *Diminished scar size* over a period of months or years. An increase in scar size indicates keloid formation.

CLINICAL GUIDELINES

Assessing Treated Wounds

Appearance

- Inspect color of wound and surrounding area and approximation of wound edges.

Size

- Note size and location of dehiscence, if present. For wounds healing by *secondary intention*, measure the length, width, and depth in centimeters (see Chapter 30, page 791).

Drainage

- Observe location, color, consistency, odor, and degree of saturation of dressings. Note number of gauzes saturated or diameter of drainage on gauze.

Swelling

- Wearing sterile gloves, palpate wound edges for tension and tautness of tissues; minimal to moderate swelling is normal in early stages of wound healing.

Pain

- Expect severe to moderate postoperative pain for 3 to 5 days; persistent severe pain or sudden onset of severe pain may indicate internal hemorrhaging or infection.

Drains or Tubes

- Inspect drain security and placement, amount and character of drainage, and functioning of collecting apparatus, if present.

LABORATORY DATA

Laboratory data can often support the nurse's clinical assessment of the wound's progress in healing. A *decreased leukocyte count* can delay healing and increase the possibility of infection. *Blood coagulation studies* are also significant. Prolonged coagulation times can result in excessive blood loss and prolonged clot absorption. Hypercoagulability can lead to intravascular clotting. Intra-arterial clotting can result in a deficient blood supply to the wound area. *Serum protein analysis* provides an indication of the body's nutritional reserves for rebuilding cells. *Wound cultures* can either confirm or rule out the presence of infection. Sensitivity studies are helpful in the selection of appropriate antibiotic therapy. The nurse obtains a wound culture whenever an infection is suspected. Procedure 44–1 provides guidelines to obtain a wound culture.

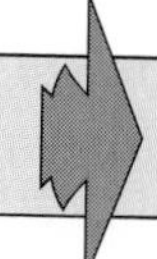

PROCEDURE 44–1 OBTAINING A SPECIMEN OF WOUND DRAINAGE

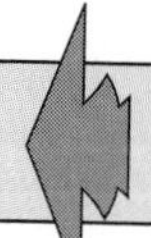

PURPOSES

- To identify the microorganisms causing an infection and the antibiotics to which they are sensitive
- To evaluate the effectiveness of antibiotic therapy

ASSESSMENT FOCUS

Pain at the wound site; clinical signs of infection (eg, fever, chills); appearances of the wound and the character and amount of wound drainage.

EQUIPMENT

- ☐ Clean disposable gloves
- ☐ Sterile gloves
- ☐ Moisture-resistant bag
- ☐ Sterile dressing set
- ☐ Normal saline and irrigating syringe
- ☐ Culture tube with swab and culture medium (aerobic and anaerobic tubes are available) and/or sterile syringe with needle for anaerobic culture
- ☐ Completed labels for each container
- ☐ Completed requisition to accompany the specimens to the laboratory

INTERVENTION

1. Remove any moist outer dressings that cover the wound.

- Put on disposable gloves.
- Remove the outer dressing, observe any drainage on it. Hold the dressing so that the client does not see the drainage. *The appearance of the drainage could upset the client.*
- Discard the dressing in the moisture-resistant bag. Handle it carefully so that the dressing does not touch the outside of the bag. *Touching the outside of the bag will contaminate it.*
- Remove gloves and dispose of them properly.

2. Open the sterile dressing set using sterile technique.

- See Procedure 27–2 on page 694.

3. Assess the wound.

- Put on sterile gloves.
- Assess the appearance of the tissues in and around the wound and the drainage. Infection can cause reddened tissues with a thick discharge, which may be foul-smelling, whitish, or colored.
- Determine the amount of the drainage, for example, one 2×2 gauze saturated with pale yellow drainage.

4. Clean the wound. Cuzzell (1993, p. 49) recommends the following:

- Irrigate the wound with normal saline until all visible exudate has been washed away.
- Avoid irrigating with an antiseptic solution before obtaining the swab for culture. *Antiseptic solutions may destroy the organisms desired for culture and cause a false-negative culture report.*
- After irrigating, apply a sterile gauze pad to the wound. *This absorbs excess saline and exposes the culture site.*
- If a topical antimicrobial ointment or cream is being used to treat the wound, use a swab to re-

PROCEDURE 44–1 *continued*

move it. *Residual antiseptic must be removed prior to culture.*

- Remove sterile gloves.

5. Obtain the culture.

- Open a specimen tube, and place the cap upside down on a firm, dry surface so that the inside will not become contaminated *or*, if the swab is attached to the lid, twist the cap to loosen the swab. Hold the tube in one hand, and take out the swab in the other.
- Rotate the swab back and forth over clean areas of granulation tissue from the sides or base of the wound. *Microorganisms most likely to be responsible for a wound infection reside in viable tissue, where bacterial toxins are more readily absorbed into the bloodstream* (Cuzzell 1993, p. 49).
- Do *not* use pus or pooled exudate to culture. *These secretions contain a mixture of contaminants that are not the same as those causing the infection.*
- Avoid touching the swab to intact skin at the wound edges. *This prevents the introduction of superficial skin organisms into the culture.*
- 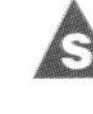 Return the swab to the culture tube, taking care not to touch the top or the outside of the tube. *The outside of the container must remain free of pathogenic microorganisms to prevent their spread to others.*
- Crush the inner ampule containing the medium for organism growth at the bottom of the tube. *This ensures that the swab with the specimen is surrounded by culture medium.*
- Twist the cap to secure it.
- If a specimen is required from another site, repeat the above steps. Specify the exact site (eg, inferior drain site or lower aspect of incision) on the label of each container, if not labeled previously. Be sure to put each swab in the appropriately labeled tube.

6. Dress the wound.

- Apply any ordered medication to the wound.
- Cover the wound with sterile dressings. See Procedure 44–2.

7. Arrange for the specimen to be transported to the laboratory immediately. Be sure to include the completed requisition.

8. Document all relevant information.

- Record on the client's chart the taking of the specimen and source.
- Include the date and time; the examination requested; the appearance of the wound; the color, consistency, amount, and odor of any drainage; and any discomfort experienced by the client.

Variation: Obtaining a Specimen for Anaerobic Culture, Using a Sterile Syringe and Needle

- Insert a sterile 10-mL syringe (without needle) into the wound, and aspirate 1 to 5 mL of drainage into the syringe.
- Attach the #21 gauge needle to the syringe, and expel all air from the syringe.
- Immediately inject the drainage into the anaerobic culture tube.

  or

  If a rubber stopper or cork is available, insert the needle into the rubber stopper or cork to prevent the entry of air.
- Label the tube or syringe appropriately.
- Send the syringe of drainage to the laboratory immediately.

EVALUATION FOCUS
The character of the drainage (amount, color, consistency, and odor); any client discomfort; appearance of the wound.

DIAGNOSING

Nursing diagnoses for clients who have wounds or who are at risk of sustaining wounds largely reflect the need to support wound healing, to prevent complications, and to teach the client self-care. Depending on the assessment data obtained and the client's health status, some of the following NANDA diagnoses may be appropriate: **High risk for infection, Pain, High risk for impaired skin integrity, Anxiety,** and **Body image disturbance.** Examples of these diagnoses, with possible contributing factors, are shown below. Defining characteristics and related factors are discussed elsewhere in this book.

- **High risk for infection** related to impaired skin integrity (eg, surgical incision, leg ulcer, Penrose drain)

- **Pain** related to
  a. Infected surgical incision
  b. Joint swelling secondary to knee injury
- **High risk for impaired skin integrity** related to
  a. Exposure to secretions (eg, from draining fistula, ostomy, Penrose drain)
  b. Altered nutrition: less than body requirements
  c. Impaired physical mobility
- **Body image disturbance** related to
  a. Altered body structure (eg, loss of breast, extensive scarring associated with burns)
  b. Altered body function (eg, ostomy)
- **Anxiety** related to knowledge deficit (care of incision and drain)

PLANNING

There are many different kinds of wounds, and clients have many different needs; therefore, the nurse needs to individualize the care plan to accommodate these factors. Generally, the nurse focuses on interventions that promote wound healing, prevent infection, promote health and coping, and prevent further injury or complications.

Examples of outcome criteria follow.

The client

- Maintains normal or baseline vital signs.
- Achieves timely wound healing, as manifested by decreasing inflammation and wound drainage and absence of purulent drainage.
- Accomplishes activities of daily living with minimal or no pain.
- Maintains adequate dietary intake for healing.
- Maintains intact skin around drainage site.
- Resumes normal activities within specified period.
- Demonstrates wound care as instructed.
- Reports understanding of discharge instructions.
- States signs of complications that require notification of the nurse or physician.

A critical pathway can also be useful for planning client care (see p. 1393).

IMPLEMENTING

Nursing interventions for wounds involve preventing infection, cleaning wounds, dressing wounds, and supporting wounds.

PREVENTING WOUND INFECTION

There are two main aspects to controlling wound infection: preventing microorganisms from entering the wound and preventing the transmission of bloodborne pathogens to or from the client to others. See the box below.

CLEANING WOUNDS

Wound cleaning has traditionally involved the removal of debris (ie, foreign materials, excess slough, necrotic tissue, bacteria, and other microorganisms). Formerly, antimi-

CDC GUIDELINES FOR PREVENTING INFECTION AND THE TRANSMISSION OF BLOODBORNE PATHOGENS

General Precautions

- Wear gloves when touching blood and body fluids, mucous membranes, or nonintact skin of all clients, and when handling items or surfaces soiled with blood or body fluids.
- Wash hands thoroughly after removing gloves, and if contaminated with blood or body fluids.
- Take precautions to prevent injuries by needles, sharp instruments, or sharp devices.
- Avoid direct client care if you have open or weeping lesions or dermatitis.
- Wear gloves, surgical masks, and protective eyewear as appropriate if procedures commonly cause droplets or splashing of blood or body fluids.

Wound Care

- Wash hands before and after caring for surgical wounds.
- Touch an open or fresh surgical wound only when wearing sterile gloves or using sterile forceps. After the wound is healed over (sealed), sterile gloves are no longer required.
- Remove or change dressings over open and closed wounds when they become wet.
- Take a specimen of any drainage from the wound that is suspected of being infected. Send the specimen to the laboratory for culture and Gram stain.

Sources: JS Garner, CDC guidelines for the prevention and control of nosocomial infections: Guideline for prevention of surgical wound infections, 1985, *American Journal of Infection Control,* April 1986, 14:71–80; Centers for Disease Control, Recommendations for prevention of HIV transmission in health care settings, *Morbidity and Mortality Weekly Report,* 1987, 36:55.

crobial solutions, such as povidone-iodine (Betadine), 3% hydrogen peroxide, 70% alcohol, and Dakin's solution were commonly used. However, these solutions have been reported to have caustic effects on granulation tissue and the skin (Rodeaver 1989, p. 19). The choice of cleaning agent and method depend largely on agency protocol and the physician's preference. Recommended guidelines for cleaning wounds are shown in the box below.

A major principle of cleaning wounds is to clean from "clean to dirty." In many wounds, however, it may be difficult to differentiate which is which. Various methods for cleaning wounds are described in the literature. Because these methods vary so considerably, a need for further research is indicated. Variations include the following:

- Holding cleaning sponges with forceps, versus holding the sponges with a sterile gloved hand
- Cleaning from the wound in an outward direction to avoid transferring organisms from the surrounding skin into the wound, versus cleaning in any direction unless there are obvious signs of infection (eg, pus)
- Cleaning the skin first and in a direction away from the wound, versus cleaning the wound first and then the surrounding skin
- *Not* cleaning the wound at all if it appears to be clean

Commonly used methods to clean a surgical wound and drain site are shown in Figure 44–1 on page 1368.

CLINICAL GUIDELINES

Cleaning Wounds

- Use physiologic solutions, such as isotonic saline or lactated Ringer's solution, to clean or irrigate wounds. If antimicrobial solutions are used, make sure they are well diluted.
- When possible, warm the solution to body temperature before use. This prevents lowering of the wound temperature, which slows the healing process.
- If a wound is grossly contaminated by foreign material, bacteria, slough, or necrotic tissue, clean the wound at every dressing change. Foreign bodies and devitalized tissue act as a focus for infection and can delay healing.
- If a wound is clean, has little exudate, and reveals healthy granulation tissue, avoid repeated cleaning. Unnecessary cleaning can delay wound healing by traumatizing newly produced, delicate tissues, reducing the surface temperature of the wound and removing exudate which itself may have bactericidal properties.
- Use gauze squares. Avoid using cotton balls and other products that shed fibers onto the wound surface. The fibers become embedded in granulation tissue and can act as foci for infection. They may also stimulate "foreign body" reactions, prolonging the inflammatory phase of healing and delaying the healing process.
- Consider cleaning superficial noninfected wounds by irrigating them with normal saline rather than using mechanical means (ie, using gauze and forceps). The hydraulic pressure of an irrigating stream of fluid dislodges contaminating debris, reduces bacterial colonization, and is less irritating (Glide 1992, p. 78).
- To retain wound moisture, avoid drying a wound after cleaning it.

Sources: DB Doughty, Principles of wound healing and wound management. In RA Bryant, editor, *Acute and Chronic Wounds: Nursing Management* (St Louis: Mosby-Year Book, 1992), p. 51; JZ Cuzzell and NA Stotts. Wound care: Trial and error yields knowledge, *American Journal of Nursing*, October 1990, 90:54; and S Glide, Cleaning choices, *Nursing Times*, May 6–12, 1992, 88:74, 76, 78.

DRESSING WOUNDS

Dressings are applied for the following purposes:

- To protect the wound from mechanical injury
- To protect the wound from microbial contamination
- To provide or maintain high humidity of the wound
- To provide thermal insulation
- To absorb drainage and/or debride a wound
- To prevent hemorrhage (when applied as a pressure dressing or with elastic bandages)
- To splint or immobilize the wound site and thereby facilitate healing and prevent injury
- To provide psychologic (aesthetic) comfort

Types of Dressing Various dressing materials are available to cover wounds. The type of dressing used depends on (a) the location, size, and type of the wound; (b) the amount of exudate; (c) whether the wound requires debridement, is infected, or has sinus tracts; and (d) such considerations as frequency of dressing change, ease or difficulty of dressing application, and cost.

Gauze Dry sterile gauze dressings are commonly used to cover surgical incisions. Several sizes of gauze are available (Figure 44–2, p. 1368). The standard sizes are 10 × 10 cm (4 × 4 in) and 10 × 20 cm (4 × 8 in). The size and number of pads used depend on the nature of the wound, the amount of exudate, and the location of the wound. These decisions are left to the nurse's judgment. Sometimes the gauze is precut halfway through one side to make it fit around a drain, or it is folded in a special way.

Telfa gauze is a special type. It has a shiny, nonadherent surface on one or both sides and is applied with the shiny surface on the wound. Exudate seeps through this surface

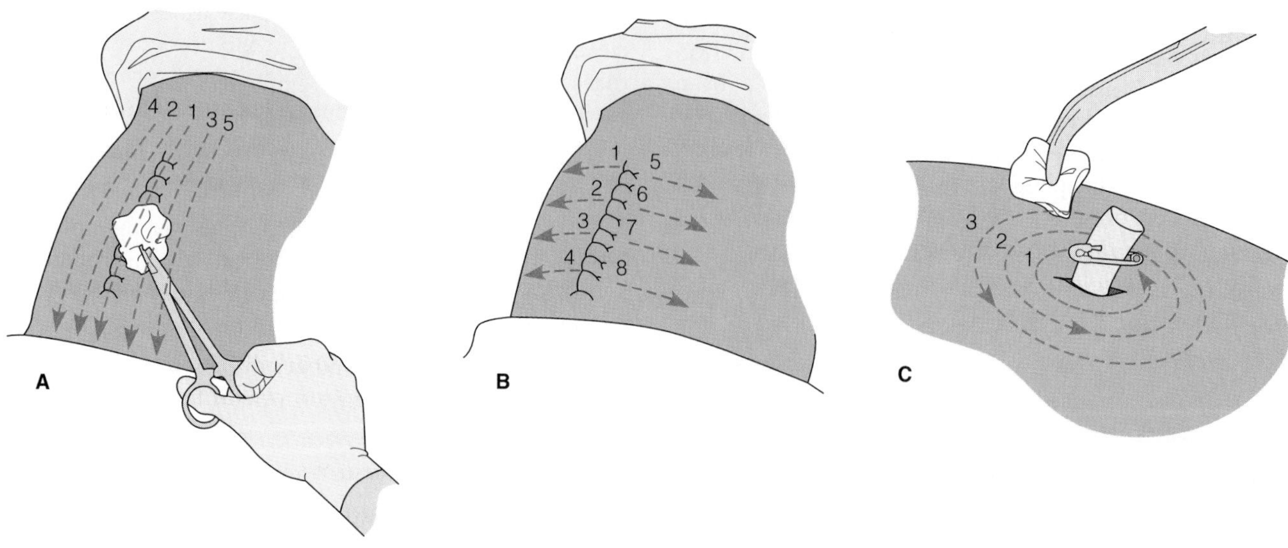

Figure 44–1 Methods of cleaning surgical wounds: *A,* cleaning the wound from top to bottom, starting at the center; *B,* cleaning a wound outward from the incision; *C,* cleaning around a drain site. For all methods, a clean sterile swab is used for each stroke.

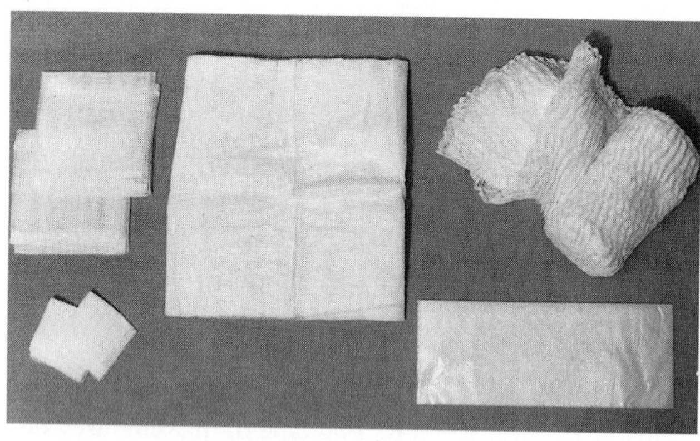

Figure 44–2 Some frequently used dressing materials (clockwise from bottom left): 2 × 2 gauze, 4 × 4 gauze, surgipad or abdominal pad, roller gauze, and nonadherent absorbent dressing.

and collects on the absorbent material on the other side or is sandwiched between the two nonadherent surfaces. Because the dressing does not adhere, it does not cause injury to the wound when removed.

Larger and thicker gauze dressings, called *surgipads* or *abdominal pads,* are used to cover small gauzes. They not only hold the other gauzes in place but also absorb and collect excess drainage. Surgipads are more absorbent on one side, and this side is placed toward the wound; the less absorbent, more protective side is placed outward to protect the wound from external contamination. The outer side is often indicated with a blue stripe.

Gauze dressings also vary by mode of application. These include dry-to-dry, wet-to-dry, wet-to-damp, and wet-to-wet. Each has specific purposes. See Table 44–2.

Synthetic Dressings Prior to the 1960s, many open wounds were treated by exposure to the air to encourage scab formation. Studies conducted since then have revealed that superficial wounds heal faster when kept moist than when kept dry. Studies have also shown that a moist environment speeds up collagen synthesis (Cuzzell & Stotts 1990, p. 54). As a result of these discoveries, a variety of occlusive and semiocclusive wound dressings has been developed, including thin films, hydrocolloids, and foams.

The purposes, absorbency, thickness, and ability to support debridement of these dressings vary. However, all dressings hydrate the wound and insulate and protect it from environmental contamination. See Table 44–3 on page 1370.

Securing Dressings The nurse tapes the dressing over the wound, ensuring that the dressing covers the entire wound and does not become dislodged. The correct type of tape must be selected for the purpose. Elastic tape can provide pressure; nonallergenic tape is used when a client is allergic to other tape. The nurse follows these steps:

1. Place the tape so that the dressing cannot be folded back to expose the wound. Place strips at the ends of the dressing, and space tapes evenly in the middle (Figure 44–3).

Table 44–2 Modes of Applying Gauze Dressings

Dressing	Description	Purpose
Dry-to-dry	A layer of wide-mesh cotton gauze lies next to the wound surface. A second layer of dry absorbent cotton or Dacron is on top.	Necrotic debris and exudate are trapped in the interstices of the contact (gauze) layer. These are removed when the dressing is removed.
Wet-to-dry	Next to the wound surface is a layer of wide-mesh cotton gauze saturated with saline or an antimicrobial solution. This layer is covered by a moist absorbent material, that is, moistened with the same solution.	Necrotic debris is softened by the solution and then adheres to the mesh gauze as it dries. It is removed when the dressing is removed. Also, moisture helps dilute viscous exudate.
Wet-to-damp	A variation of the wet-to-dry dressing, this dressing is removed before it has completely dried.	The wound is debrided when the gauze is removed.
Wet-to-wet	A layer of wide-mesh gauze saturated with antibacterial or physiologic solution lies next to the wound surface. Above is a second layer of absorbent material saturated with the same solution. The entire dressing is kept moist with a wetting agent.	The wound surface is continually bathed. Moisture dilutes viscous exudate.

2. Ensure that the tape is long and wide enough to adhere to several inches of skin on each side of the dressing, but not so long or wide that the tape loosens with activity (Figure 44–3).
3. Place the tape in the opposite direction from the body action, for example, across a body joint or crease, not lengthwise (Figure 44–4, p. 1371).

After surgery, an elastic adhesive tape may be applied over wounds because of its ability to compress and thereby control hemorrhage. The original tape is removed during the initial dressing change, and a lighter dressing is applied. The nurse secures the dressing at both ends and across the middle and uses tape of a sufficient width for the dressing and the wound.

Montgomery straps (tie tapes) are commonly used for wounds requiring frequent dressing changes (Figure 44–5, p. 1371). These straps prevent skin irritation and discomfort caused by removing the adhesive each time the dressing is changed. Nonallergenic tie tapes are available

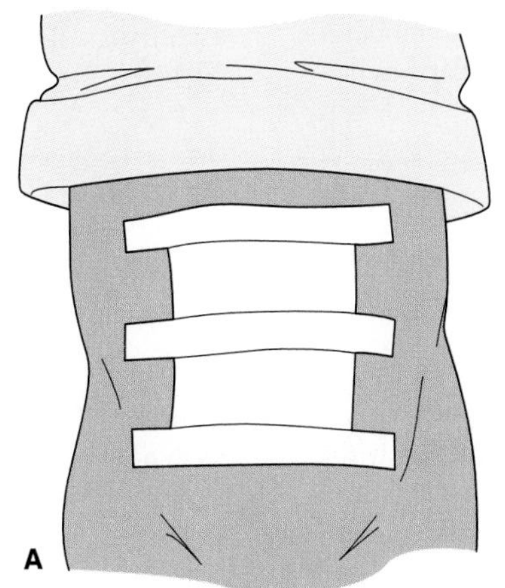

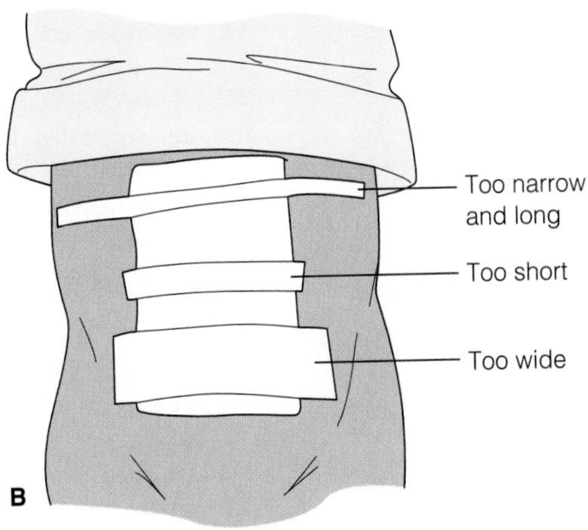

Figure 44–3 The strips of tape should be placed at the ends of the dressing and must be sufficiently long and wide to secure the dressing. The tape should adhere to intact skin.

Table 44–3 Selected Types of Wound Dressings

Dressing	Description	Purpose	Examples
Transparent adhesive films	Adhesive plastic semipermeable *nonabsorbent* dressings that allow exchange of oxygen between the atmosphere and wound bed. They are impermeable to bacteria and water.	To provide protection against contamination and friction; to maintain a clean moist surface that facilitates cellular migration; to provide insulation by preventing fluid evaporation; and to facilitate wound assessment	Op-Site, Tegaderm, Bio-occlusive, ACU-derm
Impregnated nonadherent dressings	Woven or nonwoven cotton or synthetic materials that are impregnated with petrolatum, saline, zinc-saline, antimicrobials, or other agents. Require secondary dressings to secure them in place, retain moisture, and provide wound protection.	To cover, soothe, and protect partial- and full-thickness wounds without exudate	Vaseline gauze, Carragauze, Dermagran Wet Dressing, Xeroform
Hydrocolloids	Waterproof adhesive wafers, pastes, or powders. Wafers, designed to be worn for up to seven days, consist of two layers. The inner adhesive layer has particles that absorb exudate and form a hydrated gel over the wound; the outer film provides a seal.	To absorb exudate; to produce a moist environment that facilitates healing but does not cause maceration of surrounding skin; to protect the wound from bacterial contamination, foreign debris, and urine or feces; and to prevent shearing	DuoDERM, Comfeel, Tegasorb, Restore
Hydrogels	Glycerin or water-based *nonadhesive* jellylike sheets, granules, or gels that are oxygen permeable, unless covered by a plastic film. May require secondary occlusive dressing. Have replaced enzyme dressings.	To liquefy necrotic tissue or slough, rehydrate the wound bed, and fill in dead space	Aquasorb, ClearSite, Elasto-Gel, Intrasite
Polyurethane foams	Nonadhesive, *nonadherent,* hydrocolloid dressings that need to have their edges taped down or sealed. Require secondary dressings to obtain an occlusive environment. Surrounding skin must be protected to prevent maceration.	To absorb light to moderate amounts of exudate; to debride wounds	Lyofoam, Allevyn, Nuderm, Flexan
Exudate absorbers	Nonadherent dressings of powder, beads or granules, or paste that conform to the wound surface and absorb up to 20 times their weight in exudate; require a secondary dressing.	To provide a moist wound surface by interacting with exudate; to form a gelatinous mass; to absorb exudate; to eliminate dead space or pack wounds, and to support debridement	Debrisan, Triad paste, Sorbsan

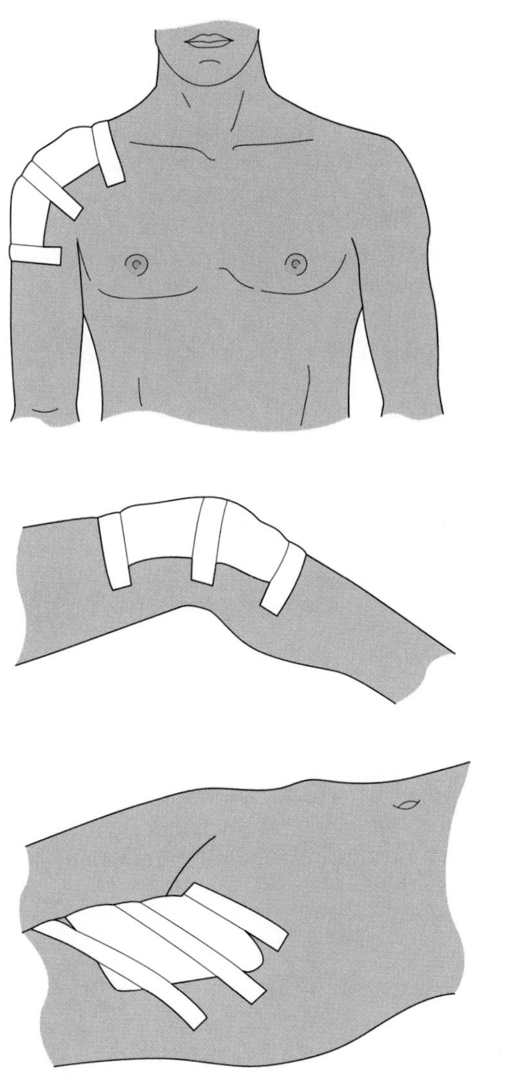

Figure 44–4 Dressings over moving parts must remain secure in spite of the movement. Place the tape over a joint at a right angle to the direction the joint moves.

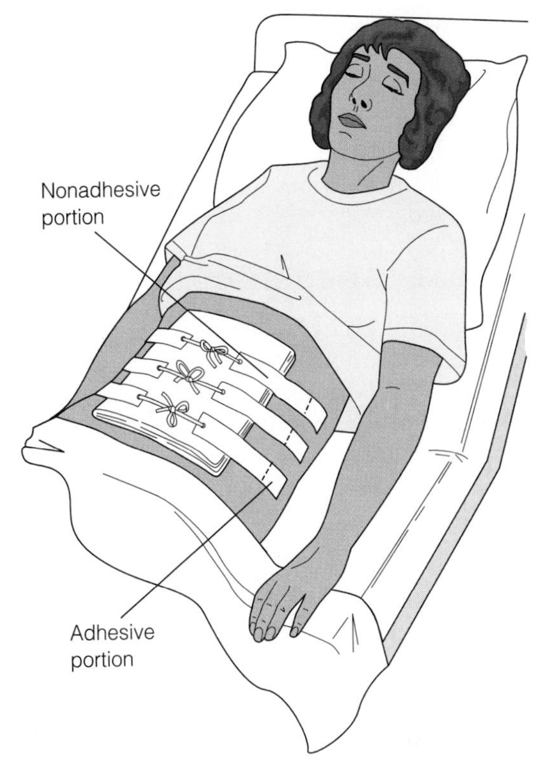

Figure 44–5 Montgomery straps, or tie tapes, are used to secure large dressings that require frequent changing.

for people with sensitive skin. If these are not available, the nurse can protect the skin by applying tincture of benzoin to the site where the adhesive is to be placed.

THE RYB COLOR CODE

To guide wound care, the nurse can use the RYB color code of wounds developed by Marion Laboratories, Inc. (Stotts 1990, p. 59). This concept is based on the color of an open wound—red, yellow, or black (RYB)—rather than the depth or size of a wound. On this scheme, the goals of wound care are to *protect* (cover) red, *cleanse* yellow, and *debride* black. The RYB code can be applied to any wound allowed to heal by *secondary intention.*

Wounds that are *red* are usually in the late regeneration phase of tissue repair (ie, developing granulation tissue) and are clean and uniformly pink in appearance. They need to be protected to avoid disturbance to regenerating tissue. Examples are superficial wounds, skin donor sites, and partial-thickness or second-degree burns. The nurse protects red wounds by (a) gentle cleansing, (b) avoiding the use of dry gauze or wet-to-dry saline dressings, (c) applying a topical antimicrobial agent, (d) applying a transparent film or hydrocolloid dressing, and (e) changing the dressing as infrequently as possible.

Yellow wounds are characterized primarily by liquid to semiliquid "slough" that is often accompanied by purulent drainage. The nurse *cleanses* yellow wounds to absorb drainage and remove nonviable tissue. Methods used may include applying wet-to-wet dressings; irrigating the wound; using absorbent dressing materials such as impregnated nonadherent, hydrogel dressings, or other exudate absorbers; and consulting with the physician about the need for a topical antimicrobial to minimize bacterial growth.

Black wounds are covered with thick necrotic tissue, or eschar. Examples are full-thickness or third-degree burns and gangrenous ulcers. Black wounds require **debridement** (removal of the infected and necrotic material). Debridement may be achieved surgically by the physician or by a process called **autolytic debridement,** in which the wound is covered with an occlusive or semiocclusive dressing to provide a moist environment. The body's own defense mechanisms clean the wound of necrotic debris. When the eschar is removed, the wound is treated as yellow, then red. When more than one color is present, the nurse treats the most serious color first, that is, black, then yellow, then red.

SURGICAL DRESSINGS

Not all surgical dressings require changing. Sometimes, surgeons in the operating room apply a dressing that remains in place until the sutures are removed, and no further dressings are required. In most, situations, however, surgical dressings are changed regularly to prevent the growth of microorganisms.

In some instances, a client may have a Penrose drain inserted (see p. 1377). In this situation, the main surgical incision is considered cleaner than the surgical stab wound made for the drain insertion, because there usually is considerable drainage. The main incision is therefore cleaned first, and *under no circumstances are materials used to clean the stab wound used subsequently to clean the main incision.* In this way, the main incision is kept free of the microorganisms around the stab wound. Cleaning a wound and applying a sterile dressing are detailed in Procedure 44–2.

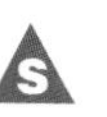

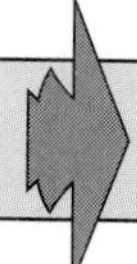

PROCEDURE 44–2 CLEANING A WOUND AND APPLYING A STERILE DRESSING

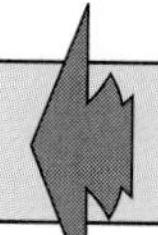

Before changing a dressing, determine any specific orders about the wound or dressing.

PURPOSES

- To promote wound healing by primary intention
- To prevent infection
- To assess the healing process
- To protect the wound from mechanical trauma

ASSESSMENT FOCUS

Allergies to wound cleaning agents; the appearance and size of the wound; the amount and character of exudate; complaints of discomfort; the time of the last pain medication; signs of systemic infection (eg, elevated body temperature, diaphoresis, malaise; leukocytosis).

EQUIPMENT

- ☐ Bath blanket (if necessary)
- ☐ Moistureproof bag
- ☐ Mask (optional)
- ☐ Acetone or another solution (if necessary to loosen adhesive)
- ☐ Clean disposable gloves
- ☐ Sterile gloves
- ☐ Sterile dressing set; if none is available, gather the following sterile items from a central supply cart
  - Drape or towel
  - Gauze squares
  - Container for the cleaning solution
  - Cleaning solution (eg, normal saline)
  - Two pairs of forceps (thumb or artery)
  - Gauze dressings and surgipads
  - Applicators or tongue blades to apply ointments
- ☐ Additional supplies required for the particular dressing (eg, extra gauze dressings and ointment or powder, if ordered)
- ☐ Tape, tie tapes, or binder

INTERVENTION

1. Prepare the client, and assemble the equipment.

- Acquire assistance for changing a dressing on a restless or confused adult. *The person might move and contaminate the sterile field or the wound.*
- Assist the client to a comfortable position in which the wound can be readily exposed. Expose only the wound area, using a bath blanket to cover the client, if necessary. *Undue exposure is physically and psychologically distressing to most people.*
- Make a cuff on the moistureproof bag for disposal of the soiled dressings, and place the bag within reach. It can be taped to the bedclothes or bedside table. *Making a cuff helps keep the outside of the bag free from contamination by the soiled dressings and*

PROCEDURE 44–2 ***continued***

prevents subsequent contamination of the nurse's hands or of sterile instrument tips when discarding dressings or sponges. Placement of the bag within reach prevents the nurse from reaching across the sterile field and the wound and potentially contaminating these areas.

- Put on a face mask, if required. *Some agencies require that a mask be worn for surgical dressing changes to prevent contamination of the wound by droplet spray from the nurse's respiratory tract.*

2. Remove binders and tape.

- Remove binders, if used, and place them aside. Untie tie tapes, if used.
- If adhesive tape was used, remove it by holding down the skin and pulling the tape gently but firmly toward the wound. *Pressing down on the skin provides countertraction against the pulling motion. Tape is pulled toward the incision to prevent strain on the sutures or wound.*
- Use a solvent to loosen tape, if required. *Moistening the tape with acetone or a similar solvent lessens the discomfort of removal, particularly from hairy surfaces.*

3. Remove and dispose of soiled dressings appropriately.

- Put on clean disposable gloves, and remove the outer abdominal dressing or surgipad.
- Lift the *outer* dressing so that the underside is away from the client's face. *The appearance and odor of the drainage may be upsetting to the client.*

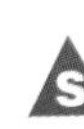

- Place the soiled dressing in the moistureproof bag without touching the outside of the bag. *Contamination of the outside of the bag is avoided to prevent the spread of microorganisms to the nurse and subsequently to others.*
- Remove the *under* dressings, taking care not to dislodge any drains. If the gauze sticks to the drain, support the drain with one hand and remove the gauze with the other.
- Assess the location, type (color, consistency), and odor of wound drainage, and the number of gauzes saturated or the diameter of drainage collected on the dressings.
- Discard the soiled dressings in the bag as before.
- Remove gloves, dispose of them in the moistureproof bag, and wash hands.

4. Set up the sterile supplies.

- Open the sterile dressing set, using surgical aseptic technique.
- Place the sterile drape beside the wound.
- Open the sterile cleaning solution, and pour it over the gauze sponges in the plastic container.
- Put on sterile gloves.

5. Clean the wound, if indicated.

- Clean the wound, using your gloved hands or forceps and gauze swabs moistened with cleaning solution.
- If using forceps, keep the forceps tips lower than the handles at all times. *This prevents their contamination by fluid traveling up to the handle and nurse's wrist and back to the tips.*
- Use the cleaning methods discussed earlier (Figure 44–1, p. 1368) or one recommended by agency protocol.
- Use a separate swab for each stroke, and discard each swab after use. *This prevents the introduction of microorganisms to other wound areas.*
- If a drain is present, clean it after the incision. Clean the skin around the drain site by swabbing in half or full circles from around the drain site outward, using separate swabs for each wipe (Figure 44–1, p. 1368).
- Support and hold the drain erect while cleaning around it. Clean as many times as necessary to remove the drainage.
- For irregular wounds, such as a decubitus ulcer, clean from the center of the wound outward, using circular strokes.
- Dry the surrounding skin with dry gauze swabs as required. Do not dry the incision or wound itself. *Moisture facilitates wound healing.*

6. Apply the ordered powder or ointment.

- Shake powders directly onto the wound. Antibiotic powders may be ordered.
- Use sterile applicators or tongue blades to apply ointments. *Ointments can protect the skin from irritation if drainage is profuse.*

7. Apply dressings to the drain site and the incision.

- Place a precut 4 × 4 gauze snugly around the drain (Figure 44–6), or open a 4 × 4 gauze to 4 × 8,

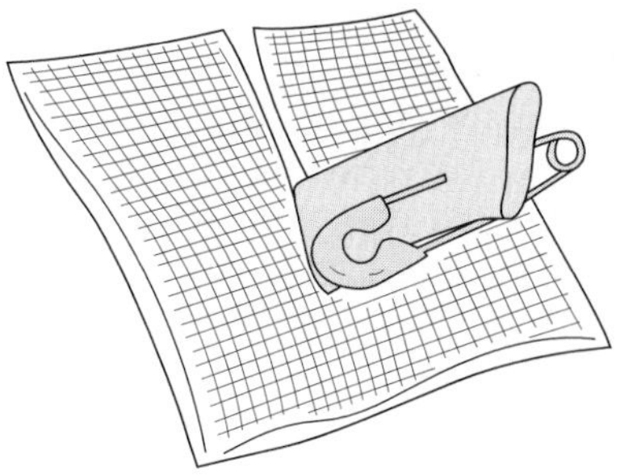

Figure 44–6 Precut gauze in place around a drain.

PROCEDURE 44–2 CLEANING A WOUND AND APPLYING A STERILE DRESSING *continued*

fold it lengthwise to 2 × 8, and place the 2 × 8 around the drain so that the ends overlap. *This dressing absorbs the drainage and helps prevent it from excoriating the skin. Using precut gauze or folding it as described, instead of cutting the gauze, prevents any threads from coming loose and getting into the wound, where they could cause inflammation and provide a site for infection.*

- Apply the sterile dressings one at a time over the drain and the incision. Place the bulk of the dressings over the drain area and below the drain, depending on the client's usual position. *Layers of dressings are placed for best absorption of drainage, which flows by gravity.*
- Apply the final surgipad, remove gloves, and dispose of them. Secure the dressing with tape or ties.

8. Document the procedure and all nursing assessments.

EVALUATION FOCUS
Amount of granulation tissue or degree of healing; amount of drainage and its color, consistency, and odor; presence of inflammation; degree of discomfort associated with the incision or drain site.

TRANSPARENT WOUND BARRIERS

Transparent wound barriers such as Op-Site, Tegaderm, and Bio-occlusive are often applied to wounds including ulcerated or burned skin areas. These dressings offer several advantages:

- They act as temporary skin.
- They are nonporous, self-adhesive dressings that do not require changing as other dressings do. They are often left in place until healing has occurred or as long as they remain intact.
- Because they are transparent, the wound can be assessed through them.
- Because they are occlusive, the wound remains moist and retains the serous exudate, which promotes epithelial growth, hastens healing, and reduces the risk of infection.
- Because they are elastic, they can be placed over a joint without disrupting the client's mobility.
- They adhere only to the skin area around the wound and not to the wound itself, because the wound is kept moist.
- They allow the client to shower or bathe without removing the dressing.
- They can be removed without damaging wound tissues.

Procedure 44–3 describes how to apply a moist transparent wound barrier.

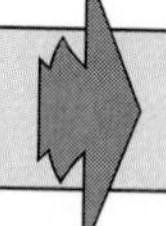

PROCEDURE 44–3 APPLYING A MOIST TRANSPARENT WOUND BARRIER

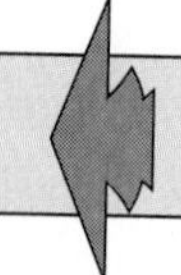

Before applying or changing a moist transparent wound barrier, (a) verify the physician's order regarding frequency and type of dressing change, and (b) determine agency protocol about solutions used to clean the wound.

PURPOSES

- To contain exudate and prevent wound infection
- To provide a moist wound environment and promote wound healing
- To protect the wound from trauma
- To facilitate assessment of wound healing

ASSESSMENT FOCUS
See Procedure 44–2 on page 1372.

PROCEDURE 44–3 *continued*

EQUIPMENT

- ☐ Disposable gloves
- ☐ Soap and water
- ☐ Razor (optional) or clippers
- ☐ Alcohol or acetone
- ☐ Moistureproof bag
- ☐ Sterile gloves
- ☐ Sterile gauze and the wound-cleaning agents specified by the physician or agency (eg, sterile saline)
- ☐ Wound barrier
- ☐ Scissors
- ☐ Paper tape
- ☐ Sterile #26 gauze needle and syringe

INTERVENTION

1. Obtain assistance as needed.

- If the size of the wound necessitates it, acquire the assistance of a co-worker to help apply the dressing.

2. Thoroughly clean the skin area around the wound.

- Put on disposable gloves.
- Clean the skin well with soap and water.
- Clip the hair about 5 cm (2 in) around the wound area if indicated.
- Rub the area with alcohol or acetone, and allow it to dry. *Alcohol or acetone defats the skin. Defatted, clean, dry skin ensures better adhesion of the dressing.*
- Remove gloves, and dispose of them in the moistureproof bag.

3. Clean the wound if indicated.

- Put on sterile gloves.
- Clean the wound with the prescribed solution.

4. Assess the wound.

- See page 1362.

5. Apply the wound barrier.

- Remove part of the paper backing on the dressing. If you have an assistant, remove all of the paper backing; the two of you should hold the colored tabs attached to the dressing.
- Apply the dressing at one edge of the wound site, allowing at least 2.5-cm (1-in) coverage of the skin surrounding the wound.
- Gently lay or press the barrier over the wound. Keep it free of wrinkles, but avoid stretching it too tightly. *A stretched dressing restricts mobility.*
- Cut off the colored tabs after the wound is completely covered.
- Remove and discard gloves.

6. Reinforce the dressing as needed.

- Apply paper or other porous tape to the edges of the dressing.

7. Assess the wound at least daily.

- Determine the extent of serous fluid accumulation under the dressing, wound healing, and the need to repair the dressing.
- If excessive serum has accumulated, use a sterile #26 gauge needle to aspirate the fluid. Then patch the needle hole.
- If the dressing is leaking, remove it, and apply another dressing.

8. Document the procedure and all nursing assessments.

EVALUATION FOCUS
Amount of granulation tissue or degree of healing; amount of serous fluid under dressing (see step 7); degree of discomfort associated with wound care.

HYDROCOLLOID DRESSINGS

Hydrocolloid dressings (see Table 44–3), such as DuoDERM, are used to (a) protect granulation tissue from excessive drying and trauma, (b) absorb slight to moderate amounts of wound drainage, and (c) liquefy necrotic tissue by autolysis (Fowler et al 1991a, p. 63). They are frequently used over venous stasis ulcers and pressure ulcers. These dressings offer several advantages:

- They last a long time.
- They do not need a "cover" dressing and are water resistant, so the client can shower or bathe.
- They can be molded to uneven body surfaces.
- They act as temporary skin and provide an effective bacterial barrier.
- They decrease pain and thus reduce the need for analgesics.

- They absorb *some* drainage and therefore can be used on draining wounds.
- They contain wound odor.

These dressings have certain limitations, however (Fowler et al 1991a, p. 63):

- They are opaque and obscure wound visibility.
- They have a limited absorption capacity.
- They can facilitate anaerobic bacterial growth.
- They can soften and wrinkle at the edges with wear and movement.
- They can be difficult to remove and may leave a residue on the skin.

Because of these limitations, hydrocolloid dressings should not be used for infected wounds or those with deep tracts or fistulas.

Procedure 44–4 describes how to apply hydrocolloid dressings.

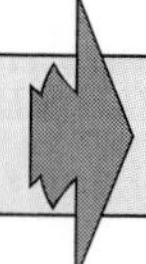

PROCEDURE 44–4 APPLYING A HYDROCOLLOID DRESSING

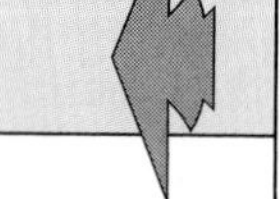

A hydrocolloid dressing should be changed whenever it becomes dislodged, leaks, or develops an odor. If the wound has substantial drainage or yellow slough, it may need to be changed every 24 to 72 hours. If it is applied to liquefy necrotic material, the change may need to be done more frequently. When drainage subsides, the dressing may be left in place for 3 to 7 days.

PURPOSES

- To maintain a moist wound surface and promote healing
- To prevent the entrance of microorganisms into the wound
- To minimize wound discomfort
- To promote autolysis of necrotic material by white blood cells
- To decrease the frequency of dressing changes

ASSESSMENT FOCUS

See Procedure 44–2 on page 1372.

EQUIPMENT

- ☐ Disposable gloves
- ☐ Moistureproof bag
- ☐ Soap and water
- ☐ Dressing set
- ☐ Sterile normal saline or other cleaning agent used by the agency
- ☐ Sterile gloves
- ☐ Hydrocolloid dressing of appropriate size
- ☐ Tape

INTERVENTION

1. Remove the old dressing.

- Put on disposable gloves.
- Pull the dressing off gradually in the direction of hair growth. *This minimizes skin irritation.*
- Dispose of the soiled dressing into the moistureproof bag.

2. Clean the skin area around the wound.

- Gently wash the skin surrounding the wound with soap and water, and dry it thoroughly with gauze squares.
- Leave the residue that is difficult to remove on the skin. It will wear off in time. *Attempts to remove residue can irritate the surrounding skin.*

3. Clean the wound if indicated.

- Open the sterile dressing supplies.
- Pour saline or other cleaning agent into the sterile container.
- Put on sterile gloves.
- Clean the wound with the prescribed solution.

4. Assess the wound.

- See page 1362.

5. Apply the dressing.

- Follow the manufacturer's instructions.
- Remove the sterile gloves by pulling them inside out. *This decreases the risk of microorganism transmission.*
- Optional: Tape all four sides of the dressing as required or ac-

PROCEDURE 44–4 *continued*

cording to agency protocol. *Taping prevents the dressing from sticking to bed linens and the edges from lifting.*

6. Assess and change the dressing as indicated.

- Inspect the dressing at least daily for leakage, dislodgement, odor, and wrinkling.
- Change the dressing if the above signs are present.

7. Document the technique and all nursing assessments.

EVALUATION FOCUS
Amount of granulation tissue or degree of healing; amount and character of any drainage; level of discomfort associated with wound care.

WOUND DRAINS AND SUCTION

Surgical **drains** are inserted to permit the drainage of excessive serosanguineous fluid and purulent material and to promote healing of underlying tissues. These drains may be inserted and sutured through the incision line, but they are most commonly inserted through stab wounds a few centimeters away from the incision line so that the incision itself may be kept dry. Without a drain, some wounds would heal on the surface and trap the discharge inside, and an abscess might form. These drains, for example, the **Penrose drain,** have an open end that drains onto a dressing.

Drains vary in length and width. The length can be 25 to 35 cm (10 to 14 in), and the width 1.2 to 4 cm (0.5 to 1.5 in). To facilitate drainage and healing of tissues from the inside to the outside, or from the bottom to the top, the physician may order that the drain be pulled out or shortened 2 to 5 cm (1 to 2 in) each day. When a drain is completely removed, the remaining stab wound usually heals within a day or two. In some agencies, this shortening procedure is performed only by physicians; in others, it is ordered by the physician and performed by nurses. When changing a dressing of a draining wound, the nurse should be careful not to dislodge the drain. Shortening the drain is usually done when the dressing is changed. Steps involved in shortening a drain are shown in the box on the next page.

A *closed wound drainage system* consists of a drain connected to either an electric suction or a portable drainage suction, such as a Hemovac (Figure 44–7) or Jackson-Pratt. The closed system eliminates the possible entry of microorganisms into the wound through the drain. The drainage tubes are sutured (stitched) in place and connected to a reservoir. For example, the Jackson-Pratt drainage tube is connected to a reservoir that maintains constant low suction. These portable wound suctions also provide for accurate measurement of the drainage.

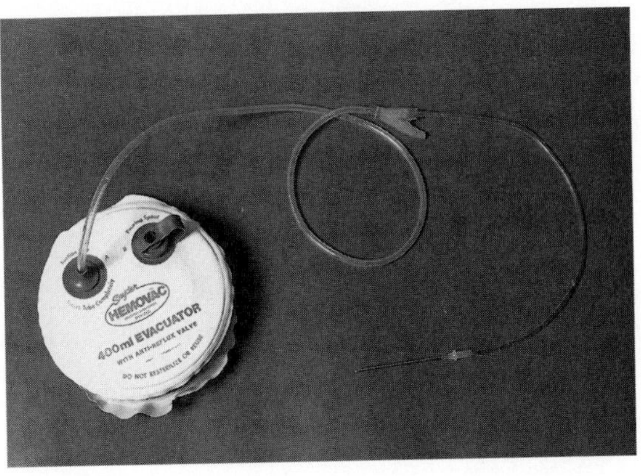

Figure 44–7 Closed wound drainage system (Hemovac).

The surgeon inserts the wound drainage tube during surgery. Generally, the suction is discontinued from 3 to 7 days postoperatively or when the wound is free from drainage. Nurses are responsible for maintaining the patency of the tube used for wound suction, which hastens the healing process by draining excess exudate that might otherwise interfere with the formation of granulation tissue.

Closed wound drainage systems have directions for use printed on the drainage container. When emptying the container, the nurse should wear gloves and avoid touching the drainage port.

WOUND IRRIGATION AND PACKING

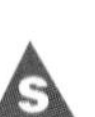

An **irrigation (lavage)** is the washing or flushing out of an area. Sterile technique is required for a wound irrigation, because there is a break in the skin integrity.

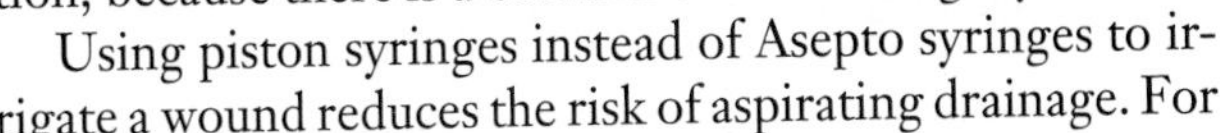

Using piston syringes instead of Asepto syringes to irrigate a wound reduces the risk of aspirating drainage. For

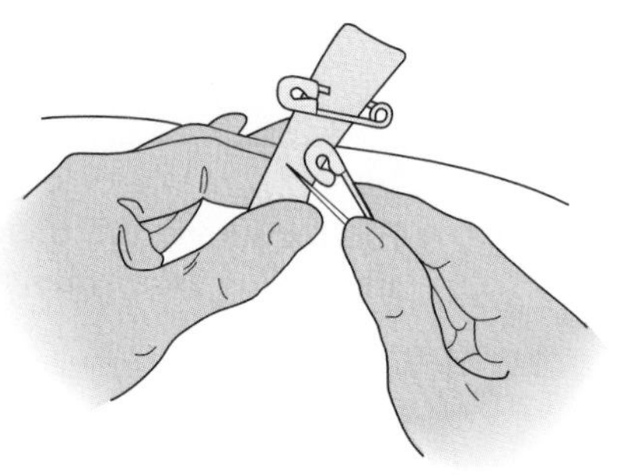

Figure 44–8 Pinning a drain.

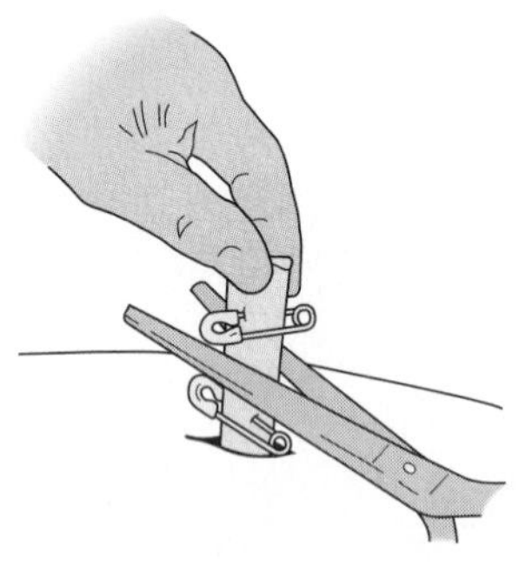

Figure 44–9 Shortening a drain.

CLINICAL GUIDELINES

Shortening a Drain

- Remove dressings, put on sterile gloves, and clean the incision (Procedure 44–2, p. 1372).
- Clean the drain site appropriately (Figure 44–1, p. 1368). Assess the amount and character of drainage, including odor, thickness, and color.
- If the drain has *not* been shortened before, cut and remove the suture. The drain is sutured to the skin during surgery to keep it from slipping into the body cavity.
- Firmly grasp the drain by its full width at the level of the skin, and pull the drain out the required length. Grasping the full width of the drain ensures even traction.
- Insert a sterile safety pin through the base of the drain as close to the skin as possible by holding the drain tightly against the skin edge and inserting the pin above your fingers (Figure 44–8). The pin keeps the drain from falling back into the incision. Holding the drain securely in place at the skin level and inserting the pin above the fingers prevents the nurse from pulling the drain further out or pricking the client during this step.
- With the sterile scissors, cut off the excess drain so that about 2.5 cm (1 in) remains above the skin (Figure 44–9). Discard the excess in the waste bag.
- Apply dressings to the drain site and the incision.

deep wounds with small openings, a sterile straight catheter may also be necessary. Frequently used irrigation solutions are sterile normal saline, lactated Ringer's solution, and antibiotic solutions. See Procedure 44–5 for the steps involved in irrigating a wound.

Gauze **packing** is placed in wounds to facilitate the formation of granulation tissue and healing by secondary intention. Generally, moistened 4 × 4 non-cotton-filled gauze dressings are used. Cotton fibers are contraindicated because they can pull loose and remain in the wound, encouraging bacterial growth and contamination. Two techniques used to pack acute or chronic wounds are the *wet-to-dry* technique and the *wet-to-damp* technique.

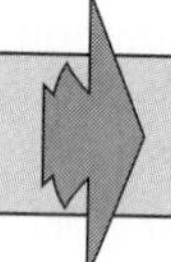

PROCEDURE 44–5 IRRIGATING A WOUND

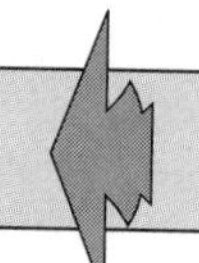

Before irrigating a wound, determine (a) the type of irrigating solution to be used, (b) the frequency of irrigations, and (c) the temperature of the solution.

PURPOSES

- To clean the area
- To apply heat and hasten the healing process
- To apply an antimicrobial solution

ASSESSMENT FOCUS

Appearance and size of the wound; the character of the exudate; the time of the last pain medication; clinical signs of systemic infection; allergies to the wound irrigation agent or tape.

Procedure 44–5 *continued*

Equipment

- ☐ Sterile dressing equipment and dressing materials
- ☐ Sterile irrigating syringes, (eg, a 50-mL piston syringe)
- ☐ Sterile basin for the irrigating solution
- ☐ Sterile basin to receive the irrigation returns
- ☐ Irrigating solution, usually 200 mL (6.5 oz) of solution warmed to body temperature, according to the agency's or physician's choice
- ☐ Disposable gloves
- ☐ Sterile gloves
- ☐ Moistureproof sterile drape
- ☐ Sterile straight catheter, if needed

INTERVENTION

1. Verify the physician's order.

- Confirm the type and strength of the solution.

2. Prepare the client.

- Assist the client to a position in which the irrigating solution will flow by gravity from the upper end of the wound to the lower end and then into the basin.
- Place the waterproof drape over the client and the bed.

- Put on disposable gloves; remove the old dressing, and clean the wound. See Procedure 44–2, page 1372.
- Assess the wound and drainage.
- Remove and discard disposable gloves.

3. Prepare the equipment.

- Wash hands, then open the sterile dressing set and supplies.
- Pour the ordered solution into the solution container.
- Put on sterile gloves.
- Position the sterile basin below the wound to receive the irrigating fluid.

4. Irrigate the wound.

- Using the syringe, gently instill a steady stream of irrigating solution into the wound. Make sure all areas of the wound are irrigated.
- If you are using a catheter, insert the catheter into the wound until resistance is met. Do not force the catheter. *Forcing the catheter can cause tissue damage.*
- Continue irrigating until the solution becomes clear (no exudate is present). *The irrigation washes away tissue debris and drainage so that later returns are clearer.*

- Dry the area around the wound. *Moisture left on the skin promotes the growth of microorganisms and can cause skin irritation.*

5. Assess and dress the wound.

- Assess the appearance of the wound, noting in particular the type and amount of exudate and the presence and extent of granulation tissue.
- Pack the wound if ordered (see p. 1378).
- Apply a sterile dressing to the wound as described in Procedure 44–2 on p. 1372.

6. Document all relevant information.

- Document the irrigation, the solution used, the appearance of the irrigation returns, and nursing assessments. Note the presence of any exudate and sloughing tissue.

Evaluation Focus

Character of irrigation returns; the extent of wound healing (ie, the amount of granulation tissue); the degree of discomfort associated with wound irrigation; color and amount of exudate.

In the *wet-to-dry* technique, wounds are packed with wet dressings and allowed to dry between dressing changes every 4 to 6 hours. The wet gauze traps necrotic material in its spaces as it dries. Wet-to-dry dressings are intended to debride a wound, that is, to remove dead tissue and drainage with removal of the packing material. It is now believed that the removal of dry gauzes may also disrupt new granulation tissue and retard healing. In addition, the procedure can be painful.

The *wet-to-damp* technique for packing is now replacing the wet-to-dry technique (Wound-Care Update 1991, p. 50). In this technique, moist gauzes are packed in the wound to absorb exudate but they are not allowed to dry before removal. Clinical guidelines for applying wet-to-damp dressings are shown in the accompanying box.

SUTURES

Sutures are threads used to sew body tissues together. Sutures used to attach tissues beneath the skin are made of an absorbable material that disappears in several days. Skin sutures, by contrast, are made of a variety of nonabsorbable materials, such as silk, cotton, linen, wire, nylon, and Dacron (polyester fiber). Silver wire clips are also available. Usually, skin sutures are removed 7 to 10 days after surgery.

There are various methods of suturing. Skin sutures can be broadly categorized as either *interrupted* (each stitch is tied and knotted separately) or *continuous* (one thread runs in a series of stitches and is tied only at the beginning and at the end of the run). Common methods of suturing are illustrated in Figure 44–10).

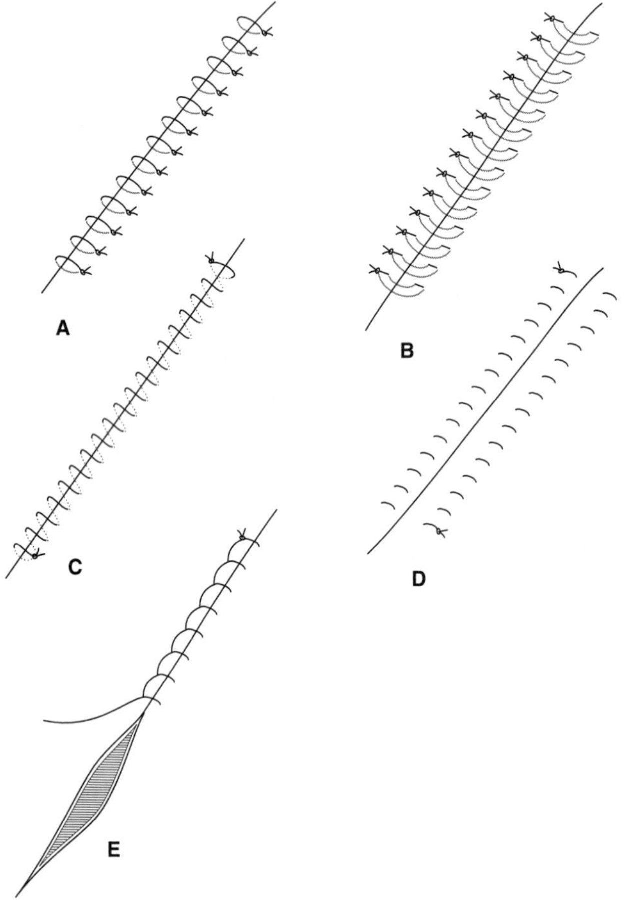

Figure 44–10 Common sutures: *A*, plain interrupted; *B*, mattress interrupted; *C*, plain continuous; *D*, mattress continuous; *E*, blanket continuous.

CLINICAL GUIDELINES

Applying Wet-to-Damp Dressings

- Open the packages of the sterile dressing set, fine-mesh gauze, and sterile solution container.
- Pour the ordered solution into the solution container.
- Put on sterile gloves.
- Place the fine-mesh gauze dressings into the solution container, and thoroughly saturate them with solution. The entire gauze must be moistened to enhance its absorptive abilities.
- If agency protocol indicates, clean the wound gently, using a circular motion. Work outward from the center of the wound to its edge and beyond. Use a separate gauze swab for each cleaning stroke.
- Wring out the packing material so that it is *slightly* moist. Avoid packing that is too wet. An excessively wet wound bed increases the risk for bacterial growth and may macerate surrounding skin.
- Pack the moistened dressings into all depressions and grooves of the wound, ensuring that all *exposed surfaces* are covered. If necessary, use forceps to feed the gauze gradually into deep depressed areas. Necrotic tissue is usually more prevalent in depressed wound areas and needs to be covered with the gauze.
- Avoid applying packing too tightly. A tight application inhibits wound edges from contracting and compresses capillaries.
- To prevent maceration of the surrounding skin, pack only to the edge of the wound, without overlapping the skin.
- If necessary, protect surrounding skin with a skin barrier (eg, skin sealant or hydrocolloid dressing).
- Apply a secondary dressing (eg, 4 × 4 gauze) over the wet dressings to absorb excess exudate.
- Cover all the dressings with a surgipad or abdominal pad. The pad protects the wound from external contaminants.
- Remove gloves inside out and discard them.

To remove the dressings, wear disposable gloves. If packing material adheres to any tissue during removal, soak it with normal saline. This facilitates removal and preserves new granulation tissue.

Retention sutures (stay sutures) are very large sutures used in addition to skin sutures for some incisions (Figure 44–11). They attach underlying tissues of fat and muscle as well as skin and are used to support incisions in obese individuals or when healing may be prolonged. They are frequently left in place longer than skin sutures (14 to 21

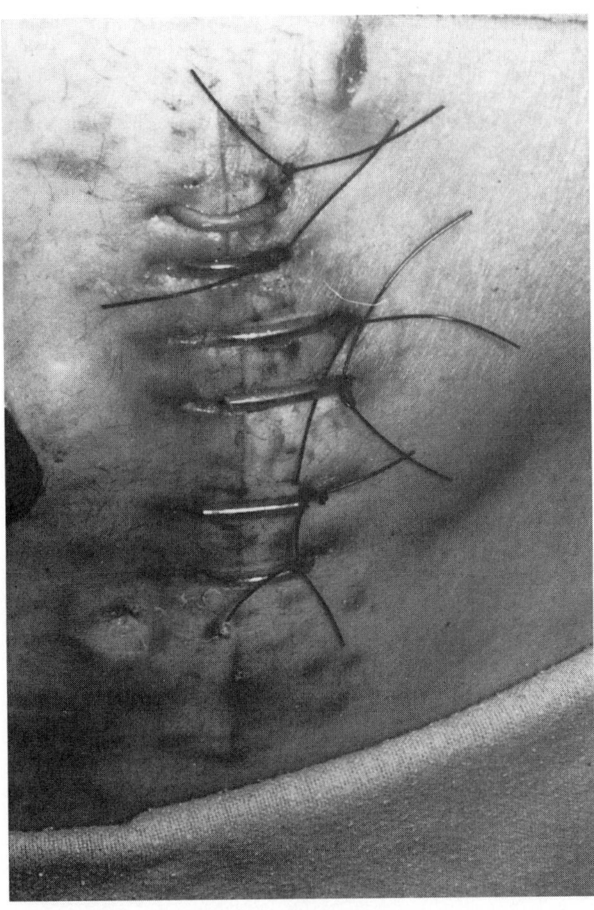

Figure 44–11 A surgical incision with retention sutures.

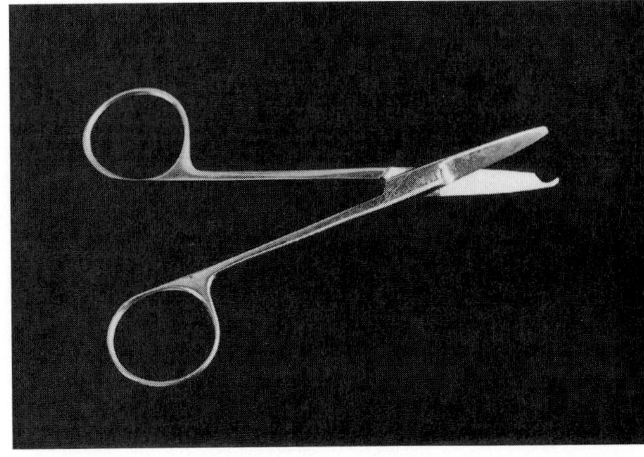

Figure 44–12 Suture scissors.

days) but in some instances are removed at the same time as the skin sutures. To prevent these large sutures from irritating the incision, the surgeon may place rubber tubing over them or a roll of gauze under them extending down the incision line.

The physician orders the removal of sutures. In some agencies, only physicians remove sutures; in others, registered nurses and nursing students with appropriate supervision may do so. Agency policies about removal of retention sutures vary. The nurse should verify whether they are to be removed and who may remove them.

Sterile technique and special suture scissors are used in suture removal. The scissors have a short, curved cutting tip that readily slides under the suture (Figure 44–12). Wire clips or staples are removed with a special instrument that squeezes the center of the clip to remove it from the skin (Figure 44–13). Guidelines for removing sutures follow.

- Before removing skin sutures, verify (a) the orders for suture removal (in many instances, only *alternate* interrupted sutures are removed one day, and the remaining sutures are removed a day or two later); and (b) whether a dressing is to be applied following the suture removal. Some physicians prefer no dressing; others prefer a small, light gauze dressing to prevent friction by clothing.
- Inform the client that suture removal may produce slight discomfort, such as a pulling or stinging sensation, but should not be painful.
- Remove dressings and clean the incision in accordance with agency protocol. Cleaning the suture line with an antimicrobial solution before and after suture removal may be required as a prophylactic measure to prevent infection.
- Put on sterile gloves. 
- Remove *plain interrupted sutures* as follows:
  a. Grasp the suture at the knot with a pair of forceps.

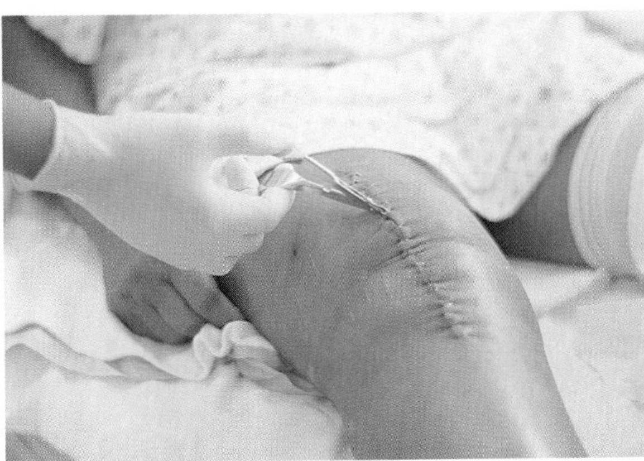

Figure 44–13 Removing surgical clips.

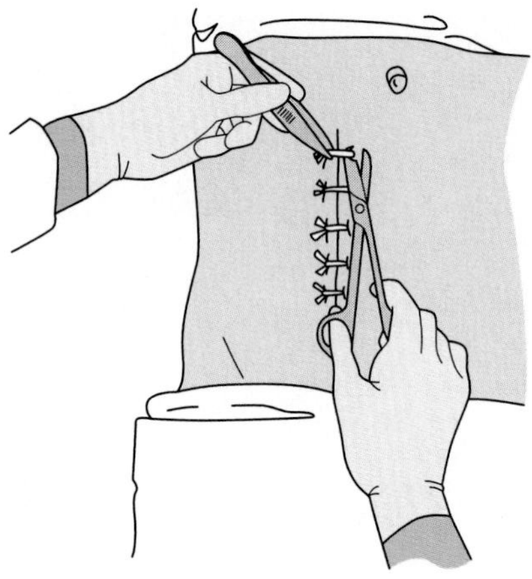

Figure 44–14 Removing a plain interrupted skin suture.

b. Place the curved tip of the suture scissors under the suture as close to the skin as possible, either on the side opposite the knot (Figure 44–14) or directly under the knot. Cut the suture. Sutures are cut as close to the skin as possible on one side of the visible part because the suture material that is visible to the eye is in contact with resident bacteria of the skin and must not be pulled beneath the skin during removal. Suture material that is beneath the skin is considered free from bacteria.

c. With the forceps, pull the suture out in one piece. Inspect the suture carefully to make sure that all suture material is removed. Suture material left beneath the skin acts as a foreign body and causes inflammation.

- Remove *mattress interrupted sutures* as follows:
  a. When possible, cut the visible part of the suture close to the skin at *A* and *B* in Figure 44–15, opposite the knot, and remove this small visible piece. Discard it as described below. In some sutures, the visible part opposite the knot may be so small that it can be cut only once.
  b. Grasp the knot (*C*) with forceps. Remove the remainder of the suture beneath the skin by pulling out in the direction of the knot.

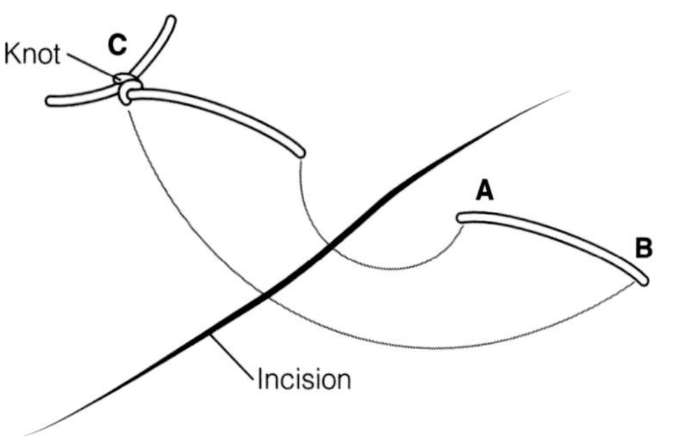

Figure 44–15 Mattress interrupted sutures.

- Discard the suture onto a piece of sterile gauze or into the moistureproof bag, being careful not to contaminate the forceps tips.
- Continue to remove *alternate* sutures, that is, the third, fifth, seventh, and so forth. Alternate sutures are removed first so that remaining sutures keep the skin edges in close approximation and prevent any dehiscence from becoming large.
- If no dehiscence occurs, remove the remaining sutures. If dehiscence does occur, do not remove the remaining sutures, and report the dehiscence to the nurse in charge.
- If a little wound dehiscence occurs, apply a sterile butterfly tape over the gap:
  a. Attach the tape to one side of the incision.
  b. Press the wound edges together.
  c. Attach the tape to the other side of the incision (Figure 44–16). The butterfly tape holds the wound edges as close together as possible and promotes healing.

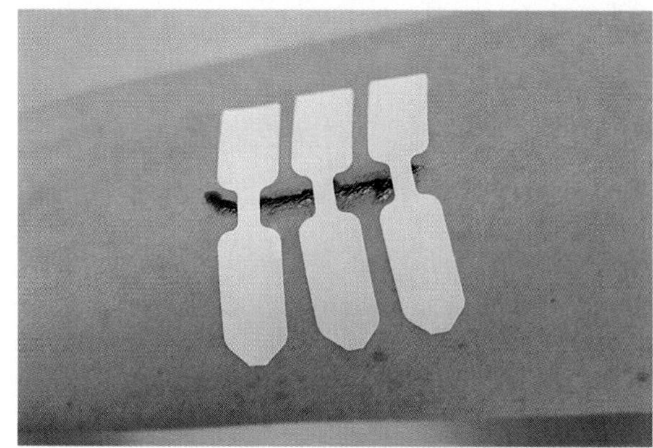

Figure 44–16 Butterfly tapes.

- If a large dehiscence occurs, cover the wound with sterile moist saline gauze, and report the problem immediately to the nurse in charge or physician.
- Reapply a dressing, if indicated.
- Instruct the client about follow-up wound care, such as contacting the physician if wound discharge appears.

HEAT AND COLD APPLICATIONS

Heat and cold are applied to the body for local and systemic effects. See Table 44–4 for the effects of heat and cold.

Physiologic Responses

Local Effects of Heat Heat is an old remedy for aches and pains; people often equate heat with comfort and relief. Heat causes **vasodilation** and increases blood flow to the affected area, bringing oxygen, nutrients, antibodies, and leukocytes. Heat accelerates the inflammatory process by increasing both the action of phagocytic cells that ingest microorganisms and other foreign material and the removal of the waste products of infection and metabolic processes. Vasodilation produces skin redness and warmth that can be assessed by touch.

Application of heat promotes soft tissue healing and increases suppuration. The increase in blood flow also dissipates the heat, that is, draws it away from the affected area. A possible disadvantage of heat is that it increases capillary permeability, which allows extracellular fluid and substances such as plasma proteins to pass through the capillary walls and may result in **edema** or an increase in preexisting edema. Heat is often used for clients with musculoskeletal problems such as joint stiffness from arthritis, contractures, and low back pain; and for those with open wounds needing debridement.

Heat can be applied to the body in both dry and moist forms. Dry heat is applied locally, for heat conduction, by means of a hot water bottle, electric pad, aquathermia pad, or disposable heat pack. Moist heat can be provided, through conduction, by compress, hot pack, soak, or sitz bath.

Local Effects of Cold Cold therapy is more recent than heat therapy. Generally, its physiologic effects are opposite to the effects of heat. Cold lowers the temperature of the skin and underlying tissues and causes **vasoconstriction.** Vasoconstriction reduces blood flow to the affected area and thus reduces the supply of oxygen and metabolites, decreases the removal of wastes, and produces skin pallor, or a bluish discoloration, and coolness. Vasoconstriction and its consequent lowered blood flow to an area help control bleeding after injury. Prolonged exposure to cold results in impaired circulation, cell deprivation, and subsequent damage to the tissues from lack of oxygen and nourishment. The signs of tissue damage due to cold are a bluish-purple mottled appearance of the skin, numbness, stiffness, pallor, and sometimes blisters and pain. Cold is most often used for sports injuries (eg, sprains, strains, fractures) to limit post injury swelling and bleeding.

Systemic Effects of Heat and Cold Heat applied to a localized body area, particularly a large body area, may increase cardiac output and pulmonary ventilation. These increases are a result of excessive peripheral vasodilation, which diverts large supplies of blood from the internal organs and produces a drop in blood pressure. A significant drop in blood pressure can cause fainting. Clients who have heart or pulmonary disease and who have circulatory disturbances such as arteriosclerosis are more prone to this effect than healthy persons.

Table 44–4 Physiologic Effects of Heat and Cold

Heat	Cold
Vasodilation	Vasoconstriction
Increases capillary permeability	Decreases capillary permeability
Increases cellular metabolism	Decreases cellular metabolism
Relaxes muscles	Relaxes muscle by decreasing muscle contractility
Increases inflammation; increases blood flow to an area, bringing phagocytes	Slows bacterial growth, decreases inflammation
Decreases pain by relaxing muscles	Decreases pain by numbing the area, slowing the flow of pain impulses, and by increasing the pain threshold
Sedative effect	Local anesthetic effect
Reduces joint stiffness by decreasing viscosity of synovial fluids	Decreases bleeding

With extensive cold applications and vasoconstriction, a client's blood pressure can increase, because blood is shunted from the cutaneous circulation to the internal blood vessels. This shunting of blood, a normal protective response to prolonged cold, is the body's attempt to maintain its core temperature. Shivering, another generalized effect of prolonged cold, is a normal response as the body attempts to warm itself.

Thermal Tolerance Various parts of the body differ in tolerance to heat and cold. The physiologic tolerance of individuals also varies. See the box on page 1384.

Specific conditions necessitate precautions in the use of hot or cold applications:

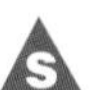

- *Neurosensory impairment.* Persons with sensory impairments are unable to perceive that heat is damaging the tissues and are at risk for burns or are unable to perceive discomfort from cold and prevent tissue injury.
- *Impaired mental status.* People who are confused or have an altered level of consciousness need monitoring during applications to ensure safe therapy.

VARIABLES AFFECTING PHYSIOLOGIC TOLERANCE TO HEAT AND COLD

- *Body part.* The back of the hand and foot are not very temperature-sensitive. In contrast, the inner aspect of the wrist and forearm, the neck, and the perineal area are temperature-sensitive.
- *Size of the exposed body part.* The larger the area exposed to heat and cold, the lower the tolerance.
- *Individual tolerance.* Tolerance to heat and cold is to some degree affected by age and condition of the skin, nervous system, and circulatory system. The very young and the very old generally have the lowest tolerance. Persons who have neurosensory impairments may have a high tolerance, but the risk of injury is greater.
- *Length of exposure.* People feel hot and cold applications most while the skin temperature is changing. After a period of time, tolerance increases.
- *Intactness of skin.* Injured skin areas are more sensitive to temperature variations.

- *Impaired circulation.* Persons with peripheral vascular disease, diabetes, or congestive heart failure lack the normal ability to dissipate heat via the blood circulation, which puts them at risk for tissue damage with heat and cold applications.
- *Immediately after injury or surgery.* Heat increases bleeding and swelling.
- *Open wounds.* Cold can decrease blood flow to the wound, thereby inhibiting healing.

Adaptation of Thermal Receptors Heat and cold receptors adapt to temperature changes. When they are subjected to an abrupt change in temperature the receptors are strongly stimulated initially. This strong stimulation declines rapidly during the first few seconds and then more slowly during the next half hour or more as the receptors adapt to the new temperature (Guyton 1991, p. 530).

Nurses and clients need to understand this adaptive response when applying heat and cold. Clients may be tempted to change the temperature of a thermal application because of the change in thermal sensation following adaptation. Increasing the temperature of a hot application after adaptation can result in serious burns. Decreasing the temperature of a cold application can result in pain and serious impairment of circulation to the body part. See Table 44–5 for temperatures of hot and cold applications.

Rebound Phenomenon The rebound phenomenon occurs at the time the maximum therapeutic effect of the hot or cold application is achieved and the opposite effect begins. For example, heat produces maximum vasodilation in 20 to 30 minutes; continuation of the application beyond 30 to 45 minutes brings tissue congestion, and the blood vessels then *constrict* for reasons unknown. If the heat application is continued further, the client is at risk for burns, since the constricted blood vessels are unable to dissipate the heat adequately via the blood circulation.

With cold applications, maximum vasoconstriction occurs when the involved skin reaches a temperature of 15 C (60 F). Below 15 C, vasodilation begins. This mechanism is protective: It helps to prevent freezing of body tissues normally exposed to cold, such as the nose and ears. It also explains the ruddiness of the skin of a person who has been walking in cold weather.

An understanding of the rebound phenomenon is essential for the nurse and client. Thermal applications must be halted *before* the rebound phenomenon begins.

Applying Heat and Cold Heat and cold can be applied in dry and moist forms. Hot water bags, aquathermia pads, electric pads, and chemical heat pads provide localized heat by conduction. Heat lamps and heat cradles apply dry heat by radiation. Hot compresses, sitz baths, and soaks provide moist heat by conduction.

For all local applications of heat, the nurse needs to follow these guidelines:

- Determine whether the agency requires the client to sign a form before local applications of heat.
- Determine the client's ability to tolerate the therapy.

Table 44–5 Temperatures for Hot and Cold Applications

Description	Temperature	Application
Very cold	Below 15 C (59 F)	Ice bags
Cold	15 to 18 C (59 to 65 F)	Cold pack
Cool	18 to 27 C (65 to 80 F)	Cold compresses
Tepid	27 to 37 C (80 to 98 F)	Alcohol sponge bath
Warm	37 to 40 C (98 to 105 F)	Warm bath, aquathermia pads
Hot	40 to 46 C (105 to 115 F)	Hot soak, irrigations, hot compresses
Very hot	above 46 C (above 115 F)	Hot water bags for adults

- Identify conditions that might contraindicate treatment (eg, bleeding).
- Explain the application to the client.
- Assess the skin area to which the heat will be applied. Circulatory impairment (as evidenced, for example, by cyanosis or coldness) decreases heat tolerance. Abrasions may also decrease tolerance.
- Ask the client to report any discomfort.

- Return to the client 15 minutes after starting the heat, and observe the local skin area for any untoward signs (eg, redness). Stop the heat if any problems occur.
- Apply the heat for the time required. Extended use of heat will trigger the rebound phenomenon discussed earlier.
- Remove the equipment at the designated time, and dispose of it appropriately.
- Examine the area to which the heat was applied, and record the client's response.

Dry Heat and Cold

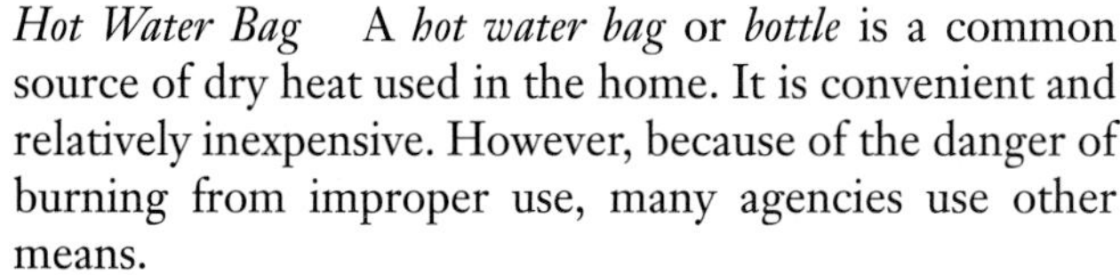

Hot Water Bag A *hot water bag* or *bottle* is a common source of dry heat used in the home. It is convenient and relatively inexpensive. However, because of the danger of burning from improper use, many agencies use other means.

The following temperatures of the water in the bag are considered safe in most situations and provide the desired effect: normal adult, 52 C (125 F); debilitated or unconscious adult, 40.5 to 46 C (105 to 115 F); child under 2 years, 40.5 to 46 C (105 to 115 F).

To apply a hot water bag, the nurse carries out the following steps:

- Measure the temperature of the water using a bath thermometer. Make sure the correct temperature is used.
- Fill the bag about two-thirds full.
- Expel the remaining air, and secure the top. By removing the air, the bag can be molded to the body part.
- Dry the bag and hold it upside down to test for leakage.
- Wrap the bag in a towel or cover, and place it on the body site.
- Remove after 30 to 45 minutes or in accordance with agency protocol. Maximum effect occurs in 20 to 30 minutes. Prolonged application initiates the rebound phenomenon.

Aquathermia Pad The *aquathermia* or *aquamatic pad* (also referred to as a *K-pad*) is a pad constructed with tubes containing water. The pad is attached by tubing to an electrically powered control unit that has an opening for water and a temperature gauge (Figure 44–17). Some aquathermia pads have an absorbent surface through which moist heat can be applied. The other surface of the pad is waterproof. These pads are disposable.

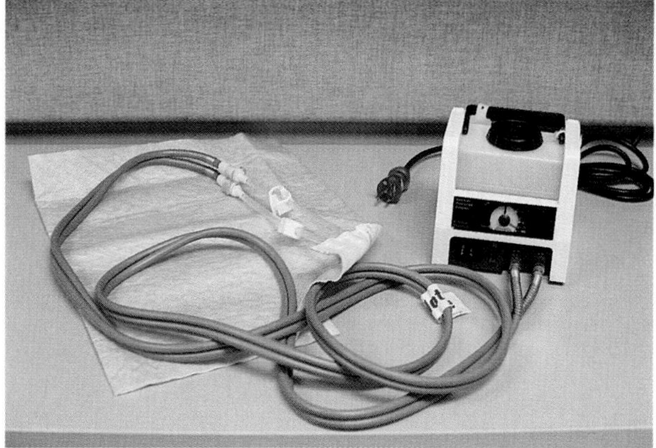

Figure 44–17 An aquathermia heating unit.

To apply an aquathermia pad, the nurse carries out the following steps:

- Fill the reservoir of the unit two-thirds full of *distilled* water.
- Set the desired temperature using a key. Check the manufacturer's instructions. Most units are set at 40.5 C (105 F) for adults.
- Cover the pad, and plug in the unit. Some manufacturers suggest warming the pad before applying it.
- Apply the pad to the body part. The treatment is usually continued for 10 to 15 minutes. Check orders and agency protocol.

Hot and Cold Packs Commercially prepared *hot* and *cold packs* (Figure 44–18, p. 1386) provide heat or cold for a designated time. Directions on the package tell how to initiate the heating or cooling process, for example, by striking, squeezing, or kneading the pack.

Electric Pads *Electric pads* provide a constant, even heat, are light-weight, and can be molded to a body part. Electric pads, however, can burn if the setting is too high. In some agencies, the controls on the pads are set to a specific temperature to prevent burning the client. Some models have waterproof covers for use when the pad is placed over a moist dressing.

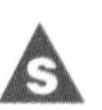

In applying electric pads, the nurse follows these guidelines:

- Do not insert sharp objects (eg, pins) into the pad. The pin could damage a wire and cause an electric shock.
- Ensure that the body area is dry unless there is a waterproof cover on the pad. Electricity in the presence of water can cause a shock.
- Use pads with a preset heating switch so a client cannot increase the heat. After adapting to the temperature,

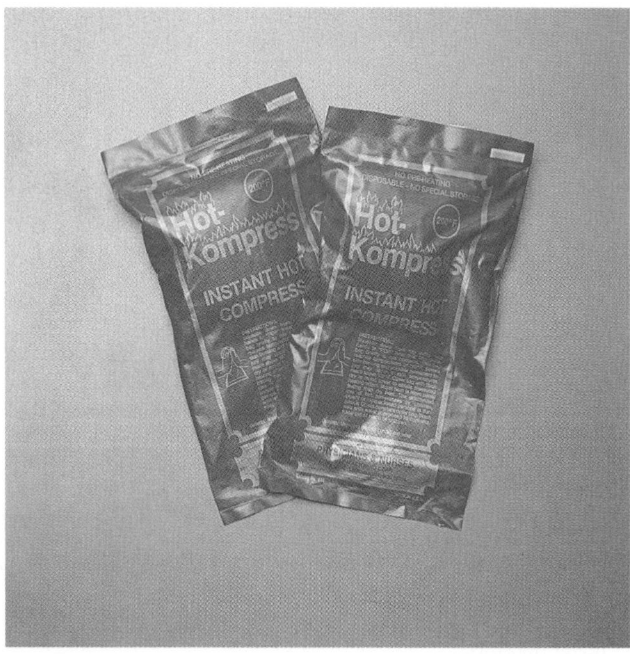

Figure 44–18 Commercially prepared disposable hot packs.

the client may feel the temperature is not warm enough.

- Do not place the pad under the client. Heat will not dissipate, and the client may be burned.

Heat Cradle A *heat cradle* is a metal frame with a row of 25-watt light bulbs. The cradle is placed over the client and usually covered with a bath blanket or sheet. The client must be assessed every 10 minutes for any untoward reactions. Heat is provided by radiation.

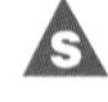

Heat Lamp Many *heat lamps* are gooseneck lamps with a 60-watt bulb. The lamp is placed 45 to 60 cm (18 to 24 in) from the area to be heated. The lamp provides heat by radiation.

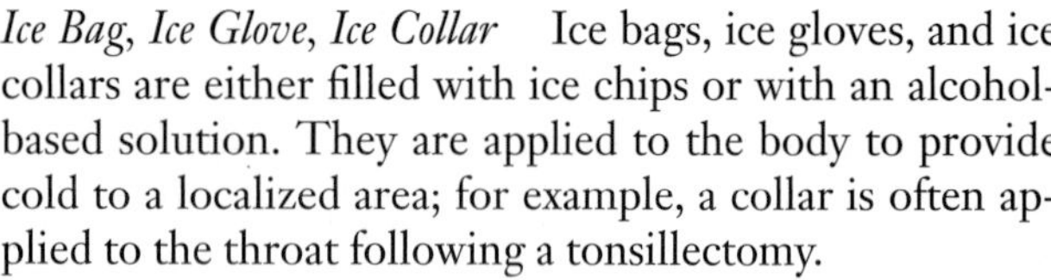

Ice Bag, Ice Glove, Ice Collar Ice bags, ice gloves, and ice collars are either filled with ice chips or with an alcohol-based solution. They are applied to the body to provide cold to a localized area; for example, a collar is often applied to the throat following a tonsillectomy.

Moist Heat and Cold

Compresses Compresses can be either warm or cold. A *compress* is a moist gauze dressing applied frequently to an open wound. When hot compresses are ordered, the solution is heated to the temperature indicated by the order or according to agency protocol, for example, 40.5 C (105 F). When there is a break in the skin or when the body part (eg, an eye) is vulnerable to microbial invasion, sterile technique is necessary; therefore, sterile gloves are needed to apply the compress, and all materials must be sterile. If a sterile thermometer is not available, the nurse can pour a small amount of the solution into a clean basin, measure the temperature, and then discard the solution (because it is no longer sterile). The nurse adjusts the temperature of the solution accordingly.

Hot compresses usually are applied to hasten the suppurative process and healing. Cold compresses are applied either to decrease or prevent bleeding or to reduce inflammation.

To apply a sterile compress, the nurse carries out the following steps:

- Add the ordered sterile solution to the dressing set.
- After removing the old dressing, clean the wound according to agency protocol.
- Put on sterile gloves.
- If the compress solution is irritating to tissues, protect the surrounding skin with sterile petroleum jelly.

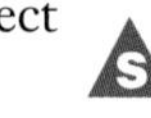

- Soak gauze in the solution, then wring it out so that it does not drip.
- Apply the gauze to the area, and pack the gauze snugly against all wound surfaces.
- Cover the gauze with dressings and a piece of plastic.
- Secure the dressings with ties or tapes.
- Apply a hot water bag or ice bag according to agency protocol.
- Remove the compress at the designated time (ie, 15 to 30 minutes).
- Dress the wound.
- Document the procedure, including the appearance of the wound, and drainage, and type and amount of solution used.

Packs A *pack* is a moist cloth applied to the body area. Packs may be hot or cold. They are usually unsterile; after application, they are often covered with a moisture-resistant material (eg, plastic wrap) to contain moisture and prevent the transfer of airborne microorganisms to the area. Hot packs are applied to relieve muscle spasm or pain, to reduce the pressure of accumulated fluid in a tissue or joint, and to reduce congestion in an underlying organ. Cold packs are used to prevent swelling of the tissues.

Soak A *soak* refers to immersing a body part (eg, an arm) in a solution or to wrapping a part in gauze dressings and then saturating the dressing with a solution. Sterile technique is generally indicated for open wounds, such as a burn or an unhealed surgical incision. Determine agency protocol regarding the temperature of the solution.

Sitz Bath A *sitz bath*, or hip bath, is used to soak a client's pelvic area. The client sits in a special tub or chair and is usually immersed from the midthighs to the iliac crests or umbilicus. Special tubs or chairs are preferred because when the legs are also immersed, as in a regular bathtub, blood circulation to the perineum or pelvic area is decreased. Disposable sitz baths are also available.

The temperature of the water should be from 40 to 43 C (105 to 110 F), unless the client is unable to tolerate the heat. Determine agency protocol. Some sitz tubs have temperature indicators attached to the water taps. The duration of the bath is generally 15 to 20 minutes, depending on the client's health.

To provide a sitz bath, the nurse carries out the following steps:

- Assist the client into the tub, and provide support for comfort. Provide support for the client's feet; a footstool can prevent pressure on the backs of the thighs.
- Provide a bath blanket for the client's shoulders, and eliminate drafts to prevent chilling.

- Observe the client closely during the bath for signs of faintness, dizziness, weakness, accelerated pulse rate, and pallor.
- Maintain the water temperature.
- Following the sitz bath, assist the client out of the tub. Help the client to dry.

Cooling Sponge Bath The purpose of a cooling sponge bath is to reduce a client's fever by promoting heat loss through conduction and vaporization. The bath consists of water or a combination of alcohol and water that is below body temperature. Alcohol evaporates at a low temperature and therefore removes body heat rapidly. However, alcohol-and-water sponge baths are less frequently used than in the past because alcohol has a drying effect on the skin. The temperatures for cooling sponge baths range from 18 to 32 C (65 to 90 F). A *tepid* sponge bath generally refers to one in which the water temperature is 32 C (90 F) throughout the bath. For a *cool* sponge bath, the water temperature is 32 C (90 F) at the beginning of the bath and is gradually lowered to 18 C (65 F) by adding ice chips during the bath. A fan is sometimes used to increase air movement around the client, which lowers the body temperature through convection. In this case, drafts are not usually eliminated during the sponge bath. Cool sponge baths are used with extreme caution because of potential deleterious effects, such as shock.

The decision to give a tepid sponge bath is generally made only after a marked fever is noted or a temperature increase of 1 to 2 C or 2 to 3 F. Some agencies require a physician's order; others permit a decision by a nurse.

To provide a cooling sponge bath, the nurse takes the following steps:

- Determine the client's temperature, pulse, and respirations.
- Assess the client for other signs of fever: skin warmth, flushing, complaints of heat or chilling, diaphoresis, and so on. See Chapter 21, page 428.
- Protect the client's bed with moistureproof material.
- Prepare ice bags or cold packs. See agency protocol.
- Sponge the face, arms, legs, back, and buttocks. The chest and abdomen are not usually sponged. Each area is sponged slowly and gently. Rubbing may increase heat production.
- Leave each area wet, and cover with a damp towel.
- Place ice bags and cold packs, if used, or a cool cloth on the forehead for comfort and in each axilla and at the groin. These areas contain large superficial blood vessels that help the transfer of heat.
- Sponge one body part and then another. The sponge bath should take about 30 minutes. A bath given more quickly tends to increase the body's heat production by causing shivering.
- Discontinue the bath if the client becomes pale or cyanotic or shivers, or if the pulse becomes rapid or irregular.
- Pat each area dry.
- Reassess the vital signs at 15 minutes and after completing the sponge bath.

Hyperthermia and Hypothermia Blankets *Hyperthermia* and *hypothermia blankets* are used to increase or decrease a client's body temperature. The blanket has an associated control panel on which the desired temperature is set and the client's core temperature registers. Details about how to manage clients with hyperthermia and hypothermia blankets are provided in the *Procedures Supplement* that accompanies this book.

SUPPORTING AND IMMOBILIZING WOUNDS

Bandages and binders serve various purposes:

- Supporting a wound (eg, a fractured bone)
- Immobilizing a wound (eg, a strained shoulder)
- Applying pressure (eg, elastic bandages apply pressure to the lower extremities to improve venous blood flow)
- Securing a dressing (eg, for an extensive abdominal surgical wound)
- Retaining splints (this applies chiefly to bandages)
- Retaining warmth (eg, a flannel bandage on a rheumatoid joint)

There are several types of bandages and binders and several ways in which they are applied. When correctly applied, they promote healing, provide comfort, and can

CLINICAL GUIDELINES

Bandaging

- Whenever possible, bandage the part in its normal position, with the joint slightly flexed to avoid putting strain on the ligaments and the muscles of the joint.
- Pad between skin surfaces and over bony prominences to prevent friction from the bandage and consequent abrasion of the skin.
- Always bandage body parts by working from the distal to the proximal end to aid the return flow of venous blood.
- Bandage with even pressure to prevent interference with blood circulation.
- Whenever possible, leave the end of the body part (eg, the toe) exposed so that you will be able to determine the adequacy of the blood circulation to the extremity.
- Cover dressings with bandages at least 5 cm (2 in) beyond the edges of the dressing to prevent the dressing and wound from becoming contaminated.
- Face the client when applying a bandage to maintain uniform tension and the appropriate direction of the bandage.

prevent injury. Clinical guidelines for bandaging are provided in the box above.

Bandages A bandage is a strip of cloth used to wrap some part of the body. Bandages are available in various widths, most commonly 1.5 to 7.5 cm (0.5 to 3 in), and are usually supplied in rolls for easy application to a body part.

Many types of materials are used for bandages. Gauze is one of the most commonly used; it is light and porous and readily molds to the body. It is also relatively inexpensive, so it is generally discarded when soiled. Gauze is frequently used to retain dressings on wounds and to bandage the fingers, hands, toes, and feet. It supports dressings and at the same time permits air to circulate; it can also be impregnated with petroleum jelly or other medications for application to wounds.

Many kinds of elasticized bandages are applied to provide pressure to an area. They are commonly used as tensor bandages or as partial stockings to provide support and improve the venous circulation in the legs. Some elasticized bandages have an adhesive backing and can be secured to the skin; these are most frequently used to retain dressings and at the same time provide some support to a wound.

Plastic adhesive bandages are also used to retain dressings. They are waterproof and thus retain wound drainage or keep the area dry. They have some elastic properties and therefore provide some pressure.

The width of the bandage used depends on the size of the body part to be bandaged. For example, a 2.5-cm (1-in) bandage is used for a finger, a 5-cm (2-in) bandage for an arm, and a 7.5-cm or 10-cm (3-in or 4-in) bandage for a leg. The larger the circumference of the part, the wider the bandage. Padding (eg, abdominal pads and gauze squares) is frequently used to cover bony prominences, such as the elbow, or to separate skin surfaces, such as the fingers.

Before applying a bandage, the nurse needs to know its purpose and to assess the area requiring support. See the box below for assessment guidelines.

Basic Turns for Roller Bandages

Circular Turn *Circular turns* are used chiefly to anchor bandages and terminate bandages. Circular turns are also used to bandage certain areas, such as the proximal aspect of a finger or a wrist. Instructions for circular turns are as follows:

- Apply the end of the bandage to the part of the body to be bandaged.
- Encircle the body part a few times or as often as needed, each turn directly covering the previous turn (Figure 44–19). This provides even support to the area.

CLINICAL GUIDELINES

Assessing Before Applying Bandages or Binders

- Inspect and palpate the area for swelling.
- Inspect for the presence of and status of wounds (open wounds will require a dressing before a bandage or binder is applied).
- Note the presence of drainage (amount, color, odor, viscosity).
- Inspect and palpate for adequacy of circulation (skin temperature, color, and sensation). Pale or cyanotic skin, cool temperature, tingling, and numbness can indicate impaired circulation.
- Ask the client about any pain experienced (location, intensity, onset, quality).
- Assess the ability of the client to reapply the bandage or binder when needed.
- Assess the capabilities of the client regarding activities of daily living (eg, to eat, dress, comb hair, bathe) and assess the assistance required during the convalescence period.

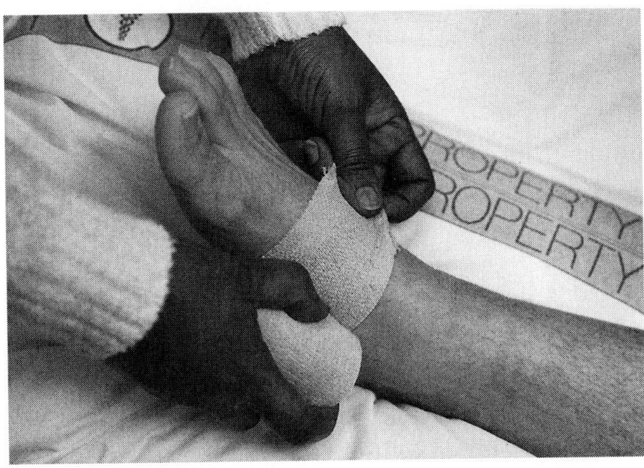

Figure 44–19 Starting a bandage with two circular turns.

- Secure the end of the bandage with tape, metal clips, or a safety pin over an uninjured area. Clips and pins can be uncomfortable when situated over an injured area.

Spiral Turn *Spiral turns* are used to bandage parts of the body that are fairly uniform in circumference, such as the upper arm or upper leg.

- Make two circular turns to anchor the bandage.
- Continue spiral turns at about a 30-degree angle, each turn overlapping the preceding one by two-thirds the width of the bandage (Figure 44–20).
- Terminate the bandage with two circular turns, and secure the end as described for circular turns.

Spiral Reverse Turn *Spiral reverse turns* are used to bandage cylindrical parts of the body that are not uniform in circumference, such as the lower leg or forearm.

- Anchor the bandage with two circular turns, and bring the bandage upward at about a 30-degree angle.
- Place the thumb of the free hand on the upper edge of the bandage (Figure 44–21, *A*, p. 1390). The thumb will hold the bandage while it is folded on itself.
- Unroll the bandage about 15 cm (6 in), then turn the hand so that the bandage falls over itself (Figure 44–21, *B*).
- Continue the bandage around the limb, overlapping each previous turn by two-thirds the width of the bandage. Make each bandage turn at the same position on the limb so that the turns of the bandage will be aligned (Figure 44–21, *C*).
- Terminate the bandage with two circular turns, and secure the end as described for circular turns.

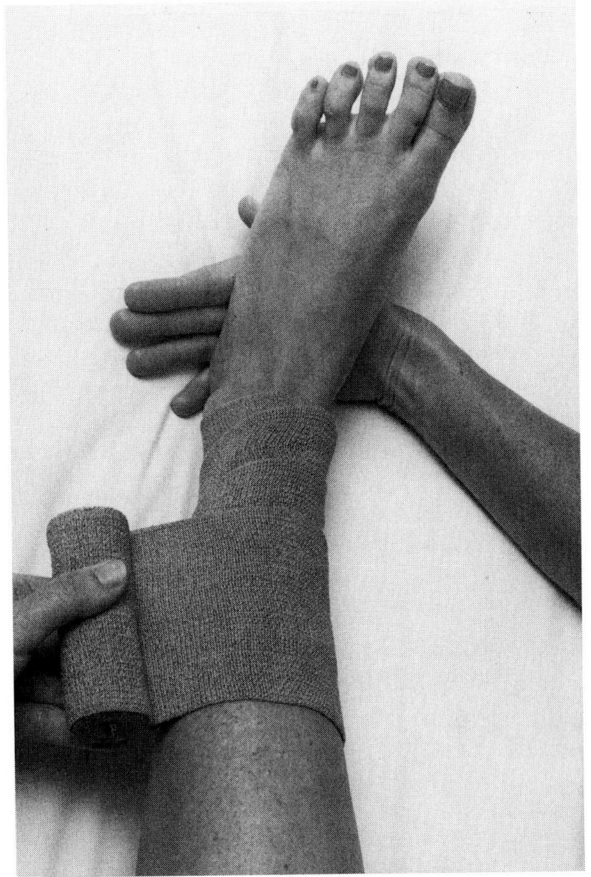

Figure 44–20 Applying spiral turns.

Recurrent Turn *Recurrent turns* are used to cover distal parts of the body, such as the end of a finger, the skull, or the stump of an amputation

- Anchor the bandage with two circular turns.
- Fold the bandage back on itself, and bring it centrally over the distal end to be bandaged (Figure 44–22, p. 1390).
- Holding it with the other hand, bring the bandage back over the end to the right of the center bandage but overlapping it by two-thirds the width of the bandage.
- Bring the bandage back on the left side, also overlapping the first turn by two-thirds the width of the bandage.
- Continue this pattern of alternating right and left until the area is covered. Overlap the preceding turn by two-thirds the bandage width each time.
- Terminate the bandage with two circular turns (Figure 44–23, p. 1390). Secure the end appropriately.

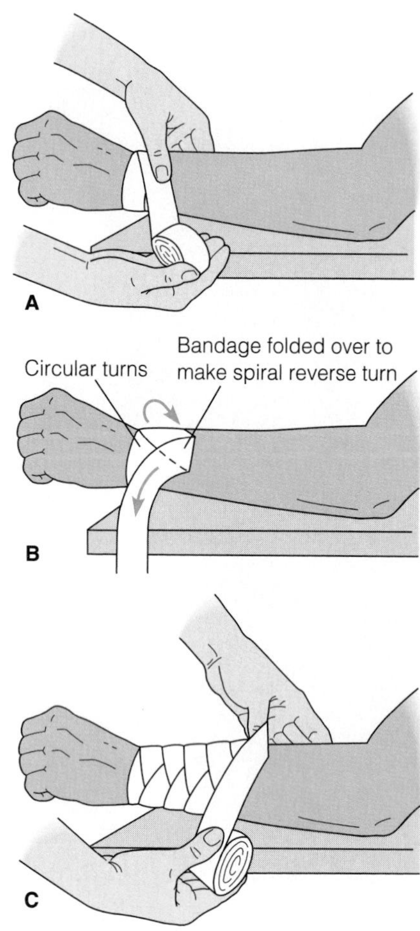

Figure 44–21 Applying spiral reverse turns.

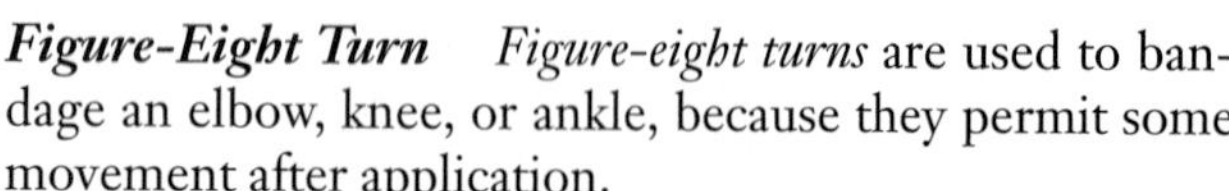

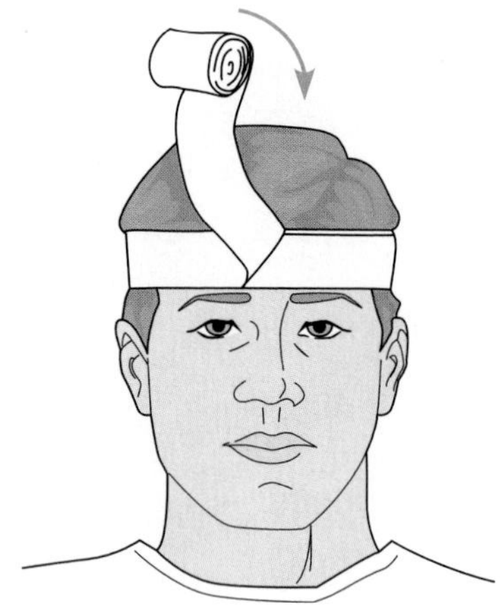

Figure 44–22 Starting a recurrent bandage with two circular turns.

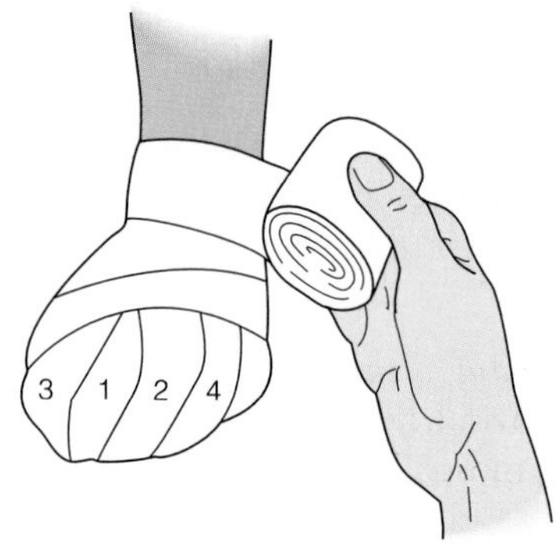

Figure 44–23 Completing a recurrent bandage with two circular turns.

Figure-Eight Turn *Figure-eight turns* are used to bandage an elbow, knee, or ankle, because they permit some movement after application.

- Anchor the bandage with two circular turns.
- Carry the bandage above the joint, around it, and then below it, making a figure eight (Figure 44–24).
- Continue above and below the joint, overlapping the previous turn by two-thirds the width of the bandage.
- Terminate the bandage above the joint with two circular turns, and secure the end appropriately.

Thumb Spica The *spica* bandage is a variation of the figure-eight bandage. It is commonly used to bandage the hip, groin, shoulder, breast, or thumb. A 2.5-cm (1-in) bandage is frequently used for a thumb spica, and a 7.5-cm (3-in) bandage for a hip or shoulder spica. To apply:

- Anchor the bandage with two circular turns around the wrist.
- Bring the bandage down to the distal aspect of the thumb, and encircle the thumb. Leave the tip of the thumb exposed if possible. This enables the nurse to check blood circulation to the thumb.
- Bring the bandage back up and around the wrist, then back down and around the thumb, overlapping the previous turn by two-thirds the width of the bandage.
- Repeat the above two steps, working up the thumb and hand until the thumb is covered (Figure 44–25).
- Anchor the bandage with two circular turns around the wrist, and secure the end appropriately.

Binders A **binder** is a type of bandage designed for a specific body part; for example, the triangular binder (sling) fits the arm. Binders are used to support large areas of the body, such as the abdomen, arm, or chest.

Triangular Arm Binder (Sling) A *triangular arm binder* or *sling* is usually applied as a full triangle to support

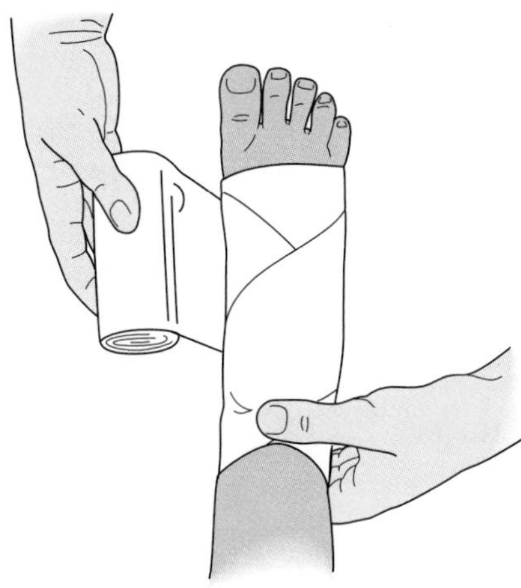

Figure 44–24 Applying a figure-eight bandage.

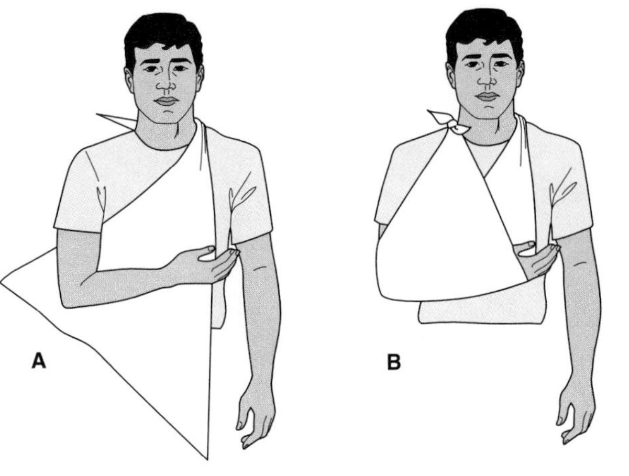

Figure 44–26 Large arm sling.

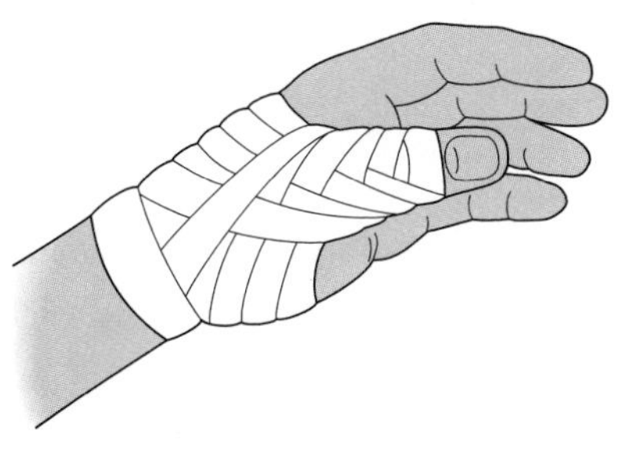

Figure 44–25 A thumb spica bandage.

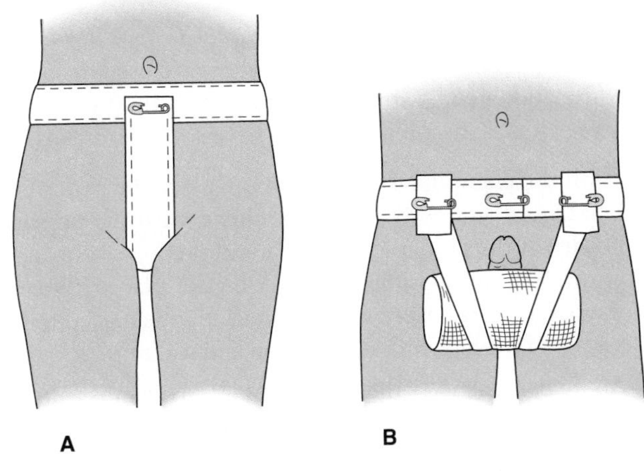

Figure 44–27 T-binders: *A*, single tail; *B*, two tails.

the arm, elbow, and forearm of the client or to reduce or prevent swelling of a hand. Most agencies use commercial strap slings.

- Place one end of the unfolded triangular binder over the shoulder of the uninjured side so that the binder falls down the front of the chest of the client with the point of the triangle (apex) under the elbow of the injured side.
- Take the upper corner, and carry it around the neck until it hangs over the shoulder on the injured side (Figure 44–26, *A*).
- Bring the lower corner of the binder up over the arm to the shoulder of the injured side. Using a square knot, secure this corner to the upper corner at the side of the neck on the involved side.
- Fold the sling neatly at the elbow, and secure it with safety pins or tape. It may be folded and fastened at the front (Figure 44–26, *B*).

T-Binder (Single or Double) T-binders are used to retain pads, dressings, or packs in the perineal area. Single T-binders are often used for females, and double T-binders for males to prevent undue pressure on the penis. The double T-binder can also provide greater support for large dressings on both males and females.

- Bring the waist tails around the client, overlap them, and secure them with a pin placed horizontally. The pins placed horizontally allow comfort when bending at the waist and moving.
- Bring the center tail up between the legs (Figure 44–27, *A*). The two tails of the double T-binder are brought up on either side of the penis (Figure 44–27, *B*). When dressings are in place, wear disposable gloves to prevent contact with body exudate.

- Fasten the ties at the waist with a safety pin placed horizontally.

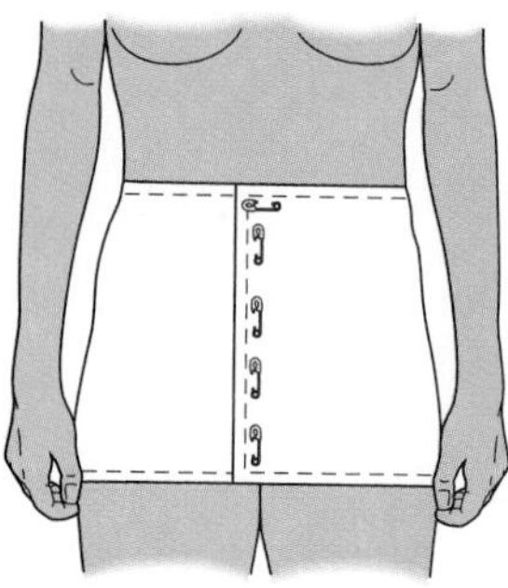

Figure 44–28 A straight abdominal binder.

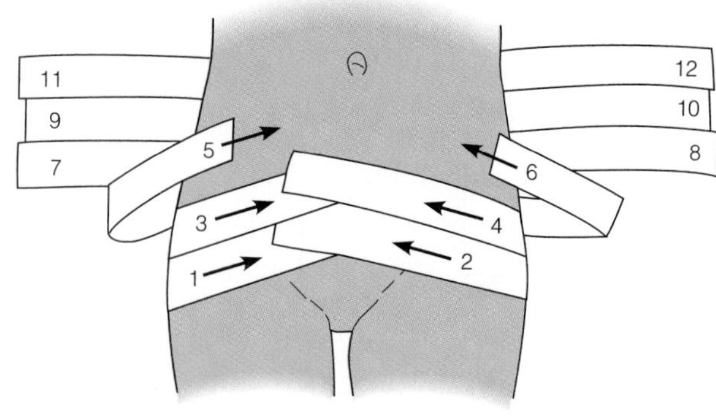

Figure 44–29 Scultetus (many-tailed) binder.

Straight Abdominal or Scultetus (Many-Tailed) Binders Straight abdominal and scultetus binders are used to support the abdomen. A straight binder is also used to support the chest. Chest binders often have shoulder straps.

- With the client in a supine position, place the abdominal binder smoothly under the client, with the upper border of the binder at the waist and the lower border at the level of the gluteal fold. A binder placed above the waist can interfere with respiration; one placed too low can interfere with elimination and walking.
- Apply padding over the iliac crests if the client is thin.
- For a straight abdominal binder, bring the ends around the client, overlap them, and secure them with pins or Velcro (Figure 44–28).
- For a scultetus binder, bring the tails over to the center from alternate sides (Figure 44–29). The last tail is secured with a safety pin or Velcro. Each tail should overlap the preceding one by about half the width of the tail for maximum support. In thin people, the tails may extend beyond the other side and require folding back.
  a. For clients who have had abdominal surgery, lace the tails from the bottom up. This provides maximum upward support.
  b. For the postpartum client, lace the tails from the top down. This provides downward pressure on the uterus.

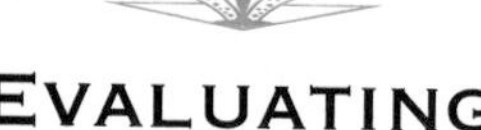

EVALUATING

To evaluate the effectiveness of nursing interventions and the achievement of client outcomes, the nurse obtains data relevant to the outcome criteria established in the planning phase. To elicit such data, the nurse may do the following:

- Assess the client's vital signs at specified intervals
- Inspect the wound and drainage site each time it is cleaned or dressed
- Observe the client's ability to perform self-care
- Ask the client about degree of pain experienced
- Monitor the client's food and fluid intake
- Watch the client demonstrate required home wound care
- Question the client about discharge instructions and symptoms or signs warranting notification of health personnel

If outcomes are not achieved, the nurse should explore the reasons. Questions the nurse might consider include the following:

- Was the client's nutritional intake adequate to support healing?
- Did the client have adequate circulation to the wound site?
- Was the wound supported and immobilized effectively?
- Were stringent aseptic practices implemented when cleaning and changing dressings to prevent infection?
- Was the client receiving anti-inflammatory medications that interfere with healing?
- Are more frequent dressing changes required because of excessive drainage?
- Was the appropriate dressing applied to keep the wound moist and/or absorb exudate?

CRITICAL PATHWAY FOR JOSÉ ALONZO

ASSESSMENT DATA

Nursing Assessment

José Alonzo is a 42-year-old construction worker who was injured at work when a wheelbarrow filled with cement rolled into him and pushed him off a four-foot ledge. He suffered several bruises and one 9 cm (3.5 in) laceration on the anterior aspect of the lower left leg. The laceration was covered with a sterile compression dressing at the scene by paramedics. Prior to irrigation and cleansing with normal saline and peroxide, the wound contained particles of cement and dirt. Dr James sutured the wound with silk suture and discharged Mr Alonzo to home care. Mr Alonzo is to return to the outpatient clinic for suture removal in 10 days. He asks the nurse whether he can use an aloe herbal ointment on the wound and drink a healing herbal tea that his wife makes.

Physical Examination

Height: 177.8 cm (5′10″)
Weight: 72.7 kg (160 lb)
Temperature: 37 C (98.6 F)
Pulse rate: 88 bpm
Respirations: 24 per minute
Blood pressure: 136/90 mm Hg

CRITICAL PATHWAY FOR WOUND MANAGEMENT AT HOME

Expected length of treatment: 7 to 10 days

	Date ________ **Outpatient setting**	**Date ________** **Daily for 10 days (Client activities)**
Daily outcomes	Client verbalizes understanding of teaching including: wound care, signs and symptoms to report, follow-up care.	At time of suture removal ▪ client is afebrile. ▪ client has a dry, clean wound with edges well-approximated, healing by first intention.
Knowledge deficit	Provide simple, brief instructions regarding injury and treatment. Encourge client to ask questions and seek assistance. Assess the client's knowledge about wound care. Review written instruction sheet for wound care with client and provide copy.	Follow written discharge teaching regarding wound care/dressing change. Call physician with questions/problems and return to office in 10 days for suture removal.
Diet	Instruct client about foods high in protein and vitamin C and encourage adequate intake.	Diet high in protein and vitamin C. Cultural remedies that will not interfere with healing.
Wound care	Irrigate and cleanse wound with normal saline and peroxide. Surgical consultation for wound closure. Following wound closure, apply dry sterile dressing.	Change dressing daily and prn to keep dressing dry and clean. Inspect wound daily and report any signs and symptoms of infection (redness, pain, warmth, drainage, redness, or fever).
Medications	Tetanus toxoid if indicated.	Only if ordered.

CHAPTER HIGHLIGHTS

- Wounds are described as intentional or unintentional; closed or open; and clean, clean-contaminated, contaminated, or dirty (infected). Wounds are also classified by depth as partial-thickness or full-thickness. In addition, wounds are classified according to how they are acquired, as incisions, contusions, abrasions, punctures, lacerations, and penetrating wounds.
- The wound-healing process has three phases: inflammatory, proliferative, and maturation.
- There are three types of healing, which are distinguished by the amount of tissue loss: primary intention healing, secondary intention healing, and tertiary intention healing.
- Major types of wound exudate are serous, purulent, and sanguineous (hemorrahagic). Exudate can be a combination of two or three (eg, serosanguineous.) The process of pus formation is referred to as suppuration.
- Factors affecting wound healing include developmental stage, nutritional status, life-style, medications, and the presence of infection.
- The main complications of wound healing are hemorrhage and possible hypovolemic shock, infection, dehiscence, and evisceration, each of which is identifiable by specific clinical signs and symptoms.
- Wound assessment is an ongoing process to evaluate healing; the nurse assesses wounds by visual inspection, palpation, and the sense of smell. Essential data for treated wounds include wound appearance, size, drainage, swelling, pain, and the presence of tubes and drains.
- Laboratory data that may be used to assess the progress of wound healing include leukocyte count, blood coagulation studies, serum protein analysis, and wound cultures. Nurses are usually responsible for obtaining specimens of wound drainage for culture.
- Nursing diagnoses related to wound care include **High risk for infection, Pain, High risk for impaired skin integrity, Anxiety,** and **Body image disturbance.**
- The care of wounds varies considerably in accordance with the type of wound, size and location, amount of exudate, presence of complicating factors, and, sometimes, the personal preference of the physician.
- Major nursing responsibilities related to wound care include preventing infection, preventing further tissue damage, preventing hemorrhage, promoting healing, and preventing skin excoriation around draining wounds.
- Wound care may involve cleaning wounds, changing dressings, maintaining drains, irrigating, inserting packing, applying heat and cold, and applying bandages and binders.
- Various dressing materials are available to protect wounds and to keep the wound bed moist, thus facilitating healing.
- Dry sterile gauze dressings are commonly applied to surgical incisions to absorb drainage. Wet-to-damp gauze dressings are replacing wet-to-dry dressings as a means of removing exudate and debriding wounds.
- Several synthetic dressings have been developed for use with specific wounds. These include transparent adhesive films, impregnated nonadherent dressings, hydrocolloids, hydrogels, polyurethane foams, and exudate absorbers. The nurse must be aware of the specific purposes of each and their indications for use.
- The type of dressing used depends on (a) location, size, and type of the wound; (b) amount of exudate; (c) whether or not the wound requires debridement, is infected, or has sinus tracts; and (d) such considerations as frequency of dressing change, ease or difficulty of dressing applications, and cost.
- The RYB color code of wounds can assist nurses to provide appropriate nursing interventions for wounds that heal by secondary intention. In this scheme, the nurse protects *red*, cleanses *yellow*, and debrides *black*.
- Before changing dressings, the nurse needs to ascertain the physician's orders, the presence of drains, the amount of wound drainage, and the cleaning solutions to be used.

- Various methods are used to suture wounds. The nurse must become familiar with agency policies about who removes sutures.
- Heat and cold produce specific local physiologic and systemic responses that account for their therapeutic effects.
- Various parts of the body differ in tolerance to heat and cold. The physiologic tolerance of individuals also varies. Specific conditions such as neurosensory and circulatory impairments necessitate precautions when applying heat or cold.
- When applying heat and cold, clients and nurses need to be aware of the effects of thermal receptor adaptation and the rebound phenomenon.

READINGS AND REFERENCES

SUGGESTED READINGS

Motta, GJ. December 1993. How moisture-retentive dressings promote healing. *Nursing93* 23:26–34.

The author discusses characteristics, indications, functions, advantages, disadvantages, and change frequency of each type of moisture-retentive dressing. The term *moisture-retentive* is preferred to *occlusive* to describe dressings that maintain a moist wound environment.

Willey, T. February 1992. Use a decision tree to choose wound dressings. *American Journal of Nursing* 92:43–46.

Numerous products are now available to aid wound healing. Knowing which dressing to use and when to use it can be a mystery for those who lack the opportunity and time to study wound care and thoroughly evaluate the products. A decision-making tree is provided to help the nurse select an appropriate dressing.

RELATED RESEARCH

Frey, KA, Briggs, J, and Broadhead, WE. December 1990. Postdischarge, postoperative nosocomial infection surveillance using random sampling. *American Journal of Infection Control* 18:383–85.

Zoutman, D, Pearce, P, McKenzie, M, and Taylor, G. August 1990. Surgical wound infections occurring in day surgery patients. *American Journal of Infection Control* 18:277–82.

SELECTED REFERENCES

Bale, S and Harding, KG. February 1990. Using modern dressings to effect debridement. *Professional Nurse* 5:244, 246, 248.

Barnes, HR. March 1993a. Alternating transparent and hydrocolloid dressings. A difficult case. *Nursing93* 23:59–61.

______. June 1993b. Wound care: Fact and fiction about hydrocolloid dressings. *Journal of Gerontological Nursing* 19:23–26.

Bruno, P. December 1979. The nature of wound healing: Implications for nursing practice. *Nursing Clinics of North America* 14:667–82.

Bryant, RA. 1992. *Acute and Chronic Wounds: Nursing Management.* St Louis: Mosby-Year Book.

Carpenito, LJ. 1992. *Nursing Diagnosis: Application to Clinical Practice.* 4th ed. Philadelphia: Lippincott.

Centers for Disease Control: Recommendations for prevention of HIV transmission in health care settings. *Morbidity and Mortality Weekly Report* 1987:36:55.

Chaloner, D. March 27–April 2, 1991. Treating a cavity wound. *Nursing Times* 87:67, 69.

Cooper, DM. March 1990a. Optimizing wound healing: A practice within nursing's domain. *Nursing Clinics of North America* 25:165–81.

______. March 1990b. Wound healing. *Nursing Clinics of North America* 25:163–64.

Cutting, K and Harding, K. December 12–18, 1990. Dressing cavities. *Nursing Times* 86:62, 64.

Cuzzell, JZ. October 1988. The new RYB color code: Next time you assess an open wound, remember to protect red, cleanse yellow, and debride black. *American Journal of Nursing* 88:1342–46.

______. May 1993. The right way to culture a wound. *American Journal of Nursing* 93:48–50.

Cuzzell, JZ and Stotts, NA. October 1990. Wound care: Trial and error yields to knowledge. *American Journal of Nursing* 90:53–63.

Fowler, E, Cuzzell, JZ, and Papen, JC. February 1991a. Healing with hydrocolloid. *American Journal of Nursing* 91:63–64.

______. March 1991b. Healing with thin film dressings. *American Journal of Nursing* 91:36, 38.

Garner, JS. April 1986. CDC guidelines for the prevention and control of nosocomial infections: Guideline for prevention of surgical wound infections, 1985. *American Journal of Infection Control* 14:71–80.

Glide, S. May 6–12, 1992. Cleaning choices. *Nursing Times* 88:74, 76, 78.

Gordon, M. 1993. *Manual of Nursing Diagnosis 1993–1994.* 6th ed. St Louis: Mosby-Year Book.

Griffiths, G. September 4–10, 1991. Choosing a dressing. *Nursing Times* 87:84, 86, 88, 90.

Guyton, AC. 1991. *Textbook of Medical Physiology.* 8th ed. Philadelphia: WB Saunders.

Jones, PL and Millman, A. March 1990. Wound healing and the aged patient. *Nursing Clinics of North America* 25:263–77.

Kim, MJ, McFarland, GK, and McLane, AM. 1993. *Pocket Guide to Nursing Diagnoses.* 5th ed. St Louis: Mosby-Year Book.

Kloth, LC, McCullogh, JM, and Feedar, JA. 1990. *Wound Healing: Alternatives in Management.* Philadelphia: FA Davis.

Krasner, D. May 1992a. Wound measurements: Some tools of the trade. *American Journal of Nursing* 92:89–90.

______. December 1992b. The 12 commandments of wound care. *Nursing92* 22:34–42.

Lederer, JR, Marculescu, GL, Mocnik, B, and Seaby, N. 1993. *Care Planning Pocket Guide—A Nursing Diagnosis Approach.* 5th ed. Redwood City, CA: Addison-Wesley Nursing.

Lehman, JF, editor. 1990. *Therapeutic Heat and Cold.* 4th ed. Baltimore: Williams and Wilkins.

McConnell, EA. June 1990. Clinical do's and don'ts . . . How to tape a dressing. *Nursing90* 20:23.

McDowell, S. July 1991. Are we using too much Betadine? *RN* 54:43–45.

McFarland, GK and McFarlane, EA. 1993. *Nursing Diagnosis and Intervention: Planning for Patient Care.* 2d ed. St Louis: Mosby-Year Book.

Modic, BM. December 1990. Myths and facts . . . about chronic wound care. *Nursing90* 20:68.

Moody, M. May 6–12, 1992. Wound care. Looking for non-adherence. *Nursing Times* 88:65,68.

Morison, MJ. February 1989. Wound cleansing—which solution? *Professional Nurse* 4:220–22, 224–25.

Motta, GJ. December 1993. How moisture-retentive dressings promote healing. *Nursing93* 23:26–34.

Neuberger, GB and Reckling, JB. February 1985. A new look at wound care. *Nursing85* 15:34–42.

Nichols, RL. January/February 1982. Techniques known to prevent post-operative wound infection. *Infection Control* 3:34–37.

North American Nursing Diagnosis Association. 1992. *NANDA Nursing Diagnoses: Definitions and Classification 1992–1993.* Philadelphia: NANDA.

Resnick, B. February 1993. Wound care for the elderly. *Geriatric Nursing* 14:26–29.

Rodeaver, G. 1989. Controversies in topical wound management. *Wounds* 1:19–27.

Schumann, D. December 1979. Preoperative measures to promote wound healing. *Nursing Clinics of North America* 14:683–99.

Stotts, NA. February 1990. Seeing red, yellow, and black. The three-color concept of wound care. *Nursing90* 20:59–61.

Thomas, S. November 7–13, 1990. Making sense of . . . Hydrocolloid dressings. *Nursing Times* 86:36–38.

Tudor, R and Gupta, R. May 6–12, 1992. Healing physiology. *Nursing Times* 88:70, 72, 74.

Van Rijswijk, L and Cuzzell, JZ. June 1991. Managing full-thickness wounds. *American Journal of Nursing* 91:18, 22.

Weber, BA. October 1991. Timely tips on adhesive tape. *Nursing91* 21:52–53.

Willey, T. February 1992. Use a decision tree to choose wound dressings. *American Journal of Nursing* 92:43–46.

Wound-care update 91. April 1991. *Nursing91* 21:47–50.

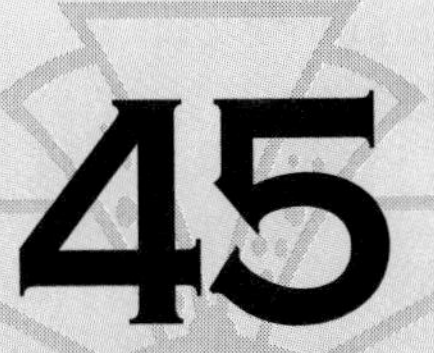

45 Perioperative Nursing

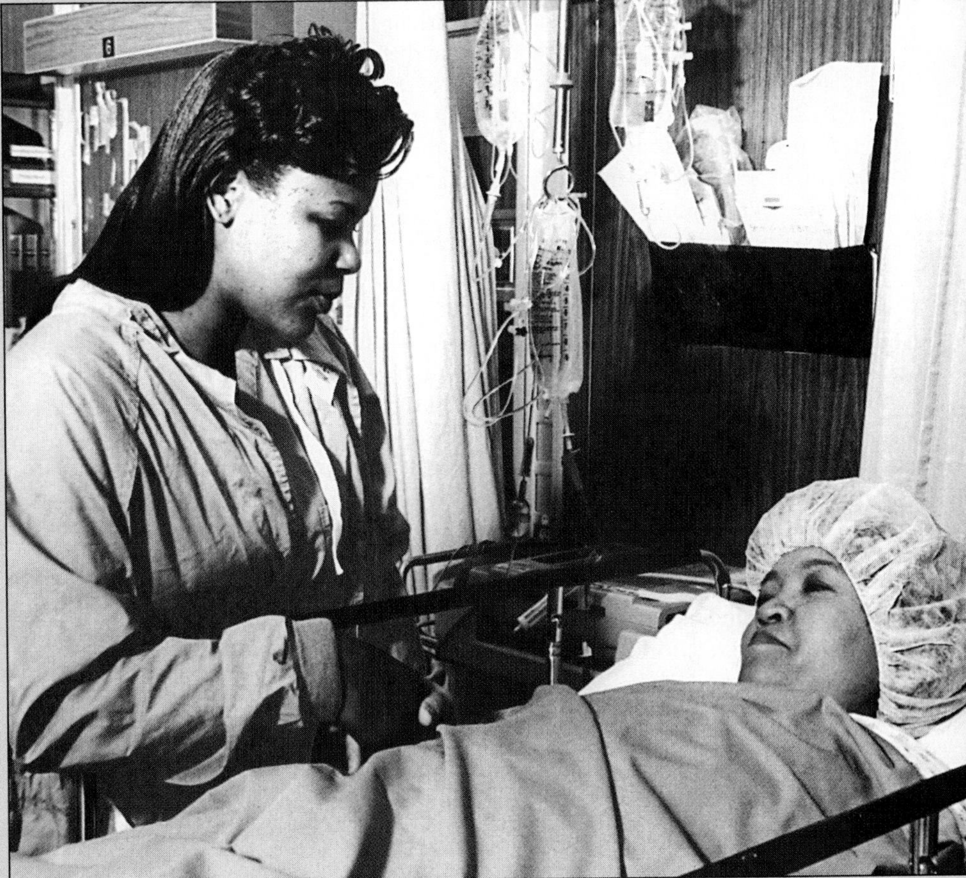

Objectives

- Describe the phases of the perioperative period
- Identify various types of surgery according to degree of urgency, degree of risk, and purpose.
- Differentiate various types of anesthesia.
- Identify essential aspects of preoperative assessment.
- Give examples of pertinent nursing diagnoses for surgical clients.
- Identify the essential nursing responsibilities included in planning perioperative nursing care.
- Describe how to teach clients to move, perform leg exercises, and perform coughing and deep breathing exercises.
- Identify essential aspects of perioperative physical preparation.
- Identify the essentials of preoperative skin preparation.
- Identify essential nursing assessments and interventions during the immediate postanesthetic phase.
- Identify essential nursing assessments and interventions during the ongoing postoperative phase.
- Discuss the importance of documentation with reference to preoperative, intraoperative, and postoperative recording.
- Identify potential postoperative complications and describe nursing interventions to prevent them.
- Identify outcome criteria by which to evaluate the effectiveness of perioperative nursing interventions.
- Identify essential aspects of managing gastrointestinal suction.

Surgery is a unique "human" experience that can be described as a planned alteration that encompasses three phases: preoperative, intraoperative, and postoperative. All three phases are referred to as the *perioperative period.*

The **preoperative phase** begins when the client decides to have surgery and ends when the client is transferred to the operating room bed. The nursing activities associated with this phase include assessment of the client, identification of potential or actual health problems, planning specific care based on the individual's needs, and preoperative teaching involving the client and support persons.

The **intraoperative phase** begins when the client is transferred to the operating room bed and ends when the client is admitted to the postanesthesia area. The nursing activities related to this phase include a variety of specialized procedures designed to create and maintain a safe, therapeutic environment for the client and the health care personnel providing the care.

The **postoperative phase** begins with the admission of the client to the postanesthesia area and ends with the discharge of the client from the hospital or facility providing the continuing care. The nursing activities include, monitoring the client's response (physiologic and psychologic) to the surgery, teaching and providing support to the client and support persons. The goal is to assist the client to achieve the most optimal health status possible.

The desired client outcomes of any surgical experience include

- The client will be free from injury related to positioning, retained foreign objects, chemical, physical, or electrical hazards.
- The client will be free from infection.
- The client's fluid and electrolyte balance will be maintained.
- The client's skin integrity will be maintained.
- The client will demonstrate an understanding of the physiologic and psychologic responses to the planned surgery.
- The client will participate in a rehabilitation process following surgery (AORN, 1993, pp 89–90).

Traditionally clients entered hospitals for 3 to 10 days during which the three phases of care occurred. More recently an increasing number of operations are carried out as day surgery. The client comes to the hospital either the evening before or the day of surgery, has the operation, and leaves the same day. In these instances, the three phases of the perioperative period are shortened and the postoperative phase often continues at home.

Preoperative Phase

Types of Surgery

Surgical procedures are commonly grouped according to (a) urgency, (b) risk, and (c) purpose.

Degree of Urgency Surgery can be classified as elective or emergency. **Elective surgery** may be planned weeks or months ahead and is based on the client's choice. It is performed for the client's well-being though often not absolutely necessary for life. **Emergency surgery** is performed to preserve the client's life, body part, or body function. Examples are to control internal hemorrhage or breast surgery for a malignancy.

Degree of Risk Surgery is classified as major or minor according to the degree of risk to the client. **Major surgery** involves a high degree of risk, for a variety of reasons: it may be complicated or prolonged; large losses of blood may occur; vital organs may be involved; or postoperative complications may be likely. Examples are organ transplant, open heart surgery, and removal of a kidney. In contrast, **minor surgery** normally involves little risk, produces few complications, and is often performed in a "day surgery." Examples are breast biopsy, removal of tonsils, and knee surgery.

Purpose Surgical procedures are also categorized according to their purpose (see the box on p. 1399).

Surgery involving any of these categories may be either **elective** or **emergent** depending on the extenuating circumstances and related pathophysiology.

Types of Anesthesia

Anesthesia is classified as *general* or *regional.* Anesthetic agents are administered by an anesthesiologist, physician, or nurse-anesthetist. **General anesthesia** is the loss of all sensation and consciousness. A general anesthetic acts by blocking awareness centers in the brain so that amnesia (loss of memory), analgesia (insensibility to pain), hypnosis (artificial sleep), and relaxation (rendering a part of the body less tense) occur. General anesthetics are usually administered by intravenous infusion or by inhalation of gases delivered through a mask or through an endotracheal tube inserted into the trachea. Often, an intravenous drug such as thiopental sodium (Pentothal) is used to render the client unconscious and is then supplemented with other agents to produce surgical anesthesia.

General anesthesia has certain advantages. Because the client is unconscious rather than awake and anxious, respiration and cardiac function are readily regulated. Also,

CATEGORIES OF SURGERY BY PURPOSE

Category I	Surgery involving the loss of a body part, organ, or function.
Category II	Surgery involving the removal of a tumor, cyst, or foreign body.
Category III	Surgery performed for diagnostic purposes.
Category IV	Surgery for insertion, removal, or application of a prosthesis, graft, transplanted organ, or therapeutic device.
Category V	Surgery for reconstruction or cosmetic revision.
Category VI	Surgery to establish drainage or reestablish a passageway.

Source: SS Fairchild, *Perioperative Nursing: Principles and Practice* (Boston: Jones & Bartlett, 1993), pp. 431–32.

the anesthesia can be adjusted to the length of the operation and the client's age and physical status. Its chief disadvantage is that it depresses the respiratory and circulatory systems. Some clients become more anxious about a general anesthetic than about the surgery itself. Often this is because they fear losing the capacity to control their own bodies.

Regional anesthesia is the temporary interruption of the transmission of nerve impulses to and from a specific area or region of the body. The client loses sensation in an area of the body but remain conscious. Several techniques are used (Fairchild 1993, pp. 90–91):

- **Topical (surface) anesthesia** is applied directly to the skin and mucous membranes, open skin surfaces, wounds, and burns. The most commonly used topical agents are cocaine (4 to 10% solution), lidocaine (Xylocaine), and benzocaine. Topical anesthetics are readily absorbed and act rapidly.
- **Local anesthesia** (infiltration) is injected into a specific area and is used for minor surgical procedures such as suturing a small wound or performing a biopsy. Lidocaine or tetracaine 0.1% may be used.
- A **nerve block** is a technique in which the anesthetic agent in injected into and around a nerve or small nerve group that supplies sensation to a small area of the body. Major blocks involve multiple nerves or a *plexus* (eg, the brachial plexus anesthetizes the arm); minor blocks involve a single nerve (eg, a facial nerve).
- An **intravenous block (Bier block)** is used most often for procedures involving the arm, wrist, and hand. An occlusion tourniquet is applied to the extremity to prevent infiltration and absorption of the injected intravenous agent beyond the involved extremity.
- **Spinal anesthesia** is also referred to as **subarachnoid block** (SAB). It requires a lumbar puncture through one of the interspaces between lumbar disk 2 (L_2) and the sacrum (S_1). An anesthetic agent is injected into the spinal canal (subarachnoid space). Spinal anesthesia is often categorized as low, mid, and high spinals. *Low spinals* (saddle or caudal blocks) are primarily used for surgeries involving the perineal or rectal areas. *Mid spinals* (below the level of the umbilicus—T_{10}) can be used for hernia repairs or appendectomies, while the *high spinal* (reaching the nipple line—T_4) can be used for surgeries such as cesarean sections.
- **Epidural (peridural) anesthesia** is the injection of an anesthetic agent into the epidural space, the area inside the spinal column but outside the dura mater.

PREOPERATIVE CONSENT

Prior to any surgical procedure, clients must sign a surgical consent form. This requirement protects clients from having any surgical procedure they do not want or do not know about. It also protects the hospital and the health personnel from a claim by client or family that permission was not granted. The consent form becomes a part of the client's record and goes to the operating room with the client.

Obtaining legal, informed consent to perform surgery is the responsibility of the surgeon. Informed consent is possible only when the client is told, in advance, of the character and importance of the surgery, its probable consequences, the chances for success, and alternative measures. Often a nurse is responsible for witnessing a consent. Nurses must be aware of their responsibilities regarding consents and of the particular hospital's policies. See Chapter 12, page 228, for information about informed consent.

ASSESSING

Preoperative assessment includes collection of a database used during postoperative evaluation and clinical assessment of the client for identification of surgical risk factors. The nurse also ensures that scheduled screening tests are completed, preparing the client beforehand and monitoring afterward when necessary.

Nursing History The nursing history obtained before surgery provides client data that help the nurse to plan preoperative and postoperative care. Although forms vary considerably among agencies, essential preoperative information that should be included is summarized in the box on page 1400.

Assessing Surgical Risk The degree of risk involved in a surgical procedure is affected by the client's age, nutritional status, fluid and electrolyte status, general health, use of medications, and mental health attitude.

Age Very young and elderly clients are greater surgical risks than children and adults. A neonate's physiologic response to surgery is substantially different from an adult's. Factors that affect the risk are the neonate's circulation, which is largely central, and renal function, which is not fully developed until about 6 months of age. The neonate can respond to an additional need for oxygen only with an increased respiratory rate, and limited blood volume results in a limited fluid reserve.

Elderly persons are frequently at additional risk from surgery because of impaired circulation due to arteriosclerosis and limited cardiac function. Energy reserves are often limited, and hydration and nutritional status may be poor. In addition, the older person may be highly sensitive to medications such as morphine sulfate and barbiturates, frequently used preoperatively and postoperatively.

Nutritional Status Two nutritional problems that can increase surgical risk are obesity and malnutrition due to protein, iron, and vitamin deficiencies. Surgery for obese clients is often deferred, except in emergencies. The obese often have overtaxed hearts and elevated blood pressures. In addition, incisions in overly fatty tissue are difficult to suture and prone to infection.

Nutritional deficiencies are particularly common among elderly clients and chronically ill clients. Protein and vitamins are needed for wound healing; vitamin K is essential for blood clotting.

Fluid and Electrolyte Status Dehydration and hypovolemia predispose a client to problems during surgery. Electrolyte imbalances often accompany fluid imbalances. Imbalances in calcium, magnesium, potassium, and hydrogen ions are of particular concern during surgery. See Chapter 38.

General Health Surgery is least risky when the client's general health is good. Any infection or pathophysiology increases the risk. Of particular concern are upper respiratory tract infections, which together with a general anesthetic can adversely affect respiratory function. Common health problems that increase surgical risk and may lead to the decision to postpone or cancel surgery are listed in the box on page 1401.

Medications The regular use of certain medications can increase surgical risk. For example

- *Anticoagulants* increase blood coagulation time.
- *Tranquilizers* may cause hypotension and thus contribute to shock.
- *Central nervous system depressants* decrease central nervous system responses.

Since some medications interact adversely with other medications and with anesthetic agents, preoperative assessment should include careful collection of a medication history. 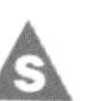 Clients may be unaware of the potential adverse interactions of medications and may fail to report the use of medications for conditions unrelated to the indication for surgery. The astute nurse interviewer may question the client and family about the use of commonly prescribed medications (and over-the-counter preparations) for specific conditions mentioned during the nursing history.

Mental Health and Attitude Extreme anxiety can increase surgical risk. The level of anxiety does not always correspond to the seriousness of the surgical procedure. The surgeon needs to know if a person fears death during

PREOPERATIVE NURSING HISTORY

- *Physical condition.* General appearance (ie, skin coloring, weight, hydration status, and energy level).
- *Mental attitude.* Mild anxiety is a normal response to surgery; severe anxiety can increase surgical risk.
- *Understanding of surgical procedure.* A well-informed client knows what to expect and in general accepts and copes more effectively with surgery and convalescence.
- *Previous experience.* May influence the physical and psychologic responses to the planned surgery.
- *Expected outcomes.* May alter a client's body image and life-style to varying degrees.
- *Medications.* List all current medications. Certain medications, such as anticonvulsants and insulin, must be continued throughout the operative period to prevent adverse effects. A physician's order to this effect is required, however.
- *Smoking.* Smokers' lung tissue may be chronically irritated, and a general anesthetic agent irritates it further.
- *Alcohol.* Heavy, consistent use can lead to problems during anesthesia, surgery, and recovery.
- *Coping resources.* Employing previously effective coping mechanisms or developing new strategies (eg, diversional activities such as reading and relaxation exercises) may be helpful.
- *Self-concept.* A healthy, positive self-concept predisposes clients to approach a surgical experience with confidence that they can handle it successfully.
- *Body image.* Possible disfigurement or change in physical identity may be a concern prior to surgery. Providing accurate information often allays fears based on misconceptions.

Critical Thinking Challenge

What Would You Do?

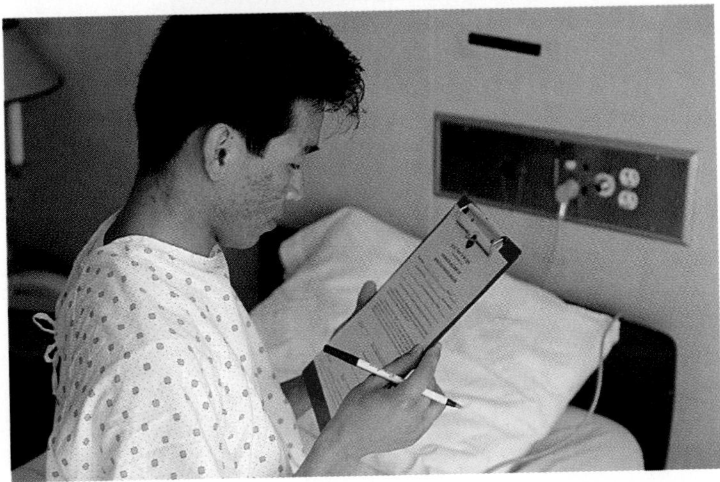

Luis Manrique is a 26-year-old client who is scheduled for surgery. During your assessment, you notice that Mr Manrique has difficulty communicating in English. You are concerned about whether he fully understands the proposed surgery.

What would you do?

surgery. In some instances, professional counseling and a delay in surgery are indicated.

Clients who have shown poor psychologic adjustment for some time may not be able to cope with the additional stress of surgery. People who cope only minimally in a stable, familiar environment can develop emotional problems postoperatively.

Screening Tests The physician orders preoperative radiologic and laboratory tests and examinations. Abnormalities may warrant treatment prior to surgery. The nurse's responsibility is to check the orders carefully, to see that they are carried out, and to ensure that the results are obtained prior to surgery. See Table 45–1 on page 1402 for routine preoperative screening tests. In addition to these routine tests, diagnostic tests directly related to the client's disease are usually appropriate (eg, stomach roentgenography to clarify the pathologic condition before gastric surgery).

Diagnosing

Examples of nursing diagnoses for the preoperative client are as follows:

Knowledge deficit (preoperative routines and postoperative exercises and activities)

Fear related to

- Effects of surgery on ability to function in usual roles
- Outcome of exploratory surgery for malignancy

Health Problems that Increase Surgical Risk

- *Cardiac conditions* such as angina pectoris, recent myocardial infarction, severe hypertension, and severe congestive heart failure. Well-controlled cardiac problems generally pose minimal operative risk.
- *Blood coagulation disorders* that may lead to severe bleeding, hemorrhage, and subsequent shock.
- *Upper respiratory tract infections or chronic obstructive lung diseases* such as emphysema. These conditions, especially when exacerbated by the effects of general anesthesia, adversely affect pulmonary function. They also predispose the client to postoperative lung infections.
- *Renal disease* that impairs the regulation of the body's fluids and electrolytes (eg, renal insufficiency).
- *Diabetes mellitus*, which predisposes the client to wound infection and delayed healing.
- *Liver disease* (eg, cirrhosis), which impairs the liver's abilities to detoxify medications used during surgery, produce the prothrombin necessary for blood clotting, and metabolize nutrients essential for healing.
- *Uncontrolled neurologic disease* such as epilepsy.

Table 45–1 Routine Preoperative Screening Tests

Test	Rationale
Urinalysis	To detect urinary tract infections and glucose in the urine
Chest roentgenography	To identify lung pathology and heart size and location
Electrocardiography (usual for clients who have cardiac pathology)	To determine cardiac pathology
Complete blood count (CBC)	To determine Hgb, Hct, RBC (ie, the blood's ability to carry oxygen), and WBC (which signals infection when elevated)
Blood grouping and cross-matching	To establish blood type for possible blood transfusion
Serum electrolytes (Na^+, K^+, Mg^{2+}, Ca^{2+}, H^+)	To determine electrolyte imbalances
Fasting blood sugar	To detect presence of glucose in the blood, which may indicate metabolic disorders (eg, diabetes mellitus)
Blood urea nitrogen (BUN) or creatinine	To assess urinary excretion

- Risk of death
- Loss of control during anesthesia or waking up during anesthesia
- Perceived inadequate postoperative analgesia

Sleep pattern disturbance related to

- Hospital routines
- Psychologic stress

Anticipatory grieving related to

- Perceived loss of body part associated with planned surgery

Ineffective individual coping related to

- Conflicting values (eg, need for blood transfusion versus the religious values of a Jehovah's Witness)
- Lack of clear outcomes of surgery
- Unresolved past negative experience with surgery

Definitions and defining characteristics of these diagnoses are detailed in other chapters of this book.

PLANNING

The duration of the preoperative period often affects preoperative care and planning. When the preoperative period lasts several days, nurses can draw up a nursing care plan and a *teaching plan.* When the preoperative period is just an hour, only the essentials can be carried out. In this case, the learning needs of the client must be met prior to admission to the clinical agency during the postoperative period. An increasing number of clients are coming to the hospital for preoperative teaching and tests before admission.

Planning for the preoperative period should involve the client and support persons. The following are essential nursing responsibilities.

- Ensure appropriate physical preparation to prevent aspiration, injury, infection, and other complications associated with anesthesia

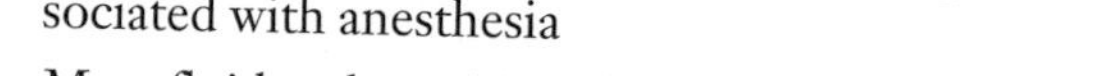

- Meet fluid and nutritional needs
- Promote rest
- Promote the client's peace of mind
- Identify and meet the learning needs of clients and support persons
- Protect the client's personal property during the intraoperative period

The overall goal in the preoperative period should reflect that the client is physically and psychologically prepared for surgery. Examples of outcome criteria to evaluate achievement of these goals and the effectiveness of nursing interventions follow.

The client

- Describes in general terms the proposed surgical procedure, reason for it, subsequent therapy, and expected length of stay in hospital.
- Verbalizes understanding of events (eg, transfer to postanesthesia room or intensive care unit) and therapeutic devices (eg, monitoring equipment, infusions) in all perioperative phases.
- States reasons for preoperative and postoperative procedures (eg, skin prep, bowel prep) and practices (eg, deep breathing, coughing, turning, leg exercises).
- Demonstrates deep breathing, coughing, splinting, leg exercises, and moving techniques as taught.
- Verbalizes expectations and understanding of usual postoperative pain control and activity.
- Verbalizes feelings about surgery and its expected outcomes.
- Reports feelings of achieving adequate rest and sleep.
- Demonstrates balanced fluid intake and output.

- Remains free from infection, as manifested by baseline temperature and pulse rate.

A critical pathway can also be useful for planning client care (see p. 1420).

IMPLEMENTING

Preoperative Teaching An explanation of the surgical experience informs the client and support persons about the perioperative period. Usually, people are anxious at this time, and many have misconceptions about surgery and surgical care. Clients often ask nurses about the operation after the surgeon has gained informed consent and left the client's room. The surgeon should be notified if the client is anxious about the procedure or has questions about the surgery that the nurse cannot answer.

Clients and their support persons need to know the time and type of surgery. The surgeon usually arranges the date and may specify it in the orders. The exact time may not be known until the surgical schedule for the hospital is distributed. If a nurse does not know the exact time of surgery, the nurse should say so and inform the client and support persons as soon as the time is decided.

The nurse needs to listen attentively and carefully to help the client identify specific concerns or fears and talk them through. Typical questions are: What will happen during surgery? How will I feel after the operation? What will the surgeon find? How long will the hospital stay be? Some clients may worry about finances. Those whose surgery involves disfigurement may have problems with their self-image.

This is also the time to clarify any misconceptions the client may have. Providing accurate information and

PREOPERATIVE INSTRUCTIONS

Preoperative Regimen

- Explain the need for preoperative tests (eg, laboratory, X-ray, ECG).
- Discuss bowel preparation, if required.
- Discuss skin preparation, including operative area and preoperative bath or shower with antimicrobial agents.
- Discuss preoperative medications.
- Explain individual therapies ordered by the physician, such as intravenous therapy, the insertion of a urinary catheter or nasogastric tube, use of a spirometer or intermittent positive pressure breathing (IPPB) machine, or antiemboli stockings.
- Discuss the visit by anesthetist.
- Explain the need to restrict food and oral fluids at least 8 hours before surgery.
- Provide a general timetable for perioperative events.
- Discuss the need for the removal of jewelry, makeup, and all prostheses (eg, eyeglasses, hearing aids, complete or partial dentures, wig) immediately before surgery.
- Confirm time of surgery.
- Inform client about the preoperative holding area, and give the location of the waiting room for support persons.

Postoperative Regimen

- Discuss postanesthesia recovery room routines and emergency equipment.
- Review type and frequency of assessment activities.
- Teach deep-breathing and coughing exercises, leg exercises, ways to turn and move (see Procedure 45–1), and splinting techniques.
- Discuss pain management.
- Explain usual activity restrictions and precautions used to help clients get up for the first time postoperatively.
- Describe usual dietary alterations.
- Discuss postoperative dressings and drains.
- Provide an explanation and tour of intensive care unit if client is to be transferred there postoperatively.

Day-Surgery Clients

- Confirm place and time of surgery, including when to arrive (eg, 1 to 1½ hours before scheduled surgery) and where to register (eg, reception desk).
- Discuss what to wear (eg, clients having hand surgery should wear a garment with large sleeve openings to fit over a bulky dressing; all clients need to leave valuables at home).
- Explain the need for someone to accompany the client home, and arrange a place for pickup.
- Review available medical and insurance forms.
- Review with the client any tests ordered and need for a urine specimen the morning of surgery.
- Communicate by telephone the evening before surgery to confirm time of surgery and arrival time, and call again the evening after surgery to assess progress.

acting supportively will help the client deal with identified concerns. The nurse should not dismiss the client's concerns by saying, "Everything will be all right." Unknowns or misconceptions can produce unrealistic fears and anxiety.

The client also may have specific learning needs regarding postoperative care. For example, learning to attend to a colostomy requires preparation *before* surgery. Pain is common postoperatively; learning *beforehand* methods that will minimize the pain (eg, by holding a pillow against the abdomen when moving after abdominal surgery) reassures the client. It also is important that clients know they will receive analgesics postoperatively to minimize discomfort.

When children are involved, the nurse should provide explanations in a language they can understand and at a rate that keeps their attention and does not overwhelm them. It will also help to show the child the anesthetic equipment and the postanesthesia room ("wake-up room") before surgery, explaining all postoperative care and discomfort clearly and simply (eg, "You will have a sore tummy."). Confirm when the parents will visit, because this is the most essential piece of information the nurse can give the child.

A summary of preoperative instructions required for all clients is shown in the box on page 1403. Clients need to be informed about the activities to expect, when to expect them, and why they are being done. The nurse should explain the "sequence of events" in lay terms and clarify any questions at this time. Procedure 45–1 provides guidelines for teaching moving, leg exercises, deep-breathing exercises, and coughing.

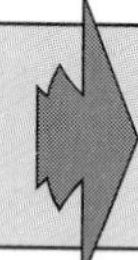

PROCEDURE 45–1 TEACHING MOVING, LEG EXERCISES, DEEP-BREATHING EXERCISES, AND COUGHING

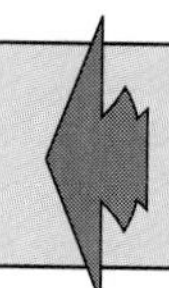

Before commencing to teach moving, leg exercises, deep-breathing exercises, and coughing, determine (a) the type of surgery, (b) the time of the surgery, (c) the name of the surgeon, (d) the preoperative orders, (e) the agency's practices for preoperative care, and (f) the learning needs of the client. Also, verify that the physician has completed the medical history and physical examination and that the consent form has been signed by the client or the family.

PURPOSES

Moving

- To maintain blood circulation
- To stimulate respiratory function
- To decrease stasis of gas in the intestine
- To facilitate early ambulation

Leg Exercises

- To stimulate blood circulation, thereby preventing thrombophlebitis and thrombus formation

Deep Breathing and Coughing

- To facilitate lung aeration, thereby preventing atelectasis and pneumonia
- To promote blood circulation to and from the lungs, thereby preventing pulmonary embolism

ASSESSMENT FOCUS
Vital signs; discomfort; temperature and color of feet and legs; breath sounds; presence of dyspnea or cough.

INTERVENTION

1. Show the client ways to turn in bed and to get out of bed.

- Instruct a client who will have a right abdominal incision or a right-sided chest incision to turn to the left side of the bed and sit up as follows:
  a. Flex the knees.
  b. Hold the left arm and hand or a small pillow against the incision to splint the wound.
  c. Turn to the left while pushing with the right foot and grasping a partial side rail on the left side of the bed with the right hand.
  d. Come to a sitting position on the side of the bed by using the right arm and hand to push down against the mattress.
- Ask a client with left abdominal or left-sided chest incision to perform the same procedure but splint with the right arm and turn to the right.
- For clients with orthopedic surgery (eg, hip surgery), use special

PROCEDURE 45–1 *continued*

aids, such as a trapeze, to assist with movement.

2. Teach the client the following three leg exercises.

- Alternate dorsiflexion and plantar flexion of the feet. See Table 34–2, page 886. *This exercise is sometimes referred to as calf pumping, since it alternately contracts and relaxes the calf muscles, including the gastrocnemius muscles.* See Figure 45–1.

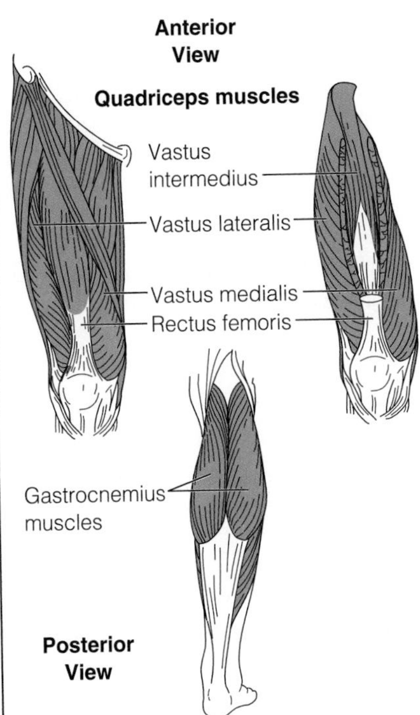

Figure 45–1 Leg muscles: anterior and posterior views.

- Flex and extend the knees, and press the backs of the knees into the bed while dorsiflexing the feet (Figure 45–2). Instruct clients who cannot raise their legs to do isometric exercises that contract and relax the muscles.
- Raise and lower the legs alternately from the surface of the bed. Extend the knee of the moving leg (Figure 45–3). *This exercise contracts and relaxes the quadriceps muscles.*

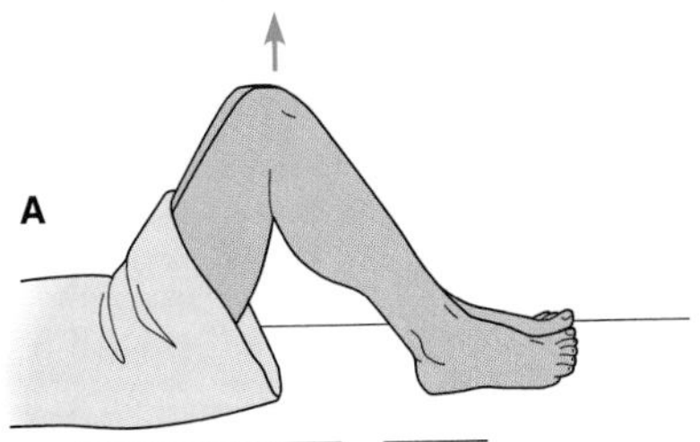

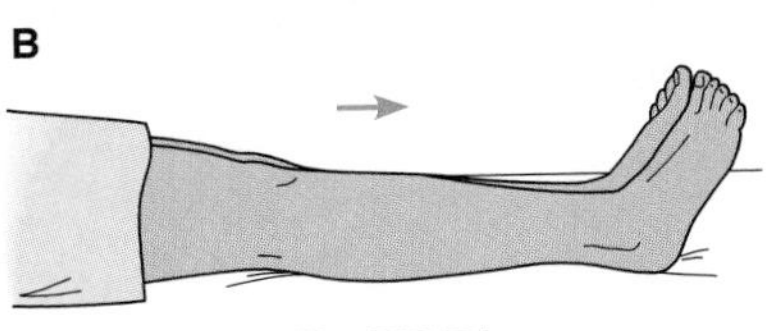

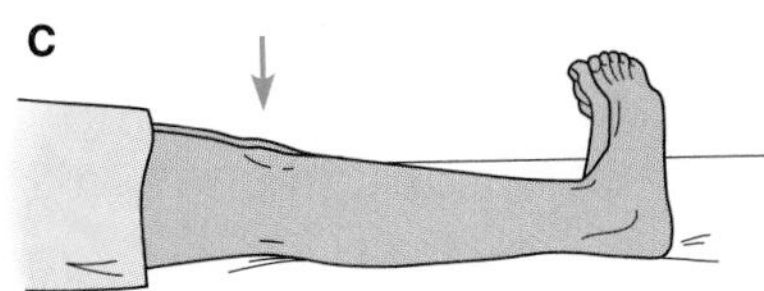

Figure 45–2 Flexing and extending the knees.

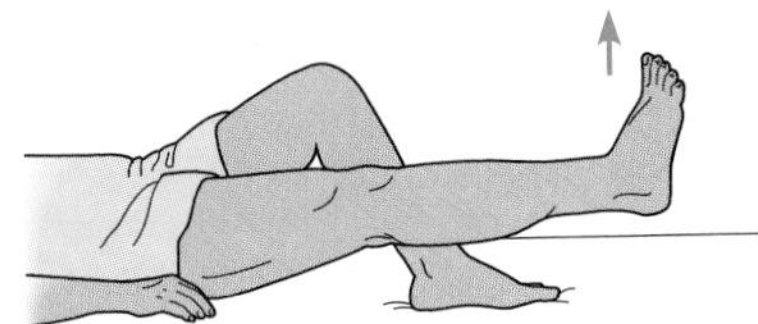

Figure 45–3 Raising and lowering the legs.

3. Demonstrate deep-breathing (diaphragmatic) exercises as follows.

- Place your hands palms down on the border of your rib cage, and inhale slowly and evenly through the nose until the greatest chest expansion is achieved (Figure 45–4).

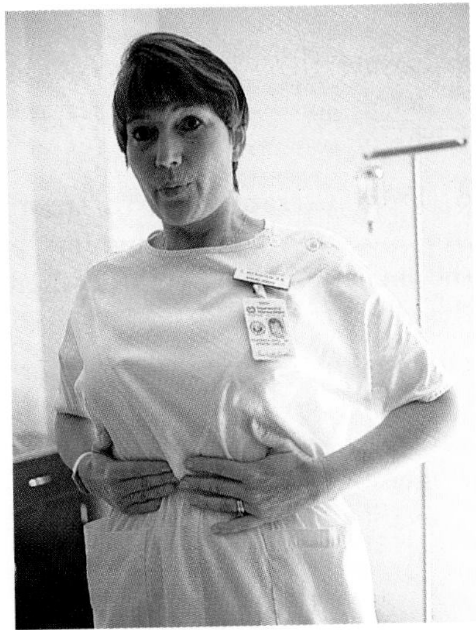

Figure 45–4 Demonstrating deep breathing.

- Hold your breath for 2 to 3 seconds.
- Then exhale slowly through the mouth.
- Continue exhalation until maximum chest contraction has been achieved.

4. Help the client perform deep-breathing exercises.

- Ask the client to assume a sitting position.
- Place the palms of your hands on the border of the client's rib cage to assess respiratory depth.
- Ask the client to perform deep breathing, as described in step 3.

5. Instruct the client to cough voluntarily after a few deep inhalations.

- Ask the client to inhale deeply, hold the breath for a few seconds, and then cough once or twice.

PROCEDURE 45–1 TEACHING MOVING, LEG EXERCISES, DEEP-BREATHING EXERCISES, AND COUGHING *continued*

- Ensure that the client coughs deeply and does not just clear the throat.

6. Demonstrate ways to splint the abdomen when coughing, if the incision will be painful when the client coughs.

- Show the client how to support the incision by placing the palms of the hands on either side of the incision site or directly over the incision site, holding the palm of one hand over the other. *Coughing uses the abdominal and other accessory respiratory muscles. Splinting the incision may reduce pain while coughing if the incision is near any of these muscles.*
- Show the client how to splint the abdomen with clasped hands and a firmly rolled pillow held against the client's abdomen (Figure 45–5).

7. Inform the client about the expected frequency of these exercises.

- Instruct the client to start the exercises as soon after surgery as possible.

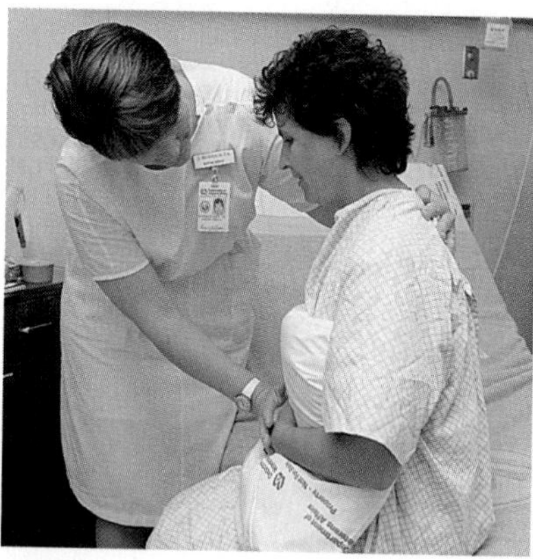

Figure 45–5 Splinting an incision with a pillow.

- Encourage clients with abdominal or chest surgery to carry out deep breathing and coughing at least three or four times daily and at each session to take a minimum of five breaths. Note, however, that the number of breaths and frequency of deep breathing varies with the client's condition. People who are susceptible to pulmonary problems may need deep-breathing exercises every hour. People with chronic respiratory disease may need special breathing exercises (eg, pursed-lip breathing, abdominal breathing, exercises using various kinds of incentive spirometers). See Chapter 39, pages 1145 and 1147.

8. Document the teaching and all assessments.

EVALUATION FOCUS
Client's demonstrated ability to perform moving, leg exercises, deep-breathing and coughing exercises.

Physical Preparation Preoperative preparation includes the following areas: nutrition and fluids, elimination, hygiene, rest, medications, care of valuables and prostheses, special orders, and surgical skin preparation. In many agencies on the day of surgery, a preoperative checklist is used. The nurse checks the agency's forms and follows appropriate recording procedures. It is essential (a) that all pertinent records (laboratory records, X-ray films, consents) be assembled and completed so that operating and recovery room personnel can refer to them and (b) that all physical preparation is completed to ensure client safety.

Nutrition and Fluids Adequate hydration and nutrition promote healing. Nurses need to record any signs of malnutrition or fluid imbalance. If the client is on intravenous fluids or on measured fluid intake, nurses must ensure that the fluids are carefully measured.

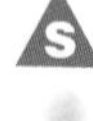

Because anesthetics depress gastrointestinal functioning and because there is a danger the client may vomit and aspirate vomitus during administration of a general anesthetic, the client usually fasts at least 6 to 8 hours before surgery, although in some instances clear liquids such as water, apple juice, and black coffee are permitted up to 2 hours before surgery. The surgical client and support persons need to understand the necessity of fasting. Usually, the nurse removes food and fluids from the bedside and places a fasting sign at the bed the evening before surgery. The client can use a mouthwash if the mouth feels dry but must not swallow any. If the client ingests food or fluids during the fasting period, the nurse must notify the surgeon.

Elimination Enemas before surgery are no longer routine, but cleansing enemas may be ordered if bowel surgery is planned. The enemas help prevent postoperative constipation and contamination of the surgical area by feces. After surgery involving the intestines, peristalsis often doesn't return for 24 to 48 hours.

Prior to surgery a retention catheter may be ordered to ensure that the bladder remains empty. This helps prevent inadvertent injury to the bladder, particularly during pelvic surgery. If the client does not have a catheter, it is important to empty the bladder prior to receiving preoperative medications. The bladder must be empty during the operation.

Hygiene In some settings, clients are asked to bathe or shower using an antimicrobial agent the evening or morning of surgery (or both). The bath includes a shampoo whenever possible. Immediately before surgery, the client's nails should be trimmed and free of polish and all cosmetics removed so that the nail beds, skin, and lips are visible when circulation is assessed during and following surgery.

Surgical caps may be donned the day of surgery by clients in some hospitals. The surgical caps contain the client's hair and any microorganisms on the hair and scalp.

On the day of surgery, the nurse removes, or asks the client to remove, all hair pins and clips; these may cause pressure or accidental damage to the scalp when the client is unconscious. Long hair can be braided and fastened with elastic bands to keep it in place.

Rest Nurses should do everything to help the client sleep the night before surgery. Often a sedative is ordered. Adequate rest helps the client manage the stress of surgery.

Medications Preoperative medications also may be ordered for the day of surgery. Usually a narcotic (eg, morphine) and a medication to dry the secretions of the mouth and respiratory tract (eg, atropine) are given by injection. Sometimes, the surgeon orders oral sedatives (eg, secobarbital) or tranquilizers to be administered before the injectable medications are given. A narcotic, sedative, or tranquilizer calms the client before general anesthesia and enhances a smooth anesthesia induction. Atropine or a similar drying drug minimizes the danger of aspirating secretions into the lungs. A newer trend is to give *no* preoperative medications, but if these are ordered, nurses need to administer them exactly at the time specified. Giving preoperative medications on time is essential because of their desired effect in combination with the anesthetic.

After giving the preoperative medications, the nurse informs the client that the medication will cause drowsiness and instructs the client to remain quietly in bed. The nurse raises the side rails and lowers the bed for safety, placing the call light within reach. Also, the nurse explains that scopolamine or atropine may cause thirst and that although a mouthwash may be used, no fluids should be swallowed.

Valuables and Prostheses Valuables such as jewelry and money should be labeled and placed in safekeeping if support persons cannot take them home. In most hospitals, valuables can be kept in special envelopes and locked in a storage area on the unit. If a client wishes not to remove a wedding band, the nurse can tape it in place. Wedding bands must be removed, however, if there is danger of the fingers swelling after surgery. Situations warranting removal of a wedding band include surgery of or cast application to an arm and a mastectomy that involves removal of the lymph nodes. (Mastectomies may cause edema of the arm and hand.)

All prostheses (artificial body parts, such as partial or complete dentures, contact lenses, artificial eyes, and artificial limbs), as well as eyeglasses, wigs, false eyelashes, and hearing aids, must be removed before surgery. The nurse also checks for the presence of chewing gum or loose teeth, a common problem with 5- or 6-year-olds undergoing tonsillectomy. In some hospitals, dentures are placed in a locked storage area; in others they are placed in labeled containers and kept at the client's bedside. Partial dentures can become dislodged and obstruct an unconscious client's breathing. Loose teeth can become dislodged and aspirated during anesthesia. Other prostheses may become damaged.

Special Orders The nurse checks the surgeon's orders for special requirements (eg, the insertion of a nasogastric tube prior to surgery, the administration of medications, such as insulin, or the application of antiemboli stockings). For the technique of inserting a nasogastric tube, see Procedure 37–1, page 1047.

Skin Preparation In most agencies, skin preparation is carried out during the intraoperative phase. See also page 1409.

Antiemboli Stockings Antiemboli (elastic) stockings are indicated for clients who have problems with circulation in their feet and legs. The elastic material compresses the veins of the legs and thereby facilitates the return of venous blood to the heart. They also improve arterial circulation to the feet and prevent edema of the legs and feet. These stockings are frequently applied preoperatively as well as postoperatively.

There are several types of stockings. One type extends from the foot to the knee and another from the foot to midthigh. These stockings usually have a partial foot that exposes either the heel or toes so that extremity circulation can be assessed. Elastic stockings usually come in small, medium, and large sizes. The box on page 1408 summarizes the assessments the nurse should make before applying antiemboli stockings.

Follow the steps below to apply antiemboli stockings:

- Apply stockings in the morning, if possible, before the client arises. *In sitting and standing positions, the veins can become distended and edema occurs; the stockings should be applied before this happens.*
- Wash the legs and feet daily.

INDICATIONS FOR ANTIEMBOLI STOCKINGS

- *Inadequate arterial blood circulation:* cool skin temperature in a warm environment; pallor; shiny, taut skin; mild edema.
- *Insufficient venous blood return:* thickening of the skin; increased pigmentation around the ankles; pitting edema (edema in which firm finger pressure on the skin produces an indentation, or pit, that remains for several seconds); peripheral cyanosis.
- *Altered posterior tibial* and *dorsalis pedis pulses:* rates, volumes, and rhythms.
- *Pain in the calf of the leg:* the nurse dorsiflexes the client's foot abruptly and firmly while the client's knee is straight or slightly flexed to assess pain in the calf (Homans' sign). The presence of pain is a positive Homans' sign.
- *Distended superficial veins in the legs:* veins normally appear distended in a dependent position but collapse when the limb is elevated.

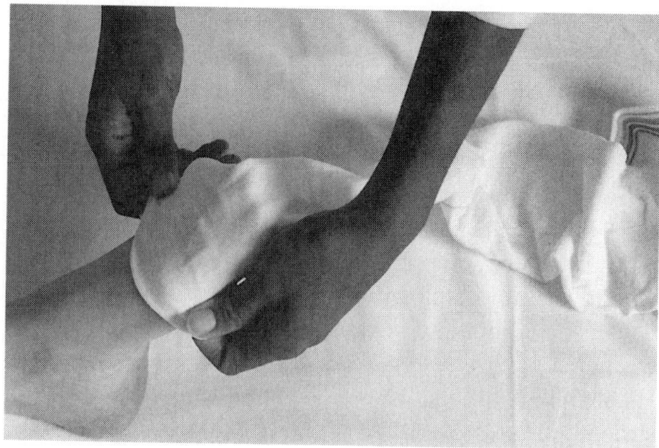

Figure 45–6 Applying the inverted stocking over client's toes.

- Assist the client who has been ambulating to lie down and elevate the legs for 15 to 30 minutes before applying the stockings. *This facilitates venous return and reduces swelling.*
- Assist the client to a lying position in bed.
- Dust the ankle with talcum powder, and ask the client to point the toes. *These measures ease application.*
- Turn the stocking inside out by inserting your hand into the stocking from the top and grabbing the heel pocket from the inside. The foot portion should now be inside the stocking leg.
- Remove your hand, and, with the heel pocket downward, hook your index and middle fingers of both hands into the foot section.
- Face the client, and slip the foot portion of the stocking over the client's foot, toes, and heel (Figure 45–6). As you move up the foot, stretch the stocking sideways.
- Support the client's ankle with one hand while using the other hand to pull the heel pocket under the heel.
- Center the heel in the pocket.
- Gather the remaining portion of the stocking up to the toes, and pull only this part over the heel. With the foot already covered, the remainder of the stocking should slide easily over it.
- At the ankle, grasp the gathered portion between your index and middle fingers, and pull the stocking up the leg to the knee. You may need to support the ankle with one hand and use the other hand to stretch the stocking and distribute it evenly.
- For *thigh-* or *waist-length stockings,* ask the client to straighten the leg while stretching the rest of the stocking over the knee.
- Ask the client to flex the knee while pulling the stocking over the thigh. Stretch the stocking from the top (front and back) to distribute it evenly over the thigh. The top should rest 2.5 to 7.5 cm (1 to 3 in) below the gluteal fold.
- For a *waist-high stocking,* ask the client to stand and continue extending the stocking up to the top of the gluteal fold.
- Apply the adjustable belt that accompanies thigh- and waist-length stockings, making sure that it does not interfere with any incision or external device (eg, drainage tube or catheter).
- Adjust the foot section by tugging on the toe section to ensure toe comfort and smoothness of the stocking. Make sure a toe window is properly positioned.
- Document the application of the stockings as well as skin temperature and color, presence of edema, posterior tibial and dorsalis pedis pulses, presence of any pain (ie, in calf), appearance of leg veins.
- Remove stockings once every shift or every 12 hours for about 30 minutes. Wash the stockings and air dry according to the manufacturer's instructions. This permits the nurse to observe the circulatory status of the legs and the condition of the skin. Test for Homans' sign indicating the possible presence of deep phlebitis. See the box on page 525 of Chapter 22.

EVALUATING

To evaluate the achievement of the preoperative client's goals, the nurse collects data in relation to the outcome criteria. Evaluative activities may include

- Asking the client (a) to describe the proposed surgery, the reason for it, and expected length of stay; (b) to describe events that will occur in intraoperative and postoperative periods; and (c) to give reasons for specific preoperative and postoperative procedures.
- Listening attentively while encouraging the client to verbalize feelings about (a) the surgery and expected outcomes and (b) obtaining sufficient rest and sleep.
- Asking the client to demonstrate deep breathing, coughing, splinting, leg exercises, and moving techniques.
- Measuring vital signs and fluid intake and output.

The plan of care is effective and goals/outcomes are met if the client is physically and emotionally prepared for surgery.

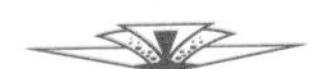

INTRAOPERATIVE PHASE

During the intraoperative phase, the perioperative nurse performs several nursing activities designed to provide the client with comprehensive, safe, and effective care during the surgical procedure. These activities include

- Assessing the client's physiologic and psychologic status
- Reviewing the results of the diagnostic tests and lab studies
- Positioning the client for surgery
- Performing the surgical skin prep
- Assisting in preparing the sterile field
- Opening and dispensing sterile supplies during surgery
- Monitoring and maintaining a safe, aseptic environment
- Managing catheters, tubes, drains and specimens
- Performing sponge, sharp, and instrument counts
- Administering medications and solutions to the sterile field
- Documenting the nursing care provided and the client's response to the nursing interventions

SURGICAL SKIN PREPARATION

Surgical skin preparation involves cleaning the surgical site, removing hair only if necessary, and applying an antimicrobial agent. In most hospitals skin preparation is done by operating room personnel close to the time of surgery. The purpose of a surgical skin preparation is to reduce the risk of postoperative wound infection. This is done by

- Removing soil and transient microbes from the skin.
- Reducing the resident microbial count to subpathogenic amounts in a short period of time and with the least amount of tissue irritation.
- Inhibiting rapid rebound growth of microbes.

Before skin preparation, the nurse must ensure that the operative site and surrounding areas are clean. The Association of Operating Room Nurses states that cleansing can be accomplished before surgery by having the client shower, by washing the operative site in the client unit, and/or by washing the operative site immediately before applying the antimicrobial agent in the operating room (AORN 1992, p. 937).

The nurse also carefully inspects the prospective surgical area for growths, moles, rashes, pustules, irritations, exudate, abrasions, bruises, or any broken or ischemic areas. These should be recorded and reported to the surgeon. In addition, the nurse must determine whether the client is allergic to any of the solutions used in the skin preparations (eg, a depilatory).

The kind and extent of skin preparation depends on the type of surgery. Agencies have protocols to follow regarding skin preparation areas. The area needs to be large enough to accommodate extension of the incision, additional incisions, and all potential drain sites.

Hair removal at the operative site is not recommended unless the hair interferes with the surgical procedure (eg, craniotomy). If hair removal is required, it should be performed by skilled personnel in a client care area outside the room where the surgery is to be performed. Because shaving can disrupt skin integrity, clippers or chemical depilatory agents are the preferred methods of hair removal.

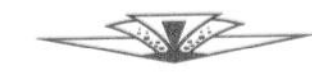

POSTOPERATIVE PHASE

Nursing during the postoperative phase is especially important for the client's recovery. Anesthesia impairs the ability of clients to respond to environmental stimuli and to help themselves, although the degree of consciousness of clients will vary. Moreover, surgery itself traumatizes the body by decreasing its energy and resistance.

IMMEDIATE POSTANESTHETIC PHASE

Immediate postanesthetic care is usually provided in a postanesthetic room (PAR) or recovery room (RR). Recovery room nurses have specialized skills to care for clients recovering from anesthesia and surgery. Once the health status has stabilized, the client is returned to the nursing unit or, in the case of a day-surgery client, to the day-surgery area before discharge. Recovery room assessment is summarized in the accompanying box.

During the immediate postanesthetic stage, an unconscious client is positioned on the side, with the face slightly down. A pillow is not placed under the head. In this position, gravity keeps the tongue forward, preventing occlusion of the pharynx and allowing drainage of mucus or vomitus out of the mouth rather than down the respiratory tree. Clients who have had spinal anesthetics may need to remain flat for a specified period.

The nurse ensures maximum chest expansion by elevating the client's upper arm on a pillow. The upper arm is supported because the pressure of an arm against the chest reduces chest expansion potential. Once the reflexes return, the client can usually assume a back-lying position. An artificial airway is maintained in place, and suction is supplied until reflexes for controlling coughing and swallowing return. Generally, the client spits out an oropharyngeal airway when coughing returns. Endotracheal tubes are not removed until clients are awake and able to maintain their own airways. Before any artificial airway is removed, suction is applied to the airway and the pharynx. The client is then helped to turn, cough, and take deep breaths, provided that vital signs are stable. See Chapter 39 for information about artificial airways.

The return of the client's reflexes, such as swallowing and gagging, indicates that anesthesia is ending. Time of recovery from anesthesia varies with the kind of anesthetic agent used, its dosage, and the individual's response to it. Nurses should arouse clients by calling them by name, and in a normal tone of voice repeatedly telling them that the surgery is over and that they are in the RR.

Once the health status has stabilized, the client is returned to the nursing unit or, in the case of a day-surgery client, to the day-surgery area.

According to Fairchild (1993, p. 357) clients are usually discharged from the PAR when

- They are conscious and oriented.
- They are able to maintain a clear airway and deep breath and cough freely.
- Vital signs have been stable and/or consistent with preoperative vital signs for at least 30 minutes.
- Protective reflexes (eg, gag, swallowing) are active.
- They are able to move four extremities.
- Urinary intake and output is adequate (urinary output at least 30mL/h)
- They are afebrile or a febrile condition has been attended to.
- Dressings are dry and intact; no overt drainage.

RECOVERY ROOM ASSESSMENT

- Adequacy of airway
  - Suction airway as indicated
- Adequacy of ventilation
  - Respiratory rate, rhythm and depth
  - Use of accessory muscles
  - Breath sounds
- Cardiovascular status
  - Pulse rate, rhythm, and volume
  - Blood pressure
  - Capillary filling
- Level of consciousness
  - Not responding
  - Arousable on calling
  - Fully awake
  - Oriented to time, person, and place
- Presence of protective reflexes (eg, gag, cough)
- Activity, ability to move extremities
- Skin color (pink, pale, dusky, blotchy, cyanotic, jaundiced)
- Fluid status
  - Intake and output
  - Status of IV infusions (rate, amount in container, patency of tubing)
  - Signs of dehydration or fluid overload (see Chapter 38)
- Condition of operative site
  - Status of dressing
  - Drainage (amount, type and color)
- Patency of and character and amount of drainage from catheters, tubes, and drains
- Discomfort (ie, pain) (type, location, and severity), nausea, vomiting
- Safety (ie, necessity for side rails, call bell within reach)

ONGOING POSTOPERATIVE CARE

Preparing for the Postoperative Client While the client is in the operating room, the client's bed and room are prepared for the postoperative phase. In some agencies, the client is brought back to the unit on a stretcher and transferred to the bed in the room. In other agencies, the client's bed is brought to the recovery room (RR), and the client is transferred there. In the latter situation, the bed needs to be made with clean linens as soon as the client goes to the operating room so that it can be taken to the RR at any time. In addition, the nurse must obtain and set up special equipment as needed, such as an intravenous pole, suction, oxygen equipment, and orthopedic appliances (eg, traction). If these are not requested on the client's record, the nurse should consult with the recovery room nurse or surgeon.

Assessing

As soon as the client returns to the nursing unit, the nurse conducts an initial assessment. The sequence of these activities varies with the situation. For example, the nurse may need to check the physician's stat orders before conducting the initial assessment; in such a case, nursing interventions to implement the orders can be carried out at the same time as assessment.

Consult the surgeon's postoperative orders to learn the following:

- Food and fluids permitted by mouth
- Intravenous solutions and intravenous medications
- Position in bed
- Medications ordered (eg, analgesics, antibiotics)
- Laboratory tests
- Intake and output, which in some agencies are monitored for all postoperative clients.
- Activity permitted, including ambulation

The nurse also checks the PAR record for the following data:

- Operation performed
- Presence and location of any drains
- Anesthetic used
- Postoperative diagnosis
- Estimated blood loss
- Medications administered in the recovery room

Many hospitals have postoperative protocols for regular assessment of clients. In some agencies, assessments are made every 15 minutes until vital signs stabilize, every hour thereafter the same day, and every 4 hours for the next 2 days. It is very important that the assessments be made as often as the client's condition requires. The nurse assesses the following:

- *Level of consciousness* and orientation to time, place, and person. Most clients are fully conscious but drowsy when returned to their unit. Assess reaction to verbal stimuli and ability to move extremities.
- *Vital signs.* Take the client's vital signs (temperature, pulse, respiration, and blood pressure) every 15 minutes until stable or in accordance with agency protocol. Compare initial findings with PAR data. In addition, assess the client for signs of common circulatory problems; hemorrhage, shock, cardiac arrest, and postoperative hypotension. See Table 45–2 on page 1413. Disruption of sutures and insecure ligation of blood vessels can cause hemorrhage. Shock occurs as a result of massive hemorrhage or cardiac insufficiency. Signs of shock are summarized in Table 45–2.
- *Skin color and temperature*, particularly that of the lips and nail beds. The color of the lips and nail beds are indicators of **tissue perfusion** (passage of blood through the vessels). Pale, cyanotic, cool, and moist skin may be a sign of circulatory problems.
- *Fluid balance.* Assess the type and amount of intravenous fluids, flow rate, and infusion site. Monitor the client's fluid intake and output. In addition to watching for shock, the nurse assesses the client for signs of circulatory overload (see Chapter 38). During surgery, aldosterone production increases, and, as a result, the body conserves sodium and fluid. Therefore, care must be taken not to overload the body with fluid. On the other hand, it is extremely important for the nurse to ensure that replacement of fluids lost during surgery is sufficient to maintain blood pressure.
- *Position and safety.* Ensure the client is in the appropriate position according to the physician's orders. In addition, following spinal anesthesia, the client may need to remain flat for a specified period. Place clients who are not fully conscious in the side-lying position to prevent aspiration of secretions. Elevate side rails and place the bed in the low position.
- *Dressing and bedclothes.* Inspect the client's dressings and the bedclothes underneath the client. Excessive bloody drainage on dressings or on bedclothes, often appearing underneath the client, can indicate hemorrhage. The amount of drainage on dressings is recorded by describing the diameter of the stains.
- *Drains and tubes.* Determine color, consistency, and amount of drainage from all tubes and suction apparatuses. All tubes should be patent, and tubes and suction equipment should be functioning. Drainage bags must be hanging properly.
- *Pain and comfort level.* Assess for location and intensity of pain and any side effects such as nausea and vomiting. Medicate the client as indicated. Determine what analgesics were given in the PAR and the time they were given. In terms of comfort level, ensure that the client is warm and feels comfortable. Notify support persons of the client's return from surgery and allow them to be with the client after initial assessments are performed.

Document the client's time of arrival and all assessments. Many agencies have progress flow records for this purpose. Alter the frequency, parameters, and priorities to meet the individual needs of the client.

DIAGNOSING

Because surgery can involve many body systems both directly and indirectly and is a complex experience for the client, the nursing diagnoses focus on a wide variety of actual, high risk, and collaborative problems. Examples are shown below:

Actual or High Risk Diagnoses

- **High risk for infection** related to
  - Impaired skin integrity (surgical incision)
  - Knowledge deficit (wound or drainage tube care)
- **High risk for injury** related to
  - Inability to adapt to environmental hazards secondary to anesthetized status
  - Impaired physical mobility secondary to incisional pain and imposed restrictions to movement (eg, intravenous line, cast)
- **High risk for fluid volume deficit** related to
  - Excessive wound drainage
  - Inadequate fluid intake
- **Pain** related to
  - Activity and surgical incision
- **Ineffective airway clearance** related to
  - Effects of anesthesia (eg, diminished cough reflex, retained secretions)
  - History of smoking
- **Ineffective breathing pattern** related to
  - Pain in high abdominal incision
  - Effects of analgesic on ventilation
- **Self-care deficit: Bathing/hygiene, dressing/grooming, toileting** related to
  - Imposed activity restrictions
  - Devices restrictive to movement
- **Altered health maintenance** related to
  - Knowledge deficit (wound care and activity restrictions after discharge)
- **Self-esteem disturbance** related to
  - Altered body image associated with mutilating surgery
- **Collaborative problems**
  Most people recover from surgery without incident. Complications or problems are relatively rare, yet nurses must be aware of such possibilities and their clinical signs. Examples of collaborative problems are
  - Potential complication: Hypostatic pneumonia
  - Potential complication: Atelectasis
  - Potential complication: Pulmonary embolism
  - Potential complication: Hemorrhage
  - Potential complication: Hypovolemic shock
  - Potential complication: Thrombophlebitis
  - Potential complication: Urinary retention
  - Potential complication: Paralytic ileus
  - Potential complication: Wound infection
  - Potential complication: Wound dehiscence

  See Table 45–2 for descriptions, causes, clinical signs, and preventive interventions.

PLANNING

Postoperative care planning and discharge planning begin in the preoperative phase when preoperative teaching is implemented. Client goals during the postoperative period include

- Being free of surgical complications
- Experiencing minimal discomfort
- Achieving adequate rest
- Being free of injury
- Maintaining a healthy attitude toward self
- Resuming the highest possible level of wellness

Examples of outcome criteria to evaluate the achievement of goals and the effectiveness of nursing interventions follow.

The client

- Maintains normal baseline vital signs.
- Performs deep-breathing exercises and voluntary coughing every 2 hours when awake, as instructed.
- Has adequate respiratory excursion (depth).
- Has clear lung sounds on auscultation.
- Performs specified leg exercises at least every 4 hours when awake, as instructed.
- Has negative Homans' sign.
- Has balanced fluid intake and output.
- Has good tissue turgor of the skin.
- Has clear amber urine.
- Experiences no burning sensation or urgency when voiding.
- Has active bowel sounds within 48 hours.
- Resumes normal defecation within 3 days.
- Is free of purulent wound drainage.
- Ambulates, performs self-care activities, and rests with minimal or no pain.
- Reports satisfactory sleep pattern each night.
- Reports feelings of increasing wellness each day.

Table 45–2 Potential Postoperative Problems

Problem	Description	Cause	Clinical Signs	Preventive Interventions
Respiratory				
Pneumonia	Inflammation of the alveoli	Commonly *Diplococcus pneumoniae*, a resident bacteria in the respiratory tract	Elevated temperature, cough, expectoration of blood-tinged or purulent sputum, dyspnea, chest pain	Deep-breathing exercises and coughing, moving in bed, early ambulation
Lobar pneumonia	Involves one or more lobes			
Bronchopneumonia	Originates in bronchi and involves patches of lung tissue	Poor lung expansion and circulation, resulting in stagnation of secretions		
Hypostatic pneumonia	Poor or stagnant circulation causing inflammation of lung tissue			
Atelectasis	Collapse of the alveoli, with retained secretions	Mucous plugs blocking bronchial passageways, inadequate lung expansion, analgesics, immobility	Marked dyspnea, cyanosis, pleural pain, prostration, tachycardia, increased respiratory rate, fever, productive cough, ausculatory crackling sounds	Deep-breathing exercises and couging, turning, early ambulation, adequate fluid intake
Pulmonary embolism	Blood clot that has moved to the lungs and obstructs a pulmonary artery, thus inhibiting blood flow to one or more lung lobes	Stasis of venous blood from immobility, venous injury from fractures or during surgery, use of oral contraceptives high in estrogen, preexisting coagulation or circulatory disorder	Sudden chest pain, shortness of breath, cyanosis, shock (tachycardia, low blood pressure)	Deep-breathing exercises and coughing, turning, ambulation, antiemboli stockings
Circulatory				
Hemorrhage	Bleeding internally or externally	Disruption of sutures, insecure ligation of blood vessels	Rapid weak pulse, increasing respiratory rate, restlessness, lowered blood pressure, cold clammy skin, thirst, pallor, reduced urine output	Early recognition of signs
Hypovolemic shock	Markedly reduced volume of circulating blood resulting in inadequate tissue perfusion	Hemorrhage	Same as Hemorrhage	Early recognition of signs
Thrombophlebitis	Inflammation of the veins, usually of the legs and associated with a blood clot	Slowed venous blood flow due to immobility or prolonged sitting; trauma to vein, resulting in inflammation and increased blood coagulability	Aching, cramping pain; affected area is swollen, red, and hot to touch; vein feels hard; discomfort in calf when foot is dorsiflexed or when client walks (Homans' sign)	Early ambulation, leg exercises, antiemboli stockings, adequate fluid intake

➤

Table 45–2 Potential Postoperative Problems *continued*

Problem	Description	Cause	Clinical Signs	Preventive Interventions
***Circulatory** continued*				
Thrombus	Blood clot attached to wall of vein or artery (most commonly the leg veins)	Venous statis; vein injury resulting from surgery of legs, pelvis, abdomen; factors causing increased blood coagulability (eg, use of estrogen)	Same as for Pulmonary Embolism; if lodged in heart or brain, cardiac or neurologic signs	Same as for Thrombophlebitis
Embolus	Clot that has moved from its site of formation to another area of the body (eg, the lungs, heart, or brain)	Same as for Thrombus	Same as for Thrombus	Same as for Thrombophlebitis
Urinary				
Urinary retention	Accumulation of urine in the bladder and inability of the bladder to empty itself	Depressed bladder muscle tone from narcotics and anesthetics; handling of tissues during surgery on adjacent organs (rectum, vagina)	Fluid intake larger than output; inability to void or frequent voiding of small amounts, bladder distension, suprapubic discomfort, restlessness	Monitoring of fluid intake and output, interventions to facilitate voiding
Urinary infection	Inflammation of the bladder	Immobilization and limited fluid intake	Burning sensation when voiding, urgency, cloudy urine, lower abdominal pain	Adequate fluid intake, early ambulation, good perineal hygiene
Gastrointestinal				
Constipation	Infrequent or no stool passage for abnormal length of time (eg, within 48 hours after solid diet started)	Lack of dietary roughage, analgesics (decreased intestinal motility)	Absence of stool elimination, abdominal distention, and discomfort	Adequate fluid intake, high-fiber diet, early ambulation
Singultus	Intermittent spasms of the diaphragm	Irritation of the phrenic nerve—for a variety of reasons (eg, abdominal distention)	Hiccups	Prevent the cause
Tympanites	Retention of gases within the intestines	Slowed motility of the intestines due to handling of the bowel during surgery and the effects of anesthesia	Obvious abdominal distention, abdominal discomfort (gas pains), absence of bowel sounds	Early ambulation, IV fluid progressing to clear fluids, full fluids and regular diet when peristalsis returns
Nausea and vomiting		Pain, abdominal distention, ingesting food or fluids before return of peristalsis, certain medications, anxiety	Complaints of feeling sick to the stomach, retching or gagging	IV fluids until peristalsis returns; then clear fluids, full fluids, and regular diet; antimetic drugs if ordered; analgesics for pain

Table 45–2 *continued*

Problem	Description	Cause	Clinical Signs	Preventive Interventions
Wound				
Wound infection	Inflammation and infection of incision or drain site	Poor aseptic technique; laboratory analysis of wound swab identifies causative microorganism	Purulent exudate, redness, tenderness, elevated body temperature, wound odor	Keeping wound clean and dry, surgical aseptic technique when changing dressings
Wound dehiscence	Separation of a suture line before the incision heals	Malnutrition (emaciation, obesity), poor circulation, excessive strain on suture line	Increased incision drainage, tissues underlying skin become visible along parts of the incision	Adequate nutrition, appropriate incisional support and avoidance of strain
Wound evisceration	Extrusion of internal organs and tissues through the incision	Same as for Wound Dehiscence	Opening of incision and visible protrusion of organs	Same as for Wound Dehiscence
Psychologic				
Postoperative depression	See Clinical Signs	Physical feelings of weakness, surprise nature of emergency surgery, news of malignancy, severely altered body image, or other personal matter	Anorexia, tearfulness, loss of ambition, withdrawal, rejection of others, feelings of dejection, sleep disturbances (insomnia, excessive sleeping)	Adequate rest, physical activity, opportunity to express anger and other negative feelings

IMPLEMENTING

Nursing interventions designed to promote client recovery and prevent complications include (a) appropriate client positioning, (b) encouraging deep-breathing and coughing exercises, (c) leg exercises, (d) early ambulation, (e) adequate hydration, (f) diet, (g) promoting urinary elimination, (h) administering analgesics, and (i) wound care.

Positioning Position the client as ordered. Clients who have had spinal anesthetics usually lie flat for 8 to 12 hours. Agencies often have protocols regarding this practice. An unconscious or semiconscious client is placed on a side, if possible, or in a position that allows fluids to drain from the mouth. Otherwise, follow the client's preference. Most people prefer a back-lying position.

Deep-Breathing and Coughing Exercises Deep-breathing exercises help remove mucus, which can form and remain in the lungs due to the effects of general anesthetic and analgesics. These drugs depress the action of both the cilia of the mucous membranes lining the respiratory tract and the respiratory center in the brain. By increasing lung expansion and preventing the accumulation of secretions, deep breathing helps prevent pneumonia, which may result from stagnation of fluid in the lungs. See Table 45–2, page 1413. Deep breathing frequently initiates the coughing reflex. Voluntary coughing in conjunction with deep breathing facilitates the movement and expectoration of respiratory tract secretions.

Encourage the client to do deep-breathing and coughing exercises hourly, or at least every 2 hours, during waking hours for the first few days. Assist the client to a sitting position in bed or on the side of the bed. The client can splint the incision with a pillow when coughing, or the nurse can splint the incision for the client to reduce discomfort. To assist clients who have difficulty with deep-breathing and coughing exercises, check about the use of incentive spirometers (see Chapter 39). Clients unable to cough up secretions may require suction (see Chapter 39).

Leg Exercises Encourage the client to do leg exercises every hour, or at least every 2 hours, during waking hours. Muscle contractions compress the veins, preventing the stasis of blood in the veins, a cause of **thrombus** formation and subsequent **thrombophlebitis** and **emboli.** See Table 45–2, pages 1413 and 1414. Contractions also promote arterial blood flow.

Moving and Ambulation Turn the client from side to side at least every 2 hours. Turning allows alternating maximum expansion of the uppermost lung. Avoid placing pillows or rolls under the client's knees because pressure on the popliteal blood vessels can slow the blood circulation to and from the lower extremities. Clients who had practiced turning before surgery usually find it easier to do after surgery. The client should ambulate as soon as possible after surgery in accordance with the surgeon's orders. Generally, clients begin ambulation the evening of the day of surgery or the first day after surgery, unless the surgeon orders otherwise. Early ambulation prevents respiratory, circulatory, urinary, and gastrointestinal complications. It also prevents general muscle weakness. See Table 47–2, pages 1413 and 1414. Schedule ambulation for periods after the client has taken an analgesic or when the client is comfortable. Ambulation should be gradual, starting with the client sitting on the bed and dangling the feet over the side. A client who cannot ambulate should be periodically assisted to a sitting position in bed, if allowed, and turned frequently. The sitting position permits the greatest lung expansion.

Hydration Maintain intravenous infusions as ordered. Intravenous infusions are given to balance loss of body fluids during surgery (eg, blood loss, perspiration, vomiting, and fasting). Only small sips of water should be offered to clients who can have fluids by mouth, until they establish tolerance. Large amounts of water can induce vomiting, since anesthetics and narcotic analgesics temporarily inhibit the motility of the stomach. Ice chips, if permitted, may be offered. The client who cannot take fluids by mouth *may* be allowed to suck ice chips; check the surgeon's orders. Provide mouth care and place a mouthwash at the client's bedside. Postoperative clients often complain of thirst and a dry, sticky mouth. These discomforts are a result of the preoperative fasting period, preoperative mediations (such as atropine or scopolamine), and loss of body fluid.

Measure the client's fluid intake and output for at least 2 days or until fluid balance is stable and without an intravenous infusion. Ensuring adequate fluid balance is important. Sufficient fluids keep the respiratory mucous membranes and secretions moist, thus facilitating the expectoration of mucus during coughing. Also, an adequate fluid balance will prevent dehydration and the resulting concentration of the blood that, along with venous stasis, is conducive to thrombus formation.

Diet The surgeon orders the client's postoperative diet. Depending on the extent of surgery and the organs involved, some clients may be given intravenous fluids and nothing by mouth for a few days, whereas others may progress from a diet of clear liquids to full fluids, to a light diet, and then to a regular diet within a few days, provided that gastrointestinal functioning is normal. Assess the return of peristalsis by auscultating the abdomen. Gurgling and rumbling sounds indicate peristalsis (see Chapter 22). Anesthetic agents, narcotics, handling of the intestines during abdominal surgery, changes in fluid and food intake, and inactivity all inhibit peristalsis. Therefore, bowel sounds should be carefully assessed every 4 to 6 hours. Oral fluids and food are usually started after the return of peristalsis. Assist very weak clients to eat.

Observe the client's tolerance of the food and fluids ingested and note and report the passage of flatus or abdominal distention.

Urinary Elimination Provide measures that promote urinary elimination. For example, help male clients stand at the bedside, ensure that clients are free from pain, ensure that fluid intake is adequate, and help clients walk. Determine whether the client has any difficulties voiding and assess the client for bladder distention (see Figure 22–69, p. 538). Report to the surgeon if a client does not void within 8 hours following surgery, unless another time frame is specified.

Anesthetic agents temporarily depress urinary bladder tone, which usually returns within 6 to 8 hours after surgery. Surgery in the pubic area, vagina, or rectum, during which the surgeon may manipulate the bladder, often causes urinary retention. If all measures to promote voiding fail, a urinary catheterization is often ordered. See Chapter 41. Measure the liquid intake and output of all clients with urinary catheters or other drainage devices. Generally I & O records are kept for at least 2 days and until the client reestablishes fluid balance without a catheter in place.

Pain Give analgesics *before* activities (eg, ambulation or meals) or rest periods (eg, at bedtime) and assess the effectiveness of the analgesics. Watch the client for signs indicating acute pain: pallor, perspiration, tension, and reluctance to perform deep-breathing and coughing exercises or to move or ambulate. Do not assume that the pain is caused by the incision (other causes include tight dressings, irritation from drainage tubes, or muscle strains resulting from positioning on the operating table).

Pain is usually greatest 12 to 36 hours after surgery, decreasing on the second or third day. Analgesics are usually administered every 3 or 4 hours the first day; by the third day most clients require only oral analgesics. Analgesics are also administered in infusions. Some may refuse to take analgesics on a regular schedule because they are not in severe pain. Inform the client that analgesics are most effective if given *before* pain becomes severe. Because tension increases pain perception and responses, provide comfort measures to relax the client (eg, back rubs, position changes, rest periods, and diverting activities).

Wound Care Inspect dressings regularly to ensure that they are clean, dry, and intact. Excessive drainage can indicate hemorrhage, infection, or dehiscence. See Table

45–2, page 1415. Change dressings, using sterile technique as required, when they are soiled with drainage or in accordance with the orders or agency protocol.

Maintain closed wound drainage (eg, the *Hemovac* is used to apply suction to wounds). See Chapter 44. Report wound separations promptly to the nurse in charge and the surgeon. If a large dehiscence or evisceration occurs, cover the wound with sterile, moist saline towels or dressings.

Suction The manner in which suction is applied to drainage tubes depends on the type of equipment available in the agency and the amount of suction required. The following are most commonly used:

- *Portable electric motor suction.* Portable electric units are plugged into wall outlets. They have an on-off switch, a motor that generates negative pressure, and a drainage bottle that needs to be monitored regularly to prevent overflow of drainage into the motor, which can cause irreparable damage to the apparatus.
- *Gomco thermotic pump.* The Gomco pump is electrically operated but consists of a pump rather than a motor. It provides intermittent suction by alternating the air pressure (ie, expanding and contracting the air). As the pressure alternates, red and green lights flash on and off. The amount of suction is regulated by a "high" or "low" pressure button. The pump is commonly used to suction gastrointestinal tubes.
- *Wall suction.* Some agencies have wall units with piped-in negative pressure available, consisting of a suction pressure regulator and a drainage receptacle, which needs to be checked regularly to prevent overflow.

Some clients return from surgery with a gastric or intestinal tube in place and orders to connect the tube to suction. For more information about gastrointestinal tubes, see Chapter 37. The suction ordered can be continuous or intermittent. Intermittent suctioning is less likely to harm the mucous membrane lining near the tip of the suction tube.

Nasogastric tubes are generally irrigated (a) before and after tube feedings or the installation of medications, and (b) as ordered to prevent clogging. Check agency policies. Nasogastric irrigation may require a physician's order. Excessive irrigation can lead to metabolic alkalosis.

Procedure 45–2 describes the management of gastrointestinal suction.

Text continued on page 1420

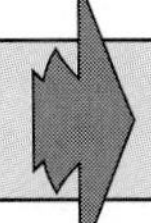

PROCEDURE 45–2 MANAGING GASTROINTESTINAL SUCTION

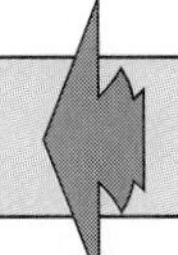

Before initiating gastric suction, determine (a) whether the suction is continuous or intermittent; (b) the ordered suction pressure (a low suction pressure is between 80 and 100 mm Hg, and a high pressure is between 100 and 120 mm Hg); and (c) whether there is an order to irrigate the gastrointestinal tube and, if so, the type of solution to use.

PURPOSES

- To relieve abdominal distention
- To maintain gastric decompression after surgery
- To remove blood and secretions from the gastrointestinal tract
- To relieve discomfort (ie, when a client has a bowel obstruction)
- To maintain the patency of the nasogastric tube

ASSESSMENT FOCUS

Presence of abdominal distention on palpation; auscultated bowel sounds; abdominal discomfort; vital signs for baseline data.

EQUIPMENT

Initiating Suction

- ☐ Gastrointestinal tube in place in the client
- ☐ Basin
- ☐ 50-mL syringe with an adapter
- ☐ Stethoscope
- ☐ Suction device for either continuous or intermittent suction
- ☐ Connector and connecting tubing
- ☐ Disposable gloves

Maintaining Suction

- ☐ Graduated container as required to measure gastric drainage
- ☐ Basin of water
- ☐ Cotton-tipped applicators
- ☐ Ointment or lubricant
- ☐ Disposable gloves

Irrigation

- ☐ Disposable gloves
- ☐ Stethoscope
- ☐ Disposable irrigating set containing a sterile 50-mL syringe, moisture-resistant pad, basin, and graduated container
- ☐ Sterile normal saline (500 mL) or the ordered solution

PROCEDURE 45–2 MANAGING GASTROINTESTINAL SUCTION *continued*

INTERVENTION

Initiating Suction

1. Position the client appropriately.

- Assist the client to semi-Fowler's position if it is not contraindicated because of health. *In semi-Fowler's position the tube is not as likely to lie against the wall of the stomach and will therefore suction most efficiently. Semi-Fowler's position also prevents reflux of gastric contents, which could lead to aspiration.*

2. Confirm that the tube is in the stomach.

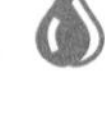

- Don gloves.
- Aspirate stomach contents and check their acidity.
- Insert air into the tube with the syringe and listen with a stethoscope over the stomach (just below the xiphoid process) for a swish of air.
- Use other methods in accordance with agency protocol. See Chapter 37, pages 1044 to 1045.

3. Set and check the suction.

- Adjust the suction machine for the recommended suction pressure, in accordance with agency policy or the physician's order. Some suctions are preset and cannot be adjusted. If using a Gomco thermotic pump, the suction is usually set on intermittent "low" suction for a single-lumen nasogastric tube or on "high" suction for a double-lumen nasogastric tube (eg, Salem sump tube).
- Turn on the suction machine and check that the suction is working. The Gomco thermotic drainage pump has a red indicator light in the middle of the front panel; it blinks continuously when the machine is functioning. When using other machines, test for proper suctioning by holding the open end of the suction tube to the nurse's ear. Suctioning is confirmed by a sucking noise.

4. Establish gastric suction.

- Connect the gastrointestinal tube to the tubing from the suction by using the connector.
- If a Salem sump tube is in place, connect the larger lumen to the suction equipment. This double-lumen tube has a smaller tube running inside the primary suction tube. *The smaller tube provides a continuous flow of atmospheric air through the drainage tube at its distal end and prevents excessive suction force on the gastric mucosa at the drainage outlets. Damage to the gastric mucosa is thus avoided.*

- Always keep the air vent tube of a Salem sump tube open when suction is applied. *Closing the vent would stop the sump action and cause mucosal damage.*
- After suction is applied, watch the tubing for a few minutes until the gastric contents appear to be running through the tubing into the receptacle. A Salem sump tube makes a soft, hissing sound when it is functioning correctly.
- If the suction is not working properly, check that the rubber stopper in the collection bottle and all tubing connections are tightly sealed and that the tubing is not kinked.
- Coil and pin the tubing on the bed so that it does not loop below the suction bottle. *If the tubing falls below the suction bottle, the suction may be obstructed because of the pressure required to push the fluid against gravity.*

5. Assess the drainage.

- Observe the amount, color, odor, and consistency of the drainage. Normal gastric drainage has a mucoid consistency and is either colorless or yellow-green because of the presence of bile. A coffee-grounds color and consistency may indicate bleeding.
- Test the gastric drainage for pH and blood (by using Hematest) when indicated. A person who has had gastrointestinal surgery can be expected to have some blood in the drainage.

Maintaining Suction

6. Assess the client and the suction system regularly.

- Assess the client every 30 minutes until the system is running effectively and then every 2 hours, or as the client's health indicates, to ensure that the suction is functioning properly. If the client complains of fullness, nausea, or epigastric pain or if the flow of gastric secretions is absent in the tubing or in the collection bottle, ineffective suctioning or blockage of the nasogastric tube is likely.
- Inspect the suction system for patency of the system (eg, kinks or blockages in the tubing) and tightness of the connections. *Loose connections can permit air to enter and thus decrease the effectiveness of the suction by decreasing the negative pressure.*

7. Relieve blockages if present.

- Don gloves.
- Milk the suction tubing.
- Check the suction equipment. To do this, disconnect the nasogastric tube from the suction over a collecting basin (to collect gastric drainage), and then, with the suc-

PROCEDURE 45–2 ***continued***

tion on, place the end of the suction tubing in a basin of water. If water is drawn into the drainage bottle, the suction equipment is functioning properly, but the nasogastric tube is either blocked or positioned incorrectly.

- Reposition the client (eg, to the other side) if permitted. *This may facilitate drainage.*
- Rotate the nasogastric tube, and reposition it. This step is contraindicated for clients with gastric surgery. *Moving the tube may interfere with gastric sutures.*

- Irrigate the nasogastric tube as agency protocol states or on the order of the physician. See steps 11 to 13.

8. Prevent reflux into the vent lumen of a Salem sump tube. Reflux of gastric contents into the vent lumen may occur when stomach pressure exceeds atmospheric pressure. In this situation gastric contents follow the path of least resistance and flow out the vent lumen rather than the drainage lumen. To prevent reflux

- Place the vent tubing above the client's midline. *A vent lumen placed below the midline acts as a siphon and allows gastric contents to flow through the air vent lumen.*
- Always keep the drainage receptacle below the client's midline. *A drainage receptacle placed above midline and the fluid level in the client's stomach will cause reflux of gastric contents through the air vent lumen.* To avoid reflux when wall suction units are used, place the drainage container on the side of the bed or on the floor and attach a connecting tube from the drainage container to the wall outlet.
- Keep the drainage lumen free of particulate matter that may obstruct the lumen. See irrigating a nasogastric tube in steps 11 to 13.

9. Ensure client comfort.

- Clean the client's nostrils every 3 hours or as needed, using the cotton-tipped applicators and water. Apply a water-soluble lubricant or ointment.

- Provide mouth care every 3 hours as needed. Some postoperative clients are permitted to suck ice chips or a moist cloth to maintain the moisture of the oral mucous membranes.

10. Empty the drainage receptacle every 8 hours, or whenever it becomes three-quarters full.

- Clamp the nasogastric tube, and turn off the suction.
- Don gloves.
- If the receptacle is graduated, determine the amount of drainage.
- Disconnect the receptacle.
- If not already measured, empty the contents into a graduated container and measure.
- Inspect the drainage carefully for color, consistency, and presence of substances (eg, blood clots).
- Rinse the receptacle with warm water.
- Reattach the receptacle to the suction.
- Turn on the suction and unclamp the nasogastric tube.
- Observe the system for several minutes to make sure function is reestablished.
- Go to step 14.

Irrigating a Gastrointestinal Tube

11. Prepare the client and the equipment.

- Place the moisture-resistant pad under the end of the gastrointestinal tube.
- Turn off the suction.
- Don gloves.
- Disconnect the gastrointestinal tube from the connector.
- Determine that the tube is in the stomach. See step 2 above and Chapter 37, page 1045. *This ensures that the irrigating solution enters the client's stomach.*

12. Irrigate the tube.

- Draw up the ordered volume of irrigating solution in the syringe; 30 mL of solution per instillation is usual, but up to 60 mL may be given per instillation if ordered.
- Attach the syringe to the nasogastric tube, and slowly inject the solution.

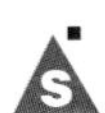

- Gently aspirate the solution. *Forceful withdrawal could damage the gastric mucosa.*
- If you encounter difficulty in withdrawing the solution, inject 20 mL of air and aspirate again, and/or reposition the client or the nasogastric tube. *Air and repositioning may move the end of the tube away from the stomach wall.* If aspirating difficulty continues, reattach the tube in intermittent low suction, and notify the nurse in charge or physician.
- Repeat the above steps until the ordered amount of solution is used.
- Note: A Salem sump tube can also be irrigated through the vent lumen without interrupting suction. However, only small quantities of irrigant can be injected via this lumen compared to the drainage lumen.

PROCEDURE 45–2 MANAGING GASTROINTESTINAL SUCTION *continued*

- After irrigating a Salem sump tube, inject 10 to 20 mL of air into the vent lumen while applying suction to the drainage lumen. *This tests the patency of the vent and ensures sump functioning.*

13. Reestablish suction.

- Reconnect the nasogastric tube to suction.
- If a Salem sump tube is used, inject the air vent lumen with 10 mL of air after reconnecting the tube to suction.
- Observe the system for several minutes to make sure it is functioning.

14. Document all relevant information.

- Record the time suction was started. Also record the pressure established, the color and consistency of the drainage, and nursing assessments.
- During maintenance, record assessments, supportive nursing measures, and data about the suction system.
- When irrigating the tube, record verification of tube placement; the time of the irrigation; the amount and type of irrigating solution used; the amount, color and consistency of the returns; the patency of the system following the irrigation; and nursing assessments.

EVALUATION FOCUS
Relief of abdominal distention or discomfort; bowel sounds; character and amount of gastric drainage; integrity of nares; hydration of oral mucous membranes; patency of tube; system functioning.

EVALUATING

To evaluate goal achievement and the effectiveness of nursing interventions, the nurse collects data related to the outcome criteria. Data collection for the postoperative client may include the following:

- Measurement of vital signs and fluid intake and output
- Auscultation of the lungs for breath sounds and the abdomen for bowel sounds
- Inspection of the client's wound and urine
- Observing the client when performing deep-breathing, coughing, and leg exercises
- Asking the client about problems with pain, voiding, defecation, or sleep
- Observing how well the client performs activities
- Performing other specific assessments, such as testing tissue turgor or testing for the presence of Homans' sign.

The following are examples of evaluative statements: "Bilateral lung sounds are clear"; "Wound is dry, with only slight inflammation around suture line"; "Client states, 'I can get out of bed more easily today—my stomach isn't as sore.' "

CRITICAL PATHWAY FOR GEORGE HANSEN

ASSESSMENT DATA

Nursing Assessment
George Hansen is a 22-year-old college student who was admitted to the surgical unit with a diagnosis of appendicitis. He was in good health until about 3 days ago, when he started experiencing nausea, anorexia, and vague abdominal discomfort. He was brought to the emergency department by his roommate today with pain in the right lower quadrant. He has been scheduled for an appendectomy later today. He has been medicated with meperidine 75 mg IM for pain. His abdomen has been shaved and prepped for surgery. Mr Hansen has never been hospitalized and expresses concern about the operation. He asks the nurse if he will be asleep during the procedure and if there will be much pain afterward. He is drowsy but startles easily and appears anxious. He asks the nurse to stay with him.

Physical Examination
Height: 188 cm (6′2″)
Weight: 68.2 kg (150 lb)
Temperature: 37.2 C (99.6 F)
Pulse rate: 92 bpm
Respirations: 26 per minute
Blood pressure: 122/84 mm Hg

Diagnostic Data
Hgb: 16g/dL
Hct: 48%
WBC: 18,000/µL
Urine: normal

Critical Pathway for Client Following Appendectomy

Expected length of stay 3 days following surgery

	Date ________ Preoperative day	Date ________ 1st Postoperative day
Daily outcomes	Client ▪ verbalizes understanding of preoperative teaching including turning, coughing, deep breathing, incentive spirometer, mobilization, possible tubes (Nasogastric tube [NG] and intravenous), pain management (PCA or prn medications). ▪ verbalizes ability to cope.	Client will ▪ be afebrile. ▪ have clean, dry wound with edges well-approximated, healing by first intention. ▪ recover from anesthesia as evidenced by: VS return to baseline, awake, alert, and oriented. ▪ verbalize understanding and demonstrate cooperation with turning, coughing, deep breathing, and splinting. ▪ tolerate ordered diet without nausea and vomiting. ▪ verbalize control of incisional pain. ▪ verbalize ability to cope.
Tests and treatments	CBC. Urinalysis. Emergency surgery. Baseline physical assessment: with a focus on respiratory status and gastrointestinal function.	CBC. Electrolytes if on NG suction. Vital signs and O_2 saturation, neurovascular assessment, dressing and wound drainage assessment q15min × 4; q30min × 4; q1h × 4; and then q4h if stable. Assess respiratory status and gastrointestinal function q4h and prn. Incentive spirometer q2h. Intake and output q shift. Assess voiding: if unable to void, try suggestive voiding techniques or catheterize q8h or prn if still unable to void.
Knowledge deficit	Orient to room and surroundings. Provide simple, brief instructions. Review preoperative preparation including hospital and surgical routines. Discuss surgery and specific postoperative care: turning, coughing, deep breathing, incentive spirometer, mobilization, possible tubes (Nasogastric tube [NG] and intravenous), pain management (PCA or prn medications).	Reorient to room and postoperative routine. Review plan of care and importance of early mobilization. Begin discharge teaching regarding wound care/dressing change.
Psycho-social	Assess anxiety related to diagnosis and pending surgery. Assess fears of the unknown and surgery. Encourage verbalization of concerns. Provide information regarding surgical experience. Minimize external stimuli (eg, noise, movement).	Assess level of anxiety. Encourage verbalization of concerns. Provide information. Provide ongoing support and encouragement.

➤

	Preoperative day *continued*	**1st Postoperative day** *continued*
Diet	NPO. Baseline nutritional assessment.	Advance to clear liquids, if NG not ordered or discontinued.
Activity	Provide safety precautions. Bedrest or bathroom privileges with assistance.	Provide safety precautions. Bathroom privileges with assistance. Ambulate 4 times with assistance.
Medications	After diagnosis made: IM or IV analgesics IV fluids	IM or IV/PCA analgesics IV antibiotics IV fluid or intermittent IV device
Transfer/ discharge plans	Assess discharge plans and support system at college or home.	Determine needs at time of discharge. Begin home care teaching.

	Date ________ **2d Postoperative day**	**Date ________** **3d Postoperative day**
Daily outcomes	Client will ▪ be afebrile. ▪ have clean, dry wound with edges well-approximated, healing by first intention. ▪ demonstrate cooperation with turning, coughing, deep breathing, and splinting. ▪ tolerate ordered diet without nausea and vomiting. ▪ ambulate 4 times per day. ▪ verbalize control of incisional pain. ▪ verbalize ability to cope. ▪ verbalize beginning understanding of home care instructions.	Client ▪ is afebrile. ▪ has a dry, clean wound with edges well-approximated, healing by first intention. ▪ manages pain with nonpharmacologic measures. ▪ is independent in self-care. ▪ is fully ambulatory. ▪ has resumed preadmission urine and bowel elimination pattern. ▪ verbalizes home care instructions. ▪ tolerates usual diet. ▪ verbalizes ability to cope with ongoing stressors.
Tests and treatments	Vital signs and dressing and wound drainage assessment q4h. Assess respiratory status and gastrointestinal function q4h. Incentive spirometer q2h until fully ambulatory. Intake and output shift. Assess voiding pattern q shift.	Vital signs, dressing and wound drainage assessment q4h. Assess respiratory status and gastrointestinal function.
Knowledge deficit	Initiate discharge teaching regarding wound care, diet, and activity. Review written discharge instructions.	Complete discharge teaching to include wound care, diet, follow-up care, signs and symptoms to report, activity, and medications: dose, frequency, route, and side effects. Provide client with written discharge instructions.

	2d Postoperative day *continued*	**3d Postoperative day** *continued*
Psycho-social	Encourage verbalization of concerns. Provide ongoing support and encouragement.	Encourage verbalization of concerns. Provide ongoing support and encouragement.
Diet	If tolerating clear liquids or NG removal, advance diet to full liquids to regular diet to tolerance.	Regular diet as tolerated.
Activity	Provide safety precautions. Ambulate independently at least 4 times.	Fully ambulatory.
Medications	PO analgesics IV antibiotics Intermittent IV device	PO analgesics D/C intermittent IV device
Transfer/ discharge plans	Complete discharge plans. Continue home care instructions.	Complete discharge instructions.

CHAPTER HIGHLIGHTS

- Surgery is a unique human experience that creates stress and necessitates physical and psychologic changes.
- The perioperative period includes three phases: preoperative, intraoperative, and postoperative.
- Surgical procedures are categorized by degree of urgency, degree of risk, and purpose.
- Anesthesia may be general or regional. Regional anesthesia includes topical, local, nerve block, intravenous block, spinal anesthesia (subarachnoid block), and epidural.
- Clients must agree to surgery and sign an informed consent.
- Nurses should assess the risk factors prior to a client's surgery whenever possible.
- Nursing history data are an important source for planning preoperative and postoperative care.
- Preoperative nursing interventions to prepare the client for surgery and the postoperative period include preoperative teaching, physical preparation, and promoting the client's peace of mind.
- Preoperative teaching should include moving, leg exercises, and coughing and deep-breathing exercises. Many aspects of preoperative teaching are intended to prevent postoperative complications.
- Physical preparation includes the following areas: nutrition and fluids, elimination, hygiene, rest, medications, care of valuables and prostheses, special orders, and surgical skin preparation.
- Antiemboli stockings may be required by some clients to facilitate venous return.
- A surgical skin preparation should be carried out as close to the time of surgery as possible and is commonly performed during the intraoperative phase.
- A preoperative checklist provides a guide to and documentation of a client's preparation before surgery.
- Immediate postanesthetic care focuses on assessment and monitoring parameters to prevent complications from anesthesia or surgery.

- Ongoing postoperative care includes many of the same assessments conducted in the PAR and interventions designed to promote client recovery and prevent complications.
- Ongoing postoperative interventions include (a) appropriate client positioning, (b) encouraging deep-breathing and coughing exercises, (c) leg exercises, (d) early ambulation, (e) adequate hydration, (f) diet, (g) promoting urinary elimination, (h) administering analgesics, and (i) wound care.

READINGS AND REFERENCES

SUGGESTED READINGS

Cahill-Wright, C. December 1991. Managing postoperative pain. *Nursing91* 21:42–45.

Cahill-Wright writes about the personal experience of pain and provides pain assessment guidelines. The positive and negative aspects of narcotics are discussed together with the importance of timing for pain control.

Lawler, M. November 1991. Managing other complications beyond the respiratory system. *Nursing91* 21:40–46.

The author writes that perioperative medications and physical and emotional stress can put a client at risk of many different complications. Problems of central nervous system, cardiovascular system, gastrointestinal system, and renal system are included.

RELATED RESEARCH

Raleigh, EH, Lepcyzyk, M, and Rowley, C. August 1990. Significant others benefit from preoperative information. *Journal of Advanced Nursing* 15:841–45.

Yount, ST, Edgell, Sr, J, and Jakovec, V. February 1990. Preoperative teaching: A study of nurses' perceptions. *AORN Journal* 51:572, 574–75, 577–79.

REFERENCES

Association of Operating Room Nurses. November 1992. Recommended practices: Skin preparation of patients. *AORN Journal* 56:937–41.

———. 1993. *AORN Standards and Recommended Practices for Perioperative Nursing.* Denver: Association of Operating Room Nurses, Inc.

Erickson, R. July 1982. Tube talk principles of fluid flow in tubes. *Nursing82* 12:54–61.

Fairchild, SS. 1993. *Perioperative Nursing: Principles and Practice.* Boston: Jones & Bartlett.

Garner, JS. April 1986. CDC guidelines for the prevention and control of nosocomial infections: Guideline for prevention of surgical wound infections, 1985. *American Journal of Infection Control* 14:71–80.

Jackson, MF. October 1989. Implications of surgery in very elderly patients. *AORN Journal* 50:859, 862–64, 866.

Kam, BW and Werner, PW. May 1990. Self-care theory: Application to perioperative nursing. *AORN Journal* 51:1365–67.

Kneedler, JA and Dodge, GH. 1994. *Perioperative Patient Care: The Nursing Perspective*, 3d ed. Boston: Jones & Bartlett.

Leckrone, L. July 1991. Preparing your patient for surgery. *Nursing91* 21:46–49.

Lierman, J. February 1988. Preoperative assessment: Can we afford to do without them? *AORN Journal* 47:586, 588, 590.

McConnell, EA. September 1975. All about gastrointestinal intubation. *Nursing75* 5:30–37.

———. March 1977. After surgery. *Nursing77* 7:32–39.

———. September 1977. Ensuring safer stomach suctioning with a Salem sump tube. *Nursing77* 7:54–57.

———. April 1979. Ten problems with nasogastric tubes . . . and how to solve them. *Nursing79* 9:78–81.

Mott, SR, James, SR, and Sperhac, AM. 1990. *Nursing Care of Children and Families*, 2d ed. Redwood City, CA: Addison-Wesley Nursing.

Page, SM and Beresford, LA. February 1988. Planning and documentation: Addressing patient needs in a day surgery setting. *AORN Journal* 47:526, 528, 530, 532–35, 537.

Reeder, JM. December 1989. Ethical dilemmas in perioperative nursing practice. *Nursing Clinics of North America* 24:999–1007.

APPENDICES

A Nursing Organizations
B ANA Human Rights Guidelines for Research

STUDENT GALLERY

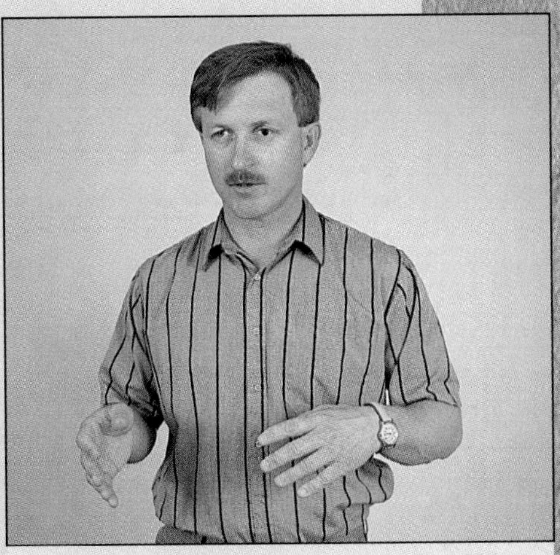

Ted Woirhaye
University of Nebraska
Omaha, Nebraska

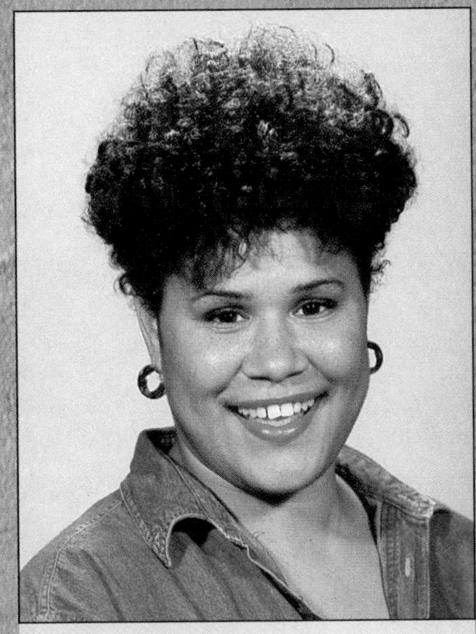

Beryl Hocke
James Cook University
Townsville, Australia

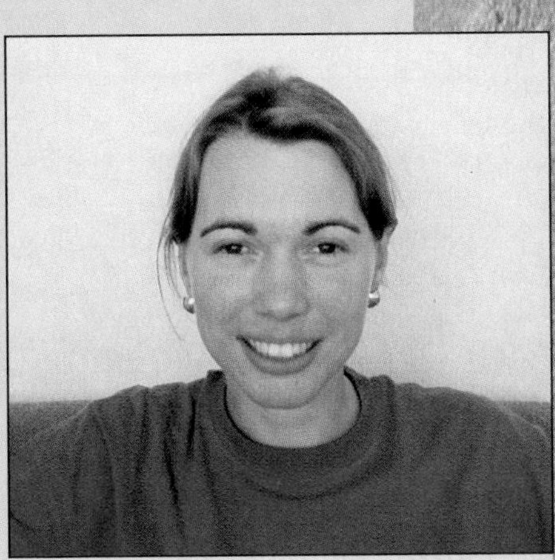

Lesley Blake
Berkshire College of Nursing and Midwifery
England, UK

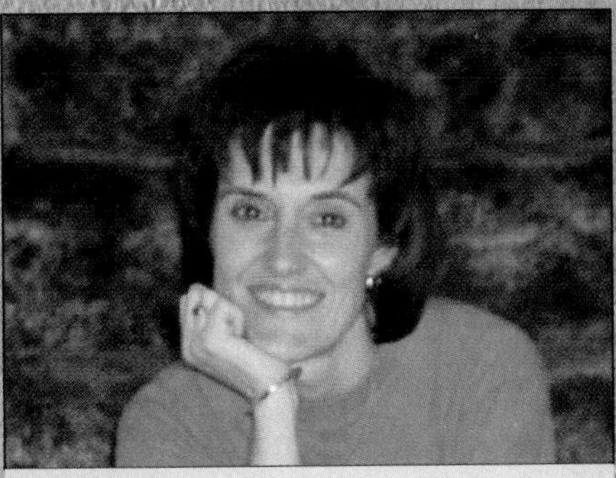

Karen Whiting
Mohawk College
Hamilton, Ontario, Canada

Appendix A

Nursing Organizations and Publications

International

Organization	Publications
International Committee of Catholic Nurses 43, Square Vergote 1040 Brussels, Belgium	
International Council of Nurses (ICN) 3, place Jean-Marteau 1201 Geneva, Switzerland	*International Nursing Review*
North American Nursing Diagnosis Association (NANDA) St Louis University Department of Nursing 3525 Caroline St. St Louis, MO 63104	*Nursing Diagnosis*
Sigma Theta Tau International Honor Society of Nursing 550 W. North St. Indianapolis, Indiana 46202	*Image: Journal of Nursing Scholarship; Reflections*
World Federation of Neurosurgical Nurses Avenue Appia 1211 Geneva 27 Switzerland	
World Health Organization (WHO) Avenue Appia 1211 Geneva 27, Switzerland	

United States

Related to Scholarship

Organization	Publications
Alpha Tau Delta 14631 N. 2nd Dr. Phoenix, AZ 85023	*Captions of Alpha Tau Delta*
American Academy of Nursing (AAN) 600 Maryland Ave. SW Suite 100 West Washington, DC 20024-2671	*Nursing Outlook*
Sigma Theta Tau (see above)	

Related to Ethnic Origin

Organization	Publications
American Indian Nurses Association (AINA) PO Box 1588 Norman, OK 73071	*Newsletter of the AINA*
National Association of Hispanic Nurses 1501 Sixteenth St. NW Washington, DC 20036	*Newsletter*
National Black Nurses Association, Inc. 1012 Tenth St. NW Washington, DC 20001	*Journal of National Black Nurses Association*

General

Organization	Publications
American Nurses Association (ANA) 600 Maryland Ave. SW Suite 100 West Washington, DC 20024-2671	*American Journal of Nursing; The American Nurse*
Committee on Nursing of the Catholic Hospital Association 1438 S. Grand Blvd. St Louis, MO 63104	
National Center for Nursing Ethics PO Box 2237 Cincinnati, OH 45201	
National League for Nursing (NLN) 350 Hudson St. New York, NY 10014	*Nursing and Health Care*
National Student Nurses Association (NSNA) 555 W. 57th St. New York, NY 10019	*Imprint*

Related to Occupation or Specialty

Organization	Publications
American Association of Critical Care Nurses (AACN) 101 Columbia Aliso Viejo, CA 92656-1491	*Heart and Lung*

Organization	Publications
American Association for the History of Nursing PO Box 90803 Washington, DC 20090-0803	*The Bulletin*
American Association of Neuroscience Nurses (AANN) 224 N. Des Plaines Suite 601 Chicago, IL 60661	*Journal of Neuroscience Nursing*
American Association of Nurse Anesthetists (AANA) 222 S. Prospect Ave. Park Ridge, IL 60068-4001	*American Association of Nurse Anesthetists Journal*
American Association of Occupational Health Nurses 50 Lenox Pointe Atlanta, GA 30324	*AAOHN Journal; AAOH News*
American Burn Association Burn Treatment Center Crozier-Chester Medical Center 15th and Upland Ave. Chester, PA 19013	
American College of Nurse-Midwives (ACNM) 1522 K St. Suite 1000 Washington, DC 20005	*Journal of Nurse Midwifery*
American Geriatric Society Room 1470 10 Columbus Circle New York, NY 10019	
American Holistic Nurses Association 4101 Lake Boone Tr. Suite 201 Raleigh, NC 27607	*Journal of Holistic Nursing; Beginnings*
American Nephrology Nurses Association (ANNA) N. Woodbury Rd. Box 56 Pitman, NJ 08071	
American Public Health Association Public Health Nursing Section 1015 15th St. NW Washington, DC 20005	*American Journal of Public Health; The Nation's Health*
American Radiological Nurses Association c/o E. Deutsch 502 Forest Court Carrboro, NC 27510	*ARNA Images*
American Society of Ophthalmic Registered Nurses (ASORN) PO Box 193030 San Francisco, CA 94119	*Insight*
American Society of Plastic and Reconstructive Surgical Nurses N. Woodbury Rd. Box 56 Pitman, NJ 08071	*Journal of Plastic and Reconstructive Surgical Nursing*
American Society of Post-Anesthesia Nurses (ASPAN) 11512 Allecingie Pkwy. Richmond, VA 23235	*Breathline; Journal of Post-Anesthesia Nursing*
American Urological Association Allied 11512 Allecingie Pkwy. Richmond, VA 23235	*Urologic Nursing*
Association of Operating Room Nurses, Inc. (AORN) 2170 S. Parker Rd. Suite 300 Denver, CO 80231-5711	*AORN Journal*
Association of Pediatric Oncology Nurses (APON) 11512 Allecingie Pkwy. Richmond, VA 23235	*APON Newsletter*
Association for Practitioners in Infection Control 505 E. Hawley St. Mundelein, IL 60060	
Association of Rehabilitation Nurses 5700 Old Orchard Rd., 1st fl. Skokie, IL 60077-1057	*Rehabilitation Nursing*
Dermatology Nurses Association N. Woodbury Rd. Box 56 Pitman, NJ 08071	*DNA Focus*
Drug and Alcohol Nursing Association Box 92 Lonely Cottage Dr. Upper Black Eddy, PA 18972	*DANA Newsletter*
Emergency Nurses Association (ENA) 216 Higgins Rd. Park Ridge, IL 60068	
Flight Nurse Section Aerospace Medical Association Washington National Airport Washington, DC 20001	

Organization	Publications
International Association for Enterostomal Therapy 1701 Lake Avenue Glenview, IL 60025	*Journal of Enterostomal Therapy*
National Association of Neonatal Nurses 1304 Southpoint Blvd. Suite 280 Petaluma, CA 94954-6859	*Neonatal Network: The Journal of Neonatal Nursing*
National Association of Orthopedic Nurses N. Woodbury Rd. Box 56 Pitman, NJ 08071	*Orthopedic Nursing*
National Association of Pediatric Nurse Associates and Practitioners (NAPNAP) 1101 Kings Hwy. North Suite 206 Cherry Hill, NJ 08034	*The Pediatric Nurse Practitioner*
National Association of School Nurses, Inc. Lamplighter Lane PO Box 1300 Scarborough, ME 04074	*School Nurse Journal*
National Flight Nurses Association 6900 Grove Rd. Thorofare, NJ 08086	*Aeromedical Journal*
National Intravenous Therapy Association 87 Blanchard Rd. Cambridge, MA 02138	*NITA Journal; NITA Update*
National Organization for Associate Degree Nursing 11250 Roger Bacon Drive, Suite 8 Reston, VA 22090	
Nurses Association of the American College of Obstetricians and Gynecologists 409 12th St. SW Washington, DC 20024-2191	
Oncology Nursing Society 501 Holiday Dr. Pittsburgh, PA 15220	*Oncology Nursing Forum*
Society for Peripheral Vascular Nursing PO Box 11356 Baltimore, MD 21239	*SPVN Journal*
Transcultural Nursing Society College of Nursing & Health Madonna University 36600 Schoolcraft Rd. Livonia, MI 48150	*Journal of Transcultural Nursing*

Miscellaneous

Organization	Publications
The American Assembly for Men in Nursing PO Box 31753 Independence, OH 44131	
Gay Nurses Alliance PO Box 530 Back Bay Annex Boston, MA 02117	
National Male Nurses Association 2308 State St. Saginaw, MI 48602	
National Nurses for Life 1998 Menold Allison Park, PA 15104	
Nurses Christian Fellowship 6400 Schroeder Rd. PO Box 7895 Madison, WI 53707-7895	*Journal of Christian Nursing*
Nurses' Environmental Health Watch, Inc. 181 Marshall St. Duxbury, MA 03443	
Nurses House, Inc. 350 Hudson St. New York, NY 10014	

CANADIAN

Organization	Publications
Canadian Association of Critical Care Nurses (CACCN) 73 Pembroke St. West Pembroke, Ontario K8A 5M5	*Canadian Critical Care Journal*
Canadian Association of Enterostomal Therapy (CAET) Ottawa General Hospital 50 The Driveway Ottawa, Ontario K2P 1E2	
Canadian Association of Nephrology Nurses and Technicians 2175 Sheppard Ave. East Suite 110 Willowdale, Ontario M2J 1W8	

Organization	Publications
Canadian Council of Cardiovascular Nurses c/o Heart Stroke Foundation 160 George St. Suite 200 Ottawa, Ontario K1N 9M2	*Canadian Journal of Cardiovascular Nursing*
Canadian Gerontological Nursing Association PO Box 368 Postal Station K Toronto, Ontario M4P 2G7	*Perspectives*
Canadian Intravenous Nurses Association 200-4433 Sheppard Ave. East Agincourt, Ontario M1S 1V3	*Canadian Intravenous Nurses Association Journal*
Canadian Nurses Association 50 The Driveway Ottawa, Ontario K2P 1E2	*The Canadian Nurse*
Canadian Nurses Foundation 50 The Driveway Ottawa, Ontario K2P 1E2	
Canadian Nurses Respiratory Society Nurses Section Canadian Lung Association 908-75 Albert Street Ottawa, Ontario K1P 5E7	
Canadian Orthopedic Nurses Association 43 Wellesley St. East Toronto, Ontario M4Y 1H1	*CONA Journal ACIIO*
Canadian University Nursing Students Association School of Nursing Université de Montréal C.P. 6128 Montreal, Quebec H3T 1J4	
Dynamics of Critical Care Association of Canada CNSC 200-4433 Sheppard Ave. East Agincourt, Ontario M1S 1V3	
Operating Room Nurses Association of Canada 213-52377 Range Rd. Sherwood Park, Alberta T8G 1B9	*Canadian Operating Room Nurse Journal*
Psychiatric Nurses Association of Canada 1854 Portage Ave. Winnipeg, Manitoba R3J 0G9	*Canadian Journal of Psychiatric Nursing*
Registered Nurses of Canadian Indian Ancestry 500-275 Portage Ave. Winnipeg, Manitoba R3B 2B3	
TPN Nurses Association of Canada PO Box 62 Station K Toronto, Ontario M4P 2G1	

Appendix B

American Nurses Association Human Rights Guidelines for Nurses in Clinical and Other Research

The guidelines in this table attempt to specify several important entities: (1) the type of activities involved, (2) the rights to be protected, (3) the persons to be safeguarded, and (4) the mechanisms necessary to ensure that protection is adequate.

Guideline 1: Employment in Settings Where Research Is Conducted

Conditions of employment in settings in which clinical or other research is in progress need to be spelled out in detail for all potential workers. . . . Anyone employed in work that carries the potential of risk to others needs to be advised as to the types of risks involved, the ways of recognizing when risk is present, and the proper actions to take to counteract harmful effects and unnecessary danger.

Guideline 2: Nurses' Responsibilities for Vigilant Protection of Human Subjects' Rights

In all instances the prospective subject must be given all relevant information prior to participation in activities that go beyond established and accepted procedures necessary to meet the subject's personal needs. . . . Nurses must be increasingly vigilant in their concern for subjects and patients who by reason of their situation and/or illness are not able to protect themselves effectively from externally imposed threat or injury. They must be sensitive to the tendency toward exploitation of "captive" populations such as students, patients, and inmates in institutions and prisons. All proposals to be used need to be discussed with the prospective subject and with any worker who is expected to participate as a subject or data collector or both. Special mechanisms must be developed to safeguard the confidentiality of information and protect human dignity.

Guideline 3: Scope of Application

The persons to whom these human rights guidelines apply include all individuals involved in research activities and include the following groups: patients, donors of organs and tissue, informants, normal volunteers including students, and vulnerable populations that are "captive" audiences, such as the mentally disordered, mentally retarded, and prisoners.

Guideline 4: Nurses' Responsibility to Support the Accrual of Knowledge

Just as nurses have an obligation to protect the human rights of patients, so do they also have an obligation to support the accrual of knowledge that broadens the scientific underpinnings of nursing practice and the delivery of nursing services.

Guideline 5: Informed Consent

To safeguard the basic rights of self-determination, nurses must obtain consent from the prospective subject or the subject's legal representative to participate in research of unusual clinical activities. The subject needs to receive:

- A description of any benefit to the subject or the development of new knowledge that might be expected
- An offer to discuss or answer any questions about the study
- A clear statement to the subject that the subject is free to discontinue participation at any time the subject wishes to do so
- Full freedom from direct or indirect coercion and deception

Guideline 6: Representation on Human Subjects Committee

There is increasing public support for systematic accountability to ensure that individual rights are not denied to human subjects who participate in research studies. In most instances, the protective mechanism takes place through a committee judged competent to review studies and other investigative activities that involve human subjects. The profession of nursing has an obligation to publicly support the inclusion of nurses as regular members of institutional review committees of this kind.

Source: Adapted and summarized with permission from the American Nurses Association, *Human Rights Guidelines for Nurses in Clinical and Other Research* (ANA Publication No. D-46 5M 7/75, 1975). Also found in ANA, *Guidelines in Nursing Research* (Kansas City, MO: ANA, 1975).

Glossary

Abdominal paracentesis removal of fluids from the peritoneal cavity

Abduction movement of a bone away from the midline of the body

Abortion termination of a pregnancy before the fetus reaches the stage of viability, may be accidental, spontaneous, or induced

Abrasion wearing away of a structure, such as the skin or teeth

Abscess a localized collection of pus and disintegrating body tissues

Acapnia a decreased level of carbon dioxide in the blood

Accountable (accountability) being responsible for one's actions and accepting the consequences of one's behavior

Accreditation the process by which a voluntary organization or governmental agency appraises and grants accredited status to institutions, programs, or services that meet predetermined criteria

Acculturation (assimilation) (of a group) the blending of attitudes and beliefs; process by which members of a foreign culture learn the values and behaviors of a culture to which they have immigrated

Acholic clay colored and free from bile

Acidosis (acidemia) a condition that occurs with increases in blood carbonic acid or with decreases in blood bicarbonate; blood pH below 7.35

Acne an inflammatory condition of the sebaceous glands

Acromegaly a disorder caused by excessive growth hormone secretion

Active assistive range-of-motion (ROM) exercise the client with the nurse's assistance uses a stronger, opposite arm or leg to move each of the joints of a limb incapable of active motion

Active immunity a resistance of the body to infection in which the host produces its own antibodies in response to natural or artificial antigens

Active range-of-motion (ROM) exercise isotonic exercise in which the client moves each joint in the body through its complete range of movement, maximally stretching all muscle groups within each plane, over the joint

Active transport movement of substances across cell membranes against the concentration gradient

Acupuncture a Chinese practice of piercing specific superficial nerves with needles, often to treat pain

Acute sharp or severe; describing a severe condition with a sudden onset and short course (as opposed to chronic)

Adaptation the process of modifying to meet new, changing, or different conditions

Adaptive behavior the responses by which the whole person copes with internal and external environmental stimuli

Adaptive mechanisms learned behaviors that assist an individual to adjust to the environment

Adduction movement of a bone toward the midline of the body

Adherent (cohesive) sticking together, clinging

Adhesion a fibrous band or structure by which parts are abnormally held together

Adipose fat; of a fatty nature

ADLs, activities of daily living the tasks of daily life, such as eating, bathing and dressing

Advance medical directive a statement the client makes prior to receiving health care specifying the client's wishes regarding health care decisions

Adventitious breath sounds abnormal or acquired breath sounds

Advocate an individual who pleads the cause of another or argues or pleads for a cause or proposal

Aerobic requiring oxygen

Aerobic exercise any activity during which the body takes in more or an equal amount of oxygen than it expends

Affect feelings, emotions

Agglutination the process of clumping together

Agglutinin a specific antibody formed in the blood

Agglutinogen a substance that acts as an antigen and stimulates the production of agglutinins

Agnostic a person who doubts the existence of God or a supreme being or believes the existence of God has not been proved

Agonist a drug that interacts with a receptor to produce a response

AIDS (acquired immune deficiency syndrome) an immunodeficiency syndrome which is caused by the human immunodeficiency virus (HIV) and results in the high susceptibility to opportunistic infections (eg, pneumocycstic carinii pneumonia [PCP]), malignancies (eg, Kaposi's sarcoma), and neurologic disorders (eg, leukoencephalopathy)

Albinism the complete or partial lack of melanin in the skin, hair, and eyes

Albumin the main protein found in the blood, also found in breast milk

Albuminuria the presence of albumin in the urine

Algor mortis the gradual decrease of the body's temperature after death

Alignment (posture) the proper relationship of body segments to one another

Alkalosis (alkalemia) a condition that occurs with increases in blood bicarbonate or decreases in blood carbonic acid; blood pH above 7.45

Alopecia the loss of scalp hair (baldness) or body hair

Alternating pressure mattress (airbed) a specialized mattress which is attached to a motor that lowers or raises the air pressure inside the mattress, designed to decrease pressure on bony prominences

Alzheimer's disease a progressive, chronic, organic mental disorder

AMA (against medical authority) when a client leaves the agency without permission of the physician

Amblyopia reduced visual acuity in one eye

Ambu bag (resuscitation bag) a device used to provide oxygen to a client when they are unable to breathe for themselves

Ambulation the act of walking

Ampule a small glass container for individual doses of liquid medications

Anabolism a process in which simple substances are converted by the body cells into more complex substances (eg, building tissue, positive nitrogen balance)

Anaerobe an organism that does not require oxygen to live

Anaerobic not requiring oxygen to live

Analgesic a medication used to alter the perception and interpretation of pain

Anal intercourse a type of genital intercourse in which the penis is inserted into the anus

Anaphylaxis (anaphylactic shock, anaphylactic reaction) a severe allergic reaction

Anemia a condition in which the blood is deficient in red blood cells or hemoglobin

Aneroid containing no liquid

Anesthesia loss of sensation or feeling; induced loss of the sense of pain

Aneurysm dilation or outpouching of the wall of an artery or vein

Angiography a diagnostic procedure enabling X-ray visual examination of the vascular system after injection of a radiopaque dye

Anion ion which carries a negative charge; chloride, bicarbonate, phosphate, sulfate

Anisocoria unequal pupils

Ankylosis permanent fixation of a joint

Anorexia lack of appetite

Anorexia nervosa a disease characterized by a prolonged inability or refusal to eat, rapid weight loss, and emaciation in persons who continue to believe they are fat

Anoscopy visual examination of the anal canal using an anoscope (a lighted instrument)

Anoxemia (hypoxemia) a condition in which the level of oxygen in the blood is below normal

Anoxia systemic absence or reduction of oxygen in the body tissues below physiologic levels

Antecubital fossa or space the point on the arm located in front of the elbow

Anterior toward, or at the front of

Anthropometric measurements measurements of the size and composition of the body (eg, height, weight, skin fold)

Antibiotic a natural or synthetic substance that has the capacity to inhibit the growth of or kill other microorganisms

Antibody (immunoglobulin) a protective protein substance produced in the body to counteract antigens

Antidiuretic hormone (ADH) a hormone that is stored and released by the posterior pituitary gland and that controls water reabsorption from the kidney tubules; also referred to as vasopressin

Antigen a substance capable of inducing the formation of antibodies

Antimicrobial destructive to or preventing the development of microorganisms

Antipyretic a substance that is effective in relieving fever

Antiseptic an agent that inhibits the growth of some microorganisms

Anuria the failure of the kidneys to produce urine, resulting in a total lack of urination or output of less than 100 mL per day in an adult

Anxiety a state of mental uneasiness, apprehension, or dread producing an increased level of arousal caused by an impending or anticipated threat to self or significant relationships

Apathy lack of interest or feeling

Apgar a scoring system to assess newborn babies

Aphasia inability to communicate through speech, writing, or signs, caused by dysfunction of brain centers

Apical pulse a central pulse located at the apex of the heart

Apical-radial pulse measurement of the apical beat and the radial pulse at the same time

Apnea a complete absence of respirations

Apothecary a system of medication measurement that derives from old England

Approximate (referring to wound or incision edges) to bring close together

Aquathermia to treat with warm water

Areflexia absence of reflexes

Arm muscle circumference (AMC) considered an index of the body's protein reserves, calculated from the triceps skinfold and mid-upper-arm circumference

Arrhythmia (dysrhythmia) a pulse with an abnormal rhythm

Arterial blood pressure the measure of the pressure exerted by the blood as it pulsates through the arteries

Arteriosclerosis a condition in which the elastic and muscular tissues of the arteries are replaced with fibrous tissue

Ascites the accumulation of fluid in the abdominal cavity

Asepsis freedom from infection or infectious material

Asphyxia inadequate intake of oxygen

Aspirate to remove gases or fluids from a cavity by using suction

Assault an attempt or threat to touch another person unjustifiably

Assessing the process of collecting, organizing, validating, and recording data (information) about a client's health status

Assimilation (of a group) see Acculturation

Assumptions statements of fact or suppositions that people accept as the underlying theoretical foundation for conceptualizations about a phenomenon

Astigmatism an uneven curvature of the cornea that prevents horizontal and vertical rays from focusing on the retina

Astringent an agent that causes contraction or shrinkage of tissue; usually applied topically

Ataxia impaired muscle coordination

Atelectasis a condition that occurs when ventilation is decreased and pooled secretions accumulate in a dependent area of a bronchiole and block it

Atheist one who denies the existence of God

Athlete's foot a fungal infection of the foot caused by tinea pedis

Atomizer a device that produces large droplets for inhalation

Atony lack of normal muscle tone

Atrophic vaginitis vaginal atrophy characterized by thinning and drying of the vaginal wall, loss of elasticity, and decreased lubrication

Atrophy wasting away; decrease in size of organ or tissue (eg, muscle)

Audit (nursing) a process in which the nursing interventions are monitored and measured against established standards

Auditory related to or experienced through hearing

Auscultation the process of listening to sounds produced within the body

Auscultatory gap the temporary disappearance of sounds normally heard over the brachial artery when the sphygmomanometer cuff pressure is high and the sounds reappear at a lower level

Autonomy the state of being independent and self-directed without outside control, to make one's own decisions

Autopsy (postmortem examination) an examination of the body after death to determine the cause of death and to learn more about a disease process

Awareness the ability to perceive environmental stimuli and body reactions and to respond appropriately through thought and action

Axillary line an imaginary line extending vertically from the anterior fold of the axilla

Babinski (plantar) reflex in infants up to 1 year, the normal fanning out of toes and dorsiflexion of the big toe elicited by stroking the sole of the foot; after 1 year the normal flexing of the toes at this stroking

Bactericide an agent capable of killing some microorganisms (bacteria)

Bacteriocin substance produced by certain bacteria that kills other strains of bacteria

Bacteriostatic agent an agent that prevents the growth and reproduction of some microorganisms

Bacteriuria bacteria in the urine

Barium a metallic element commonly used in solution as a contrast medium for X-ray filming of the gastrointestinal tract

Barium enema X-ray filming of the large intestine using a contrast medium; also called a lower gastrointestinal series or lower GI series

Barium swallow X-ray filming of the esophagus, stomach, and duodenum; also referred to as an upper gastrointestinal series or upper GI series

Barrel chest a variation of chest shape where the ratio of the anteroposterior to lateral diameter is 1:1

Barrier technique (reverse isolation) interventions used to protect clients who are highly susceptible to infection (eg, clients with AIDS, burns)

Basal metabolic rate (BMR) the rate of energy utilization in the body required to maintain essential activities such as breathing

Baseline data all information known about a client when the client first enters the health care agency

Base of support the area on which an object rests

Battery the willful or negligent touching of a person (or the person's clothes or even something the person is carrying), which may or may not cause harm

Beau's lines transverse white lines or grooves in the nail resulting from severe injury or illness

Belief (opinion) interpretations or conclusions that one accepts as true

Beneficence the moral obligation to do good or to implement actions that benefit clients and their support persons

Bereavement a subjective response of a person who has experienced the loss of a significant other through death

Bevel a slanting edge

Bilateral affecting two sides

Bilirubin orange pigment in the bile

Binder a type of bandage applied to large body areas (abdomen or chest) or for a specific body part (arm sling); used to provide support

Binocular vision ability to focus on images with both eyes

Bioethics ethical rules or principles that govern right conduct concerning life

Biofeedback a stress management technique that brings under conscious control bodily processes normally thought to be beyond voluntary command

Biopsy the removal and examination of tissue from the living body

Biorhythm an inner rhythm that appears to control a variety of biologic processes

Biot's respirations shallow breaths interrupted by apnea

Biotransformation process by which a drug is converted to a less active form; also called detoxification

Bleb (wheal) a small, smooth, slightly raised area on the skin, usually filled with fluid

Blood volume expanders solutions used to increase the volume of blood following severe loss of blood

Body image how a person perceives the size, appearance, and functioning of their body and its parts

Body language nonverbal communication using gestures, body movements, touch and physical appearance

Body mass index (BMI) indicates whether weight is appropriate for height

Body mechanics the efficient and coordinated use of the body to produce motion and maintain balance during activity

Body temperature the balance between the heat produced by the body and the heat lost from the body

Boundary the real or imaginary line that differentiates one system from another system or a system from its environment

Bowel diversion the surgical creation of an ostomy to enable the excretion of fecal waste while at the same time rerouting the feces away from a specific segment of the intestine

Bowel incontinence (fecal incontinence) refers to loss of voluntary ability to control fecal and gaseous discharges through the anal sphincter

Brachial pulse a pulse located on the inner side of the biceps muscle just below the axilla; usually palpated medially in the antecubital space

Bradycardia abnormally slow pulse rate, less than 60 per minute

Bradykinin an amino acid chain that causes powerful vasodilation, increased capillary permeability, smooth muscle contraction, and stimulation of pain receptors

Bradypnea abnormally slow respiratory rate, usually less than 10 respirations per minute

Bronchial sounds normal loud, harsh, hollow blowing sounds heard by auscultation over the trachea and main bronchi

Bronchodilator an agent that dilates the bronchi of the lungs

Bronchogram an X-ray film of the bronchial tree taken after injection of an iodized oil dye as a contrast medium

Bronchophony an increase in vocal resonance; an abnormal voice sound heard on auscultation of the chest wall

Bronchopneumonia an infection that originates in the bronchi and involves patches of lung tissue

Bronchoscope a lighted instrument used to visualize the bronchi of the lungs

Bronchoscopy visual examination of the bronchi using a bronchoscope

Bronchovesicular sounds combination of bronchial and vesicular sounds heard by auscultation over parts of the chest where a bronchus is near lung tissue

Bruit a blowing or swishing sound created by turbulence of blood flow

Bruxism grinding of the teeth during sleep

Bryant's traction a type of traction used to stabilize fractured femurs or correct congenital hip dislocation in young children

Buccal pertaining to the cheek

Buck's extension a type of simple traction used to immobilize fractures of the hip and reduce muscle spasm before surgical repair

Buffer an agent or system that tends to maintain constancy or that prevents changes in the chemical concentration of a substance

Bulimia an uncontrollable compulsion to eat large amounts of food and then expel it by self-induced vomiting or by taking laxatives

Bunion lateral deviation of the big toe with swelling or callus formation over the metatarsophalangeal joint

Cafe-au-lait spots spots of patchy pigmentation of skin, usually light brown in color

Calculus a stone composed of minerals that is formed in the body (eg, a renal calculus formed in the kidney)

Calipers an instrument used to measure the thickness of folds of skin or to measure electrocardiogram wave forms

Callus (bone) early bone, formed following fracture of a bone, normally ultimately replaced by hard bone

Callus (skin) a thickened portion of the skin

Caloric value the amount of energy that nutrients or foods supply to the body

Calorie (C, Cal, kcal) a unit of heat energy equivalent to the amount of heat required to raise the temperature of 1 kg of water 1 C

calorie see Small calorie

Cannula a tube with a lumen (channel) that is inserted into a cavity or duct and is often fitted with a trocar during insertion

Canthus the angle formed by the upper and lower eyelids; each eye has an inner and an outer canthus

Carbohydrate a nutrient composed of carbon, hydrogen, and oxygen (eg, starches and sugars)

Carbonic acid the compound formed when carbon dioxide combines with water

Cardiac arrest the cessation of heart function

Cardiac monitor a machine used to enable continual observation or monitoring of the electrical function of the heart

Cardiac output the amount of blood ejected by the heart with each ventricular contraction

Cardiopulmonary resuscitation (CPR) artificial stimulation of the heart and lungs; also referred to as basic life support (BLS)

Caries (dental) tooth cavities

Carina the ridge or junction where the main bronchi meet the trachea

Carminative an agent that promotes the passage of flatus from the colon

Carrier a person or animal that harbors a specific infectious agent and serves as a potential source of infection, yet does not manifest any clinical signs of disease

Case management a method for delivering nursing care in which the nurse is responsible for a case load of clients across the health care continuum

CAT scan see Tomography

Catabolism a destructive process in which complex substances are broken down into simpler substances (eg, breakdown of tissue)

Cataracts opacity of the lens or capsule of the eye

Cathartic (laxative) a drug that induces evacuation of feces from the large intestine

Catheter a tube of rubber, plastic, metal, or other material used to remove or inject fluids into a cavity such as the bladder

Cation ion that carries a positive charge; sodium, potassium, calcium, magnesium

Caudal anesthetic an anesthetic injected into the caudal canal, below the spinal cord

Cavity a hollow space within the body or one of its organs

Cellular fluid see Intracellular fluid

Cellulitis inflammation of cellular tissue

Celsius (Centigrade) a thermometer scale used to measure heat; the freezing point of water is 0 C and the boiling point is 100 C

Center of gravity the point at which the mass (weight) of the body is centered

Central venous line a catheter inserted into a large vein located centrally in the body (eg, the superior vena cava, right atrium)

Central venous pressure (CVP) the measurement of the pressure of the blood, in millimeters of water, within the vena cava or the right atrium of the heart

Cephalocaudal proceeding in the direction from head to toe

Cerebral death the higher brain center or cerebral cortex is irreversibly destroyed

Certification the voluntary practice of validating that an individual nurse has met minimum standards of nursing competence in a specialty area

Cerumen the wax-like substance secreted by glands in the external ear canal

Cervical head halter traction a device that provides skin-encircling traction on the cervical spine to relieve muscle spasm and nerve compression, related to cervical injuries in the neck, upper arms, or shoulders

Chancre a papular lesion (sore) occurring at the entry of infection in some diseases; the primary lesion of syphilis

Change agent a person (or group) who initiates changes or who assists others in making modifications in themselves or in the system

Chaplain one who serves the spiritual needs of clients

Chart (medical record) a written account of a client's health history, current health status, treatment, and progress

Charting (recording) the process of making written entries about a client on the medical record

Chemical restraints medications used to control socially disruptive behavior

Chemical thermogenesis the stimulation of heat production in the body through increased cellular metabolism caused by increases in thyroxine output

Chemoreceptor a receptor that is sensitive to chemical substances

Cheyne-Stokes respirations rhythmic waxing and waning of respirations from very deep breathing to very shallow breathing with periods of temporary apnea, often associated with cardiac failure, increased intracranial pressure, or brain damage

Choanal atresia congenital occlusion of the opening between the nasal cavities and the nasopharynx

Cholangiography (cholangiogram) an X-ray film of the biliary tract taken after the injection of a dye

Cholecystogram (cholecystography, oral cholecystography) an X-ray film of the gallbladder after ingestion of a contrast dye

Cholesterol a lipid that does not contain fatty acid but possesses many of the chemical and physical properties of other lipids

Chronic illness illness that lasts for an extended period of time, usually greater than 6 months

Chronologic charting recording of data in sequence as time moves forward

Chvostek's sign an indication of tetany, spasm of facial muscles in response to a tap over the facial nerve

Cicatrix scar

Circadian rhythm rhythmic repetition of certain phenomena each 24 hours

Circa dies about a day

Circulatory overload a state in which the intravascular fluid compartment contains more fluid than normal

Circolectric bed a therapeutic bed that enables a variety of client positions

Circumcision surgical removal of part or all of the foreskin of the penis; usually performed during infancy

Circumduction movement of the distal part of the bone in a circle while the proximal end remains fixed

Circumference the outer measurement or perimeter (eg, the distance around the chest)

Citric acid cycle (Krebs cycle) a complex series of chemical reactions involving the oxidative metabolism of pyruvic acid and the liberation of energy

Clapping (percussion, cupping) (in physiotherapy) the forceful striking of the chest with cupped hands to loosen secretions in the lungs

Clean free of potentially infectious agents

Clergy priests, rabbis, ministers, church elders, deacons, and other spiritual advisors

Client advocate an individual who pleads the cause of clients' rights

Climacteric the point in development when reproduction capacity in the female terminates (menopause) and the sexual activity of the male decreases (andropause)

Closed bed an unoccupied bed with the top covers drawn up to the head of the bed under the pillows

Closed questions restrictive questions requiring only a short answer

Closed system a system that does not exchange energy, matter, or information with its environment

Closed wound a tissue injury without a break in the skin

Clubbing (of a nail) elevation of the proximal aspect of the nail and softening of the nail bed

Coagulate to clot

Coarctation (of the aorta) severe narrowing of the aorta

Code of Ethics a formal statement of a group's ideals and values; a set of ethical principles shared by members of a group, reflecting their moral judgments and serving as a standard for professional actions

Cognitive (skills) referring to intellectual processes such as remembering, thinking, perceiving, abstracting, and generalizing

Cohabiting (communal) family a family made up of unrelated individuals or families living under one roof

Cohesive (adherent) sticking together, clinging

Coinsurance an insurance plan where the client pays a percentage of the payment and some other group (eg, employer, government) pays the additional percentage

Coitus (copulation) a type of genital intercourse in which the penis is inserted into the vagina

Collaborative nursing intervention (action) those activities performed either jointly with another member of the health care team or as a result of a joint decision by the nurse and another health care team member

Collagen a protein found in connective tissue; a whitish protein substance that adds tensile strength to a wound

Collective bargaining the formalized decision-making process between representatives of management and representatives of labor to negotiate wages and conditions of employment

Colloid substances, such as large plasma protein molecules, that do not readily dissolve in true solution

Colonization the presence of organisms in body secretions or excretions in which strains of bacteria become resident flora but do not cause illness

Colonoscope a lighted instrument used to visualize the interior of the colon

Colonoscopy visual examination of the interior of the colon with a colonoscope

Colostomy an opening into the colon (large bowel)

Comatose a state of unconsciousness in which the person shows no response to maximum painful stimuli, absence of reflexes, and absence of muscle tone in the extremities

Combustible able to burn; flammable

Comedo a blackhead or whitehead; a plug of dried sebum in a sebaceous gland

Commode a portable, chairlike structure used as a toilet

Communicable disease (infectious disease) a disease that can spread from one person to another

Compartment syndrome the condition in which increased pressure in a limited space compromises or reduces the circulation and function of the tissues within the space

Compensation defense mechanism in which a person substitutes an activity for one that they would prefer doing or cannot do

Compliance (of arteries) the distensibility of the arteries (ie, their ability to contract and expand)

Compliance (client) the extent to which an individual's behavior coincides with medical or health advice

Compound fracture fracture in which there is an open wound over the broken bone, or where bone fragments protrude through the skin

Compress a moist gauze dressing applied frequently to an open wound, sometimes medicated

Compromised host any person at increased risk for an infection

Computerized axial tomography (CAT) see Tomography

Concave hollowed or rounded inward

Concept abstract idea or mental image of phenomena or reality

Conceptual framework a group of related concepts

Conceptual model a graphic illustration of the relationships between concepts

Conceptualization the intellectual process of forming a concept

Condom a sheath or cover, usually made of rubber or plastic, worn over the penis during coitus to prevent conception or infection; urinary condoms are used to catch urine

Conduction the transfer of heat from one molecule to another in direct contact

Confer to consult another person or persons for advice, information, ideas, or instructions

Confidentiality the right of a client or research subject that any information revealed by that individual will not be made public or available to others

Conformity actions in accordance with specified standards

Confusion a mental state in which a person appears bewildered and may make inappropriate statements and answers to questions

Congenital existing at, and often before, birth

Congestion excessive accumulation of blood or fluid in a part of the body

Congruence in communication, when words and behavior coincide or are unified

Conjunctivitis inflammation of the bulbar and palpebral conjunctiva

Consciousness a person's normal state of awareness of the environment, self, and others

Consensual reaction (eyes) a reaction in which one pupil constricts quickly in response to a bright light and the other pupil constricts also, but more slowly

Consent permission given voluntarily by a person in his or her right mind; informed consent requires that the individual is knowledgeable about the consent and understands it

Constipation passage of small, dry, hard stool or passage of no stool for an abnormally long time

Consultation a process in which two or more people deliberate with one another to seek advice or clarification

Consumer an individual, a group of people, or a community that uses a service or commodity

Continuum a grid or graduated scale

Contraception the prevention of fertilization of the ovum by any method

Contract a written or verbal agreement between two or more people to do or not do some lawful act

Contraction an intermittent tightening and shortening of uterine muscle fibers which cause cervical dilation and effacement during labor

Contracture permanent shortening of a muscle and subsequent shortening of tendons and ligaments

Contraindicate not indicated or inappropriate

Contusion a closed wound that occurs as a result of a blow from a blunt instrument; a bruise

Convection the dispersion of heat by air currents

Conversion a defense mechanism in which a mental conflict is converted into a physical symptom

Convex curved or rounded like the external surface of a sphere

Coping the process through which the individual manages the demands of the person-environment relationship that are appraised as stressful

Coping behavior behavior learned in response to stress; immediate response to a threatening situation

Coping mechanisms physical or emotional adaptive or defensive abilities

Cordotomy (chordotomy) surgical severing of the spinothalamic portion of the anterolateral tract of the spinal cord, usually for the purpose of relieving pain

Core temperature the temperature of the deep tissues of the body (eg, thorax, abdominal cavity); relatively constant at 37 C (98.6 F)

Corn a conical, circular, painful, raised area on the toe or foot

Coroner a public official, not necessarily a physician, appointed or elected to inquire into the causes of death

Corticoid a term applied to hormones of the adrenal cortex or substances with similar activity

Cortiosone a hormone produced by the adrenal cortex that has anti-inflammatory properties and is involved in the metabolism of glycogen to glucose

Costal breathing (thoracic breathing) breathing involving the external intercostal muscles and other accessory muscles, such as the sternocleidomastoid muscles

Costovertebral angle the angle formed by a rib and the spine

Counseling the process of helping a client to recognize and cope with stressful psychologic or social problems, to develop improved interpersonal relationships, and to promote personal growth

Countertraction a force that counteracts the direct pull of traction

Covert data (symptoms, subjective data) information (data) apparent only to the person affected that can be described or verified only by that person

CPR see Cardiopulmonary resuscitation

Crackles (rales) bubbling or rattling sounds audible by ear or stethoscope on inhalation; they are a result of fluid in the lungs

Creatinine a nitrogenous waste that is excreted in the urine

Credé's maneuver manual exertion of pressure on the bladder to force urine out

Credentialing the process of determining and maintaining competence in practice; includes licensure, registration, certification, and accreditation

Crepitation (1) a dry, crackling sound like that of crumpled cellophane, produced by air in the subcutaneous tissue or by air moving through fluid in the alveoli of the lungs; (2) a crackling, grating sound produced by bone rubbing against bone

Criterion a standard or model that can be used in judging

Critical pathways multidisciplinary guidelines for client care based on specific medical diagnoses designed to achieve predetermined outcomes

Cross contamination the transfer or microorganisms from one surface to another

Crutch palsy a weakness of the muscles of the forearm, wrist, and hand caused by prolonged pressure of the crutch on the axillary nerve

Cryotherapy therapeutic use of cold

Cryptorchidism failure of the testes to descend from the abdominal cavity to the scrotal sacs

Crystalloid salts that dissolve readily in true solutions

Cue(s) any piece of information or data that influences decisions

Cultural heritage values and beliefs unique to a particular culture that influence the family's structure, methods of interaction, health care practices, and coping mechanisms

Culture a world view and set of traditions used and transmitted from generation to generation by a particular group, includes related attitudes and institutions

Curet a spoon-shaped instrument used for removing material from a body cavity

Cushing's syndrome a disorder in which there is increased adrenal hormone production

Cyanosis bluish discoloration of the skin and mucous membranes caused by reduced oxygen in the blood

Cyst an enclosed cavity or sac lined by epithelium and containing liquid or semisolid material

Cystectomy removal of the bladder

Cystitis inflammation of the urinary bladder

Cystocele protrusion of the urinary bladder through the vaginal wall

Cystoscope a lighted instrument used to visualize the interior of the urinary bladder

Cystoscopy visual examination of the urinary bladder with a cystoscope

Cytology the study of the origin, structure, function, and pathology of cells

Dacryocystitis inflammation of the lacrimal sac

Dandruff a dry or greasy, scaly material shed from the scalp

Data information

Database (baseline data) all information about a client, includes nursing health history and physical assessment, physician's history and physical examination, laboratory and diagnostic test results

Debilitated having lost strength

Debridement removal of infected and necrotic tissue

Deceased dead; a person who is dead

Deciduous teeth temporary teeth that are shed

Decubitus ulcer see Pressure sores

Deductive reasoning making specific observations from a generalization

Defamation a communication that is false, or made with careless disregard for the truth, and results in injury to the reputation of another

Defecation expulsion of feces from the rectum and anus

Defervescence the stage of abatement of a fever

Defense (adaptive) mechanisms any reaction that serves to protect against something physically or psychologically harmful

Defining characteristics client signs and symptoms that must be present to validate a nursing diagnosis

Dehydration insufficient fluid in the body

Delegate to assign responsibility and authority for performing specific tasks to another

Delirious experiencing mental confusion, restlessness, and incoherence

Dementia a global impairment of cognitive function that usually is progressive and may be permanent, interferes with normal social and occupational activities

Demineralization excessive loss of minerals or inorganic salts

Demise death

Demography the study of population, including statistics about distribution by age and place of residence, mortality, and morbidity

Demulcent a drug that coats the intestine, thus protecting the lining

Denial a defense mechanism in which painful or anxiety-producing aspects of reality are blocked out of consciousness

Dental caries tooth decay

Dental plaque deposits on the teeth that serves as a medium for bacterial growth

Denver Developmental Screening Test (DDST) a screening test used to assess children from birth to 6 years of age

Dentifrice a paste or powder used to clean or polish the teeth

Dentures a natural or artificial set of teeth; usually the term designates artificial replacements for natural teeth

Deontology an approach to moral theory which proposes that the morality of a decision is not determined by the consequences; it emphasizes duty, rationality, and obedience to rules

Dependent edema edema of the lowest or most dependent parts of the body

Dependent nursing intervention (action, function) those activities carried out on the order of the physician, under the physician's supervision, or according to specified routines

Depilatory a cream used to remove body hair

Depression feelings of sadness and dejection, often accompanied by physiologic change such as a decreased functional activity

Dermatitis inflammation of the skin

Dermatologic preparation a medication applied to the skin

Development an individual's increasing capacity and skill in functioning, related to growth

Developmental crisis a crisis that occurs as a result of stressors related to development

Developmental tasks skills and behavior patterns learned during stages of development

Deviance behavior that goes against social norms

Diagnosing the process that results in a diagnostic statement or nursing diagnosis that provides the basis for the selection of nursing interventions for the client

Diagnosis a statement or conclusion concerning the nature of some phenomenon

Diagnostic label (problem statement) title used in writing a nursing diagnosis; taken from the North American Nursing Diagnosis Association's (NANDA) standardized taxonomy of terms

Diagnostic related groups (DRGs) a Medicare payments system to hospitals and physicians which establishes fees according to diagnosis

Dialyzing membrane a membrane that permits water molecules and crystalloids in true solution to move through it but not particles in a colloid dispersion

Diapedesis the movement of blood corpuscles through a blood vessel wall

Diaphoresis profuse perspiration

Diaphragmatic breathing (abdominal breathing) breathing that involves the contraction and relaxation of the diaphragm

Diarrhea defecation of liquid feces and increased frequency of defecation

Diastole the period during which the ventricles relax

Diastolic pressure the pressure of the blood against the arterial walls when the ventricles of the heart are at rest

Dilemma a situation involving a choice between equally satisfactory or unsatisfactory alternatives or a difficult problem that seems to have no satisfactory solution

Diplopia double vision

Directed thinking a pattern of thinking that is purposeful and is used for forming judgments, problem-solving, and decision-making

Discharge planning the process of anticipating and planning for client needs after discharge

Discrimination the differential treatment of individuals or groups based on categories such as race, ethnicity, gender, social class, age, or exceptionality

Disease an alteration in body function resulting in a reduction of capacities or shortening of the normal life span

Disengagement any withdrawal from usual social patterns

Disequilibrium a disturbed state of equilibrium (balance), either mental or physical

Disinfectant agent that destroys all microorganisms

Disorientation a state of mental confusion; loss of bearings, time, and place

Displacement a defense mechanism in which an emotional reaction is transferred from one object to another less threatening object

Distal farthest from the point of reference

Distention (abdominal) see Tympanites

Distraction a mechanism for relieving pain where the person's attention is drawn away from the pain

Diuresis (polyuria) the production of abnormally large amounts of urine by the kidneys without an increased fluid intake

Diuretic an agent that increases urine secretion

DNR (do not resuscitate, no code) a physician's order that requires that no effort be made to resuscitate the client with terminal or irreversible illness in the event of a respiratory or cardiac arrest

Dorsal toward, or at the back of

Dorsal flexion (dorsiflexion) movement of the ankle so that the toes are pointing upward

Dorsal (supine) position back-lying position without a pillow

Dorsal recumbent position a back-lying position with the head and shoulders slightly elevated

Douche vaginal irrigation; washing of the vagina by a liquid at a low pressure

Drain a substance or appliance that assists in the discharge of serosanguinous fluid and purulent material from a wound and promotes healing of underlying tissues

Drainage a discharge from a wound or cavity

Drawsheet (half sheet) a special sheet, made of cotton, plastic, or rubber, that is placed across the center of the foundation of the bed and used to facilitate moving bed-bound clients

Dressing a material used to cover and protect a wound

Drip factor (drop factor) the number of drops per milliliter of solution delivered for a particular drip chamber before calculating the drip rate

Droplet nuclei residue of evaporated droplets that remains in the air for long periods of time

Drug (medication) a chemical compound taken for disease prevention, diagnosis, cure, or relief or to affect the structure or function of the body

Drug abuse excessive intake of a substance either continually or periodically

Drug dependence inability to keep the intake of a drug or substance under control

Drug habituation a mild form of psychologic dependence on a drug

Drug interaction the beneficial or harmful interaction of one drug with another drug

Drug misuse improper use of common medications in ways that can lead to acute and chronic toxicity

Drug tolerance a condition in which successive increases in the dosage of a drug are required to maintain a given therapeutic effect

Drug toxicity the quality of a drug that exerts a deleterious effect on an organism or tissue

DT diphtheria vaccine and tetanus toxoid

DTP (DPT) Diphtheria toxoid, tetanus toxoid, and pertussis vaccine

Duchenne muscular dystrophy a genetically acquired disease that causes gradual progressive muscle wasting

Dullness a thudlike sound produced during percussion by dense tissue of body organs such as the liver, spleen, or heart

Dumping syndrome a condition experienced by jejunostomy clients when hypertonic foods and liquids suddenly distend the jejunum

Dunlop's traction (side-arm traction) combined horizontal and vertical adaptation of Buck's extension traction to the humerus and forearm

Duodenocolic reflex a mass peristaltic movement of the colon stimulated by the presence of chyme in the duodenum

Duration (of sound) the length of time that a sound is heard

Dynamic equilibrium tendency of the body to maintain a state of balance or equilibrium while continually changing

Dynorphins compounds found in the pituitary gland, hypothalamus, and spinal cord that seem to have an analgesic effect

Dysmenorrhea painful menstruation

Dyspareunia pain experienced by a woman during intercourse

Dyspepsia indigestion

Dysphagia difficulty or inability to swallow

Dysphasia difficulty speaking

Dysphoria disquiet, restlessness

Dyspnea difficult or labored breathing

Dysrhythmia (arrhythmia) a pulse with an irregular rhythm

Dysuria painful or difficult voiding

Ecchymosis A bruise that changes in color from blue-black to greenish brown or yellow

Ecology the study of the relationship of humans with the environment

Ectropion eversion or outturning of the eyelid

Edema the presence of excess interstitial fluid in the body

Edentulous without teeth

Efferent conveying away from the center

Effleurage a stroking massage technique

Effluent urine or feces discharged through a stoma

Egg crate mattress a specialized foam rubber mattress designed to provide support while relieving pressure on the body's bony prominences

Ego includes consciousness and memory which serves to mediate between primitive instinctual drives (id), internal social prohibitions (superego), and reality

Egocentricity concern about oneself

Ego integrity feeling satisfied with one's life-style and accepting the inevitability of one's life cycle

Egophony a type of bronchophony in which the voice has a nasal, bleating quality

Ejaculation expulsion of seminal fluid and sperm

Electrocardiogram (ECG, EKG) a graph of the electrical activity of the heart

Electroencephalogram (EEG) a graph of the electrical activity of the brain

Electrolyte a chemical substance that develops an electric charge and is able to conduct an electric current when placed in water; an ion

Electromyogram (EMG) a record of the electrical potential created by the contraction of a muscle

Electron a negatively charged electric particle

Emaciated excessively thin

Embolus a blood clot (or a substance such as air) that has moved from its place of origin and is causing obstruction to circulation elsewhere (plural: emboli)

Emmetropic normal refraction so that the eyes focus images on the retina

Emollient an agent that soothes and softens skin or mucous membrane; often an oily substance

Empathy the ability to discriminate what the other person's world is like and to communicate to the other this understanding in a way that shows that the helper understands the client's feelings and the behavior and experience underlying these feelings

Emphysema a chronic pulmonary condition in which the alveoli are dilated and distended

Empirical by observation or experience

Emulsion a preparation in which one liquid is distributed throughout another

Endemic present in a community all the time

Endogenous developing from within

Endogenous opioids chemical regulators in the body that may modify pain

Endorphins a polypeptide found throughout the body that is thought to relieve pain

Endoscope an instrument used for examining the interior of a hollow organ (eg, the bladder, rectum, stomach, or bronchi)

Endotracheal tube a tube which is inserted through the mouth or nose into the trachea

Enema a solution introduced into the rectum and sigmoid colon to remove feces and/or flatus

Engorgement excessive fullness of an organ or passage

Enkephalins a pentapeptide naturally occurring in the brain that has opiate like effects

Enteric referring to the intestines

Enteric-coated tablets and capsules surrounded with a special coating that prevents release of the drug until it is in the intestines

Enteric feeding a feeding administered directly into the small intestine through a tube

Enteritis inflammation of the small intestine

Enterocele any hernia of the intestine through the vaginal mucosa

Enterostomal therapist a person who specializes in ostomy care

Enterostomy an opening through the abdominal wall into the intestines

Entropion inversion or inturning of the eyelid

Enuresis bedwetting; involuntary passing of urine in children after bladder control is achieved

Environment all the conditions, circumstances, and influences surrounding and affecting the development of an organism or person

Enzyme a biologic catalyst that speeds up chemical reactions

Epidemic the occurrence of a disease in many people at the same time or in rapid succession in an area

Epidemiology the study of the occurrence and distribution of disease

Epispadias opening of the urethra on the upper side of the penis

Epistaxis nose bleed

Equilibrium a state of balance

Erogenous sexually sensitive

Eructation belching; the expulsion of swallowed gases through the mouth

Erythema a redness associated with a variety of skin rashes

Erythrocyte red blood cell

Erythropoiesis the formation of red blood cells

Eschar thick necrotic tissue produced by burning, by a corrosive application, or by death of tissue associated with loss of vascular supply, bacterial invasion, and putrefaction

Esophagoscopy visual examination of the interior of the esophagus with a lighted instrument

Ethics the rules or principles that govern right conduct

Ethnic (Ethnicity) belonging to a specific group of individuals who share a common social and cultural heritage

Ethnocentrism the belief that one's own culture is superior to all others

Ethnoscience the systematic study of the way of life of a designated cultural group to obtain accurate data regarding behavior, perceptions, and interpretations of the universe

Etiology the causal relationship between a problem and its related or risk factors

Eupnea normal, quiet breathing

Euthanasia (mercy killing) the act of painlessly putting to death persons suffering from incurable or distressing disease

Evaluation a planned, ongoing, purposeful activity in which client and health care professionals determine the client's progress toward goal achievement and the effectiveness of the nursing care plan

Evaporation conversion of a liquid into a vapor

Eversion turning the sole of the foot outward by moving the ankle joint

Evisceration extrusion of the internal organs

Exacerbation the period during a chronic illness when symptoms reappear after remission

Excise to cut off or out

Excoriation loss of the superficial layers of the skin

Excretion elimination of a waste product produced by the body cells from the body

Exhalation (expiration) the movement of gases from the lungs to the atmosphere

Exogenous developing from without

Exophthalmus a protrusion of the eyeballs with elevation of the upper eyelids, resulting in a startled or staring expression

Exotoxin a toxic substance formed by bacteria and found outside the bacterial cell

Expectorate to cough and spit up mucus or other materials

Expert witness one who has special training, experience, or skill in a relevant area and is allowed by the court to offer an opinion on some issue within that area of expertise

Expiration (exhalation) the outflow of air from the lungs to the atmosphere

Expiratory reserve volume the maximum amount of air exhaled after a normal exhalation

Expired dead

Expressive language skills ability to use or to speak words

Extended family family that includes the relatives of the nuclear family (eg, grandparents, aunts, uncles)

Extension increasing the angle of a joint

External cardiac massage rhythmic massage of the heart muscle over the sternum during resuscitation

External respiration the interchange of oxygen and carbon dioxide between the alveoli of the lungs and the pulmonary blood

Extracellular outside the cell

Extracellular fluid (ECF) fluid found outside the body cells

Extrapolating inferring facts or data from known facts or data

Extrathecal outside the sheath (eg, outside the spinal canal)

Extravasation the escape of blood from a vessel into the body tissues

Exudate material, such as fluid and cells, that has escaped from blood vessels during the inflammatory process and is deposited in tissue or on tissue surfaces

Face mask a mask covering the client's nose and mouth, used to deliver oxygen and/or other gases

Face tent a device that covers the face, used to deliver oxygen to the client when a face mask is not tolerated

Fahrenheit a thermometer scale used to measure heat; the freezing point of water is 32 F and the boiling point is 212 F

False imprisonment the unlawful restraint or detention of another person against his or her wishes

Family-centered nursing nursing that considers the health of the family as a unit in addition to the health of individual family members

Fantasy an adaptive mechanism in which wishes and desires are imagined as fulfilled

Fasciculation an abnormal contraction or shortening of a bundle of muscle fibers

Fasting abstinence from eating

Fat embolism fat globules that are released into the blood circulation from bone marrow and from local tissue trauma

Fear an emotional response to an actual, present danger

Febrile pertaining to a fever; feverish

Fecal impaction a mass or collection of hardened, puttylike feces in the folds of the rectum

Fecal incontinence (bowel incontinence) loss of voluntary ability to control fecal and gaseous discharges through the anal sphincter

Feces (stool) body wastes and undigested food eliminated from the rectum

Feedback (homeostasis) the mechanism by which some output of a system is returned to the system as input

Feedback (communication) the response or message that the receiver returns to the sender during communication

Fenestrated drape a drape with an opening in its center

Fetus the unborn offspring in the postembryonic stage of development

Fever elevated body temperature

Fiber an indigestible carbohydrate derived from plants

Fibrillation involuntary contractions of a muscle; cardiac arrhythmia characterized by extremely rapid, irregular, and ineffective contractions of the atria or ventricles

Fibrin an insoluble protein formed from fibrinogen during the clotting of blood

Fibrous tissue common connective tissue composed of elastic and collagen fibers

Fidelity a moral principle which obligates the individual to be faithful to agreements and responsibilities one has undertaken

FiO_2 fraction of inspired oxygen

First intention healing primary wound healing; occurs when tissue surfaces have been approximated

Fissure a cleft or groove

Fistula an abnormal communication or passage usually between two organs or between an organ and the body surface

Fixation (psychologic) immobilization or the inability of the personality to proceed to the next developmental stage because of anxiety

Flaccid weak or lax

Flaccid paralysis impaired muscle function with loss of muscle tone

Flail chest the ballooning out of the chest wall through fractured rib spaces during exhalation

Flatness an extremely dull sound produced, during percussion, by very dense tissue, such as muscle or bone

Flatulence the presence of excessive amounts of gas in the stomach or intestines

Flatus gas or air normally present in the stomach or intestines

Flexion decreasing the angle of a joint (between two bones); the act of bending

Flora collective vegetation in a given area

Flowmeter a device used to control the flow of oxygen delivery

Flowsheet a record of the progress of specific or specialized data such as vital signs, fluid balance, or routine medications; often charted in graph form

Fluoroscopy An examination using a fluoroscope, which views internal structures using X-rays

Flushing (of the skin) transient redness of the skin, often of the face and neck; it may be generalized or restricted to a particular area

Focus charting a method of charting that uses key words or foci to describe what is happening to the client

Fomite an inanimate object other than food that can harbor disease producing microorganisms and transmit an infection

Footboard a board placed at the foot of the client bed to support the feet and prevent foot drop; may also be used to keep bed covers off the client's feet

Footdrop plantar flexion of the foot with permanent contracture of the gastrocnemius (calf) muscle and tendon

Forceps an instrument with two blades and a handle used to grasp sterile supplies and to compress or grasp tissues

Forensic medicine the application of medical knowledge to the law

Formulary a collection or list of prescriptions and formulas

Fowler's position a bed sitting position with the head of the bed raised to 45 degrees

Fracture a break in the continuity of a bone

Fremitus vibrations felt through the chest wall by palpation

Frenulum a midline fold connecting the undersurface of the tongue to the floor of the mouth

Frequency (of urination) voiding at more frequent intervals than usual

Friction rubbing; the force that opposes motion

Friction strokes a massage technique in which strong circular massage is followed by centripetal stroking

Fulcrum the fixed point of a lever

Full disclosure provision of complete and truthful information to a client participating in a research study

Functional hemoglobin the ratio of oxygen bound to hemoglobin compared to the amount of hemoglobin that is available for binding

Functional nursing a model for delivering nursing care which focuses on the tasks to be completed

Functional residual capacity volume of air remaining in the lungs after a normal expiration

Funnel chest (pectus excavatum) a congenital defect of the chest where the sternum is depressed, narrowing the anteroposterior diameter

Gait the way a person walks

Gastric pertaining to the stomach

Gastrocolic reflex increased peristalsis of the colon after food has entered the stomach

Gastroenteritis inflammation of the stomach and the intestines

Gastroscopy visual examination of the stomach with a lighted instrument (gastroscope)

Gastrostomy an opening through the abdominal wall into the stomach

Gastrostomy feeding the instillation of liquid nourishment via a tube that enters the stomach through a surgical opening in the abdominal wall

Gavage administration of nourishment to the stomach through a nasogastric or orogastric tube; tube feeding

Gender behavior behavior with masculine or feminine connotations

Gender identity a person's sense of being masculine or feminine, as distinct from being male or female

Gender role the outward expression of a person's sense of maleness or femaleness, the expression of what is perceived as gender-appropriate behavior

General adaptation syndrome (GAS, stress syndrome) (Selye) a general arousal response of the body to a stressor that is characterized by certain physiologic events and that is dominated by the sympathetic nervous system

Generativity (Erikson) concern for establishing and guiding the next generation

Generic name (of drug) a drug name not protected by trademark and usually describing the chemical structure of the drug

Genupectoral position kneeling position with torso at a 90-degree angle to hips

Genu valgum (knock-knee) a condition in which knees are very close to each other and the ankles are apart

Genu varum (bowleg) a condition of curving out of the legs

Geriatrics the branch of medicine pertaining to elderly people

Germicidal possessing the ability to kill microorganisms

Gerontology the study of all aspects of the aging process, including biologic, psychologic, and sociologic

Gingiva the gum tissue

Glaucoma a disturbance in the circulation of aqueous fluid; causes an increase in intraocular pressure

Glossitis inflammation of the tongue

Glucagon a hormone produced by the alpha cells of the islands of Langerhans in the pancreas; it stimulates the breakdown of liver glycogen

Glucocorticoid a hormone produced by the adrenal glands that influences the metabolism of glucose, protein, and fat

Glucometer a device used to measure the amount of glucose in a blood sample

Gluconeogenesis the process by which the liver converts proteins and fats into glucose

Glycogen the chief carbohydrate stored in the body, particularly in the liver and muscles

Glycogenesis formation of glycogen

Glycogenolysis the breakdown of glycogen to reform glucose

Glycolysis the release of energy through the breakdown of glucose

Glycosuria the presence of glucose in the urine; glucosuria

Goniometer a device used to measure the angle of a joint in degrees

Governance the establishment and maintenance of social, political, and economic arrangements by which practitioners control their practice, self-discipline, working conditions, and professional affairs

Granulation tissue young connective tissue with new capillaries formed in the wound healing process

Graphesthesia ability to recognize a figure traced on the skin with the tip of a finger, blunt pencil, or similar object

Grief emotional suffering often caused by bereavement

Grievance any dispute, difference, controversy, or disagreement arising out of the terms and conditions of employment

Ground (electrical) to transmit electric current from an object or surface to the ground

Group dynamics (process) forces that determine the behavior of the group and the relationships among the group members

Growth physical change and increase in size

Guided imagery a relaxation technique using self-chosen positive images to achieve specific health-related goals (ie, stress reduction, pain control)

Guilt the painful emotion associated with transgression of moral-ethical beliefs

Gurgles see Rhonchi

Gustatory referring to the sense of taste

Gynecology the branch of medicine that deals with processes of the female reproductive tract

Half-life (of a drug) the time interval required for the body's elimination processes to reduce the concentration of the drug in the body by one-half

Halitosis bad breath

Hallucinate to perceive through the senses something unreal; such as hearing voices or seeing things that do not exist

Hallucinogens drugs that cause distortion of the sensory perception

Halo ring a type of traction consisting of a circular metal band secured by two anterior and two posterior pins that penetrate the skull only a fraction of an inch, used to immobilize fractures of the cervical and upper thoracic vertebrae

Halo-thoracic vest traction a device where a halo ring is attached to a plaster cast or plastic vest by metal rods, used to immobilize fractures of the cervical and upper thoracic vertebrae

Hangnail a shred of epidermal tissue at either side of the nail

Haustrum a saclike formation of a part of the colon, produced by contraction of both the longitudinal and the circular muscles (plural: haustra)

Health a state of being physically fit, mentally stable, and socially comfortable; it encompasses more than the state of being free of disease

Health behavior the action a person takes to understand his or her health state, maintain an optimal state of health, prevent illness and injury, and reach his or her maximum physical and mental potential

Health beliefs concepts about health that an individual believes are true

Health care proxy a legal statement that appoints a proxy to make medical decisions for the client in the event the client is unable to do so

Health care system the totality of services offered by all health disciplines

Health care team health personnel from different disciplines who coordinate their skills to assist a client and/or support persons, commonly includes nurses, physicians, pharmacists, dietitians, physiotherapists

Health Maintenance Organization (HMO) a group health care agency that provides basic and supplemental health maintenance and treatment services to voluntary enrollees

Health practice an activity that a person carries out as a result of his or her health beliefs and definition of health

Health problem any condition or situation in which a client requires help to promote, maintain, or regain a state of health or to achieve a peaceful death

Health promotion any activity undertaken for the purpose of achieving a higher level of health and well-being

Health risk appraisal (HRA) tool that indicates a client's risk of diseases or injury over time by comparing the client with a large national sample with similar demographic data

Health status the health of a person at a given time

Heave an abnormal lateral movement of the chest related to enlargement of the left ventricle

Heimlich maneuver subdiaphragmatic abdominal thrusts used to clear an obstructed airway

Hemangioma a large, persistent, bright red or dark purple vascular area of the skin

Hematemesis the vomiting of blood

Hematocrit the proportion of red blood cells (erythrocytes) to the total blood volume

Hematoma a collection of blood in a tissue, organ, or space due to a break in the wall of a blood vessel

Hematuria the presence of blood in the urine

Hemiplegia loss of movement on one side of the body

Hemoglobin the red pigment in red blood cells that carries oxygen

Hemoglobinuria the presence of hemoglobin in the urine

Hemolysis rupture of red blood cells

Hemopneumothorax a collection of blood and air or gas in the pleural cavity

Hemoptysis the presence of blood in the sputum

Hemorrhage excessive loss of blood from the vascular system

Hemorrhoids distended veins in the rectum

Hemostasis cessation of bleeding

Hemostat (artery forceps) a small pair of forceps used to constrict blood vessels

Hemothorax a collection of blood in the pleural cavity

Heparin a substance that prevents coagulation of blood

Heparin lock (intravenous lock) the airtight cap covering the end of a client's intravenous or central venous tubing

Herbalist an herb doctor; one who prescribes herbs for treating people

Hering-Breuer reflex a reflex that inhibits inspiration

Hernia a protrusion of the organ or tissue through an abdominal or inguinal opening

Hesitancy (of urination) delay and difficulty initiating voiding

Heterosexual a person whose primary sexual orientation is to a member of the opposite sex

High-Fowler's position a bed-sitting position in which the head of the bed is elevated 90 degrees

Hirsutism abnormal hairiness, particularly in women

Holism all living organisms are seen as interacting, unified wholes that are more than the sums of their parts

Holistic health a model of health based on the belief that the whole is more than the sum of its parts

Homans' sign calf pain produced by dorsiflexion of the foot

Homeodynamics the continual exchange of energy between humans and the external environment

Homeostasis (negative feedback) the tendency of the body to maintain a state of balance or equilibrium while continually changing; a mechanism in which deviations from normal are sensed and counteracted

Homogeneity a high degree of likeness of attitudes and beliefs among members of a group

Homosexual a person whose primary sexual orientation is to a member of the same sex

Hordeolum (sty) a redness, swelling, and tenderness of the hair follicle and glands that empty at the edge of the eyelids

Horizontal recumbent back-lying position with legs extended; small pillow under the head

Hospice the delivery of care for terminally ill clients either in health care facilities or in the client's home

Hot pack (foment) hot, moist cloth applied to an area of the body

Human needs physiologic or psychologic conditions that an individual must meet to achieve a state of health or well-being

Humanism concern for human attributes

Humidifier a device that adds water vapor to inspired air

Humidity the amount of moisture in the air, expressed as a percentage

Hydration the act of combining or being combined with water

Hydrocephalus a condition in which there is excessive cerebrospinal fluid within the skull

Hydrolysis the process of splitting a molecule in the presence of digestive enzymes with the addition of water

Hydrometer (urinometer) an instrument used to measure the specific gravity of urine

Hydrostatic pressure the pressure a liquid exerts on the sides of the container that holds it; also called filtration force

Hygiene the science of health and its maintenance

Hyperalgesia extreme sensitivity to pain

Hyperalimentation (Total Parenteral Nutrition, TPN) see Total Parenteral Nutrition

Hypercalcemia an excess of calcium in the blood plasma

Hypercalciuria excessive calcium in the urine

Hypercapnea (hypercarbia) accumulation of carbon dioxide in the blood

Hyperchloremia an excess of chloride in the blood plasma

Hyperemia increased blood flow to an area

Hyperesthesia greater than normal sensation

Hyperextension further extension between two bones or stretching out of a joint

Hyperglycemia an excessive concentration of sugar in the blood

Hyperhidrosis excessive perspiration

Hyperkalemia an excess of potassium in the blood plasma

Hyperlipidemia elevated concentration of lipids in the plasma

Hypermagnesia an excess of magnesium in the blood plasma

Hypernatremia an excess of sodium in the blood plasma

Hyperopia (farsightedness) abnormal refraction in which light rays focus behind the retina

Hyperphosphatemia an excess of phosphate in the blood plasma

Hyperplasia an abnormal increase in the number of cells in a tissue or an organ

Hyperpnea an abnormal increase in the rate and depth of respirations

Hyperpyrexia see Hyperthermia

Hyperreflexia an exaggeration of the reflexes

Hyperresonance an abnormal booming sound produced during percussion of the lungs

Hypersensitivity an exaggerated response of the body to a foreign substance

Hypersomnia excessive sleep

Hypertension an abnormally high blood pressure; over 140 mm Hg systolic and/or 90 mm Hg diastolic

Hyperthermia (hyperpyrexia) an extremely high body temperature (eg, 41 C [105.8 F])

Hypertonicity excessive muscle tone or activity

Hypertonic solution a fluid possessing a greater concentration of solutes than plasma

Hypertrophy enlargement of a muscle or organ

Hyperventilation very deep, rapid respirations

Hypervolemia an abnormal increase in the body's blood volume; circulatory overload

Hypnotic (drug) a drug that induces sleep

Hypoalbuminemia reduction in the level of albumin in the blood

Hypocalcemia deficiency of calcium in the blood plasma

Hypocarbia (hypocapnia) depressed level of carbon dioxide in the blood plasma

Hypochloremia deficiency of chloride in the blood plasma

Hypodermic (subcutaneous) under the skin

Hypodermoclysis the introduction of fluid in the subcutaneous tissues

Hypoesthesia (hypesthesia) less than normal sensation

Hypoglycemia a reduced amount of glucose in the blood

Hypokalemia deficiency of potassium in the blood plasma

Hypomagnesia deficiency of magnesium in the blood plasma

Hyponatremia deficiency of sodium in the blood plasma

Hypophosphatemia deficiency in phosphate in the blood plasma

Hypopnea low rate of alveolar ventilation

Hypoproteinemia small amounts of protein in the blood plasma

Hypospadias opening of the urethra on the underside of the penis

Hypostatic pneumonia an infection of lung tissue resulting from poor circulation or stagnation of secretions

Hypotension an abnormally low blood pressure; less than 100 mm Hg systolic in an adult

Hypothermia a core body temperature below the lower limit of normal

Hypotheses statements of the relationship between two or more concepts (singular: hypothesis)

Hypotonicity decreased muscle tone

Hypotonic solution a fluid possessing a lesser concentration of solutes than plasma has

Hypoventilation very shallow respirations

Hypovolemia an abnormal reduction in blood volume

Hypovolemic shock a state of shock caused by a reduction in the volume of circulating blood

Hypoxemia see Anoxemia

Hypoxia insufficient oxygen anywhere in the body

Iatrogenic caused by the physician or medical therapy

Id the source of instinctive and unconscious psychologic urges

Identification perceiving one's self as similar to and behaving like another person

Idiosyncratic effect a different, unexpected or individual effect from the normal one usually expected from a medication; the occurrence of unpredictable and unexplainable symptoms

Ileal conduit most commonly used urinary diversion procedure

Ileostomy an opening into the ileum (small bowel)

Illicit drug a drug that is sold illegally; a street drug

Illness a highly personal state in which the person feels unhealthy or ill, may or may not be related to disease

Illness behavior the course of action a person takes to define the state of his or her health and pursue a remedy

Illusion a false interpretation of some stimulus

Imitation copying the behaviors and attitudes of another person

Immobility prescribed or unavoidable restriction of movement in any area of a person's life

Immunity a specific resistance of the body to infection; it may be natural, endowed resistance or resistance developed after exposure to a disease agent

Immunization the process of becoming immune or rendering someone immune

Immunoglobulin (immune bodies, antibodies) a part of the body's plasma proteins

Immunologic reaction (allergic reaction) production of antibodies in response to an antigen

Impaction a condition of being firmly wedged or lodged; in reference to feces, a collection of hardened puttylike feces in the folds of the rectum

Impaired nurse a nurse whose practice has deteriorated because of chemical abuse

Imperforate abnormally closed; used to describe an opening, such as the anus or the hymen, that is not open

Implementing the phase of the nursing process in which the nursing care plan is put into action

Implied consent consent that is assumed in an emergency when consent cannot be obtained from the client or a relative

Impotence (erectile dysfunction) the inability to achieve or maintain an erection sufficient for sexual satisfaction for the self and/or partner

Incentive spirometer (sustained maximal inspiration device, SMI) a device that measures the flow of air through a mouthpiece

Incident report an agency record of an accident or incident

Incision a cut or wound that is intentionally made (eg, during surgery)

Incontinence involuntary urination

Incubation period the time between entrance of microorganism into the body and the onset of symptoms of the infection

Independent nursing action (intervention or function) an activity that the nurse is licensed to initiate as a result of the nurse's own knowledge and skills

Inductive reasoning making generalizations from specific data

Induration hardening

Inertia inactivity; inability to move spontaneously

Infarct a localized area of necrosis (dead cells) usually owing to obstructed arterial blood flow to the part

Infection the disease process produced by microorganisms

Inferences interpretation or conclusions made based on cues or observed data

Inferior situated below

Infestation invasion of the body by insects, mites, or ticks

Infiltration the diffusion or deposition into tissue of substances that are not normal to it

Inflammation local and nonspecific defensive tissue response to injury or destruction of cells

Informed consent a client's agreement to accept a course of treatment or a procedure after receiving complete information, including the risks of treatment and facts relating to it, from the physician

Infradian rhythm a biorhythm that cycles monthly, such as the human menstrual cycle

Infrared heat a radiant type of heat capable of penetrating body tissues to a depth of 10 mm; sources include heat lamps and incandescent light bulbs

Infusion the introduction of fluid into vein or part of the body

Infusion controller a device used with intravenous infusions to control the infusion rate by using gravitational force

Infusion pump a device used with intravenous fluids to deliver a desired infusion rate by exerting positive pressure on the tubing or on the fluid

Ingestion the act of taking in food or medication

Inhalation (inspiration) the act of breathing in; the intake of air or other substances into the lungs

Inhalation (aerosol) therapy deliverance of droplets of medication or moisture suspended in a gas, such as oxygen, by inhalation through the nose or mouth

Inorganic substances substances not derived from hydrocarbons and not of organic origin

Inquest a legal inquiry into the cause or manner of a death

Insensible heat loss heat loss that occurs from evaporation (vaporization) of moisture from the respiratory tract, mucosa of the mouth, and the skin

Insensible perspiration unnoticeable sweating that evaporates immediately once it reaches the surface of the skin

In situ in place; localized

Insomnia inability to obtain a sufficient quality or quantity of sleep

Inspection visual examination to detect features detectable to the eye

Inspiration see inhalation

Inspiratory capacity the maximum amount of air inhaled after a normal expiration

Inspiratory reserve volume the maximum amount of air inhaled after a normal inspiration

Instillation application of a medication into a body cavity or orifice

Integumentary system the skin, hair, and nails

Intensity (amplitude) the loudness or softness of a sound

Intercostal between the ribs

Intercostal retractions indrawing between the ribs

Intermittent (quotidian) fever a body temperature that alternates at regular intervals between periods of fever and periods of normal temperature

Intermittent positive pressure breathing (IPPB) delivery of oxygen into the lungs at positive pressure and release of the pressure passively during expiration

Internal respiration the interchange of oxygen and carbon dioxide between the circulating blood and the cells of the body tissues

Internal rotation a turning toward the midline (eg, rotation of the hip joint)

Interstitial between the cells of the body's tissues

Interstitial fluid fluid that surrounds the cells, includes lymph

Intervertebral between the vertebrae, as in intervertebral disks

Intra-arterial into an artery

Intra-cardiac into the heart muscle

Intracellular within a cell or cells

Intracellular fluid (ICF) fluid found within the body cells, also called cellular fluid

Intractable pain pain that is resistant to cure or relief

Intradermal (intracutaneous) under the epidermis; into the dermis

Intralipid therapy the infusion of essential fatty acids or fat emulsions through a central venous line

Intramuscular into the muscle

Intraoperative period the phase during surgery; begins when the client is transferred to the operating room bed, and ends when the client is admitted to the recovery room

Intraosseous into the bone

Intrapleural within the pleural cavity

Intrapleural pressure pressure within the pleural cavity

Intrapulmonic pressure pressure within the lungs

Intraspinal (intrathecal) into the spinal canal

Intrauterine within the uterus

Intravascular within a blood vessel

Intravascular fluid plasma

Intravenous within a vein

Intravenous cholangiogram an X-ray film of the bile ducts after a contrast dye has been administered intravenously

Intravenous lock see Heparin lock

Intravenous push (IVP, bolus) the direct intravenous administration of a medication that cannot be diluted or that is needed in an emergency

Intravenous pyelography (IVP); intravenous urography (IVU) X-ray filming of the kidney and ureters after injection of a radiopaque material into the vein

Intubation the insertion of a tube

Inversion a turning inward

Ion an atom or group of atoms that carry a positive or negative electric charge; an electrolyte

Iritis inflammation of the iris

Iron deficiency anemia a form of anemia caused by inadequate supply of iron for synthesis of hemoglobin

Irradiation exposure to penetrating rays, such as X rays, gamma rays, infrared rays, or ultraviolet rays

Irrational confused as to time, place, or person

Irrigation (lavage) a flushing or washing-out of a body cavity, organ, or wound with a specified solution

Ischemia deficiency of blood supply caused by obstruction of circulation to the body part

Isolation practices that prevent the spread of infection and communicable disease

Isometric (static, setting) exercise tensing of a muscle against an immovable outer resistance, which does not change muscle length or produce joint motion

Isotonic (dynamic) exercise exercise in which muscle tension is constant and the muscle shortens to produce muscle contraction and movement

IV filters devices attached to intravenous infusion tubing to filter or remove air, particulate matter, and microbes to prevent contamination

Jaundice a yellowish color of the sclera, mucous membranes, or skin

Jejunostomy an opening through the abdominal wall into the jejunum

Jejunostomy feeding the instillation of liquid nourishment via a tube that enters the jejunum through a surgical opening into the abdominal wall

JVD jugular venous distention

Kegel's exercises pelvic floor or perineal muscle tightening exercises

Keratotic spots horny growths, such as warts or calluses

Ketone any compound containing the carbonyl group, CO, and having hydrocarbon groups attached to the carbonyl group

Ketone bodies products of incomplete fat metabolism which appear in the urine

Ketosis a condition in which excessive ketones are formed in the body

Kilocalorie see Calorie

Kilogram a unit of weight equal to 1000 grams or approximately 2.2 pounds

Kinesiology the study of the motion of the human body

Kinesthesia the ability to perceive extent, direction, or weight of movement

Knee-chest position see Genupectoral position

Koplick's spots red spots on the buccal mucosa; associated with measles

Korotkoff's sounds a series of five sounds produced by blood within the artery with each ventricular contraction

Kussmaul breathing (Kussmaul-Kien respiration) deep rapid breathing; a dyspnea occurring in paroxysms often preceding diabetic coma; air hunger

Kwashiorkor a condition occurring in children, after weaning, as a result of protein and calorie malnutrition; evidenced by growth failure, potbelly, edema, and mental apathy

Kyphosis excessive convex curvature of the thoracic spine

Lacerate to tear, rather than cut, a body tissue

Lacrimation tearing of the eyes

Lanugo the fine , woolly hair or down on the shoulders, back, sacrum, and earlobes of the unborn child that may remain for a few weeks after birth

Large calorie see Calorie

Laryngeal stridor a harsh, crowing sound heard during expiration when there is a laryngeal obstruction

Laryngoscopy visual examination of the larynx with a laryngoscope

Lateral to the side, away from the midline

Lateral position a side-lying position

Lavage an irrigation or washing of a body organ, such as the stomach

Laxative a medication that stimulates bowel activity

Learning a change in human disposition or capability that persists over a period of time and cannot be solely accounted for by growth

Lentigo senilus small brown areas that appear on the hands and arms of an elderly client

Lesion the traumatic or pathologic interruption of a tissue or the loss of function of a body part

Lethargy drowsiness; sleeping much of the time when not stimulated

Leukocyte white blood cell

Leukocytosis an increase in the number of white blood cells

Leukoplakia white patches or spots on the mucous membrane of the tongue or cheek

Lever a rigid bar that moves on a fixed axis called a fulcrum

Levin tube a single-lumen nasogastric tube

Liable being legally responsible to account for one's obligations and actions and to make financial restitution for wrongful acts

Libido urge or desire for sexual activity

Lice parasitic insects that infest mammals

Life-style the values and behaviors adopted by a person in daily life

Life-style assessment appraisal of the personal life-style and habits of the client as they affect health

Lift an abnormal anterior movement of the chest related to enlargement of the right ventricle

Line of gravity an imaginary vertical line running through the center of gravity

Liniment a topical liquid applied to the skin frequently to stimulate circulation or to relieve pain

Lipid an organic substance that is greasy and insoluble in water

Lipofuscin an insoluble lipid pigment present in cardiac and smooth muscle cells

Lithotomy position a back-lying position in which the feet are supported in stirrups

Livor mortis discoloration of the skin caused by break down of the red blood cells; occurs after blood circulation has ceased; appears in the dependent areas of the body

Local adaptation syndrome (LAS) the reaction of one organ or body part to stress

Locus of control (LOC) a concept about whether clients believe their health status is under their own or other's control

Long board (Smooth mover, Easyglide) a lacquered or smooth polyethylene board with handholds along its edges used to facilitate moving the client from bed to stretcher or stretcher to bed

Longevity life expectancy

Lordosis an exaggerated concavity in the lumbar region of the vertebral column

Loss an actual or potential situation in which a valued ability, object, or person is inaccessible or changed so that it is perceived as no longer valuable

Lotion a liquid that often carries an insoluble powder

Louse a parasitic insect that infests mammals (plural: lice)

Low-Fowler's (semi-Fowler's) position a bed-sitting position in which the head of the bed is elevated between 15 and 45 degrees, with or without knee flexion

Lumbar puncture (LP, spinal tap) insertion of a needle into the subarachnoid space at the lumbar region

Lumen a channel within a tube

Lung compliance expansibility of the lung

Lung recoil the tendency of lungs to collapse away from the chest wall

Lymphadenitis inflammation of the lymph nodes

Lymphangitis the inflammation of a lymphatic vessel or vessels

Lymphocyte mononuclear leukocyte formed chiefly by lymphoid tissue

Lysis (of a fever) the gradual reduction of an elevated body temperature to normal

Lysozyme an enzyme in saliva and tears that functions as an antibacterial agent

Maceration the wasting away or softening of a solid as if by the action of soaking; often used to describe degenerative changes and eventual disintegration

Macrocephaly abnormally large head circumference

Macrognathia abnormally large jaw

Macrophage a large phagocytic cell that destroys microorganisms or harmful cells

Malaise a general feeling of being unwell

Malignancy abnormal tissue with a tendency to grow and invade other tissues

Malingering pretending to be ill rather than facing something unpleasant

Malnutrition a disorder of nutrition; insufficient nourishment of the body cells

Malpractice the negligent acts of persons engaged in professions or occupations in which highly technical or professional skills are employed

Malocclusion malposition and imperfect contact of the mandibular and maxillary teeth

Mammography X-ray study of breast tissue

Managed care a method of organizing care delivery that emphasizes communication and coordination of care among all health care team members

Manager one who is appointed to a position in an organization which gives the power to guide and direct the work of others

Manometer an instrument used to measure the pressure of fluids or gases

Margination the aggregating or lining up of substances along a surface or edge (eg, the lining up of white blood cells against the wall of a blood vessel during the inflammatory process)

Mastication the act of chewing

Mastitis inflammation of the breast

Masturbation manual self-stimulation of the genital organs or other erogenous areas

Matriarchy a system of social organization in which the mother is the head of the house or family

Matrilineal relating to descent through the female line

Maturation the process of becoming mature or fully developed; development of inherited traits

Maturity the state of maximal function and integration; the state of being fully developed

Mean blood pressure the midway point between the systolic and diastolic pressures

Meatus an opening, passage, or channel

Medial toward the middle or midline

Mediastinal shift a lateral movement of the organs in the mediastinum (ie, the heart and major vessels)

Medicaid a United States federal public assistance program paid out of general taxes and administered through the individual states to provide health care for those who require financial assistance

Medical asepsis all practices intended to confine a specific microorganism to a specific area, limiting the number, growth, and spread of microorganisms

Medical examiner a physician who usually has advanced education in pathology or forensic medicine who determines causes of death

Medicare a national and state health insurance program for United States residents over 65 years of age

Medication (drug) a substance administered for the diagnosis, cure, treatment, mitigation, or prevention of disease

Meditation mental exercise that directs the mind to think inwardly by closing the sense organs to external stimulation

Melanin the pigment that gives color to the skin

Menarche onset of menstruation

Meniscus the crescent-shaped upper surface of a column of fluid

Menopause cessation of menstruation

Menses menstrual flow

Mentor a person who serves as an experienced guide, adviser, or advocate and assumes responsibility for promoting the growth and professional advancement of a less experienced individual

Metabolism the sum of all the physical and chemical processes by which living substance is formed and maintained and by which energy is made available for use by the organism

Metacarpal referring to the part of the hand between the wrist and the fingers

Microcephaly abnormally small head circumference

Microorganism minute living body visible only under a microscope

Micturition see Urination

Midclavicular line an imaginary line that runs inferiorly and vertically from the center of the clavicle

Midsternal line an imaginary line that runs vertically through the middle of the sternum

Midwife a female who practices the art of aiding in the delivery of infants; may be a nurse who has received special training in obstetrics and is qualified to deliver infants

Milk, milking (a tube) the compression and movement of fingers along the length of a tube in order to move its contents toward an opening for removal

Milliequivalent (mEq) one-thousandth of an equivalent, which is the chemical combining power of a substance

Milliliter (mL) a unit of volume in the metric system approximating 1 cubic centimeter

Millimol one-thousandth of a mol

Minim the basic unit of measure in the apothecary system, equal to 0.0616 mL

Miosis constricted pupils

Miter a method of folding the bedclothes at the corners to secure them in place while the bed is occupied

MMR combined measles, mumps, and rubella vaccine

Mobility ability to move about freely

Modeling observing the behavior of people who have successfully achieved a goal that one has set for oneself and, through observing, acquiring ideas for behavior and coping strategies

Mol a molar solution of a substance

Mongolian spots blue-gray areas of discoloration of the skin of the lower back, thighs, and sometimes shoulders of the infant and small children; more often seen in non-white children.

Monocyte mononuclear leukocyte formed in the bone marrow

Monotheism belief in the existence of one God

Montgomery straps tie tapes used to hold dressings in place

Morality a doctrine or system denoting what is right and wrong in conduct, character, or attitude

Morbidity incidence of disease

Mores values of members in a group

Morgue a place where dead bodies are temporarily kept before release to a mortician

Moro's reflex the startle reflex of infants, in which the arms and legs are extended outward and retracted in response to a sudden stimulus such as a loud noise

Mortality death rate

Mortician a person trained in the care of the dead; also called an undertaker

Mourning the process through which grief is eventually resolved or altered

Mucous membrane epithelial tissue that forms mucus, concentrates bile, and secretes or excretes enzymes

Mucus the lubricating, free slime of the mucous membranes

Multigravida a woman who has been pregnant more than once

Multilumen catheter a catheter which has more than one channel, each channel or lumen has a separate port located along or at the catheter tip

Multiparous a female who has more than one child

Murmurs (cardiac) an adventitious or abnormal sound heard on auscultation of the heart during systole and diastole

Mydriasis enlarged pupils

Mydriatic a medication that dilates the pupils of the eyes

Myelogram (myelography) an X-ray film of the spinal cord, nerve roots, and vertebrae after injection of a contrast medium into the subarachnoid space

Myocardial infarction cardiac tissue necrosis owing to obstruction of blood flow to the heart

Myopia (nearsightedness) abnormal refraction in which light rays focus in front of the retina

Myotonia increased muscle tension

Myxedema (hypothyroidism) underactivity of the thyroid

Narcolepsy a condition in which an individual experiences an uncontrollable desire for sleep or attacks of sleep during the day

Narcotic a strong analgesic

Narcotic agonist-antagonist a drug with properties that simulate a narcotic and with properties that act against the effects of a narcotic

Nasal cannula (nasal prongs) a device used to administer low-flow oxygen

Nasogastric tube a plastic or rubber tube inserted through the nose into the stomach for the purpose of feeding or irrigating the stomach

Naturopath a nonmedical practitioner who uses such things as light, heat, and water in therapy, but not drugs

Nausea the urge to vomit

Nebulization the conversion of a fine mist or spray from a liquid

Nebulizer a device which produces a fine mist; atomizer or sprayer

Necrosis death of tissue cells caused by inadequate blood supply

Negative feedback see Homeostasis

Negative nitrogen balance a nitrogen output that exceeds nitrogen intake

Negligence failure to behave in a reasonable and prudent manner; an unintentional tort

Neoplasm any growth that is new and abnormal

Nephritis inflammation of a kidney

Nerve block chemical interruption of a nerve pathway effected by injecting a local anesthetic

Nerve conduction study a procedure to determine the excitability and conduction velocity of motor and sensory nerves and the presence of disease of the peripheral nerves

Networking a process by which people development linkages throughout the profession to communicate, share ideas and information, and offer support and direction to each other

Neurologic pertaining to the nervous system

Nitrogen balance the state of protein nutrition

Nociceptor a pain receptor

Nocturia (nycturia) increased frequency of urination at night that is not a result of increased fluid intake

Nocturnal enuresis involuntary urination at night

Noncompliance failure to follow the prescribed treatment plan

Nonmaleficence the duty to do no harm

Nonproductive cough a dry, harsh cough without secretions

Non-rapid-eye-movement sleep see NREM sleep

Nonverbal communication (body language) communication other than words, including gestures, posture and facial expressions

Norm an ideal or fixed standard; an expected standard of behavior of group members

Normal saline an isotonic concentration of salt (NaCl) solution

Nosocomial referring to or originating in a hospital or similar institution (eg, a nosocomial infection)

NREM (non-rapid-eye-movement) sleep a deep restful sleep state; also called slow wave sleep

Nursing diagnosis the nurse's clinical judgment about individual, family, or community responses to actual and potential health problems/life processes to provide the basis for selecting nursing interventions to achieve outcomes for which the nurse is accountable

Nursing process a systematic rational method of planning and providing nursing care

Nursing standards optimum levels of nursing care against which actual performance of a nurse is compared

Nutrient an organic and inorganic substance found in food; nutrients are digested and absorbed in the gastrointestinal tract and then used in the body's metabolic processes

Nutritive value the nutrient content of a specified amount of food

Nystagmus involuntary rapid movement of the eyeball

-ostomy a suffix denoting the formation of an opening or outlet

Obese (obesity) to weigh greater than 20% of the ideal for height and frame

Objective data (signs, overt data) information (data) that is detectable by an observer or can be tested against an accepted standard; can be seen, heard, felt, or smelled

Obligatory heat the heat produced by the body as a result of the metabolism of food

Obligatory loss the essential fluid loss required to maintain body functioning

Obstetrics the branch of medicine dealing with the birth process and related events that precede and follow it

Obtunded difficult to arouse from sleep; requiring shaking or a painful stimulus to awaken

Obturator a disc or instrument that closes an opening (eg, the obturator of a tracheostomy set fits inside and closes off the end of the outer tube)

Occlusive closed

Occult hidden

Occupational therapist one who assists clients with impaired function to gain the skills required to perform activities of daily living

Occupied bed a bed currently being used by a client

Olfactory referring to the sense of smell

Oliguria production of abnormally small amounts of urine by the kidney

Oncotic pressure pulling force exerted by colloids that help maintain the water content of blood

Opaque not admitting the passage of light

Open system a system in which energy, matter, and information move into and out of the system through the system boundary

Ophthalmoscope an instrument used to examine the interior of the eye

Oral referring to the mouth

Organic referring to an organ or organs; in chemistry, referring to compounds containing carbon; arising from an organism

Orgasm climax of sexual excitement

Orientation awareness of time, place, and person

Orifice an external opening of a body cavity

Orthopnea ability to breathe only when in an upright position (sitting or standing)

Orthopneic position a sitting position to relieve respiratory difficulty in which the client leans over and is supported by an overbed table across the lap

Orthostatic hypotension decrease in blood pressure related to positional or postural changes from lying to sitting or standing positions

Osmol the number of particles in 1 gram molecular weight of a disassociated solute

Osmolarity (osmolality) the concentration of solutes in solution; the osmolar concentration of a solution expressed in osmols per liter of solution

Osmosis passage of a solvent through a semipermeable membrane from an area of lesser solute concentration to one of greater solute concentration

Osmotic pressure pressure exerted by the number of nondiffusable particles in a solution; the amount of pressure needed to stop the flow of water across a membrane

Osteoarthritis noninflammatory degenerative joint disease

Osteoporosis demineralization of the bone

Otoscope an instrument used to examine the ears

Outward rotation a turning away from the midline

Overt data see Objective data

Oxidation a chemical process by which a substance combines with oxygen; energy is released, and other substances are formed

Oxygen analyzer a device used to measure the concentration of oxygen being received by the client

Oxyhemoglobin the compound of oxygen and hemoglobin

Pace number of steps taken per minute or the distance taken in one step when walking

Pack an unsterile hot or cold moist cloth applied to an area of the body

Packing filling an open wound or cavity with a material such as gauze

$Paco_2$ partial pressure of carbon dioxide (arterial blood)

Pain reaction the autonomic nervous system and behavioral responses to pain

Pain threshold (pain sensation) the amount of pain stimulation a person requires before feeling pain

Pain tolerance the maximum amount and duration of pain that an individual is willing to endure

Palliative affording relief but not cure

Pallor the absence of underlying red tones in the skin and may be most readily seen in the buccal mucosa

Palpation the examination of the body using the sense of touch

Pandemic an epidemic disease that is widespread

Pao_2 partial pressure of oxygen (arterial blood)

Pap (Papanicolaou) smear a method of taking a sample of cervical cells for microscopic examination to detect malignancy

Papule a superficial, circumscribed elevation of the skin

Paracentesis the insertion of a needle into a cavity (usually the abdominal cavity) to remove fluid

Paradoxical breathing the ballooning out of the chest wall during expiration and depression or sucking inward of the chest wall during inspiration

Paralysis the impairment or loss of motor function of a body part

Paramedical having a connection with medicine

Paraphrasing (restating) actively listening for the client's basic message and then repeating those thoughts and/or feelings in similar words

Paraplegia paralysis of the lower part of the body (including the legs) affecting both motor function and sensation

Parasite a microorganism that lives in or on another from which it obtains nourishment

Parenteral drug administration occurring outside the alimentary tract; injected into the body through some route other than the alimentary canal (eg, intramuscularly)

Paresis paralysis

Paresthesia an abnormal sensation of burning or prickling

Paronychia infection of the tissue surrounding the nail

Parotitis inflammation of the parotid salivary gland

Paroxysm a sudden attack or sharp recurrence; a spasm

Partial pressure the pressure exerted by each individual gas in a mixture according to its percentage concentration in the mixture

Passive euthanasia allowing a person to die by withholding or withdrawing measures to maintain life

Passive immunity a resistance of the body to infection in which the host receives natural or artificial antibodies produced by another source

Passive range-of-motion (ROM) exercise exercise in which another person moves each of the client's joints through their complete range of movement, maximally stretching all muscle groups within each plane over each joint

Passivity lethargy; receptivity to outside influence; lack of energy or will

Patent open, unobstructed; not closed

Pathogenic capable of producing disease

Patient controlled analgesia (PCA) a pain management technique that allows the client to take an active role in managing pain

Patient Self Determination Act (PSDA) legislation requiring that every competent adult be informed in writing upon admission to a health care institution about his or her rights to accept or refuse medical care and to use advance directives

Patriarchy a social system in which the father is the head of the household or family

Patrilineal relating to descent through the male line

Pco_2 partial pressure of carbon dioxide (venous blood)

Peak plasma level (of drug) the concentration of a drug in the blood plasma that occurs when the elimination rate equals the rate of absorption

Pectoriloquy exaggerated bronchophony

Pediculosis infestation with head lice

Penrose drain a flexible rubber drain

Perception the ability to interpret the environment through the senses

Percussion (clapping, cupping) (in physiotherapy) the forceful striking of the chest with cupped hands to loosen secretions in the lungs

Percussion (in assessment) a method in which the body surface is struck to elicit sounds that can be heard or vibrations that can be felt

Perfusion passage of blood constituents through the vessels of the circulatory system

Perineum the area between the anus and the posterior (back) aspect of the genitals

Periodontal disease (pyorrhea) disorder of the supporting structures of the teeth

Periorbital around the eye socket

Peripheral at the edge or outward boundary

Peripheral pulse a pulse located in the periphery of the body (eg, foot, wrist)

Peristalsis wavelike movements produced by circular and longitudinal muscle fibers of the intestinal walls; it propels the intestinal contents onward

Peristomal around a stoma

Peritoneal dialysis the instillation and drainage of a solution (dialysate) from the peritoneal cavity

Personal space the distance people prefer in interactions with others

Personality the outward expression of the inner self

Perspiration the fluid secreted by the sweat glands for excreting waste products and cooling the body

PES format the three essential components of nursing diagnostic statements including the terms describing the problem, the etiology of the problem, and the defining characteristics or cluster of signs and symptoms

Petechiae pinpoint red areas in the skin

Petrissage a massage technique consisting of kneading or large, quick pinches of the skin, subcutaneous tissue, and muscle

pH a measure of the relative alkalinity or acidity of a solution; a measure of the concentration of hydrogen ions

Phagocyte a white blood cell; it ingests microorganisms, other cells, and foreign particles

Phagocytosis the process by which cells engulf microorganisms, other cells, or foreign particles

Phantom pain pain that remains after the perceived location has been removed, such as pain perceived in a foot after the leg has been amputated

Pharmacokinetics the study of the absorption, distribution, biotransformation, and excretion of drugs

Pharmacology the scientific study of the actions of drugs on living animals and humans

Pharmacopoeia a book containing a list of drug products used in medicine, including their descriptions and formulas

Phlebitis inflammation of the vein

Phlebotomy opening a vein to remove blood

Photophobia intolerance to light

Photosensitive sensitive to light

Phrenic referring to the diaphragm

Physical restraints any manual method or physical or mechanical device, material, or equipment attached to the client's body that restrict the client's movement

Physiologic dependence biochemical changes occurring in the body as a result of excessive use of a drug

Physiologic homeostasis the internal environment of the body is relatively stable and constant

Pica a craving for unnatural foods, often during pregnancy, some psychologic conditions, or extreme malnutrition

Pigeon chest (pectus carinatum) a permanent deformity of the chest characterized by a narrow transverse diameter, and increased anteroposterior diameter, and a protruding sternum

Pitch the frequency or number of the vibrations heard during auscultation

Pitting edema edema in which firm finger pressure on the skin produces an indentation (pit) that remains for several seconds

Placebo any form of treatment (eg, medication) that produces an effect in the client because of its intent rather than its chemical or physical properties

Plantar flexion movement of the ankle so that the toes point downward

Plantar reflex see Babinski reflex

Plantar wart a wart on the sole of the foot

Plaque an invisible soft film consisting of bacteria, molecules of saliva, and remnants of epithelial cells and leukocytes that adheres to the enamel surface of teeth

Plasma the fluid portion of the blood in which the blood cells are suspended

Pleural rub (friction rub) a coarse, leathery, or grating sound produced by the rubbing together of the pleura

Pleximeter in percussion, the middle finger of the dominant hand placed firmly on the client's skin

Plexor in percussion, the middle finger of the nondominant hand or a percussion hammer used to strike the pleximeter

Plexus a network (eg, of nerves or veins)

Plumbism lead poisoning

Pneumonia inflammation of the lung tissue

Pneumothorax accumulation of gas or fluid in the pleural cavity

PO_2 partial pressure of oxygen (venous blood)

Point of maximal impulse (PMI) the point where the apex of the heart touches the anterior chest wall

Polydipsia excessive thirst

Polyuria (diuresis) the production of abnormally large amounts of urine by the kidneys without an increased fluid intake

POMR (POR) see Problem-oriented medical record

Port (portal) an opening or entrance

Portal of entry in communicable disease, the opening through which infectious organisms invade the body (eg, urinary tract, respiratory tract, open wound)

Positive reinforcement giving rewards such as praise for a learner's achievements

Positive nitrogen balance nitrogen input exceeding nitrogen output

Posterior toward, or at the back of

Postural drainage the drainage, by gravity, of secretions from various lung segments

Posture the bearing and position of the body; the relative arrangements of the various parts of the body

Power capacity to influence another person in some way or to produce change

Powerlessness perceived lack of control over events

Preceptor an experienced nurse who assists the novice nurse in improving nursing skill and judgment

Precordium an area of the chest overlying the heart

Preferred provider organization (PPO) a group of physicians or a hospital that provides companies with health services at a discounted rate

Preoperative period the period before an operation; begins when the decision for surgery has been made and ends when the client is transferred to the operating room bed

Presbycusis loss of hearing related to aging

Presbyopia loss of elasticity of the lens and thus loss of ability to see close objects as a result of the aging process

Prescription the written direction for the preparation and administration of a drug

Pressure sores (decubitus ulcers, bedsores, distortion sores) reddened areas, sores, or ulcers of the skin occurring over bony prominences

Primary care the point of entry into the health care system at which initial health care is given

Primary (source) data data or information which is obtained from the client

Primary intention healing (primary union, first intention healing) healing that occurs in a wound in which the tissue surfaces are or have been approximated and there is minimal or no tissue loss; it is characterized by the formation of minimal granulation tissue and scarring

Primary memory short-term memory

Primary prevention activities directed toward the protection from or avoidance of potential health risks

Priority setting the process of establishing a preferential order for nursing strategies

Privacy a deserved degree of social retreat that provides a comfortable feeling

Privileged communication information given to a professional who is forbidden by law from disclosing the information in a court without the consent of the person who provided it

PRN an order which enables the nurse to give a medication or treatment when, in the nurse's judgment, the client needs it

Problem-oriented medical record (POMR or POR) data about the client are recorded and arranged according to the client's problems, rather than according to the source of the information

Process a series of actions directed toward a particular result; in anatomy, a prominence or projection (eg, of a bone)

Process recording the verbatim (word-for-word) account of a conversation

Proctoscopy visual examination of the interior of the rectum with a lighted instrument (proctoscope)

Proctosigmoidoscopy visual examination of the rectum and the sigmoid colon with a lighted instrument (proctosigmoidoscope)

Prodromal period the time from the onset of nonspecific symptoms to the appearance of specific symptoms

Professional socialization the process in which the knowledge, skills, and attitudes characteristic of a profession are acquired

Prognosis the medical opinion about the outcome of a disease

Progressive relaxation a formalized relaxation technique designed to reduce stress and chronic pain

Projection a defense mechanism by which a person attributes his or her own undesired characteristics to another

Proliferation rapid reproduction of parts or cells

Pronation moving the bones of the forearm so that the palm of the hand faces downward when held in front of the body

Prone position face-lying position, with or without a small pillow

Prophylaxis preventive treatment; prevention of disease

Proprioceptor a sensory receptor that is sensitive to movement and the position of the body

Prospective payment system (PPS) federal plan that establishes Medicare reimbursement rates in advance of hospitalization and according to diagnostic related groups (DRG's)

Prostatectomy the removal of the prostate

Prosthesis an artificial part (eg, a glass eye, an artificial limb, or dentures)

Prostration extreme exhaustion

Proteinuria the presence of protein in the urine

Protocol a predetermined and preprinted plan specifying the procedure to be followed in a particular situation

Protraction moving a part of the body forward in the same plane parallel to the ground

Proxemics the study of distance between people in their interactions

Proximal closest to the point of reference

Pruritis itching

Psychologic dependence (on a drug) a state of emotional reliance on a drug to maintain one's well-being; a feeling of need or craving for a drug

Psychologic homeostasis emotional or psychologic balance or state of mental well-being

Psychomotor referring to motor actions, such as hand and finger movements

Psychosomatic concerning the mind and the body; emotional disturbances manifested by physiologic symptoms

Ptosis eyelids that lie at or below the pupil margin

Ptyalism excessive secretion of saliva

Puberty the first stage of adolescence in which sexual organs begin to grow and mature

Pulmonary capacities the combinations of two or more pulmonary volumes

Pulmonary embolus a blood clot that has moved to the lungs

Pulse the wave of blood within an artery that is created by contraction of the left ventricle of the heart

Pulse deficit the difference between the apical pulse and the radial pulse

Pulse oximeter a noninvasive device that measures the arterial blood oxygen saturation by means of a sensor attached to the finger

Pulse pressure the difference between the systolic and the diastolic blood pressure

Pulse rate the number of pulse beats per minute

Pulse rhythm the pattern of the beats and intervals between the beats

Pulse tension the elasticity of the arteries

Pulse volume the strength or amplitude of the pulse, the force of blood exerted with each beat

Purulent containing pus

Purulent exudate an exudate consisting of leukocytes, liquefied dead tissue debris, and dead and living bacteria

Pus a thick liquid associated with inflammation and composed of cells, liquid, microorganisms, and tissue debris

Pustule a visible collection of pus within the epidermis

Putrid rotten

Pyelogram an X-ray film of the kidney and ureter, showing the pelvis of the kidney

Pyogenic pus-producing

Pyorrhea purulent periodontal disease

Pyrexia (hyperthermia) a body temperature above the normal range; fever

Pyrogen a substance that produces a fever

Pyuria the presence of pus in the urine

Quality (of sound) a subjective description of a sound (eg, whistling, gurgling)

Quality assurance the evaluation of nursing services provided and the results achieved against an established standard

Race classification of people according to shared biologic characteristics and physical features

Racism assumption of inherent racial superiority or inferiority and the consequent discrimination against certain races

Radial pulse the pulse point located where the radial artery passes over the radius of the arm

Radiating pain pain perceived at the source and in surrounding or nearby tissues

Radiation the transfer of heat from the surface of one object to the surface of another without contact between the two objects

Radiopaque able to block the passage of radiant energy, such as X-rays

Rales (crackles) bubbling or rattling sounds, audible by ear or stethoscope on inhalation; they are a result of fluid in the lungs

Range of motion (ROM) the degree of movement possible for each joint

Rapport a relationship between two or more people of mutual trust and understanding

Rationale the scientific reason for selecting a specific action

Rationalization the attempt to justify behavior by logical reasoning and explanation

Reaction formation a defense mechanism in which one behaves exactly opposite to the way one is feeling

Rebound phenomenon (thermal) the time when the maximum therapeutic effect of a hot or cold application is achieved and the opposite effect begins

Receptor (sensor) the terminal of a sensory nerve that is sensitive to specific stimuli

Reconstitution the technique of adding a solvent to a powdered drug to prepare it for injection

Recording (charting) the process of making written entries about a client on the medical record

Rectal referring to the distal portion of the large intestine

Rectocele (proctocele) a protrusion of part of the rectum into the vagina

Reduced hemoglobin hemoglobin that has released its oxygen

Reduction the realignment of fractured bone fragments to their normal position

Referred pain pain perceived to be in one area but whose source is another area

Referring the transfer of a client's care to another person

Reflex an automatic response of the body to a stimulus

Reflux backward flow

Regeneration (tissue) renewal, regrowth, the replacement of destroyed tissue cells by cells that are identical or similar in structure and function

Regimen a regulated pattern of activity

Regression a defense mechanism in which one adapts behavior that was comforting earlier in life to overcome the discomfort and insecurity of the present situation

Regurgitation the spitting up or backward flow of undigested food

Rehabilitation the process of restoring clients to useful function in physical, mental, social, economic, and vocational areas of their lives

Reliability the degree to which an instrument produces consistent results on repeated use

Remission a period during a chronic illness when there is a lessening of severity or cessation of symptoms

REM sleep (paradoxical sleep) sleep during which the person experiences rapid eye movements

Renal relating to the kidney

Renal calculi calcium crystals or stones in the renal system

Renal dialysis a process in which blood flows from an artery through an artificial membrane that removes impurities; the blood then returns to the client through a vein

Renin a substance secreted by the kidneys when blood sodium levels are low; it controls aldosterone secretion

Repression a defense mechanism in which painful thoughts, experiences, and impulses are removed from awareness

Research process a series of steps or phases that are dynamic, flexible, and expandable, aimed toward generating useful knowledge

Reservoir a source of microorganisms

Resident flora microorganisms that normally reside on the skin, mucous membranes, and inside the respiratory and gastrointestinal tracts

Residual urine the amount of urine remaining in the bladder after a person voids

Residual volume (air) the amount of air remaining in the lungs after a person exhales both tidal and expiratory reserve volumes

Resistive exercise exercise in which the client contracts a muscle against an opposing force (eg, a weight)

Resonance a low-pitched, hollow sound prouced over normal lung tissue when the chest is percussed

Respiration the act of breathing; transport of oxygen from the atmosphere to the body cells and transport of carbon dioxide from the cells to the atmosphere

Respiratory acidosis (hypercapnia) a state of excess carbon dioxide in the body

Respiratory alkalosis a state of excessive loss of carbon dioxide from the body

Respiratory arrest the sudden cessation of breathing

Respiratory excursion (chest expansion) the amount of chest expansion or movement from full expiration to full inspiration

Respiratory quality (character) refers to those aspects of breathing that are different from normal, effortless breathing, includes the amount of effort exerted to breathe and the sounds produced by breathing

Respiratory rhythm (pattern) refers to the regularity of the expirations and the inspirations

Restitution an adaptive mechanism in which one performs restorative acts to relieve guilt

Restraints protective devices used to limit physical activity of the client or a part of the client's body

Resuscitate to restore life; to revive

Resuscitation bag (Ambu bag) a device used to provide oxygen to a client when they are unable to breathe for themselves

Retching the involuntary attempt to vomit without producing emesis

Retention (urinary) the accumulation of urine in the bladder and the inability of the bladder to empty itself

Retention sutures (stay sutures) large sutures used in addition to skin sutures to attach underlying tissues of fat and muscle as well as skin; used to support incisions in obese individuals or when healing may be prolonged

Retraction (mobility) moving a part of the body backward in same plane parallel to the ground

Retrograde pyelography an X-ray film taken after a contrast medium is injected through ureteral catheters into the kidneys

Retroperitoneal behind the peritoneum

Reverse Trendelenburg's position a position with the head of the bed raised and the foot lowered, while the bed foundation remains unbroken

Rhinitis inflammation of the mucous membrane of the nose

Rhonchi (gurgles) coarse, dry, wheezy, or whistling sounds, more audible during exhalation, as the air moves through tenacious mucus or a constricted bronchus

Rights privileges that individuals possess unless revoked by law or given up voluntarily

Rigidity stiffness or inflexibility of a muscle

Rigor mortis the stiffening of the body that occurs after death

Rinne test a hearing test that compares bone and air conduction of sound

Risk factors factors that cause a client to be vulnerable to developing a health problem

Roentgenogram a film produced by photography with X-rays

Role the set of expectations about how a person occupying a specific position behaves

Role conflict a clash between the beliefs or behaviors imposed by two or more roles fulfilled by one person

Romberg's sign inability to maintain balance while standing with the feet together

Rotation movement of the bone around its central axis either toward the midline of the body (internal rotation) or away from the midline of the body (external rotation)

S_1 the first heart sound which occurs when the atrioventricular valves (mitral and tricuspid) close

S_2 the second heart sound which occurs when the semilunar valves (aortic and pulmonic) close

Salem sump tube a double-lumen nasogastric tube

Sanguineous containing blood

Sanguineous exudate an exudate containing large amounts of red blood cells

Satiety a feeling of fullness as a result of satisfying the desire for food

Saturated fat a fat whose molecular structure is saturated with hydrogen, such as fats in meat, butter, and eggs

Scabies a contagious skin infestation caused by an arachnid, the itch mite

Scan a noninvasive type of X-ray procedure capable of distinguishing minor differences in the radiodensity of soft tissues

Scar (cicatrical) tissue defense fibrous tissue derived from granulation tissue

Scientific method a logical, systematic approach to solving problems

Sclerosis a process of hardening that occurs from inflammation and disease of the interstitial substance; the term is used to describe hardening of nervous tissues and arterioles

Scoliosis an abnormal lateral deviation of the spine

Screening examination (review of systems) a brief review of essential functioning of various body parts or systems

Seborrheic dermatitis a chronic disease of the skin, characterized by scaling and crusted patches on various body areas (eg, the scalp)

Sebum the oily, lubricating secretion of glands in the skin called sebaceous glands

Secondary care health care focusing on preventing complications of disease conditions

Secondary data data or information that is obtained from a source other than the client (eg, family, friends, medical records)

Secondary intention healing (secondary union) healing that occurs in a wound in which the tissue surfaces are not approximated and there is extensive tissue loss; it is characterized by the formation of excessive granulation tissue and scarring

Secondary memory long-term memory

Secondary prevention activities designed for early diagnosis and treatment of disease or illness

Sedative an agent that tends to calm or tranquilize

Self-actualization (Maslow) the highest level of personality development in which people reach their full potential

Self-care activities performed by individuals in their own behalf to maintain health and well-being

Self-concept the collection of ideas, feelings, and beliefs one has about oneself

Self-determination the right of clients to feel free from undue influence

Self-esteem the value one has for oneself; self-confidence

Self-expectancy (self-ideal) what a person wants to become; the power a person perceives he or she has to meet self-expectations

Self-identity the conscious sense of individuality and uniqueness that evolves throughout life

Self-image a person's perception of self at a specific time or over a period of time

Semi-Fowler's (low-Fowler's) position a bed-sitting position in which the head of the bed is elevated 15 to 45 degrees, with or without knee flexion

Semiprone position (Sims' position) side-lying position with lowermost arm behind the body and uppermost leg flexed

Senescence the process of growing old

Sensitivity quick response, often referring to the response of microorganisms to an antibiotic

Sensoristasis the need for sensory stimulation

Sensory adaptation ability of sensory receptors to adapt partially or completely to a repeated stimulus

Sensory deficit partial or complete impairment of any sensory organ

Sensory deprivation (input deficit) insufficient sensory stimulation for a person to function

Sensory memory momentary perception of stimuli by the senses

Sensory overload an overabundance of sensory stimulation

Sensory perception the organization and translation of stimuli into meaningful information

Sensory reception process of receiving environmental stimuli

Septic produced by putrefaction or decomposition

Serosanguineous composed of serum and blood

Serous of or like serum

Serum (blood) the clear liquid portion of the blood that does not contain fibrinogen

Sexual identity (core-gender identity) a person's inner feeling or sense of being male or female; more commonly indicates a person's sexual orientation

Sexuality the collective characteristics that mark the differences between the male and female, the constitution and life of the individual as related to sex

Sexually transmitted (venereal) disease a disease that can be passed on through intercourse with an infected person

Shearing force a combination of friction and pressure which when applied to the skin results in damage to the blood vessels and tissues

Shiatsu (acupressure) form of massage in which firm, gentle pressure is applied to the acupuncture points of the body

Shock acute circulatory failure

Sick role behavior actions directed at getting well taken by a person who considers him- or herself ill

Side rails (safety rails) movable rails attached to the sides of hospital beds and stretchers designed to decrease the risk of client falls

Sigmoidoscopy visual examination of the interior of the sigmoid colon with a lighted instrument (sigmoidoscope)

Significant other an individual or group who takes on special importance for a person

Sims' position (semiprone position) side-lying position with lowermost arm behind the body and uppermost leg flexed

Singultus hiccups

Sleep apnea periodic cessation of breathing during sleep

Small calorie (c, cal) the amount of heat required to raise the temperature of 1 g of water 1 C

Soak refers to immersing a body part in a solution or wrapping the part in gauze dressings and then saturating the dressing with a solution

SOAP an acronym for a charting method that follows a recording sequence of *s*ubjective data, *o*bjective data, *a*ssessment, and *p*lanning

Socialization a process by which a person learns the ways of a group or society in order to become a functioning participant

Social support network others outside the immediate family unit who provide strength, encouragement, and assistance to the family, especially during a crisis

Sociogram a diagram of the flow of verbal communication within a group during a specified period

Solute a substance dissolved in a liquid

Solvent the liquid in which a solute is dissolved

Somatic referring to the body, referring to the structures of the body wall in contrast to the viscera

Somnambulism sleepwalking

Sordes accumulation of foul matter (food, microorganisms and epithelial elements) on the teeth and gums

Source oriented clinical record (source oriented medical record) a record in which each person or department makes notations in a separate section or sections of the client's chart

Souffle a blowing sound heard by auscultation

Spastic describing the sudden, prolonged involuntary muscle contractions of clients with damage to the central nervous system

Specific gravity the weight or degree of concentration of a substance compared with that of an equal volume of another, such as distilled water, taken as a standard

Spectrophotometry a means of measuring the amount of red and infrared light absorbed by oxygenated and deoxygenated hemoglobin in arterial blood, used in the pulse oximetry

Speculum a funnel-shaped instrument used to widen and examine canals of the body (eg, the vagina or nasal canal)

Spermicide a substance which kills sperm

Sphygmomanometer an instrument used to measure blood pressure

Spirometry the measurement of pulmonary volumes and capacities using a spirometer

Splint a rigid bar or appliance used to stabilize or immobilize a body part

Splinter hemorrhages (nails) red or brown longitudinal streaks in the nail

Spore a round or oval structure enclosed in a tough capsule

Sprain injury of the ligaments and associated structure of a joint by wrenching or twisting; associated structures include tendons, muscles, nerves, and blood vessels

Sputum the mucous secretion from the lungs, bronchi, and trachea

Stamina staying power or endurance

Stance the manner in which a person stands

Standard (norm) a generally accepted rule, model, pattern, or measure

Stasis stagnation or stoppage of flow of body fluids, such as intestinal fluids, urine , or blood

Stasis dermatitis inflammation of the skin in the lower extremities caused by poor venous circulation

STAT indicates an order that is to carried out immediately and only once

Station (mobility) the way a person stands

STD (sexually transmitted disease) infectious diseases transmitted through sexual contact

Stereognosis the ability to recognize objects by touching and manipulating them

Stereotyping assuming that all members of a culture or ethnic group are alike

Sterile free from microorganisms, including spores

Sterile field a specified area that is considered free from microorganisms

Sterilization a process that destroys all microorganisms, including spores

Stertor snoring or sonorous respiration, usually due to a partial obstruction of the upper airway

Stethoscope an instrument used to listen to various sounds inside the body, such as the heartbeats

Stoma an artificial opening in the abdominal wall; it may be permanent or temporary

Stomatitis inflammation of the oral mucosa

Stool (feces) waste products excreted from the large intestine

Strabismus squinting or crossing of the eyes; uncoordinated eye movements

Strain (of a muscle) overexertion or overstretching of a muscle or part of a muscle

Stress (as a stimulus) an event or set of circumstances causing a disrupted response; the disruption caused by a noxious stimulus or stressor

Stressor any factor that produces stress or alters the body's equilibrium

Striae skin streaked with reddish or whitish lines on various parts of the body (eg, breasts, abdomen, thighs, upper arms) as a result of skin stretching from pregnancy, obesity, tumor, or edema

Stricture a narrowing of a passageway or canal

Stridor a harsh, crowing sound made on inhalation caused by constriction of the upper airway

Stroke volume the amount of blood ejected from the heart with each ventricular contraction

Stupor a condition of partial or nearly complete unconsciousness; stuporous clients are never fully awakened even when painfully stimulated

Stylet a metal or plastic probe inserted into a needle or cannula to render it stiff and to prevent occlusion of the needle by particles of tissue

Sublingual under the tongue

Subcostal below the ribs

Subcutaneous (hypodermic) beneath the layers of the skin

Sublimation the channeling of sexual and aggressive desires into socially acceptable forms of behavior

Sublingual under the tongue

Suborbital beneath the cavity or orbit

Subscapular below the scapula

Substance P a neurotransmitter in the dorsal horn of the spinal cord that enhances transmission of pain impulses

Substernal retractions indrawing beneath the breastbone

Substitution replacing one thing with another; an adaptive mechanism in which unattainable or unacceptable goals are replaced with ones that are attainable or acceptable

Suctioning the aspiration of secretions by a catheter connected to a suction machine or wall outlet

Sudoriferous glands a gland of the dermis that secretes sweat

Sulcular technique (Bass method) a technique of brushing the teeth under the gingival margins

Superego the conscience of personality; the source of feelings of guilt, shame, and inhibition

Supination moving the bones of the forearm so that the palm of the hand faces upward when held in front of the body

Supine (dorsal) position a back-lying position; lying on the back with the face upward without support for the head and shoulders

Support system the people and activities that can assist a person at a time of stress

Suppository a solid, cone-shaped, medicated substance inserted into the rectum, vagina, or urethra

Suppression the willful exclusion of a thought or feeling from consciousness; the sudden stoppage of a secretion or an excretion (eg, urine)

Suppuration the formation of pus

Supraclavicular retractions indrawing above the clavicles

Suprapubic above the pubic arch

Surface temperature the temperature of the skin, the subcutaneous tissue, and fat; variable in response to environmental temperature changes

Surgical asepsis (sterile technique) those practices that keep an area or object free of all microorganisms

Susceptible host any person who is at risk for infection

Sutures (of the skull) junction lines of the skull bones

Sutures (wound) the surgical stitches used to close accidental or surgical wounds, can also refer to the material used to sew the wound

Symbolization an adaptive mechanism by which objects are used to represent ideas or emotions too painful for a person to express; the creation of a mental image to stand for something

Symmetry correspondence in shape, size, and relative position of parts on opposite sides of a body

Synapse the junction between two neurons, where nerve impulses are transmitted from one to another

Syncope faintness

Syndrome a group of signs and symptoms resulting from a single cause and constituting a typical clinical picture (eg, the shock syndrome)

Synergist an agent that enhances the action of another so that their combined effect is greater than the effect of either

Synthesis putting together the parts into the whole

Syringe an instrument used to inject or withdraw liquids

Systole the period during which the ventricles contract

Systolic pressure the pressure of the blood against the arterial walls when the ventricles of the heart contract

Tachycardia an abnormally rapid pulse rate, greater than 100 beats per minute

Tachypnea abnormally fast respirations, usually more than 24 respirations per minute

Tactile related to touch

Tactile (vocal) fremitus vibrations, palpable with the palms of the hands originating in the larynx and transmitted to the chest wall during speech

Tartar a visible, hard deposit of plaque and dead bacteria that forms at the gum lines

Taxonomy a classification system or set of categories, such as nursing diagnoses, arranged on the basis of a single principle or consistent set of principles

Td combined tetanus and diphtheria toxoid used for people over 6 years of age; has less diphtheria toxoid than DT

Technical skills "hands-on" skills such as those required to manipulate equipment, administer injections, and move or reposition patients

Tenacious sticky, adhesive

Tenesmus straining; painful, ineffective straining during defecation or urination

Tension the elasticity of the arteries

Territoriality a concept of the space and things that individuals consider their own

Tertiary care rehabilitation or long-term care

Tertiary prevention activities designed to restore disabled individuals to their optimal level of functioning

Tetany a syndrome manifested by muscle twitching, cramps, convulsions, and sharp flexion of the wrist and ankle joints

Therapeutic healing; supportive of health

Therapeutic communication an interactive process between nurse and client that helps the client overcome temporary stress, to get along with other people, to adjust to the unalterable, and to overcome psychological blocks which stand in the way of self-realization

Therapeutic touch (TT) a process by which energy is transmitted or transferred from one person to another with the intent of potentiating the healing process of one who is ill or injured

Therapy remedial treatment

Thermography the use of an infrared camera to photograph the surface of the body, thus indicating surface temperatures

Thoracentesis (thoracocentesis) insertion of a needle into the pleural cavity for diagnostic or therapeutic purposes

Thrill a vibrating sensation over a blood vessel which indicates turbulent blood flow

Throat culture a specimen collected from the mucosa of the oropharynx and tonsillar regions using a culture swab

Thrombocytopenia an abnormal reduction in the number of platelets in the blood

Thrombophlebitis inflammation of a vein followed by formation of a blood clot

Thrombosis the development of a blood clot

Thrombus a solid mass of blood constituents in the circulatory system; a clot (plural: thrombi)

Tic a repetitive twitching of the muscles, often of the face or upper trunk

Tick a parasite that bites into tissue and suck blood

Tidal volume the volume of air that is normally inhaled and exhaled

Tinea pedis (Athlete's foot) a fungal infection of the foot

Tinnitus a ringing or buzzing in the ears that is purely subjective

Tissue perfusion passage of fluid (eg, blood) through a specific organ or body part

Tolerance the ability to endure without ill effects; the term is often used with reference to taking medications

Tomography (computerized axial tomography, CAT) a scanning procedure during which a narrow X-ray beam passes through the body part from different angles; see also Scan

Tonicity the normal condition of tension or tone (eg, of a muscle)

Tonometer an instrument used to assess the pressure inside the eye

Tonus the slight, continual contraction or tension of muscles

Topical applied externally (eg, to the skin or mucous membranes)

TOPV trivalent oral polio vaccine

Torsion twisting

Tortuous twisted

Total lung capacity the maximum volume to which the lungs can be expanded

Total Parenteral Nutrition (TPN, hyperalimentation) is the intravenous infusion of water, protein, carbohydrates, electrolytes, minerals, and vitamins through a central vein

Tourniquet a device (eg, a rubber strip) that is wrapped around a body extremity to compress the blood vessels

Toxemia a generalized intoxication due to the absorption of toxins in the body

Toxin a poison produced by some microorganisms, animals, and plants

Toxoid a modified exotoxin that is no longer toxic but still has the ability to stimulate the production of antibodies

Tracheal lavage the insertion of sterile normal saline through a tracheostomy tube into the trachea

Tracheal tug an indrawing and downward pulling of the trachea during inhalation

Tracheostomy a surgical incision in the trachea below the first or second tracheal cartilage

Tracheostomy tube a tube inserted into the trachea through a surgical incision

Traction exertion of a pulling force either manually or by a device in order to stabilize and immobilize a fracture

Traction tape (strap) adhesive or nonadhesive tape, made of various materials (elastic, porous) which is applied lengthwise along a limb and attached to a spreader bar

Transabdominal through or across the abdomen or abdominal wall

Transcutaneous electric nerve stimulation (TENS) a noninvasive, nonanalgesic pain control technique that allows the client to assist in the management of acute and chronic pain

Transdermal a method of medication administration in which medication is applied to the skin in a gel and is then absorbed

Transferrin a blood protein that binds with iron and transports it throughout the body

Transfusion (blood) the introduction of whole blood or its components into the venous circulation

Trapeze bar a triangular handgrip suspended from an overbed frame, used by the client

Trauma injury

Tremor an involuntary trembling of a limb or body part

Trocar a sharp pointed instrument that fits inside a cannula and is used to pierce body tissues

Trochanter roll a rolled towel support placed against the hips to prevent external rotation of the legs

Trousseau's sign an indicator of tetany; muscular spasm that results when pressure is applied to nerves and vessels of the upper arm

Tuning fork an instrument shaped like a two-pronged fork and made of metal; the prongs vibrate when struck

Turgor normal fullness and elasticity

Tympanites (distension) when the presence of excessive flatus leads to stretching and inflation or distention of the intestines

Tympany a musical or drumlike sound produced during percussion over an air filled stomach and abdomen

Ulcer a localized open sore or lesion characterized by sloughing of necrotic skin tissue or mucous membrane

Ultradian rhythm a biologic cycle completed in minutes or hours

Ultrasonography the use of ultrasound to produce an image of an organ or tissue

Ultrasound a noninvasive diagnostic technique that uses sound waves to measure the acoustic density of tissues

Ultraviolet radiation radiation having wavelengths shorter than violet rays and longer than X-rays; has powerful chemical properties

Unconscious incapable of responding to sensory stimuli; insensible

Unilateral affecting one side

Unpalatable distasteful, unpleasant to the taste

Unsterile containing microorganisms; unsterile material may be clean or contaminated

Untoward adverse, undesirable

Urban relating to or constituting a city

Urea a substance found in urine, blood, and lymph; the main nitrogenous substance in blood

Ureterostomy an opening into the ureter

Urethritis inflammation of the urethra

Urgency (of urination) the feeling that one must urinate

Urinal a receptacle used to collect urine

Urinalysis laboratory analysis of the urine

Urinary diversion the surgical rerouting of the urine produced in the kidneys to a site other than the bladder

Urinary incontinence a temporary or permanent inability of the external sphincter muscles to control the flow of urine from the bladder

Urinary pH the measurement of the concentration of hydrogen ions in the urine which indicates its acidity or alkalinity

Urinary reflux backward flow of urine

Urinary retention the accumulation of urine in the bladder and inability of the bladder to empty itself

Urinary stasis stagnation of urinary flow

Urinary suppression the sudden stoppage of urine secretion or excretion

Urination (micturition, voiding) the process of emptying the bladder

Urine the fluid of water and waste products excreted by the kidneys

Urinometer (hydrometer) an instrument used to measure the specific gravity of urine

Urography X-ray of any part of the urinary tract after the introduction of a radiopaque dye

Urostomy (ureterostomy) see Urinary diversion

Urticaria an allergic reaction marked by smooth, reddened, slightly elevated patches of skin and intense itching

Uterine prolapse a displacing of the uterus as it pulls downward through the vaginal orifice

Vaccine a suspension of killed, attenuated, or living microorganisms administered to prevent or treat an infectious disease

Vacutainer a device used in the collection of blood specimens that allows the collection of multiple specimens with one needle stick

Vaginismus the irregular and involuntary contraction of the muscles around the outer third of the vagina when coitus is attempted

Validation the determination that the diagnosis accurately reflects the problem of the client, that the methods used for data gathering were appropriate, and that the conclusion or diagnosis is justified by the data

Validity the degree to which an instrument measures what it is intended to measure

Valsalva maneuver forceful exhalation against a closed glottis, which increases intrathoracic pressure and thus interferes with venous return to the heart

Value something of worth; a belief held dearly by a person

Value conflict situation in which two or more values are incongruent

Values clarification a process by which individuals define their own values

Value system the organization of a person's values along a continuum of relative importance

Vaporization continuous evaporation of moisture from the respiratory tract and from the mucosa of the mouth and from the skin

Variable data information (data) which changes over time (eg, blood pressure, temperature)

Varicose veins (varicosities) enlarged, twisted superficial veins, most commonly seen in the lower extremities

Vasoconstriction a decrease in the caliber (lumen) of blood vessels

Vasodilation an increase in the caliber (lumen) of blood vessels

Vasopressor an agent that causes the blood pressure to rise

Vasospasm spasm or constriction of the blood vessels

Vasovagal syncope a sudden fainting caused by hypotension induced by the response of the nervous system to abrupt vagal stimulation

Vector an insect or other animal that transfers microorganisms from a reservoir to a host

Vellus fine, nonpigmented body hair

Venipuncture puncture of a vein for collection of a blood specimen or for infusion of therapeutic solutions

Ventilation the movement of air in and out of the lungs; the process of inhalation and exhalation

Ventral toward, or at the front of; anterior

Ventriculogram an X-ray film of the ventricles of the brain taken after the introduction of an opaque medium

Ventriculography radiologic examination of the ventricles of the brain following the insertion of air or a radiopaque medium

Vermin external animal parasites (eg, ticks, lice, and fleas)

Vertex the top of the head

Vertigo dizziness

Vesicular sounds normal, quiet, rustling or swishing respiratory sounds heard over the terminal bronchioles and alveoli during auscultation

Vial a glass medication container with a sealed rubber cap, for single or multiple doses

Vibration a series of vigorous quiverings produced by hands that are placed flat against the chest wall to loosen thick secretions

Virulence ability to produce disease

Virus minute infectious agents smaller than bacteria

Visceral referring to viscera

Viscosity the physical property that results from friction of molecules in a fluid, the greater the viscosity, the "thicker" the fluid

Viscous thick, sticky

Visual acuity the degree of detail the eye can discern in an image

Visual fields the area an individual can see when looking straight ahead

Vital capacity the maximum amount of air that can be exhaled after a maximum inhalation

Vital signs (cardinal signs) measurements of physiologic functioning, specifically temperature, pulse, respiration, and blood pressure

Vitiligo patches of hypopigmented skin, caused by the destruction of melanocytes in the area

Vocal resonance vibrations of the larynx transmitted during speech through the respiratory system to the chest wall

Voiding see Urination

Volatile evaporating readily

Volume-control set a small fluid container attached below the primary infusion container used to administer intermittent intravenous medications

Vomitus material vomited; emesis

Walker a metal, rectangular frame used as an aid to ambulation

Weber's test a test that assesses lateralization of bone conduction of sound

Well-being a subjective perception of balance, harmony, and vitality

Wheal see Bleb

Wheezing a rasping or whistling sound in breathing caused by constriction in the upper airway

Wound a break in the continuity of a body tissue

Xerography type of X-ray procedure used in examining different body tissues (eg, breast tissue)

X rays electromagnetic radiation with extremely short wavelengths

Photographic Credits

Unit Openers (Units 1, 2, 3, 5, 6, 7, 9, 10) B Proud Photography.

Chapter Openers **1:** The Bettmann Archive. **2:** Sharon Beals. **3:** Elena Dorfman. **4:** Richard Tauber. **5–8:** Suzanne Arms. **9:** Richard Tauber. **10:** Tom Ferentz. **11:** Richard Tauber. **12:** Elena Dorfman. **13:** Tom Ferentz. **14:** Jane Wattenberg. **15:** Elena Dorfman. **16:** Karen Stafford. **17:** © Frank Siteman/Jeroboam, Inc. **18:** Sharon Beals. **19:** Elena Dorfman. **20:** Richard Tauber. **21:** Elena Dorfman. **22:** Tom Ferentz. **23:** Kim Raftery. **25:** Suzanne Arms. **26:** Dore Gardner. **27:** Alain McLaughlin. **28–29:** Elena Dorfman. **30:** Alain McLaughlin. **31:** Richard Tauber. **32:** Judy Braginsky. **33:** Karen Stafford. **34:** © Frank Smith/Jeroboam, Inc. **35–36:** Judy Braginsky. **37:** Karen Stafford. **38:** Judy Braginsky. **39:** Suzanne Arms. **40:** Richard Tauber. **41:** Tom Ferentz. **42:** Richard Tauber. **43:** Elena Dorfman. **44:** Judy Braginsky. **45:** Elena Dorfman.

Critical Thinking Challenges **Chapters 11, 16, 19, 34:** Elena Dorfman. **Chapters 17, 18, 29:** Alain McLaughlin. **Chapters 26, 27, 37, 40, 43, 45:** Richard Tauber.

Chapter 1 Timeline Images, Page 4: Left, Alinari/Art Resource, NY. Center, Courtesy of Parke-Davis, A Division of Warner-Lambert Co. Right, Foto Marburg/Art Resource, NY. Page 5: Left, © Robert Hoesch-Milano/Elena Dorfman. Center, The Bettmann Archive. Right, The Bettmann Archive. Page 6: Left, The Bettmann Archive. Center, Courtesy of Hotel Dieu de Montreal. Right, Reprinted with permission from Abbey Press, St. Meinrad, IN 47577. All rights reserved. Page 7: Left, Library Council of New South Wales, Australia. Center, Courtesy of Morriand-Spingam Research Center, Howard University. Right, The Bettmann Archive. Page 8: Left, National Library of Medicine, Bethesda, MD. Center, The Bettmann Archive. Right, The Bettmann Archive. Page 9: Left, National Portrait Gallery, Smithsonian Institution/Art Resource, NY. Center, National Portrait Gallery, Smithsonian Institution/Art Resource, NY. Right, Courtesy of International Council of Nursing. Page 10: Left, Library Council of New South Wales, Australia. Center, Archives and Special Collections on Women in Medicine, Medical College of Pennsylvania. Right, The Schlesinger Library, Radcliffe College. Page 11: Left, Schomberg Center for Research in Black Culture. Center, The Bettmann Archive. Right, Courtesy of Canadian Nurses Association. Page 12: Center, University of Iowa, College of Nursing, Iowa City, IA. Right, Courtesy of American Nursing Association. Page 13: Left, Courtesy of the International Council of Nurses. Center, Courtesy of the University of California at San Francisco Library/Elena Dorfman. Right, National Postal Museum, Smithsonian Institution, Washington, D.C. Page 14: Left, Courtesy of Canadian Nursing Association. Center, Courtesy of National League for Nursing. Right, The Bettmann Archive. Page 15: Left, Courtesy of Milbank Memorial Library, Teacher's College, Columbia University. Center, Courtesy of Sigma Theta Tau. Right, Frontier Nursing Service. Page 16: Left, The Bettmann Archive. Center, Courtesy of National Student Nurses Association. Right, The Bettmann Archive. Page 17: Left, Courtesy of National Black Nurses Association. Center left, The Bettmann Archive. Center right, Courtesy of Louden Associates. Right, Courtesy of Ildaura Murillo-Rohde. Page 18: Left, The Bettmann Archive. Center, Courtesy of National Institute of Nursing Research. Right, Courtesy of United States Public Health Service. Page 19: Left, Courtesy of American Nurses Association. Center, Courtesy of American Nurses Association. Right, Courtesy of Sigma Theta Tau.

Chapter 2 2–1, Top right: Alain McLaughlin. 2–1, Bottom right, bottom middle, bottom left, top left: Elena Dorfman.

Chapter 3 Table 3–1, Page 47 : Top, The Bettmann Archive. Middle, Courtesy of Sigma Theta Tau. Bottom, Courtesy of Sigma Theta Tau. Page 48: Top, Courtesy of Sigma Theta Tau. Middle, Courtesy of Dorothea E. Orem. Bottom, Courtesy of Sigma Theta Tau. Page 49: Top, Courtesy of Betty Neuman. Bottom, Courtesy of Dorothy E. Johnson.

Chapter 9 9–2: © Mike English, MD/Medichrome.

Chapter 10 10–1: Alain McLaughlin.

Chapter 13 13–1: Elena Dorfman.

Chapter 14 14–5: Alain McLaughlin. 14–6, 7: Elena Dorfman. 14–8: Robert Brenner/PhotoEdit.

Chapter 15 15–2: Left, Courtesy of Armida Quinonez. Right, Bill Aron/PhotoEdit. 15–3, 4: Alain McLaughlin.

Chapter 18 18–1: William Thompson. 18–3: Judy Braginsky. 18–4: Alain McLaughlin.

Chapter 19 19–1, 3: Alain McLaughlin. 19–2: Elena Dorfman. 19–4: Photo Researchers.

Chapter 20 20–1: Alain McLaughlin.

Chapter 21 21–5, 6, 15, 18, 22: Elena Dorfman. 21–8: Alain McLaughlin. 21–11, 16: Richard Tauber.

Chapter 22 22–1, 2, 3, 10, 11, 12, 13, 14, 16, 20, 21, 22, 23, 27, 28, 29, 30, 34, 35, 42, 46, 56, 57, 66, 67, 68, 69, 70, 71, 72, 73: Richard Tauber. 22–77: Elena Dorfman. Table 22–4: Elena Dorfman.

Chapter 24 24–1, 2: Richard Tauber. 24–4, 7: Jane Wattenberg. 24–5: Michael Newman/PhotoEdit. 24–6: Elena Dorfman.

Chapter 25 25–1: Elena Dorfman. 25–2: David Young-Wolff/PhotoEdit. 25–3: Tony Freeman/PhotoEdit.

Chapter 26 26–1: Top left, Bottom left, Joel Gordon. Top right, Patricia J. Bruno. Bottom, right, Adam Smith Productions/Westlight. 26–2: Westlight. 26–3: Joel Gordon.

Chapter 27 27–3, 4, 5, 6, 17, 18: Elena Dorfman. 27–7, 8, 19, 20, 21, 22: Alain McLaughlin. 27–30, 31, 32, 33, 34: William Thompson.

Chapter 28 28–2, 3, 4, 5, 6: Ambularm Co. 28–7, 8, 12: Richard Tauber.

Chapter 29 29–18, 20, 21: Richard Tauber. 29–19: Tom Ferentz. 29–22, 36, 37: Alain McLaughlin. 29–24, 25: William Thompson.

Chapter 30 30–4: Tom Ferentz.

Chapter 34 34–19, 25, 26, 32, 40, 41, 43, 55, 56, 57: Richard Tauber. 34–33, 42: William Thompson. 34–38: Tom Ferentz.

Chapter 36 36–11: William Thompson. 36–12: Richard Tauber.

Chapter 37 37–2, 3, 4: Elena Dorfman. 37–6: Alain McLaughlin. 37–8, 9: Richard Tauber. 37–10: Elena Dorfman. 37–11, 14, 16: William Thompson.

Chapter 38 38–11, 29: William Thompson. 38–16, 17, 23, 25: Tom Ferentz. 38–24: Richard Tauber.

Chapter 39 39–1, 2, 4, 5, 6, 7, 16, 17, 32, 33: Richard Tauber. 39–9, 12, 13, 15, 18, 19, 20, 28, 31, 35: William Thompson. 39–29, 30: Tom Ferentz. 39–37: Elena Dorfman.

Chapter 40 40–9: Richard Tauber. 40–13: Judy Braginsky. 40–15, 16, 17, 19, 20: William Thompson.

Chapter 41 41–6, 9, 10, 11: William Thompson.

Chapter 42 42–2: Elena Dorfman. 42–3: Richard Tauber.

Chapter 43 43–11, 38, 57, 58, 59: Richard Tauber. 43–15, 19, 20, 21, 22, 28, 41, 44, 45, 46, 47, 49, 51, 52, 53, Elena Dorfman. 43–17: Courtesy of On•Gard Systems. 43–50: Courtesy of Becton Dickinson and Company. InterLink is a trademark of Baxter Healthcare Corporation. 43–54, 55, 61: William Thompson.

Chapter 44 44–13, 16, 17, 18: Richard Tauber. 44–19, 20: William Thompson.

Chapter 45 45–4, 5: Elena Dorfman. 45–6: William Thompson.

Art Credits

Chapter 4 4–1: GTS Graphics.

Chapter 5 5–1: Nea Hanscomb. 5–2: GTS Graphics. Nursing Process Art (pages 79–80): Nea Hanscomb.

Chapter 6 6–1, 2: Nea Hanscomb.

Chapter 7 7–1: Nea Hanscomb. 7–2: GTS Graphics.

Chapter 8 8–1, 2: Nea Hanscomb.

Chapter 9 9–1, 3, 4, 5, 6, 7, 9, 10: GTS Graphics. 9–8: Nea Hanscomb.

Chapter 12 12–1: Nea Hanscomb. 12–2, 3: GTS Graphics.

Chapter 13 13–2, 4, 5, 6: Nea Hanscomb. 13–3, 7: GTS Graphics.

Chapter 14 14–1: Kristen N. Mount. 14–2, 3, 4, 9: Nea Hanscomb.

Chapter 15 15–1, 5: Nea Hanscomb.

Chapter 16 Table 16–1: Nea Hanscomb.

Chapter 18 18–2: Nea Hanscomb.

Chapter 21 21–1, 2, 3, 4, 7, 9: Nea Hanscomb. 21–10, 13, 14: Romaine LoPrete. 21–12: GTS Graphics. 21–17, 21, 23, 24, 25: Linda Harris. 21–19, 20: Kristen N. Mount.

Chapter 22 22–4, 7, 8, 18, 19, 25, 26, 32, 52, 61, 62, 79, 80: Christopher Burke. 22–5, 6, 24, 33, 38, 40, 41, 47, 48, 49, 54, 74, 75, 78, 81, 82: Kristen N. Mount. 22–15, 51: Nea Hanscomb. 22–17, 31, 36, 37, 39, 43, 44, 45, 50, 55, 60, 63, 65, 76: Romaine Lo Prete. 22–53: Linda Harris. 22–58, 59, 64: Precision Graphics. Table 22–2: Precision Graphics.

Chapter 24 24–3: Kristen N. Mount.

Chapter 27 27–1, 2: Nea Hanscomb. 27–9: Precision Graphics. 27–10, 11, 12, 13, 14, 15, 16, 23, 24, 25, 26, 27, 28, 29: Linda Harris.

Chapter 28 28–1, 9: Linda Harris. 28–10, 11, 16, 17: Precision Graphics. 28–14, 15: Nea Hanscomb.

Chapter 29 29–1, 6, 7, 13, 14, 15, 30, 31: Linda Harris. 29–2, 3, 8, 9, 10, 11, 12, 16, 17, 23, 26, 27: Precision Graphics. 29–4, 5: Christopher Burke. 29–28, 29, 32, 33, 34, 35: Nea Hanscomb. Table 29–12: Nea Hanscomb.

Chapter 30 30–1: Precision Graphics. 30–2: Christopher Burke. 30–3: GTS Graphics.

Chapter 32 32–1: Christopher Burke. 32–2, 3: Nea Hanscomb.

Chapter 34 34–1, 2, 3, 4, 5, 10, 11, 12, 14, 15, 16, 17, 18, 21, 22, 23, 24, 27, 28, 29, 36, 47, 48, 53, 54: Precision Graphics. 34–6, 7, 8, 9: Romaine LoPrete. 34–13, 20, 35, 37, 44: Linda Harris. 34–30, 49, 50, 51, 52: Nea Hanscomb. Table 34–2: Precision Graphics.

Chapter 35 35–1: GTS Graphics. 35–2: Nea Hanscomb.

Chapter 36 36–1: Precision Graphics. 36–2, 3, 4, 5: Christopher Burke. 36–6: Linda Harris. 36–7, 8, 10: Nea Hanscomb. 36–9, 13: GTS Graphics.

Chapter 37 37–1: Robert Voights. 37–5: GTS Graphics. 37–7: Nea Hanscomb. 37–12: Christopher Burke. 37–13, 15: Precision Graphics.

Chapter 38 38–1, 2, 3, 4, 5, 6, 7, 9, 12, 13, 14, 21, 22, 26, 28, 30, 31, 32, 33: Nea Hanscomb. 38–8: GTS Graphics. 38–10, 15, 18, 20: Linda Harris. 38–27: Precision Graphics.

Chapter 39 39–3, 21, 25: Christopher Burke. 39–8, 11, 27, 36: Nea Hanscomb. 39–10, 34: Linda Harris. 39–14, 22, 23, 24, 26: Precision Graphics.

Chapter 40 40–1, 2, 4, 5, 11: Christopher Burke. 40–3, 7, 8, 14: Nea Hanscomb. 40–6, 10, 12, 18: Linda Harris.

Chapter 41 41–1, 2, 3, 4, 5, 17, 21, 22, 23: Christopher Burke. 41–7: Linda Harris. 41–8, 15, 16, 18, 19: Precision Graphics. 41–12, 13, 14, 20: Nea Hanscomb.

Chapter 42 42–1: Christopher Burke.

Chapter 43 43–1, 6, 10, 12, 13, 16, 18, 23, 37, 43, 48, 56: Nea Hanscomb. 43–2, 3, 24, 25, 26, 60: Precision Graphics. 43–4, 5, 7, 42: GTS Graphics. 43–8, 9: Linda Harris. 43–27, 29, 30, 31, 32, 33, 34, 35, 36, 39, 40, 62, 63, 65, 66, 67: Christopher Burke. Table 43–10: Nea Hanscomb.

Chapter 44 44–1, 3, 4, 5, 14, 22, 26: Precision Graphics. 44–6, 8, 9, 21, 23, 24, 25, 27, 28, 29: Linda Harris. 44–10, 15: Nea Hanscomb.

Chapter 45 45–1: Christopher Burke. 45–2, 3: Linda Harris.

Index

NOTE: A *t* following a page number indicates tabular material and an *f* following a page number indicates an illustration.

continued

continued

continued

continued

continued

continued

continued

continued

continued

continued

continued

continued

continued

continued

continued

Nursing Diagnoses

North American Nursing Diagnosis Association (NANDA)
Current as of October, 1994

Activity Intolerance
Activity Intolerance, High Risk for
Adjustment, Impaired
Airway Clearance, Ineffective
Anxiety
Aspiration, High Risk for
Body Image Disturbance
Body Temperature, High Risk for Altered
Breastfeeding, Effective
Breastfeeding, Ineffective
Breastfeeding, Interrupted
Breathing Pattern, Ineffective
Cardiac Output, Decreased
Caregiver Role Strain
Caregiver Role Strain, High Risk for
Communication, Impaired Verbal
Constipation
Constipation, Colonic
Constipation, Perceived
Coping, Defensive
Coping, Ineffective Individual
Decisional Conflict (specify)
Denial, Ineffective
Diarrhea
Disuse Syndrome, High Risk for
Diversional Activity Deficit
Dysreflexia
Family Coping: Compromised, Ineffective
Family Coping: Disabling, Ineffective
Family Coping: Potential for Growth
Family Processes, Altered
Fatigue
Fear
Fluid Volume Deficit
Fluid Volume Deficit, High Risk for
Fluid Volume Excess
Gas Exchange, Impaired
Grieving, Anticipatory
Grieving, Dysfunctional
Growth and Development, Altered
Health Maintenance, Altered
Health-Seeking Behaviors (specify)
Home Maintenance Management, Impaired
Hopelessness
Hyperthermia
Hypothermia
Incontinence, Bowel
Incontinence, Functional
Incontinence, Reflex
Incontinence, Stress
Incontinence, Total
Incontinence, Urge
Infant Feeding Pattern, Ineffective
Infection, High Risk for
Injury, High Risk for
Knowledge Deficit (specify)
Noncompliance (specify)
Nutrition, Altered: Less than Body Requirements
Nutrition, Altered: More than Body Requirements
Nutrition, Altered: Potential for More than Body Requirements
Oral Mucous Membrane, Altered
Pain
Pain, Chronic
Parental Role Conflict
Parenting, Altered
Parenting, High Risk for Altered
Peripheral Neurovascular Dysfunction, High Risk for
Personal Identity Disturbance
Physical Mobility, Impaired
Poisoning, High Risk for
Post-Trauma Response
Powerlessness
Protection, Altered
Rape Trauma Syndrome
Rape Trauma Syndrome, Compound Reaction
Rape Trauma Syndrome, Silent Reaction
Relocation Stress Syndrome
Role Performance, Altered
Self-Care Deficit
- Bathing/Hygiene
- Feeding
- Dressing/Grooming
- Toileting

Self-Esteem, Chronic Low
Self-Esteem, Situational Low
Self-Esteem Disturbance
Self-Mutilation, High Risk for
Sensory-Perceptual Alterations (specify) (visual, auditory, kinesthetic, gustatory, tactile, olfactory)
Sexual Dysfunction
Sexuality Patterns, Altered
Skin Integrity, High Risk for Impaired
Skin Integrity, Impaired
Sleep Pattern Disturbance
Social Interaction, Impaired
Social Isolation
Spiritual Distress
Suffocation, High Risk for
Swallowing, Impaired
Therapeutic Regimen, Ineffective Management of
Thermoregulation, Ineffective
Thought Processes, Altered
Tissue Integrity, Impaired
Tissue Perfusion, Altered (specify type) (renal, cerebral, cardiopulmonary, gastrointestinal, peripheral)
Trauma, High Risk for
Unilateral Neglect
Urinary Elimination, Altered
Urinary Retention
Ventilation, Inability to Sustain Spontaneous
Ventilatory Weaning Response, Dysfunctional
Violence, High Risk for: Self-Directed or Directed at Others